C Hamilton

848-218-0585

UFLACKER'S

ATLAS *of* Vascular Anatomy

AN ANGIOGRAPHIC APPROACH

THIRD EDITION

THIRD EDITION

UFLACKER'S

ATLAS of Vascular Anatomy

AN ANGIOGRAPHIC APPROACH

Andre Uflacker, MD
Assistant Professor
Vascular and Interventional Radiology
Medical University of South Carolina
Charleston, South Carolina

Marcelo Guimaraes, MD, MBA, FSIR
Director, Vascular & Interventional Radiology
Professor Surgery and Radiology
Medical University of South Carolina
Charleston, South Carolina

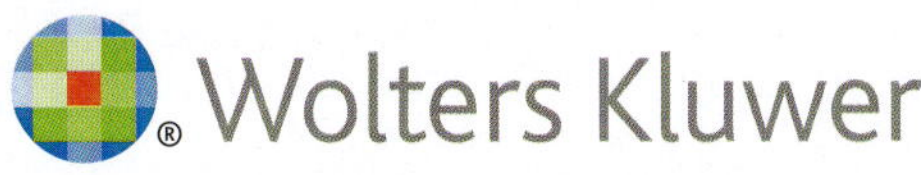

Philadelphia • Baltimore • New York • London
Buenos Aires • Hong Kong • Sydney • Tokyo

Acquisitions Editor: Sharon Zinner
Development Editor: Liz Schaeffer
Editorial Coordinator: Ashley Pfeiffer
Editorial Assistant: Nicole Dunn
Marketing Manager: Julie Sikora
Senior Production Project Manager: Alicia Jackson
Design Coordinator: Holly McLaughlin
Manufacturing Coordinator: Beth Welsh
Prepress Vendor: TNQ Technologies
3rd edition

9 8 7 6 5 4 3 2 1

Printed in China

Library of Congress Cataloging-in-Publication Data

ISBN-13: 978-1-4963-5601-7

Cataloging-in-Publication data available on request from the Publisher.

shop.lww.com

CCS0120

"Variability is the law of life,"
Sir William Osler

To Curry and Hugo, with all my gratitude
and
To my parents, Helena and Renan, and to Barbara and Duke, for these gifts
Andre

To Julia and Mateus: life is a wonderful journey. You have the opportunity to live it meaningfully with integrity, creativity, courage, dedication, passion, persistency, and patience.
As you cannot predict the future, dare to create it!
It is your choice!

To my wife Rossana: many thanks for your unconditional love and support.
To my parents Marilene and Allan: thanks for being outstanding parents.
Marcelo

CONTRIBUTORS

Illustrations by

José Falcetti
Director, Center for Medical Arts, Hospital das Clinicas
Faculdade de Medicina da Universidade de São Paulo
Functional Neurosurgery
São Paulo, SP, Brazil

Body Scientific International
Grayslake, Illinois

Andre Uflacker, MD
Assistant Professor
Vascular and Interventional Radiology
Medical University of South Carolina
Charleston, South Carolina

With Contributions by

Arindam Chatterjee, MD
Assistant Professor of Radiology
Division of Neuroradiology
Medical University of South Carolina
—Arteries of the Head and Neck
—Veins of the Head and Neck

Pal Spruill Suranyi, MD, PhD, FNASCI
Professor of Radiology and Medicine
Department of Radiology and Radiological Science
Divisions of Cardiovascular and Thoracic Imaging
Department of Medicine, Division of Cardiology
Medical University of South Carolina
—The Heart and Coronary Arteries
—The Heart Venous Circulation

PREFACE TO THIRD EDITION

We are pleased to provide an update to the *Atlas of Vascular Anatomy* in the form of its third edition. This work has its roots in the stacks of type-written pages, cut film, and the original illustrations of José Falcetti, which were painstainkingly labeled by my father, Renan Uflacker, using cut pieces of paper, tape, and glue. Ever grateful to stand on the shoulders of this giant, we are lucky that technology has continued to evolve and that we are able to add to this work.

The development of 3D cinematic volume-rendered reconstructions would have shocked Renan and José with their beauty, as they allowed only the most accurate and highest quality material to go on print. We hope that the cinematic reconstructions provided herein are a useful adjunct to the understanding and teaching of vascular anatomy, and that they help kindle the love for the discipline in the coming generations of students, clinicians, researchers, and academics. These images would not have been possible without the assistance of my colleagues at the University of Virginia, who took the time to teach me the intricacies of the software used to create them, and without the dedication of that institution to scholarship, which allowed me the required time and resources.

As our understanding of anatomy and technical expertise evolve, the clinical application of this knowledge presents itself in sometimes surprising areas. One of the best examples of this is the advent of Prostatic Artery Embolization, which has reignited interest in pelvic vascular anatomy. We have provided an updated discussion of the pelvic arteries, with a fresh understanding of the incredible complexity of this territory, where variability truly is law.

The evolution of imaging technology now allows the appreciation of a multitude of variants outside of the cadaver lab or the operating room. Cinematic reconstructions have been added to several chapters, but particularly in the neurovascular and cardiac anatomy chapters. We hope that these images provide the reader with an enhanced understanding of the often-complex anatomy of those systems with renderings that are often akin to virtual cadaveric dissections.

This preface would not be complete without acknowledging the two people who made it possible, Renan Uflacker and José Falcetti. Renan's death in 2011 left us in uncharted territory, and it was only through the guidance of his love of medicine and anatomy that we were able to get back on the course that landed us here. He will be forever missed and remembered.

José was a tremendous artist and medical illustrator who created the color plates for the first edition of the *Atlas*, which we maintain as an essential part of this work. I approached José with a proposal to create new illustrations for this edition in 2017 and found him genuinely elated to see this project still alive. Unfortunately, José succumbed to leukemia in May of 2018, before we could complete our work. His original illustrations provide the perfect standard for the art found in this book. His artistic genius thus lives on, guiding every decision we have made with regards to art in this volume. We would like to thank the staff of Lippincott Williams & Wilkins for their patience and attention to detail in producing this work. We would also like to thank you, our reader, whether you are a student, trainee, seasoned clinician, researcher, or artist. Finally, we would like to thank our patients, for whom this book was ultimately made, and without whom its creation would have been impossible.

Andre Uflacker, MD
Co-Editor

Renan Uflacker has trained directly or indirectly hundreds of Vascular Interventionalists around the world. The *Atlas of Vascular Anatomy* is one of many contributions that he left in 2011 to future generations of interventionalists to come. Considering Renan as an intellectual father, to whom I will be always grateful, I felt the urge to give continuity to his work on vascular anatomy. I believe that one of our tasks in life is to demonstrate gratitude in a genuine way, so it was a natural choice to include Andre Uflacker (his son) on this humbling task.

It is important to recognize that Andre not only worked as a co-editor but was fundamental for the completeness and quality of the third edition. Andre is also a talented artist. Several drawings of this edition were created by him.

This project was only possible with Andre's dedication and hard work and after the incredible LWW staff support. I am grateful that we were able to give continuity to Renan's vascular anatomy project and to keep his intellectual and scientific spirit strong amongst ourselves.

Marcelo Guimaraes, MD, MBA, FSIR
Co-Editor

Acknowledgment of Prior Contributors

The authors would like to acknowledge the contributions of prior authors who have worked in the first and second editions of this text. These authors set the standards against which we measured the quality of our material. It was an honor to build upon their work, and we will be forever grateful.

Carlos Jader Feldman, MD
Chief, Department of Radiology
Hospital Hernesto Dornelles
Porto Alegre, RS, Brazil
—Vascular Anatomy of the Lower Genital Tract

Ronie L. Piske, MD
Interventional Neuroradiologist
Med–Imagem Hospital
Beneficência
Poruguesa, São Paulo, SP, Brazil
—Arteries of the Head and Neck
—Veins of the Head and Neck

Francisco J.B. Sampaio, MD, PhD
Professor of Anatomy and Urology
Head, Department of Anatomy
State University of Rio de Janeiro
Rio de Janeiro, RJ, Brazil
—Kidney Arterial Vascularization
—Kidney Venous Drainage
—Lymphatic Drainage of the Kidney
—Periprostatic Venous Plexus

J. Bayne Selby, MD
Professor of Radiology
Medical University of South Carolina
Charleston, SC
—The Heart and Coronary Arteries
—The Heart Venous Circulation
—Pulmonary Arterial Circulation
—Pulmonary Venous Circulation

Luiz Maria Yordi, MD
Chief, Department of Hemodynamic and Cardiovascular Radiology
Hospital São Francisco
Porto Alegre, RS, Brazil
—The Heart and Coronary Arteries
—The Heart Venous Circulation

CONTENTS

1

The Fetal Circulation and Vascular Embryology

Early in fetal life, fetal blood reaches the placenta through the two umbilical arteries and returns to the fetus by the two umbilical veins. Later, the right umbilical vein disappears and the left vein persists as the single returning vessel. Fetal blood receives oxygen and nutrients by close contact with maternal blood in the placenta. The umbilical vein (persistent left umbilical vein) enters the abdomen at the umbilicus and runs along the edge of the falciform ligament to the hepatic visceral surface, where it sends branches to the left hepatic lobe and joins the left branch of the portal vein. At the opposite side of these anastomoses arises the ductus venosus, which joins the inferior vena cava, conveying the oxygen-rich blood that comes from the maternal placenta. The fetal portal vein is small, and the right and left branches function as branches of the ductus venosus, carrying oxygenated blood to the liver. Oxygenated blood mixes with a small amount of oxygen-poor blood from the caudal portion of the fetus in the inferior vena cava. Blood from the inferior vena cava and ductus venosus enters the right atrium and hits the interatrial membrane and is directed through the foramen ovale into the left atrium, guided by a valve in the most central aspect of the inferior vena cava, the Eustachian valve. In the left atrium, oxygen-rich blood mixes with a small amount of nonoxygenated blood from the pulmonary vein. From the left atrium, blood enters the left ventricle and, subsequently, the aorta. A small portion of oxygenated blood, instead of crossing the foramen ovale, joins blood flow from the superior vena cava and, after passing through the right atrium, enters the right ventricle of the heart. Inflow from the superior vena cava and, to a lesser extent, from the umbilical vein is diverted to the pulmonary artery, thereby supplying the lungs. Most of this blood flow is shunted through the ductus arteriosus directly into the descending aorta, where it joins the stream of blood ejected from the left ventricle. Most of the oxygenated blood from the left ventricle reaches the heart and cerebral circulation, providing higher oxygen content to these organs, rather than to structures less sensitive to hypoxia in the abdomen and extremities. The blood in the descending aorta is poorer in oxygen and is partly distributed to the lower limbs and viscera of the abdomen and pelvis, but most of it returns to the placenta via the umbilical arteries arising from the internal iliac arteries (Fig. 1.1).

After birth, the ductus venosus closes rapidly and is transformed into the ligamentum venosum upon obliteration, connecting with the ligamentum teres (round ligament), at the site of the occluded umbilical vein. The round ligament reaches the umbilicus, as well as the lateral umbilical ligaments, remnants of the umbilical arteries, which reach the internal iliac arteries, and typically arise from the common trunk of the superior vesical artery. After closure of the ductus venosus and umbilical vein, the liver is supplied by oxygenated blood from the abdominal aorta through the celiac trunk and from the portal vein.

With the first breath, the newborn's pulmonary vascular resistance reduces markedly, and the pressure changes cause a hemodynamic shift between the right and left atria in a manner such that no blood passes through the foramen ovale. In most individuals the foramen ovale closes within the first year of life, at first by apposition and later by fusion of the interatrial septa. In adults, the fossa ovalis indicates the location of the foramen. The ductus arteriosus closes by muscular contraction and is obliterated by intimal proliferation, and its remnant is called the ligamentum arteriosum.

Development of the Systemic Arterial Circulation

The embryologic development of the arterial circulation is complex, and an extensive discussion is outside the scope of this chapter. However, a brief description of the development of the systemic arteries is described with particular focus on the resulting anatomical morphology.

The truncus arteriosus continues as the aortic sac from which symmetrical aortic arches arise and extend dorsally to the paired dorsal aortae. Eventually six paired aortic arches develop, although not all are present at any one time. Portions of these arches regress and disappear (Fig. 1.2). The aortic sac becomes the ascending aorta, while its right and left horns become the brachiocephalic artery and the proximal aortic arch, respectively. The first and second aortic arches contribute little to adult structures, whereas the third arch becomes the common carotid arteries and the proximal internal carotid arteries. The common carotid arteries give rise to the external carotid artery, whereas the fourth aortic arch becomes the proximal right subclavian artery and on the left, the distal aortic arch, between the left carotid artery and the left subclavian artery (left seventh intersegmental artery). The fifth arches involute entirely without derived adult structures. The sixth aortic arches become the right and left pulmonary arteries, with the distal left sixth arch becoming the ductus arteriosus. The distal right sixth arch involutes; although if it persists, it may develop into a right patent ductus arteriosus. During development of the aorta, seven pairs of cervical intersegmental arteries form, with the most important one being the seventh. The seventh cervical intersegmental artery gives rise to the arteries of the upper extremity and the vertebral artery.

The remnants are:

- Arch I: Part of the maxillary arteries
- Arch II: Part of the stapedial arteries
- Arch III: The common carotid arteries
- Arch IV: The aortic arch and part of the right subclavian artery
- Arch V: No derivatives
- Arch VI: The proximal part of the left pulmonary artery and distal part of the ductus arteriosus (left), and the proximal part of the right pulmonary artery (right). The distal part usually disappears. If present, it represents a right patent ductus arteriosus.

Early in embryonic development, the two dorsal aortae begin to fuse in the abdomen, with the fusion progressing toward the thorax. The right dorsal aorta in the thorax gradually regresses, leaving only the left dorsal aorta as the descending thoracic aorta. Several variants of the aortic anatomy can be seen with their corresponding developmental etiology in Fig. 1.3.

Neurovascular Development

The blood supply to the brain and spinal cord is derived from dorsal intersegmental arteries. The 4 mm embryo has developed paired plexiform longitudinal neural arteries, which anastomose with the primitive carotid arteries via the trigeminal arteries and the otic arteries, the proatlantal arteries, and with the aortic arches via the hypoglossal arteries, and the primitive C1 segmental arteries. It is from these early anastomoses that variant carotid-vertebral anastomoses arise (Fig. 1.4A). In the 5 to 6 mm embryo, there is regression of the otic and hypoglossal arteries (Fig. 1.4B). At this stage, the caudal division of the primitive internal carotid artery begins to form the precursor of the posterior communicating artery. At the 7 to 12 mm stage, there is fusion of the primitive cervical segmental arteries into the vertebral artery, which remains with a plexiform junction with the basilar artery. This allows for variable patterns of inferior cerebellar artery formation. After this stage, the anterior and posterior circulations are usually distinct. Persistence of one or more of these carotid-vertebral anastomoses may give rise to the variants depicted on Fig. 1.5.

Development of the Visceral Arteries

The paired dorsal aortae fuse caudally to form the descending aorta in the fourth week of development, giving the lateral and ventral segmental arteries and the dorsal intersegmental arteries. The distal end of the descending aorta develops into the median sacral artery. The lateral segmental arteries supply the diaphragm, the kidneys, adrenal glands, and gonads. These primitive vessels go on to form the phrenic, renal, suprarenal, and gonadal arteries.

The ventral segmental arteries form the vitelline arteries, the umbilical arteries, and the chorionic arteries. The vitelline arteries supply the yolk sac and primitive gut. The celiac artery supplies the foregut; the superior mesenteric artery, the midgut; and the inferior mesenteric artery, the hindgut. The segmental nature of these vessels during development may give rise to anatomical variants such as a celiacomesenteric trunk and varying types of anastomoses between these main three trunks.

Development of the Peripheral Arteries

Approximately 30 pairs of primitive arteries arise serially at segmental levels running between somites. In the thoracic region, these arteries become the posterior intercostal arteries. In the abdominal region, the primitive dorsal arteries become the first through fourth lumbar arteries. In the pelvic region, the dorsal arteries become the sacral arteries.

In the lower extremity (Fig. 1.6A), the axial artery of the lower limb continues from the internal iliac artery, a branch of the fifth lumbar intersegmental artery. The fifth intersegmental artery joints with the umbilical arteries to form the common iliac arteries. At 36 days of gestation, the sciatic artery is the main branch supplying the lower extremity limb bud, arising from the umbilical artery. The external iliac artery and the femoral arteries have already branched from the common iliac artery, which go on to develop the common femoral artery, the superficial femoral artery, and the proximal profunda femoris artery. The sciatic artery communicates with the popliteal artery above the knee, and it begins to involute leaving the popliteal artery as the main artery supplying the distal limb bud. Segments of the remaining sciatic artery form the part of the popliteal artery, the profunda femoris artery, and the peroneal artery (Fig. 1.6B). The proximal segment of the sciatic artery in the pelvis forms the inferior gluteal artery.

The popliteal artery is derived from the deep and superficial popliteal arteries, which arise from the sciatic artery and the femoral artery, respectively. The distal deep popliteal artery regresses, whereas the proximal deep popliteal artery and the superficial popliteal artery merge posterior to the popliteus muscle. Persistence of the distal deep popliteal artery anterior to the popliteus muscle may result in popliteal entrapment syndrome. The distal sciatic artery persists as the peroneal artery and also gives rise to a branch that becomes the anterior tibial artery. Some authors describe the saphenous artery as being a branch of the femoral artery whose proximal segment regresses, with the distal segment anastomosing with the peroneal artery and giving rise to the posterior tibial artery. The posterior tibial artery has also been described as a continuation of the popliteal artery from the developing iliofemoral system.

In the upper extremity (Fig. 1.7), the arterial supply is derived from the seventh cervical intersegmental artery which gives rise to the axial artery that supplies the upper limb bud. The axial artery becomes the brachial artery and later, the deep palmar arch. At 41 days of gestation, the arterial supply to the upper limb bud is provided by the interosseous artery, the median artery, and a developing ulnar artery. By day 46, the interosseous artery begins to regress, the radial artery is developing from the brachial artery, and the median and ulnar arteries are the primary arterial vessels to the developing hand. The radial and ulnar arteries develop as branches from the axial artery to supply the forearm as the interosseous and median arteries involute. The median artery may persist in up to 12% of the population. The radial artery may have a proximal origin in the brachial artery, which is seen in up to 14.2% of the population.

Development of the Systemic Venous Circulation

By the fourth week of development, the embryo has begun the formation of multiple paired venous precursors which regress and develop to form the systemic venous circulation. The sinus venosus is the common structure into which blood flow from these precursors drain, and its left horn eventually forms the coronary sinus, which receives blood from the left anterior cardinal vein. Paired anterior cardinal veins develop into jugular, subclavian, brachiocephalic, and left superior intercostal veins, as well as the superior vena cava (from the right anterior cardinal vein).

The right and left vitelline veins go on to form the hepatic veins and the hepatic segment of the inferior vena cava, and the portal and mesenteric veins. Paired umbilical veins drain directly into the right and left horns of the sinus venosus until the right umbilical vein regresses, and the left umbilical vein fuses with the vitelline veins, which have joined to become the hepatocardiac channel, and anastomosed with right subcardinal vein. This anastomosis forms the segment of the inferior vena cava between the hepatic and renal veins. The right and left subcardinal veins fuse to form the juxtarenal segment of the inferior vena cava, into which the bilateral renal, right gonadal, and right adrenal veins drain. The infrarenal inferior vena cava is derived from the anastomosis of the subcardinal veins with the sacrocardinal veins, from which the iliac veins arise. As the posterior cardinal veins regress, they are replaced by the supracardinal veins, which then form the azygos, hemiazygos, accessory hemiazygos, right superior intercostal, and intercostal veins (Fig. 1.8).

Development of the Portal Venous Circulation

By the end of the third week of gestation, the embryo has two extraembryonic venous systems (the paired vitelline veins and the paired umbilical veins) and one intraembryonic system (the cardinal veins), forming the sinus venosus as the common confluence of all three systems (Fig. 1.9A). At this stage, the umbilical veins are paired and return oxygenated blood from the placenta through the hepatic primordium through branches draining directly into the developing liver and into the sinus venosus through bilateral branches that run along the liver. By the end of the fourth week of gestation, major changes have undergone in the vitelline and umbilical veins.

Four vitelline anastomoses have formed between the left and right vitelline veins, and the segments of the bilateral vitelline veins that run through the fetal liver resolve into a plexus of small vessels that connect with the hepatic sinusoids. The right umbilical vein regresses almost entirely, with only a segment draining into the left umbilical vein persisting in the anterior abdominal wall. The left umbilical vein's terminal branch, which anastomoses with the sinus venosus, regresses, and the left umbilical vein's hepatic branch enlarges and connects with the intervitelline anastomoses within the fetal liver. At this point, all of the oxygenated blood returning from the placenta passes through the liver, until the formation of the ductus venosus shortly thereafter.

During the fifth week, the portal vein emerges from the vitelline system, the ductus venosus forms, and persistence of the subhepatic intervitelline anastomosis creates the portal sinus, which anastomoses the umbilical vein with the newly formed portal vein. The main portal vein terminates in the right angle of the subhepatic intervitelline anastomosis. This is followed by emergence of two large intrahepatic vessels, which is known as the ramus angularis on the left side. Branches then emerge from the trunk of the portal vein and portal sinus tributaries, eventually communicating with the sinusoidal network. The portal vein branches within the hepatic parenchyma become enveloped by a rim of mesenchyme, which will give rise to the portal spaces and the intrahepatic branches of the hepatic arterial bed. At this point, the umbilical vein is still the predominant source of blood flow to the developing liver, delivering oxygenated blood to the sinusoidal network through the portal sinus.

The left angle of the portal sinus develops the ductus venosus, which connects with the inferior vena cava. The ductus venosus is a branchless channel, with a wall rich in elastic fibers and smooth muscle. It is thought to form from a small vessel connecting the subhepatic and subdiaphragmatic intervitelline anastomoses. Upon regression of the left and right intrahepatic vitelline veins, the whole umbilical circulation is transferred to the liver, and this vessel rapidly enlarges, becoming the ductus venosus. At the end of the sixth week of gestation, the intrauterine pattern of the hepatic circulation is complete. Approximately 80% of the blood flow to the liver at this stage is derived from the umbilical vein, with the left lobe receiving 100% of its flow from the umbilical vein and the right lobe receiving about 50% from the umbilical vein and 50% from the portal vein.

Upon birth, there is rapid involution of the ductus venosus and the left umbilical vein, which become the ligamentum venosum and the ligamentum teres, respectively. In summary, the main portal vein is derived from the right vitelline vein and the middle intervitelline anastomosis. The superior mesenteric vein arises from the left vitelline vein. The right portal vein is derived in part from the right vitelline vein and its intrahepatic branches at the right angle of the subhepatic intervitelline anastomosis. The left portal vein results from the persistence of the portal sinus (the subhepatic intervitelline anastomosis) and the ramus angularis, at the left angle of the confluence of left umbilical vein with the left vitelline vein.

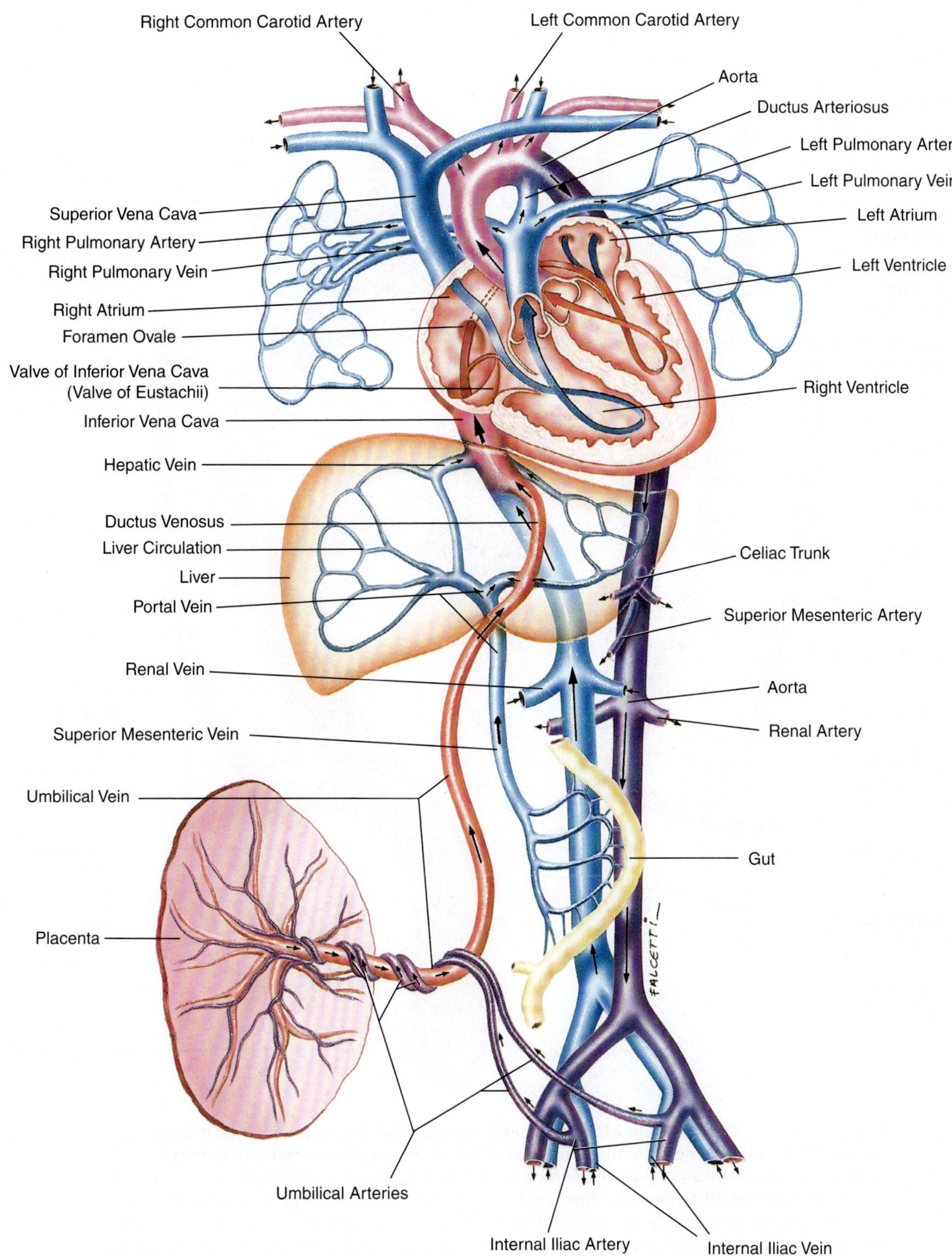

Figure 1.1. Fetal circulation. The fetus receives oxygenated blood from the placenta through the umbilical vein. Part of the received blood passes through the hepatic sinusoids, whereas most of the incoming blood passes through the ductus venosus directly into the inferior vena cava. In the inferior vena cava, oxygen-rich blood from the placenta mixes with blood from the caudal portions of the fetus. The mixed stream of blood enters the right atrium and crosses the interatrial membrane through the foramen ovale into the left atrium. At the left atrium, the blood is mixed again with poorly oxygenated blood from the pulmonary veins and then passes through the left ventricle to the aorta. The blood from the superior vena cava and a small amount of blood from the inferior vena cava is diverted into the pulmonary artery, where the blood is shunted into the descending thoracic aorta through the ductus arteriosus. The resultant mixed blood goes into the abdominal aorta, to the circulation of the viscera and lower extremities, eventually reaching the placenta through the umbilical arteries, for oxygenation.

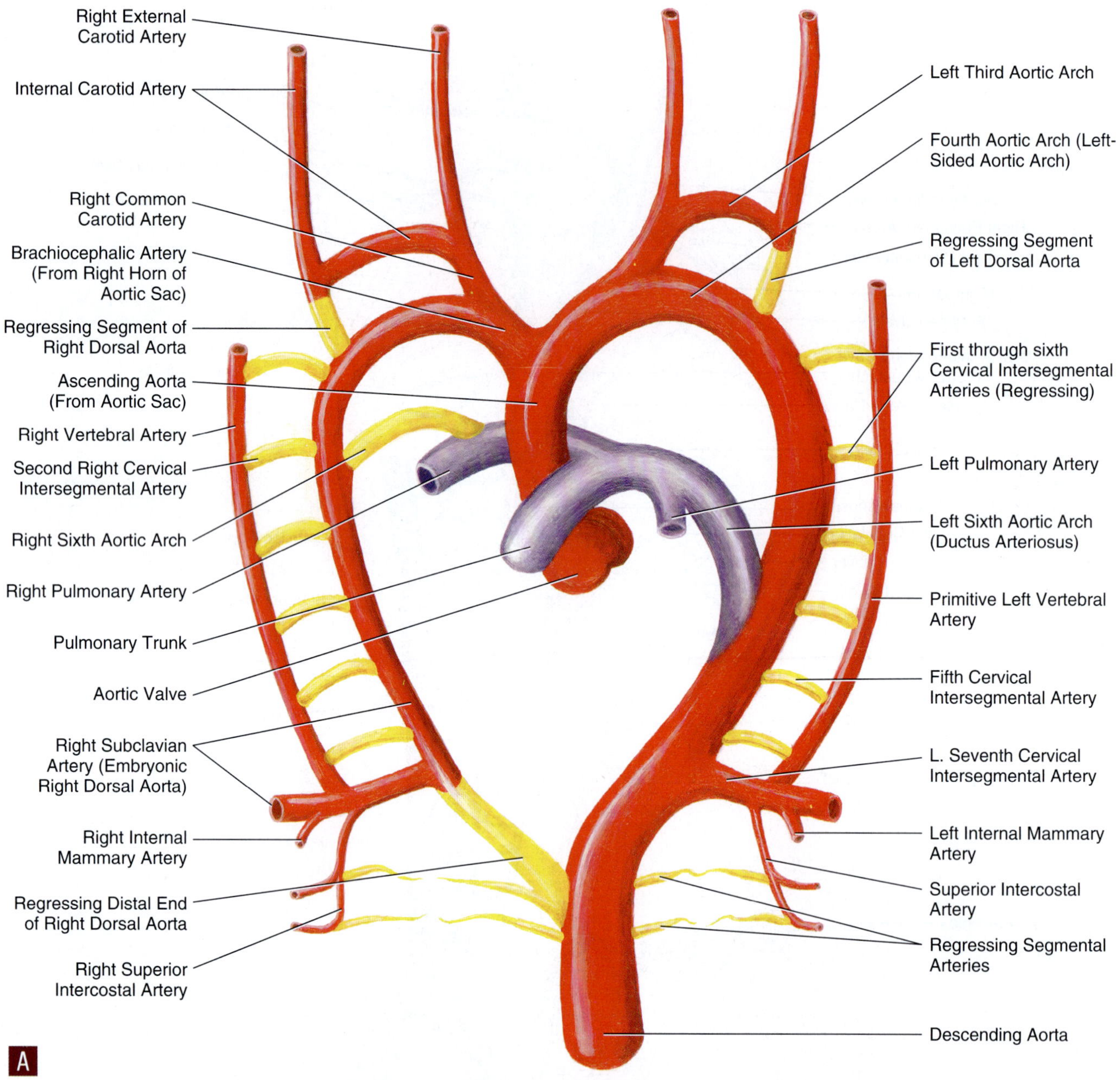

Figure 1.2. Development of the aorta and branches. A, The segments that normally regress are in yellow. The pulmonary artery and ductus arteriosus are depicted in purple. Bilateral aortic arches arise from the aortic sac and pass posteriorly into the dorsal aorta. The first (I) and second (II) arches have involuted (not shown). The branches of the third (III) arch form the internal carotid arteries. The left fourth (IV) aortic arch persists as the aortic arch and the sixth (VI) persists as the ductus arteriosus. The proximal right fourth (IV) arch and a portion of the right dorsal aorta form the right subclavian artery. The subclavian arteries are derived from the seventh cervical intersegmental arteries. Following birth, normal patterns of the aortic arch and pulmonary trunk persist. The ductus arteriosus remains as the only remnant of the sixth (VI) arch. B, Anterior and lateral views of the developing aortic arches and their relationships with the pharyngeal pouches and the developing lung in an 11 mm embryo. The arterial trunk has differentiated into the pulmonary and aortic trunks. The first, second, and fifth aortic arches have regressed.

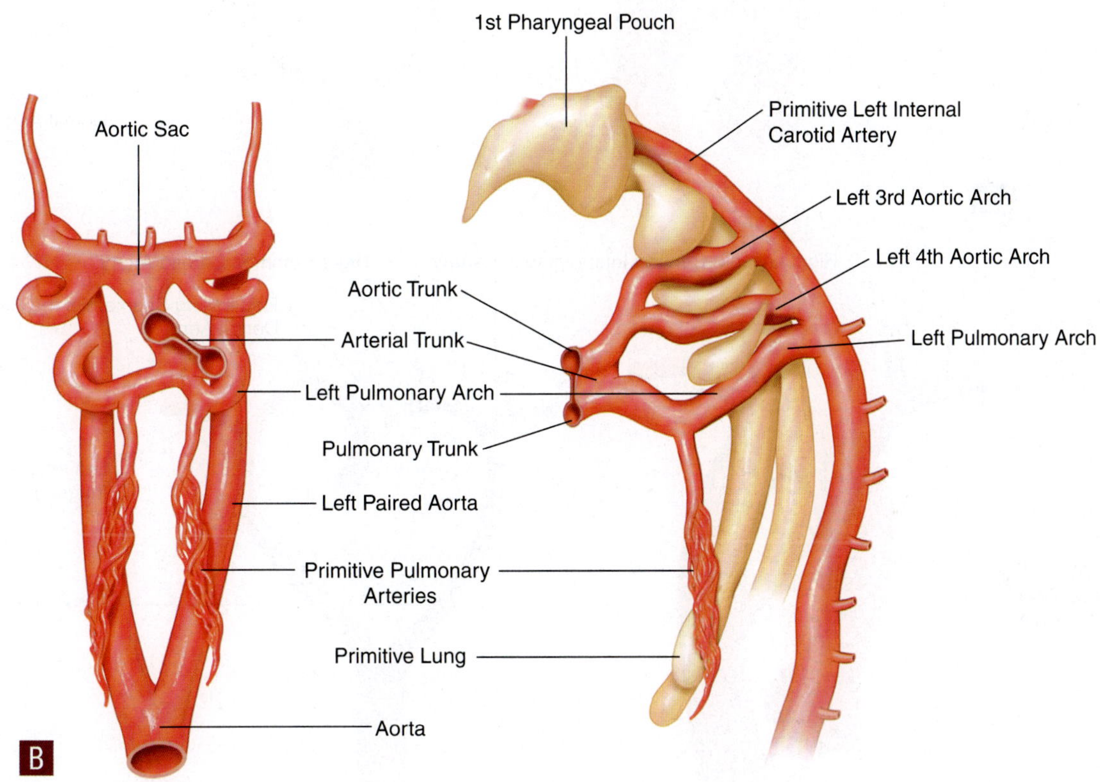

Figure 1.2. *Continued*

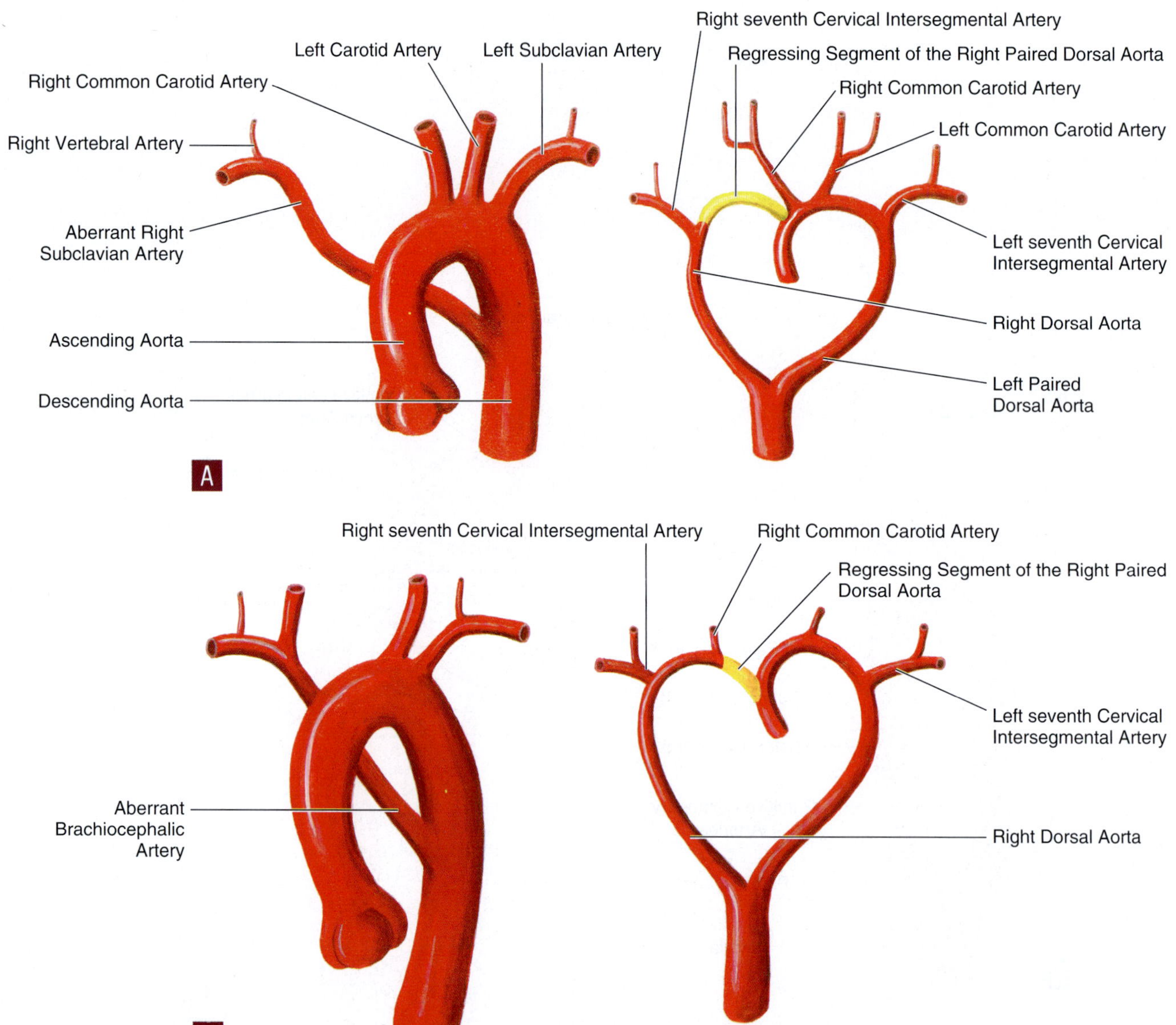

Figure 1.3. Aortic branching variants and their corresponding embryological origins. A, An aberrant right subclavian artery arises because of the interruption of the embryonic right paired dorsal aorta proximal to the right seventh cervical intersegmental artery. B, Interruption of the right paired dorsal aorta proximal to the right common carotid artery gives rise to an aberrant brachiocephalic artery. C, Right-sided aortic arch with mirror image branching arises from regression of the left-sided dorsal aortal distal to the left seventh cervical intersegmental artery. D, Regression of the left fourth arch proximal to the seventh left cervical intersegmental artery gives rise to a right-sided aortic arch with aberrant left subclavian artery. E, Regression of the left fourth arch at the level of the left horn of the aortic sac gives rise to a right-sided aortic arch with an aberrant left brachiocephalic artery.

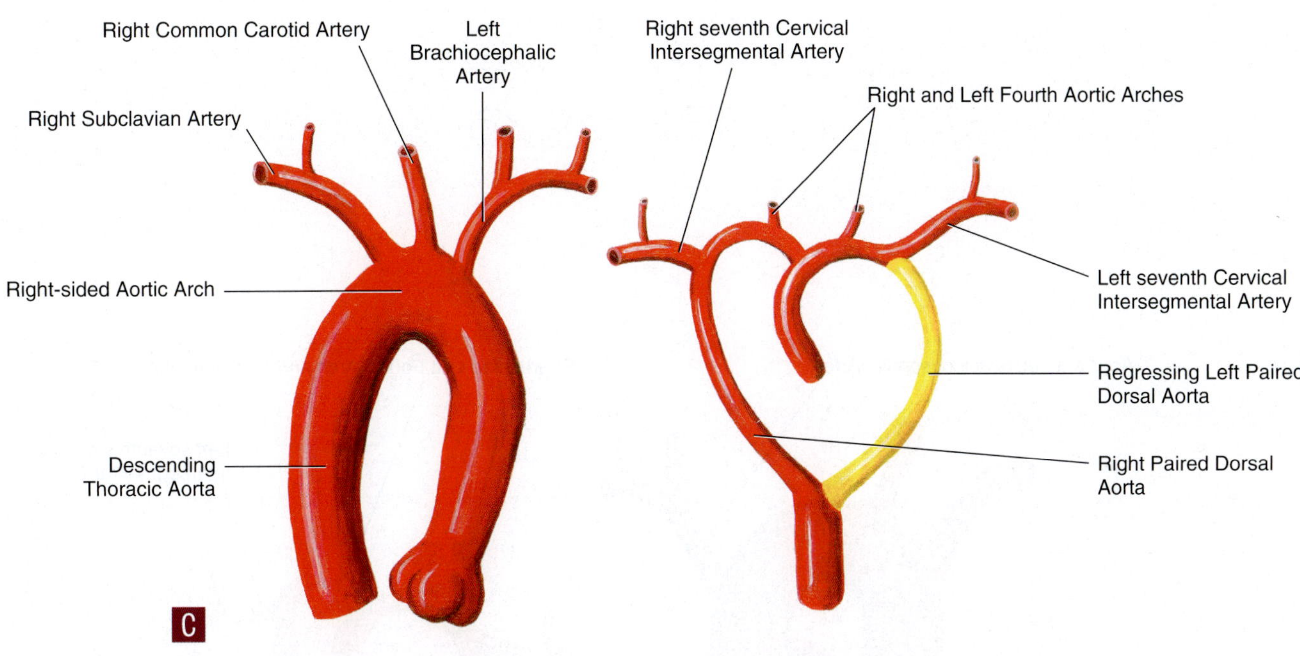

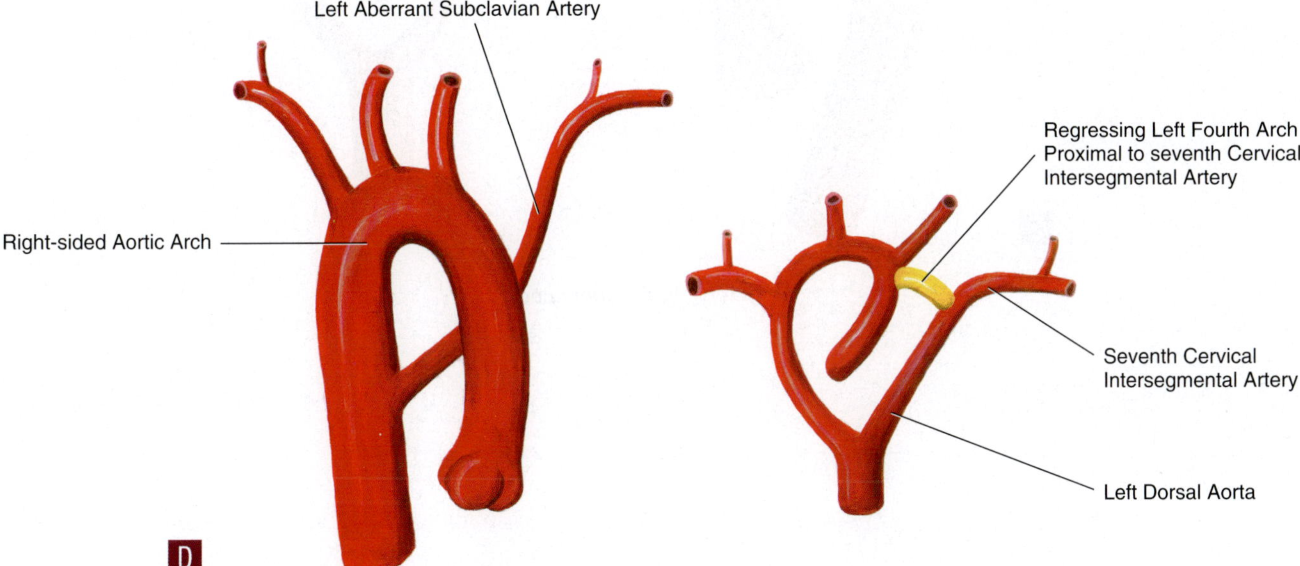

Figure 1.3. *Continued*

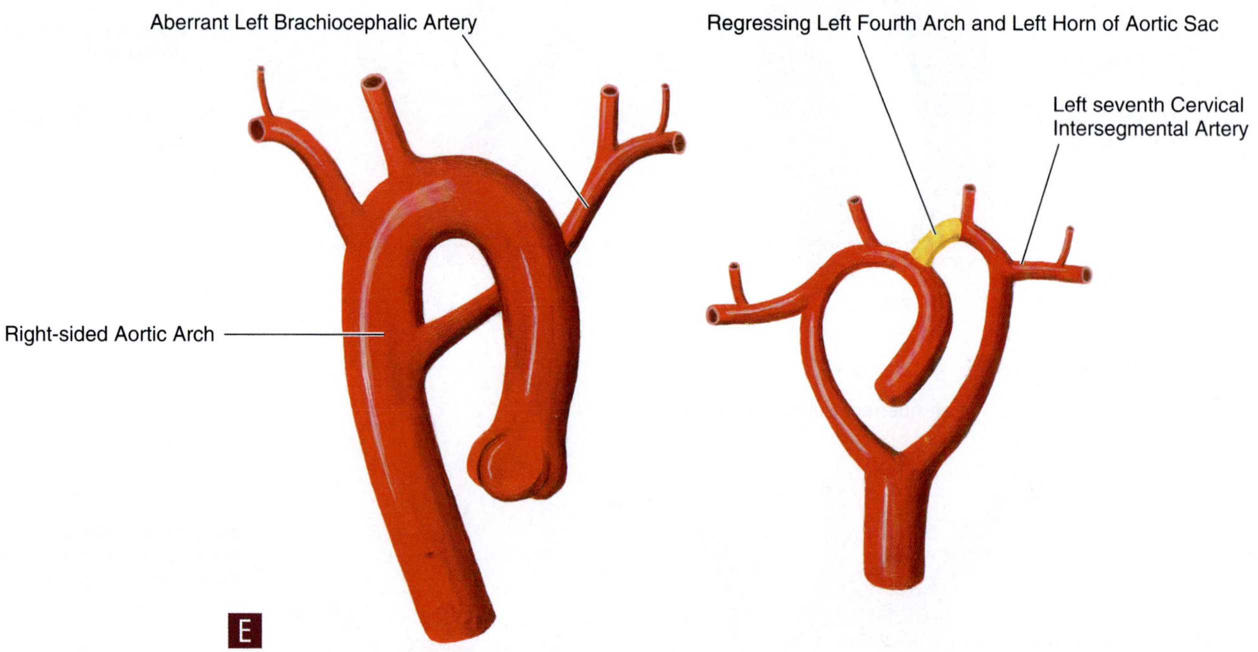

Figure 1.3. *Continued*

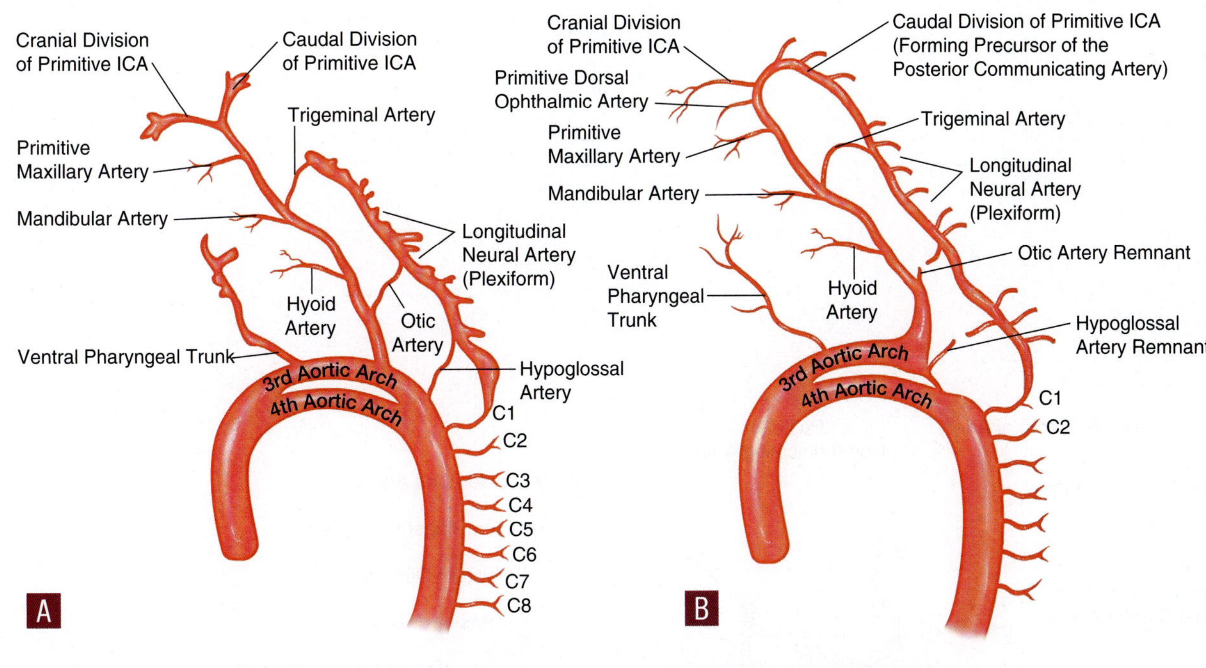

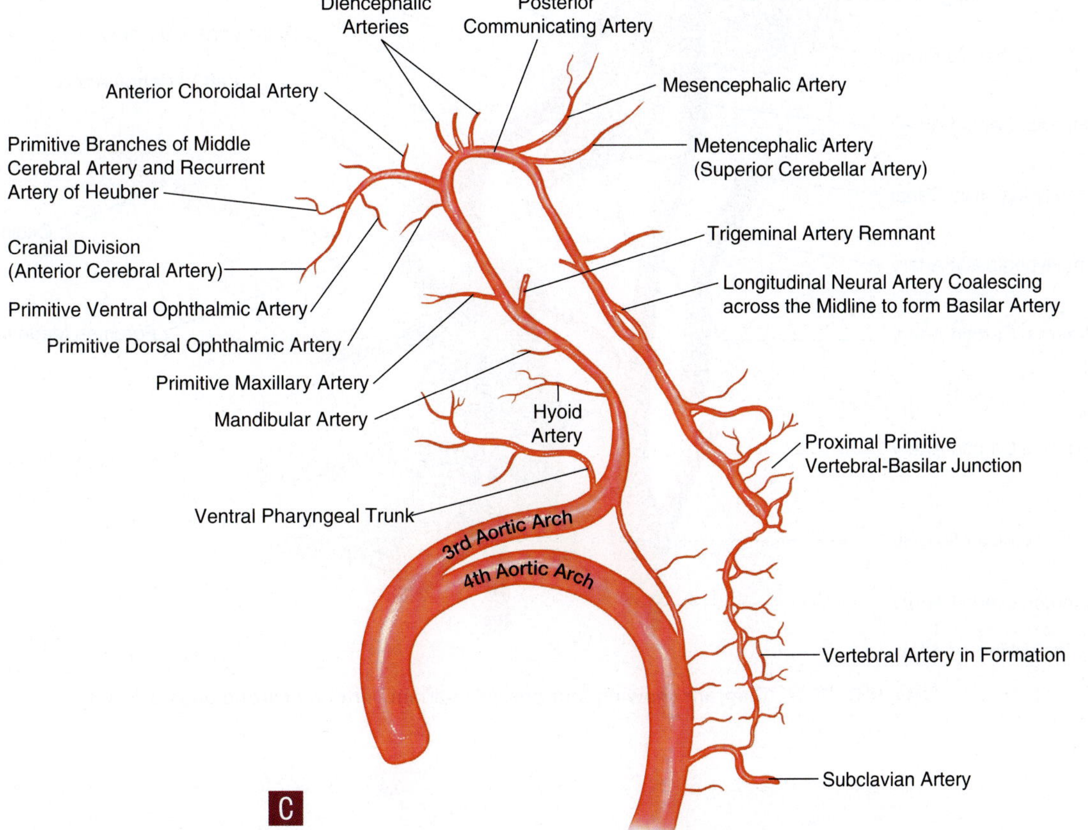

Figure 1.4. Neurovascular development, with the evolution of the anterior and posterior circulations. **A**, A 4 mm embryo has multiple connections between the developing internal carotid artery and the longitudinal neural artery, which include the trigeminal, otic, and the hypoglossal arteries. At this stage, the vertebral artery is still underdeveloped. **B**, By the 6 mm stage, the otic and hypoglossal arteries have begun regressing, and the caudal division of the primitive internal carotid artery has anastomosed with the longitudinal neural artery, forming the precursor of the posterior communicating artery. **C**, The trigeminal artery has regressed by 12 mm, and the vertebral artery has begun to form. All but the seventh cervical intersegmental arteries have regressed, which gives rise to the subclavian arteries. At this stage, the longitudinal neural artery coalesces to form the basilar artery. The vertebrobasilar junction is still plexiform, allowing variable patterns of the inferior cerebellar artery.

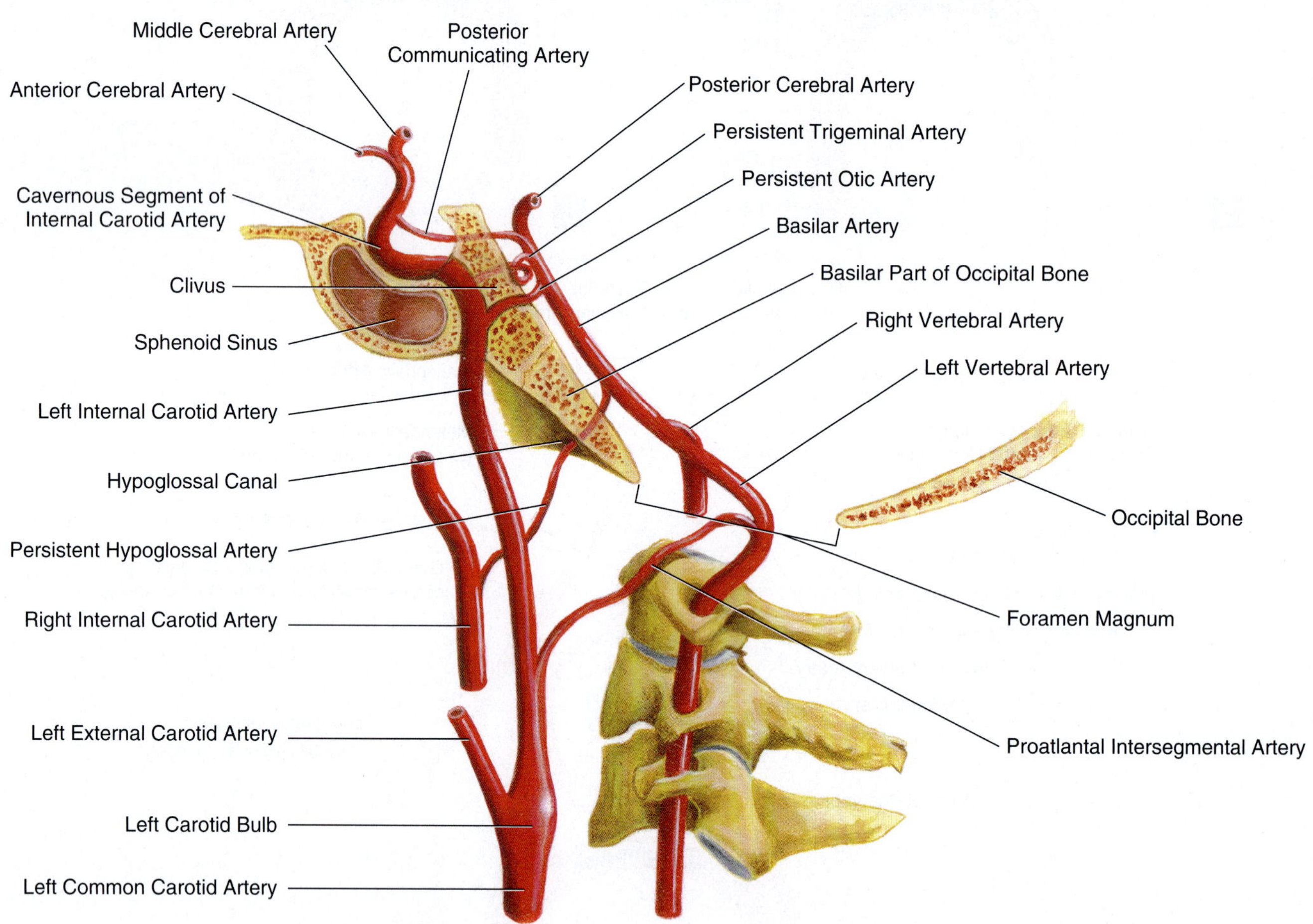

Figure 1.5. Diagram showing four possible variant vertebral carotid anastomoses.

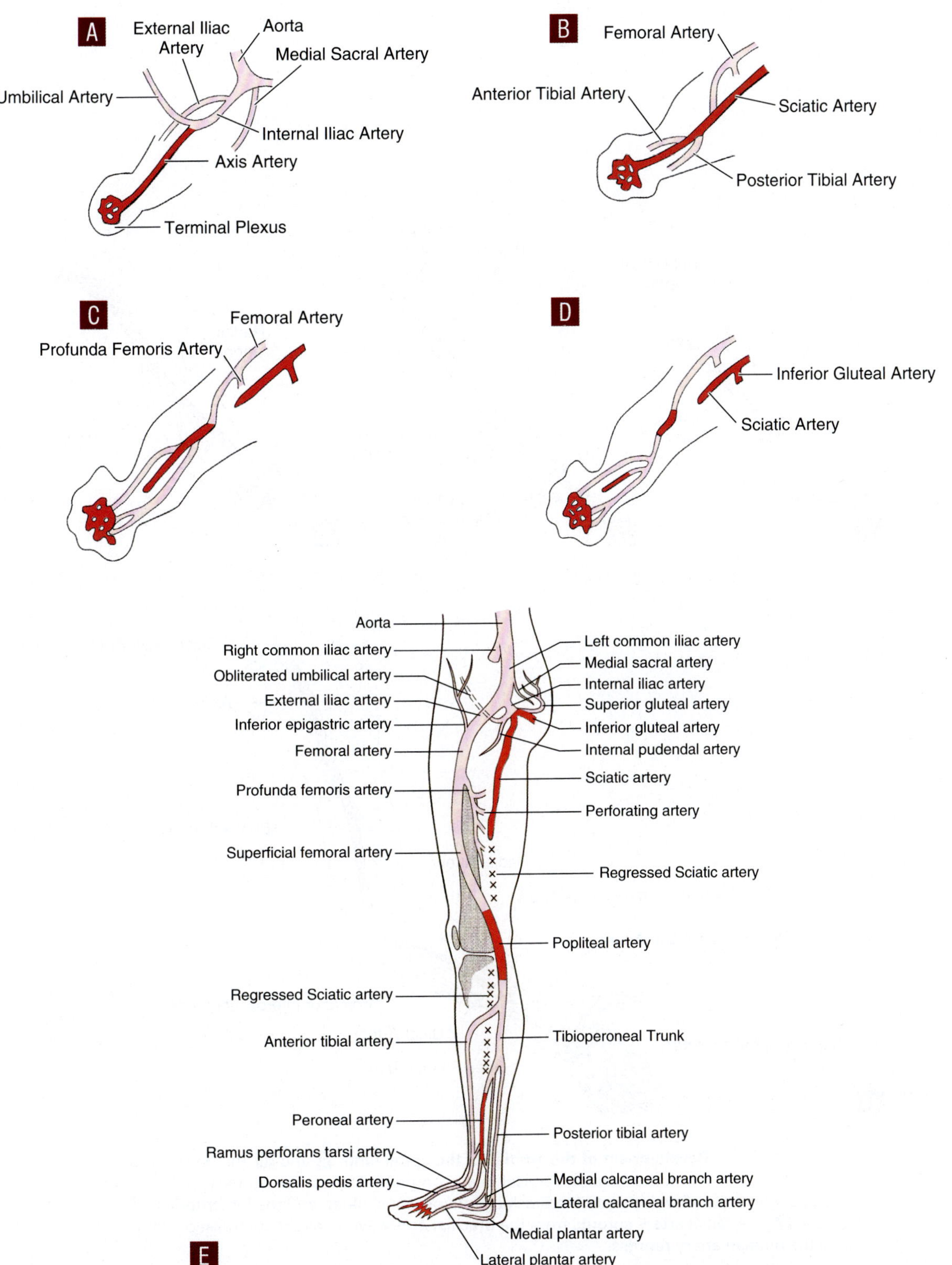

Figure 1.6. **Development of the arteries of the lower limb.** The lower limb bud is vascularized by the sciatic artery which arises from the umbilical artery (A). The external iliac artery and the femoral arteries have already branched from the common iliac artery, which go on to develop the common femoral artery, the superficial femoral artery, and the proximal profunda femoris artery (B). The sciatic artery regresses and its major remnants are the inferior gluteal artery and the distal segment of the peroneal artery (C and D). Additional remnants of the sciatic artery are segments of the profunda femoris and the popliteal arteries (E).

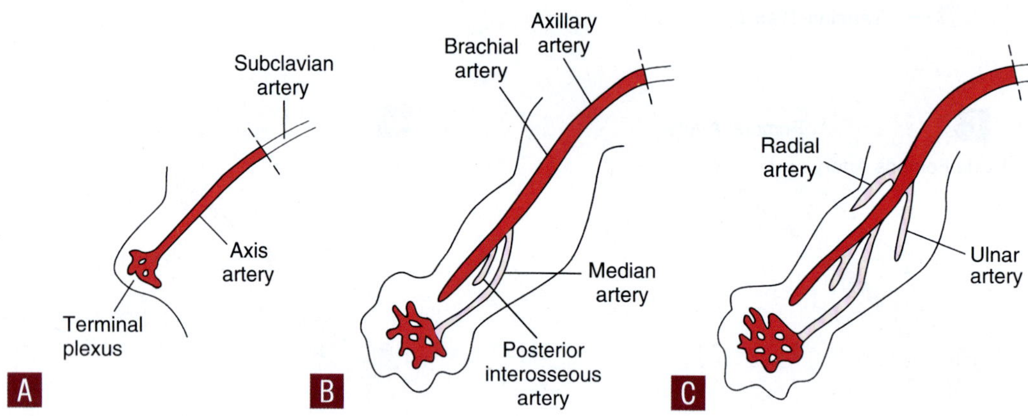

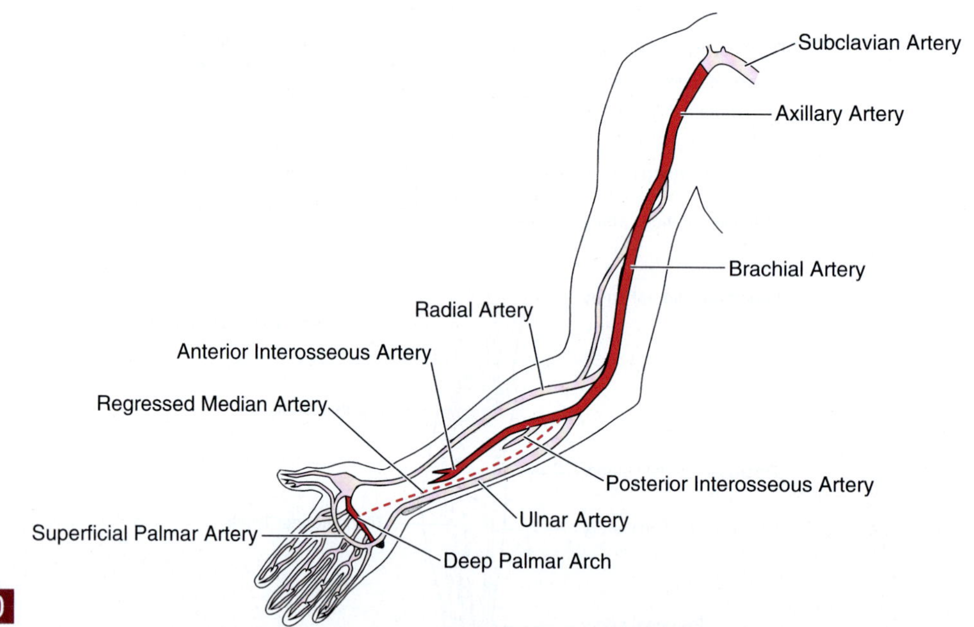

Figure 1.7. Development of the arteries of the upper limb. A and B, the upper limb vasculature arises from the seventh cervical intersegmental arteries. The primary axial artery of the upper limb bud develops into the brachial, interosseous, ulnar, and median arteries. C and D, The radial artery sprouts from the brachial artery, whereas the interosseous artery and the median artery regress.

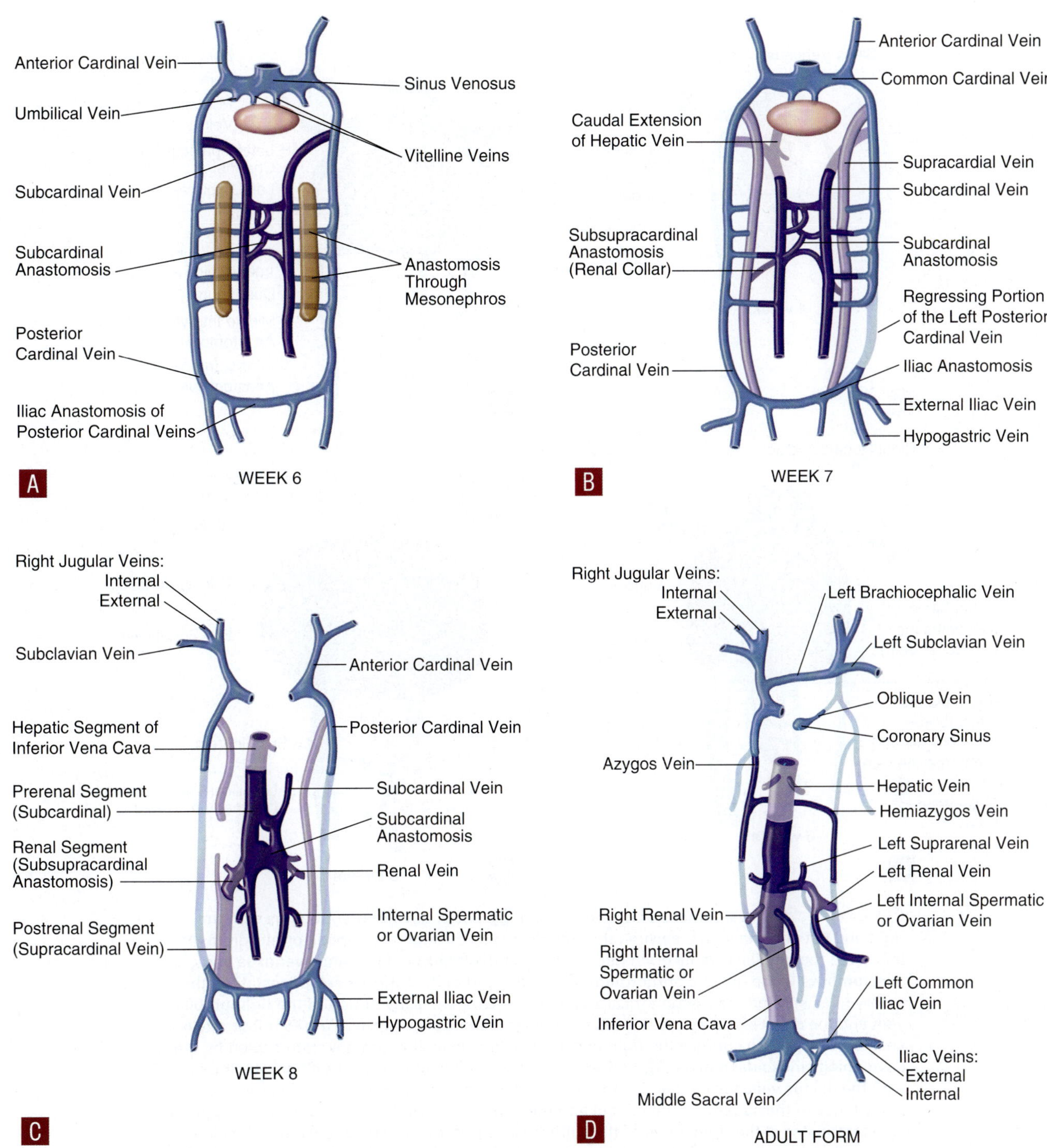

Figure 1.8. Development of the systemic veins. **A**, At week 6, the sinus venosus is the common confluence of the anterior cardinal veins, the umbilical veins, the posterior cardinal veins, and the vitelline veins. The subcardinal veins anastomose through the subcardinal anastomosis at the midline, and through the posterior cardinal veins through the developing mesonephros. **B**, At week 7, the supracardinal veins develop, as well as subsupracardinal anastomoses. **C**, By week 8, the posterior cardinal veins begin to regress. **D**, In the adult form, the inferior vena cava is a continuous channel from the iliac veins to the right atrium. Light blue indicates regressed structures.

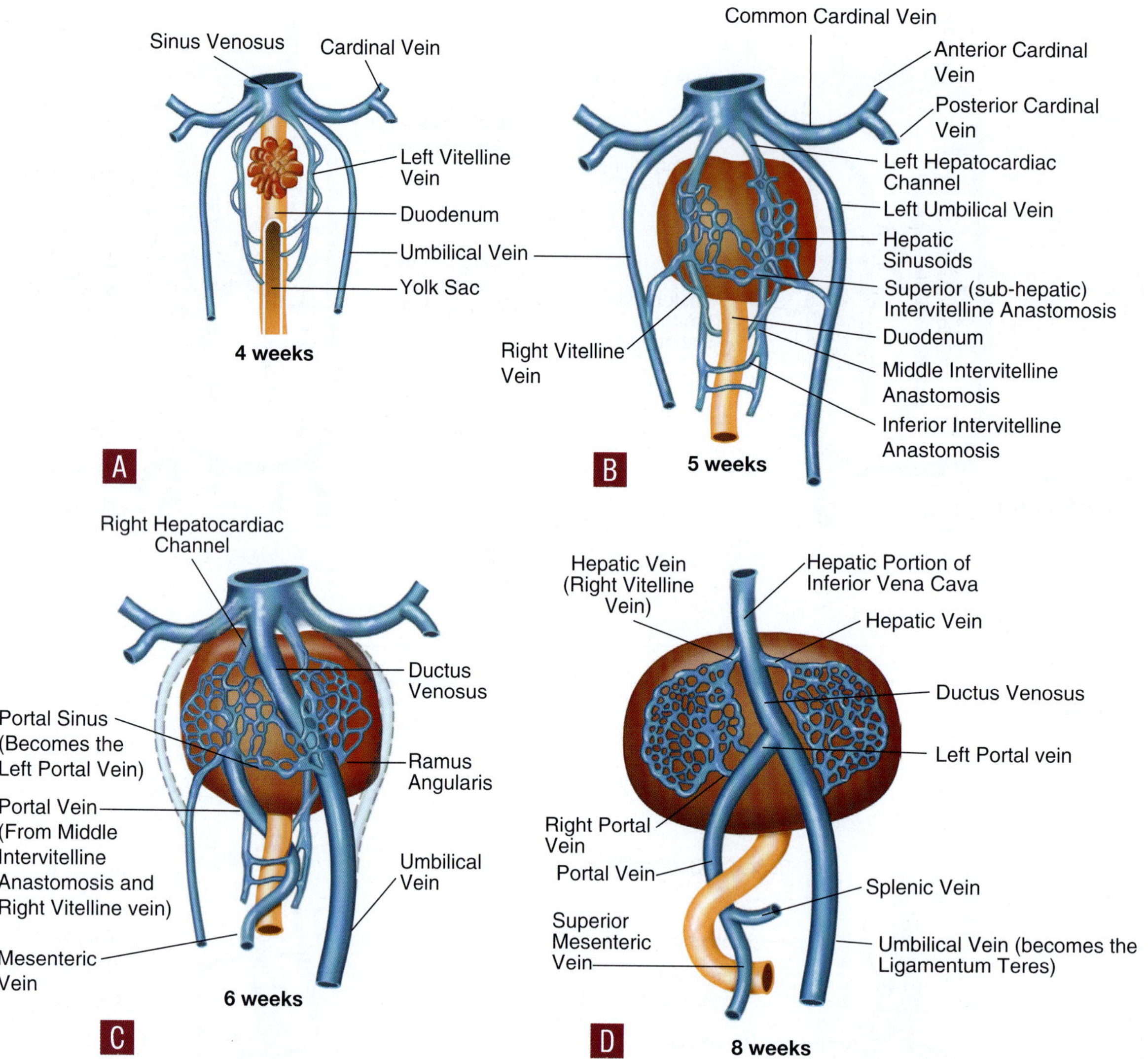

Figure 1.9. **Development of the portal vein.** **A**, portal development begins with the right and left vitelline veins reaching the sinus venosus through the hepatic primordium. At this stage the umbilical veins drain into the right and left horns of the sinus venosus and give anastomoses to the hepatic primordium. **B**, By the end of the fourth week of gestation, the embryo has entered the "symmetrical stage," in which there is involution of the right umbilical vein and the distal extrahepatic segment of the left umbilical vein. There are four intervitelline anastomoses, which connect the right and left vitelline veins that are now interrupted by the developing sinusoidal plexus. **C**, At 6 weeks, the definitive fetal circulation has developed, with the ductus venosus connecting the umbilical vein to the inferior vena cava. There is persistence of the superior (subhepatic) and the middle intervitelline anastomoses. The portal vein terminates at the right angle of the subhepatic anastomosis, which becomes the sinus intermedius (portal sinus). The central aspect of the left vitelline vein and the peripheral right vitelline vein have regressed, and development of the ramus angularis is observed on the left side of the sinus intermedius, with corresponding large intrahepatic veins forming at the right angle of the sinus intermedius. **D**, At birth, the mature portal vein is now present, with the ligamentum venosum and the ligamentum teres. The right portal vein is derived from intrahepatic branches of the right angle of the sinus intermedius. The left portal vein is derived from the subhepatic intervitelline anastomosis (the sinus intermedius) and the ramus angularis. The main portal vein and the superior mesenteric veins are derived from the right and left vitelline veins and the middle intervitelline anastomosis.

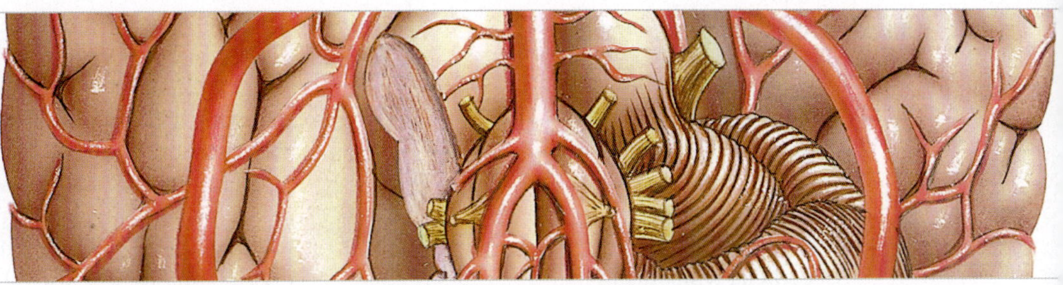

2

Arteries of the Head and Neck

Arterial perfusion of the head and neck arises entirely from the great vessel branching pattern of the aortic arch. The standard aortic arch pattern is present in approximately 70% of the population and has three great vessels: the innominate (also known as the brachiocephalic trunk), left common carotid, and subclavian arteries. The relatively short innominate artery terminally branches to form the right subclavian and right common carotid arteries. The vertebral arteries arise as branches of their respective subclavian arteries (Fig. 2.1). There are a number of variations to this standard aortic arch pattern. In 13% of the population, there is a common origin of the innominate and left common carotid arteries (Fig. 2.2A), and in approximately 9% of the population, the left common carotid artery arises as a proximal branch of the innominate (Fig. 2.2B). "Bovine arch" was historically used to describe both of these but is now considered a misnomer. The terms "variant arch with common origin of the innominate and left common carotid" or "left common carotid arising from the innominate" are favored for their more specific description of the branching pattern. Other less common variations include an origin of the left vertebral artery directly from the aortic arch (Fig. 2.2C) and an aberrant right subclavian artery that courses posterior to the esophagus (Fig. 2.2D).

Common Carotid Artery

The common carotid artery together with the vagus nerve and jugular vein are enclosed within the carotid sheath. The thoracic common carotid arteries arise from the aortic arch anterior to the trachea. The cervical common carotid continues its ascent lateral to the trachea (Figs. 2.1B and 2.3). The common carotid arteries usually have no branches but may anomalously supply the origin of the vertebral, the superior thyroid or its laryngeal branch, the ascending pharyngeal, the inferior thyroid, or occipital arteries (Fig. 2.3).

The common carotid artery terminates at its bifurcation into the external and internal carotid arteries. The carotid bifurcation has a variable location and can be as far inferiorly as the level of the cricoid cartilage or as superiorly as the hyoid but is usually at the C2-3 vertebral body level (Figs. 2.4, 2.5, 2.13, and 2.16).

External Carotid Artery

The external carotid artery arises medial and anterior to the internal carotid artery (Figs. 2.3-2.5) as the smaller terminal branch of the common carotid artery. Occasionally, it may arise lateral to the internal carotid artery, particularly in older individuals in whom chronic hypertension can lead to progressive lengthening and redundant curvature of the internal carotid artery. The external carotid artery provides vascular supply to all of the head and neck structures with the exception of the brain and eyes.

- Branches (Figs. 2.4-2.8)
  - Anterior branches
    - Superior thyroid artery
    - Lingual artery
    - Facial artery

- Posterior branches
  - Ascending pharyngeal artery
  - Occipital artery
  - Posterior auricular
- Terminal branches
  - Superficial temporal artery
  - Internal maxillary artery

Superior Thyroid Artery (Figs. 2.4-2.6)

The superior thyroidal artery is the first branch of the external carotid artery. It divides into terminal branches at the apex of the thyroid gland. It may very rarely arise from the common carotid artery.

- Branches
  - Anterior branch or superior marginal arcade
    - anastomoses with the opposite artery through the isthmus
  - Posterior branch or posterior glandular arcade
    - anastomoses with the inferior thyroid artery
  - Lateral branch or lateral glandular
    - arcade is not constant
  - Hyoid branch
    - anastomoses with the thyrolaryngeal system inferiorly with the linguofacial system superiorly
  - Sternocleidomastoid artery
  - Superior laryngeal artery
    - anastomoses with the opposite artery and the inferior laryngeal artery
  - Cricothyroid artery
    - anastomoses with the opposite artery

Ascending Pharyngeal Artery (Figs. 2.8-2.12)

The ascending pharyngeal artery arises most commonly as the second branch of the external carotid artery but may also arise from a common trunk with the occipital artery (Fig. 2.6) or from the internal carotid artery (Fig. 2.12). This critical yet modest 1 mm diameter artery ascends outside the carotid sheath vertically between the internal carotid and the side of the pharynx to the base of the skull and contributes to vascularization of the nasopharynx, oropharynx, middle ear, eustachian tube, dura around the jugular bulb, and the hypoglossal canal. It has an anterior pharyngeal division and posterior neuromeningeal division with a number of critical vertebral artery, anterior spinal artery, and internal carotid artery anastomoses.

The anterior division gives origin to pharyngeal branches (superior, middle, and inferior) (Fig. 2.9) and to the inferior tympanic artery (Fig. 2.10) which may be a single independent branch. The posterior neuromeningeal division gives origin, distally, to a jugular branch (enters the jugular foramen and feeds the IX, X, and XI cranial nerves) and a hypoglossal nerve branch (enters the hypoglossal canal supplying the hypoglossal nerve and reaches the meninges of the posterior fossa).

The hypoglossal branch may supply the odontoid arcade, which vascularizes the meninges close to the odontoid process (Fig. 2.11). The two branches of the posterior division anastomose with the clival branches of the meningohypophyseal trunk from the internal carotid artery (Fig. 2.11). Another branch of the posterior division is the musculospinal artery, oriented inferiorly and posteriorly, supplying the accessory cranial nerve and the superior sympathetic ganglion.

The posterior neuromeningeal division has critical anastomoses with the vertebral artery at the second and third cervical levels (Figs. 2.9 and 2.11) and with the anterior spinal artery (Fig. 2.9). Inadvertent embolization of the collateral vessels during diagnostic or therapeutic external carotid embolization procedures can lead to devastating spinal cord infarction or cranial nerve dysfunction.

The anterior branch of the ascending pharyngeal artery anastomosis with the internal carotid artery is from a connection with the inferior tympanic artery and caroticotympanic artery (Fig. 2.10). Individuals with agenesis of the high cervical segment of the internal carotid artery develop compensatory collateral flow through this anastomosis, resulting in an "aberrant course of the internal carotid artery." This can be seen as a vessel overlying the cochlear promontory in the mesotympanum, a pulsatile red mass behind the tympanic membrane seen on otoscopy and can present with pulsatile tinnitus.

Lingual Artery (Figs. 2.4, 2.5, 2.13-2.15)

The lingual artery is the third branch of the external carotid artery and main arterial supply of the intrinsic tongue musculature and the sublingual gland. It arises from the anteromedial aspect of the proximal external carotid artery, between the origin of the ascending pharyngeal artery and the facial artery. It may have a common origin with the facial artery with a linguofacial trunk in 10% of the population. This artery runs obliquely superior and medially, curving inferiorly and anteriorly forming a characteristic U-shaped loop (Figs. 2.5 and 2.13). It courses anteriorly and finally ascends superiorly under the surface of the tongue.

The lingual artery may be divided into three parts. The first is in the carotid triangle. The second traverses the upper border of the hyoid bone, deep to the hypoglossal membrane and the submandibular gland. The sublingual artery supplies the sublingual gland and neighboring muscles and mucous membrane of the mouth and gums. It anastomoses with the submental artery arising from the facial artery. A medial mandibular branch supplies the anterolateral surface of the body of the mandible. Depending on the hemodynamic balance of the region, the lingual artery, through its anastomotic branches, can take over the supply of the gland and the mandible and occasionally part of the submental territory (Figs. 2.14 and 2.15). The hypoglossal membrane separates the artery from the hypoglossal nerve and its vena comitans. The third part of the lingual artery is the dorsal lingual artery which courses along the tongue with the lingual nerve until the tip of the tongue where it anastomoses with the contralateral artery (Figs. 2.14 and 2.15).

- Branches
  - Suprahyoid branch
    - small and anastomoses with the contralateral artery
  - Sublingual artery
    - anastomosis with the submental artery from the facial artery
  - Dorsal lingual artery
    - the largest branch supplying the tongue

Facial Artery (Figs. 2.5, 2.6, 2.8, 2.13, 2.16-2.21)

The facial artery originates from the anterior aspect of the external carotid artery typically as the fourth branch within the carotid triangle, just above the lingual artery and the greater cornu of the hyoid bone. The facial artery courses medial to the ramus of the mandible causing a groove on the posterior border of the submandibular gland. It then runs inferiorly and anteriorly around the lower border of the mandible becoming superficial and subcutaneous. At this point, the main facial trunk can have two different courses, a more posterolateral or jugal course, or a more anteromedial or labial course (Figs. 2.13, 2.16, and 2.17). The facial artery turns superiorly along the side of the nose terminating at the medial palpebral commissure where it supplies the lachrymal sac and can anastomose with the dorsal nasal branch of the ophthalmic artery.

The ascending palatine artery arises close to the origin of the facial artery and runs superiorly along the side of the pharynx in the tonsillar pillar where it divides into two branches: the levator veli palatini muscle and soft palate (Fig. 2.9) where it anastomoses with a branch of the descending palatine artery while the other branch penetrates the superior constrictor and supplies the tonsils and the auditory tube. Anastomoses are with the tonsillar, accessory meningeal, and ascending pharyngeal artery and with its counterpart on the other side. The ascending palatine artery or artery of the soft palate may arise directly from the external carotid artery (Figs. 2.19 and 2.20), from the ascending pharyngeal artery (Fig. 2.9), or from the accessory meningeal artery.

The facial artery supplies the muscles and tissues of the face, the submandibular gland, the tonsil, and the soft palate. The branches may be separated in cervical and facial groups. There are abundant anastomoses of the facial artery with the contralateral branches. There are also anastomoses in the neck with the sublingual branch of the lingual artery and with the palatine branch of the maxillary. Anastomoses are also present in the face with the mental branch of the inferior alveolar artery, the transverse facial branch of the superficial temporal artery, the infraorbital branch of the maxillary, and the dorsal nasal branch of the ophthalmic artery. The territory vascularized by the facial artery is in hemodynamic equilibrium with the adjacent arteries that are part of the facial artery territory (Figs. 2.17-2.20)

- Branches
  - Cervical branches
    - Ascending palatine artery (Fig. 2.20)
    - Tonsillar artery supplies the tonsil and root of the tongue (Figs. 2.18 and 2.19).
    - Glandular branches
      - These are several branches supplying the submandibular salivary gland, lymph nodes, and neighboring muscles and skin (Figs. 2.17-2.19).
    - Submental artery
      - The largest cervical branch. It supplies the musculocutaneous region of the mandible and chin and anastomoses with the sublingual branch of the lingual artery and mylohyoid of the inferior alveolar artery. It divides into superficial and deep branches (Fig. 2.14). The submental artery may replace the entire facial trunk when it is hypoplastic.
  - Facial branches (Figs. 2.17-2.19)
    - Inferior labial artery
      - Arises at the angle of the mouth and extends near the edge of the lower lip between the muscle and mucous membrane. There is anastomosis with the contralateral artery and the mental branch of the submental artery (Fig. 2.19).
    - Superior labial artery
      - Courses along the edge of the upper lip between the muscle and mucous membrane having anastomoses with the contralateral artery. It gives off a septal branch to the lower and frontal part of the nasal septum, and an alar branch to the ala of the nose.
    - Lateral nasal branch
      - Also called the angular artery. This vessel ascends along the side of the nose. It supplies the alar artery and the nasal arcade at the dorsum of the nose, anastomosing with the contralateral artery, the septal and alar branches of the superior labial artery, and with the dorsal nasal ramus of the ophthalmic artery and the infraorbital branch of the maxillary artery.
    - Inferior masseteric artery
      - Arises from the facial artery after it has passed under the mandible. It anastomoses with the middle and superior masseteric arteries.

- Jugal trunk
  - The buccomasseteric system or buccal branch.
    - It anastomoses with the facial artery and with the maxillary artery in the upper part of the pterygopalatine fossa. It supplies the deep muscle-mucosal structures and constitutes the preferential collateral pathway between both systems.
  - The posterior jugal artery
    - This has a superficial course connecting the lower border of the mandible with the external orifice of the infraorbital canal. Here, it anastomoses with the infraorbital artery, the superior alveolar artery, and the anterior and middle jugal branches.
  - Middle mental artery
    - Arises midway between the lateral surface of the body of the mandible.
  - Anterior jugal artery supplies the anterior part of the jugal area and anastomoses with the posterior and middle jugal arteries.

Internal Maxillary Artery (Figs. 2.5, 2.8, 2.16, 2.21-2.27)

The larger of the two terminal branches of the external carotid artery, the internal maxillary artery arises behind the neck of the mandible, and it is proximately embedded in the parotid gland. It courses adjacent to the lower margin of the lateral pterygoid muscle before coursing deep into the pterygopalatine fossa. It may be divided into three segments: mandibular, pterygoid, and pterygopalatine.

Mandibular Segment (Behind the Neck of the Mandible)

Branches of the Mandibular Segment

Deep auricular artery is small, may be a branch of the anterior tympanic artery. Supplies the outer aspect of the tympanic membrane and temporomandibular joint.

Anterior tympanic artery supplies the medial aspect of the tympanic membrane and anastomoses with the posterior tympanic branch of the stylomastoid artery.

Middle meningeal artery (largest meningeal artery) (Figs. 2.22, 2.24-2.27). This artery enters the cranial cavity through the foramen spinosum of the sphenoid bone. It runs forward and laterally in a temporal bone groove with a characteristic anterior bend, or genu, and vascularizes large areas of the supratentorial meninges and anastomoses with other meningeal branches and as a variant with the ophthalmic artery. It may give origin to the ophthalmic artery or to its glandular and muscular branches (meningolachrymal artery) (Fig. 2.26). This is a critical common variant origin of the ophthalmic artery. Inadvertent embolization of the ophthalmic artery during embolization of a distal internal maxillary artery branch can result in irreversible blindness due to occlusion of the central retinal artery which is a true-end artery with no collateral supply.

Accessory meningeal artery is most commonly a branch of the maxillary artery (Figs. 2.22, 2.25, and 2.26) or a variant more distal branch of the middle meningeal artery (Fig. 2.22B). The accessory meningeal artery enters the cranium through the foramen ovale. It has an extracranial branch that goes to the cavum at the pharyngotympanic tube level and another intracranial branch anastomosing with branches of the internal carotid, ophthalmic artery, and middle meningeal artery.

Inferior alveolar (dental) artery (Figs. 2.22 and 2.24) arises from the proximal portion of the internal maxillary artery and follows a descending direction. It enters the mandibular canal at the internal surface of the mandible together with the nerve and inferior alveolar vein. It has anastomoses with the submental artery branch of the facial artery and originates the mylohyoid branch.

Pterygoid Segment (Superficial or Deep to the Lateral Pterygoid Muscle in the Temporal Fossa)

Branches of the Pterygoid Segment

Deep temporal branches (Figs. 2.27) anterior, middle, and posterior. They supply the temporalis muscle. These vessels distinguish themselves by the straightness of their course and by the fact that their course is not altered at the base of the skull. The anterior branch anastomoses with the lachrymal artery, through the zygomatic and sphenoid bones.

Pterygoid branches supply the pterygoid muscle.

Masseteric arteries (Figs. 2.22) supply the masseter, a muscle of mastication. This muscle is supplied by four groups of vessels: superior, middle, inferior, and deep masseteric arteries.

Buccal artery (Figs. 2.22 and 2.24) runs along the buccal nerve, to the buccinator muscle, and anastomoses with branches of the facial and infraorbital arteries. This branch constitutes the most important functional anastomosis between the maxillary and facial systems. It arises from the distal maxillary artery and descends posterior to the maxillary tuberosity.

Pterygopalatine Segment (Fig. 2.21)

This segment enters the pterygopalatine fossa and terminates by dividing into several branches denominated according to the direction with which they exit the fossa.

Branches of the Pterygopalatine Segment (Figs. 2.22 and 2.23)

Posterior superior alveolar (dental) artery originates as the maxillary artery and enters the pterygopalatine fossa. Gives rise to several branches, some to the alveolar canals and others to the alveolar process to supply the gums.

Infraorbital artery artery is the most anterior branch of the maxillary artery. It defines the superior boundary of the maxillary sinus and corresponds to the most inferior part of the orbit. It enters the inferior orbital fissure and emerges with the infraorbital nerve on the face through the infraorbital foramen. On the face, there are anastomoses with terminal branches of the facial artery, a dorsal nasal branch of the ophthalmic artery, and transverse facial and buccal arteries.

Greater descending palatine artery runs through the greater palatine canal and gives off two or three lesser palatine arteries to the soft palate and tonsil. It anastomoses with the ascending palatine artery and branches of the sphenopalatine artery.

Pharyngeal branch is very small and distributes to the mucosa of the nose, pharynx, sphenoidal air sinus, and auditory tube.

Artery of the pterygoid canal is a branch of the greater palatine artery and feeder of the upper pharynx, the auditory tube, and the tympanic cavity.

Sphenopalatine artery is the terminal branch of the internal maxillary artery. It passes into the nose at the posterior part of the superior meatus. It has posterior lateral nasal branches and anastomoses with the ethmoidal arteries and the nasal branches of the greater palatine artery. The sphenopalatine artery terminates on the nasal septum as the posterior septal branches and anastomoses with the ethmoidal arteries, the terminal ascending branch of the greater palatine artery, and the septal branch of the superior labial artery.

Occipital Artery (Figs. 2.4, 2.6, 2.7, 2.16, 2.21, 2.27, 2.29-2.31)

The occipital artery is a posterior branch of the external carotid artery. It arises at the level of the facial artery. The artery runs posteriorly and superiorly, crossing the internal carotid artery, the internal jugular vein, as well as the hypoglossal, vagus, and accessory nerves. The distal artery traverses the space between the transverse process of the atlas and mastoid process of the temporal bone. It then courses along the occipital groove on the temporal bone where it is medial to the mastoid process and the attachment of the sternocleidomastoid muscle. Distally, it turns superiorly and divides into several smaller branches.

Branches

Sternocleidomastoid branches. The lower and upper branches supply the muscle.

Mastoid branch. Usually small and sometimes absent; enters through the mastoid foramen to feed the mastoid air cells and dura mater at the level of the cerebellopontine angle. Anastomoses with the middle meningeal artery.

Auricular branch. Supplies the posterior aspect of the auricle and anastomoses with the posterior auricular artery.

Muscular branches. There are several unnamed muscular branches; the most important of them follows a pattern determined by the intervertebral spaces. For each posterior space, a parasagittal branch gives rise to a posterior anastomotic radicular branch and a lateral branch. There are anastomoses with the vertebral artery in the first three cervical intervertebral spaces (Fig. 2.31).

Meningeal branches. Two branches supply the meninges of the posterior cranial fossa: (1) the artery of the falx cerebelli (Fig. 2.30)—this artery arises from the anastomoses in the first cervical space—and (2) the mastoid branch.

Posterior Auricular Artery (Figs. 2.4, 2.6, 2.22, and 2.27)

This is a small artery, arising directly from the posterior aspect of the external carotid artery. It supplies muscles and the parotid gland, and it has three main branches. There is hemodynamic equilibrium between the posterior auricular artery, the occipital artery, and superficial temporal arteries.

Branches

Stylomastoid artery. This artery enters the stylomastoid foramen and supplies the tympanic cavity, the mastoid antrum, the mastoid air cells, and the semicircular canals. In early life, the posterior tympanic artery forms a vascular arcade surrounding the tympanic membrane.

Auricular branch. Supplies the auricularis posterior.

Occipital branch. Anastomoses with the occipital artery.

Superficial Temporal Artery (Figs. 2.5-2.7, 2.16, 2.21, 2.25-2.27, and 2.29)

The superficial temporal artery is one of the terminal branches of the external carotid artery. It arises close to the parotid gland, behind the neck of the mandible, and has an anterior and a posterior branch. This artery supplies the parotid gland, the temporomandibular joint, the masseter, the auricula, and the skin and scalp.

Branches

Transverse facial artery (Figs. 2.22A, 2.24, and 2.25). This vessel arises from the parent artery inside the parotid gland. It divides into numerous branches that extend to the parotid gland and duct, the masseter, and the skin. It has anastomosis with the facial, masseteric, buccal, lachrymal, and infraorbital arteries.

Anterior auricular branch. This supplies the lobule, the anterior part of the auricle, and the external acoustic meatus.

Zygomatico-orbital artery (Figs. 2.6 and 2.25). This occasionally is a branch of the middle temporal artery and supplies the orbicular muscles and anastomoses with branches of the ophthalmic, lachrymal, and palpebral arteries.

Middle temporal artery (Figs. 2.6 and 2.25). This anastomoses with the deep temporal branches of the maxillary artery.

Frontal (anterior) branch. This runs superiorly and anteriorly over the frontal bone. It is tortuous and anastomoses with the contralateral frontal branch.

Parietal (posterior) branch. This courses superiorly and posteriorly along the side of the calvarium. It has anastomoses with the posterior auricular and occipital arteries.

Internal Carotid Artery

The internal carotid artery originates from the bifurcation of the common carotid artery as described in the introductory common carotid artery section. It typically lies posterior and lateral to the external carotid artery. It may, however, have a course anterior and medial to the external carotid artery. At the carotid bifurcation, the vessel dilates posteriorly at the carotid sinus which is the origin of the internal carotid artery (Figs. 2.1B, 2.3, 2.5, 2.6, 2.13, 2.16, and 2.21). The Hering nerve is a small branch of the glossopharyngeal nerve that innervates the vessel-wall baroreceptors of the carotid sinus and carotid body which communicates with the vagus nerve and sympathetic trunk to help respond to both increases and decreases in blood pressure through the vasomotor center in the brainstem.

The internal carotid artery has three main segments: cervical, petrous, and intracranial segments.

Cervical Segment (Fig. 2.1B)

At the cervical segment, the internal carotid artery is vertically oriented, from the origin to the carotid canal at the base of the skull. It is located in the carotid sheath along with the jugular vein and vagus nerve which lies behind and between these two vessels forming a neurovascular bundle. Elongation, loops, and tortuosity can be an acquired change that occurs in the elderly especially in the setting of hypertension. These changes are accentuated by flexion of the neck and straightened by extension of the neck.

Petrous Segment (Figs. 2.32, 2.33, 2.37, 2.38, and 2.40)

There is a vertical and a horizontal subsegment of the petrous segment of the internal carotid artery. The vertical portion passes inside the petrous temporal bone for about 1 cm and then courses anteriorly and medially. The horizontal portion passes anteriorly and medially within the petrous temporal bone to emerge near the apex of the bone.

Intracranial Segment (Figs. 2.28, 2.32, 2.34, and 2.37)

The intracranial portion of the internal carotid artery may be divided into three segments: the precavernous segment, the cavernous segment, and the supraclinoid segments.

The precavernous segment courses superiorly, anteriorly, and medially from the apex of the petrous temporal bone to the lower and posterior aspects of the sella turcica before entering the cavernous sinus. This segment of the internal carotid artery is also called ganglionar segment because it medially abuts the Gasserian ganglion (trigeminal ganglion).

The cavernous segment lies within the cavernous sinus and ascends a short distance lateral to the lower and posterior aspects of the sella. At the carotid sulcus, this segment passes anteriorly on the inferior and lateral aspects of the sella and then curves superiorly, medial to the anterior clinoid process. Within the cavernous sinus, the sixth (VI) nerve courses along the lateral aspect of the artery. The third (III), the fourth (IV), the ophthalmic (V1), and the maxillary (V2) nerves are relatively protected within the lateral wall of the cavernous sinus.

The supraclinoid segment courses superiorly after entering the dura medial to the anterior clinoid process where it is posterior and lateral to its terminal bifurcation. The optic nerve lies medial to the lower supraclinoid segment.

Branches

Mandibular artery
Caroticotympanic branch
Meningohypophyseal trunk
- Basal tentorial branch
- Inferior hypophyseal artery
- Clival branches

Inferolateral trunk
- Marginal tentorial branch
- Branches to the Gasserian ganglion; IV, V, and VI nerves; and to the wall of cavernous sinus. Branches to the orbit
- Superior hypophyseal branches
- Ophthalmic artery
- Posterior communicating artery
- Anterior choroidal artery
- Middle mental artery

Anterior cerebral artery (terminal branch of internal carotid artery)
Middle cerebral artery (terminal branch of internal carotid artery)

Mandibular Artery

It arises from the petrous segment, either in the foramen lacerum or in the horizontal portion at the carotid canal.

Caroticotympanic Branch

Arises from the posterior, distal, and vertical petrous segment of the internal carotid artery. This small branch penetrates the tympanic cavity and anastomoses with the inferior tympanic branch of the ascending pharyngeal artery (Fig. 2.10), the anterior tympanic branch of the maxillary artery, and the stylomastoid artery.

Meningohypophyseal Trunk (Figs. 2.37 and 2.38)

The branches of the meningohypophyseal trunk arise from the posterior aspect of the internal carotid artery. The tentorial branch, inferior hypophyseal artery, and clival branches arise from the dorsal main stem.

Branches

Basal tentorial branch. Enters the tentorium anterior to the apex of the petrous bone and continues in the tentorium near the tentorium attachment to the petrous bone (tentorial basal), supplying the adjacent tentorium, or at the free edge of the tentorium (marginal of tentorium).

Clivus branches. Supply the dura of the dorsum sellae and clivus. Anastomosis with the contralateral corresponding arteries.

Inferior hypophyseal artery (Fig. 2.42). Supplies the posterior lobe of the gland.

Inferolateral Trunk (Fig. 2.37)

The inferolateral trunk arises more anteriorly from the lateral and inferior aspects of the internal carotid artery. It passes downward and laterally over the lateral aspect of the sixth nerve and further downward through lateral or under the fifth nerve. It also gives branches to the Gasserian ganglion; the fourth, fifth, and sixth nerves; and the wall of the cavernous sinus. The main vessel supplies the dura in the floor of the middle fossa and anastomoses with branches of the middle meningeal artery and accessory meningeal artery, whereas other small branches course anteriorly through the superior orbital fissure or directly through the greater wing of the sphenoid to the orbit where they anastomose with branches of the ophthalmic artery.

Superior Hypophyseal Branches (Fig. 2.37A)

These are branches of the internal carotid artery at the level of the supraclinoid segment or posterior communicating artery. They supply the pituitary stalk and the anterior lobe of the pituitary gland.

Ophthalmic Artery (Figs. 2.3, 2.26, 2.28, 2.37, and 2.38)

The ophthalmic artery arises immediately above the superior limit of the cavernous sinus. It is the first major branch of the internal carotid artery. In approximately 80% of the population, the origin of the ophthalmic artery is in the subdural space at the level where the internal carotid artery exits the cavernous sinus, penetrating the dura. In 6%, it may be slightly distal to this site by approximately 1 mm. In 7%, it may be extradural, arising from the intracavernous portion of the internal carotid artery (Fig. 2.38). In 2%, it arises from the internal carotid artery at the level it penetrates the dura.

Alternate supply of the ophthalmic artery Numerous smaller fetal collateral vessels supply the ophthalmic artery bed. The collateral blood supply to the orbit is adequate to prevent permanent blindness after occlusion of the internal carotid and ophthalmic artery in about 90% of patients.

Functionally and embryologically, there are two groups of arteries supplying the orbit: one that supplies the optic nerve and the globe originating from the anterior cerebral artery and internal carotid artery (dorsal ophthalmic artery). The other group supplies the remaining orbital structures, including, such as muscles, eyelids, lachrymal gland, and meninges originating from the stapedial system and provides an origin for the middle meningeal artery and internal maxillary artery (ventral ophthalmic artery).

***Alternate ophthalmic artery origin from the middle meningeal artery* (Fig. 2.26).** This is the most common anomalous origin of the ophthalmic artery present in about 1% of cases due to embryologic regression of the dorsal ophthalmic artery.

***Alternate ophthalmic artery origin from the intracavernous segment of the internal carotid artery* (Fig. 2.38).** Anomalous development of anastomosis between the ophthalmic artery and the internal carotid artery through the superior orbital fissure due to regression of the meningolachrymal segment and dorsal ophthalmic artery.

From the ascending pharyngeal artery. This is the pharyngomeningolachrymal artery.

Course of the ophthalmic artery

Intracranial course
Intracanalicular course
Intraorbital course

Intracranial and intracanalicular course segments:

1. Short limb
2. Angle A (90°-135°)
3. Long limb
4. Angle B (90°-210°)
5. Distal part (to the apex of the orbit)

Intraorbital course. Courses inferolaterally to the optic nerve until it crosses over or under the optic nerve to proceed medially. It may be subdivided into three segments.

1. *First part.* The angle (120°-135°) (between the first and second parts)
2. *Second part* (crosses over or under the optic nerve). The bend (between the second and third parts)
3. *Third part.* Medial to the optic nerve

Terminal segment of the ophthalmic artery The ophthalmic artery terminates at the superomedial angle of the orbital opening.

Branches of the ophthalmic artery There are three groups of branches from the ophthalmic artery.

Ocular group

Central retinal artery
Anterior ciliary (medial and lateral posterior ciliary and anterior ciliary arteries)
Choroid plexus of the eyeball (supplied by the ciliary arteries)

Orbital group

Lachrymal artery
Muscular arteries
Orbital periosteum and areolar tissue arteries

Extraorbital group

Posterior ethmoidal artery
Anterior ethmoidal artery
Supraorbital artery
Medial palpebral artery
Dorsal nasal artery (terminal branches)
Supratrochlear artery (terminal branches)

Posterior Communicating Artery (Figs. 2.1A, 2.3, 2.32B, 2.37B, 2.38, and 2.40C)

The posterior communicating artery joins the posterior cerebral artery to the internal carotid artery, representing an embryologic caudal division of the carotid system. Late in the fetal life, the posterior communicating artery involutes and the posterior cerebral artery shifts its dependence from the carotid to the basilar posterior system. The posterior communicating artery originates posterior to the internal carotid artery above the oculomotor nerve (third cranial nerve) and anastomoses with the posterior cerebral artery. The caliber of the posterior communicating artery and posterior cerebral artery P1 segment is in balance to supply the more distal P2 segment. The posterior half of the posterior communicating artery has several small central branches that perforate the posterior perforated substance and supply the medial surface of the thalamus and the walls of the third ventricle. A slight posterior dilation of the internal carotid artery at the expected origin of the posterior communicating artery is classified as an infundibulum if it is less than 3 mm and has a pyramidal shape (Fig. 2.40B). A posterior communicating artery infundibulum is not considered to be at an increased risk for hemorrhage and is not considered to be an aneurysm.

Anterior Choroidal Artery (Figs. 2.37B, 2.41, 2.45, and 2.47)

The anterior choroidal artery originates from the posterior aspect of the internal carotid artery, a few millimeters distal to the origin of the posterior communicating artery and before the internal carotid bifurcation. It may, however, arise from the posterior communicating artery, from the middle cerebral trunk, or before the posterior communicating artery (Fig. 2.45). This artery courses posteroinferiorly and medially immediately below the optic tract. It then passes posteriorly and laterally and crosses the optic tract from the medial to the lateral side. The artery continues laterally across the wing of the ambient cistern to enter the choroidal fissure and joins the choroidal plexus within the supracornual cleft.

Two segments of the anterior choroidal artery are the cisternal segment and the plexal segment.

The cisternal segment has 3 to 10 branches. The proximal branches are small, perforating vessels that supply the posterior two-thirds of the optic tract, perforating substance and globus pallidus and genus of the internal capsule (Fig. 2.47). Lateral and inferiorly directed branches supply part of the piriform cortex and uncus of the temporal lobe (Fig. 2.45). Medially directed branches enter the midbrain to supply part of the middle third of the cerebral peduncle, which contains the corticospinal fibers. A distal group of branches supplies the inferior half of the posterior limb of the internal capsule, retrolenticular fibers of the internal capsule, and the hilum of the lateral geniculate body. These distal branches anastomose with tributaries from the lateral choroidal branch of the posterior cerebral artery.

The plexal segment begins where this vessel enters the supracornual recess of the temporal horn and supplies the plexus only in the temporal horn but may occasionally supply the entire plexus in the temporal horn and atrium. The size and extent of distribution is in equilibrium with the posterior choroidal branches of the ipsilateral posterior cerebral artery. A few branches of the posterior choroidal artery may arise from the anterior choroidal artery. Branches of the posterior cerebral artery may arise from the anterior choroidal artery and feed that territory (Fig. 2.45).

Anterior Cerebral Artery (Figs. 2.3, 2.32, 2.33-2.35, 2.37, 2.38, 2.43, 2.46, and 2.47)

The anterior cerebral artery complex is composed of the anterior cerebral artery, the anterior communicating artery, and the pericallosal artery and its orbital, frontopolar, and callosomarginal branches. The horizontal portion of the anterior cerebral artery arises anteriorly as the smaller of the two terminal branches of the internal carotid artery. It courses anteriorly and medially to the interhemispheric fissure, passing over the optic nerve and chiasm and below the medial olfactory stria with a slightly posterior convex curve. In the interhemispheric fissure, it is joined by the opposite anterior cerebral artery through the anterior communicating artery. The anterior cerebral artery may be hypoplastic, and, in that case, the contralateral anterior cerebral artery supplies both pericallosal arteries through the anterior communicating artery. The horizontal segment or segment A1 may be duplicated by a fenestration of the artery.

The anterior cerebral artery gives origin to two groups of small arteries: an inferior and a superior group. The small inferior group of branches supplies the superior surface of the optic nerve and chiasm and the superior group is formed by the medial striate arteries, including the artery of Heubner. There are 5 to 10 small arteries that supply the anterior hypothalamus, the septum pellucidum, the medial portion of the anterior commissure, the pillars of the fornix, and the anterior inferior part of the striatum. The recurrent artery of Heubner (Fig. 2.46) originates from the horizontal segment of the anterior cerebral artery or from the initial portion of segment A2 close to the anterior communicating artery. It has a course parallel to the horizontal segment in anterior perforated substance feeding a variable extension of the base nuclei. When fully developed, it may be described as the accessory middle cerebral artery reaching the territory of the middle cerebral artery receiving a few of its branches.

Anterior Communicating Artery (Fig. 2.46)

The anterior communicating artery is a few millimeters in length and communicates between both anterior cerebral arteries in the interhemispheric fissure (Fig. 2.46). It completes the anterior portion of the circle of Willis. The anterior communicating artery is usually single but may be duplicated or triplicated. It may be hypoplastic or very robust simulating an aneurysm.

Several small branches may arise from the anterior communicating artery to the infundibulum, chiasm, and preoptic areas of the hypothalamus. Occasionally, the anterior middle cerebral artery or median artery of the corpus callosum may originate from the anterior communicating artery.

Pericallosal Artery (Figs. 2.3 and 2.47)

It is the portion of the major anterior cerebral artery complex distal to the anterior communicating artery. The artery ascends in front of the lamina terminalis, between the two hemispheres along the longitudinal fissure, making a curve around the genus of the corpus callosum in the pericallosal cistern (Fig. 2.47).

Segments

Infracallosal segment. Ascends in front of the lamina terminalis to the level of the genu of the corpus callosum.

Precallosal segment. Curved portion of the artery around the genu of the corpus callosum.

Supracallosal segment. Lies in the pericallosal cistern and passes posteriorly toward the splenium, generally following the upper surface of the corpus callosum.

The posterior length of the pericallosal artery depends on the size of the callosomarginal artery and the posterior pericallosal branch of the posterior cerebral artery. The posterior pericallosal branch may be the terminal portion of the pericallosal artery and may not originate from the posterior cerebral artery. Several large cortical branches arise from the convexity of the pericallosal artery to supply the white matter of the medial part of the orbital gyri, the gyrus rectus, the olfactory bulb and tract, the medial surface, and a strip of the lateral surface of the frontal and parietal lobes. Multiple small branches arising from the concavity of the pericallosal artery supply the corpus callosum, septum pellucidum, and columns of the fornix. The distribution pattern of the anterior cerebral artery is variable, and specific branch identification is defined by the territory perfused (Fig. 2.47).

Branches of the Pericallosal Artery (Fig. 2.47)

Orbital artery (frontobasilar artery). First branch of the pericallosal artery. Usually arises from the infracallosal segment of the pericallosal artery or from a common trunk that also gives rise to the frontopolar artery. The anterior course of the orbital artery lies in the medial or inferior surface of the frontal lobe and supplies the medial basal region of the frontal lobe, including the gyrus rectus, the medial part of the medial gyri, and the olfactory bulb and tract.

Frontopolar artery. Usually the second branch of the pericallosal artery, arising from the infracallosal segment. It may arise as a common trunk with the frontobasilar artery or from the callosomarginal artery. This artery passes in anteriorly along the medial surface of the brain hemisphere along a gentle curve in the direction of the frontal pole to supply the anterior portion of the medial and lateral surfaces of the superior frontal gyrus.

Callosomarginal artery. It may be a single vessel or a group of several ascending vessels arising from the pericallosal artery. This artery courses over the cingulate gyrus at the cingulate sulcus. When this branch is a single trunk, it follows a course roughly parallel to that of the pericallosal artery. The branches of the callosomarginal artery ascend on the medial surface of the hemisphere and continue to the lateral convexity for approximately 2 cm, supplying premotor, motor, and sensory areas.

Branches

Anterior internal frontal artery
Middle internal frontal artery
Posterior internal frontal artery
Paracentral artery

Cortical Branches of the Anterior Cerebral Artery

Eight territories of vascular supply are identified regarding the cortical branches of the anterior cerebral artery (Fig. 2.3).

Orbitofrontal
Frontopolar
Anterior internal frontal
Middle internal frontal
Posterior internal frontal
Paracentral
Superior internal parietal
Inferior internal parietal

The distribution of the cortical branches of the anterior cerebral artery is based on the anatomy of the medial surface of the cerebral hemisphere. The medial surface supplied by the anterior cerebral artery is compartmentalized by several named sulci or fissures. The sulci and fissures are the subfrontal sulcus (frontopolar artery), cingulate sulcus (callosomarginal artery), marginal limb of the cingulate sulcus (paracentral artery and/or superior internal parietal artery), paracentral sulcus (posterior internal frontal artery), central sulcus (paracentral artery branch), subparietal sulci, and parieto-occipital fissure.

The subfrontal sulcus is constant and located at the inferior limit of the superior frontal gyrus. The gyrus rectus lies beneath the subfrontal sulcus. Superior to the subfrontal sulcus is the large superior frontal gyrus, which is subdivided by many inconstant and unnamed sulci. The paracentral sulcus marks the posterior limit of the superior frontal gyrus and the limit between it and the paracentral lobule. The paracentral lobule is variable in size and is divided from above by the central sulcus, which extends from the lateral surface of the hemisphere. The marginal limit of the cingulate sulcus separates the paracentral lobule from the precuneus, or quadrilateral lobe, which is bounded inferiorly by the subparietal sulcus and posteriorly by the parieto-occipital fissure.

The cortical arteries arise from either the pericallosal artery or a marginal trunk of the pericallosal artery. The size of the pericallosal artery varies inversely with that of the callosomarginal trunk. The cortical arteries are named according to their territories of supply.

Orbitofrontal artery (Fig. 2.43). This is the first cortical branch of the anterior cerebral artery. It arises independently from the pericallosal artery in the majority of the cases. It may share a common origin with the frontopolar artery or arise as a branch of a callosomarginal trunk together with two or more other cortical branches. The orbitofrontal artery supplies the gyrus rectus and the medial half of the inferior surface of the frontal lobe.

There are anastomoses with the orbitofrontal branch of the middle cerebral artery in the area of the H-shaped sulcus. In lateral projection, angiograms this branch projects at the level or underneath the level of the ophthalmic artery (Fig. 2.47).

Frontopolar artery (Fig. 2.47). Arises from the pericallosal artery or callosomarginal trunk in opposition to the anterior genu of the corpus callosum and courses anteriorly in and along the subfrontal sulcus. The origin may be in common with the orbitofrontal artery as well as with the anterior and middle internal frontal arteries in less than 50% of cases. This is invariably a single artery with two branches. It supplies the inferior portion of the superior frontal gyrus.

Anterior internal frontal artery. This artery arises directly from the pericallosal artery in approximately half of cases. It may be a common origin with any other cortical branch except the internal parietal artery or have a common origin with the frontopolar artery and middle internal frontal arteries. The artery supplies the anterior third of the internal surface of the superior frontal gyrus.

Middle internal frontal artery. Originates, most commonly from the pericallosal artery. Less frequently arises from the callosomarginal trunk, in combination with the other internal frontal arteries. Supplies the middle third of the internal surface of the superior frontal gyrus.

Posterior internal frontal artery. It is a branch of the callosomarginal trunk in more than 50% of cases, most often in combination with the middle internal frontal and paracentral arteries. In the remaining cases, it is a branch of the pericallosal artery. Before emerging from the medial surface of the hemisphere, the posterior internal frontal artery gives off a branch that lies in the paracentral sulcus. It supplies the posterior third of the medial aspect of the superior frontal gyrus.

Paracentral artery. This may be small in caliber but is invariably present. In about 50% of cases, it arises from the pericallosal artery. It may originate from a common trunk with the posterior internal frontal artery, the superior internal parietal artery, or both. It courses in the marginal limb of the cingulate sulcus but may occasionally run in the paracentral sulcus. It supplies the paracentral lobule and sends a branch from the medial surface of the brain in the central sulcus.

Superior internal parietal artery. This is usually the largest cortical branch of the anterior cerebral artery. It arises directly from the pericallosal artery in about 75% of cases. In the remaining 25% of cases, it shares an origin with the posterior internal frontal, paracentral, or inferior internal parietal arteries. It courses in the marginal limb of the cingulate sulcus and supplies the upper two-thirds of the precuneus. This territory extends posteriorly to include approximately 80% of the precuneus where the artery anastomoses with the parieto-occipital branches of the posterior cerebral artery.

Inferior internal parietal artery. This is the last cortical branch of the anterior cerebral artery and arises at the point before the pericallosal artery courses around the splenium of the corpus callosum. It may be multiple and supplies the inferior third of the precuneus and extends posteriorly as far as the superior internal parietal artery.

Middle Cerebral Artery (Figs. 2.1A, 2.32-2.35, 2.37, 2.43, 2.48, and 2.49)

The middle cerebral artery originates as a terminal division of the internal carotid artery. The middle cerebral artery is on average 20% larger than the anterior cerebral artery and is located below the medial part of the anterior perforated substance at the medial end of the lateral cerebral fissure. An accessory middle cerebral artery may be found in about 3% of cases, below the bifurcation of the internal carotid artery. More rarely the accessory middle cerebral artery may originate from the anterior cerebral artery, and its embryologic origin is likely to be related to the recurrent artery of Heubner. The anterior choroidal artery may rarely arise from the middle cerebral artery.

The middle cerebral artery is divided into the M1, M2, and M3 segments. The M1 horizontal segment supplies the basal ganglia, the orbital surface of the frontal lobe, and the temporal pole. The M2 sylvian segment supplies the insular cortex. The M3 cortical branches supply the lateral convexities of the cerebrum.

Horizontal M1 Segment of the Middle Cerebral Artery

The horizontal or M1 segment of the middle cerebral artery begins at the internal carotid bifurcation, runs laterally in the lateral cerebral fissure, and ends at its bifurcation or trifurcation usually as it enters the sylvian fissure. The M1 segment bifurcates or trifurcates usually near the island of Reil. There is often an earlier branch (Fig. 2.46).

The segment M1 presents three main groups of branches.

Lenticulostriate branches
Orbitofrontal branch
Anterior temporal arteries

Lenticulostriate branches (Fig. 2.43). These 6 to 12 branches usually arise from the posterosuperior aspect of the M1 segment of the middle cerebral artery, entering the anterior perforated substance. They may be divided into lateral and medial groups that arise from the proximal segments for M1 and A1. Occasionally, they arise from an early branch of the middle cerebral artery. The lenticulostriate arteries supply most of the head of the caudate nucleus, most of the putamen, the lateral one-third of the globus pallidus, and the superior half of the anterior limb of the internal capsule. The recurrent artery of Heubner is one of the larger medial striate arteries. Rarely, the recurrent artery of Heubner may give origin to orbital branches, supplying portions of the frontal lobe.

Orbitofrontal branch. This branch arises from the anterior surface of the M1 segment of the middle cerebral artery and courses anteriorly, superiorly, and laterally to supply the inferior and lateral surface of the frontal lobe. The size of this artery is inversely proportional to the size of the frontopolar branch of the pericallosal artery.

Anterior temporal arteries. These arteries arise from the anterior surface of the M1 segment, opposite to the lenticulostriate arteries, and courses over the temporal lobe. They may have a common trunk with the orbitofrontal artery or the posterior temporal artery.

These anterior temporal arteries usually have two branches: a small branch that passes inferiorly and anteriorly to supply the pole and a recurrent branch that runs laterally and posteriorly in the sylvian fissure or in the lateral aspect of the temporal lobe. The caliber of these branches is in equilibrium with the posterior temporal artery.

M2 Sylvian Segment of the Middle Cerebral Artery (Figs. 2.32A, 2.33, 2.34, 2.43, and 2.49)

The insula is a triangular territory of the cerebral cortex along the medial aspect of the sylvian fissure enclosed by the operculum. This cortex is outlined by branches of the middle cerebral artery (ascending branches or ascending frontal artery complex) before they exit through the sylvian fissure to supply the cortex over the cerebral convexity. The term ascending frontal artery complex includes the operculofrontal or candelabra group and the arteries of the central sulcus. The arteries in the insula are triangular when viewed laterally. The inferior point of the triangle is formed by the horizontal segment of the middle cerebral artery; the anterior superior point is formed by the most anterior artery in the insula as it begins to loop inferiorly to leave the sylvian fissure; the posterior superior point is formed by the most posterior artery as it begins to loop inferiorly to leave the insula. The posterior superior point is also called the sylvian point. The superior border of the triangle is drawn by connecting the arteries in the superior limiting sulcus before they loop inferiorly to leave the sylvian fissure.

In frontal projection, the insular branches of the middle cerebral artery curve gently outward until they reach the superior limiting sulcus (Figs. 2.43 and 2.49A). The anterior portion of the insula is more medially located than the posterior portion.

The candelabra group may bifurcate or trifurcate symmetrically in the proximal part of its course in the form of a candelabrum. These arteries supply Broca's area. The posterior branches always supply the premotor area and may supply accessory branches to the motor strip.

M3 Cortical Branches of the Middle Cerebral Artery (Figs. 2.37B, 2.47-2.49B)

The middle cerebral artery M3 segments supply the entire superficial lateral surface of the cerebral hemisphere in the frontal, temporal, parietal, and occipital lobes. Most commonly, 12 branches of the middle cerebral artery may be identified. These branches arise separately from the M2 segment of the middle cerebral artery in a bifurcation or trifurcating divisional pattern.

Branches

Orbitofrontal artery
Prefrontal artery
Precentral artery
Central arteries
Anterior parietal artery
Posterior parietal artery
Angular artery (terminal artery)
Temporo-occipital artery
Posterior temporal artery
Middle temporal artery
Anterior temporal artery
Temporal polar artery

Orbitofrontal artery. This artery arises directly from the M2 segment of the middle cerebral artery or from a common trunk with the prefrontal artery. When the M2 segment bifurcates or trifurcates early, the orbitofrontal artery originates from the more anterior trunk of the middle cerebral artery. It supplies the orbital aspect of the middle and inferior frontal gyri and sometimes the inferior part of the pars orbitalis of the inferior frontal gyrus.

Prefrontal artery. Constitutes the anterior part of the operculofrontal or candelabra group. This supplies the lateral aspect of the frontal lobe anterior to the sylvian triangle, including the pars marginalis of the inferior frontal gyrus and the pars orbitalis and pars opercularis of the inferior frontal gyrus. It may have a common origin with the orbitofrontal artery or the precentral artery. It emerges from the sylvian fissure at the level of the pars orbitalis of the inferior frontal gyrus. In lateral angiograms, it has an inclined path anterior and superior beyond the anterior portion of the sylvian fissure. It divides into two trunks, which further divide into four to six branches supplying the middle and inferior frontal gyri.

Precentral artery. When the middle cerebral artery bifurcates, the precentral artery arises from the anterior trunk. When the middle cerebral artery trifurcates, it arises from the anterior or middle trunk. The precentral and prefrontal arteries may originate from a single trunk. The precentral artery emerges from the sylvian fissure at or behind the pars opercularis of the inferior frontal gyrus and has an almost vertical course. It is the most vertical branch of the middle cerebral artery. The two major branches usually follow the course of the precentral sulcus. It supplies the pars opercularis of the inferior frontal gyrus, the posterior part of the middle frontal gyrus, and the inferior two-thirds of the precentral gyrus.

Central arteries. The central arteries have variable origin, dependent on the division pattern of the M2 segment. When the M2 segment is a single vessel, it may originate from a common trunk with the anterior parietal artery. When the M2 segment bifurcates, it arises from the anterior trunk. When the M2 segment trifurcates, it arises from the middle trunk. The central artery may be single in two-thirds of cases and two vessels in the remaining cases. The central artery runs near the fissure of Rolando as two branches encircling the operculum. It supplies the precentral and postcentral gyri and has a slight posterior superior inclined course after emerging from the fissure.

Parietal arteries. There are two parietal arteries: the anterior and posterior. The anterior parietal artery has a variable origin. It may arise with the central artery or with the posterior parietal artery. This artery emerges from the posterior third of the sylvian fissure at the base of the ascending parietal gyrus to pass upward and posterior in the postcentral sulcus. It supplies the ascending parietal gyrus, the upper portion of the central sulcus, and the anterior part of the first two parietal gyri. The posterior parietal artery is the most posterior of the ascending branches of the middle cerebral artery. It varies in size and site of origin and may originate from the anterior or posterior trunk of a bifurcated middle cerebral artery. If the M2 segment trifurcates, it arises from the middle trunk. It emerges from the sylvian fissure at the level of the parietal operculum and passes posteriorly and superiorly in the posterior part of the parietal lobe. It supplies the posterior part of the first and second parietal gyri and the supramarginal gyrus.

Angular artery. It is the terminal and longest branch of the M2 segment. Its origin is from the posterior trunk of the M2 segment when it bifurcates and the middle or posterior trunk when it trifurcates. The artery emerges at the end of the sylvian fissure, running over the superior temporal gyrus. This is the most horizontal branch of the middle cerebral artery in lateral angiograms and the most posterior branch of the sylvian fissure in a Towne view of angiography. It supplies the posterior part of the superior temporal gyrus, the supramarginal gyrus, the angular gyrus, and the first two occipital gyri.

Temporo-occipital artery. The temporo-occipital artery may have a common origin with the angular artery and may be sometimes considered a branch of the angular artery. The size of this artery is inversely proportional to the size of the posterior temporal artery. It supplies the area posterior to and above the area usually supplied by the posterior temporal artery. It has a posterior and inferior bend after arising from the sylvian fissure.

Posterior temporal artery. The posterior temporal artery arises from the posterior trunk of the M2 segment if a bifurcation or trifurcation is present. It is a single branch in most cases and exits the sylvian fissure through the posterior part, crossing the external surface of the superior temporal gyrus. It courses through the superior temporal sulcus, crossing the middle temporal gyrus, and terminating opposite the preoccipital fissure. It supplies the middle and posterior part of the superior temporal gyrus, the posterior third of the middle temporal gyrus, and the posterior part of the inferior temporal gyrus.

Middle temporal artery. It is frequently a small artery. Leaves the sylvian fissure opposite or slightly behind the pars opercularis of the inferior frontal gyrus. The direction is similar to that of the posterior temporal artery. Supplies the temporal gyri anterior to the territory of supply of the posterior temporal artery.

Anterior temporal artery. Supplies the remainder of the anterior portion of the temporal lobe. The vessel outlines the temporal operculum. It descends posteriorly over the temporal gyri, immediately behind the temporal polar artery to terminate at the level of the middle temporal sulcus. It may originate as an early branch of the M2 segment.

Temporal polar artery. This is a relatively constant vessel that courses anteriorly to the anterior and inferior aspects of the tip of the temporal lobe to supply the anterior portions of the superior, middle, and inferior temporal gyri.

Posterior Cerebral Artery (Figs. 2.32B-2.35, 2.37B, 2.40B and C, 2.41, 2.43, 2.50, 2.51, 2.53, and 2.54)

The posterior cerebral artery generally receives the blood supply from the basilar artery. The artery is located superior to the tentorium and embryologically during early development receives blood supply from the internal carotid artery. The posterior cerebral artery shifts its origin from the carotid to the basilar system in the final stages of embryonic development, and the ultimate origin is from the basilar artery bifurcation at the interpeduncular fossa. In 25% of cases, the fetal type (Figs. 2.37B, 2.40C, 2.41, and 2.45) persists either on an individual side or bilaterally with the internal carotid artery supplying the posterior cerebral artery via a robust posterior communicating artery.

The posterior cerebral artery more typically has a communication with the basilar artery through the P1 segment of the posterior cerebral artery (Figs. 2.32B-2.34, 2.50-2.53). The posterior cerebral artery courses posteriorly in the perimesencephalic cisterns to encircle the midbrain. Terminal cortical branches supply the occipital poles, the medial and inferior portions of the occipital lobes, and the medial portions of the temporal lobes. The proximal trunk of the posterior cerebral artery is divided into peduncular, ambient, and quadrigeminal segments, corresponding to the cisterns through which the vessel passes.

Peduncular Segment

This is the proximal segment of the posterior cerebral artery, which arises from the basilar artery, and it is closely related to the anteromedial portion of the peduncle of the midbrain. The posterior communicating artery connects to the midportion of the peduncular segment. The proximal portion of the peduncular segment is closely related to the oculomotor nerve. The peduncular segment is usually horizontal, but when the basilar artery is short with a low bifurcation, the peduncular segments are directed upward in a V-like configuration (Fig. 2.51). With elongation of the basilar artery, the peduncular segments pass anteriorly and inferiorly to reach the surface of the peduncles. Asymmetry is common in more than 50% of cases.

Ambient Segment

It is the second cisternal segment of the posterior cerebral artery and courses posteriorly in the hippocampal fissure between the midbrain and the hippocampal gyrus. It parallels the basal vein, which lies superior, and courses adjacent to the trochlear nerve, at the free edge of the tentorium. The superior cerebellar artery (SCA) is inferior to the ambient segment. The relationship of this segment with the free margin of the tentorium varies. With low origin of the posterior cerebral artery, the ambient segment crosses the line of the tentorial margin from below with high origin and courses posteriorly in the hippocampal fissure above the tentorium.

Quadrigeminal Segment

It is the continuation of the posterior cerebral artery within the lateral aspect of the quadrigeminal cistern. At this level, the quadrigeminal segments approach each other and then continue posteriorly beneath the splenium of the corpus callosum to terminate in cortical branches.

Branches (Figs. 2.49-2.51)

- *Mesencephalic and thalamic branches*
  - Mesencephalic branches
    - Interpeduncular perforating branches
    - Tiny peduncular branches
    - Circumflex mesencephalic branches
  - Thalamic branches (Fig. 2.54)
    - Anterior thalamoperforating arteries
    - Posterior thalamoperforating arteries
      - Interpeduncular thalamoperforating branches
      - Thalamogeniculate perforating branches
- *Posterior choroidal branches* (Figs. 2. 44 and 2.54)
  - Medial posterior choroidal artery
  - Lateral posterior choroidal artery
- *Hippocampal branches*
- *Meningeal branches*
- *Posterior pericallosal artery*
- *Cortical branches*
  - Anterior temporal artery
  - Posterior temporal artery
  - Parieto-occipital artery
  - Calcarine artery

Mesencephalic and Thalamic Branches

Mesencephalic branches. The interpeduncular perforating branches arise from the initial posterior surface of the posterior cerebral artery. There are three to six perforating branches, which penetrate the rostral floor of the interpeduncular fossa through the posterior perforated substance. These supply the oculomotor and trochlear nuclei, the paramedian mesencephalic reticular formation, the pretectum, and the rostromedian floor of the fourth ventricle.

The tiny peduncular branches arise from the posterior cerebral artery and penetrate the cerebral peduncle. They supply the corticospinal and corticobulbar pathways as well as the substantia nigra, red nuclei, and other structures of the tegmentum (oculomotor nerve). The circumflex mesencephalic branches are a group of several small vessels of variable length, arising from the peduncular segment of the posterior cerebral artery that passes around the midbrain. These supply small perforating branches to the cerebral peduncle and substantia nigra but also the posterior tegmental structures.

Thalamic branches. The so-called thalamoperforating arteries are divided into an anterior and a posterior group.

The anterior thalamoperforating arteries comprise a group of 7 to 10 arteries, arising from the lateral aspect of the posterior communicating artery. They supply the posterior chiasm, optic tract, posterior hypothalamus, and part of the cerebral peduncle.

The posterior thalamoperforating arteries consist of two groups of arteries.

The interpeduncular thalamoperforating branches originate from the proximal peduncular segment of the posterior cerebral artery. They penetrate the thalamus via the paramedian aspect of the posterior perforate substance.

The thalamogeniculate perforating branches arise from the ambient segment of the posterior cerebral artery. There are three to six small arteries that penetrate the base of the thalamus and the geniculate bodies.

Posterior Choroidal Branches

Posterior medial choroidal artery. This artery usually arises from the proximal segment of the posterior cerebral artery and runs parallel to the posterior cerebral artery and is interposed between that artery and the midbrain to which it gives small branches. It enters the lateral portion of the quadrigeminal cistern, supplying the quadrigeminal plate and the pineal gland, and approaches midline and courses forward in the roof of the third ventricle adjacent to the internal cerebral vein. Multiple small branches of this artery reach the level of the foramen of Monro and supply the choroid plexus of the third ventricle. This also supplies the dorsal medial nucleus of the thalamus.

Posterior lateral choroidal artery. Originates from the ambient segment of the posterior cerebral artery. Variations in origin are common with 50% having multiple origins. The anterior branch supplies the anterior portion of the choroid plexus of the temporal horn of the ventricles, whereas the posterior branch supplies the choroid plexus of the trigone and lateral ventricle. The lateral choroidal artery also supplies the crus, commissure, body, and part of the anterior columns of the fornix and thalamus. The size of this vessel is usually inversely proportional to the size of the anterior choroidal artery with anastomoses between branches of this artery with branches of posteromedial and anterior choroidal arteries.

Hippocampal Branches

The arteries to the hippocampus originate from the trunk of the posterior cerebral artery near the origin of the lateral choroidal arteries.

Meningeal Branches

The meningeal branches are small and arise from the peduncular segment of the posterior cerebral artery. They course around the midbrain and supply the midline strip of the inferior surface of the tentorium opposite to the junction of the falx cerebri with the tentorium.

Posterior Pericallosal Artery

Usually arises at the level of the quadrigeminal cistern from the parieto-occipital branch of the posterior cerebral artery. It may also arise from the posterior cerebral artery, from the lateral choroidal artery, or from the posterior temporal artery. It is usually a plexus of small arteries, rather than a single vessel. This artery passes around the splenium, running anteriorly within the supracallosal cistern and anastomosing with the distal branches of the anterior pericallosal artery.

Cortical Branches (Figs. 2.44 and 2.49)

There are four main cortical branches of the posterior cerebral artery.

Anterior temporal artery. Arises as a single trunk or as multiple branches from the proximal ambient segment of the posterior cerebral artery. Runs lateral and anterior under the hippocampal gyrus supplying the inferior aspect of the anterior portion of the temporal lobe. There are anastomoses with the anterior temporal branches of the middle cerebral artery.

Posterior temporal artery. Arises from the midambient segment of the posterior cerebral artery as a single trunk in 80% of cases. May give origin to an anterior temporal branch. Courses posteriorly and laterally along the hippocampal gyrus. Several small branches originate from this artery along the inferior surface of the posterior temporal lobe and adjacent occipital lobe. The distal vessels may anastomose with branches of the calcarine artery in the posterior third of the calcarine fissure. It supplies the primary visual cortex in approximately 25% of cases.

Parieto-occipital artery. May arise independently from the posterior cerebral artery at the level of the ambient cistern. It may also originate with the calcarine artery from the bifurcation of the posterior cerebral trunk in the proximal third of the calcarine fissure. This artery originates from the quadrigeminal segment in 22% and more distally in 40% of cases. It arises as a single trunk in 95% of cases. Branches include lateral posterior choroidal arteries and branches to the hippocampus, pulvinar, and medial and lateral geniculate bodies. The main trunk of the parieto-occipital artery usually divides into a number of cortical branches that supply the medial portion of the parieto-occipital lobe, precuneus, and deep into the parieto-occipital fissure. On a lateral view arteriogram, the parieto-occipital branches course posteriorly and superiorly as the superior most of the three posterior cortical branches of the posterior cerebral artery. In the frontal projection, the proximal parieto-occipital artery is usually the most medial of the three posterior cortical branches as it surrounds the medial face of the parieto-occipital lobe.

Calcarine artery. Arises at the bifurcation of the main posterior cerebral trunk in the rostral third of the calcarine sulcus. At its origin, this artery lies just lateral to the parieto-occipital branch. After this, it follows a winding posterior course deep in the calcarine fissure. The origin of the calcarine artery is variable as is the number of trunks with one branch present in 40% and two branches in 60% of cases. This supplies part of the visual cortex.

Vertebral Artery (Figs. 2.1-2.3, 2.32-2.34, 2.35, 2.40, 2.50, 2.51, and 2.55)

The vertebral artery, in more than 80% of cases, originates at the upper posterior aspect of the first segment of the subclavian artery as the most proximal and largest branch of this artery. The most common variant has a more proximal origin. On the left, the vertebral artery originates from the arch between the left common carotid and left subclavian arteries in about 5% of cases (Fig. 2.2C). In that case, the vertebral artery enters the foramen of the transverse process of the fifth cervical vertebra, instead of the sixth cervical vertebra as usual. Other variations such as origin of the left vertebral artery distal to the left subclavian artery or from the left common carotid artery or external carotid artery are extremely rare. The right vertebral artery originating from the right common carotid artery or the aortic arch is found in less than 1% of cases. A bifid origin of the vertebral artery is also very uncommon. The size of the vertebral arteries is variable but the left is more commonly dominant. In cases of occlusion of the left subclavian artery, a steal phenomenon develops with enlargement of the right and left vertebral arteries and inversion of the flow in the left vertebral artery (Fig. 2.56). There is also reversal of the flow in the posterior brain circulation causing loss of balance or collapse, particularly when heavy exercise is performed with the left arm. The occlusion of the right subclavian artery and steal phenomenon related to the right arm is less common.

Segments of the Vertebral Artery

The first V1 segment of the vertebral artery extends from the origin to its point of entrance into the foramen of the transverse process of the sixth cervical vertebra in 87% of cases. It is directed superiorly and posteriorly to the extravertebral segment. It is surrounded by the cervical sympathetic nerve plexus and is related anteriorly to the vertebral and jugular vein and the inferior thyroid artery. The inferior thyroid artery (Fig. 2.57) and costocervical trunk may rarely originate from the proximal vertebral artery.

The second V2 segment courses cranially through the foramina of the transverse processes until it reaches the transverse process of the axis. The artery is in close contact medially with the uncinate process of the vertebral body and posteriorly with the ventral rami of the cervical nerves. In this segment it is surrounded by the vertebral venous plexus. This segment is at risk during cervical transforaminal nerve root blocks that are performed too centrally.

The third V3 segment extends from where it exits the cervical spinal transverse foramen until it enters the dura in the spinal canal. After leaving the transverse foramen, it courses laterally and posteriorly to pass through the transverse foramen of the atlas. After passing the transverse foramen of the atlas, the artery runs posteromedially at the horizontal groove on the upper surface of the posterior arch of the atlas. When it approaches the midline, it turns cephalad and perforates the posterior atlanto-occipital membrane to enter the vertebral canal. At this level, the persistence of the embryonic proatlantal intersegmental artery may result in a rare but exuberant communication between the internal or external carotid arteries and the vertebral artery (Fig. 2.31). The junction between the V3 and V4 segment where the vessel crosses into the dura is a point of relative vessel fixation to the dura. This decrease in vessel mobility leads to slight increased turbulence of blood flow and results in focal intracranial atherosclerotic calcification to accumulate at the junction. The occipital artery may arise rarely as a branch of the third segment of the vertebral artery.

The fourth V4 segment of the vertebral artery perforates the dura and runs anteromedially through the foramen magnum. At this level, the artery lies in front of the medulla oblongata and joins the contralateral vertebral artery forming the basilar artery. In 0.2%, the vertebral artery fails to join the basilar artery on one side and thus terminates in the posterior inferior cerebellar artery (PICA).

Branches

- Muscular branches
- Meningeal branches
- Spinal branches
- Radicular branches
- Proatlantal intersegmental artery
- Posterior inferior cerebellar artery

Muscular Branches

In every cervical space, the vertebral artery sends a radicular branch, following the ventral (anteriorly) and dorsal (posteriorly) nerve roots, and muscular branches creating an anastomotic network with muscular branches from the deep cervical artery, occipital artery (posteriorly), ascending cervical artery, and ascending pharyngeal artery (anteriorly). Together with the muscular and radicular branches, some branches give origin to the adjacent meninges. Some of the radicular branches give origin to the anterior and posterior radiculomedullary branches.

Meningeal Branches

Posterior meningeal branch. Arises above the level of the arch of the atlas just below the foramen magnum. It supplies the medial portion of the dura of the posterior fossa, as well as the falx cerebelli. It may extend cephalad to supply the tentorium and the falx cerebri. It may rarely arise as a branch from the PICA. It may arise from the posterior division of the ascending pharyngeal artery (neuromeningeal trunk) (Fig. 2.9) or from the occipital artery (Fig. 2.30).

Anterior meningeal branch. Originates from the distal part of the second segment of the vertebral artery. It runs medially and cephalad to enter the spinal canal to supply the medulla at the level of the foramen magnum.

Arterial arch of the odontoid (Figs. 2.9, 2.11, and 2.52). Each one of the vertebral arteries feeds the posterior meninges of the odontoid process through an arterial arch. The arterial arch of the odontoid may originate or have anastomoses with the ascending pharyngeal artery.

Spinal Branches

Anterior spinal artery (Figs. 2.1 and 2.58). The anterior spinal artery originates from both vertebral arteries near there junction to form the basilar artery. These branches join at the midline and generally fuse about 2 cm from the origin forming the anterior spinal artery. The anterior spinal artery extends the length of the spinal cord, in close relationship to the anterior median fissure with a varying caliber according to the segment observed.

Posterolateral spinal arteries. The posterior spinal arteries may originate from the PICA or from the intradural portion of the vertebral artery. They run caudally along the posterolateral aspect of the medulla and spinal cord.

Radicular Branches

Several small and posterior radicular branches enter the spinal canal via the neural foramina anastomosing with the spinal arteries. There are one to six arteries anteriorly and up to eight posteriorly.

Proatlantal Intersegmental Artery (Fig. 2.40)

This is the rare embryonic primitive cervical segmental artery that persists into adult life. When it is present, the proximal segment of the vertebral artery may be atretic. It usually joins the internal or external carotid arteries to the distal vertebral artery.

Posterior Inferior Cerebellar Artery (Figs. 2.50-2.52, 2.54, and 2.55)

The posterior inferior cerebellar artery (PICA) is the largest and most distal branch of the vertebral artery. In approximately half of cases, the PICA originates above the foramen magnum, whereas in only 4% of cases, it is identified at the level of the foramen magnum and in approximately 20% is found below. This is important to consider prior to attempting a cervical C1-C2 spinal tap performed posterior to the cervical spinal cord. The PICA is absent in about 20% of cases with its territory supplied by the anterior inferior cerebellar artery (AICA). Anastomoses between the two arteries are common. A single stem may take the place of both the AICA and PICA (Fig. 2.51).

There are many variations in the course of the PICA, and it is divided into several segments. The segmental division is intimately related to the adjacent structures that it supplies, including the medulla, the inferior portion of the fourth ventricle, the inferior vermis, the tonsils, and the inferior aspect of the cerebellar hemispheres: the anterior medullary segment, lateral medullary segment, posterior medullary segment, supratonsillar segment, and branches.

Anterior medullary segment. The PICA anterior medullary segment courses posteriorly within the medullary cistern and turns around the lower end of the olive of the medulla oblongata, adjacent to the biventral lobule. It is also called proximal cisternal segment.

Lateral medullary segment. The PICA lateral medullary segment continues posteriorly in the cerebellomedullary fissure around the lateral aspect of the medulla, and it is called the lateral medullary segment with a characteristic caudal loop.

Posterior medullary segment. The PICA posterior medullary segment reaches the posterior margin of the medulla oblongata, ascends behind the roots of the 9th and 10th cranial nerves to the anterior aspect of the superior pole of the tonsil behind the posterior medullary velum. It is also known as medullary segment.

Supratonsillar segment. The PICA supratonsillar segment continues in the posterior course over the superior pole of the tonsil. It is also known as cranial loop or choroid arch. The caudal point of the supratonsillar segment is always in apposition with the fourth ventricle to supply the choroid in the fourth ventricle.

Branches

Perforating branches. There are multiple small arterial branches that arise from the anterior, lateral, and posterior medullary segments of the PICA to supply the posterolateral aspect of the medulla. When the PICA is hypoplastic or absent, these bulbar branches originate from the vertebral artery. A small branch of the PICA may extend superiorly and lateral to the tonsil to supply the dentate nucleus of the cerebellum.

Terminal branches. In most cases, the PICA bifurcates a short distance distal to the apex of the cranial loop into two main terminal branches: the tonsillohemispheric (lateral) and the vermian (medial) branches.

Tonsillohemispheric branches. These descend along the posterior margin of the medial aspect of the tonsil and divide into tonsillar branches, extending anteriorly, and hemispheric branches coursing inferiorly and posterolaterally. There are anastomoses between the hemispheric branches and the AICA or SCA. When there are no hemispheric branches from the PICA, the hemispheric branches may arise from the AICA or the SCA.

Vermian branches. These branches pass at the inferior aspect of the inferior vermis in the sulcus valleculae between the inferior vermis and the cerebellar hemisphere. At this point, these branches form a loop of inferior and lateral convexity. In some cases, all of the vermis branches arise from a single PICA.

Meningeal branches. A posterior meningeal branch is occasionally seen arising from the PICA, rather than from the vertebral artery.

Basilar Artery (Figs. 2.1, 2.3, 2.32, 2.33, 2.35, 2.50, 2.51, and 2.53-2.55)

The basilar artery is formed by the junction of the two vertebral arteries at the level of the pontomedullary sulcus. It follows an ascending course along the shallow groove in close contact with the anterior aspect of the pons. This artery is found within the prepontine cistern posteriorly to the clivus. The distal part of the artery usually bends posteriorly and divides into the two posterior cerebral arteries just after passing between the two oculomotor nerves. Often the course of the basilar artery is tortuous and deviated from the midline in a position opposite to the more dominant vertebral artery due to increased flow in that direction.

Branches

- *Pontine branches*
  - Median branches
  - Transverse branches
- *Anterior inferior cerebellar artery* (AICA)
- *Superior cerebellar artery*
- *Pontine branches*

The basilar branches to the pons and midbrain are small arteries that arise from the lateral and posterior sides of the main vessel. They may be divided into median or paramedian branches and transverse or circumferential branches.

Median Branches

Small and numerous arteries that originate from the posterior part of the basilar artery, entering the pons at the median groove. These arteries penetrate the pons deeply, reaching the floor of the fourth ventricle.

Transverse Branches

There are several pairs of these arteries. The transverse branches arise from the lateral aspect of the basilar artery and encircle the anterior and lateral borders of the brainstem. These arteries originate several small perforating branches that penetrate the pons at right angles to the parent vessel.

Anterior Inferior Cerebellar Artery (Figs. 2.50, 2.51, and 2.54)

The AICA originates from the proximal or middle third of the basilar artery. The artery is divided into the main trunk and recurrent limb. It is further divided into two major branches: the lateral branch and medial branch. The size of the AICA is inversely proportional to the size of the PICA. When one is absent or hypoplastic, the other ipsilateral artery is larger and replaces blood flow to the normally nourished territory.

The main trunk of the AICA courses laterally and inferiorly in contact with either the dorsal or the ventral aspects of the abducens nerve. Within the cerebellopontine angle cistern, the proximal arterial trunk usually lies ventral and medial to the roots of the facial and vestibulocochlear nerves. The main trunk of the AICA supplies small branches to the lateral aspect of the pons from the middle third down to the upper part of the medulla.

The recurrent limb of the AICA arises from the area of the internal acoustic meatus and courses medially to reach the cerebellopontine angle and extends to reach the cerebellum dorsally.

The lateral branch courses laterally and curves around the flocculus coursing within the horizontal fissure between the superior and inferior semilunar lobules of the cerebellum. This artery sends hemispheric branches to the superior and inferior semilunar lobules, and the distal hemispheric branches anastomose with branches of the SCA and the PICA.

The medial branch of the AICA courses medially and inferiorly to the medial and anterior border of the cerebellum supplying the biventral lobule. This branch also anastomoses with the PICA.

The internal auditory artery originates from the proximal segment of the AICA in almost all cases or may arise from the basilar artery above the origin of the AICA. This artery supplies the structures within the meatus of the auditory canal including the nerve roots and internal ear.

Superior Cerebellar Artery (Figs. 2.50-2.52, and 2.54)

This SCA originates from the basilar artery proximal to the origin of the posterior cerebral artery. It may rarely arise from the posterior cerebral artery. The proximal trunk of the SCA runs posteriorly in the perimesencephalic cisterns, encircling the upper pons and lower mesencephalon. It supplies portions of the midbrain, the superior surface of the cerebellar hemisphere, the superior vermis, and the cerebellar nucleus.

The proximal trunk (perimesencephalic) or cisternal segment of the SCA is divided into three segments: anterior pontine, ambient, and quadrigeminal segments. It has cortical and perforating branches.

Anterior Pontine Segment

This is the proximal portion of the SCA; it courses laterally on the anterior surface of the pons in an arcuate curve. It lies inferior to the emerging roots of the oculomotor nerve separating it from the proximal segment of the posterior cerebral artery. This segment may duplicate (Fig. 2.52) or triplicate and give rise to the marginal and superior vermis branches.

Ambient Segment

This is the second portion of the SCA, beginning at the lateral border of the pons and turning posteriorly over the brachium pontis or middle cerebellar peduncle. It courses posteriorly in the infratentorial portion of the ambient cistern. This segment parallels the course of the trochlear nerve.

Quadrigeminal Segment

This is the distal segment of the SCA which lies within the lateral aspects of the quadrigeminal cistern. At this point, the two SCAs are in close apposition near the midline with anastomotic branches.

Cortical Branches

Lateral (marginal) branch. The marginal branch is the largest branch of the SCA, originating at the second portion of the SCA within the ambient cistern or more rarely from the anterior pontine segment. This artery reaches the anterolateral margin of the cerebellum coursing posterolaterally in the region of the horizontal fissure. It demarcates the superior and inferior cerebellar lobes. The hemispheric branches originate from the marginal branch of the SCA.

Hemispheric branches. There are a few hemispheric branches arising distal to the origin of the marginal branch from the ambient or second segment of the SCA when the artery courses around the posterior surface of the brainstem. These branches course superiorly reaching the superior surface of the cerebellum where they distribute radially in the direction of the horizontal fissure. They supply the dentate nucleus, and at the cortical territory, they supply the medial portion of the quadrigeminal and superior semilunar lobules and the superior half of the vermis.

Superior vermian branch (Fig. 2.53). This is the terminal branch of the SCA originating from the third or quadrigeminal segment. There are one or two vermian branches on either side. Anastomoses may be found between these branches closer to midline within the quadrigeminal cistern and between these branches and the inferior vermian branches from the PICA. They course over the vermis close to the midline.

Perforating branches. Many small branches originate from the main trunk of the SCA perforating the brainstem. These branches are more common in the interpeduncular and quadrigeminal regions. The branches to the pons and mesencephalon originate from the anterior pontine segment of the SCA. The few branches arising from the ambient segment of the SCA are also perforating and supply the lateral portion of the brainstem. The inferior colliculi are supplied by the small branches that arise from the quadrigeminal region of the SCA. Several larger branches arising from the distal ambient segment of the SCA supply the dentate nucleus and course inferiorly along the superior cerebellar peduncle.

Collateral Circulation

Collateral circulation to the brain parenchyma is highly variable. The cerebrovascular reserve of a specific territory to maintain blood perfusion is based on the extent of collateralization in the event of pathologic or iatrogenic cerebrovascular arterial occlusion. Collateral flow to the brain may occur from extracranial sources from the external carotid artery, collaterals from the internal carotid artery, or from intracranial sources by anastomoses in the subarachnoid space and the leptomeningeal pial vessels. Intracranial subarachnoid collateralization occurs through the circle of Willis in the terminal branches of the cerebral arteries and in embryonic connections between the basilar and carotid arteries.

The most common intracranial collateral pathway is the circle of Willis. Anteriorly this is from the A1 segment of the anterior cerebral arteries, the supraclinoid segment of the internal carotid arteries, and the anterior communicating artery. Laterally, this is achieved by the posterior communicating arteries and posteriorly by the P1 segment of the posterior cerebral arteries. When one of the major arteries of the circle of Willis is occluded, blood flow is shunted from the area of normal pressure circulation to the low-pressure territory thereby minimizing ischemia by maintaining hemodynamic perfusion. However, the circle of Willis is incomplete in the majority of cases.

Normal antegrade flow through the external carotid artery with retrograde flow at the ophthalmic artery may recanalize the flow at the distal internal carotid artery. Additional collateral flow may be supplied through the rete mirabile from the meningeal arteries to the cortical arteries on the surface of the brain. When the vertebral arterial system is occluded in the event of hypoplasia of the posterior communicating arteries, muscular branches of the vertebral arteries may develop and recanalize the distal vertebral arteries.

There are supratentorial cortical anastomoses between the cortical branches of the anterior, middle, and posterior cerebral arteries at the surface of the brain. Similarly, in the infratentorial territory on the surface of the cerebellum, there are cortical anastomoses between the cortical branches of the posterior inferior, anterior inferior, and superior cerebellar arteries. The deep penetrating medullary arteries that arise from this network do not anastomose with one another; therefore, occlusions of these vessels more commonly result in infarction.

Circle of Willis (Figs. 2.1, 2.32-2.34, and 2.36)

Most of cerebrovascular perfusion is supplied by the two internal carotid arteries and the central anastomosis between them called the circle of Willis. This connects the internal carotid arteries to the vertebrobasilar system supplying the remainder brain. The circle of Willis is polygonal in shape. It is located in the cisterna interpeduncularis surrounding the optic chiasm, the neural infundibular stem of the hypophysis gland, and the remaining neural structures in the interpeduncular fossa. Anteriorly, the anterior cerebral arteries are joined by the anterior communicating artery. Posteriorly, the basilar artery divides and originates the two posterior cerebral arteries, and each artery is joined to the ipsilateral internal carotid by a posterior communication artery. The preceding description, however, refers only to a minority of cases. The vessels of the circle of Willis vary in caliber and are often maldeveloped or absent. In about 60% of cases, the circle shows some variation or anomaly. Cerebral anterior and posterior communicating arteries may be absent, hypoplastic, double, or triple. The anterior communicating artery has the greatest variability in length and the posterior communicating arteries and posterior cerebral artery P1 segments demonstrate the greatest variability in diameter. Anteriorly, hypoplasia, or absence of the A1 segment of the anterior cerebral artery is more frequent than anomalies of the anterior communicating artery.

Embryonic Communications (Fig. 2.40)

The most common embryonic communication between the internal carotid artery and the basilar artery is the persistent trigeminal artery (Fig. 2.20B). This embryonic vessel communicates with the precavernous segment of the internal carotid artery and the basilar artery. The persistent hypoglossal artery connects the cervical portion of the internal carotid artery with the proximal extremity of the basilar artery after passing through the hypoglossal canal. The proatlantal intersegmental artery communicates the internal carotid artery or occipital with the vertebral artery, through the first (type I) or second cervical spaces (type II). The rarest communication is the persistent otic artery in the petrous segment of the internal carotid artery (Fig. 2.40C).

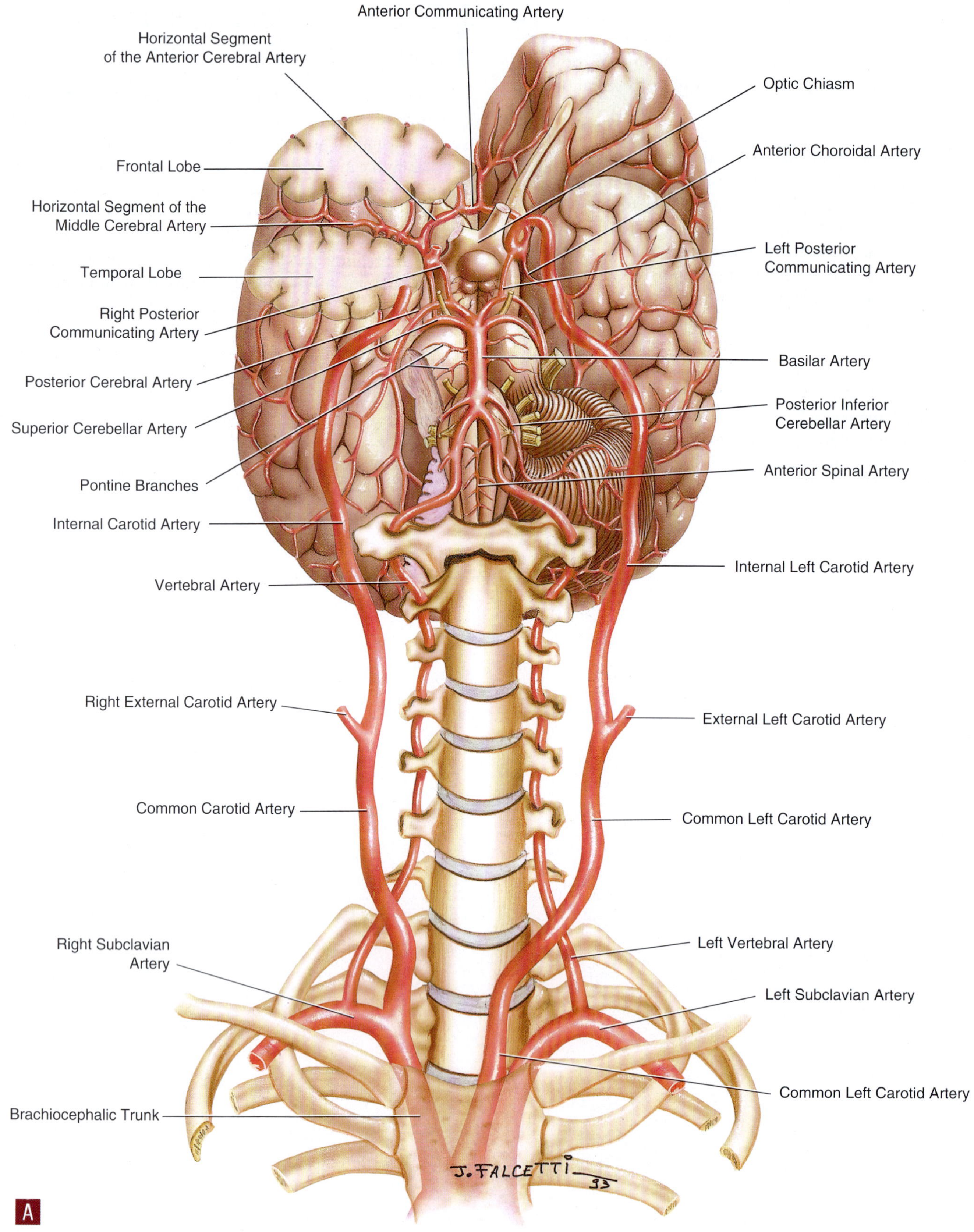

Figure 2.1. The standard aortic arch branching pattern as seen in illustration (A), noninvasively with MRA (B), and catheter-based DSA with contrast injected in the aortic arch (C). DSA, digital subtraction angiography.

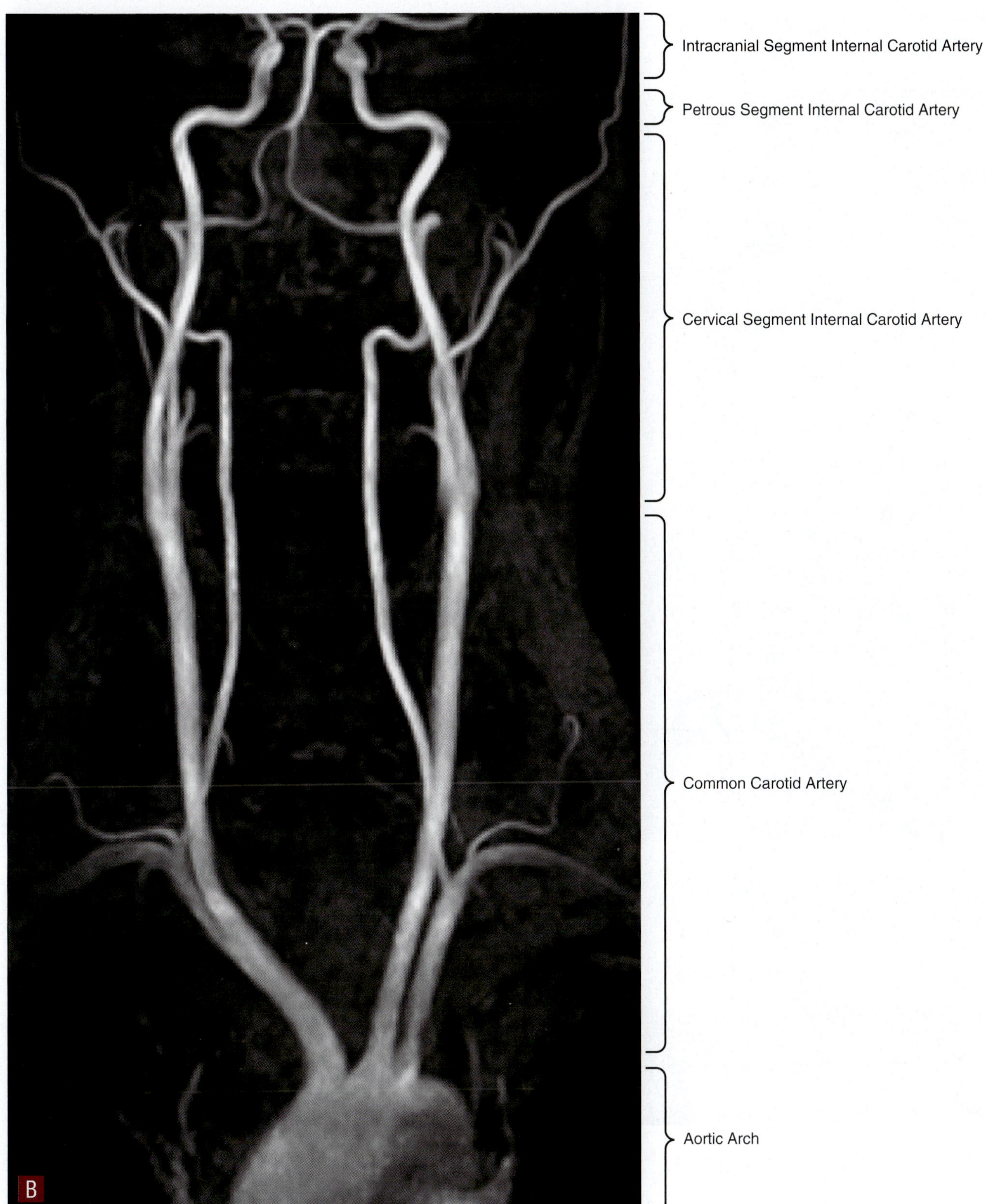

Figure 2.1. *Continued*

C

Right Internal Carotid Artery
Right External Carotid Artery
Left Internal Carotid Artery
Left External Carotid Artery
Right Common Carotid Artery
Left Vertebral Artery
Suprascapular Artery
Left Internal Mammary Artery
Left Common Carotid Artery
Brachiocephalic Trunk
Left Subclavian Artery
Aortic Arch
Descending Thoracic Aorta
Right Axillary Artery
Right Internal Mammary Artery
Right Subclavian Artery

Figure 2.1. *Continued*

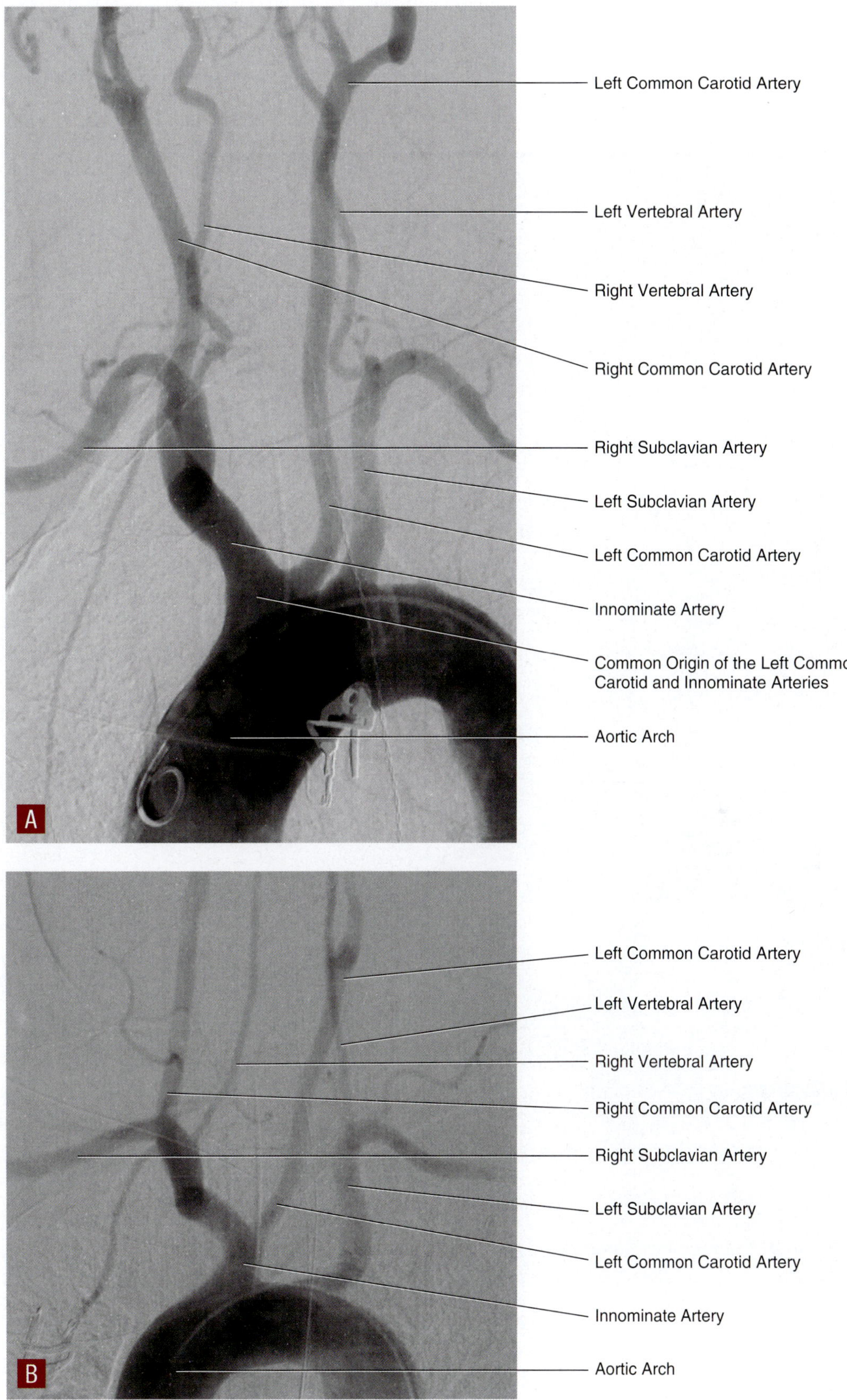

Figure 2.2. Variant aortic arch configurations seen on DSA with a common origin of the innominate and left common carotid (A), left common carotid arising as a branch of the innominate artery (B), left vertebral artery arising from the aortic arch (C), aberrant right subclavian artery (D). DSA, digital subtraction angiography.

C

Left Common Carotid Artery

Right Common Carotid Artery

Right Vertebral Artery

Right Brachiocephalic Trunk

Left Internal Mammary Artery

Left Subclavian Artery

Left Vertebral Artery
with Origin Directly from the Aorta

Aortic Arch

Right Internal Mammary Artery

Figure 2.2. *Continued*

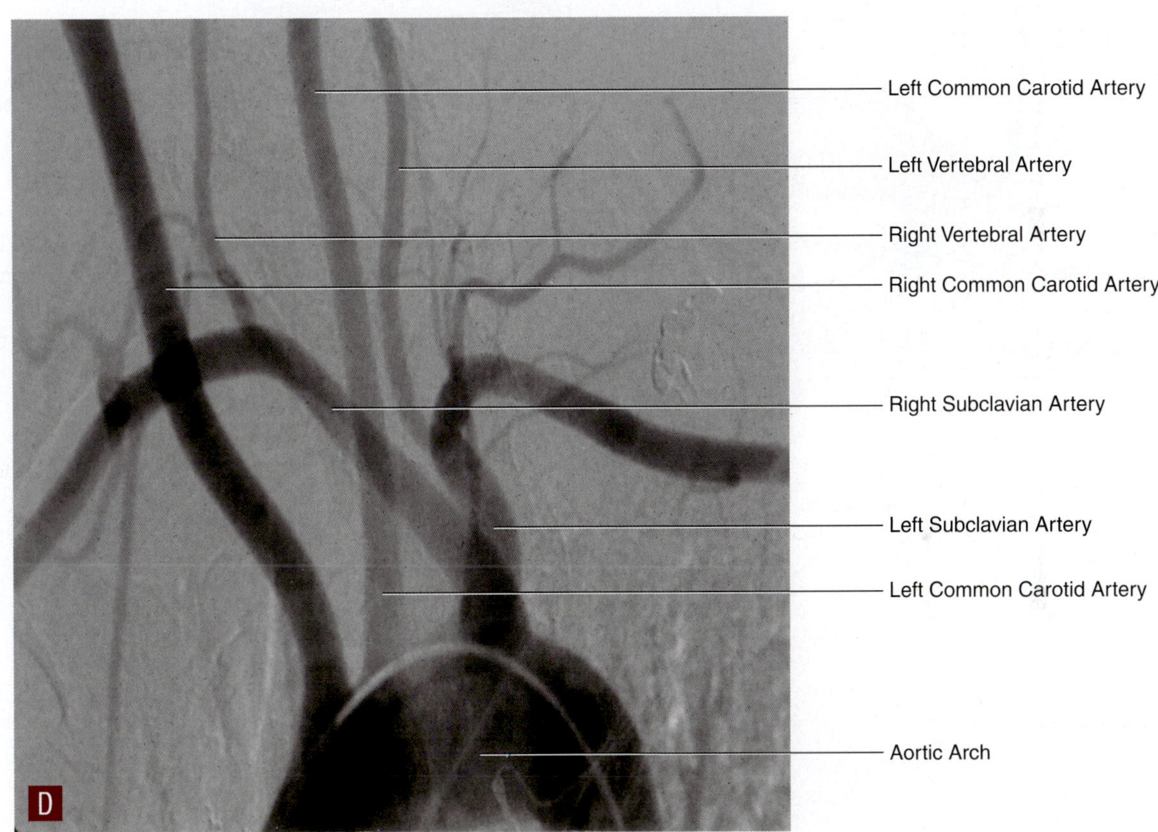

Figure 2.2. *Continued*

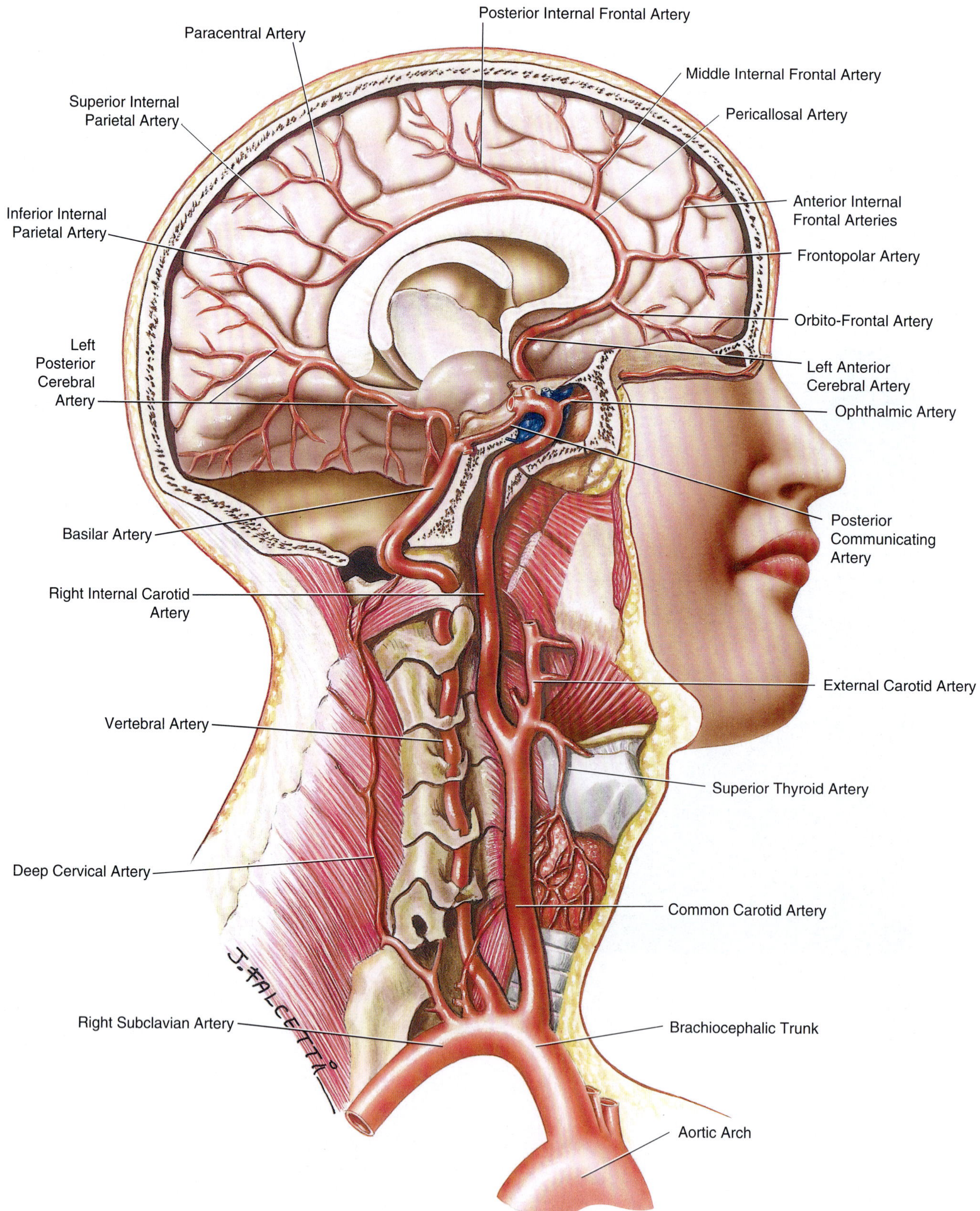

Figure 2.3. Lateral view of a schematic drawing of the carotid arteries, vertebral arteries, and intracranial vessels and their relationships to the neck and brain.

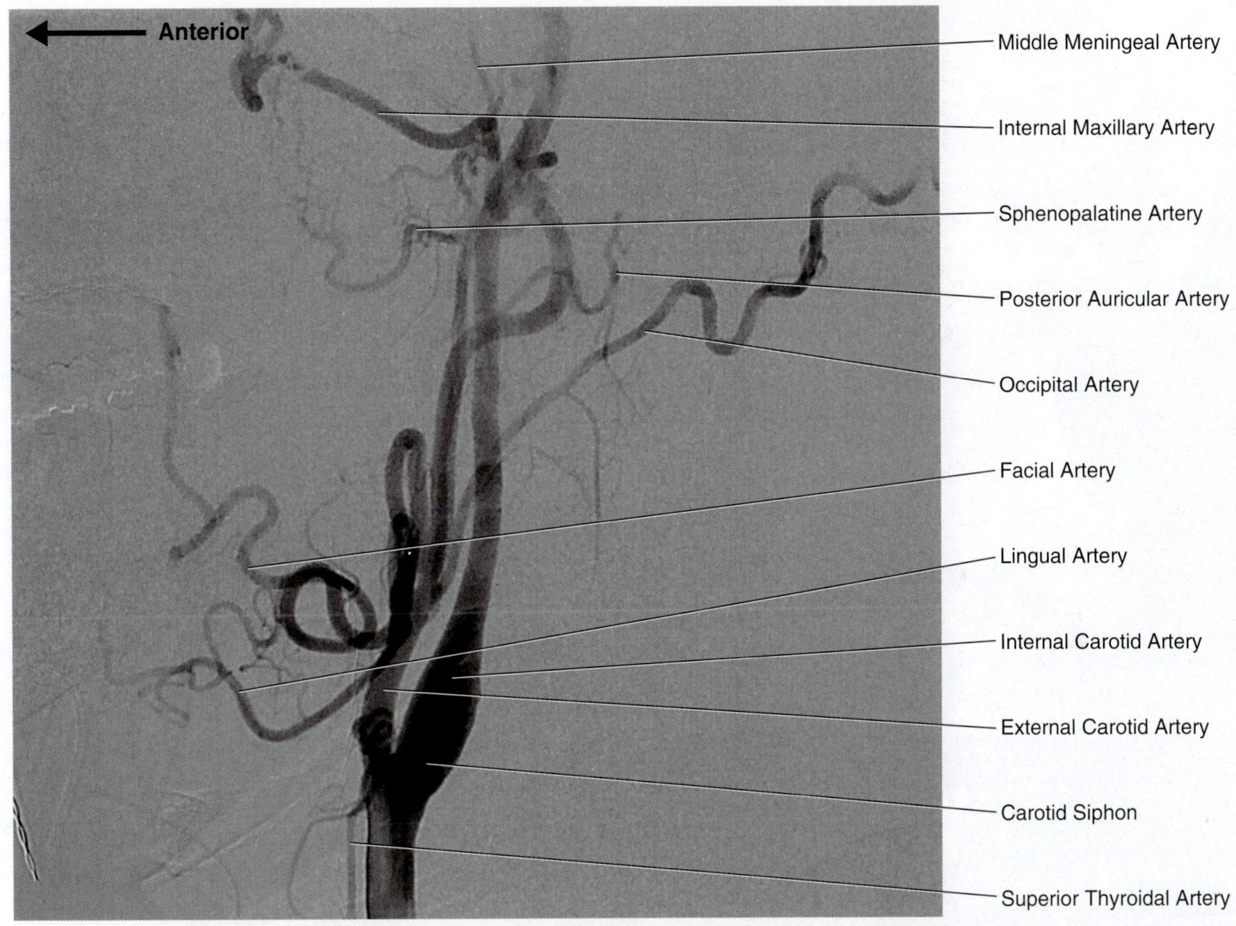

Figure 2.4. Lateral DSA of the carotid bifurcation. DSA, digital subtraction angiography.

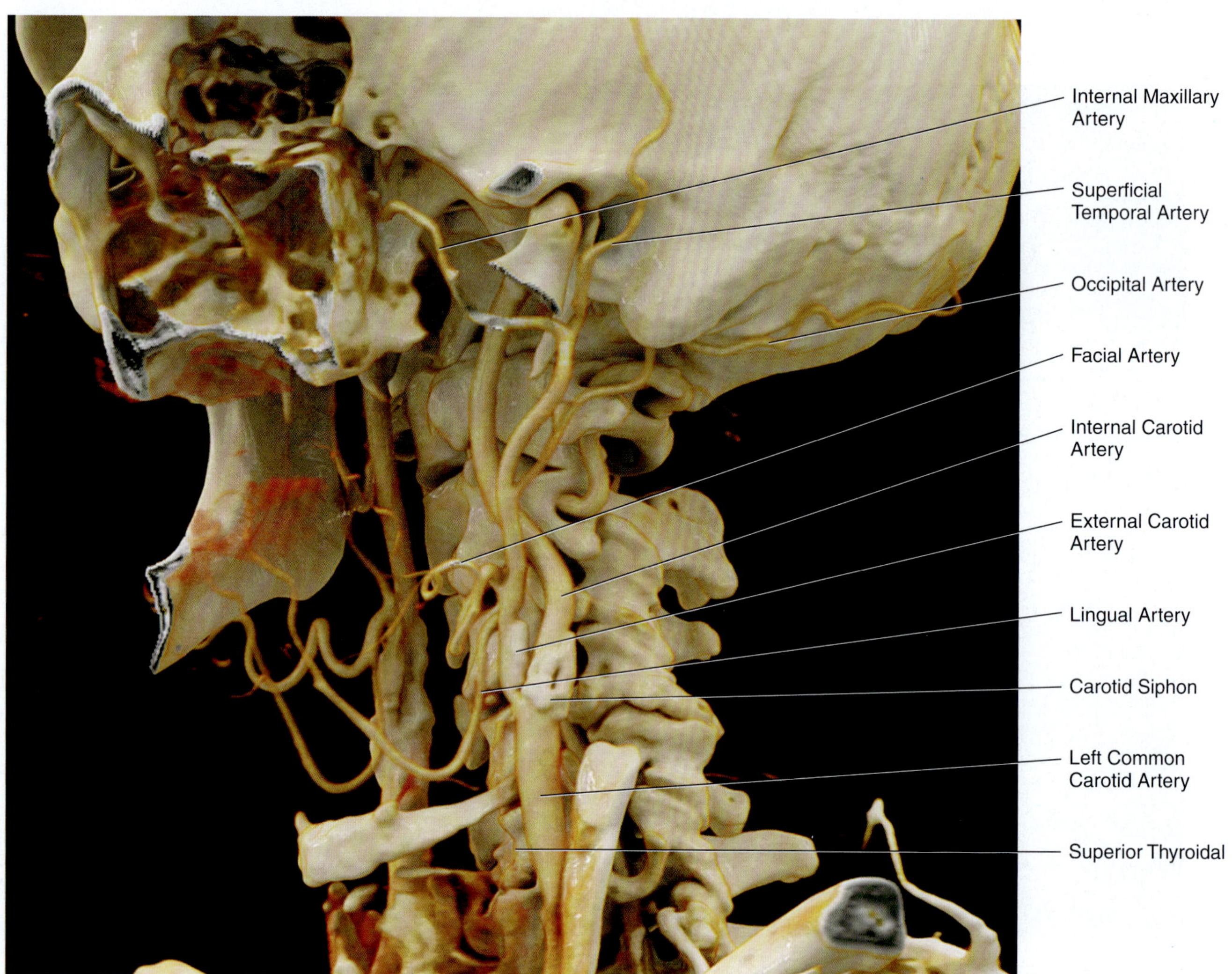

Figure 2.5. CT angiogram 3D surface-rendered view of the internal and external carotid branches and their relationship to the head and neck.

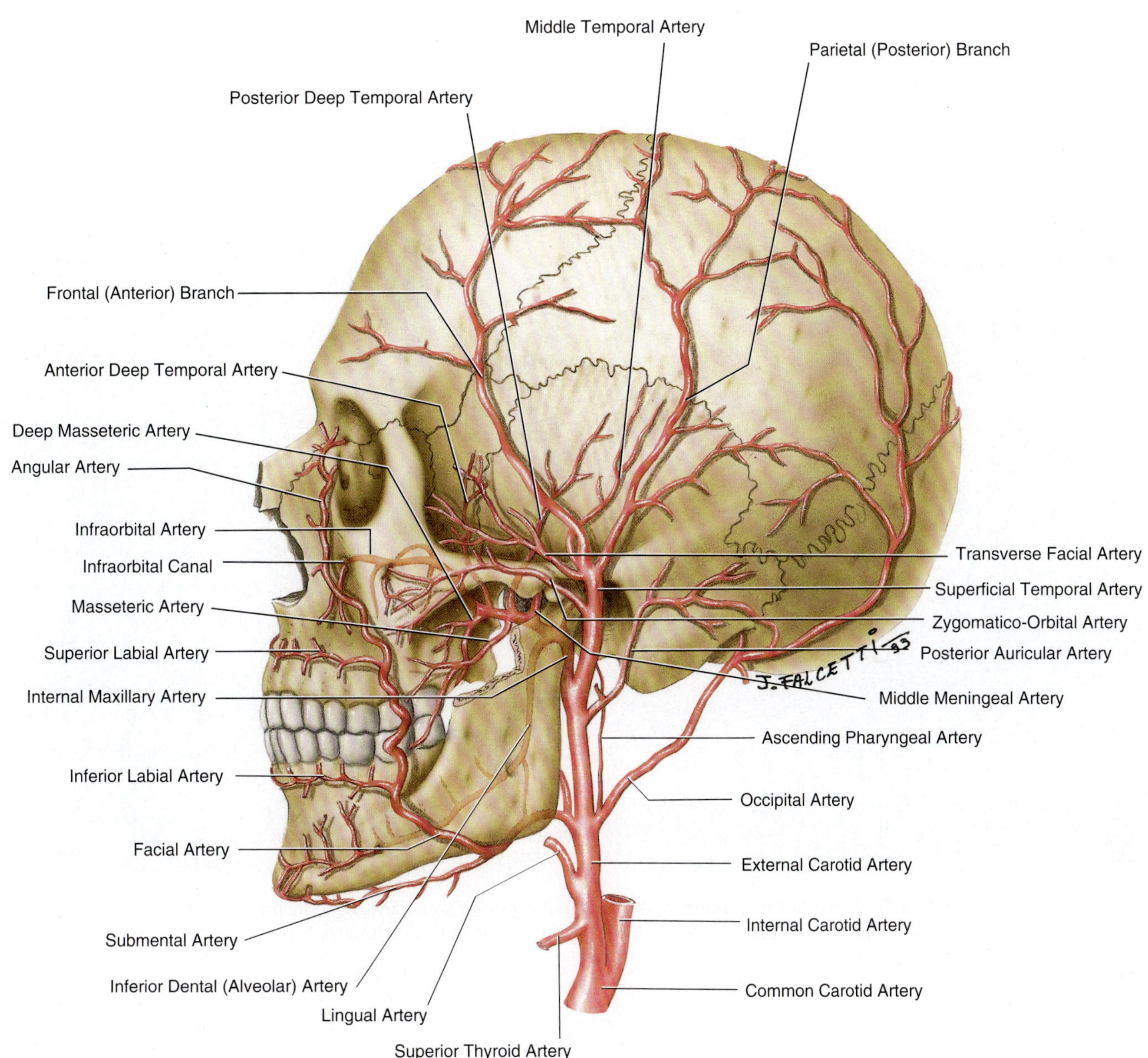

Figure 2.6. Illustration of the relationship of the external carotid artery branches and the skull. The ascending pharyngeal artery is shown arising from the occipital artery, a normal variant.

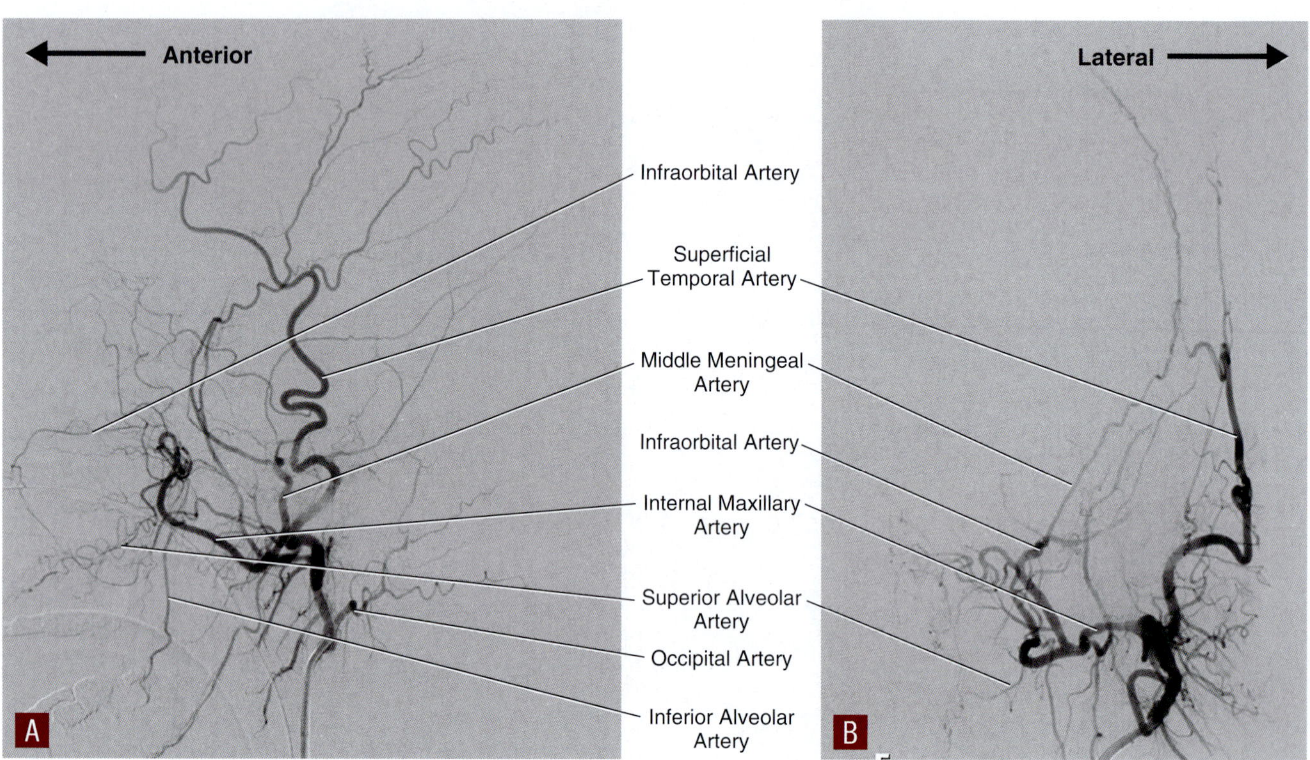

Figure 2.7. DSA with injection of the proximal external carotid artery and its branches with lateral (A) and AP (B) projections. DSA, digital subtraction angiography.

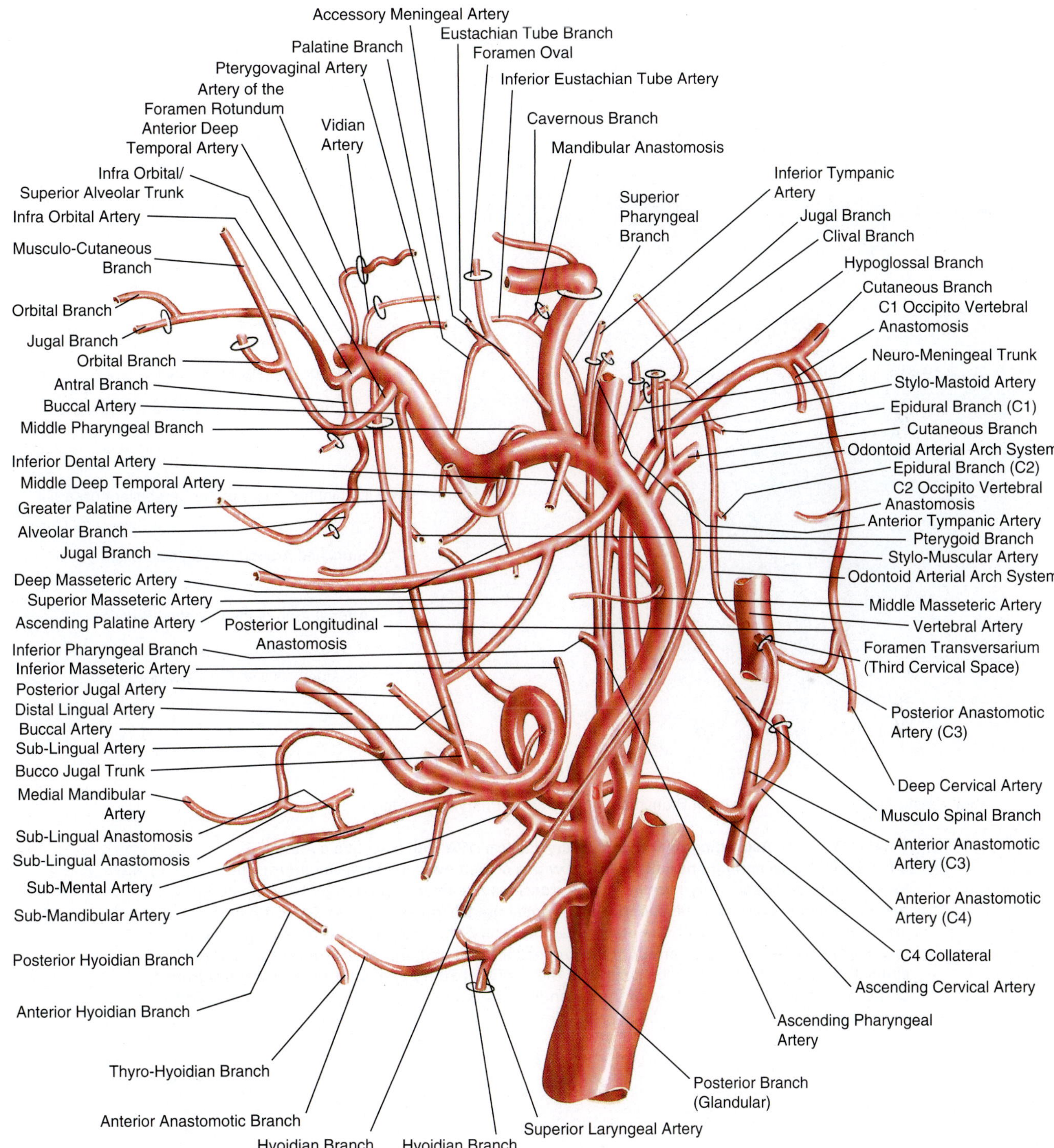

Figure 2.8. Illustration of the multiple branches of the external carotid artery and their relationship with the skull foramina.

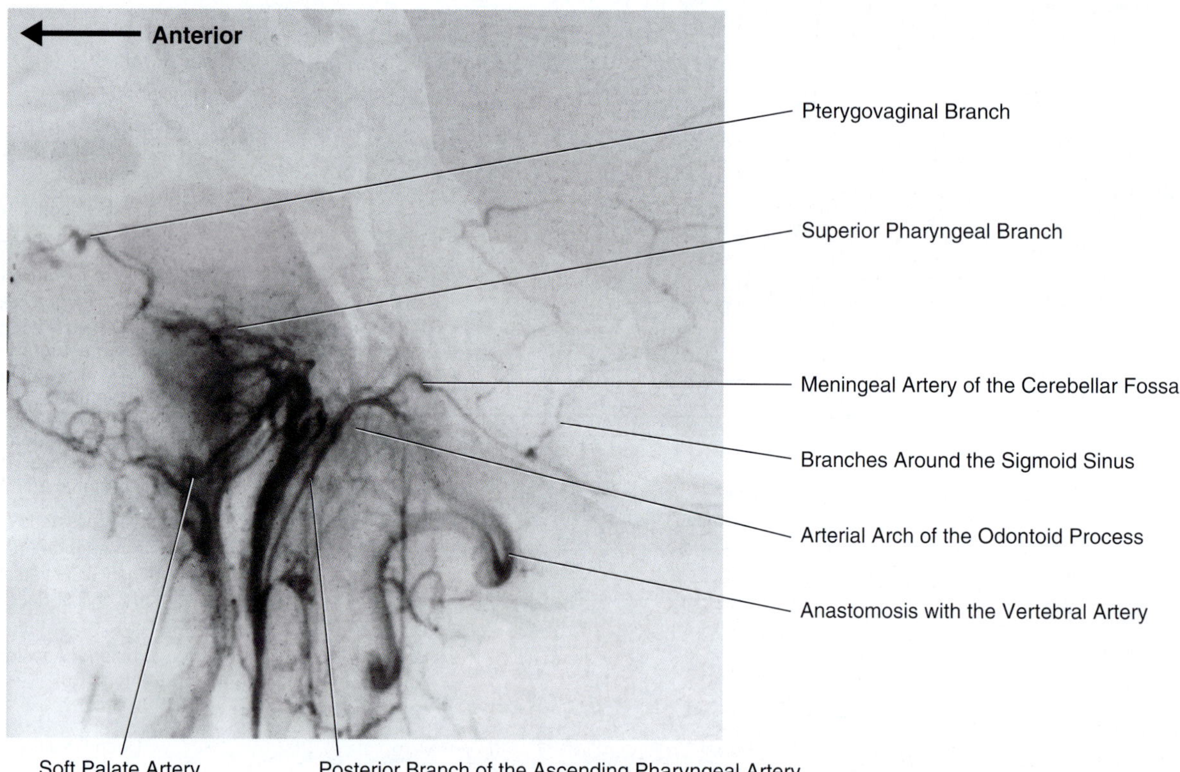

Figure 2.9. Ascending pharyngeal artery. Lateral DSA with selective contrast injection in the ascending pharyngeal artery with a screen overlay of the calvarium. The ascending pharyngeal artery has two major branches: the anterior pharyngeal and posterior neuromeningeal branches. The superior pharyngeal branch, gives origin to the soft palate artery; it has anastomosis with the pterygovaginal artery. The posterior neuromeningeal branch gives origin to the meningeal artery of the cerebellar fossa and branches around the sigmoid sinus. Critical anastomosis can be seen with the vertebral artery and anterior spinal artery from branches of the posterior division of the ascending pharyngeal artery. DSA, digital subtraction angiography.

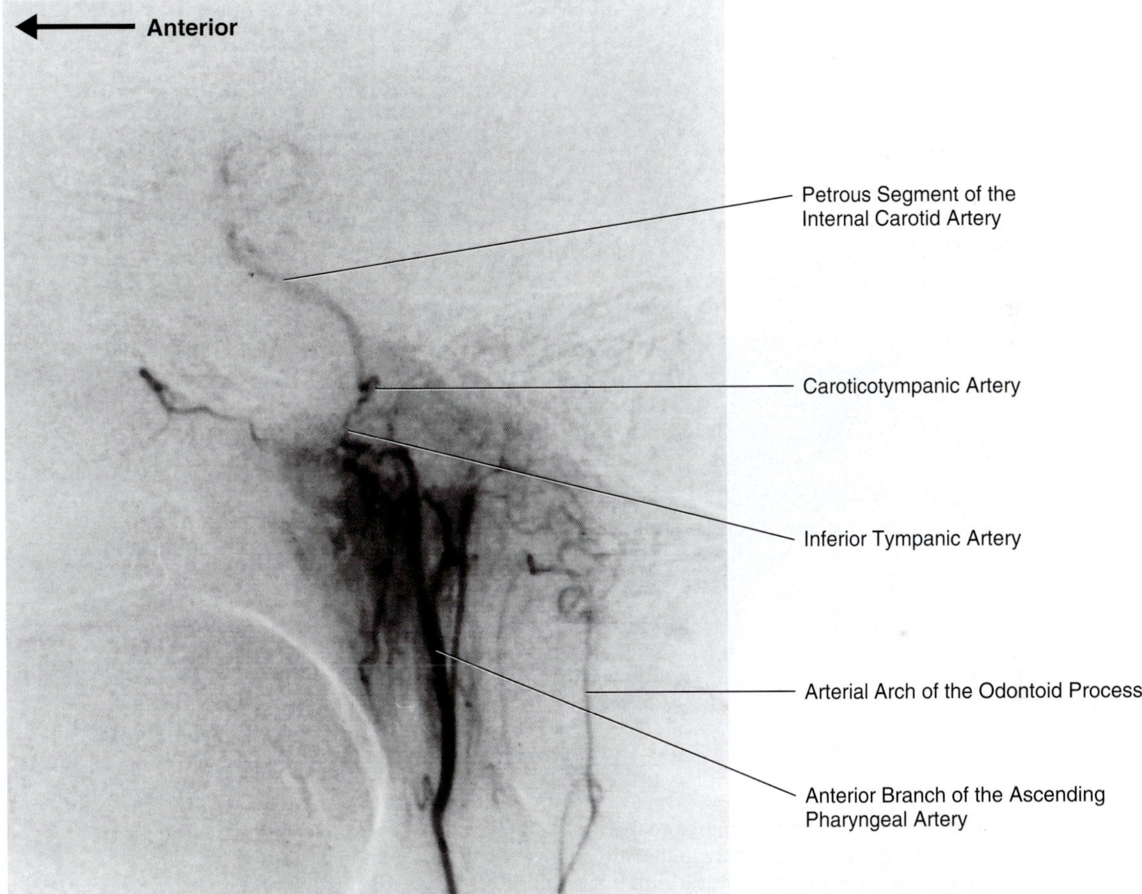

Figure 2.10. Ascending pharyngeal artery. Lateral DSA with selective contrast injection in the ascending pharyngeal artery. This angiogram demonstrates the anastomosis of the ascending pharyngeal artery with the internal carotid artery. This anastomosis consists of a connection from the anterior pharyngeal branch of the ascending pharyngeal artery to the inferior tympanic artery, the caroticotympanic artery, and ultimately to the internal carotid artery. DSA, digital subtraction angiography.

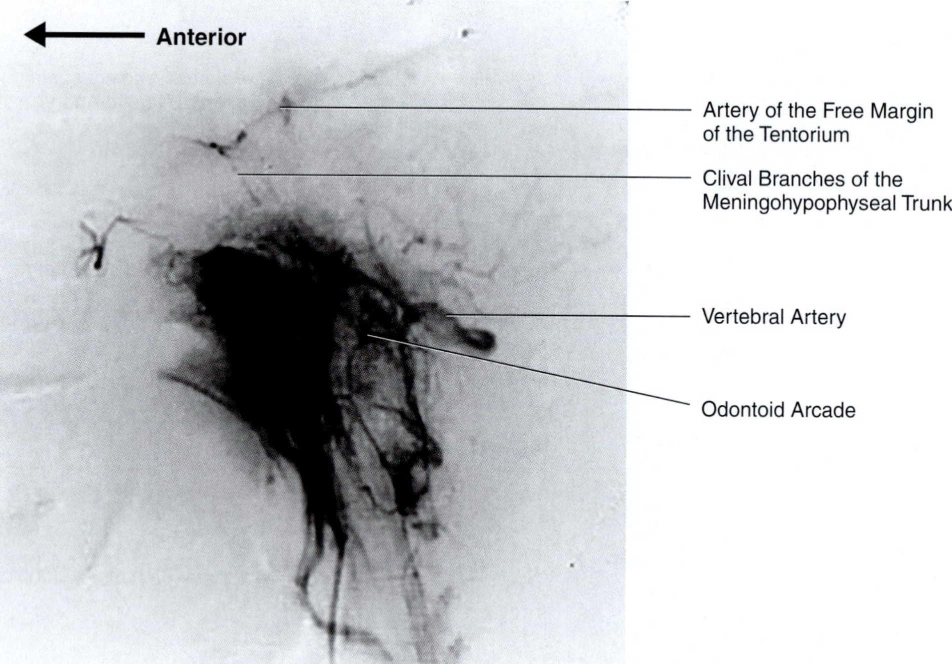

Figure 2.11. Ascending pharyngeal artery. Lateral DSA with selective contrast injection in the ascending pharyngeal artery in the late arterial phase. This demonstrates the posterior neuromeningeal branch anastomosis with the vertebral artery via the posterior arterial arch of the odontoid, the clival artery branch of the hypoglossal artery, and anastomosis with the meningohypophyseal trunk and artery of the free margin of the tentorium. DSA, digital subtraction angiography.

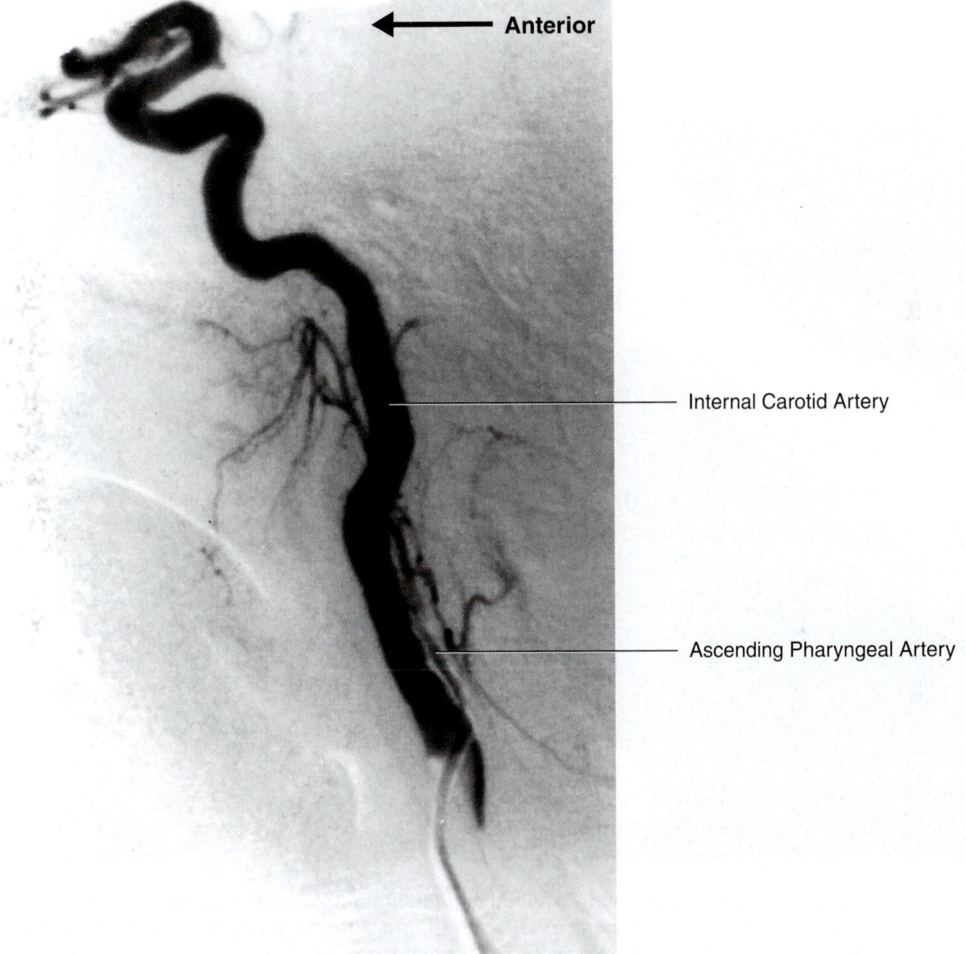

Figure 2.12. Ascending pharyngeal artery arising from the ICA. Lateral DSA with selective injection in the internal carotid artery origin demonstrating a variant origin of the ascending pharyngeal artery from the proximal ICA. DSA, digital subtraction angiography; ICA, internal carotid artery.

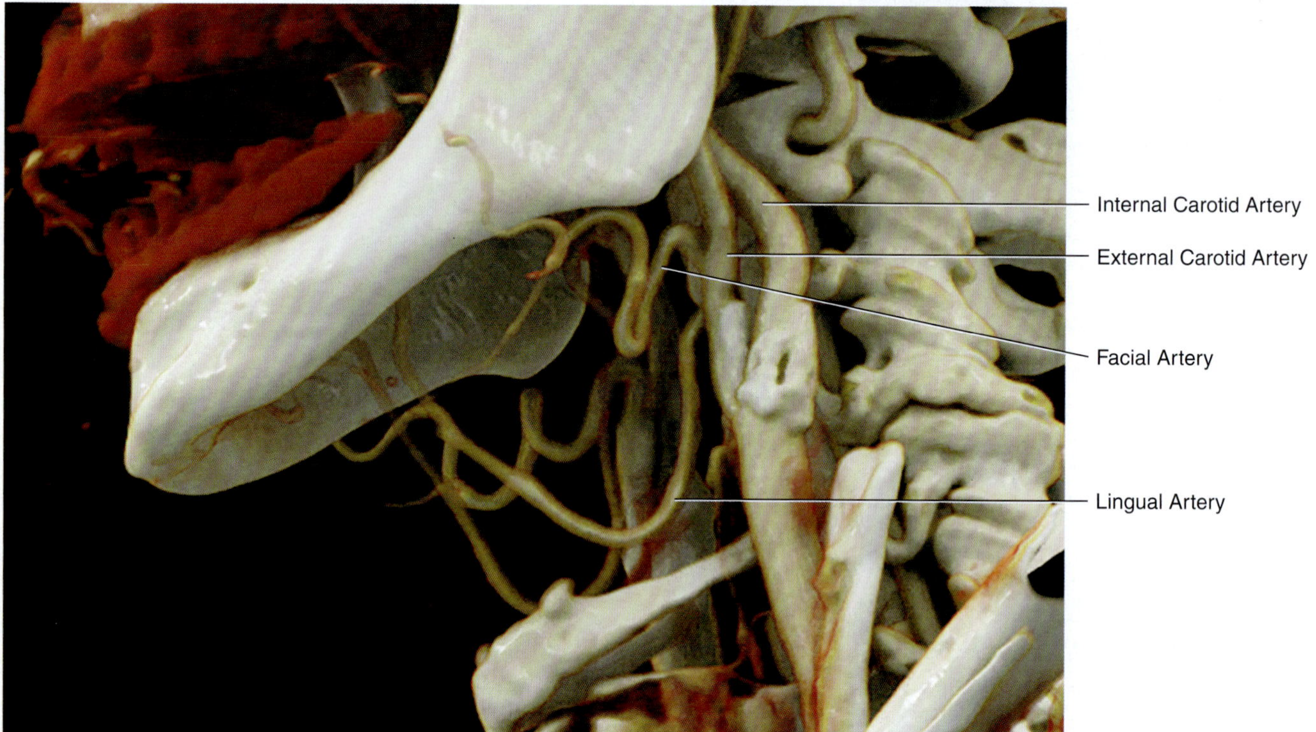

Figure 2.13. CT angiogram 3D cinematic rendering of the carotid bifurcation with the internal and external carotid arteries as well as the lingual and facial artery branches from the external carotid artery. Note the characteristic U-shaped loop of the proximal lingual artery.

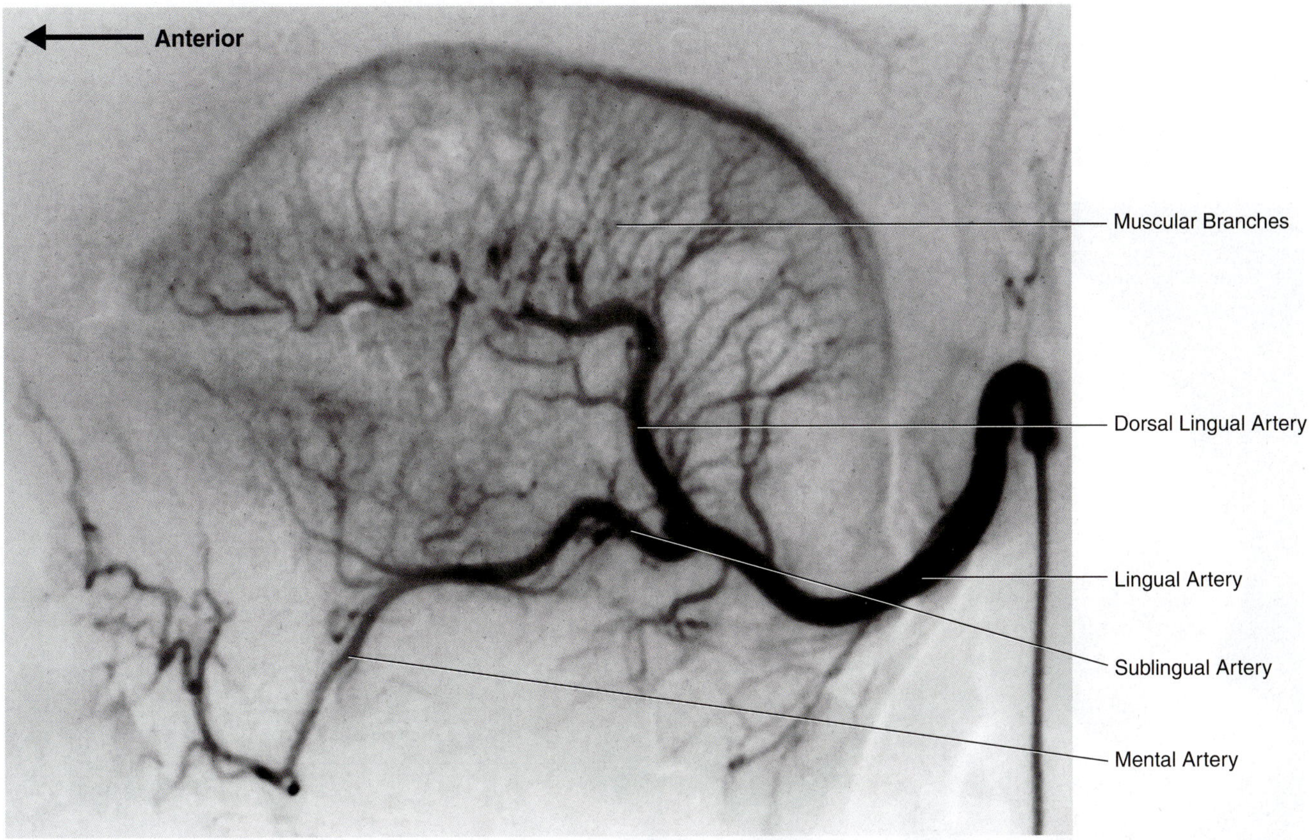

Figure 2.14. **Lingual artery.** Lateral DSA with injection of the lingual artery in the arterial phase demonstrating typical muscular branches and the prominent mental artery branch of the sublingual artery. DSA, digital subtraction angiography.

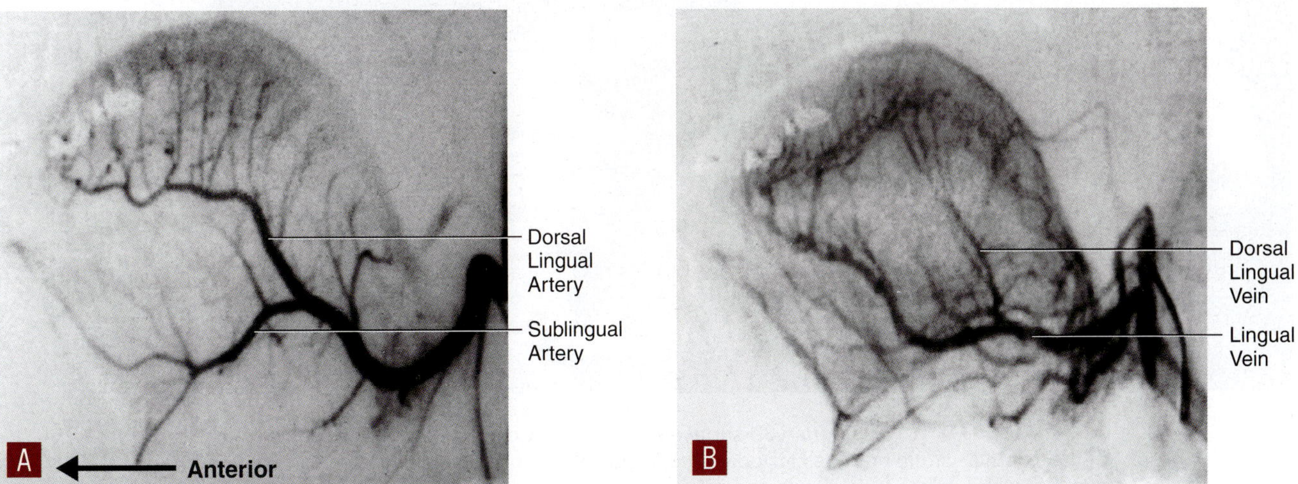

Figure 2.15. **Lingual artery in arterial and venous phases.** Lateral DSA with injection of the lingual artery in the arterial (A) phase demonstrating the dorsal artery of the tongue and the sublingual artery. The venous phase (B) demonstrates two dorsal lingual veins draining into the lingual vein. DSA, digital subtraction angiography.

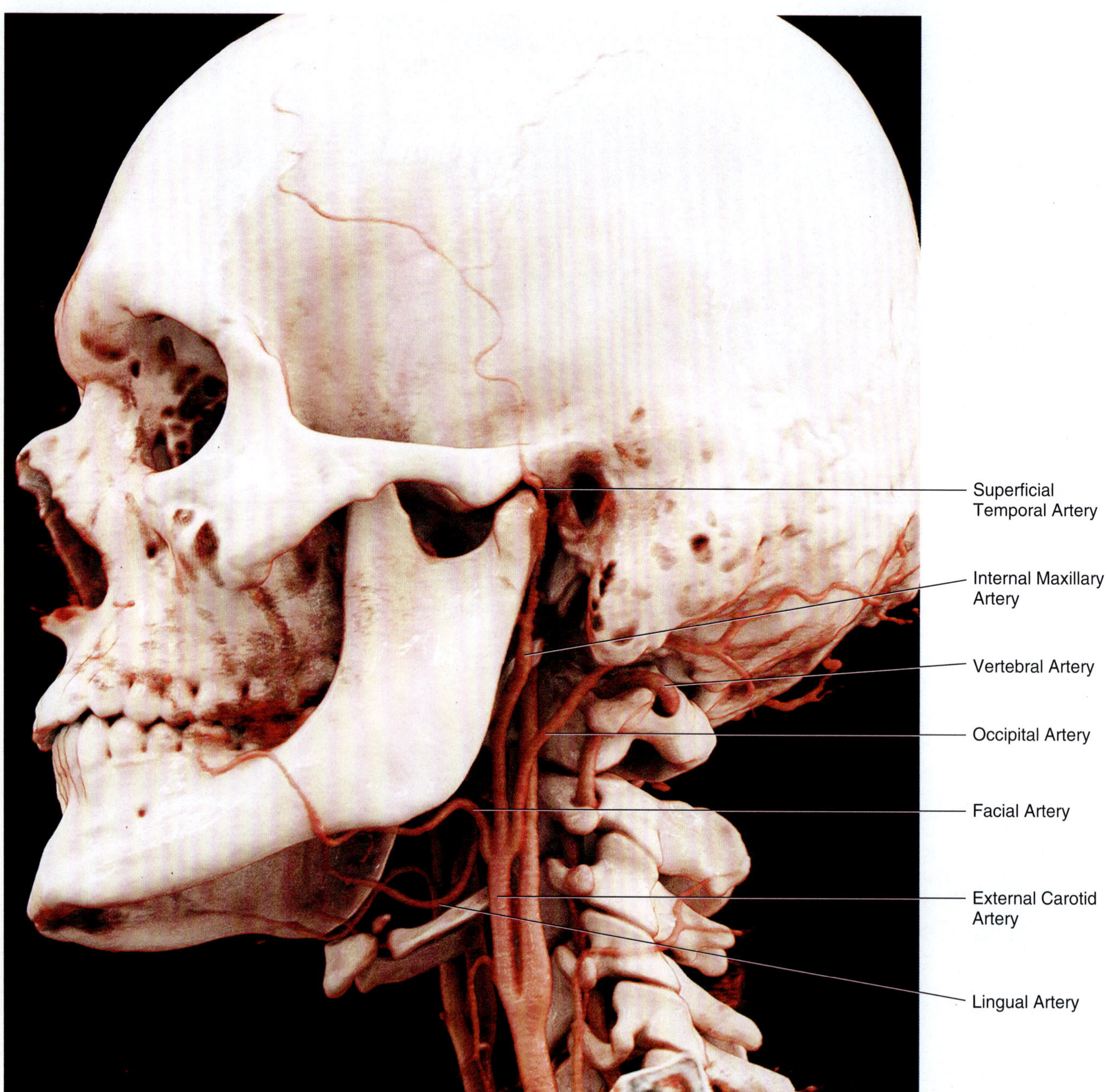

Figure 2.16. CT angiogram 3D surface-rendered view demonstrating the relationship of the external carotid branches including the lingual, facial, occipital, and internal maxillary artery branches to the facial bones and calvarium.

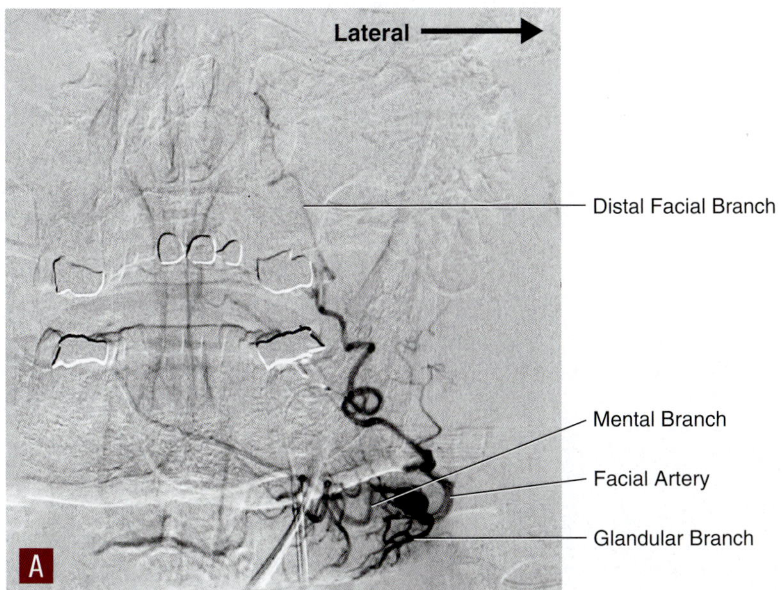

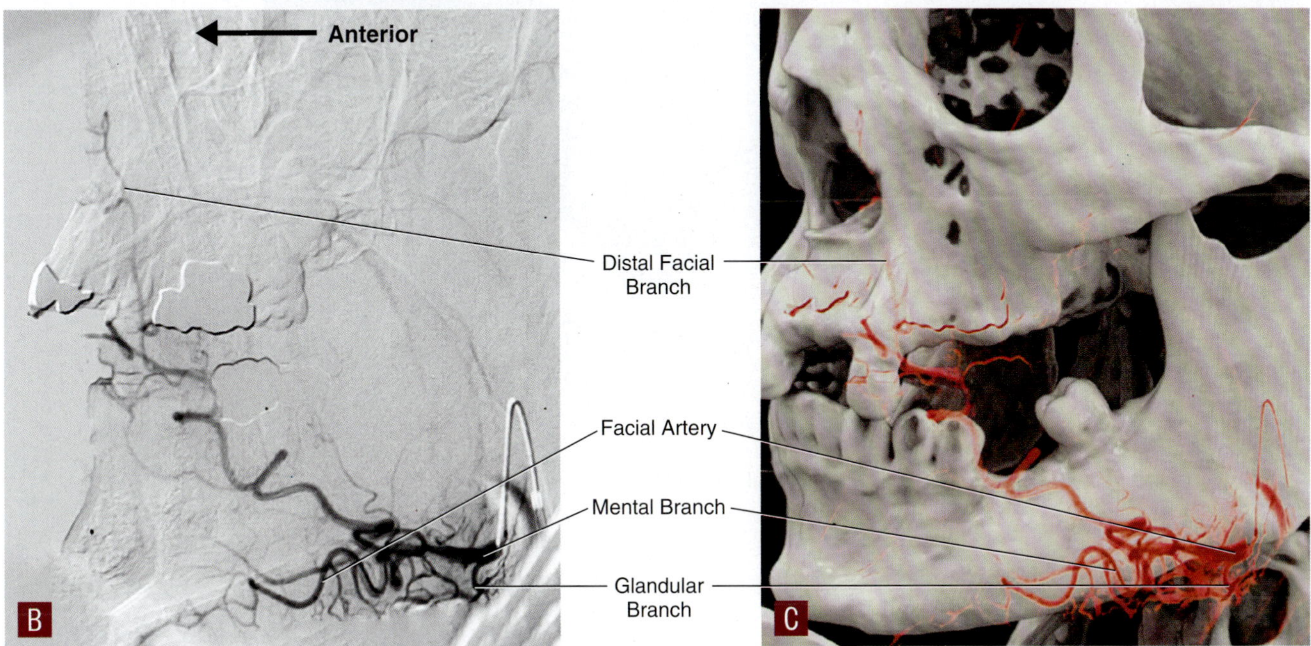

Figure 2.17. **Facial artery, AP, and lateral oblique views.** (A) AP and (B) lateral oblique DSA with injection in the facial artery origin demonstrating the glandular branch, mental branch, and distal facial branches. (C) CT angiogram 3D surface image merged with the lateral oblique DSA demonstrates the relationship of the facial artery to the mandible. DSA, digital subtraction angiography.

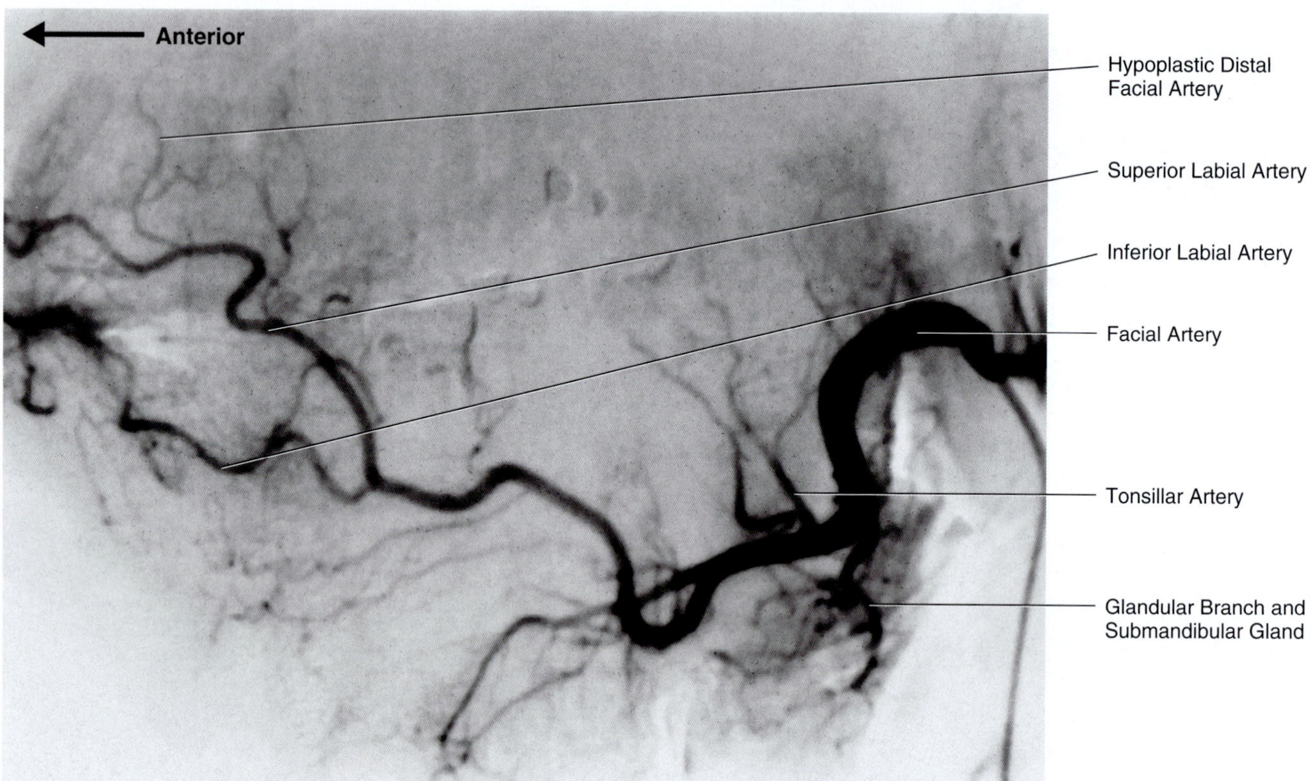

Figure 2.18. **Facial artery lateral view.** Lateral DSA with injection of the facial artery. DSA, digital subtraction angiography.

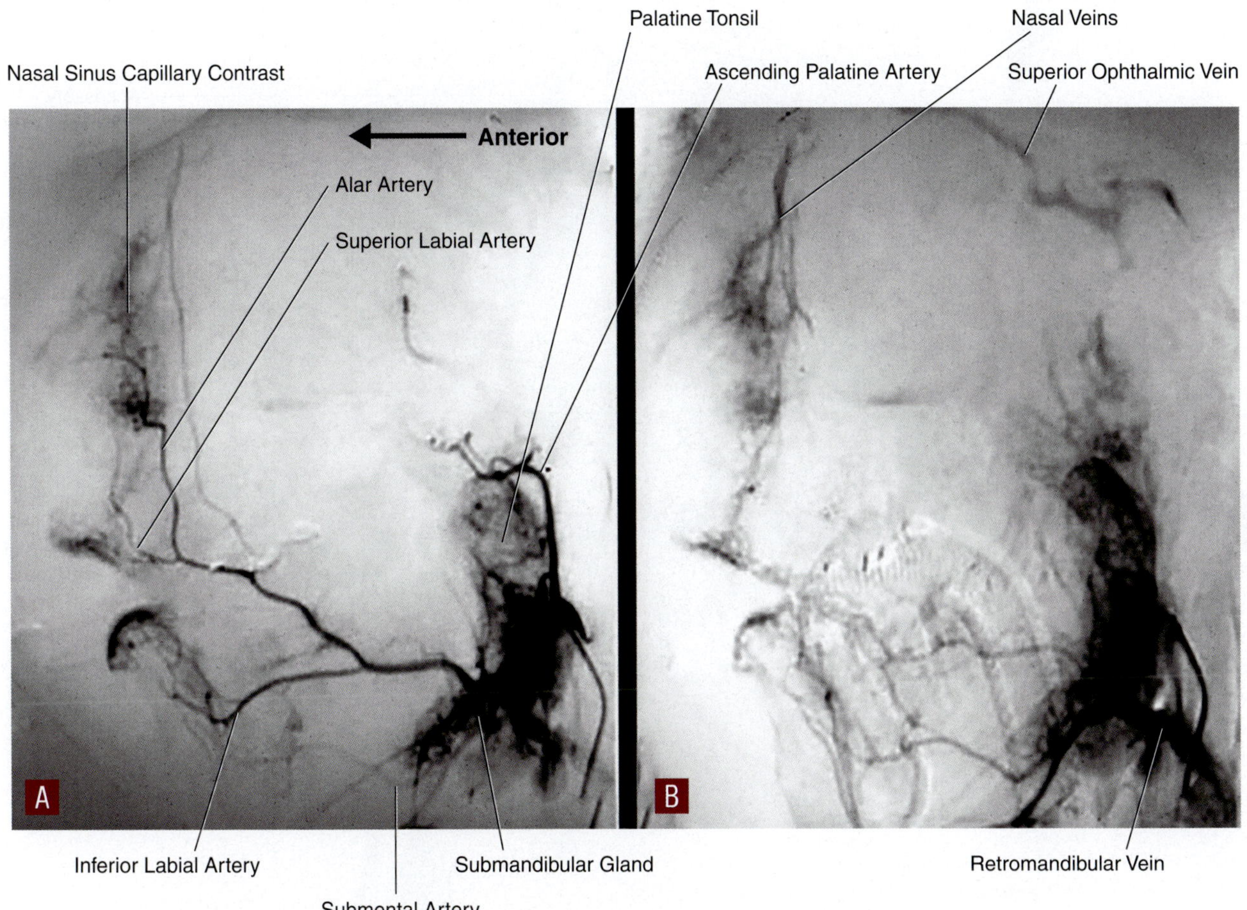

Figure 2.19. Facial artery lateral view in the late arterial and venous phases. Lateral DSA with injection of the facial artery in the late arterial (A) and venous (B) phases. **A**, In the late arterial phase, tonsillar capillary contrast is demonstrated along with nasal sinus capillary contrast from the alar artery. This alar artery can contribute to anterior nasal epistaxis that can require endovascular embolization. **B**, In the venous phase, the nasal veins are seen draining into the superior ophthalmic vein. The lips and jugal territory are seen draining into the retromandibular vein. DSA, digital subtraction angiography.

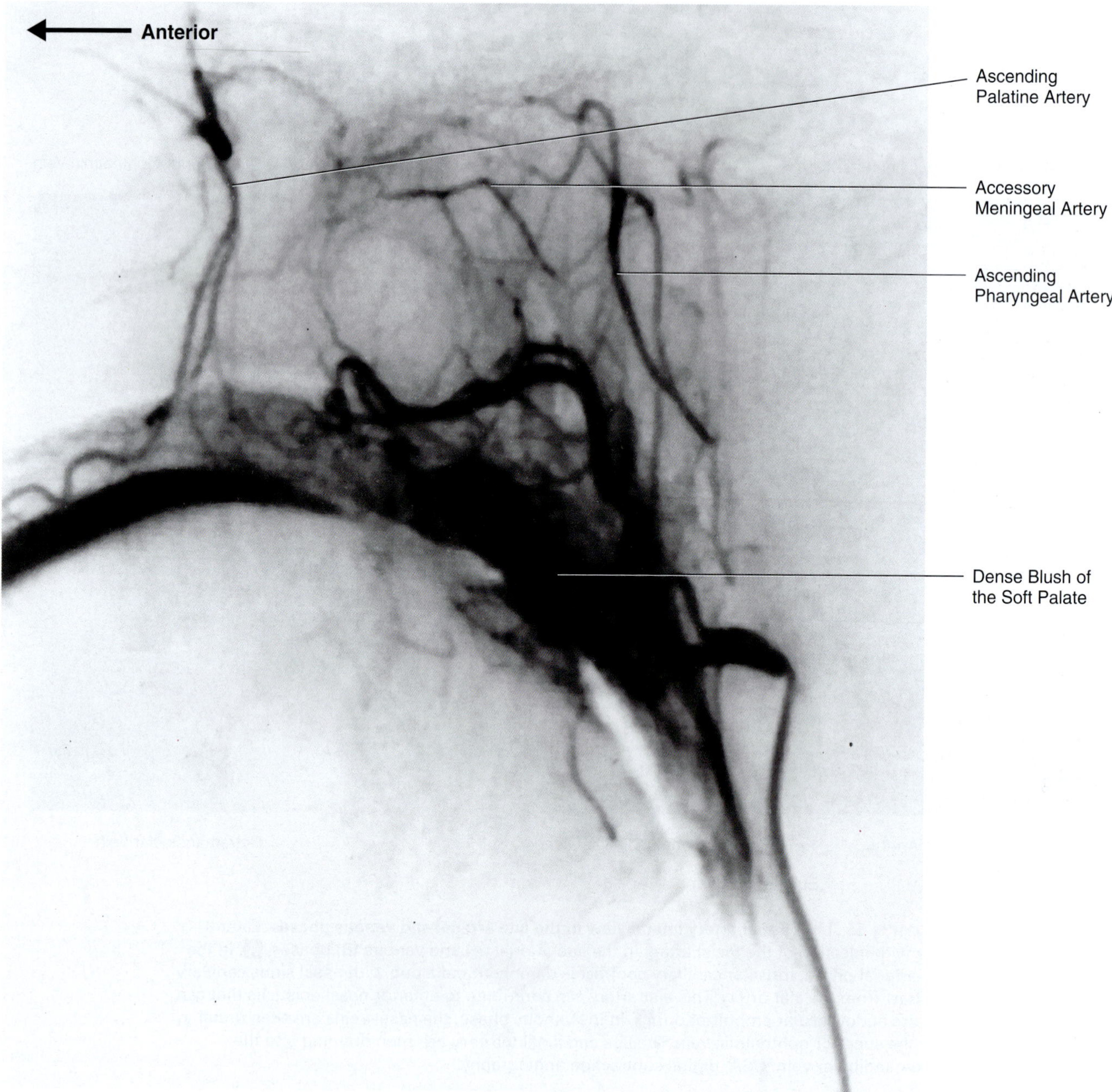

Figure 2.20. Artery of the soft palate. Lateral DSA with injection of the proximal facial artery in the late arterial phase. This demonstrates the anastomoses of the ascending palatine artery with the ascending pharyngeal artery. DSA, digital subtraction angiography.

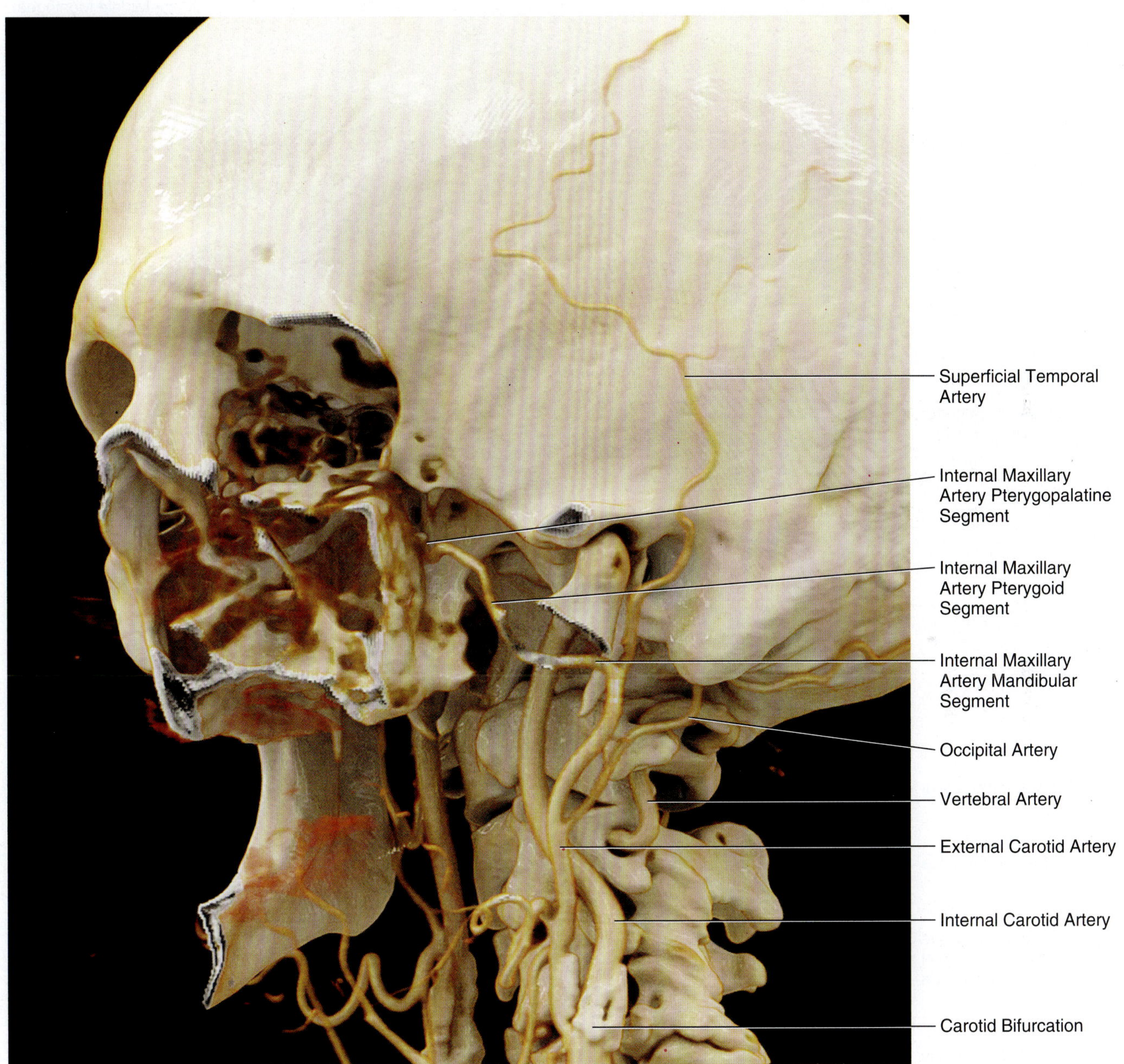

Figure 2.21. CTA 3D cinematic reconstruction. The mandible and part of the maxilla have been removed. This demonstrates the anatomic relationship of the external carotid artery terminal branches with the mandibular condyle and calvarium.

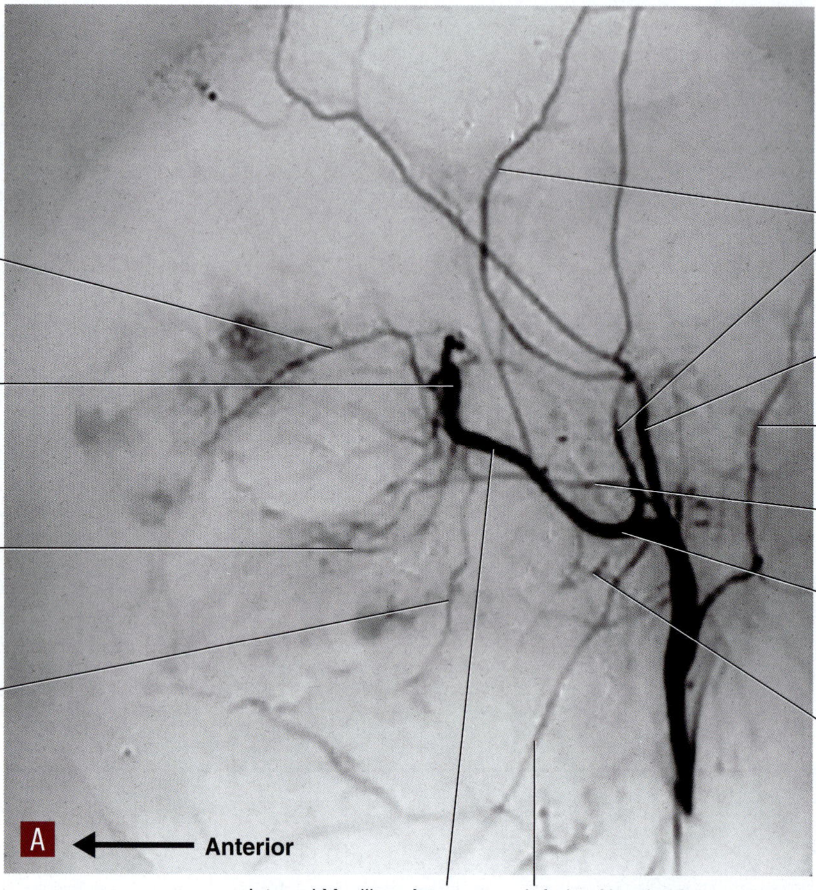

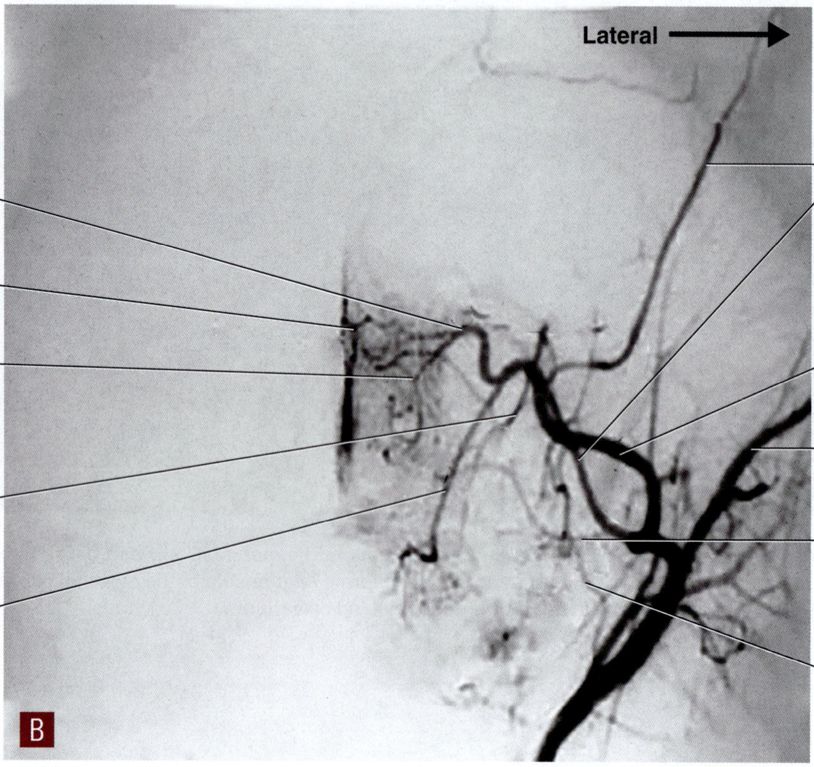

Figure 2.22. External carotid artery. Lateral (A) and AP (B) views. Lateral (A) and AP (B) DSA with injection of the distal external carotid artery. DSA, digital subtraction angiography.

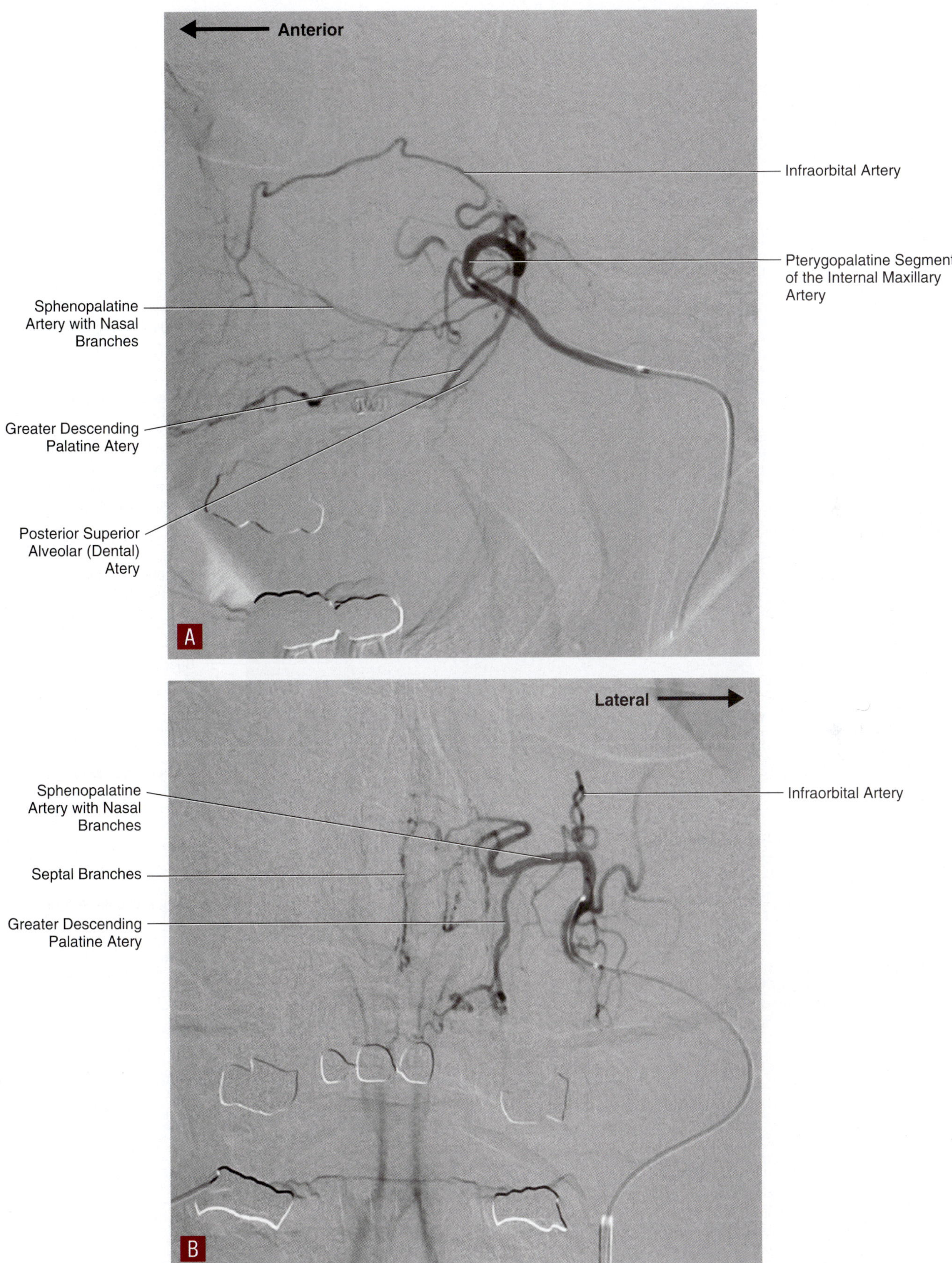

Figure 2.23. External carotid artery. Lateral (A) and AP (B) views. Lateral (A) and AP (B) DSA with injection of the distal pterygopalatine segment of the internal maxillary artery. DSA, digital subtraction angiography.

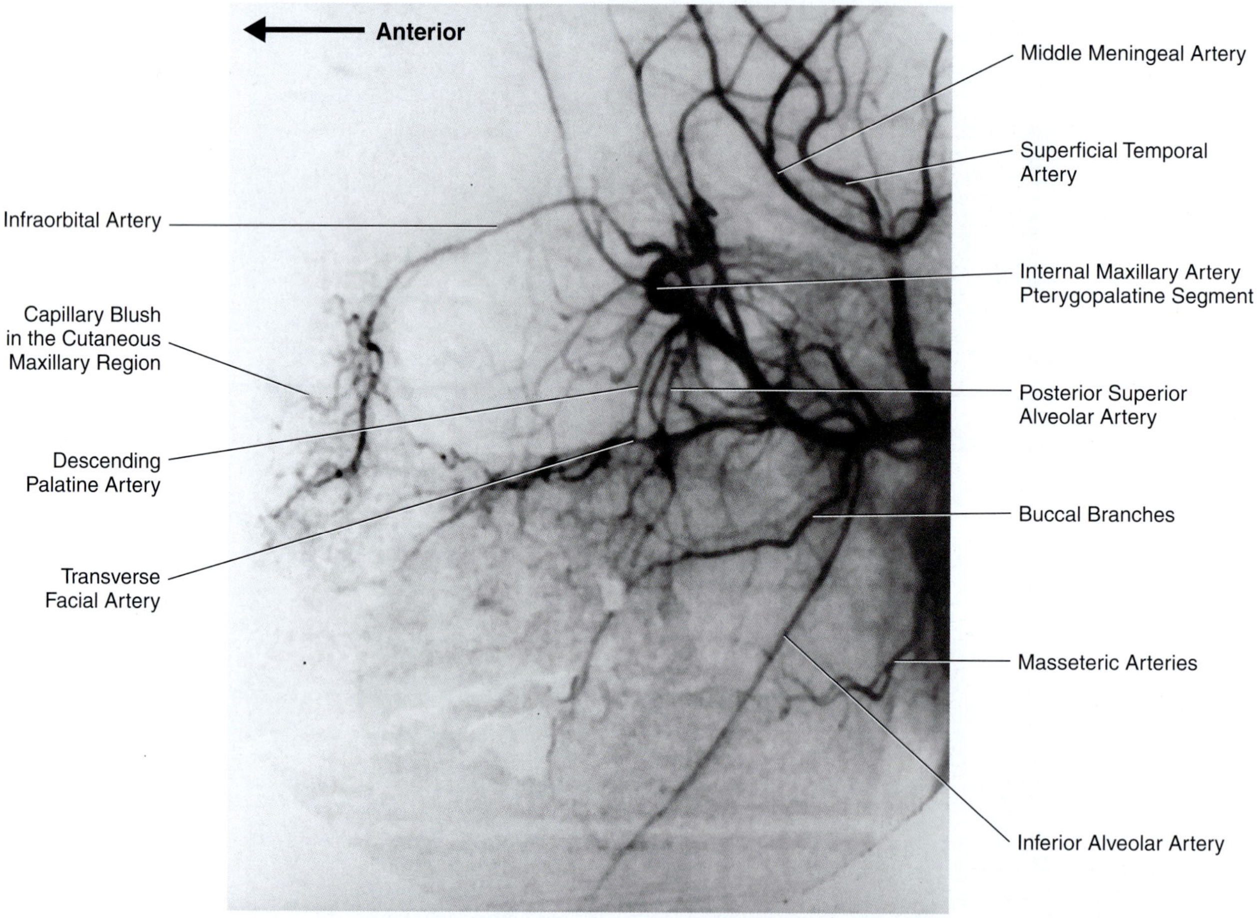

Figure 2.24. **External carotid artery.** Lateral DSA with injection of the distal external carotid artery in the late arterial phase demonstrates the cutaneous territory of the maxillary region supplied by the infraorbital artery. DSA, digital subtraction angiography.

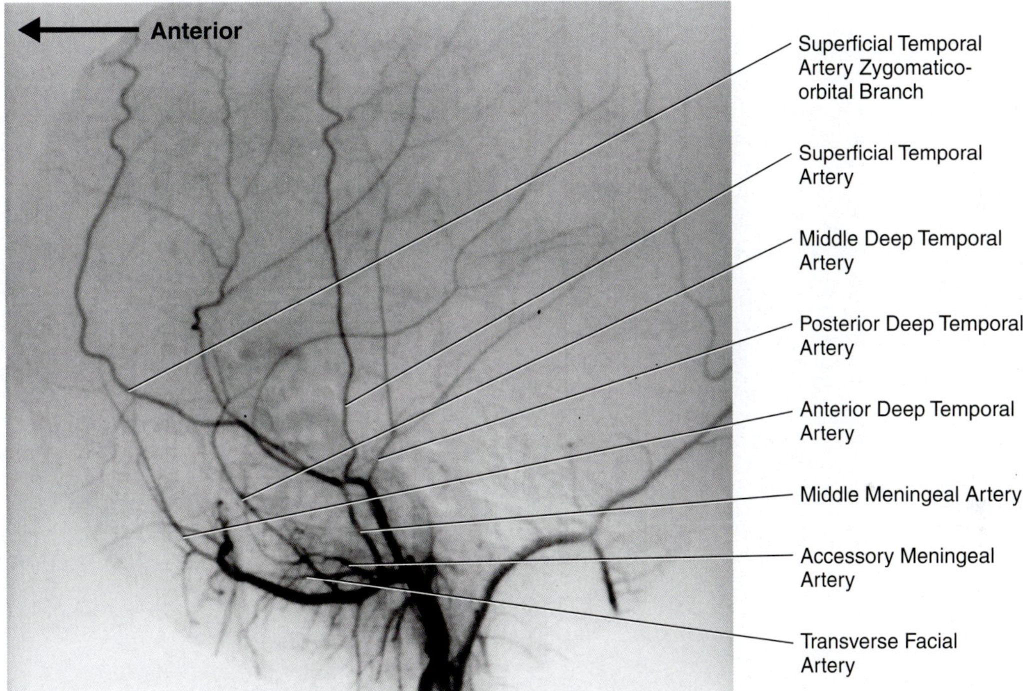

Figure 2.25. External carotid artery. Lateral DSA with injection of the distal external carotid artery with opacification of the internal maxillary artery, superficial temporal artery, and middle meningeal artery. Note the tortuous course of the superficial temporal artery and the linear course of the middle meningeal artery. DSA, digital subtraction angiography.

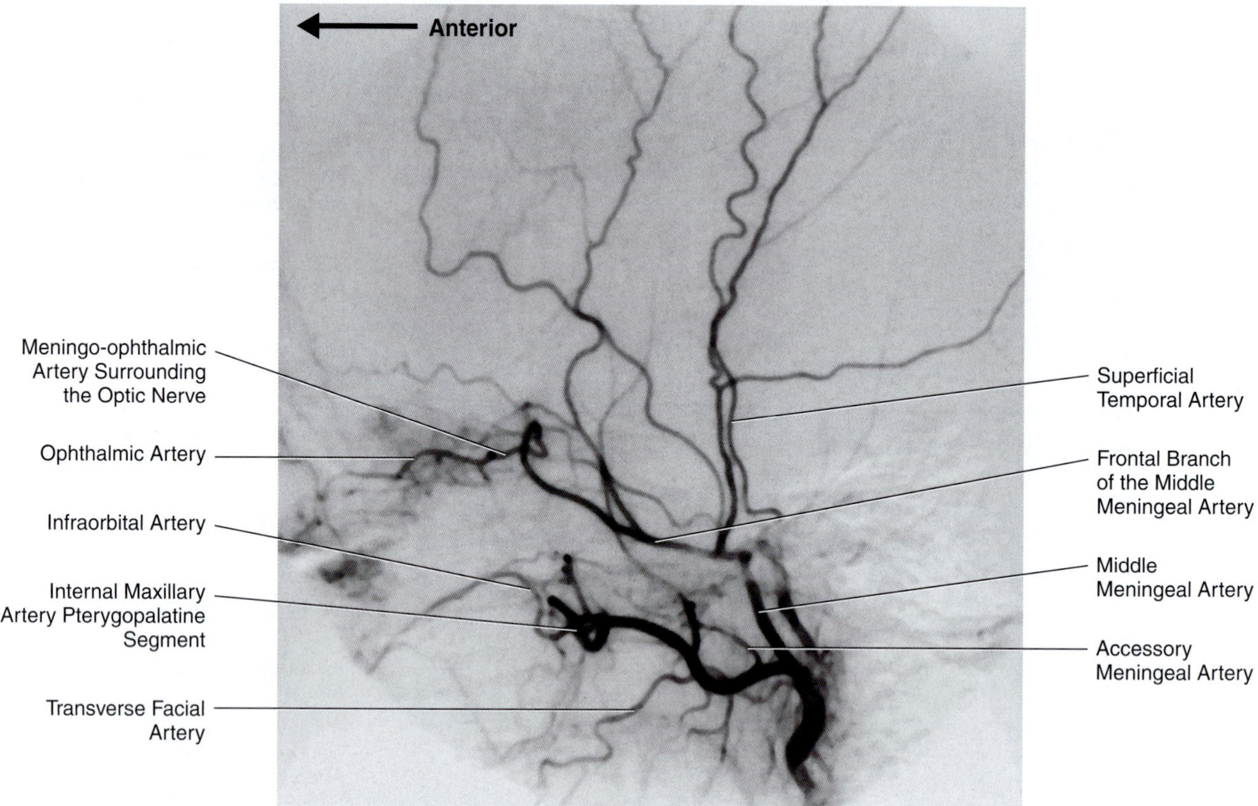

Figure 2.26. Distal branches of the external carotid artery. Lateral DSA with injection of the distal external carotid artery demonstrating an important variant ophthalmic artery origin from the frontal branch of the middle meningeal artery and surrounds the optic nerve. This variant occurs when there is persistence of the middle meningeal artery embryonic meningo-ophthalmic branch. This is a critical variant as the more distal central retinal artery represents a true-end artery with no collateral supply, and inadvertent embolization during a distal internal maxillary artery embolization with this variant results in irreversible permanent vision loss. DSA, digital subtraction angiography.

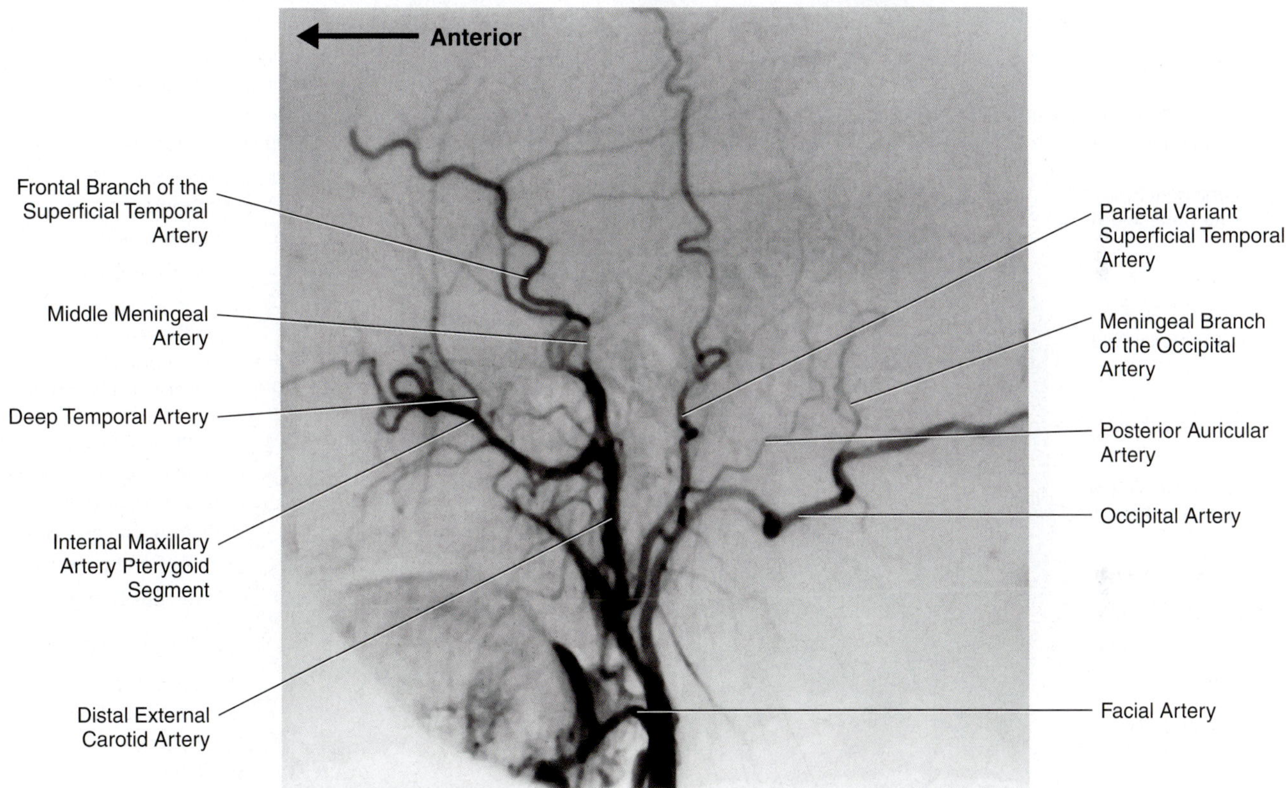

Figure 2.27. **External carotid artery.** Lateral DSA with injection of the distal external carotid artery. This demonstrates a variant double origin of the superficial temporal artery with the frontal branch arising from the distal external carotid artery and the variant parietal superficial temporal artery arising from a common origin with the posterior auricular artery. DSA, digital subtraction angiography.

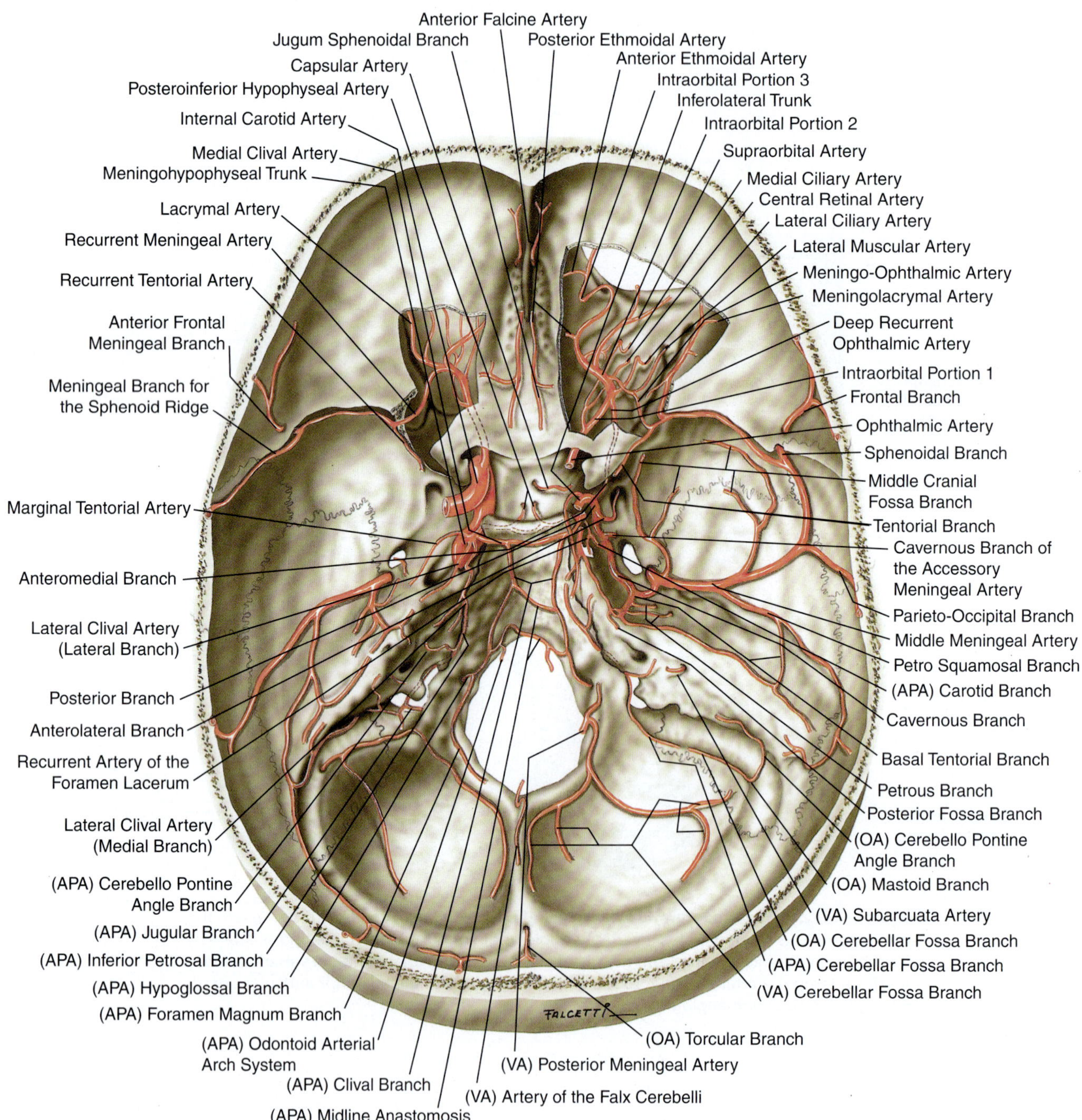

Figure 2.28. Relationship of the external carotid artery branches with the internal carotid artery. Illustration of the skull base demonstrating the anatomic relationship between the external carotid artery meningeal branches and the proximal internal carotid artery branches.

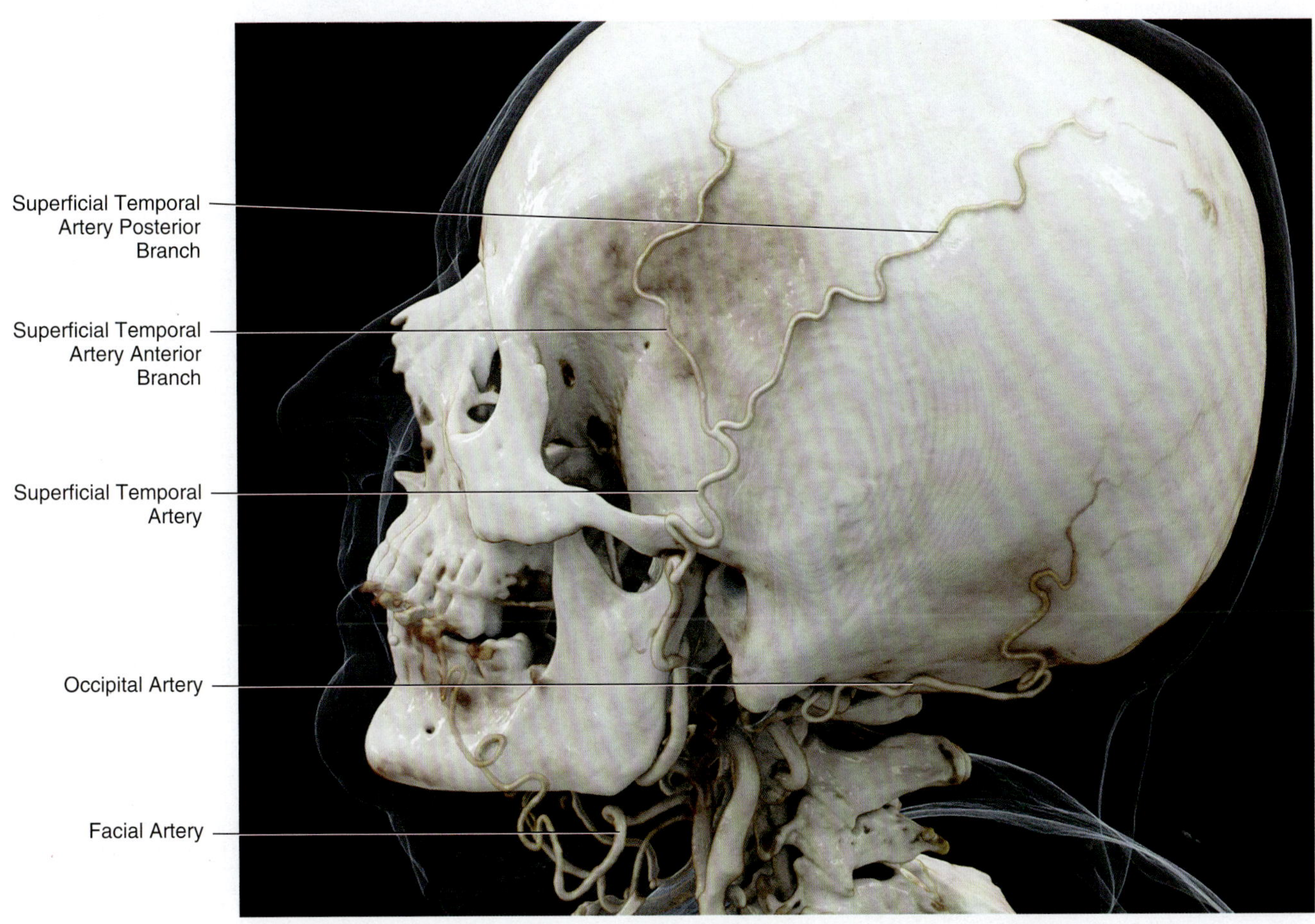

Figure 2.29. CTA 3D oblique surface reconstruction. This demonstrates the anatomic relationship of the facial artery, occipital artery, and superficial temporal artery.

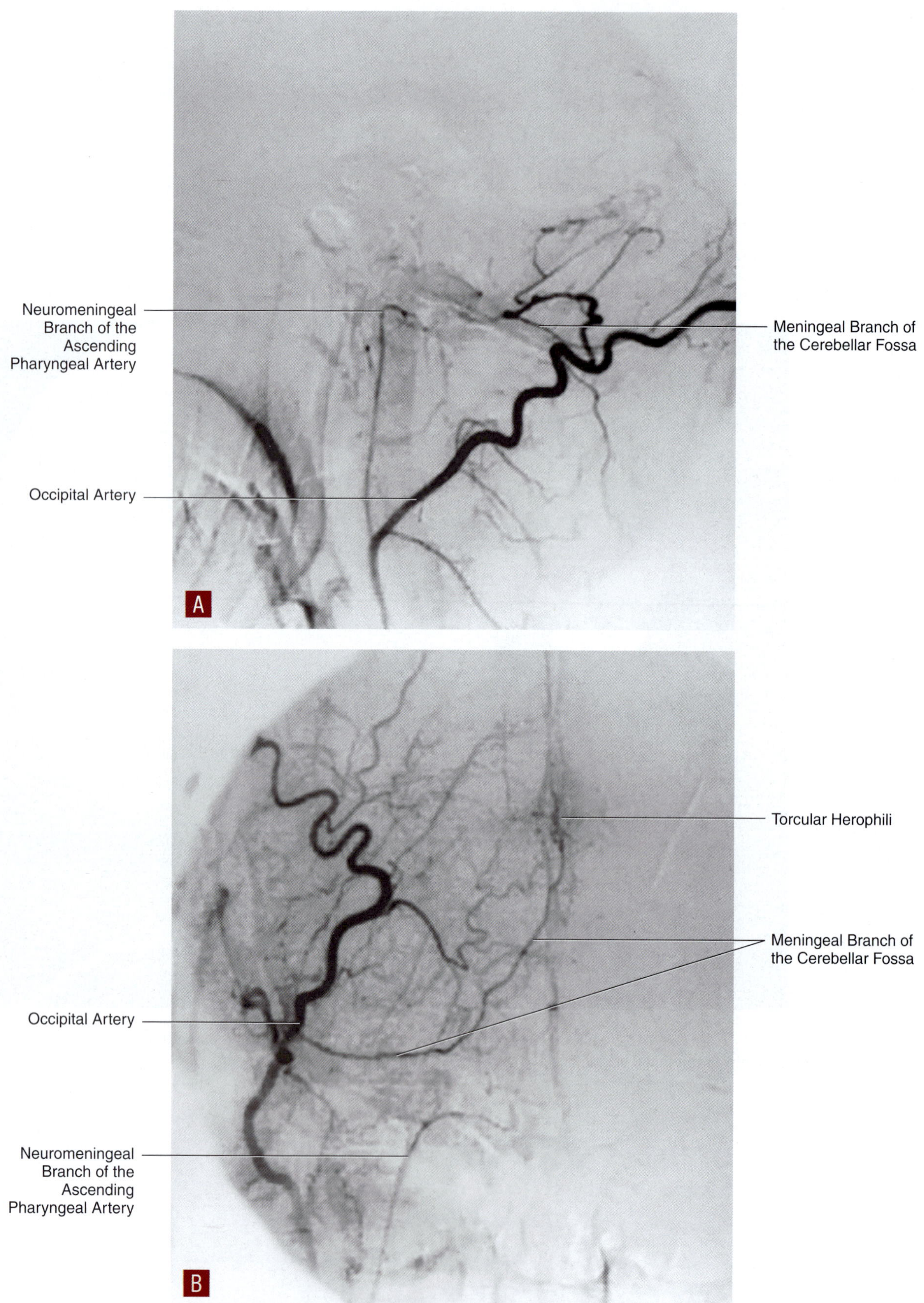

Figure 2.30. Occipital artery. DSA with injection of the occipital artery in the lateral (A) and AP (B) projections. Variant anatomy demonstrating the posterior branch of the ascending pharyngeal artery arising from the occipital artery. The meningeal branch of the cerebellar fossa is seen reaching the torcular Herophili. DSA, digital subtraction angiography.

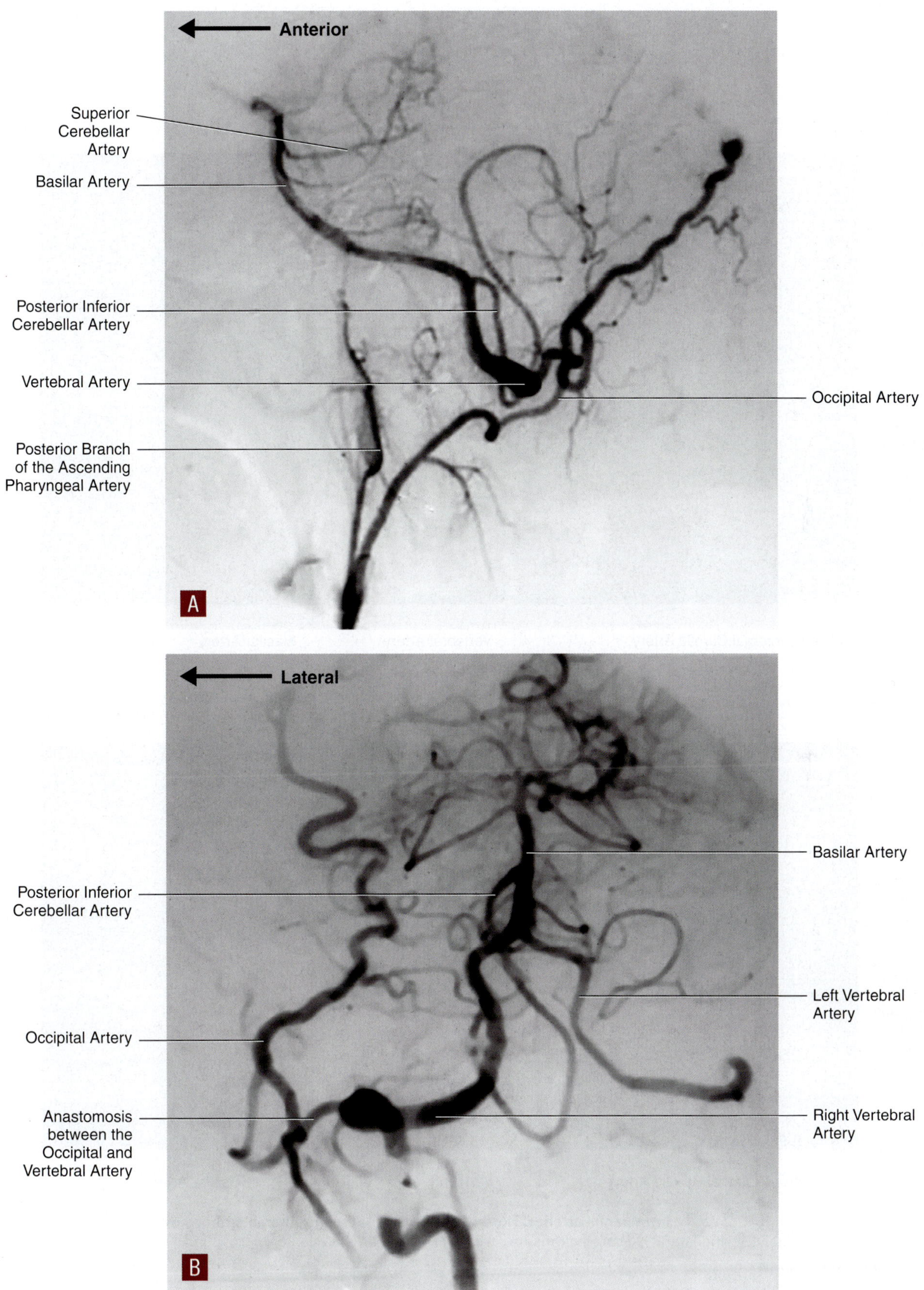

Figure 2.31. Occipital artery. Lateral (A) and AP (B) DSA with injection of the right occipital artery. This demonstrates a variant anastomosis with the right vertebral artery. DSA, digital subtraction angiography.

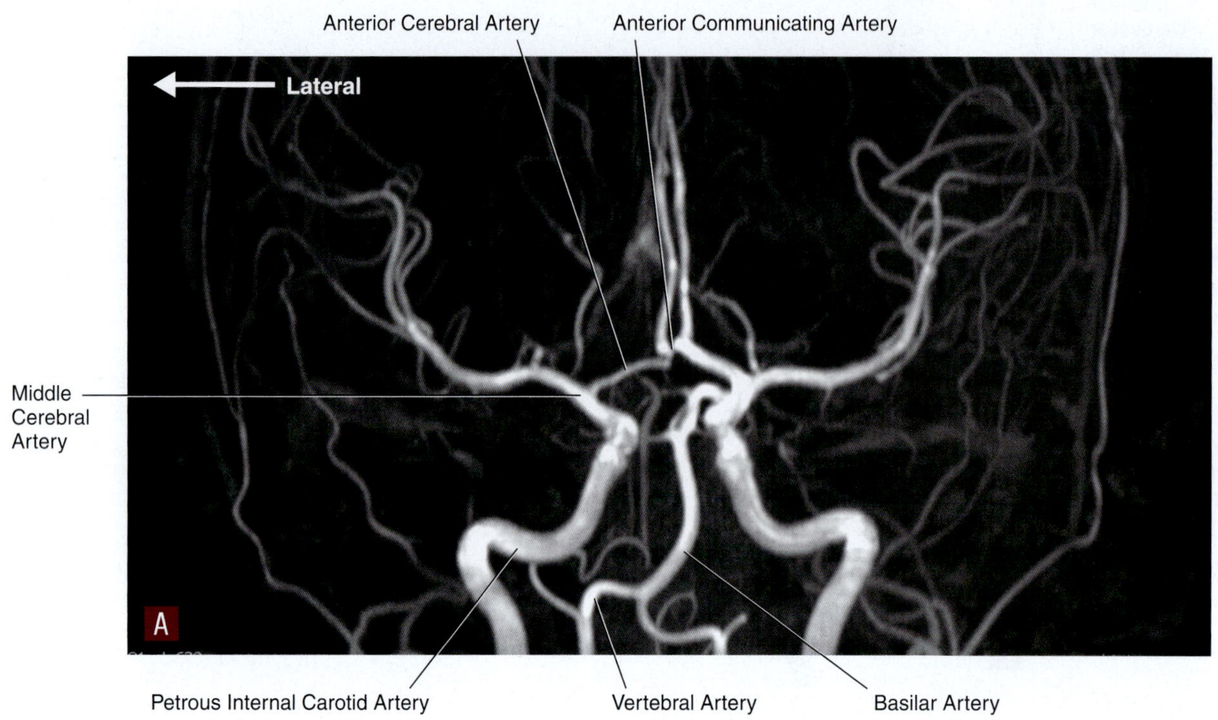

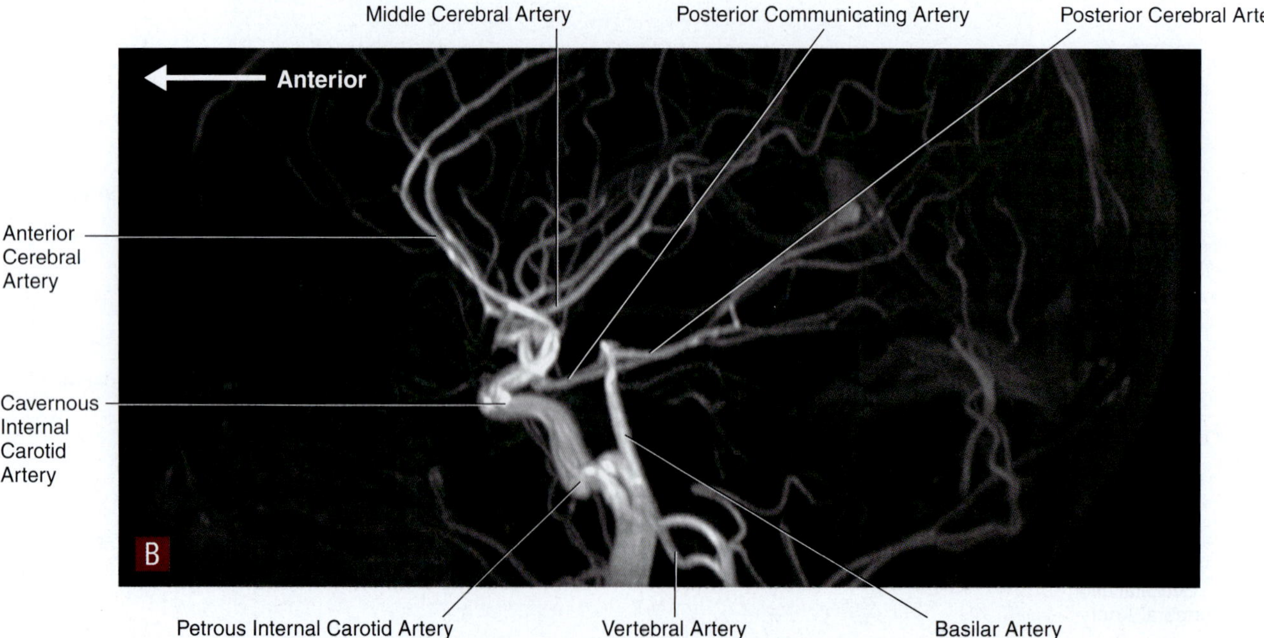

Figure 2.32. **Intracranial arteries.** Time-of-flight MRA of the intracranial arteries in the frontal (A) and lateral (B) projections.

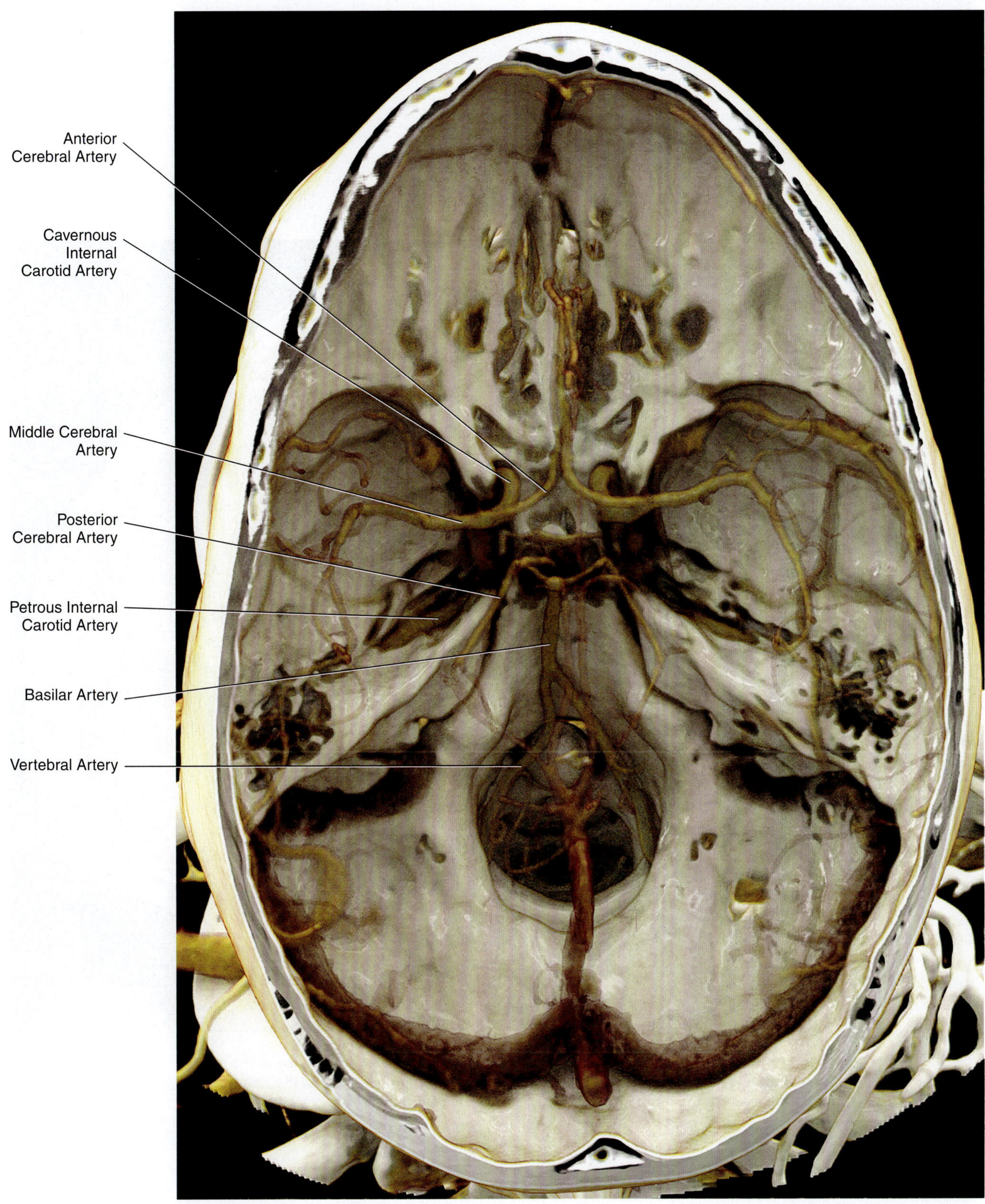

Figure 2.33. CTA 3D cinematic reconstruction. This demonstrates the relationship of the intracranial internal carotid arteries, the anterior circulation, and the posterior circulation at the skull base.

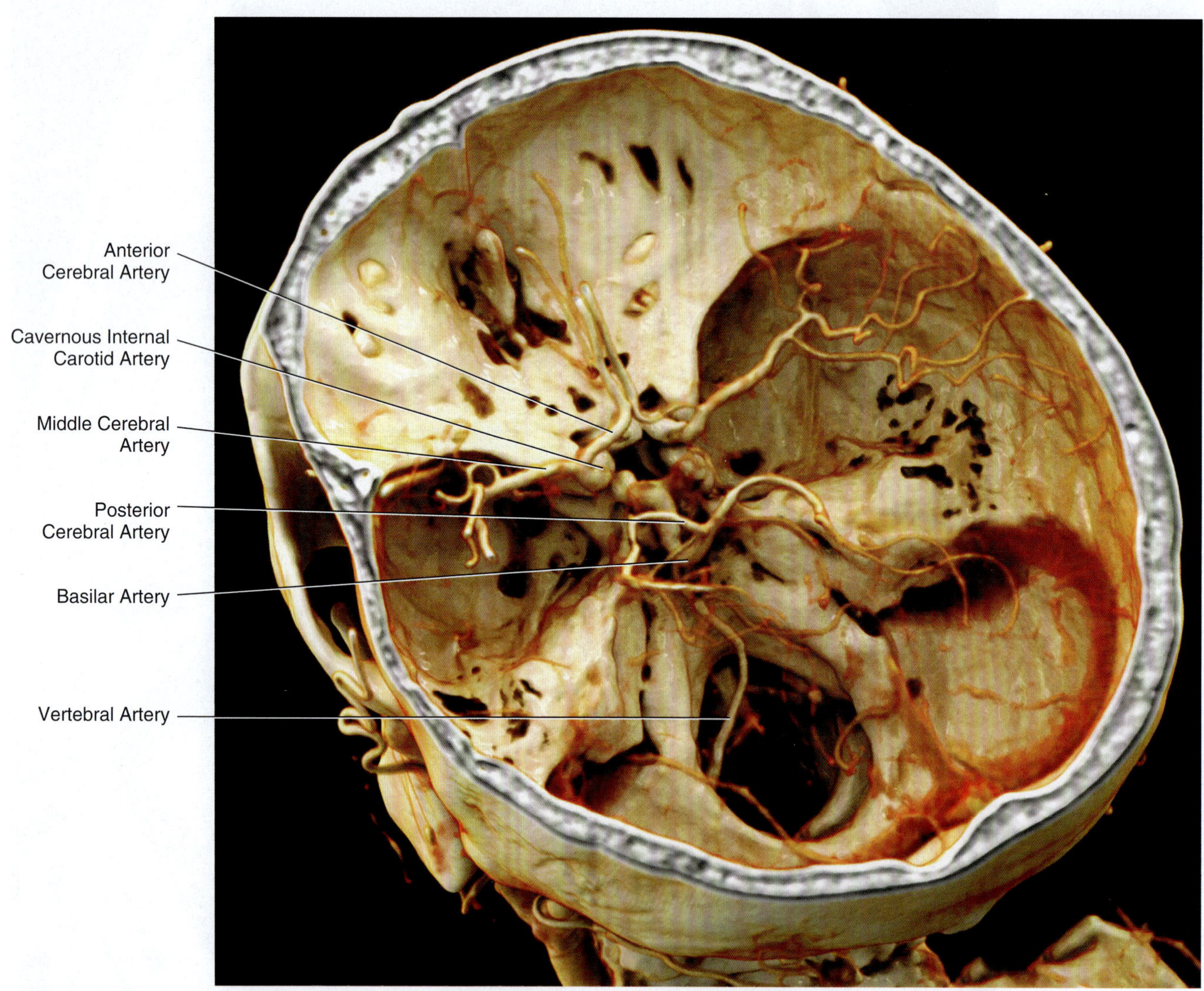

Figure 2.34. CTA 3D cinematic reconstruction, oblique view of the base of the skull. It demonstrates the relationship of the intracranial internal carotid arteries, the anterior circulation, and the posterior circulation at the skull base and the Circle of Willis.

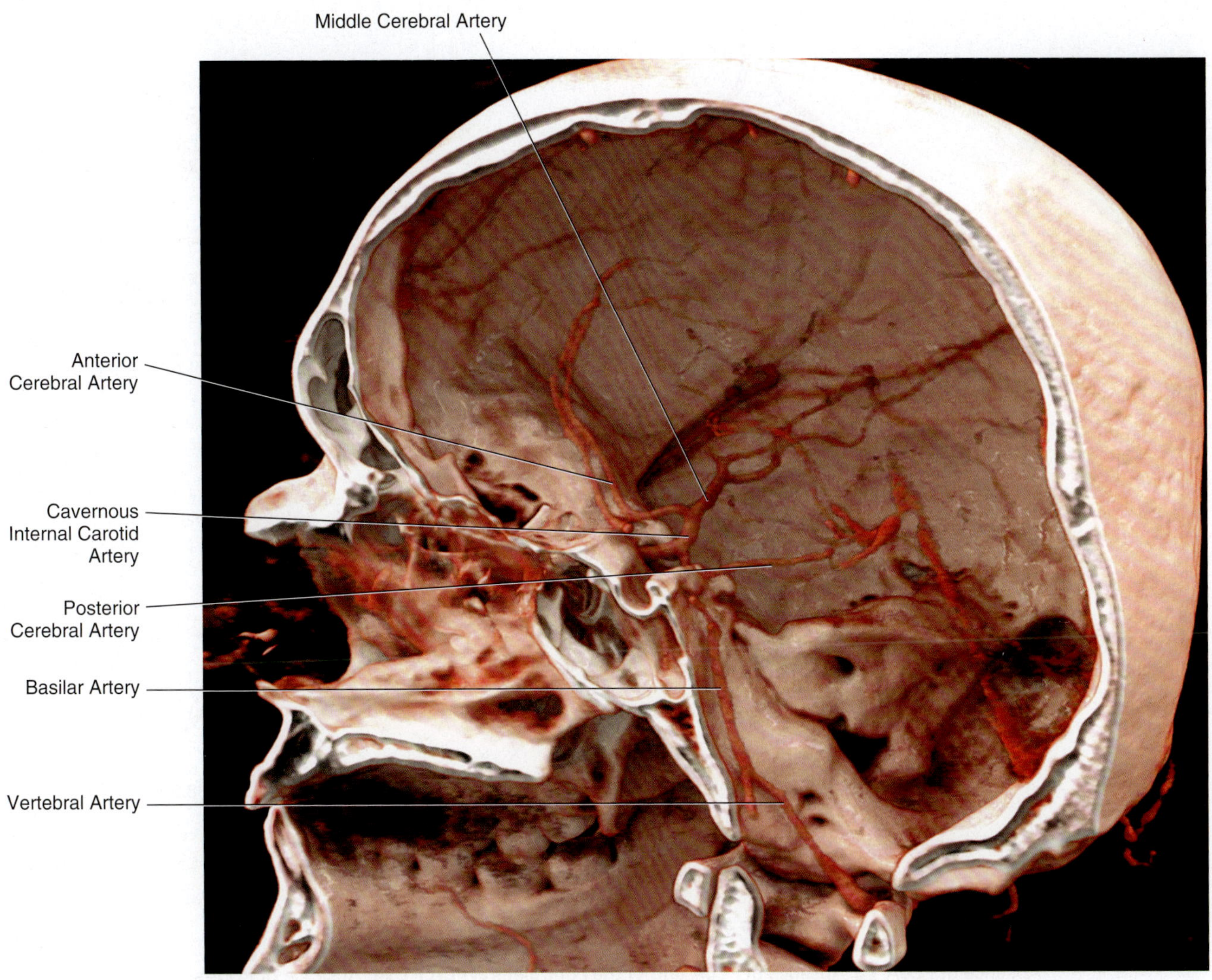

Figure 2.35. CTA 3D cinematic reconstruction, oblique lateral view of the head. It demonstrates relationship of the intracranial internal carotid and vertebral arteries, and the main arteries of the anterior and the posterior circulation.

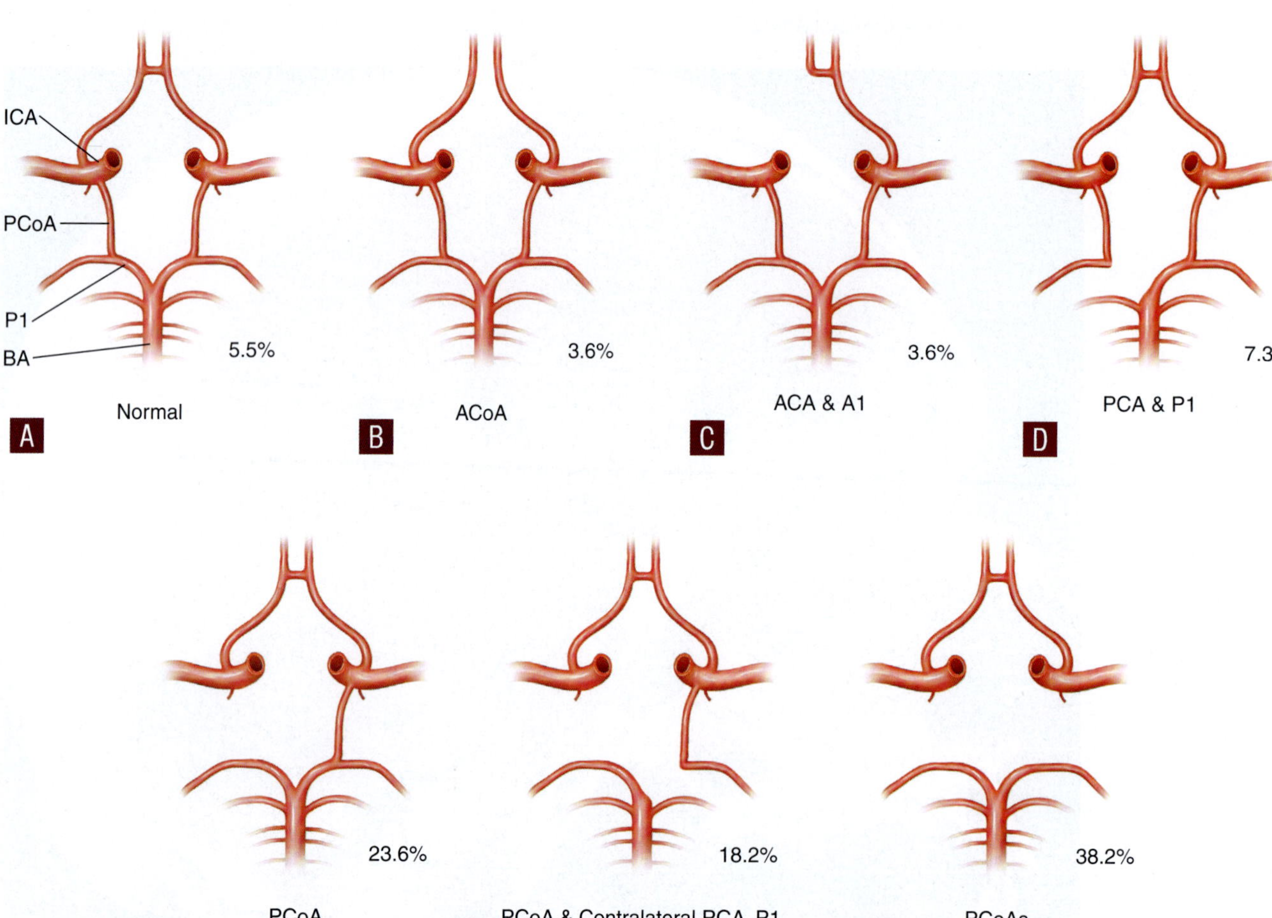

Figure 2.36. Circle of Willis and its variants. **A**, Normal anatomy with complete Circle of Willis. **B**, Absence of ACoA. **C**, Absence of ACA and A1. **D**, Absence of PCA and P1. **E**, Absence of PCoA. **F**, Absence of PCoA and of the contralateral PCA P1. **G**, Absence of PCoAs. A1, first segment of the ACA; ACA, anterior cerebral artery; AcoA, anterior Communicating Artery; BA, basilar artery; ICA, internal carotid artery; P1, first segment of the PCA; PCA, posterior cerebral artery; PCoA, posterior communicating artery.

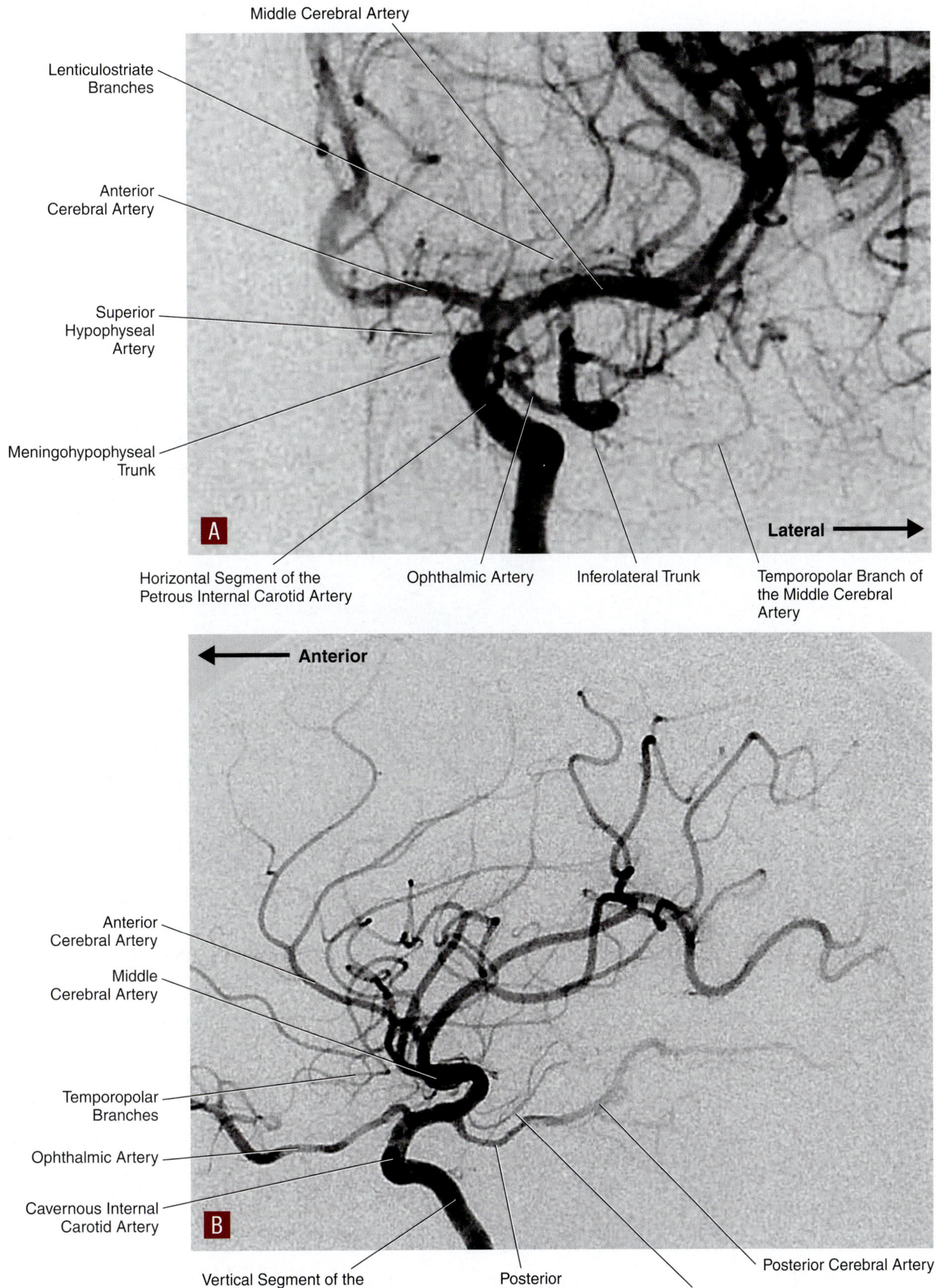

Figure 2.37. **A and B, Anterior circulation.** DSA with injection of the internal carotid artery in the AP (A) and lateral (B) projections demonstrating the anterior arterial circulation. On the lateral projection, there is filling of the posterior cerebral artery via a posterior communicating artery. DSA, digital subtraction angiography.

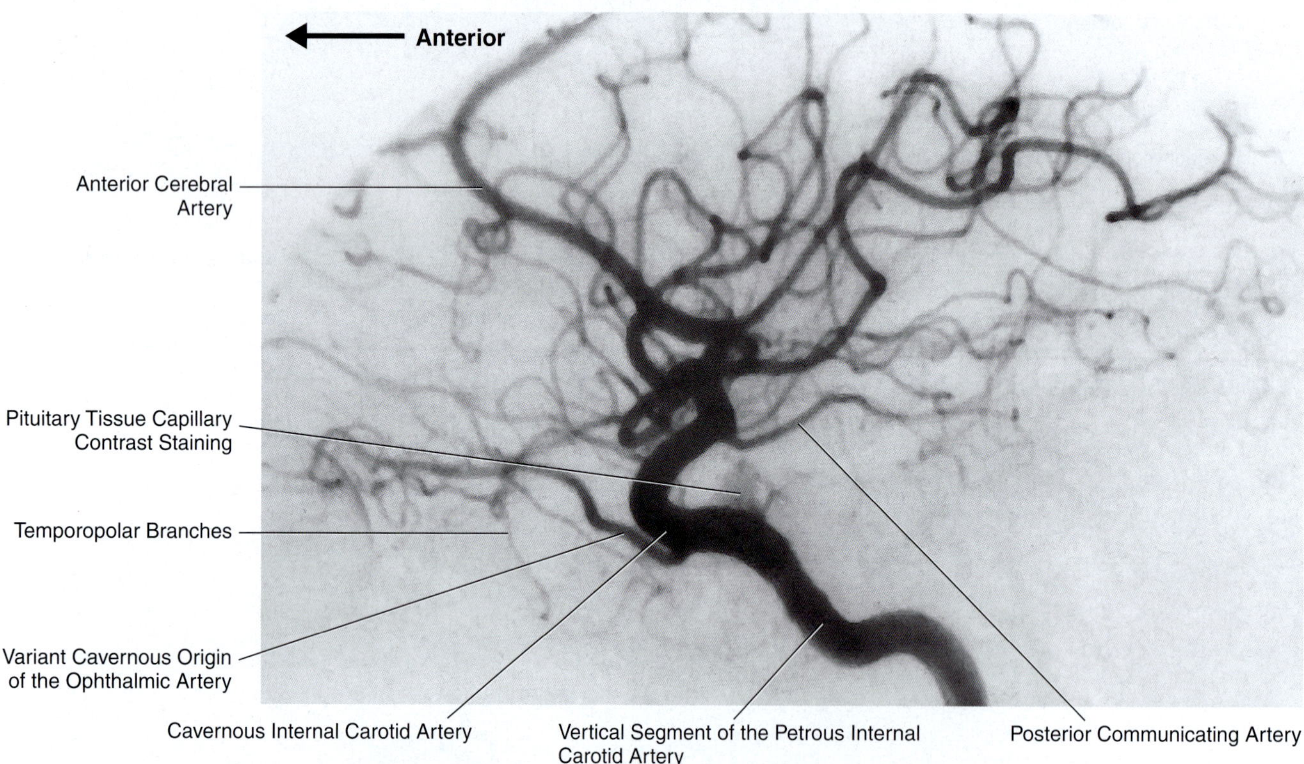

Figure 2.38. Variant ophthalmic artery cavernous origin. DSA with injection of the internal carotid artery in the lateral projection. Note the lower origin of the ophthalmic artery in the proximal cavernous segment of the internal carotid artery. This also demonstrates the normal pituitary hypophysial tissue capillary contrast staining. DSA, digital subtraction angiography.

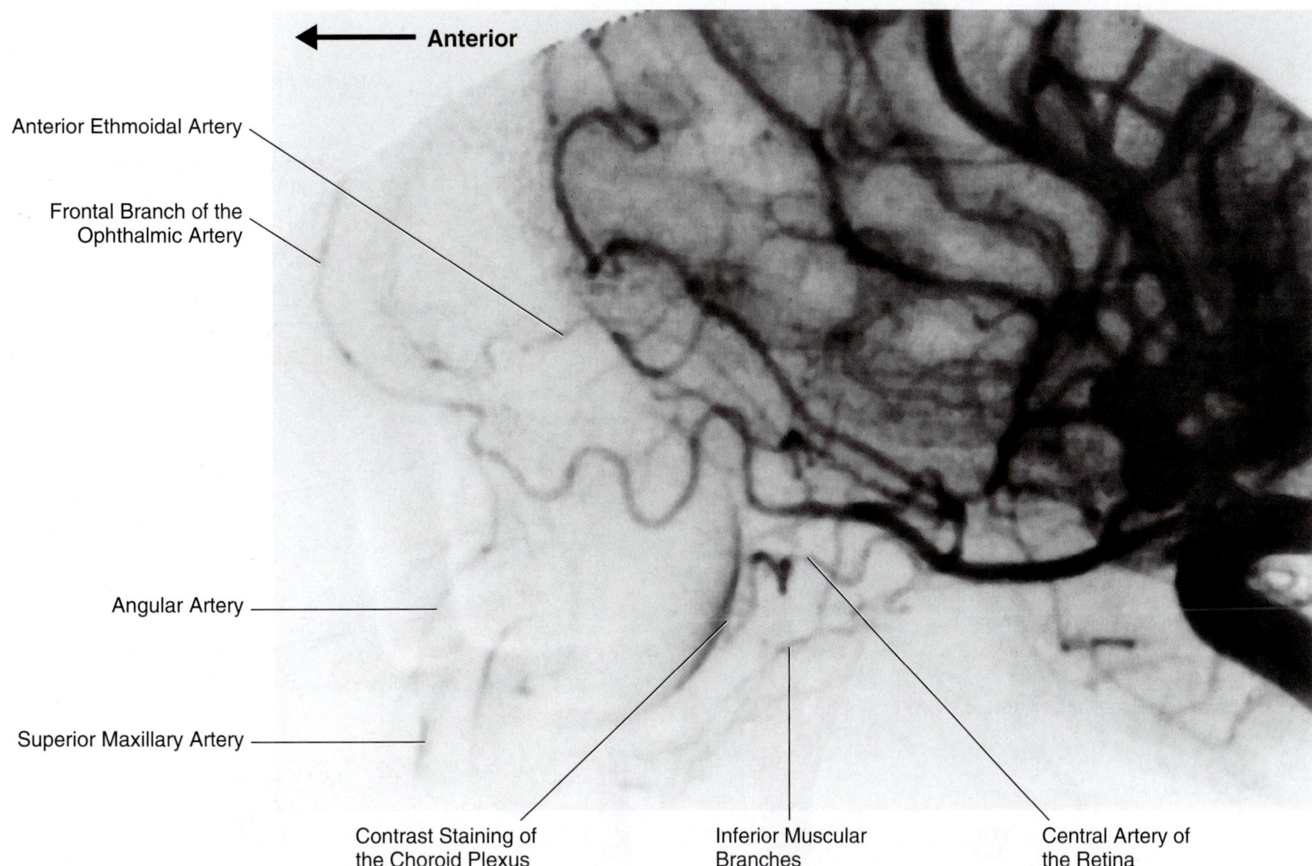

Figure 2.39. Opthalmic artery, central retinal artery, and choroid plexus of the globe. DSA with injection of the internal carotid artery in the capillary phase with a lateral projection. Note the angular artery vascularizing the superior maxillary region, the central artery of the retina, and choroid plexus of the globe contrast staining. DSA, digital subtraction angiography.

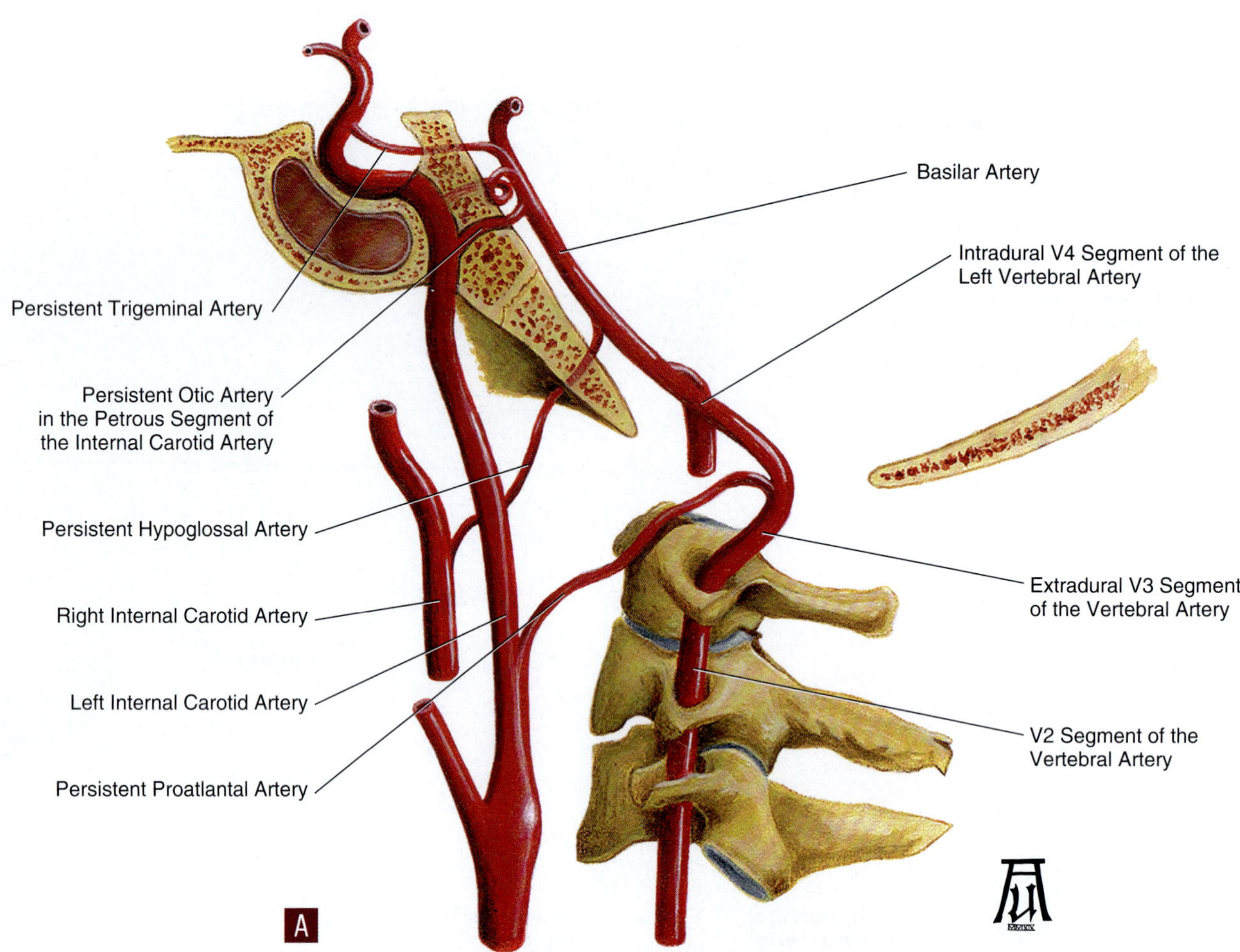

Figure 2.40. **Persistent carotid-vertebrobasilar anastomosis.** (A) Illustration of the variant anterior and posterior circulation arterial communications resulting from abnormal embryological development. (B) Lateral projection internal carotid injection DSA demonstrating a persistent primitive trigeminal artery supplying the distal basilar artery. (C) Lateral projection internal carotid injection DSA demonstrating a small persistent otic artery arising from the petrous segment of the internal carotid artery. DSA, digital subtraction angiography.

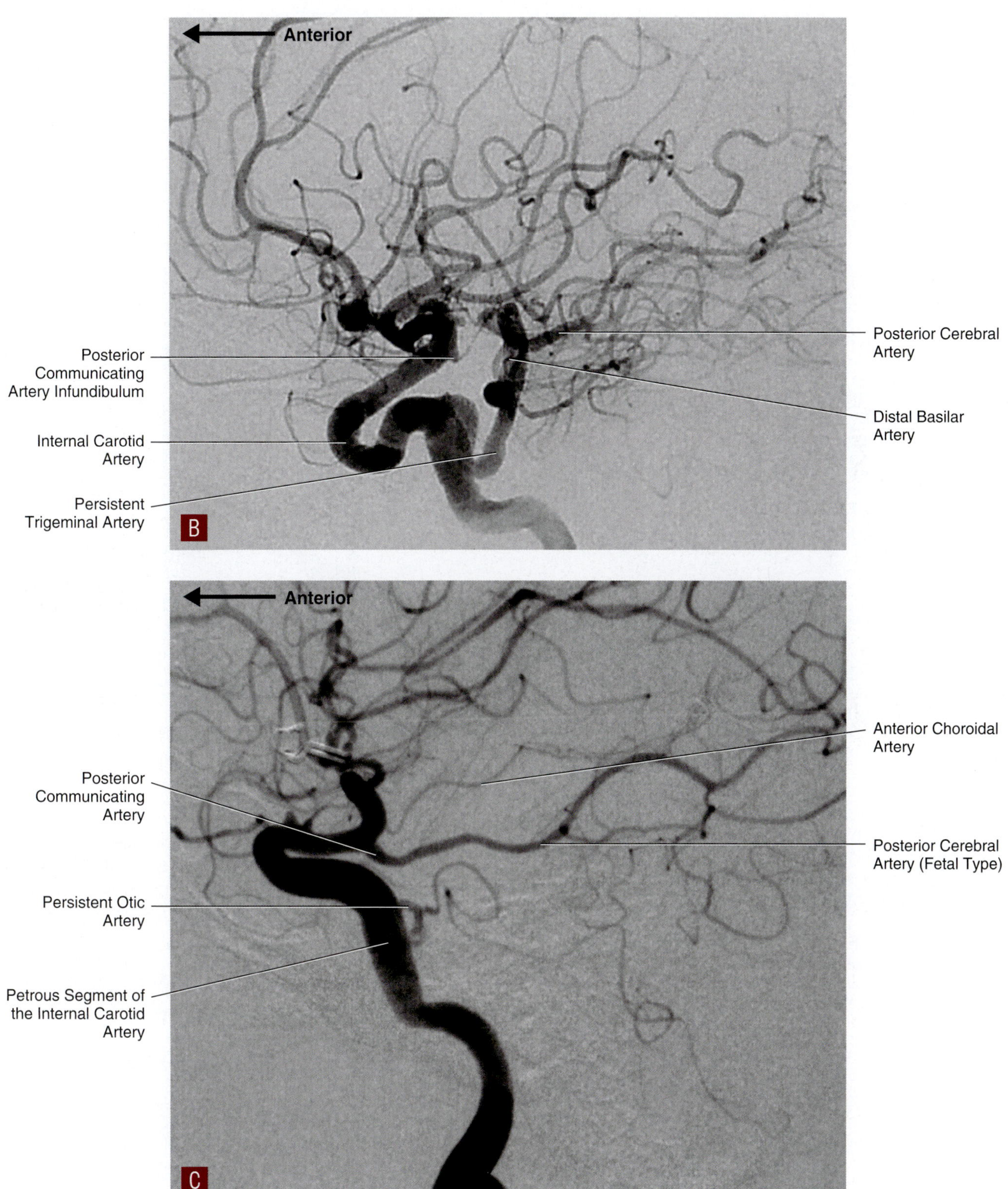

Figure 2.40. *Continued*

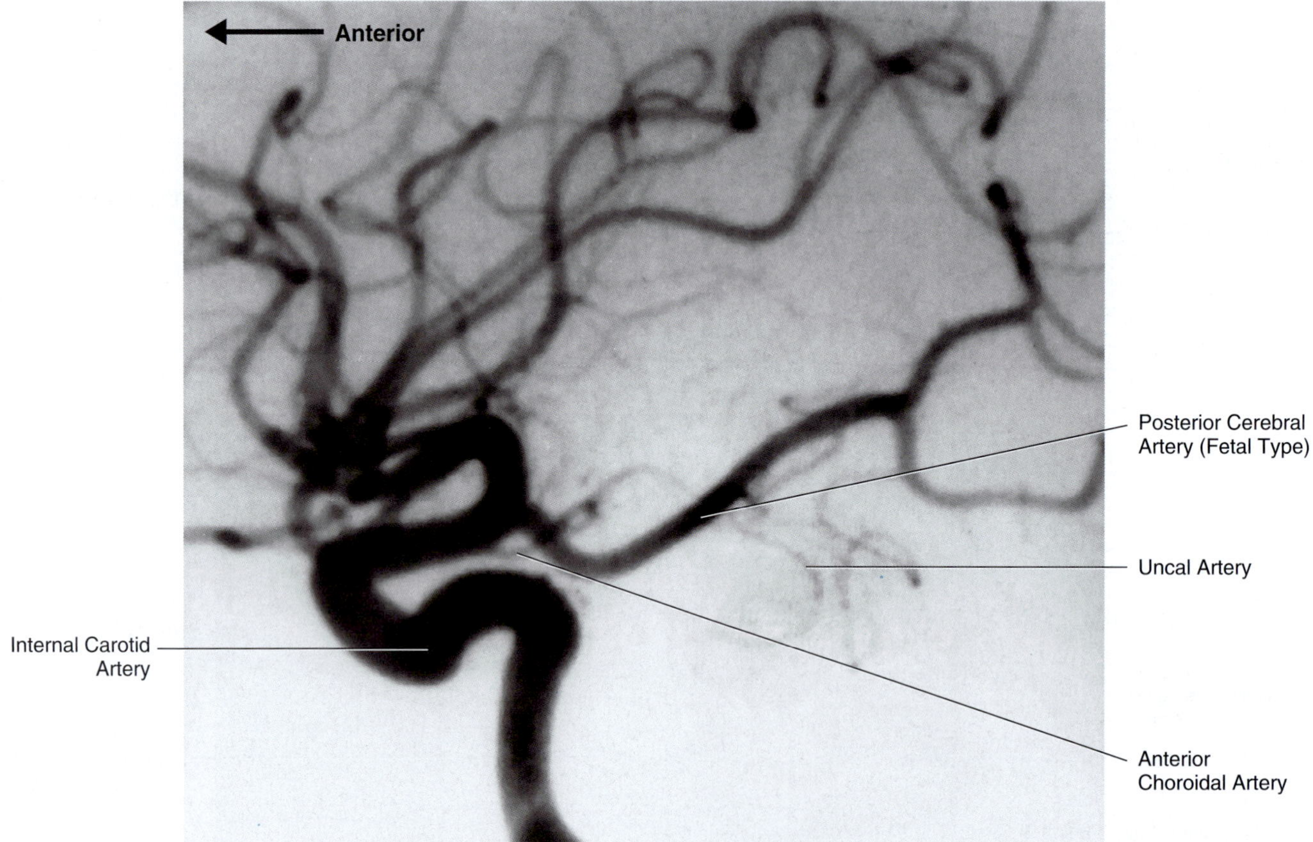

Figure 2.41. Aberrant origin of the anterior choroidal artery. Lateral DSA with injection of the internal carotid artery demonstrates an aberrant origin of the anterior choroidal artery proximal to the posterior communicating artery. DSA, digital subtraction angiography.

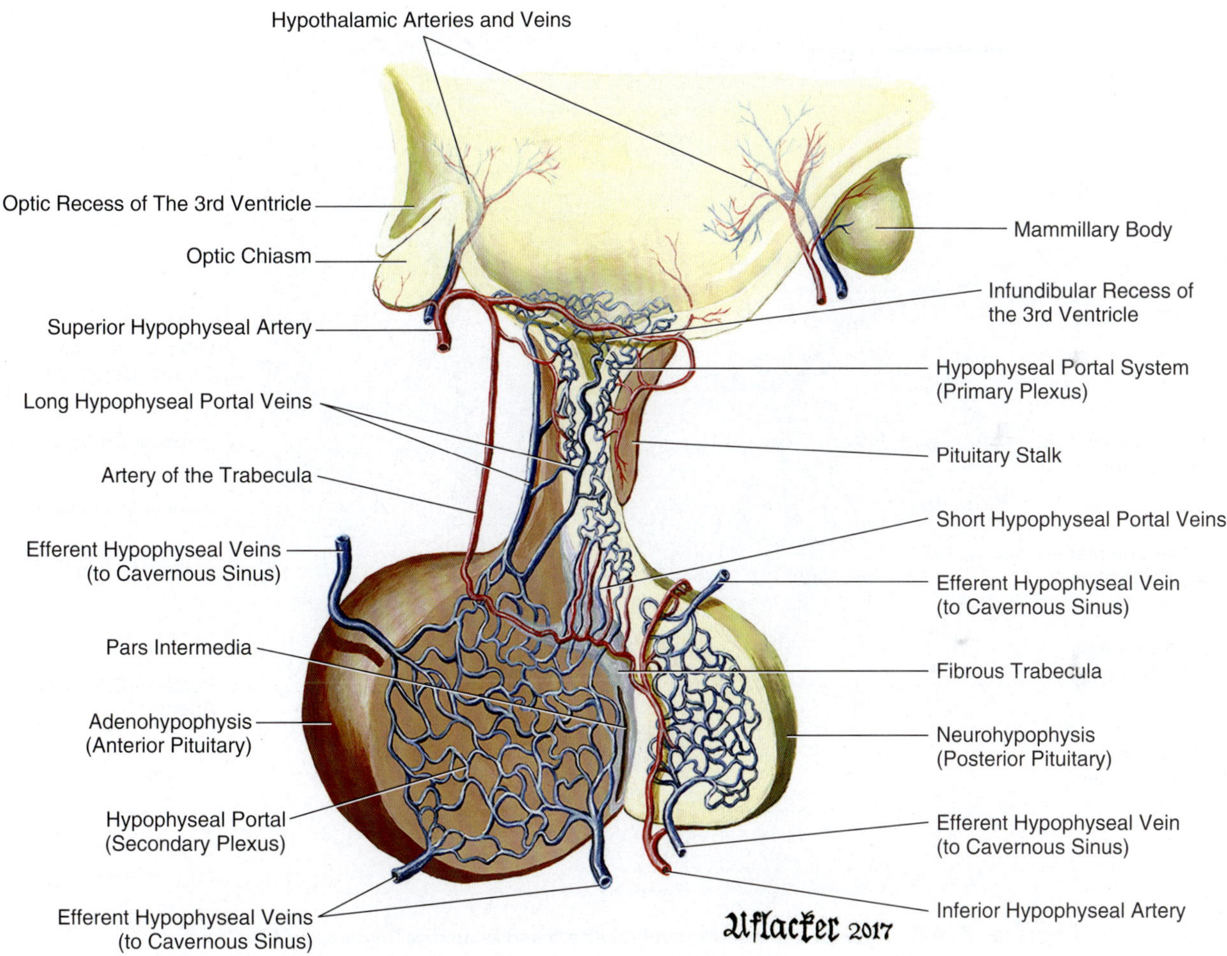

Figure 2.42. Illustration of the vasculature of the pituitary. The extensive hypothalamic and hypophyseal portal circulation demonstrates the plexus of veins in the pituitary stalk coursing from the hypothalamus to the anterior adenohypophysis of the pituitary gland. The posterior neurohypohysis of the pituitary is by comparison less vascular, with the pars intermedia between the two and the site for pars intermedia cysts.

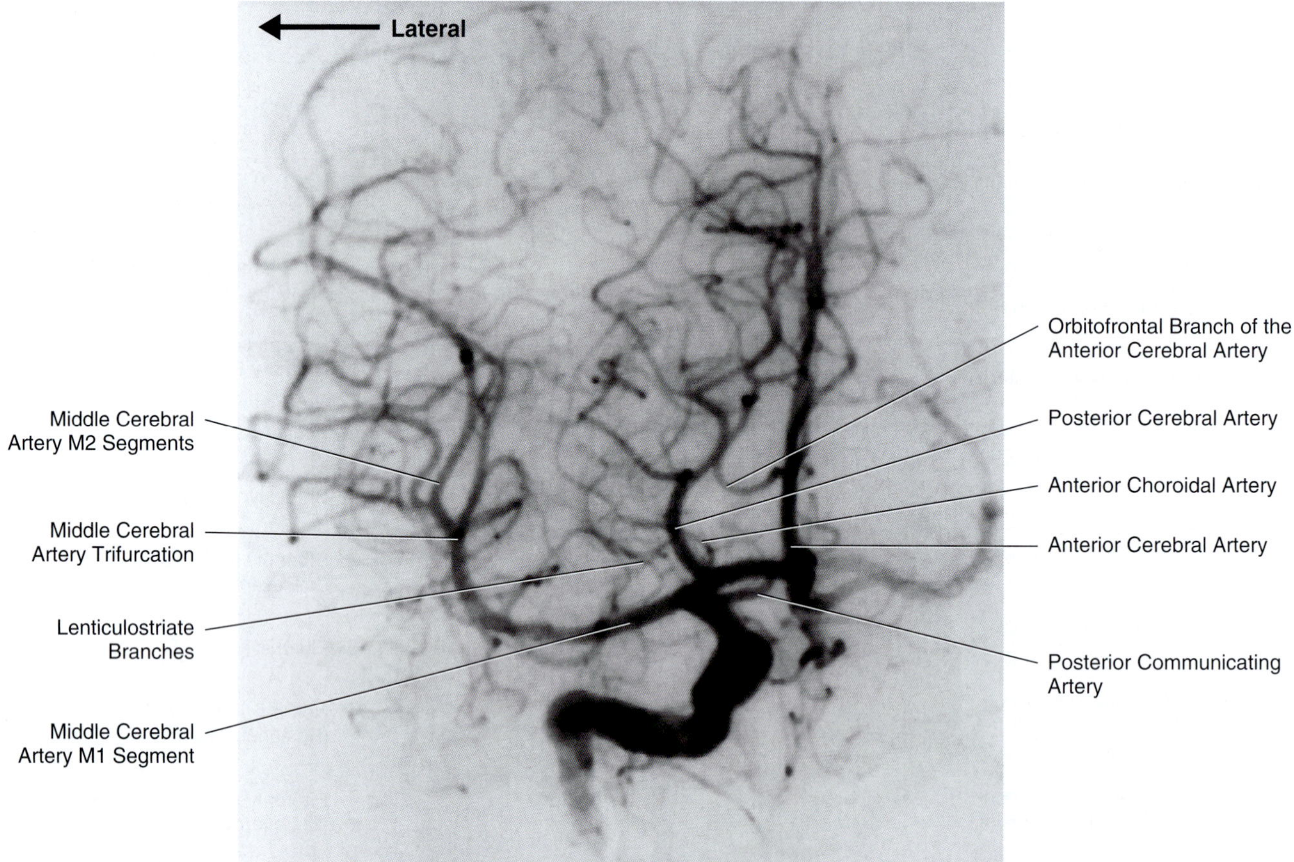

Figure 2.43. Anterior and middle cerebral artery and branches. Towne view AP projection DSA with injection of the internal carotid artery. The middle cerebral artery M1 segment is seen to its bifurcation or trifurcation point in the Sylvian fissure beyond which the M2 branches course through the Sylvian fissure along the opercular frontal, parietal, and temporal cortex. The anterior choroidal artery is seen arising from the internal carotid distal to the posterior communicating artery with a characteristic course lateral to the posterior cerebral artery. DSA, digital subtraction angiography.

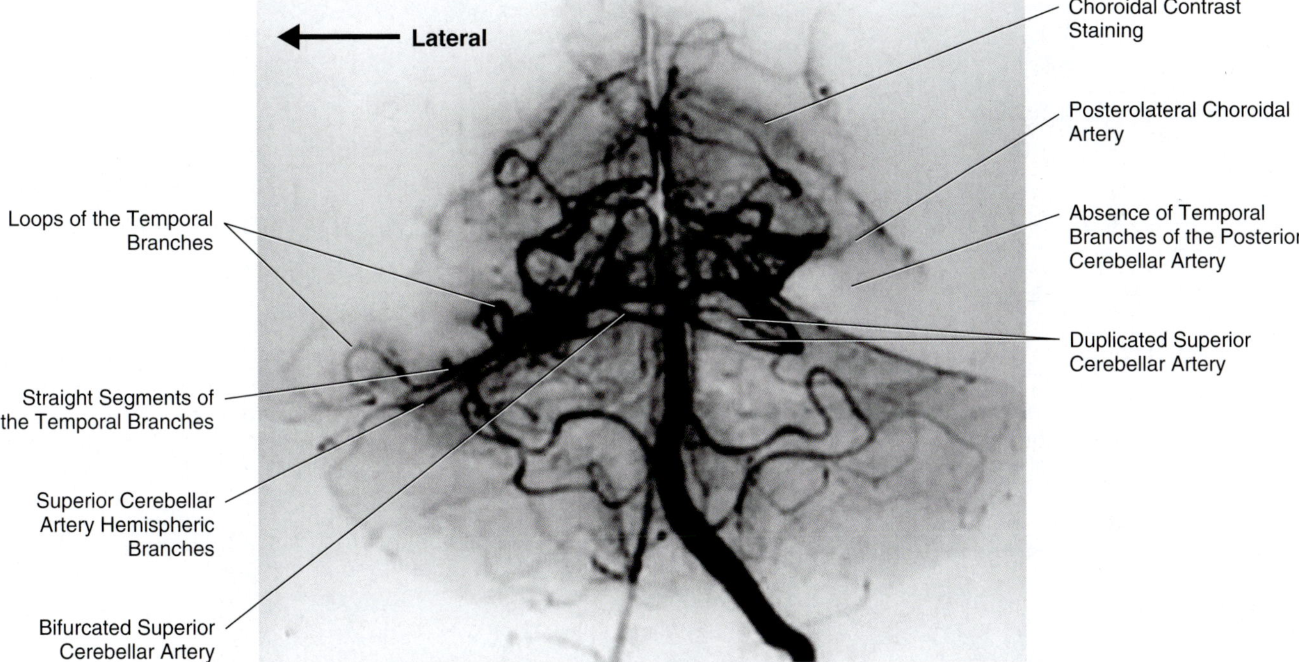

Figure 2.44. Anterior choroidal origin of the temporal branches of the posterior cerebral artery. Waters projection AP view DSA with injection of the left vertebral artery demonstrates loops of the temporal branches in the temporal sulci and the straight segments on top of the gyri. There is a parallel course of the marginal artery hemispheric branches of the superior cerebellar artery. There is a duplicated left superior cerebellar artery and no temporal branches of the posterior cerebral artery on the left. DSA, digital subtraction angiography.

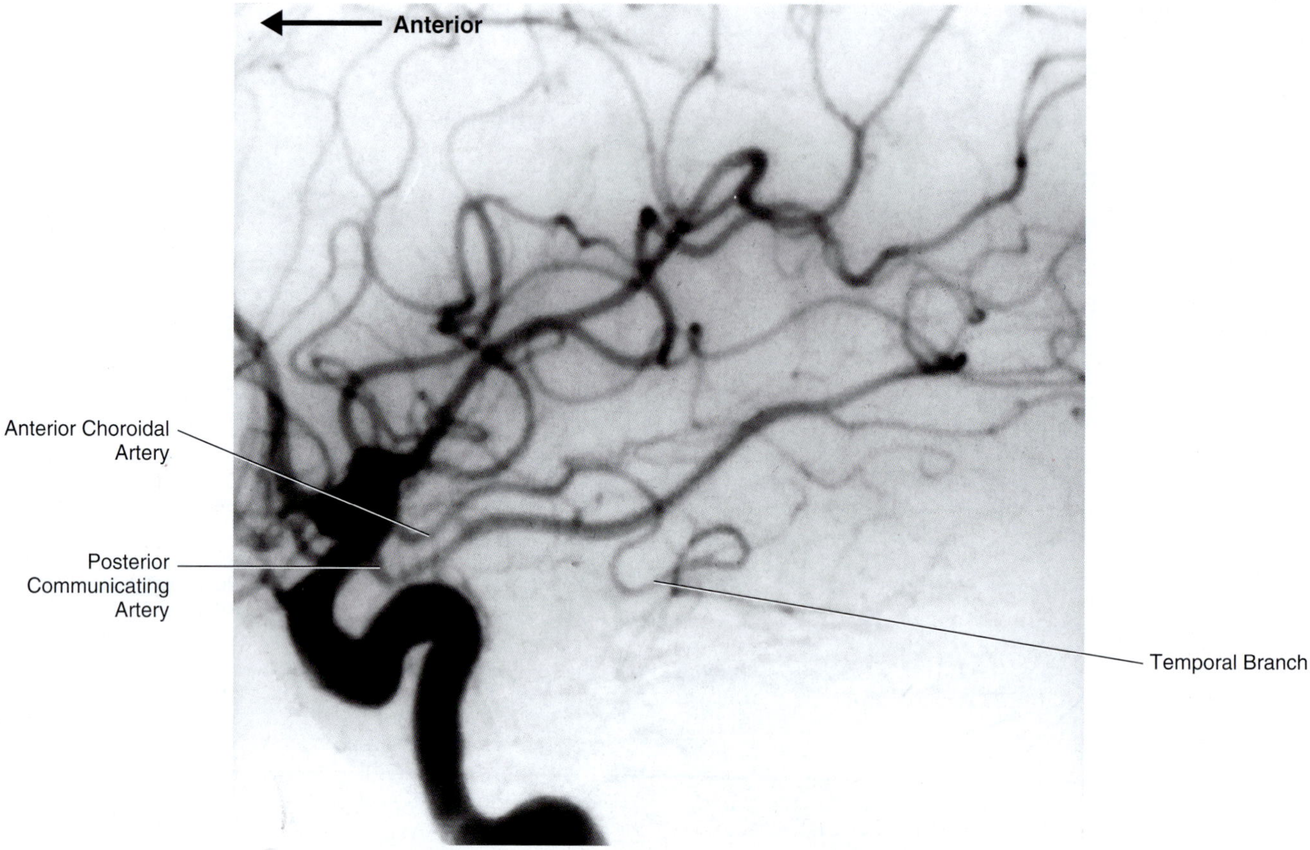

Anterior

Anterior Choroidal Artery

Posterior Communicating Artery

Temporal Branch

Figure 2.45. Internal carotid artery lateral view. Anterior choroidal artery arising from the internal carotid artery just distal to the posterior communicating artery. The anterior choroidal artery gives rise to a temporal branch.

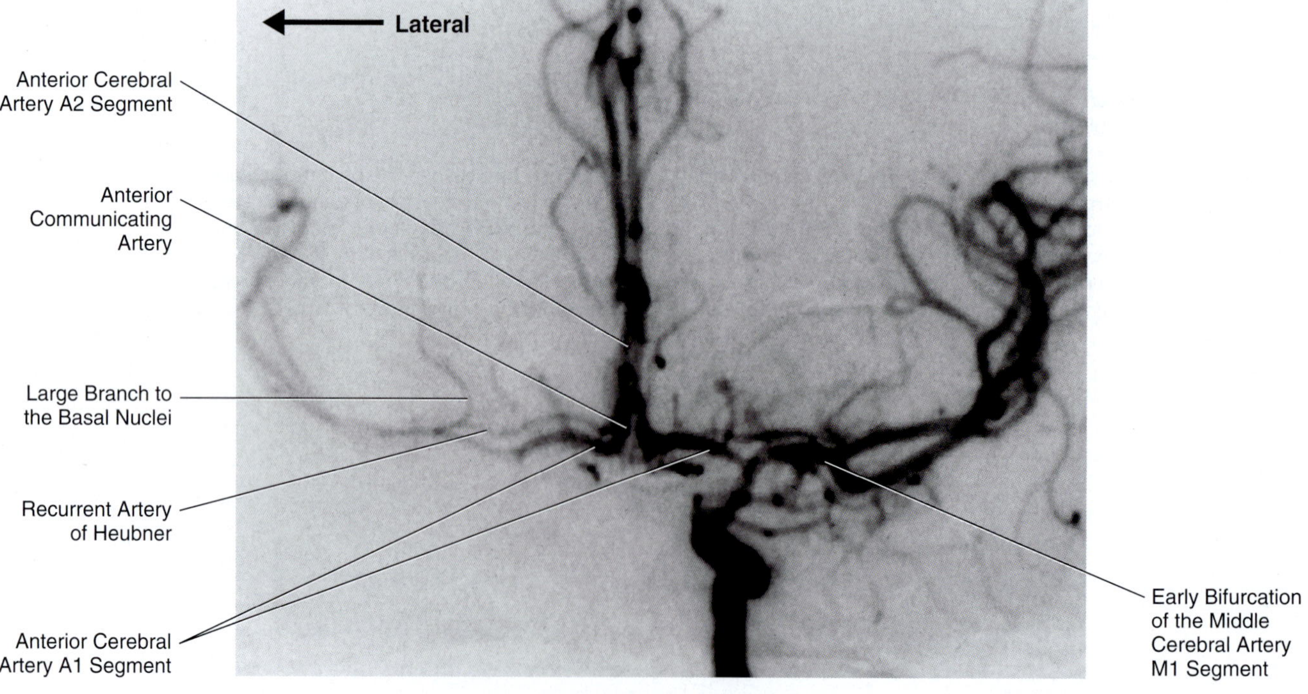

Figure 2.46. Internal carotid artery frontal view. AP projection DSA with injection of the left internal carotid artery demonstrates the recurrent artery of Heubner with large branches to the basal nuclei. DSA, digital subtraction angiography.

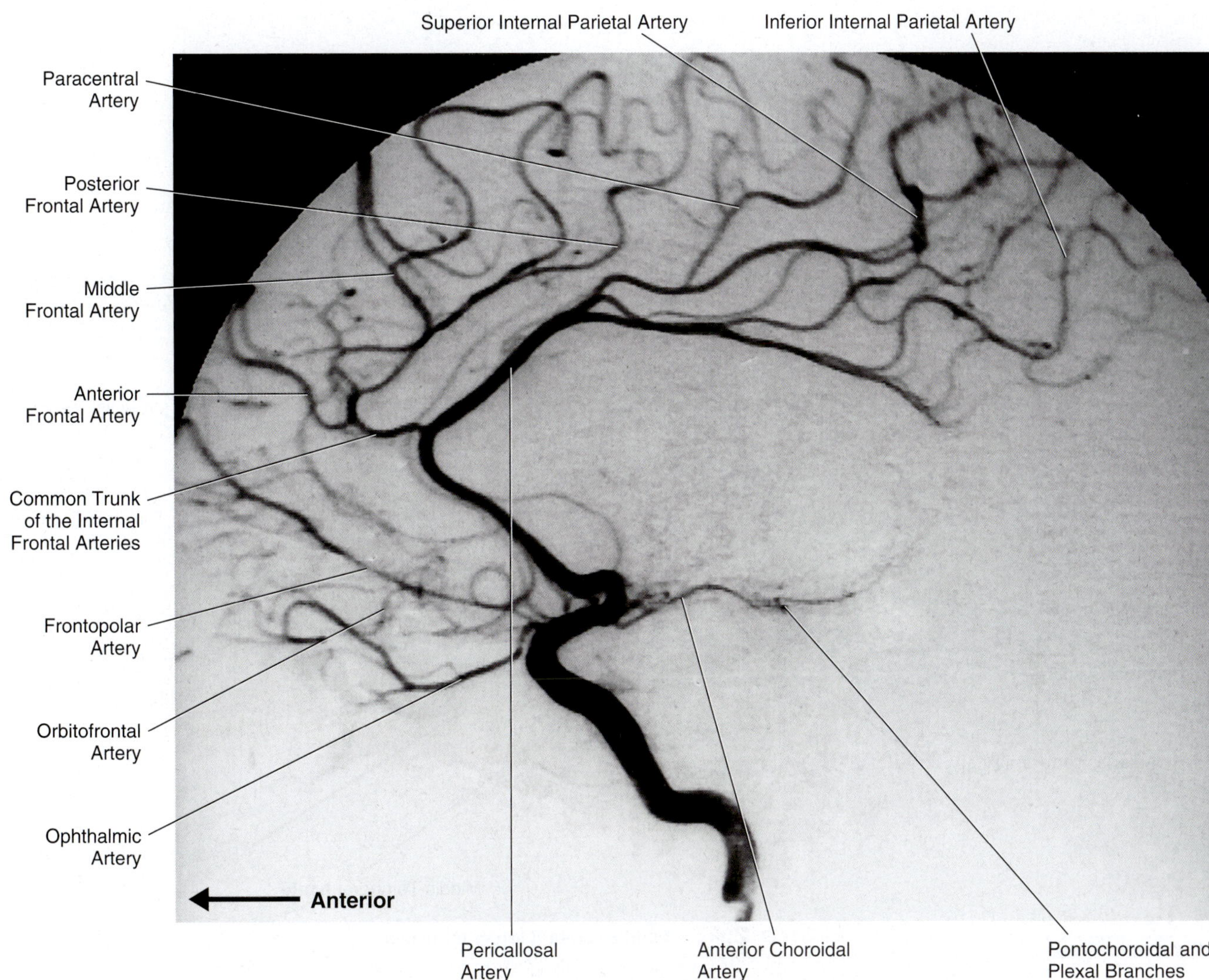

Figure 2.47. Internal carotid artery with selective opacification of the anterior cerebral artery. Lateral DSA with injection of the internal carotid artery and selective opacification of the anterior cerebral artery and its branches due to an occlusion of the middle cerebral artery. There is a pericallosal artery present but no callosomarginal artery. DSA, digital subtraction angiography.

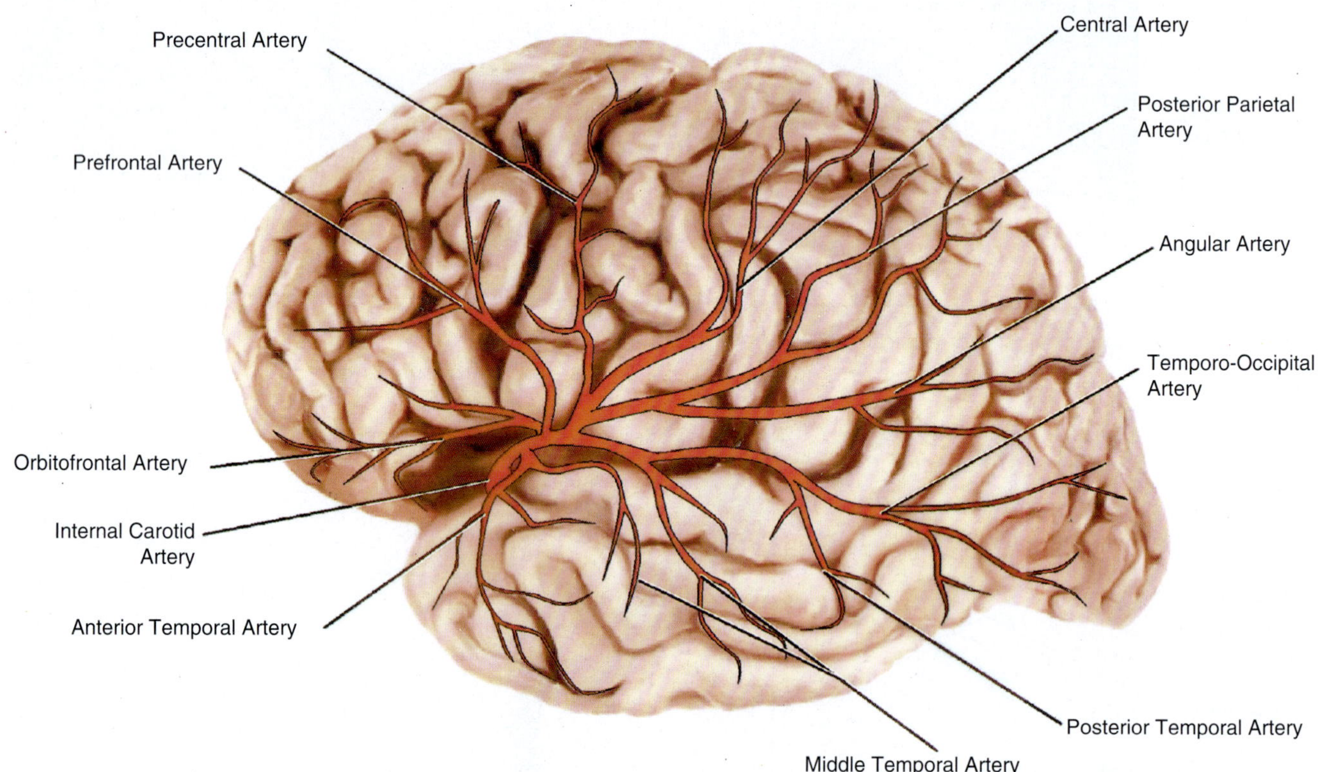

Figure 2.48. **Middle cerebral artery branches.**

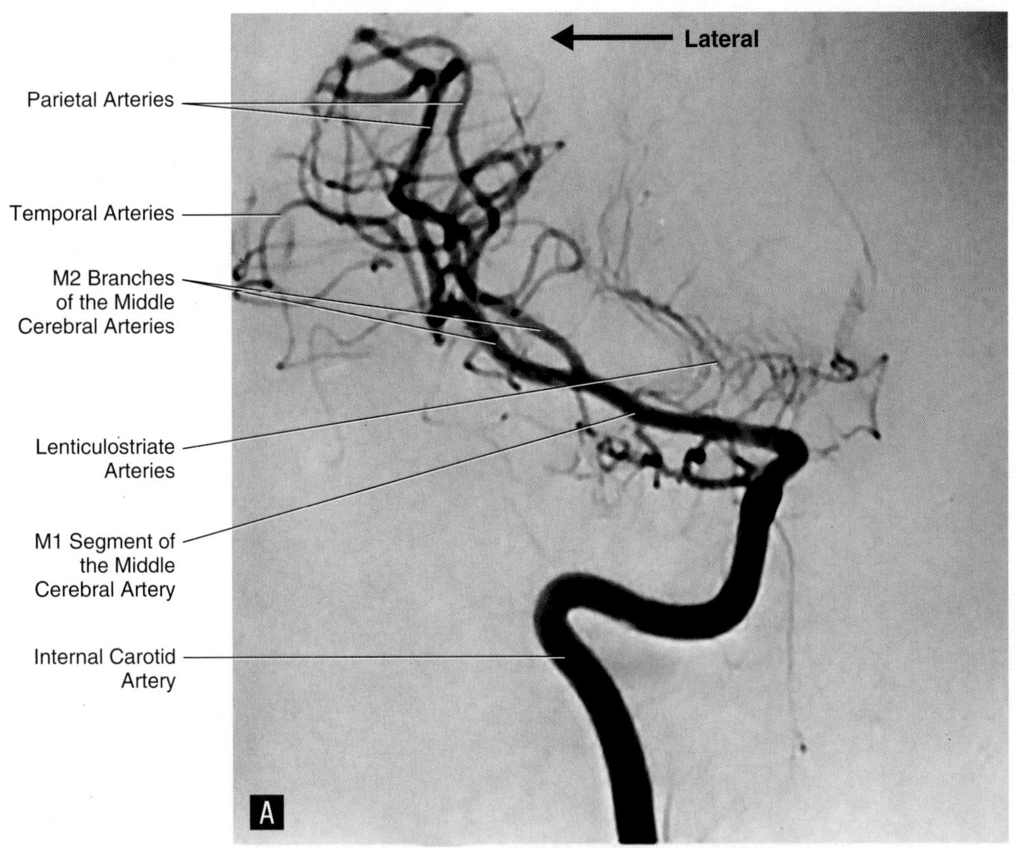

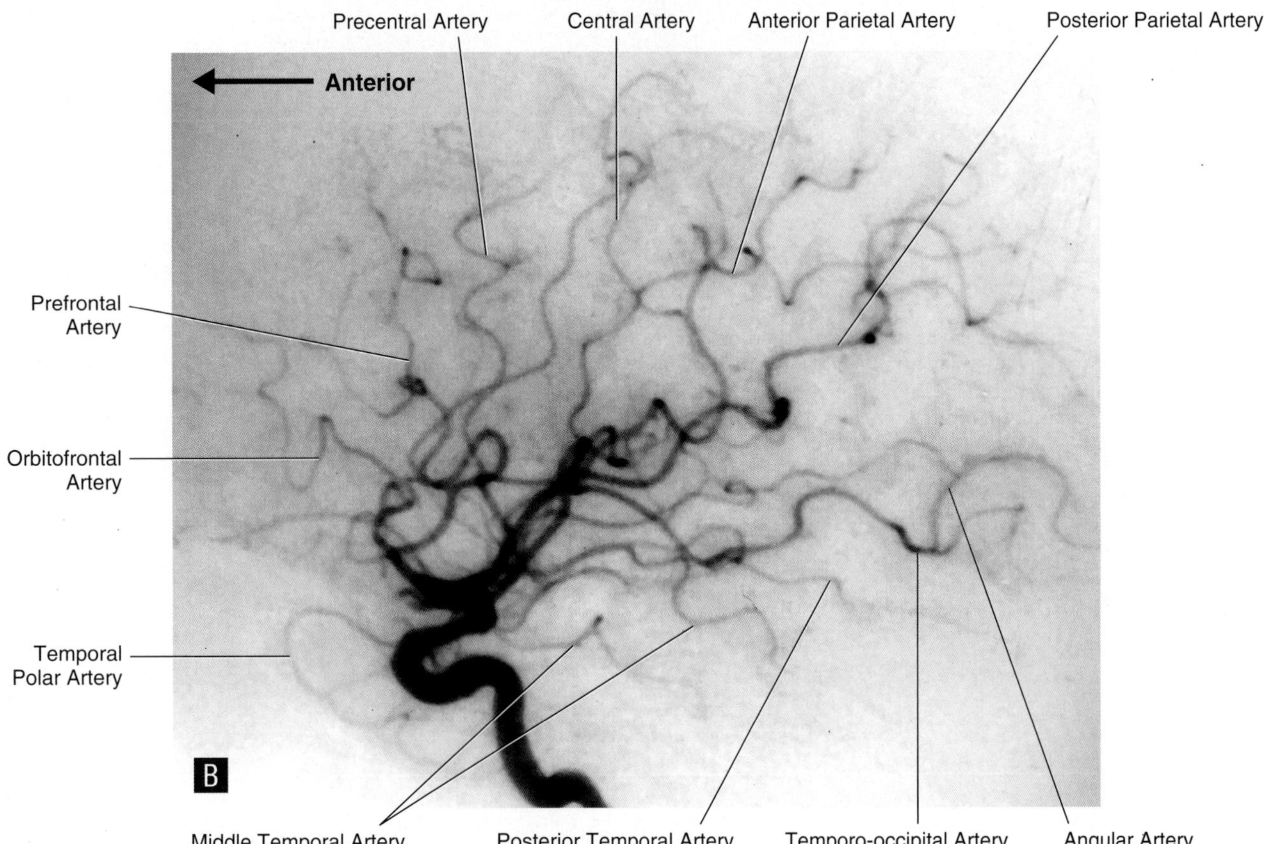

Figure 2.49. Middle cerebral artery. Frontal (A) and lateral (B) DSA with injection of the internal carotid artery with selective opacification of the middle cerebral artery and branches due to anterior cerebral artery hypoplasia. DSA, digital subtraction angiography.

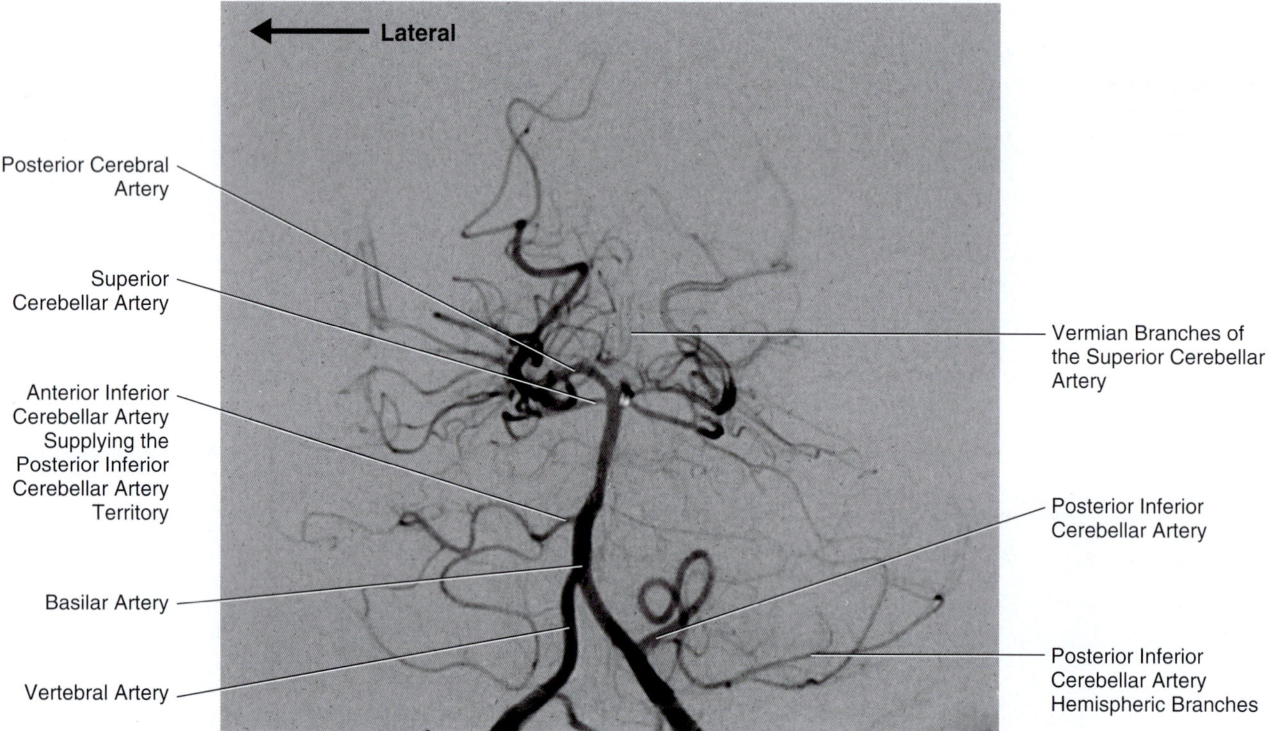

Figure 2.50. **Posterior circulation.** Towne view frontal DSA with injection of the vertebral artery. Note the contrast injection into one vertebral artery fills the opposite vertebral artery in a retrograde fashion. There is a right anterior inferior cerebellar artery supplying the right posterior inferior cerebellar artery territory with an absent right posterior inferior cerebellar artery. DSA, digital subtraction angiography.

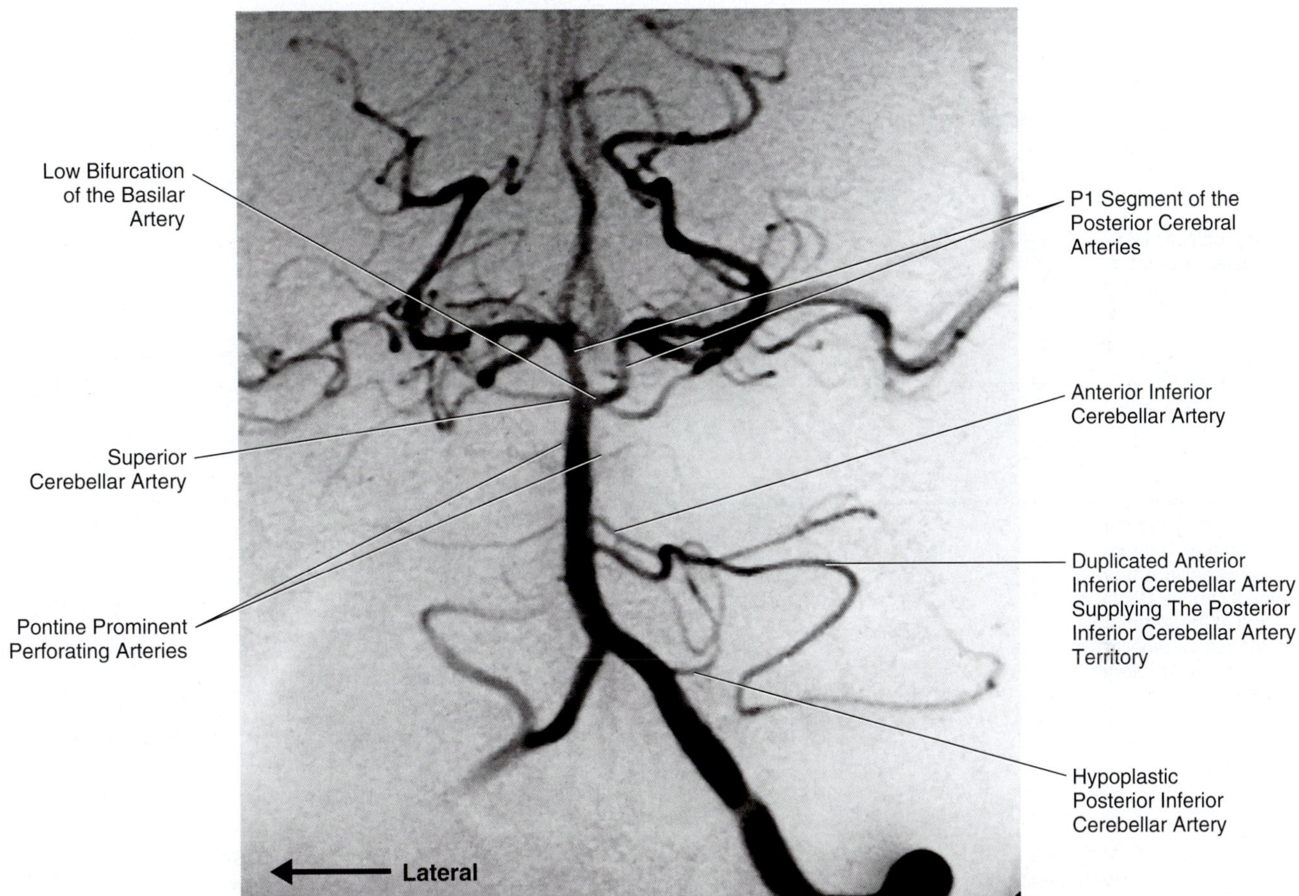

Figure 2.51. Posterior circulation with variant anatomy. Towne view frontal DSA with injection of the left vertebral artery demonstrates a low bifurcation of the basilar artery at the level of the superior cerebellar arteries. There is a duplicated left anterior inferior cerebellar artery with the inferior artery supplying the left posterior inferior cerebellar artery territory. There is compensatory hypoplasia of the left posterior inferior cerebellar artery. Two prominent pontine perforating arteries are demonstrated. DSA, digital subtraction angiography.

Lateral

Hypoplastic Right Posterior Cerebral Artery P1 Segment

Duplicated Superior Cerebellar Artery

High Intradural Origin of the Posterior Inferior Cerebellar Artery Supplying the Distal Third of the Anterior Inferior Cerebellar Artery Territory

Posterior Cerebral Artery P1 Segment

Arterial Arch of the Odontoid

Figure 2.52. Posterior circulation with variant anatomy. Waters projection frontal DSA with injection of the left vertebral artery demonstrates a duplicated right superior cerebellar artery, hypoplastic right P1 segment of the posterior cerebral artery, and a high intradural origin of the right posterior inferior cerebellar artery supplying the distal third of the anterior inferior cerebellar artery territory. The odontoid arch supplied by the vertebral arteries is also demonstrated. DSA, digital subtraction angiography.

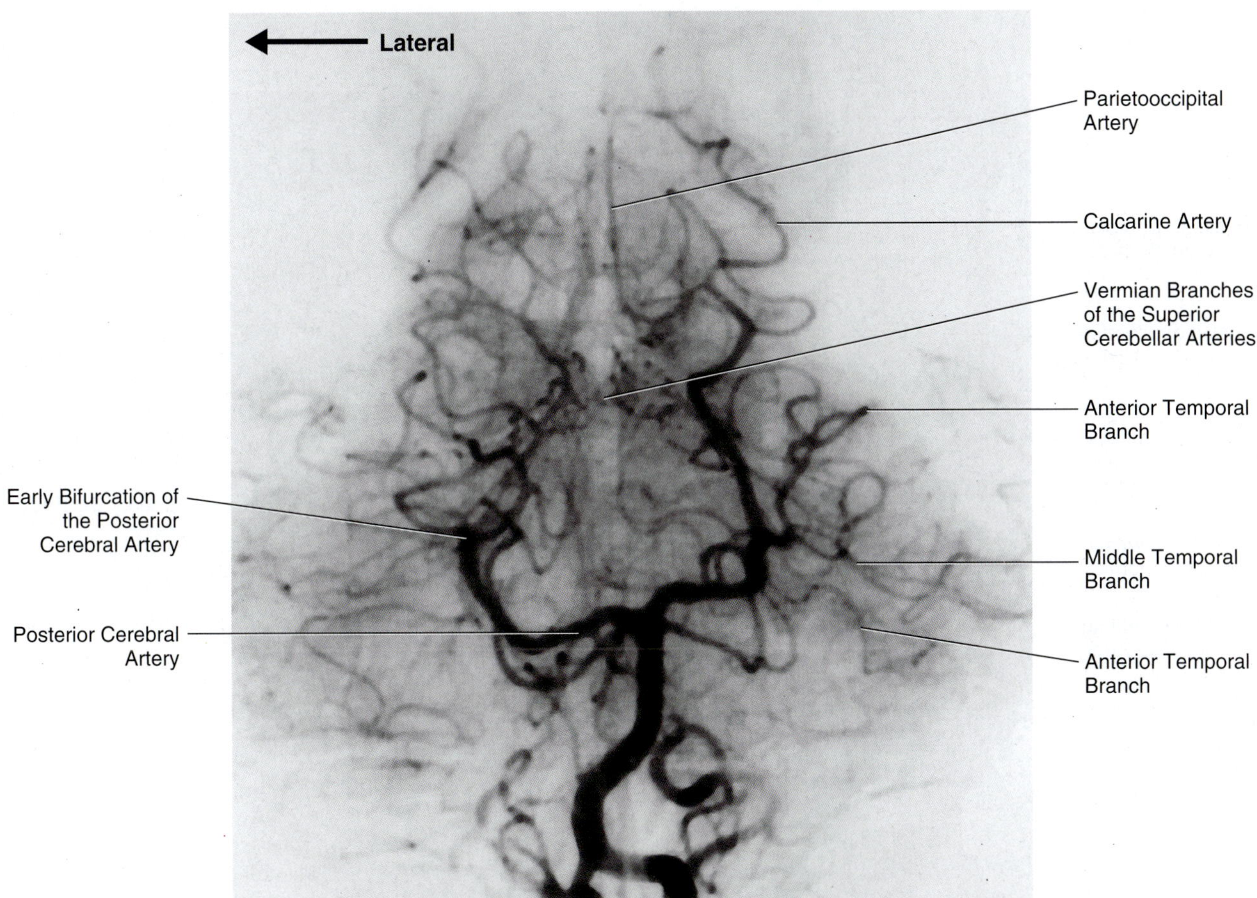

Figure 2.53. **Posterior circulation.** Towne view DSA with injection of the vertebral artery demonstrates the course of the posterior cerebral arteries and basilar tip. The posterior cerebral arteries are asymmetric with an early right bifurcation. The temporal branches, calcarine artery, and vermian branches are best seen on this Towne projection. DSA, digital subtraction angiography.

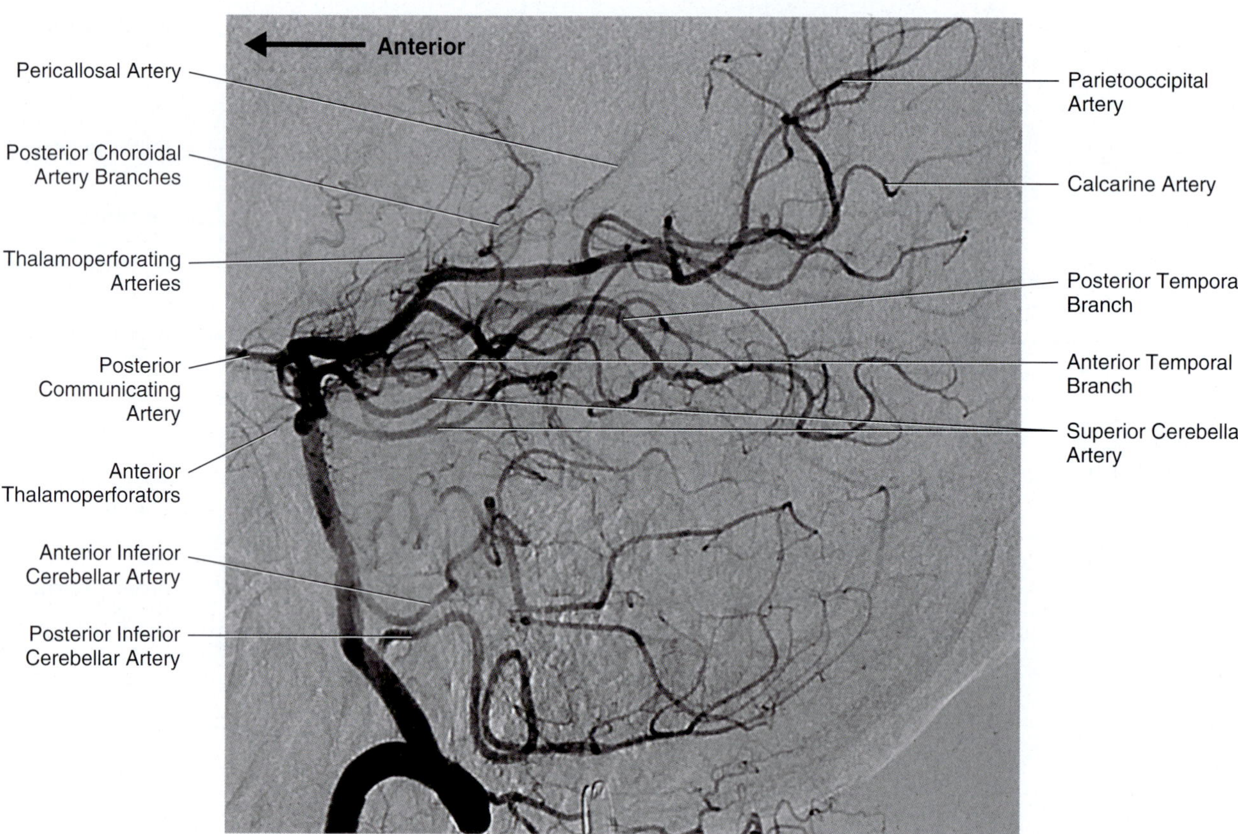

Figure 2.54. **Posterior circulation.** Lateral projection DSA with injection of the vertebral artery. DSA, digital subtraction angiography.

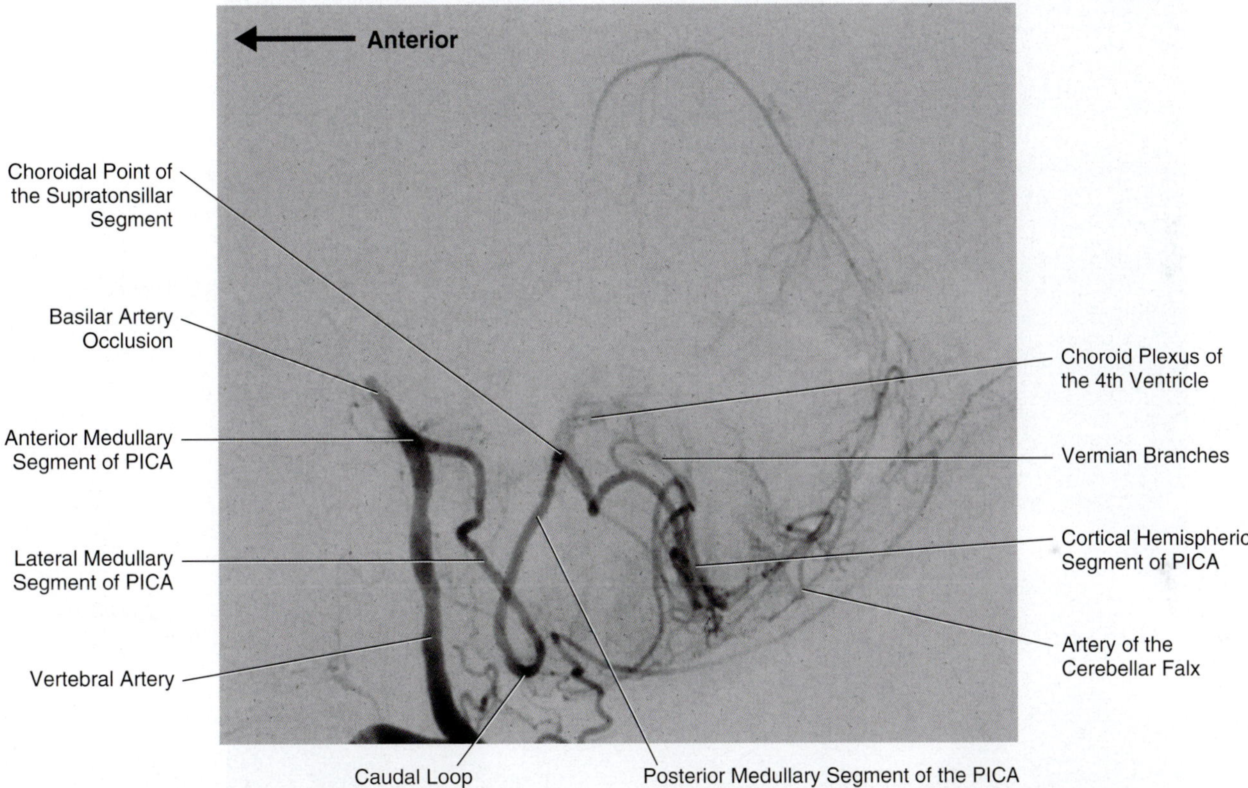

Figure 2.55. **Posterior inferior cerebellar artery.** Lateral projection DSA with injection of the vertebral artery in a person with a basilar artery occlusion. This demonstrates the segments of the posterior inferior cerebellar artery: anterior medullary, lateral medullary, posterior medullary, supratonsillar, and cortical hemispheric segments are opacified. DSA, digital subtraction angiography.

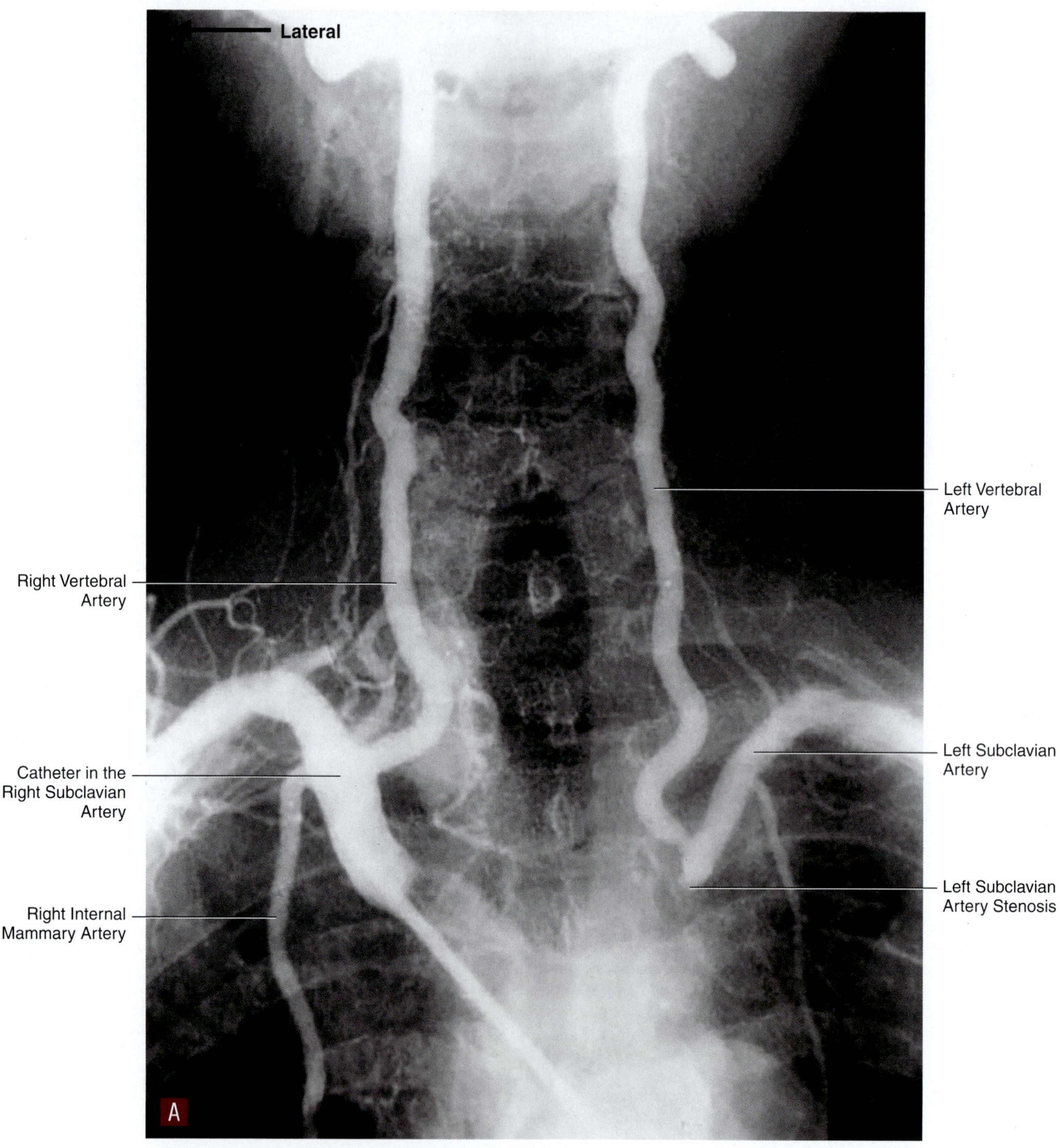

Figure 2.56. **A and B, Subclavian steal.** **A**, Frontal DSA with injection of the right subclavian artery demonstrates antegrade opacification of the right vertebral artery and retrograde flow through the left vertebral artery with severe stenosis versus occlusion of the left proximal subclavian artery. **B**, Illustration of the direction of blood flow. DSA, digital subtraction angiography.

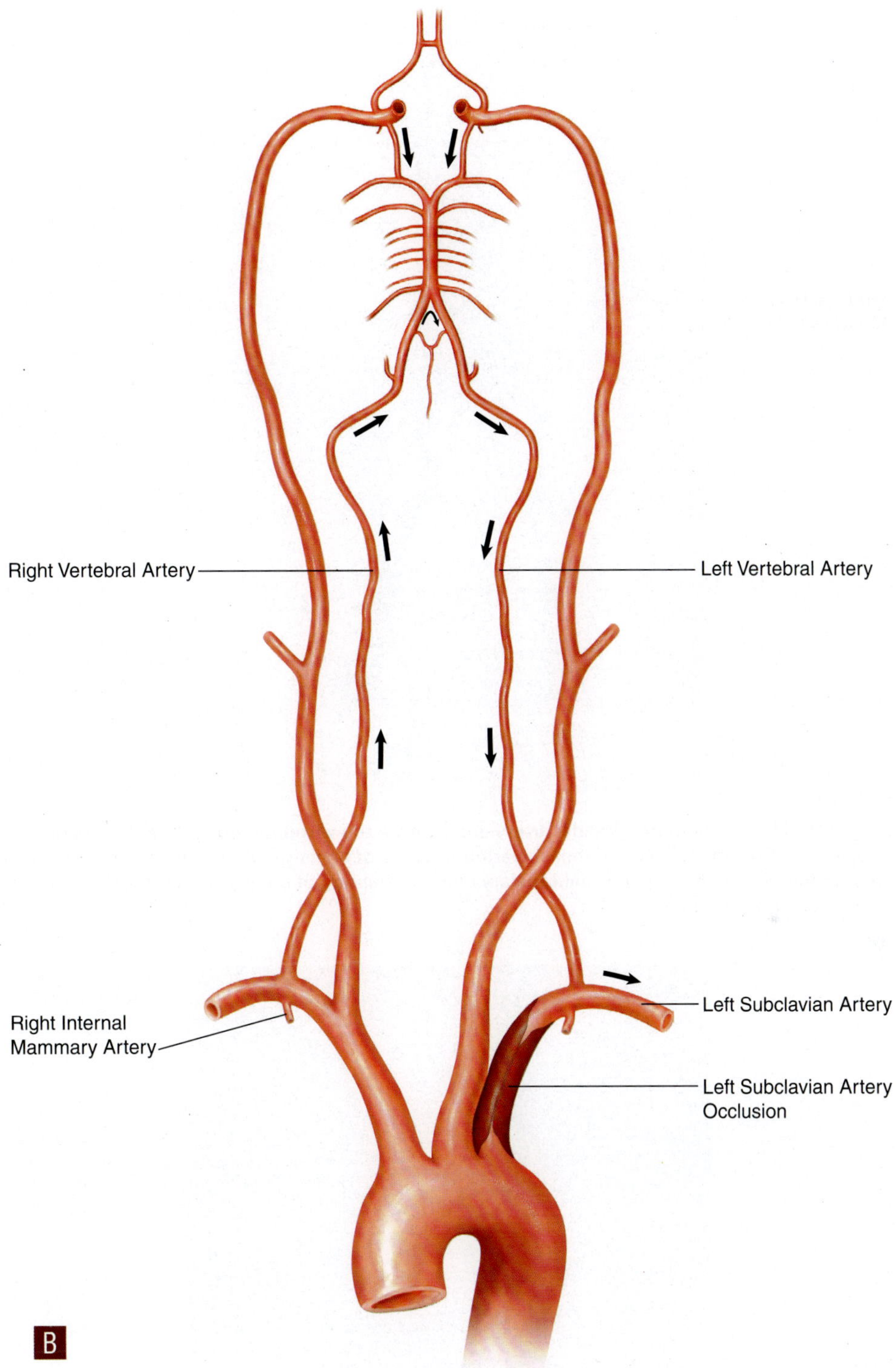

Figure 2.56. *Continued*

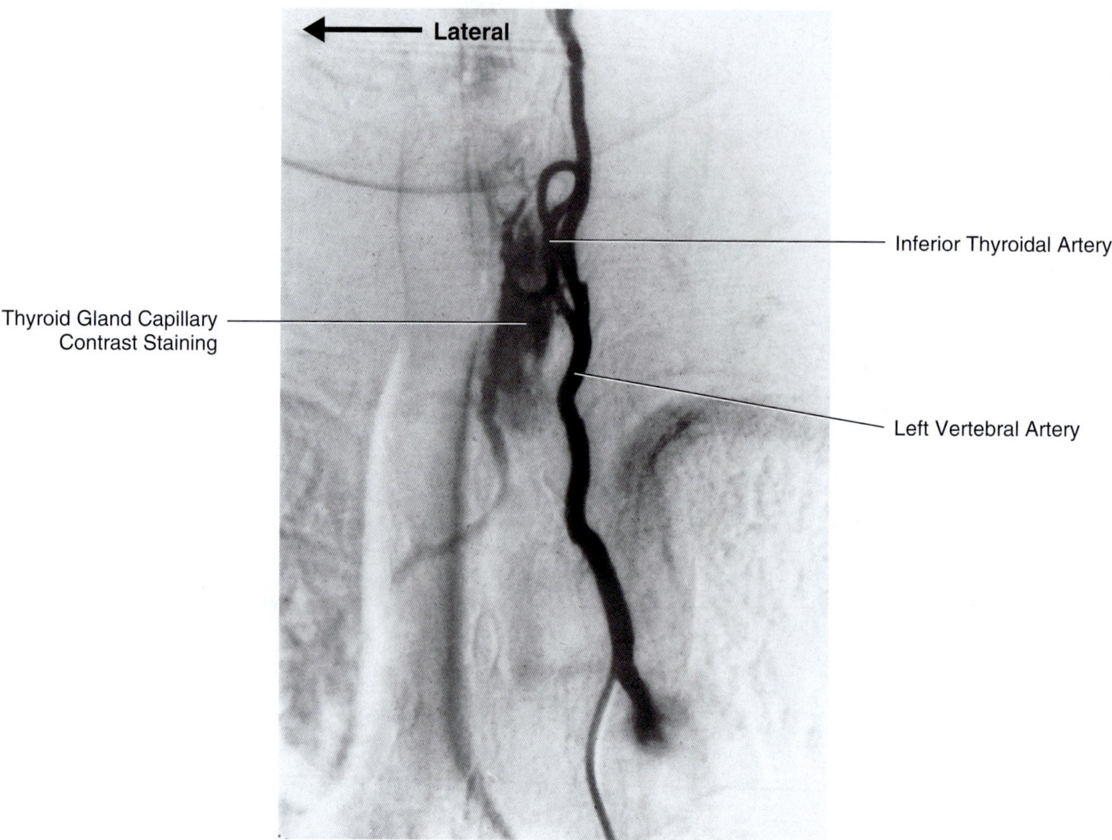

Figure 2.57. **Inferior thyroidal artery arising from the vertebral artery.** Anterior oblique projection DSA with injection of the left vertebral artery demonstrating opacification of the inferior thyroidal artery and normal capillary contrast staining of the thyroid tissue. DSA, digital subtraction angiography.

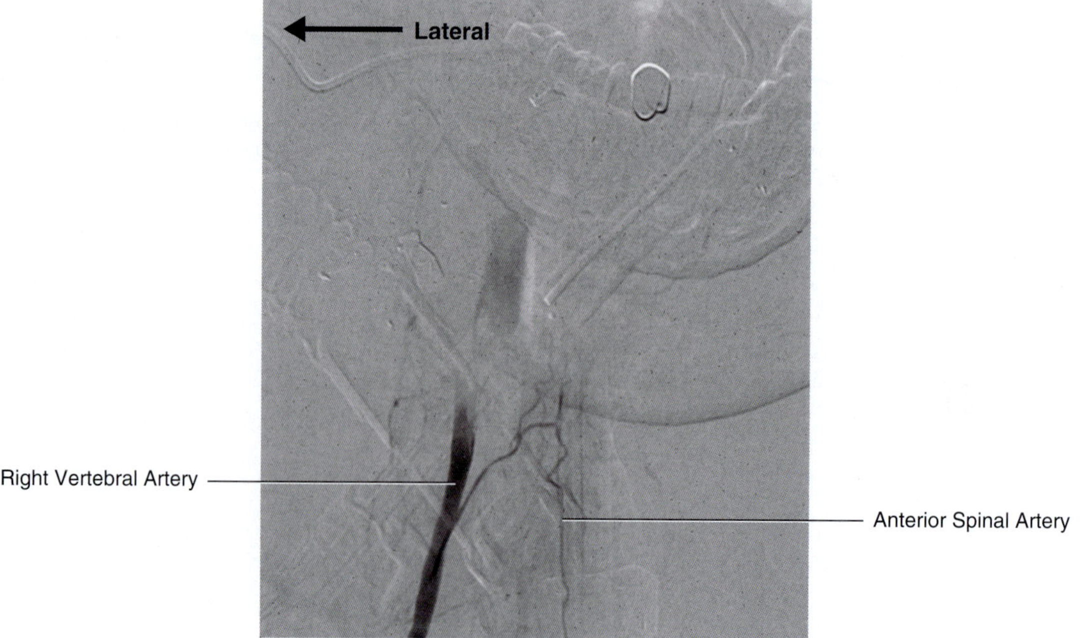

Figure 2.58. **Anterior spinal artery arising from the vertebral artery.** Anterior oblique projection DSA with injection of the right vertebral artery, demonstrating an important origin of the anterior spinal artery from the vertebral artery. Note that the more distal vertebral artery was therapeutically occluded to treat a traumatic avulsed vertebral artery. DSA, digital subtraction angiography.

3

Veins of the Head and Neck

The variability in arterial cerebrovascular anatomy is compounded in the venous system. Cross-sectional imaging studies such as CT and MRI demonstrate the global architecture of the venous system without illustrating the specific tributary drainage territories. Evaluation of a catheter-based contrast-injected venous angiographic study therefore requires knowing the capillary territory subserved by the selected arterial injection. The cerebrovascular venous system should not be considered adequately evaluated until all the possible arteries that may perfuse the venous territory have been studied. For instance, the venous drainage for the left superior precentral gyrus territory responsible for right-sided lower extremity motor function may be seen during injection of the left internal carotid artery (ICA) via the left anterior cerebral artery (ACA) in a typical circle-of-Willis, the right ICA if there is a normal variant hypoplastic left ACA, or the left ICA in a more delayed phase through the left middle cerebral artery (MCA) if compensatory MCA pial-collaterals subserve that territory with senescent stenosis of the left ACA. All this variability makes evaluation of the cerebrovascular venous system challenging but equally rewarding as mastery is gained through study of the anatomy.

I External Veins of the Head and Face

Supratrochlear Vein (Figs. 3.1 and 3.3B)

The supratrochlear vein originates in the anterior part of the head resulting from the junction of a scalp venous network, which is connected to the tributaries of the frontal superficial temporal vein (Fig. 3.2). The supratrochlear veins descend close and parallel to the midline and reach the surface of the nose, where they are joined by the nasal arch and subsequently joined by the supraorbital vein. These veins may anastomose and separate subsequently to form the facial veins. The supratrochlear veins diverge laterally and form the facial vein near the medial canthus.

Supraorbital Vein (Fig. 3.3)

This supraorbital vein originates near the zygomatic process of the frontal bone and runs medially above the orbit until it reaches the supratrochlear vein to form the facial vein near the medial canthus. A branch through the supraorbital notch anastomoses with the superior ophthalmic vein (Figs. 3.3 and 3.4).

Facial Vein (Figs. 3.1, 3.3, and 3.4)

The facial vein is formed by the junction of the supratrochlear and supraorbital veins. It descends obliquely near the side of the nose (also called angular vein at this level), turning posterolateral under the orbit, passing downwards and backwards behind the facial artery, until it reaches the mandible angle, where it is joined by the retromandibular vein (Figs. 3.1, 3.3, and 3.4). The facial vein joins the internal jugular vein near the greater horn of the hyoid bone. The facial vein is connected to the cavernous sinus by the superior ophthalmic vein (Figs. 3.3 and 3.4) or its supraorbital tributary, or by the deep facial vein to the pterygoid plexus and, hence, to the cavernous sinus. The main tributaries in the face are the superior ophthalmic vein (Figs. 3.3 and

3.4), the deep facial vein from the pterygoid venous plexus (Fig. 3.4A), the inferior palpebral vein, and the superior and inferior labial veins (Fig. 3.1). The main tributaries below the mandible are the submental, tonsillar, external palatine (peritonsillar), and submandibular veins. The vena comitans of the hypoglossal nerve and the pharyngeal and superior thyroid veins are also tributaries at the level below the mandible.

Superficial Temporal Vein (Figs. 3.1, 3.2, and 3.4)

This vein originates in the venous network of the scalp. This venous network is drained by the supratrochlear, supraorbital, posterior auricular, and occipital veins. Anterior and posterior tributaries join above the zygoma to form the superficial temporal vein and are joined by the middle temporal vein. The middle temporal vein joins the maxillary vein forming the retromandibular vein. Main tributaries are the parotid veins, temporomandibular joint rami, anterior auricular veins, transverse facial vein, and orbital veins.

Pterygoid Venous Plexus (Figs. 3.1, 3.3B, 3.4B, and 3.15)

Main tributaries are the sphenopalatine, deep temporal, pterygoid, masseteric, buccal, dental, greater palatine, and middle meningeal veins, and branches from the inferior ophthalmic artery. The plexus connects with the facial vein through the deep facial vein and with the cavernous sinus through the sphenoidal emissary foramen, foramen ovale, and foramen lacerum.

Maxillary Vein (Figs. 3.1 and 3.4B)

This is a short vein that accompanies the first part of the maxillary artery. It represents the confluence of veins from the pterygoid plexus with the superficial temporal vein to form the retromandibular vein.

Retromandibular Vein (Figs. 3.1, 3.3, and 3.4)

This vein is within the parotid gland, between the external carotid artery and, superficially, the facial nerve. It has an anterior branch forward that joins the facial vein and a posterior branch backward that forms the external jugular vein after joining the posterior auricular vein.

Posterior Auricular Vein (Figs. 3.1 and 3.4B)

The posterior auricular vein is formed in the parieto-occipital network and drains also the occipital and superficial temporal veins. It has a path of descent behind the auricle and joins the posterior division of the retromandibular vein. The vein receives tributaries from the auricle and stylomastoid vein.

Occipital Vein (Fig. 3.1)

The occipital vein originates in the posterior venous network of the scalp and, through anastomoses, joins the deep cervical and vertebral veins. The vein is a tributary of the internal jugular vein.

Veins of the Neck

The veins of the neck may be superficial and deep, but they are not entirely separable and are connected by anastomoses at various levels (Fig. 3.1).

External Jugular Vein (Figs. 3.1, 3.6, and 3.7)

The external jugular vein drains mainly the scalp and face but also some deeper tissues. It results from the union of the posterior division of the retromandibular and posterior auricular veins near the angle of the mandible. It descends superficially, covered by the platysma, superficial fascia, and skin. It ends in the subclavian vein. Main tributaries are the posterior external cervical vein, and the transverse cervical, suprascapular, and anterior jugular veins.

Posterior External Jugular Vein

The posterior external jugular vein originates in the occipital scalp and drains the skin and muscles. It joins the middle part of the external jugular vein.

Anterior Jugular Vein

The anterior jugular vein starts near the hyoid bone from the junction of the superficial submandibular veins. It descends in a direction parallel to the midline. Distally it turns lateral and deep and joins the end of the external jugular vein. It receives the laryngeal veins and a small thyroid vein. The anterior jugular vein is usually connected to the contralateral anterior jugular vein distally by the jugular arch receiving thyroid tributaries. Both veins may be replaced by a midline trunk.

Internal Jugular Vein (Figs. 3.1, 3.5-3.7, and 3.10)

The internal jugular vein drains most of the blood from the skull, brain, and superficial and deep parts of the face and neck. It originates at the jugular foramen at the cranial base, in continuation with the sigmoid sinus. The vessel is dilated at the beginning and is called the superior bulb. The vein descends along the neck in the carotid sheath, reaching the subclavian vein posteriorly to the sternal end of the clavicle, thereby forming the brachiocephalic vein. At the end, the vein is dilated at the level of the valve and is called the inferior bulb (Fig. 3.7). The internal jugular vein is directly anterior and lateral to the carotid artery. The landmark used to locate the distal portion of the internal jugular vein is the apex of the bifurcation of the two heads of the sternocleidomastoid muscle. The triangle formed by the two heads of this muscle exposes the jugular vein for percutaneous puncture (Fig. 3.6). Knowledge of this anatomic relationship is important for internal jugular vein puncture and catheterization. Fig. 3.9 shows the anatomic relationship of the internal jugular veins and the common carotid artery, viewed with the patient in the head-to-toe position, with the operator positioned at the head of the patient ready for internal jugular access. The distribution of the location of the internal jugular vein in relation to the artery is given in a clock-dial configuration and percentages shown as seen in 188 patients, who were candidates for an internal jugular puncture. The most frequent location of the left internal jugular vein is at 10 o'clock (71%) and of the right internal jugular vein is at 2 o'clock (76%).

The main tributaries of the internal jugular vein are the inferior petrosal sinus, and facial, lingual, pharyngeal, and superior and middle thyroid veins. On the left, the thoracic duct opens near the union of the left subclavian vein and internal jugular vein. The right lymphatic duct ends at the same site on the right.

Inferior Petrosal Sinus (Figs. 3.3B, 3.12, 3.13, 3.14B, 3.15, 3.17, 3.20B, 3.23, 3.25, and 3.26)

The inferior petrosal sinus leaves the skull through the anterior pars nervosa of the jugular foramen and joins the superior jugular bulb as a major drainage pathway for the cavernous sinus. The inferior petrosal sinus may be cannulated during an inferior petrosal sinus sampling procedure.

Lingual Veins

There are two main lingual veins (see Chapter 2, Fig. 2.15B). The dorsal lingual vein drains the dorsum and sides of the tongue and joins the lingual vein, which follows the lingual artery. It is a tributary of the internal jugular vein.

The deep lingual vein begins at the tip of the tongue and runs posteriorly along the inferior surface of the tongue. At the base of the tongue, it is joined by the sublingual vein from the salivary gland, forming the vena comitans nerve hypoglossi until it joins the facial, internal jugular, or the lingual veins.

Pharyngeal Veins

The pharyngeal veins begin at the pharyngeal plexus external to the pharynx. These veins receive meningeal veins and a vein from the pterygoid canal. The pharyngeal veins end in the internal jugular vein but sometimes may end in the facial, lingual, or superior thyroid veins.

Superior Thyroid Vein (Figs. 3.5 and 3.8)

The superior thyroid vein corresponds to the branches of the superior thyroid artery. It is formed by deep and superficial tributaries and is joined by the superior laryngeal and cricothyroid veins. It is a tributary of the internal jugular vein or facial vein.

Middle Thyroid Vein (Figs. 3.5 and 3.8)

The middle thyroid vein drains the inferior part of the thyroid gland and with tributaries from the larynx and trachea. It crosses anterior to the common carotid artery and is a tributary of the distal part of the internal jugular vein.

Inferior Thyroid Veins (Fig. 3.8)

The inferior thyroid veins drain the thyroid gland caudally and arise from the venous network that communicates with the middle and superior thyroid veins. These veins form a plexus anterior to the trachea. The left vein arises from this plexus and joins the left brachiocephalic vein, while the right vein descends to the right and joins the right brachiocephalic vein at the junction with the superior vena cava. Frequently, a common trunk is present from the vena cava or brachiocephalic vein.

Vertebral Vein

The vertebral vein is formed from numerous small tributaries from the internal vertebral plexuses, which arise from the vertebral canal above the posterior arch of the atlas. There are anastomoses with small veins from the muscles, and they form a vein that enters the foramen in the transverse process of the atlas and descends as a plexus around the vertebral artery. This plexus ends as the vertebral vein which emerges from the transverse foramen most commonly of the sixth cervical vertebra, descends posterior to the artery, and opens in the posterior aspect of the brachiocephalic vein. Its main tributaries are branches from the occipital vein, muscular veins from the posterior neck, veins from the internal and external vertebral plexus, and the anterior vertebral and deep cervical veins. Occasionally the first intercostal vein is a tributary of the vertebral vein.

Anterior Vertebral Vein

The anterior vertebral vein arises from a plexus around the transverse processes of the superior cervical vertebra. It runs inferiorly parallel to the ascending cervical artery and joins the terminal vertebral vein.

Deep Cervical Vein

The deep cervical vein begins in the suboccipital region in the form of communicating branches from the occipital vein and small veins from the deep muscles at the posterior aspect of the neck. It receives tributaries from the plexus around the cervical vertebrae and is a tributary for the lower vertebral veins.

Cranial and Intracranial Veins and Dural Venous Sinuses

Diploic and Meningeal Veins

Diploic Veins (Fig. 3.1)

These veins run through channels in the diploe of some of the cranial bones without valves to regulate the direction of blood flow. The diploic veins are large and have dilated segments. The walls of these veins are thin consisting of endothelium surrounded by elastic tissue. There are anastomoses of these veins with the meningeal veins, dural sinuses, and pericranial veins. The main diploic veins are the frontal diploic vein, the anterior temporal (parietal) diploic vein, the posterior temporal (parietal) diploic vein, the occipital diploic vein, and the numerous small diploic vein tributaries of the superior sagittal sinus.

Meningeal Veins

The meningeal veins are formed by the venous plexus in the dura mater and join efferent veins in the outer dural layer. These veins subsequently drain to the superior sagittal sinus, other cranial sinuses, and diploic veins.

Cerebrovascular Venous System (Figs. 3.10-3.12)

The supratentorial venous system is commonly divided into two groups: the superficial system of veins and the deep system of veins. Knowledge of these two different systems is important for the evaluation of venous occlusion in the superficial group, through the abnormal filling sequence and flow pattern, and for the thorough investigation of pathological shunts such as arteriovenous malformations and dural arteriovenous fistulas.

Superficial System of Veins (Figs. 3.10-3.12, 3.15, 3.17, 3.18, and 3.22)

Above the sylvian fissure, the lateral convexity of the brain is drained by the anterior frontal, central, and parietal veins. These veins also receive venous drainage from the medial surface of the brain from the interhemispheric fissure just before they enter the superior sagittal sinus (SSS). The largest vein draining into the SSS is known as the vein of Trolard (Figs. 3.10B, 3.17, 3.18, and 3.22) usually in the parietal region above the sylvian fissure.

The superficial middle cerebral vein is also known as the Sylvian vein (Figs. 3.12-3.14B, 3.15-3.18, and 3.20B) and has tributaries from the lateral aspect of the brain close to the sylvian fissure with a highly variable drainage pattern. The superficial middle cerebral vein may drain anteromedially via the sphenoparietal sinus into the cavernous sinus (Figs. 3.12, 3.13, 3.15-3.18, and 3.20B), posteriorly via an anastomosis through the vein of Labbe to the transverse sinus (Figs. 3.14B), or superiorly via an anastomosis through the vein of Trolard to the superior sagittal sinus.

The superficial portions of the brain, under the sylvian fissure and the inferior aspect of the temporal and occipital lobes, drain directly into the transverse sinus. The largest lateral vein under the sylvian fissure is the vein of Labbé (Figs. 3.14B, 3.16, 3.18, and 3.20B).

Deep System of Veins

The deep system of veins of the brain is formed by the internal cerebral veins, the basal veins of Rosenthal, and the thalamic veins. The site of drainage of this system is the vein of Galen and subsequently into the straight sinus.

The two internal cerebral veins (Figs. 3.10B-3.12, 3.14, 3.15, 3.17-3.20B) are approximately 2 mm from the midline. This anatomic location was historically useful for diagnosing midline shift before the broad availability of cross-sectional imaging. The internal cerebral veins drain the deep white matter including the corona radiata and centrum semiovale around the frontal horns and the body of the lateral ventricles via medial and lateral subependymal veins.

The thalamostriate (subependymal) veins (Figs. 3.12, 3.14B, 3.17-3.20A) outline the inferolateral wall of the body of the lateral ventricle. Seen from a frontal view, the distance from the superolateral corner of the thalamostriate veins and the internal cerebral vein corresponds to the width of the body of the lateral ventricles. Seen from a lateral view, the thalamostriate vein drains anteroinferiorly in a sulcus between the head of the caudate nucleus and the thalamus. The angle made by the thalamostriate vein as it drains into the internal cerebral vein is called the venous angle. A false venous angle is likely to occur when the thalamostriate vein is absent or small (Fig. 3.20B). In this situation, the thalamostriate vein is replaced by a vein 0.5 to 1 cm posterior to it. The anterior septal veins are medial subependymal veins that drain the white matter around the frontal horns of the ventricles and genu of the corpus callosum. On a lateral view, the septal veins look like an anterior extension of the internal cerebral veins (Figs. 3.14B, 3.18, 3.19B, and 3.20). The body and atrium of the lateral ventricles are drained by other medial and lateral subependymal veins. The medullary veins are small and drain into the subependymal veins. When the medullary veins are detectable, they are seen along the superior surface of the lateral ventricle.

The basal veins of Rosenthal (Figs. 3.10B-3.12, 3.14B-3.17, 3.19A, 3.20B, and 3.21) are formed in the medial portion of the lateral cerebral fissures after receiving the deep middle cerebral veins, which are lateral branches from the insulae, the superior branches from the anterior perforated substances, anterior branches from the undersurface of the frontal lobes, and medial branches from the interhemispheric fissures. The basal veins of Rosenthal leave the lateral cerebral fissures and course around the superior aspect of the uncus and pass posteriorly in the perimesencephalic cisterns to drain into the vein of Galen. The basal veins also drain the inferior portion of the ventricles through the inferior ventricular veins, the thalamus, and the hippocampus, while circling the mesencephalon. The basal veins of Rosenthal usually drain posteriorly into the vein of Galen, but when the mesencephalic portion of the vein does not follow the proper segmentation, it may drain anteriorly into the sphenoparietal sinus or the superior petrosal sinus and inferiorly into the lateral mesencephalic vein or anterior pontomesencephalic vein, or medially into the contralateral basal vein of Rosenthal through the posterior communicating vein.

The vein of Galen receives the internal cerebral veins, the basal veins of Rosenthal, the pericallosal veins, and the veins that drain the superior aspect of the posterior fossa. The vein of Galen courses beneath the splenium of the corpus callosum and then drains into the straight sinus. The posterior pericallosal vein delineates the position of the splenium of the corpus callosum.

Dural Sinuses (Figs. 3.10-3.12)

The superior sagittal sinus (SSS) is long with a triangular shape and is located within the dura at its junction with the falx cerebri along the midline. The SSS is connected laterally with the venous lacunae into which the arachnoid granulations drain cerebrospinal fluid from the extra-axial space. The SSS usually extends from the foramen cecum to the torcula herophili. In some cases, it is not formed anteriorly to the coronal suture. The frontal vein runs in the posterior direction, parallel to the midline, in the absence of the anterior SSS. The torcula herophili receives the SSS, the straight sinus, and the occipital sinus (Figs. 3.10B and 3.12) and drains into the transverse sinus. There is normal variability in size of the transverse sinuses based on the preferential drainage pattern of the SSS and the straight sinus in opposite directions. The right transverse sinus is more commonly dominant with this hypothetically attributable to venous pulse pressure during cardiac right atrial contraction. Congenital dominance of a transverse and sigmoid sinus versus an acquired stenosis can be determined by looking for a concordant asymmetric size of the bony jugular foramen on a CT scan of the head.

The cavernous sinus (Figs. 3.10B-3.14B, 3.15, 3.17, 3.20B, 3.23, 3.25, and 3.26) constitutes the lateral border of the sella turcica and contains the oculomotor, trochlear, ophthalmic, and abducens nerves, as well as the internal carotid artery. Anteriorly, the superior and inferior ophthalmic veins drain into the cavernous sinus, connecting the facial vein via the angular vein to the cavernous sinus. Anterolaterally, the cavernous sinus receives the sphenoparietal sinus. The superficial sylvian veins and the uncal veins occasionally drain into the cavernous sinus. The cavernous sinus drains posteriorly into the superior petrosal sinus which is located at the attachment of the falx to the petrous pyramid, connecting the cavernous sinus with the transverse and sigmoid sinuses (Figs. 3.10B, 3.12, 3.20B, 3.24, and 3.25). Posteroinferiorly, the cavernous sinus drains into the inferior petrosal sinus which runs along the lower border of the pyramids toward the ventromedial pars nervosa of the jugular foramen and enters the internal jugular vein, immediately below the skull base (Figs. 3.3B, 3.12-3.14B, 3.15, 3.17, 3.20B, 3.23, 3.25, and 3.26). Inferiorly, the cavernous sinus drains into the pterygoid plexus through the foramina of Vesalius (venosum), ovale, rotundum, and lacerum (Fig. 3.26A).

The bilateral cavernous sinuses are interconnected by additional sinuses (Figs. 3.13 and 3.26A). The sinus intercavernous anterior is located between the anterior surface of the anterior pituitary lobe and the anterior sella margin directly below the diaphragma sellae. The sinus intercavernous (sive coronarius) posterior in most cases is larger than the anterior intercavernous sinus. It runs posterior to the pituitary lobe and anterior to the posterior clinoid plate. The sinus intercavernous inferior is located in front of the sulcus, which delineates the border between the anterior and posterior lobes of the pituitary. The sinus may be a single channel but more often consists of multiple channels. The clival basilar plexus is a complex venous plexus along the dorsal aspect of the clivus. It extends inferiorly into the foramen magnum with the surrounding marginal sinus and continues as the internal and external vertebral venous plexus. Varying anastomoses with the cavernous sinus can be observed.

The venous drainage of the pituitary gland is complex (Fig. 2.42). Blood leaves the anterior lobe of the pituitary by numerous small hypophyseal veins. These veins empty into lateral adenohypophyseal veins, which converge into the confluent pituitary veins on the surface of the gland. The confluent pituitary veins then course laterally to join the ipsilateral cavernous sinuses. The cavernous sinuses are immediately lateral to the pituitary fossa.

Sequence of Venous Drainage

Cerebral venous drainage follows a consistent sequence. The superficial venous system fills sequentially from anterior to posterior with filling of the frontal, midfrontal, and temporal convexity surface veins first followed by the posterior frontal and parietal veins approximately half a second later. The basal vein of Rosenthal is also seen in this early venous phase, and it therefore may be considered physiologically a superficial vein despite its categorization as a deep vein based on its location. The vein of Labbe and superficial vein of Trolard also fill during this phase. While high-flow shunts such as arteriovenous malformations demonstrate venous filling in the arterial or capillary phases, low-flow shunts may be seen on the late capillary or this early venous phase with robust venous filling.

The deep venous system starts opacifying approximately 1.5 seconds later than the superficial venous system. The thalamostriate veins and the internal cerebral veins usually fill at about the same time as the parietal veins. The caudate veins and septal veins opacify late and are among the last to remain opacified in the venous phase.

Posterior Fossa Venous System (Figs. 3.23-3.25)

The superficial vessels of the posterior fossa may outline the anterior border of the brain stem, cerebellopontine angles, vermis, and cerebellar hemispheres.

From a lateral view, the anterior margin of the pons and mesencephalon is outlined by the anterior pontomesencephalic vein, the superior vermis by both the superior vermian artery and vein, and the inferior surface of the cerebellar vermis by both the inferior vermian artery and vein. The brainstem can be separated from the vermis and cerebellar hemispheres by the precentral cerebellar vein superiorly and by the posterior medullary segment of the posterior inferior cerebellar artery inferiorly.

From an anteroposterior view, the anterolateral surface of the midbrain is outlined by the posterior mesencephalic vein, whereas a rougher outline is provided by the superior cerebellar arteries. The anterior surface of the pons and its relationship to the cerebellopontine angles is outlined by the transverse pontine veins and the petrosal sinuses. The midline can be roughly approximated by studying the posterior inferior cerebellar arteries.

There are three major groups of veins in the posterior fossa, and they are identified accordingly to the direction of the flow.

The superior group drains into the vein of Galen.

The anterior group drains into the petrosal sinus. The posterior group drains into the torcula herophili and transverse sinus.

Superior Group

The precentral cerebellar vein (Figs. 3.25) originates in the precentral cerebellar fissure. It divides the posterior fossa into an anterior and a posterior compartment.

The posterior mesencephalic veins (Fig. 3.24B) drain the posterior perforated substance and the cerebral peduncles. These veins are close to the cerebral peduncles and outline the peduncles on a frontal view.

The superior vermian veins drain the superior aspect of the vermis and adjacent cerebellum. These veins outline the superior surface of the vermis.

Anterior Group

The anterior pontomesencephalic vein (Fig. 3.25) drains the interpeduncular fossa and the anterior surfaces of the pons and cerebellum. It outlines the anterior surface of the pons and is located posteriorly to the basilar artery. The anterior pontomesencephalic vein usually drains into the petrosal veins through the transverse pontine veins.

The petrosal veins (Fig. 3.25) are located in the cerebellopontine angles adjacent to the internal auditory canals. The main tributaries of the petrosal veins are the transverse pontine veins (medial branches form the pons), superior hemispheric veins, veins of the greater horizontal fissure, and inferior hemispheric veins (lateral branches from the cerebellar hemispheres), brachial veins (superomedial branches from the wings of the precentral cerebellar fissure), and inferior branches from the hemispheric veins of the lateral recess (inferomedial branches from the cerebellar pontine fissure).

Posterior Group

The inferior vermian veins (Fig. 3.23) are formed by the superior and inferior retrotonsillar tributaries. They outline the inferior surface of the vermis.

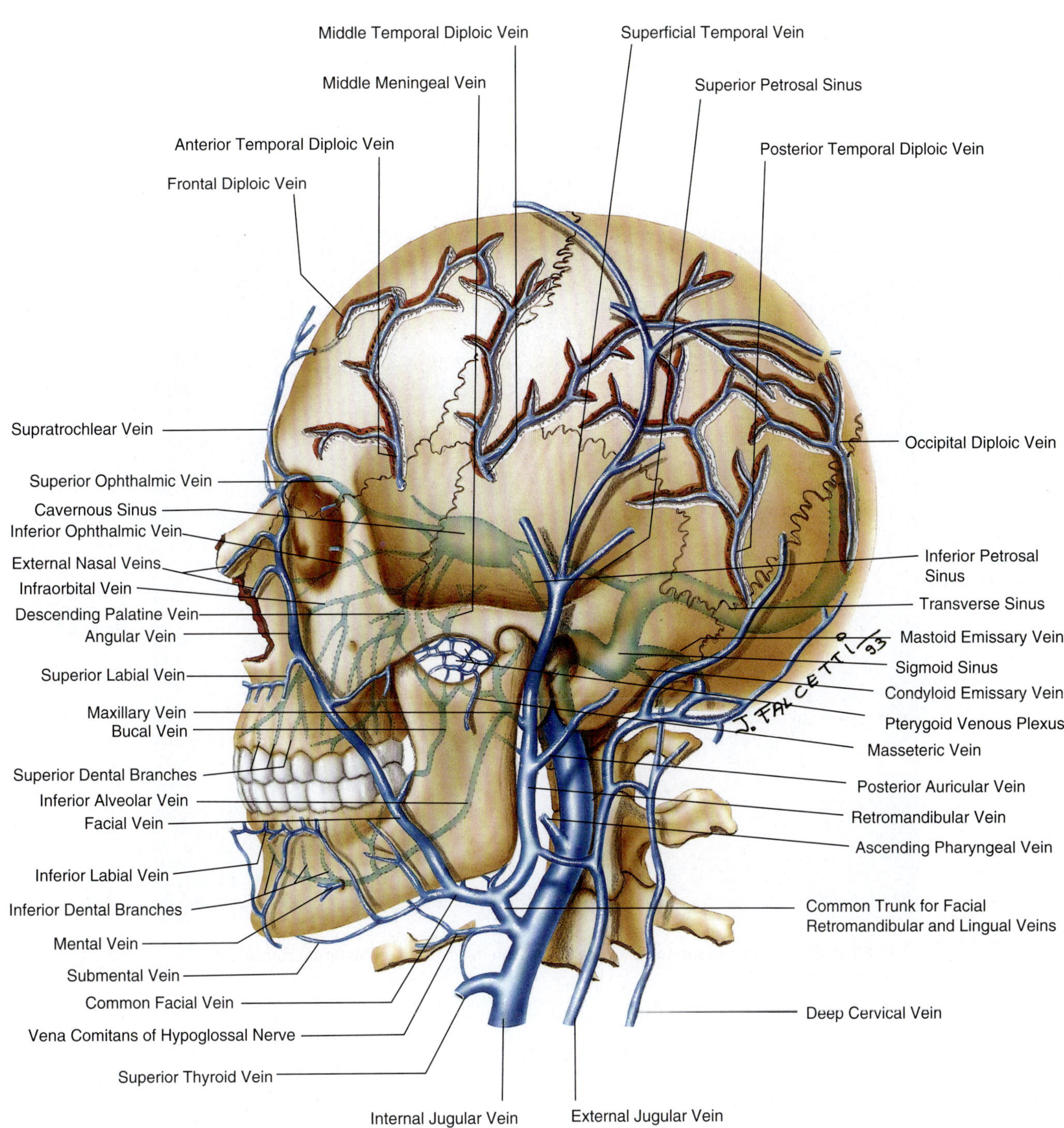

Figure 3.1. Illustration depicting the superficial veins of the head and neck. The calvarium has been removed for better visualization of the diploic veins.

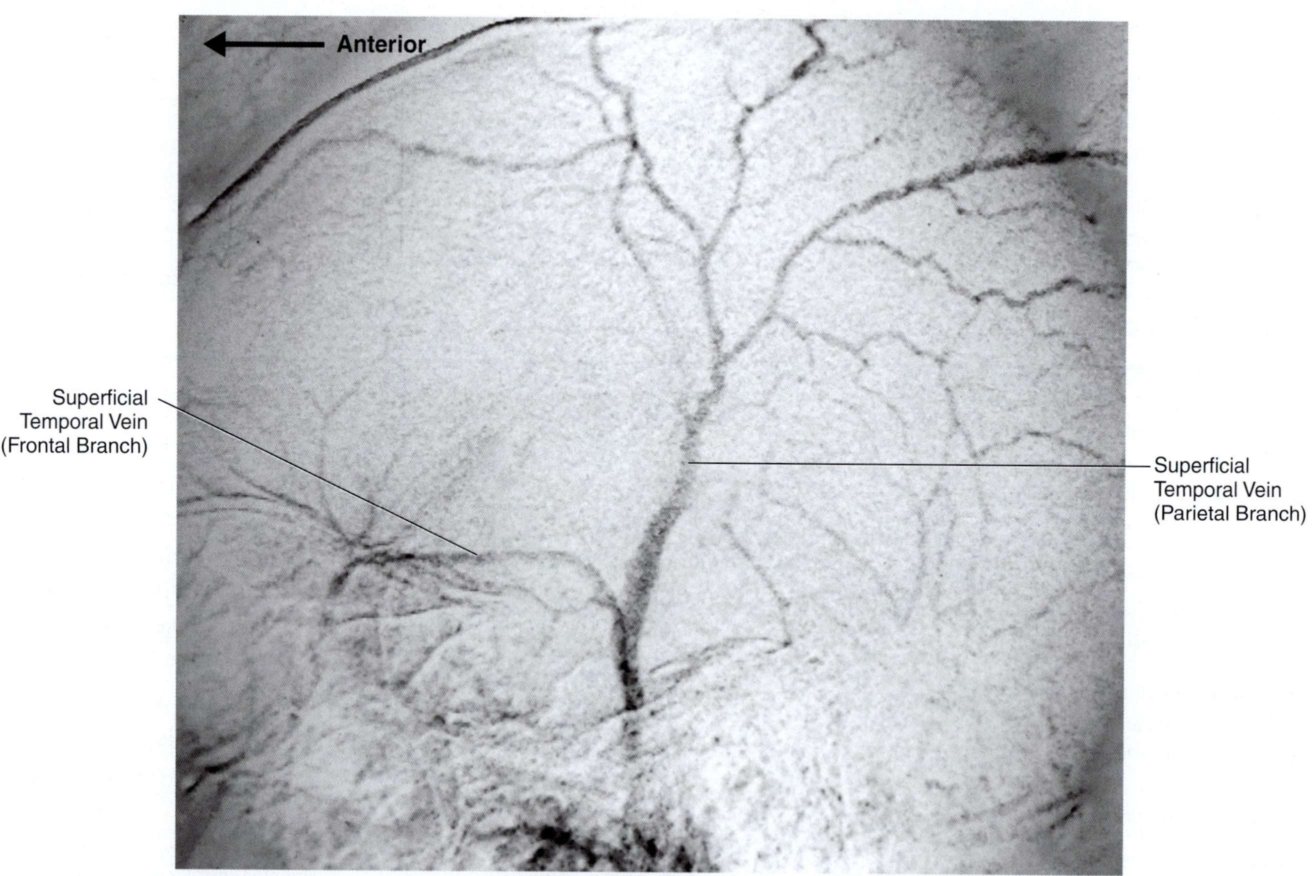

Figure 3.2. Veins of the scalp. Lateral DSA with injection of the external carotid artery in the venous phase.

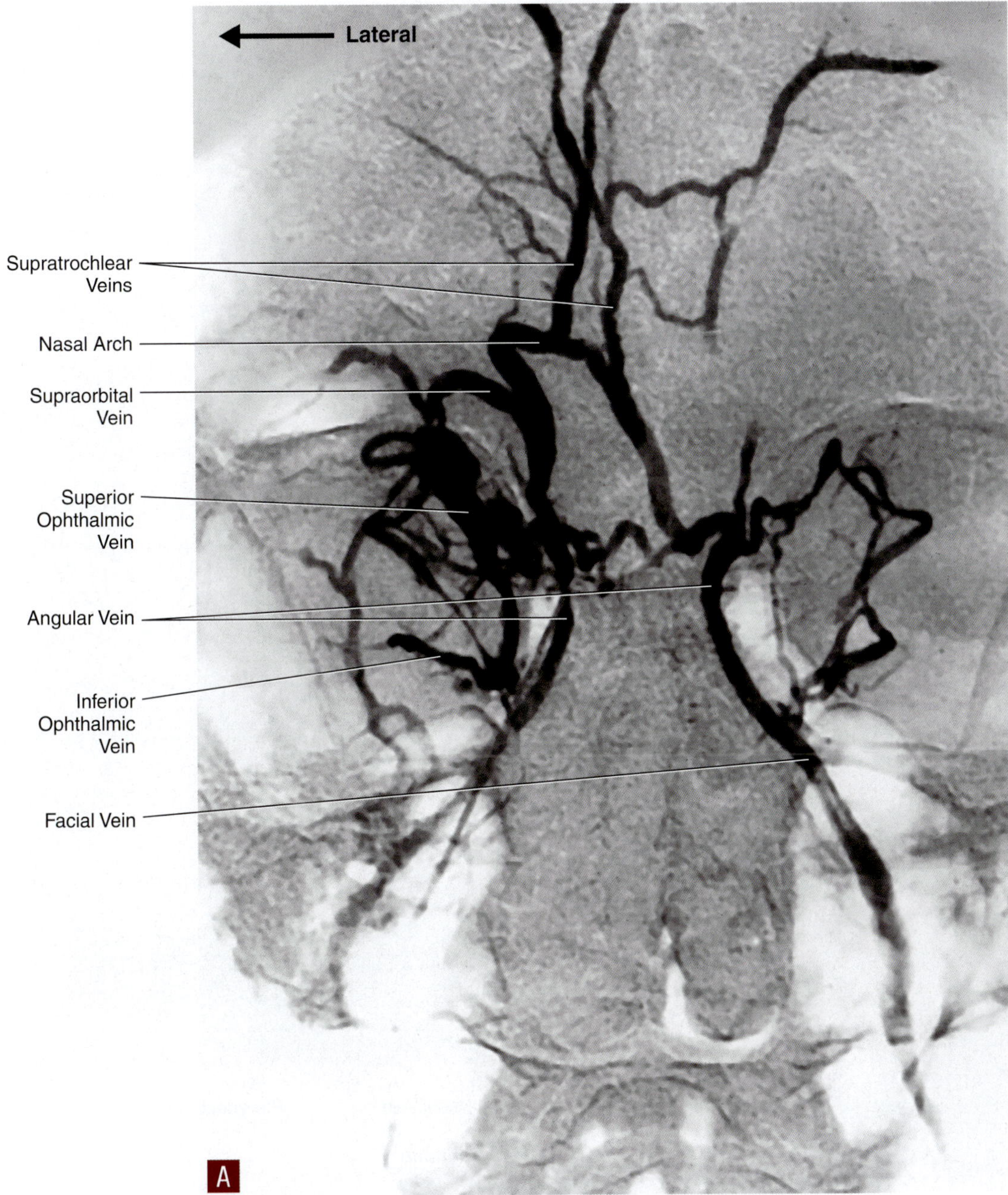

Figure 3.3. Frontal (A) and lateral (B) view of an orbital venogram showing the facial vein, supratrochlear vein, cavernous sinus, superior ophthalmic vein, and inferior ophthalmic vein.

Anterior

Supratrochlear Vein

Supraorbital Vein

Nasofrontal Vein

Angular Vein

External Nasal Vein

Facial Vein

Superior Ophthalmic Vein

Cavernous Sinus

Clival Basilar Plexus

Inferior Petrosal Sinus

B

Ethmoidal Vein

Internal Nasal Vein

Pterygoid Plexus

Figure 3.3. *Continued*

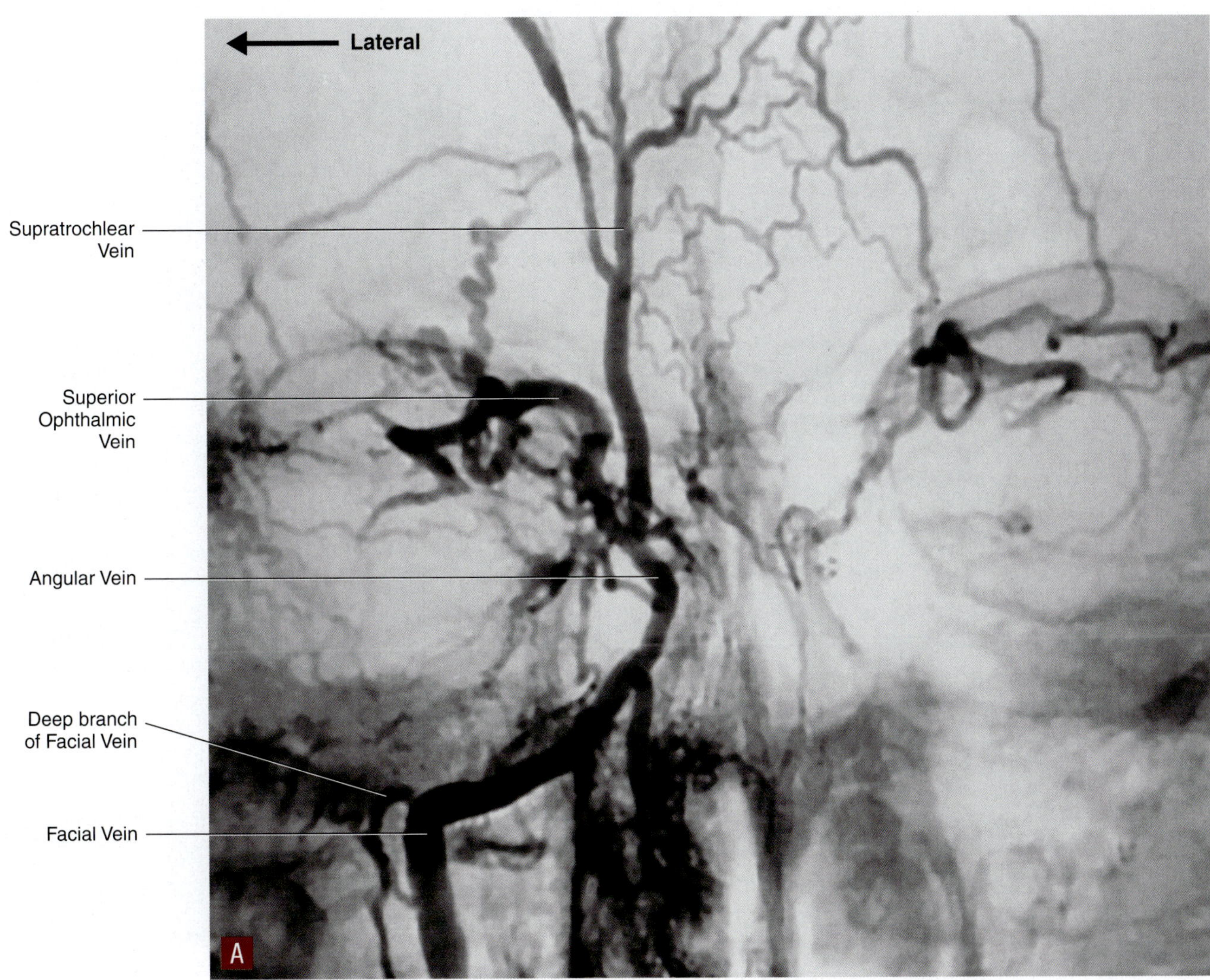

Figure 3.4. Frontal (A) and lateral (B) view of an orbital venogram demonstrating the major veins of the face.

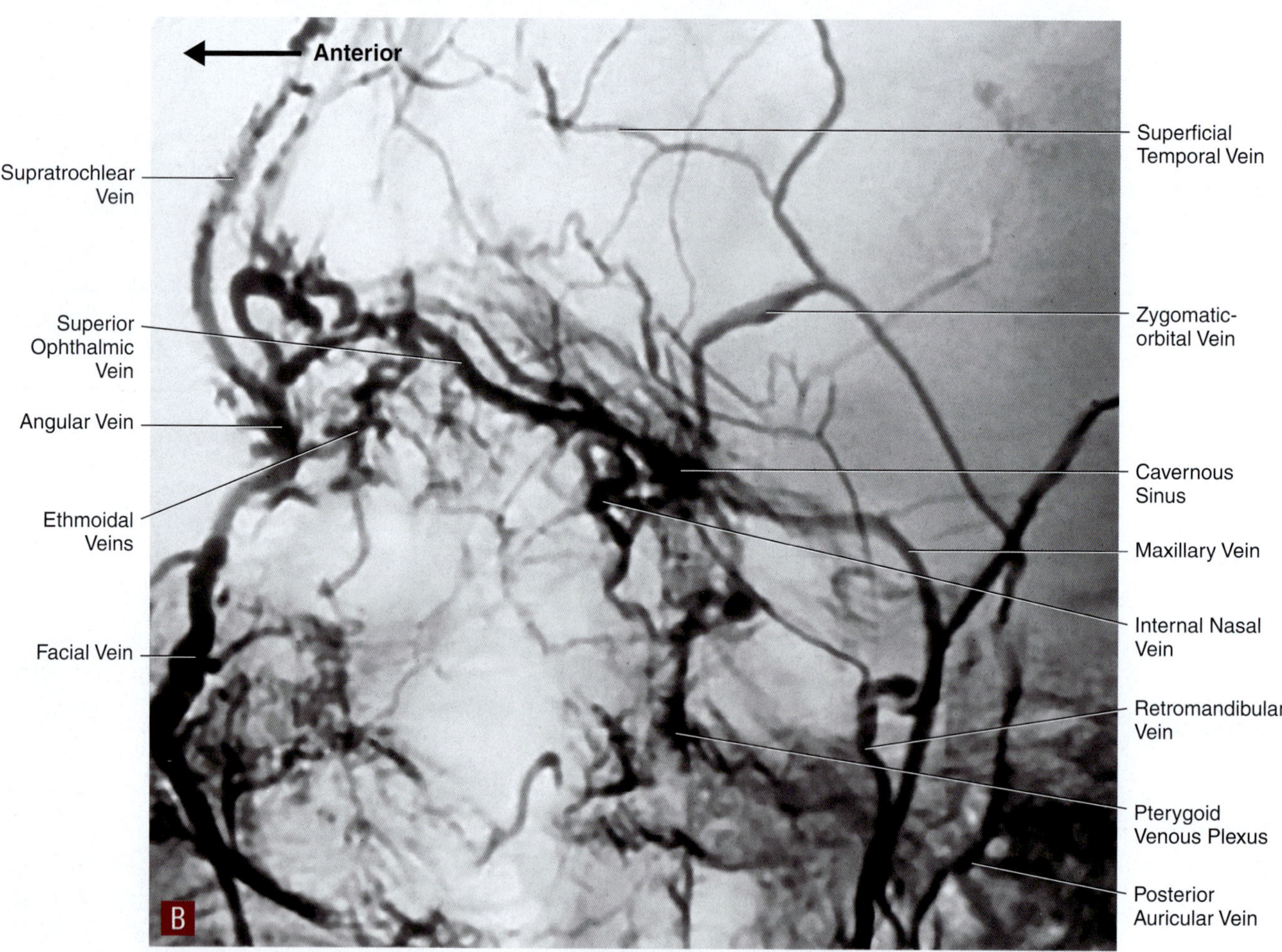

Figure 3.4. *Continued*

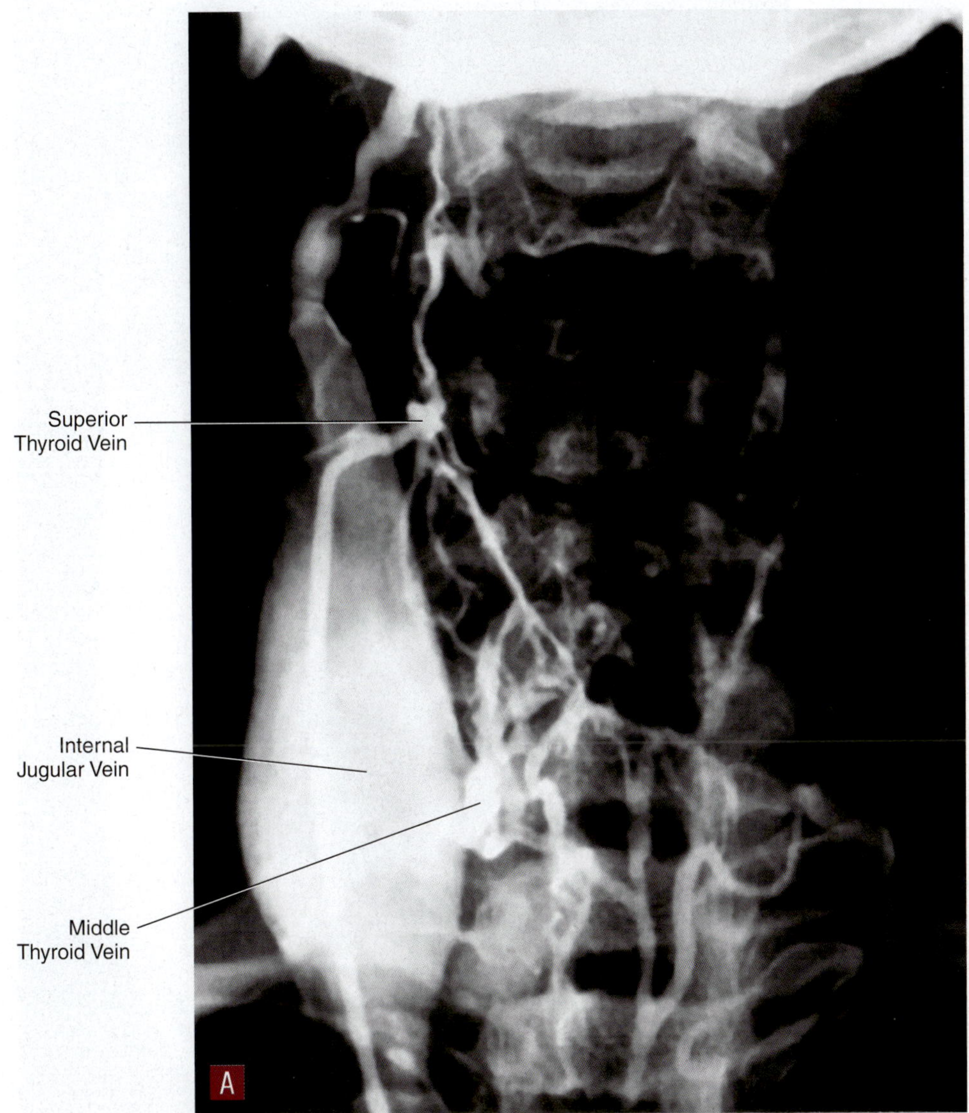

Figure 3.5. A, Venogram of the right internal jugular vein shows the dilation of the inferior bulb. Note the tributary selectively catheterized, superior thyroid vein. B, Venogram of the left internal jugular vein. Note the superior thyroid vein, tributary of the internal jugular vein.

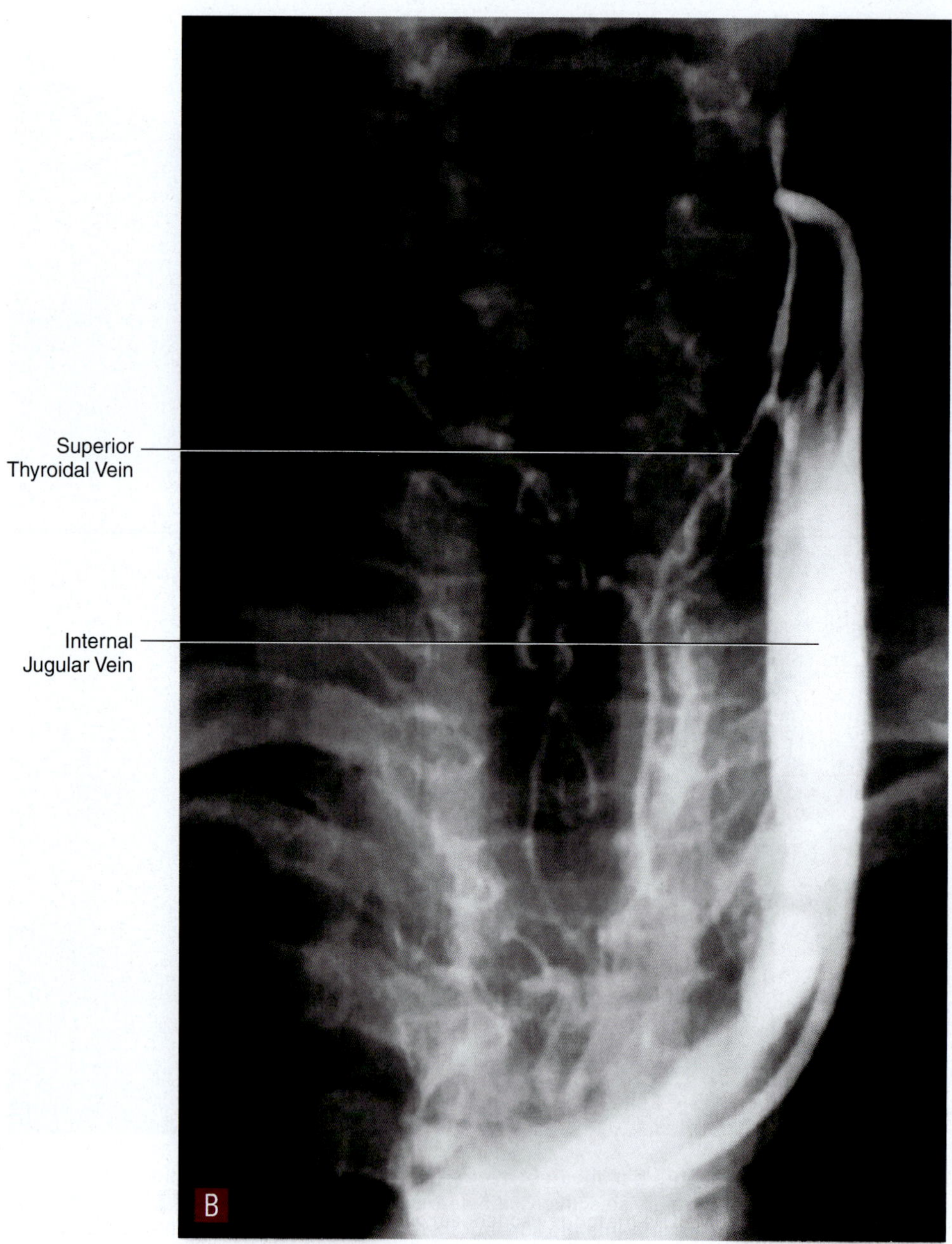

Figure 3.5. *Continued*

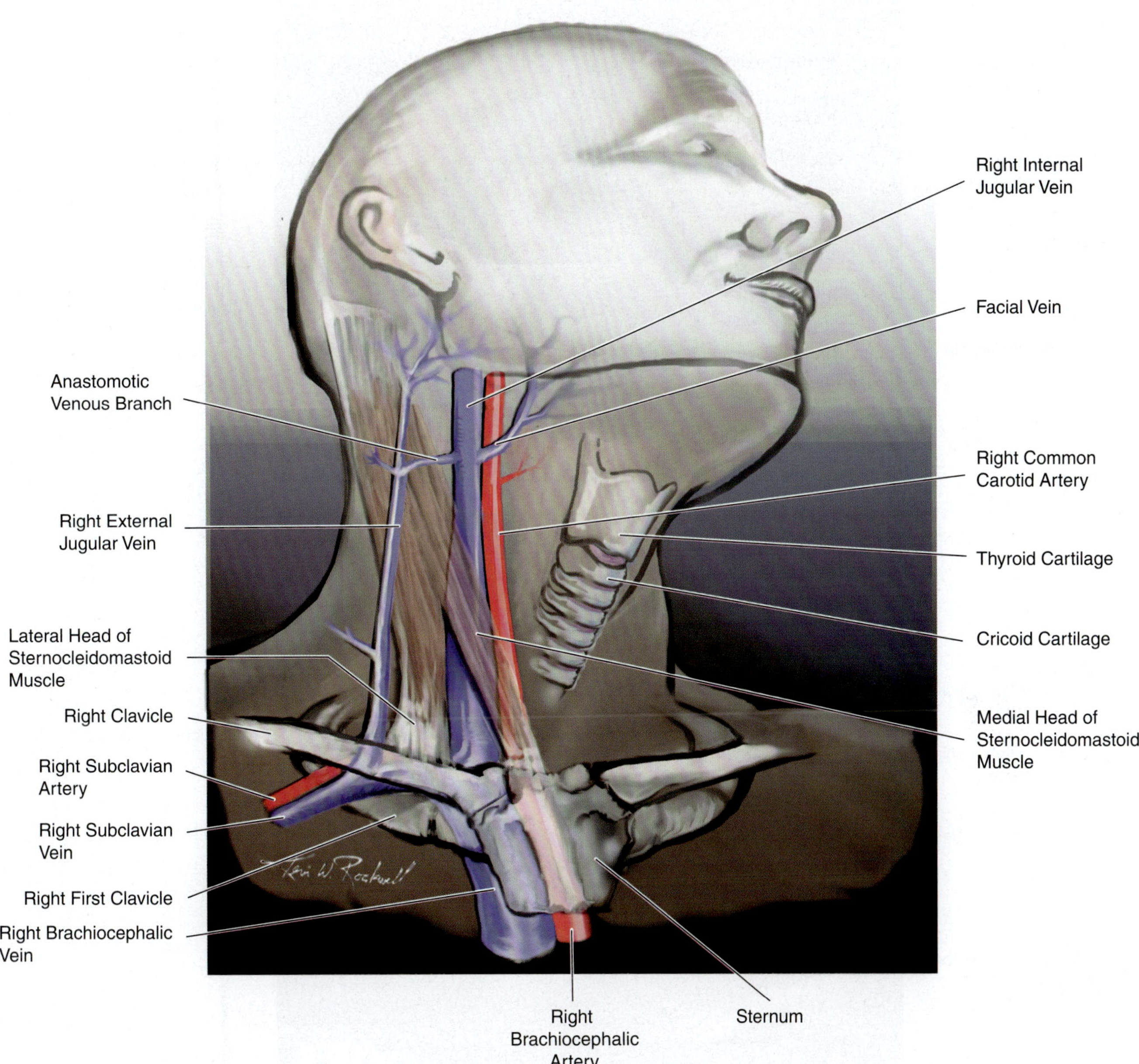

Figure 3.6. Internal jugular vein and subclavian vein anatomy at the level of the neck. Anterolateral view. Note the triangle formed by the medial and lateral heads of the sternocleidomastoid muscle showing as a window for puncture and catheterization of the internal jugular vein. The internal jugular vein is lateral and anterior to the common carotid artery.

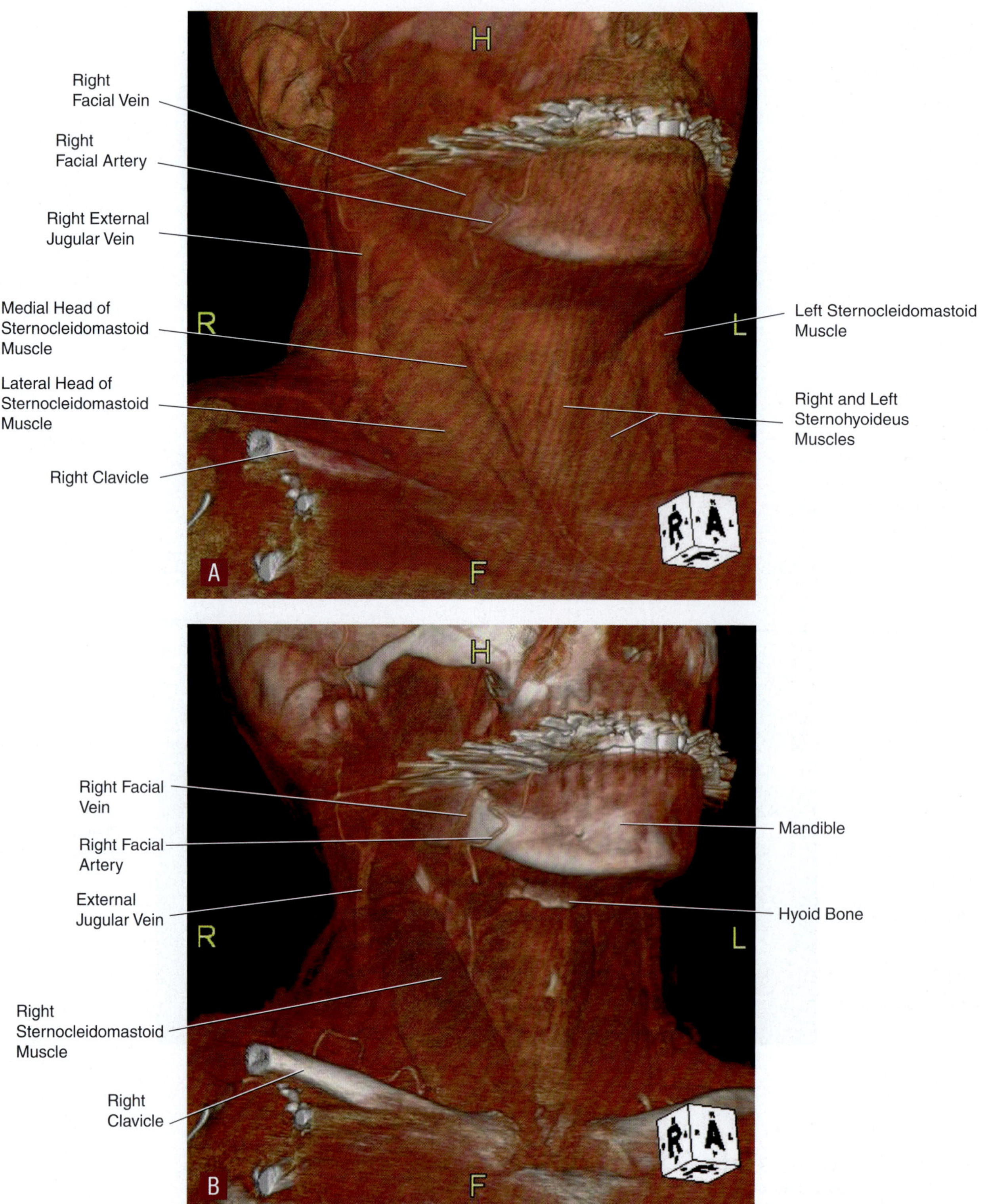

Figure 3.7. Computerized tomographic angiography of the neck showing the anatomy of the internal jugular vein, the carotid artery, and the superficial muscles. **A**, Anterolateral view of the neck showing the superficial tissues covering the right internal jugular vein and carotid. The right superficial jugular vein is barely visible. **B**, Deeper view of the soft tissues of the right neck shows the external jugular vein and part of the right facial vein and artery. The sternocleidomastoid muscle becomes visible. **C**, The relationship of the right carotid artery and internal jugular vein becomes more apparent behind the sternocleidomastoid muscle. Note the hyoid bone and the thyroid cartilage. **D**, Deeper view of the neck shows the relationship of the artery and vein. The bifurcation of the carotid is now visible and the external carotid artery is clearly delineated. Note the impression of the carotid bulb on the internal jugular vein. The thyroid lobes are visible. **E**, Deeper view shows the right internal jugular vein and the middle thyroid vein. **F**, Last image shows the right internal jugular vein faintly and the right vertebral artery becomes visible.

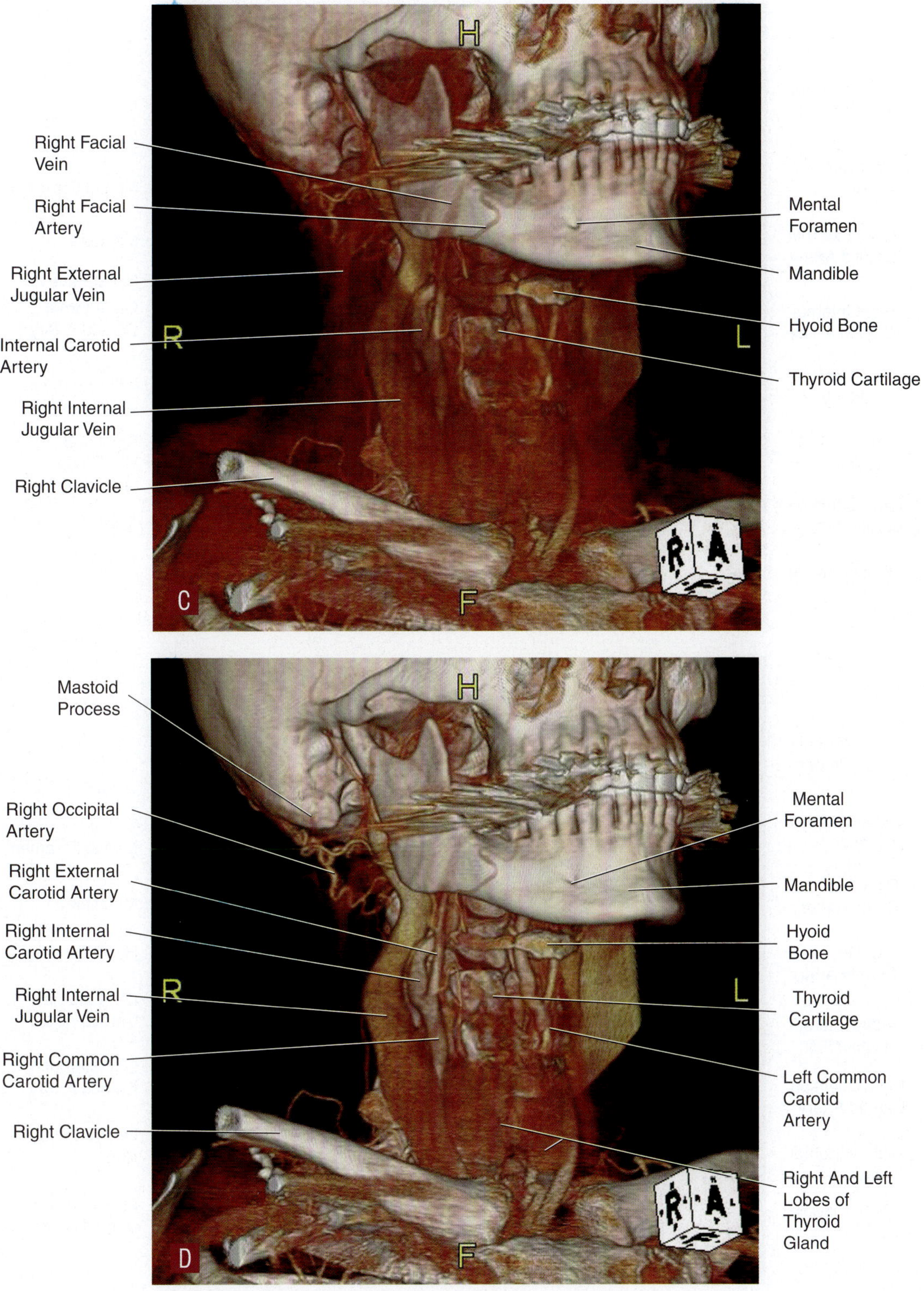

Figure 3.7. *Continued*

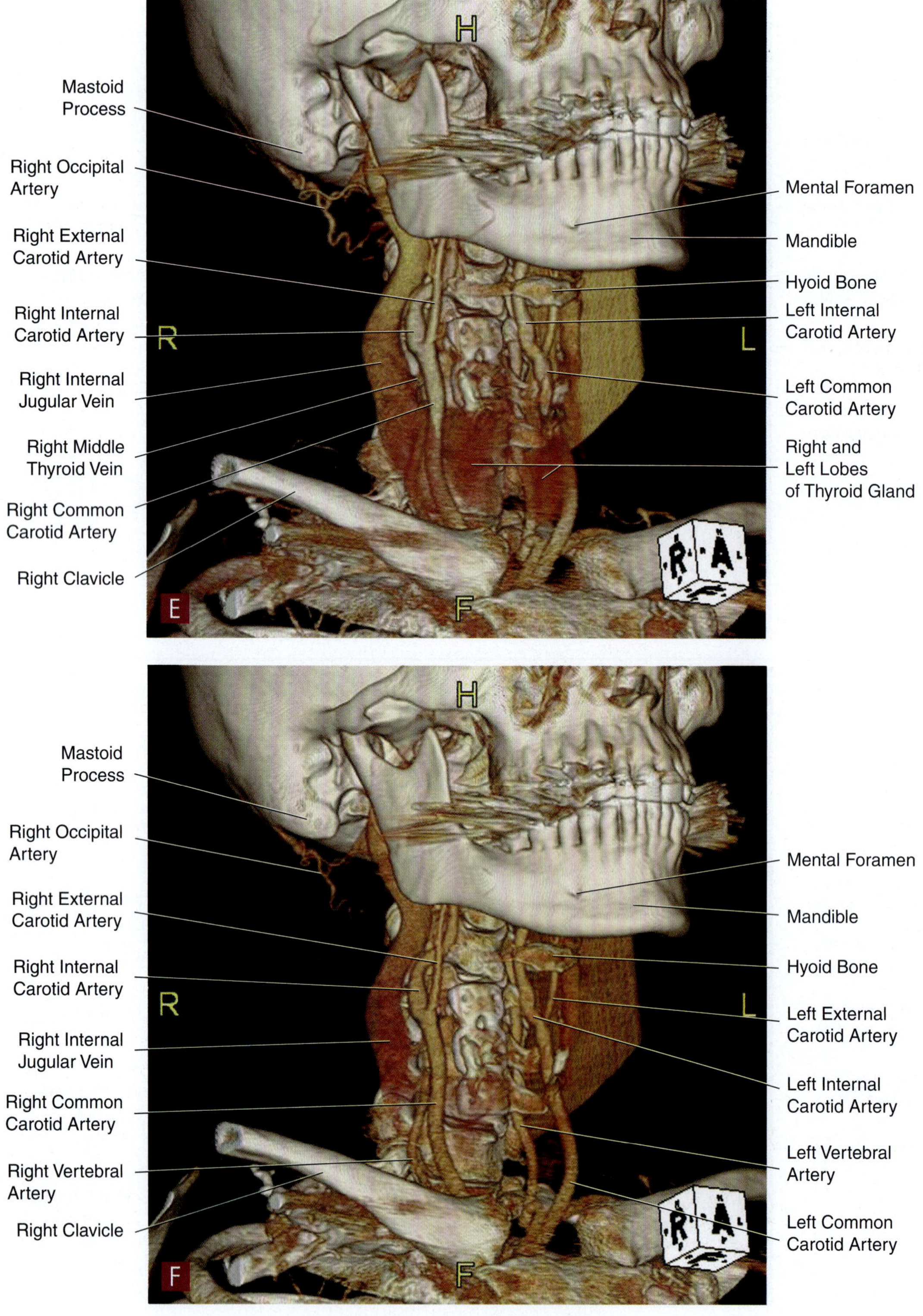

Figure 3.7. *Continued*

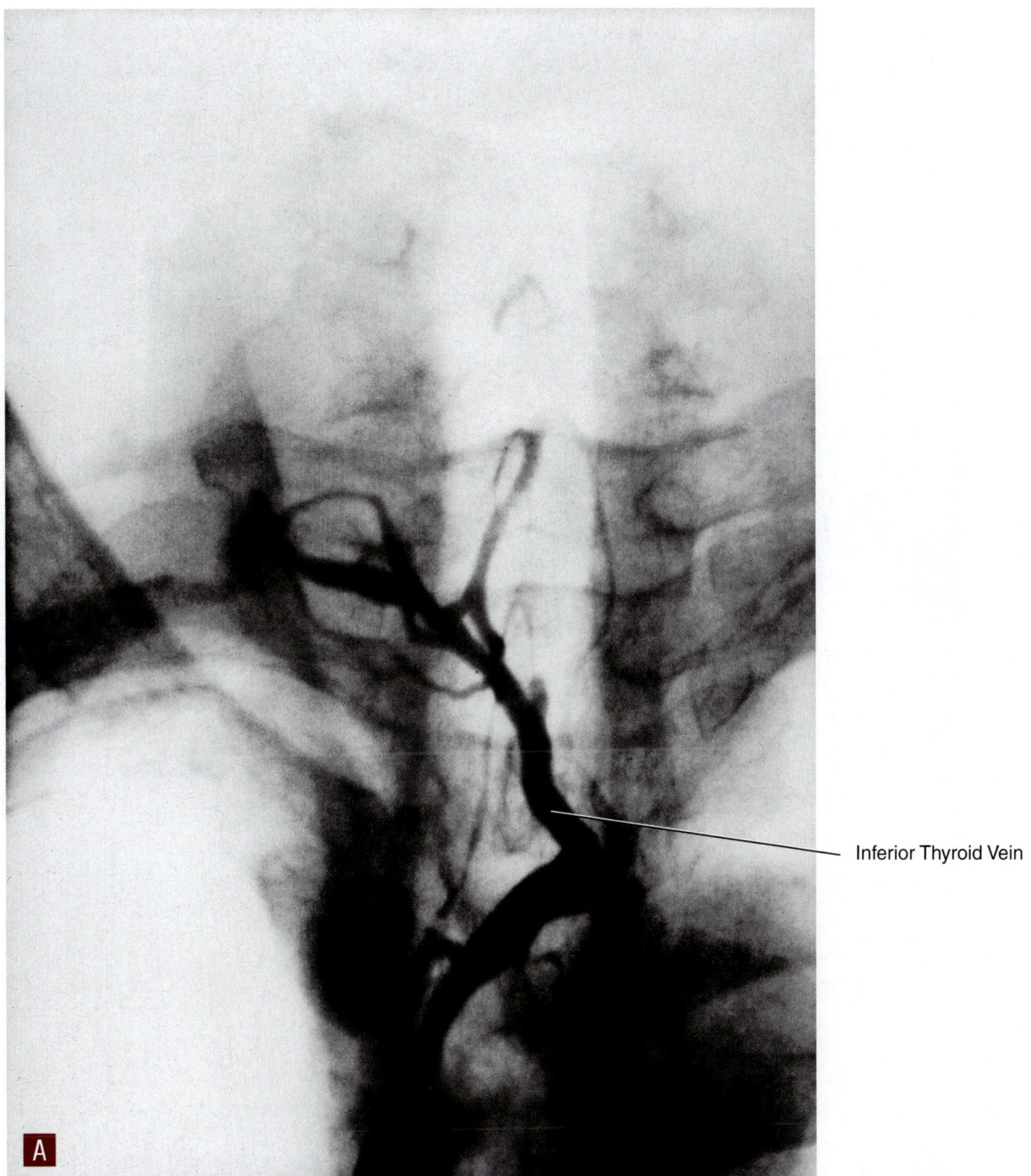

Figure 3.8. **A**, Selective injection into the inferior thyroid vein, partially filling the right middle thyroid vein retrograde. **B**, Selective injection into the left superior thyroid vein. Note filling of the middle thyroid vein and the inferior thyroid vein.

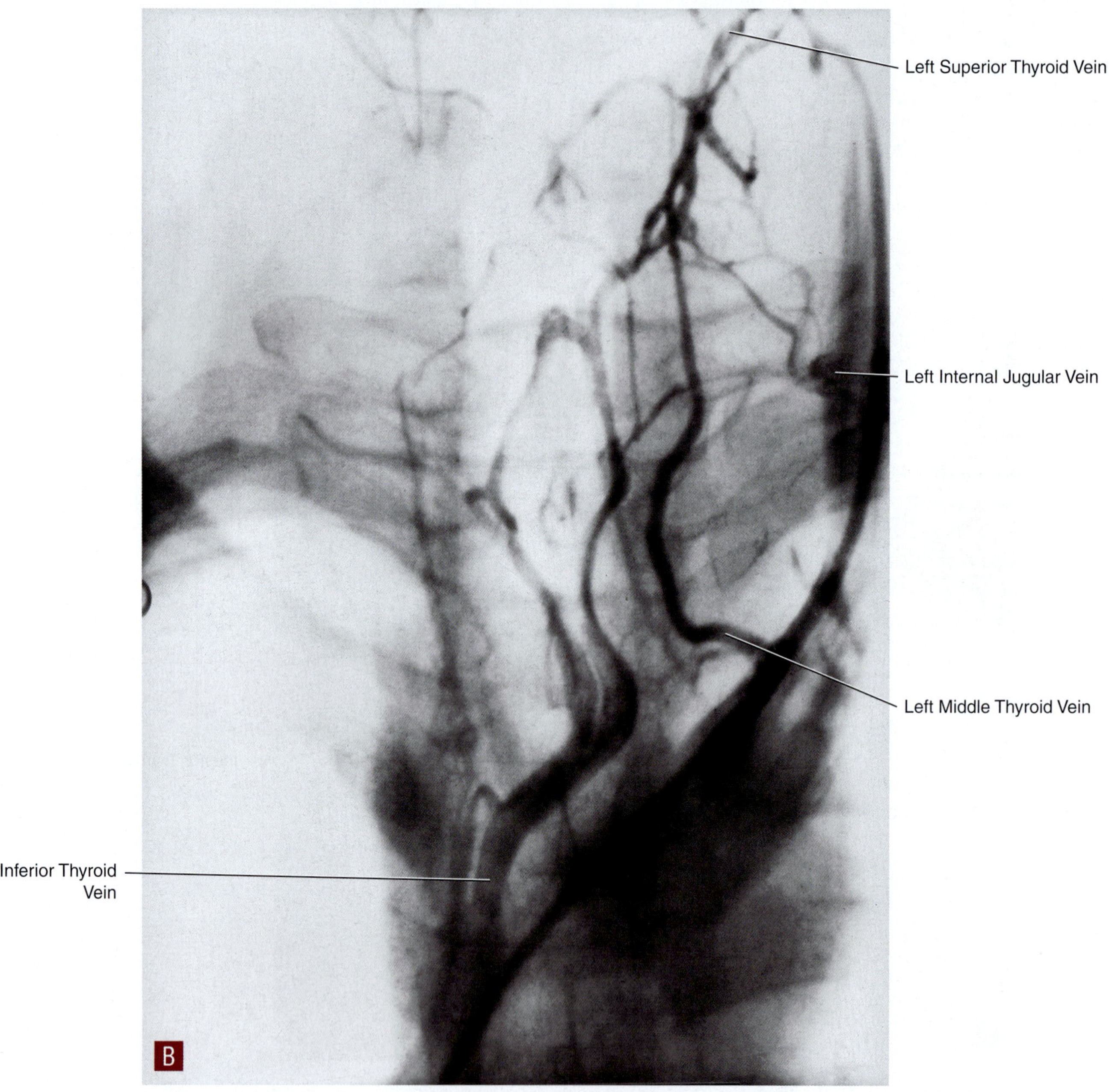

Figure 3.8. *Continued*

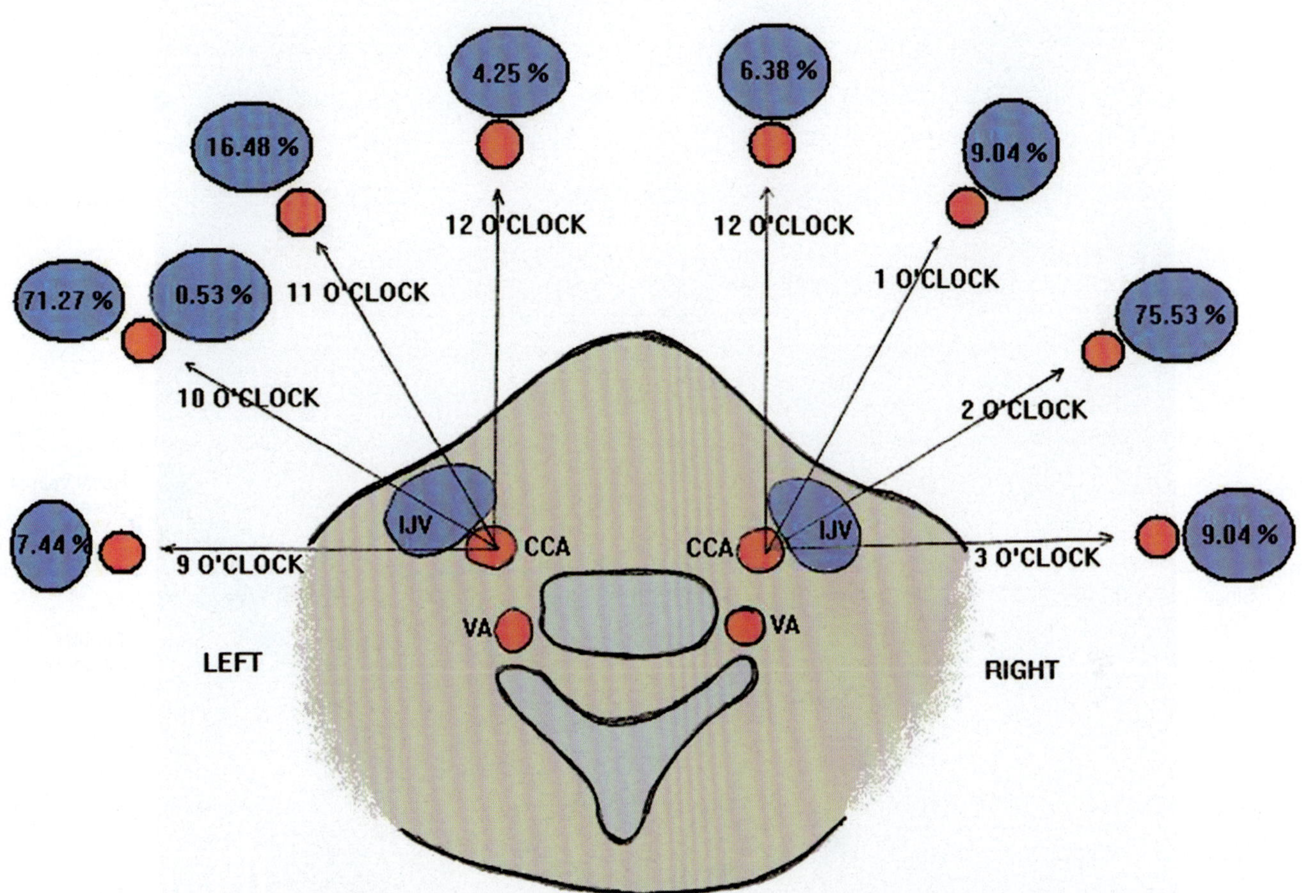

Figure 3.9. Illustration of the anatomic relationship of the internal jugular vein and the common carotid artery, viewed with the patient in the head-to-toe position, with the operator positioned at the head of the patient ready for internal jugular access. The distribution of the location of the internal jugular vein in relation to the artery is given in a clock-dial configuration and percentages shown as seen in 188 patients who were candidates for an internal jugular puncture. CCA, common carotid artery; VA, Vertebral artery.

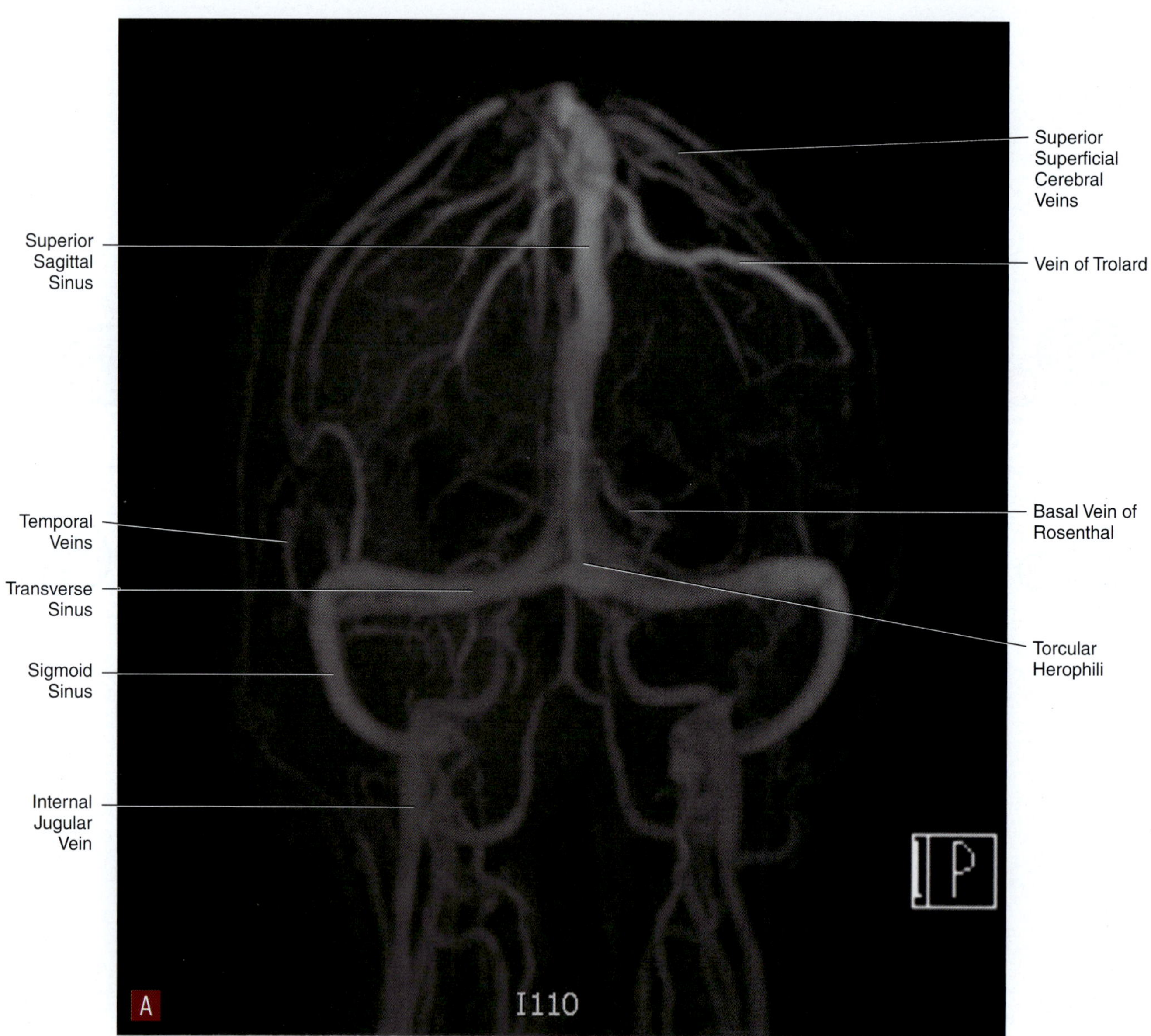

Figure 3.10. Time-of-flight magnetic resonance venogram (TOF-MRV) in the AP (A) and lateral (B) projections. Note the presence of a small amount of luminal signal from the arterial circulation.

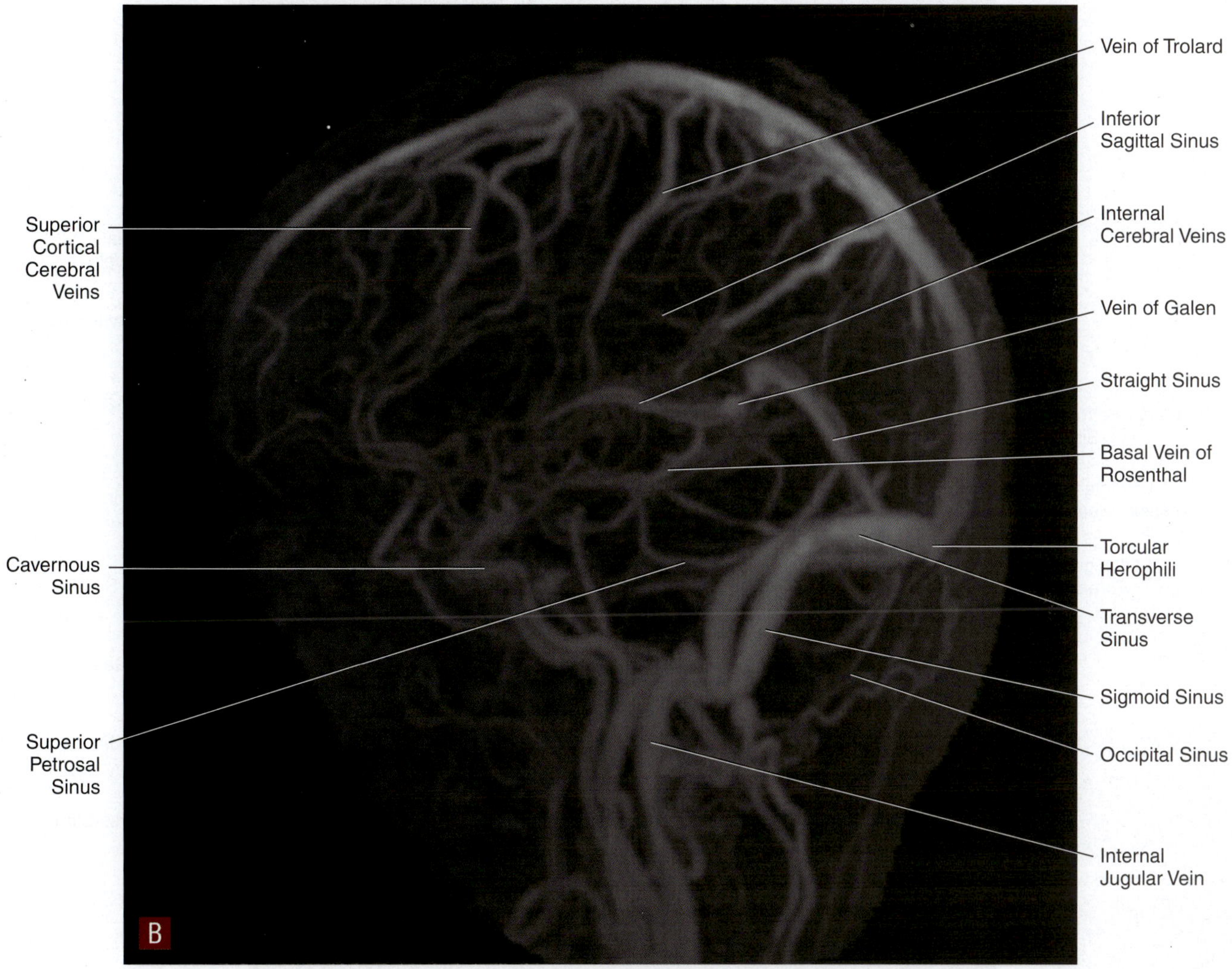

Superior Cortical Cerebral Veins
Cavernous Sinus
Superior Petrosal Sinus
Vein of Trolard
Inferior Sagittal Sinus
Internal Cerebral Veins
Vein of Galen
Straight Sinus
Basal Vein of Rosenthal
Torcular Herophili
Transverse Sinus
Sigmoid Sinus
Occipital Sinus
Internal Jugular Vein
B

Figure 3.10. *Continued*

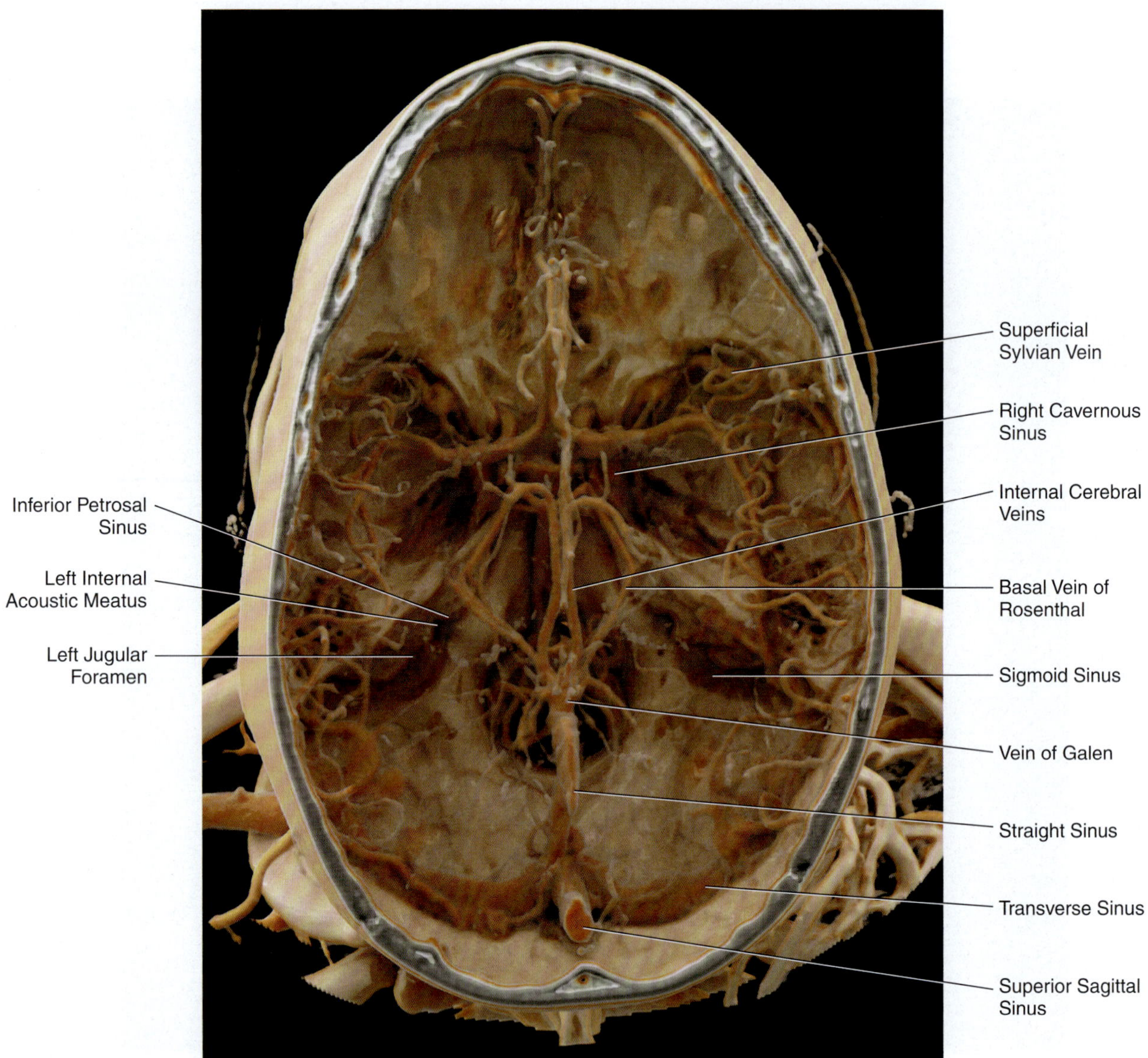

Figure 3.11. CT venogram cinematic 3D-rendered view of the skull base. The arterial and venous structures are seen with the same color because the contrast intensity in both the arteries and veins is of a similar density. This demonstrates the relationship of the large deep veins with their arterial counterparts in the skull base.

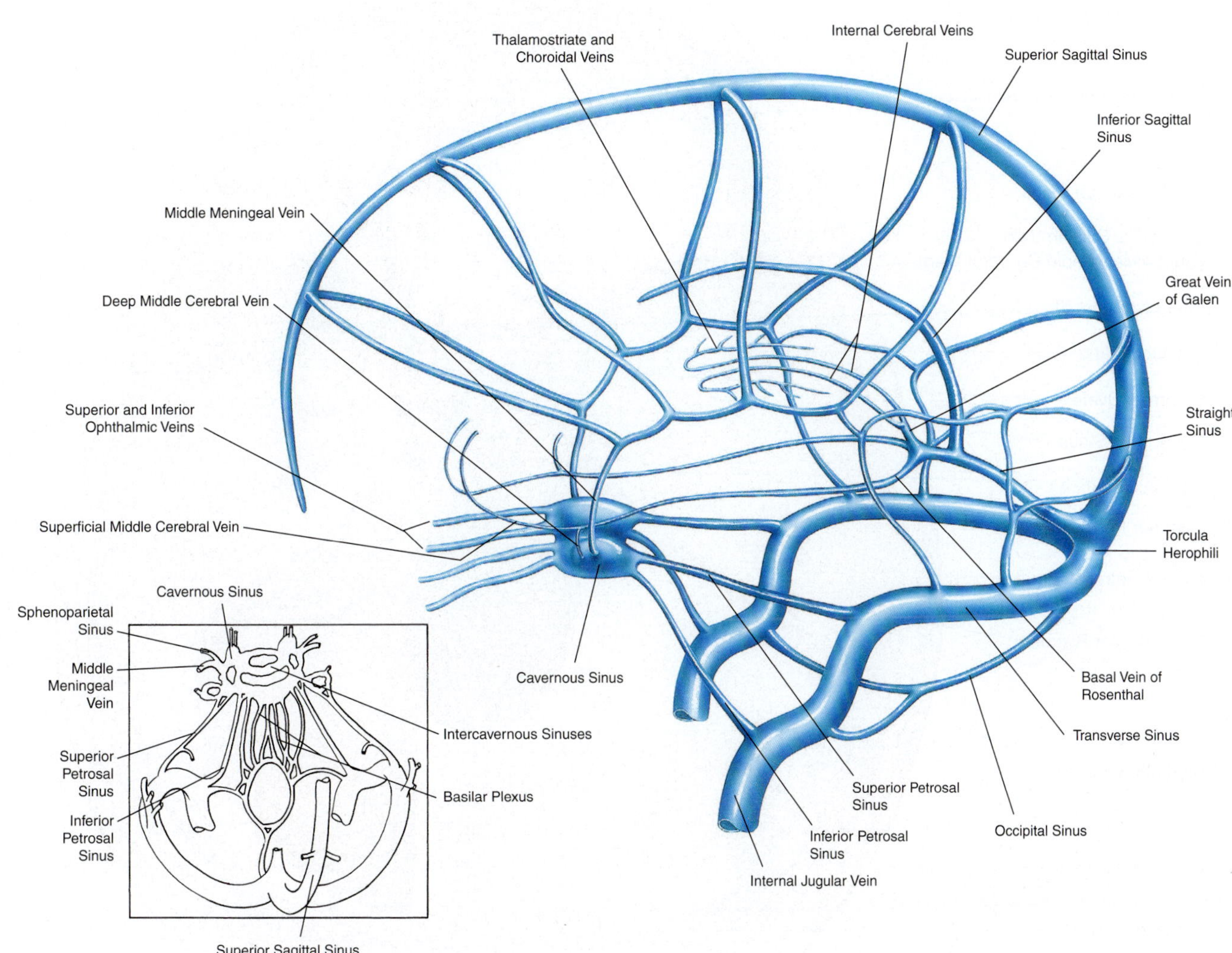

Figure 3.12. Illustration of the cerebral superficial and deep venous system.

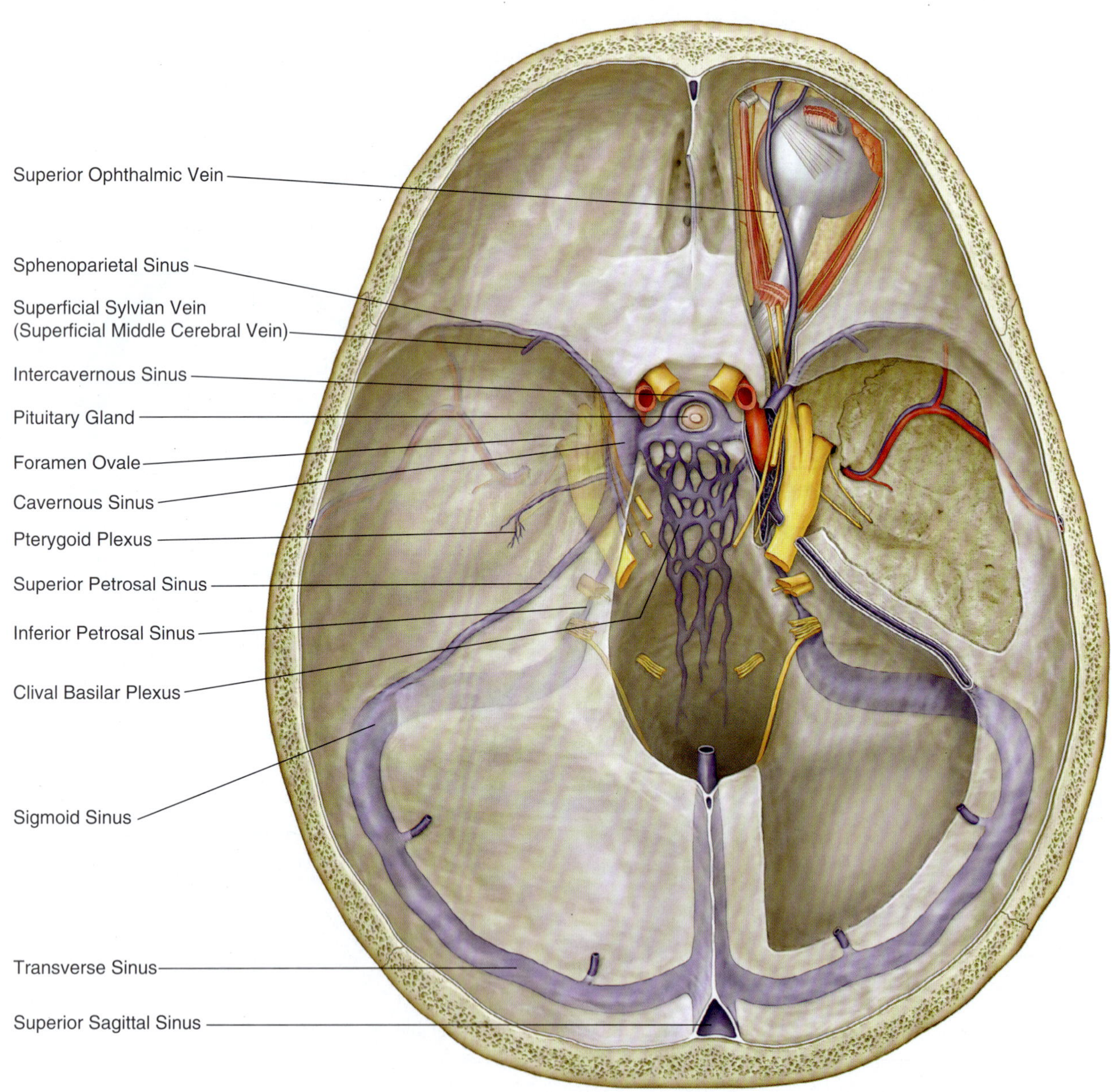

Figure 3.13. Illustration of the anatomic relationship of the cavernous sinus to the skull base venous drainage pathways.

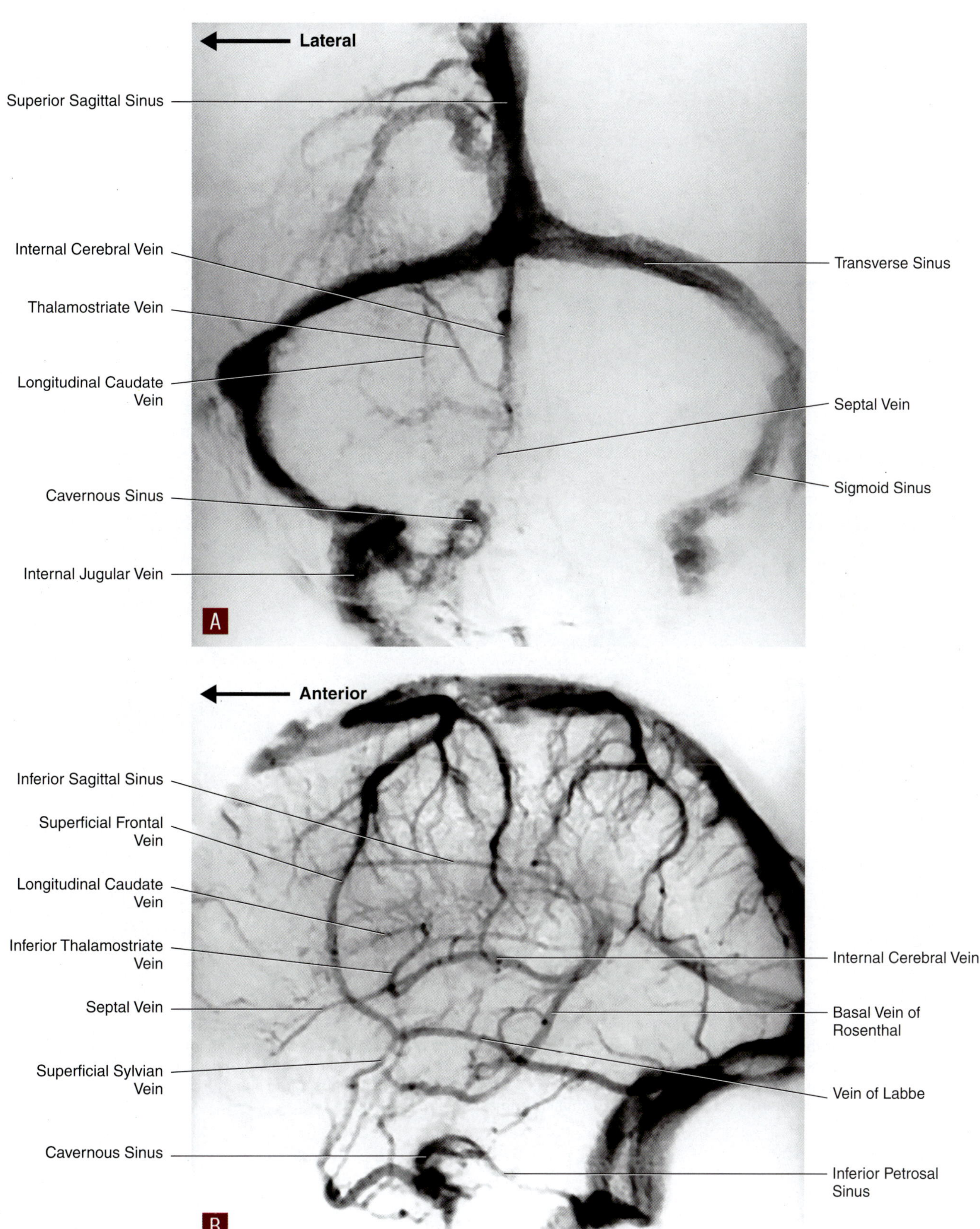

Figure 3.14. **Cerebral venous drainage.** Towne view (A) and lateral (B) projection DSA with injection of the internal carotid artery in the venous phase.

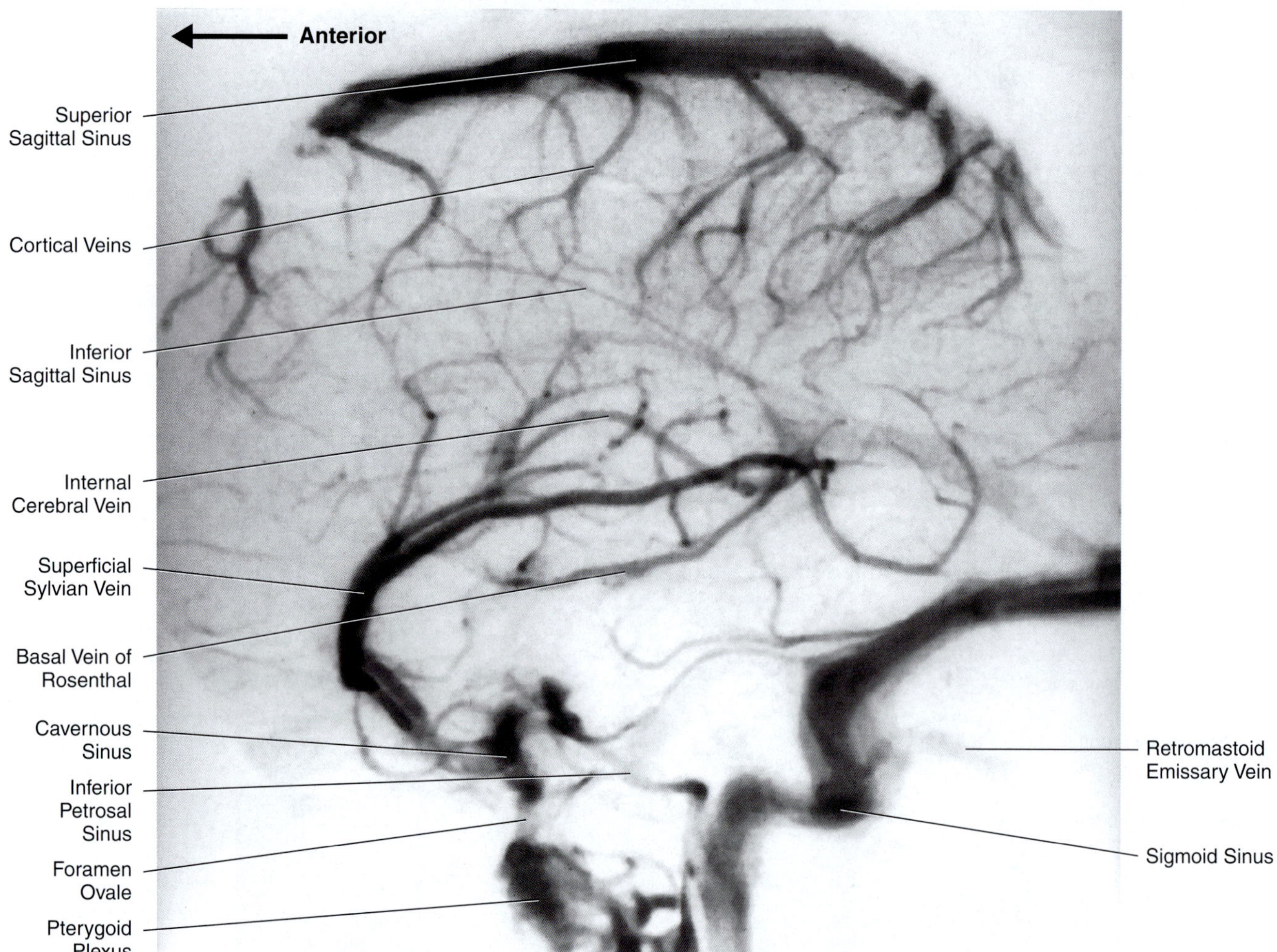

Figure 3.15. Prominent superficial sylvian venous drainage. Lateral projection DSA with injection of the internal carotid artery in the venous phase demonstrates a prominent superficial sylvian vein draining to the cavernous sinus, pterygoid plexus, and internal jugular vein via the inferior petrosal sinus. There is a small inferior sagittal sinus, more superior than usual internal cerebral vein, and a small retromastoid emissary vein.

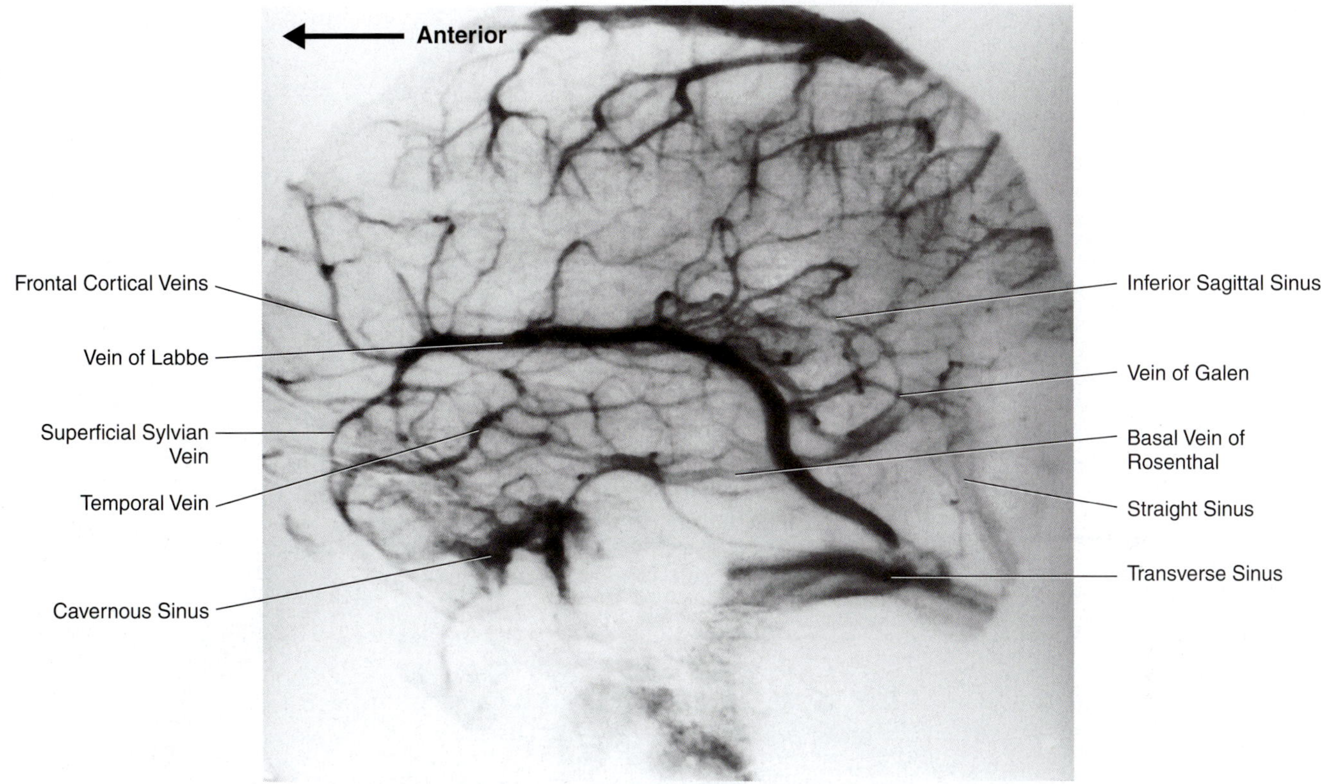

Figure 3.16. Dominant vein of Labbe. Lateral projection DSA with injection of the internal carotid artery in the venous phase demonstrates a prominent venous drainage into the vein of Labbe with frontal cortical veins seen draining into Labbe. Note the relatively decreased contrast opacification of the inferior sagittal sinus and straight sinus.

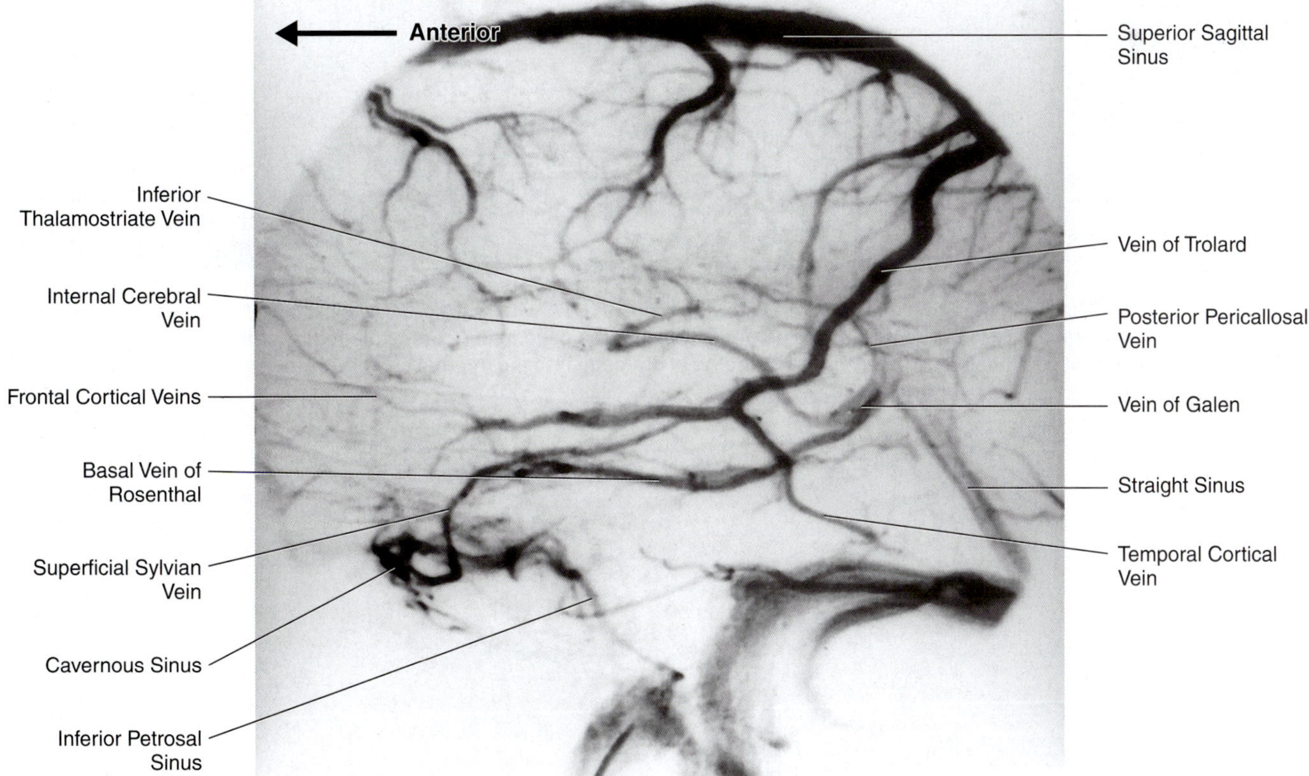

Figure 3.17. Dominand vein of Trolard. Lateral projection DSA with injection of the internal carotid artery in the venous phase demonstrates prominent venous drainage into the vein of Trolard draining into the superior sagittal sinus.

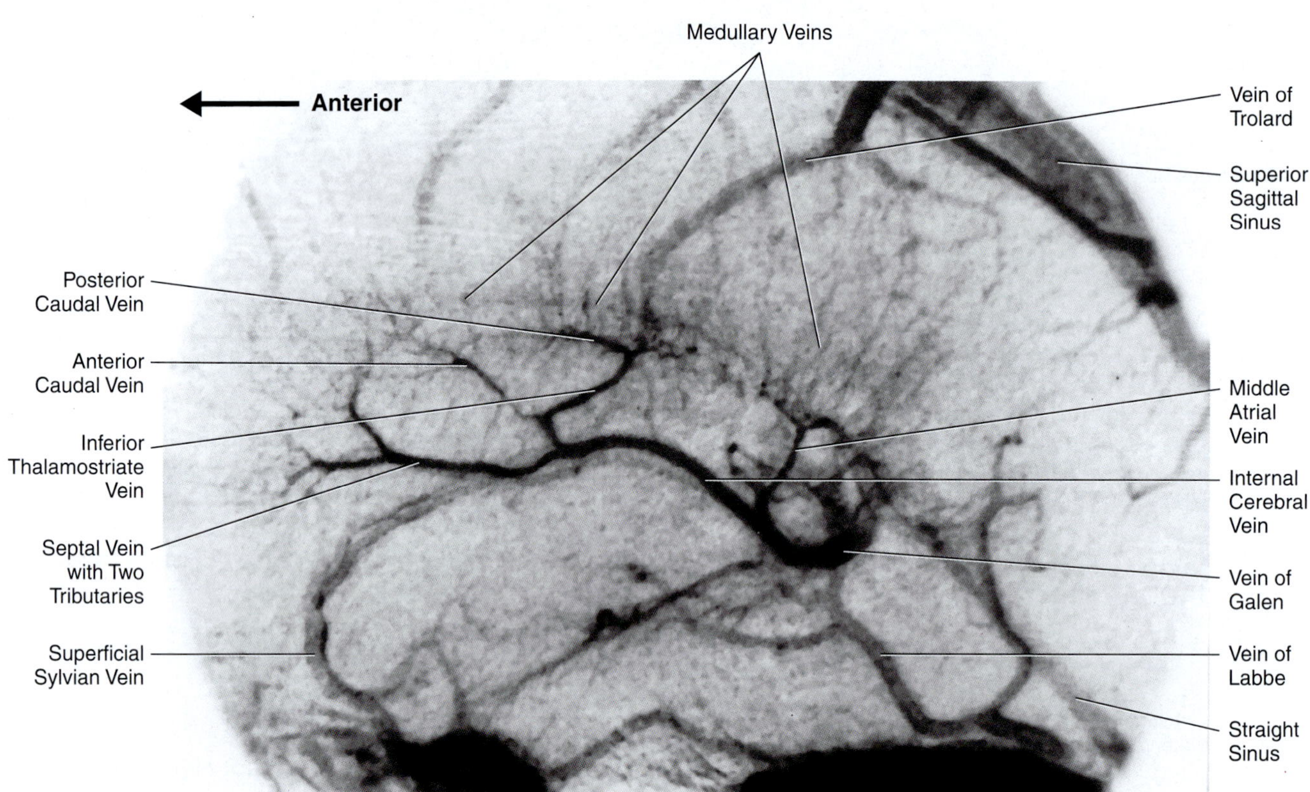

Figure 3.18. Medullary veins. Lateral projection DSA with injection of the internal carotid artery in the venous phase demonstrates the drainage pattern of the medullary veins, septal vein, thalamostriate vein, and atrial vein drainage into the internal cerebral veins.

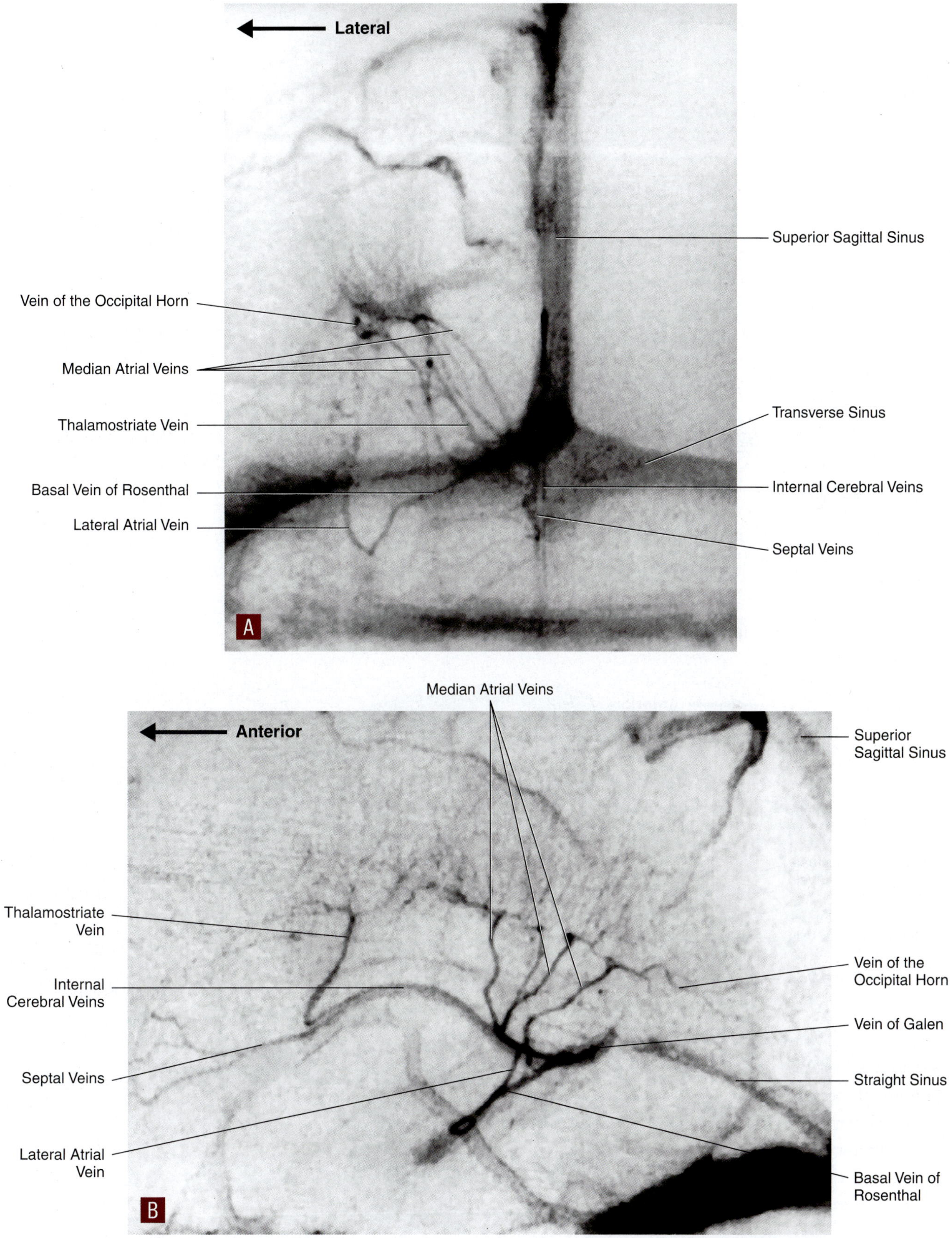

Lateral
Superior Sagittal Sinus
Vein of the Occipital Horn
Median Atrial Veins
Thalamostriate Vein
Transverse Sinus
Basal Vein of Rosenthal
Internal Cerebral Veins
Lateral Atrial Vein
Septal Veins
A

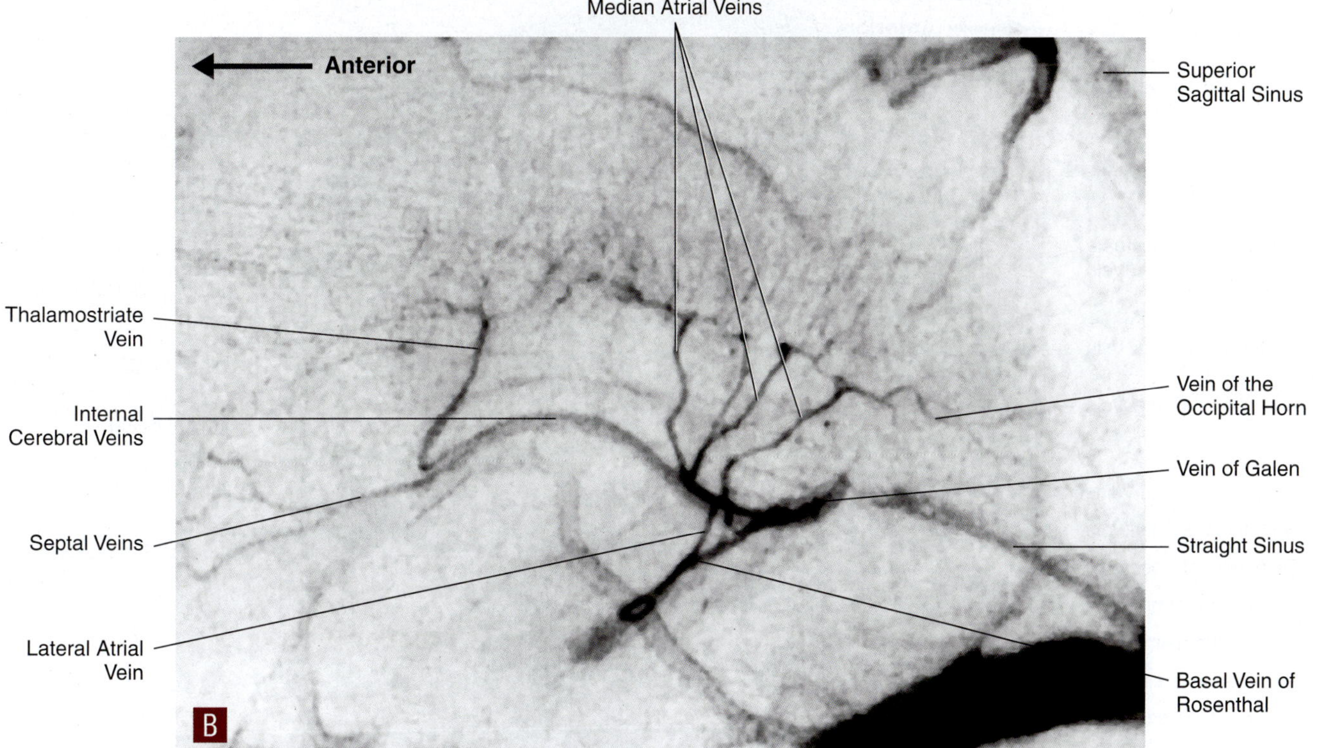

Figure 3.19. Deep venous system. Frontal (A) and lateral (B) projection DSA with injection of the internal carotid artery in the venous phase demonstrates the septal, median atrial, thalamostriate, basal vein of Rosenthal, and internal cerebral veins.

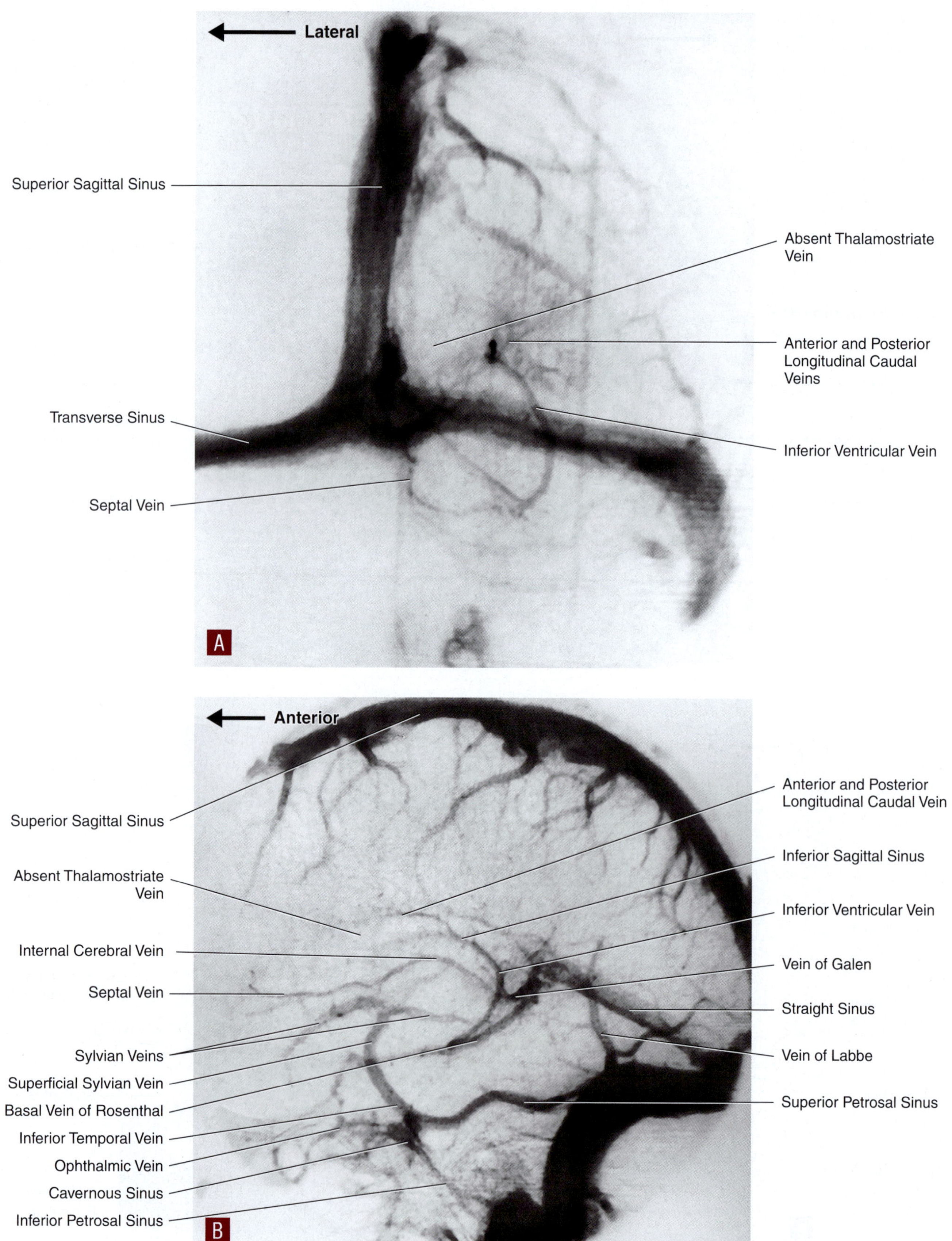

Figure 3.20. Deep venous system with an absent thalamostriate vein and dominant superficial Sylvian vein. Frontal (A) and lateral (B) projection DSA with injection of the internal carotid artery in the venous phase demonstrates the longitudinal caudal vein and inferior ventricular vein that is more pronounced with the absence of the thalamostriate vein. The lateral demonstrates the dominant superficial sylvian pattern draining through the inferior temporal vein to a large superior petrosal sinus.

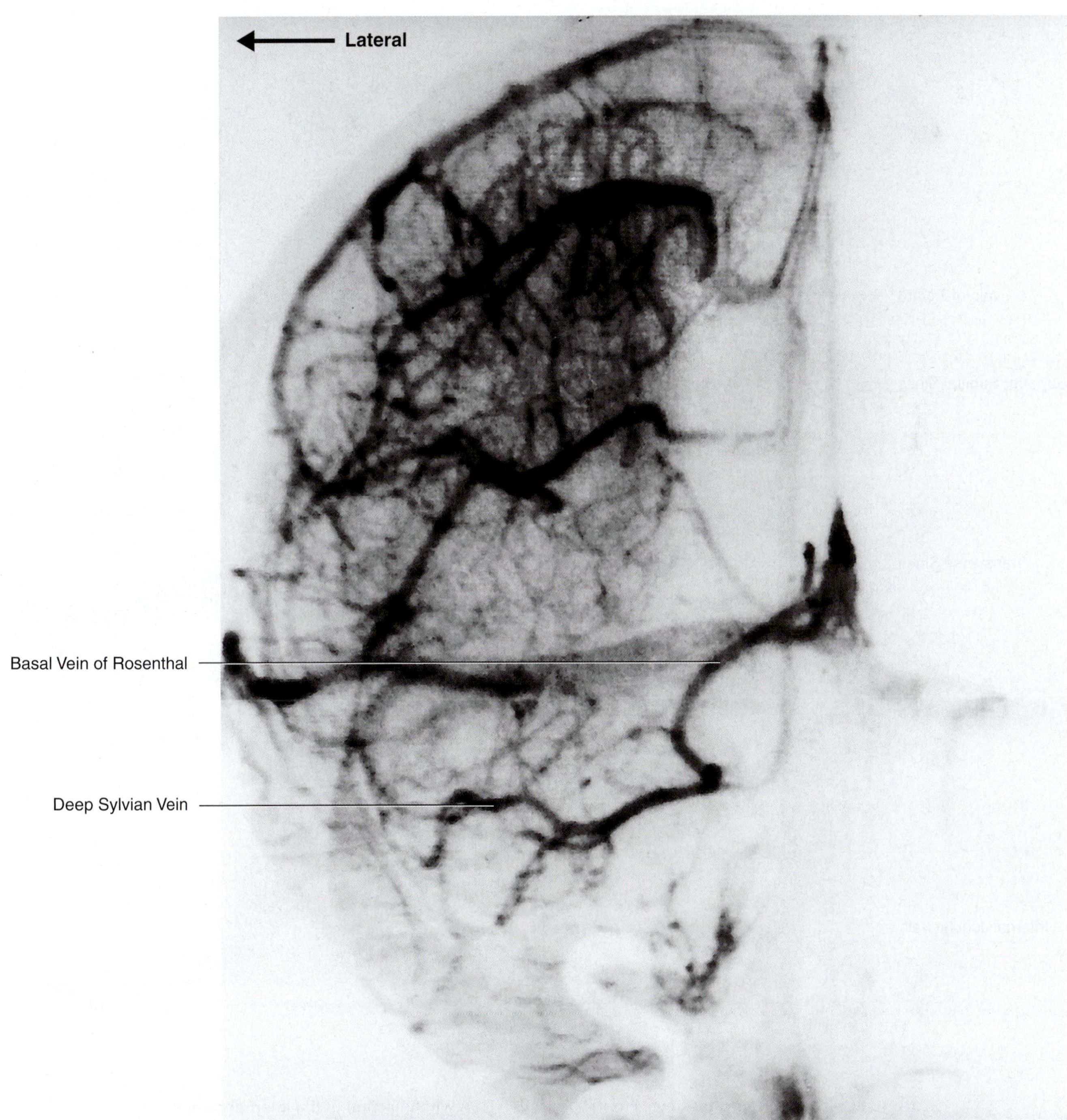

Figure 3.21. Towne view of the Basal Vein of Rosenthal. Towne view DSA with injection of the internal carotid artery in the venous phase demonstrating the typical curve of the basal vein of Rosenthal around the cerebral trunk.

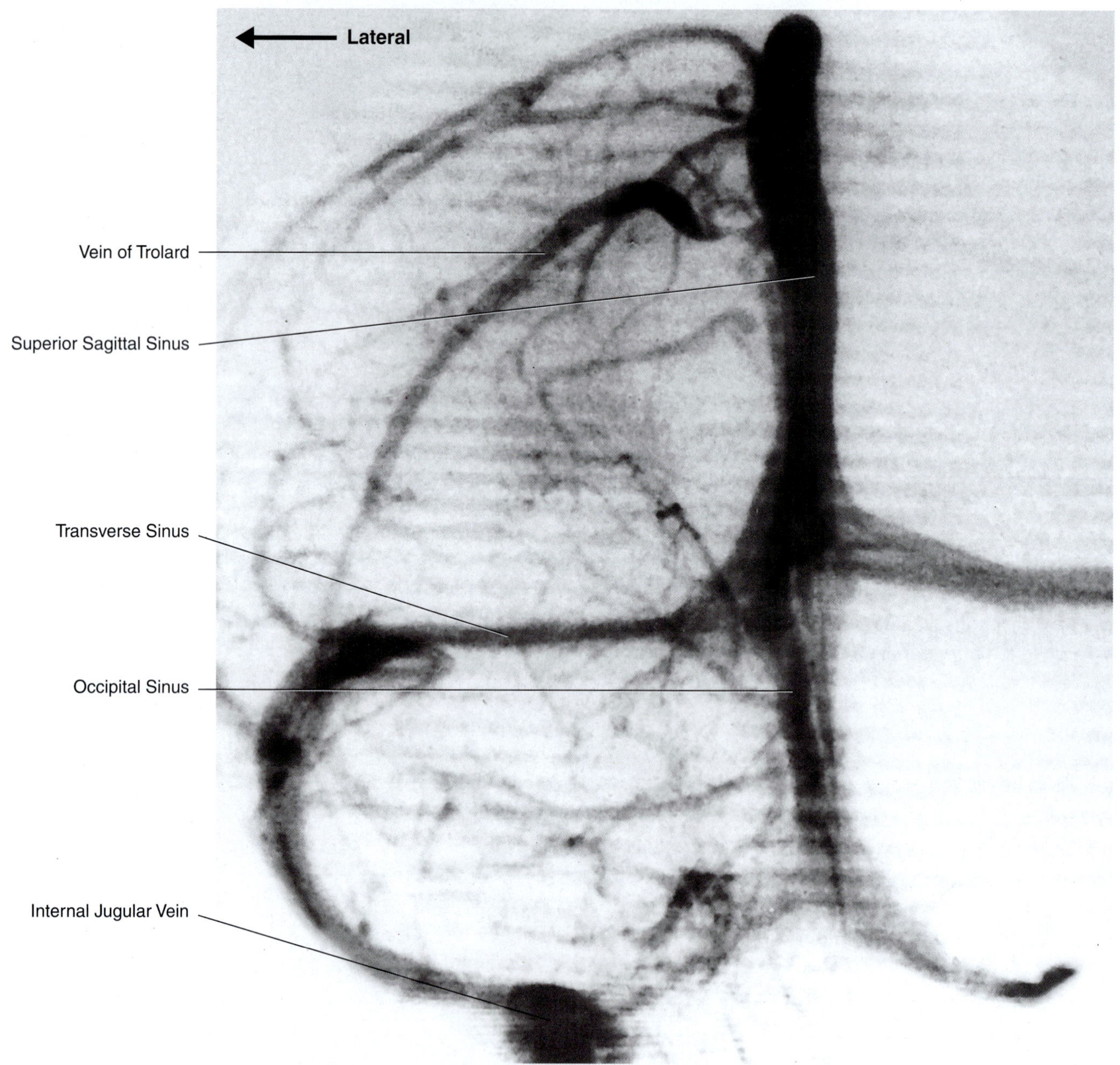

Figure 3.22. Occipital sinus. Frontal projection DSA with injection of the internal carotid artery in the venous phase demonstrating an occipital sinus draining into the internal jugular veins.

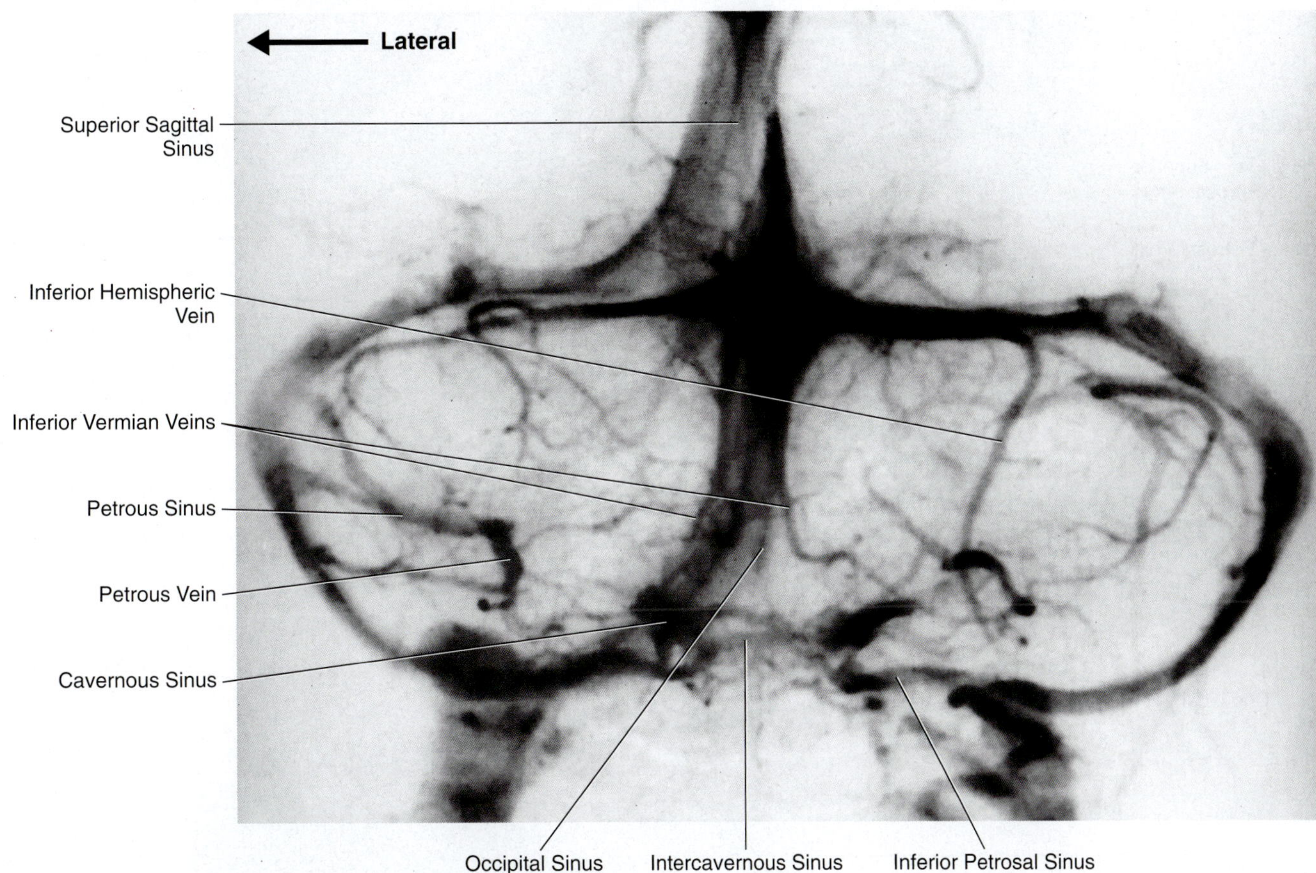

Figure 3.23. Posterior circulation venous system. Towne view DSA with injection of the vertebral artery in the venous phase. Note the inferior hemispheric vein, inferior vermian veins, petrous sinus, petrous vein, cavernous sinus and inferior petrosal sinuses.

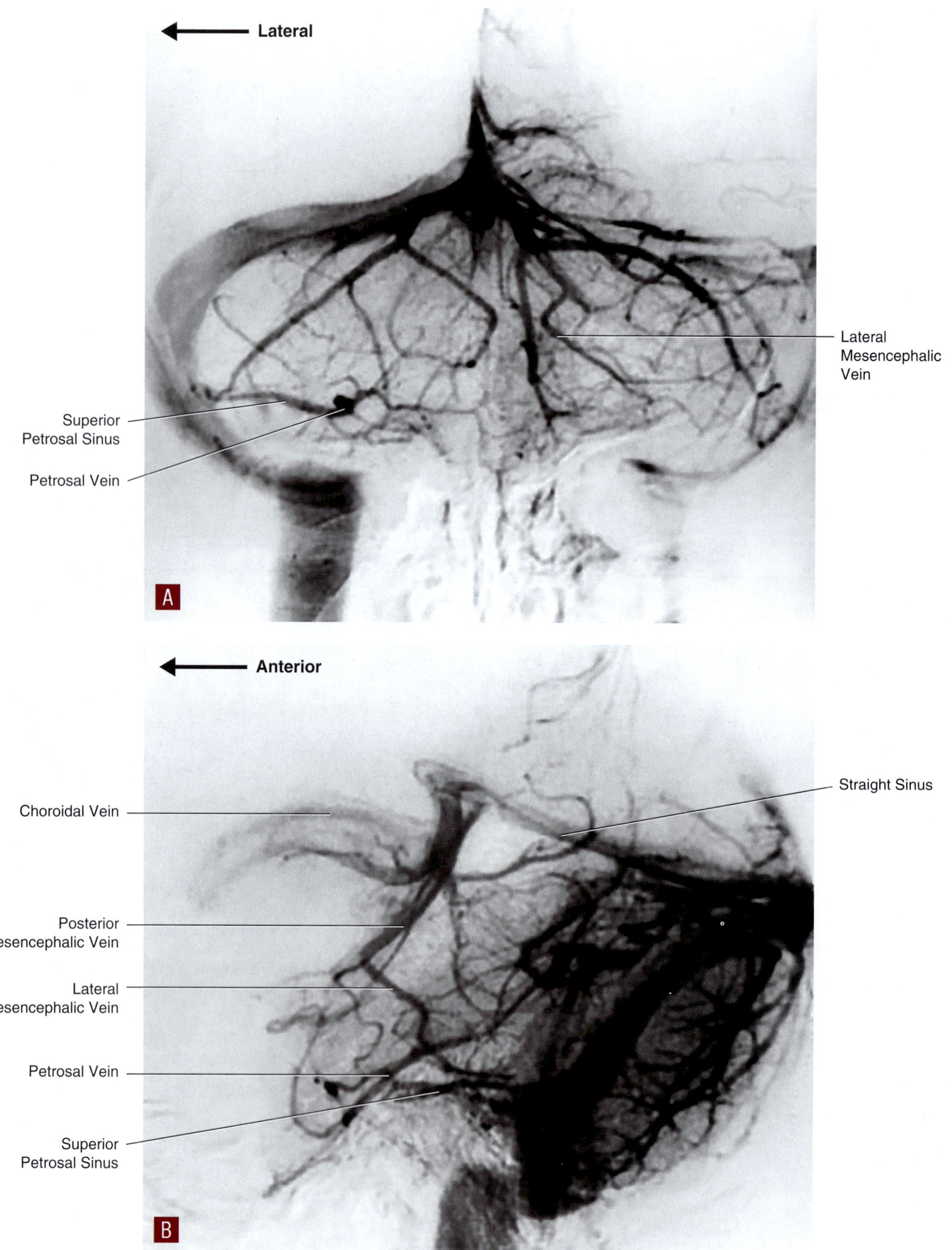

Figure 3.24. Posterior circulation venous system. Frontal (A) and lateral (B) DSA with injection of the vertebral artery in the venous phase.

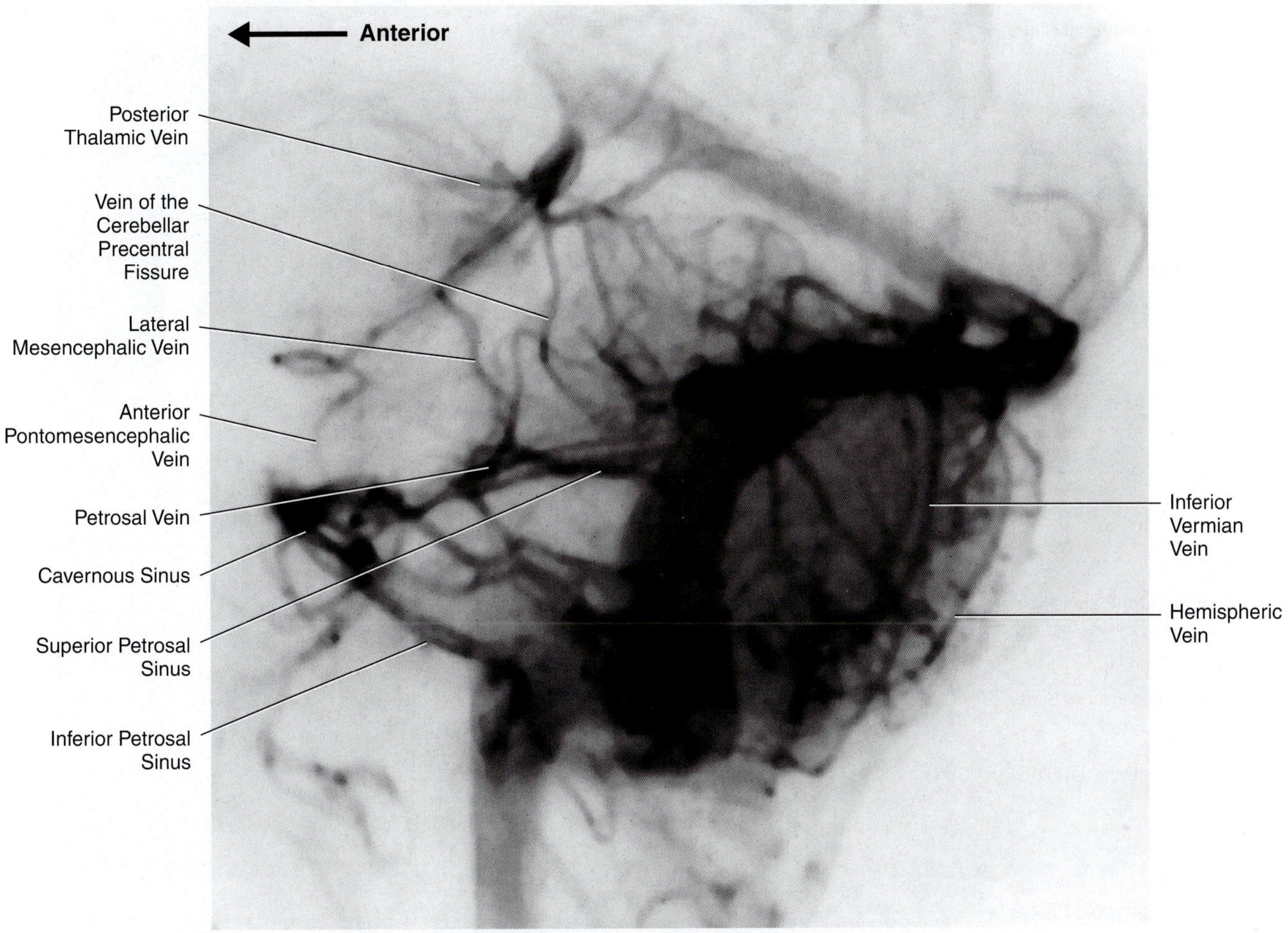

Anterior

Posterior Thalamic Vein

Vein of the Cerebellar Precentral Fissure

Lateral Mesencephalic Vein

Anterior Pontomesencephalic Vein

Petrosal Vein

Cavernous Sinus

Superior Petrosal Sinus

Inferior Petrosal Sinus

Inferior Vermian Vein

Hemispheric Vein

Figure 3.25. Posterior circulation venous system. Lateral projection DSA with injection of the vertebral artery in the venous phase demonstrating the mesencephalic and cerebellar veins.

Lateral

Cavernous Sinus

Intercavernous Sinus

Clival Basilar Plexus

Inferior Petrosal Sinus

Foramen Ovale

Pterygoid Plexus

Internal Jugular Vein

A

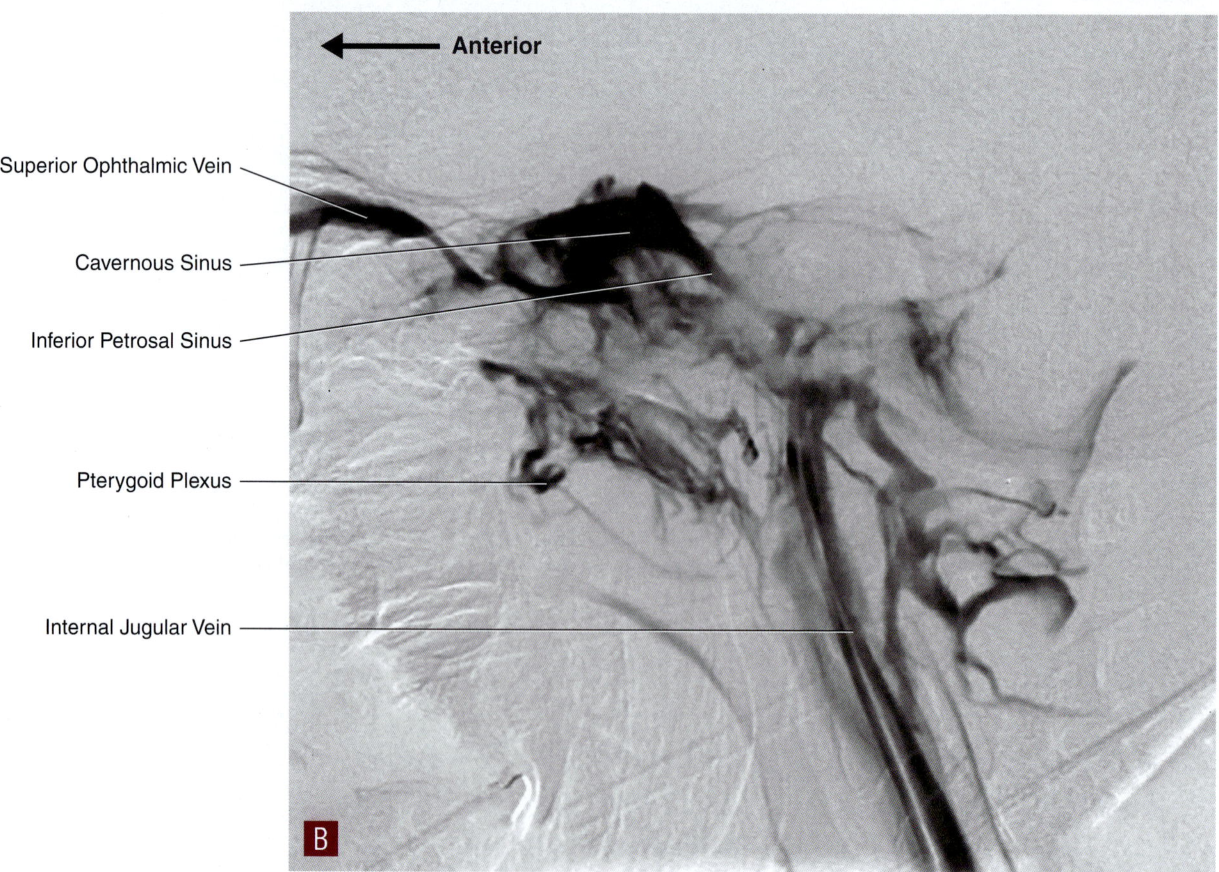

Figure 3.26. Petrosal sinuses. Frontal (A) and lateral (B) projection DSA with injection of the inferior petrosal sinus in the venous phase demonstrates retrograde filling of the intercavernous sinuses and pterygoid plexus

4

Lymphatic System of the Head and Neck

The lymph nodes of the head and neck comprise a terminal group and a number of intermediary groups. The terminal group is associated with the carotid sheath and is also called the deep cervical group. The lymphatic vessels of the head and neck drain into the cervical group, directly or indirectly. The efferents from the deep cervical lymph nodes comprise what is called the jugular trunk (Fig. 4.1).

Deep Cervical Lymph Nodes

These are the nodes located along the carotid sheath. They are divided into superior and inferior groups.

Upper Deep Cervical Lymph Nodes

These lymph nodes drain into the upper part of the internal jugular vein. Efferents from this group pass to the lower deep cervical group and extend to the jugular trunk. The jugulodigastric group of nodes is related to the drainage of the tongue.

Lower Deep Cervical Lymph Nodes

These lymph nodes are partly deep to the lower sternocleidomastoid and extend into the subclavian triangle. The jugulo-omohyoid lymph node of this group drains the tongue. The efferents from the lower deep cervical lymph nodes join the jugular trunk.

Lymphatic Drainage of the Superficial Tissues of the Head and Neck

There are several groups of lymph nodes concerned with the drainage of the superficial tissues of the head and neck. Most of the superficial tissues are drained by lymphatic vessels that drain into the neighboring groups of nodes and the efferents of which drain into the deep cervical lymph nodes.

The regional groups are as follows (Fig. 4.1):

In the Head

Occipital lymph nodes
Retroauricular (mastoid) lymph nodes
Parotid lymph nodes
Buccal (facial) lymph nodes

In the Neck

Submandibular lymph nodes
Submental lymph nodes
Anterior cervical lymph nodes
Superficial cervical lymph nodes

Lymphatic Drainage of the Scalp and Ear (Fig. 4.2)

The lymphatic vessels from the forehead, the temporal region, and the upper half of the lateral surface of the auricle and the anterior wall of the external acoustic meatus drain through the superficial parotid lymph nodes. These nodes are located in front of the tragus or on the fascia of the parotid gland and also drain the lymph from the eyelids and the skin over the zygomatic bone area. The efferents drain into the upper deep cervical lymph nodes.

The posterior aspect of the auricle and the scalp on the lateral aspect of the skull drain to the upper deep cervical lymph nodes, and some part of it drains to the retroauricular group of lymph nodes.

The retroauricular lymph nodes are superficial to the sternocleidomastoid attachment on the mastoid. The efferents drain into the upper deep cervical lymph nodes. The lobule of the auricle, the inferior meatus, and the skin over the angle of the mandible are drained by vessels that go to the superficial cervical lymph nodes or to the upper deep cervical lymph nodes.

The superficial cervical lymph nodes are located along the external jugular vein, superficial to the sternocleidomastoid. Some of the efferents of this group may join the upper deep cervical lymph nodes, and some join the lower deep cervical lymph nodes.

The occipital region is drained partly to the occipital group of lymph nodes and partly by a trunk along the posterior border of the sternocleidomastoid, which extends to the lower deep cervical lymph nodes.

Lymphatic Drainage of the Face (Fig. 4.2)

There is a lymphatic plexus in the face—including the frontal scalp, the superior and inferior eyelids, and the conjunctiva—the caruncula lacrimalis, which also drains to the superficial parotid lymph nodes and to the deep parotid lymph nodes. The more medial and inferior lymphatics follow the course of the facial vein and terminate in the submandibular group of lymph nodes.

The submandibular group of lymph nodes is located under the deep cervical fascia in the region of the submandibular gland. These nodes receive afferents from the submental, buccal, and lingual group of lymph nodes. The efferents drain into the upper and lower deep cervical lymph nodes.

The external nose, cheek and upper lip, and lateral part of the lower lip drain to the submandibular nodes. The central part of the lower lip, the floor of the mouth, and the tip of the tongue drain into the submental group of lymph nodes. This group of lymph nodes is located on the mylohyoid between the anterior bellies of the two digastric muscles. These nodes receive afferents from both sides. Efferents go to the submandibular and jugulo-omohyoid nodes.

The lymphatic drainage of the eyelid follows a path that drains into the preauricular and submandibular lymph nodes. The outer canthus usually drains into the preauricular lymph node, whereas the inner canthus drains into the submandibular lymph node. Inferior eyelid lymphatics may drain into either preauricular or submandibular lymph nodes. The efferents of these nodes drain into the upper and lower deep cervical lymph nodes (Fig. 4.3).

Lymphatic Drainage of the Superficial Tissues of the Neck

Many of the vessels draining the superficial tissues of the neck go to the upper or lower deep cervical lymph nodes. Some of these vessels drain into the superficial cervical and occipital lymph nodes.

Lymphatic Drainage of the Deeper Tissues of the Neck

The deeper tissues of the head and neck drain to the deep cervical lymph nodes directly or indirectly through one of the aforementioned groups. There are additional groups of lymph nodes concerned with the drainage of the deeper tissues, including the retropharyngeal lymph nodes, paratracheal lymph nodes, lingual lymph nodes, infrahyoid lymph nodes, and prelaryngeal and pretracheal lymph nodes.

Lymphatic Drainage of the Nasal Cavity, Nasopharynx, and Middle Ear

The lymphatic drainage of the anterior nasal cavity is through the vessels that drain the skin over the nose to the submandibular nodes. The remaining nasal cavity, paranasal tissues, nasopharynx, and pharyngeal end of the auditory tube drain to the upper deep cervical nodes directly or through the retropharyngeal lymph nodes.

Lymphatic Drainage of the Larynx, Trachea, and Thyroid Gland

There is an upper and a lower group of lymph vessels at the larynx divided by the vocal fold. The two systems anastomose on the posterior wall.

There is a dense lymphatic network in the wall of the trachea. The cervical portion is drained to the pretracheal and paratracheal nodes or directly to the nodes of the lower deep cervical group.

The thyroid gland is drained mainly to the tracheal plexus. Laterally, the gland is drained to the deep cervical lymph nodes, while some vessels may enter the thoracic duct directly.

Lymphatic Drainage of the Mouth, Teeth, Tonsil, and Tongue

The lymphatic vessels of the mouth drain to the submandibular lymph nodes, upper deep cervical lymph nodes, and retropharyngeal lymph nodes.

The teeth drain to the submandibular and deep cervical lymph nodes. The tonsil lymph vessels drain into the upper deep cervical lymph nodes. The tongue has a widely distributed lymphatic drainage but drains mainly to the anterior or middle submandibular lymph nodes, but also to the jugulo-omohyoid lymph node and jugulodigastric lymph nodes.

Lymphatic Drainage of the Pharynx and Cervical Esophagus

The pharynx and cervical esophagus drain to the deep cervical nodes directly or indirectly through the retropharyngeal and paratracheal nodes. From the epiglottis, the lymph vessels drain to the infrahyoid nodes.

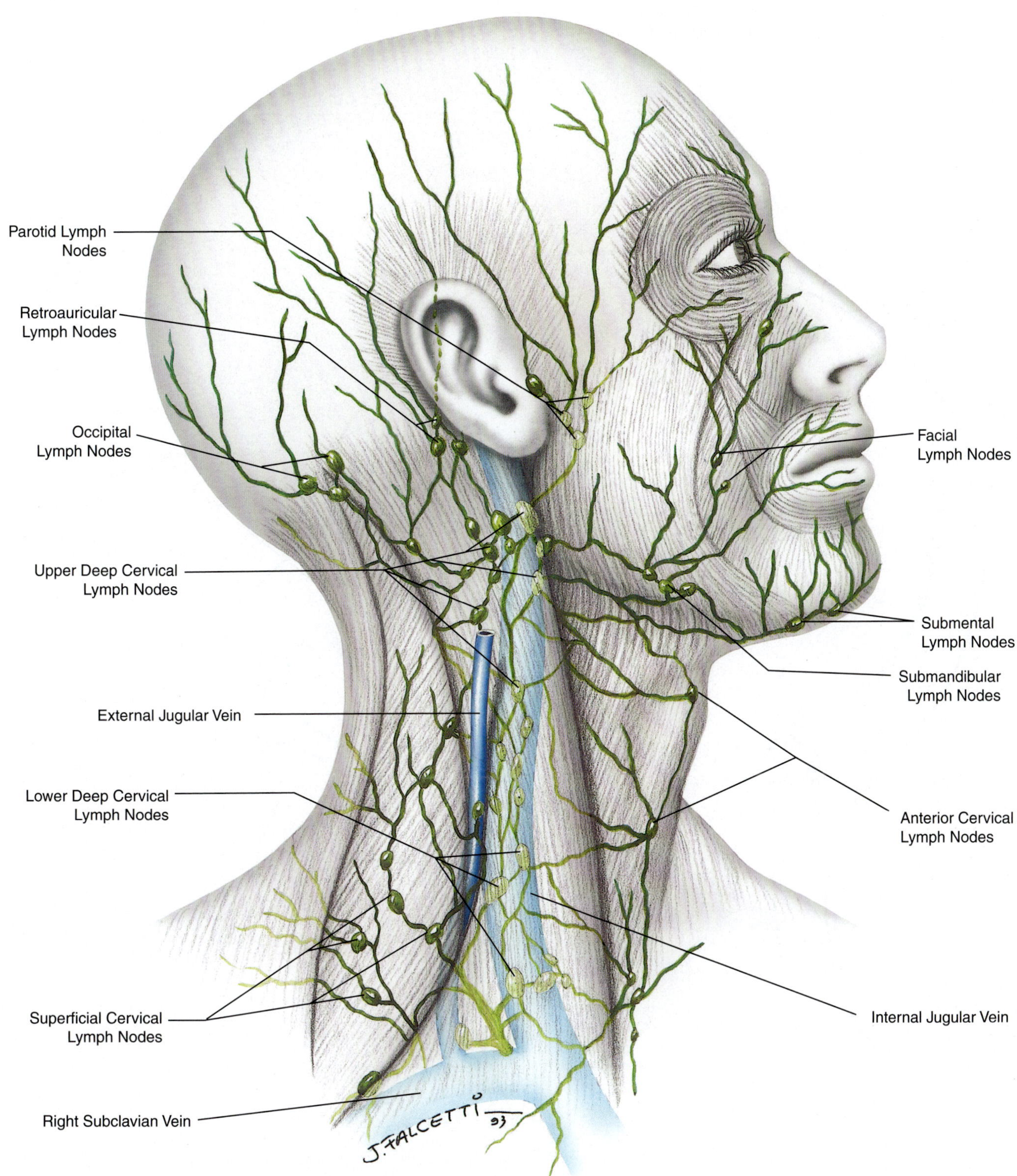

Figure 4.1. Lymphatic vessels and lymph nodes of the head and neck. Note the importance of the upper deep cervical lymph nodes and the lower deep cervical lymph nodes for the drainage of the face, scalp, and neck.

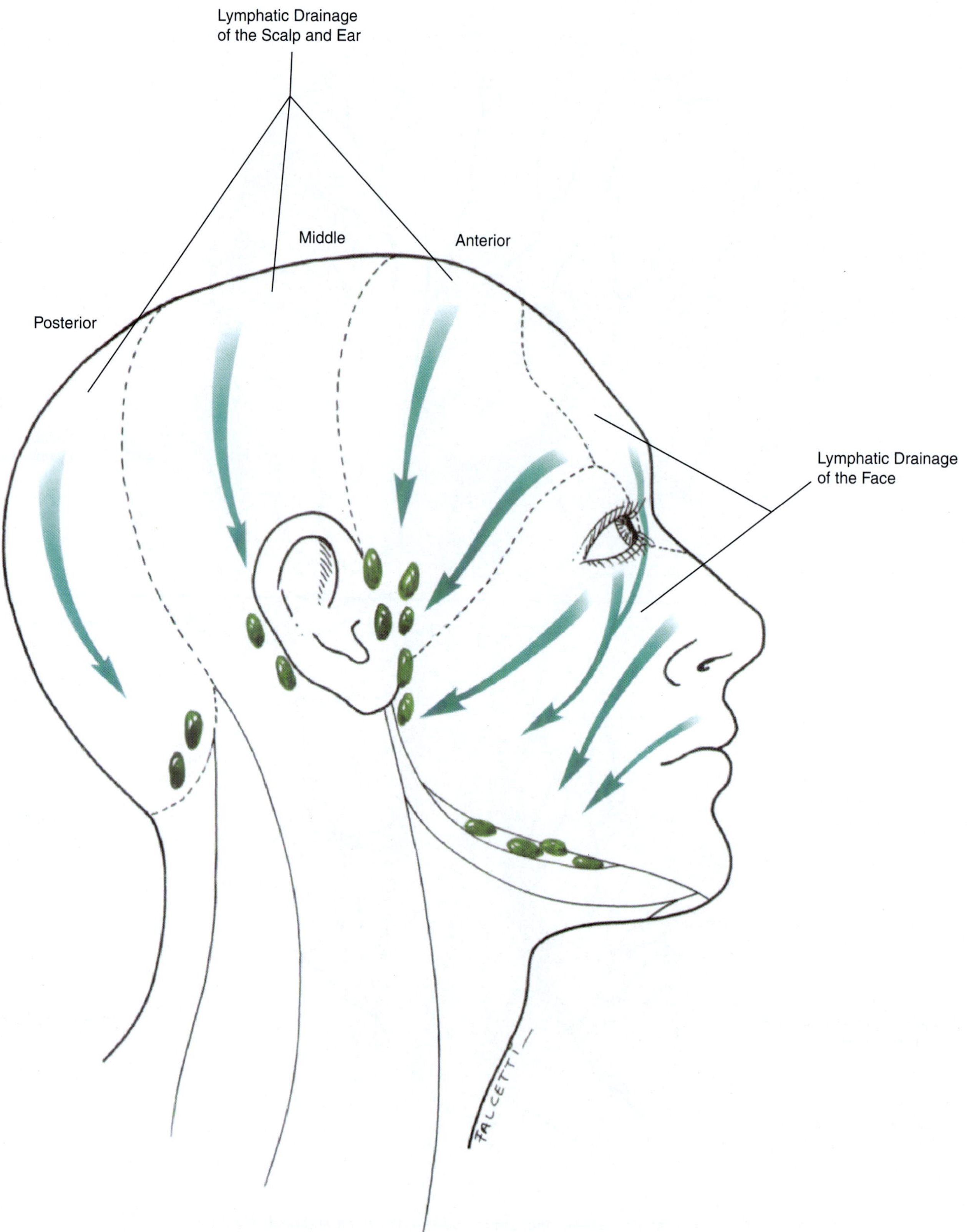

Figure 4.2. Main lymphatic drainage zones of the scalp and ear, and of the face and frontal scalp.

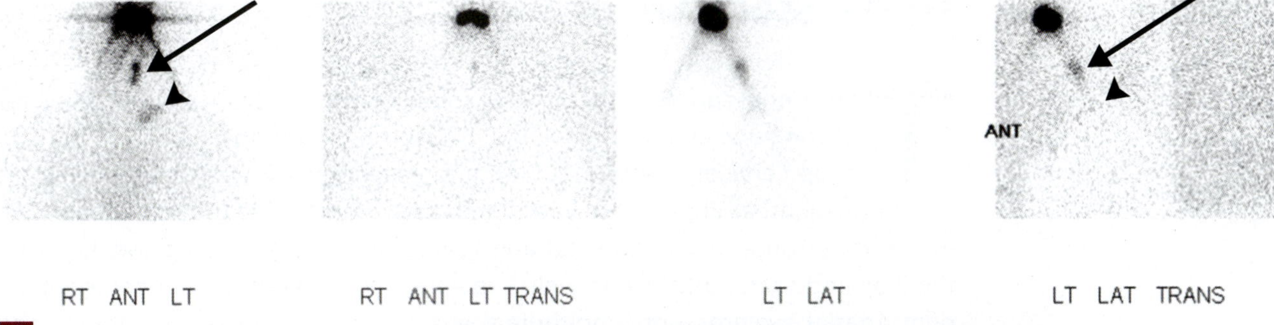

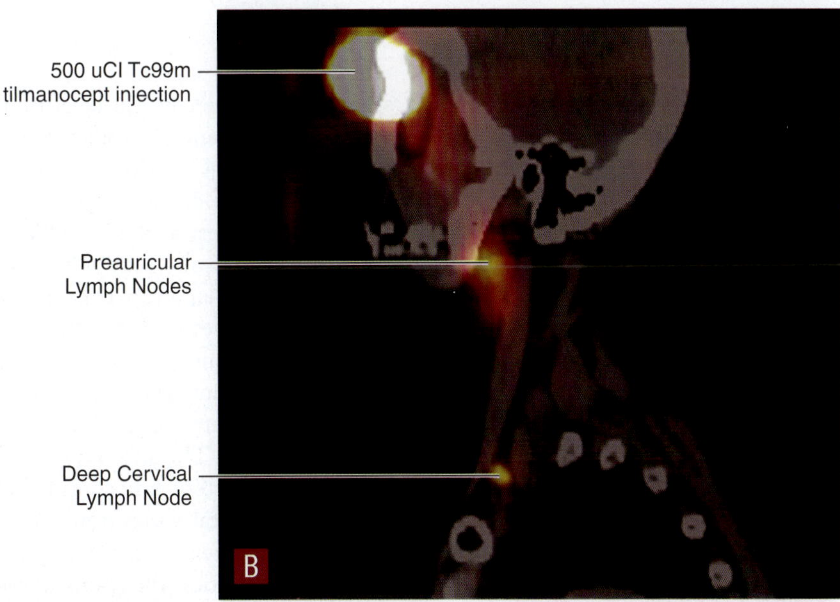

Figure 4.3. A and B. 500 uCi Tc99m tilmanocept injection of the left eyelid for lymphoscintigraphy fused with CT of the head and neck showing drainage into preauricular (solid black arrow) and lower deep cervical (arrow head) lymph nodes.

5

Arteries of the Spinal Cord and Spine

The arterial supply of the cervical spinal cord arises from several branches of the subclavian artery (Figs. 5.1 and 5.2), vertebral artery (Fig. 5.3), deep cervical artery (Fig. 5.4), and ascending cervical artery, whereas the thoracolumbar segment is vascularized by branches of the thoracoabdominal aorta through the intercostal and lumbar arteries and, occasionally, from the iliac and sacral arteries as well. The spinal cord has three almost independent arterial systems—or longitudinal anastomotic chains—one anterior and two posterior.

In the upper cervical region, the anterior spinal artery originates from the junction of the intradural segment of the vertebral arteries, just below the basilar artery. In all other segments, the arteries cross through the intervertebral foramina to reach the intrathecal level (Fig. 5.5). These are called segmental arteries (intercostal and lumbar arteries). The segmental artery divides into an anterior branch (along the costal groove) and a posterior branch to the spine. The posterior branch originates the muscular branches and the medial radiculomedullary artery. The radicular artery further bifurcates into two branches (the dorsal and ventral vertebral branches) and continues as the radicular artery, which gives off a ganglionic branch and divides into an anterior spinal radicular artery and a posterior spinal radicular artery, following each anterior and posterior nerve root. In some preferential levels, these arteries are larger and constitute the anterior and posterior radiculomedullary arteries, proceeding as direct connections within the radicular artery and the longitudinal anterior and posterior anastomotic chains on the spinal cord surface (Fig. 5.6).

The anterior spinal artery is located in the midline on the ventral aspect of the cord, lying in the groove of the anterior median fissure of the spinal cord. It is formed by the union of two branches from the terminal portion of the vertebral artery at the level of the foramen magnum. The anterior spinal artery descends as a single trunk (Fig. 5.7) in the entire length of the ventral aspect of the medulla spinalis to the conus medullaris. It is reinforced by a succession of small spinal rami at the cervical level from the vertebral arteries and by larger branches from the ascending cervical artery at the level C4–C6. Most of the tributaries in the lower two-thirds of the cervical spinal cord are derived from the deep cervical artery at the level C6–T1. The superior intercostal artery may also send a branch to the spinal arteries. The anterior spinal artery continues downward, being reinforced by branches from the thoracic and abdominal aorta down to the conus medullaris, continuing along the cauda equina, and ending as a fine artery at the filum terminale. At that level, there are anastomoses with branches from the iliolumbar artery. The anterior radicular arteries, joining the anterior spinal artery vary considerably in size, number, and location. The total varies from 3 to 15, with an average of 7. The cervical region of the spinal cord receives an average of three arteries, the thoracic region has an average of three to four, and the lumbar region has an average of one. The position of the great anterior radicular artery, also called artery of Adamkiewicz, varies from T8 to L3 (Figs. 5.8-5.10), being often the only ventral feeder to the lower thoracic and lumbosacral cord (Fig. 5.11). The size of the anterior spinal artery usually tapers gradually from the lower part of the cervical region down to the middle or lower thoracic region, also narrowing in the upper thoracic region in some cases. At the point of anastomoses with the artery of Adamkiewicz, an enlargement of the anterior spinal artery usually occurs, remaining constant in size down to the lower end of sacral region, being reduced at that point to a tiny vessel, after giving off communicating branches, called rami cruciantes, to the posterior spinal arteries. This tiny artery may have anastomoses with branches of the iliolumbar artery.

The posterolateral spinal artery arises from the posterior rami of the vertebral artery but occasionally from the posterior inferior cerebellar artery (PICA). They run along the dorsolateral surface of the spinal cord, posterior but near to the entrance of the posterior nerve roots, receiving additional supply from the posterior radicular arteries. There are free anastomoses between the posterior radicular arteries, as well as with the corresponding vessels on the opposite side, forming an arterial network between the two posterior spinal arteries. Some branches pass over the lateral surface of the spinal cord and make tiny anastomotic connections with branches from the anterior spinal artery. The posterior spinal arteries are usually distinct vessels, but they are smaller than those of the anterior aspect. At the lower end of the spinal cord, the posterior spinal arteries communicate with the anterior spinal artery via the rami cruciantes (Fig. 5.9).

The knowledge of the pelvic vasculature to the spinal cord and femoral and sciatic nerves is important for embolization procedures. The inferior and superior lateral sacral arteries, which are branches of the posterior division of the internal iliac artery, give off spinal arteries that enter the spinal canal via the anterior sacral foramina. The inferior gluteal artery, which is usually a branch of the anterior division of the internal iliac artery, supplies the sciatic nerve via the sciatic artery (Fig. 5.12). The sciatic artery is a small vessel that comes off the descending branch of the inferior gluteal artery. Occasionally, the sciatic artery plays a role as the main artery to the lower extremity in the absence of the superficial femoral artery and is extremely developed. The iliolumbar artery, another branch of the posterior division of the internal iliac artery, supplies the region of the femoral nerve as it passes over the iliac wing via an iliac branch that perforates the iliacus muscle.

There is an arterial pial plexus made by circumferential branches from the anterior and posterior spinal arteries, forming the pial arterial network. Small branches from the arterial pial plexus penetrate into the substance of the spinal cord to supply the adjacent white and gray matter (Fig. 5.6).

The nutrient vessels of the spinal cord are divided into a central and a peripheral arterial system. The central system derives from the anterior spinal artery, and the blood flow becomes centrifugal. In the peripheral system, the blood comes from the posterior spinal arteries and the pial arterial plexus, and the blood has a centripetal flow.

The gray matter of the spinal cord has a dense capillary network, most developed in the anterior and lateral gray horns, whereas the white matter is poorly supplied and the capillaries form wide meshes extended longitudinally along the nerve fibers.

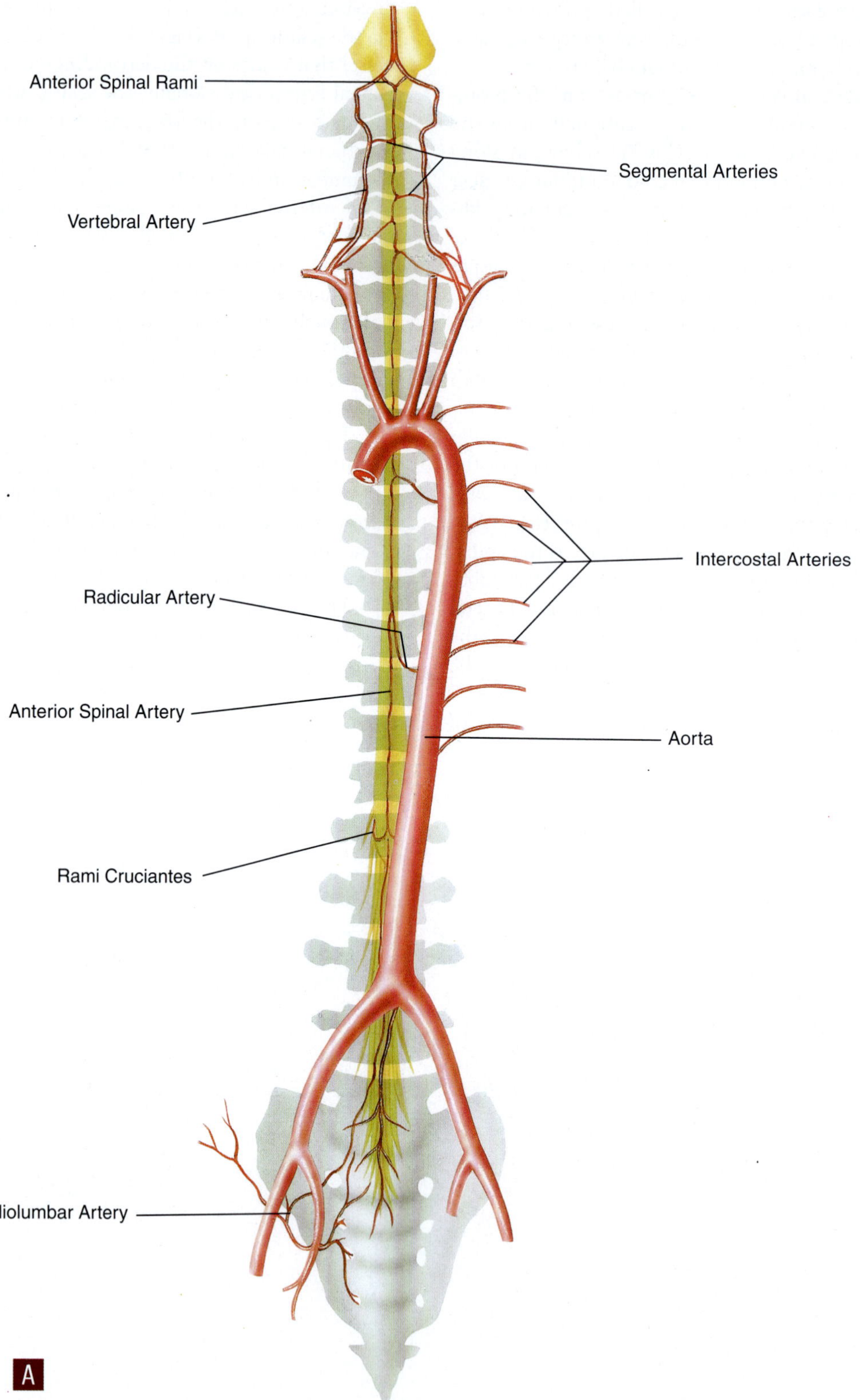

Figure 5.1. Arteries of the spinal cord and spine. A, Relationships of the spinal feeders with the vertebral levels and the aorta and branches in an anteroposterior view. B, Relationships of the spinal feeders with the vertebral levels and the aorta in a lateral view.

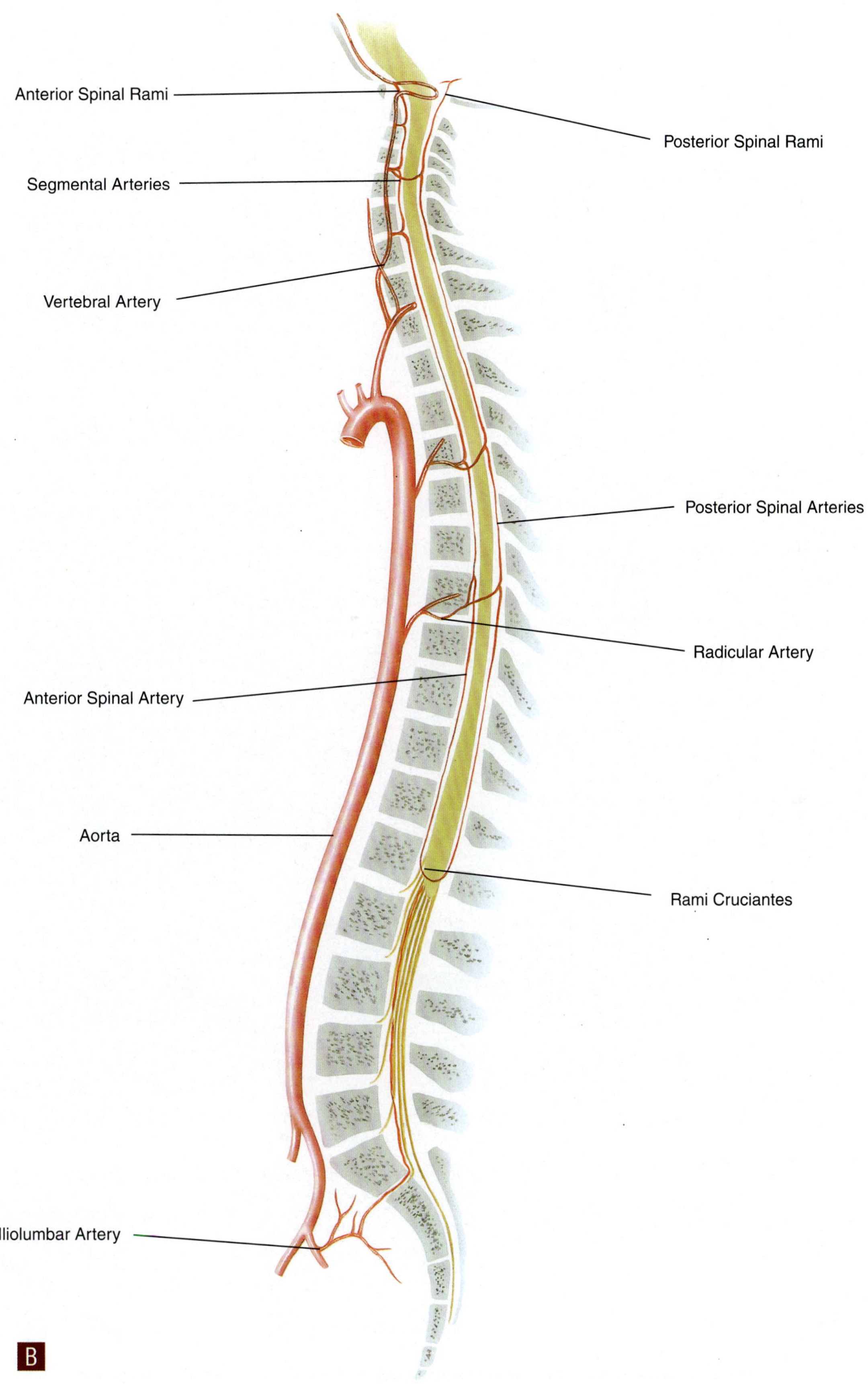

Figure 5.1. *Continued*

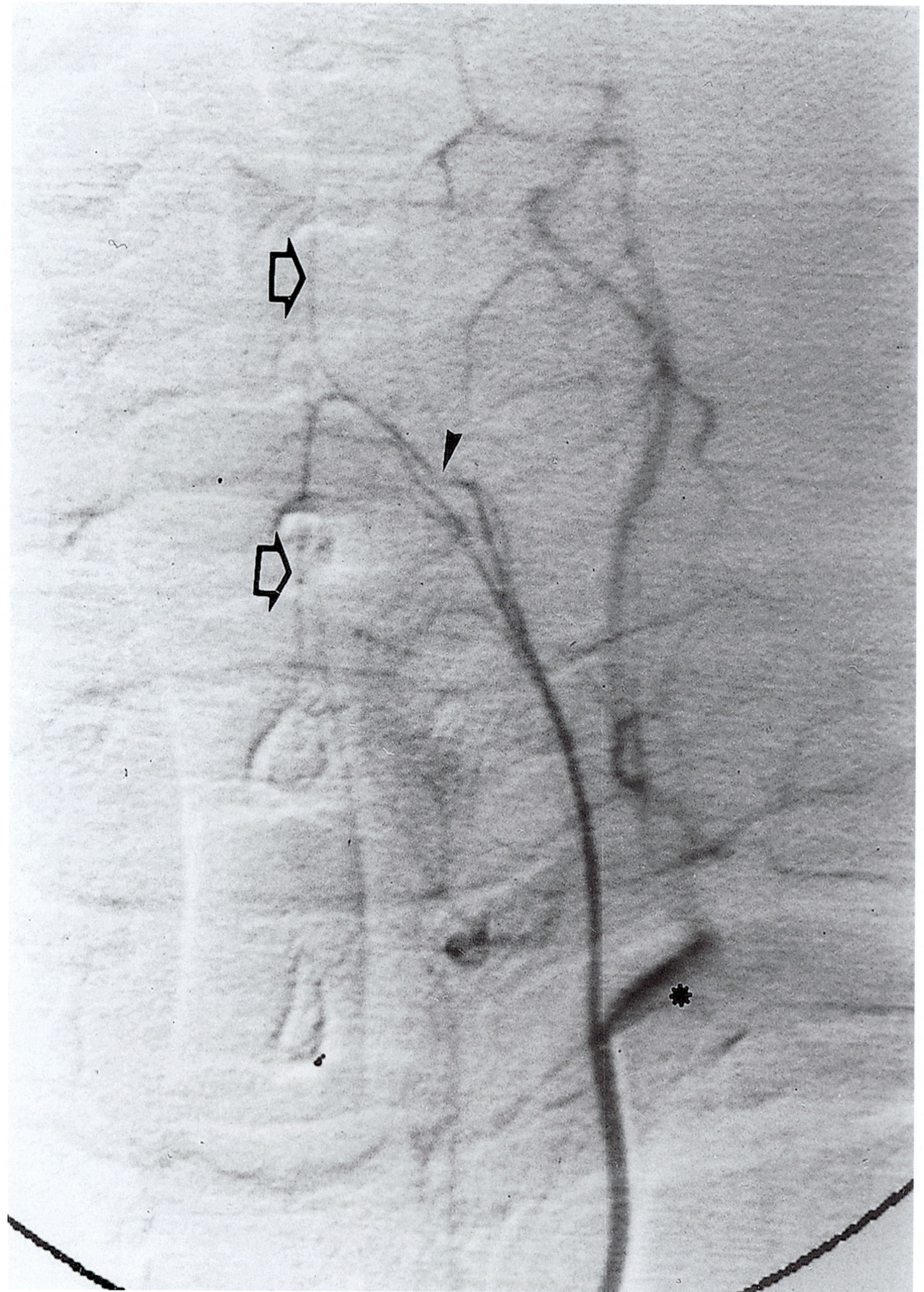

Figure 5.2. **Low anterior cervical spinal artery (open arrows) originated directly from the left subclavian artery (*).** Note narrowing of the radiculomedullary artery when entering at the dura mater (arrowhead).

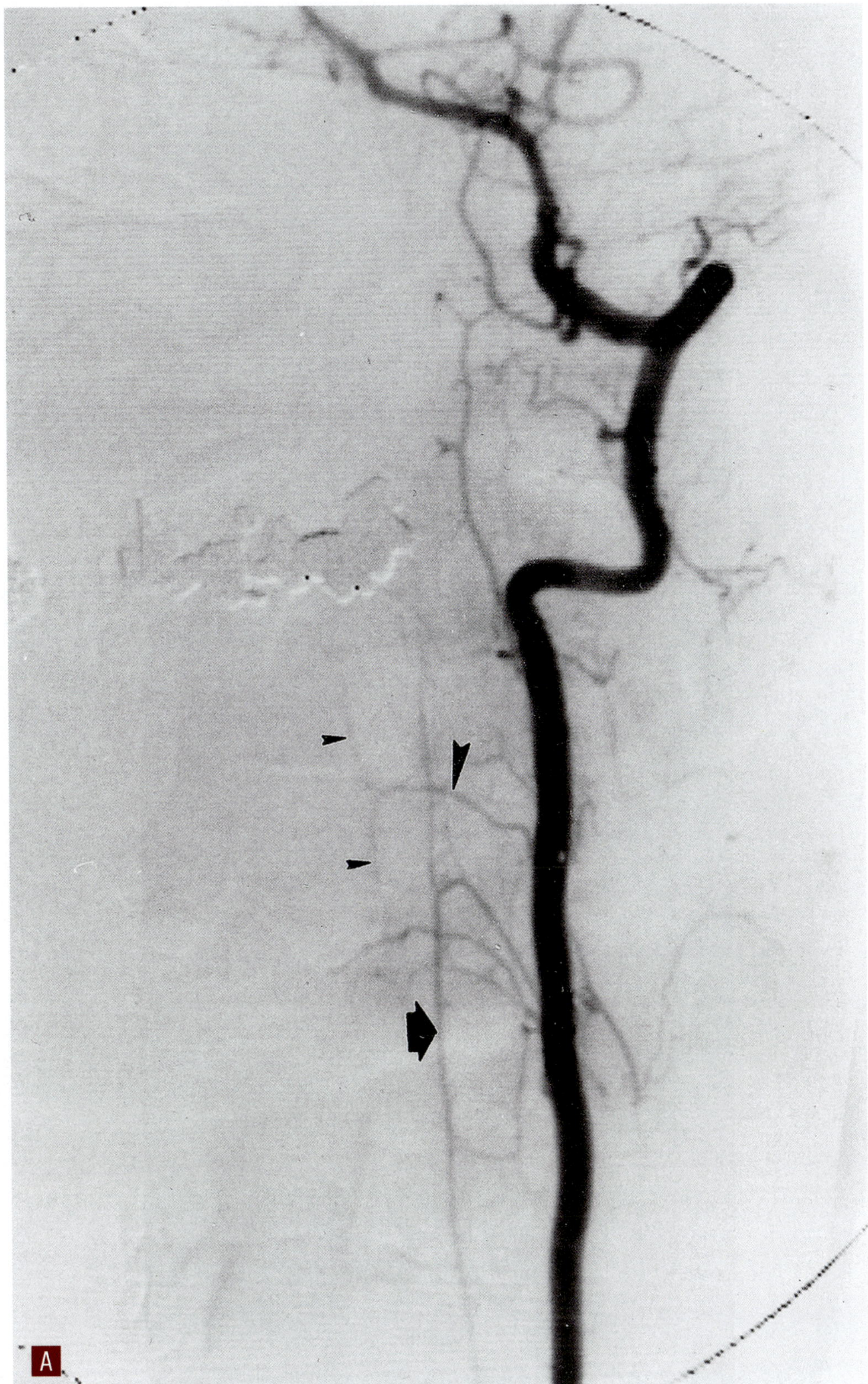

Figure 5.3. Cervical anterior and posterior spinal arteries visualized during a vertebral artery angiogram. A, The anterior spinal artery is small (small arrowhead) and the radiculomedullary artery originates in the left vertebral artery (arrowhead). The left posterior spinal artery (arrow) is larger and is also connected to the left vertebral artery. Multiple muscular arteries are observed. B, Superselective angiogram of the radiculomedullary artery (white arrow) showing the bilateral posterior spinal arteries (hollow black arrows) and the anterior spinal artery (solid black arrow).

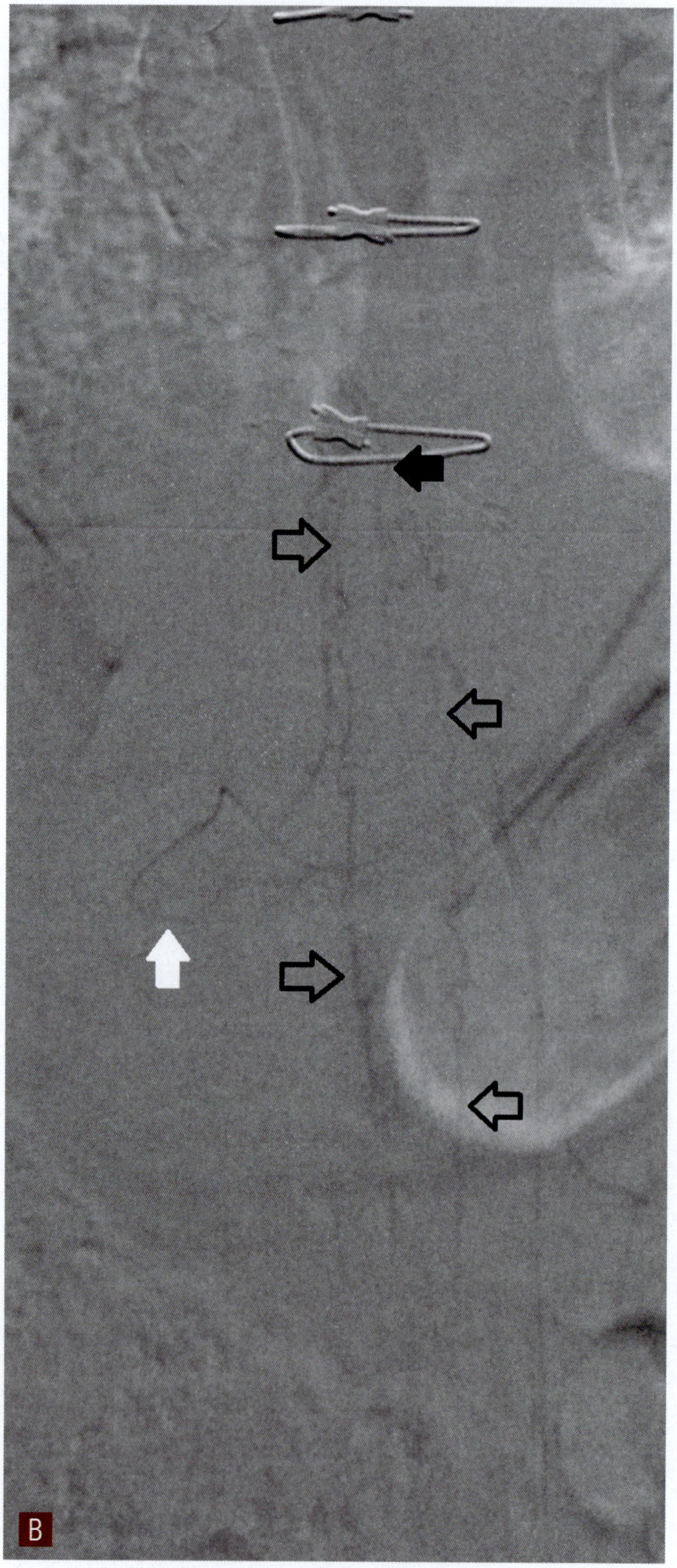

Figure 5.3. *Continued*

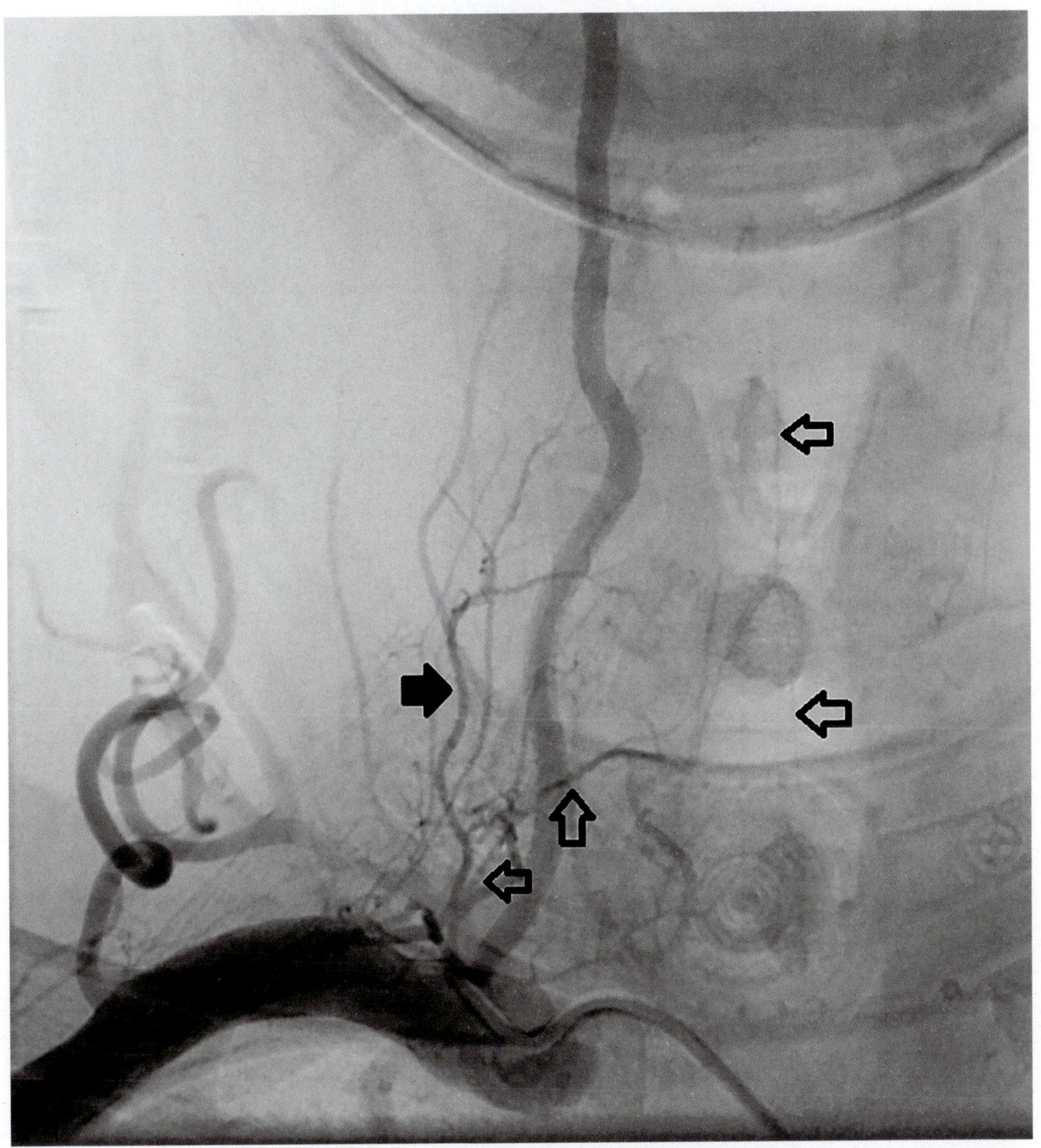

Figure 5.4. Cervical anterior spinal artery (cervical enlargement, hollow arrows) arising from the deep cervical artery (solid arrow).

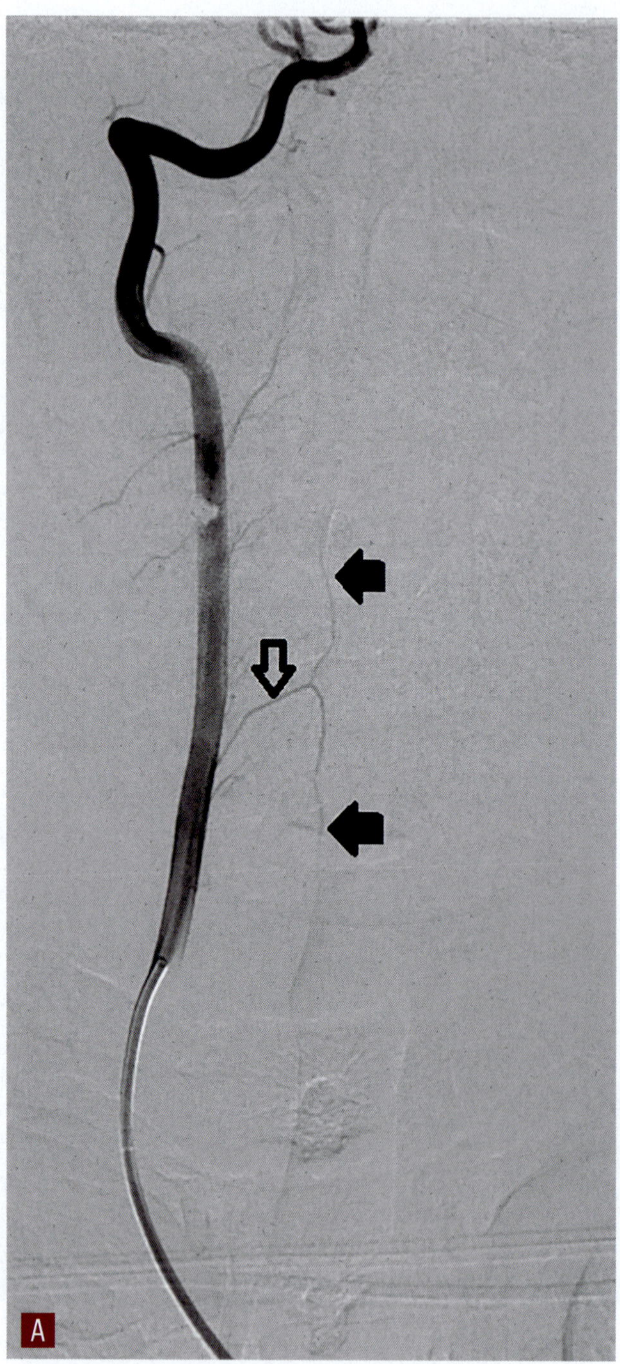

Figure 5.5. A and B, Anterior and lateral views of a vertebral artery angiogram showing the anterior spinal artery (solid arrows) and the radiculomedullary artery (open arrow).

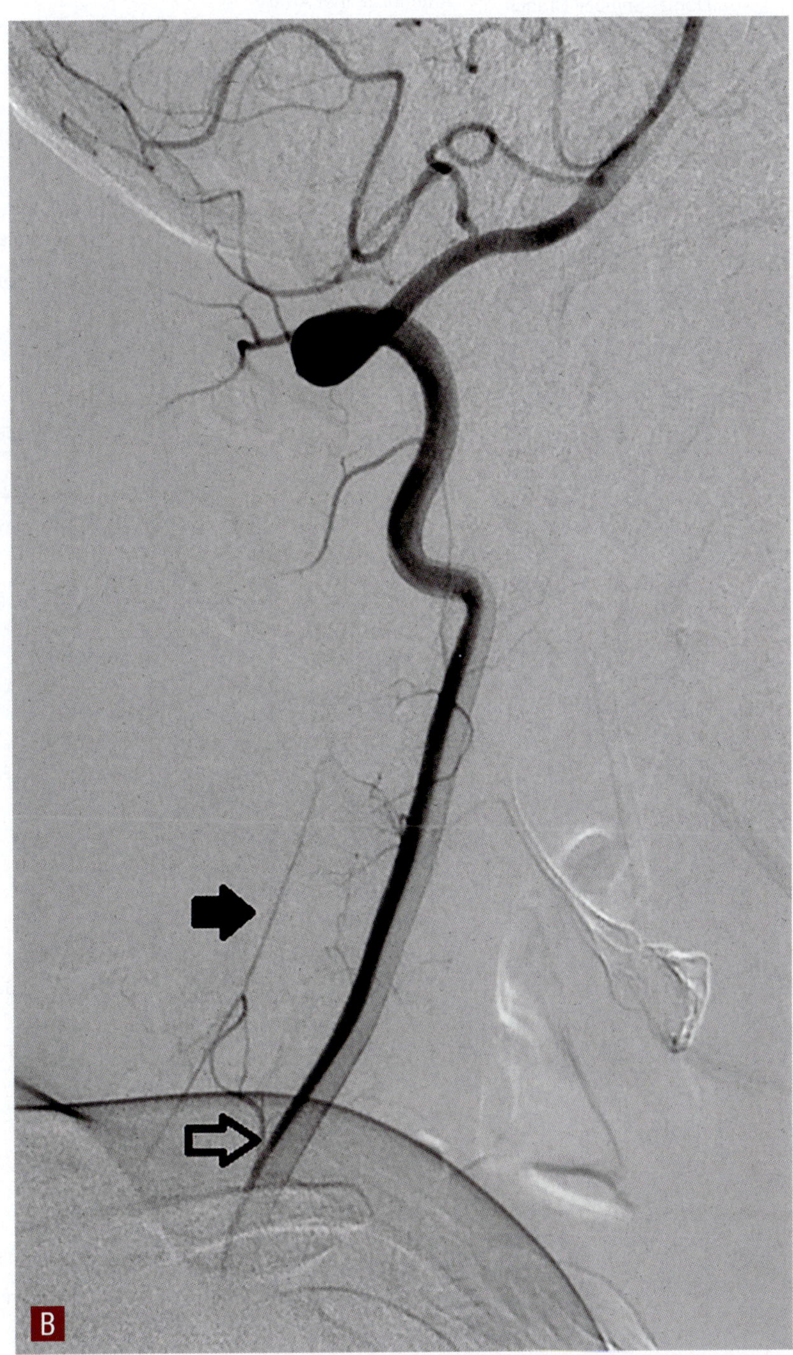

Figure 5.5. *Continued*

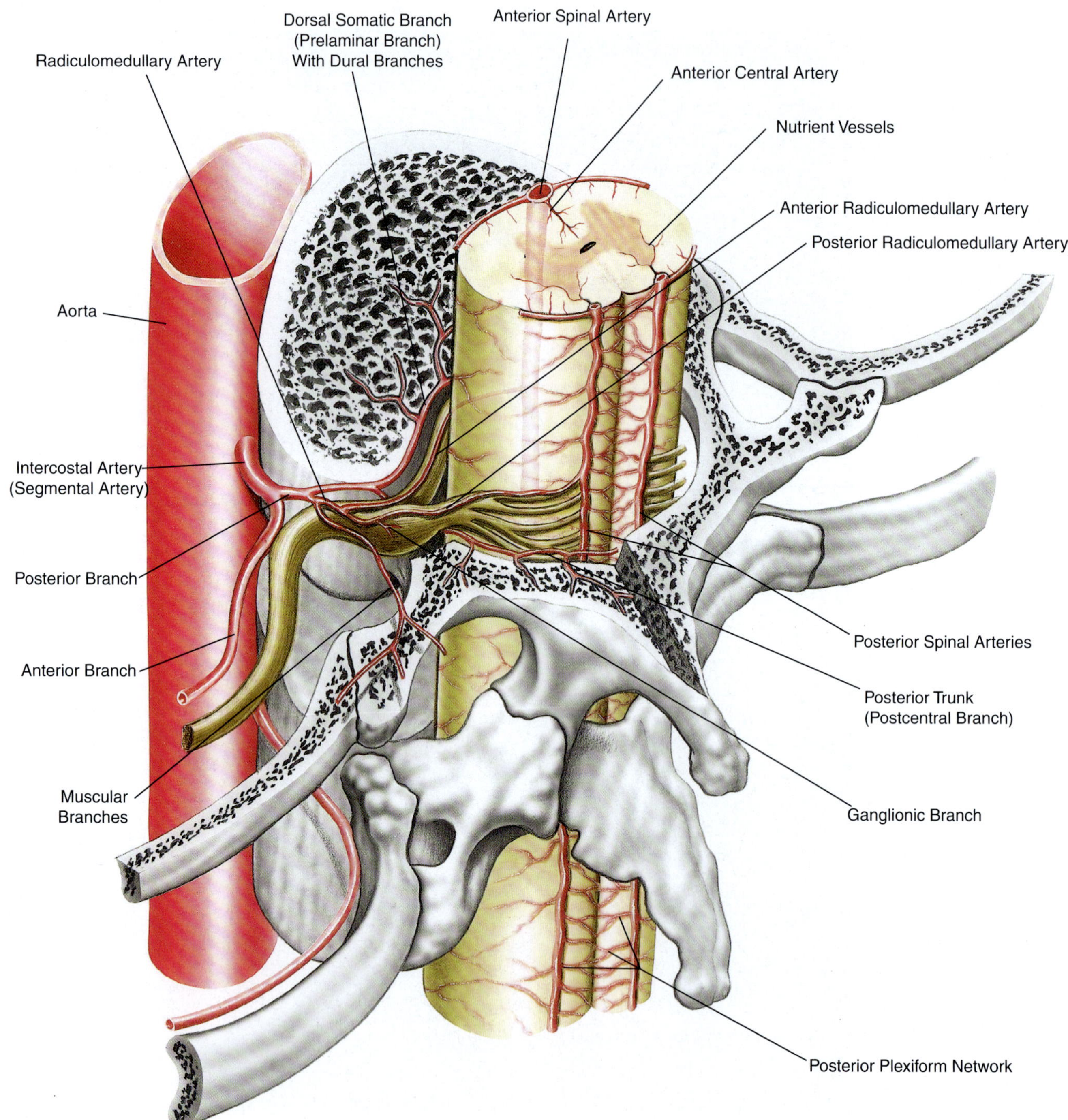

Figure 5.6. **Radiculomedullary, spinal arteries, and plexiform network.**

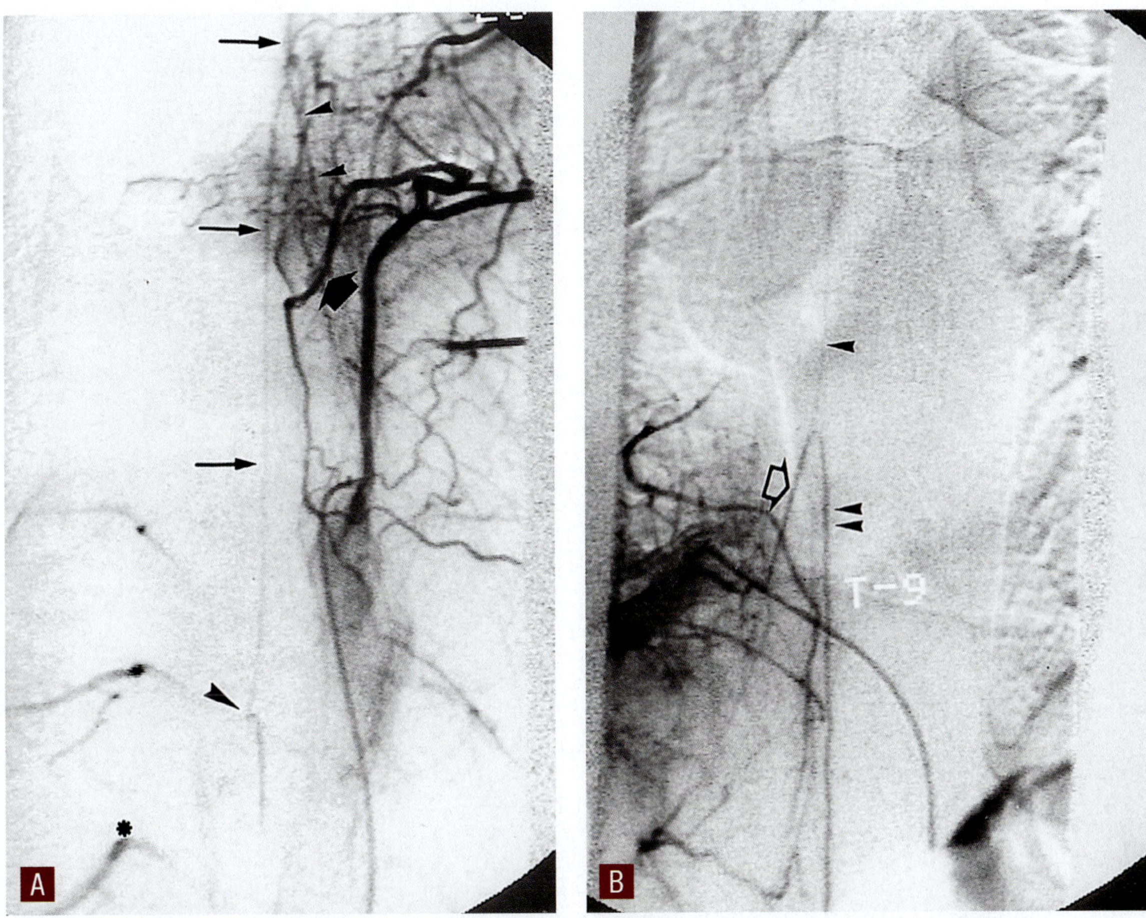

Figure 5.7. A, Injection at the fifth right posterior intercostal showing the anterior radicular artery (arrows) at the high thoracic region anastomosed with the anterior spinal artery (Adamkiewicz artery, large arrowhead). Ninth right posterior intercostal artery (*). Note the ascending direction of the radicular artery (small arrowheads), different from the descending direction of the muscular branch (large short arrow). B, Injection at the ninth right posterior intercostal artery. Anterior radiculomedullary artery (Adamkiewicz, open arrow), with the descending branch (double arrowheads) and ascending branch (arrowhead). A and B show the continuous anterior spinal axis at the thoracic region.

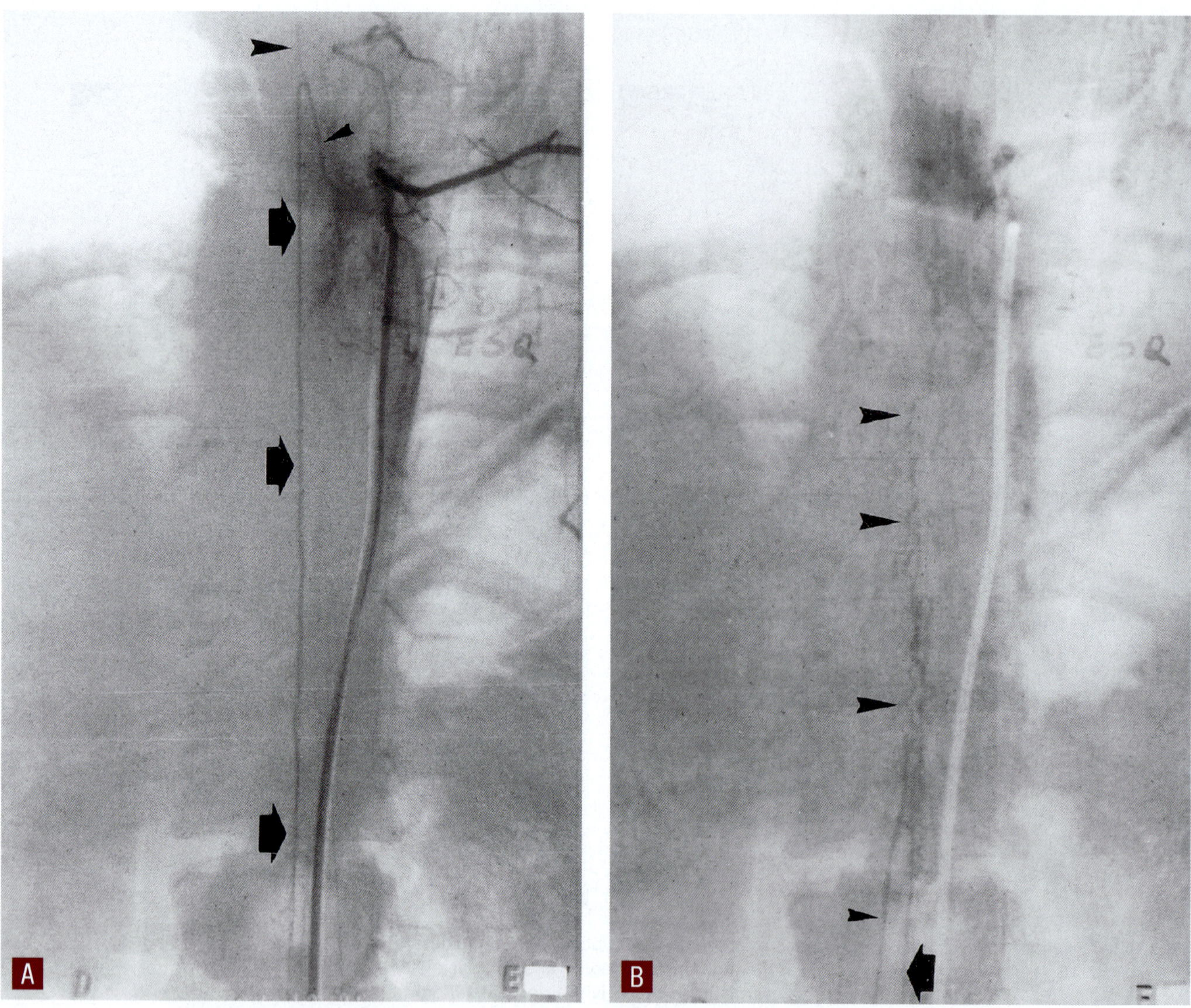

Figure 5.8. **Eighth left intercostal artery.** Anterior view. The anterior spinal artery is well visualized at the thoracolumbar segment (Adamkiewicz). Arterial phase (A) and venous (B). A, Anterior radiculomedullary artery (small arrowhead) with typical ascending curve. Anterior ascending spinal branch (large arrowhead) and descending branch, larger and longer (large arrows). B, Anterior spinal vein with the typical tortuous aspect, all along the thoracolumbar medulla (large arrowheads). Typical straight aspect of a radiculomedullary vein following a nerve root exiting the dura mater (small arrowhead). Vein of the filum terminalis (large arrow).

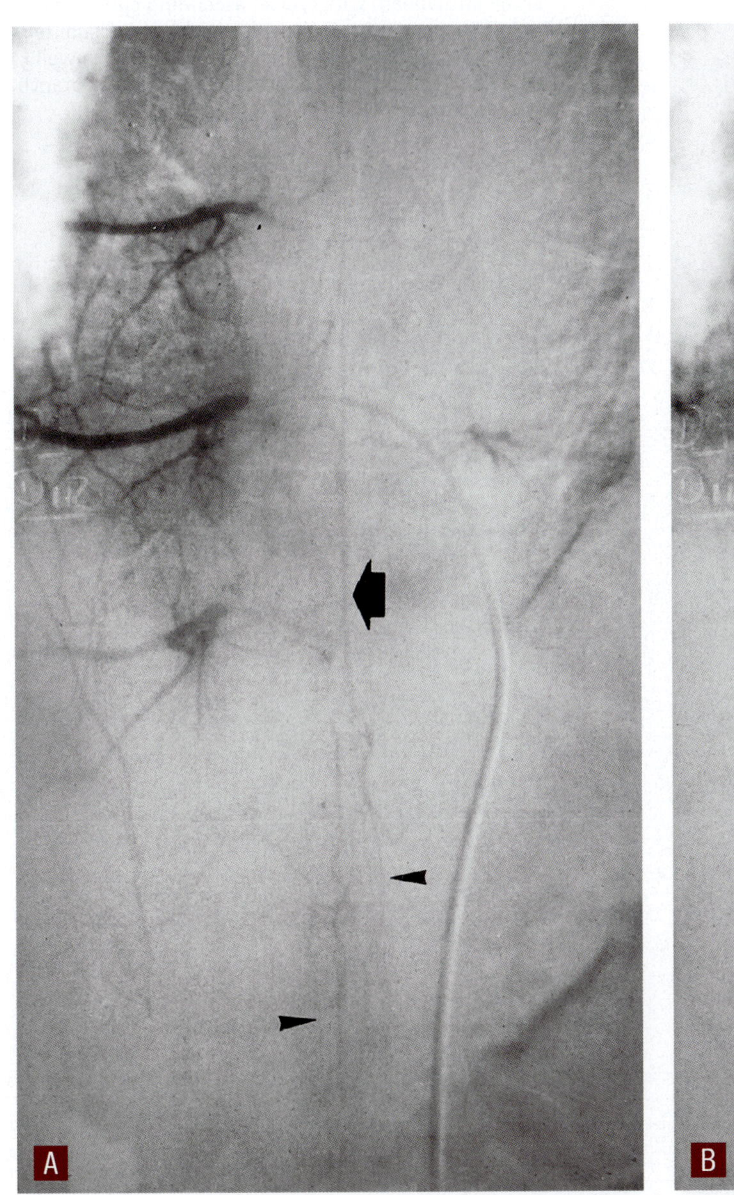

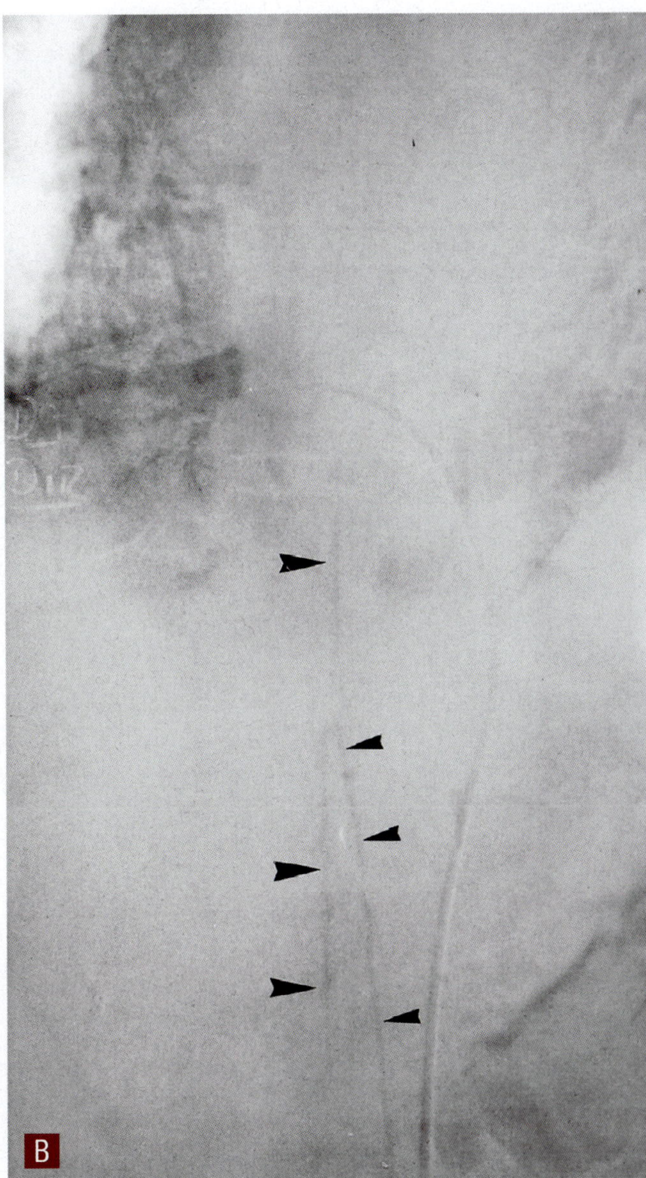

Figure 5.9. **Ninth right intercostal artery.** Anteroposterior view. Anterior spinal artery in the thoracolumbar segment. A, Arterial phase. Anterior spinal artery (large arrow) at the level of the cone fills the arterial network of the medullar cone (small arrowheads). Note a capillary blush at that level. B, Venous phase. The anterior spinal vein is single and large (large arrowheads) with a descending radicular vein long and straight, progressively leaving the midline, following a nerve root (small arrowheads).

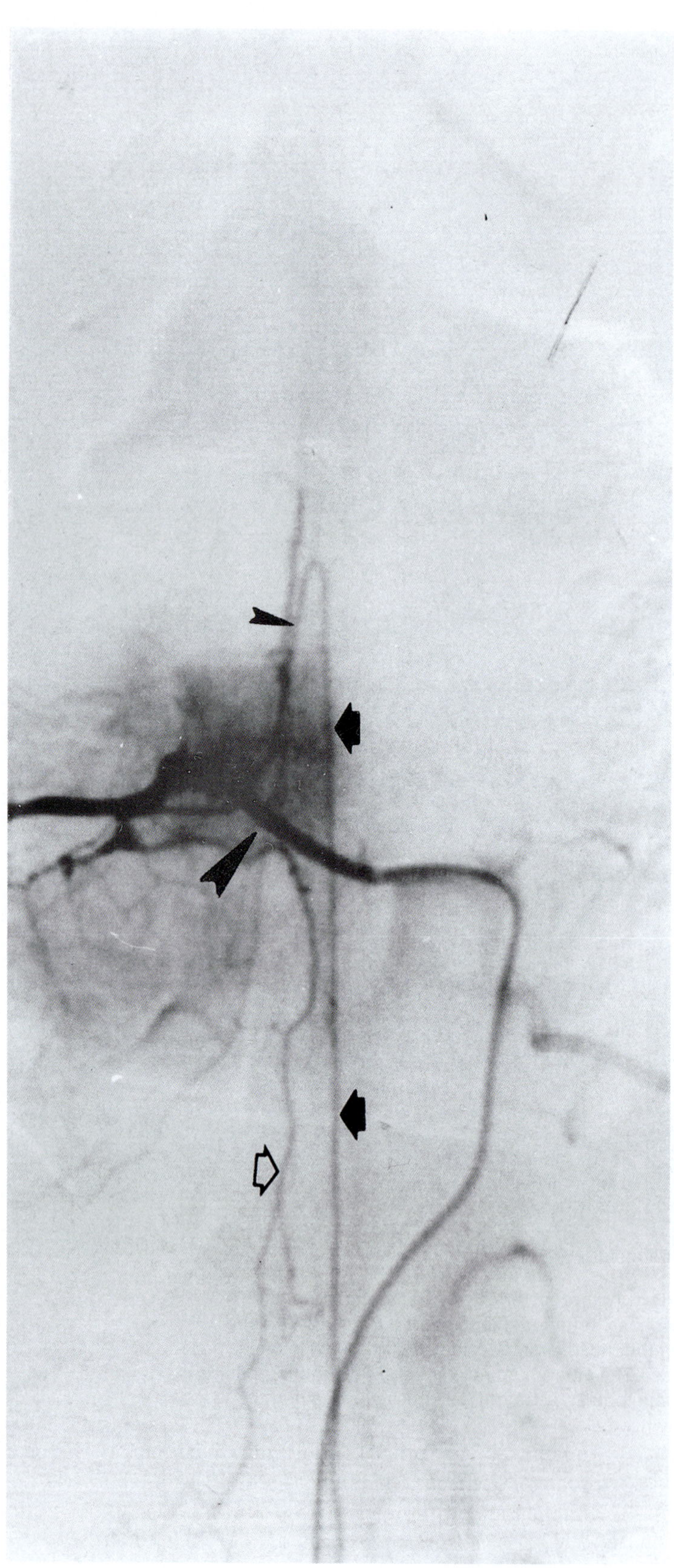

Figure 5.10. Eighth right intercostal artery (large arrowhead). Anterior view. The anterior spinal artery is well visualized at the thoracolumbar segment (Adamkiewicz). Anterior radiculomedullary artery (small arrowhead) with typical ascending curve. The anterior ascending spinal branch is not well visualized, but the descending branch, larger and longer, is well opacified (large arrows) adjacent to a muscular branch (open arrow).

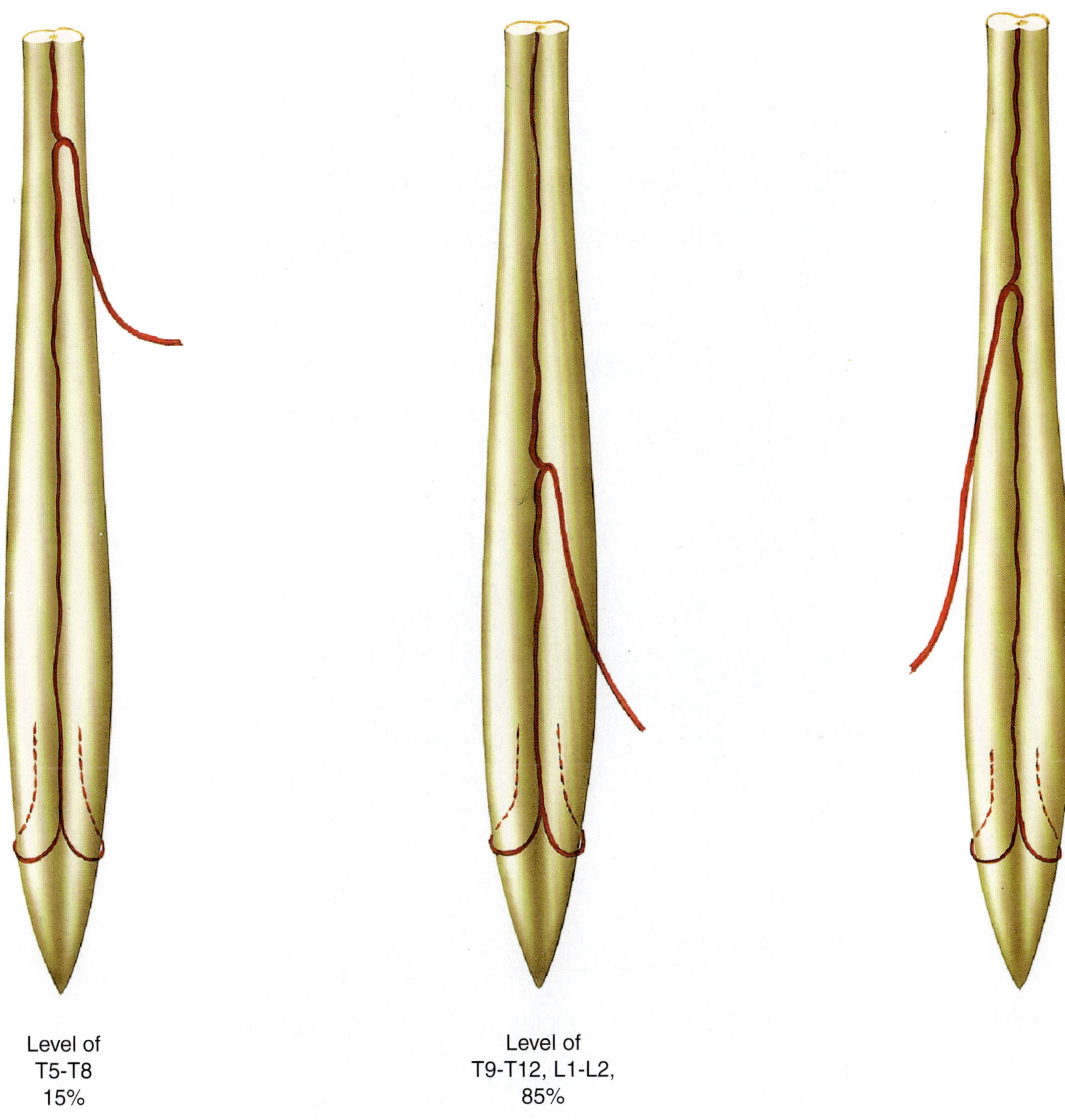

Figure 5.11. **A**, Different possible levels of origin of the anterior spinal artery (Adamkiewicz). **B**, Selective angiogram of the right L1 lumbar artery (hollow arrow) showing the artery of Adamkiewicz (solid arrow), and the L1 hemivertebral blush (arrowhead). **C**, Late phase superselective angiogram of the right-sided artery of Adamkiewicz (solid arrow) showing sharp turn as it enters the dura mater (hollow arrowhead). The descending anterior spinal artery is visualized (hollow arrow), as is the capillary blush in the spinal cord (solid arrowhead).

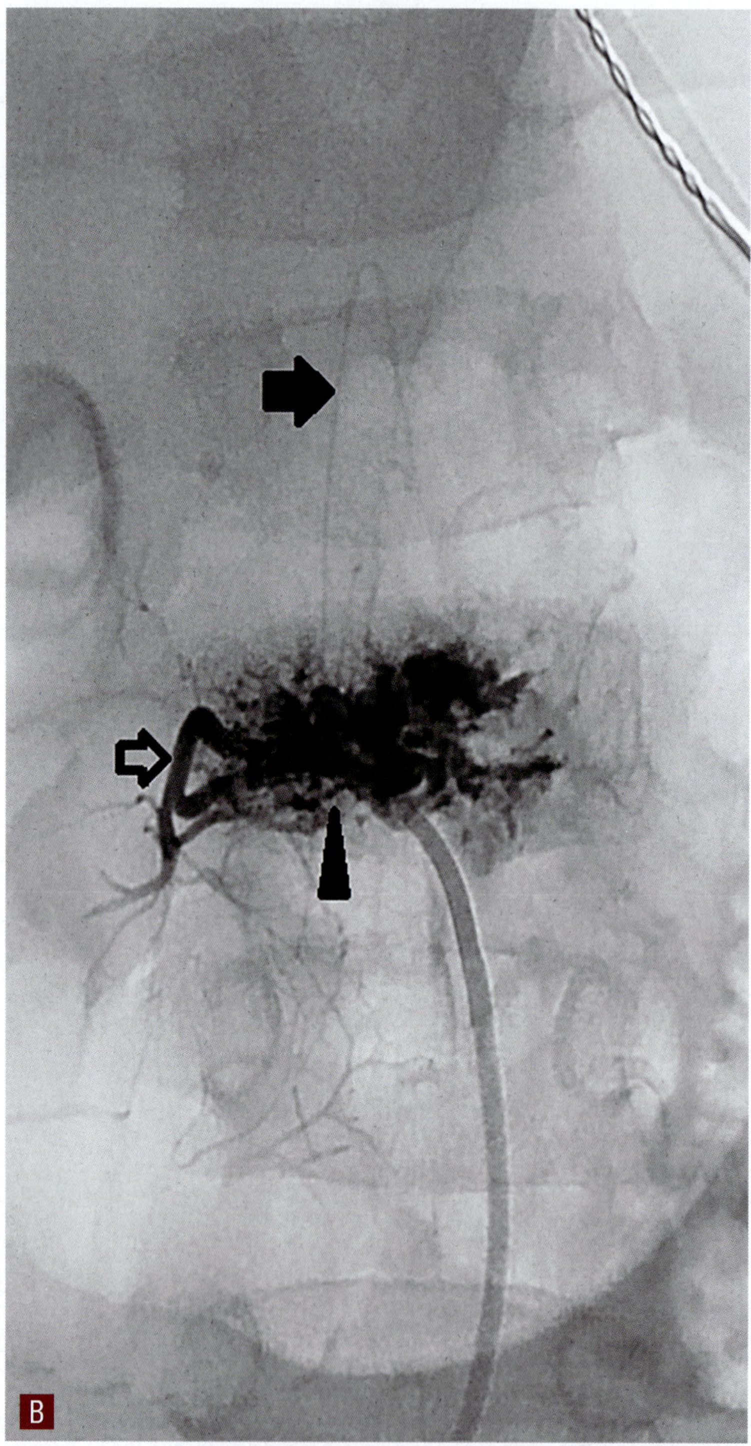

Figure 5.11. *Continued*

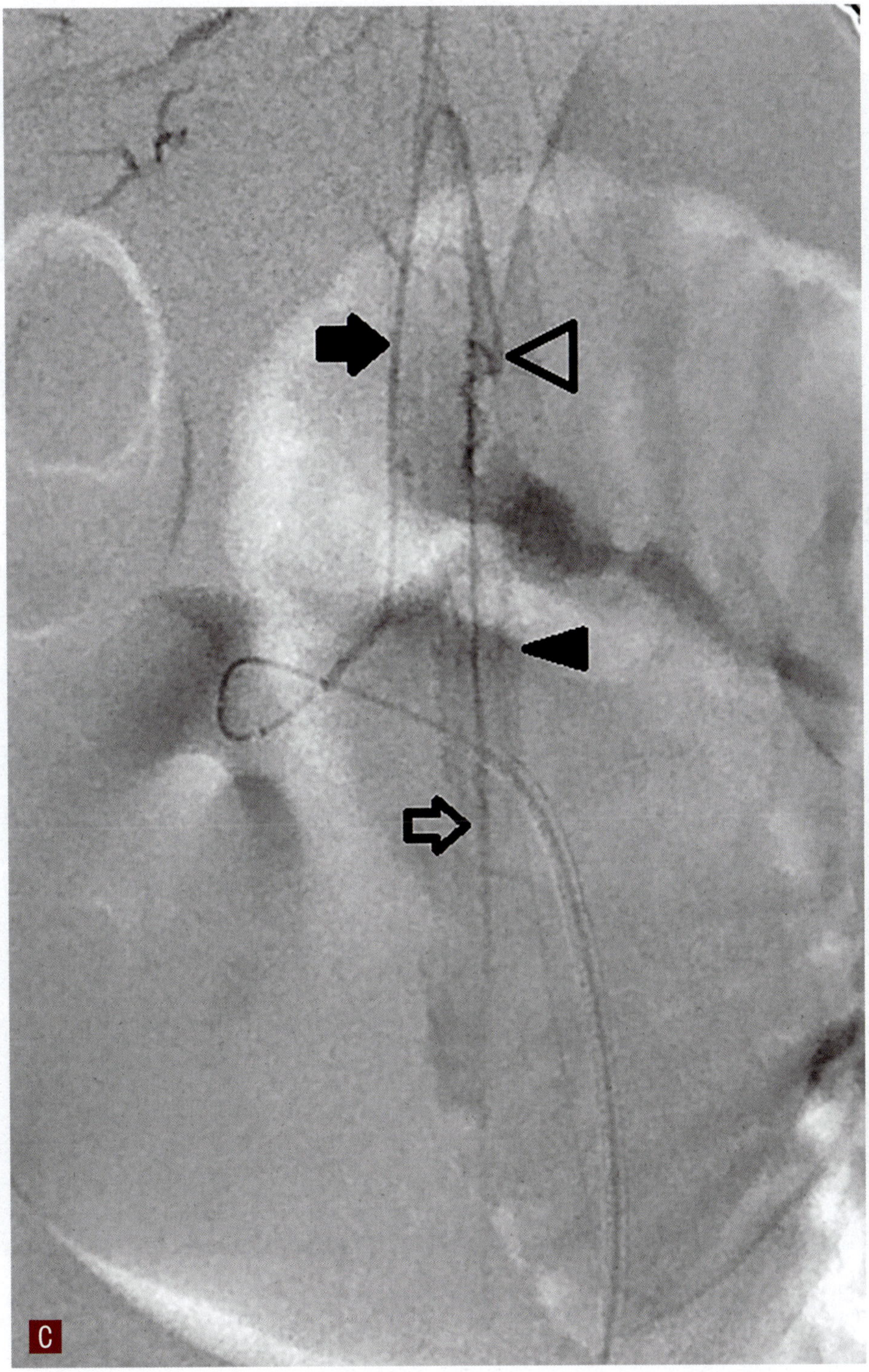

Figure 5.11. *Continued*

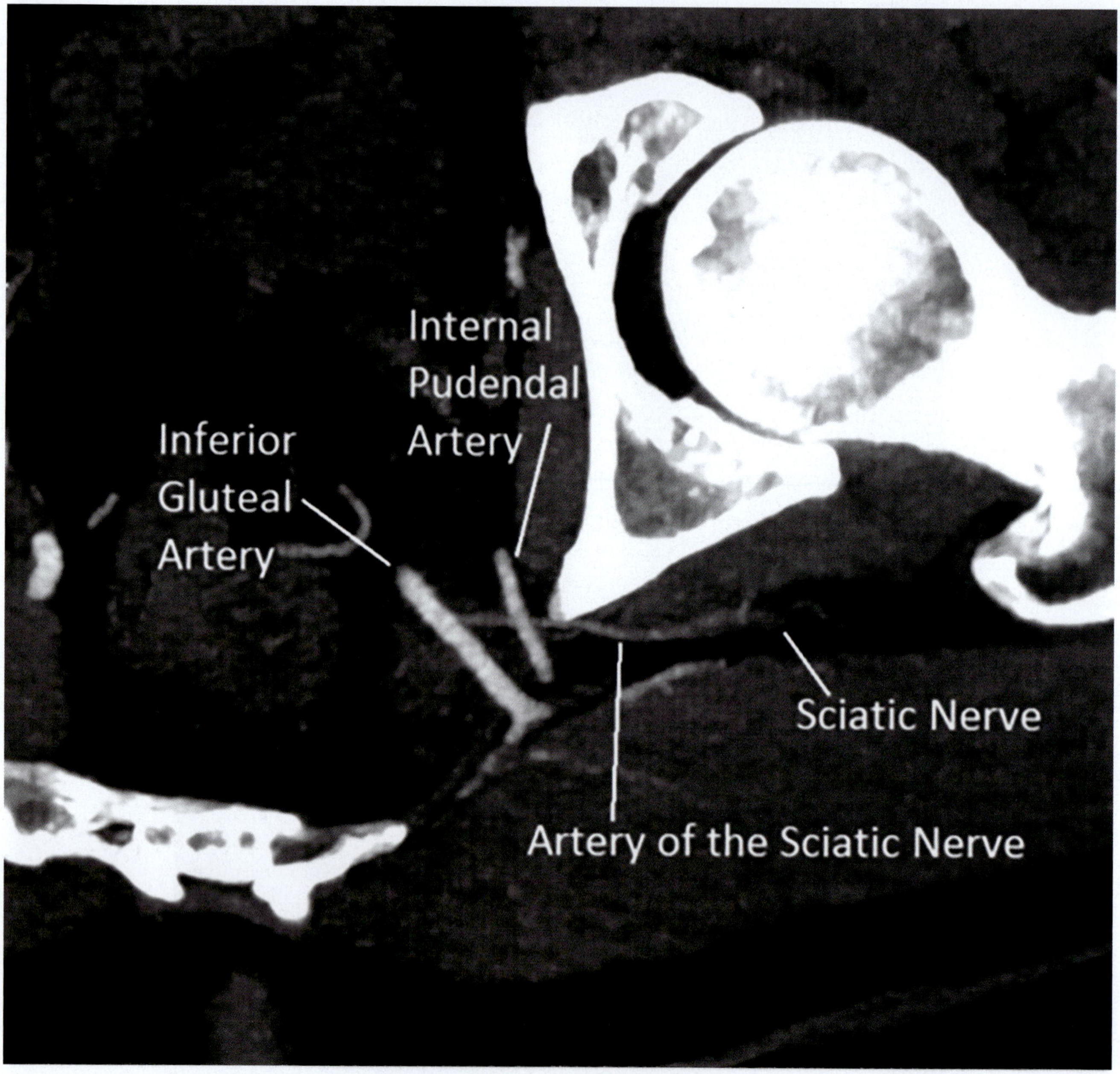

Figure 5.12. Axial pelvic CT angiogram with maximum intensity projection showing the artery of the sciatic nerve, arising from the inferior gluteal artery.

6

Veins of the Spinal Cord and Spine

Inside and outside of the vertebral canal, along the entire length of the spinal cord, there are several venous plexuses, with free anastomoses to each other and with the intervertebral veins. Two groups of venous plexuses are found on the outside of the vertebral canal: the anterior group and the posterior group. The anterior group lies anterior to the vertebral bodies and receives venous tributaries from other vertebral bodies and communicates with the basivertebral and intervertebral veins. It is most developed in the cervical region. The posterior group forms a network of venous plexuses mainly inside the spinal canal. There are three communicating valveless venous networks bearing a constant relationship to the vertebral bodies and intervertebral discs (Figs. 6.1 and 6.2). They are the intraosseous vertebral veins, the epidural venous plexus, and the paravertebral veins. Together, these valveless venous networks comprise the vertebral venous plexus, also known as the Batson plexus, which extends from the pelvis to the cranium. These veins communicate freely with sacral and intracranial veins, as well as veins of the back and thoracoabdominal wall (Fig. 6.3). The vertebral venous plexus has bidirectional flow and plays an important role in the regulation of intracranial pressure and central nervous system venous return.

Veins of the Spine

Intraosseous Vertebral Veins

These veins drain each vertebral body, emptying into a venous sinus (the basivertebral vein) at the nutrient foramen of each vertebra posteriorly (Fig. 6.2), and connect at each level with the second network, the epidural plexus (Fig. 6.3).

Epidural Venous Plexus

The epidural venous plexus is composed of two vertical channels: the anterior internal vertebral veins that course the length of the spinal canal circling around the backs of the vertebral bodies and intervertebral discs, between the dura mater and bone. Both the left and right anterior internal vertebral veins have a lateral and a medial component. The lateral component is a single channel, whereas the medial component has a variable configuration and is a rather irregular group of vessels. The medial anterior internal vertebral veins are located close to the lateral anterior internal vertebral veins at all levels of the lumbar spine, except at the level L5–S1. At this level, the medial anterior internal vertebral veins leave the lateral anterior internal vertebral veins and lie close to the midline. The anterior internal vertebral veins are medial to the pedicles and bulge laterally as they cross the intervertebral disc spaces. The anterior internal vertebral veins communicate with the basivertebral veins through the nutrient foramina (Figs. 6.2 and 6.3). There are segmental connections between the epidural venous plexus and the paravertebral veins at every level. At every intervertebral level, there are two connecting veins on each side, named the supra- and infrapedicular veins (Figs. 6.2-6.5).

There is also the posterior internal vertebral venous plexus, which is small and rudimentary, and anastomosed to the anterior internal vertebral venous plexus through the lateral transverse branches. It is located on each side in front of the vertebral arches and ligamenta flava, having anastomoses with the posterior external plexuses by veins passing through and between the ligaments (Fig. 6.2).

The internal venous plexuses form venous rings near each vertebra connected to the intervertebral veins and draining to the ascending lumbar veins at the lumbar spine level (Figs. 6.2 and 6.3). The intervertebral veins are thought to be valveless with occasional reversal of flow, explaining how pelvic neoplasms may metastasize to vertebral bodies during increased infra-abdominal pressure or postural alterations.

The anterior group venous plexus is most developed in the cervical region (Fig. 6.2). Around the foramen magnum, the epidural plexus forms a dense network connecting with the vertebral veins, occipital and sigmoid sinuses, basilar plexus, venous plexus of the hypoglossal canal, and the condylar emissary vein.

Paravertebral Veins

The paravertebral veins change names as they course along the spine. They are called vertebral veins in the neck, azygos and hemiazygos veins in the thorax (Figs. 6.4 and 6.8), ascending lumbar veins in the abdomen (Fig. 6.2), and internal iliac veins in the pelvis. The presacral veins that join the internal iliac veins reaching the epidural veins through the sacral foramina are analogous to the supra- and infrapedicular veins. The paravertebral venous system connects with the venae cavae and tributaries at any level (Figs. 6.1, 6.4, and 6.5).

Veins of the Spinal Cord

The veins of the spinal cord are small and form a tortuous and delicate venous plexus. There are two main spinal cord venous systems: the intrinsic venous system and the extrinsic venous system (Figs. 6.6 and 6.7).

Intrinsic Venous System

It is formed by three systems:

1. Network of venous capillaries largely anastomosed in the axial plane, linking sulcal and axial veins. Although with ventral and dorsal predominance in the thoracolumbar and thoracic regions, this network is spread in almost equal territories
2. Vertical anastomoses (vertical), following the white or gray matter tracts
3. Transmedullary anastomotic veins

Extrinsic Venous System

It is formed by three recognized segments:

1. Pial network
2. Longitudinal collectors
3. Radicular veins

Pial Network

The pial network collects the intrinsic venous perforators. It is a large anastomotic system surrounding the surface of the cord.

Longitudinal Collectors

Longitudinal collectors are represented by two systems. Lateral main intersegmental bridges link two adjacent radial collectors. Two main longitudinal collectors are located dorsally and ventrally to the cord. One single collector system is seen in the midline at the cervical and lumbar levels; however, at the thoracic portion, the longitudinal system may be triplicate.

Radicular Veins

These veins almost never follow the arterial contributors when exiting the spine (Fig. 6.2). The venous drainage is equally distributed between dorsal and ventral veins. A large vein is usually seen at the thoracolumbar enlargement. In 60% of cases, the radicular veins follow the nerve roots and exit the dura at the same level as that of the companion nervous structure. In 40% of cases, a distinct draining dural foramen can be found.

The spinal venous system drains into the epidural venous plexus through the radicular veins, joining the venous drainage of the bony structures of the spinal canal. Near the foramen magnum, the epidural venous plexus is connected to the inferior cerebellar veins or the inferior petrosal sinuses.

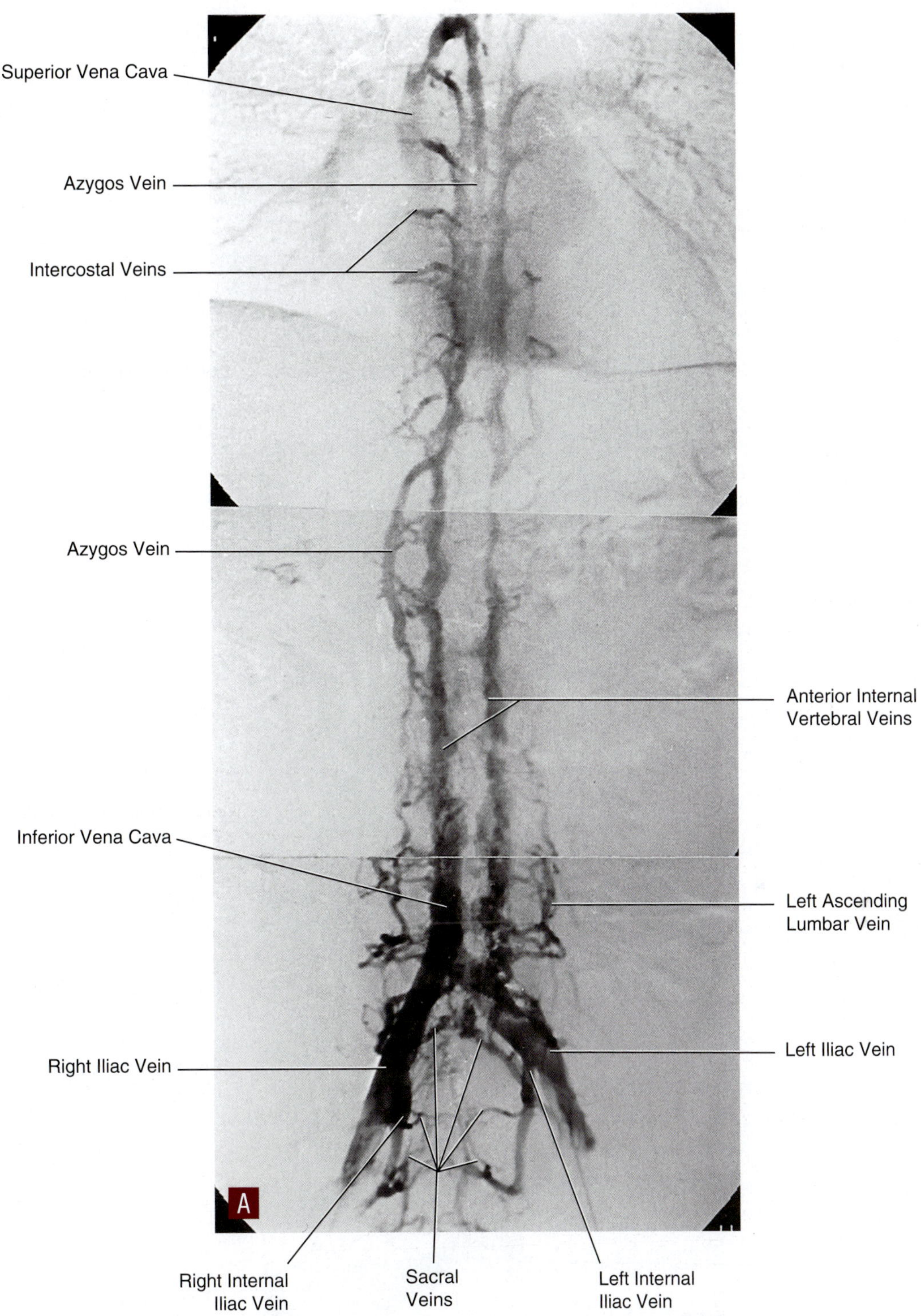

Figure 6.1. **A**, Anterior view of an angiogram of the spinal venous network, showing the three levels of spinal venous drainage: sacral, lumbar, and thoracic. The iliac veins are partially opacified as is the inferior vena cava. The ascending lumbar veins are not totally opacified. The ascending flow of contrast is through the epidural plexus. The suprapedicular and infrapedicular veins are visible throughout the length of the spine. The azygos vein is also identified. **B**, Lateral view of the epidural angiogram showing the anterior internal vertebral venous plexus and, very faintly, the posterior internal and external venous plexus. The inferior vena cava is only partially visualized because of the pathologic narrowing. The azygos vein is also depicted from its origin. Note the communication of the iliac venous system with the perivertebral venous plexus through the sacral veins, explaining the role of the vertebral veins in the spread of metastases, according to Batson.

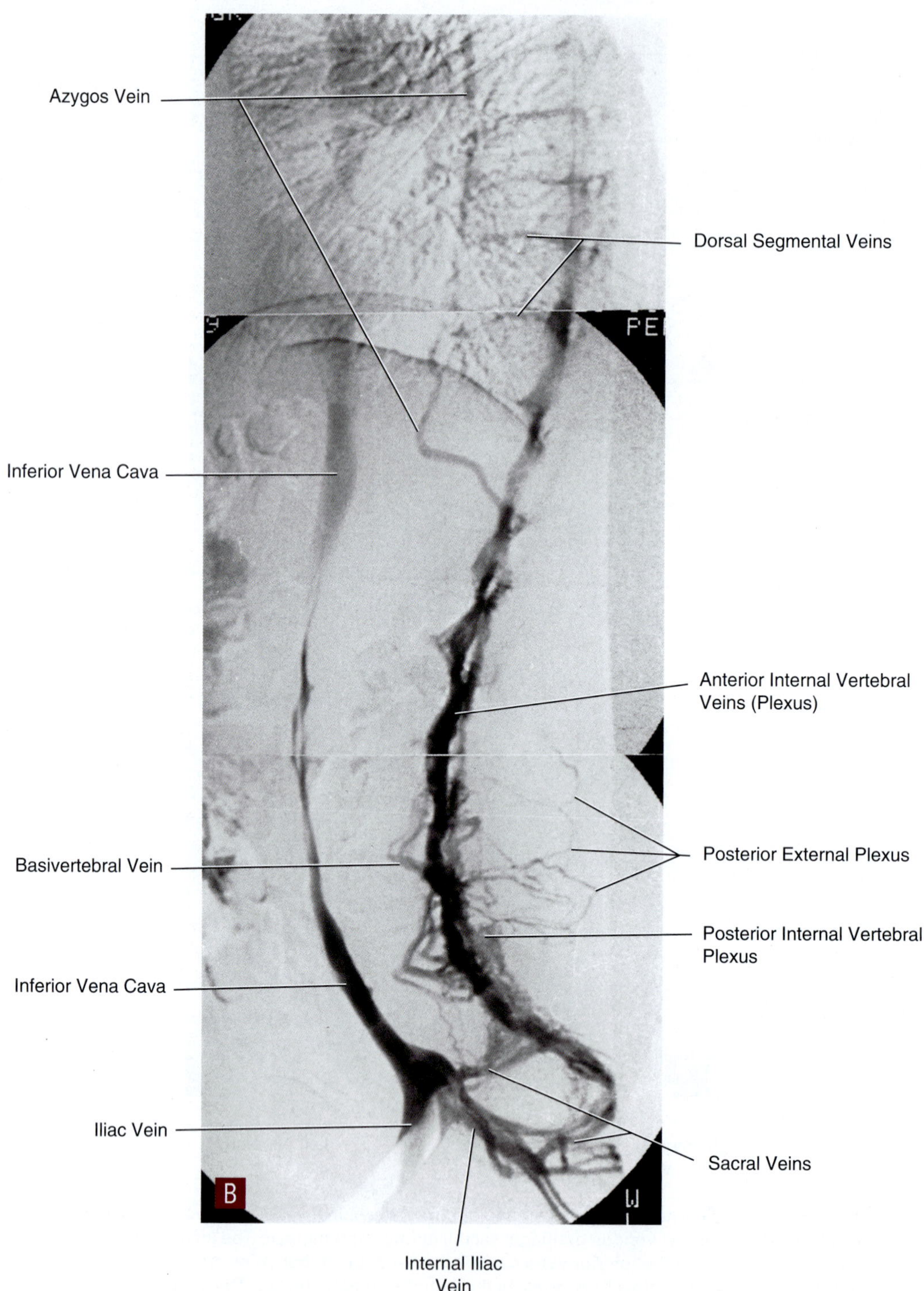

Figure 6.1. *Continued*

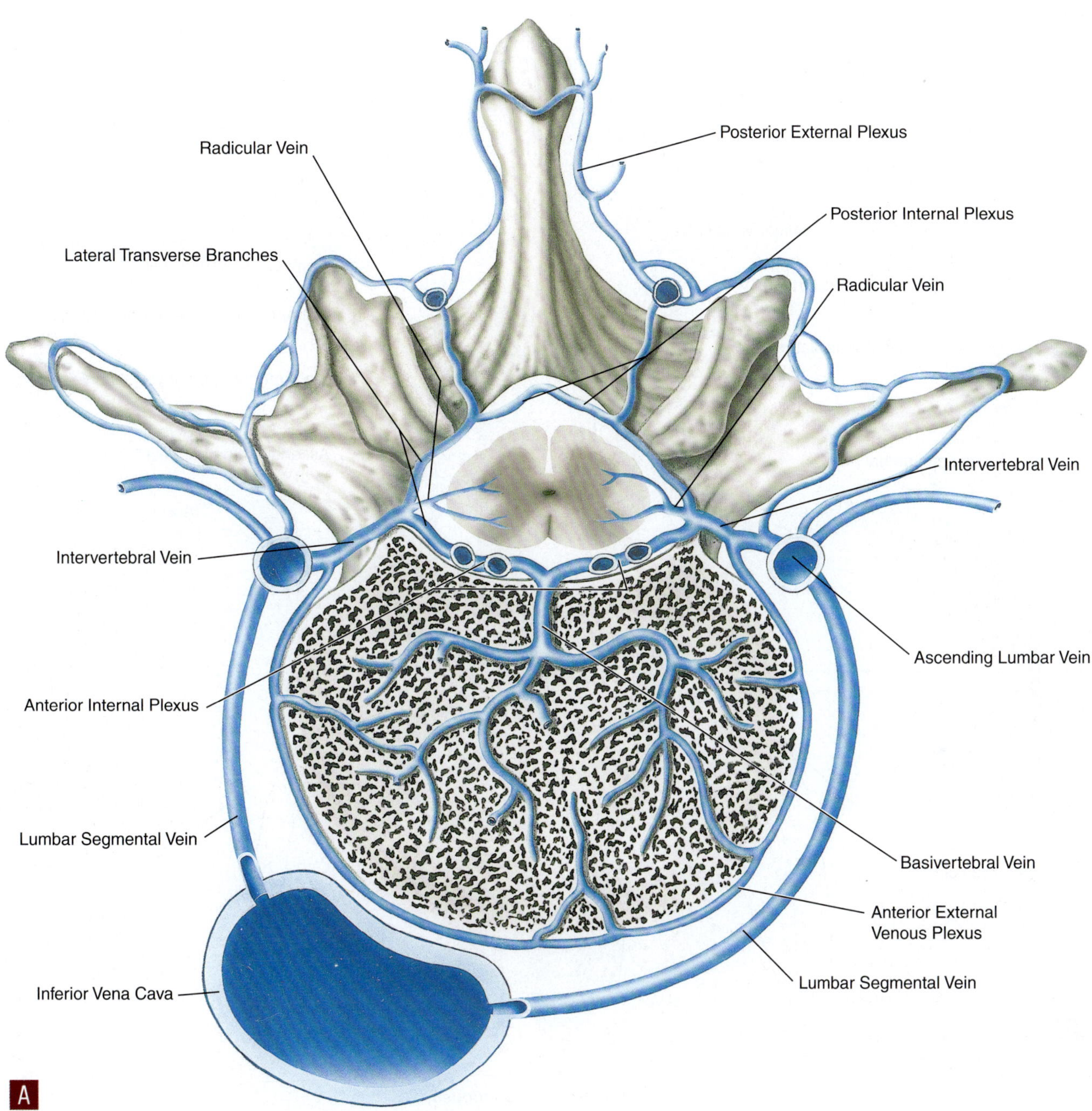

Figure 6.2. **A**, Axial view of the vertebrae showing the intimate relationship of the anterior internal venous plexus to the posterior aspect of the vertebrae. Four vertical channels are seen end-on connected by the lateral transverse branches. **B**, Anterior view of the epidural plexus and connections with the paravertebral veins. **C**, Diagram of the craniospinal venous system in a sagittal view showing the internal and external venous plexuses, and the basivertebral veins. At the level of the foramen magnum, the epidural plexus can be seen forming a dense network connecting the vertebral veins, occipital and sigmoid sinuses, the basilar plexus, and the venous plexus of the hypoglossal canal.

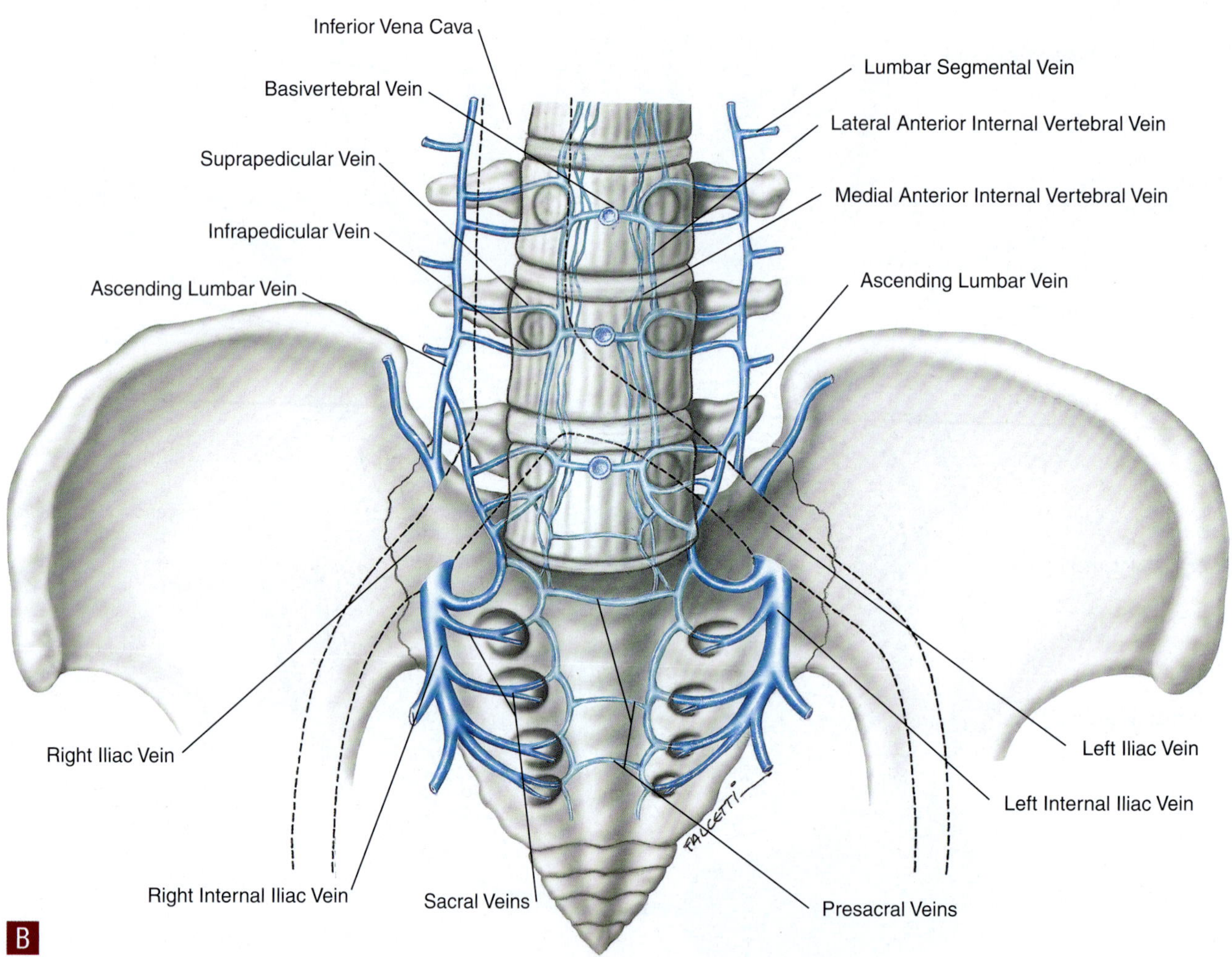

Figure 6.2. *Continued*

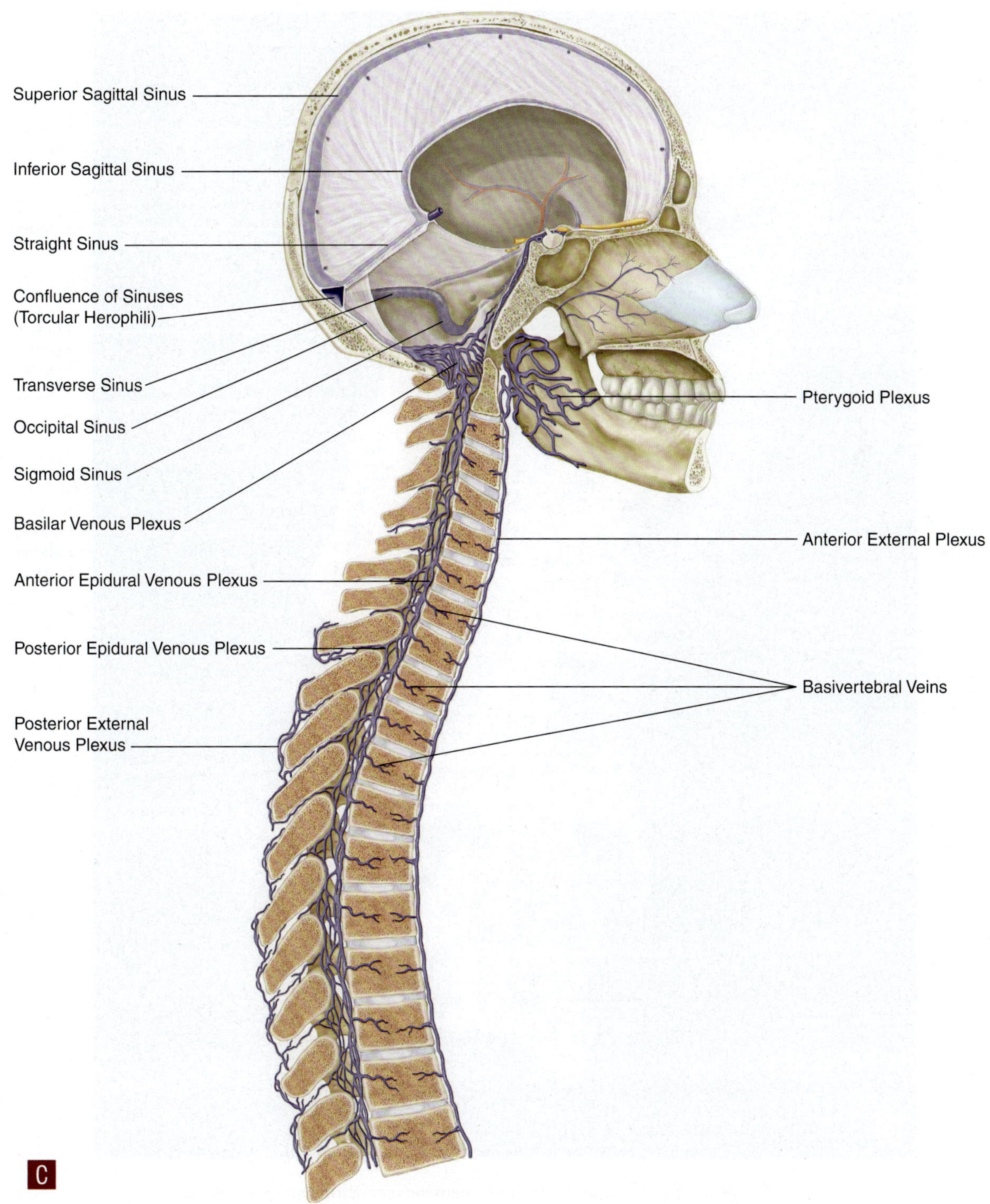

Figure 6.2. *Continued*

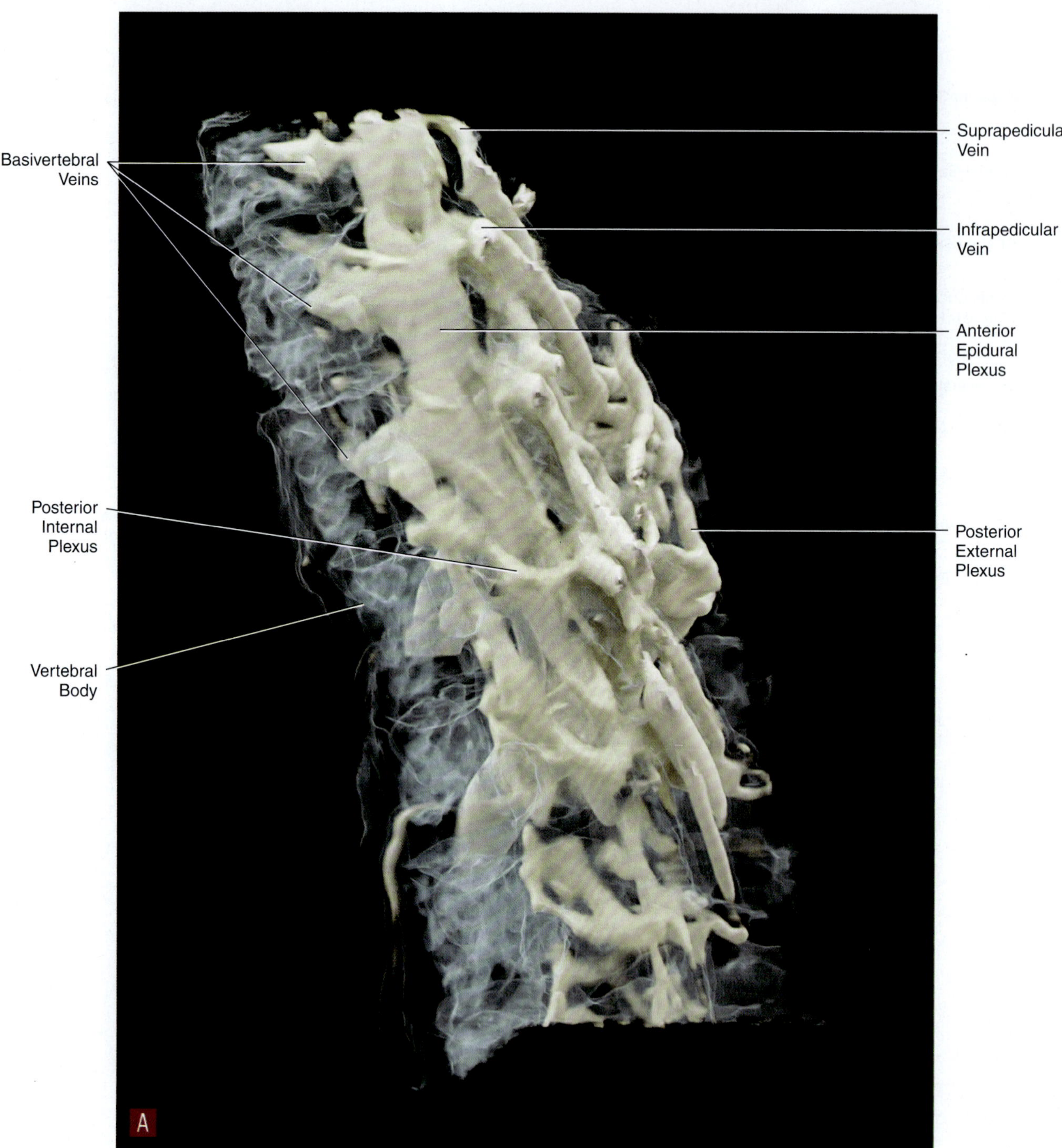

Figure 6.3. A and B, 3D volume-rendered cinematic reconstruction showing the anterior epidural venous plexus and a hypertrophic posterior external plexus in a patient with central venous occlusions.

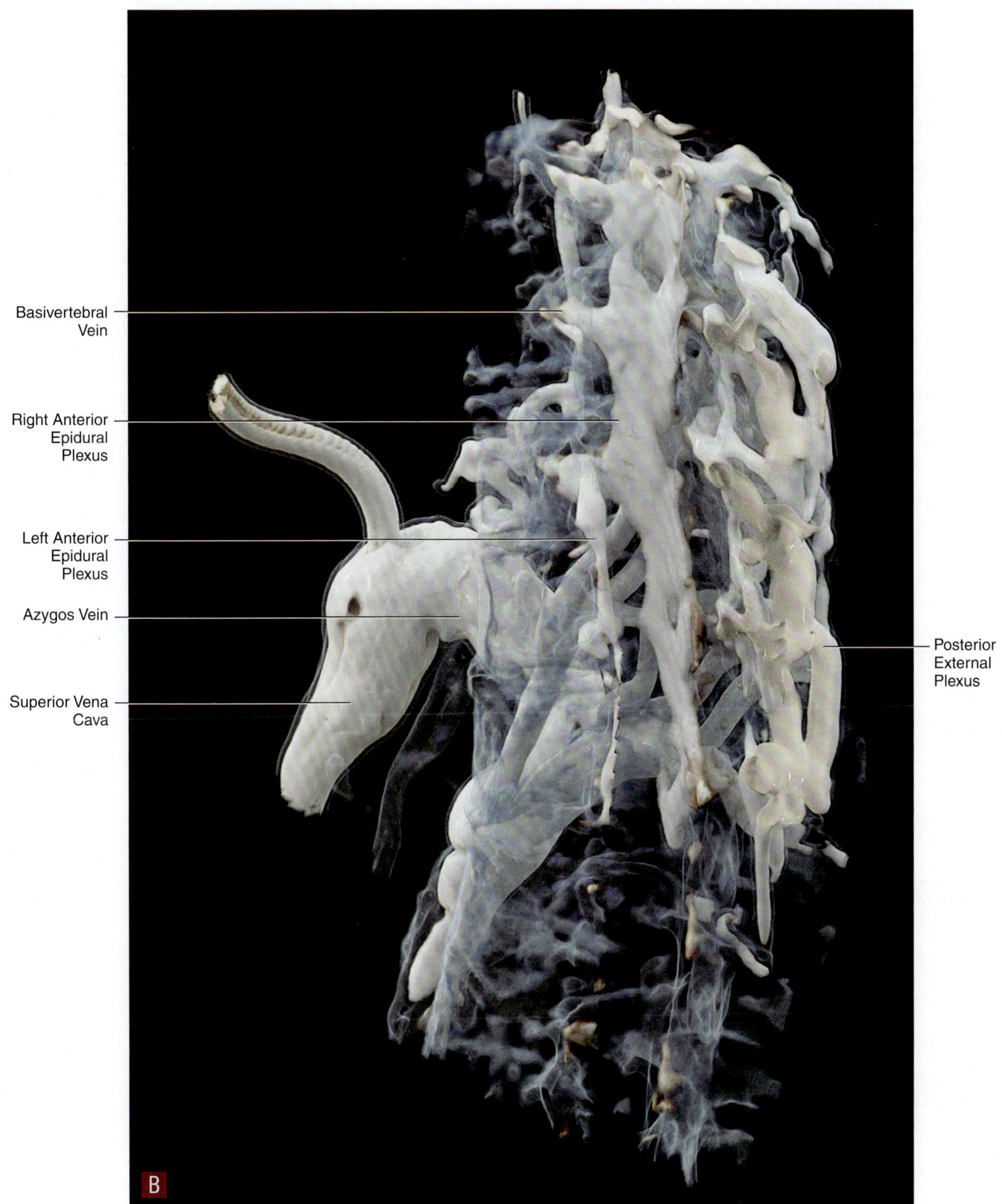

Figure 6.3. *Continued*

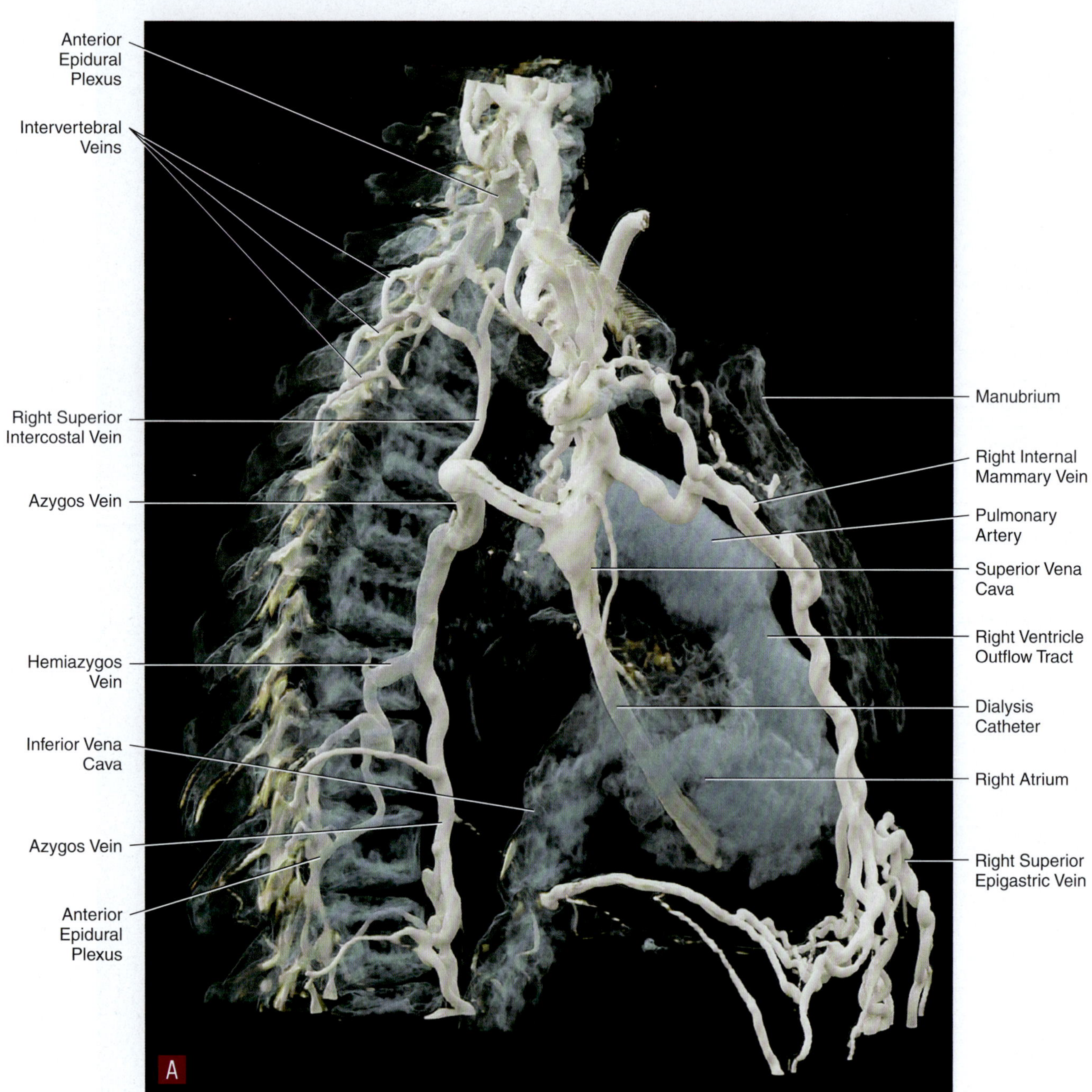

Figure 6.4. 3D volume-rendered cinematic reconstruction in a lateral and posterolateral view showing multiple collaterals in a patient with central venous occlusion. A, Lateral view demonstrating the extensive thoracic venous collateral network that drains the upper extremities into the azygos vein and the diaphragmatic veins. There is collateralization with the spinal venous plexus, including the epidural venous plexus. **B**, Posterolateral view in the same patient.

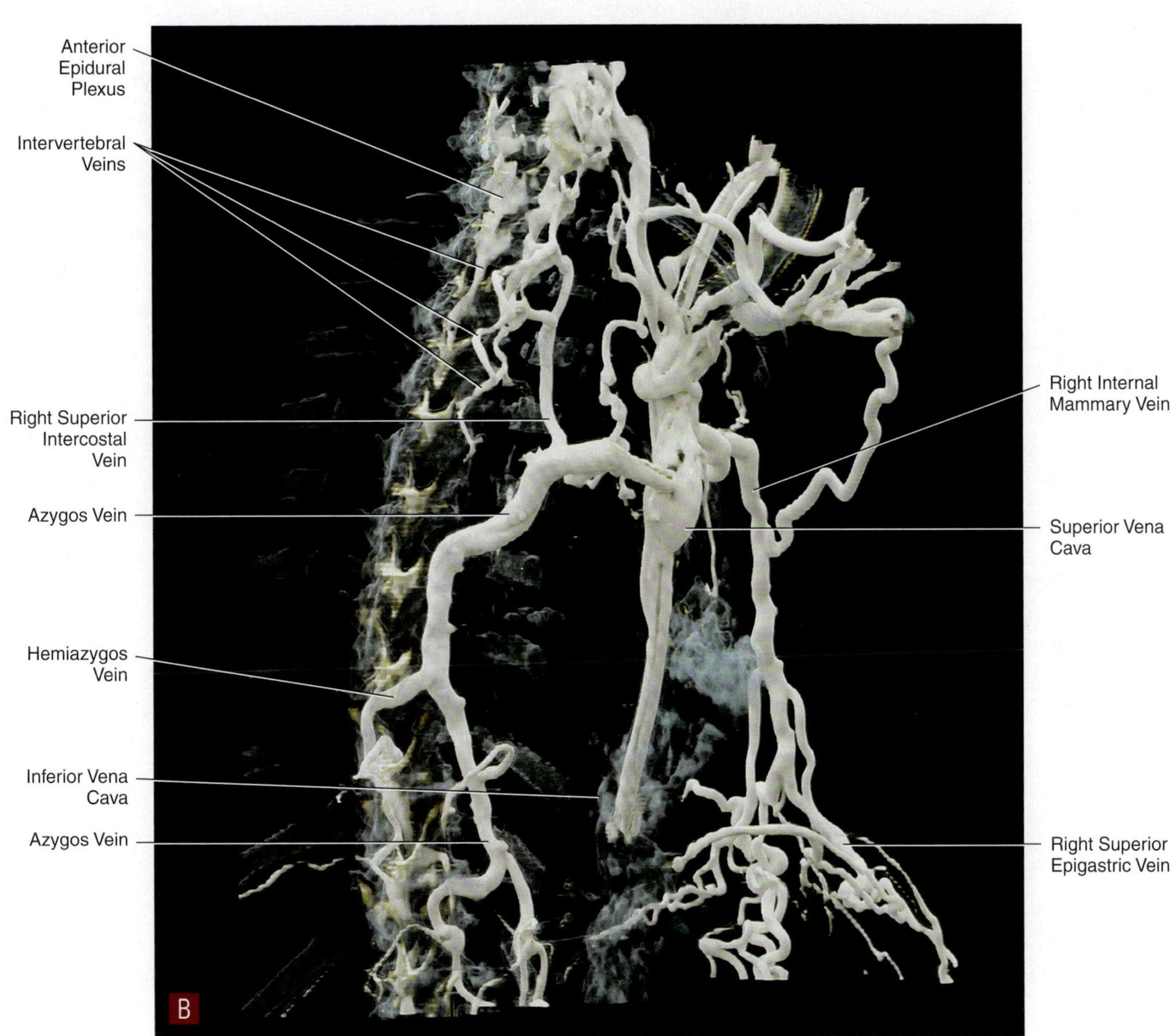

Figure 6.4. *Continued*

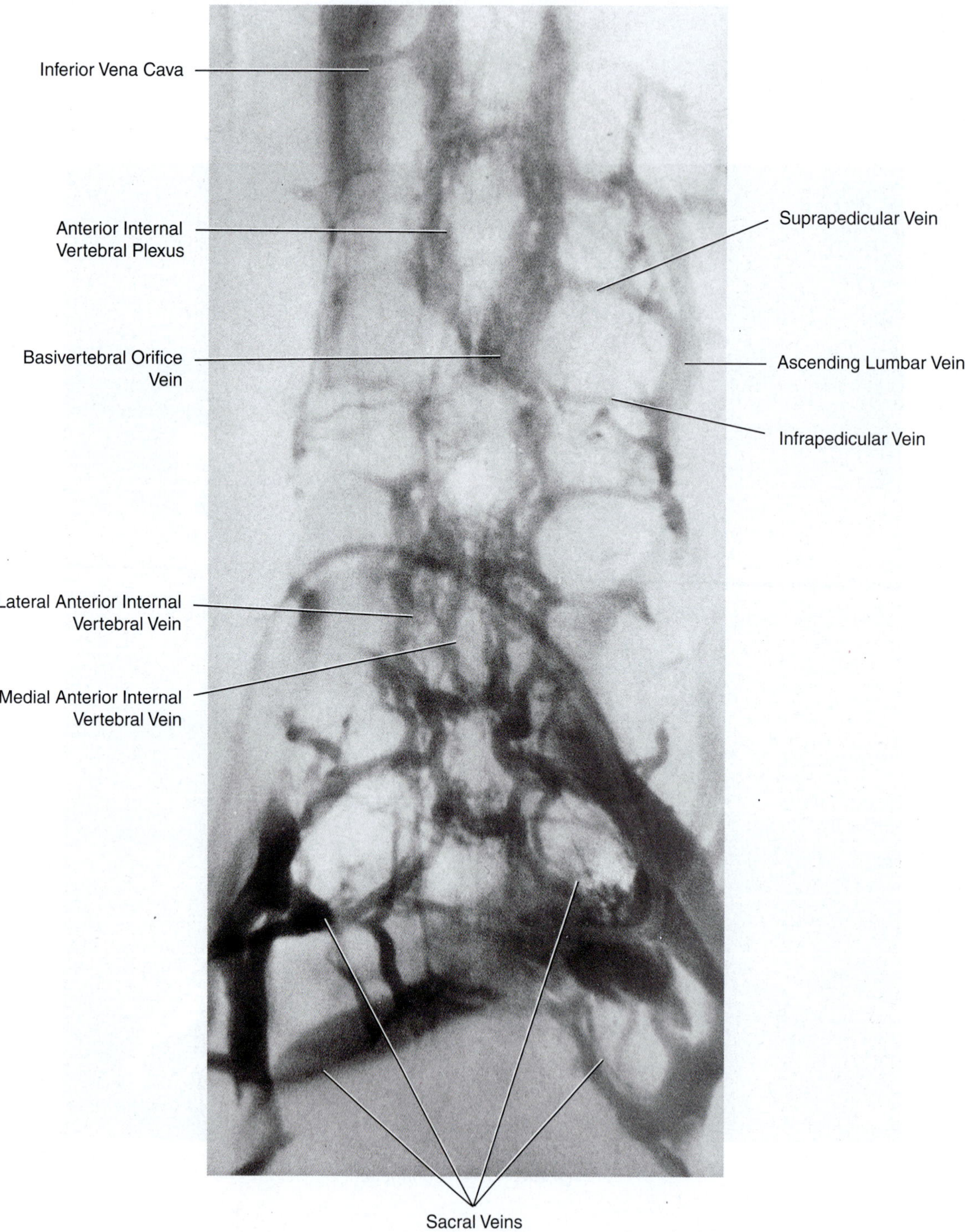

Figure 6.5. Epidural venogram. The medial anterior internal vertebral veins are plexiform with multiple irregular venous channels, and the lateral anterior internal vertebral veins are larger single vessels. At the L5–S1 level, the veins leave the lateral aspect and come closer to the midline.

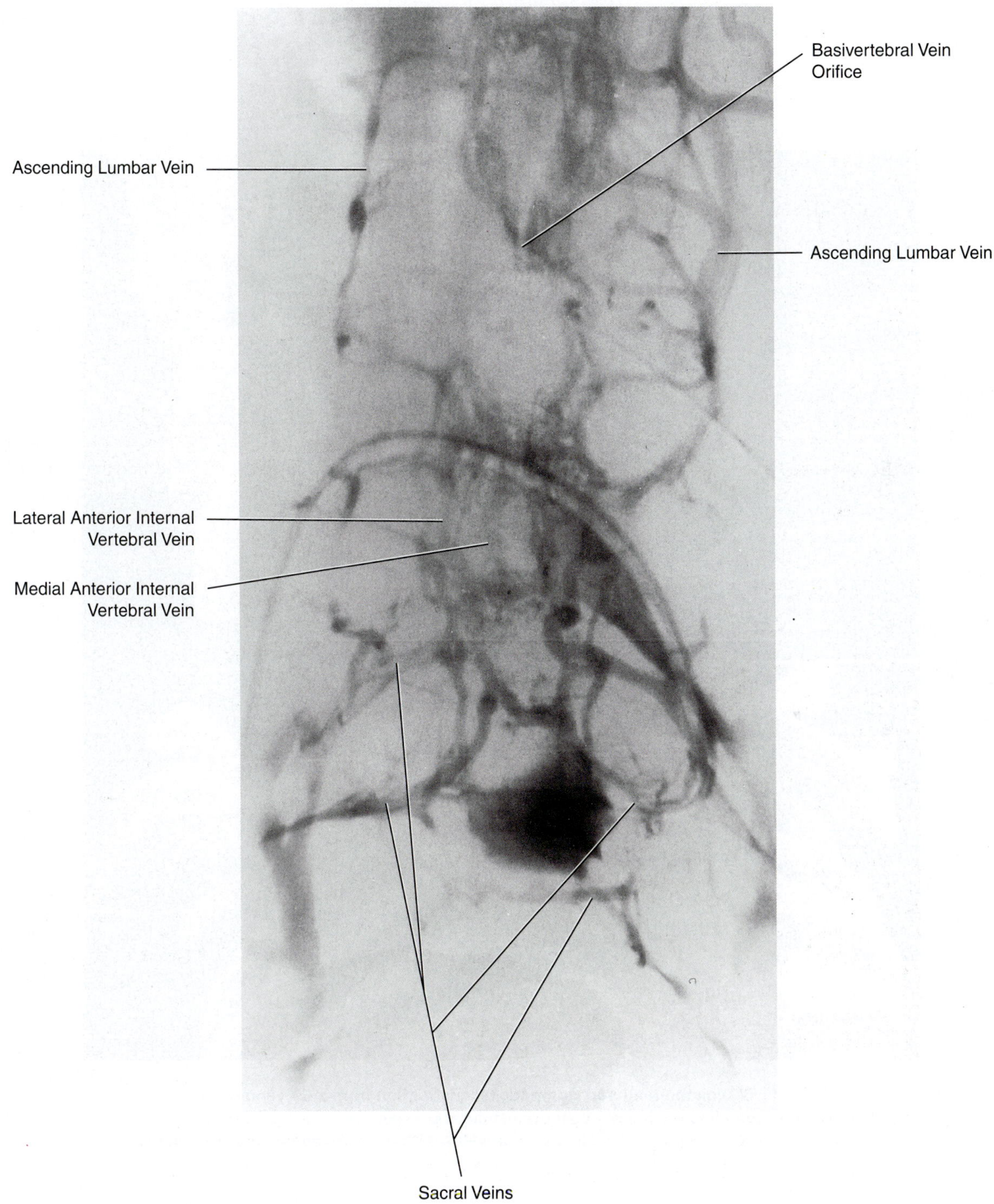

Figure 6.6. Anterior view of an epidural venogram showing the lateral and medial anterior internal vertebral veins. Note the filling defect at the level of L4–L5 due to a disc herniation.

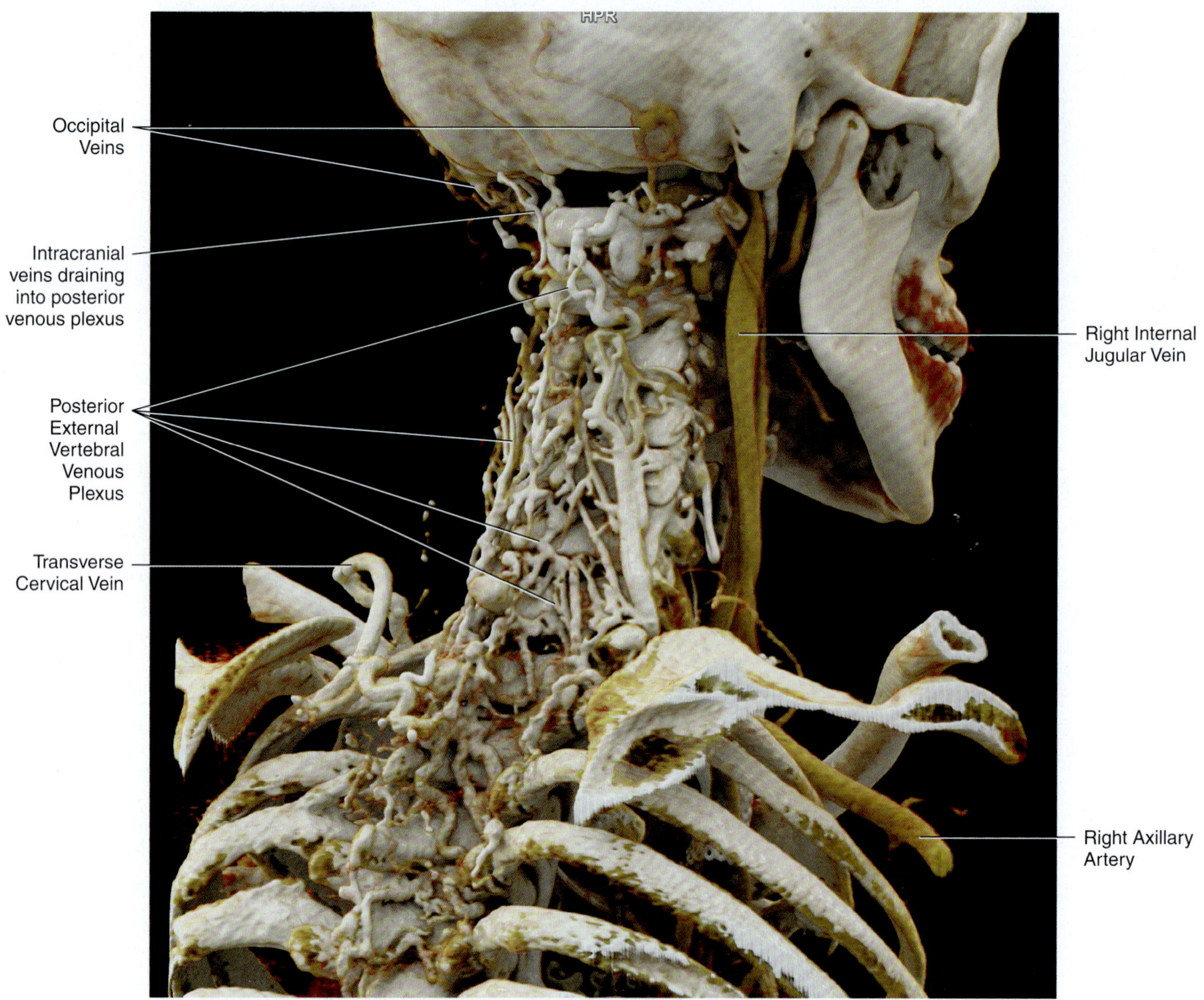

Figure 6.7. 3D volume-rendered cinematic reconstruction from a CT venogram in a patient with bilateral internal jugular vein occlusions and extensive collateralization via the posterior external venous plexus, which communicates with the intracranial and scalp veins.

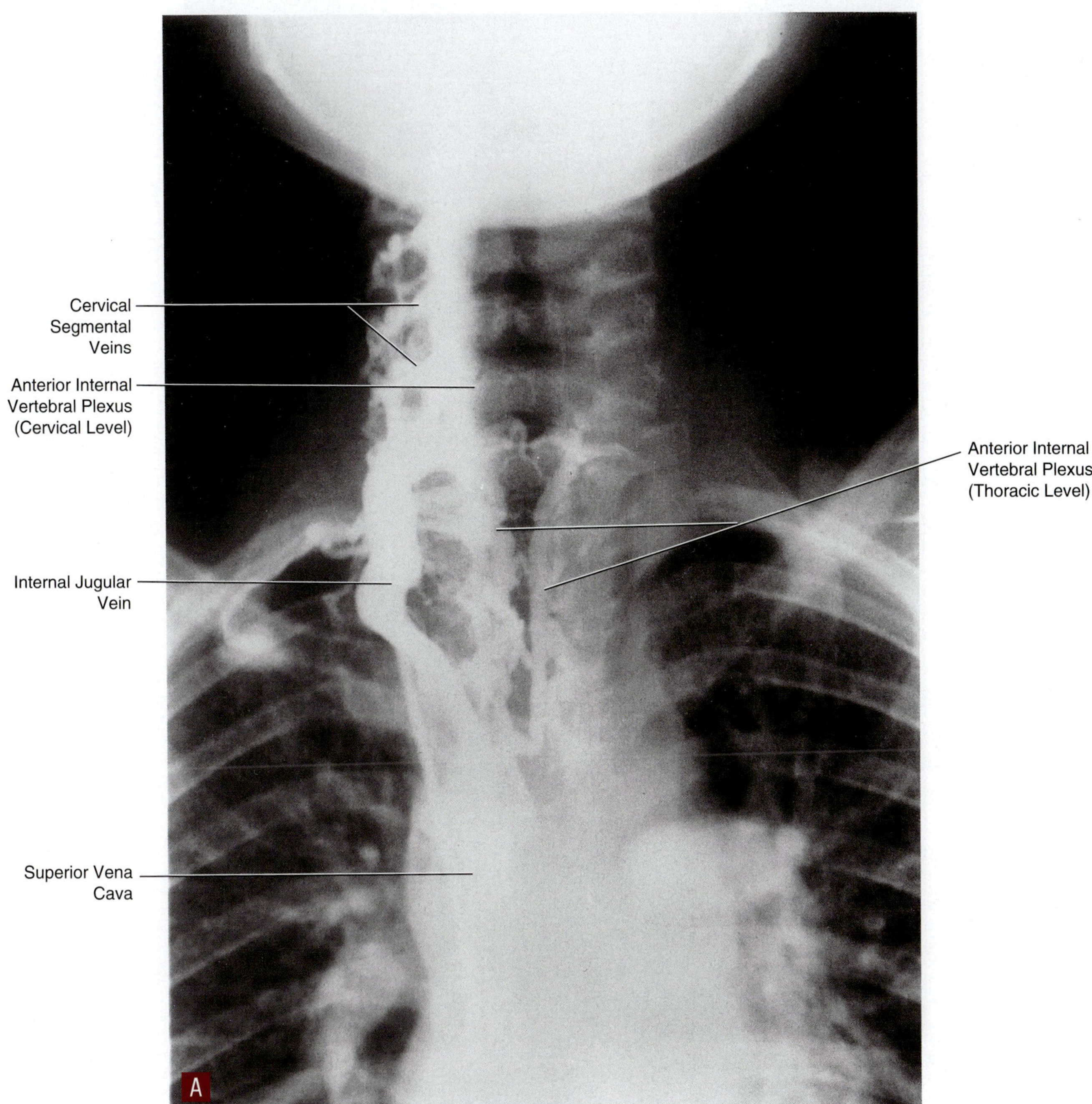

Figure 6.8. **Cervical venogram in anterior view.** **A**, The anterior group of venous plexuses is more developed in the cervical region than in the lumbar region. From the C7 level up, the spinal canal is broader and the anterior internal vertebral veins are not defined. From the C7 level down, the anterior internal vertebral veins can be observed. **B**, Venogram of the azygos vein showing retrograde filling of the paravertebral veins and partial filling of the anterior internal vertebral veins. **C**, Lateral view of the azygos vein showing the segmental veins and part of the anterior internal vertebral plexus.

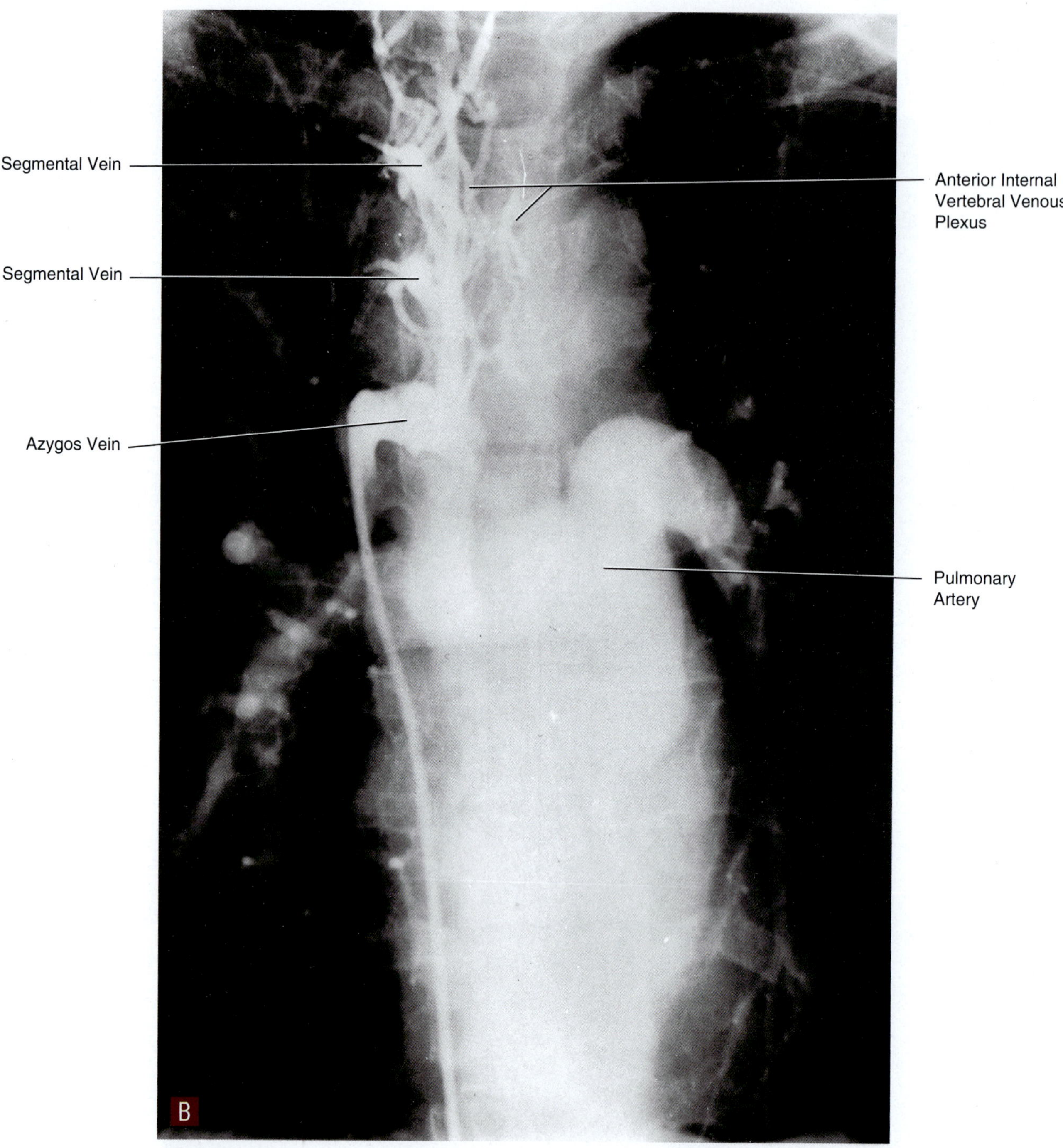

Figure 6.8. *Continued*

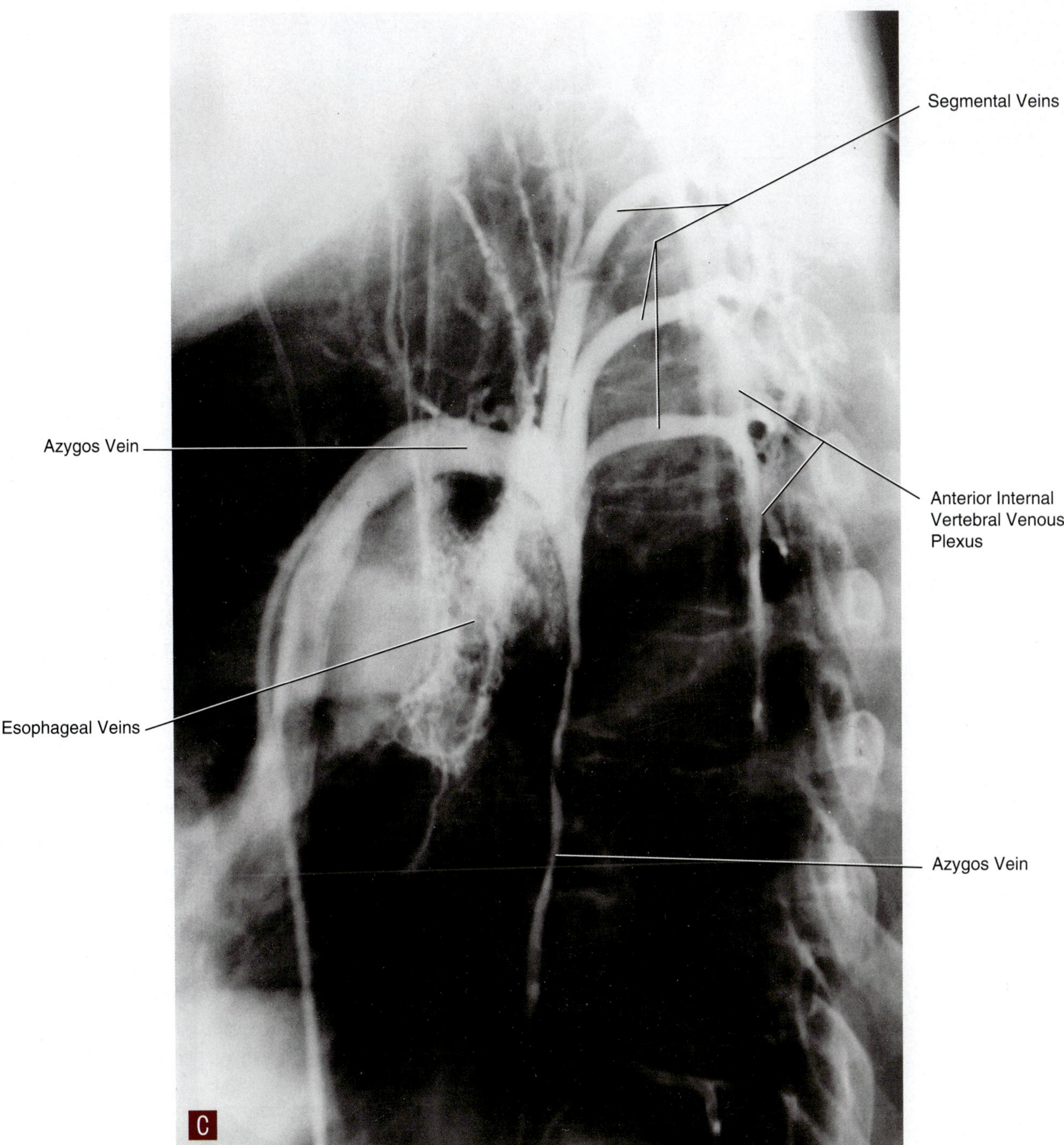

Figure 6.8. *Continued*

7

Thoracic Aorta and Arteries of the Trunk

The thoracic aorta is conventionally divided into three segments: the ascending aorta, the aortic arch, and the descending aorta, which is subsequently divided into thoracic and abdominal segments (Fig. 7.1).

The ascending aorta is about 5 cm in length and arises from the left ventricle of the heart, where the aortic valve closes it (Fig. 7.2). The aorta courses an anterior ascending tract to the right side of the chest, curving backward and crossing the mediastinum in the segment called the aortic arch, to the posterior mediastinum and to the left of the vertebral column (Fig. 7.3). The descending aorta approaches the median plane and terminates in front of the vertebral column, where it crosses the diaphragm at the aortic hiatus, where the abdominal aorta begins (Fig. 7.3).

Owing to the need for reporting the outcomes of the modern endovascular procedures performed in the thoracic aorta—the ascending aorta, aortic arch, and descending thoracic aorta were further divided into zones (Fig. 7.4). Zone 0 extends from the aortic valve to the level of the brachiocephalic trunk (including). Zone 1 extends from the edge of the brachiocephalic trunk to the left carotid artery (including). Zone 2 extends from the edge of the left carotid artery to the left subclavian artery (including). Zone 3 is the curve segment from the edge of the left subclavian artery to the beginning of the vertical descending thoracic aorta. Zone 4 includes the whole descending thoracic aorta and the segments are named T4 through T12 according to the level of the intercostal arteries. The abdominal aorta segments are named after the lumbar artery levels, from L1 to L5.

Thoracic Aorta

Aortic Vasa Vasorum

The walls of the thoracic and abdominal aorta are supplied by the vasa vasorum. The vasa vasorum system is formed by small nutrient vessels to the walls of other larger vessels. These are the vessel's vessels, which deliver blood to a capillary network within the large arterial wall. However, only part of the vessel wall is supplied by the vasa vasorum. The part of the wall that is fed by the filtration of nutrients through the vascular endothelium is called the physiologic intima. There is a "critical deepness" of vascularization, which varies according to the different arteries and species. At the thoracic aorta, the avascular zone is about 500 μm thick, whereas the avascular zone of the abdominal aorta is about 700 μm. The tunica intima and the internal third of the tunica media receive nutrients directly from the blood within the lumen of the main artery by diffusion, whereas the external two thirds of the tunica media and the tunica adventitia are fed by arterial blood from the vasa vasorum (Figs. 7.5 and 7.6).

The vasa vasorum arises from the intercostal arteries at the thoracic aorta and from the lumbar arteries at the abdominal aorta. The vasa vasorum originate at the level of the tunica adventitia with a diameter of about 350 μm. The initial trunk has a ventral direction with a length of about 4 mm. Still at the tunica adventitia, the vasa vasorum trunk with a diameter of about 150 μm divides into two secondary branches of equal diameter. These branches run parallel to the main axis of the aorta in an opposite cranial and caudal direction. From these branches, a network of smaller branches is found with a lateral and ventral distribution and with several contralateral anastomoses, forming vascular arcades on the aortic wall. The vascular disposition of the vasa vasorum follows a reticular distribution with a polygonal appearance. A rich anastomotic plexus with arterioles of first order with a diameter of 200 to 100 μm originates from the reticular vasa vasorum network. The microcirculation of the vasa vasorum is formed by vessels less than 200 μm in diameter (Fig. 7.6).

Microcirculation of the Aorta

Arterioles of first order—between 200 and 100 μm
Arterioles of second order—between 100 and 30 μm
Precapillaries or terminal—between 30 and 10 μm
Capillaries—between 3 and 10 μm
Postcapillaries venules—between 10 and 30 μm
Venules of second order—between 30 and 100 μm
Venules of first order—between 100 and 200 μm

The arterioles of second order with a diameter of 100 and 30 μm are also called arcuate arterioles. These vessels extend for sectors of the aortic circle varying from 90° to 220°, but with an average of 120°. The precapillaries, or terminal arterioles, originate from the arcuate arterioles and distribute to the junction of the medium and external third of the tunica media. The distal portion of the terminal branches does not reach the internal third of the tunica media and spreads as a tree with a flat top (Fig. 7.6). The arterial vasa vasorum is followed by the venous vasa vasorum with inverted direction of flow. Morphologically, two venous structures correspond to the arterial structure, at the precapillaries and arcuate arterioles.

Segments of the Thoracic Aorta

An important requirement for successful endografting is to select a sufficiently long segment of healthy aorta for the landing site. This position differs from case to case, but it is necessary to make it clear where the landing zone is located if data reported from various institutions are to be accurately evaluated. Balm et al. proposed distinguishing the location of an endograft deployed in the aortic arch based on lines drawn distally to each arterial branch from the arch. Although this classification tells us which branch artery is occluded by the endograft, it does not help identify the extent of the area covered by the endograft. To arrive at a more clinically useful system, an anatomic endograft landing-zone map was advocated at the First International Summit on Thoracic Aortic Endografting held in Tokyo in 2001. Use of this landing-zone map to classify the proximal deployment site of an endograft would make it possible for investigators at different institutions to evaluate indications for treatment and analyze follow-up results. In 2002, this landing-zone map was expanded to include the position of the distal end of the endograft. Since then, the map (Fig. 7.4) has achieved consensus as the standardized anatomic definition to evaluate outcomes.

Ascending Aorta

At the origin of the ascending aorta, just after the cusps of the aortic valve, there are three dilations called aortic sinuses. The coronary arteries' orifices are located high up in the aortic sinuses or even above them (Figs. 7.2, 7.7, 7.8, 7.9).

Branches

Coronary arteries are described in Chapter 13.

Aortic Arch (Figs. 7.2 and 7.11)

There are three main branches at the aortic arch. The inferior aspect of the aortic arch may show a contour abnormality which may be mistaken for a dissection in some cases but is the remnant of the ductus arteriosus, also known as a prominent ductus bump, or a ductus diverticulum (Fig. 7.2).

Branches

Brachiocephalic trunk (innominate artery) and right common carotid artery
Left common carotid artery
Left subclavian artery

The aortic arch, with age and the presence of longstanding arterial hypertension, tends to become elongated and tortuous, and the origin of the brachiocephalic vessels tends to move forward; the angle between the branches and the aortic arch becomes more acute, making selective catheterization much more difficult. The aortic arch is classified into three different types: type I, type II, and type III, according to the angle between the branches and the aortic arch. One way to determine the arch's type is to measure the diameter of the brachiocephalic artery and compare that measurement to the distance from the horizontal line traced tangential to the top of the aortic arch to the origin of the brachiocephalic trunk (Fig. 7.10). One width or less of the brachiocephalic artery is type I, two widths is type II, and three widths is type III.

Variations of the Aortic Arch

Right aortic arch (Fig. 7.12)
Double aortic arch (Fig. 7.13)
Cervical aortic arch (Fig. 7.14)

Brachiocephalic Trunk

It is the first and largest branch of the aortic arch. This trunk arises from the superior posterior aspect of the aortic arch. It ascends posterolaterally to the right. At first positioned anterior to the trachea, it gradually moves to the right. From its bifurcation originates the two terminal branches: the right subclavian and right common carotid arteries. Occasional branches are the arteria thyroidea ima (thyroid artery of Neubauer), the thymic artery, and the bronchial artery. The right vertebral artery originates from the right subclavian artery. The right subclavian artery has been described as the arterial supply of the upper limb section. The right common carotid artery is the principal terminal branch of the brachiocephalic artery.

The principal arteries of the head and neck are the common carotid arteries. These arteries ascend in the neck up to the level of the upper border of the thyroid cartilage, where they divide into two main branches, the external and internal carotid arteries. At the division of the vessel, there is a dilation known as the carotid sinus. At the bifurcation, there are terminal nerve fibers, a baroreceptor, and a chemoreceptor called the carotid body. The common carotid arteries differ in length and place of origin. While the right carotid artery originates from the brachiocephalic trunk, the left carotid artery arises directly from the arch of the aorta.

Left Common Carotid Artery (Figs. 7.15-7.18)

It is the second branch of the arch of the aorta, arising immediately behind and to the left of the brachiocephalic trunk, presenting thoracic and cervical portions. The artery courses in an upward direction, originally in front of the trachea and progressively inclining to the left side.

Left Subclavian Artery (Fig. 7.17)

It is the third branch of the arch of the aorta, arising after and behind the left common carotid artery. It is described in Chapter 15. The left vertebral artery originates from the left subclavian artery.

Variations of the Branches of Aortic Arch

There are a number of variations of the origins of the aortic arch branches. The six vessels may arise separately from the aortic arch: carotids, the subclavians, and the vertebrals, or they may arise as a single trunk or in a number of combinations (Figs. 7.19-7.24). The most common variation is a high origin of the innominate artery (to the left of the trachea) (Fig. 7.19), a common origin of the left carotid artery with the brachiocephalic trunk (bovine arch) (Fig. 7.18, 7.19, 7.22), an anomalous origin of the right subclavian artery distal to the left subclavian artery (Figs. 7.21 and 7.22), and an origin of the left vertebral artery directly from the aorta (Fig. 7.20).

65% usual pattern (Figs. 7.11 and 7.17).

27% left common carotid artery shares the brachiocephalic trunk with the right subclavian and right common carotid artery (Fig. 7.18).

2.5% the four large arteries branched separately. Independent origin of all vessels (Fig. 7.22)

5.0% variety of patterns. Right subclavian artery with origin at the distal aortic arch (Figs. 7.22 and 7.24). Common carotid trunk and right subclavian originated from the posterolateral wall of the aortic arch (Fig. 7.22). Left common carotid originating together with the brachiocephalic trunk and the right common carotid originating from the aortic arch (Fig. 7.23).

1.2% symmetrical right and left brachiocephalic trunk.
- Common carotid trunk giving off the left subclavian artery
- Common carotid trunk
- Left and right brachiocephalic arteries
- Single arch vessel
- Left brachiocephalic artery

Normally the aorta arches to the left as a persistence of the left fourth primitive arch. If the right fourth primitive arch persists instead, it will arch to the right (Fig. 7.12). If the right-sided arch with its brachiocephalic vessel origins is a mirror image of the left arch and if it descends on the right, there is a very high incidence of associated intracardiac anomalies (98%). If there is a right-sided arch with the aorta descending instead on the left or if there is an associated anomalous left subclavian artery with the anomalous right-sided aortic arch, then intracardiac anomalies are much less frequent. When there is a right aortic arch, the arrangement of the three branches may be reversed; there is a left brachiocephalic trunk, and the right common carotid artery and right subclavian artery arise independently.

The double aortic arch reflects a persistence of both primitive arches (Fig. 7.13). There are many variants of this phenomenon, with atresia between segments as well as variations in the size of the descending aorta and also in the relative size of each arch. Cervical arches arise unusually high (Fig. 7.14); they may be located in the thoracic outlet or may even extend up beyond the neck, at or above the sternal end of the clavicles. Cervical arches are the result of persistence of the third arch rather than the fourth during embryologic development. An abnormally high position of a right- or left-sided arch is often associated with anomalous brachiocephalic branch origins. See Chapter 1 (Fig. 1.2).

Descending Thoracic Aorta

The descending thoracic aorta begins as a continuation of the aortic arch, usually at the level of T4. Rarely, folding or kinking of the arch and descending aortic junction may be present without a pressure gradient, which is known as pesudocoarctation. It is thought to arise as a persistence of the left third arch, which also associated with a cervical arch (Fig. 7.14).

Pericardial Branches

These are small vessels arising from the descending aorta, supplying the posterior aspect of the pericardium.

Bronchial Arteries

The right bronchial artery usually arises together with a right intercostal artery, the third posterior intercostal artery, but other intercostal arteries may arise from that trunk. This common trunk is called intercostobronchial trunk and originates from the right lateral, anterolateral, or dorsal aspect of the descending aorta (Figs. 7.25, 7.26, 7.32B). The left bronchial arteries arise directly from the anterior aspect of the descending aorta, either as single arteries (Fig. 7.27) or as common bronchial trunks, giving branches to both sides (Fig. 7.28) and usually come off perpendicular to the aortic wall (Figs. 7.29 and 7.30). The site of origin may range from the level T4 to T9, but about 90% of the bronchial arteries arise at the level of T5 and T6.

Bronchial arteries vascularize mainly the bronchi and the peribronchial connective tissue, but also supply parts of the trachea, the esophagus, the prevertebral muscles, the vagus nerve, the visceral pleura, and the parietal leaf of the pericardium. They supply paratracheal, carinal, hilar, and intrapulmonary lymph nodes and vasa vasorum of the aorta and pulmonary arteries and veins. The peripheral bronchial artery includes various components, including arterioles, capillaries, and venous plexuses. There is a dense vascular network around the bronchi, which is an arteriolar network terminating in bronchial capillaries and numerous bronchial venous plexuses with a characteristic irregular shape and course. The vascular components of this circulation exist either in the bronchial wall or in the peribronchial connective tissue. These microvascular structures are observed along the entire length of the bronchial tree as far distally as the terminal bronchioles, with a progressive decrease in caliber and number. The connective tissue around the pulmonary arteries contains the same vascular network found in the bronchial wall.

The bronchial arteries, in addition to the vascular system around the bronchi, are also observed with direct communications of the bronchial venous plexuses with the surrounding alveolar capillaries through small venules. There is also nutrition of the visceral pleura by the bronchial arteries (Chapter 10, Fig. 10.15).

The distribution of the main bronchial arteries has been described by several authors. According to Caldwell's description, in 90% of the cases, the bronchial artery anatomy is one of the following four types.

- Type I: Two bronchial arteries on the left and one intercostobronchial trunk (ICBT) on the right (40.6%)
- Type II: One bronchial artery on the left and one ICBT on the right (21.3%)
- Type III: Two bronchial arteries on the left and two on the right, one of which is an ICBT (20.6%)
- Type IV: One bronchial artery on the left and two on the right, one of which is an ICBT (9.7%)

There is no mention of a common bronchial trunk in Caldwell's classification. According to Botenga's classification, 10 different patterns of bronchial arteries are encountered.

- Type I: One intercostobronchial trunk on the right and two bronchial arteries on the left (27.7%)
- Type II: One intercostobronchial trunk on the right and one bronchial artery on the left (17.0%)
- Type III: One intercostobronchial trunk on the right, one bronchial artery on the left, and one common bronchial trunk with one artery to the right and one to the left (17.0%)
- Type IV: One intercostobronchial trunk and one bronchial artery on the right and two bronchial arteries on the left (10.7%)
- Type V: Two bronchial arteries on the right and one bronchial artery on the left (8.5%)
- Type VI: One intercostobronchial trunk on the right and one common bronchial trunk with one artery to the right and one to the left (8.5%)
- Type VII: One common bronchial trunk (4.3%)
- Type VIII: One intercostobronchial trunk, plus one bronchial artery on the right and three bronchial arteries on the left (2.1%)
- Type IX: One intercostobronchial trunk plus two bronchial arteries on the right and one bronchial artery on the left (2.1%)
- Type X: One common bronchial trunk, with one artery to the right and to the left, and one bronchial artery to the left (2.1%)

According to Uflacker's description of the bronchial arteries anatomy, 10 different patterns may be encountered, including common bronchial trunks (Fig. 7.31).

- Pattern I: One ICBT on the right and a bronchial artery on the left (30.5%)
- Pattern II: One ICBT on the right and a common trunk with a bronchial artery on the right and one on the left (25.0%)
- Pattern III: One ICBT on the right and two bronchial arteries on the left (12.5%)
- Pattern IV: One ICBT on the right, one bronchial artery on the right, and one on the left (11.1%)
- Pattern V: One ICBT on the right, one common bronchial trunk, and one left bronchial artery (8.3%)
- Pattern VI: One ICBT on the right, one bronchial artery on the left, and one common bronchial trunk in caudal position (4.2%)
- Pattern VII: Only one common bronchial trunk (2.8%)
- Pattern VIII: One ICBT on the right, giving origin to a left bronchial artery, and one bronchial artery on the left (2.8%)
- Pattern IX: Two common bronchial trunks giving origin to bronchial arteries on the right and on the left (1.4%)

Pattern X: One ICBT on the right, one bronchial artery on the right, and one common bronchial trunk origin to arteries on the right and on the left (1.4%)

The first six patterns described comprise approximately 90% of the anatomic patterns encountered in this series.

Aberrant Origins and Anatomic Variations of the Bronchial Arteries

The bronchial arteries may arise from the aortic arch or have an aberrant origin from other arteries in the greater circulation. They may be small but important when bleeding supervenes. Aberrant, replaced, and accessory bronchial arteries are supplied from other systemic arteries, including subclavian, innominate (brachiocephalic trunk), abdominal aorta, inferior phrenic arteries, thyrocervical trunk, pericardiophrenic, internal thoracic, intercostal artery, and axillary arteries (Figs. 7.32 and 7.33).

Anastomotic Connections of the Thoracic Arteries

There are innumerable anastomotic channels in the chest (Fig. 7.34), related to the internal thoracic (mammary) arteries and systemic thoracic arteries (Fig. 7.35). Pathways are transverse anastomoses and vertical anastomoses (Figs. 7.35 and 7.36). Collaterals may develop in addition to the natural anastomoses, related to inflammatory and other pathologic problems (Figs. 7.37 and 7.38).

Radicular arteries originating from the ICBT may be present in 58.3% of the cases. The anterior spinal artery is supplied by a radiculomedullary branch, which may originate from the right ICBT in 5% of the cases in one series, usually at the level of T4–T6.

Esophageal Arteries

There are four or five esophageal arteries, arising anteriorly from the descending thoracic aorta, forming a vascular network with anastomoses superiorly with the esophageal branches of the inferior thyroid arteries and inferiorly with the phrenic arteries and branches of the left gastric artery (Figs. 7.39 and 7.40). Esophageal arteries may be branches of the bronchial arteries or may arise as a common trunk, together with bronchial arteries in a significant number of cases. Variant branches may also be encountered from other adjacent arteries including intercostal, splenic, and subclavian arteries.

Mediastinal Branches

These branches are small arteries supplying mediastinal lymph nodes and areolar tissue of the posterior mediastinum.

Phrenic Branches

These branches arise from the lower thoracic aorta and vascularize the superior diaphragmatic surface and have anastomoses with the pericardiophrenic and musculophrenic arteries.

Posterior Intercostal Arteries

There are usually nine pairs of the posterior intercostal arteries, arising from the posterior aspect of the descending thoracic aorta and distributed to the intercostal spaces (Figs. 7.37 and 7.38). The first two or three intercostal arteries usually arise from the superior intercostal artery (or trunk). The second and third right posterior intercostal arteries usually arise together with the right bronchial artery and are called the intercostobronchial trunk (Fig. 7.39). The left posterior intercostal arteries are shorter and run backward on the vertebral bodies; the right posterior intercostal arteries are longer, owing to the aortic deviation to the left, and run in front of the vertebral body, turning posteriorly following the vertebral body curvature. Reaching the ribs, the posterior intercostal arteries run along the costal grooves. The posterior intercostal vein and nerve are parallel to the artery. The last paired branches of the thoracic aorta are called subcostal arteries and run a path below the 12th ribs (Figs. 7.1, 7.3, and 7.41).

Branches

Dorsal branch (anterior)
Spinal branch (posterior)
Collateral intercostal branch
Muscular branches
Unnamed branches
Anterior branch

The posterior intercostal artery runs dorsally between the necks of adjoining ribs. It has an anterior branch (intercostal) and a posterior branch (spinal branch), which enter the vertebral canal by the intervertebral foramen to supply the vertebrae, spinal cord, and meninges.

Spinal Branch. The posterior branch of the intercostal artery originates muscular branches and the radiculomedullary arteries. The radiculomedullary artery, after originating a ganglionic branch, divides into the anterior radiculomedullary artery and the posterior radiculomedullary artery, which anastomose with the anterior spinal artery and posterior spinal artery, respectively.

Collateral Intercostal Artery. This artery arises from the posterior intercostal artery near the costal angle and descends to the upper border of the subjacent rib. It runs along the upper border of the rib and anastomoses with branches from the anterior intercostal branch of the internal thoracic artery.

Muscular Branches. These branches supply the intercostal, pectoral muscles, and serratus muscles. The muscular branches give several lateral cutaneous branches and mammary branches.

Unnamed Branches. There are several unnamed branches of the posterior intercostal artery that supply all the other tissues of the chest wall including bone, periosteum, and parietal pleura.

Anterior Intercostal Arteries. These arteries originate from the internal mammary artery (Fig. 7.41) and are usually smaller than the posterior intercostal arteries.

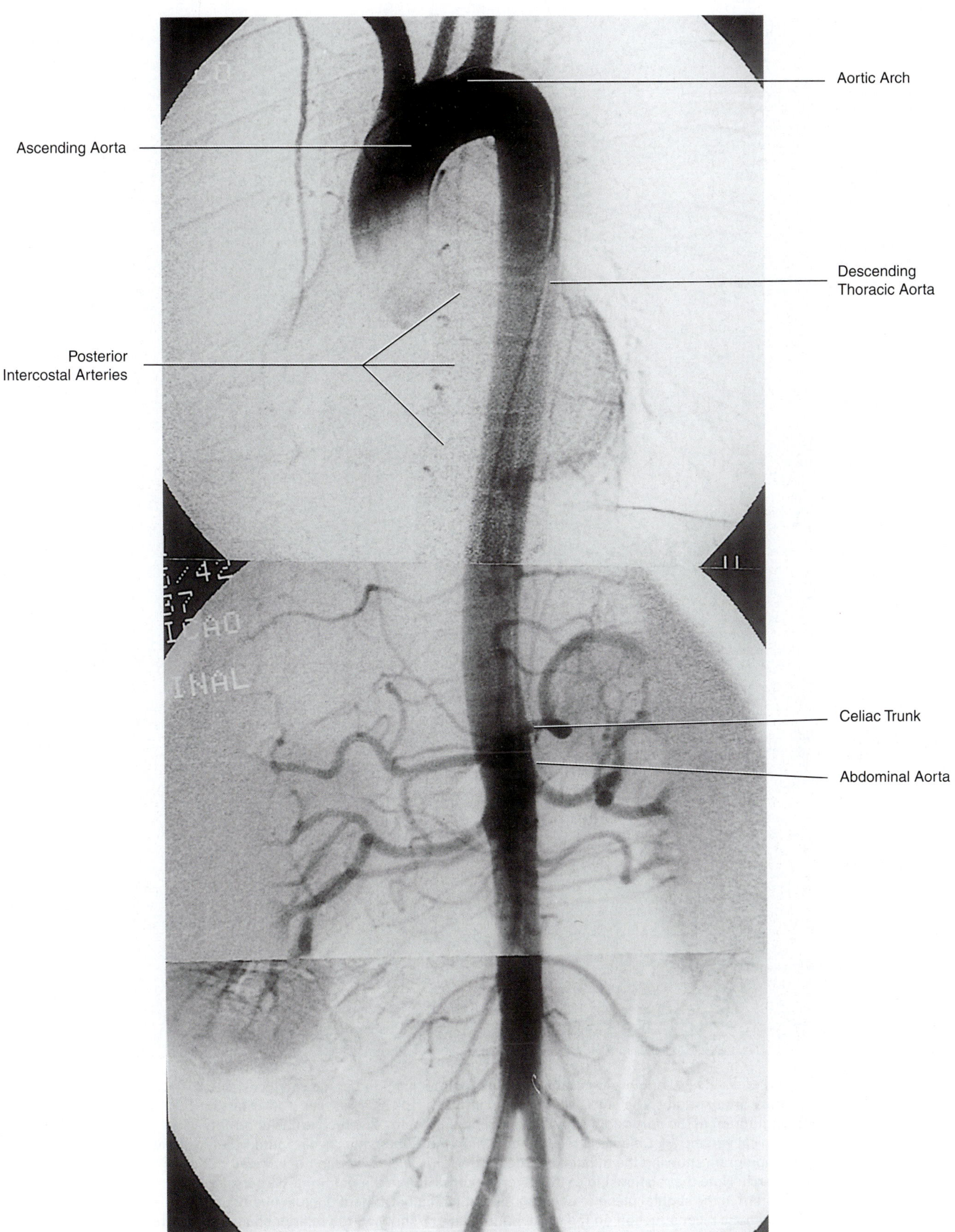

Figure 7.1. **Aortic angiogram showing the ascending thoracic aorta, the aortic arch, the descending thoracic aorta, and the abdominal aorta.** The posterior intercostal arteries and the right internal thoracic (mammary) artery are partially seen. The visceral arteries are well visualized.

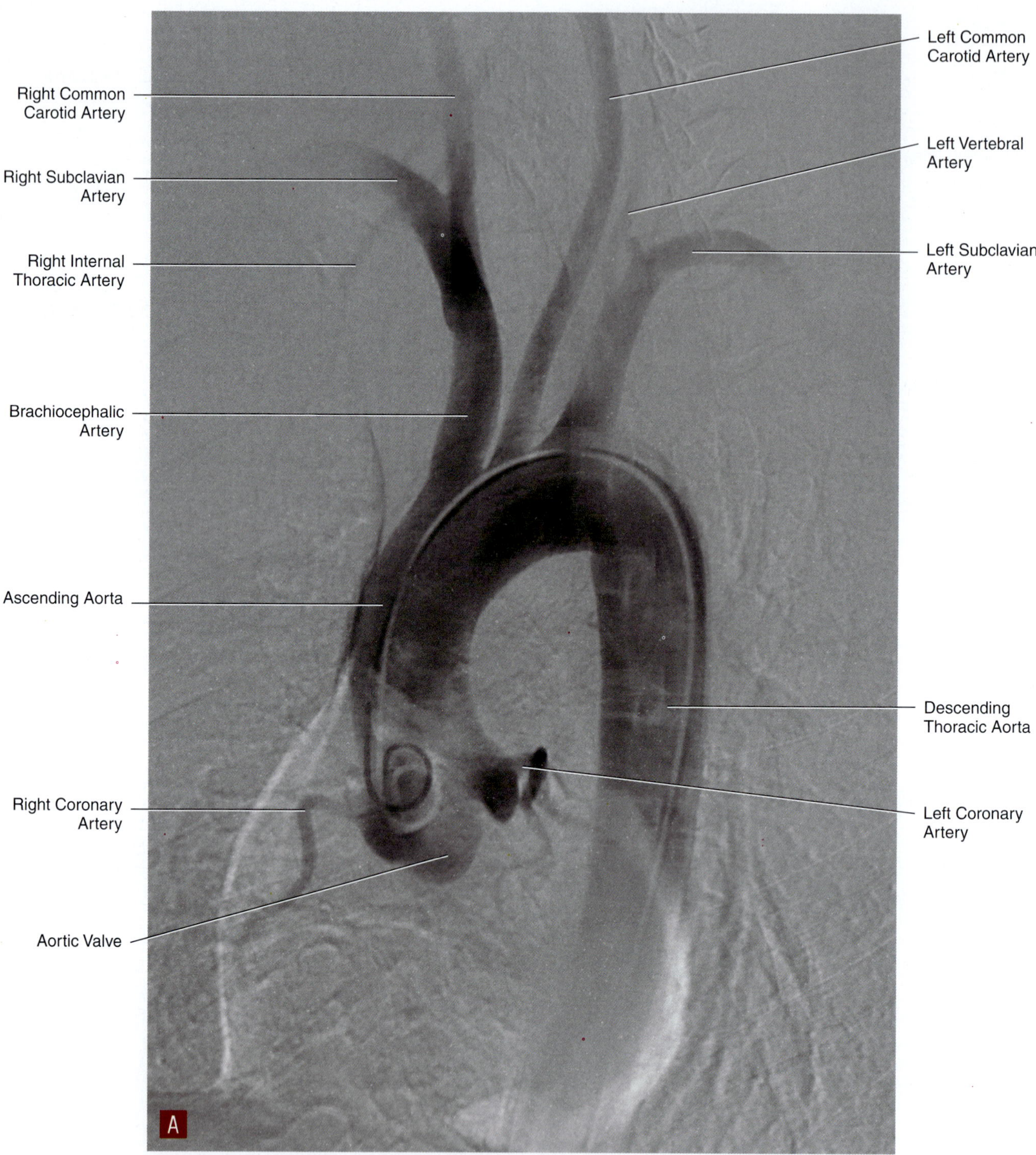

Figure 7.2. **A**, **Angiogram of the ascending aorta.** Note the aortic valve cusps and coronary artery origins. The aortic arch is seen partly en face as it courses posteriorly. **B**, Angiogram of the aortic arch showing a prominent ductus diverticulum, a common anatomical variant. **C**, Cinematic reconstruction on the same patient's computed tomography (CT) angiogram showing the ductus diverticulum near a calcification in the left wall of the aortic arch. Note the relationship of the diverticulum with the the pulmonary artery. **D**, CT angiogram in the sagittal plane of a young patient with a prominent ductus diverticulum. **E**, Cinematic reconstruction on the same patient as (**D**) showing the relationship of the ductus diverticulum with the pulmonary artery.

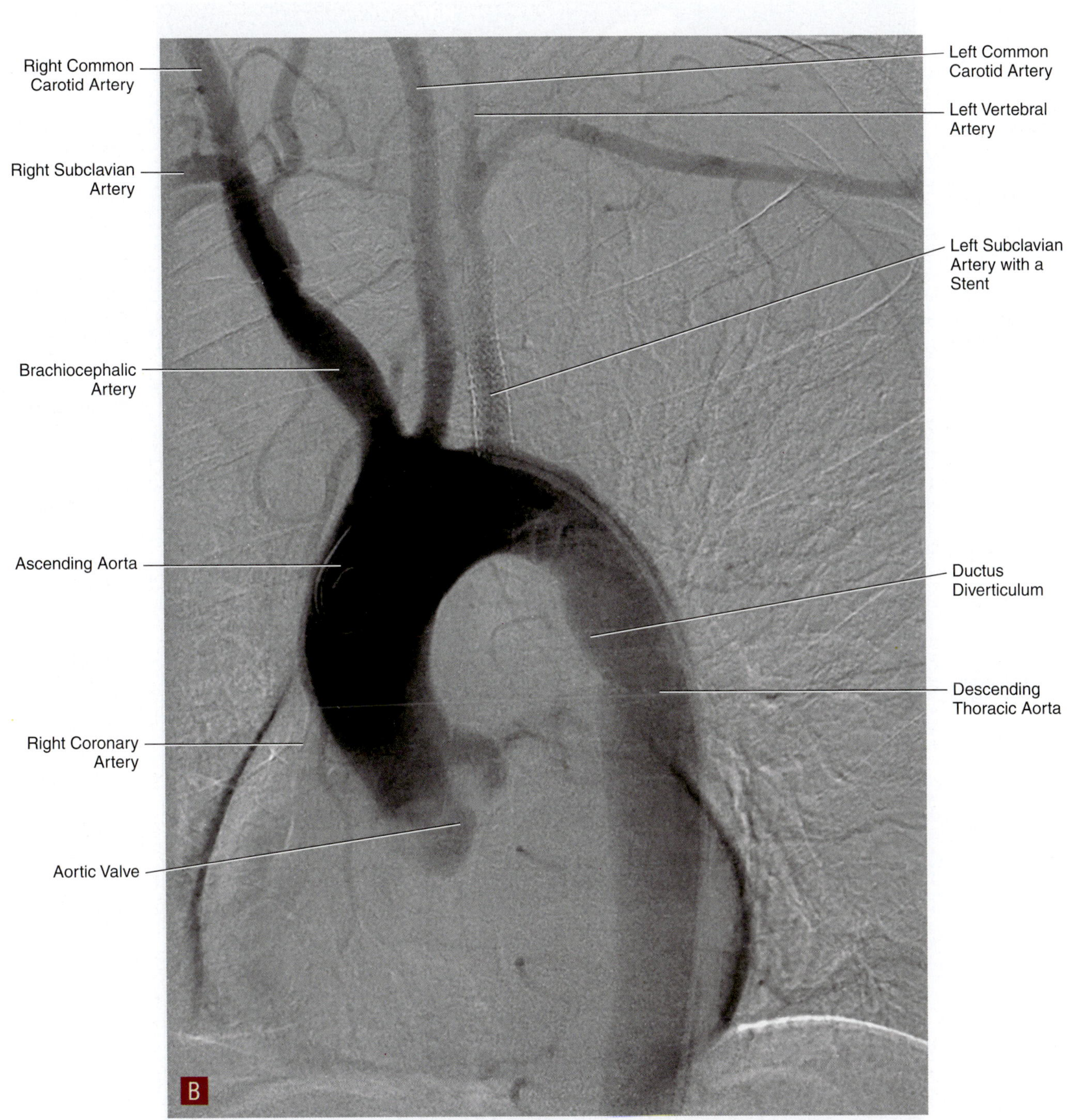

Figure 7.2. *Continued*

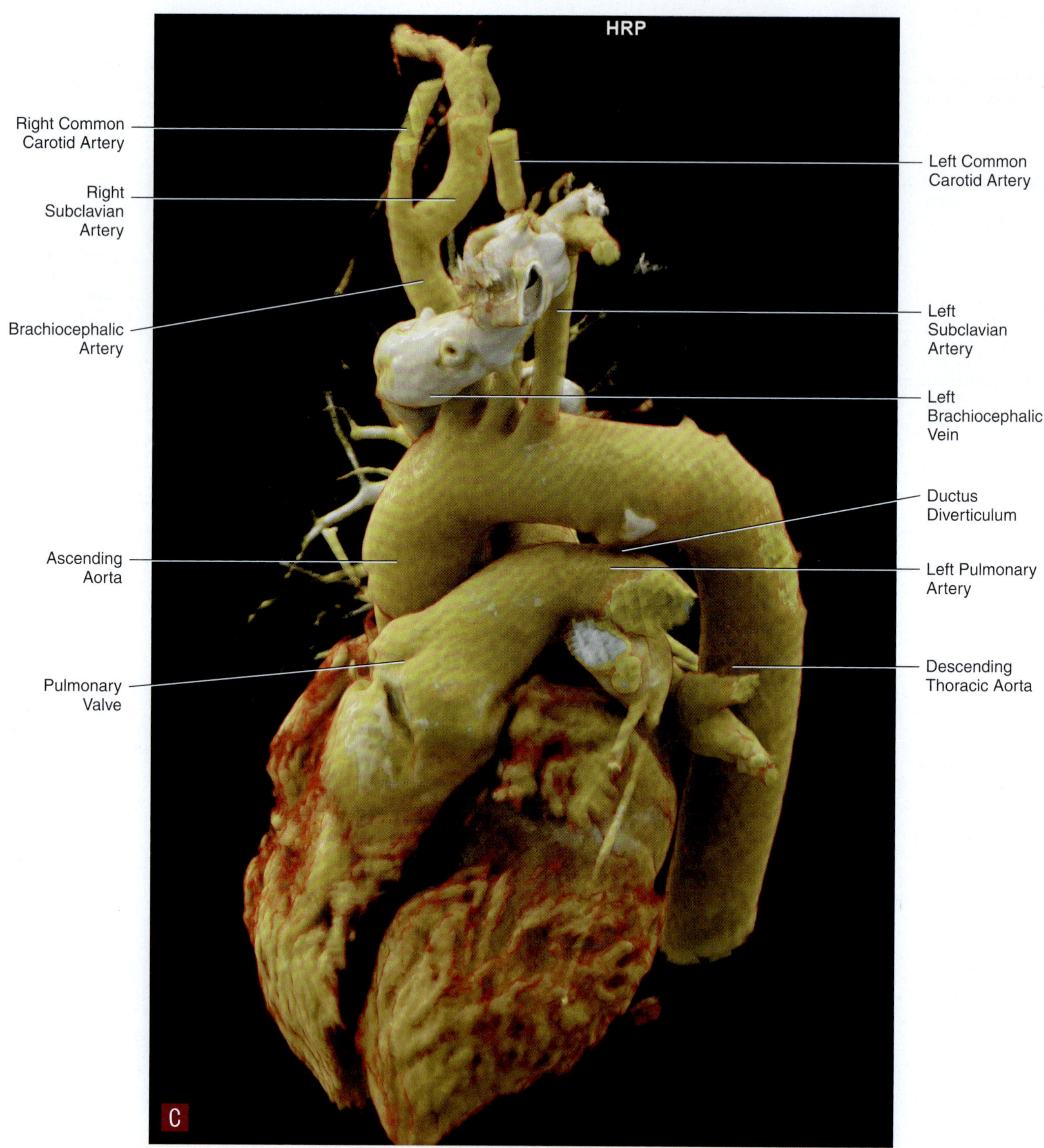

Figure 7.2. *Continued*

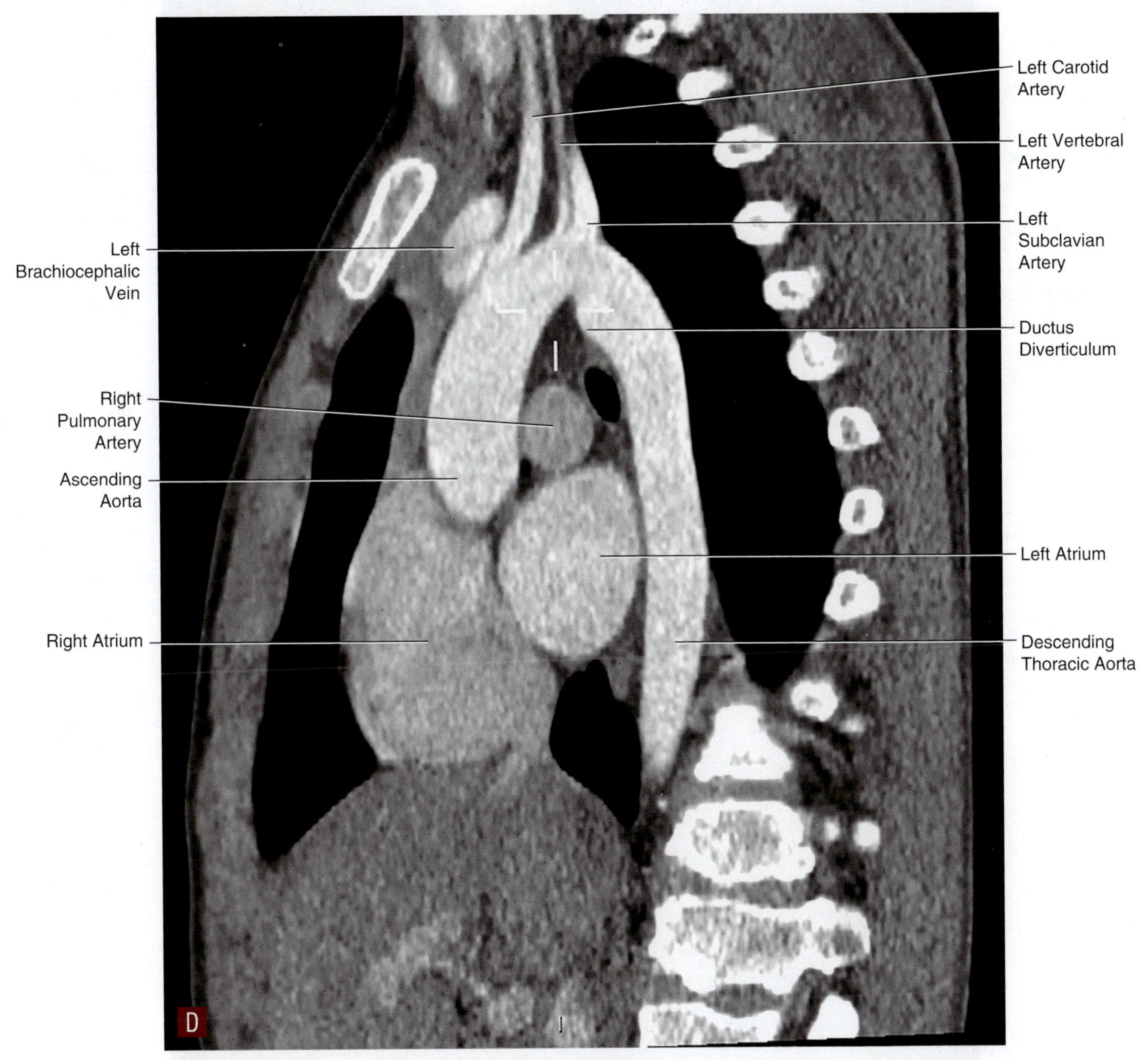

Figure 7.2. *Continued*

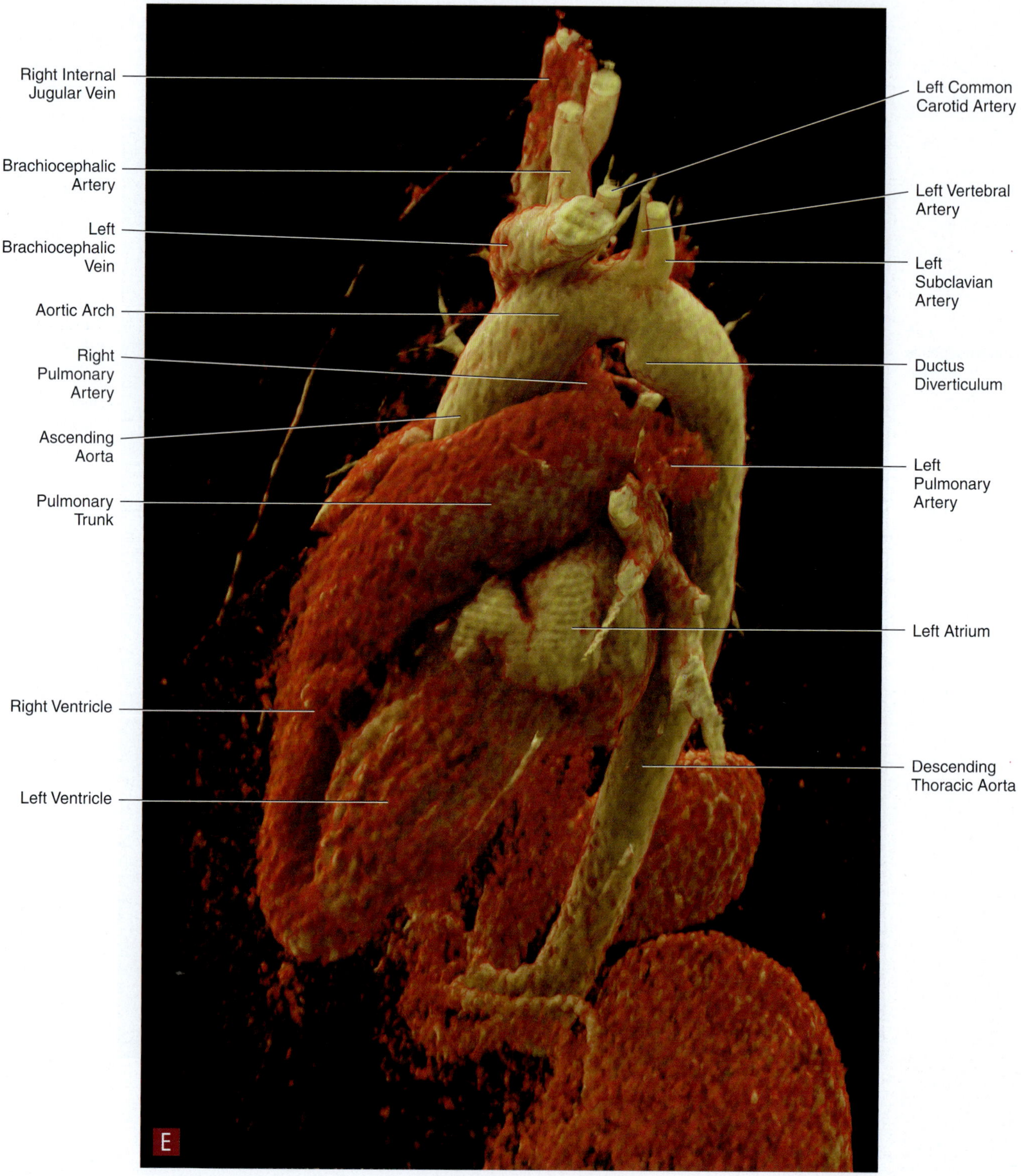

Figure 7.2. *Continued*

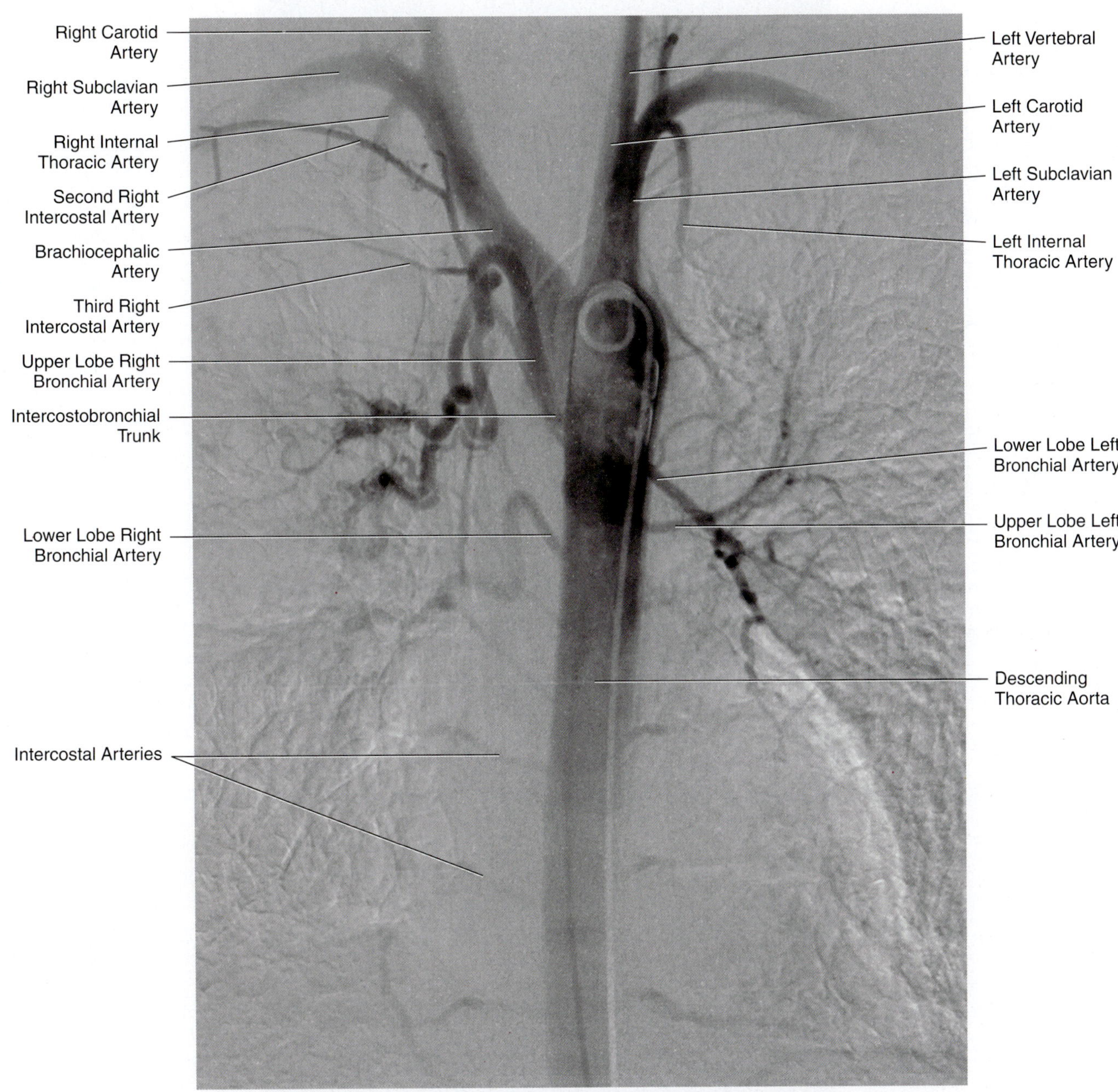

Figure 7.3. Anterior view of the angiogram of the descending thoracic aorta. Note an enlarged bronchial artery appearing bilaterally. The intercostal arteries are partially observed.

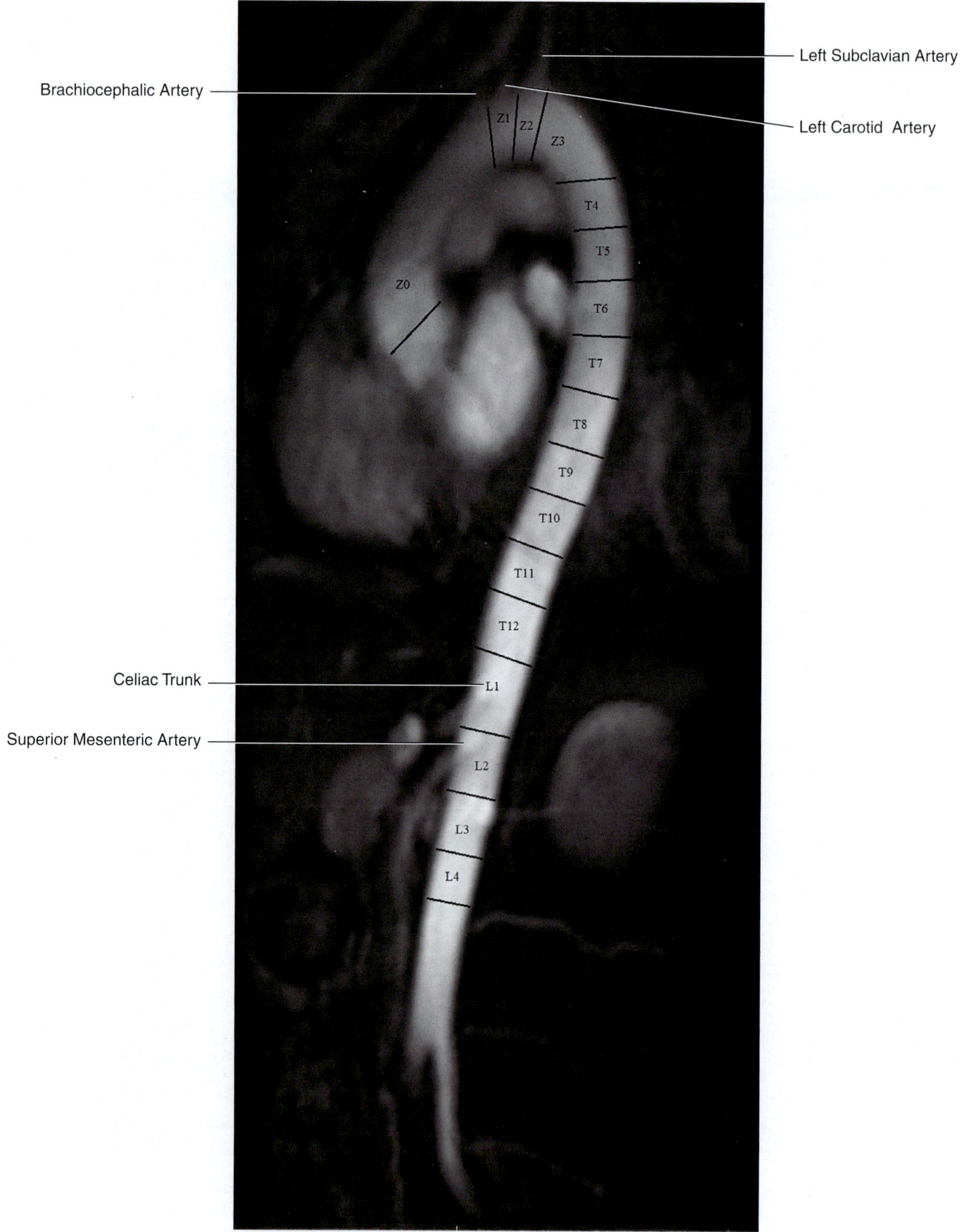

Figure 7.4. Zones of the thoracic aorta, as recently described. The location of an endograft deployed in the aortic arch based on lines drawn distally to each arterial branch from the arch. To arrive at a more clinically useful system, an anatomic endograft landing-zone map was advocated at the First International Summit on Thoracic Aortic Endografting held in Tokyo in 2001; this landing-zone map is used to classify the proximal deployment site of an endograft. In 2002, this landing-zone map was expanded to include the position of the distal end of the endograft. Since then, this map has achieved consensus as the standardized anatomic definition to evaluate outcomes. Zone Z4 includes zones T4 through T12.

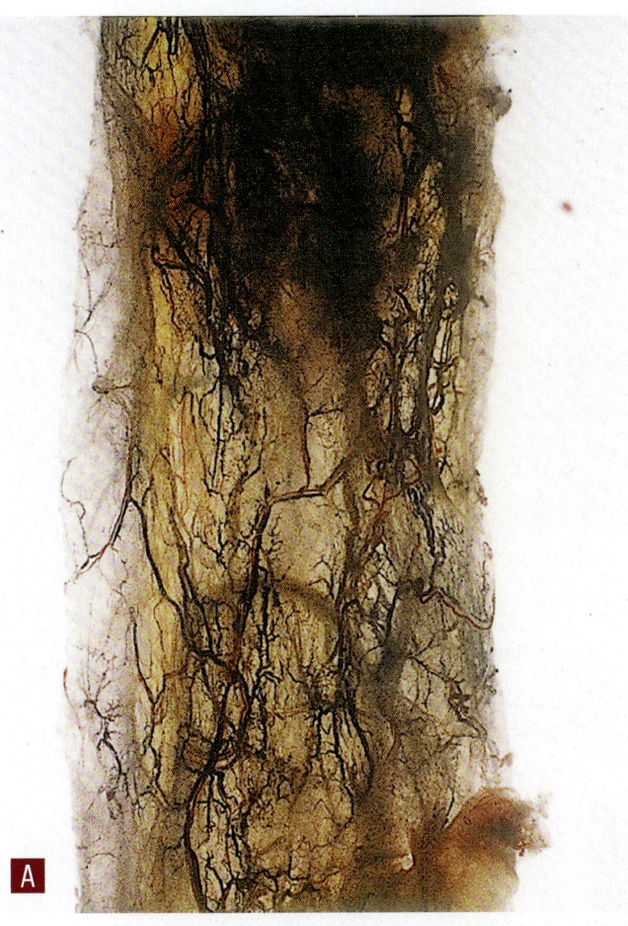

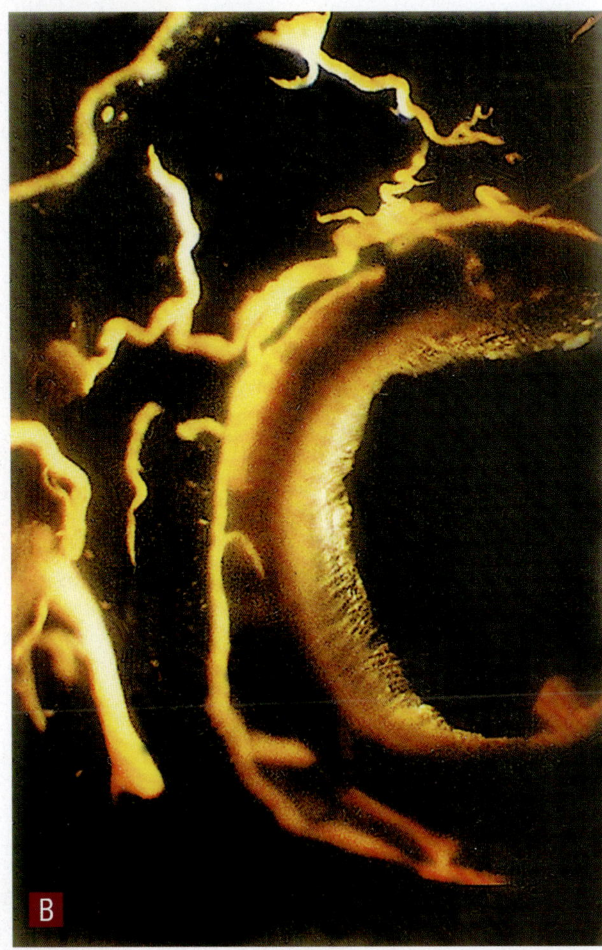

Figure 7.5. A, Diaphanography of a sagittal cut into a canine aorta, showing the arterial and venous vasa vasorum opacified by acrylic plastic. Note the reticulated pattern in a polygonal network, resulting from the bifurcation of the vasa vasorum and anastomoses with neighboring branches of vasa vasorum. The polygonal network is located mostly in the adventitia of the aorta. B, Axial cut into the aortal of a dog showing the vasa vasorum with origin in a lumbar artery. Note the multiple layers of vessels. (Provided by Dr JM Pisco, Lisbon, Portugal.)

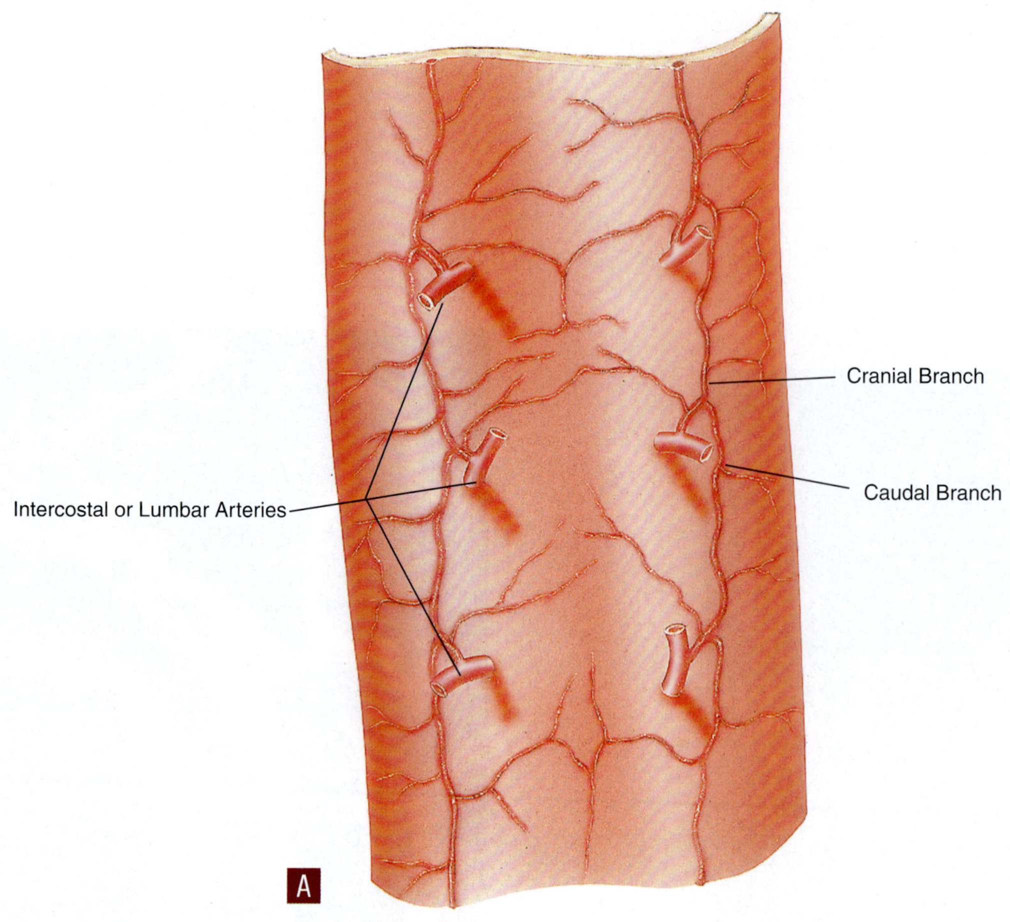

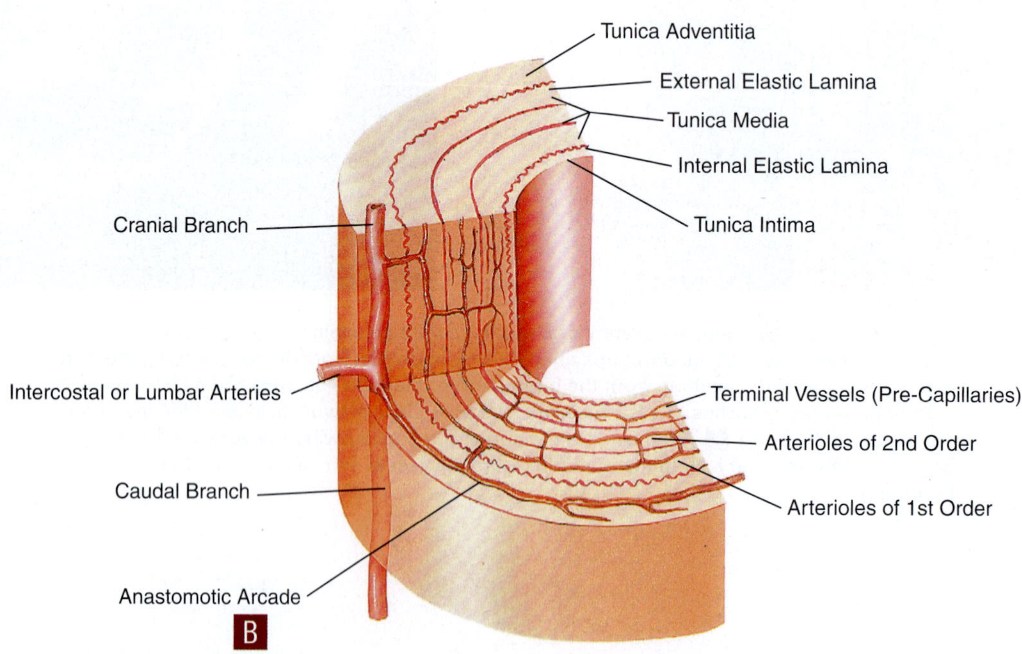

Figure 7.6. A, Sagittal cut of the aorta showing the polygonal network of vasa vasorum in the aortic wall. B, Axial cut of the aorta showing the multiple layers of vessels in the aortic wall.

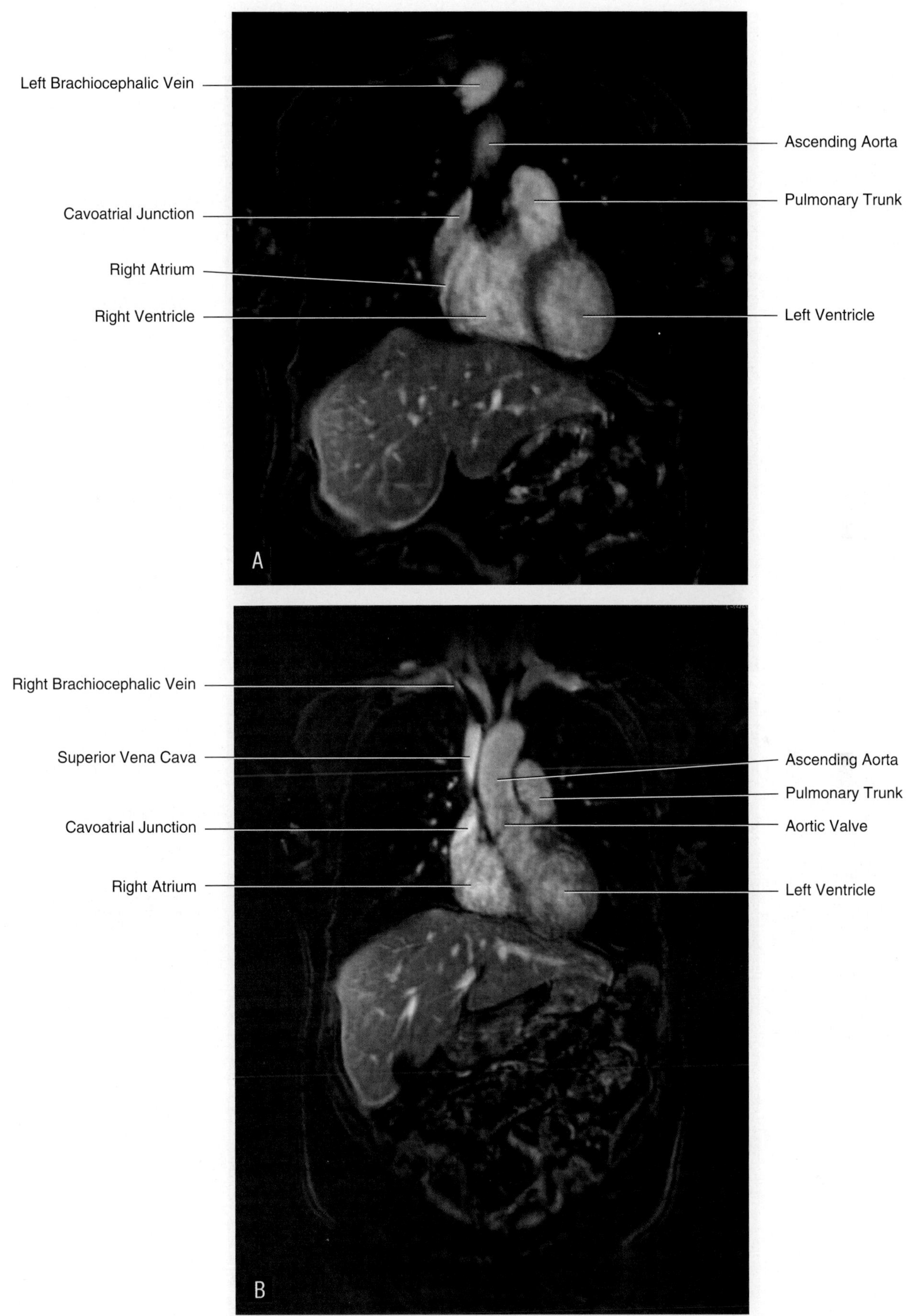

Figure 7.7. **A** – **D**, Magnetic resonance imaging (MRI) angiogram with coronal sections of the chest showing the heart and the great vessels, including the aorta.

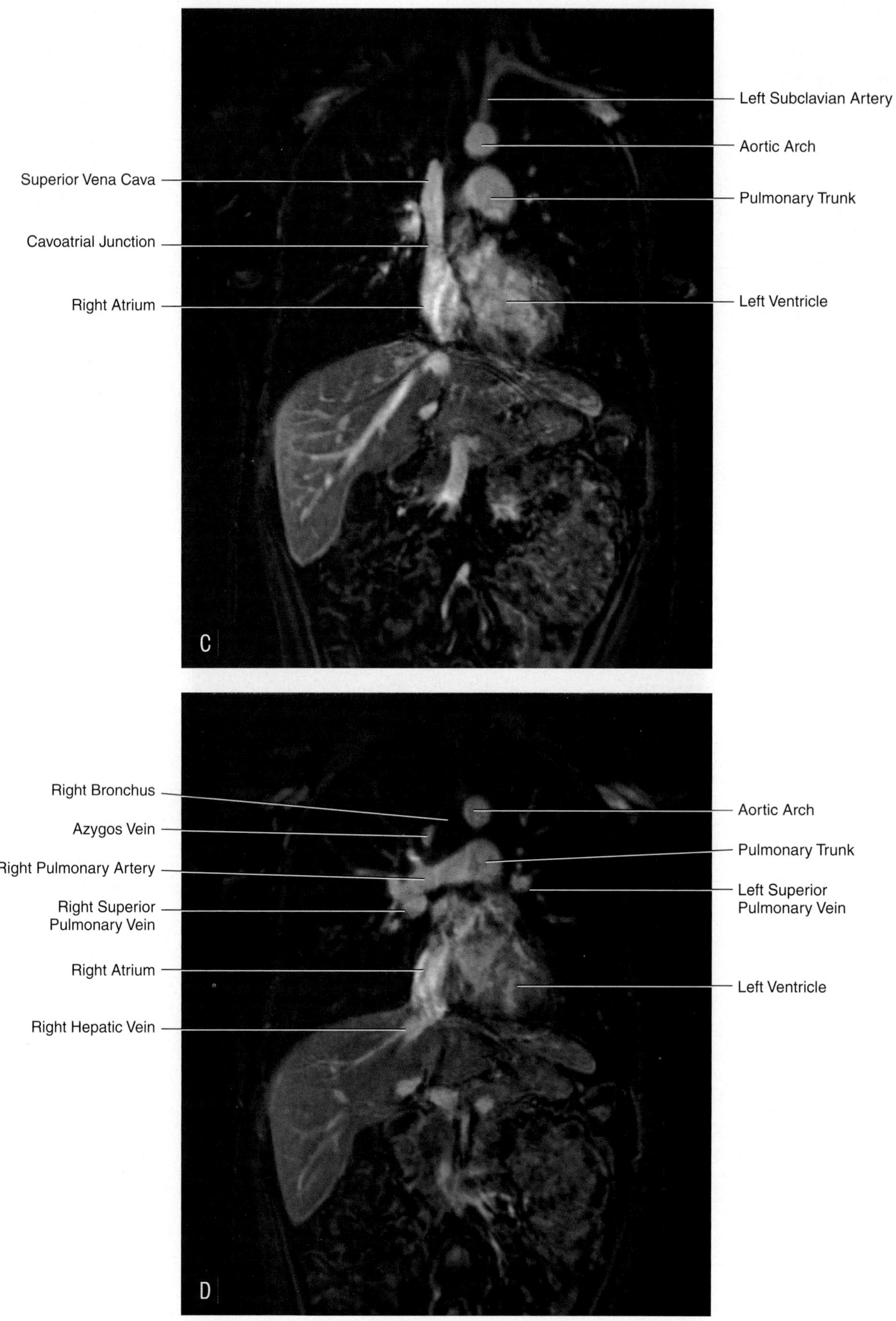

Figure 7.7. *Continued*

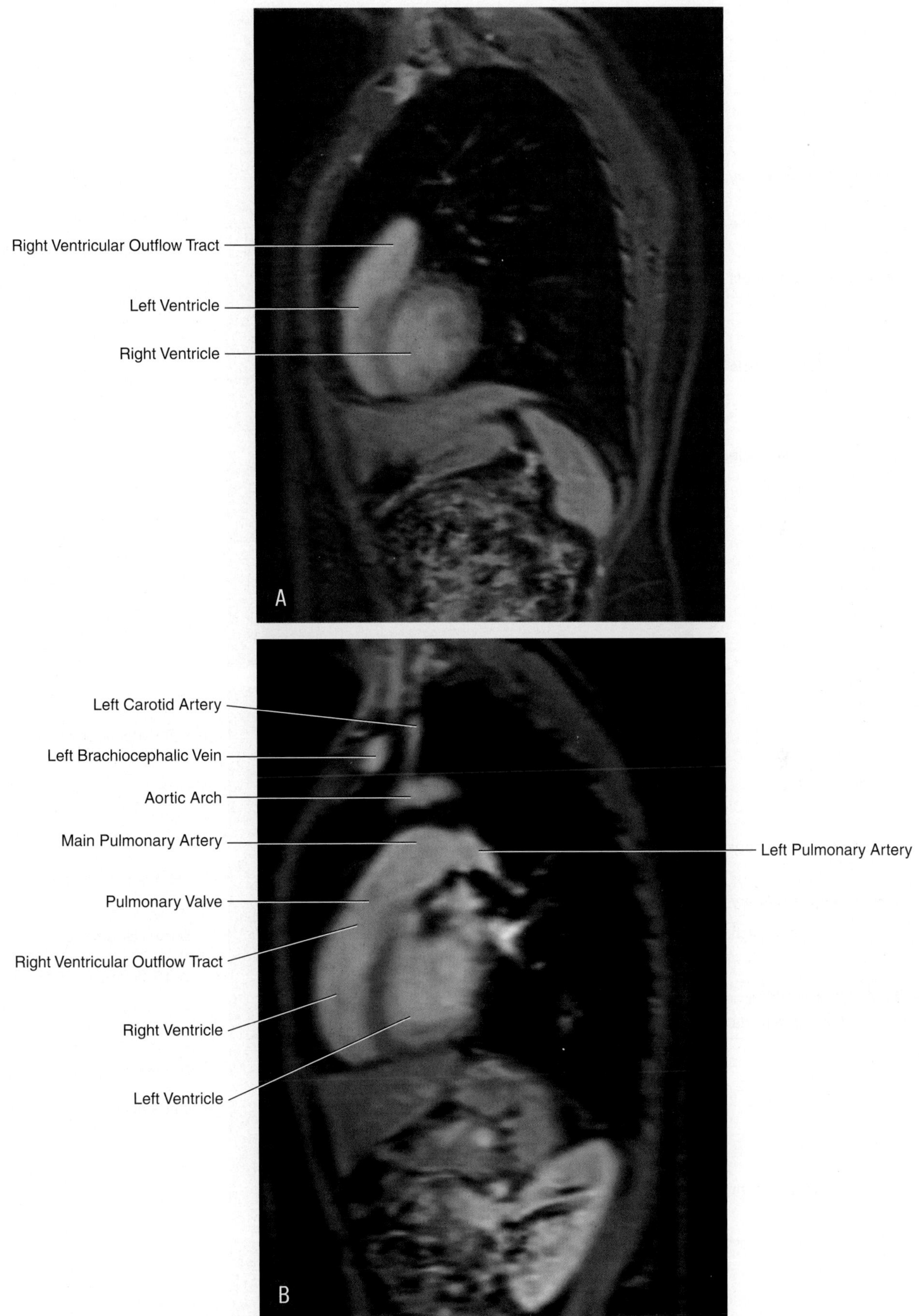

Figure 7.8. A – F, MR angiogram sagittal sections of the chest showing the heart and the great vessels, including the aorta.

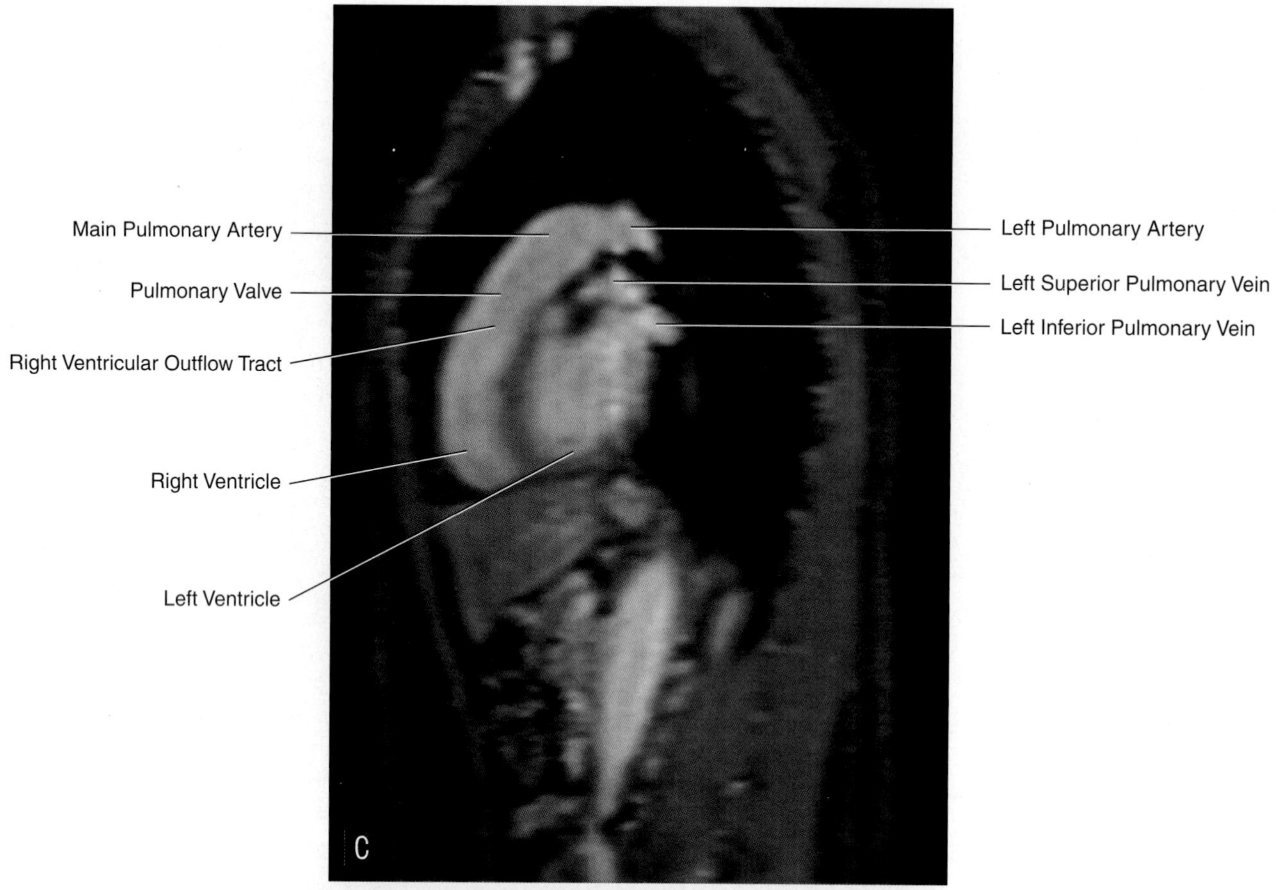

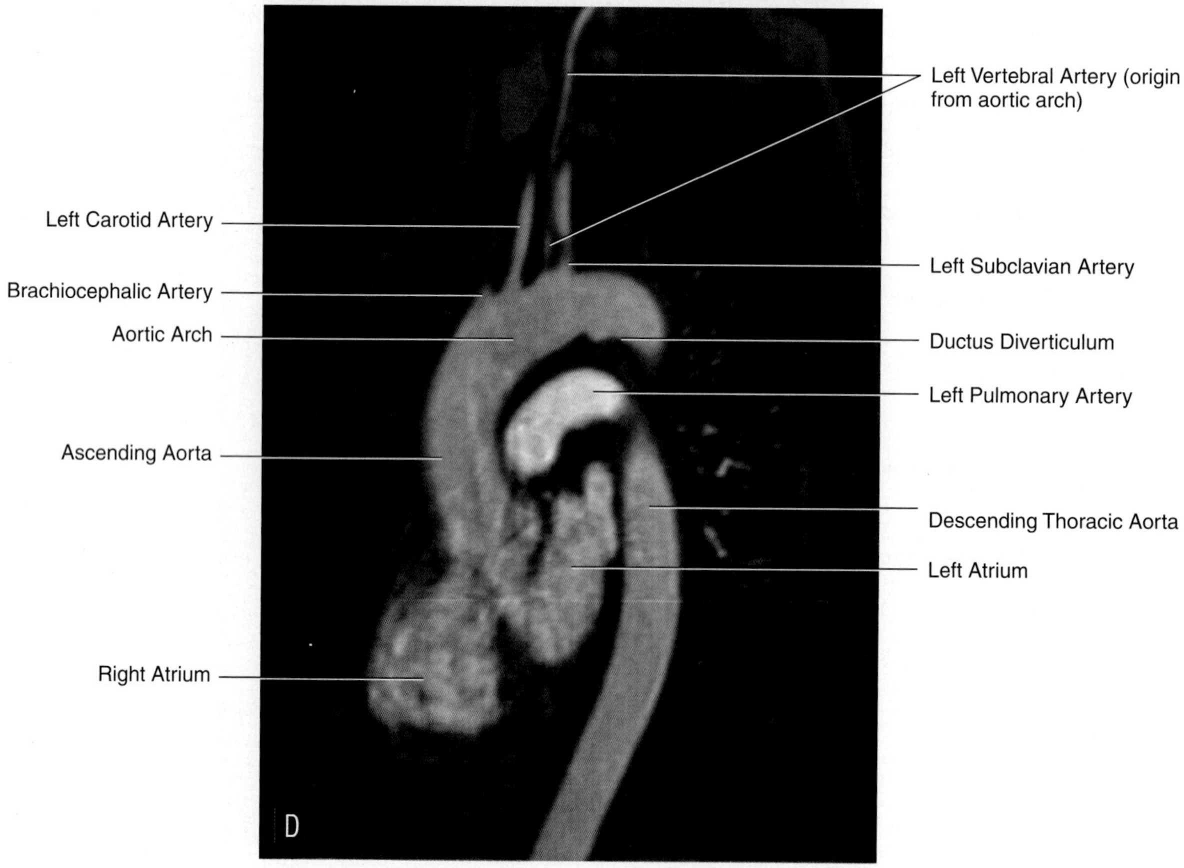

Figure 7.8. *Continued*

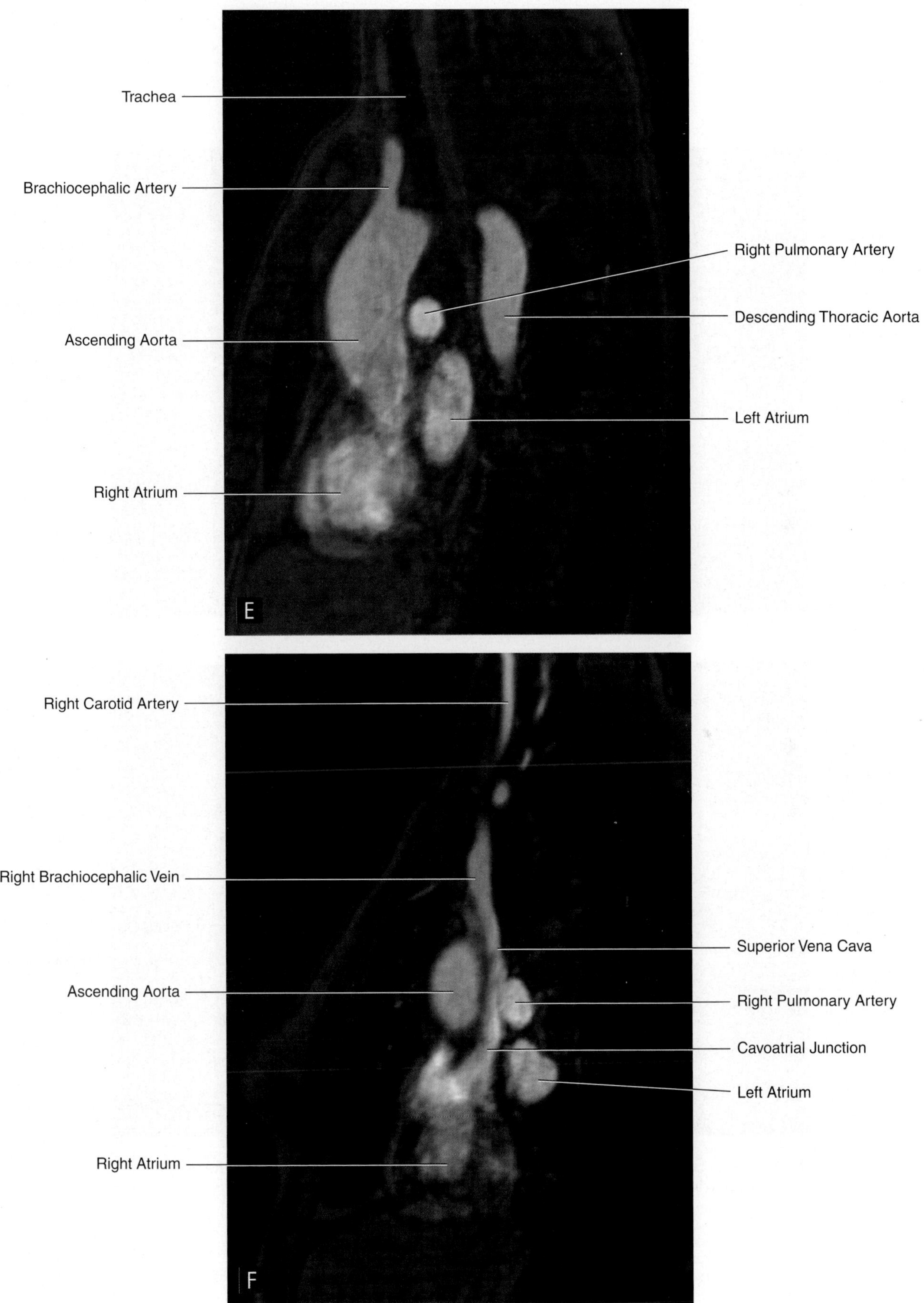

Figure 7.8. *Continued*

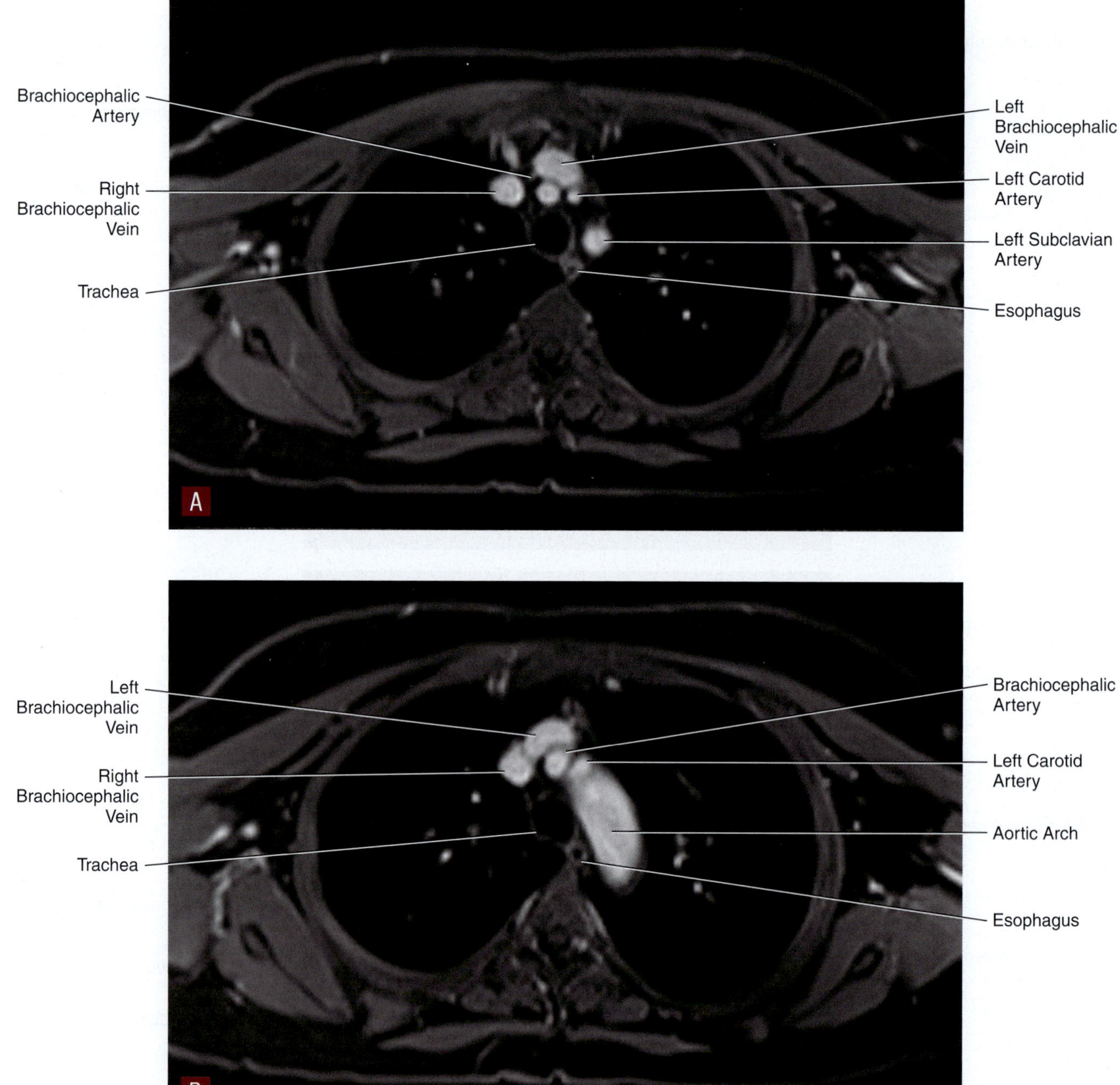

Figure 7.9. A – H, MR angiogram axial sections of the chest showing the heart and the great vessels, including the aorta.

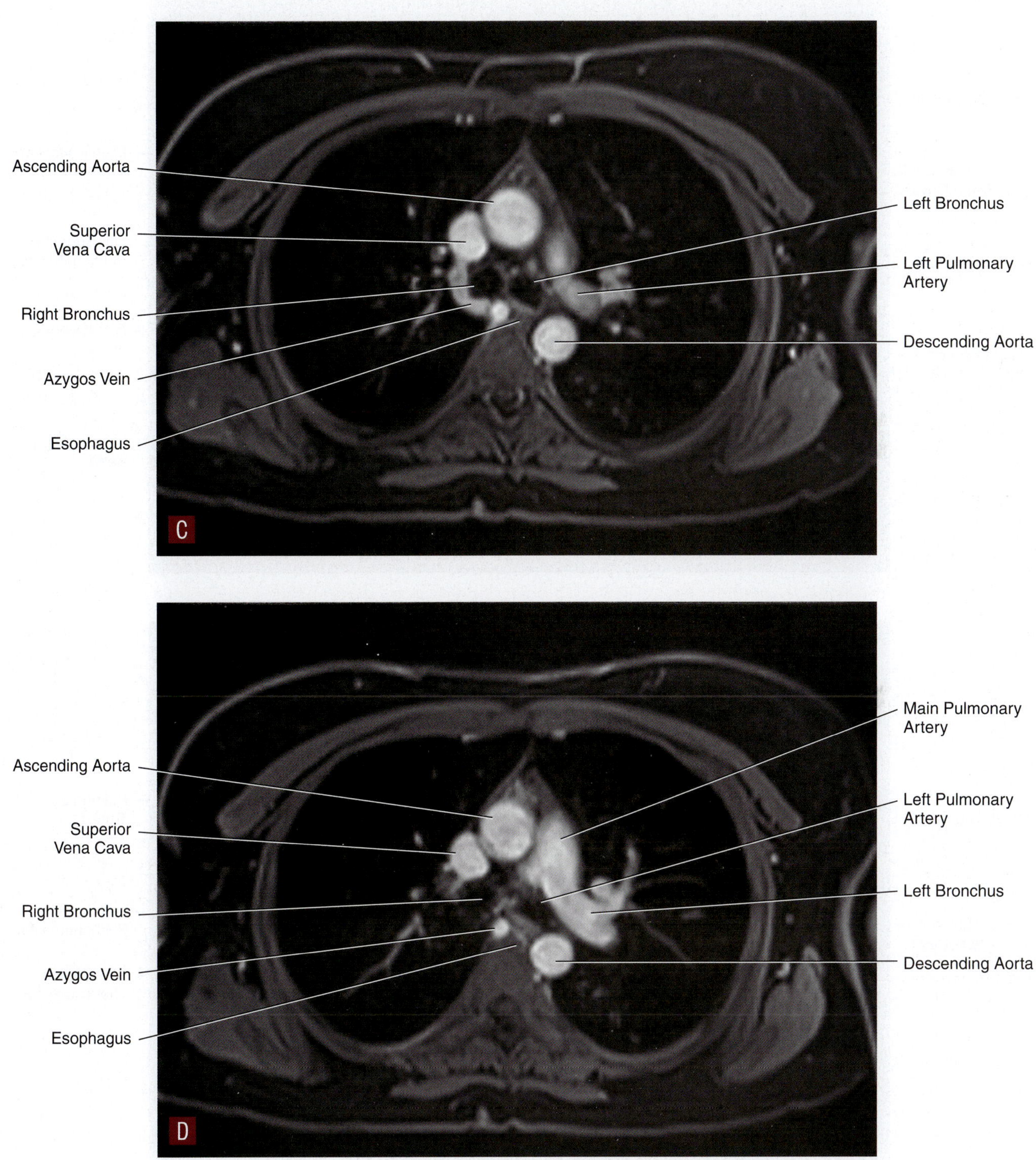

Figure 7.9. *Continued*

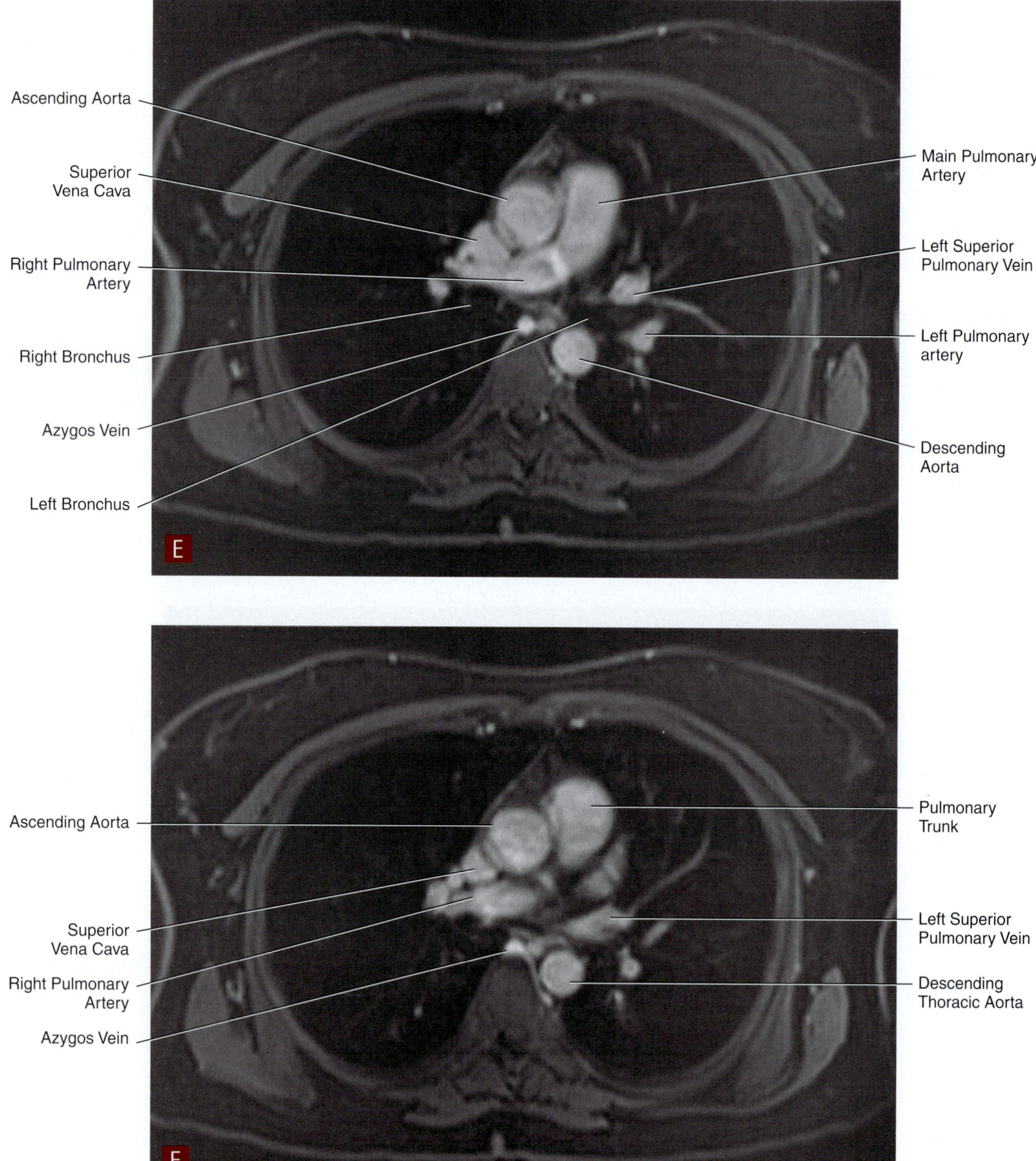

Figure 7.9. *Continued*

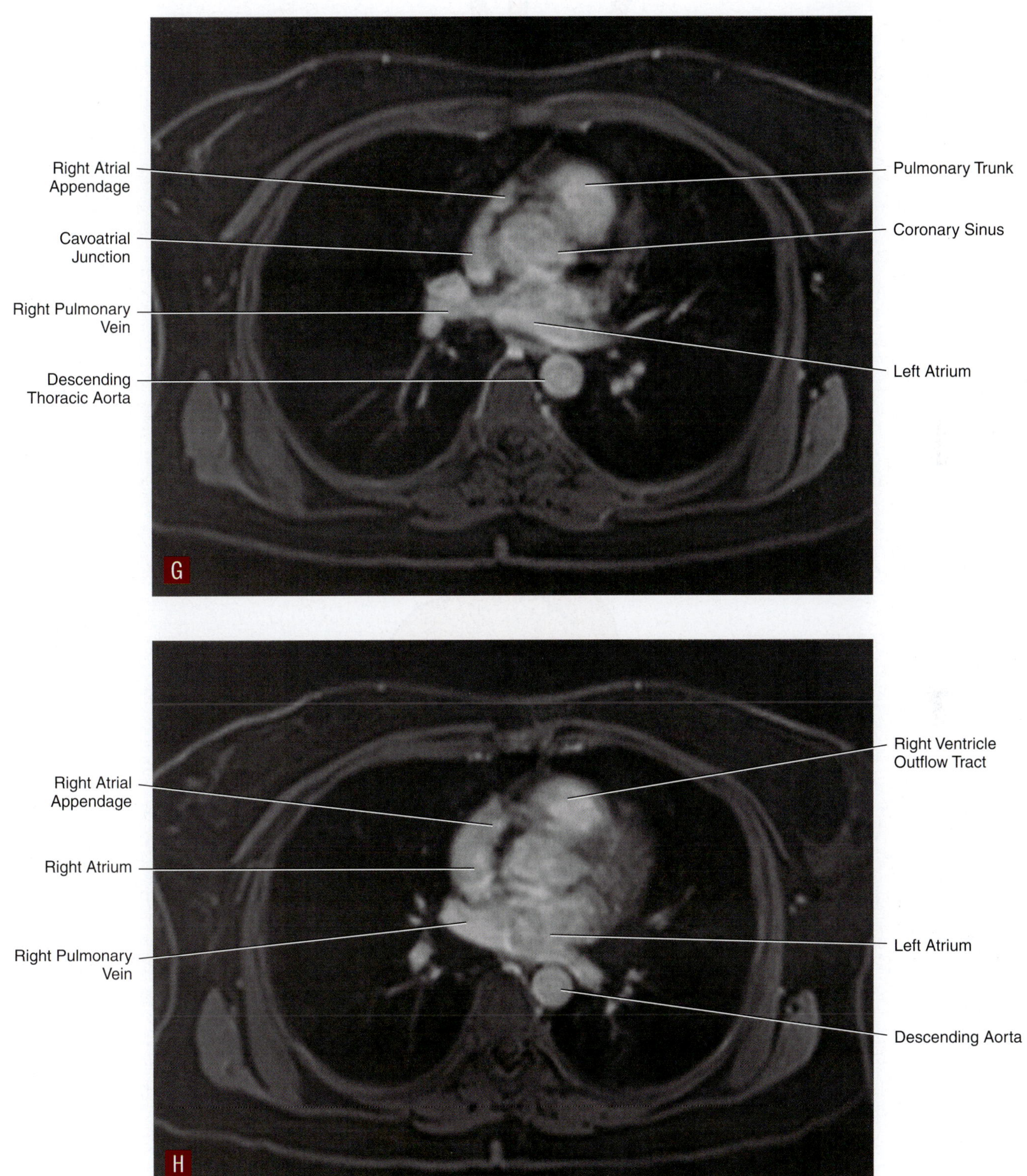

Figure 7.9. *Continued*

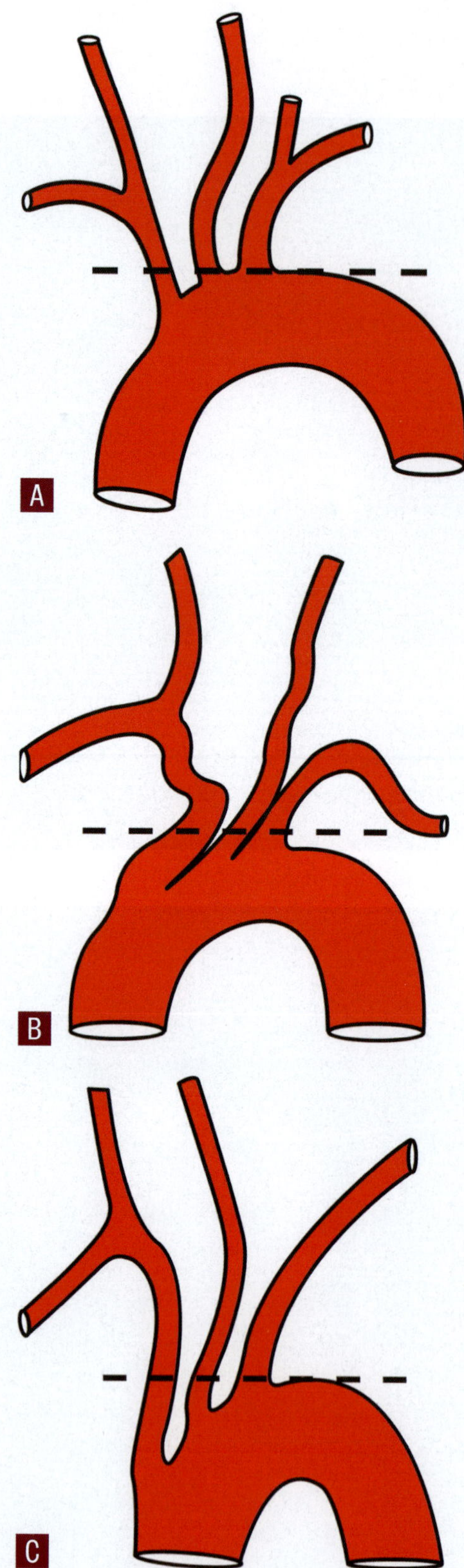

Figure 7.10. Types of aortic arches. A, Type I, the distance between the tangent to the top of the arch to the origin of the brachiocephalic trunk is equal to one width or less of the brachiocephalic trunk. B, Type II, the distance between the tangent to the top of the aortic arch to the origin of the brachiocephalic trunk is equal to two widths of the brachiocephalic trunk. C, Type III, the distance between the tangent to the top of the aortic arch to the origin of the brachiocephalic trunk is equal to three widths or more of the brachiocephalic trunk.

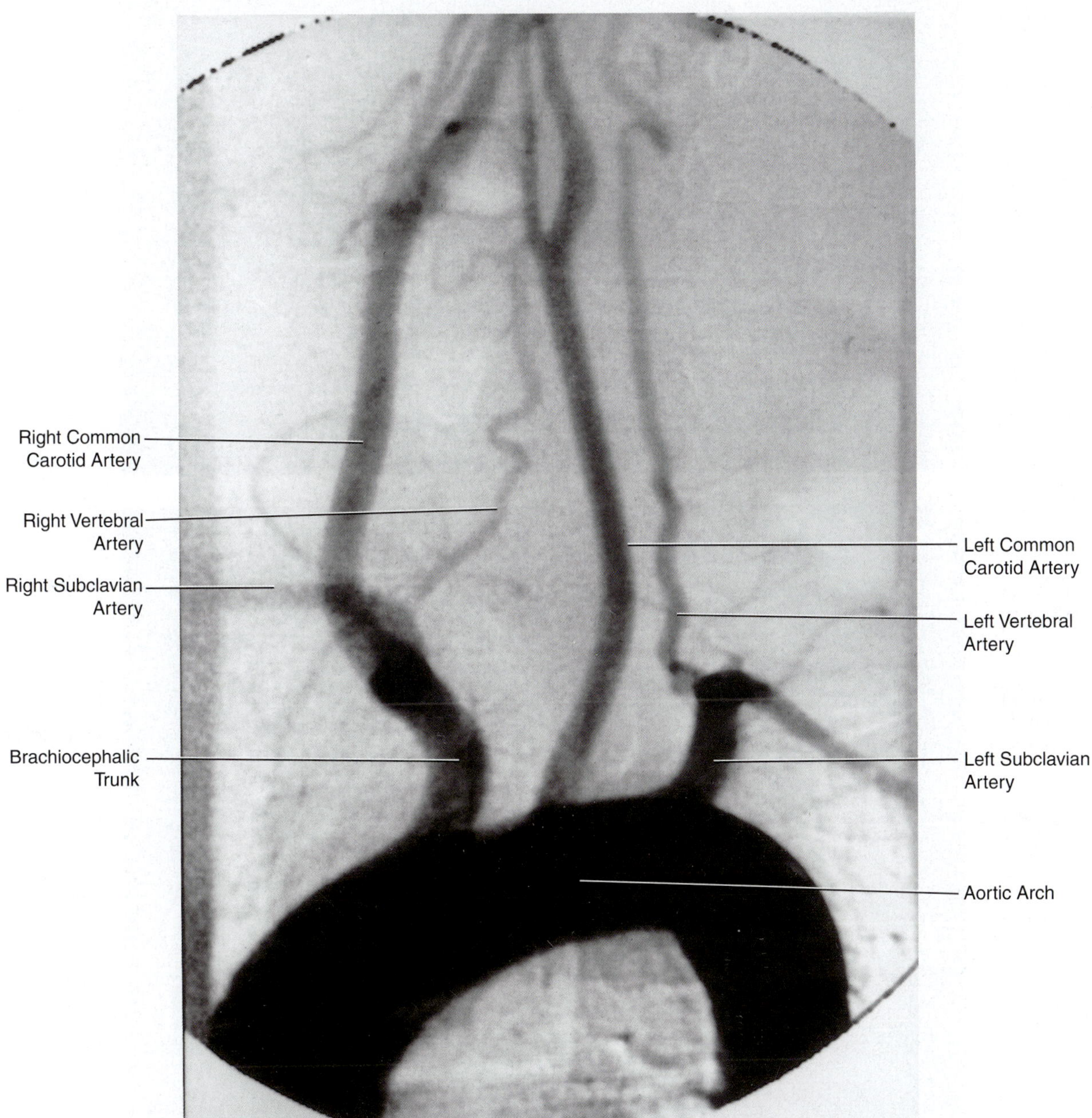

Figure 7.11. Angiogram of the aortic arch showing the usual distribution of the origins of the main branches.

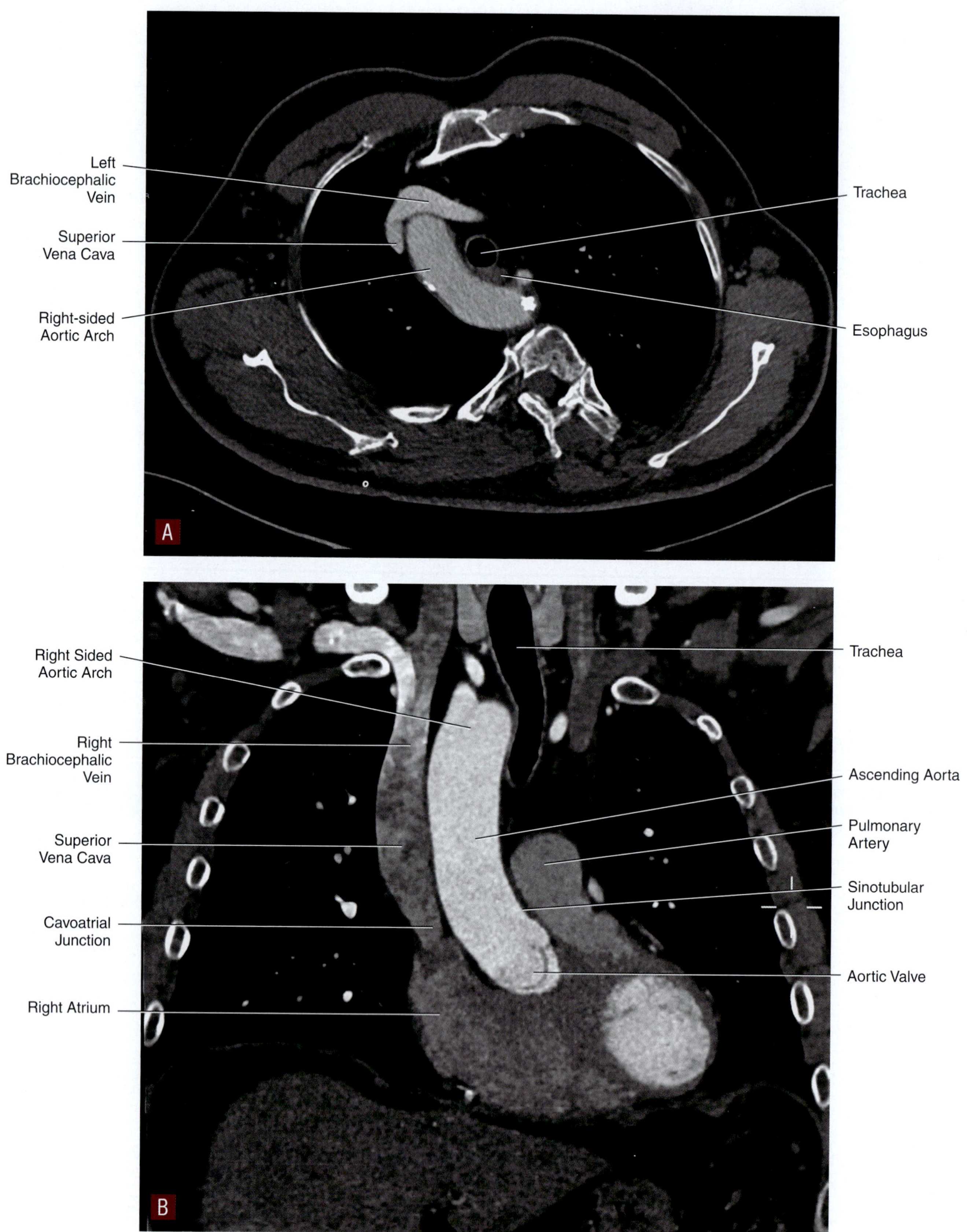

Figure 7.12. **A**, Axial computed tomography (CT) angiogram showing a right-sided aortic arch, coursing to the right of the trachea. **B**, Coronal view showing the right-sided aortic arch.

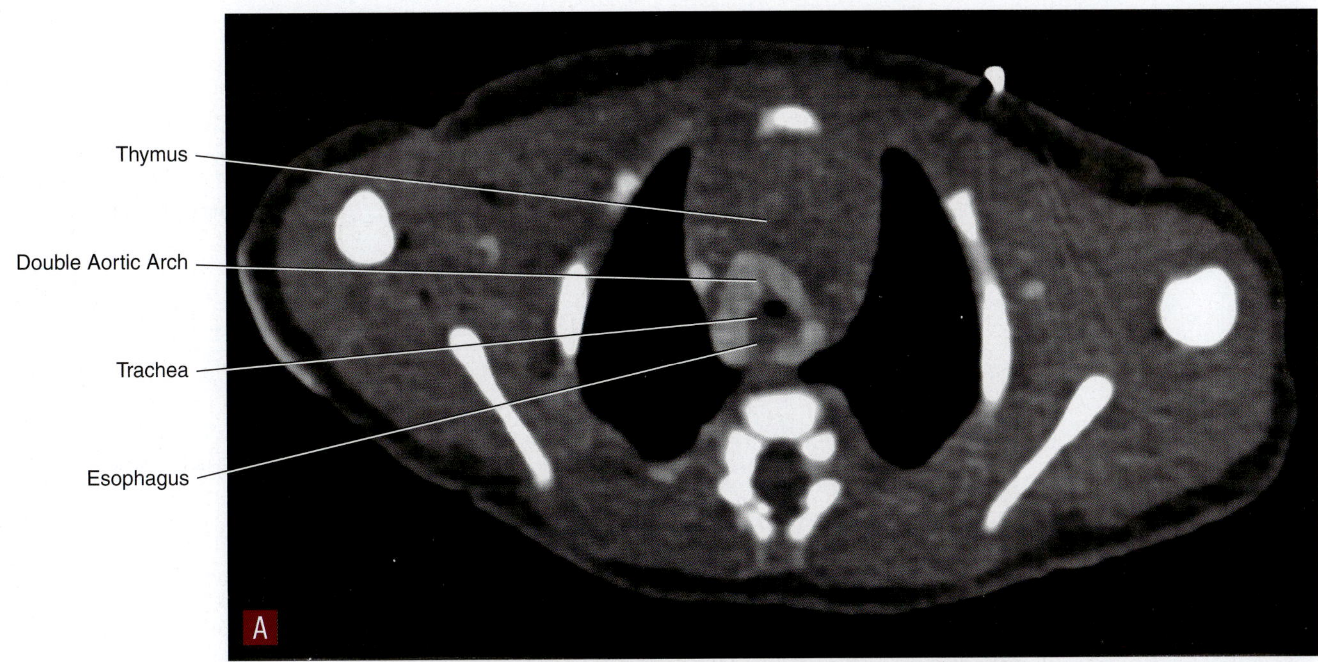

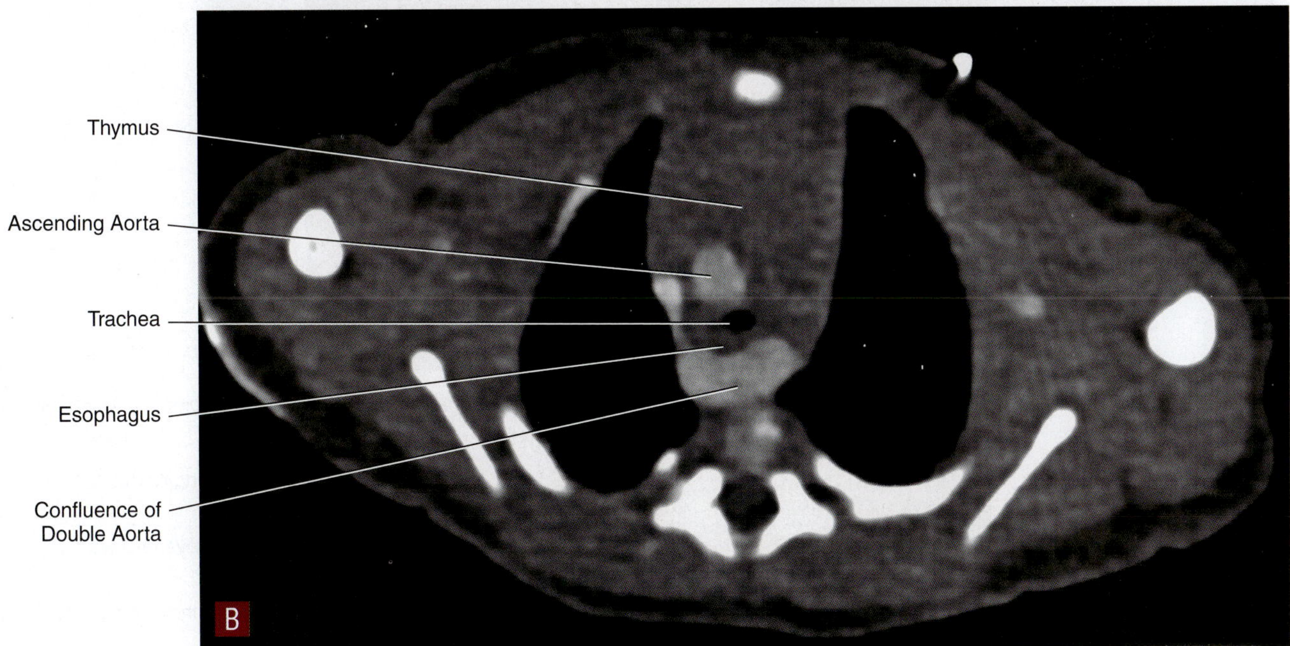

Figure 7.13. A, Axial computed tomography (CT) angiogram of a young patient with a double aortic arch. B, Axial CT angiogram of the double aortic arch showing the confluence of the right and left arches to form the descending thoracic aorta. C, Three-dimensional (3D) volume rendered reconstruction on the same patient in a left anterior oblique projection. D, 3D volume rendered reconstruction in a superior view showing the double aortic arch, with the left arch giving rise to the left brachiocephalic and carotid arteries, with mirror image branching on the right. The pulmonary arteries and the left atrium can be seen inferior to the double arch. E, Axial CT angiogram of an elderly patient with double aortic arch. F, 3D cinematic volume-rendered reconstruction in the same patient's CT angiogram in an anterior view showing the origins of the supra-aortic vessels. G, Posterolateral view, demonstrating variant anatomy of the left brachiochephalic vein posterior to the ascending aorta. H, Posterior view showing the confluence of the double aortic arch posterior to the enlarged left atrium.

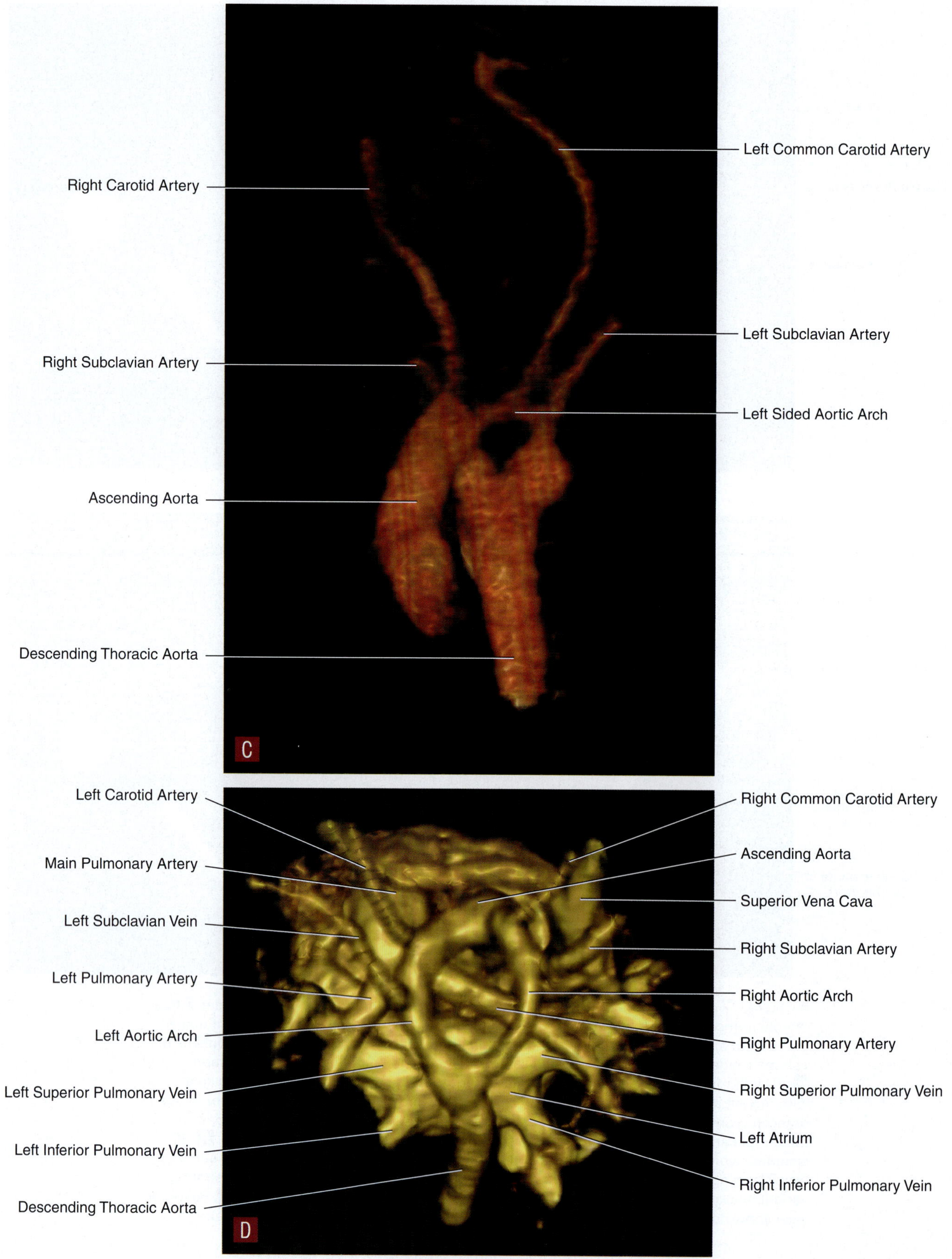

Figure 7.13. *Continued*

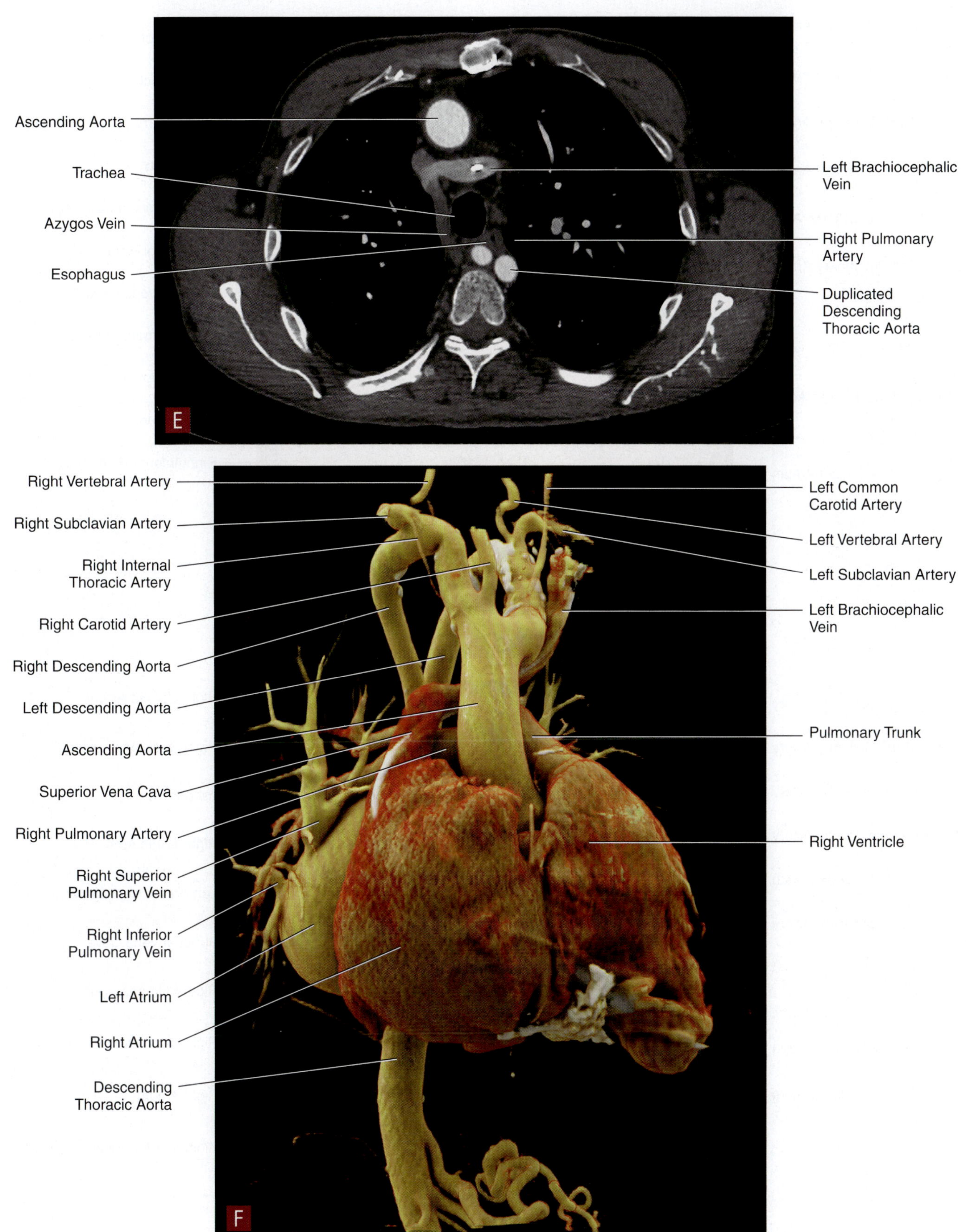

Figure 7.13. *Continued*

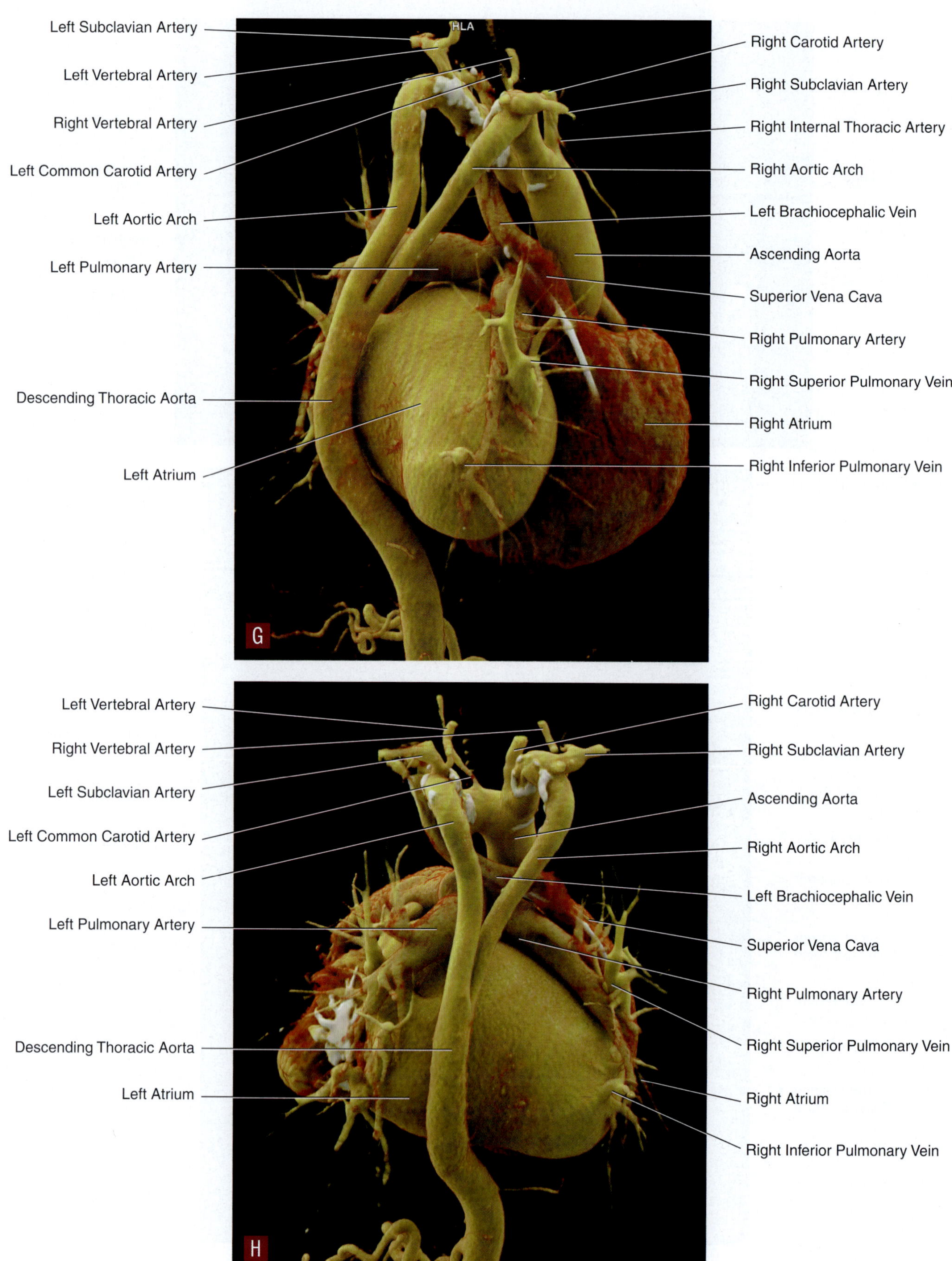

Figure 7.13. *Continued*

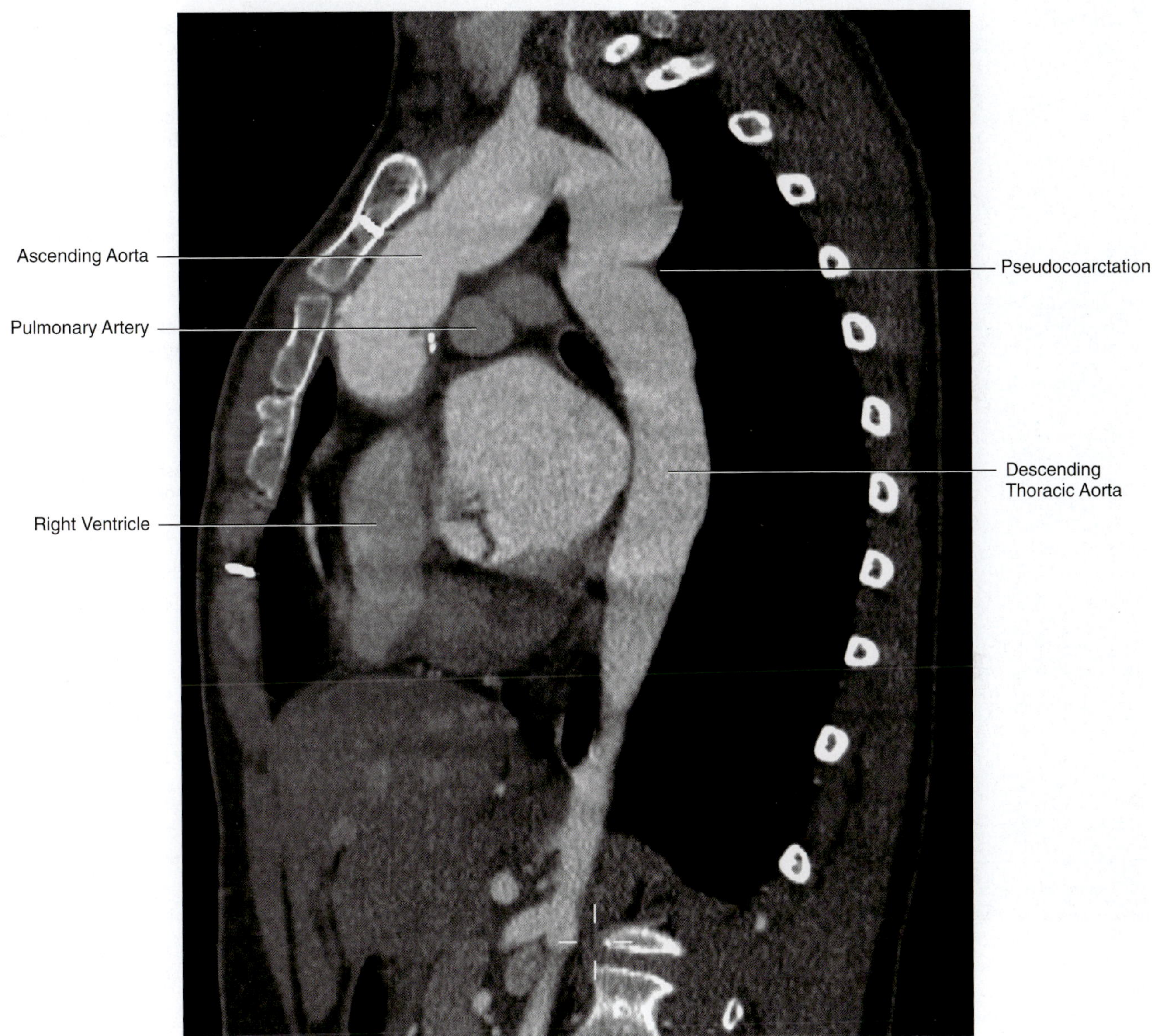

Figure 7.14. Computed tomography (CT) angiogram in a sagittal view showing a cervical aortic arch. A cervical arch extends up to or above the level of the mediastinal ends of the clavicles at the sternoclavicular joints. There is an association with pseudocoarctation, which is also seen in this example.

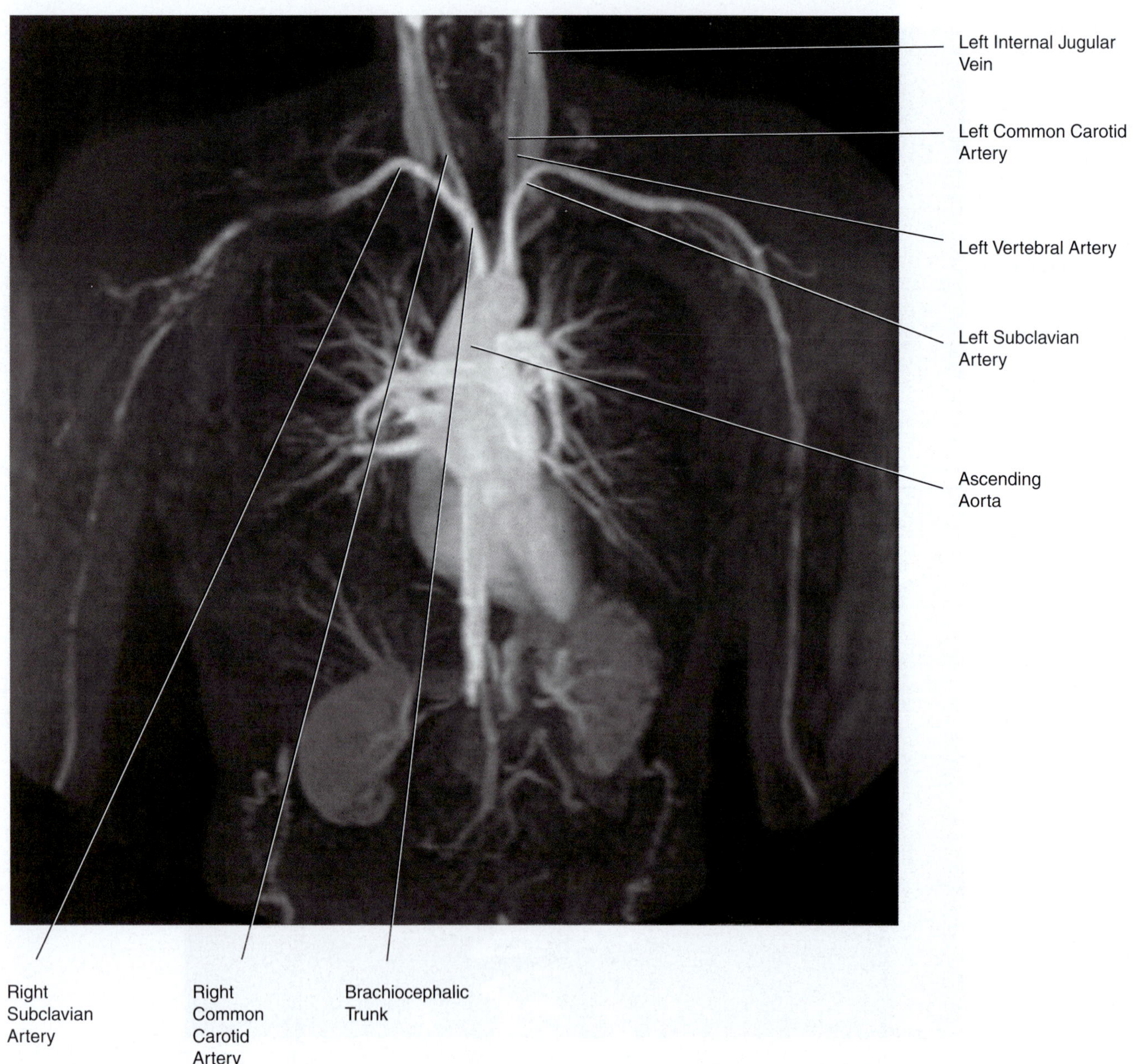

Figure 7.15. **Magnetic resonance angiography** (MRA) of the aortic arch and main vessels. Note the simultaneous visualization of the internal jugular veins and pulmonary artery circulation.

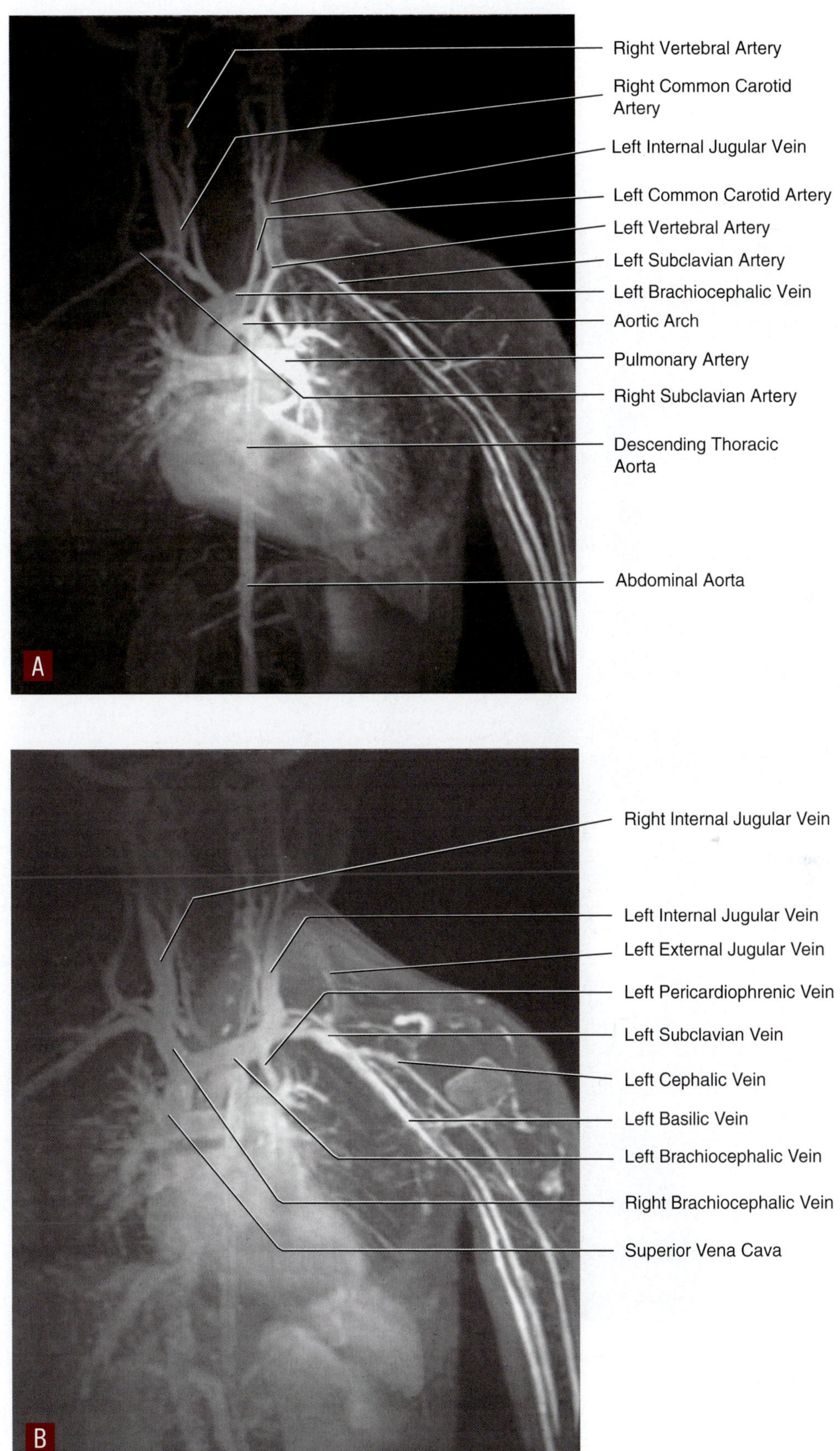

Figure 7.16. A and B, Early and late phase of magnetic resonance angiography (MRA) of the aortic arch and main vessels of the chest.

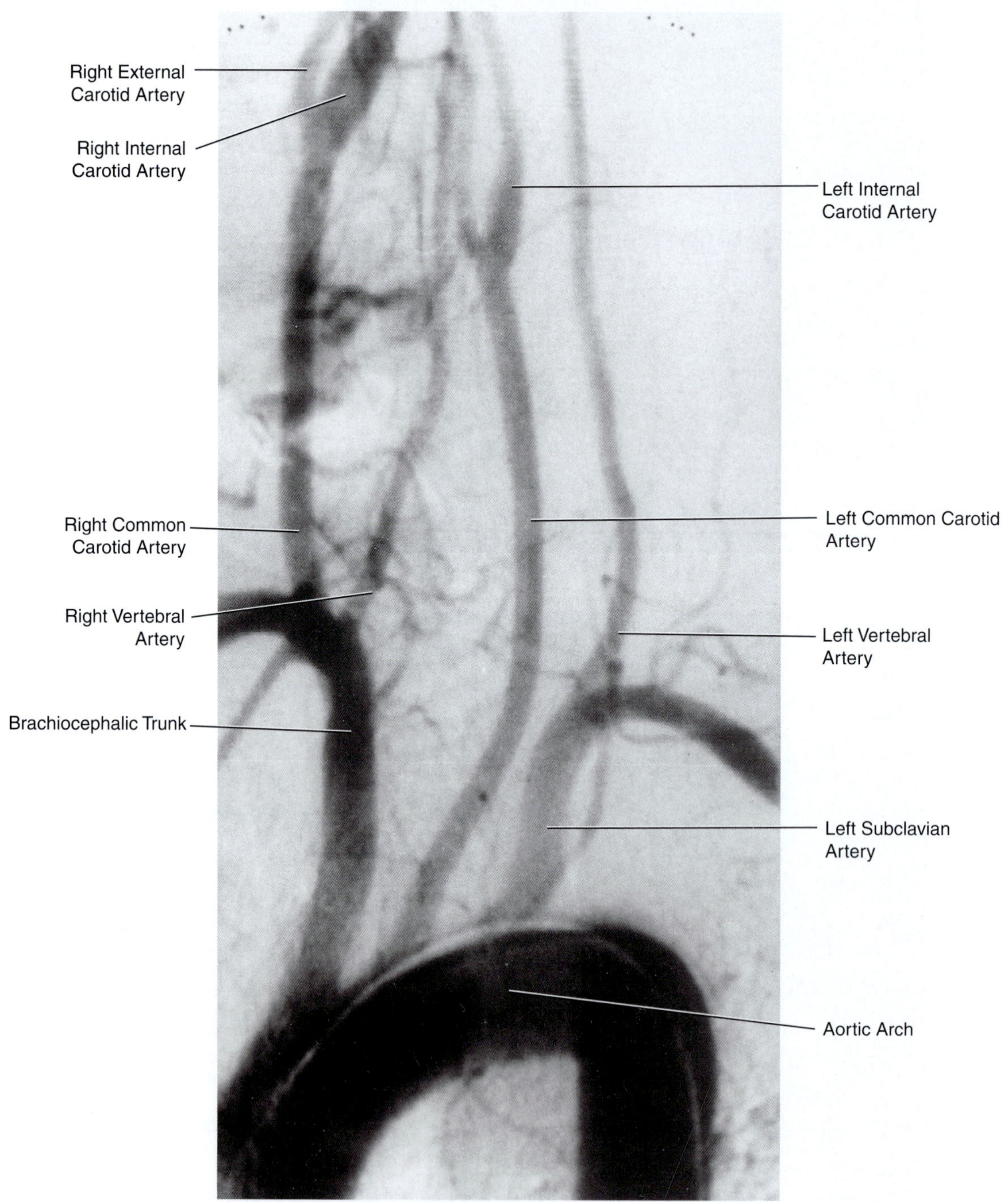

Figure 7.17. **Angiogram of the aortic arch showing the origin of the main branches of the aortic arch.**

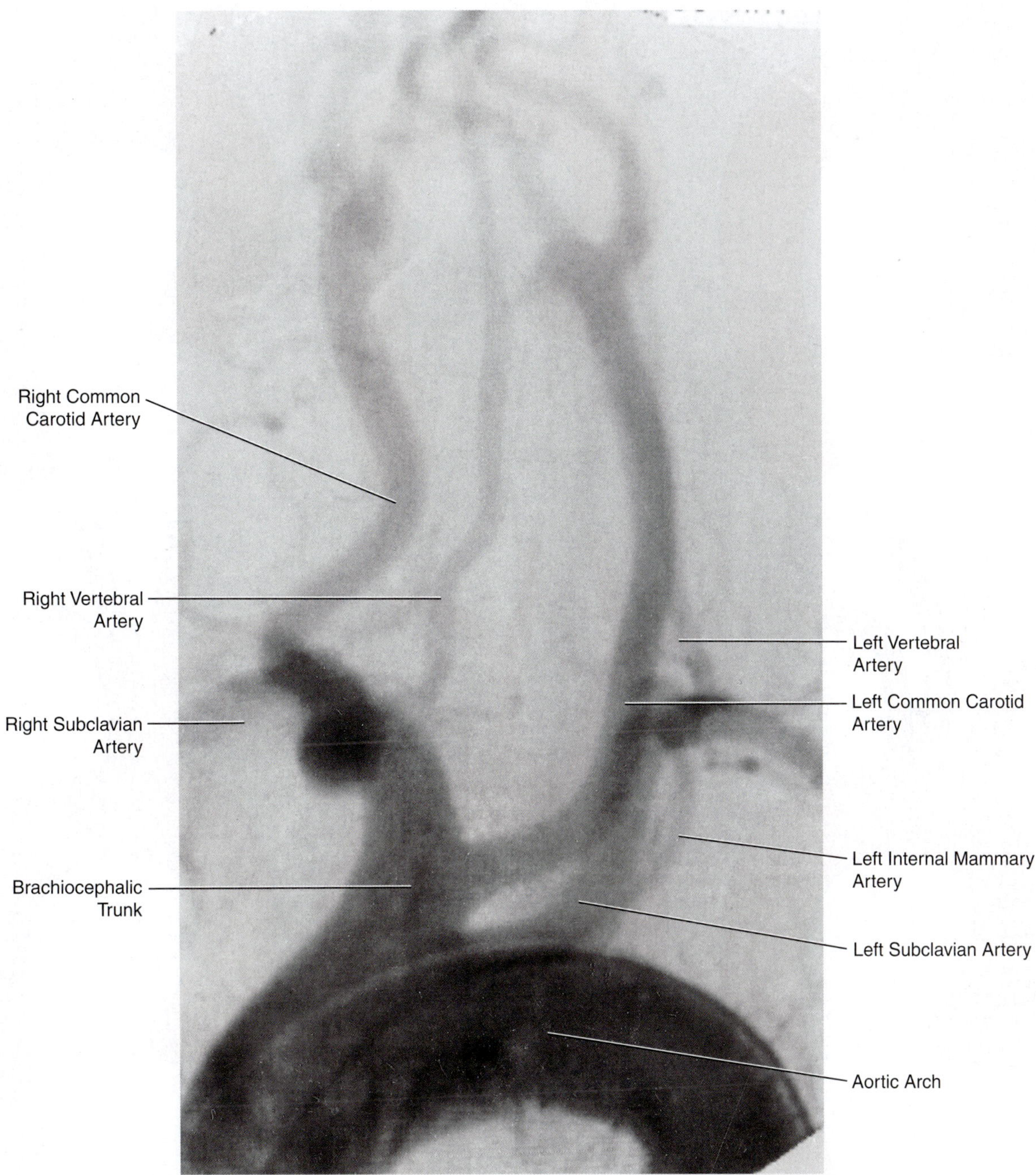

Figure 7.18. Angiogram of the aortic arch showing the common origin of the left common carotid artery and the brachiocephalic trunk, also known as a "bovine arch."

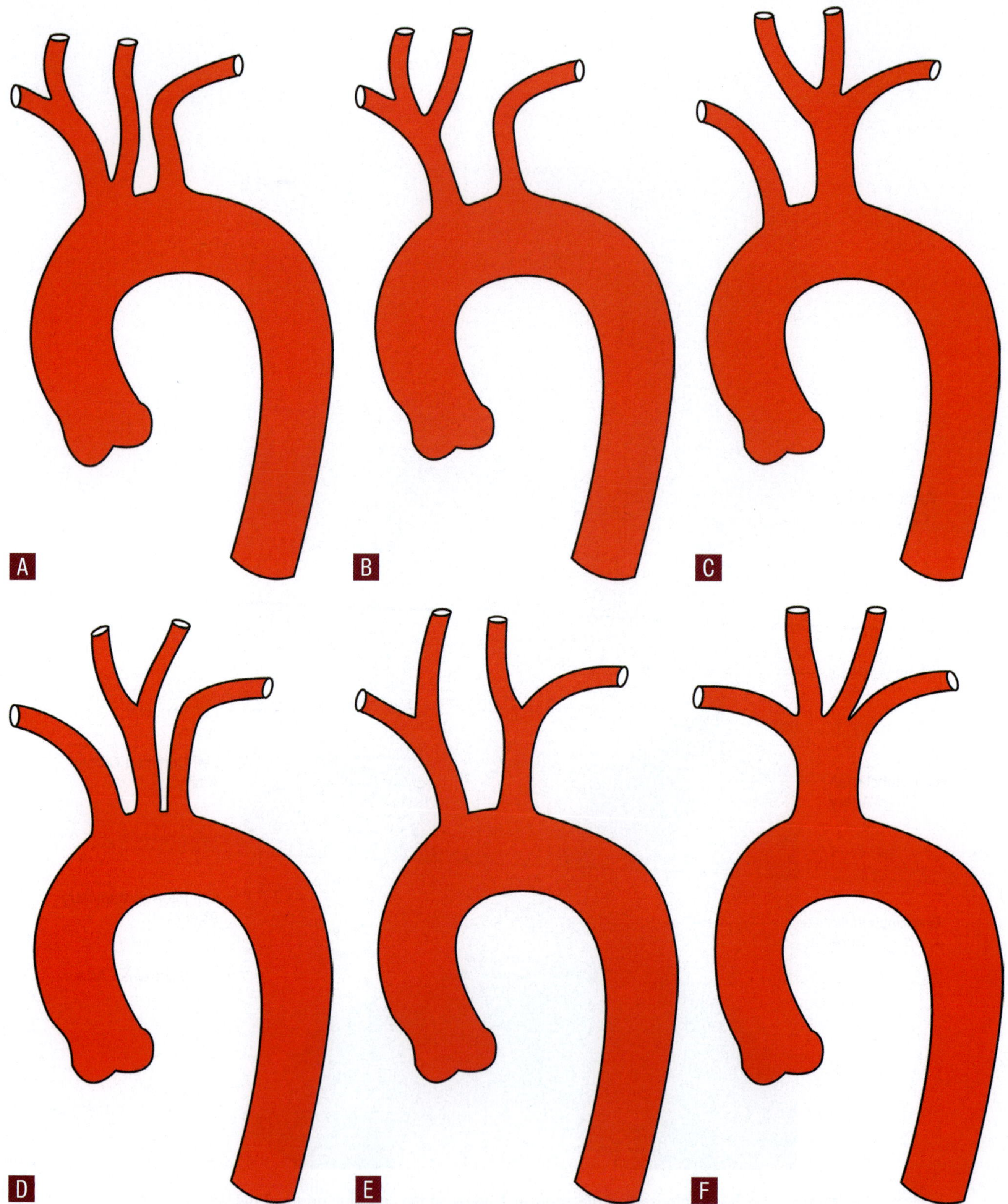

Figure 7.19. Variations in the origin of the aortic arch branches. A and B account for about 73% of all arch branch variations and 22% of the anomalies found in the general population. A, Common origin of the left common carotid artery and brachiocephalic artery (aka bovine arch). B, Origin of the left common carotid from the mid to upper brachiocephalic artery. C, Common carotid trunk giving origin to the left subclavian artery. D, Common carotid trunk, independent from both subclavian arteries. E, Left and right brachiocephalic arteries. F, Single arch vessel (aka brachiocephalic artery) originates the left common carotid and left subclavian arteries. G, Common carotid trunk originates the right subclavian artery. The left subclavian artery originates from the aortic arch. H, Independent origin of all vessels in the aortic arch. I, Left brachiocephalic artery.

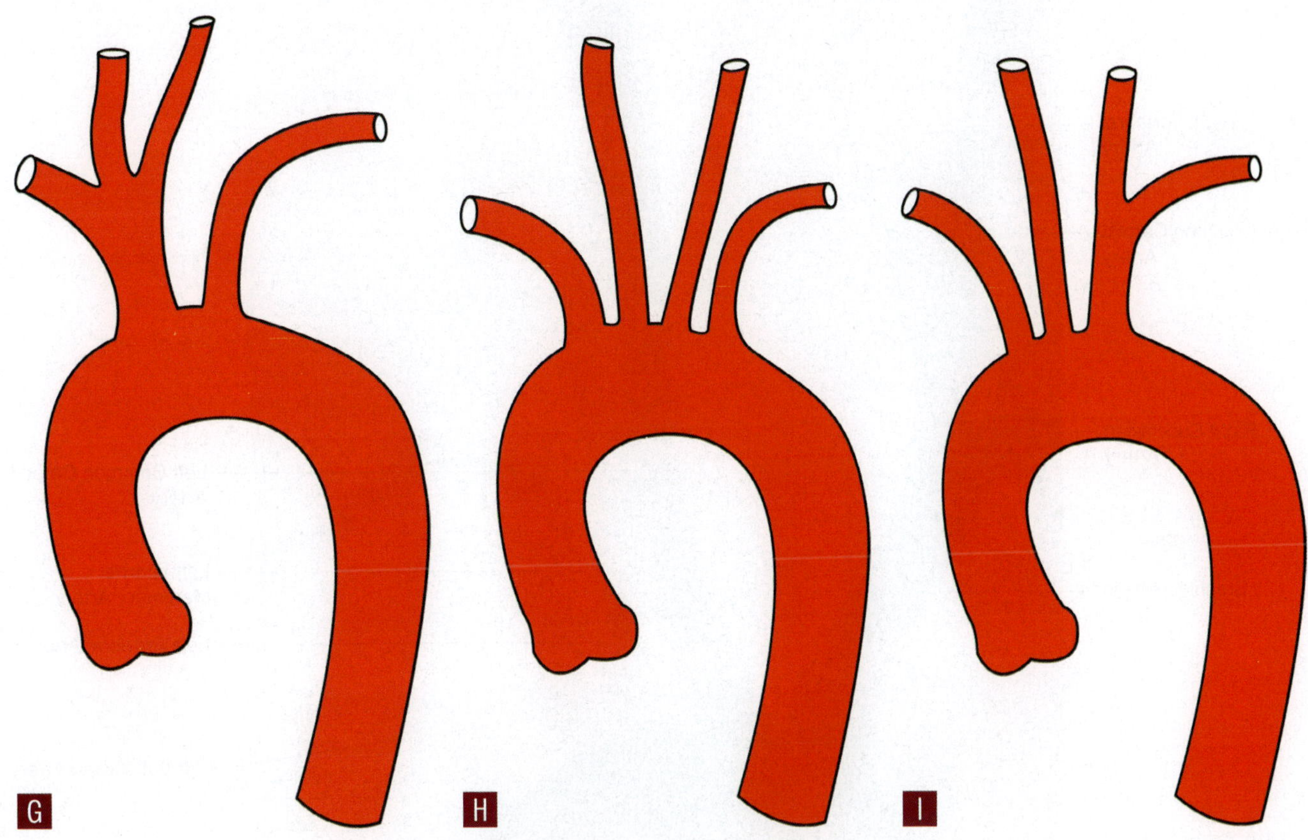

Figure 7.19. *Continued*

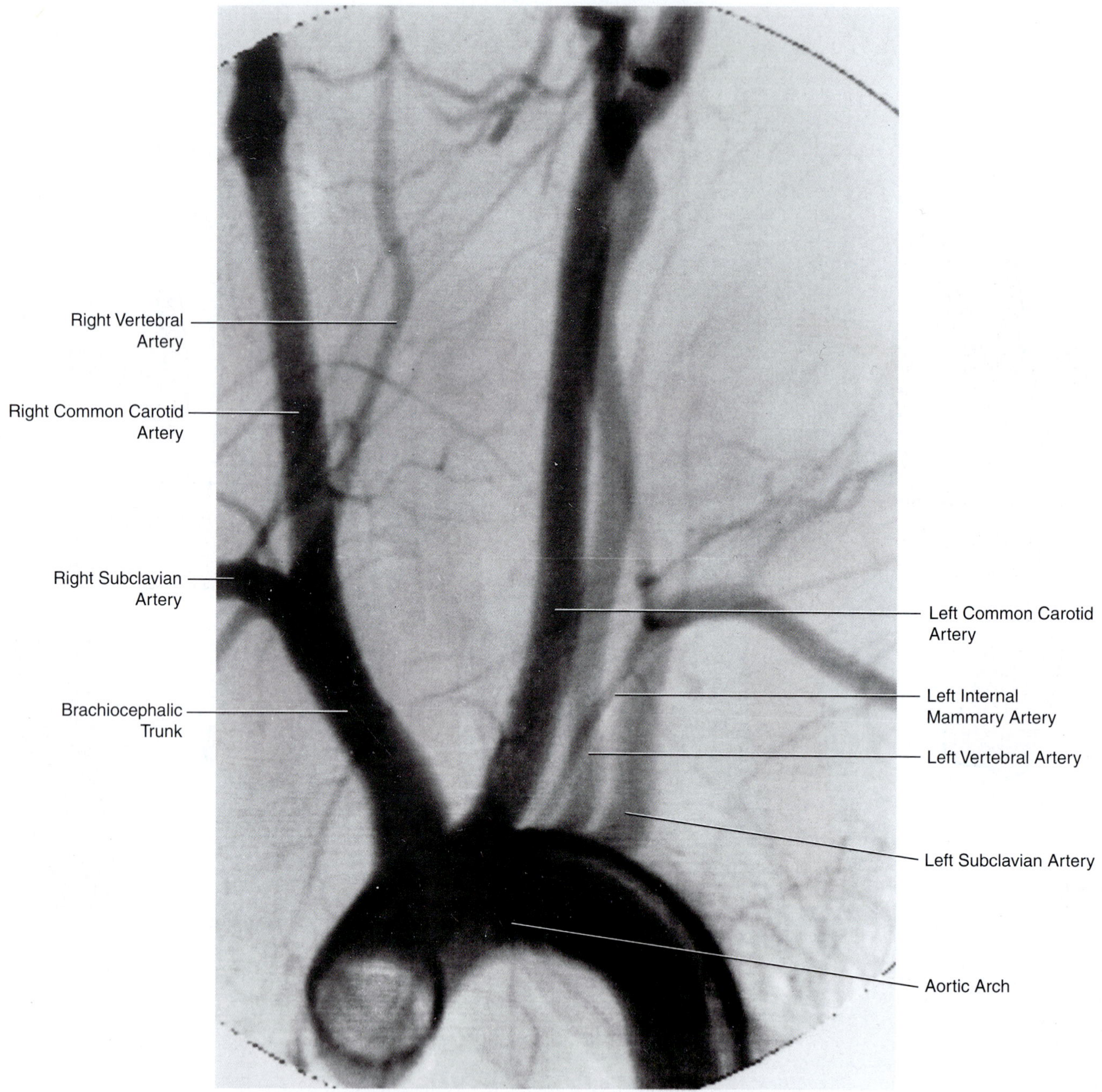

Figure 7.20. Aortic arch angiogram showing independent origin of four major branches of the arch directly from the arch. (Note the dominant left vertebral artery directly from the aorta.)

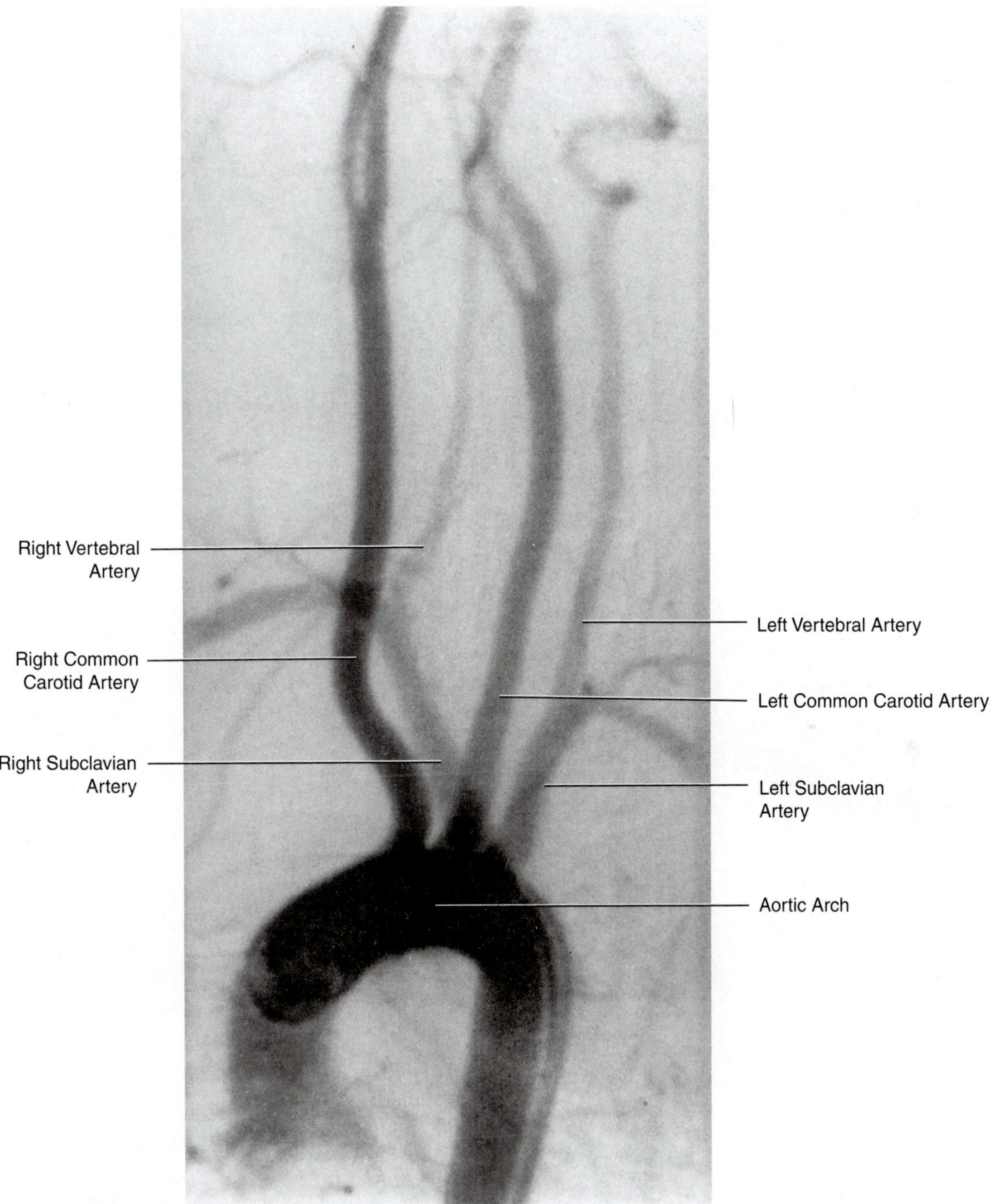

Figure 7.21. Aortic arch angiogram showing the origin of the right common carotid artery directly from the arch, as well as the left carotid artery and the left subclavian artery. Aortic arch angiogram showing an aberrant right subclavian artery arising directly from the distal aspect of the aortic arch.

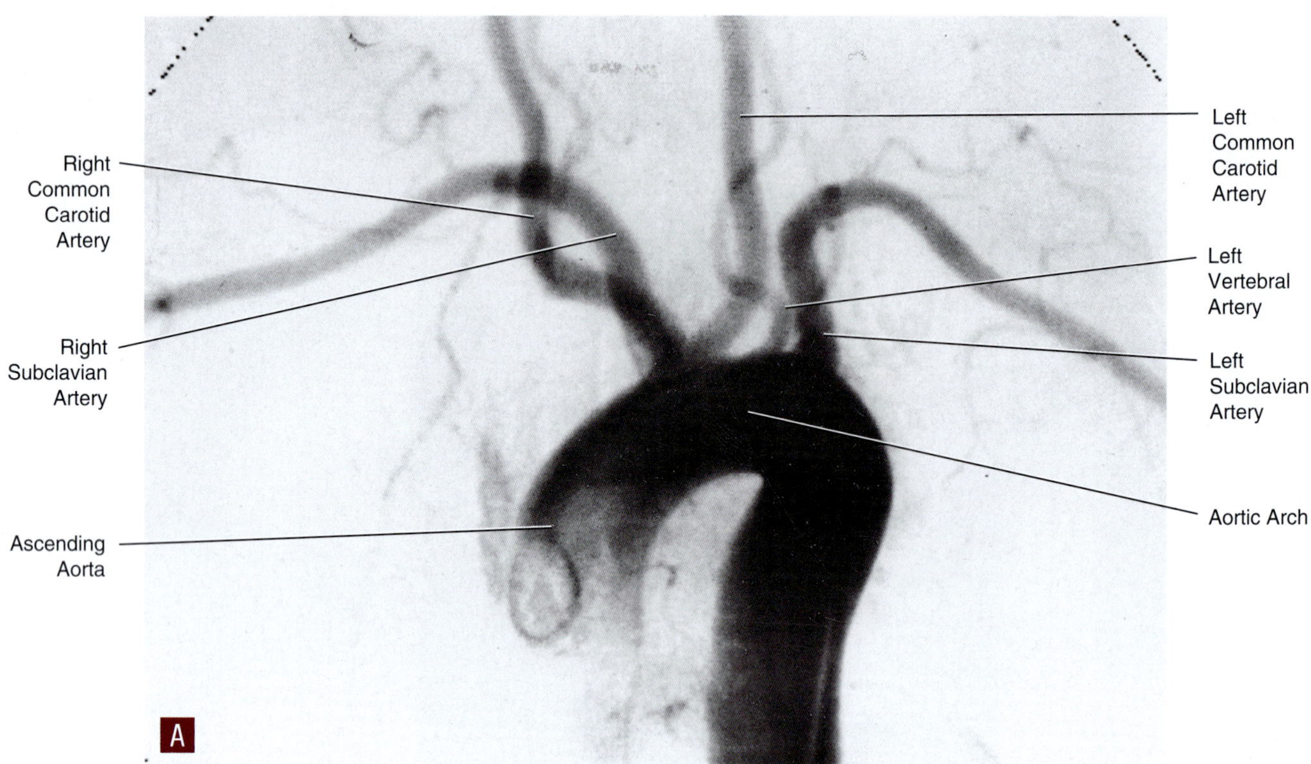

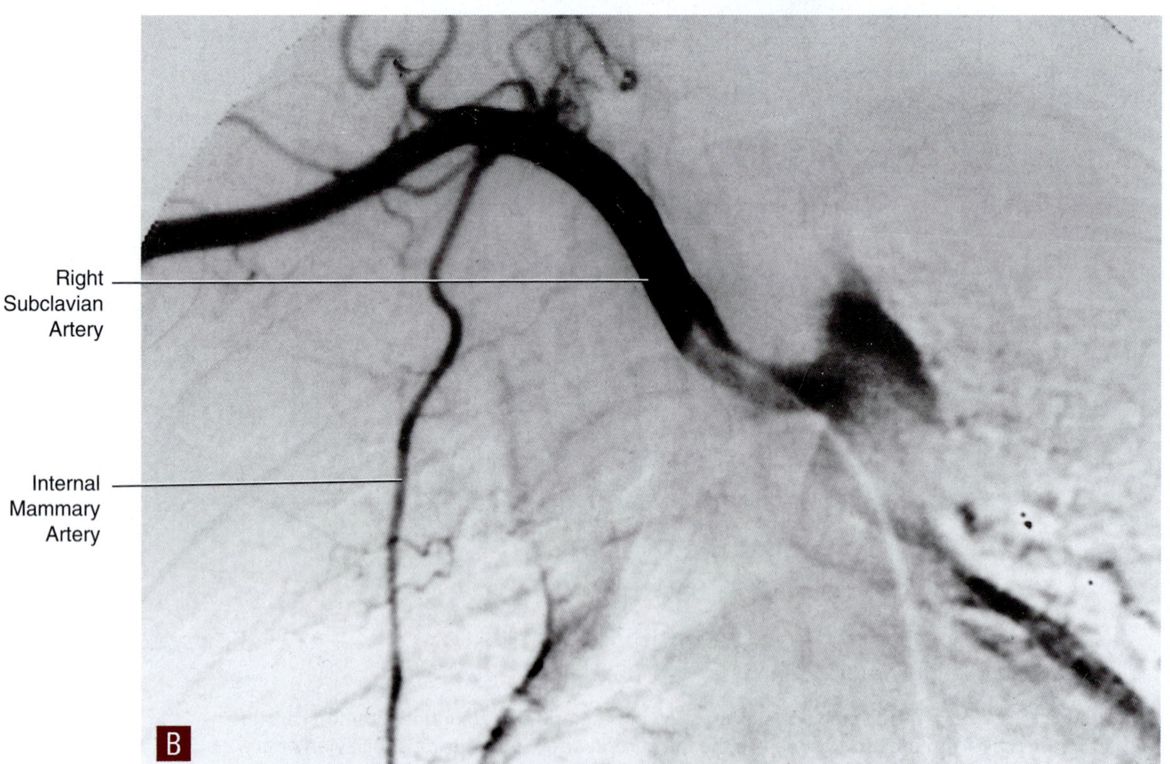

Figure 7.22. **A** and **B**, Aortic arch angiogram showing anatomic variation with the common origin of both common carotid arteries, direct origin of the left vertebral artery from the aorta, normal origin of the left subclavian artery, and independent posterolateral origin of the right subclavian artery from the arch. **C**, Computed tomography (CT) angiogram of the chest showing the anatomic variation. The posterolateral origin of the right subclavian artery. **D**, MR angiogram with another example of the posterolateral origin of the right subclavian artery.

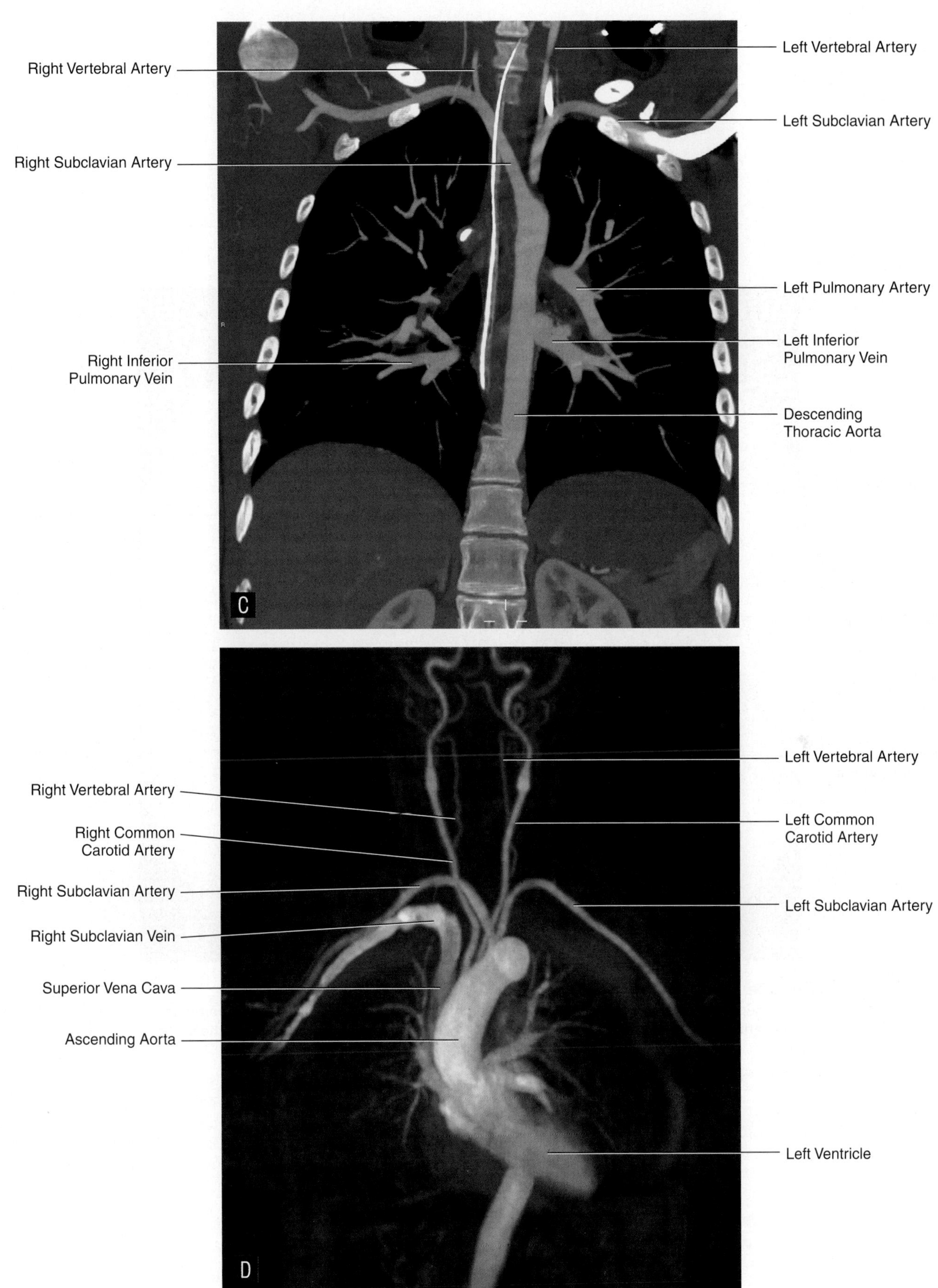

Figure 7.22. *Continued*

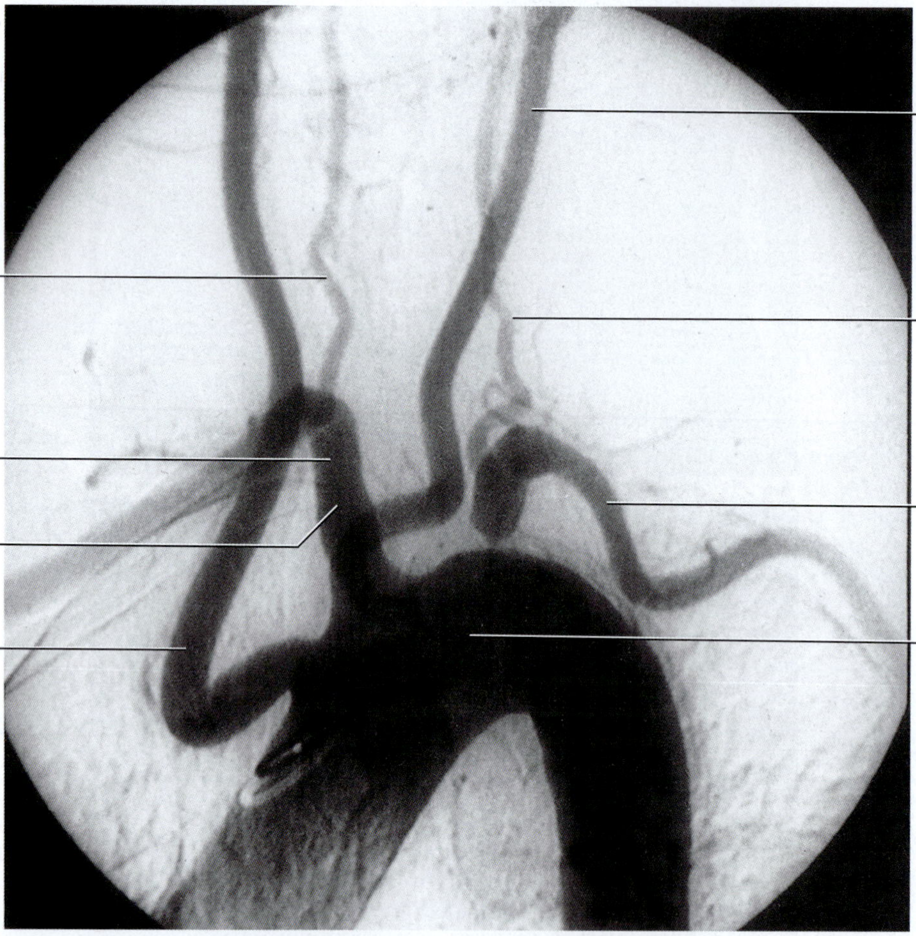

Figure 7.23. Aortic arch angiogram showing anatomic variation, with the brachiocephalic trunk giving origin to the left common carotid artery, and the right common carotid artery with independent origin directly from the aorta, as the first branch of the aortic arch.

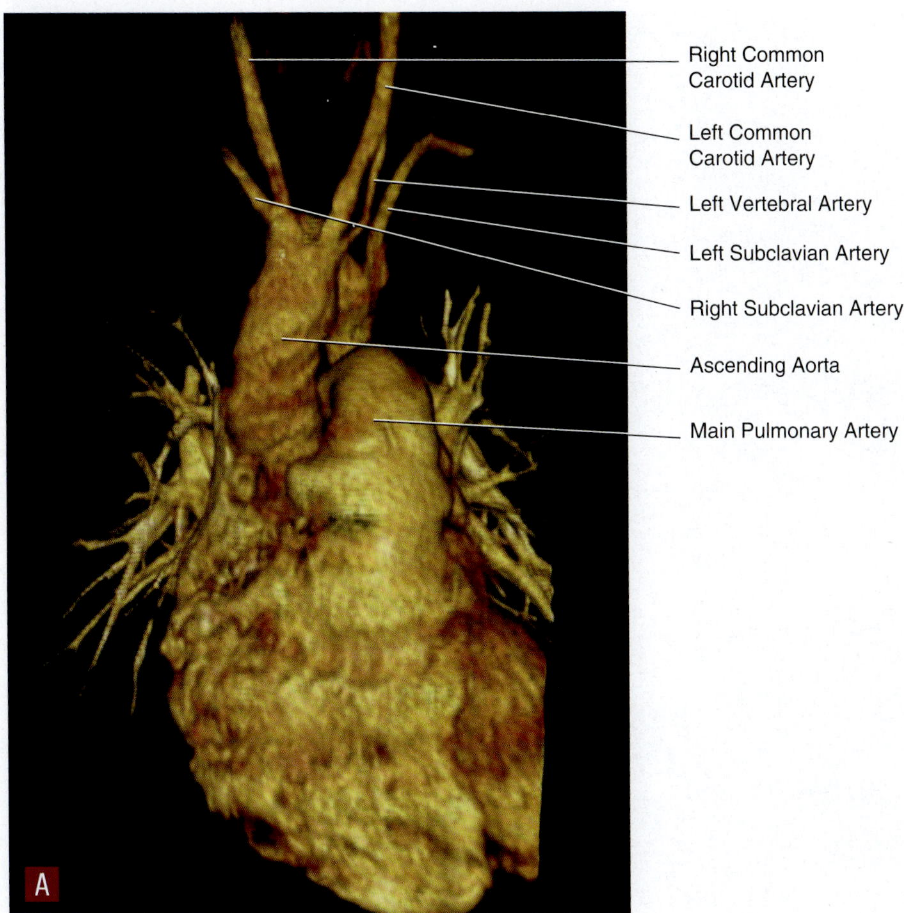

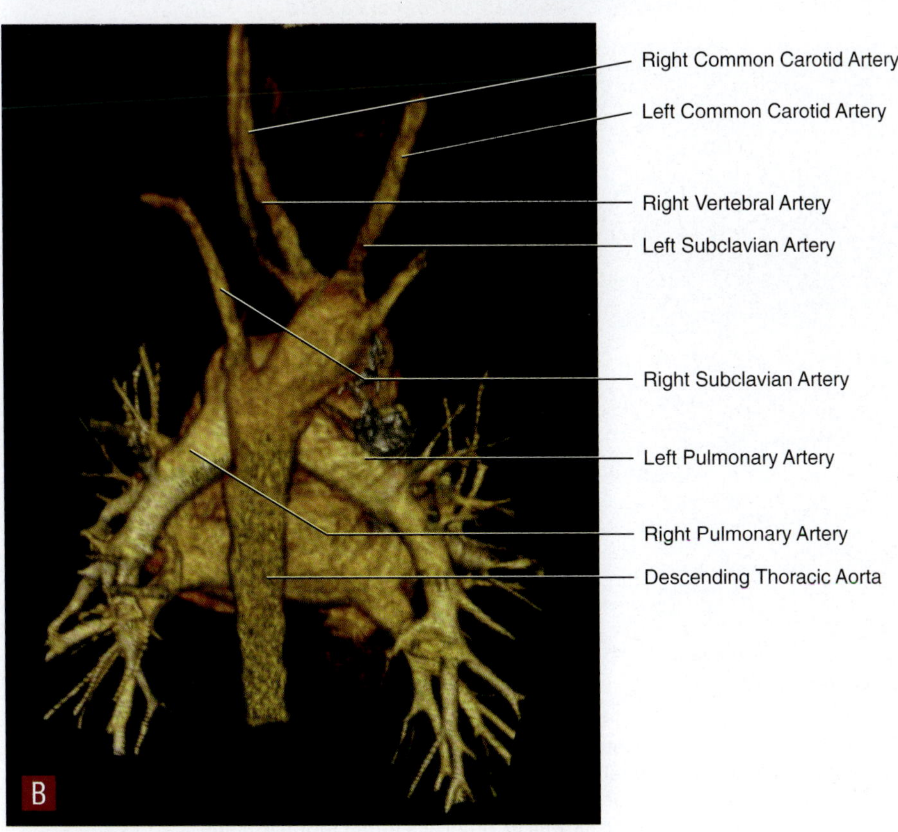

Figure 7.24. A and B, Computerized tomographic (CT) angiogram with three-dimensional (3D) reconstruction of the heart and aortic arch showing a rare variation of the aortic arch origin of the branches.

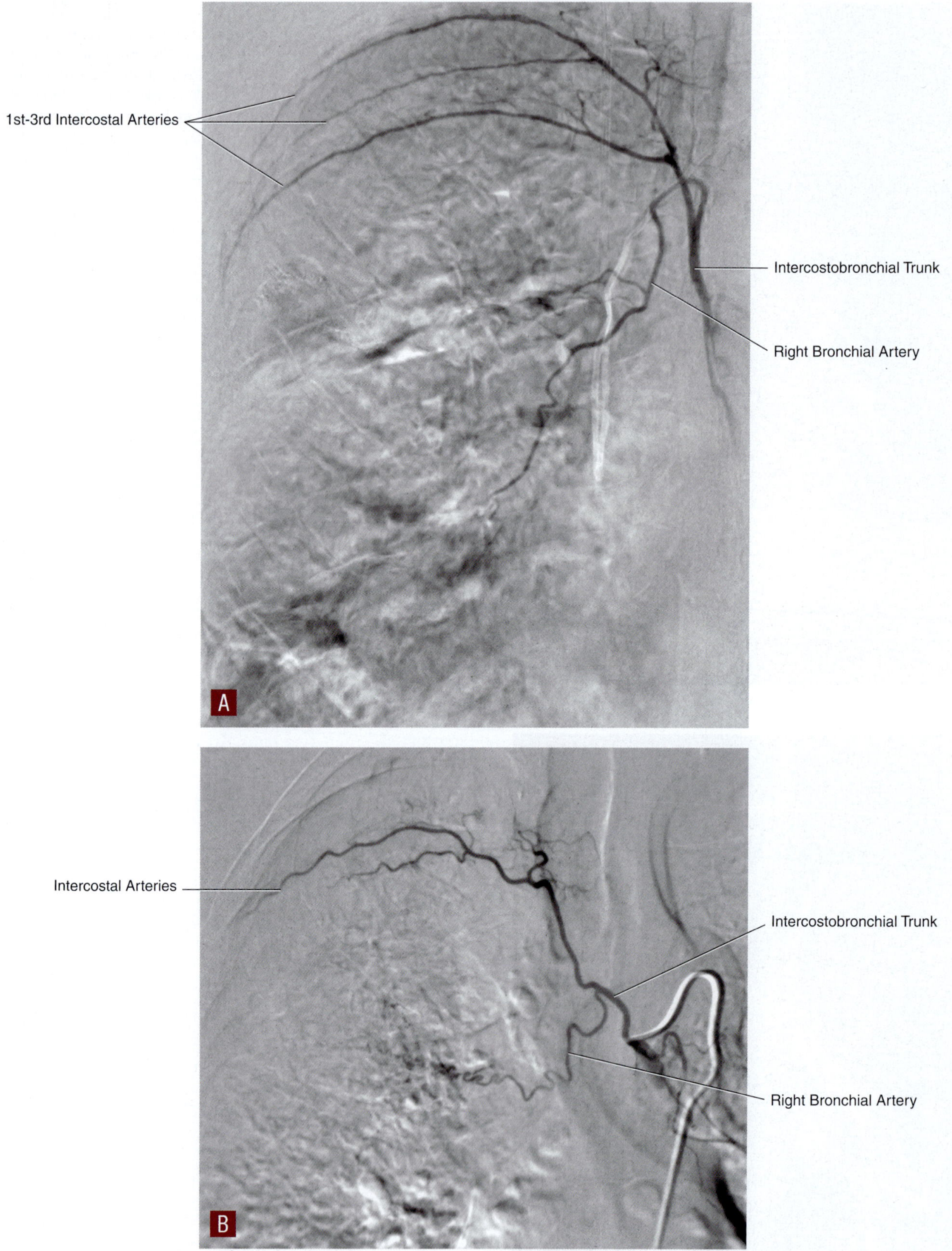

Figure 7.25. **A**, Selective angiogram of the intercostobronchial trunk showing filling of the right three first intercostal arteries and simultaneous filling of the right superior and inferior bronchial arteries. **B**, Selective angiogram of the intercostobronchial trunk showing a single bronchial artery and the third intercostal artery, as well as branches to the thoracic spine vertebral bodies.

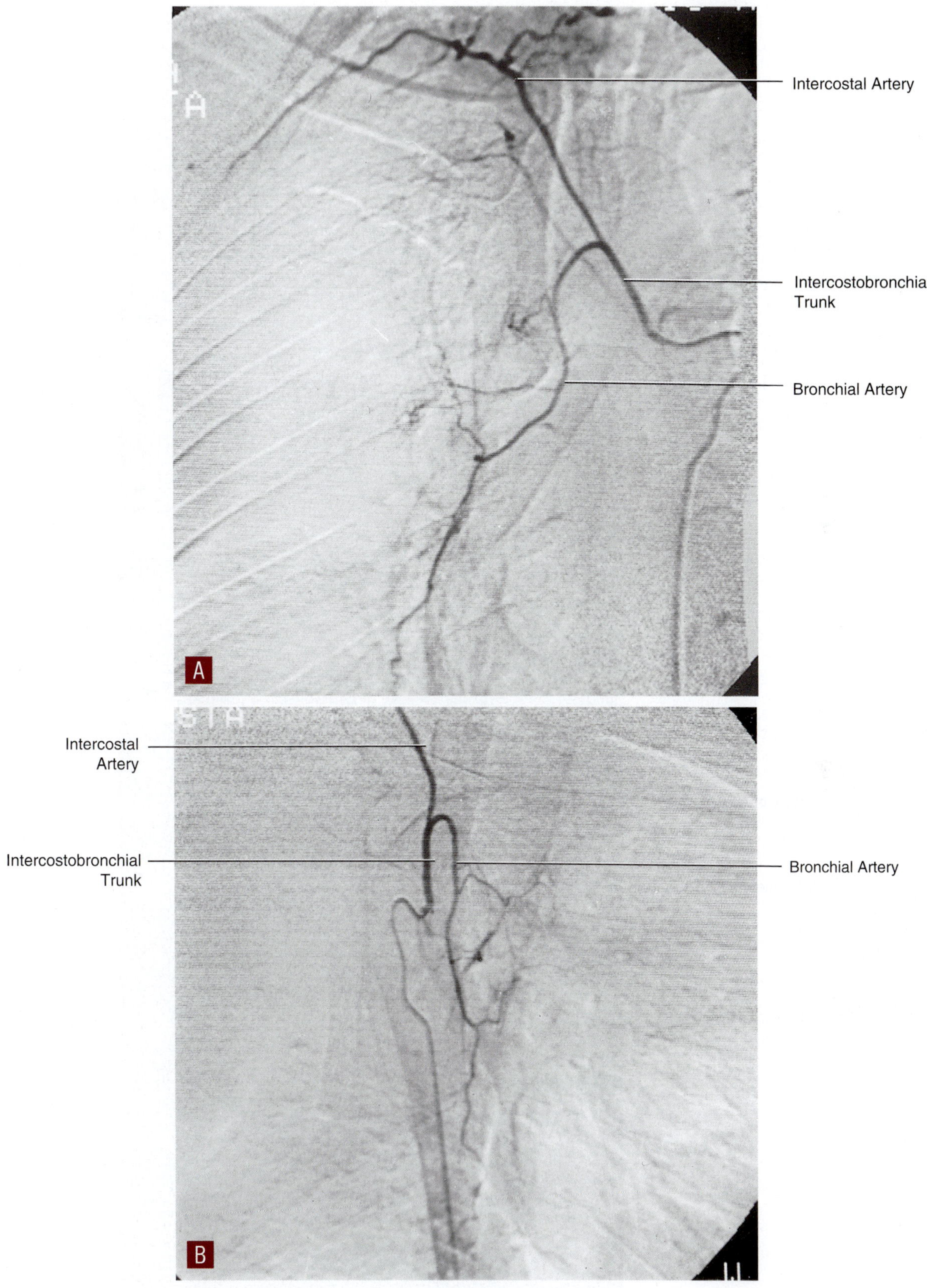

Figure 7.26. A, Anterior view of the angiogram of the intercostobronchial trunk showing filling of the second intercostal artery and right bronchial arteries. B, Lateral view of the angiogram of the same artery as in (A) showing that the intercostal artery is posterior and the bronchial arteries follow a more central or anterior direction, along with the bronchus.

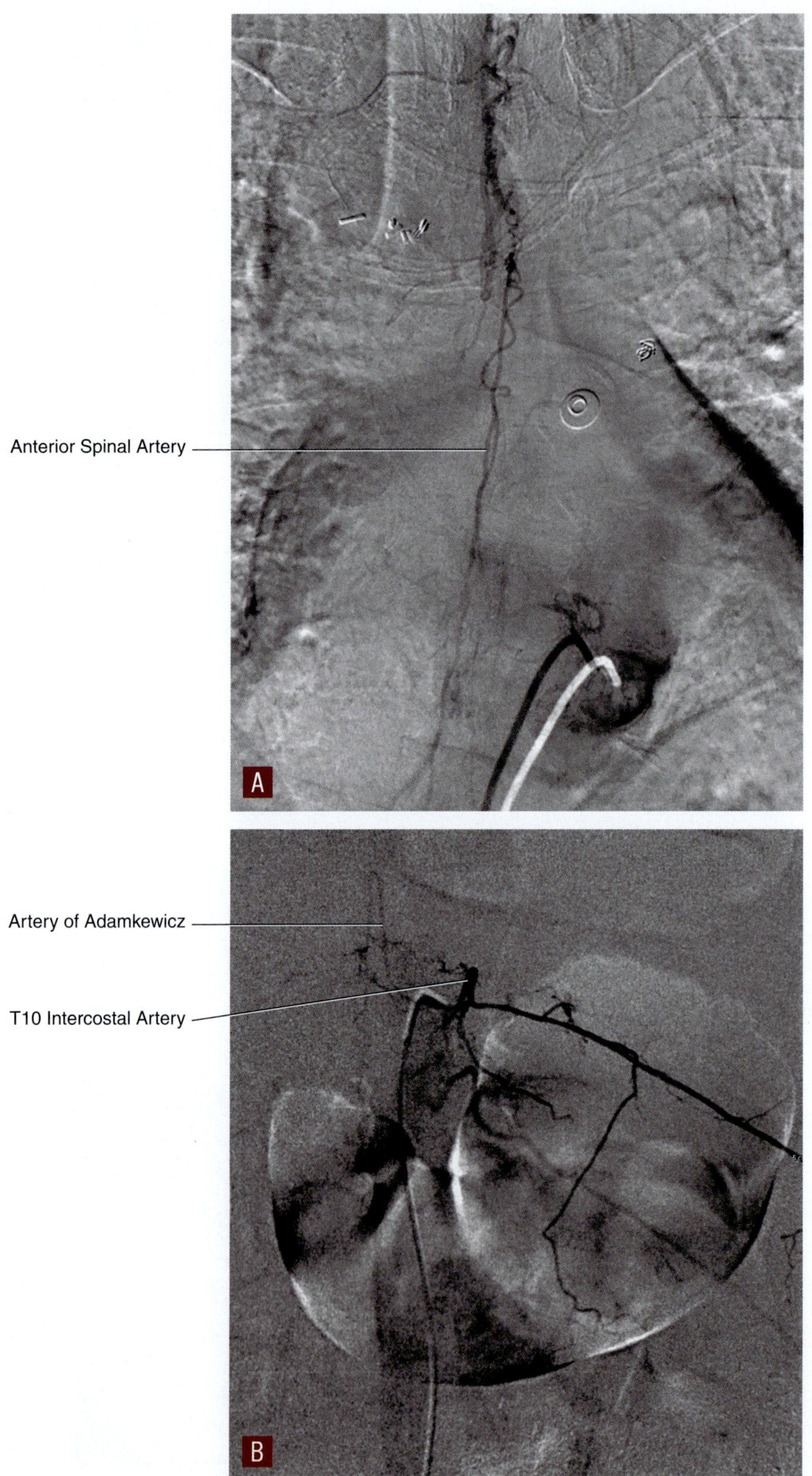

Figure 7.27. **A**, Anterior view angiogram of the left bronchial artery after embolization showing reflux of contrast into the anterior spinal artery. **B**, Left T10 intercostal artery angiogram showing a low origin of artery of Adamkewicz (anterior spinal artery) with its typical hairpin turn. This important branch arises between T9 and L2 in 85% of cases.

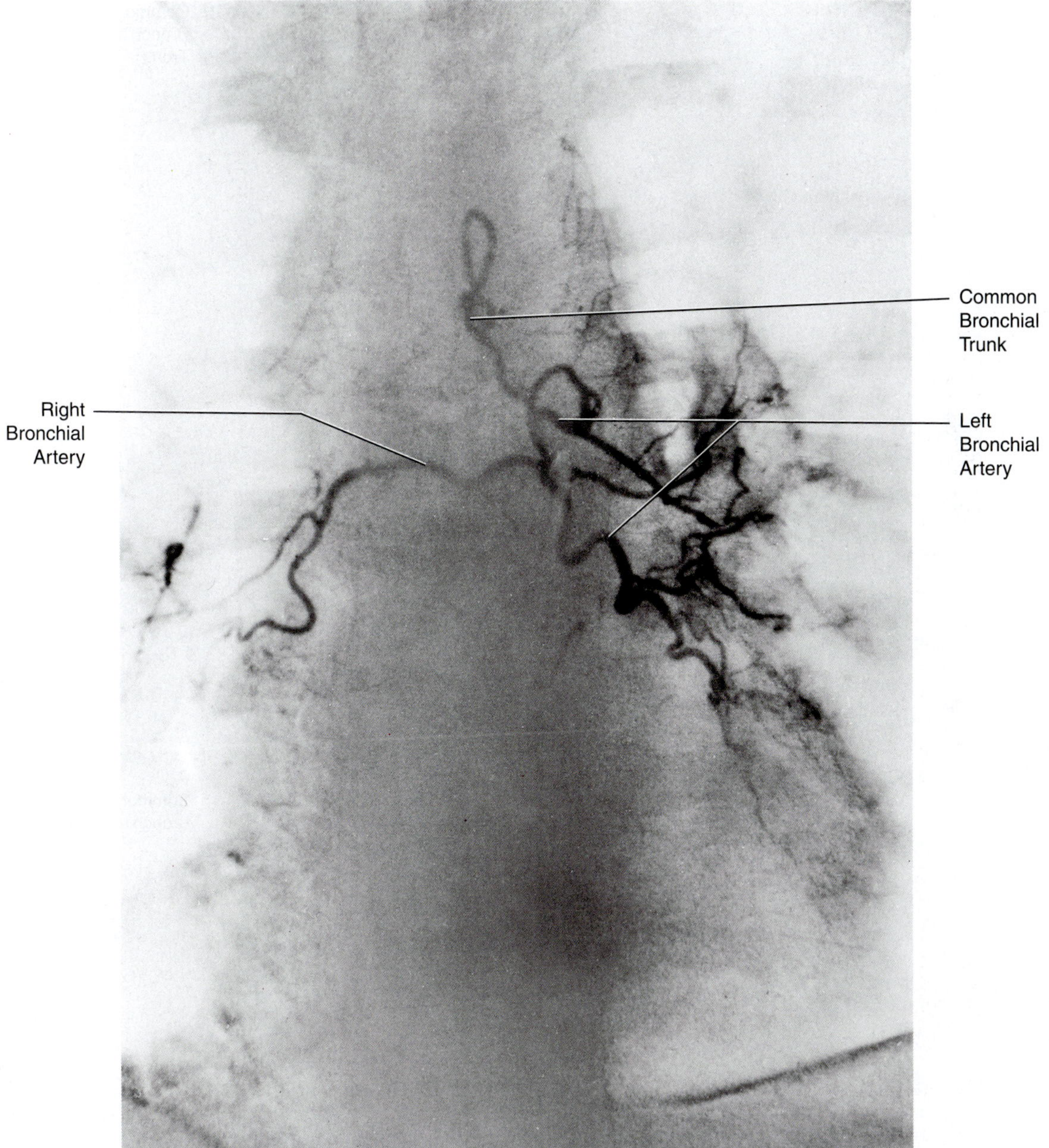

Figure 7.28. Angiogram of a bronchial artery common trunk giving origin to a right bronchial artery and a left bronchial artery. Note the right bronchial artery is inferior and on the left there are superior and inferior bronchial arteries.

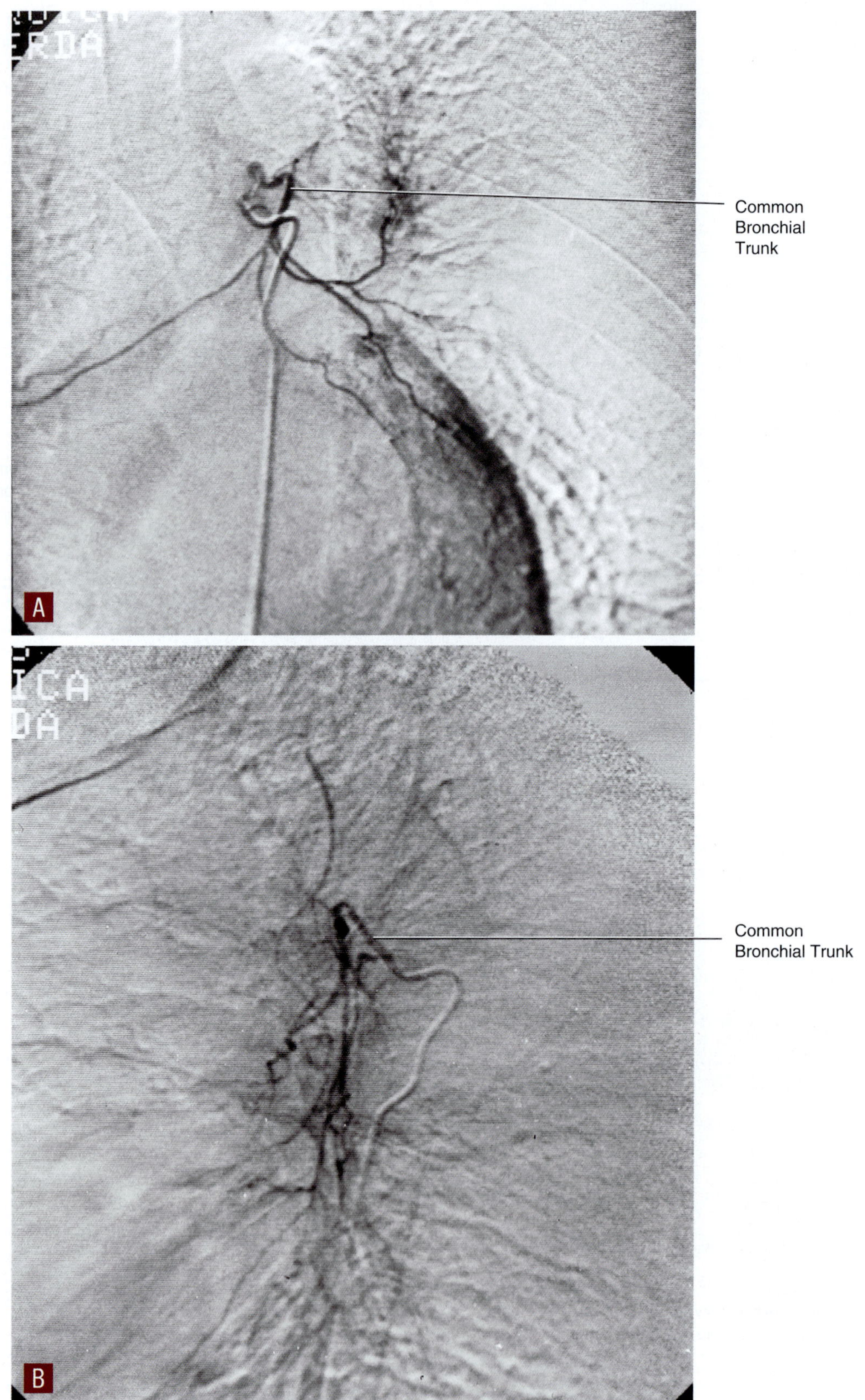

Figure 7.29. A, Selective angiogram of a common bronchial trunk showing the branches to right and left. B, Lateral view showing the right and left bronchial arteries following a central or anterior direction. The origin of the common trunk is almost perpendicular to the aortic wall.

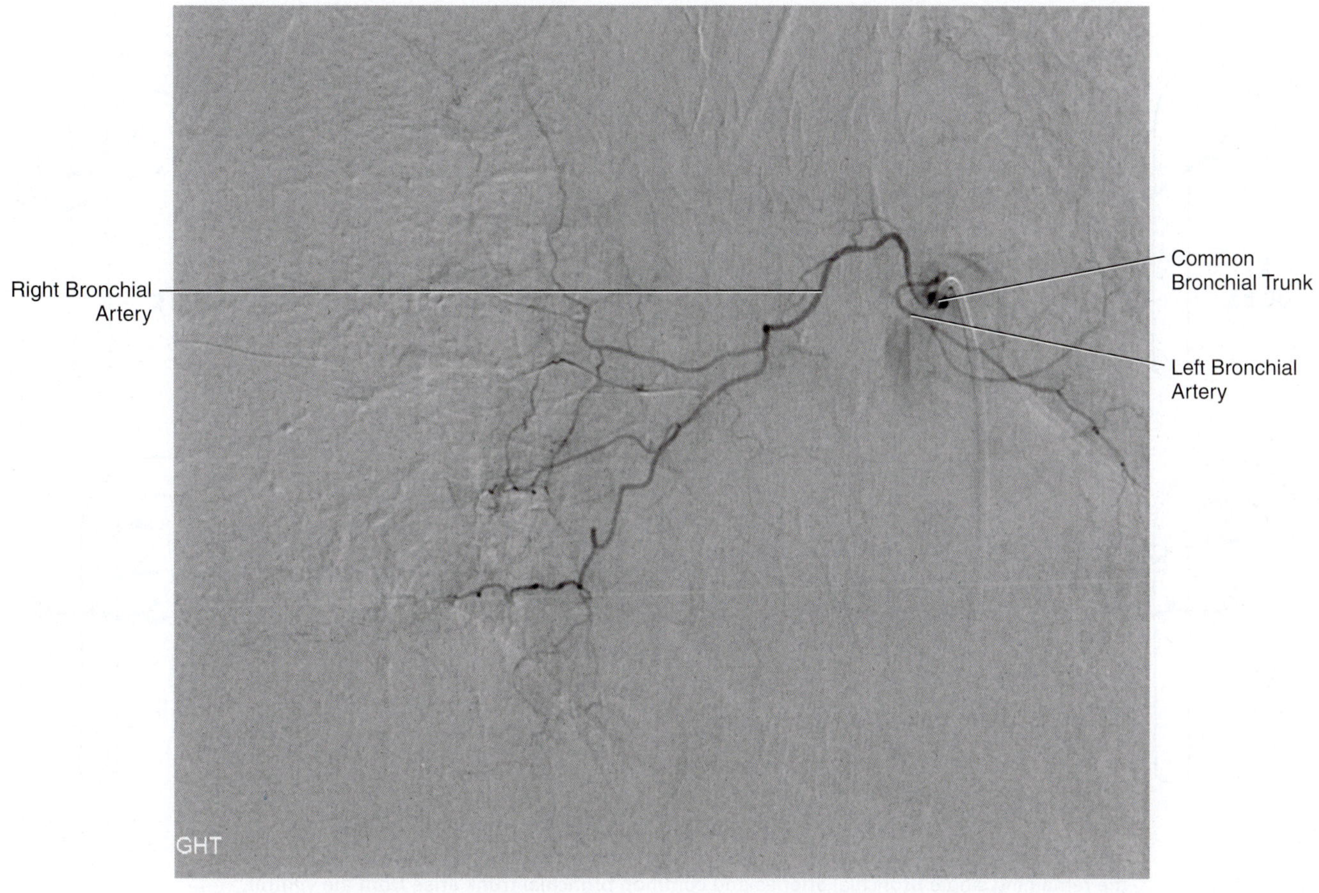

Figure 7.30. Selective angiogram of a common bronchial trunk, with inferior and superior bilateral bronchial arteries.

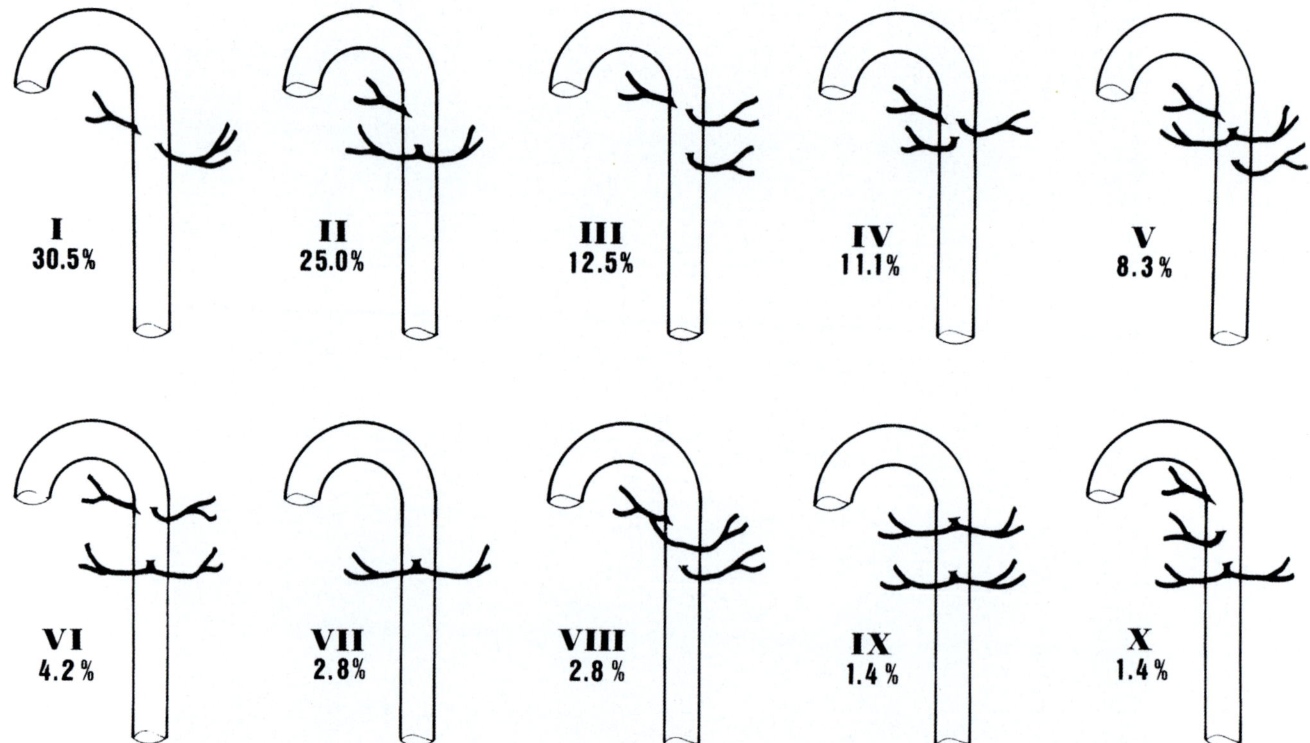

Figure 7.31. Ventral aspect of the types of bronchial arterial supply, based on the angiographic data of 72 patients. The right intercostobronchial trunk arises laterally or dorsally; the remaining single bronchial arteries and common bronchial trunk arise from the ventral aspect of the aorta. (From Uflacker, et al. *Radiology*. 1985;157:637-644.)

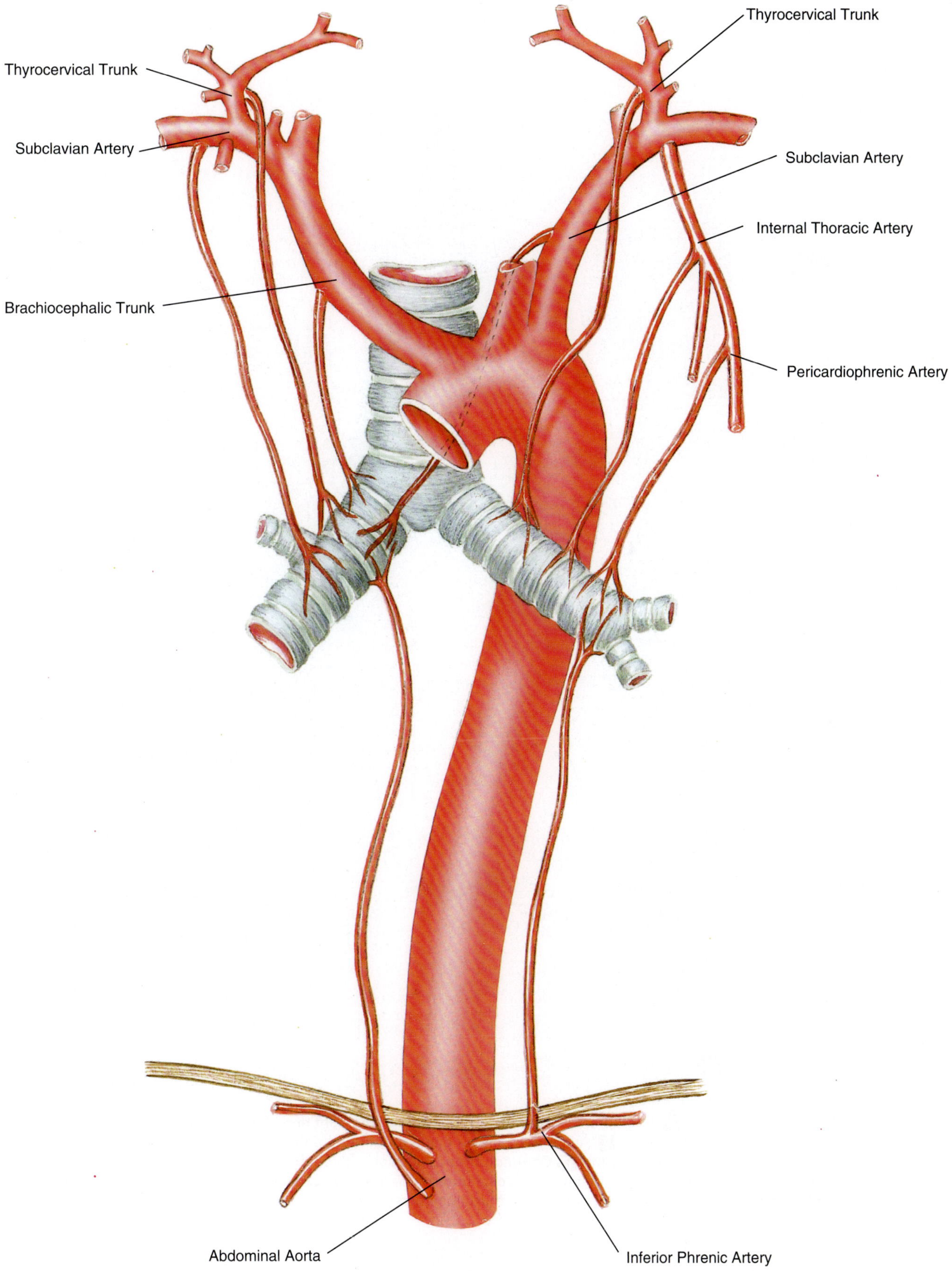

Figure 7.32. Aberrant origins and anatomic variations of the bronchial arteries.

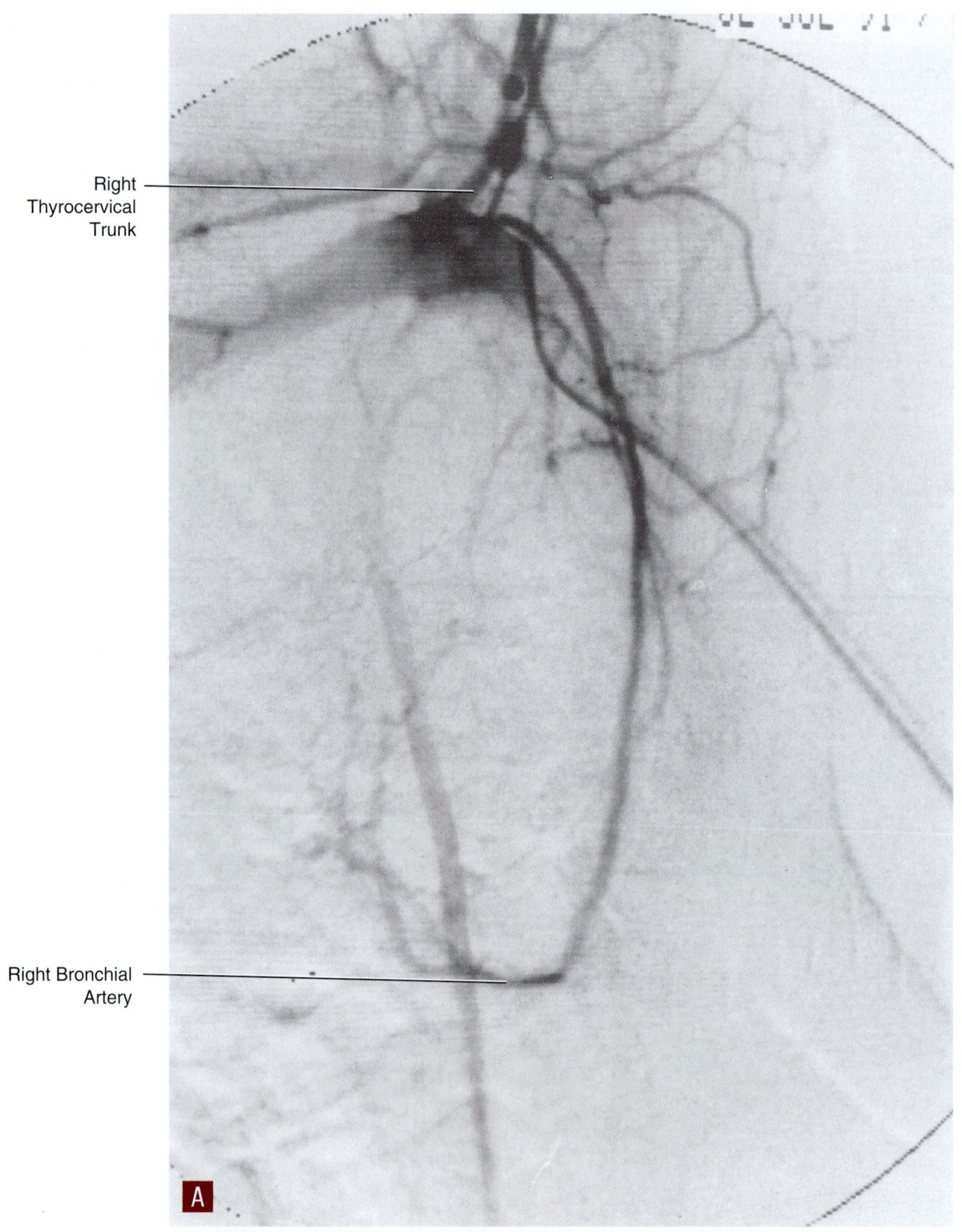

Figure 7.33. **A**, Angiogram showing aberrant origin of the right bronchial artery from the right thyrocervical trunk. **B**, Angiogram showing aberrant origin of the left bronchial artery from the right thyrocervical trunk. **C**, Common bronchial trunk with aberrant origin from the left thyrocervical trunk. (Note multiple intercostal arteries originated from the same trunk.) **D**, Left bronchial artery arising from the left third intercostal artery.

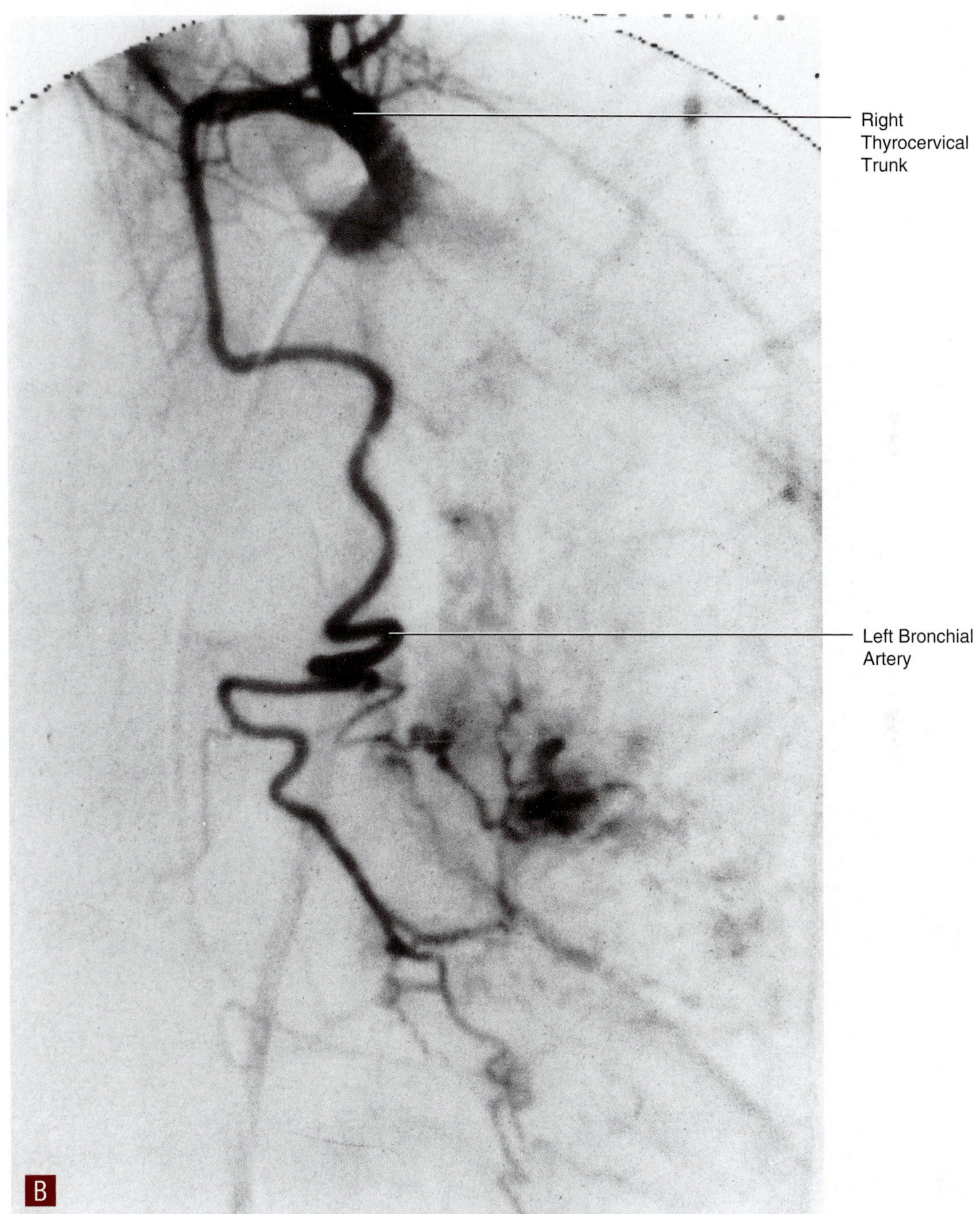

Figure 7.33. *Continued*

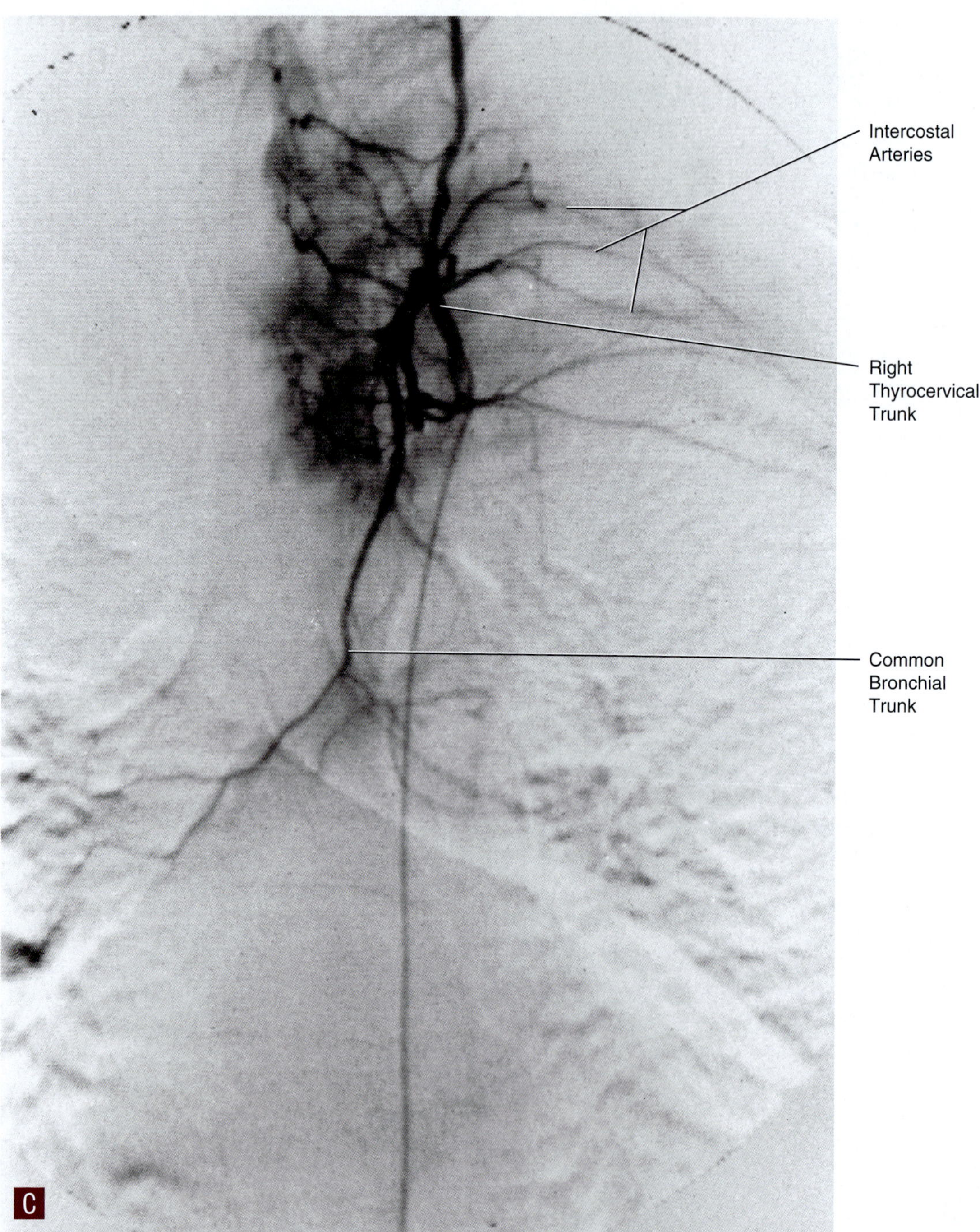

Figure 7.33. *Continued*

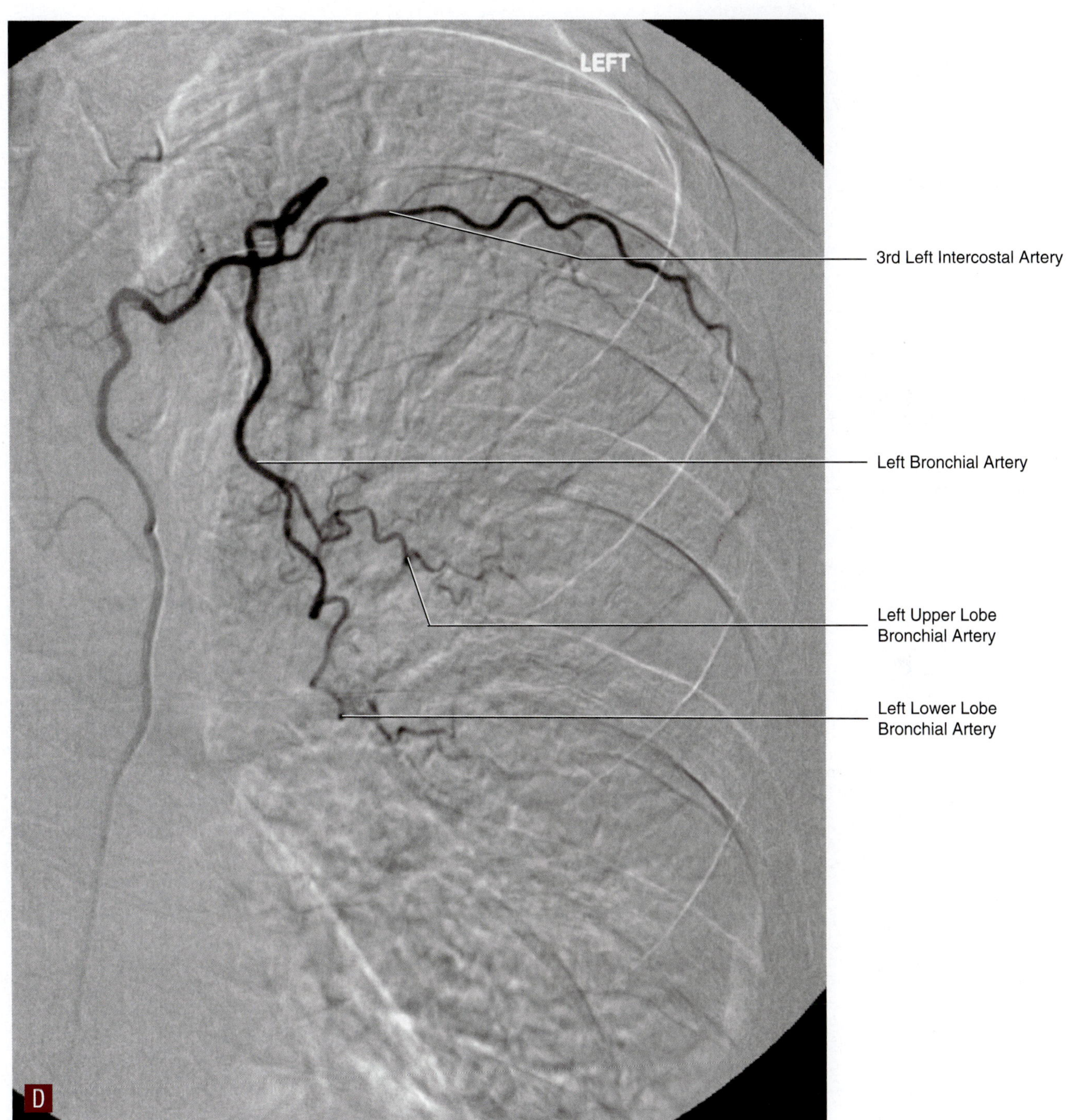

Figure 7.33. *Continued*

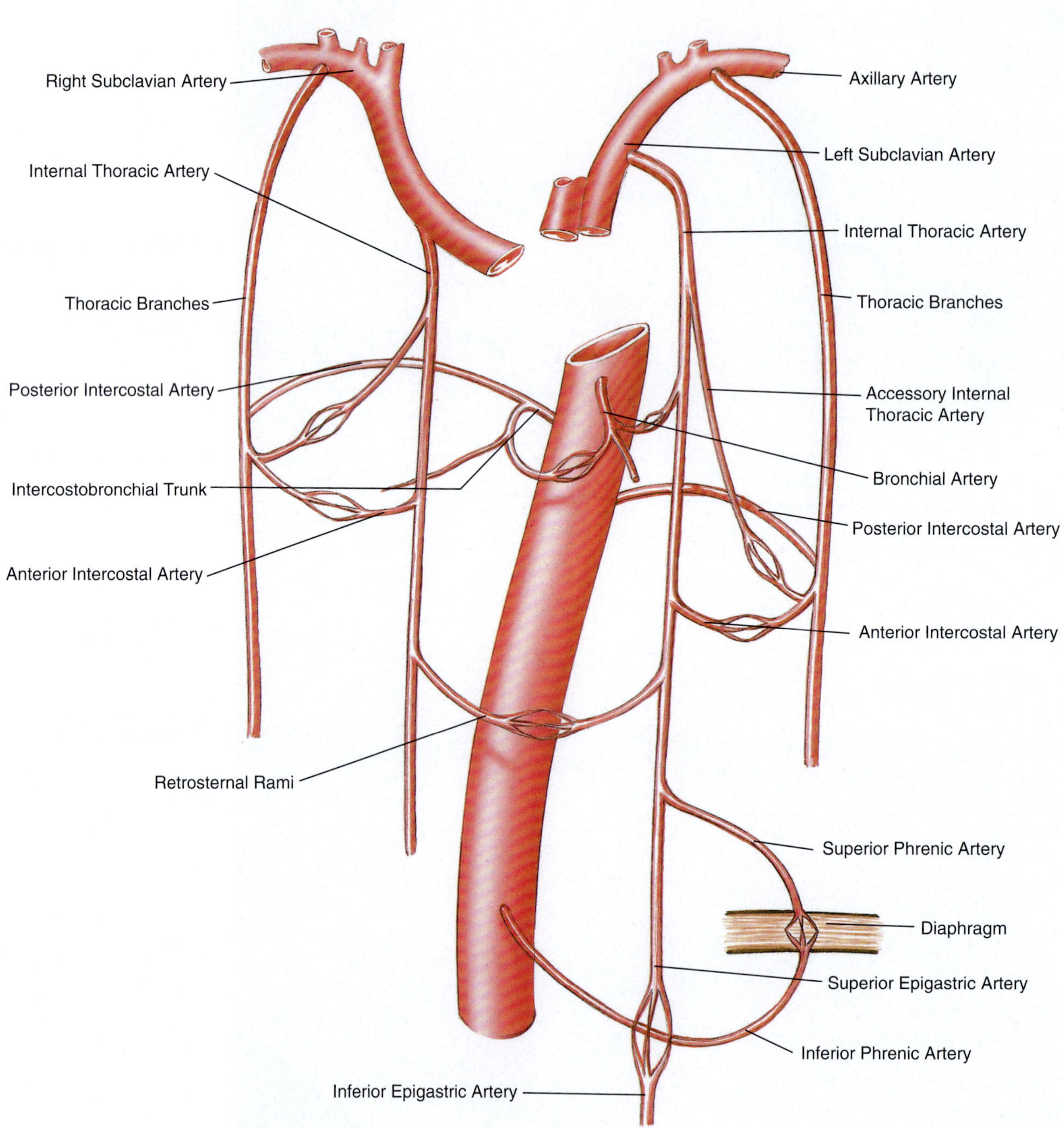

Figure 7.34. Anastomotic connections of the thoracic arteries.

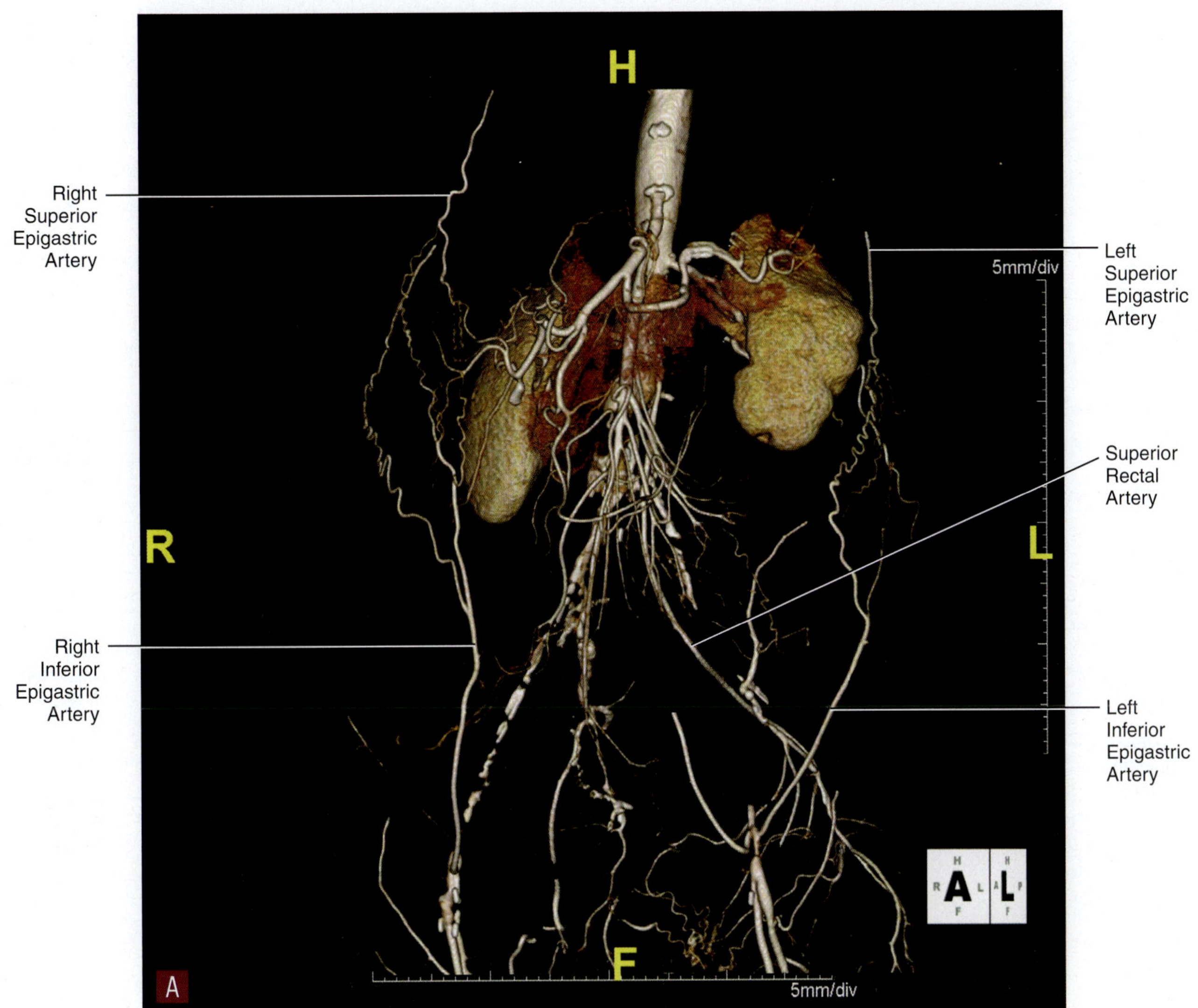

Figure 7.35. Computed tomography (CT) angiogram volume rendered reconstruction of a patient with aortoiliac occlusive disease. A, Anterior view showing distal reconstitution of the femoral arteries via the hypertrophied retiform anastomoses between the inferior and superior epigastric arteries via the internal mammary artery. B, Left lateral view showing anastomoses between the middle rectal artery and internal iliac artery, circumflex iliac artery and intercostal artery, and the inferior epigastric arteries. C, Posterior view showing iliolumbar, rectal, circumflex iliac, and intercostal anastomoses.

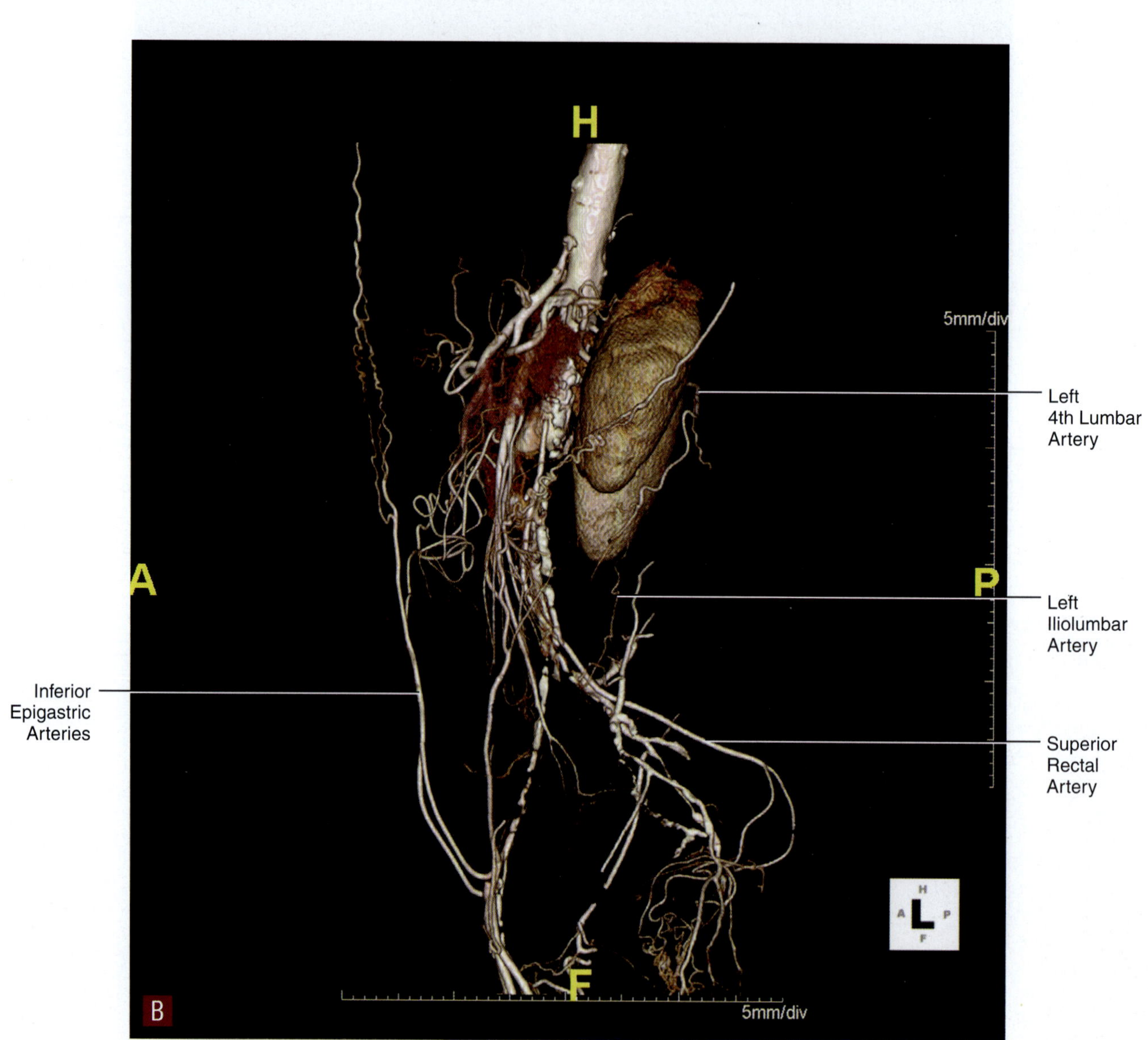

Figure 7.35. *Continued*

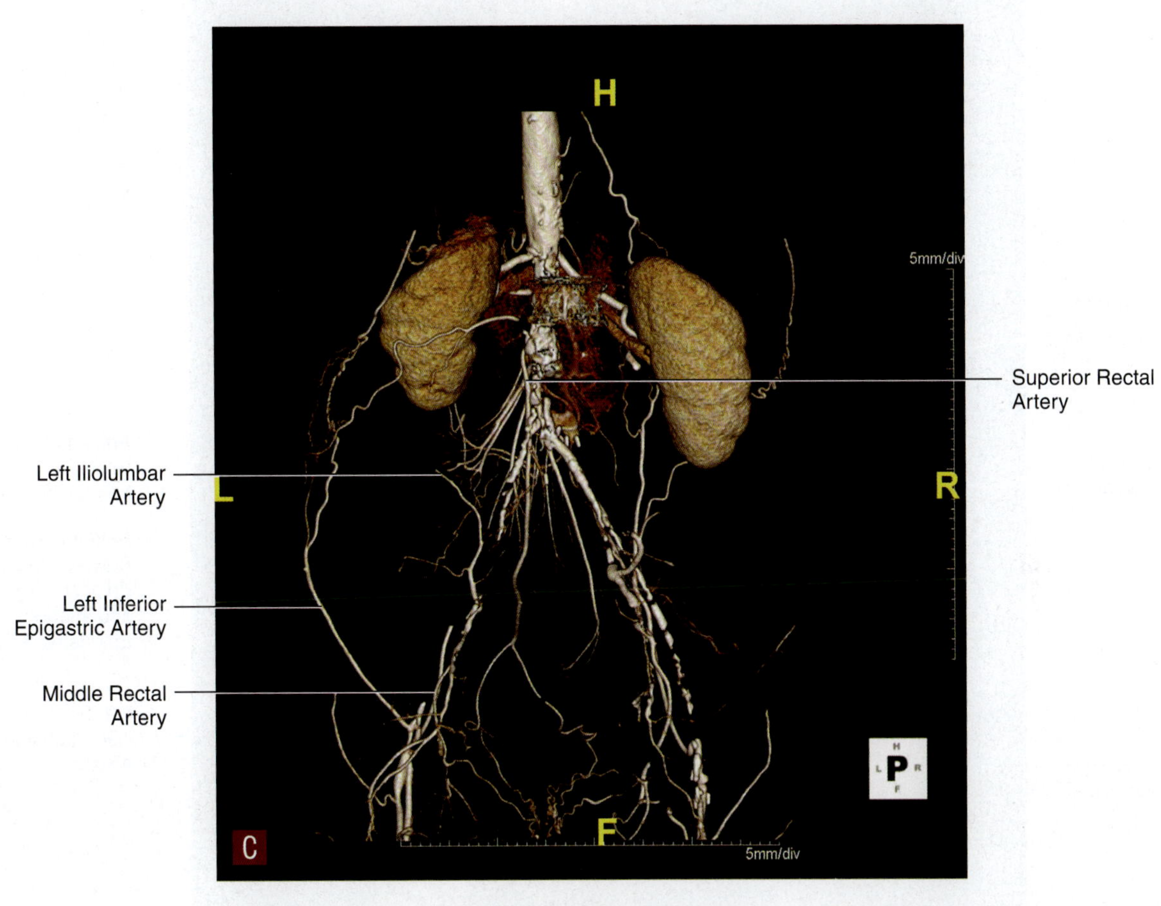

Figure 7.35. *Continued*

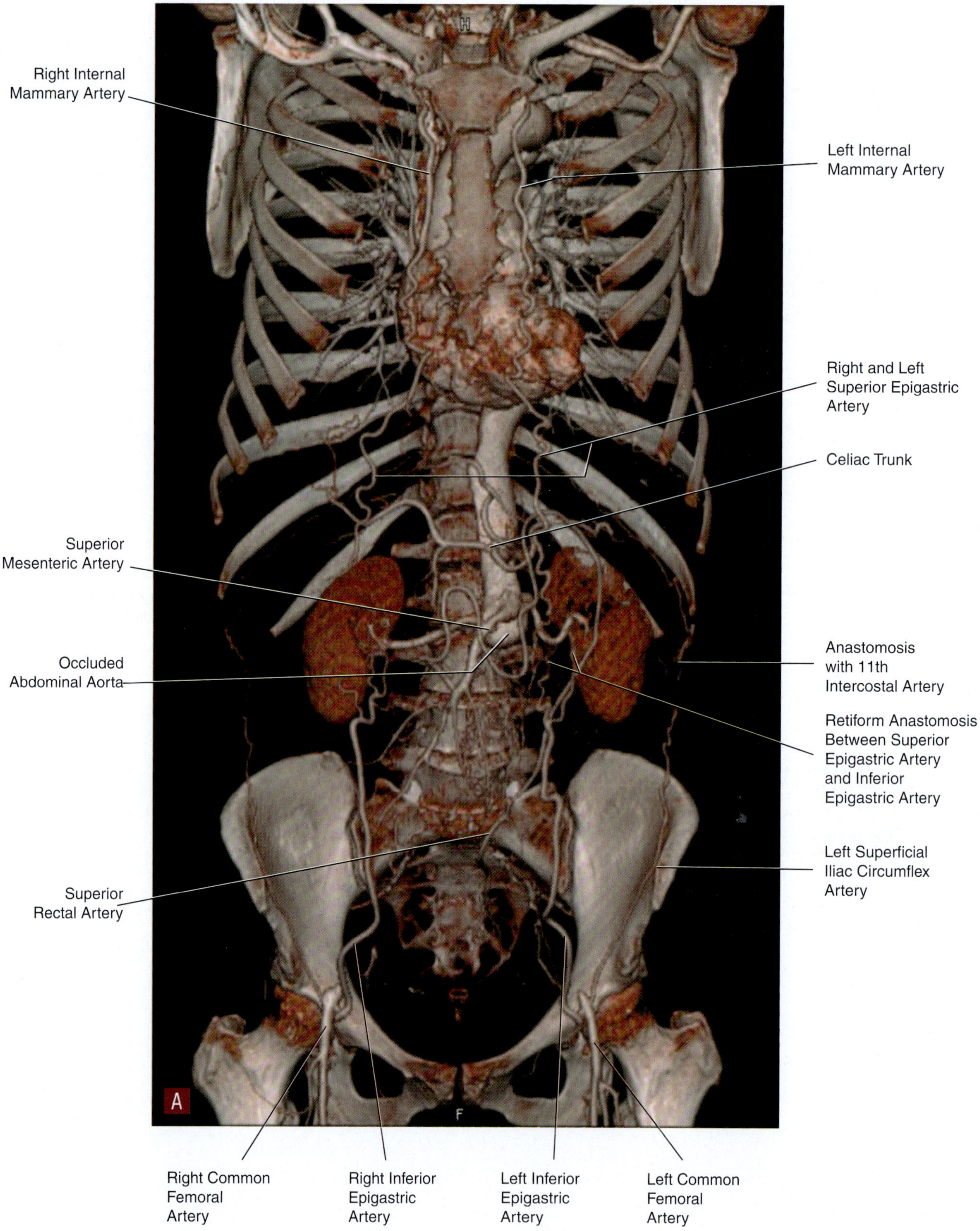

Figure 7.36. **Computerized tomographic (CT)** angiogram of the thorax and abdomen showing the thoracoabdominal arterial anastomoses through the superior epigastric arteries and the inferior epigastric arteries, connecting with the common femoral arteries through the retiform anastomosis between the two systems. Note the occluded abdominal aorta, which caused the development of the collateral circulation. **A**, Anteroposterior view. **B** and **C**, Lateral right and left views of the thoracoabdominal arterial anastomoses through the superior epigastric arteries and the inferior epigastric arteries.

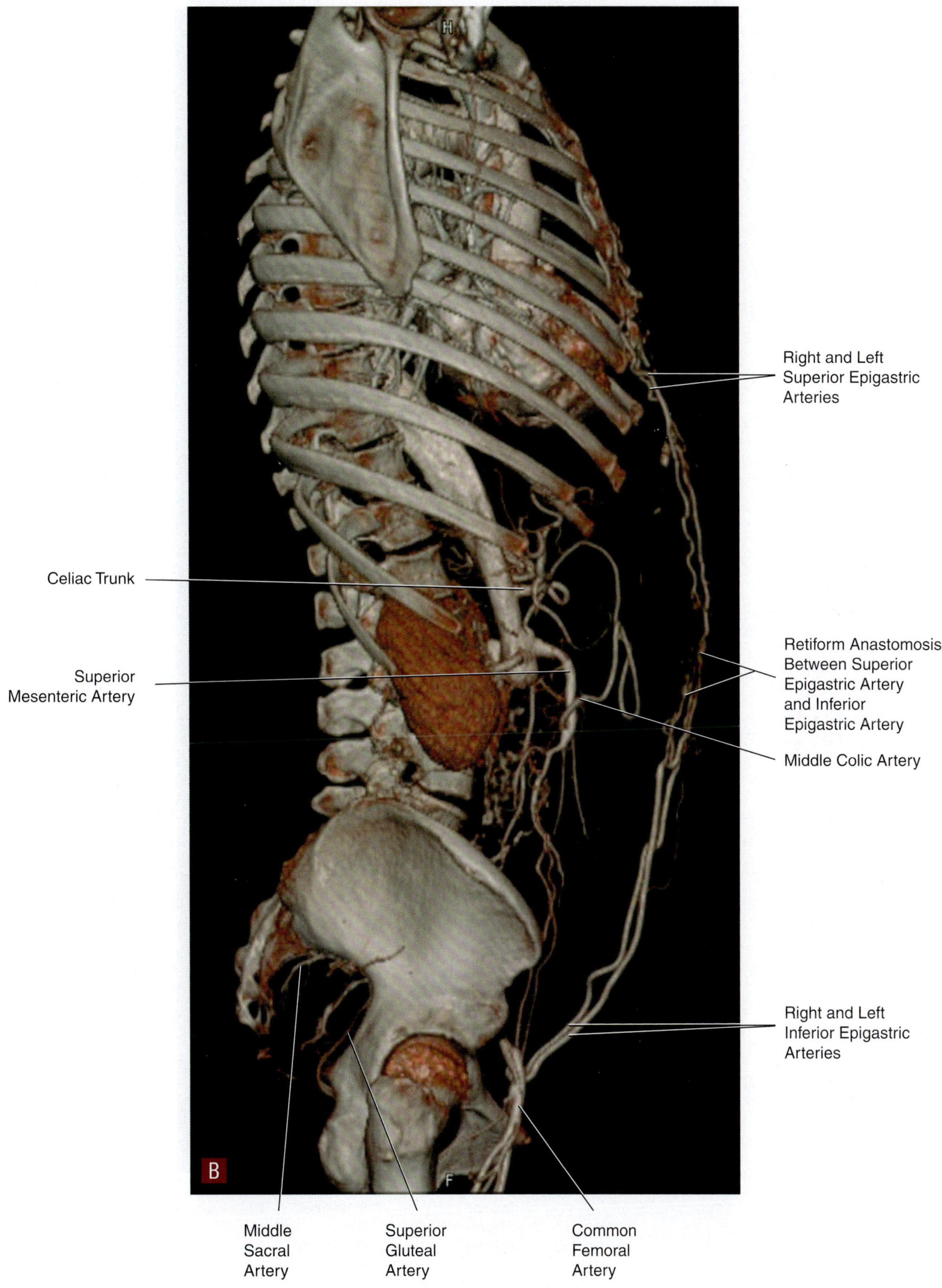

Figure 7.36. *Continued*

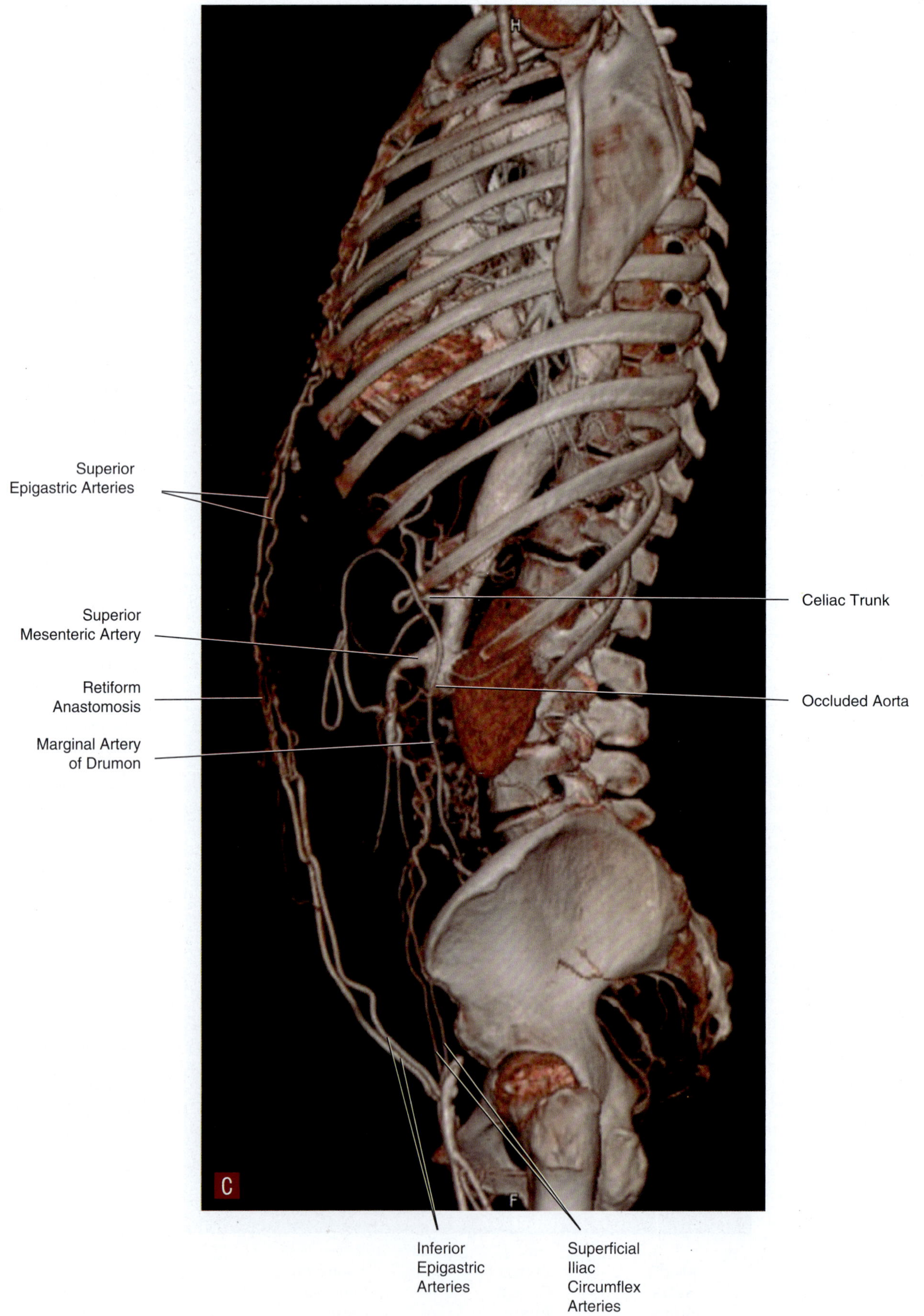

Figure 7.36. *Continued*

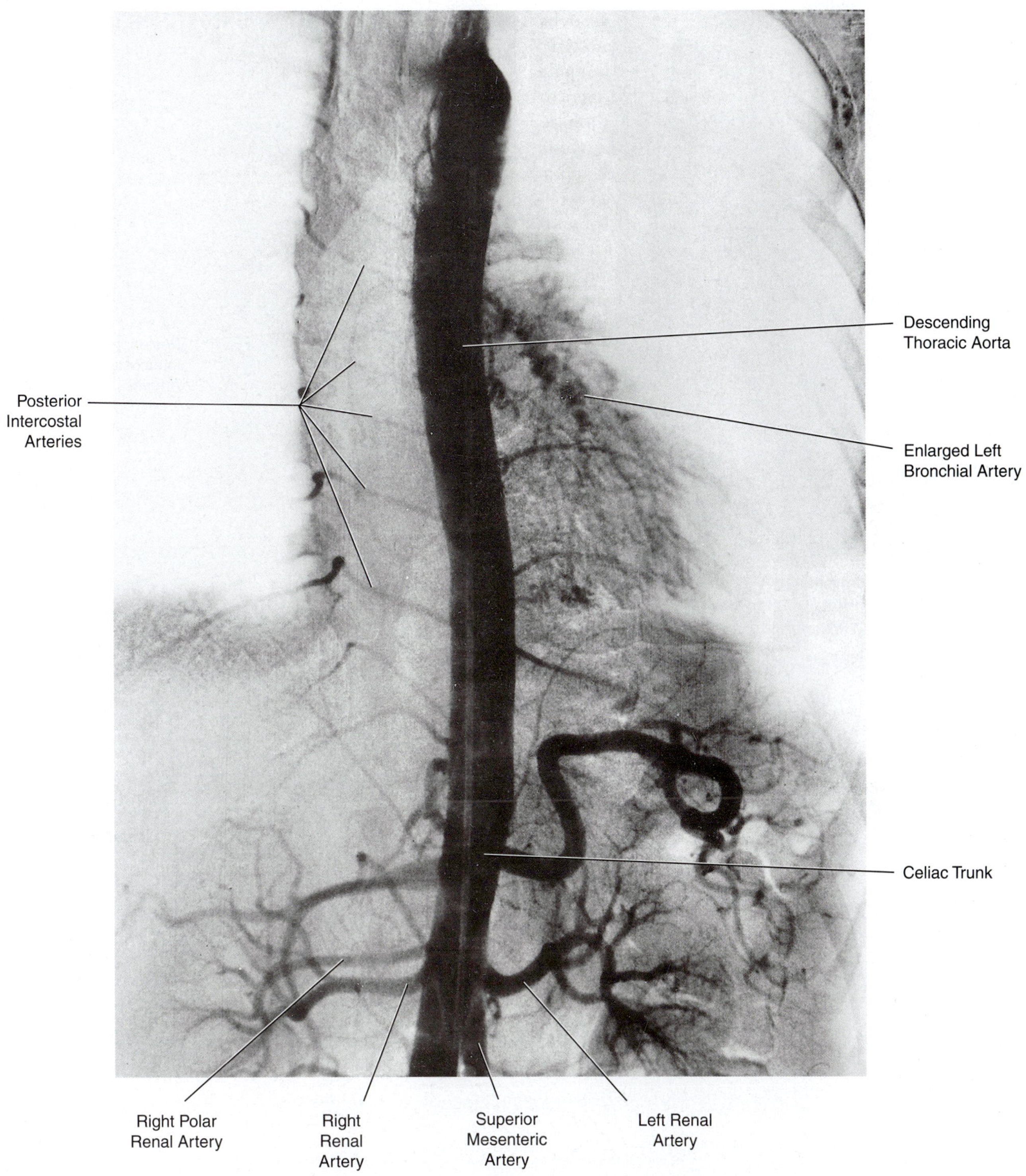

Figure 7.37. Descending thoracic aortogram showing the posterior intercostal arteries and an enlarged left bronchial artery. The visceral arteries are also seen.

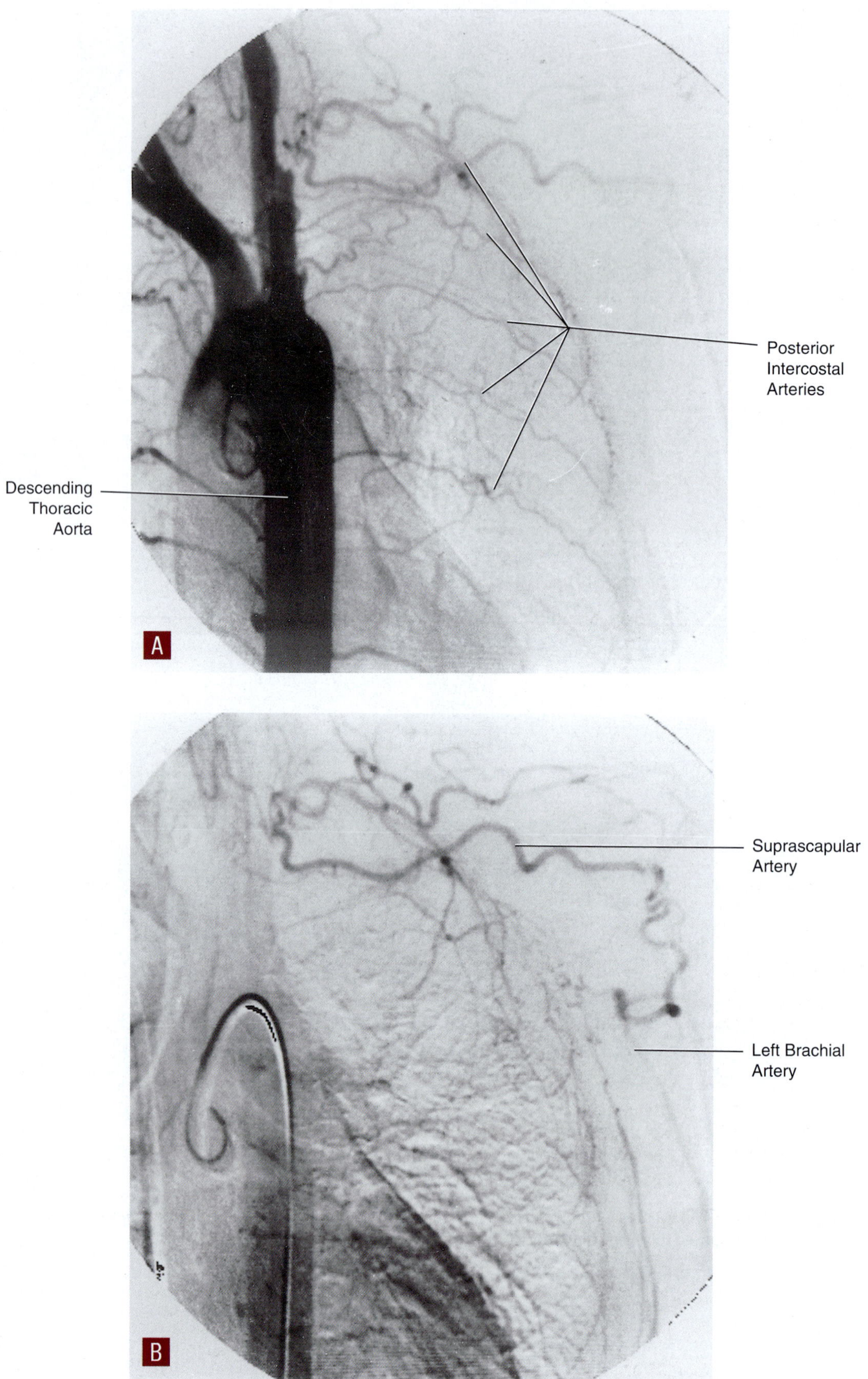

Figure 7.38. A, Thoracic aortogram showing the enlarged posterior intercostal arteries due to the occlusion of the left subclavian artery, in an attempt to reconstitute the left brachial artery. B, Later phase of the angiogram showing development of the suprascapular artery.

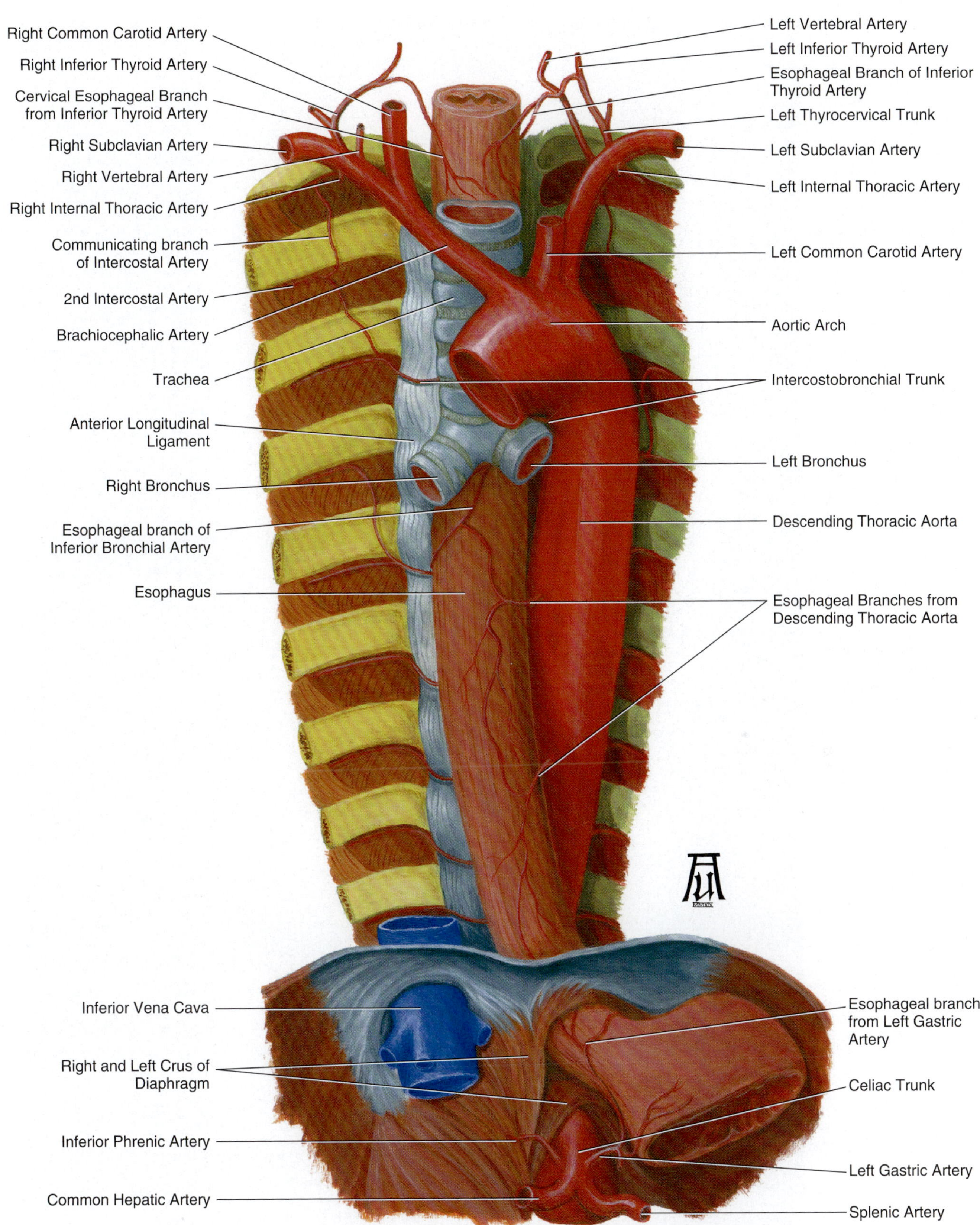

Figure 7.39. Diagram showing the arterial supply of the esophagus. Arteries from the descending thoracic aorta anastomose with branches from the inferior thyroid, inferior phrenic, bronchial, and left gastric arteries. Occasionally, esophageal arteries may arise from other adjacent vessels such as intercostal or phrenic arteries.

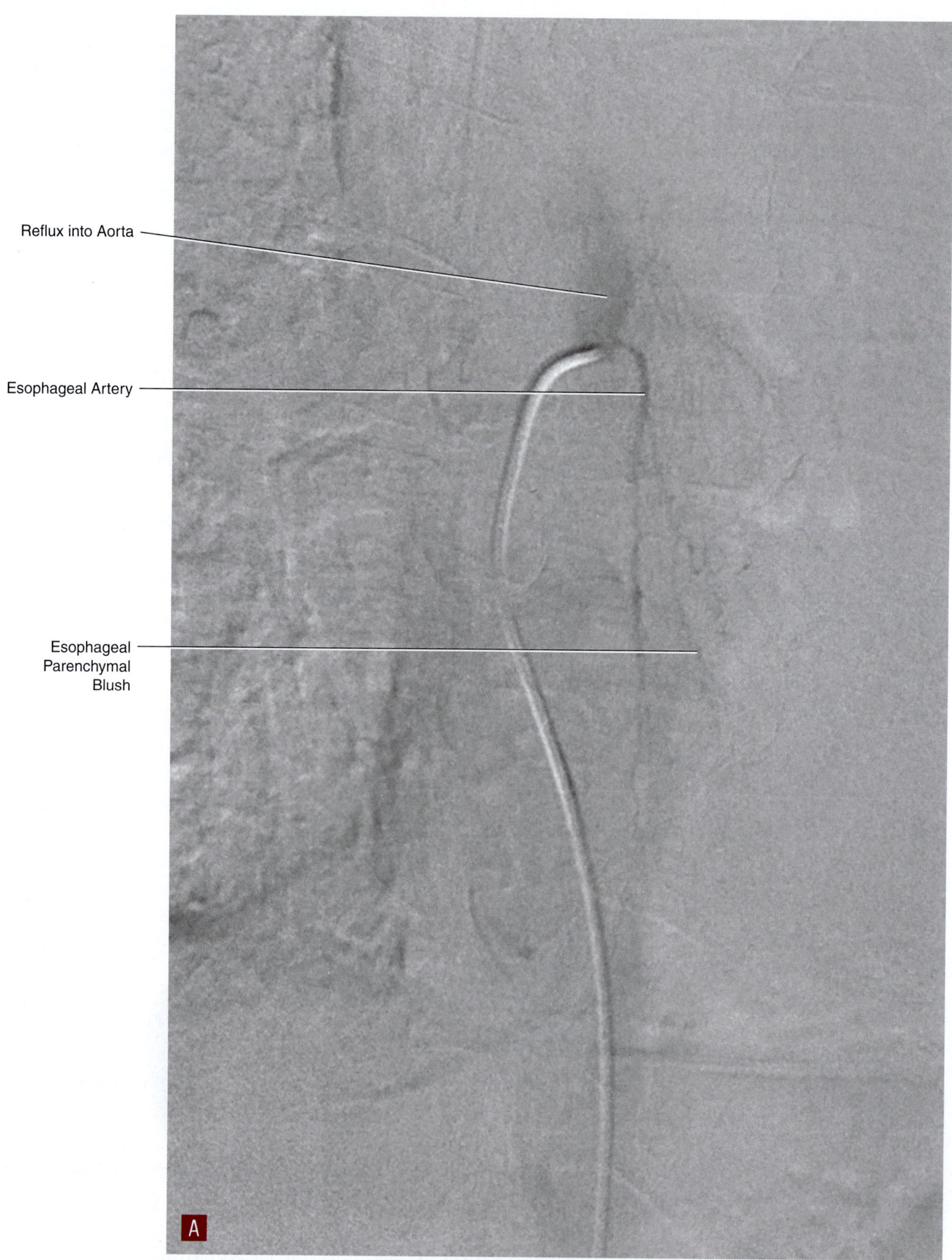

Figure 7.40. A, Selective angiogram of an esophageal branch directly from the aorta. B, Selective celiac angiogram showing a hypertrophied left gastric artery, with an esophageal branch supplying the gastroesophageal junction. C, Selective left fourth intercostal angiogram showing an esophageal branch supplying the thoracic mid portion of the esophagus. There is also a left bronchial artery, and a communicating branch with the fifth left intercostal artery.

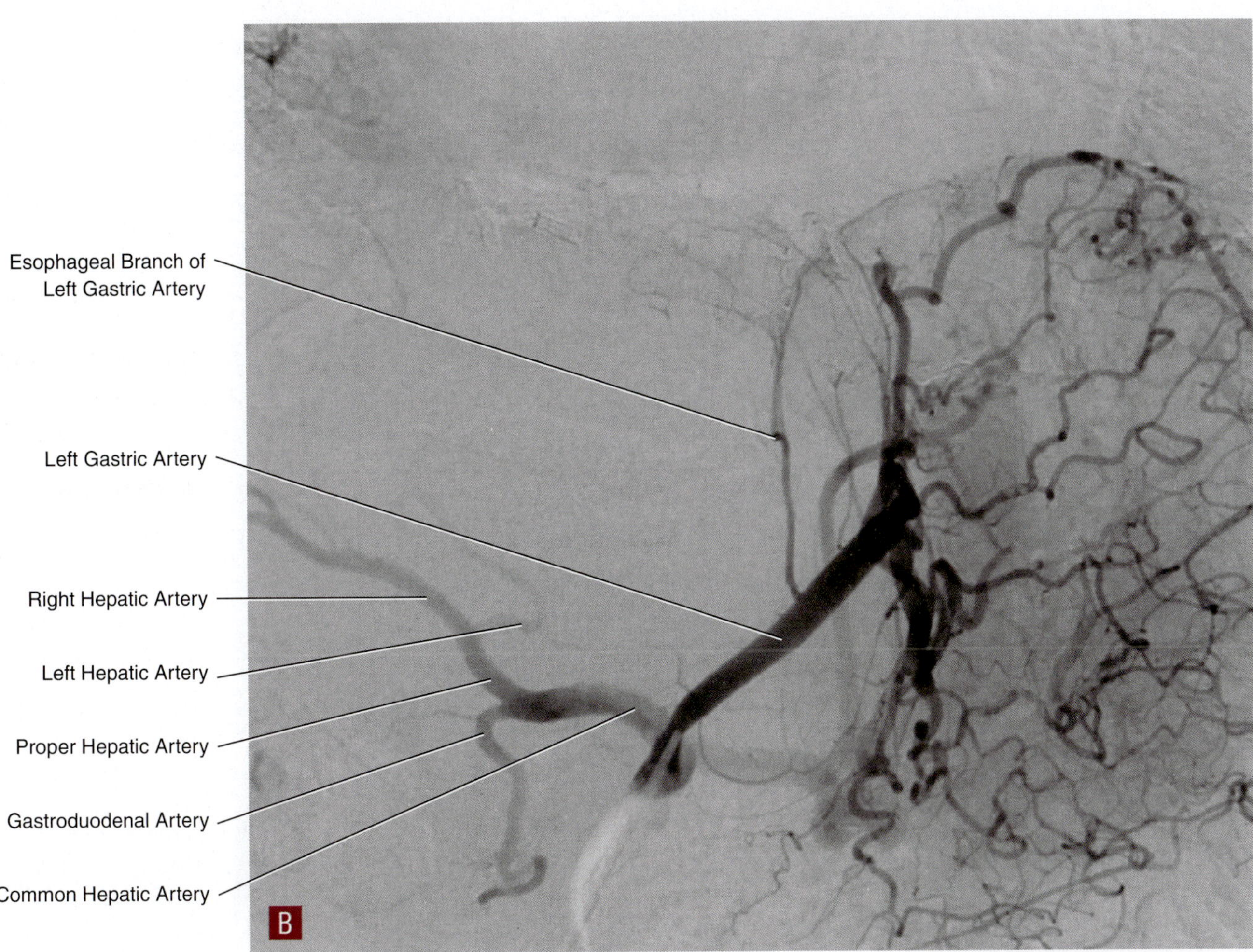

Figure 7.40. *Continued*

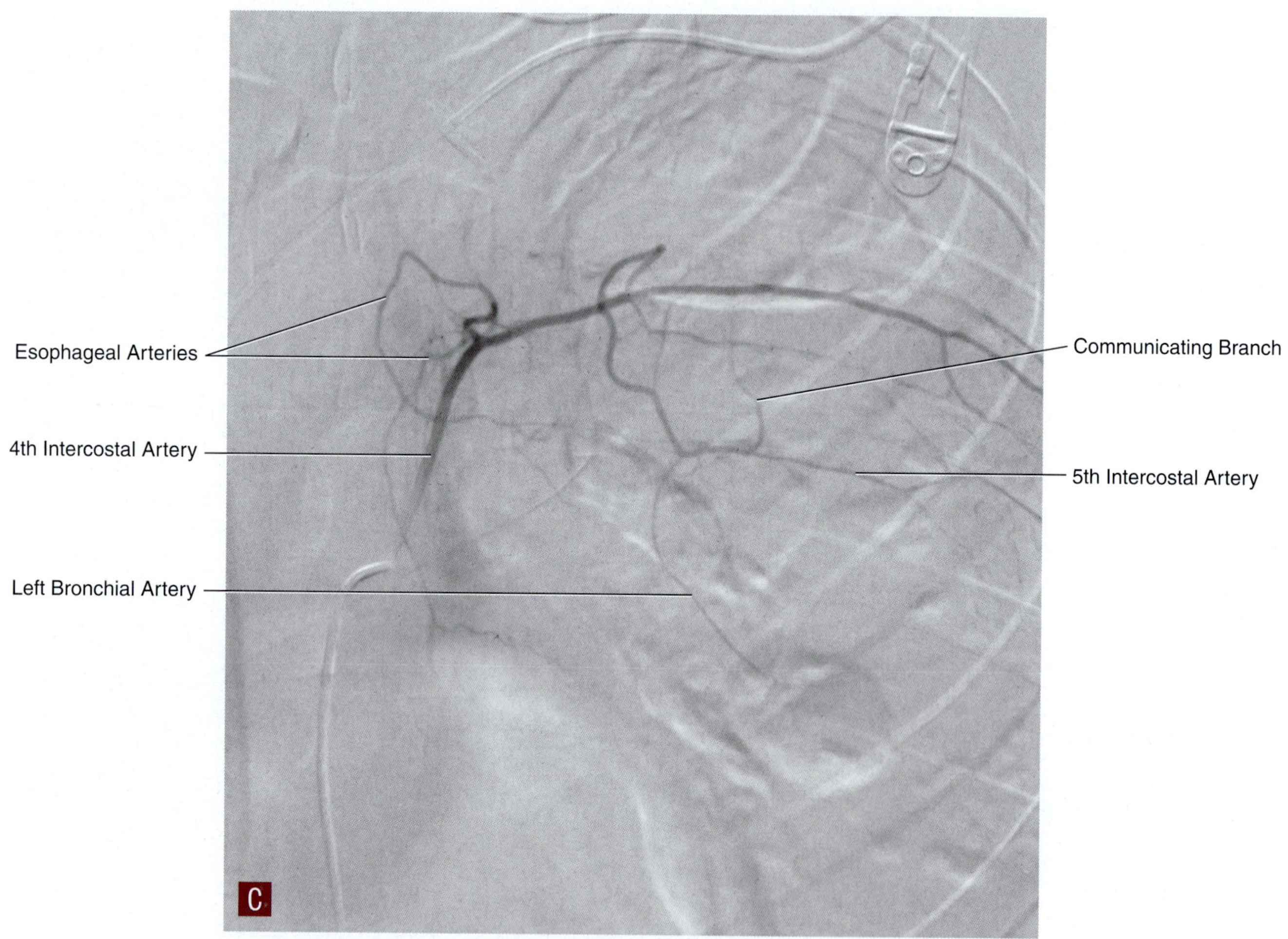

Figure 7.40. *Continued*

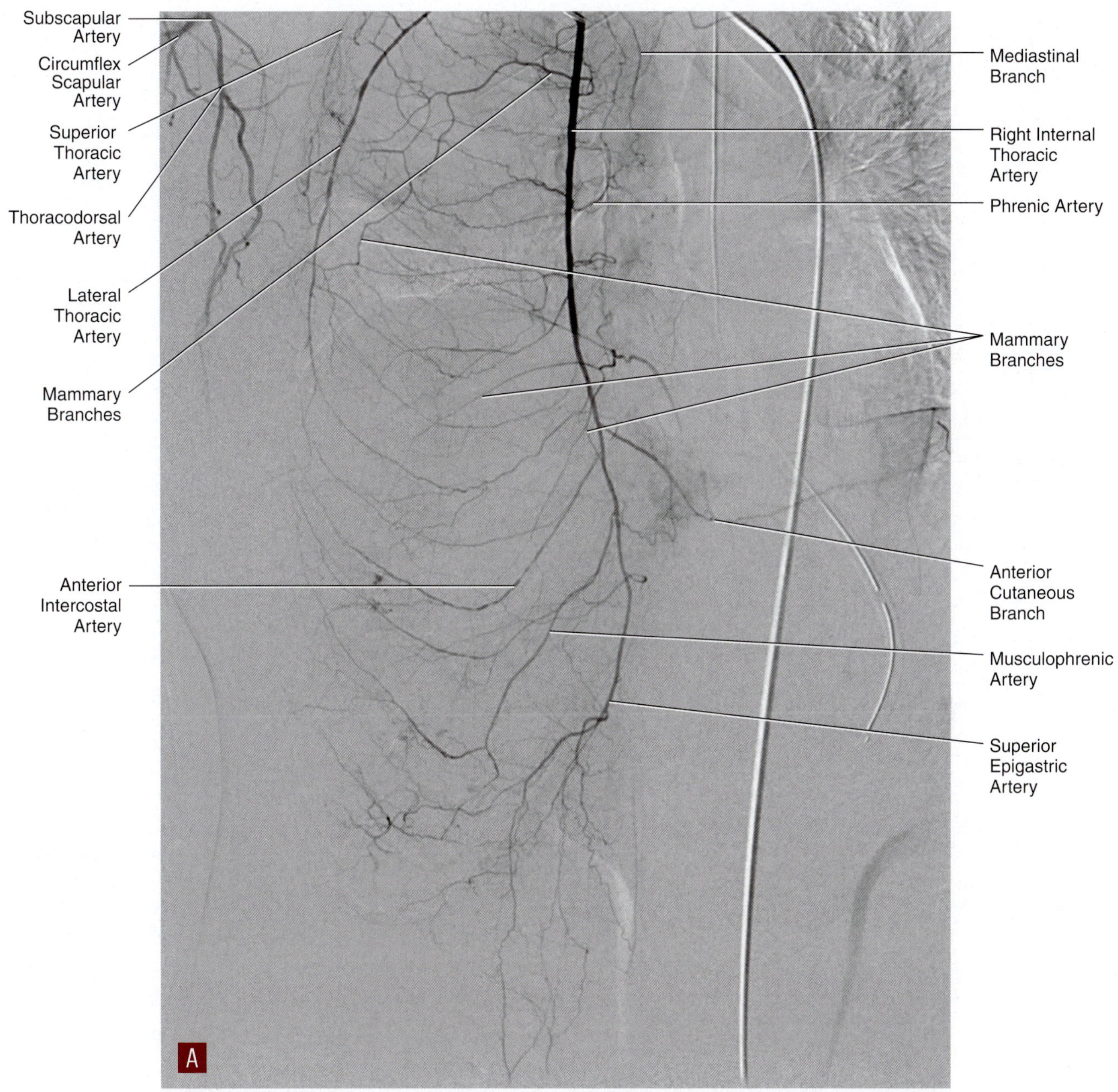

Figure 7.41. A, Selective angiogram of the right internal mammary artery, showing filling of the anterior intercostal arteries. The anterior intercostal arteries are much smaller than the posterior intercostal arteries. B, Selective angiogram of the left internal mammary artery.

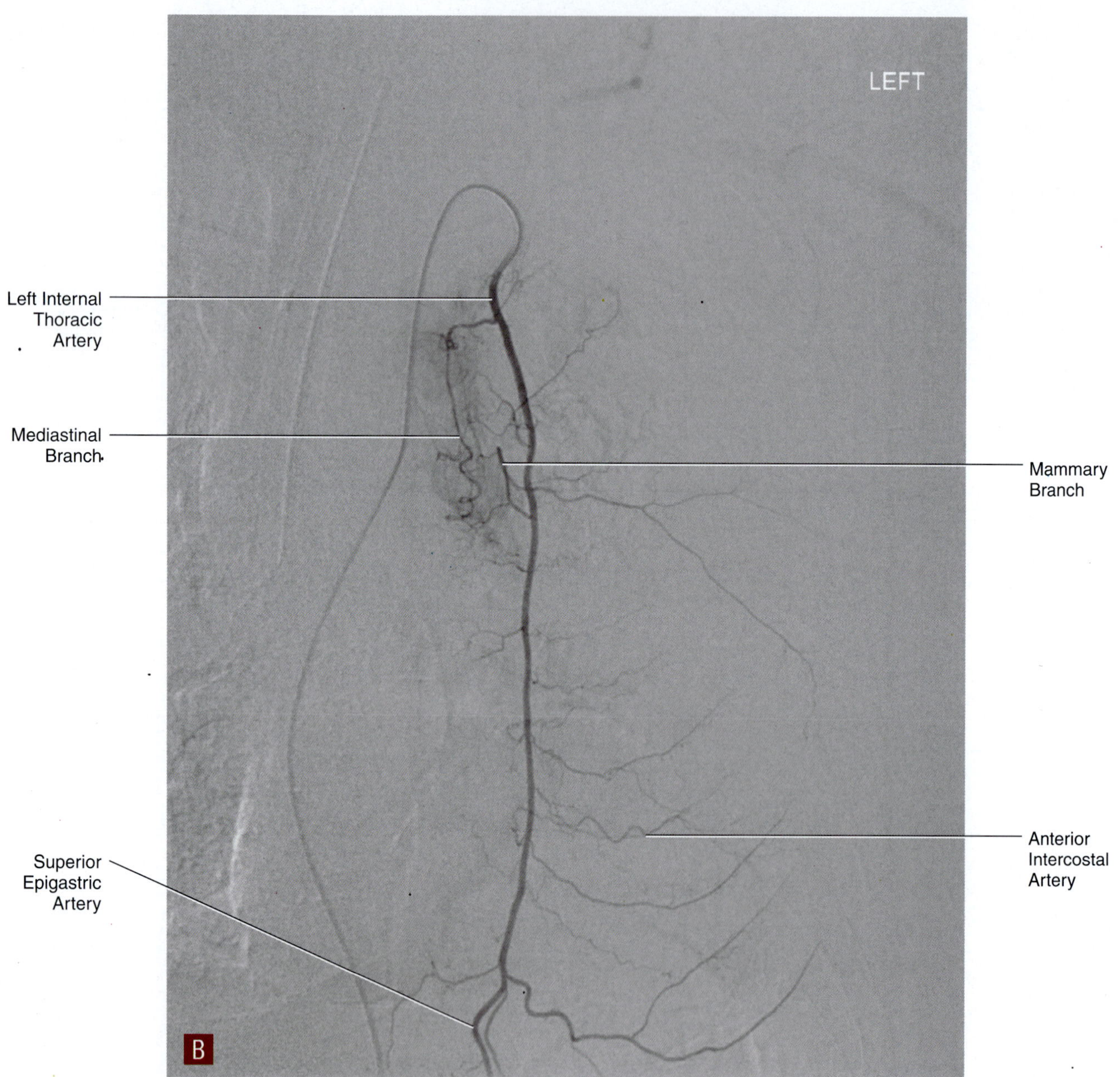

Figure 7.41. *Continued*

8

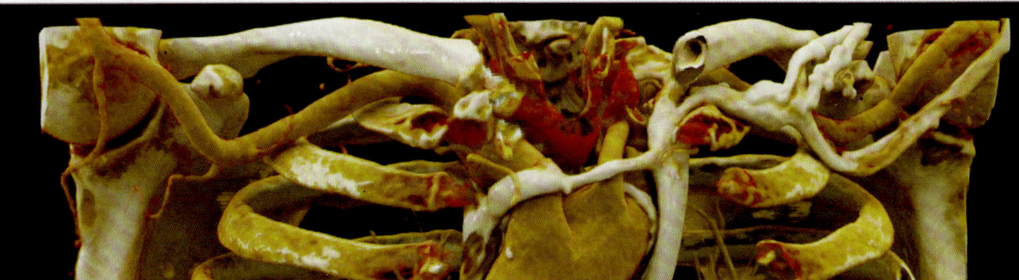

Veins of the Thorax

The brachiocephalic veins, also called the innominate veins, are large valveless veins at the upper thorax and represent united trunks of the internal jugular veins and subclavian veins (Figs. 8.1-8.6). The right brachiocephalic vein is approximately 2.5 cm long, following an almost vertical inferior direction anterior to the right brachiocephalic trunk and joining the left brachiocephalic vein, thereby forming the superior vena cava. The tributaries are the right vertebral, internal thoracic, inferior thyroid, and occasionally the first right intercostal veins (Fig. 8.7).

The left brachiocephalic vein is approximately 6 cm long, following an oblique path to the right direction to join the right brachiocephalic vein to form the superior vena cava. It is positioned anteriorly to the left subclavian and common carotid arteries. Tributaries are the left vertebral, internal thoracic, inferior thyroid, superior intercostal, thymic vein, and pericardiophrenic veins. Variations of the brachiocephalic veins include entering the right atrium separately and the configuration of a persistent left vena cava, which occurs in about 0.5% of the population (Fig. 8.8).

Brachiocephalic Veins

Internal Thoracic Veins (Mammary) (Fig. 8.9)

The internal thoracic veins are venae comitans to the internal thoracic arteries, ending in the corresponding brachiocephalic veins. Tributaries are the intercostal veins and pericardiophrenic veins.

Inferior Thyroid Veins (Fig. 8.10)

The inferior thyroid veins originate in the glandular venous plexus, having connections with the middle and superior thyroid veins. There is a pretracheal venous plexus, from which the left inferior vein descends to enter the left brachiocephalic vein, and the right inferior thyroid vein crosses the neck to open in the right brachiocephalic vein. The jugular arch, which connects the anterior jugular veins, also may receive veins from the thyroid glandular venous plexus (Figs. 8.14 and 8.15).

Superior Vena Cava (Figs. 8.11 and 8.14)

The superior vena cava is the main vein for venous drainage for the superior aspect of the body. It is around 7 cm in length and is formed by the confluence of the brachiocephalic veins. It has no valves and ends in the right atrium. The superior vena cava is in contact with the right lung, pleura, trachea, right pulmonary hilum, and aorta. Tributaries are the azygos vein and small veins from the mediastinum.

Pericardiophrenic Vein (Fig. 8.12)

The pericardiophrenic veins are the main venous drainage channel for the diaphragm and the pericardium. These veins are in contact with the pericardium and pleura.

Thymic Veins (Figs. 8.13 and 8.14)

The thymic veins are small in adults, unless there is some enlargement of the thymus gland, and typically drain into the left brachiocephalic vein.

Left Superior Intercostal Vein (Figs. 8.16 and 8.17)

The left superior intercostal vein drains the second, third, and also the fourth left posterior intercostal veins, directly to the left brachiocephalic vein. It may communicate with the accessory hemiazygos vein. In less than 5% of chest roentgrams, the left superior intercostal vein may form a contour deformity of the left lateral aspect of the aortic arch known as an "aortic nipple," which should be less than 4.5 mm in diameter (Fig. 8.17).

Azygos Vein

The azygos vein is formed by the confluence of the ascending lumbar veins, subcostal veins, and lumbar azygos. It ascends in the posterior mediastinum up to the level of the fourth vertebra, where it arches anteriorly above the right pulmonary hilum, ending in the superior vena cava. Tributaries are the posterior intercostal veins, the hemiazygos, the accessory hemiazygos veins, and the esophageal, mediastinal, and pericardial veins. The right bronchial veins also drain to the azygos vein, near the hilum. When present, the trunk formed by the subcostal and ascending lumbar veins is a major tributary of the azygos vein. The azygos vein starts laterally to the vertebral bodies but turns anterior to the thoracic spine as it approaches the vena cava (Figs. 8.16, 8.18-8.20).

Hemiazygos Vein

The hemiazygos vein starts on the left side, ascending anteriorly to the spine, crossing the column, and reaching the azygos vein. Tributaries are the lower three posterior intercostal veins, a common trunk formed by the left ascending lumbar vein, and the subcostal vein (Figs. 8.16-8.20).

Accessory Hemiazygos Vein

The accessory hemiazygos vein results from the confluence of several posterior intercostal veins, descending laterally to the thoracic spine, reaching the azygos vein. It may, however, join the hemiazygos vein (Figs. 8.16 and 8.18).

Posterior Intercostal Veins

There are 11 pairs of posterior intercostal veins. They are companions of the posterior intercostal arteries, running along the subcostal groove. On the right, the second, third, and fourth posterior intercostal veins form the right superior intercostal vein (Figs. 8.16 and 8.21).

There are anterior intercostal veins, which are small tributaries of the internal thoracic and musculophrenic veins.

Bronchial veins are also found on each side, draining blood from larger hilar structures and the bronchial tree. The right bronchial vein joins the azygos, and the left joins the left superior intercostal or hemiazygos vein.

Esophageal Veins

The esophageal veins run along the esophagus and drain to the azygos vein, and the more distal veins drain into the portal venous system through the left gastric vein (Fig. 8.22).

Veins of the Vertebral Spine (See Chapter 6)

There is a large and complex venous plexus around the vertebral column. This is also called Batson venous plexus. This plexus is internal and external to the spinal canal (Chapter 6, Fig. 6.1; Chapter 20, Fig. 20.33).

External Venous Plexuses

Anterior external venous plexus
Posterior external venous plexus
Internal vertebral venous plexus
Anterior internal venous plexus
Posterior internal venous plexus
Basivertebral veins
Intervertebral veins
Veins of the spinal cord

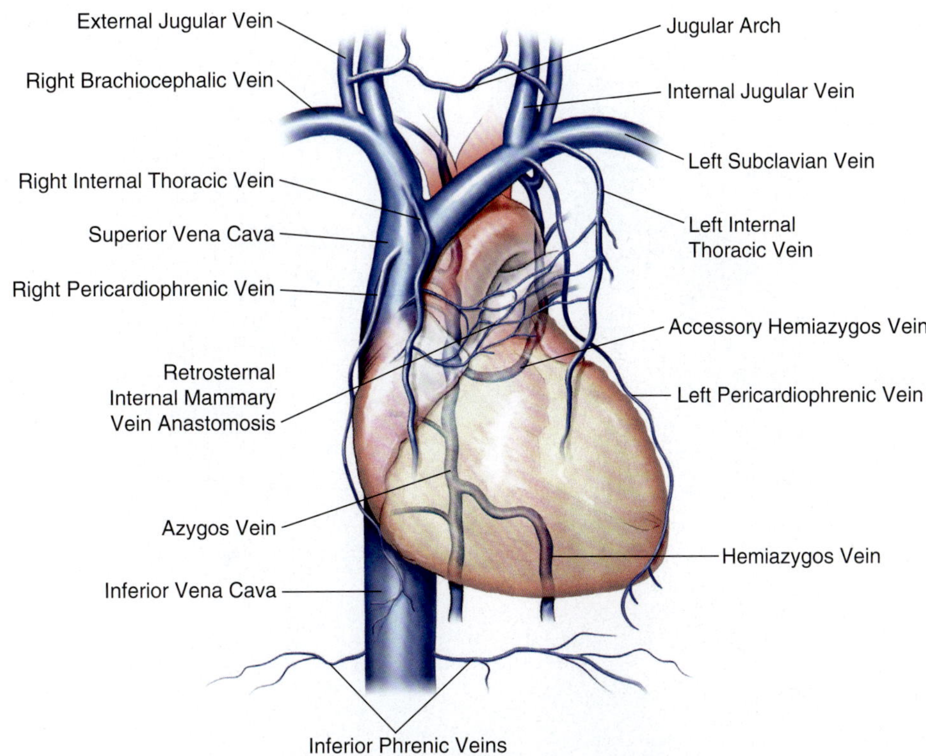

Figure 8.1. Anterior view of the thoracic veins. The right internal thoracic vein terminates more proximally on its brachiocephalic vein than does the left. The left pericardiophrenic vein terminates on the left brachiocephalic vein; it may also terminate on the internal thoracic vein or left superior intercostal vein. Note that the superior vena cava (SVC) is encased by pericardium in which can extend up to 4 cm cranially from the SVC-right atrium junction.

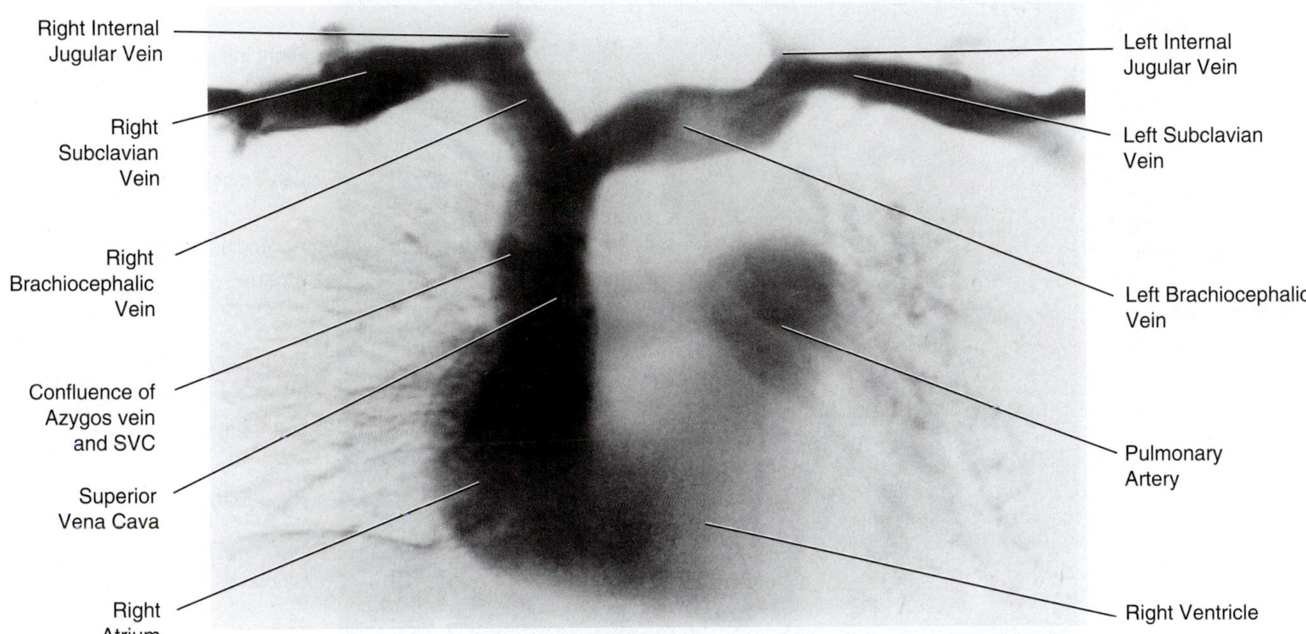

Figure 8.2. Anterior view of a venogram of the main thoracic veins. Note the vertical course of the right brachiocephalic vein and the horizontal course of the left brachiocephalic vein.

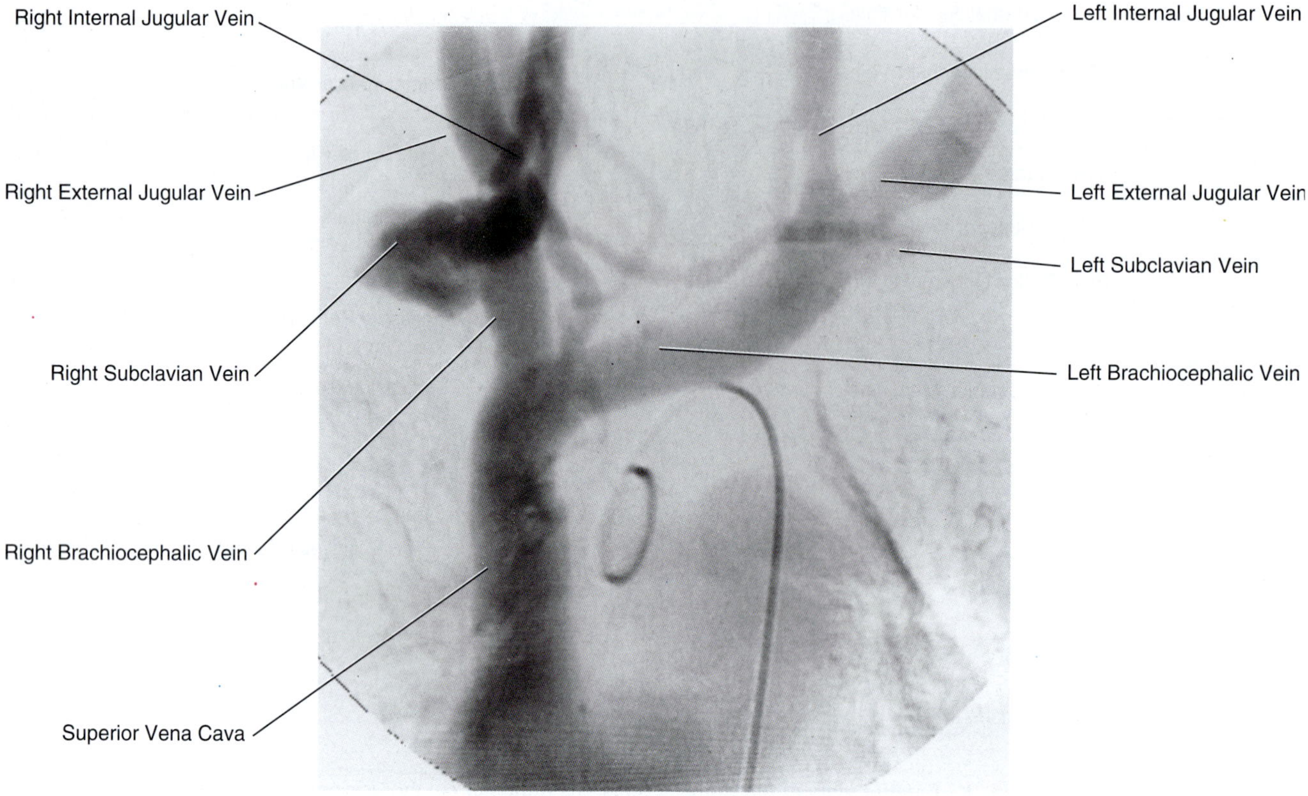

Right Internal Jugular Vein
Right External Jugular Vein
Right Subclavian Vein
Right Brachiocephalic Vein
Superior Vena Cava
Left Internal Jugular Vein
Left External Jugular Vein
Left Subclavian Vein
Left Brachiocephalic Vein

Figure 8.3. Anterior view of a venogram of the main thoracic veins showing the superior vena cava and some of the tributaries of the brachiocephalic veins.

Right Cephalic Vein
Right Subclavian Vein
Right Brachiocephalic Vein
Left Internal Jugular Vein
Right Internal Jugular Vein
Left Brachiocephalic Vein
Ascending Aorta
Superior Vena Cava
Pulmonary Artery
Left Ventricle
Right Atrium
Stomach
Portal Vein
A

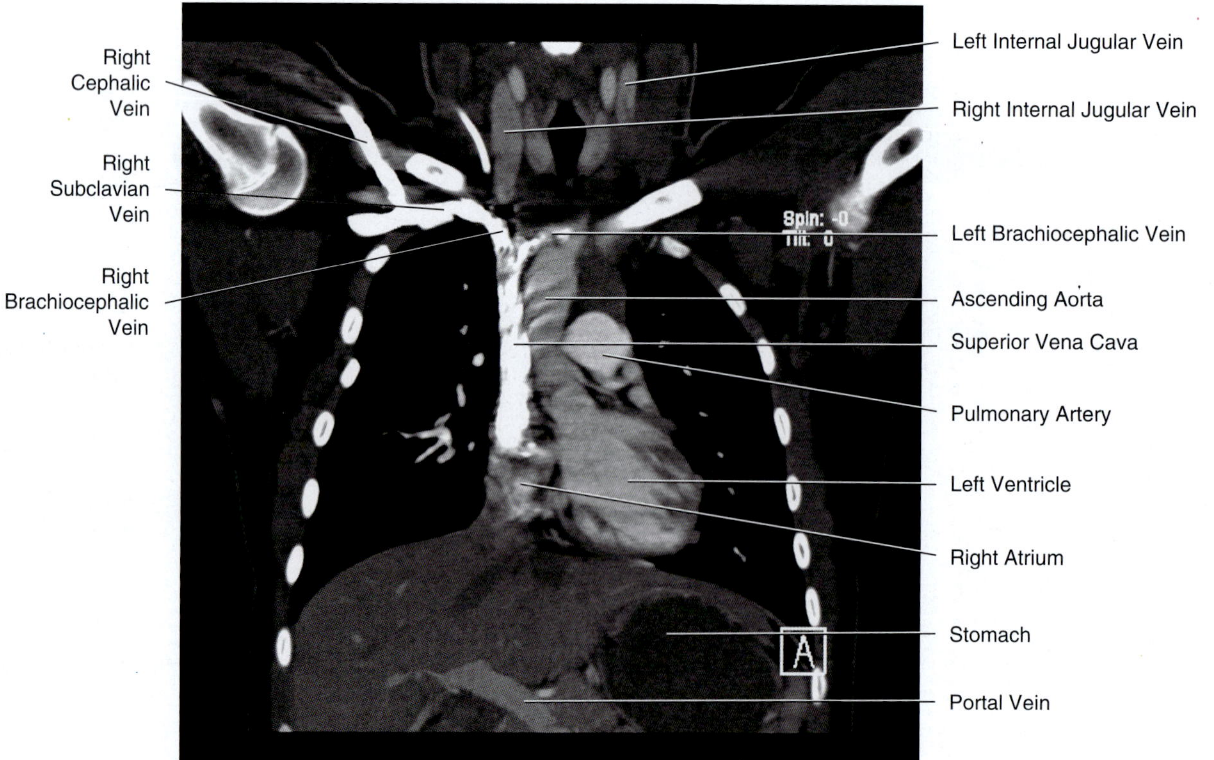

Figure 8.4. Maximum intensity projection (MIP) reconstruction in frontal view computerized tomography of the chest with a venous phase, showing the superior vena cava and the main thoracic veins.

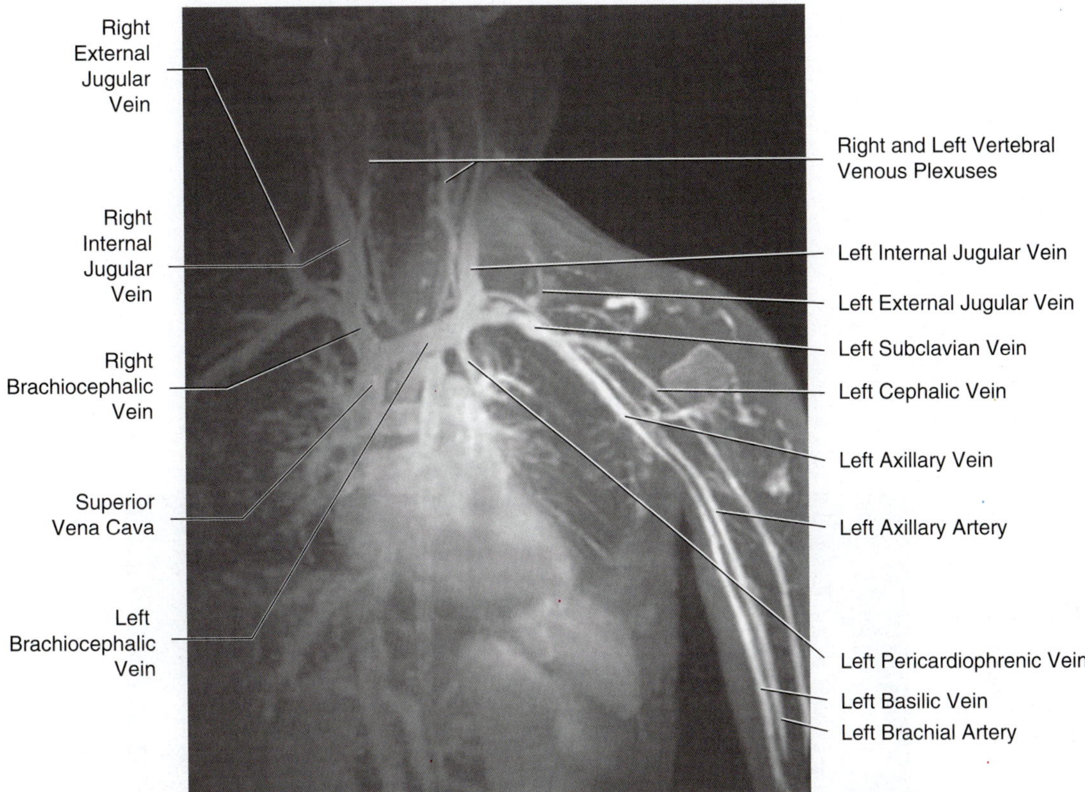

Figure 8.5. Magnetic resonance angiography (MRA) with two-dimensional (2D) reconstruction of the chest in a venous phase, showing the superior vena cava and the major veins of the chest and neck. Note the presence of the vertebral venous plexus.

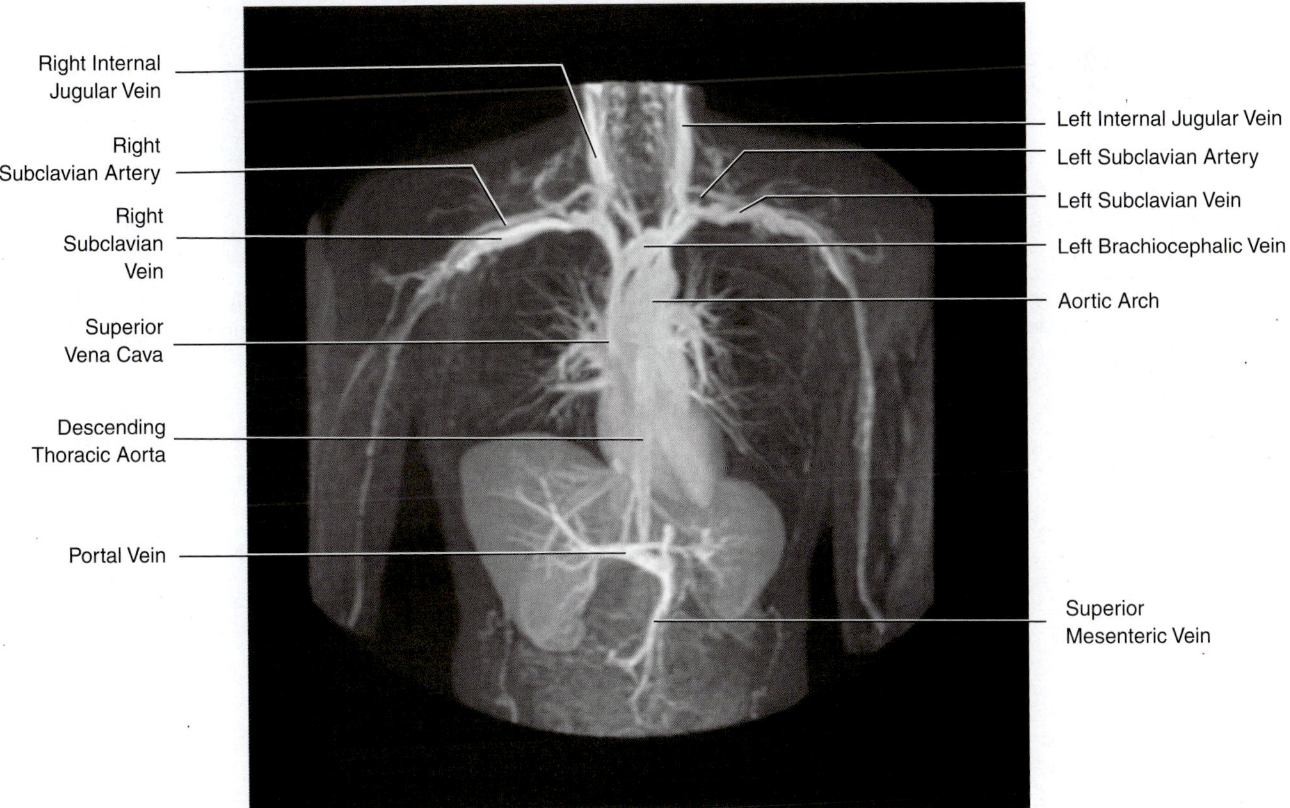

Figure 8.6. Magnetic resonance angiography (MRA) with 2D reconstruction of the chest in a venous phase, showing the superior vena cava and the arteries still opacified. Note the filling of the portal vein and hepatic veins.

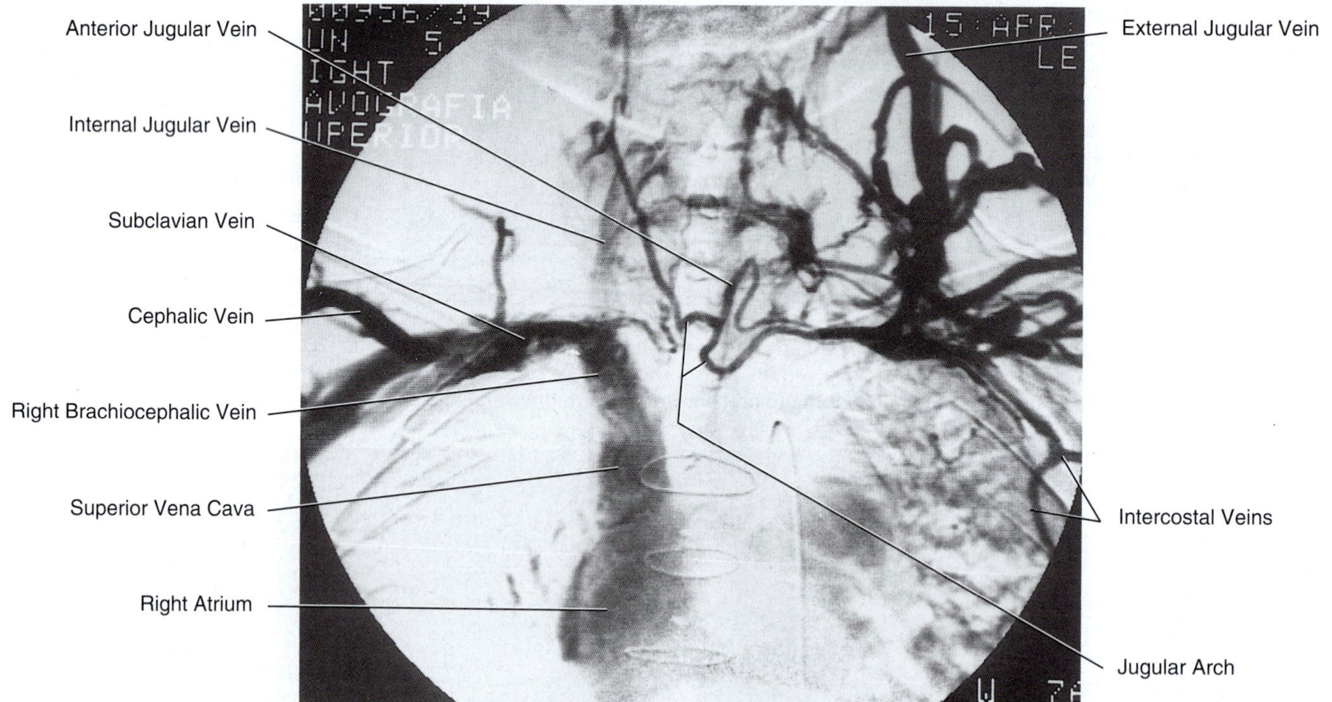

Figure 8.7. Anterior view of a venogram of the main thoracic veins. Owing to occlusion of the left brachiocephalic vein, there is marked development of collateral circulation around the neck and upper thorax.

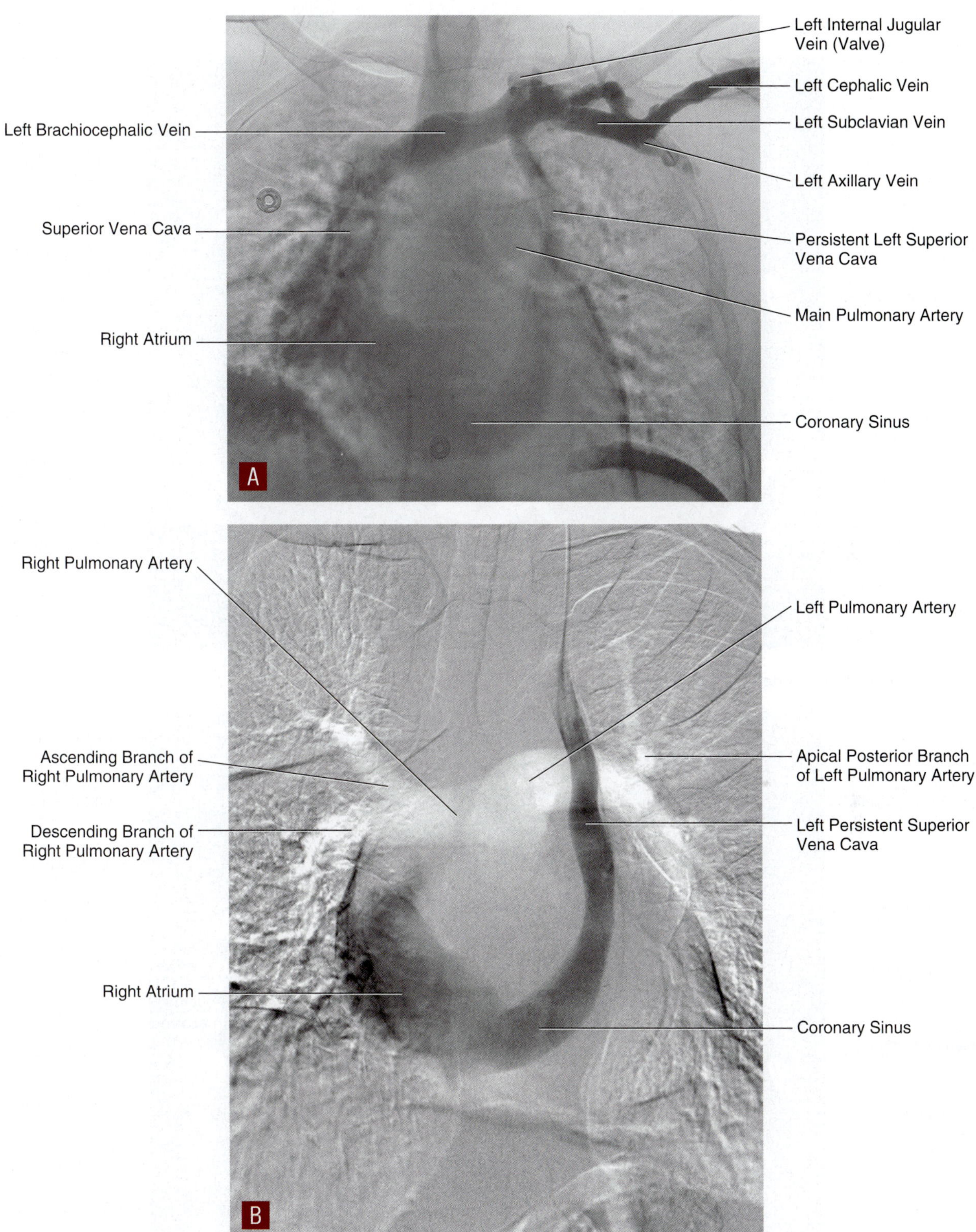

Figure 8.8. **A**, Left upper extremity venogram showing filling of the central veins through the cephalic vein with a persistent left superior vena cava (SVC) which drains into the right atrium through the coronary sinus. **B**, Venogram of a persistent left SVC during catheter placement. The coronary sinus is seen with filling of the right atrium and pulmonary arteries. **C**, Axial contrast enhanced CT showing a persistent left SVC immediately anterior to the left pulmonary artery. **D**, Coronal contrast enhanced CT showing a persistent left SVC. **E**, Volume rendered 3D reconstruction CT venogram showing the persistent left SVC coursing posterior to the main pulmonary artery, looping lateral to the aorta and left atrium. **F**, Anterior view of the volume rendered 3D CT venogram reconstruction. **G** and **H**, Cinematic volume rendered reconstruction in anterior and anterolateral views of a different patient with persistent left SVC.

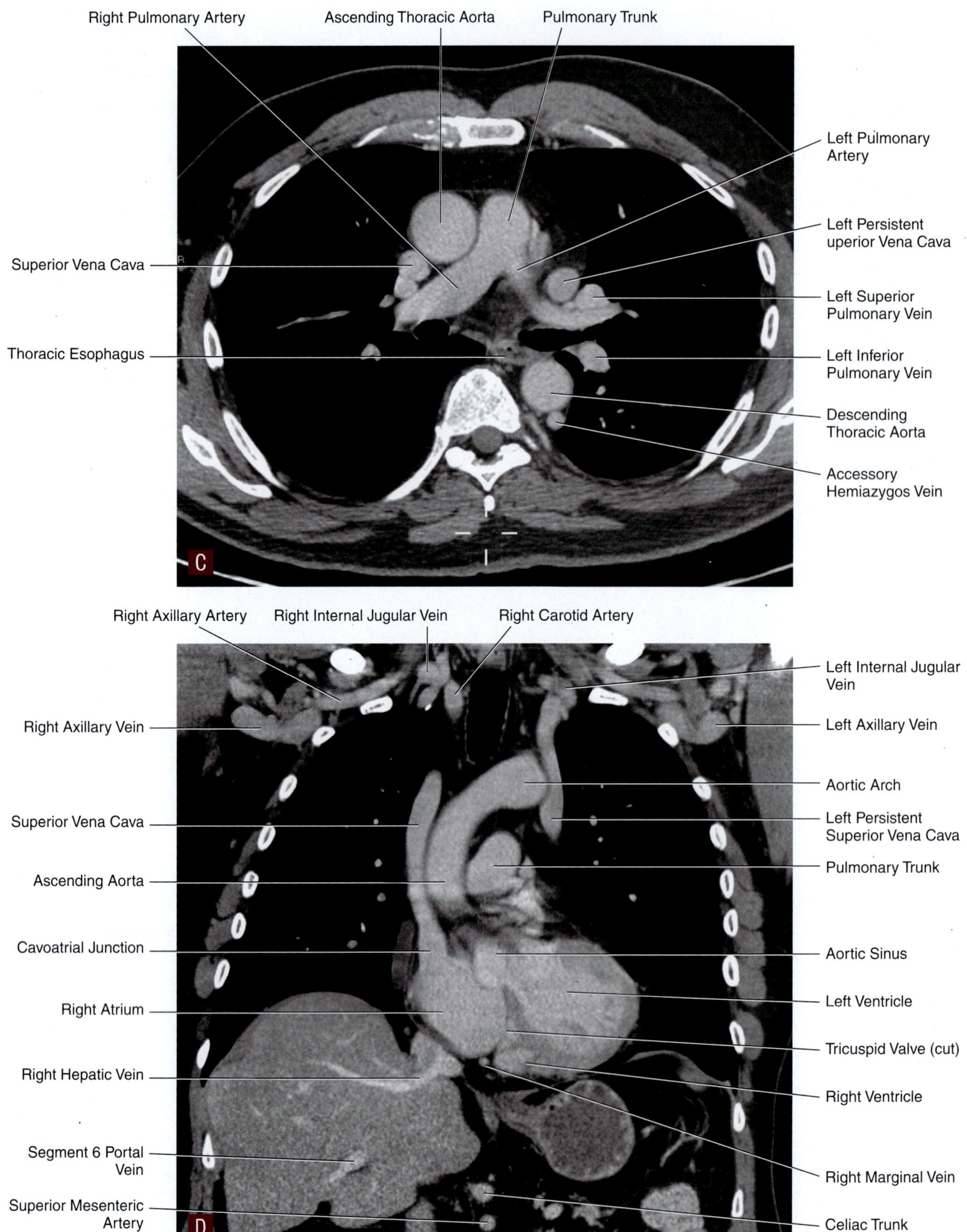

Figure 8.8. *Continued*

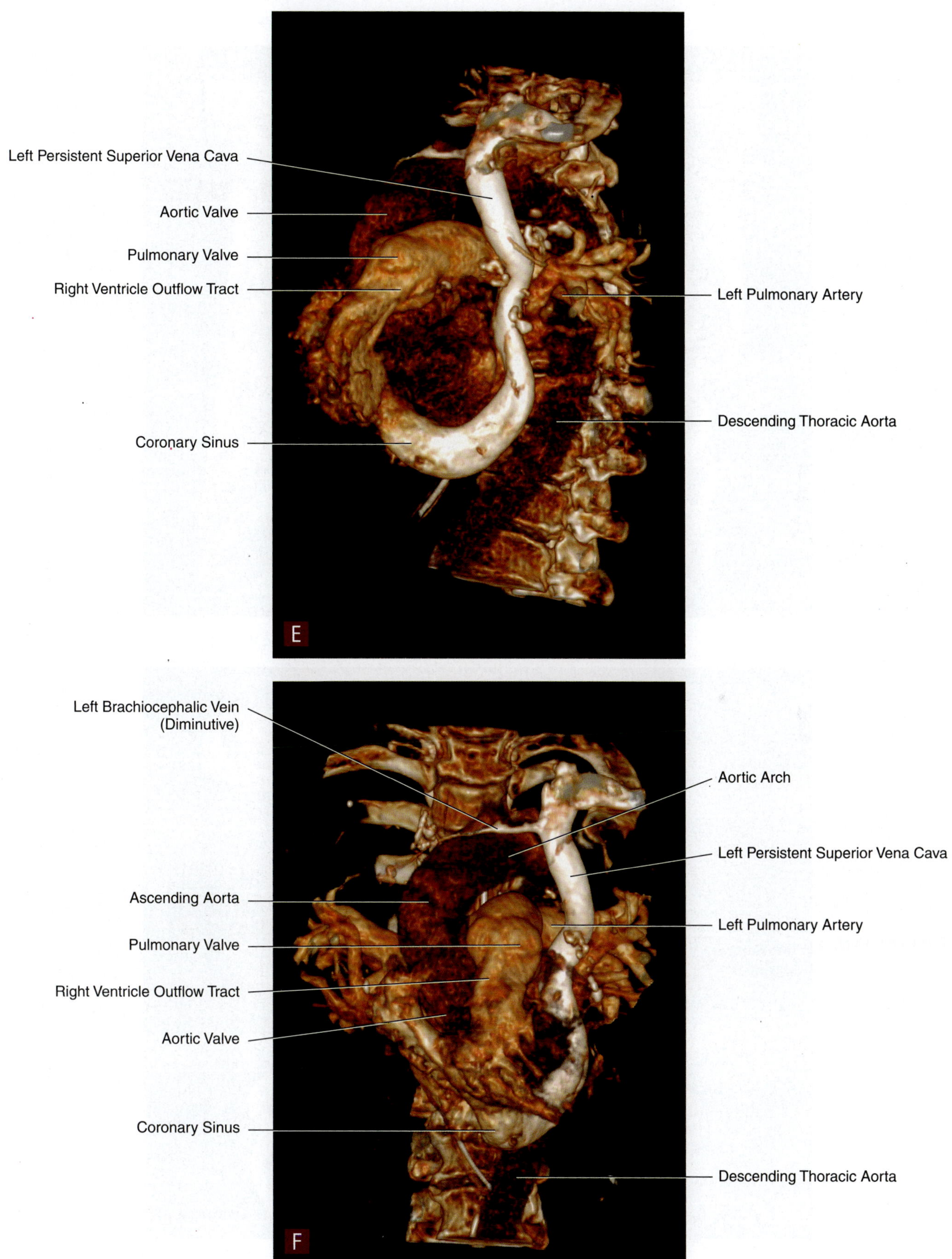

Figure 8.8. *Continued*

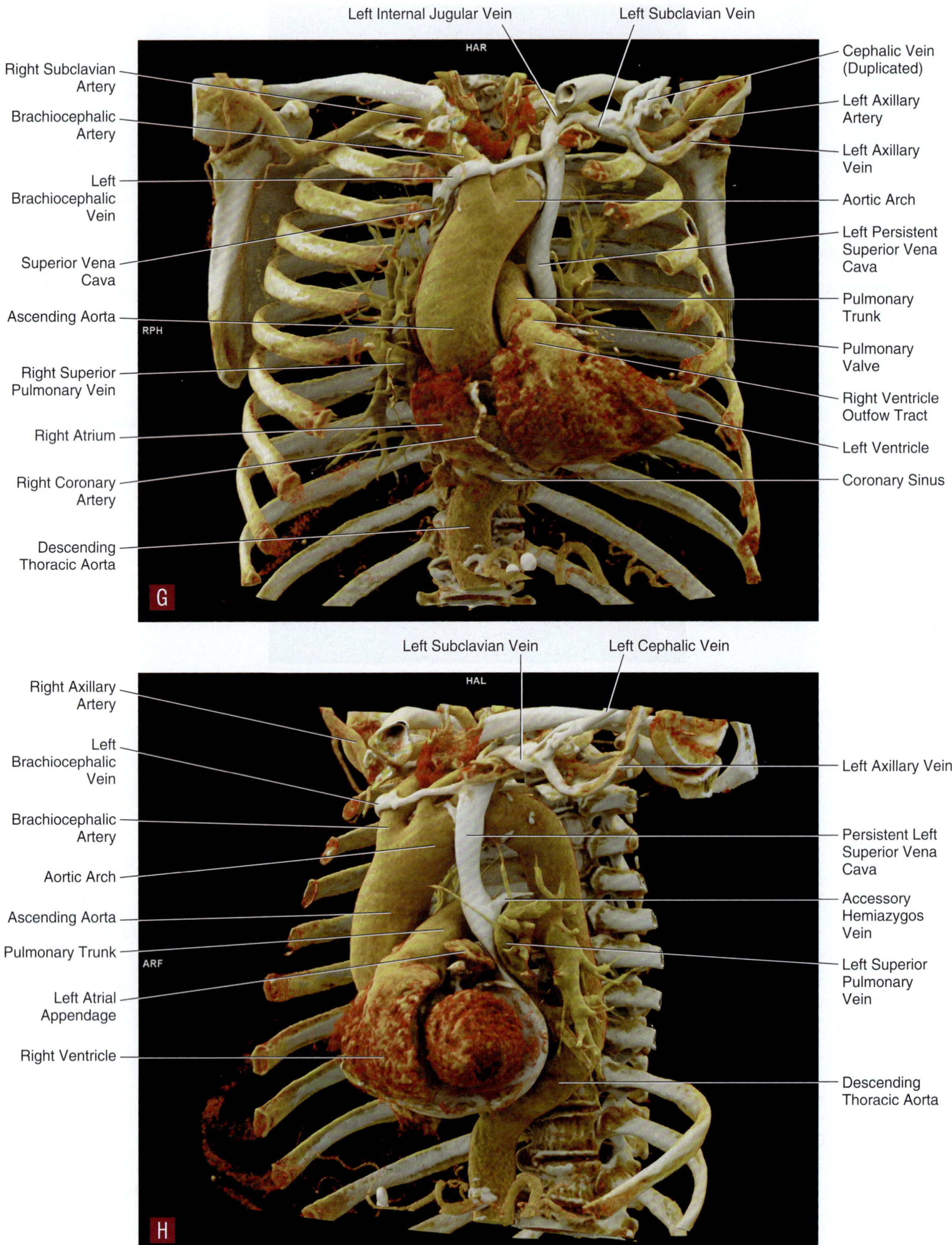

Figure 8.8. *Continued*

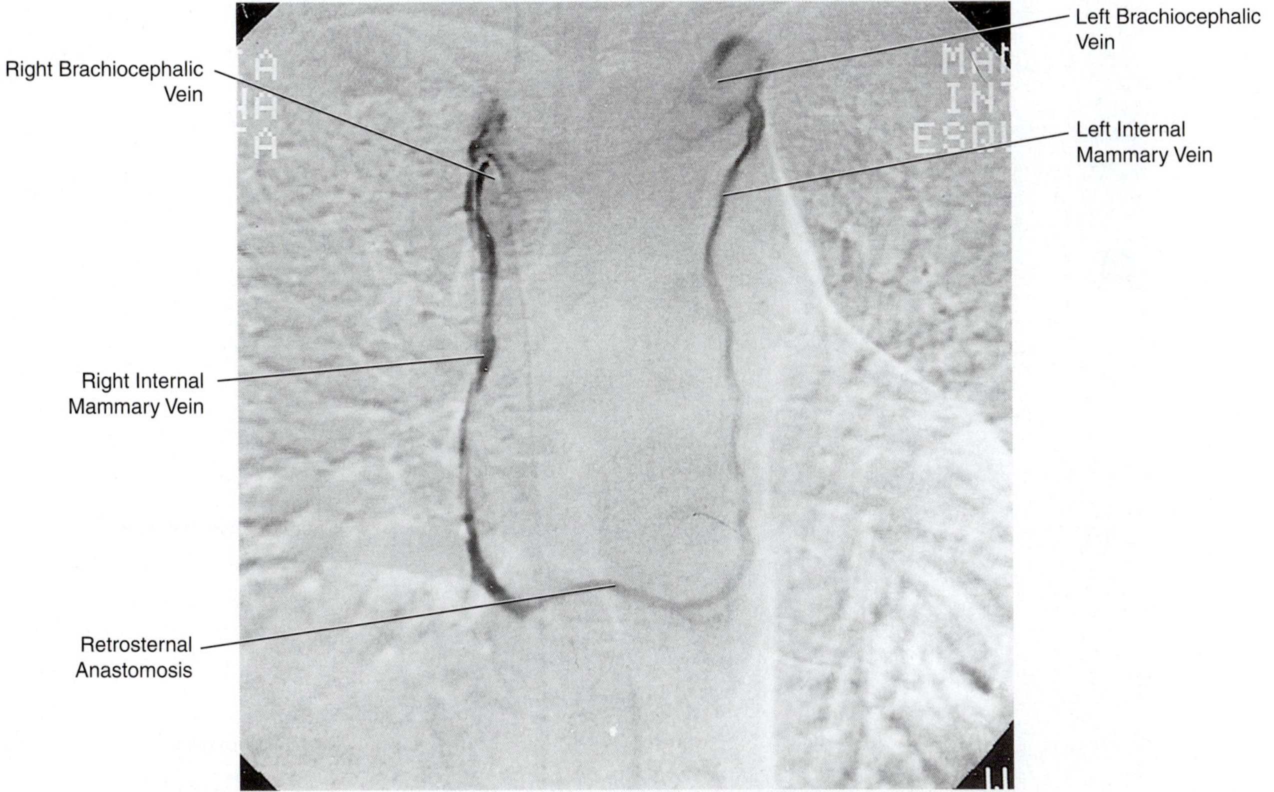

Figure 8.9. Anterior view of a venogram with selective injection at the right internal thoracic vein with contralateral filling of the left internal thoracic vein (internal mammary vein). Note the retrosternal anastomosis.

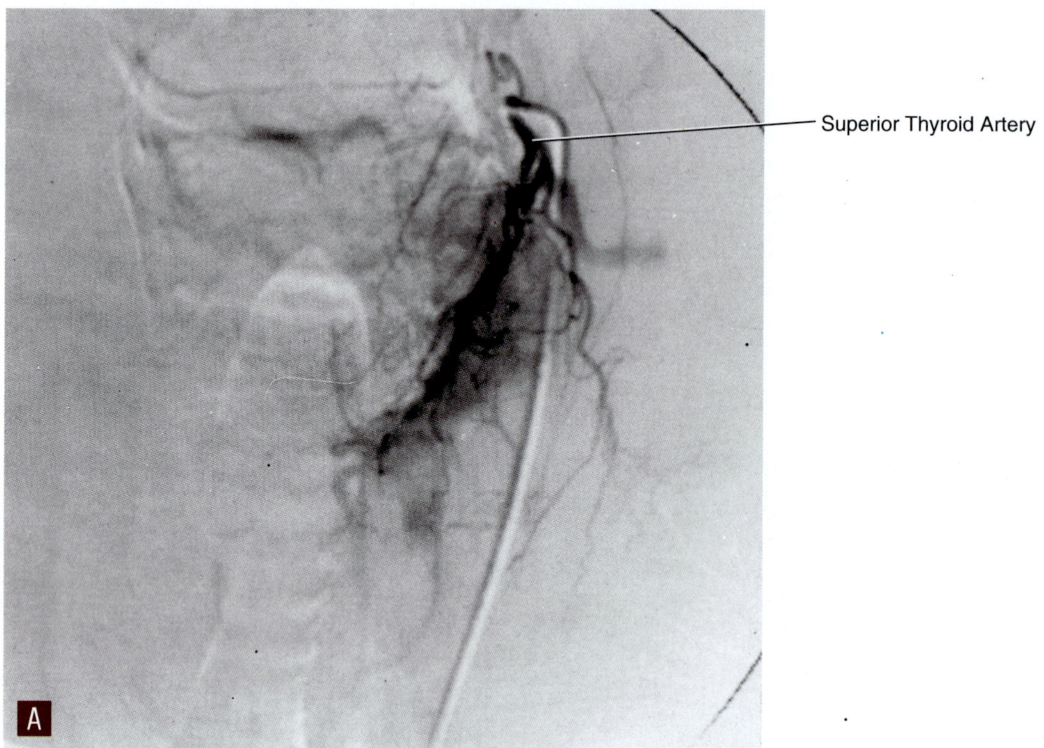

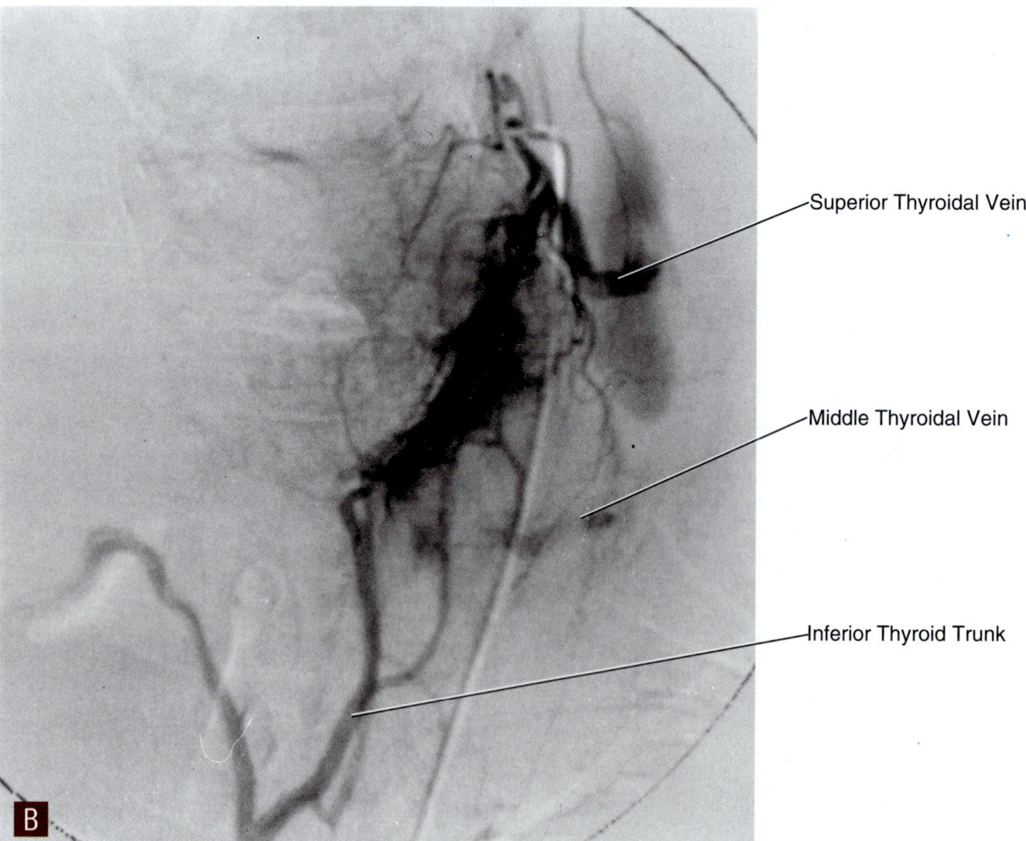

Figure 8.10. **A**, Left superior thyroid artery injection showing early filling of the upper and lower drainage veins. **B**, Late phase of the angiogram showing the thyroid venous drainage. **C**, Right-side arterial injection showing the venous drainage. **D**, Selective venogram of the inferior thyroid vein showing the thyroid venous plexus.

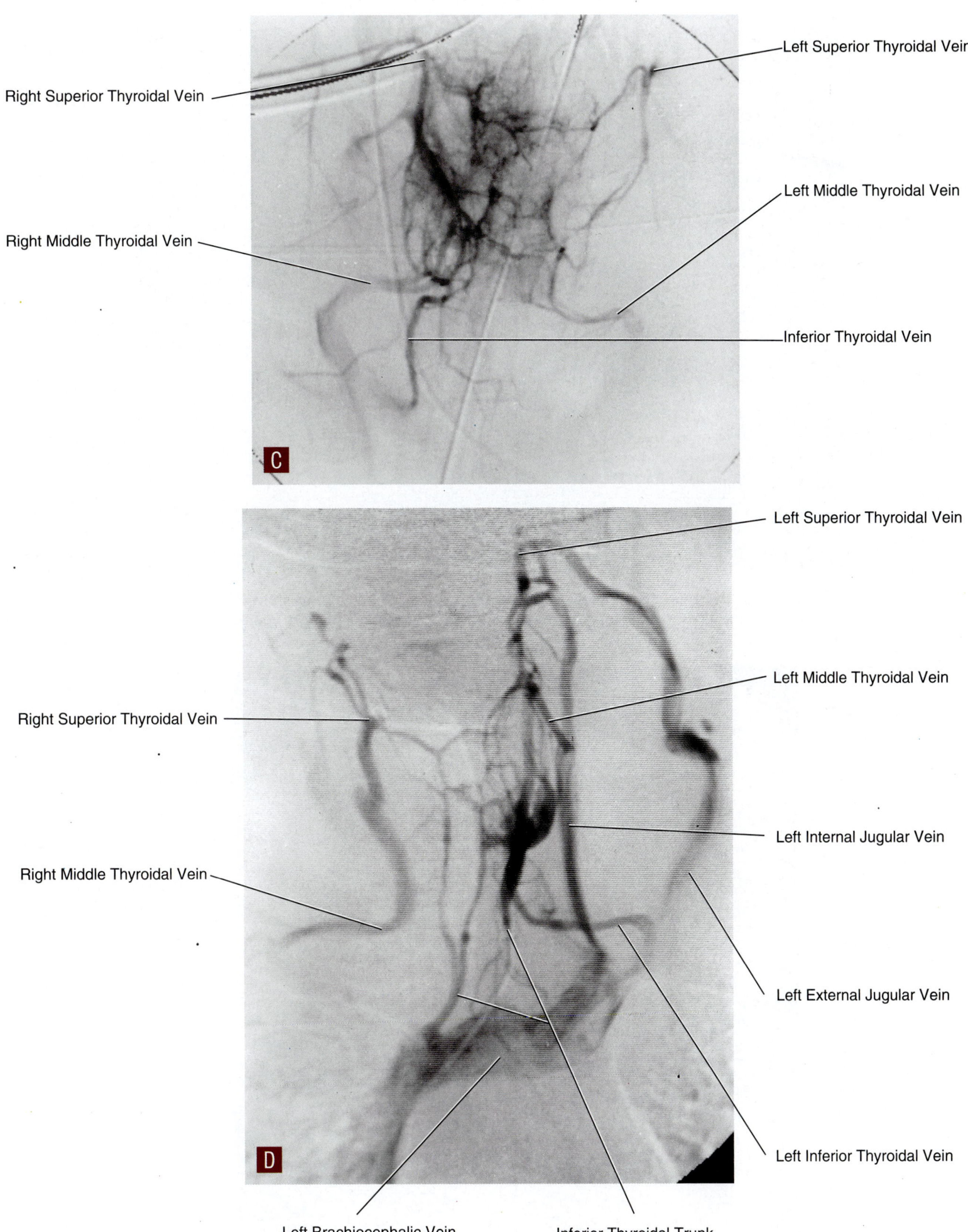

Figure 8.10. *Continued*

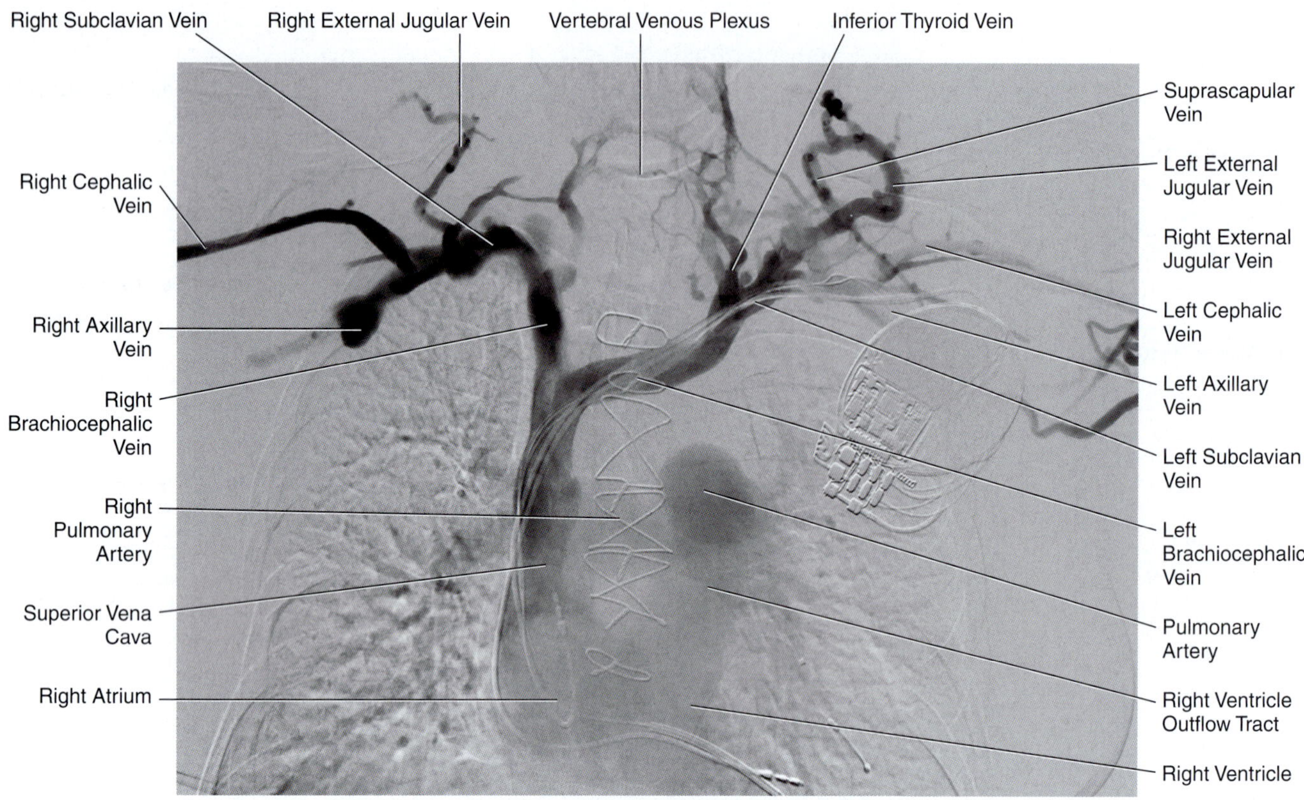

Figure 8.11. Anterior view of a venogram of the great thoracic veins showing the brachiocephalic veins, the superior vena cava, and the right atrium and right ventricle.

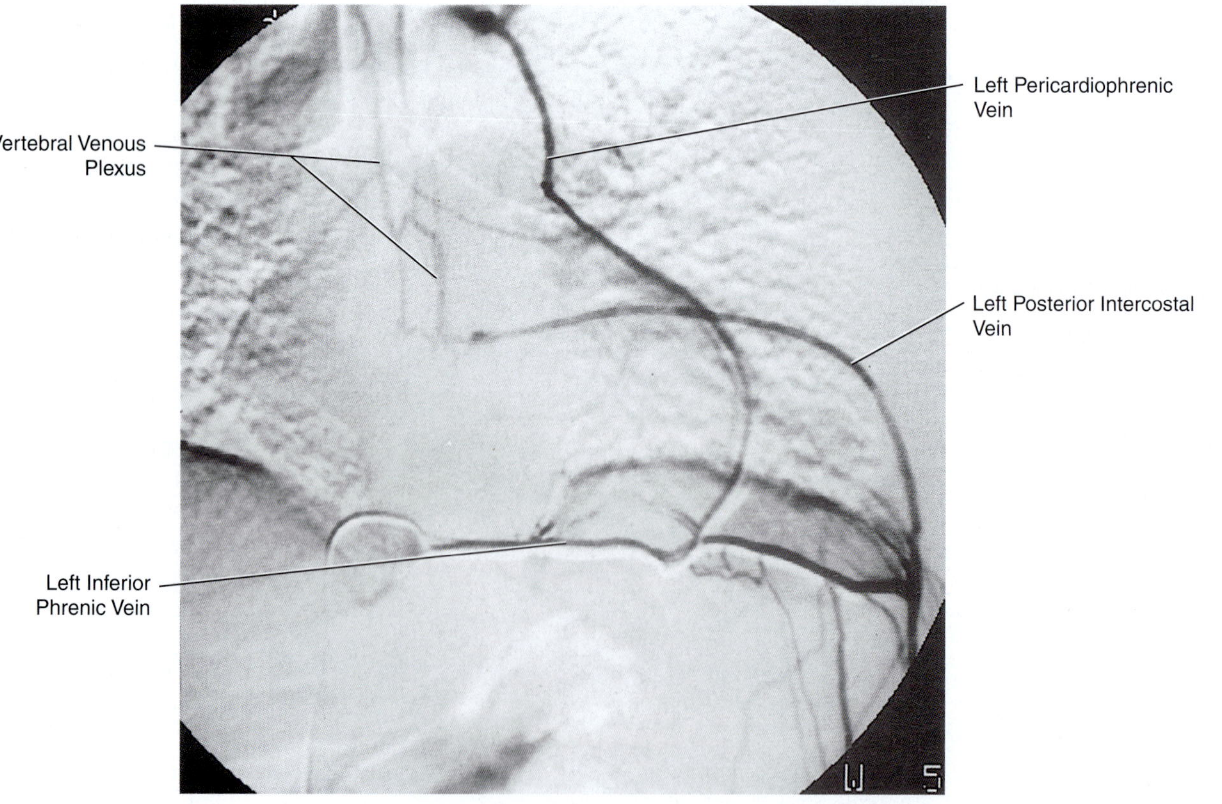

Figure 8.12. Anterior view of a venogram showing the pericardiophrenic vein, one intercostal vein, and the connections with the inferior phrenic vein catheterized from the inferior vena cava. Note the connections with the perivertebral venous plexus.

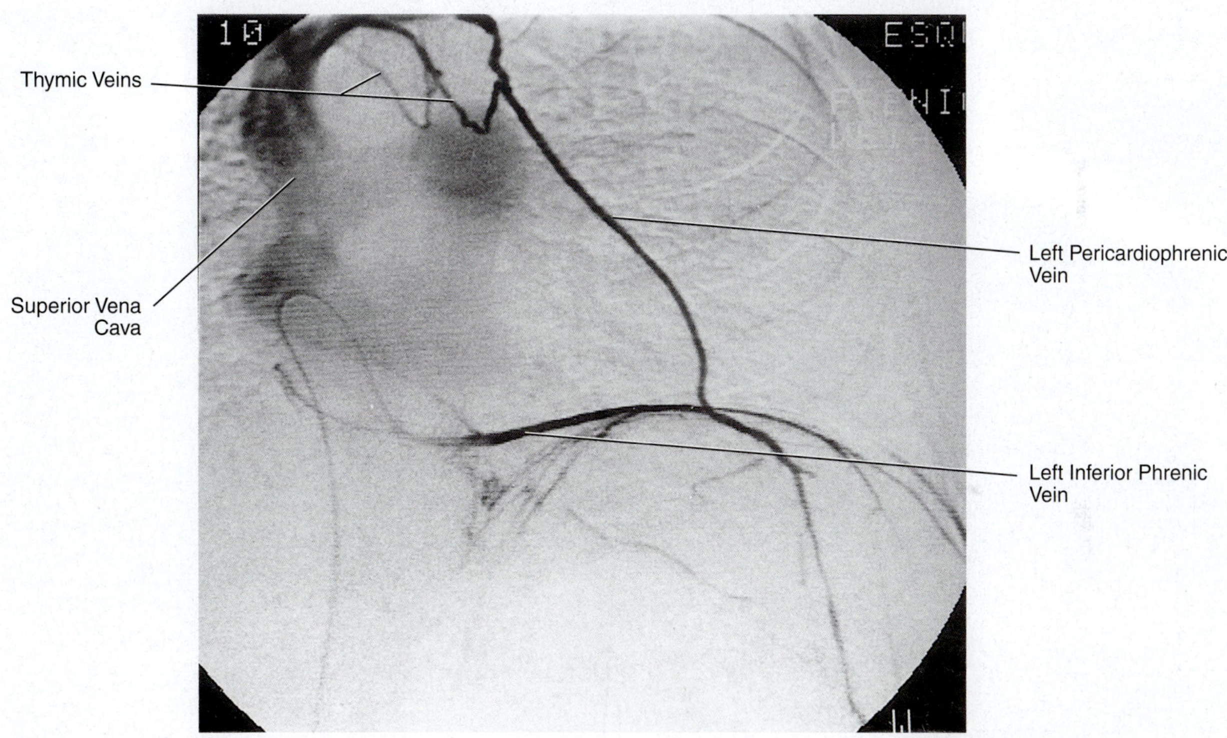

Figure 8.13. Selective injection of the inferior phrenic vein with opacification of the pericardiophrenic vein and the thymic veins in connection with the superior mediastinal venous drainage.

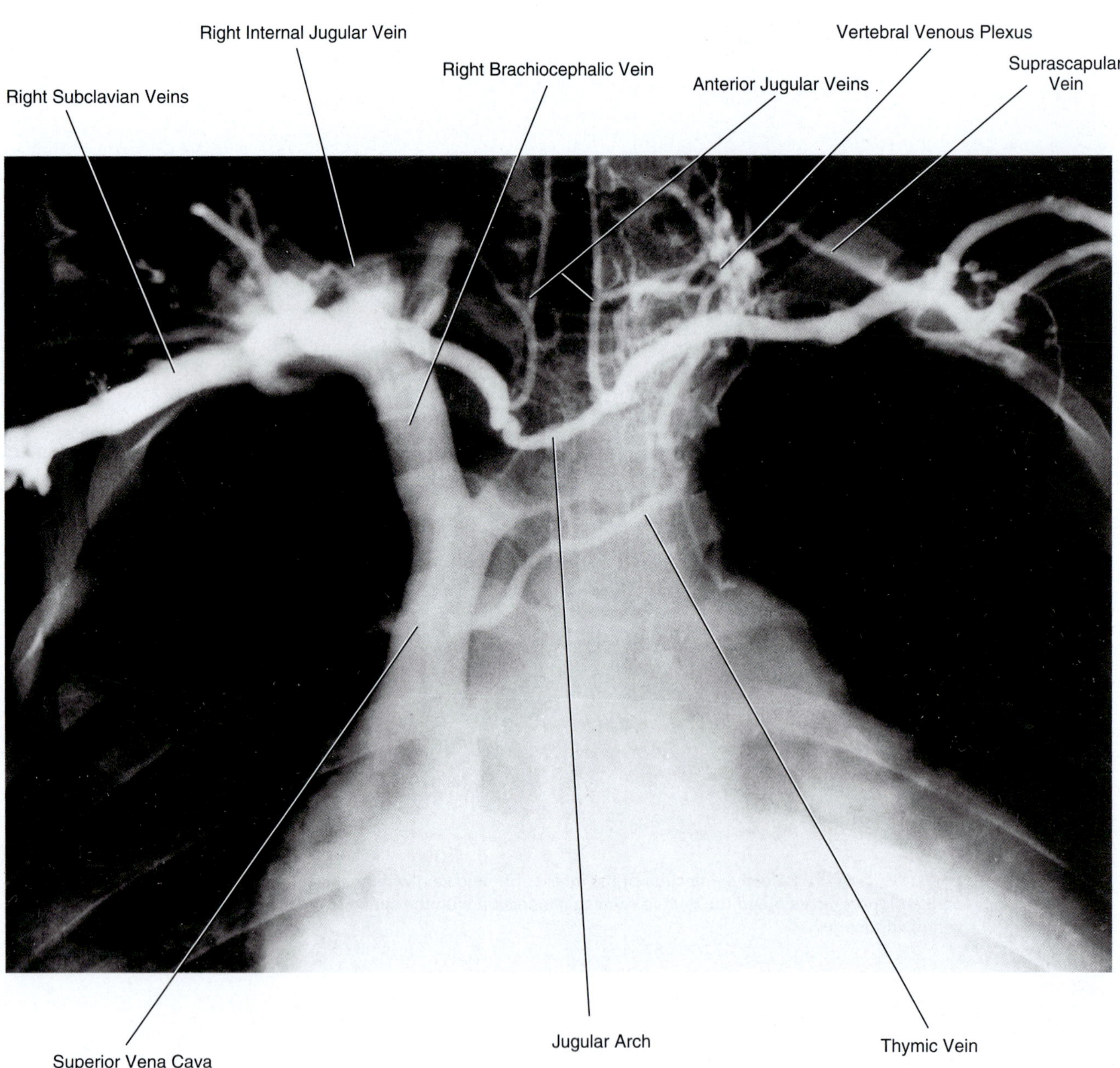

Figure 8.14. Venogram of the great venous vessels of the thorax with occlusion of the left brachiocephalic vein and development of cervical and thoracic collaterals.

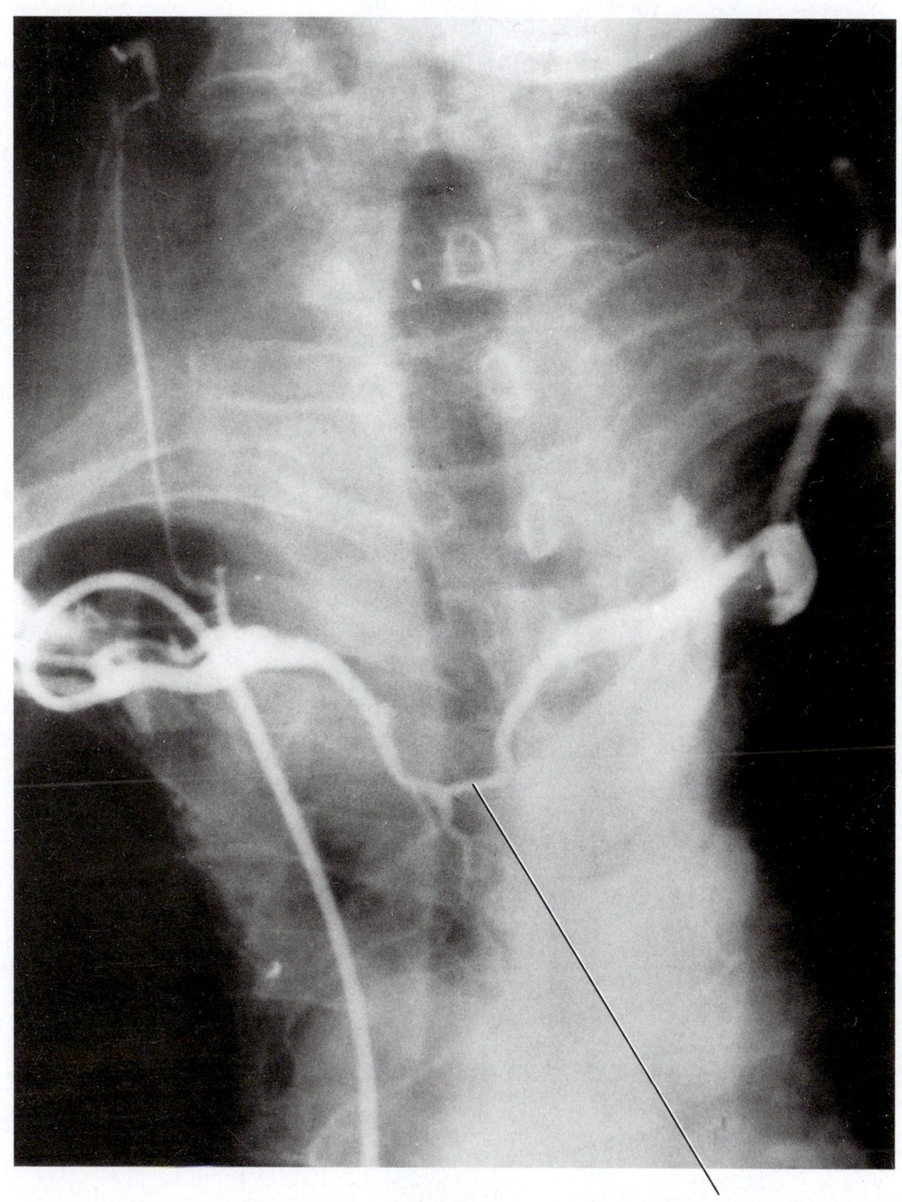

Figure 8.15. Selective venogram of the jugular arch.

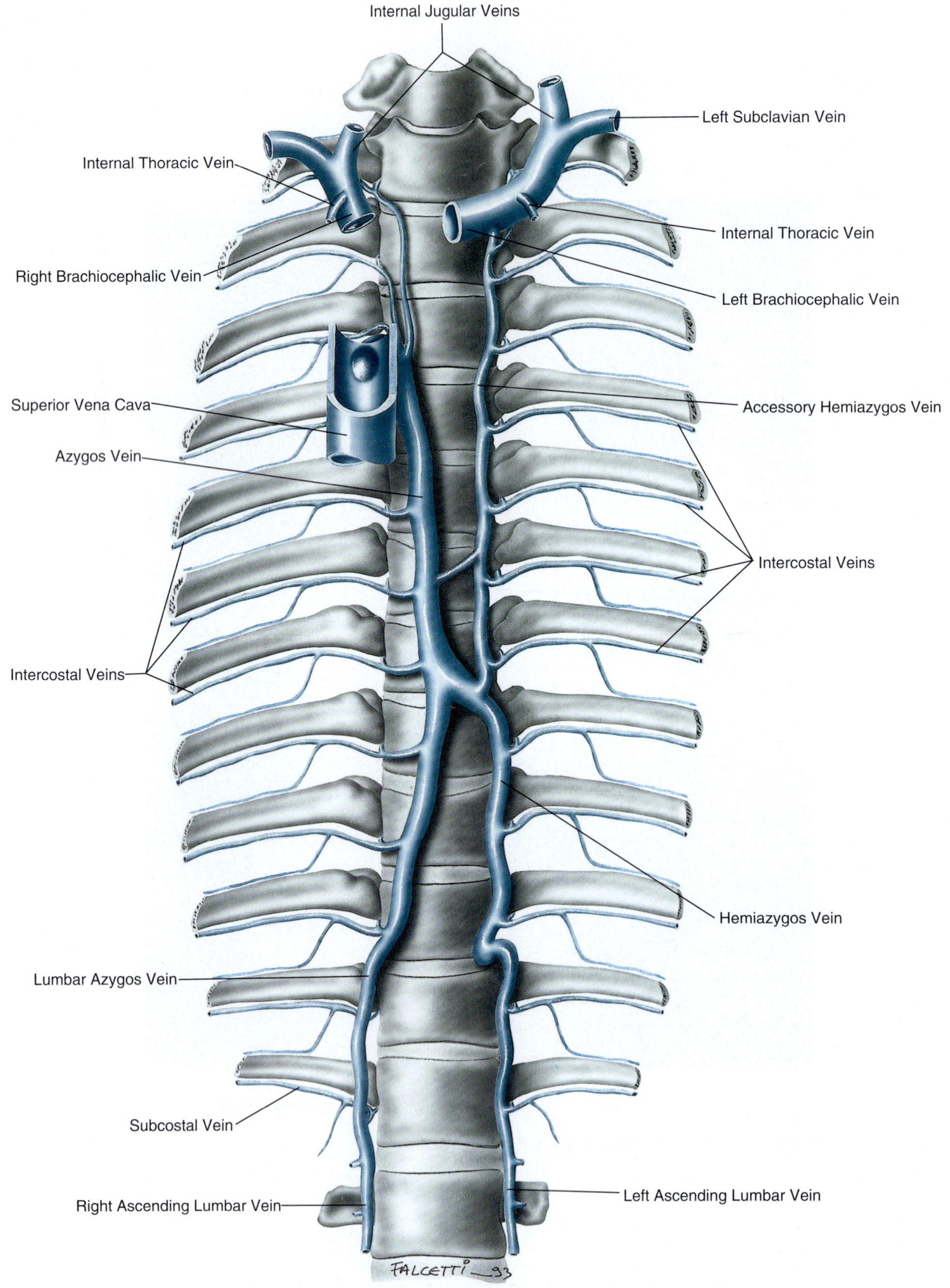

Figure 8.16. **Venous circulation of the thorax in an anterior view.**

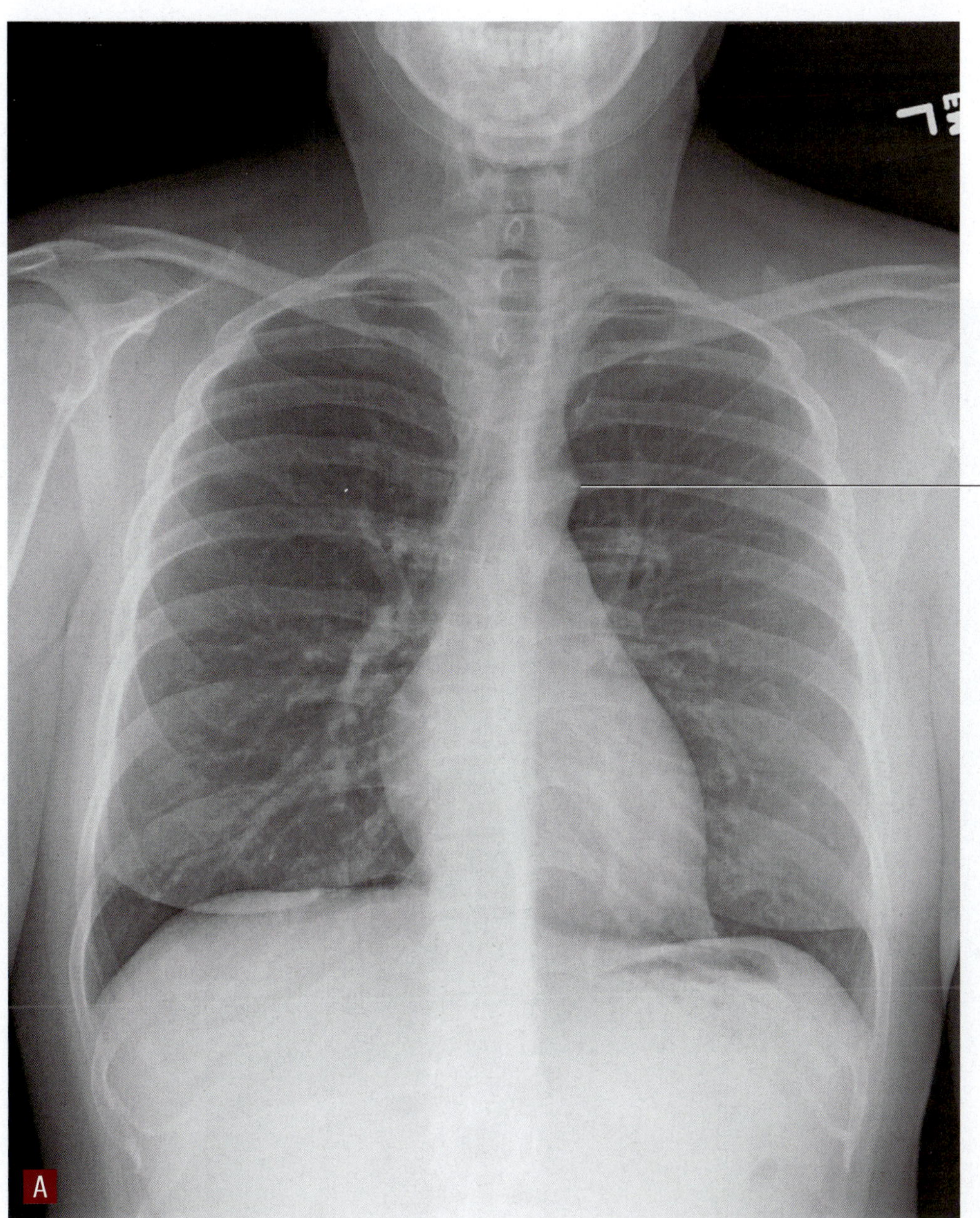

Figure 8.17. A and B, Posterior-anterior chest roentgrams showing an aortic nipple, a normal finding caused by the left superior intercostal vein.

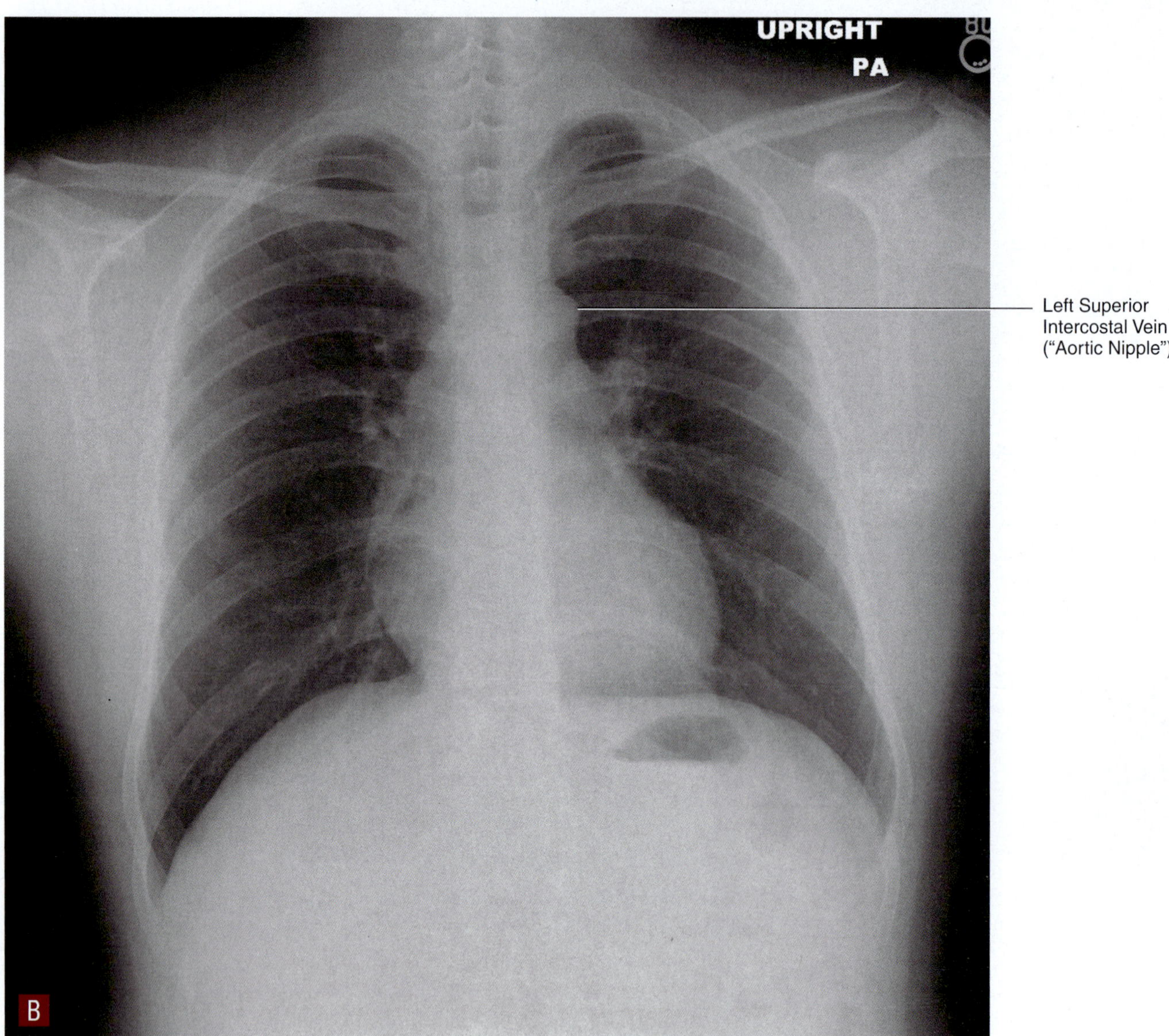

Figure 8.17. *Continued*

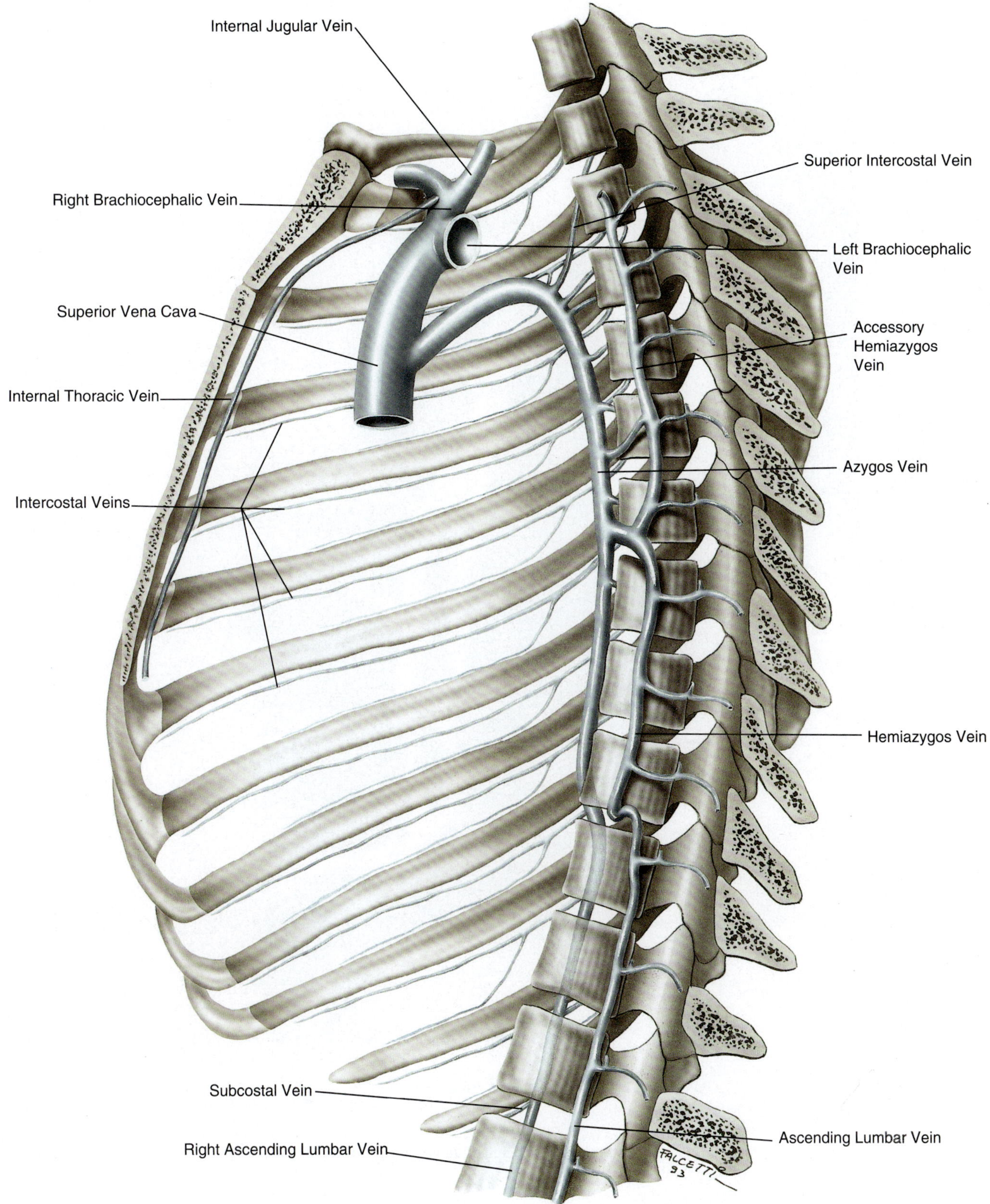

Figure 8.18. **Lateral view of the venous circulation of the thorax, especially the azygos vein.**

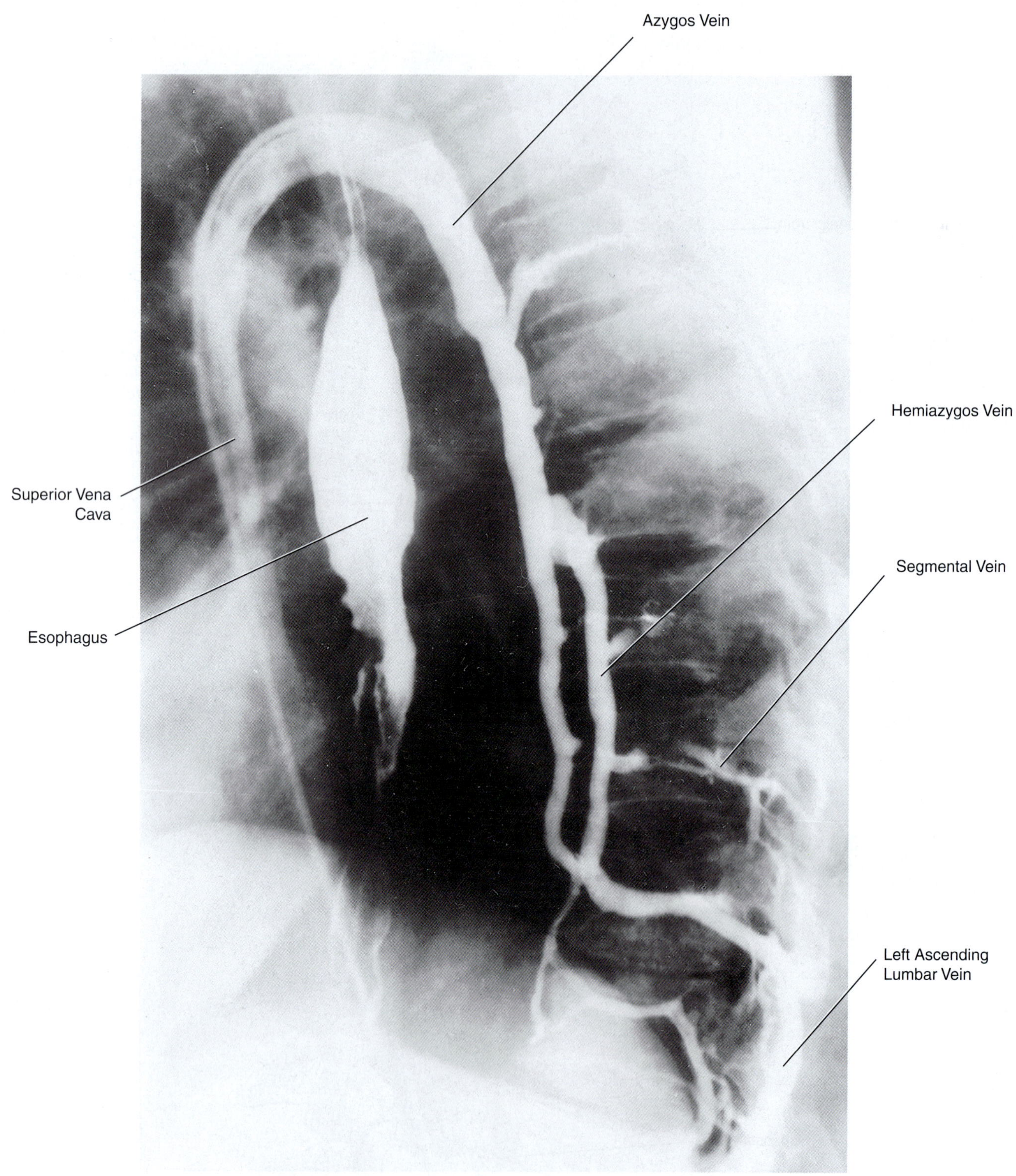

Figure 8.19. Lateral view of a selective venogram of the azygos vein.

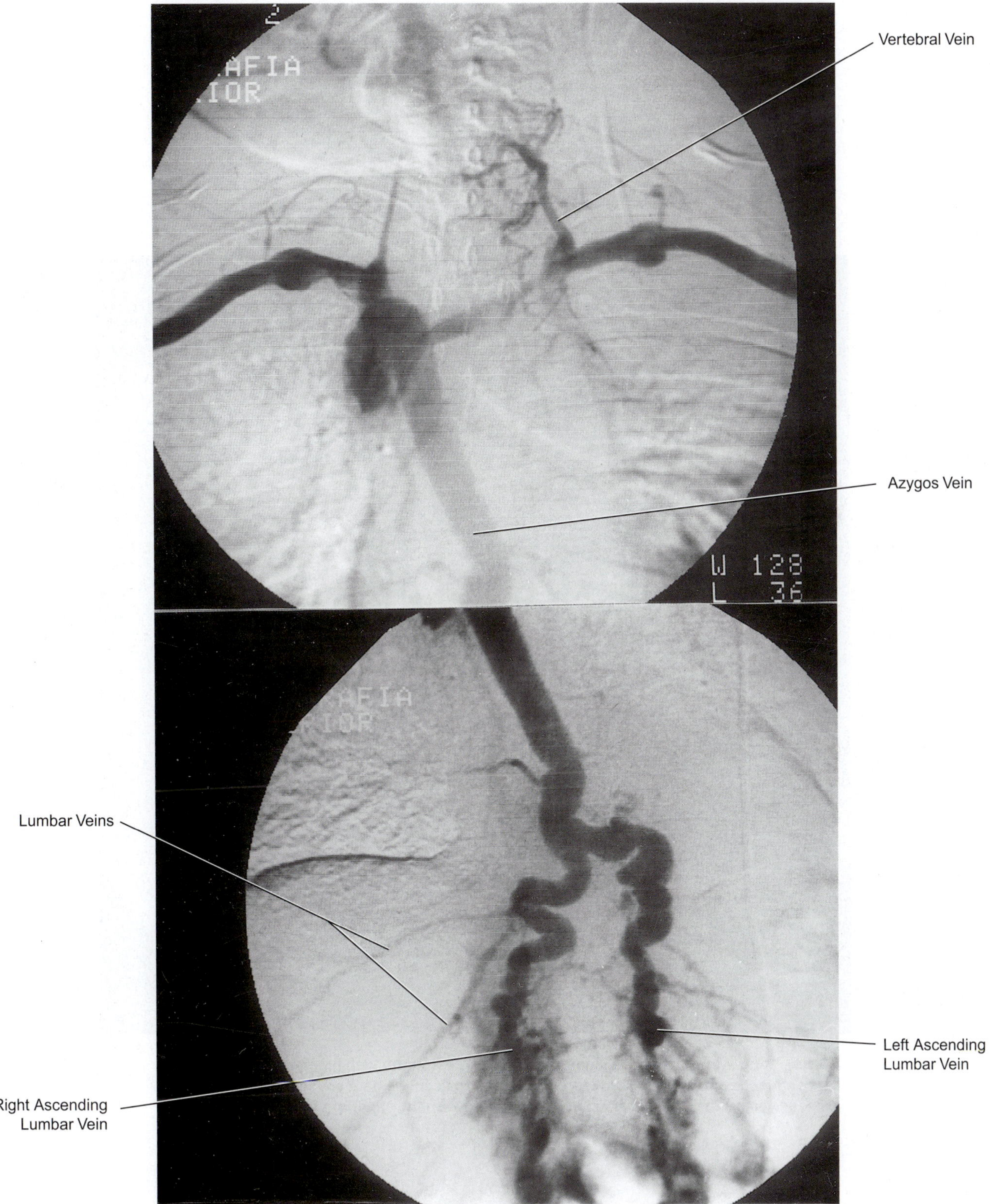

Figure 8.20. Anterior composite view of a venogram of the azygos vein in a case of occlusion of the superior vena cava, with drainage of the thorax veins through the azygos system and inferior vena cava, not demonstrated in this venogram.

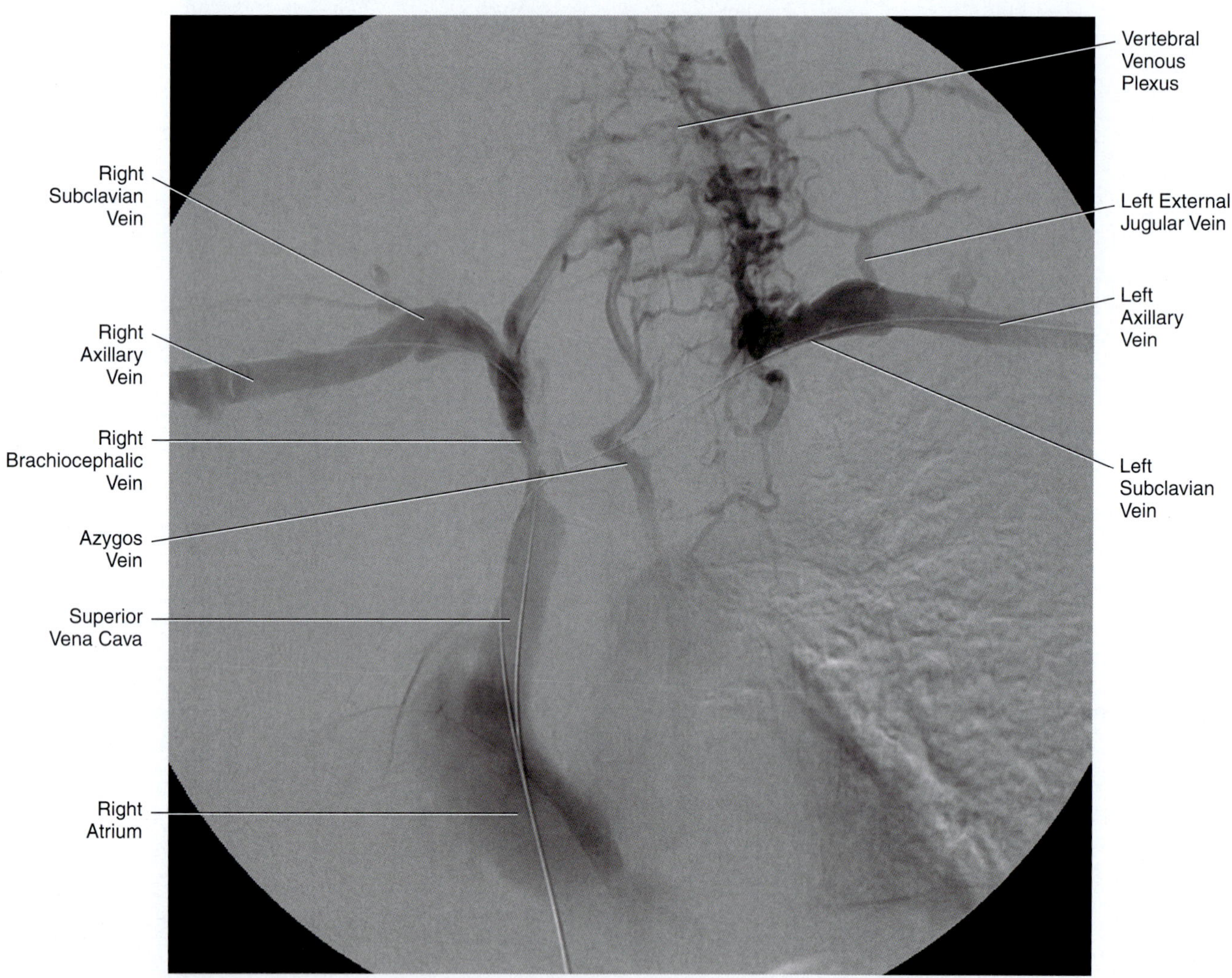

Figure 8.21. Bilateral venogram of the upper extremity with high-grade stenosis of the confluence of the brachiocephalic veins. Collaterals in the neck are seen draining into the azygous veins, which are occluded at their junction with the superior vena cava.

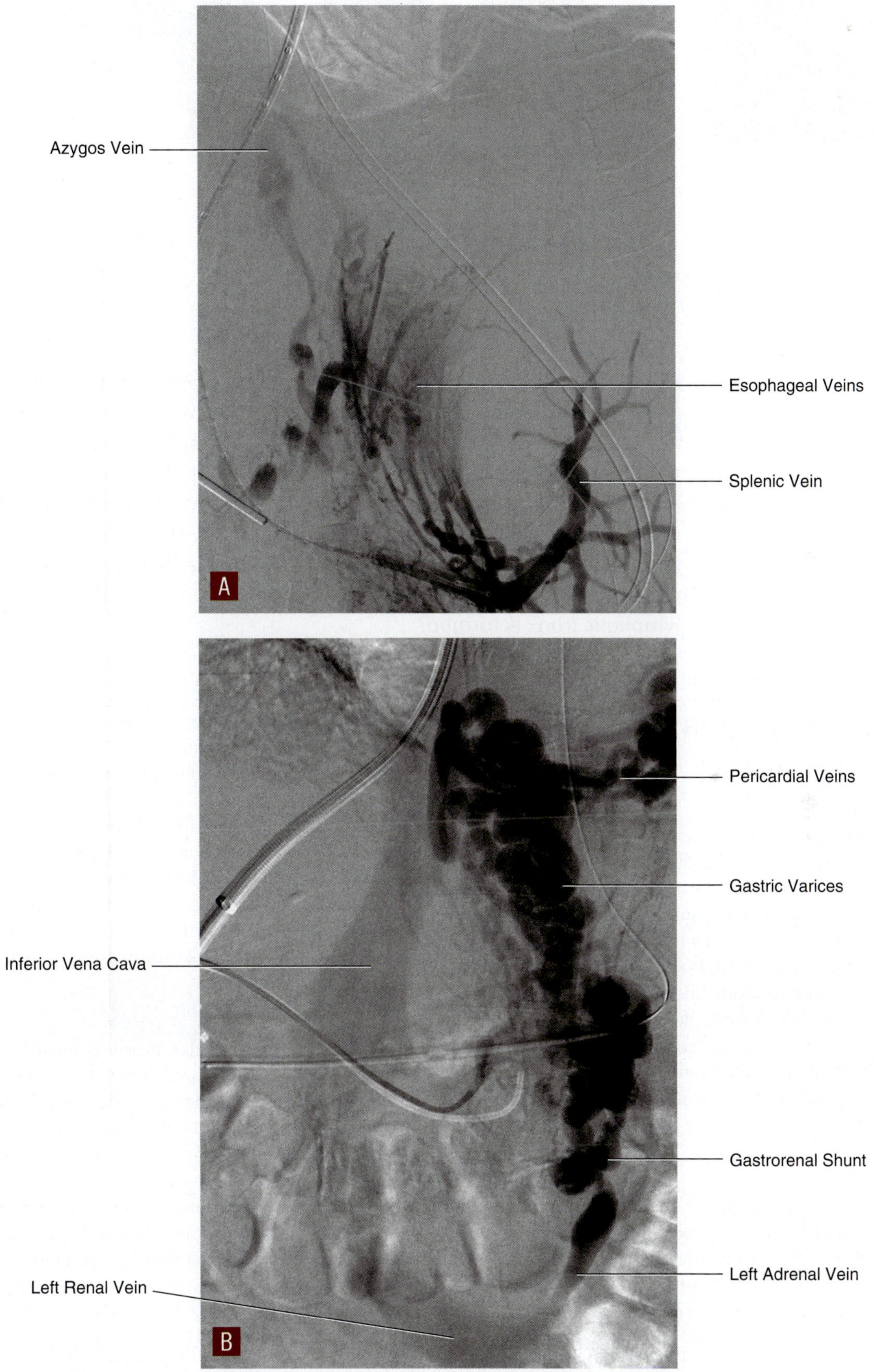

Figure 8.22. **A**, Selective venogram of the inferior esophageal veins from the splenic vein, showing drainage into the azygos vein, in a patient with portal hypertension. **B**, Selective venogram of the left gastric vein showing dilated esophageal veins draining into the pericardial and azygous veins. Gastric varices are seen communicating with the esophageal veins, which drain into the left renal vein via a gastrorenal shunt.

9

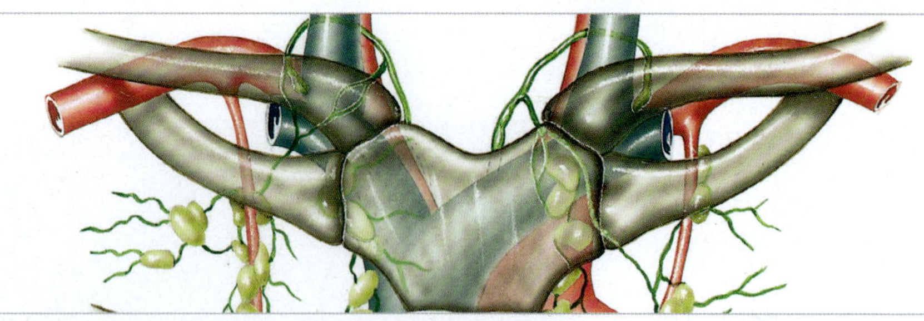

Lymphatic System of the Thorax

Peripheral lymph drainage to the venous circulation is accomplished via the right and left lymphovenous portals, which are located close to the junction of the large internal jugular and subclavian veins. On the right, there are three main lymphatic trunks; on the left, four main lymphatic trunks are identified: the three corresponding to the right and the thoracic duct, which is the largest lymphatic trunk in the body (Figs. 9.1-9.5). The anatomy of the lymphovenous portals varies. In 80% of subjects, the right trunks open independently at the jugular-subclavian junction. In one-fifth of cases, a short right lymphatic trunk is formed.

Thoracic Lymphatic Drainage

Lymphovenous Portals

On the Right

There are three main lymphatic trunks converging to the junction of the right internal jugular vein with the right subclavian vein: (1) the right jugular trunk, which runs along the ventrolateral aspect of the internal jugular vein, carrying all the lymph from the right half of the head and neck; (2) the right subclavian trunk from the right apical axillary lymph nodes, running along the axillary and subclavian vein, and carrying lymph from the upper right limb and the superficial tissues of the right chest and abdominal wall; and (3) the right bronchomediastinal trunk, which runs along the trachea, carrying lymph from the right lung, diaphragm, bronchi, and trachea.

On the Left

The left lymphovenous portal receives the volume of lymph from all over the body, except the territories mentioned for the right lymphatic trunks (Figs. 9.6-9.8). There are four main lymphatic trunks converging to the left lymphovenous portal: (1) the left jugular trunk, which runs along the ventrolateral aspect of the internal jugular vein, carrying lymph from the left half of the head and neck; (2) the left subclavian trunk draining lymph from the upper left limb and superficial tissues of the left chest and abdominal wall; (3) the left bronchomediastinal trunk, which drains more of the heart and esophagus, in addition to the lung, bronchi, and trachea; and (4) the thoracic duct, which drains the remaining territories of the body. It is formed by the abdominal confluence of the lymphatic trunks to the cisterna chyli.

Thoracic Duct

In adults, the thoracic duct measures about 38 to 45 cm in length, extending from the abdomen to the neck, transgressing the diaphragm, ascending at the posterior mediastinum right of the midline, between the descending thoracic aorta and the azygos vein and anterior of the vertebral column. In many cases, the thoracic duct starts as a wide pouch called the cisterna chyli and diminishes in caliber up to the neck, where it arches laterally to the left and anteriorly, and eventually descends in a direction to the junction of the left internal jugular and left subclavian veins, opening into the venous system through a bicuspid valve. At its terminus, the thoracic duct may be multiple, and the site or opening may be in any of the left great veins. The origin of the thoracic duct is the confluence of the four main abdominal lymph trunks (Figs. 9.1-9.3, and 9.5).

Tributaries of the Thoracic Duct Proper

Confluence of the Abdominal Lymphatic Trunks

- Lumbar lymph trunks
- Intestinal lymph trunks
    - Bilateral descending lymph trunks
    - Bilateral ascending lymph trunks
- Upper intercostal lymph trunks
- Mediastinal lymph trunks
- Left subclavian lymph trunk
- Left jugular lymph trunk
- Left bronchomediastinal lymph trunk

Lymphatic Drainage of the Thoracic Wall

Lymphatic Vessels

The superficial lymphatic vessels of the chest wall converge to the axillary nodes, subscapular nodes, pectoral nodes, and parasternal nodes (Fig. 9.9). The deeper lymphatic vessels of the chest walls drain mainly to the parasternal, intercostal, and diaphragmatic lymph nodes (Fig. 9.1).

Parasternal Lymph Nodes (Internal Thoracic)

There are four or five nodes on each side, at the anterior end of the intercostal spaces, following the path of the internal thoracic arteries and veins. They drain the internal, anterior thoracic wall, and the mammary glands. Their efferents form the bronchomediastinal trunk, together with the tracheobronchial and the brachiocephalic lymph nodes (Fig. 9.10).

Intercostal Lymph Nodes

The intercostal lymph nodes are located at the heads and necks of the ribs and receive lymphatic vessels from the posterolateral aspect of the chest and mammary gland. The lower four to seven intercostal spaces unite, forming the descending trunk, which joins the thoracic duct or the abdominal confluence of the lymphatic trunks (Figs. 9.1 and 9.9).

Diaphragmatic Lymph Nodes

There are anterior, right and left lateral, and posterior groups of diaphragmatic lymph nodes on the thoracic surface of the diaphragm.

Lymphatic Drainage of the Thoracic Contents

The lymph from the thoracic organs is drained through one of the three groups of lymph nodes in the chest before entering the thoracic duct or the right lymphatic duct: the brachiocephalic, the posterior mediastinal, or tracheobronchial lymph nodes.

Brachiocephalic Lymph Nodes

The brachiocephalic lymph nodes are located in the superior mediastinum, anterior to the brachiocephalic veins and the large arterial trunks. They receive lymph from the thymus, thyroid gland, pericardium, heart, and lateral diaphragmatic nodes. They drain to the right and left bronchomediastinal trunks after joining the efferent lymphatics from the tracheobronchial nodes.

Posterior Mediastinal Lymph Nodes

The posterior mediastinal lymph nodes are located behind the pericardium, close to the esophagus and the descending thoracic aorta. They receive afferent lymphatic vessels from the esophagus, posterior pericardium, diaphragm, and sometimes from the left lobe of the liver. Most drain into the thoracic duct.

Tracheobronchial Lymph Nodes (Chapter 12, See Fig. 12.3)

There are five foremost groups of tracheobronchial lymph nodes.

1. Paratracheal
2. Superior tracheobronchial
3. Inferior tracheobronchial (carinate nodes)
4. Bronchopulmonary (hilar nodes)
5. Pulmonary

These groups are continuous and without clear differentiation. The afferent vessels drain the lung parenchyma, the pleura, the bronchi, thoracic trachea, and heart and connect with some posterior mediastinal nodes. The efferent vessels ascend to the trachea to join the efferent vessels of the parasternal and brachiocephalic nodes, forming the right and left bronchomediastinal trunks. On the right side, the trunk may join a right lymphatic duct or another lymphatic trunk. On the left side, the trunk may connect to the thoracic duct but more often opens independently at the jugular-subclavian junction.

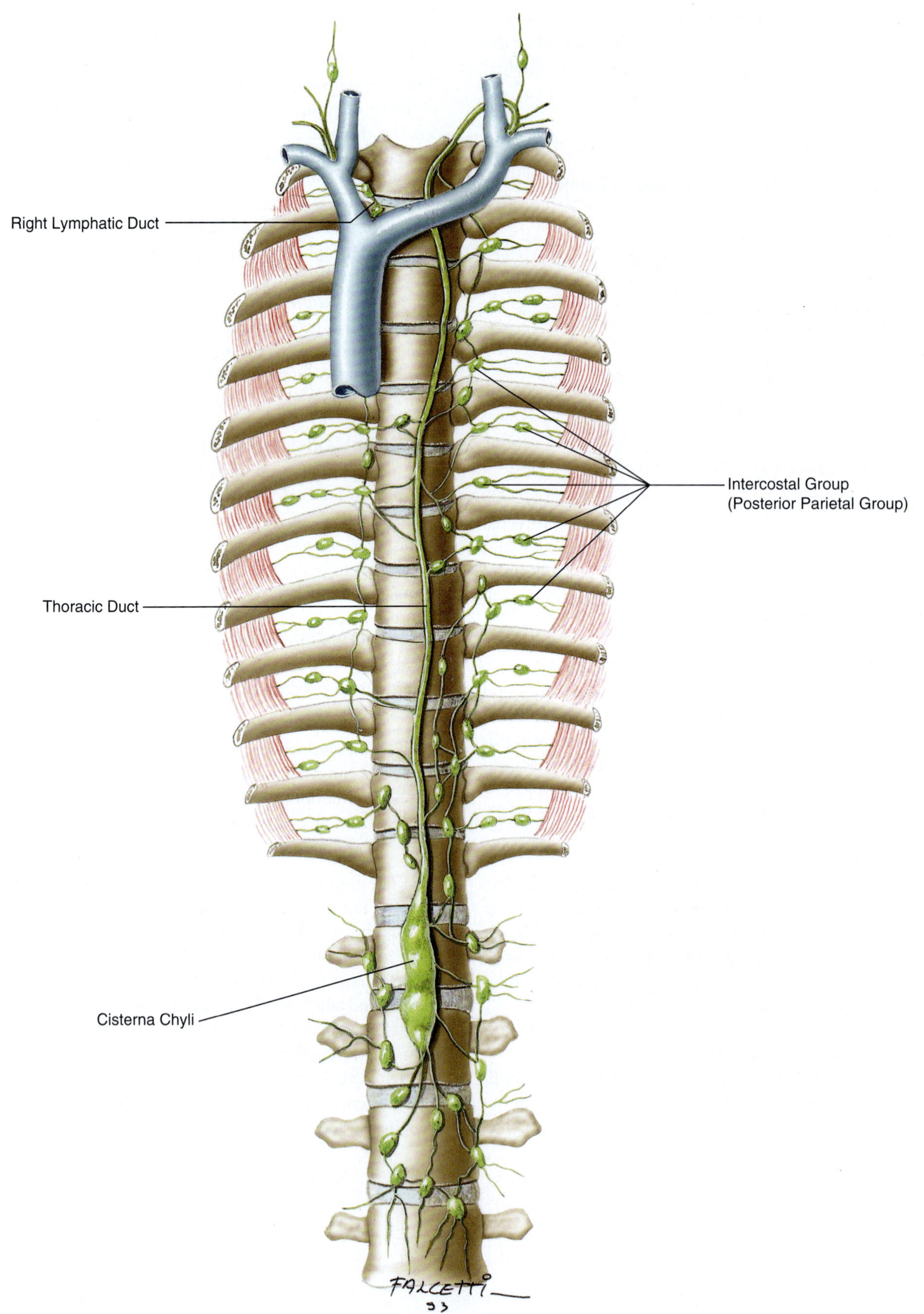

Figure 9.1. Posterior mediastinal lymphatic system with the thoracic duct, intercostal lymphatic nodes group, and the cisterna chyli. Note the right lymphatic duct entering the right subclavian vein.

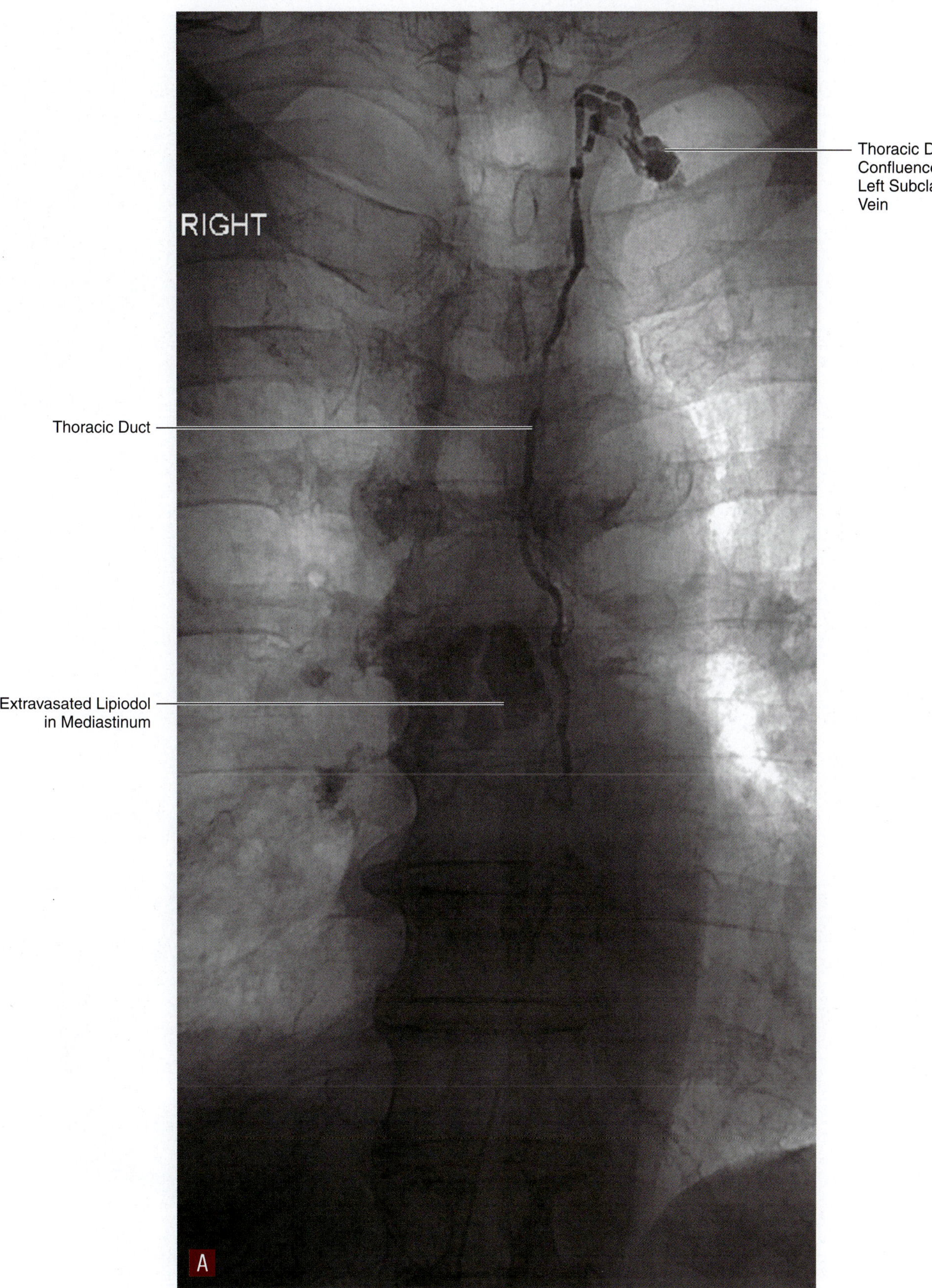

Figure 9.2. **A**, Lymphangiogram showing the thoracic duct and its confluence with the left subclavian vein. **B**, Lymphangiogram showing the confluence of the four main abdominal lymphatic trunks.

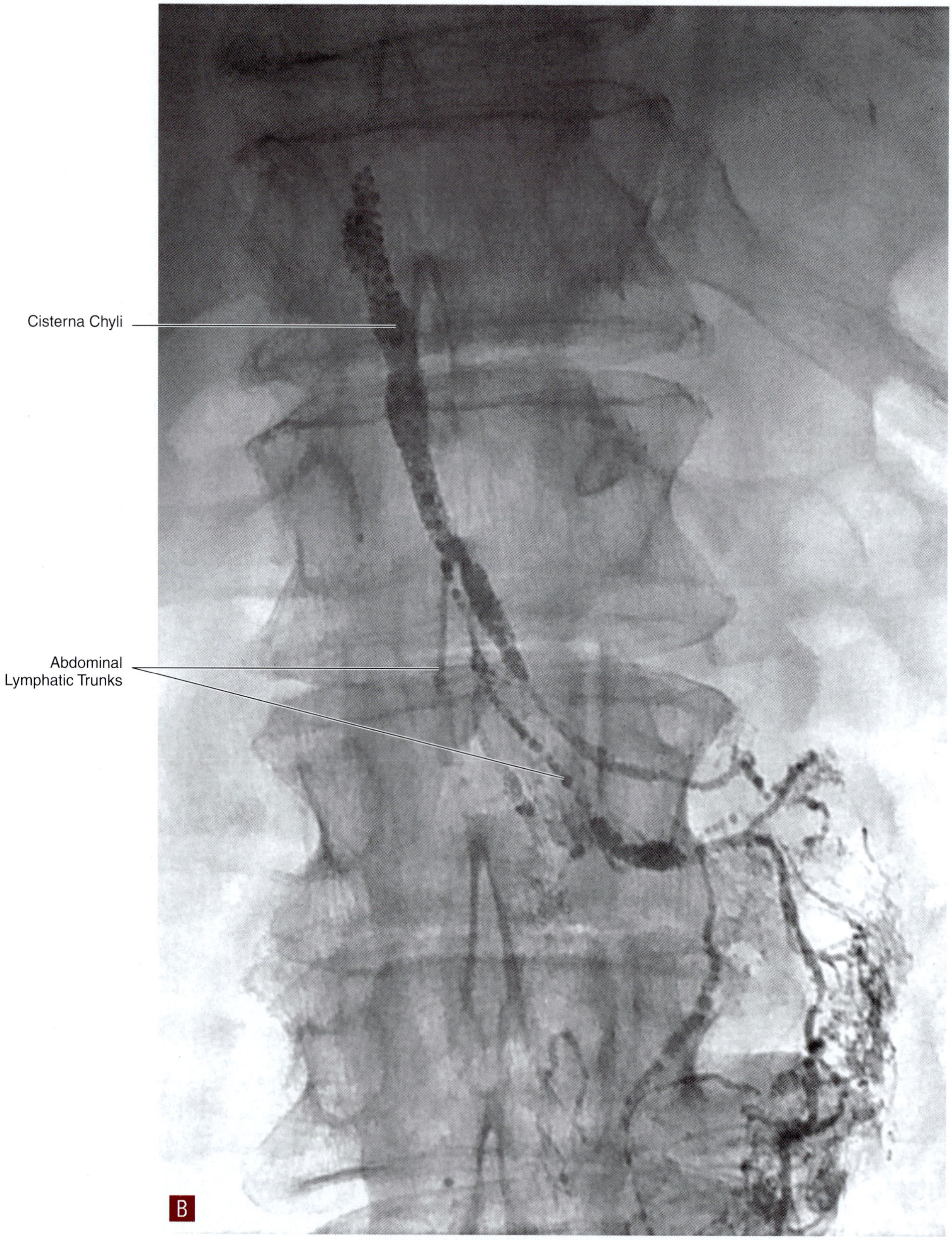

Figure 9.2. *Continued*

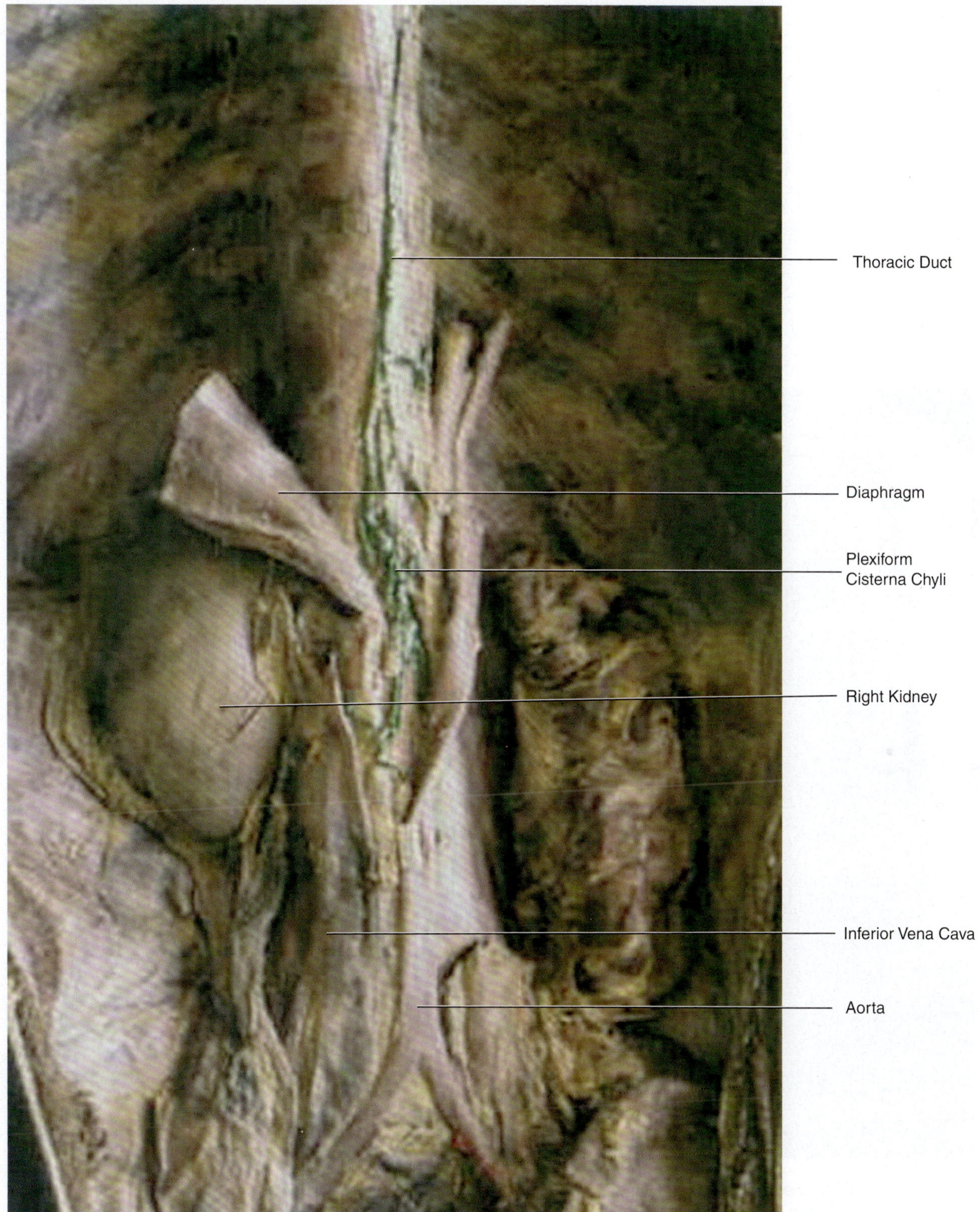

Figure 9.3. Anatomic preparation of the cisterna chyli and thoracic duct. The thoracic duct is formed from the confluence of abdominal lymphatic vessels, in this case forming a plexiform cisterna chyli. Note the position of the cisterna chyli behind the aorta (removed) and the diaphragmatic crura.

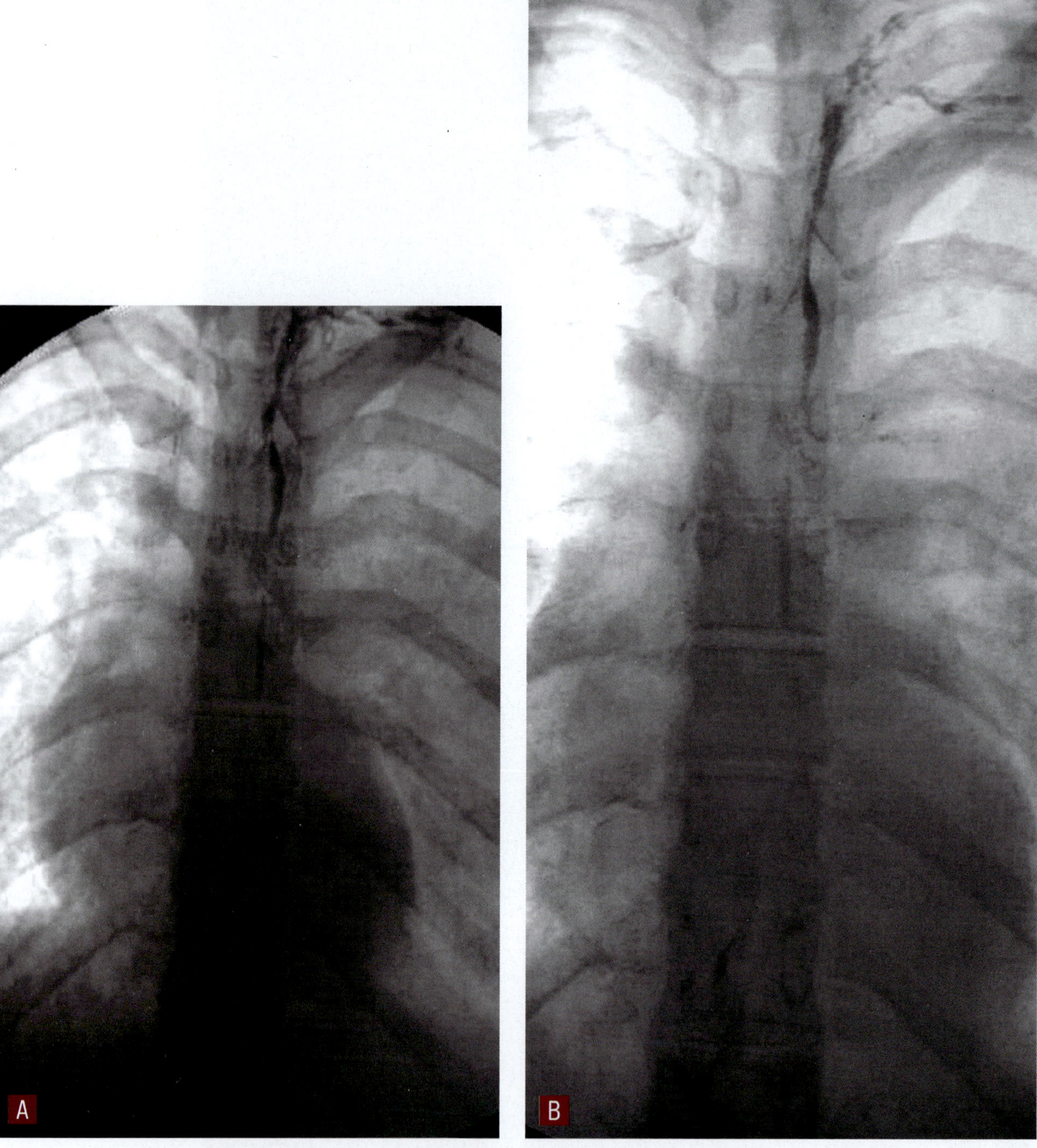

Figure 9.4. A, Lymphangiogram of the thoracic duct visualized along the mediastinum. Note the interruptions of the column of contrast. The thoracic duct has contractility due to muscles in the wall of the duct and has active ascending flow. B, Upper segment of the thoracic duct demonstrating the plexus configuration of the duct. Most commonly the duct is a single channel connected to the venous angle or the subclavian vein. The subclavian lymphatic trunk can also be visualized. Note extravasation to the mediastinum with delineation of the left bronchus.

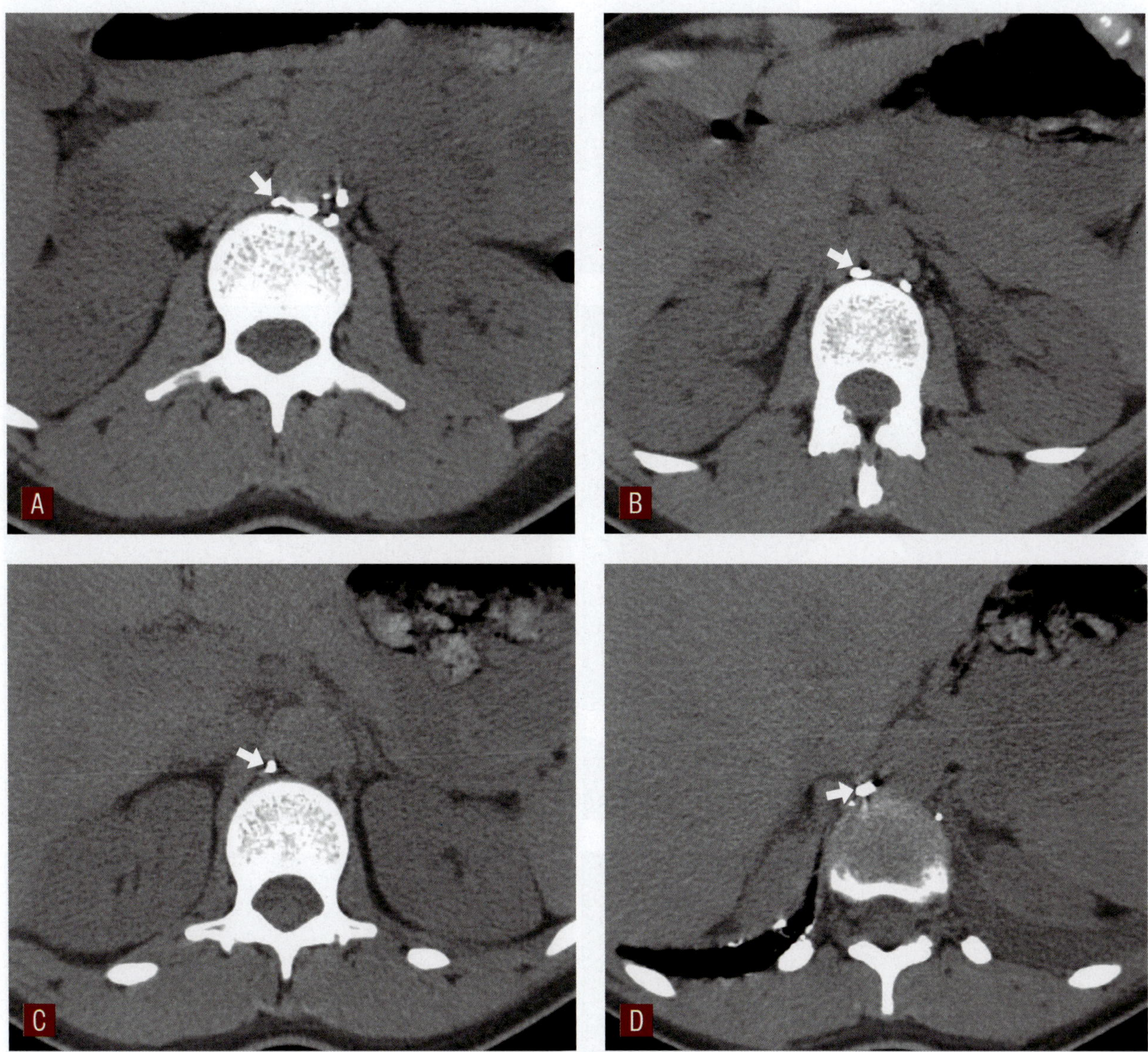

Figure 9.5. A to D, Computerized tomographic (CT) scan of the mediastinum following a lymphangiogram, showing the formation of the thoracic duct in the retroaortic space in a plexiform cisterna chyli (arrows). From E to L, note the thoracic duct following a course behind the azygous vein right to the midline (arrows). From M to P, note the duct moving to the left side of the mediastinum (arrows). From Q to S, note the thoracic duct directed forward and further to the left passing into the neck, behind the left common carotid and internal jugular vein until it reaches the subclavian vein in a wide arch. In this case, the termination of the thoracic duct seems to be plexiform (arrows).

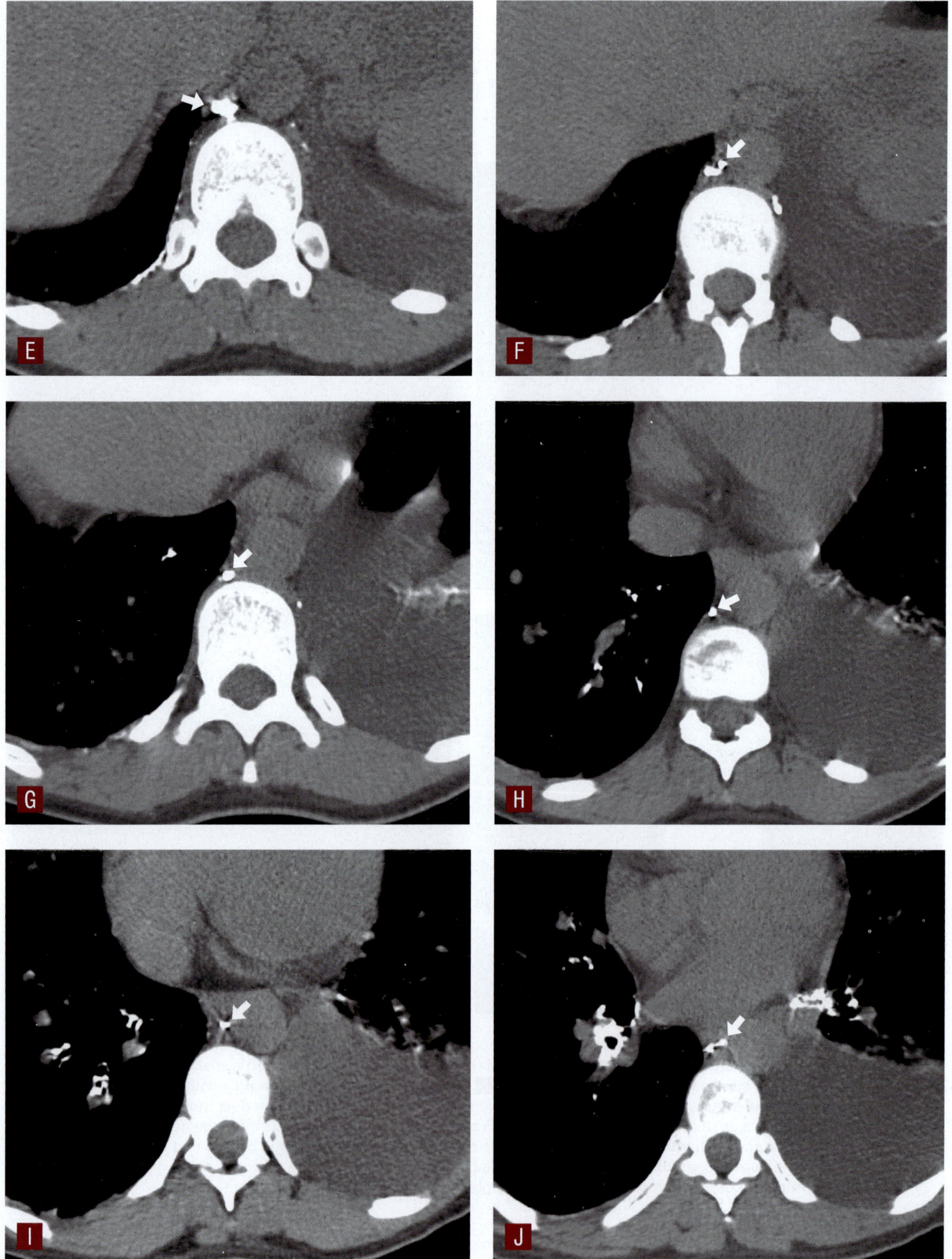

Figure 9.5. *Continued*

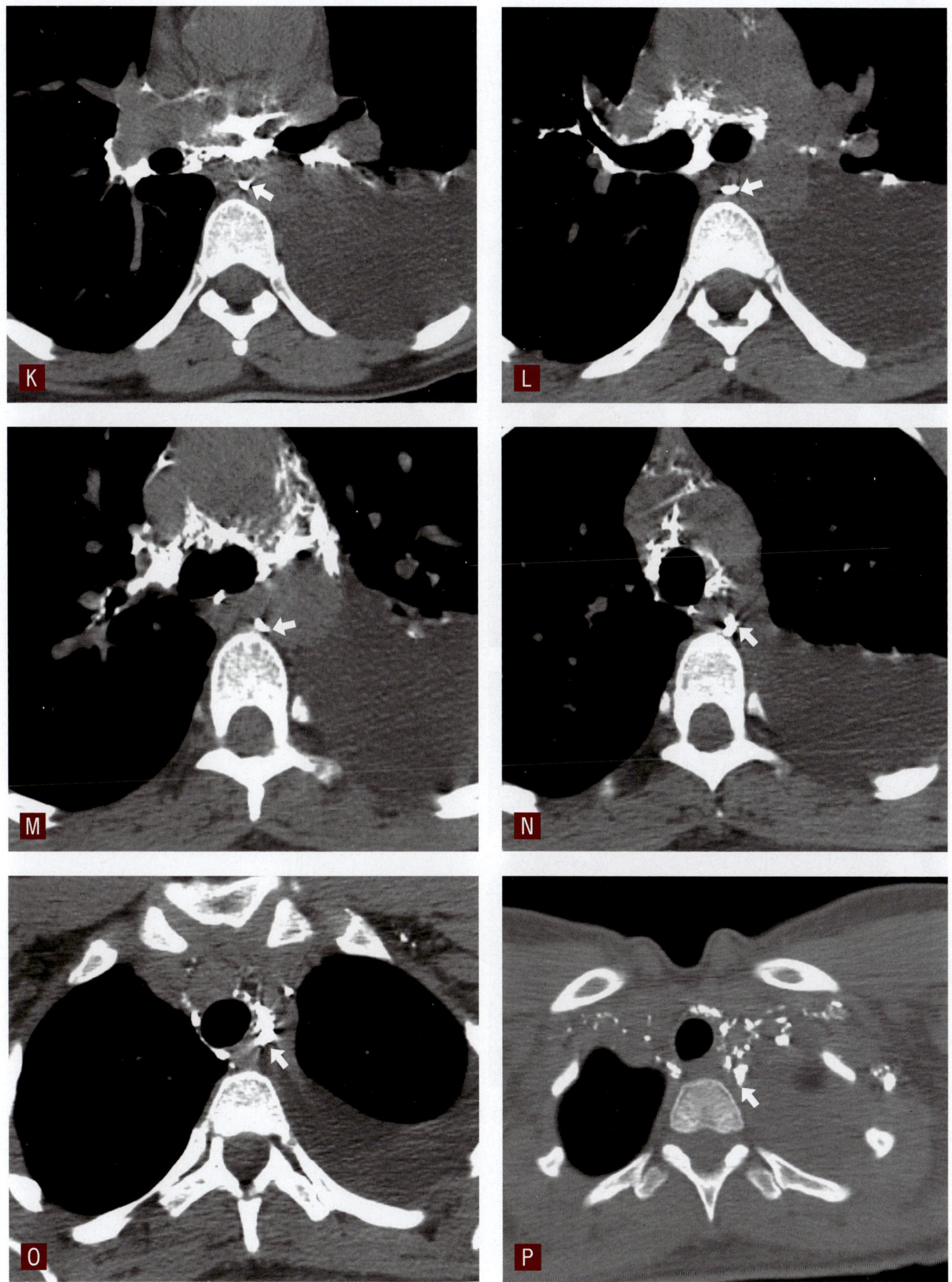

Figure 9.5. *Continued*

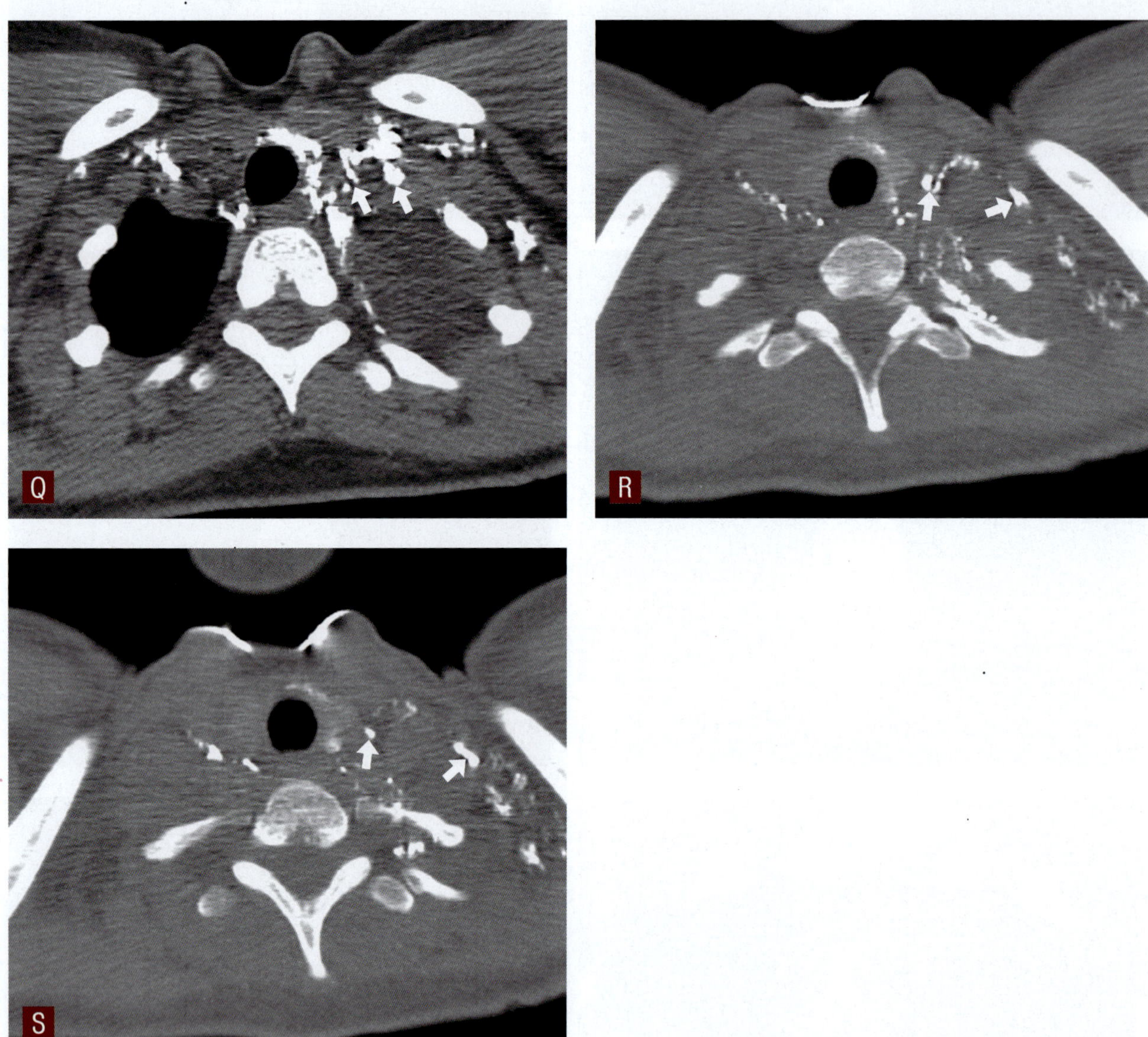

Figure 9.5. *Continued*

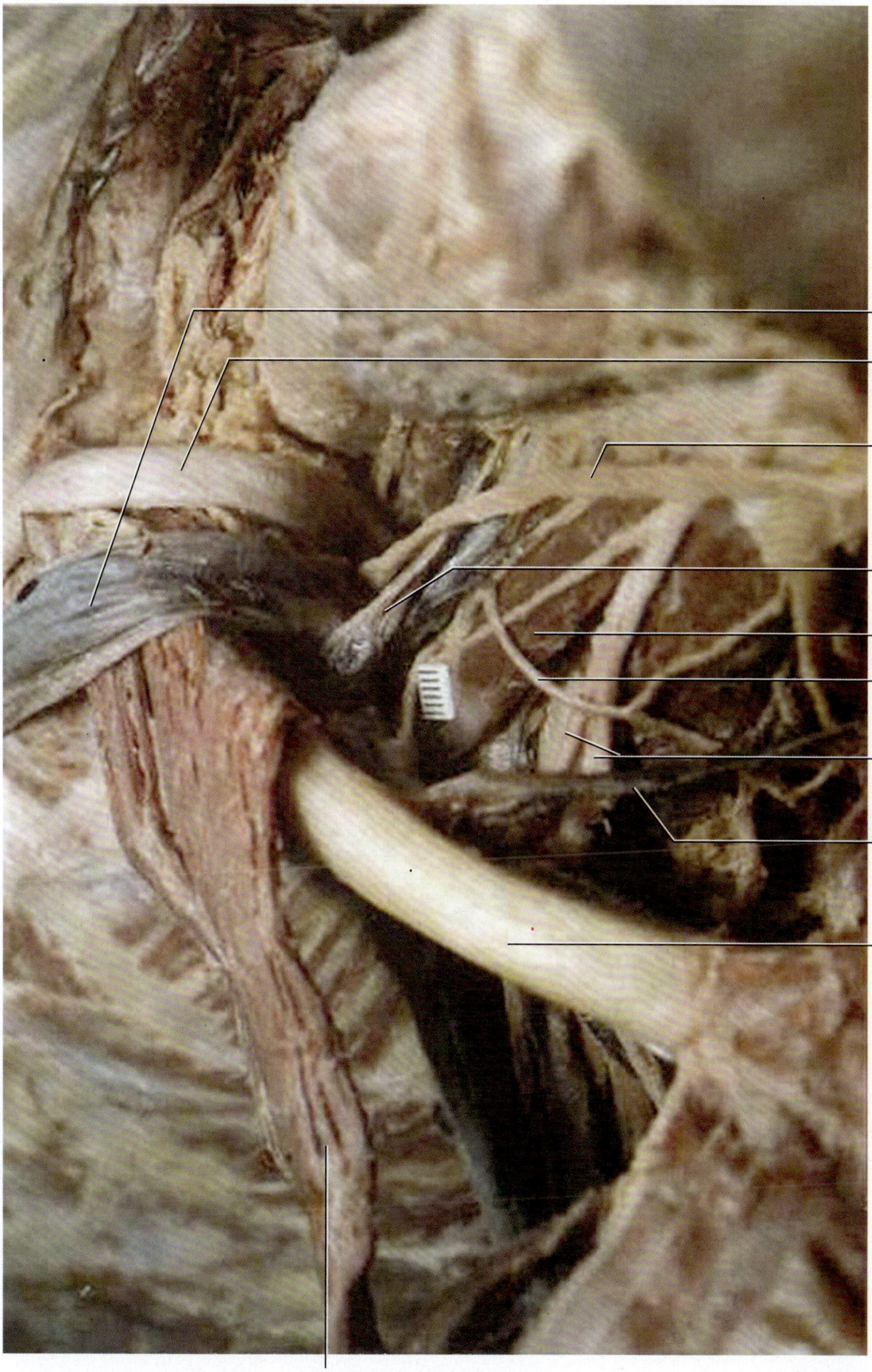

Figure 9.6. Anatomic preparation of the left supraclavicular fossa showing the relationships of the structures with the cervical segment of the thoracic duct.

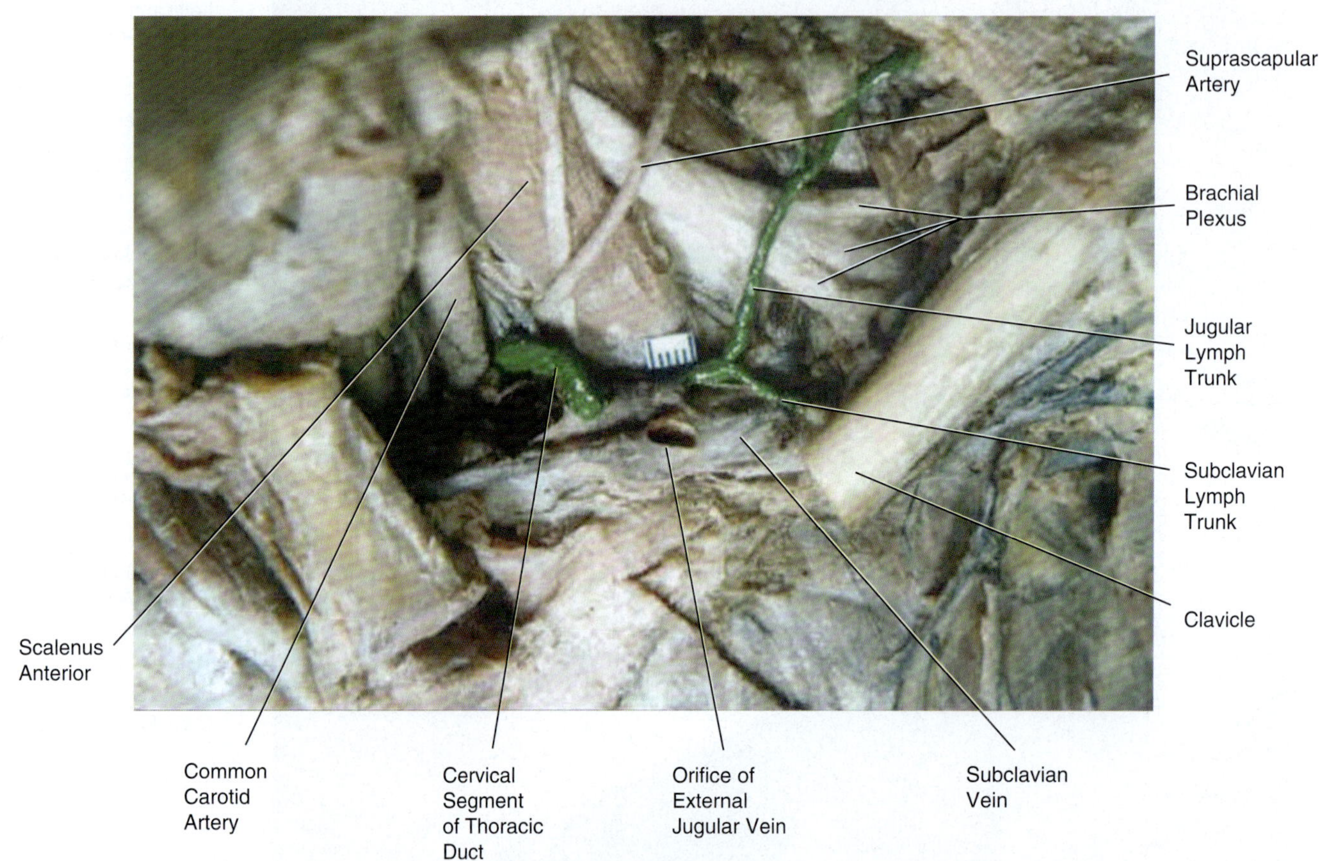

Figure 9.7. Anatomic preparation of the left supraclavicular fossa showing the thoracic duct and jugular and subclavian lymph trunks colorized in green. Note the relationship with the other structures.

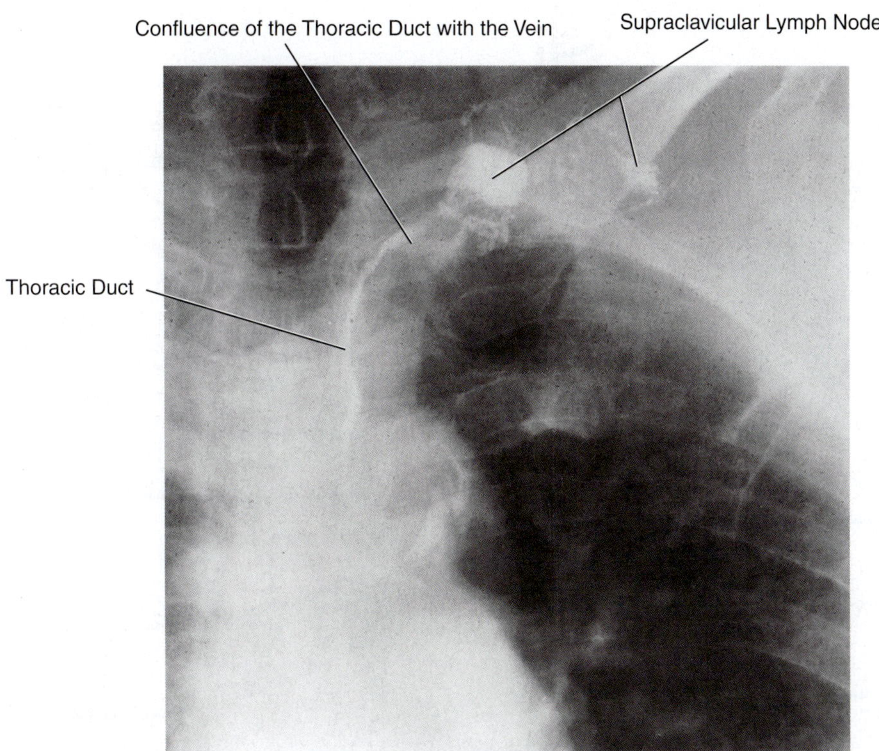

Figure 9.8. Lymphangiogram showing the thoracic duct entering the left subclavian vein at the junction with the right internal jugular vein. Note the lymph nodes opacified by the contrast.

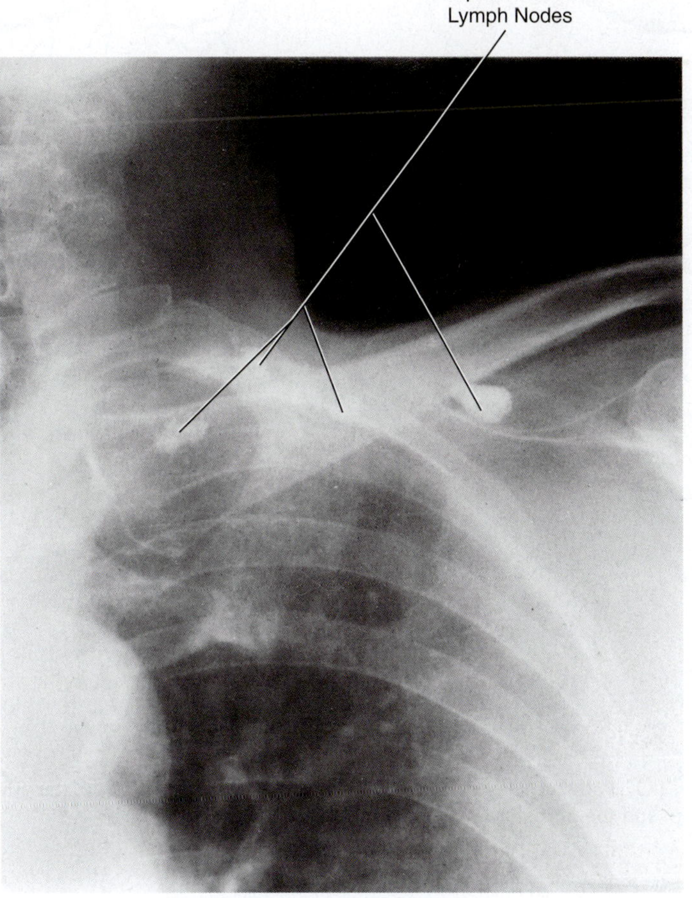

Figure 9.9. Supraclavicular lymph nodes opacified 24 hours after the lymphangiogram.

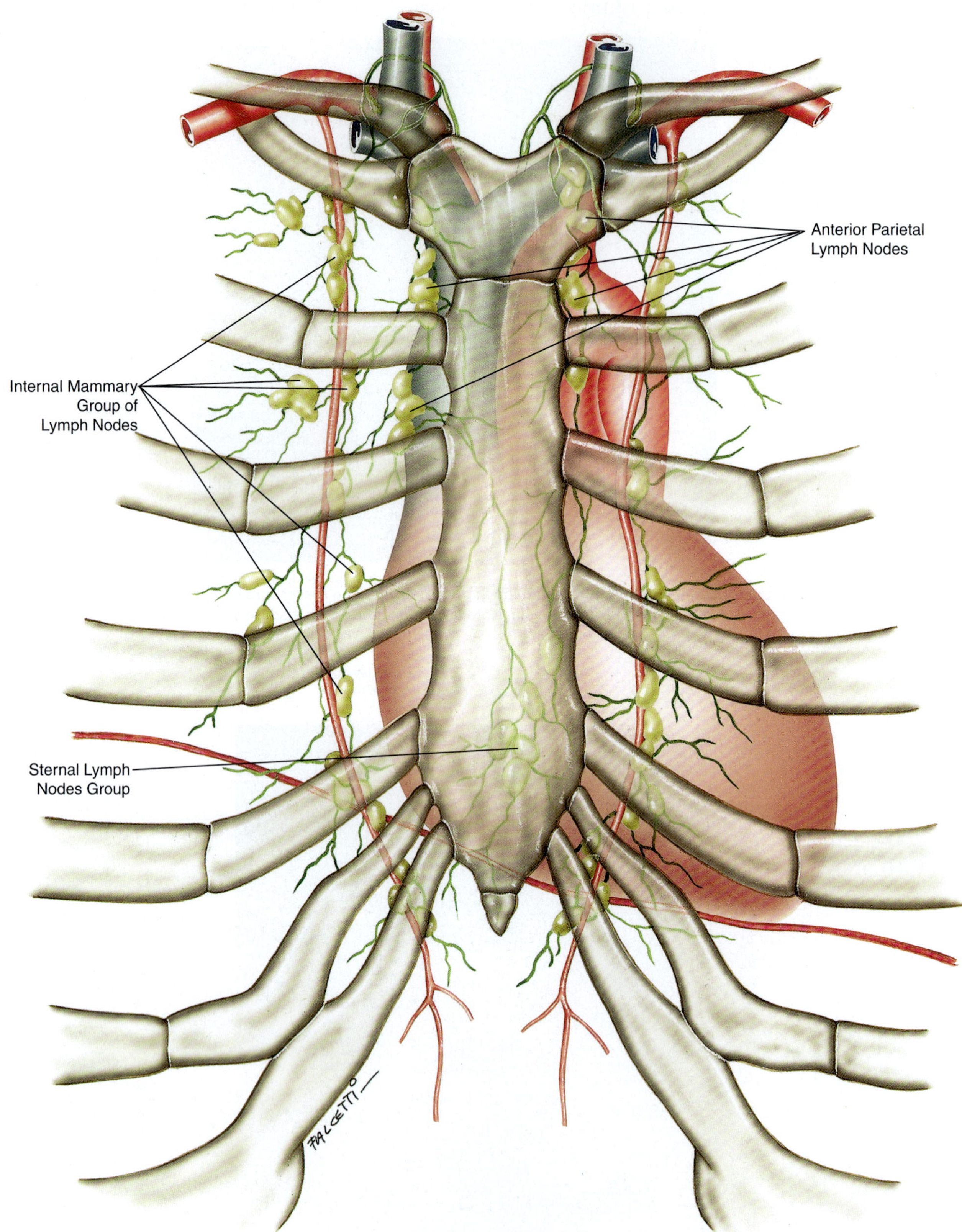

Figure 9.10. Parasternal lymph nodes, the internal mammary group, the anterior parietal group, and the retrosternal lymph node group.

10

Pulmonary Arterial Circulation

Anatomically, the pulmonary arteries are elastic, with little mural musculature down to their fifth or sixth divisions. Peripherally, the amount of smooth muscle in the walls of intrapulmonary arteries increases. The branches of 1.0 to 0.1 mm in diameter are mainly muscular. Branches less than 0.1 mm in diameter are nonmuscular and are chiefly poorly supported endothelial tubes, with profuse anastomotic, alveolar capillary networks—the principal structural elements in the walls of the respiratory membranes. The pulmonary circulation is a low-resistance, low-pressure system with high distensibility and little vasomotor control. The pulmonary resistance is about a sixth of the systemic, with a pressure averaging 22/8 mm Hg (mean, 13 mm Hg). The pulmonary blood flow can triple without significant increase in pulmonary artery pressure, owing to the high degree of distensibility of the normal pulmonary vasculature. The large and small pulmonary arteries carry about 30% of the blood in the lungs, whereas the capillaries carry around 20%.

Pulmonary Trunk

The pulmonary trunk carries deoxygenated blood from the right ventricle of the heart to the lung circulation. It is normally about 5 cm in length and 3 cm in diameter and arises from the right ventricle base above and left to the supraventricular crest. It is a short vessel, arising from the pulmonary conus of the right ventricle at the pulmonary semilunar valves. The trunk has an ascending and posterior orientation, in front of the ascending aorta toward its left aspect (Fig. 10.1). The pulmonary trunk lies totally within the pericardium. It divides into the left and right pulmonary arteries, with each artery about the same diameter. The bifurcation of the main pulmonary artery varies in appearance, its angle ranging between 100° and 180° (Fig. 10.2). The diameter of the right pulmonary artery ranges between 17 and 30 mm (mean, 23.4 mm). The caliber of the main pulmonary artery is between 20 and 30 mm (mean, 26.4 mm). The sum of the diameters of the left and right main branches is greater than the diameter of the main pulmonary artery.

Three-dimensional (3D) volume-rendered computerized tomographic (CT) images emphasize the central location of the bifurcation of the main pulmonary artery into the left and right pulmonary arteries (Fig. 10.3A). From a frontal view, the right pulmonary artery disappears from view as it passes under the aortic arch. A posterior view with the aorta and spine cut away gives a good illustration of the superior position of the pulmonary arteries in relation to the pulmonary veins (Fig. 10.3B).

Right Pulmonary Artery

The right pulmonary artery is only slightly smaller in caliber than the main artery, as seen in angiograms. It runs a horizontal, sometimes slightly downward, course across the heart image on the frontal view, to the hilum of the right lung, where it divides into superior and inferior branches. It lies behind the ascending aorta and the superior vena cava and in front of the tracheal bifurcation and esophagus (Fig. 10.4).

The right pulmonary artery divides at the right hilum into two main branches: the ascending branch, to the right upper lobe, and the descending branch, to the right middle lobe and the right lower lobe (Figs. 10.5-10.7). The ascending branch of the right pulmonary artery supplies the right upper lobe, coursing upward for a short distance, and divides into three branches: the apical segmental artery, the posterior segmental artery, and the anterior segmental artery.

The apical segmental artery divides into two major rami: the apical and the posterior rami, supplying the apical bronchopulmonary segment of the right upper lobe.

The posterior segmental artery often arises as a trifurcation, with the apical and posterior segmental arteries supplying the posterior bronchopulmonary segment of the right upper lobe. There are two main rami: a posterior ramus and a lateral ramus.

The anterior segmental artery of the right upper lobe supplies the bronchopulmonary segment of the same name and is the most inferior artery of the trifurcation of the ascending branch of the right pulmonary artery. There are two main rami: an anterior ramus and a lateral ramus.

The descending branch of the right pulmonary artery supplies the right middle and lower lobes. It originates at the bifurcation of the right pulmonary artery and is caudally oriented. The first branch is the middle lobe artery and the superior segmental artery of the right lower lobe. The next branches are the basal segmental artery and the anterior basal segmental artery. The parent vessel splits to form the posterior basal segmental artery and the lateral basal segmental artery. Each branch supplies the correspondingly named bronchopulmonary segment of the right lower lobe.

The middle lobe artery arises from the descending branch of the right pulmonary artery, at the opposite aspect of the origin of the superior segmental artery. It has an anteriorly and inferiorly oriented direction, bifurcating into a lateral and a medial segmental artery, which supply the respective bronchopulmonary segments of the right middle lobe (Fig. 10.6).

The superior segmental artery of the right lower lobe courses posteriorly upward and laterally, supplying the upper part of the right lower lobe. The medial basal segmental artery of the right lower lobe arises as the third major branch of the right pulmonary artery and just distally to the point of origin of the superior segmental artery. The anterior basal segmental artery of the right lower lobe arises from the anterolateral aspect of the descending branch of the right pulmonary artery, slightly distal to the point of origin of the medial basal segmental artery. The posterior basal segmental artery of the right lower lobe arises together with the lateral basal segment, as a bifurcation of the descending branch of the right pulmonary artery, reaching the most posterior and dependent portion of the right lower lobe. The lateral basal segmental artery of the right lower lobe arises together with the posterior basal segmental artery as a bifurcation of the descending branch of the right pulmonary artery and supplies the lateral basal bronchopulmonary segment (Fig. 10.8).

Left Pulmonary Artery

The left pulmonary artery is a short continuation of the main pulmonary artery. It runs upward, to the back and to the left, when it turns sharply to the left and caudally to the hilum of the left lung. It lies in front of the descending aorta, beneath the curve of the aortic arch, and is connected to the arch by the ligamentum arteriosum. The left pulmonary artery bifurcates in the left hilum into ascending and descending branches, which supply the left upper and lower lobes, respectively (Figs. 10.9-10.11).

The ascending branch of the left pulmonary artery arises about 2 to 4 cm from the origin of the main artery. It runs cranially and bifurcates into two segmental arteries: the posterior apical segmental artery and the anterior segmental artery to the left upper lobe (Figs. 10.12 and 10.13). The apical posterior segmental artery of the left upper lobe, the larger artery supplying to the upper lobe, is short and bifurcates into two major rami: apical and posterior, supplying the correspondingly named apical posterior bronchopulmonary segment of the left upper lobe. The apical ramus is medial and the posterior ramus is lateral. The anterior segmental artery of the left upper lobe arises as an inferior branch of the ascending branch of the left pulmonary artery and courses anteriorly. It bifurcates into the anterior and lateral rami, supplying the named portions of the anterior bronchopulmonary segment of the left upper lobe.

The descending branch of the left pulmonary artery courses downward into the lung as a smooth continuation of the main left pulmonary artery, giving origin to the lingular artery, the superior segmental artery, and to the arteries to the basal bronchopulmonary segments of the left lower lobe (Figs. 10.13-10.15).

The lingular artery arises about 2 cm distal from the origin of the ascending branch of the left pulmonary artery and laterally and immediately bifurcates in two segmental components: the superior and inferior lingular segmental arteries.

The segmental arteries to the left lower lobe are like those of the contralateral lower lobe, but there are usually three instead of four bronchopulmonary segments in the left. The superior segmental artery is posterior and arises distally to the lingular artery. The anterior and medial segmental arteries are combined and called anteromedial basal segment, being larger than the anterior or medial basal segmental artery of the right lower lobe. The posterior basal segmental artery arises with the lateral basal segmental artery as a bifurcation of the descending branch of the left pulmonary artery and proceeds inferiorly and posteriorly to the posterior bronchopulmonary segment. The lateral basal segmental artery proceeds inferiorly and laterally to supply the lateral bronchopulmonary segment.

Computerized Tomographic Appearance

As CT has become a standard method for evaluating pulmonary arterial disease, the appearance of the pulmonary arteries on axial view (cross-section) has become increasingly important. The exact appearance can vary with the orientation of the individual's heart. The main pulmonary artery, right pulmonary artery, and the left pulmonary artery run generally in the axial plane. Depending on the level of the image, one may be able to see all three of these vessels (Fig. 10.16). Above and below the hilum, the segmental branches are usually oriented longitudinally.

One reason for the increasing use of CT is that with improved spatial resolution on the newer multislice scanners, pulmonary emboli (PEs) are easy to visualize. With massive PEs, filling defects may be seen in the right and left pulmonary arteries, a so-called saddle embolus (Fig. 10.17). More often, the diagnosis is made by finding filling defects in the segmental branches. When the segmental arteries are traveling in a cephalad or caudal direction, the filling defect manifests as a low-density circle, often with a rim of contrast around the outside where some blood is reaching the periphery (Fig. 10.17). The sensitivity and specificity of the test have now risen to a level at which angiography is usually reserved for those cases where interventional treatment is being considered.

Pulmonary Microcirculation

The pulmonary circulation plays the role of a universal blood filter among the venous and arterial territories. Particles larger than 75 μm are usually retained at the level of the pulmonary arterioles. The pulmonary arterioles reduce their caliber rapidly from 100 to 50 μm. The sizes of the capillaries are about 8 to 9 μm in diameter and 6 to 18 μm in length. The size of the capillaries varies markedly according to the gravity and position of the individual. Experimentally it was established that particles as large as 400 μm could be recovered in the venous side of the pulmonary circulation, indicating precapillary shunts between pulmonary arteries and veins (Fig. 10.18).

The peripheral pulmonary artery and alveolar capillary network are large vascular beds of about 70 to 90 m^2, in the adult, allowing intimal contact of the blood circulation with the oxygen from the air in the alveoli. The process of O_2-CO_2 exchange is performed by diffusion of the gases through the alveolar and capillary membranes due to a concentration gradient. The pulmonary capillaries develop a dense network enclosed in the alveolar wall. The basic elements of this network, the capillary segments, are short cylindric tubes joined at both ends by two adjacent segments, making a network of hexagonal aspect.

The pulmonary artery, despite high volume and flow, has no capability of lung nutrition. The blood supply to the bronchial connective tissue of the lung is part of the systemic circulation. There is free communication between the capillaries of the pulmonary and bronchial systems, and these capillary beds may drain into either the systemic venous system through the azygos vein or through the pulmonary veins into the left atrium. The interrelation of the two circulations at the capillary level provides a potential shunt, which can serve to prevent elevation of capillary hydrostatic pressure, should an increase in either right or left atrial pressure occur unilaterally. The bronchial vessels can provide collateral circulation to the lungs when the pulmonary arterial supply is interrupted (Fig. 10.18).

From the lung hilum, the bronchial arteries go in two different directions. They follow the bronchial tree and the visceral pleura. The bronchial arteries are significant in size up to the terminal bronchiole, where the pulmonary artery circulation takes over the nutrition. The small arteriolar branches of the bronchial artery may, however, extend to the alveolar ducts and occasionally even into the lung parenchyma around the alveolar sacs. The bronchial arteries vascularize the bronchial walls, muscles, glands, and cartilage. The bronchial arteries supply the vasa vasorum to the walls of the pulmonary arteries and the vasa nervorum to the nerves.

The bronchial arteries are unique in that they have dual venous drainage. The blood from the bronchial arteries drains into the systemic veins, bronchial veins, tributaries of the azygos vein, or superior vena cava. From the secondary or tertiary bronchi, the blood of the bronchial arteries drains into the alveolar capillary network at precapillary, capillary, and postcapillary sites and subsequently into the pulmonary veins. Dense vascular networks around the bronchi are arteriolar networks terminating in bronchial capillaries and numerous bronchial venous plexuses with a characteristic irregular shape and course. There are connections of bronchial capillaries with the bronchial venous plexuses, and these vascular components exist either in the bronchial wall or in the peribronchial connective tissue.

These microvascular structures are observed along the entire length of the bronchial tree as far distally as the terminal bronchioles but with decreased numbers in proportion to the reduction of the caliber of the bronchi and bronchioles. The connective tissue around the pulmonary arteries contains a similar vascular network but with less numerous vessels. Most of the blood of juxtapleural bronchial arteries drains into the pulmonary capillary network. A fine vascular network exists in the mediastinal pleura, and the bronchial venous plexus in the pleura communicates with branches of the pulmonary vein. There are precapillary and postcapillary anastomoses between the bronchial artery circulation and the pulmonary arterial circulation. There are communications of bronchial venous plexuses with small branches of the pulmonary vein. Bronchial vessels around the pulmonary vein also communicate with small branches of the pulmonary vein. Therefore, all bronchial venous systems around the airway and blood vessels are connected with the pulmonary vein through small branches. There are direct communications of bronchial venous plexuses with the surrounding alveolar capillaries through small venules, also observed in both bronchi and bronchioles.

Pulmonary Artery Variants

Clinically significant pulmonary arterial variants are rare, and typically associated with congenital heart anomalies, such as Tetralogy of Fallot, in whom they are present in up to 40% of cases. When presenting in young or older adults, they are often incidentally found on cross-sectional imaging.

Interruption of the Pulmonary Artery (Fig. 10.19)

Proximal interruption of a pulmonary artery is a rare, usually isolated congenital anomaly present in about 1 in 200,000 individuals. The interruption occurs at the level of the hilum, and the affected lung is supplied by systemic collaterals. This collateral supply most frequently arises from the bronchial arteries but can also be observed from intercostal, brachiocephalic, subclavian, or internal mammary arteries. The right pulmonary artery is more frequently involved, as the interruption occurs typically contralateral to the aortic arch, with left pulmonary artery interruption being associated with right-sided aortic arch, and other congenital heart anomalies.

Anomalous Origin of the Left Pulmonary Artery

Also known as a pulmonary sling, or aberrant left pulmonary artery, this rare anomaly is characterized by a left pulmonary artery originating from the the extrapericardial segment of the right pulmonary artery. The left pulmonary artery then courses between the trachea and the esophagus before reaching the left hilum. There is an association with complete cartilaginous tracheal rings, tracheal stenosis, and cardiovascular anomalies. The occurrence is estimated at 59 cases per 1,000,000 individuals.

Idiopathic Dilation of the Pulmonary Trunk

Individuals with this rare anomaly are usually asymptomatic and incidentally detected on imaging studies, and the diagnosis is made after the exclusion of other etiologies of pulmonary arterial enlargement above 30 mm diameter. The right and/or left pulmonary arteries may be involved. Affected individuals have normal pulmonary artery pressures. The occurrence is not known.

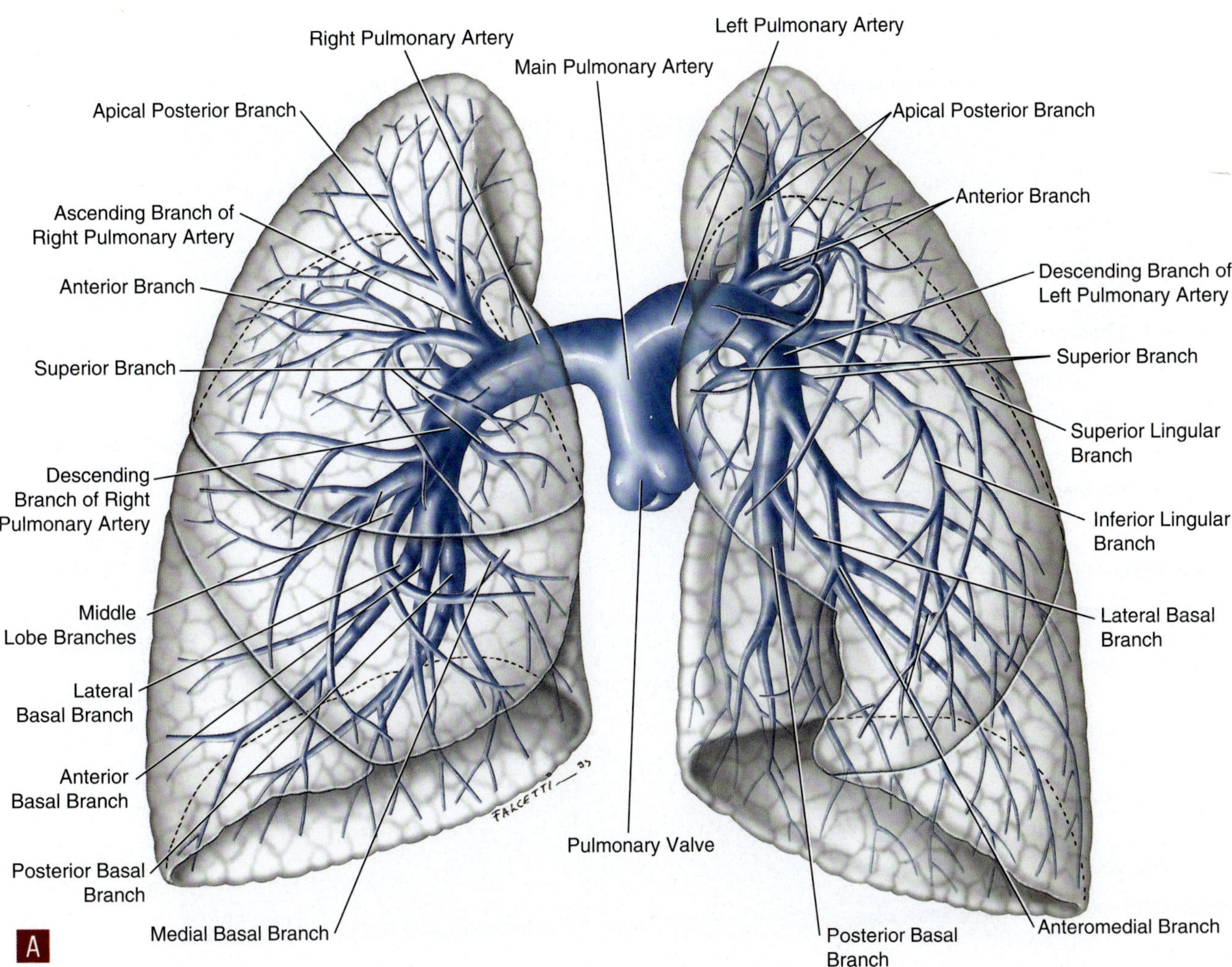

Figure 10.1. A, Diagram showing the distribution of the pulmonary artery in both lungs. B, Corresponding bilateral pulmonary angiogram.

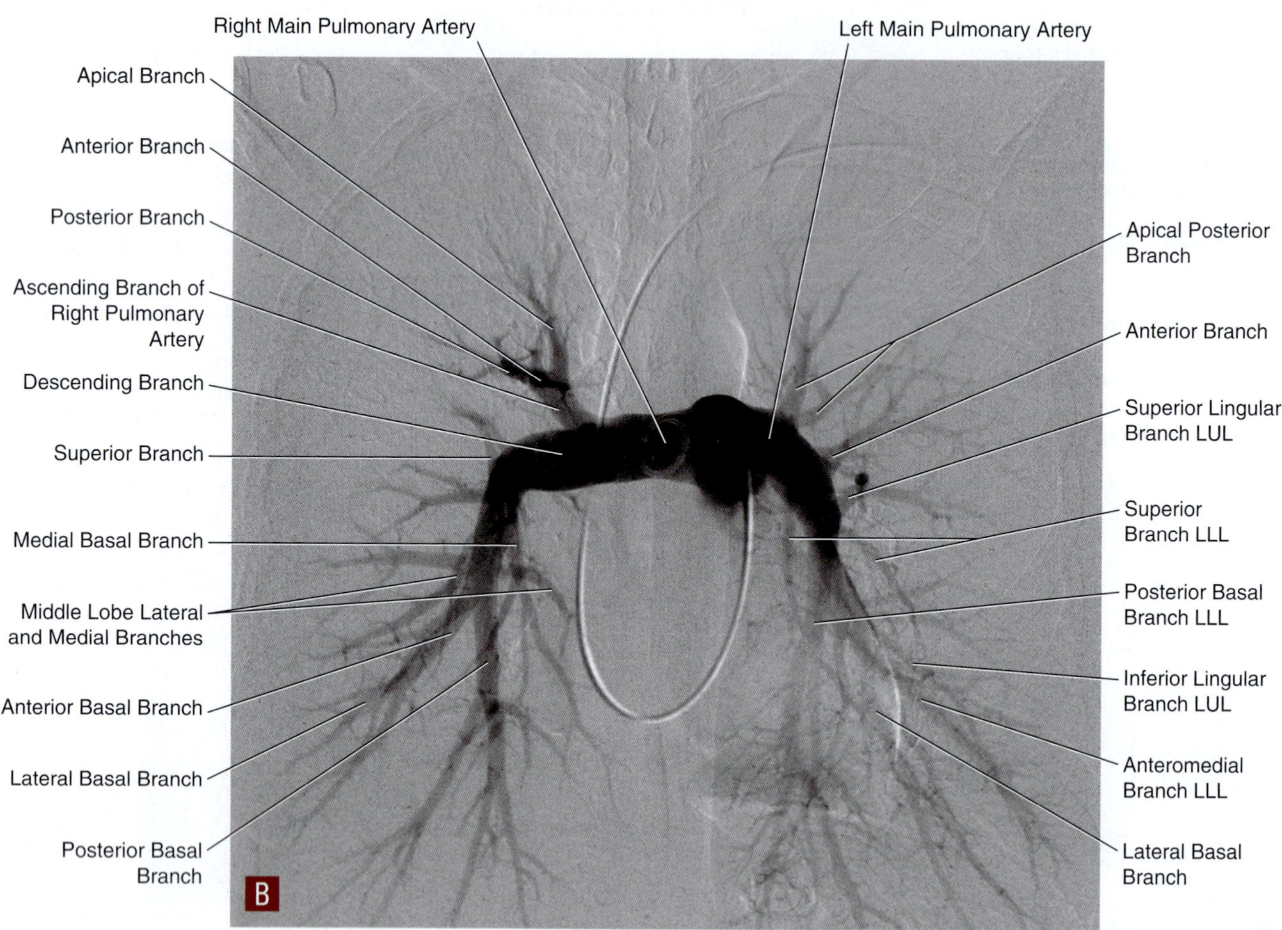

Figure 10.1. *Continued*

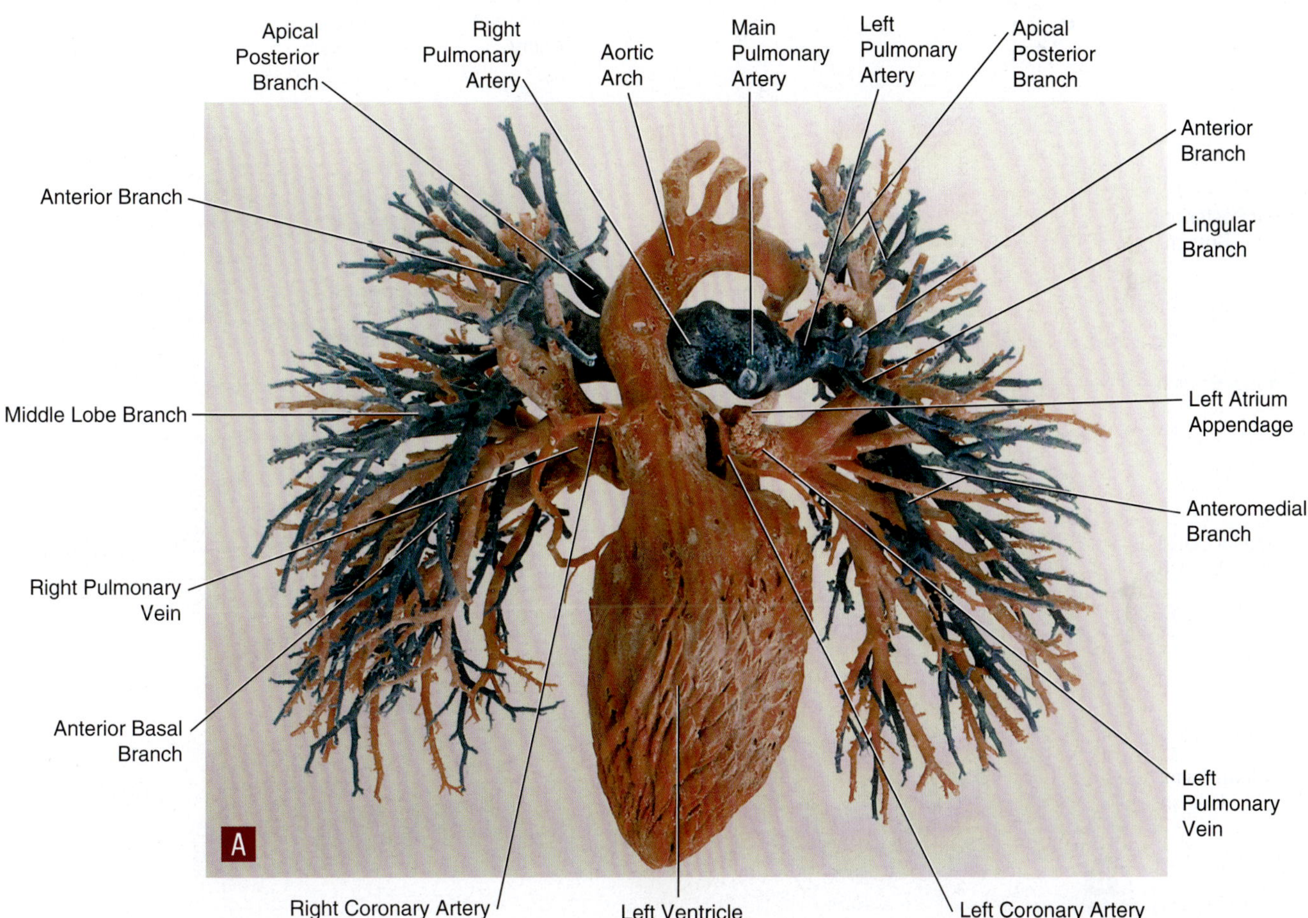

Figure 10.2. A, Anterior view of an injection cast of the pulmonary arteries, pulmonary veins, left ventricle, and aortic arch. B, Posterior view of the cast.

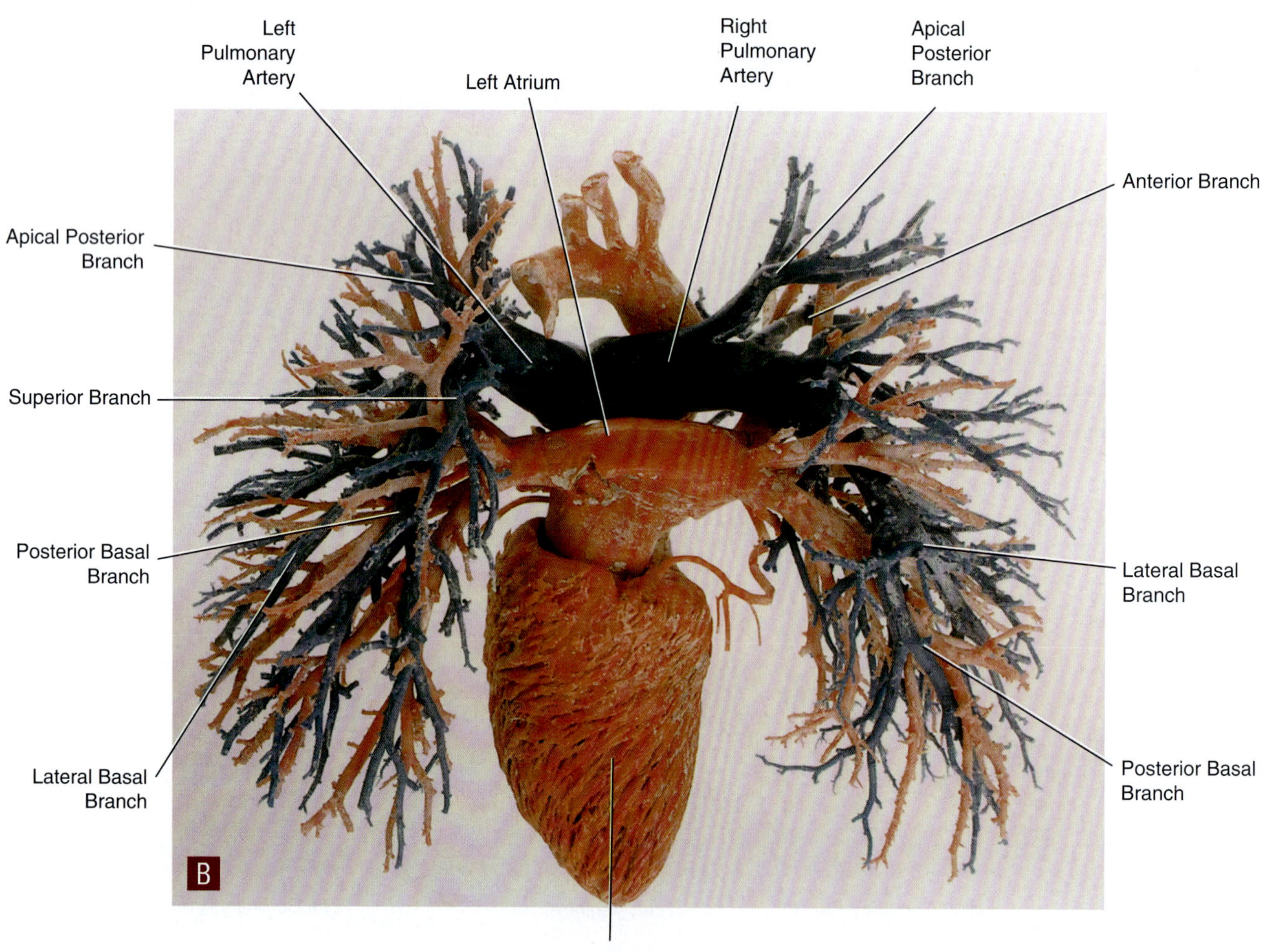

Figure 10.2. *Continued*

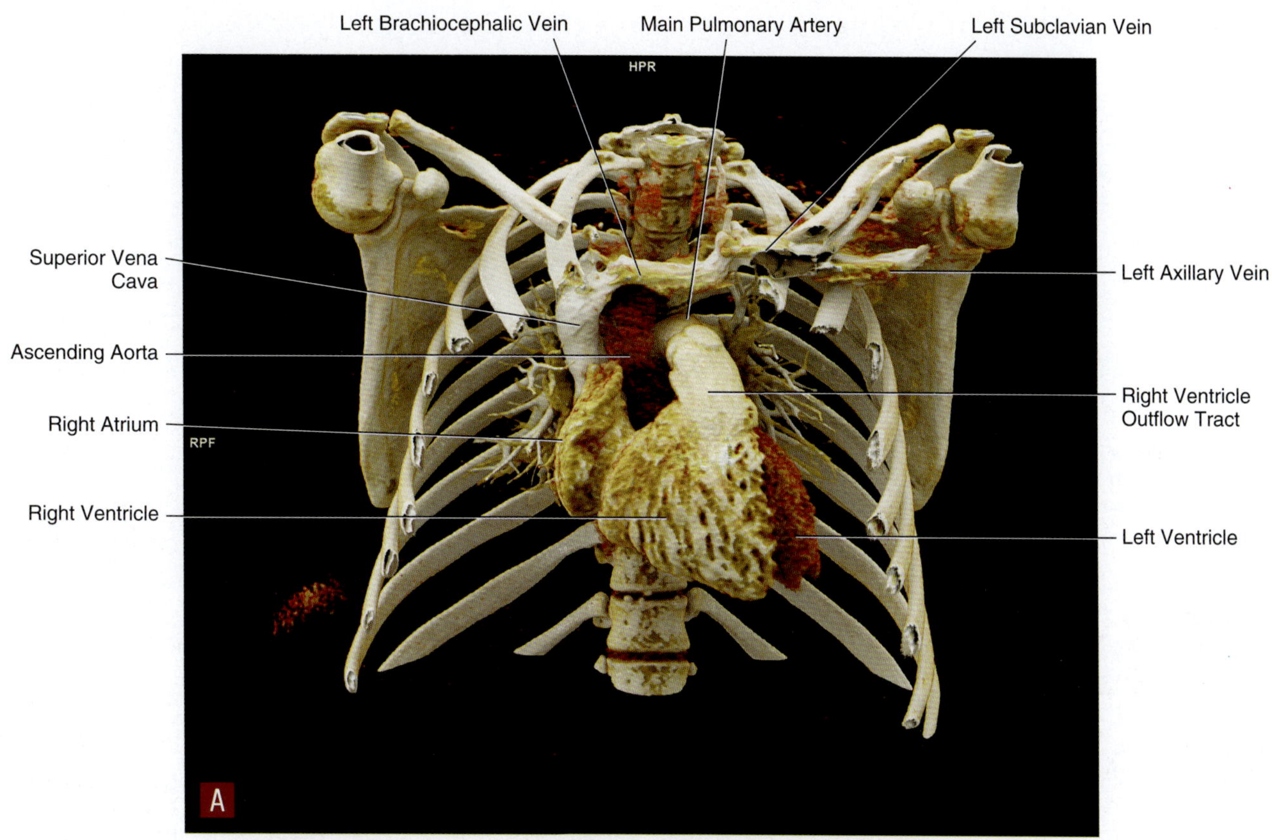

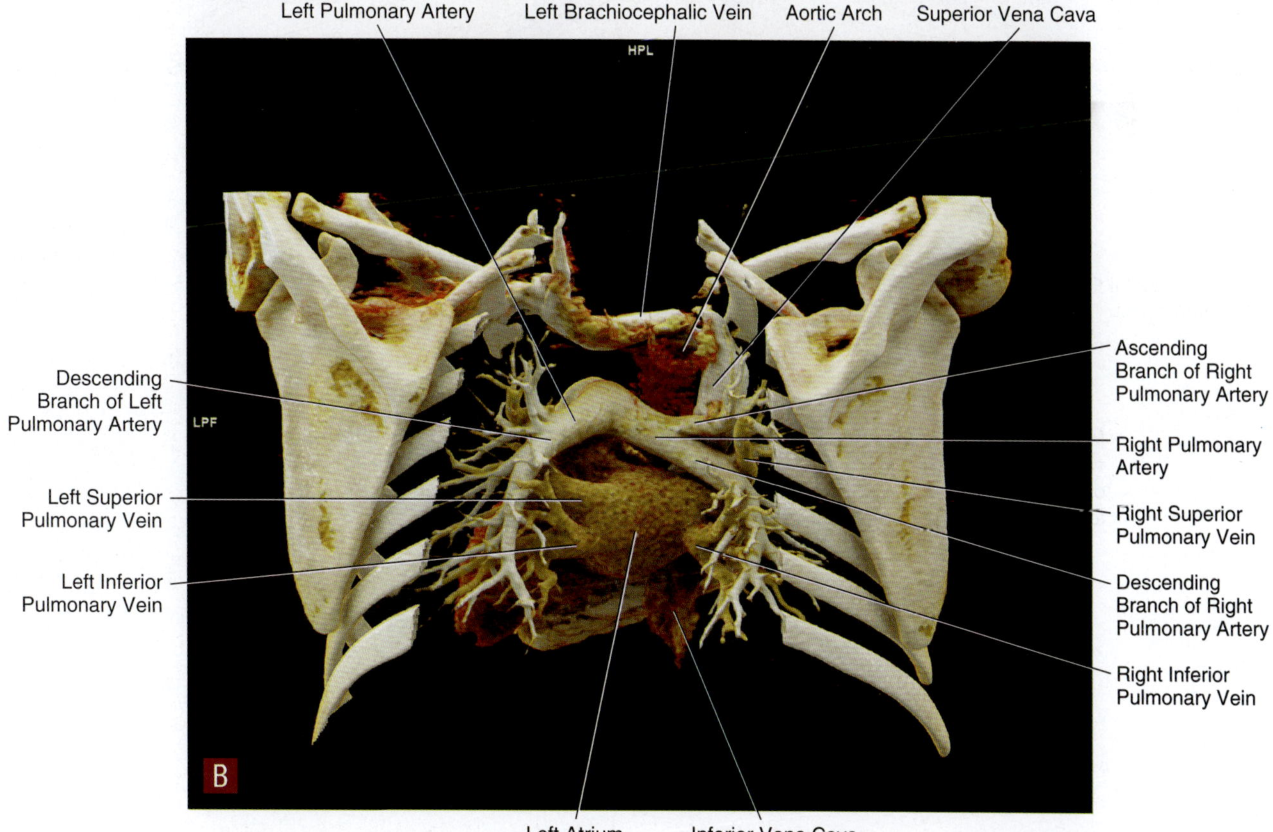

Figure 10.3. **CT angiogram cinematic rendered image.** **A**, Anterior view showing main pulmonary trunk passing posteriorly. **B**, Posterior view with aorta and spine removed. Note location of pulmonary veins draining into the left atrium at a level inferior to the pulmonary arteries.

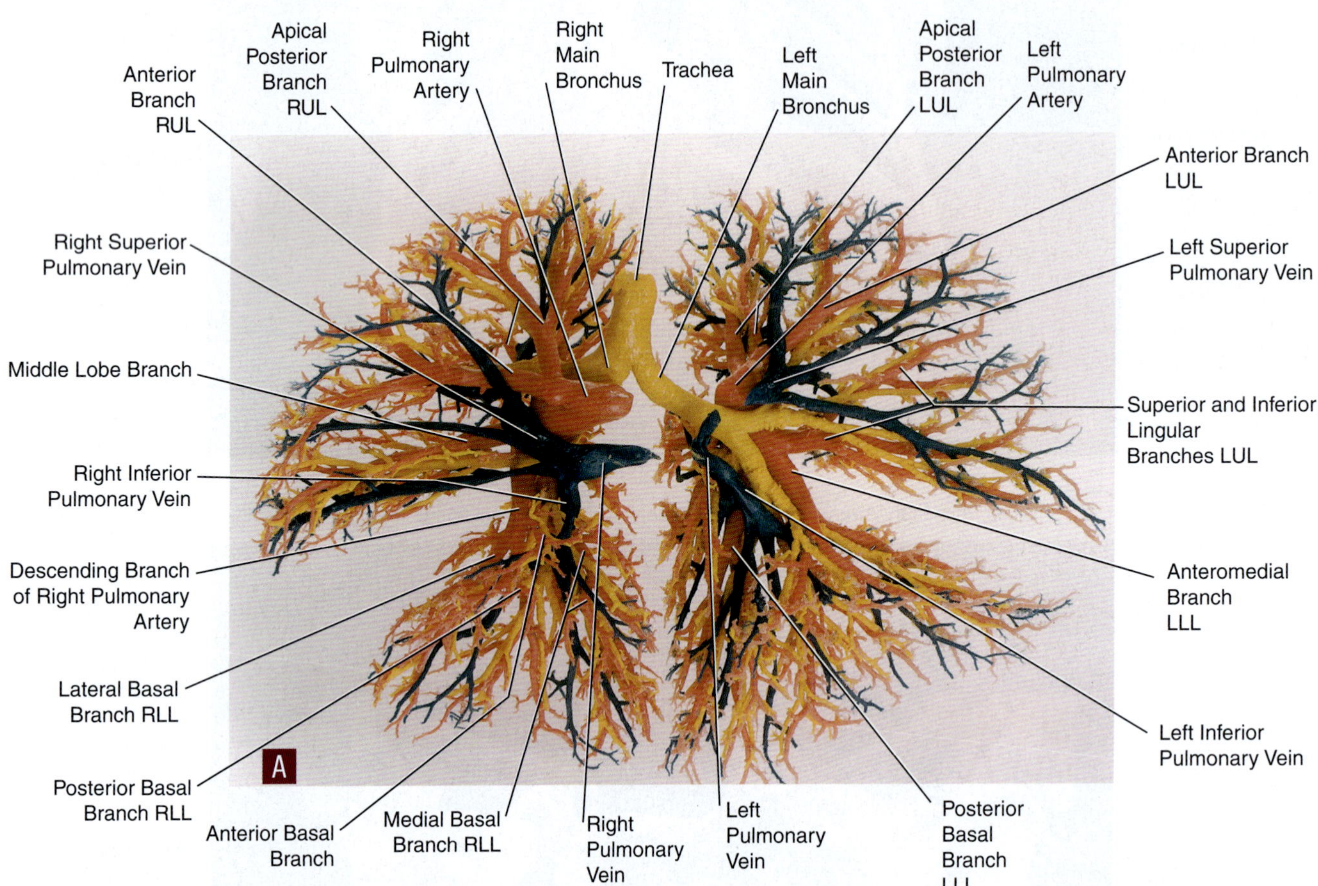

Figure 10.4. **A**, Anterior view of an injection cast of the pulmonary arteries, pulmonary veins, and tracheobronchial tree. **B**, Posterior view of the cast. Some degree of deformation of the structures is seen because of technique artifacts. AUL, apical upper lobe; LLL, left lower lobe; LUL, left upper lobe; RLL, right lower lobe; RUL, right upper lobe.

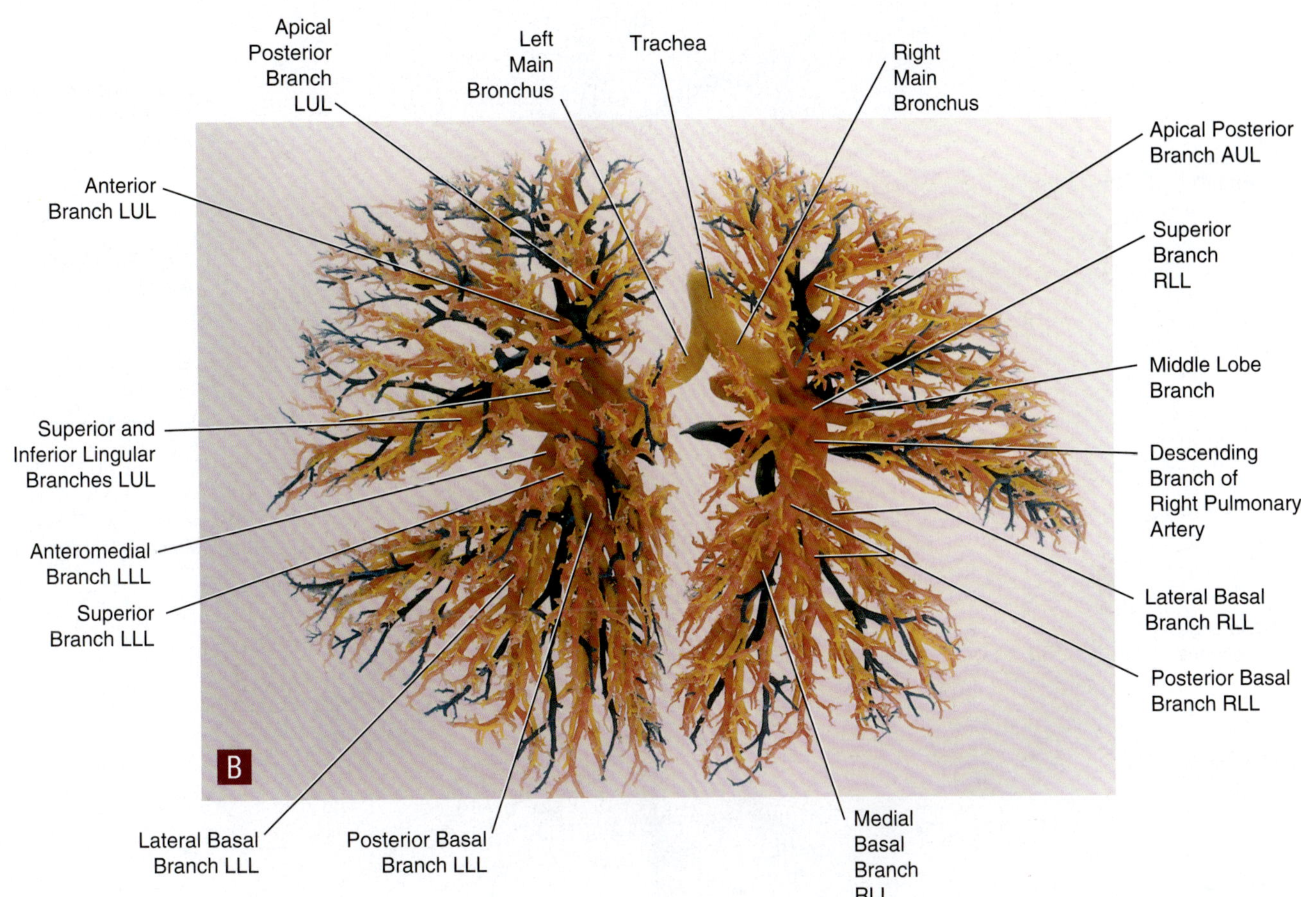

Figure 10.4. *Continued*

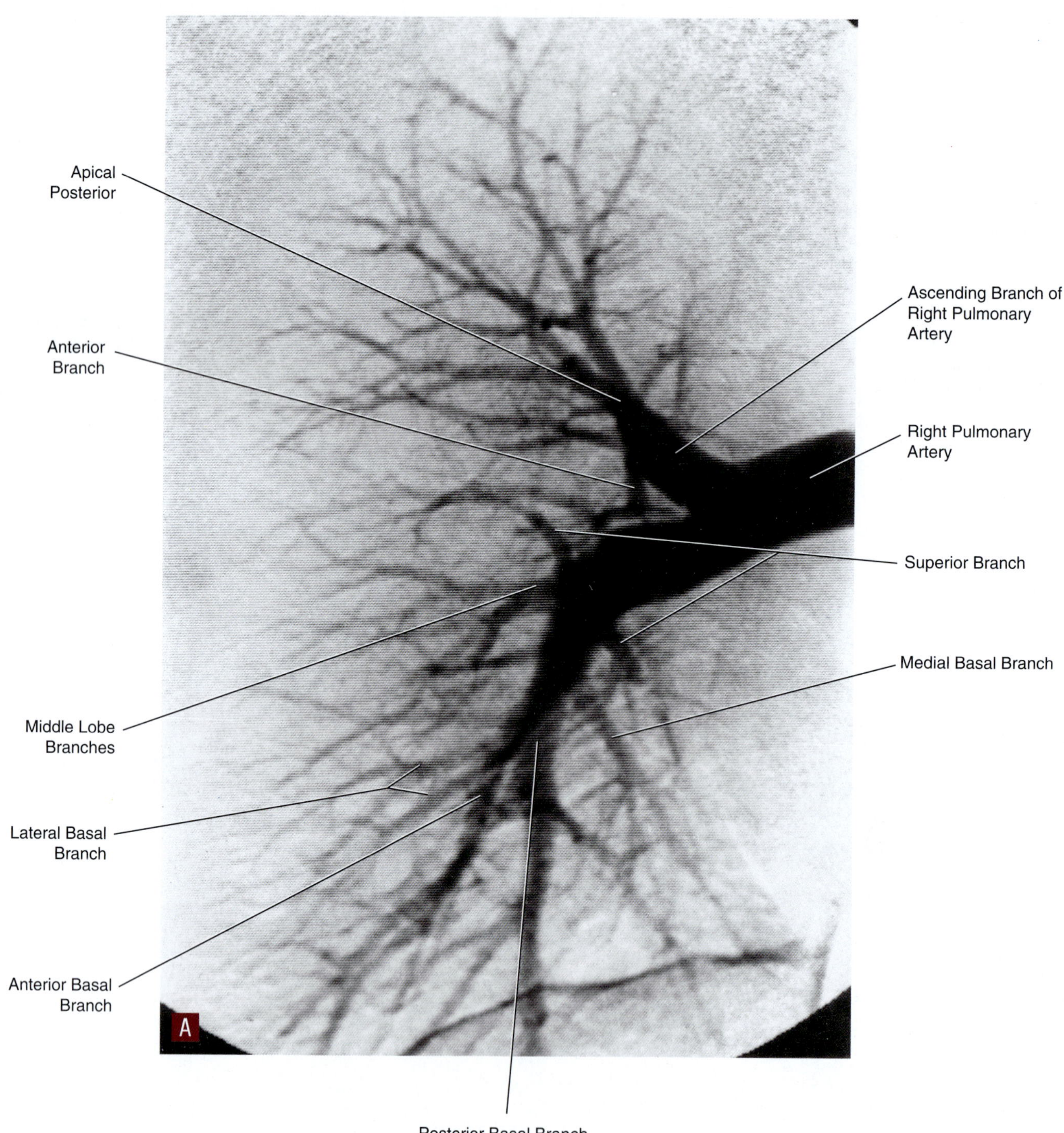

Figure 10.5. **A**, Anterior view of an angiogram of the right pulmonary artery. **B**, Late-phase angiography showing the right pulmonary veins.

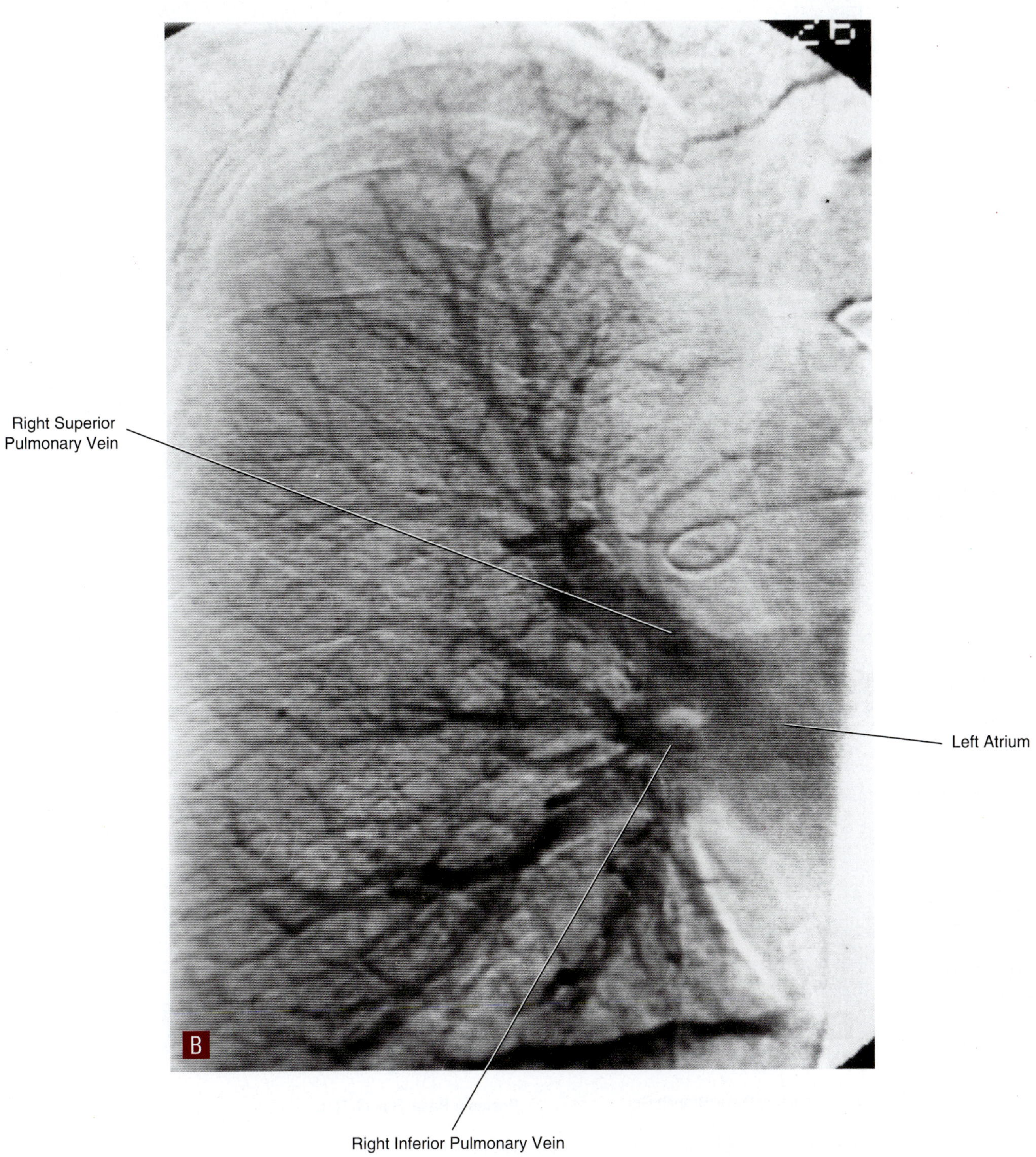

Figure 10.5. *Continued*

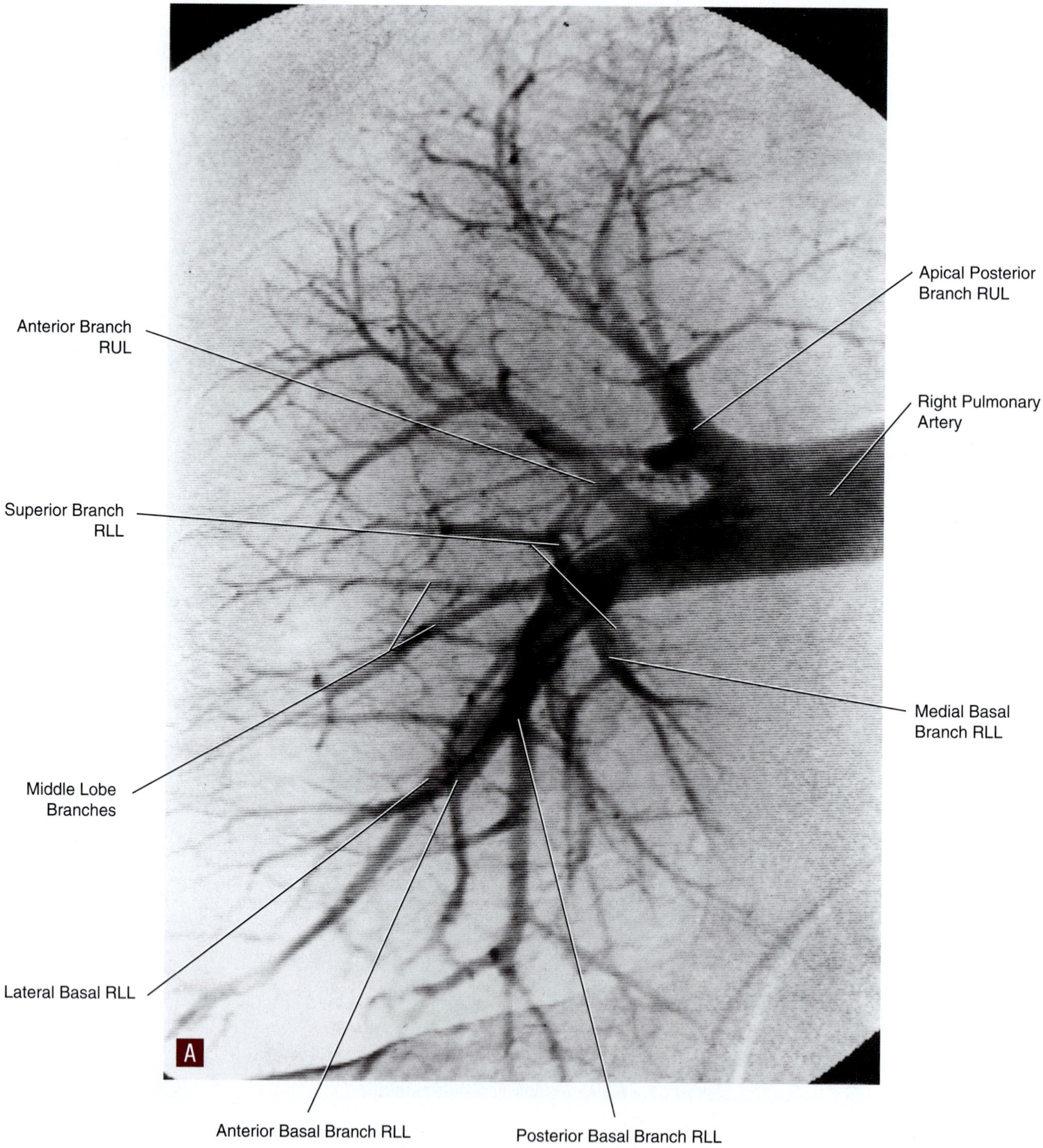

Figure 10.6. **A**, Anterior view of an angiogram of the right pulmonary artery. **B**, Late-phase angiography showing the right pulmonary veins. **C**, Right oblique view of the angiogram of the right pulmonary artery. **D**, Right oblique view of the late phase of the angiography showing the pulmonary veins. RLL, right lower lobe; RUL, right upper lobe.

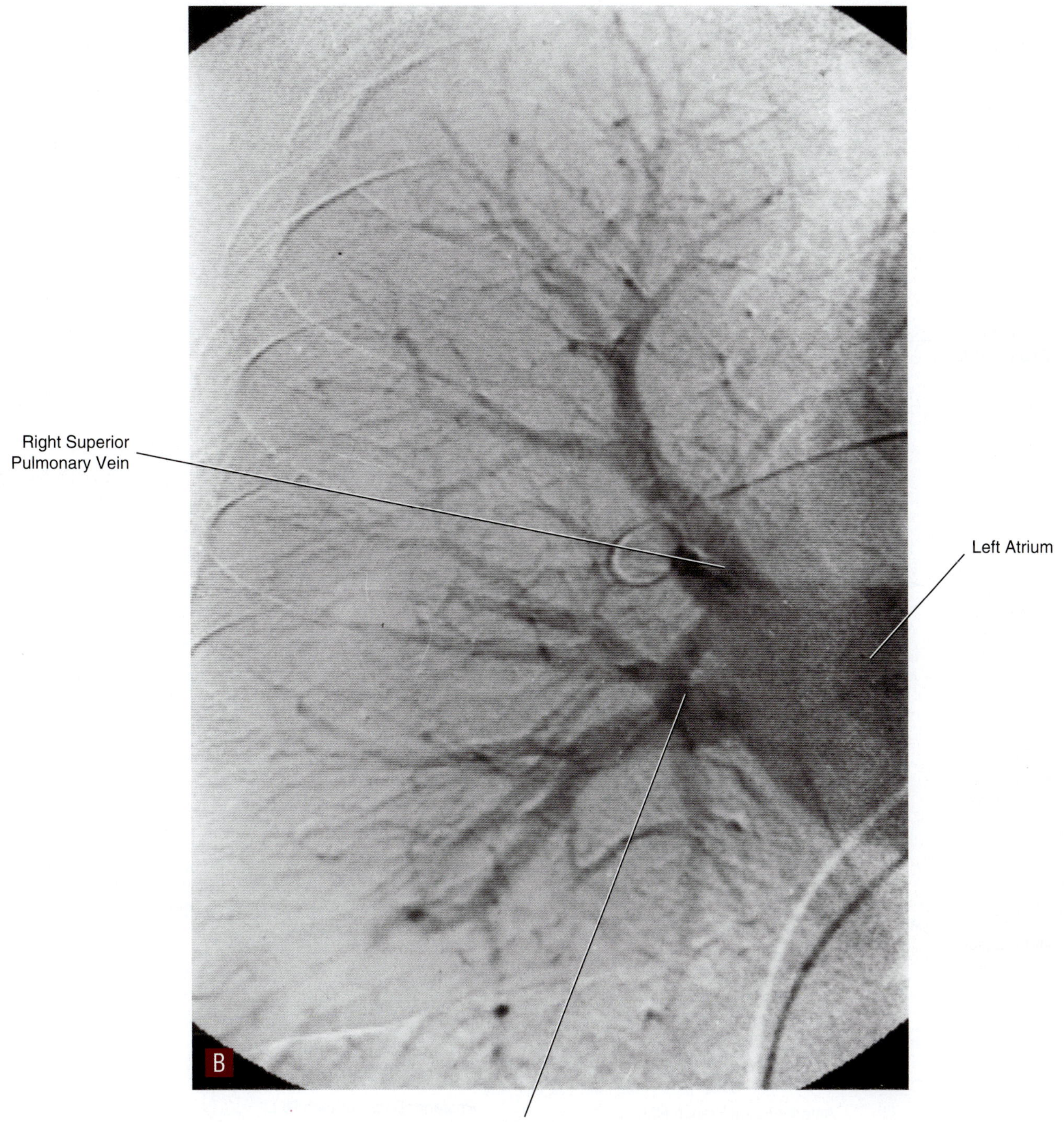

Figure 10.6. *Continued*

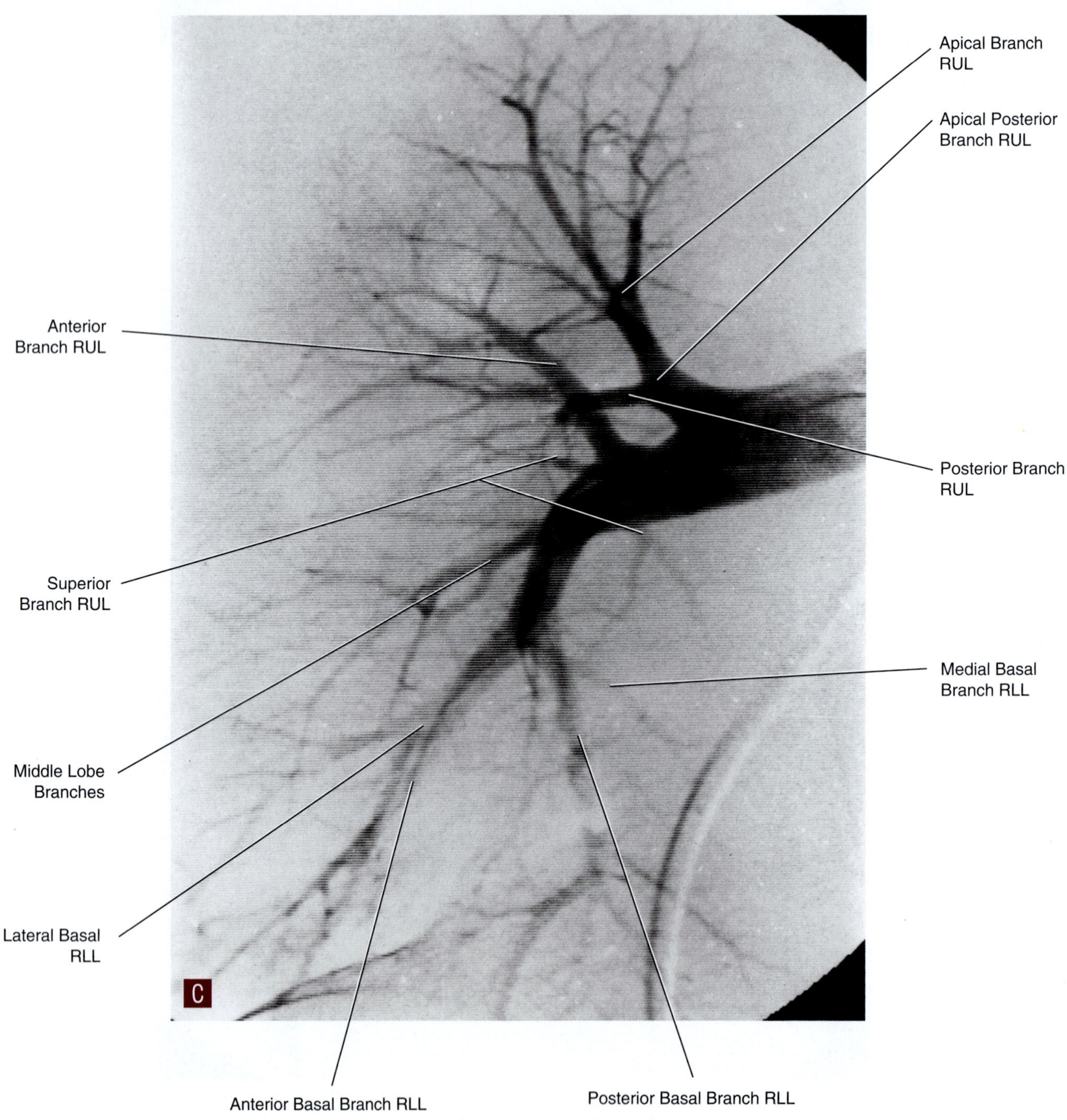

Figure 10.6. *Continued*

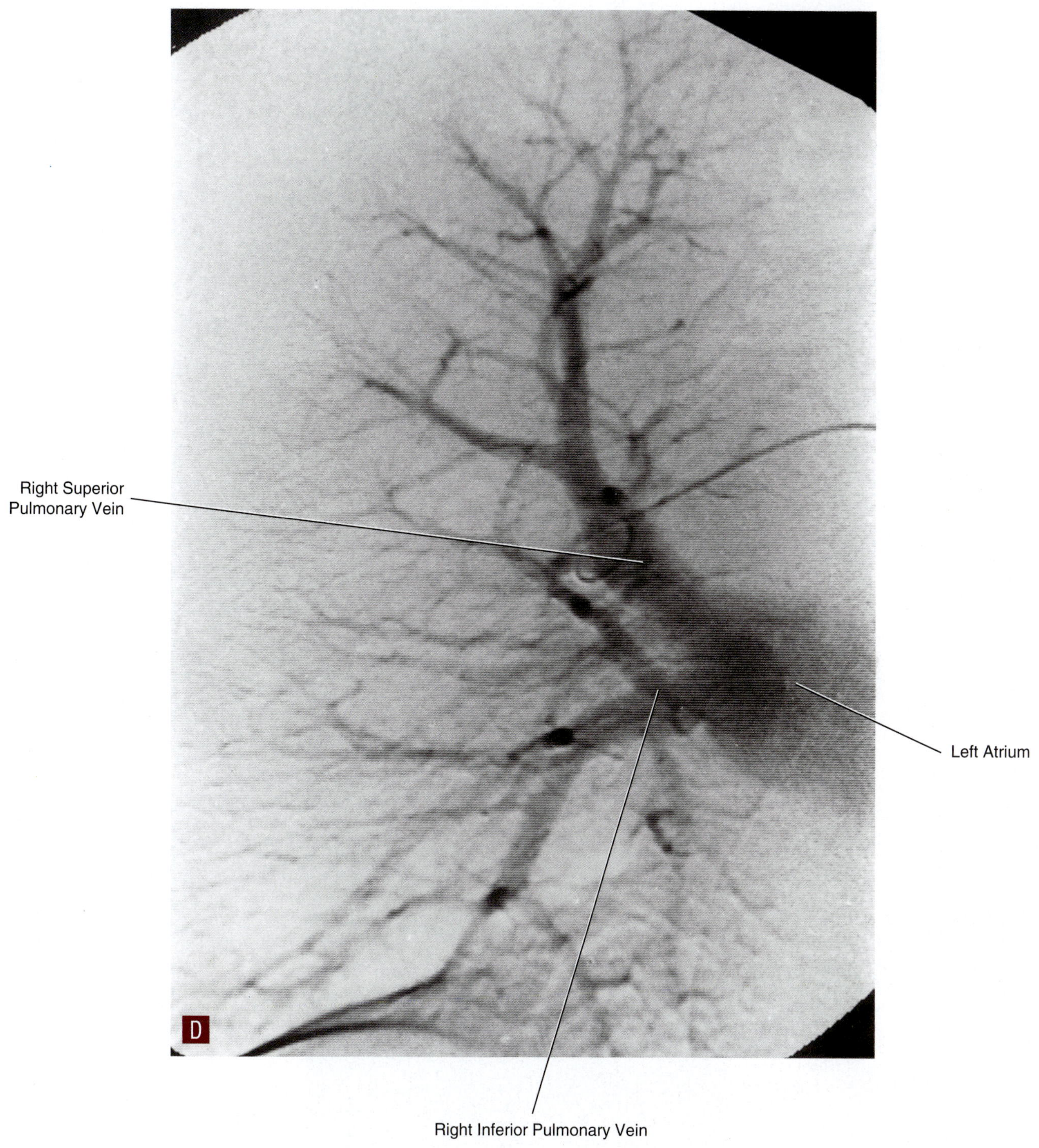

Figure 10.6. *Continued*

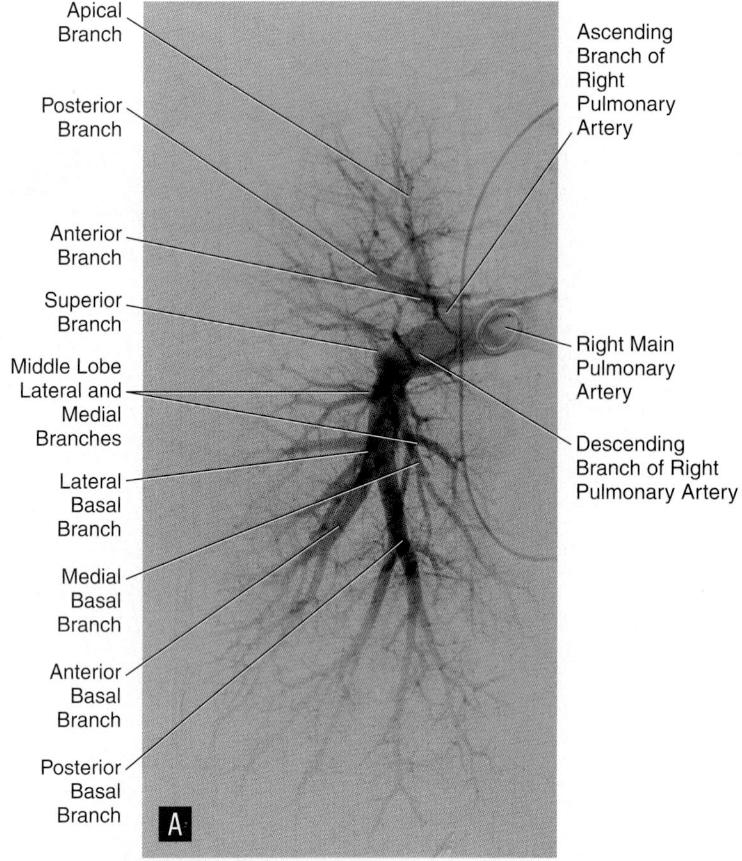

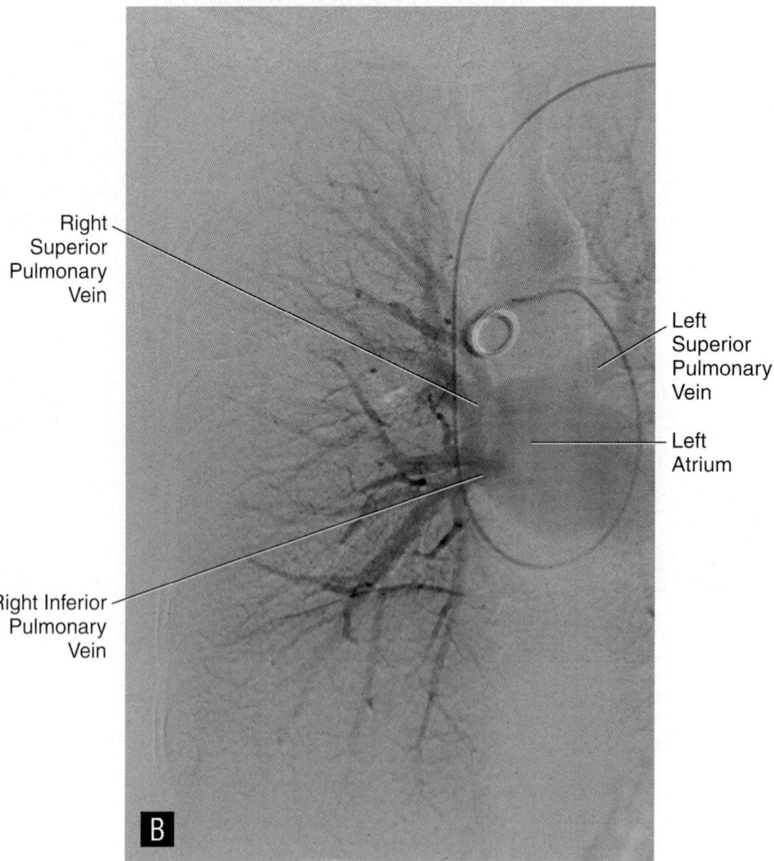

Figure 10.7. **A**, Anterior view of an angiogram of the right pulmonary artery. **B**, Late-phase angiography showing the right pulmonary veins.

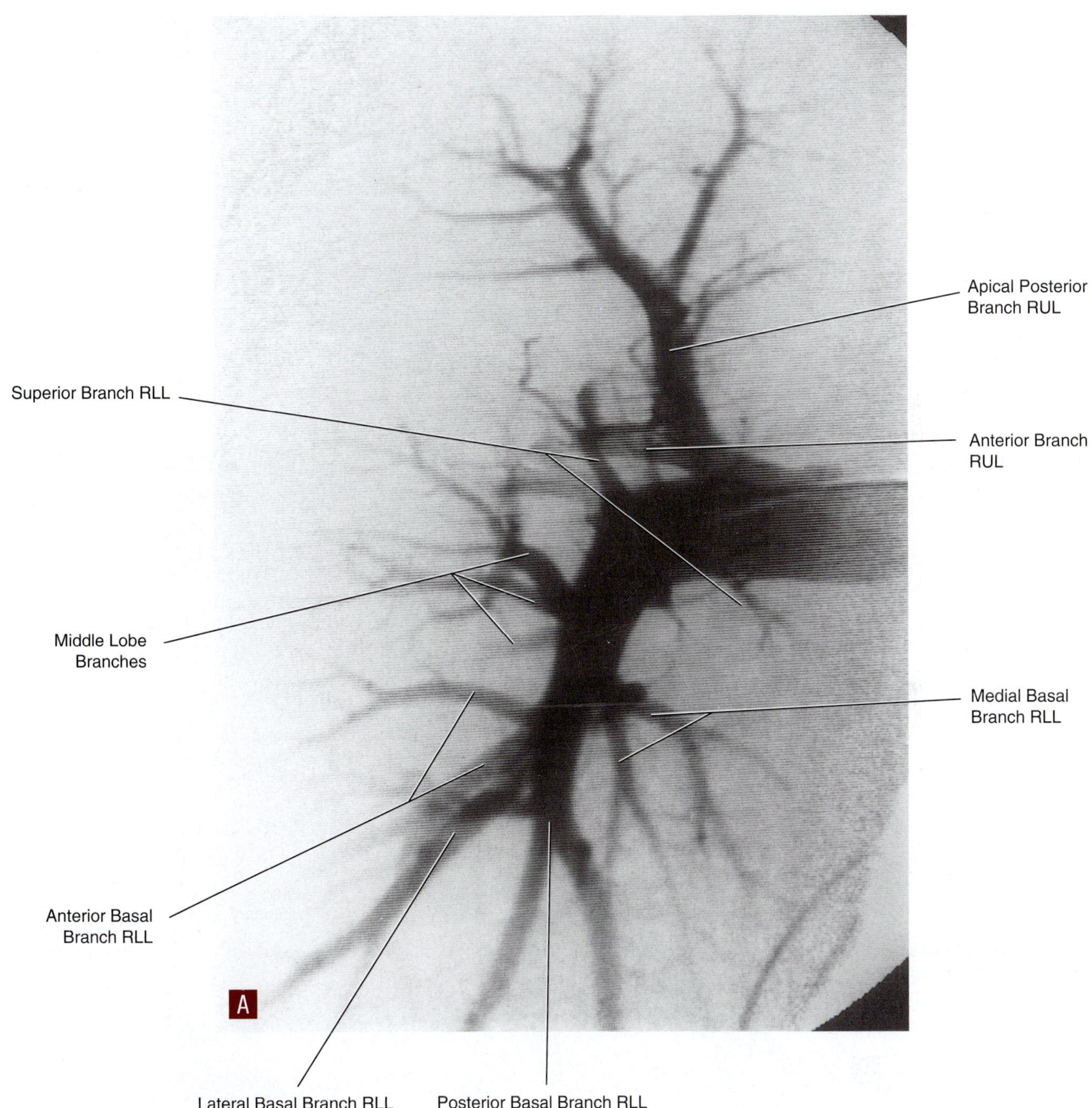

Figure 10.8. **A**, Early phase of the anterior view of an angiogram of the right pulmonary artery. **B**, Later phase of the right pulmonary angiography. **C**, Late phase of the right pulmonary angiography showing the pulmonary veins. RLL, right lower lobe; RUL, right upper lobe.

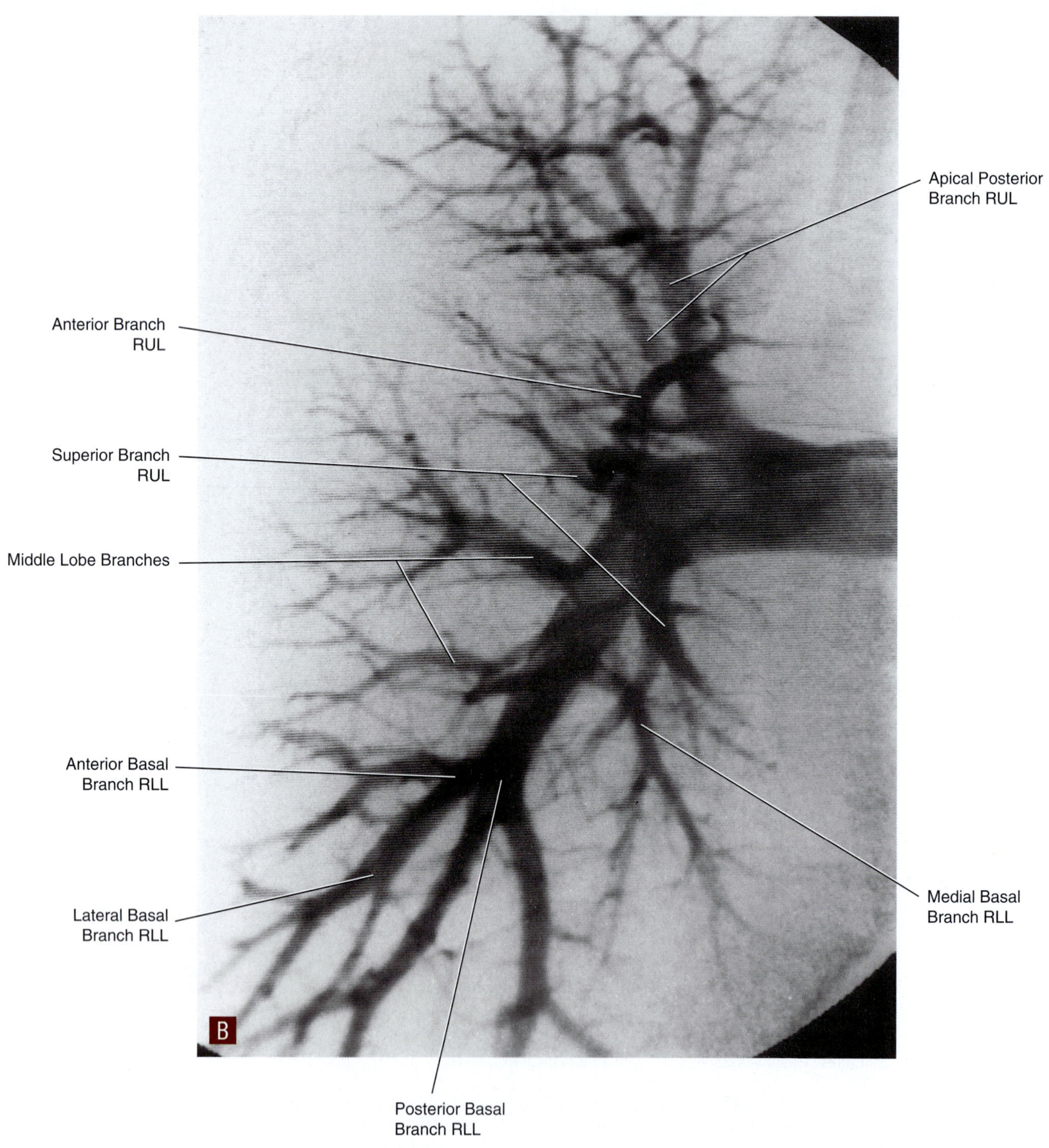

Figure 10.8. *Continued*

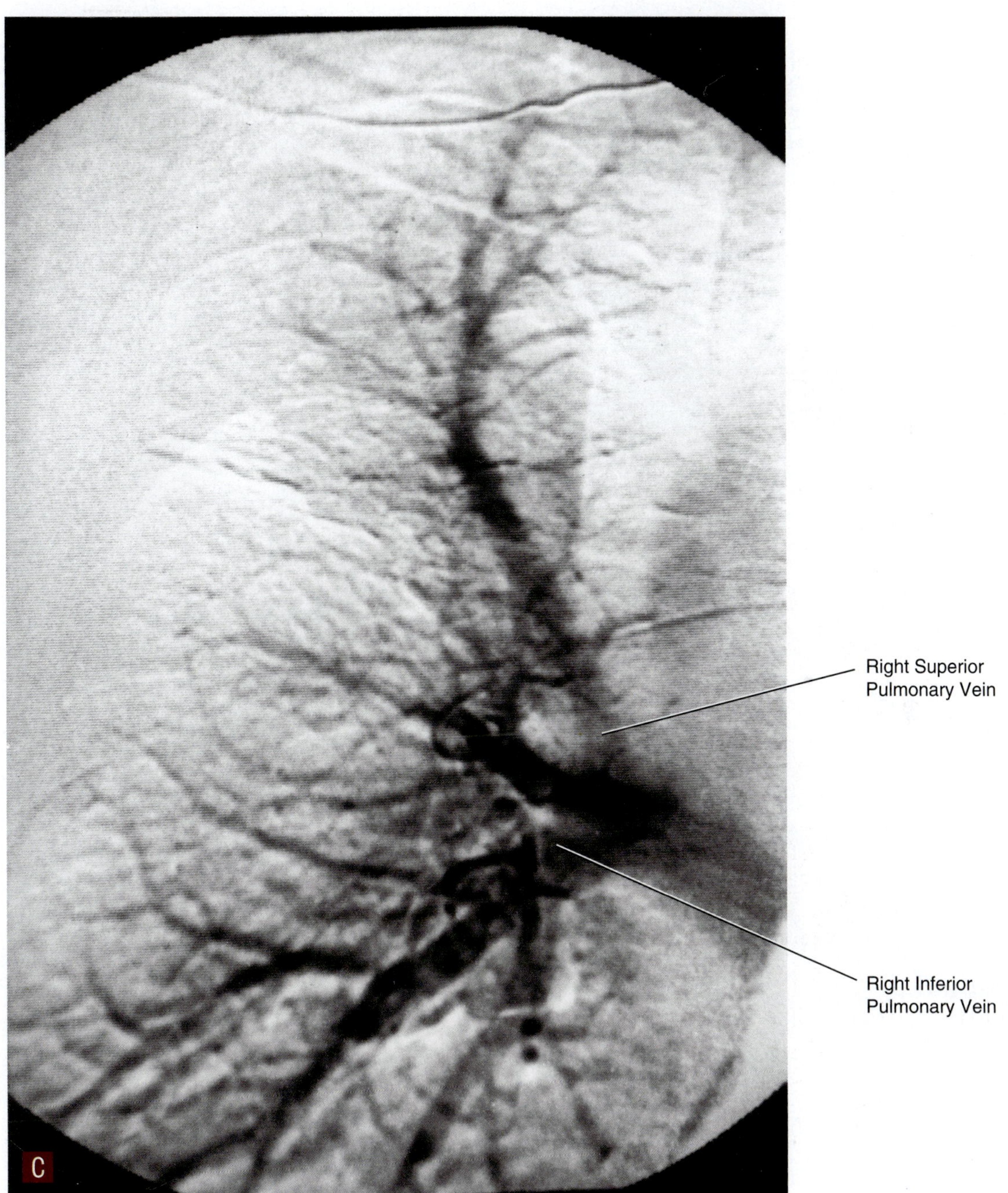

Figure 10.8. *Continued*

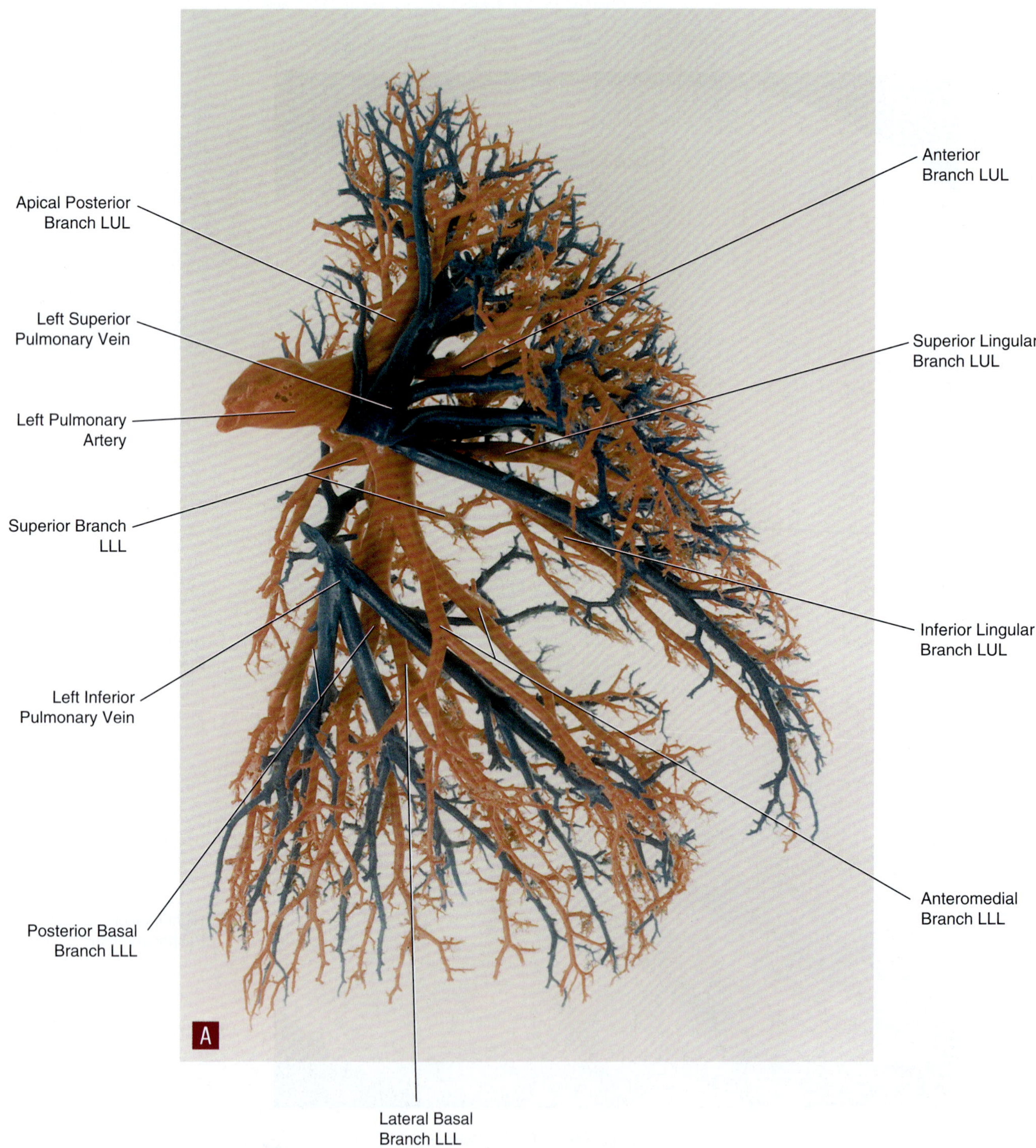

Figure 10.9. A, Anterior view of an injection cast of the left pulmonary artery and pulmonary veins. B, Posterolateral view of the cast. LLL, left lower lobe; LUL, left upper lobe.

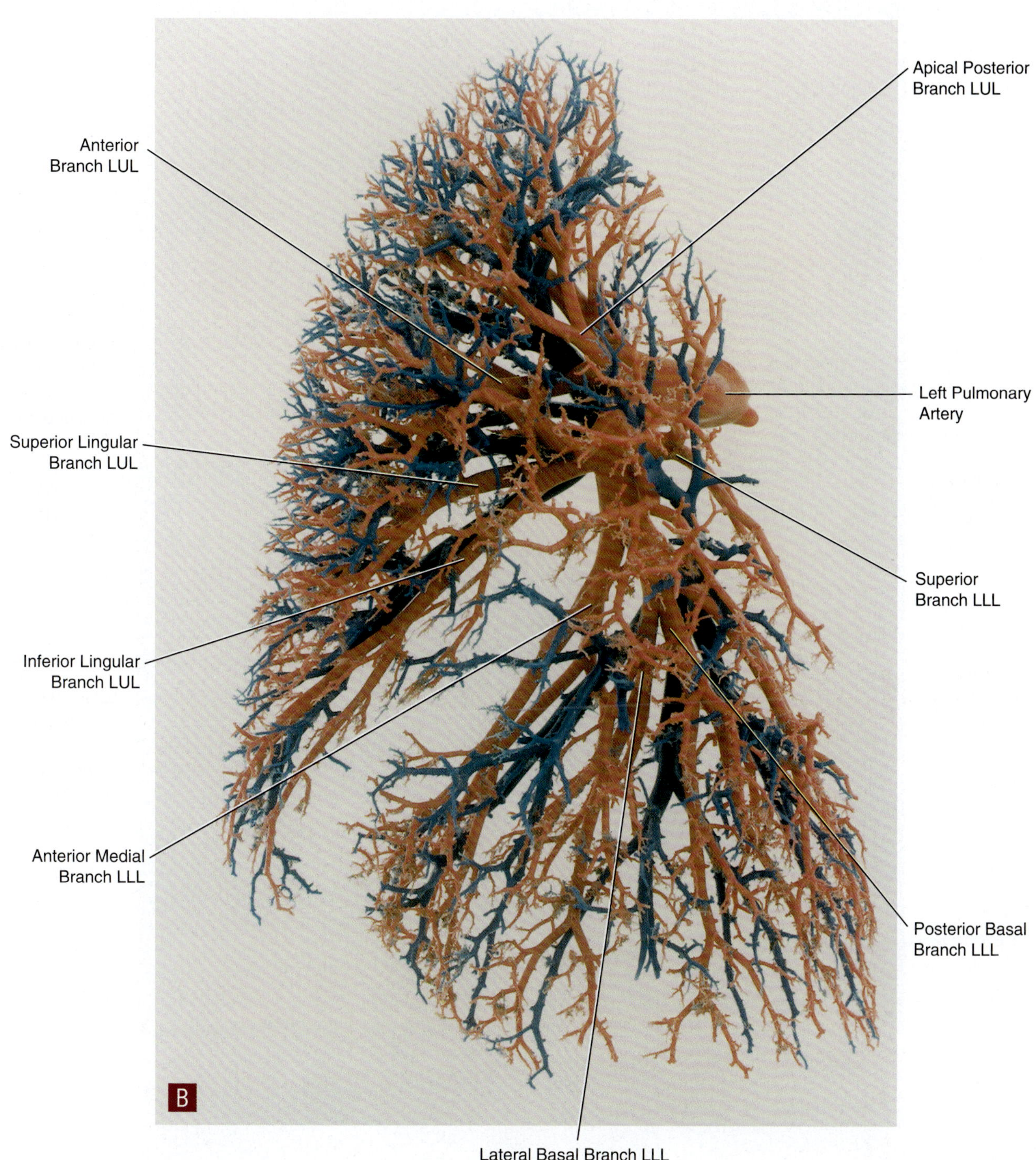

Figure 10.9. *Continued*

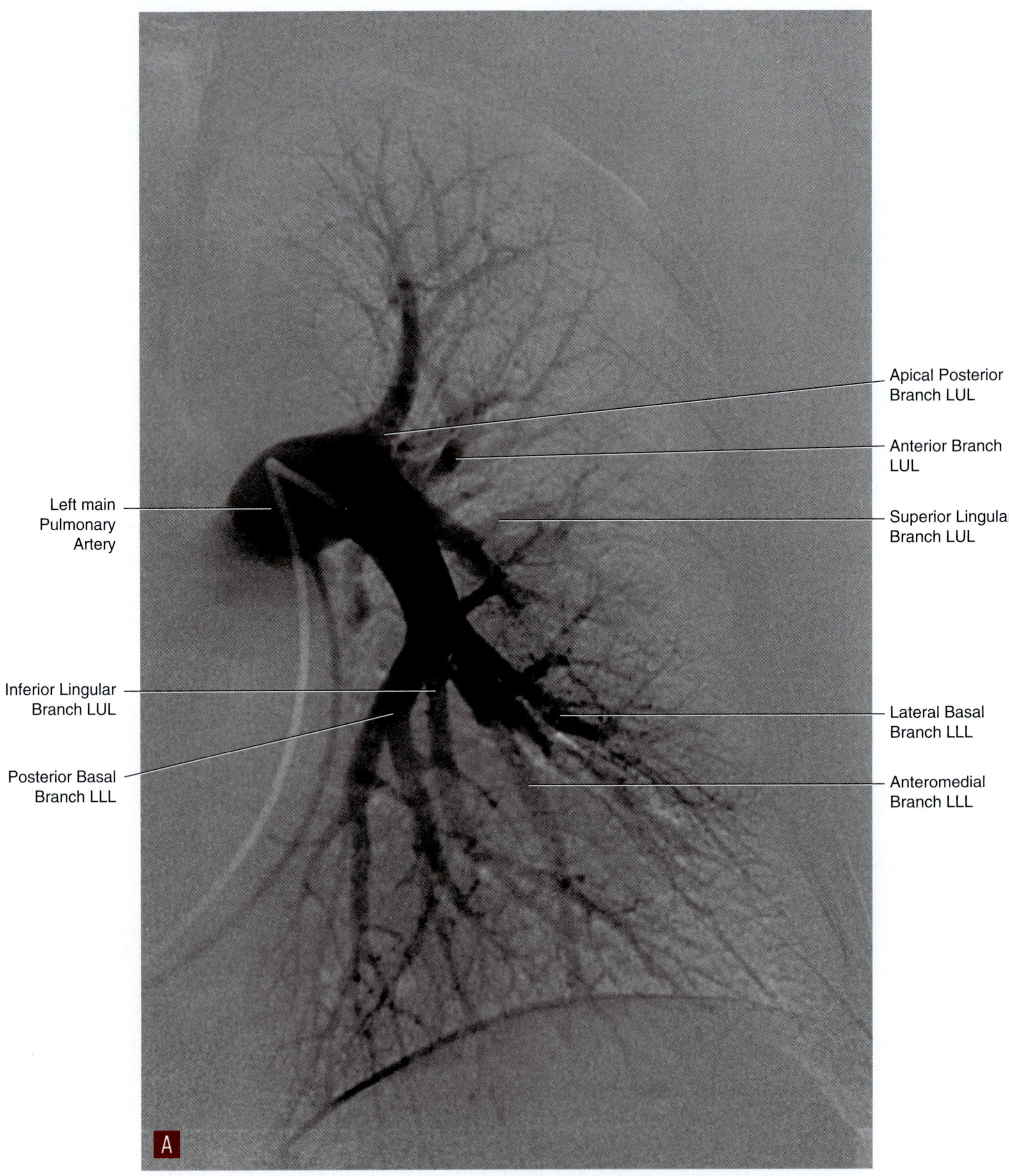

Figure 10.10. A, Anterior view of the early phase of the angiogram of the left pulmonary artery. B, Late phase of the left pulmonary angiogram showing the pulmonary veins.

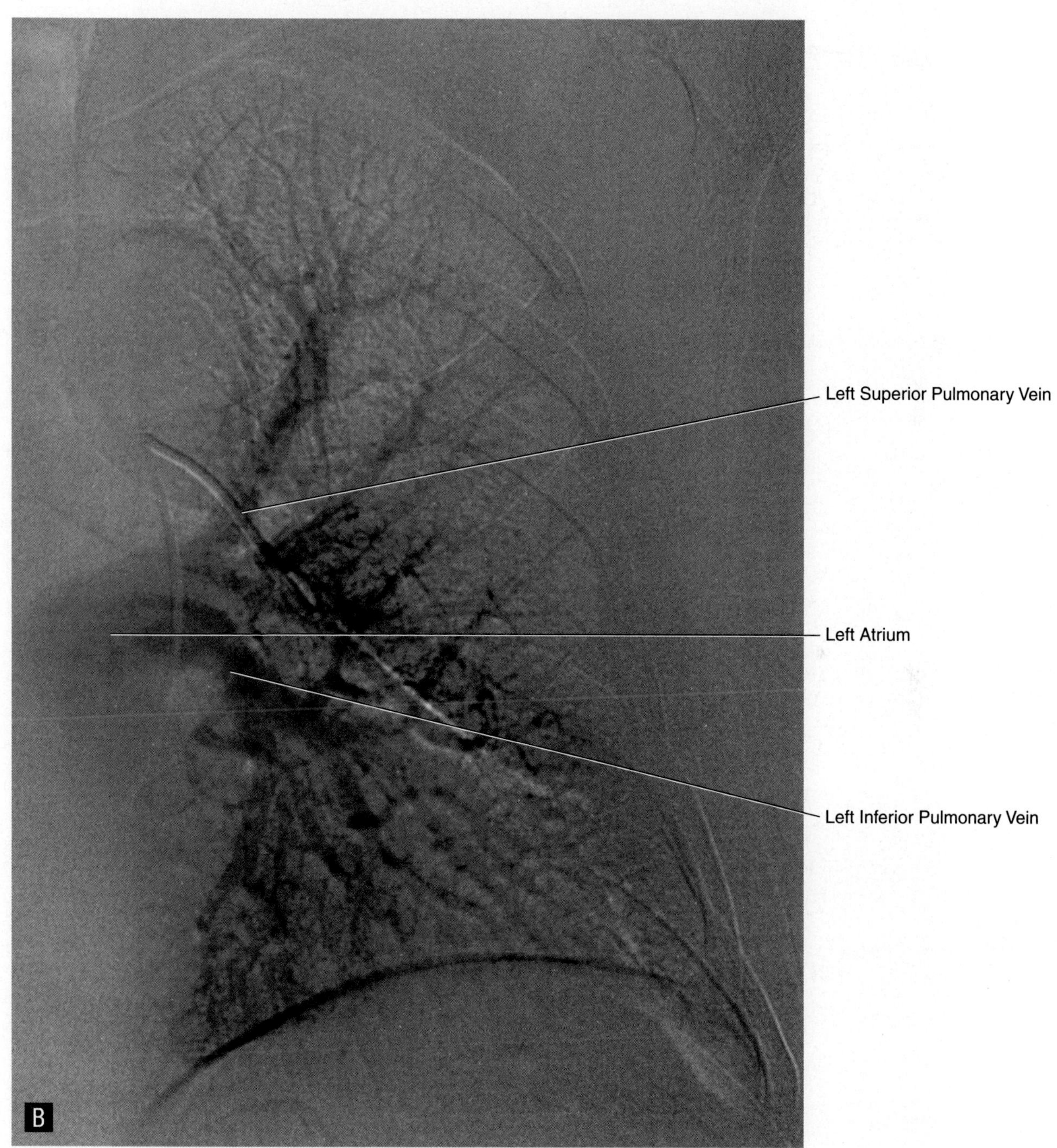

Figure 10.10. *Continued*

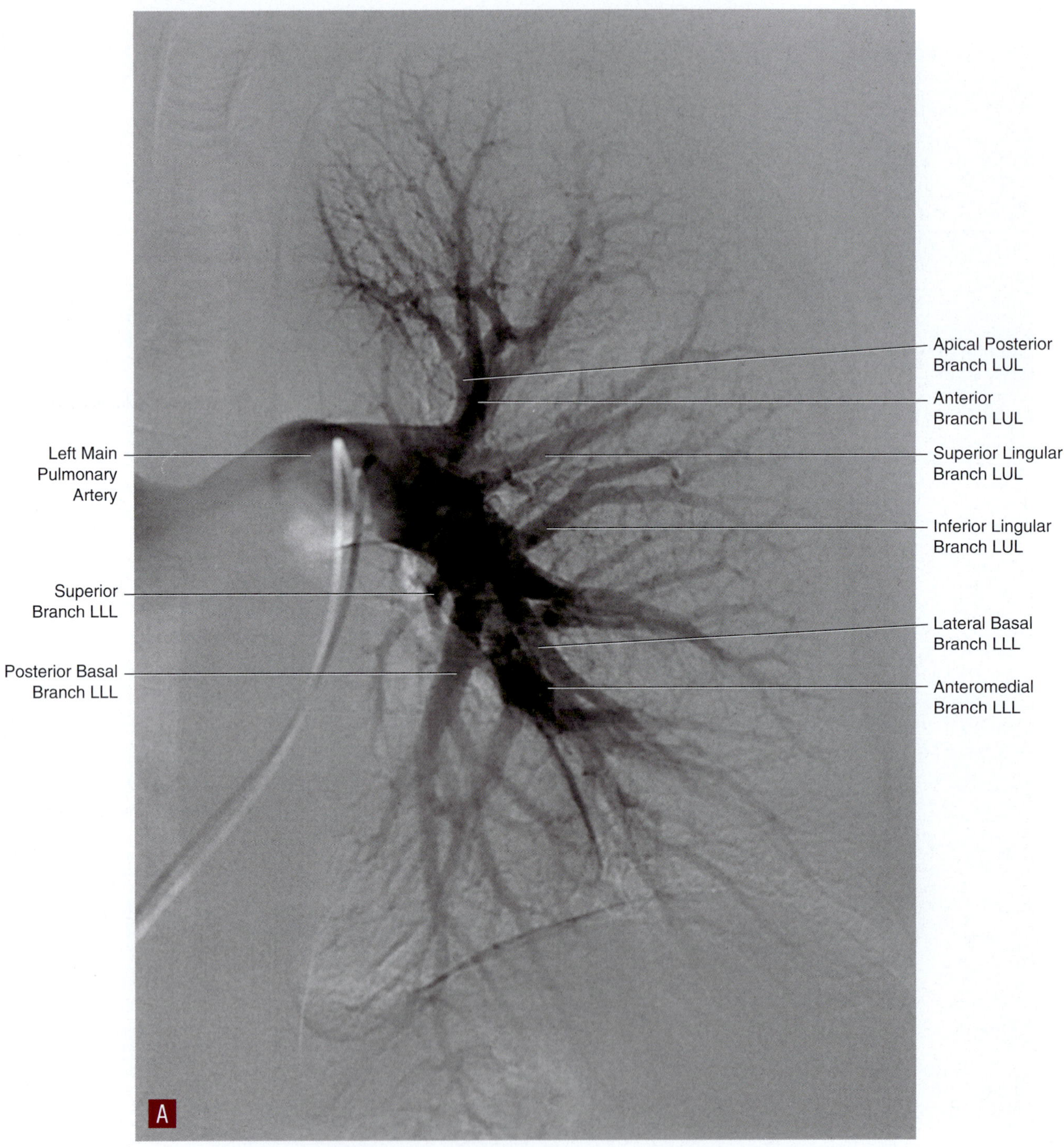

Figure 10.11. A, Left oblique angiography of the left pulmonary artery. B, Late phase of the left angiography showing the pulmonary veins.

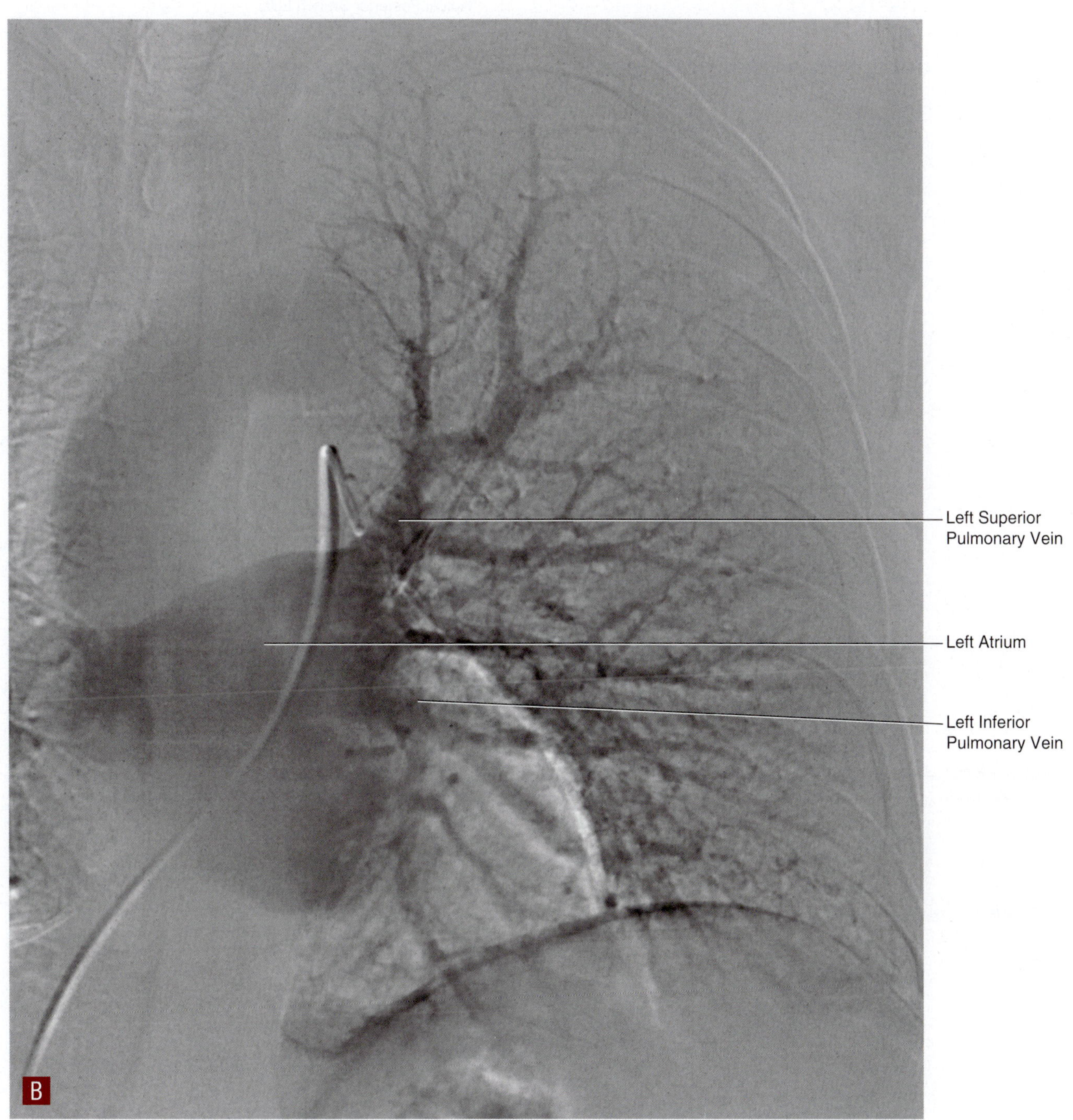

Figure 10.11. *Continued*

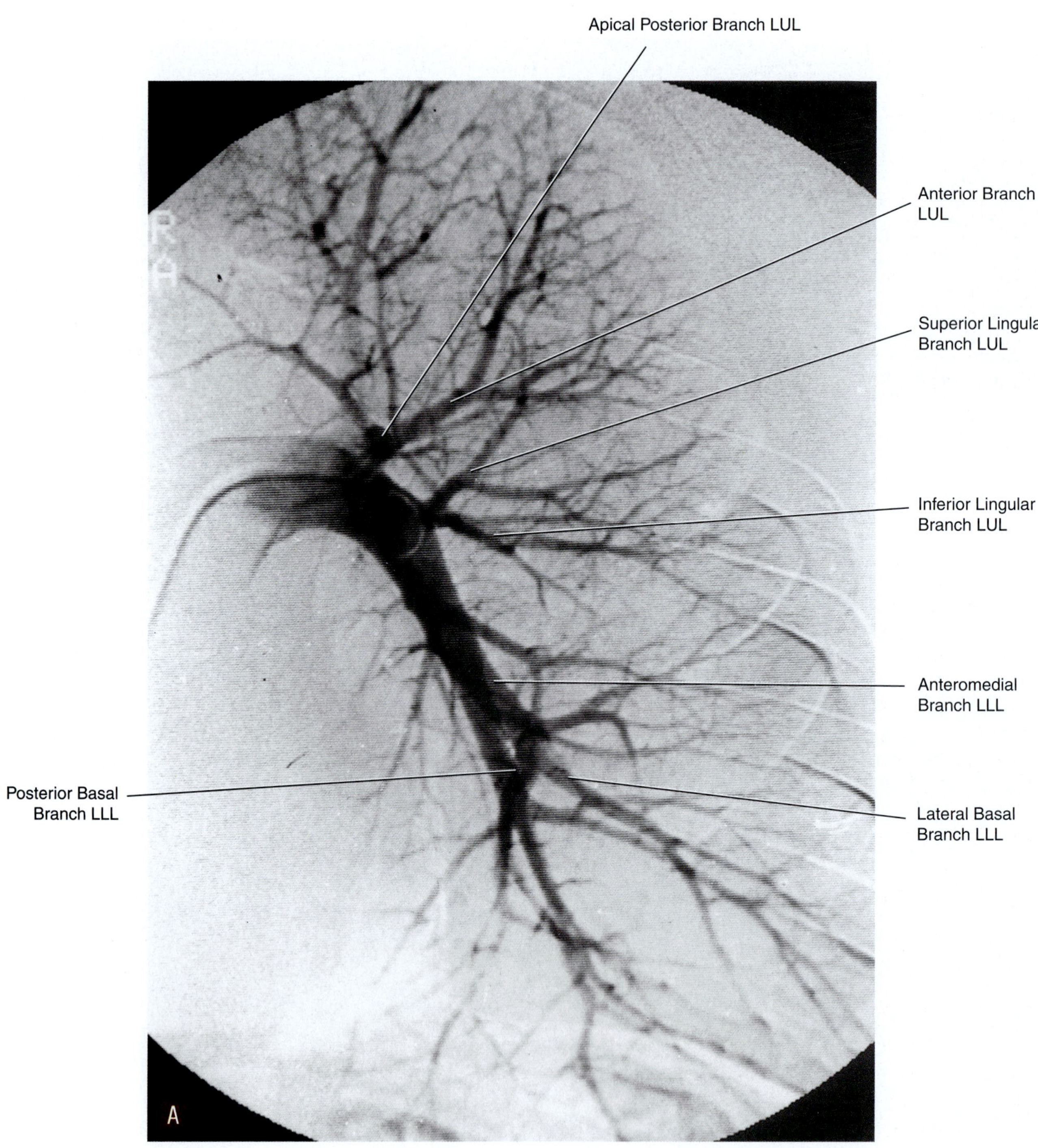

Figure 10.12. **A**, Left oblique angiography of the left pulmonary artery. **B**, Late phase of the left angiography showing the pulmonary veins. LLL, left lower lobe; LUL, left upper lobe.

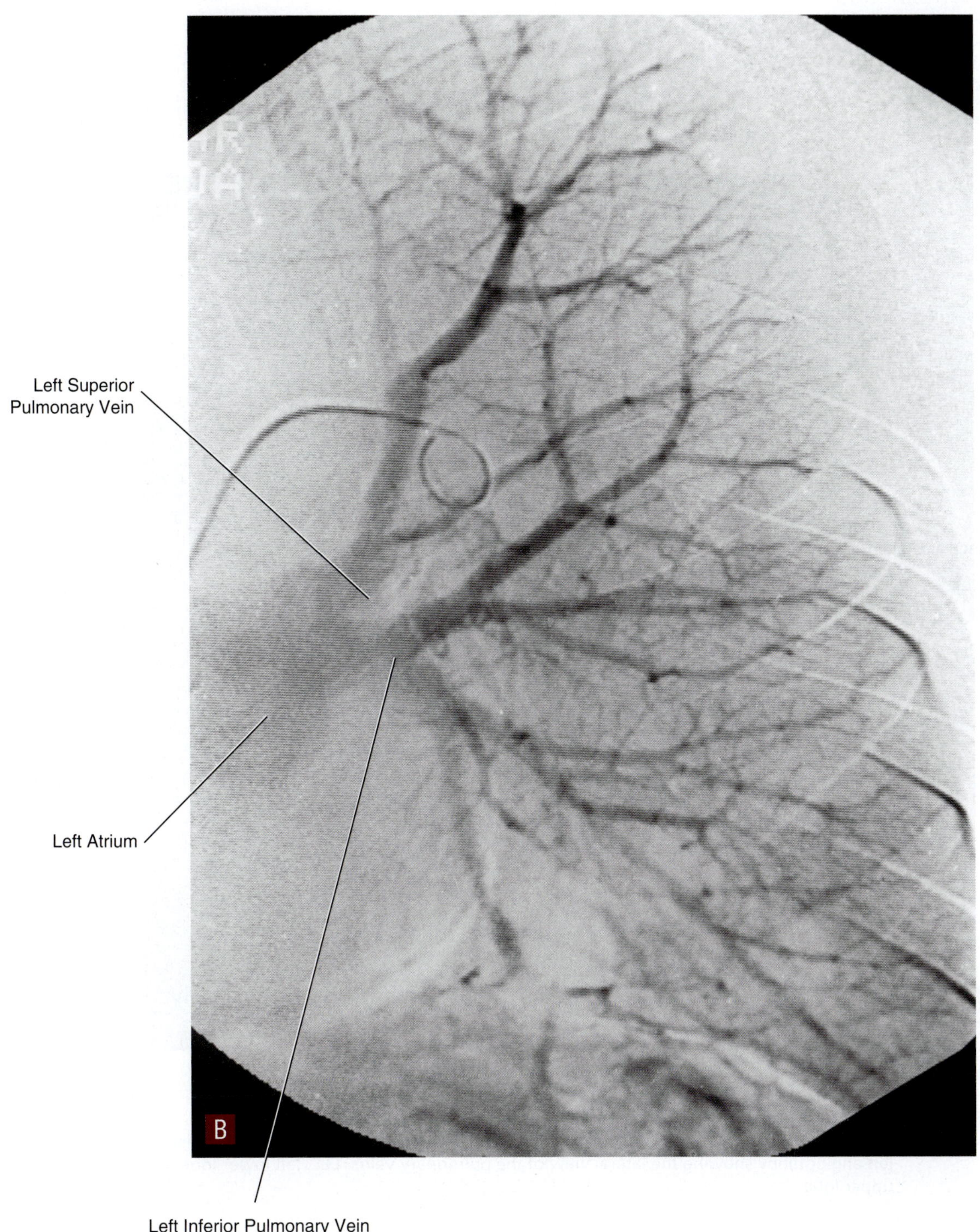

Figure 10.12. *Continued*

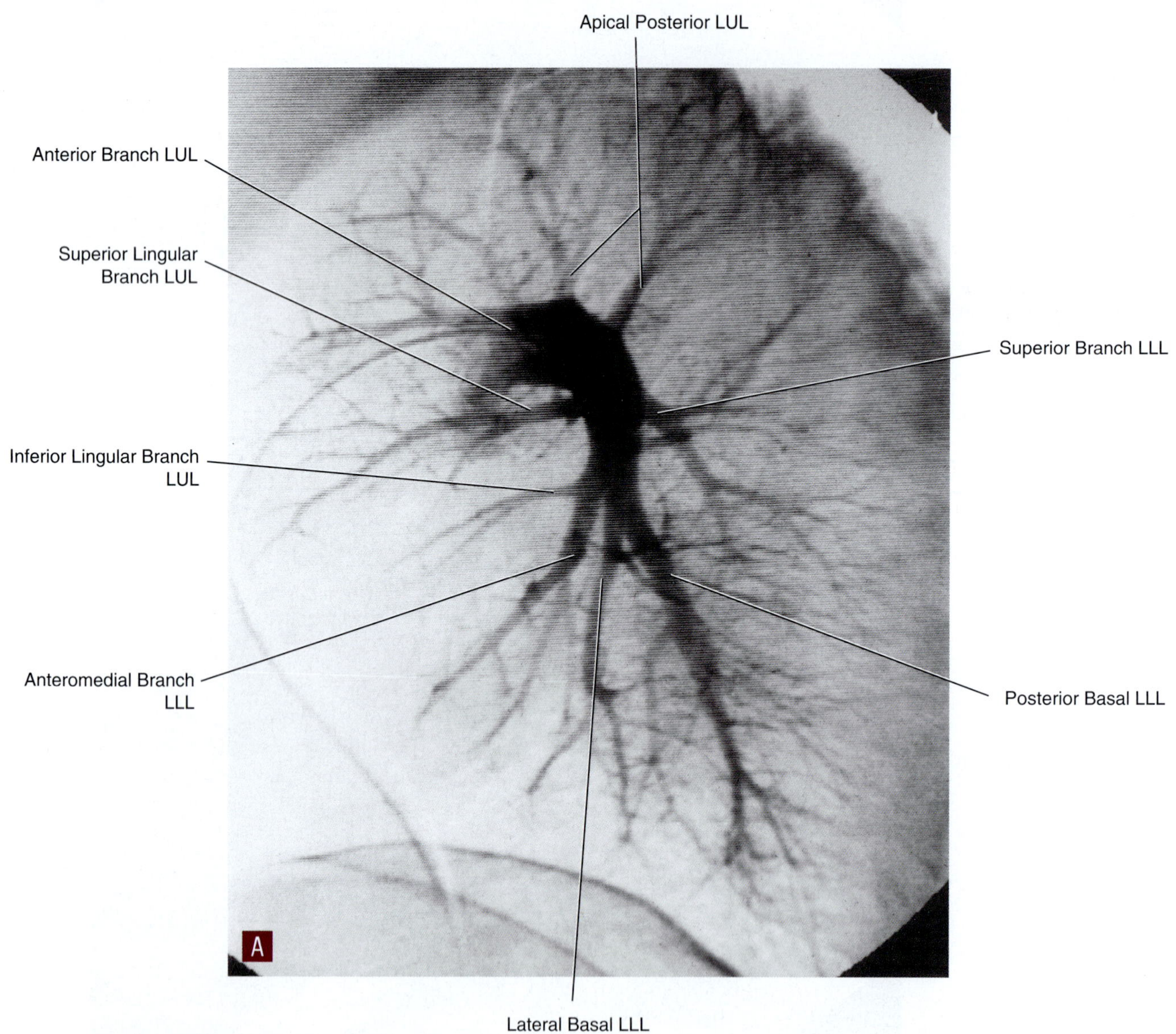

Figure 10.13. **A**, Lateral angiogram of the left pulmonary artery. **B**, Late phase of the left angiography showing the lateral view of the pulmonary veins. LLL, left lower lobe; LUL, left upper lobe.

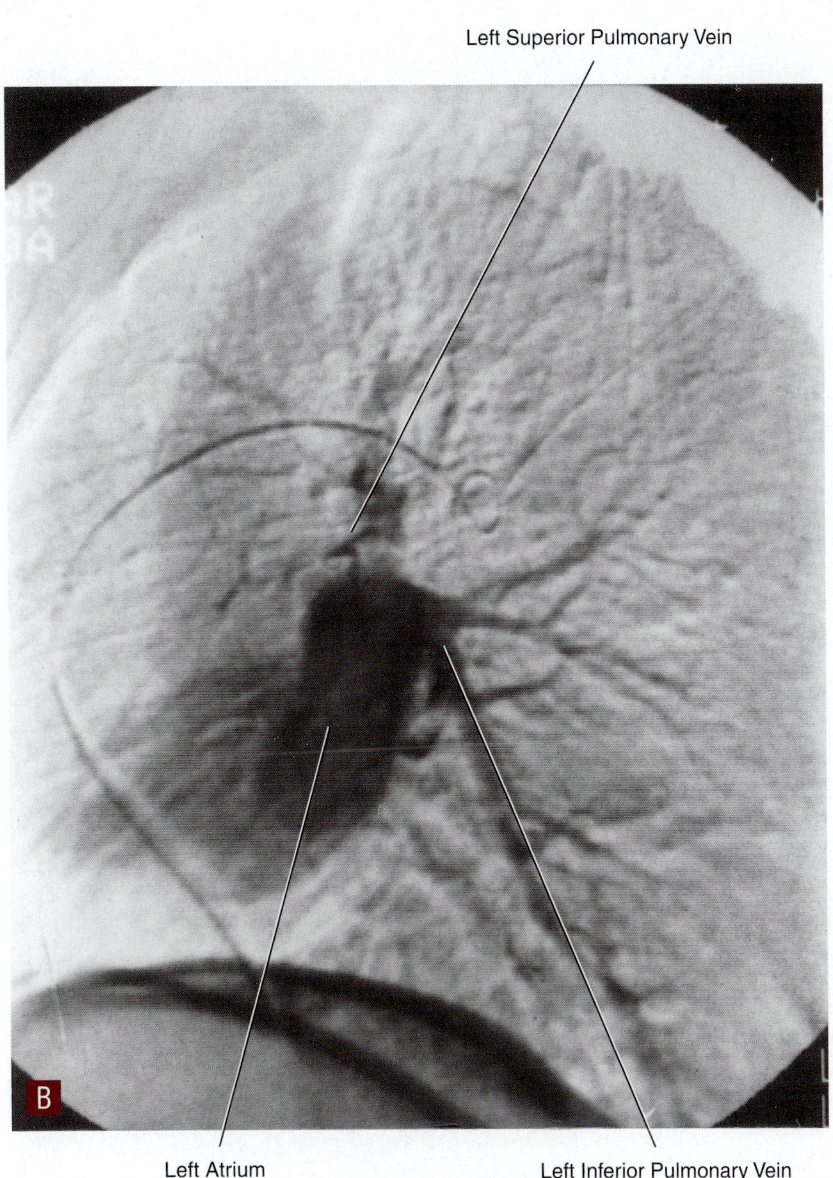

Figure 10.13. *Continued*

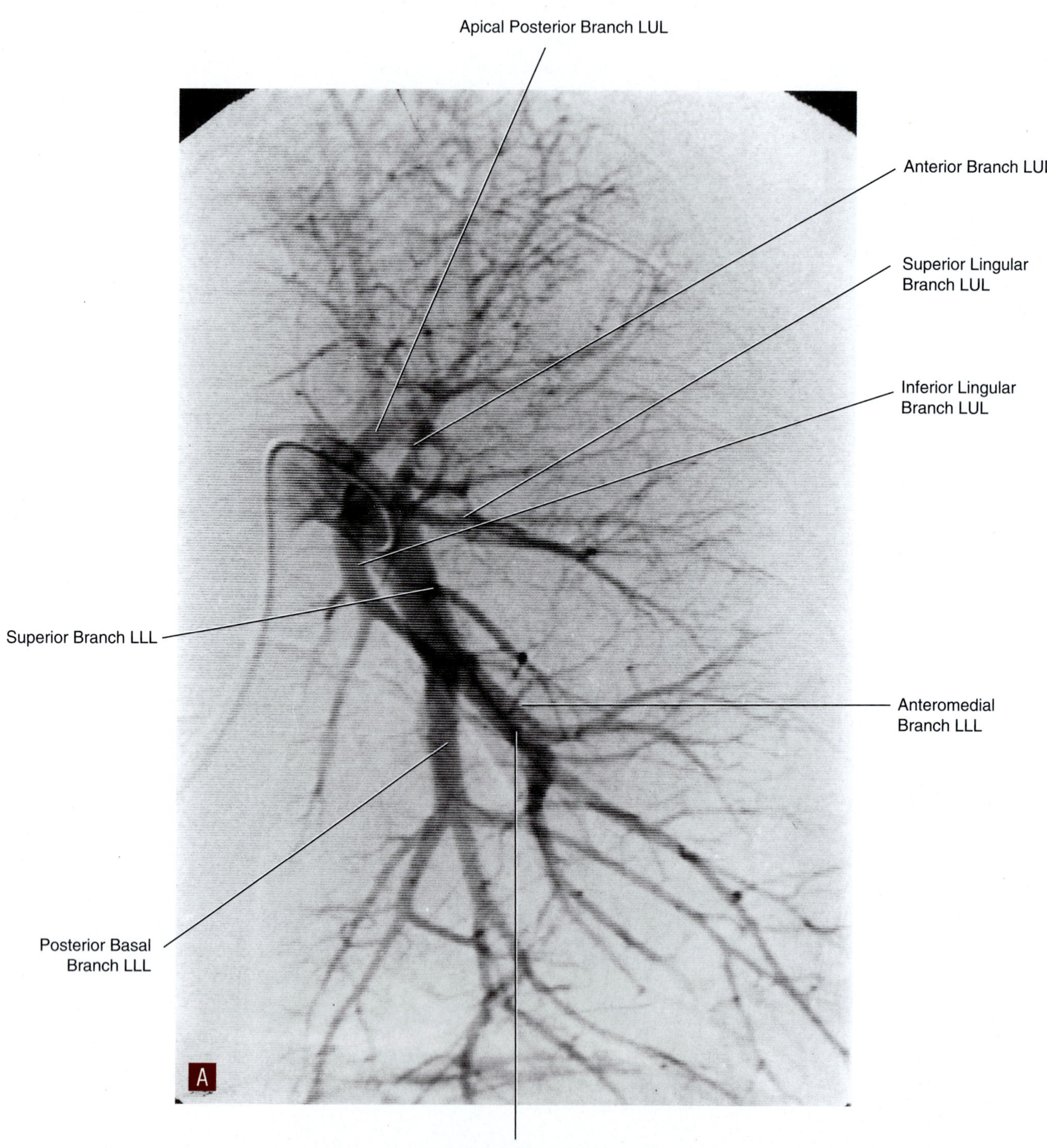

Figure 10.14. A, Anterior view of the left pulmonary artery angiography. B, Late phase of the left angiogram showing the pulmonary veins. LLL, left lower lobe; LUL, left upper lobe.

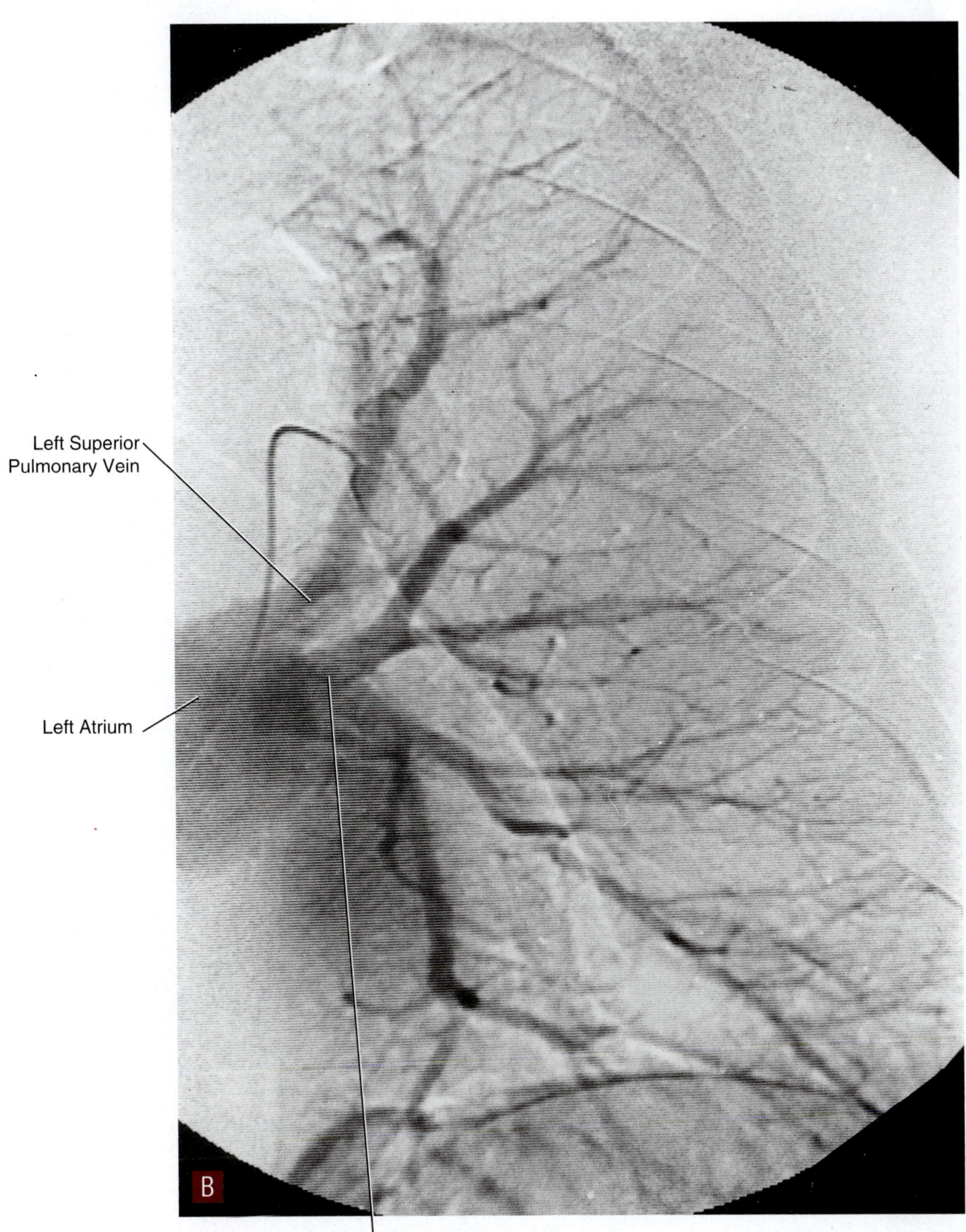

Figure 10.14. *Continued*

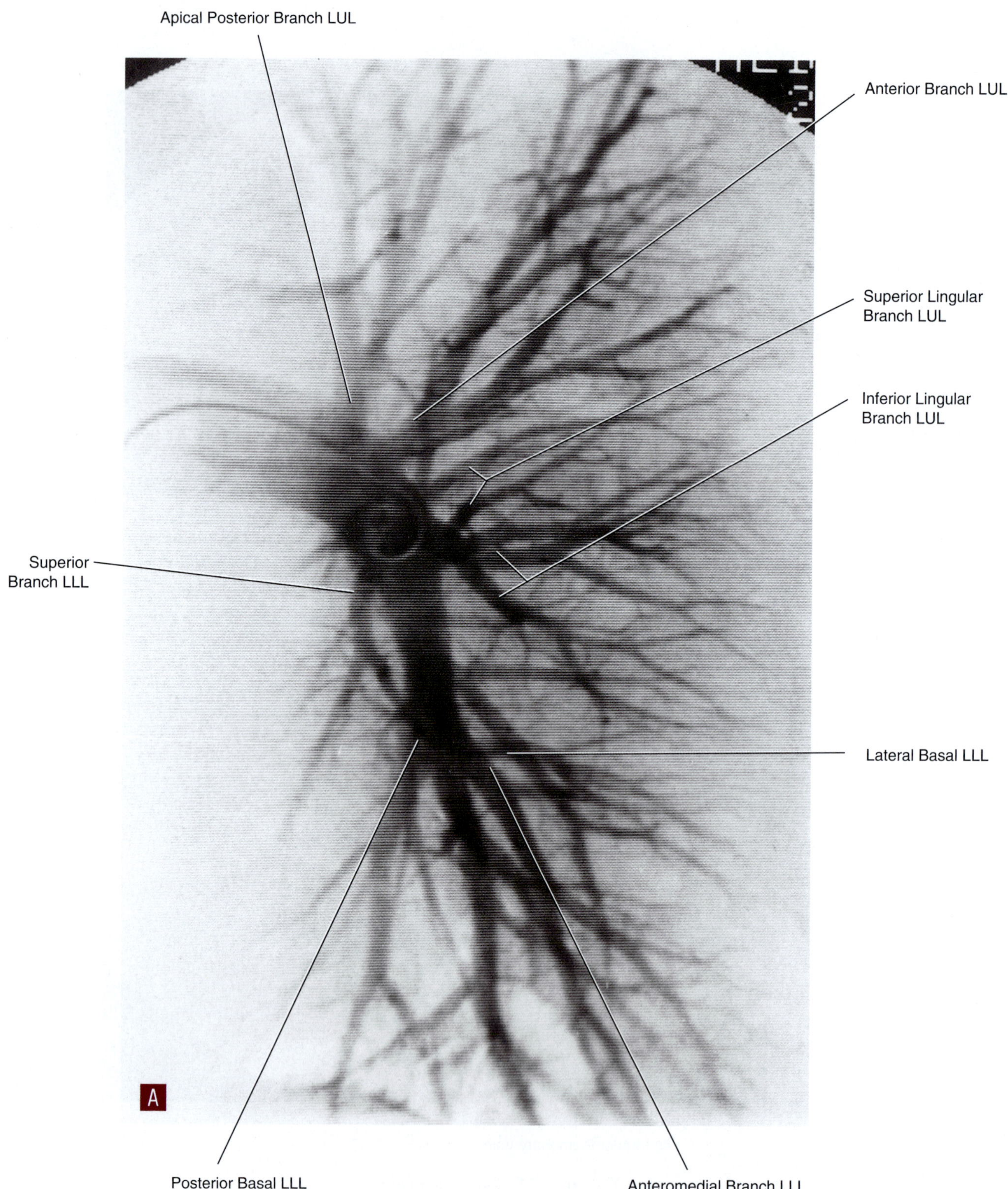

Figure 10.15. A, Anterior view of the left pulmonary artery angiography. B, Late phase of the left angiogram showing the pulmonary veins. C, Oblique view of the left pulmonary artery angiography. LLL, left lower lobe; LUL, left upper lobe.

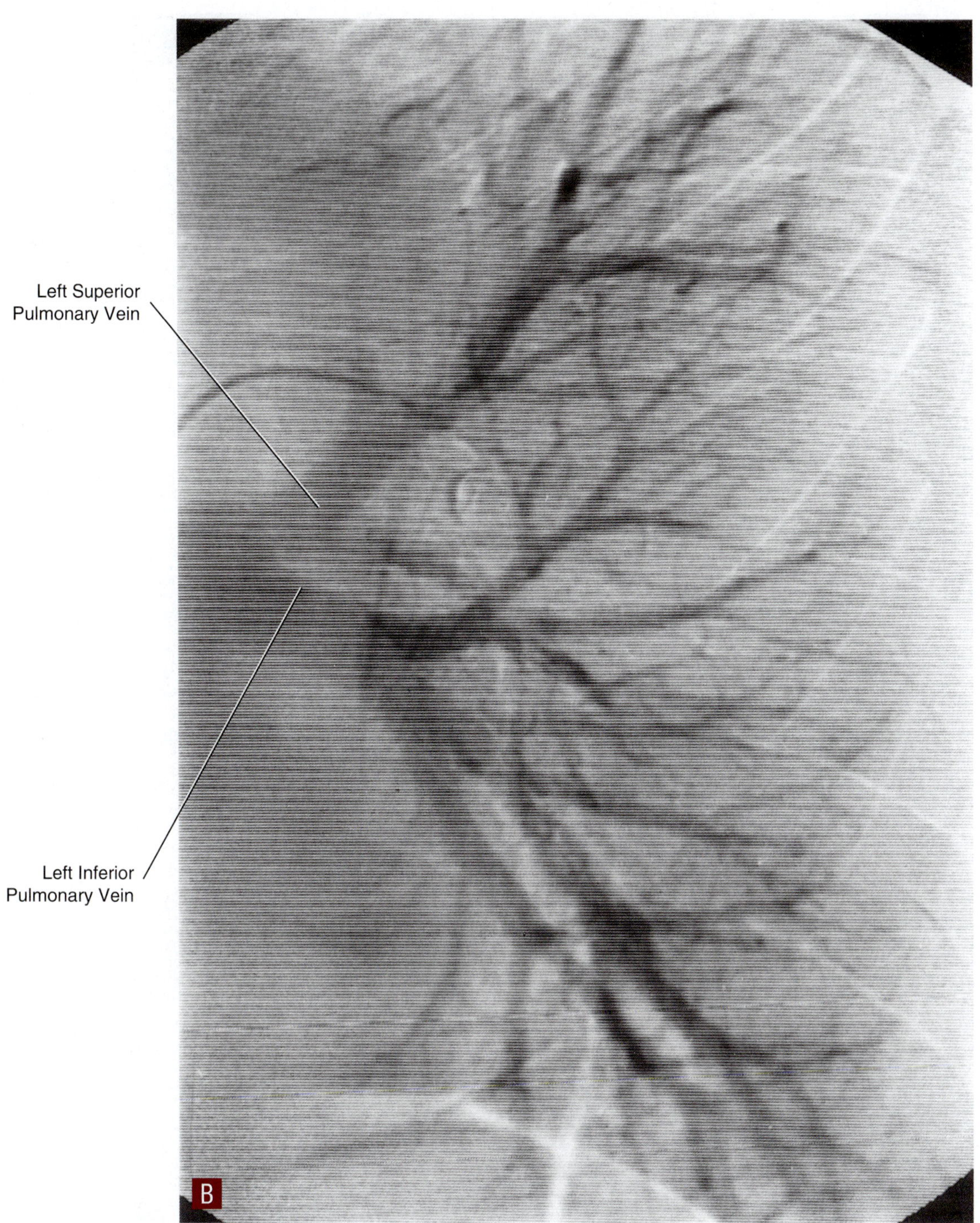

Figure 10.15. *Continued*

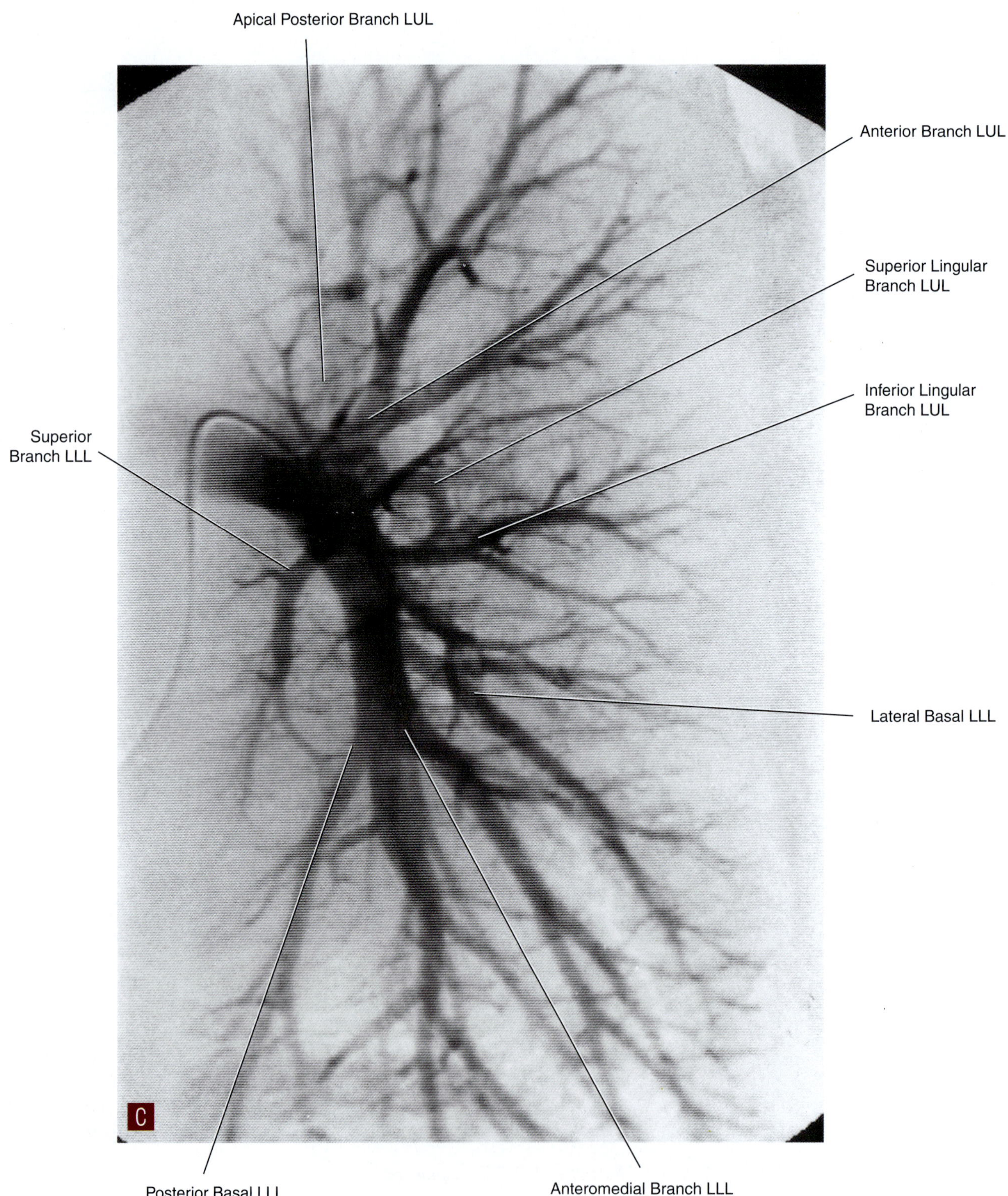

Figure 10.15. *Continued*

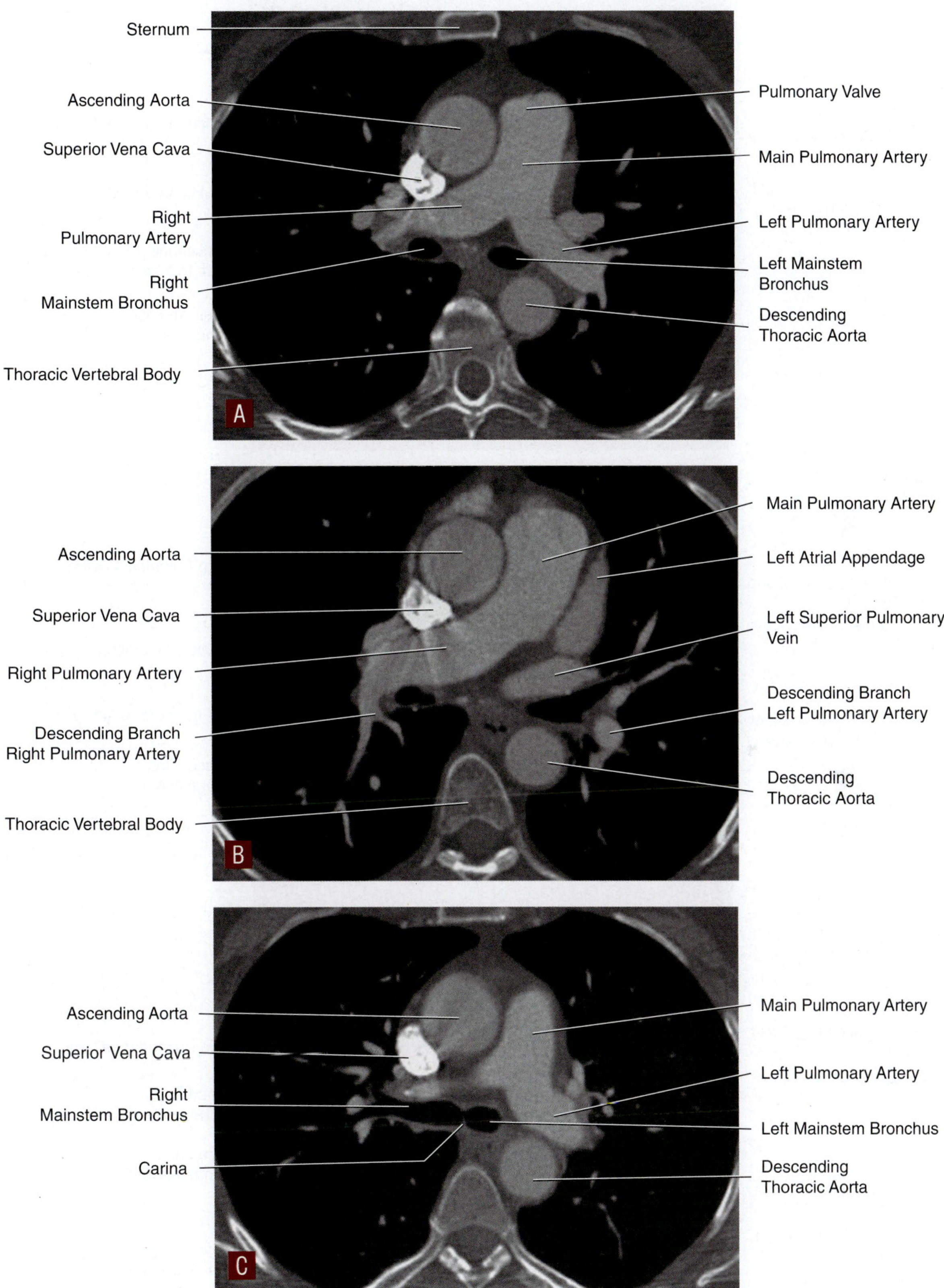

Figure 10.16. **CT axial images.** **A**, Axial image demonstrating bifurcation of the main pulmonary artery into the right and left pulmonary arteries. **B**, Slightly caudal axial image at the level of the right pulmonary artery. **C**, Slightly cranial axial image showing the left pulmonary artery passing up and over the left mainstem bronchus.

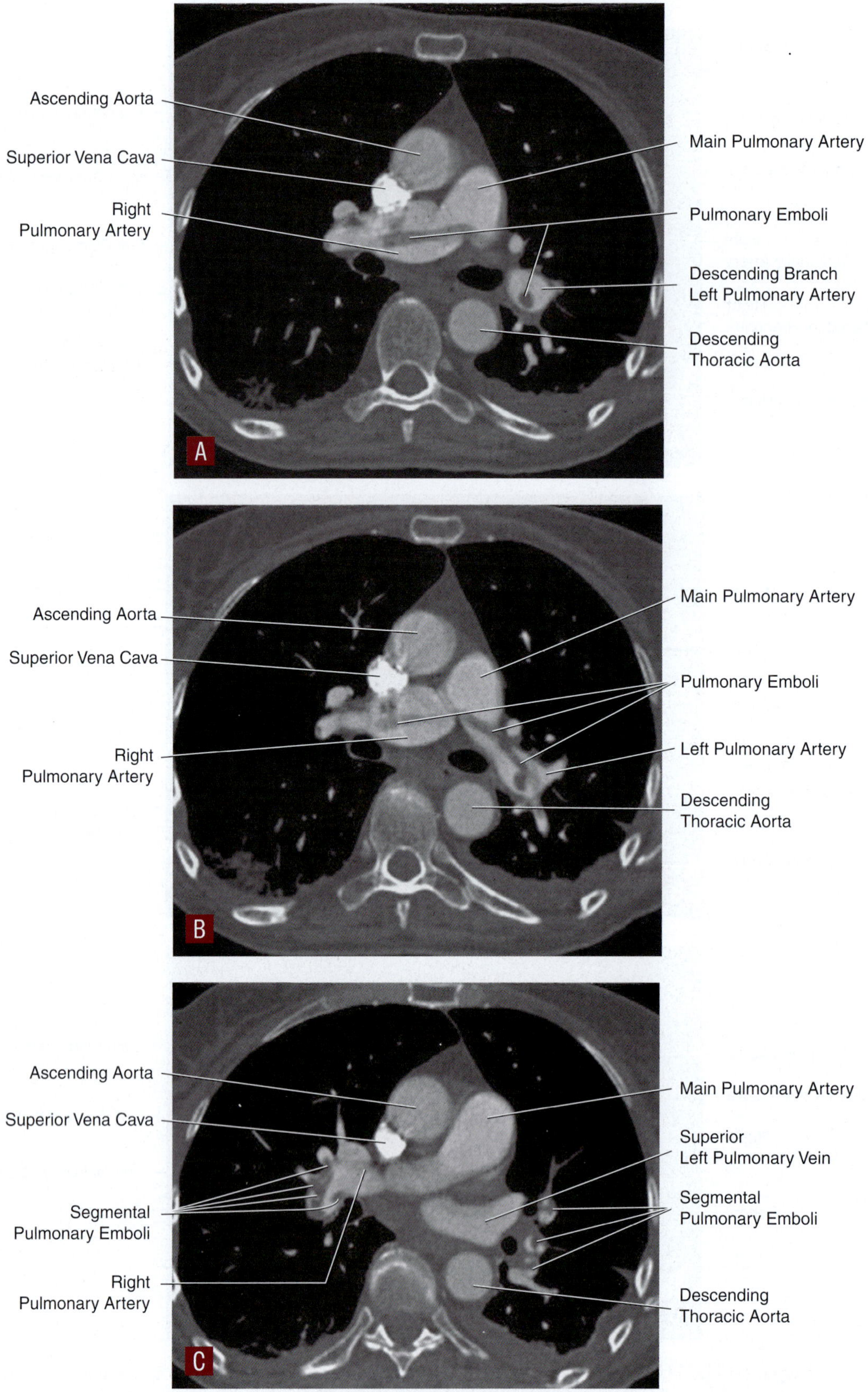

Figure 10.17. **CT axial images of pulmonary embolus.** A and B, Images at the level of bifurcation of the main pulmonary artery demonstrating a saddle embolus extending into the right and left pulmonary arteries. C, Axial image at a more caudal level showing emboli (filling defects) in the segmental pulmonary arteries.

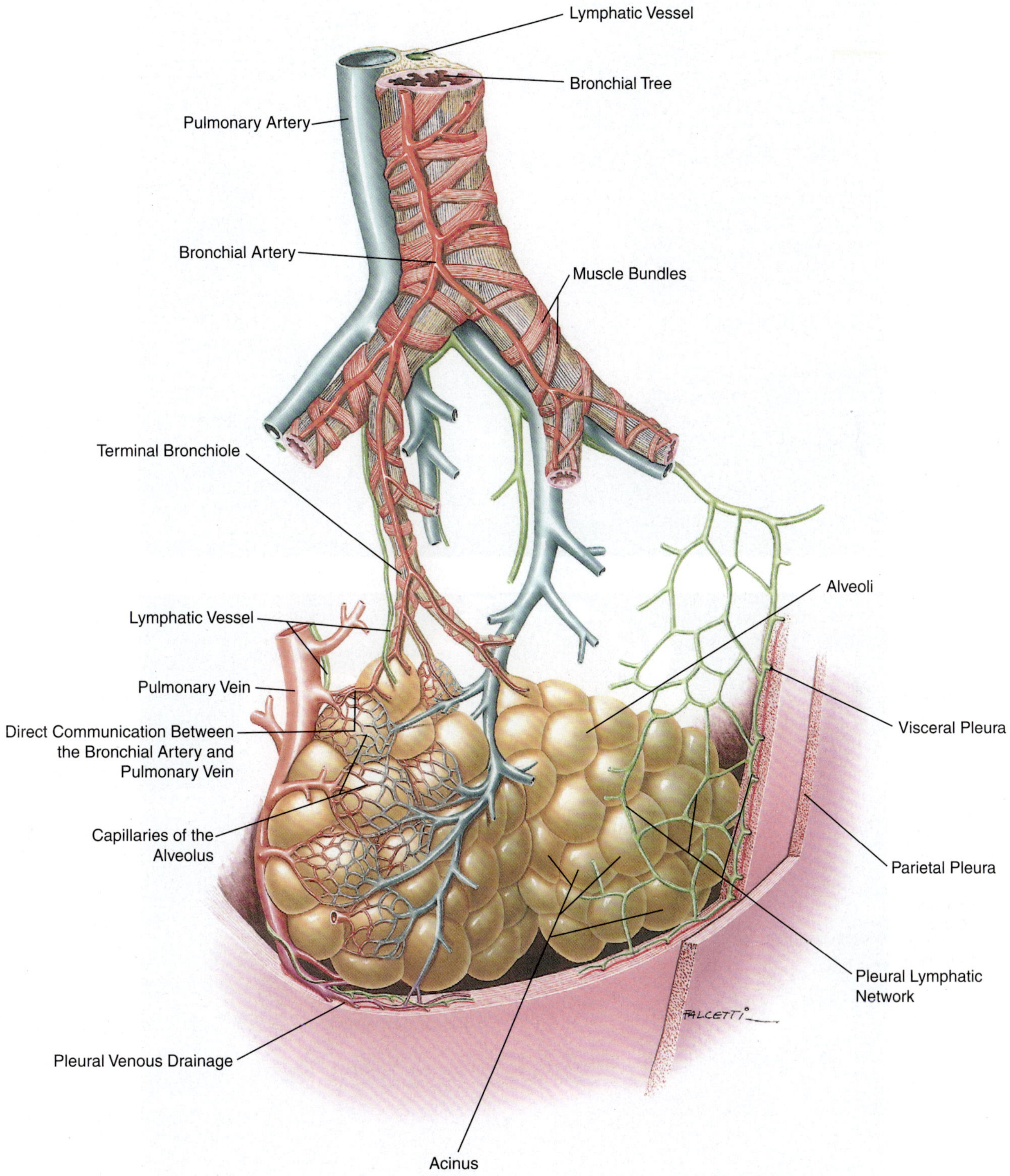

Lymphatic Vessel
Bronchial Tree
Pulmonary Artery
Bronchial Artery
Muscle Bundles
Terminal Bronchiole
Alveoli
Lymphatic Vessel
Pulmonary Vein
Visceral Pleura
Direct Communication Between the Bronchial Artery and Pulmonary Vein
Capillaries of the Alveolus
Parietal Pleura
Pleural Lymphatic Network
Pleural Venous Drainage
Acinus

Figure 10.18. Pulmonary microcirculation showing the relationships of the pulmonary artery, bronchial artery, capillaries of the alveolus, pulmonary vein, and lymphatic network.

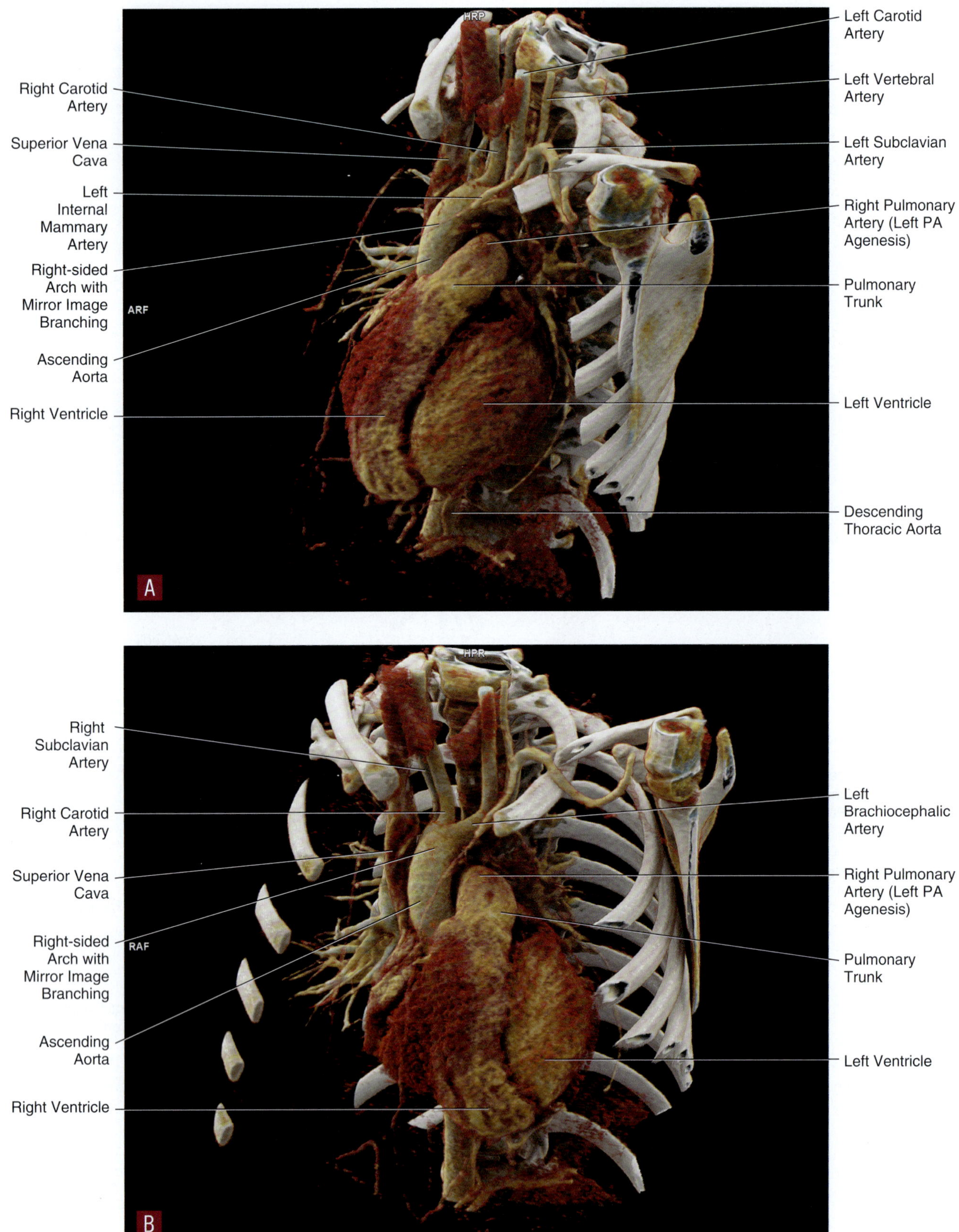

Figure 10.19. **A**, CT pulmonary angiogram cinematic-rendered reconstruction showing interruption of the left pulmonary artery. There is compensatory hypertrophy of bronchial arteries on the side with pulmonary agenesis and a right-sided arch with mirror image branching. **B**, Additional view of the cinematic reconstruction showing absence of the left main PA and right-sided arch with mirror image branching.

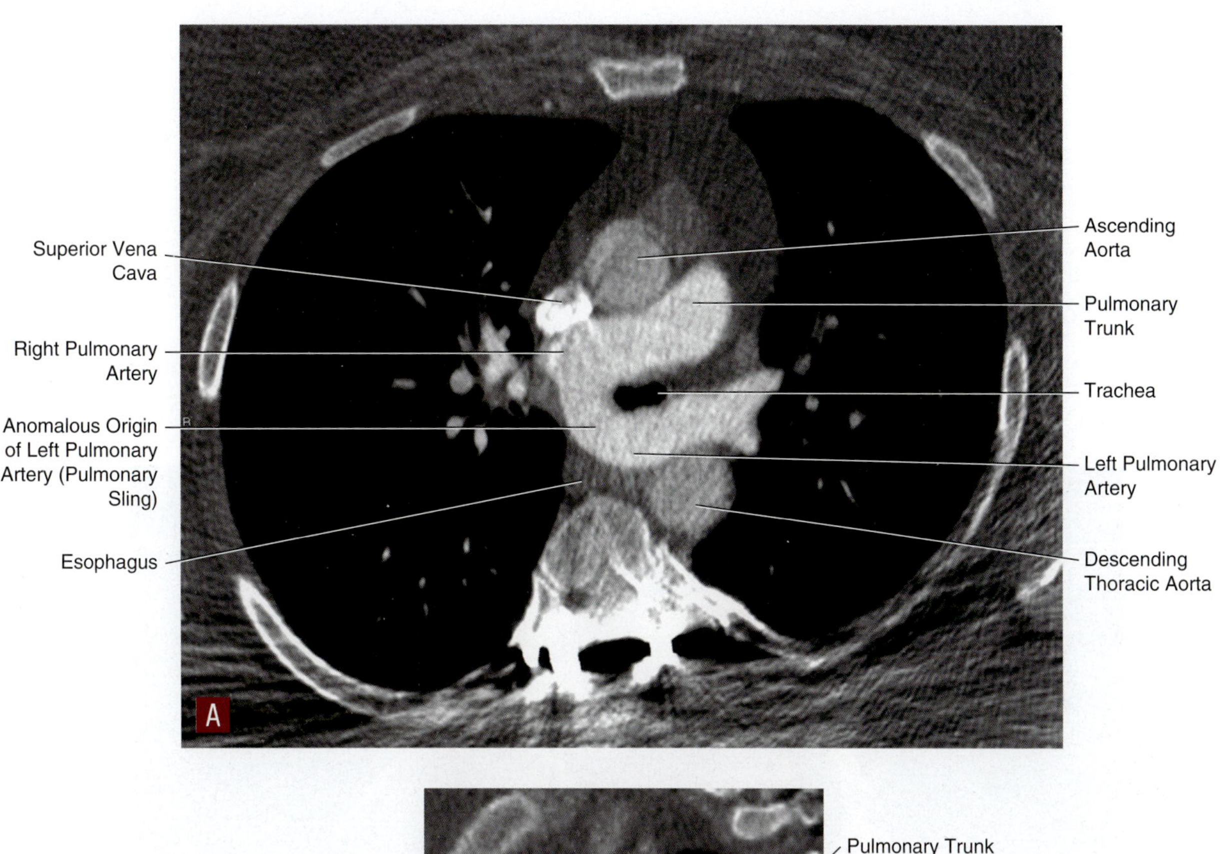

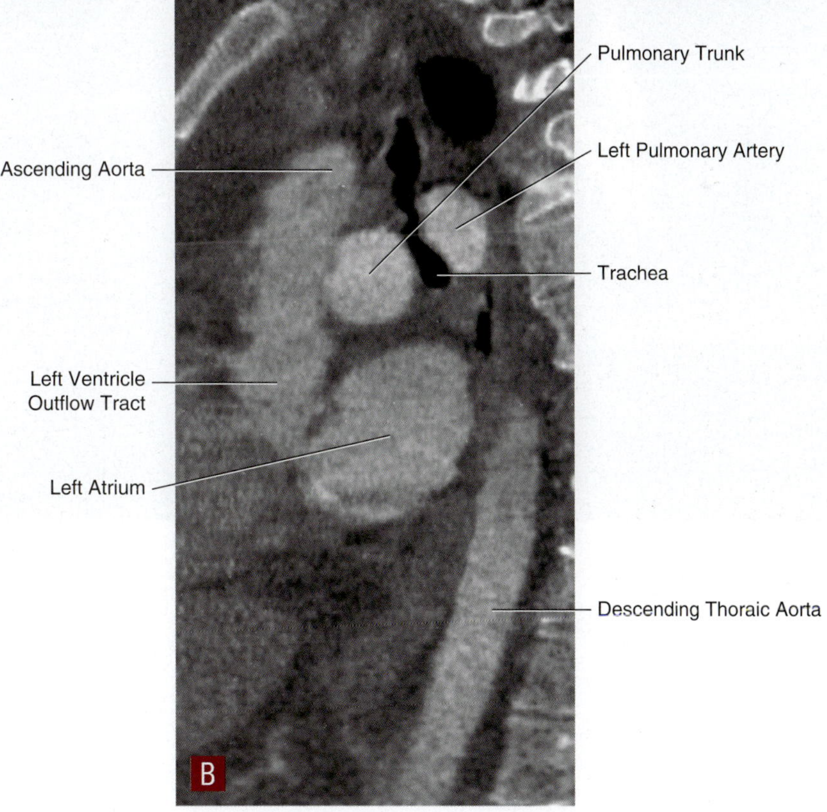

Figure 10.20. A, Axial CT pulmonary angiogram showing an anomalous origin of the left pulmonary artery, also known as a pulmonary sling. The left pulmonary artery arises from the right pulmonary artery, coursing between the trachea and descending thoracic aorta. B, Sagittal view of the same patient above demonstrating the degree of tracheal stenosis that can be seen with a pulmonary sling. C, CT pulmonary angiogram cinematic-rendered reconstruction from a right posterior lateral view showing the left pulmonary artery arising from the right pulmonary artery.

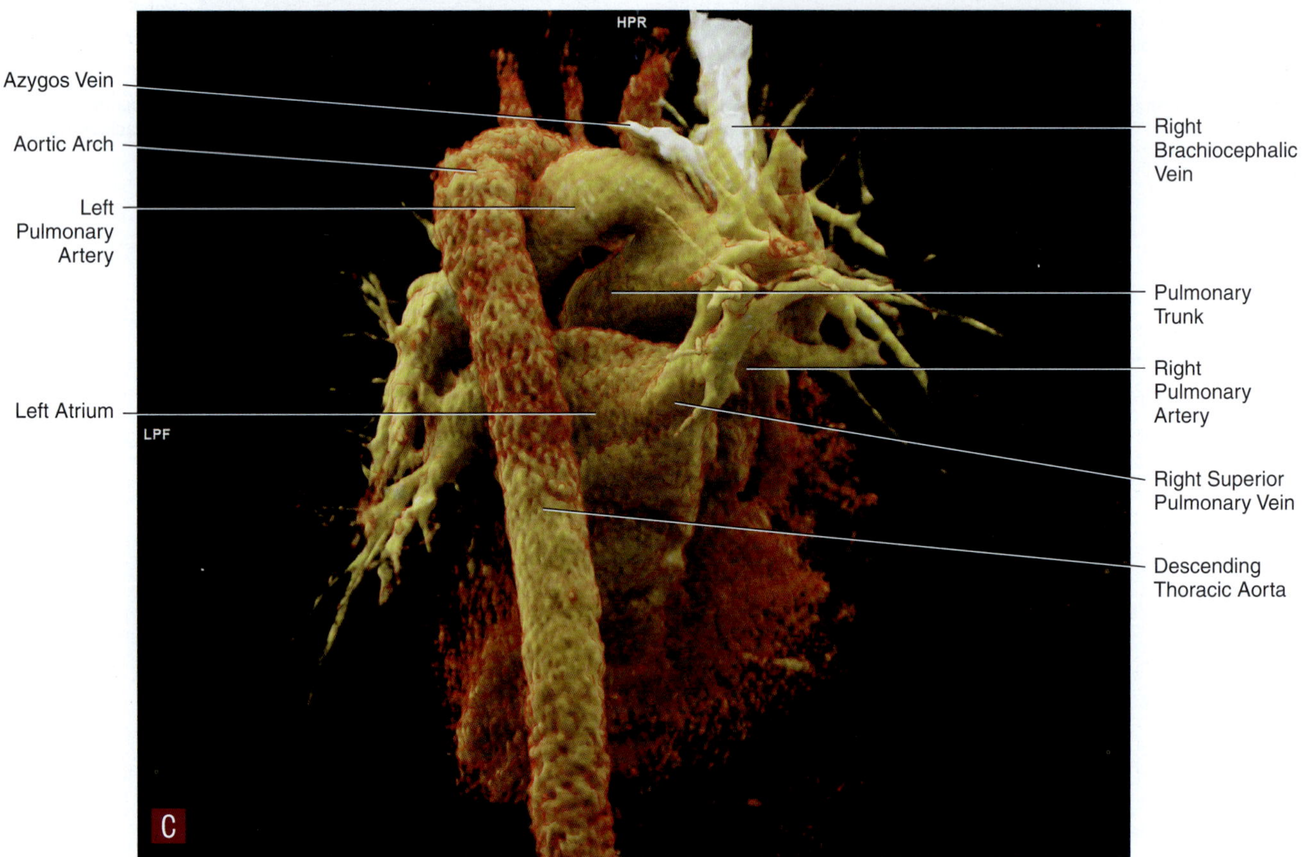

Figure 10.20. *Continued*

11

Pulmonary Venous Circulation

The pulmonary veins arise from the capillaries of the alveolar meshwork and from the capillary network of the pleura. The larger branches run within the interlobular septa and are, therefore, separate from the pulmonary bronchoarterial pathways. Histologically, the smaller pulmonary veins are identical to the arterioles. As the diameter of the veins increases, smooth muscle cells and elastic laminae are identifiable, and, at a diameter of 60 and 100 μm, they become evident as veins and enter the interlobular septa (see Chapter 10, Fig. 10.18).

There is a dense vascular network around the bronchi, which is an arteriolar network terminating in bronchial capillaries and numerous bronchial venous plexuses with a characteristic irregular shape and course. There are also connections between the bronchial capillaries with the bronchial venous plexuses. The bronchial venous plexus communicates with the smaller branches of the pulmonary vein.

Pulmonary Veins

There are usually two superior and two inferior main pulmonary veins, the former draining the middle and upper lobes on the right side and the upper lobe on the left with the inferior veins draining the lower lobes (Fig. 11.1). The pulmonary veins drain the oxygenated pulmonary blood to the left atrium. Computerized tomography is now used as an excellent way to image these structures (Fig. 11.2). As with many venous structures, there are occasional variations in this pattern. On the right side, the most common variation is to have three separate pulmonary veins with the third vein usually draining the right middle lobe. On the left side, the most common variation is a single common trunk where all the veins empty into before reaching the left atrium (Fig. 11.3). Less commonly more complex arrangements may be seen (Fig. 11.4). These patterns are usually referred to as normal variants, as the blood still follows the same pathway.

In anomalous pulmonary venous drainage, the veins drain into a different structure, usually directly to the superior vena cava or to the right atrium. This will be discussed in more detail in subsequent text. The right veins reach the hilum beneath the main pulmonary artery and posteriorly to the superior vena cava. The veins usually reach the left atrium independently as two separate veins. The left veins cross in front of the descending aorta and may enter the left atrium separately as on the right side or may join each other already within the pericardial cavity to enter the atrium as a common vein (Figs. 11.5-11.8).

The pulmonary venous system carries approximately 50% of the blood in the lungs at any given time. Knowledge of pulmonary venous anatomy has become more important with the increasing use of catheterization and ablation to treat cardiac arrhythmias. The abnormal conduction pathways that cause some arrhythmias are located near the orifice of the pulmonary veins. Treatment consists of applying radiofrequency energy around the pulmonary veins to disrupt these pathways. Knowledge of normal variants or partial anomalous venous return is important in preprocedural planning. In addition, some veins may scar down and develop narrowed areas or even close off completely (Fig. 11.9). Fortunately, these narrowed areas may be treated by stent placement if identified in time (Fig. 11.10).

Anomalous Pulmonary Venous Drainage

Total anomalous pulmonary venous return is a complex and very serious form of congenital heart disease in which all the pulmonary veins empty into the superior vena cava, inferior vena cava, or right atrium (Fig. 11.11). When partial anomalous pulmonary venous drainage exists, it usually involves part or all of one lung. In most cases, there is an associated reduction in size of the pulmonary arteries supplying the anomalous-drained lung segment (Fig. 11.12). Other anomalies of the pulmonary venous drainage are related to pulmonary sequestration, Halasz syndrome, or can be the sole anomaly. Halasz syndrome (also known as scimitar syndrome) refers to dextrocardia, hypoplasia of the right pulmonary artery, and scimitar-like pulmonary venous drainage. Scimitar-shaped partial anomalous venous return can be seen as an isolated finding outside of the syndrome above (Fig. 11.13). The venous drainage in the scimitar vein may be through the inferior vena cava and less frequently through the azygos vein, whereas the anomalous pulmonary venous drainage may be to the superior vena cava or the brachiocephalic vein.

Computerized tomography is being used increasingly to evaluate the pulmonary veins following an ablation procedure to treat arrhythmias. In this setting, it is very important to recognize partial anomalous venous return as it may be asymptomatic into adult life. Computerized tomography will show absence of the vein in its expected location but also will demonstrate the vessel draining into another vessel or chamber (Fig. 11.14).

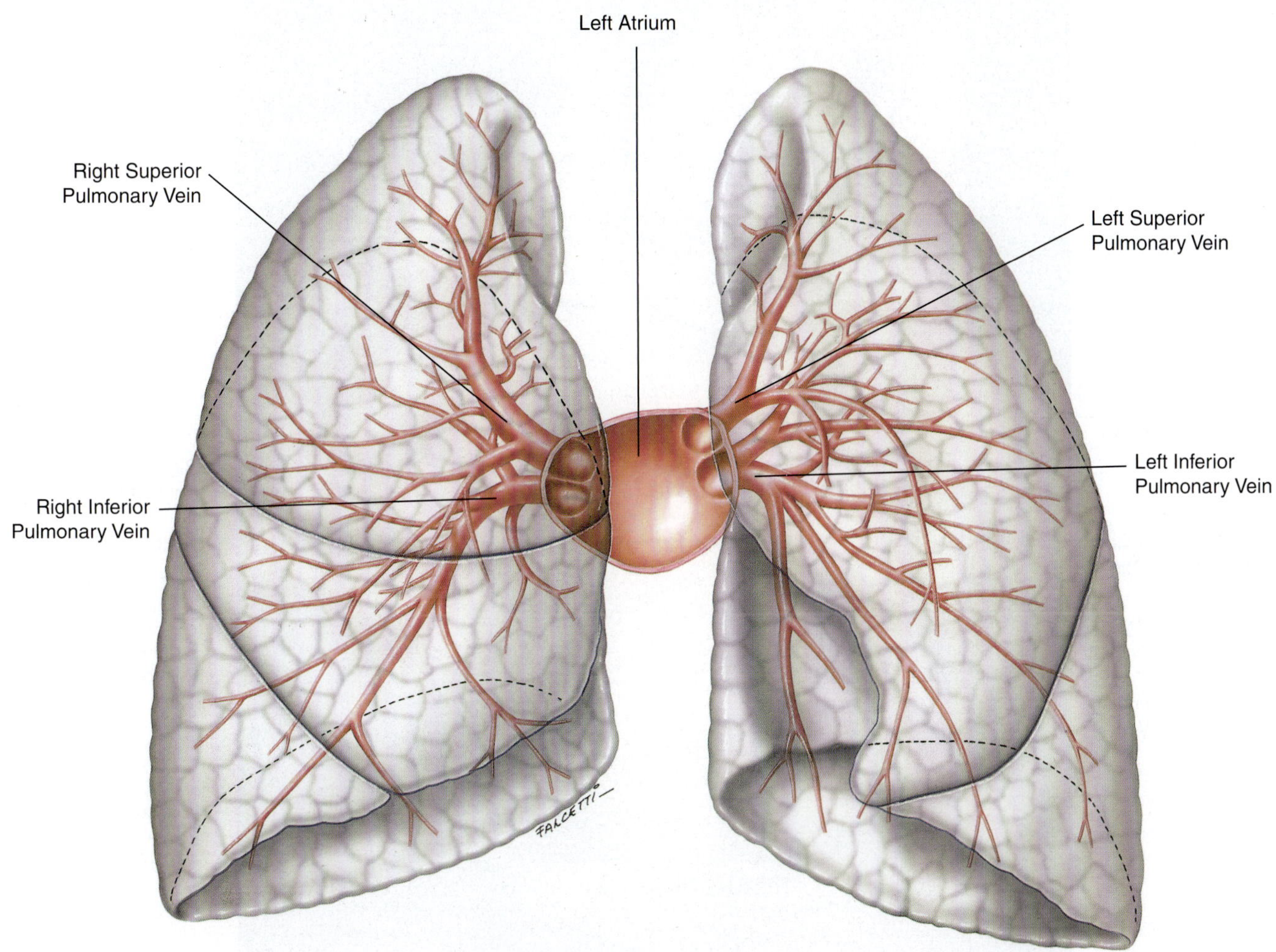

Figure 11.1. **Schematic drawing of the pulmonary veins and left atrium.** Note the two superior pulmonary veins and the two inferior pulmonary veins.

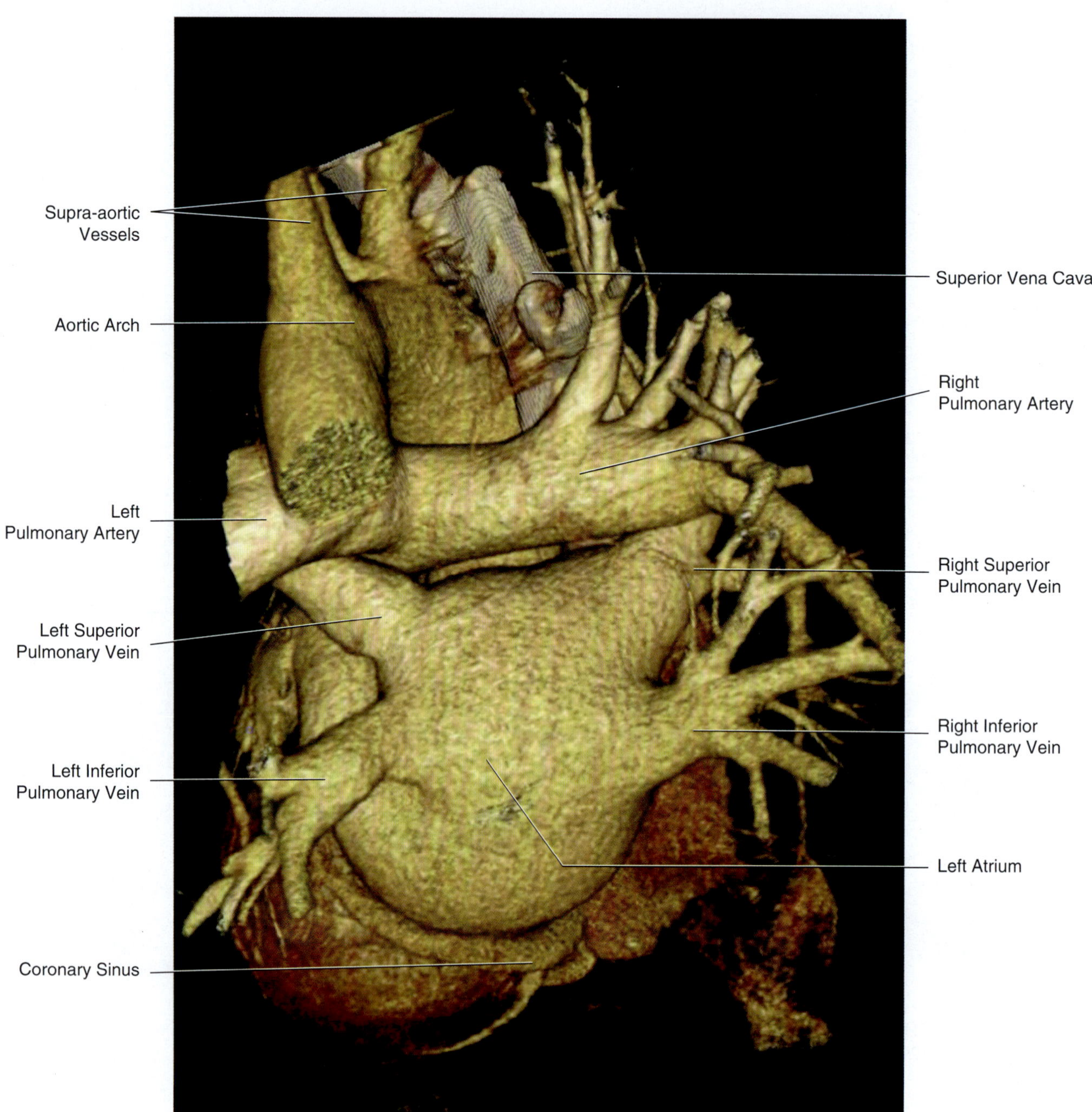

Figure 11.2. Three-dimensional (3D) computerized tomographic imaging of posterior view of the heart. Note left atrium lying caudal to the pulmonary arteries. Descending aorta has been cut away to allow better visualization of left atrium and pulmonary veins.

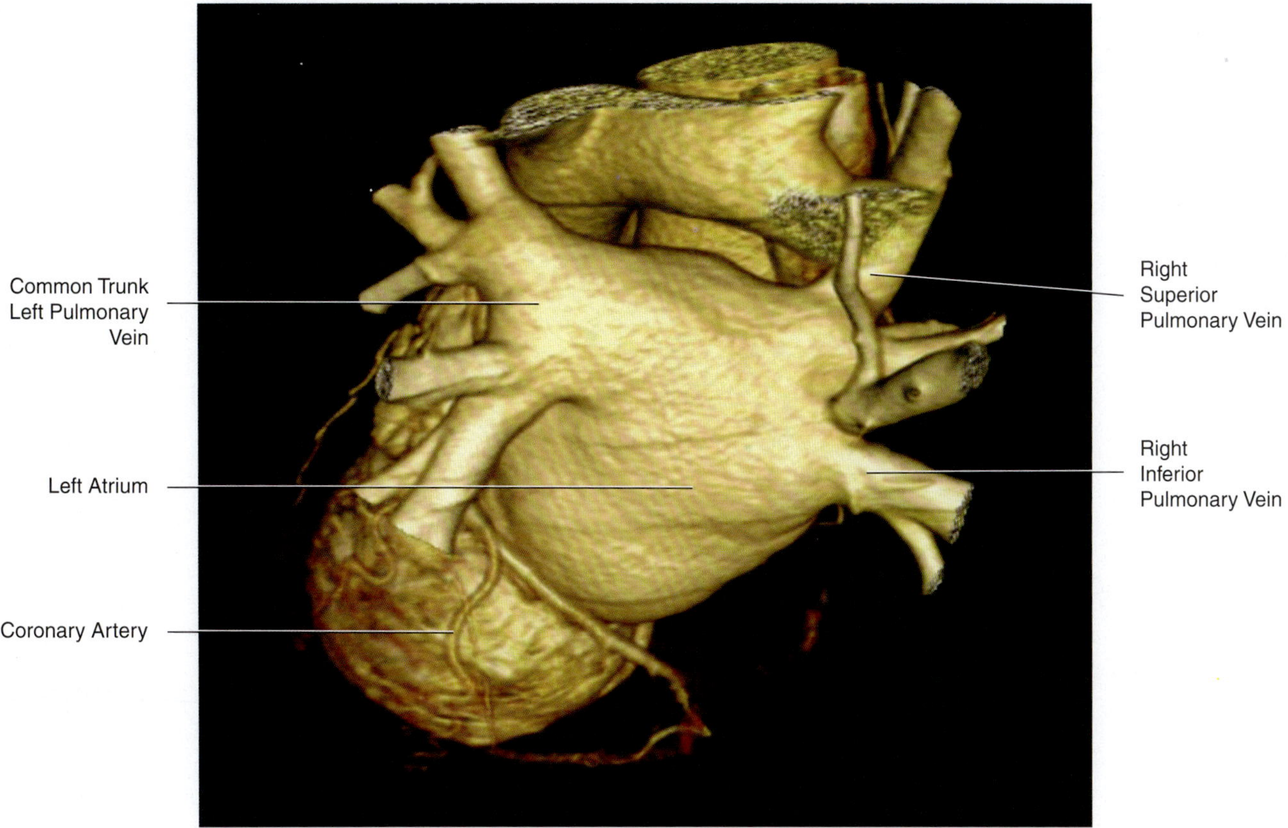

Figure 11.3. 3D computerized tomographic posterior view. Normal variant of left-sided veins joining to form a common trunk prior to entering the left atrium.

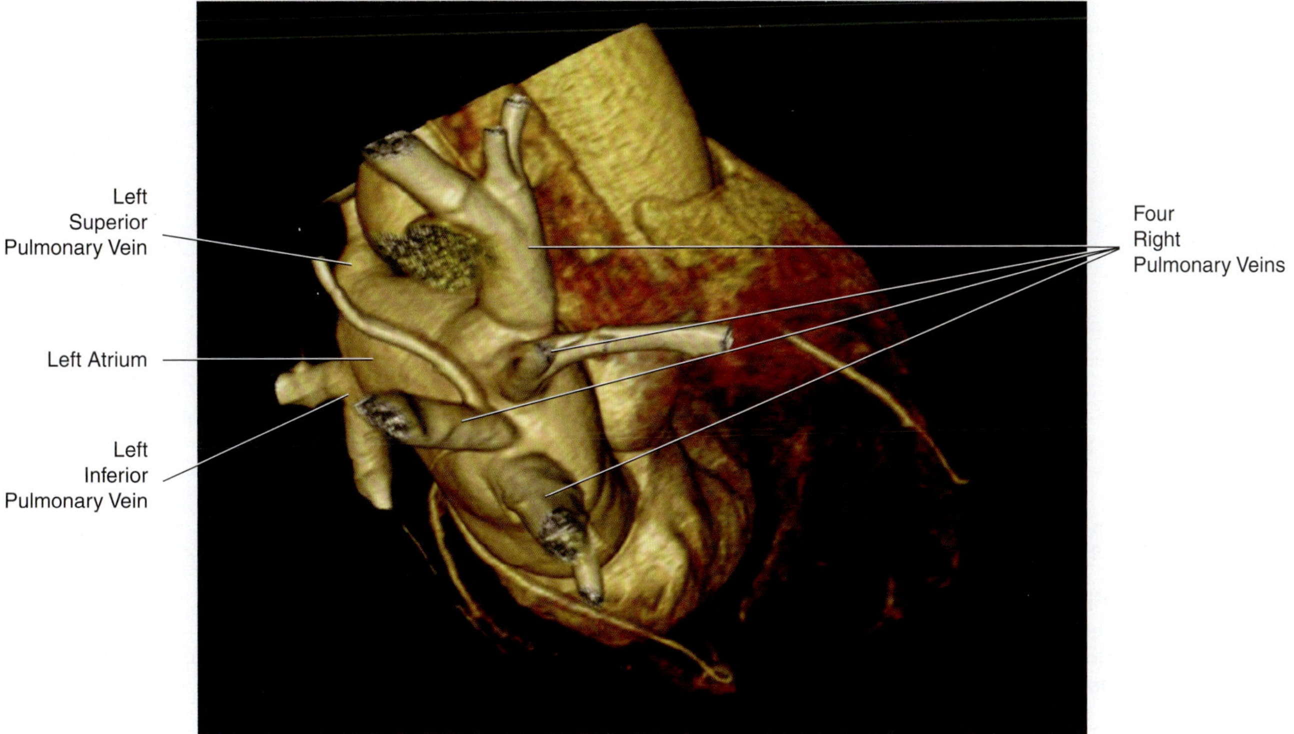

Figure 11.4. 3D computerized tomographic view from right side. Unusual variation of four right-sided veins all draining separately into the left atrium.

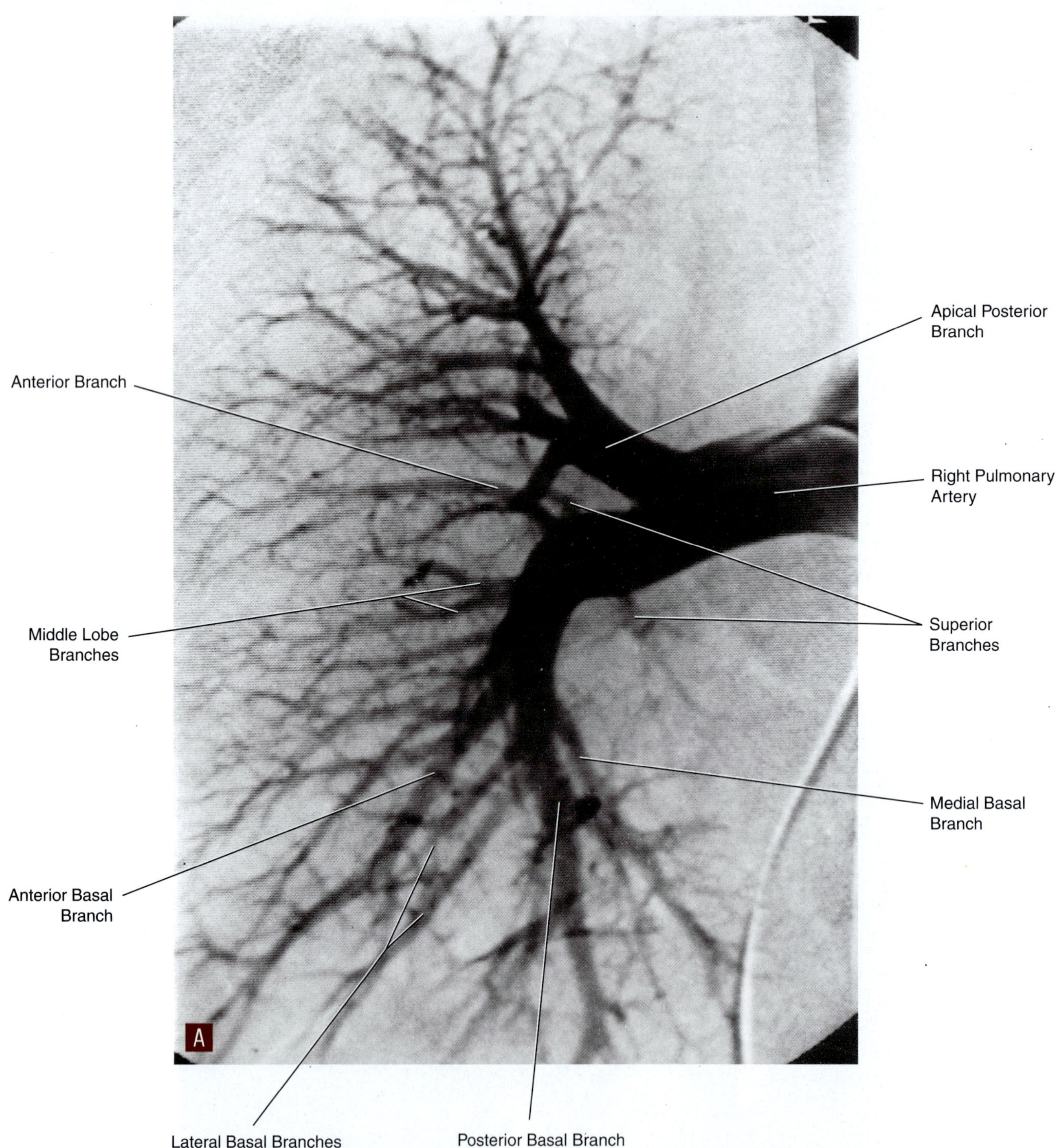

Figure 11.5. A, Right pulmonary artery angiogram showing the pulmonary artery to the superior, middle, and inferior pulmonary lobes. B, Late-phase angiogram showing the drainage of the right lung by the superior and inferior pulmonary veins. The left atrium and the ascending aortic arch are also visualized.

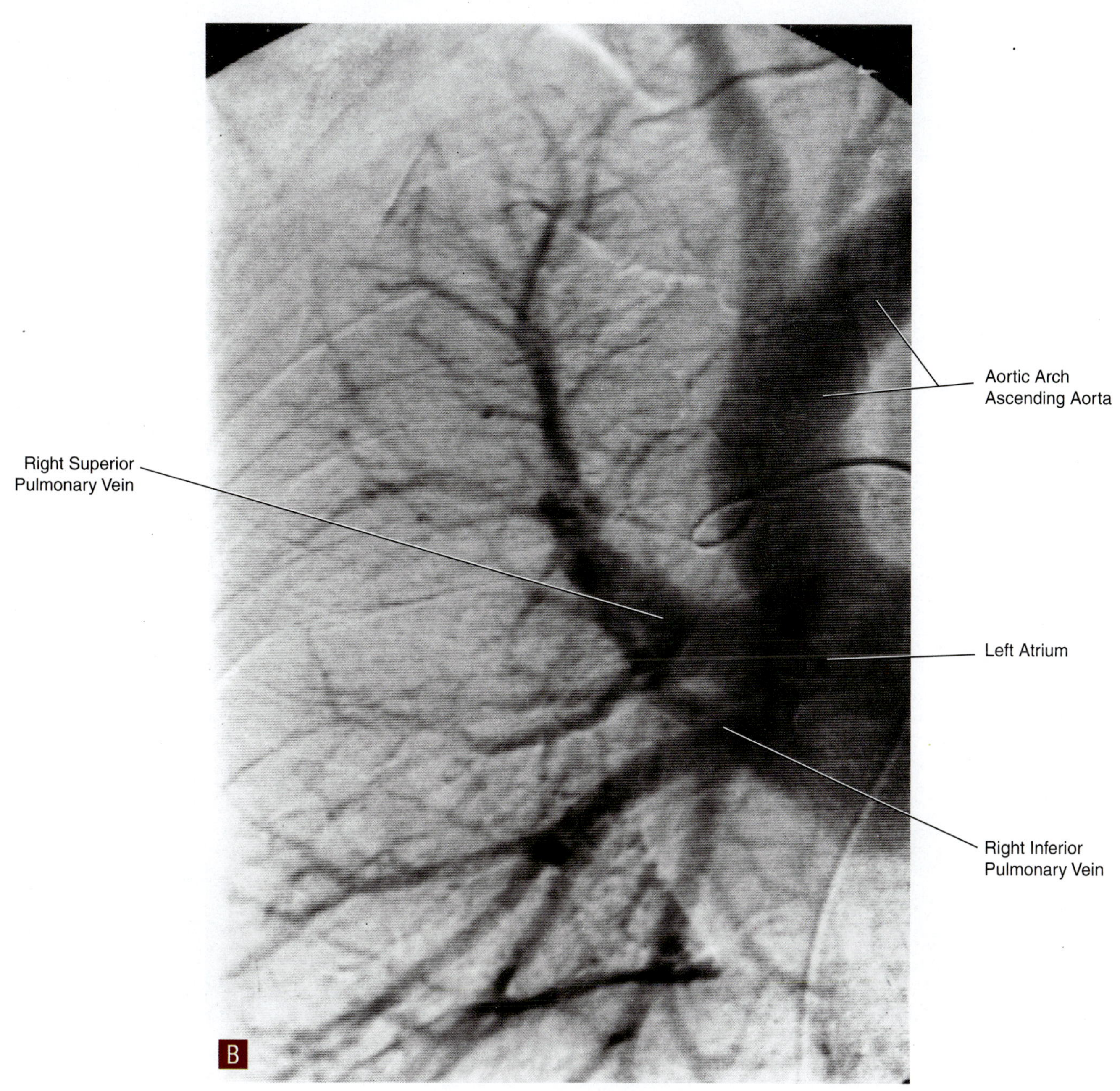

Figure 11.5. *Continued*

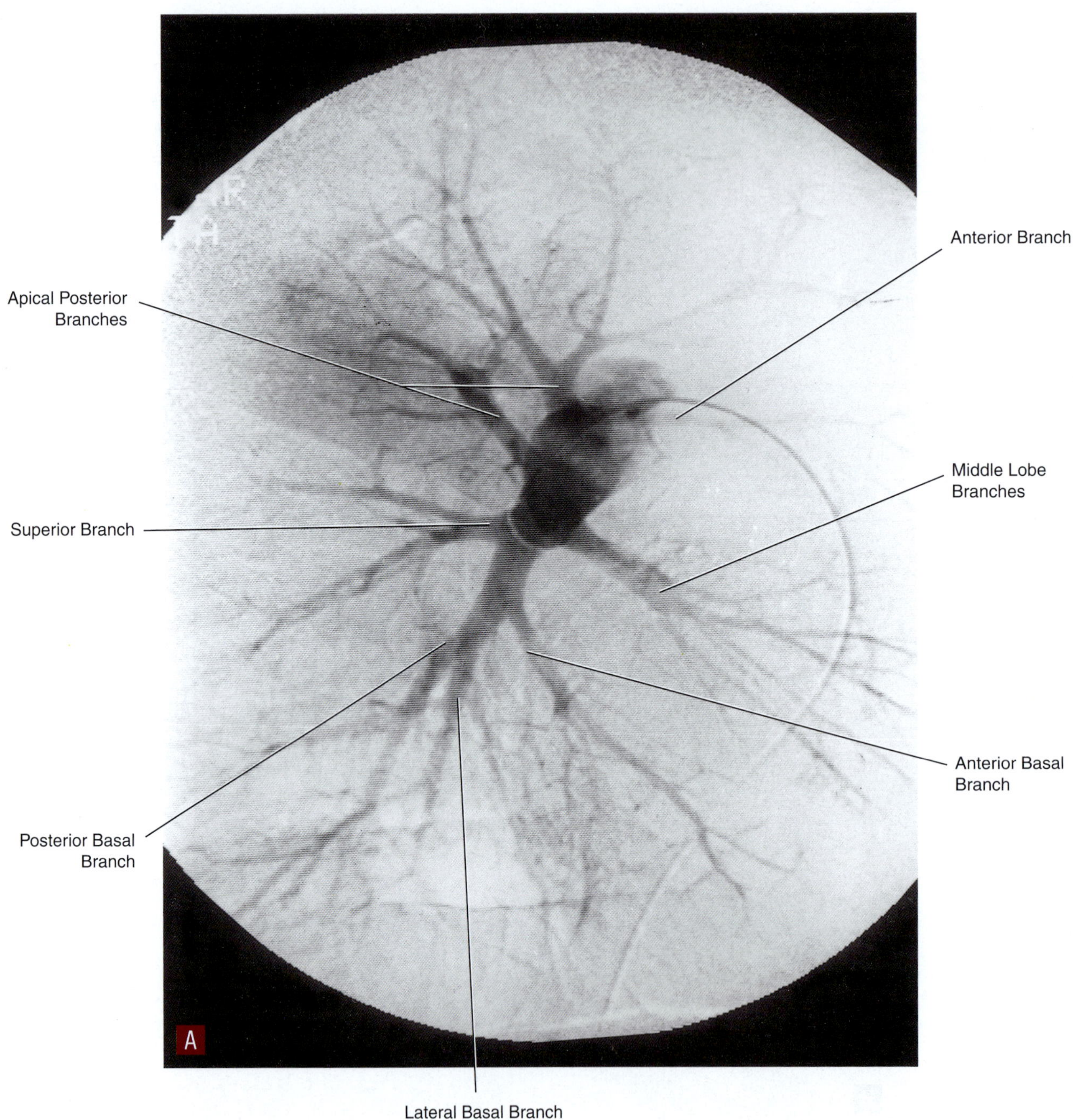

Figure 11.6. A, Lateral view of the right pulmonary artery angiogram showing the segments to the superior, middle, and inferior lobes. B, Late-phase angiogram showing the venous drainage from the superior and inferior pulmonary veins. The left atrium is also visualized.

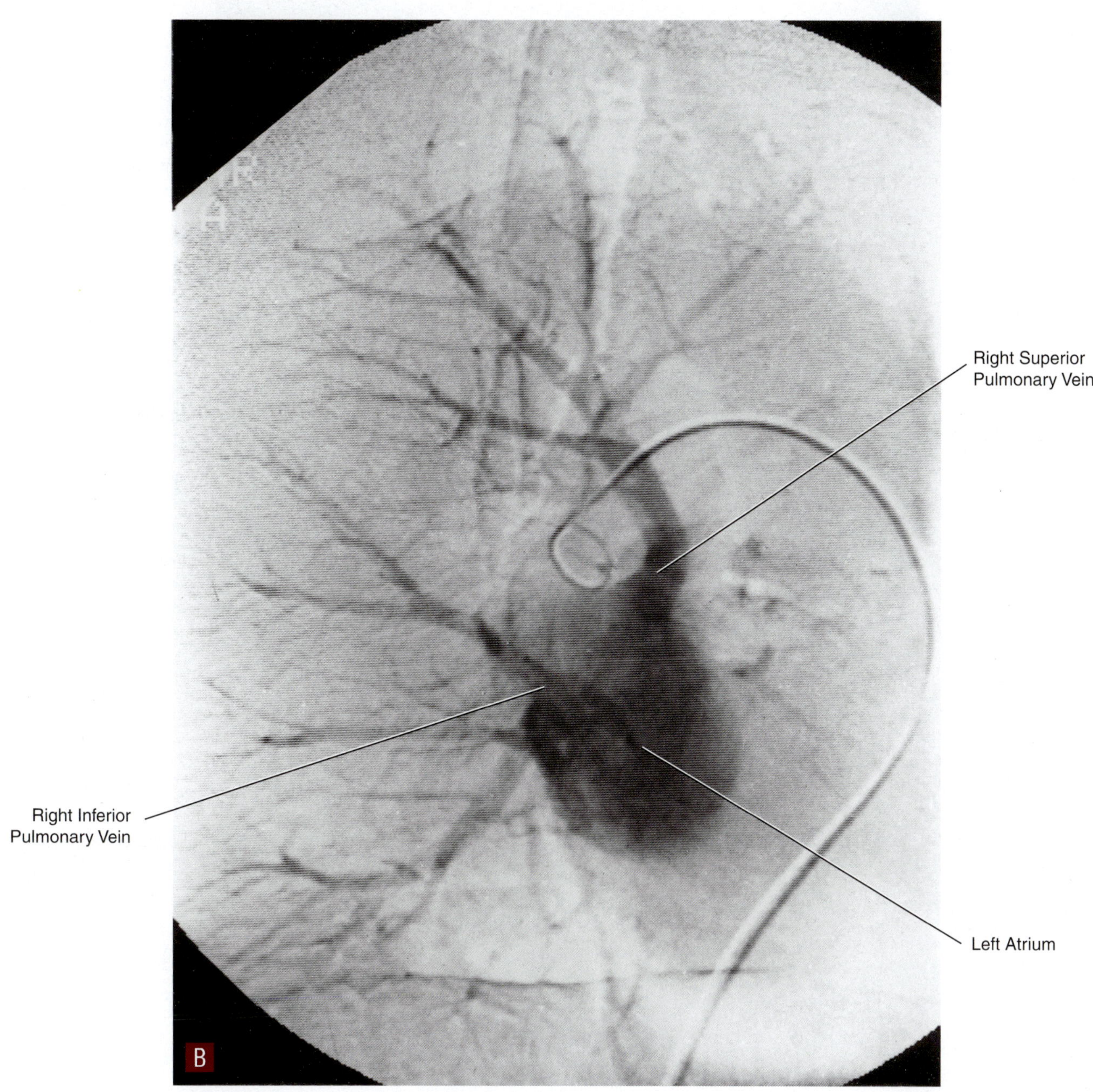

Figure 11.6. *Continued*

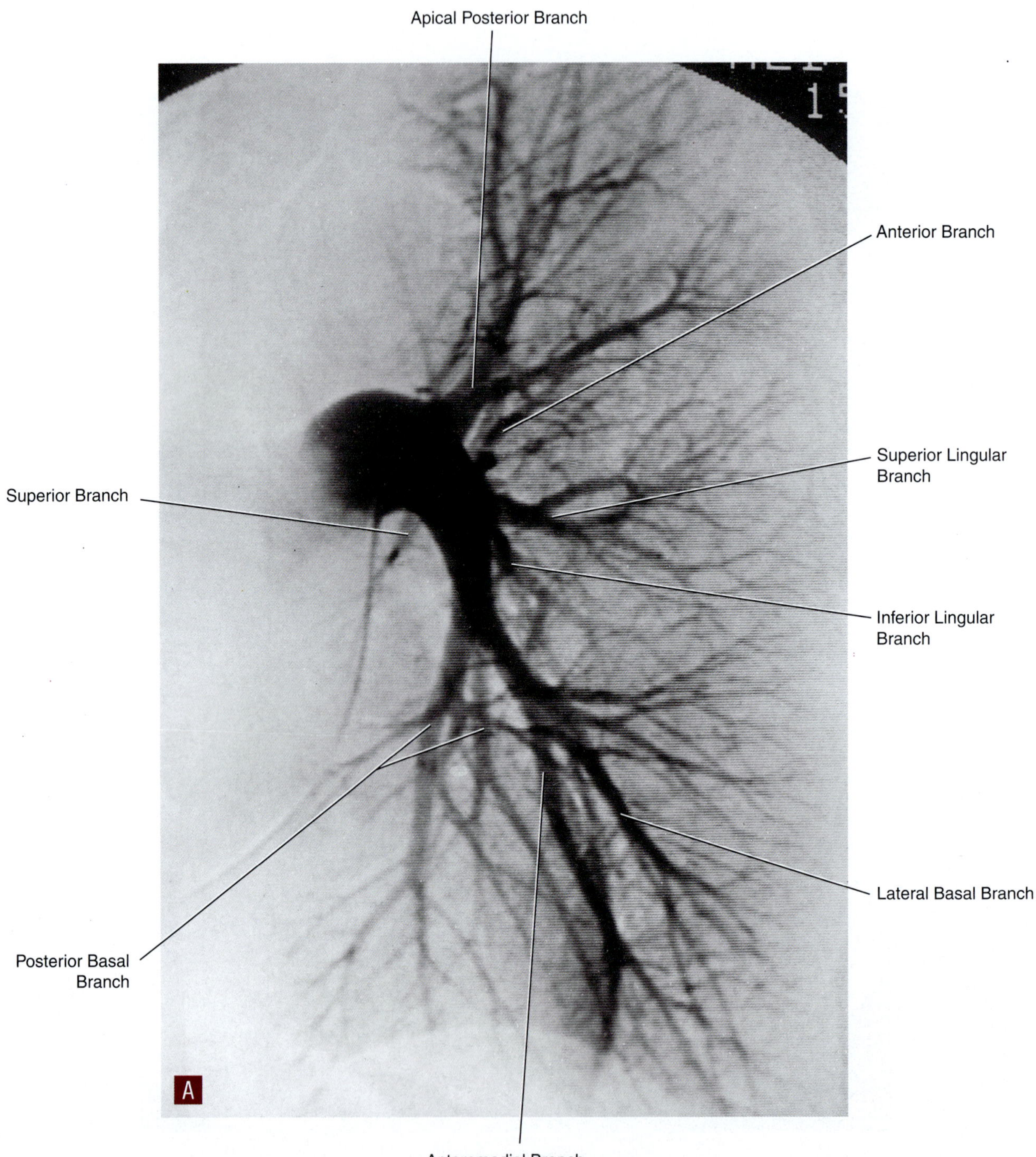

Figure 11.7. A, Anterior view of the left pulmonary artery angiogram showing the segments to the superior and inferior lobes. B, Late-phase angiogram showing the venous drainage from the superior and inferior pulmonary veins. The left atrium is partially visible.

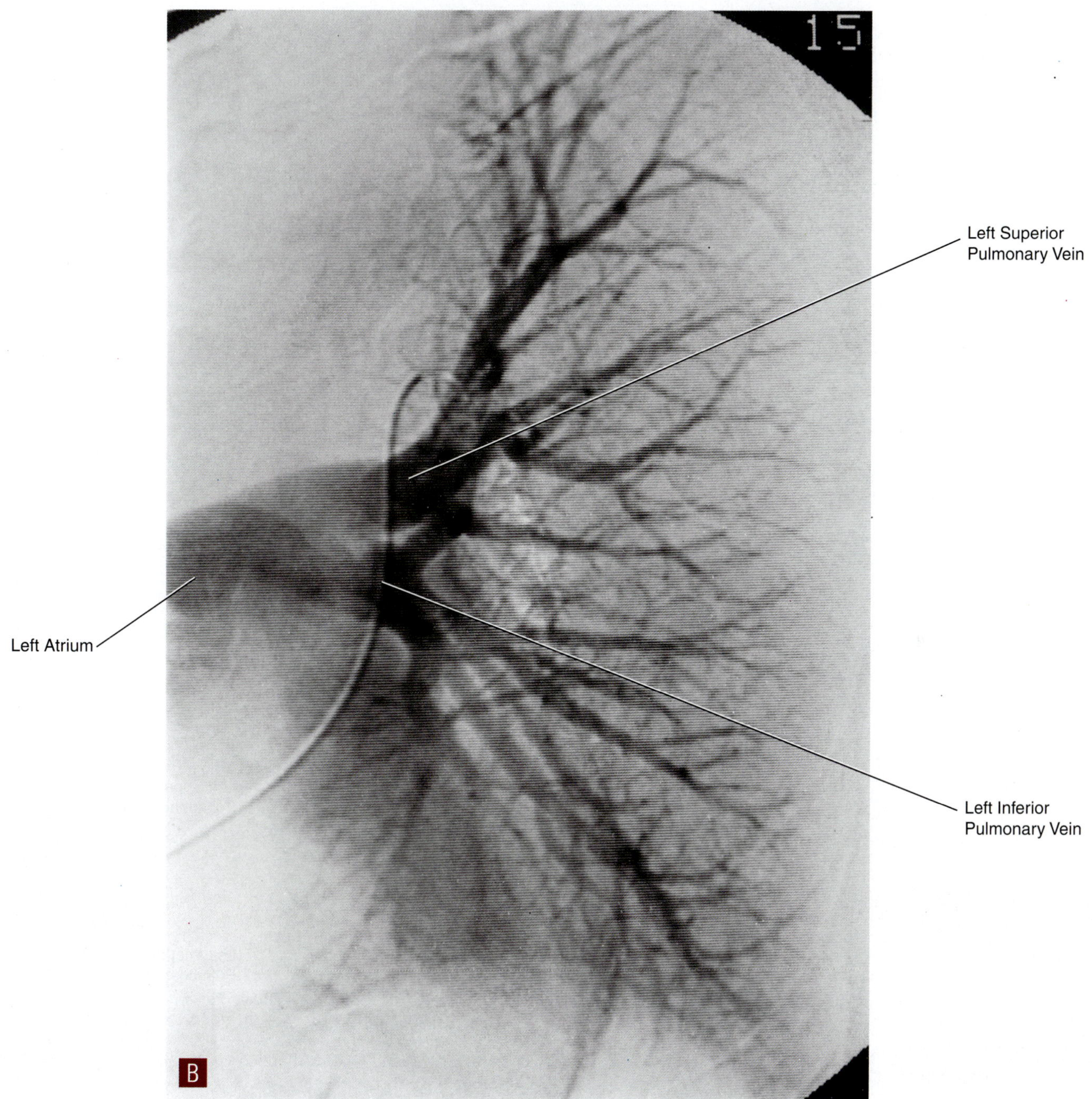

Figure 11.7. *Continued*

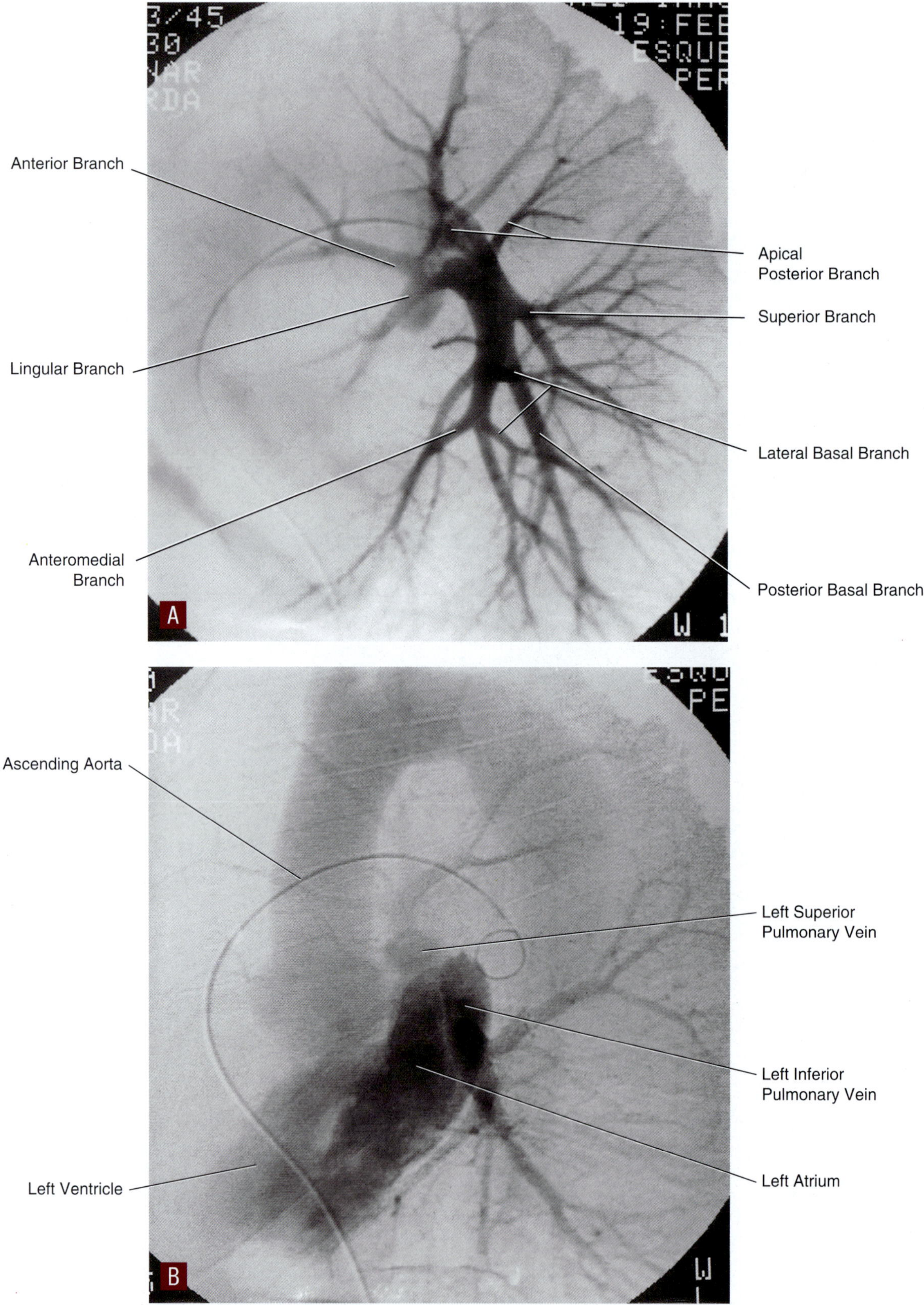

Figure 11.8. **A**, Lateral view of the left pulmonary artery angiogram showing the segments to the superior and inferior lobes. **B**, Late-phase angiogram showing the venous drainage. The left superior pulmonary vein is not seen well. The left atrium is visualized as is the left ventricle.

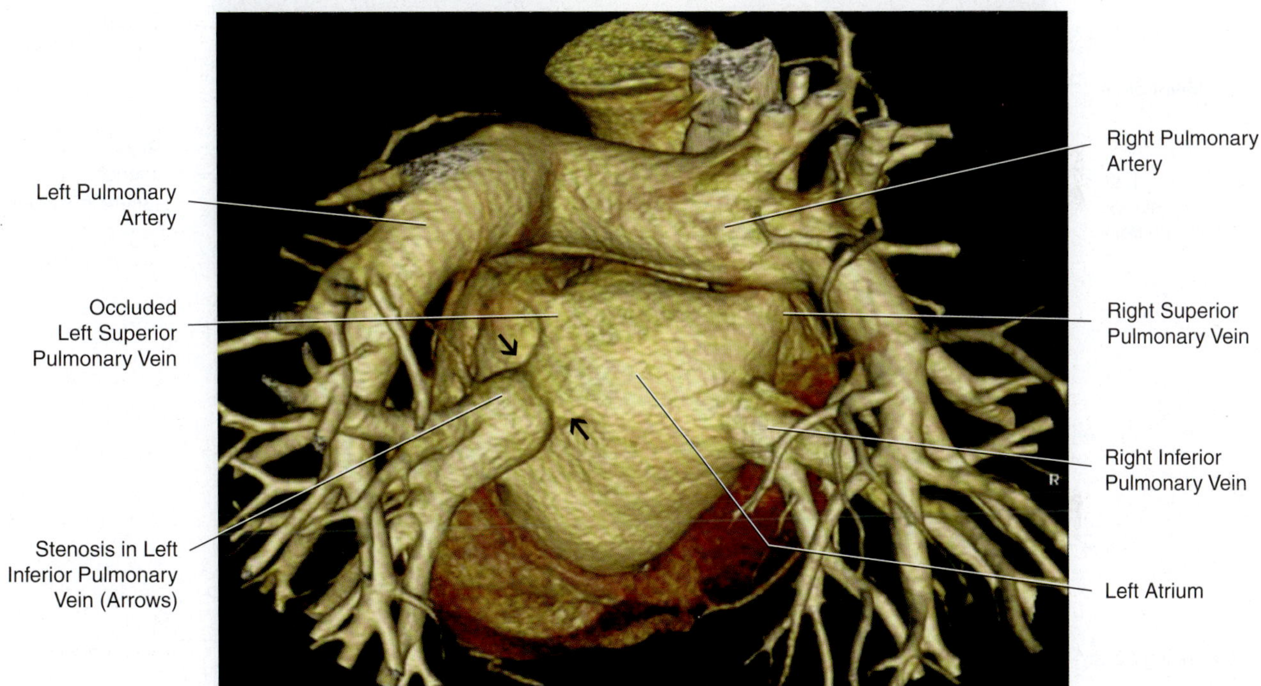

Figure 11.9. 3D computerized tomographic view in a patient treated with radiofrequency ablation for atrial fibrillation. Posterior view shows stenosis (arrows) in the left inferior vein with complete occlusion in the left superior vein. Right-sided veins are unremarkable.

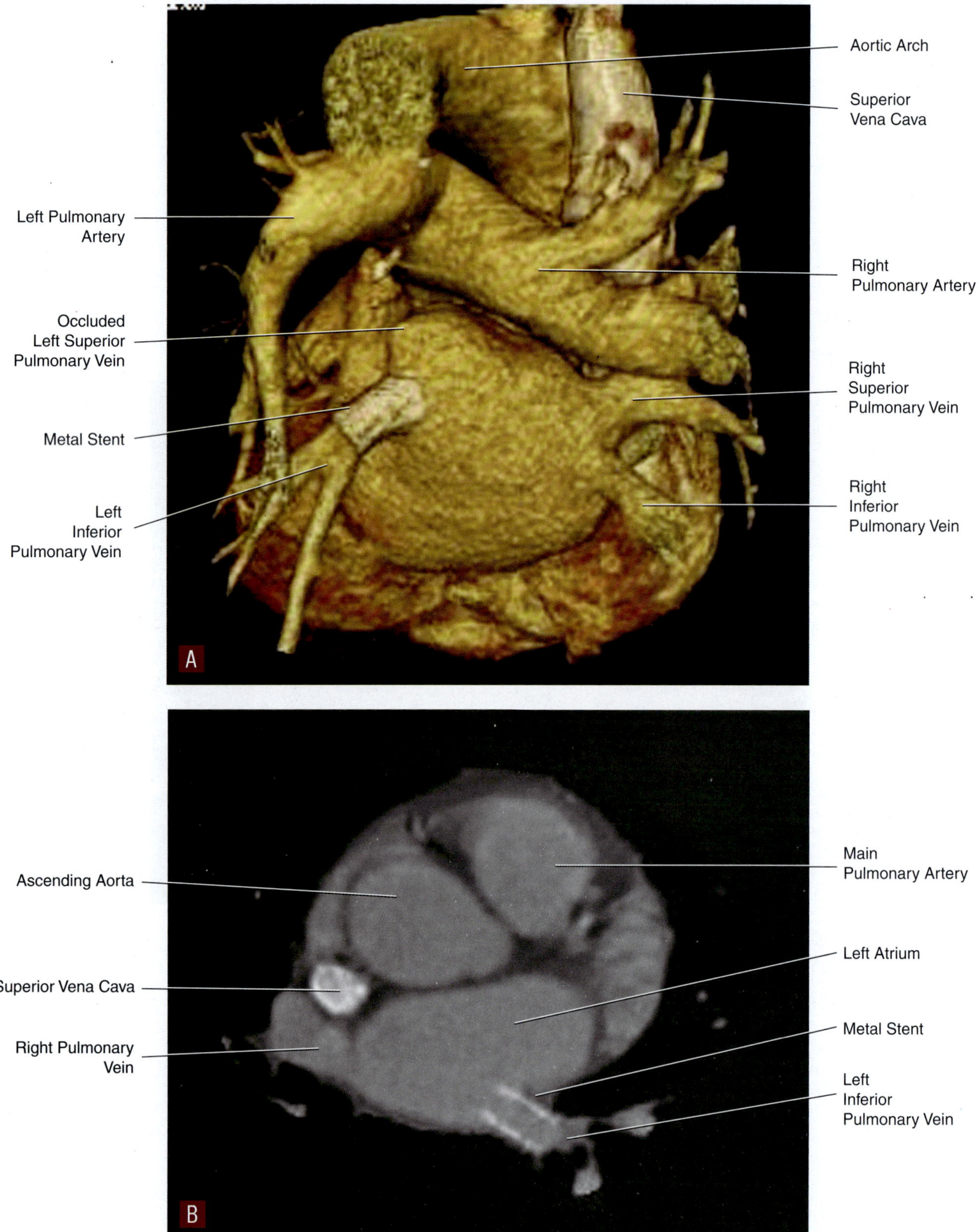

Figure 11.10. Computerized tomographic view in a patient with vein stenosis treated with a metal stent. **A**, 3D image shows the stent but does not reveal interior detail. **B**, Axial image shows widely patent stent in the left inferior pulmonary vein.

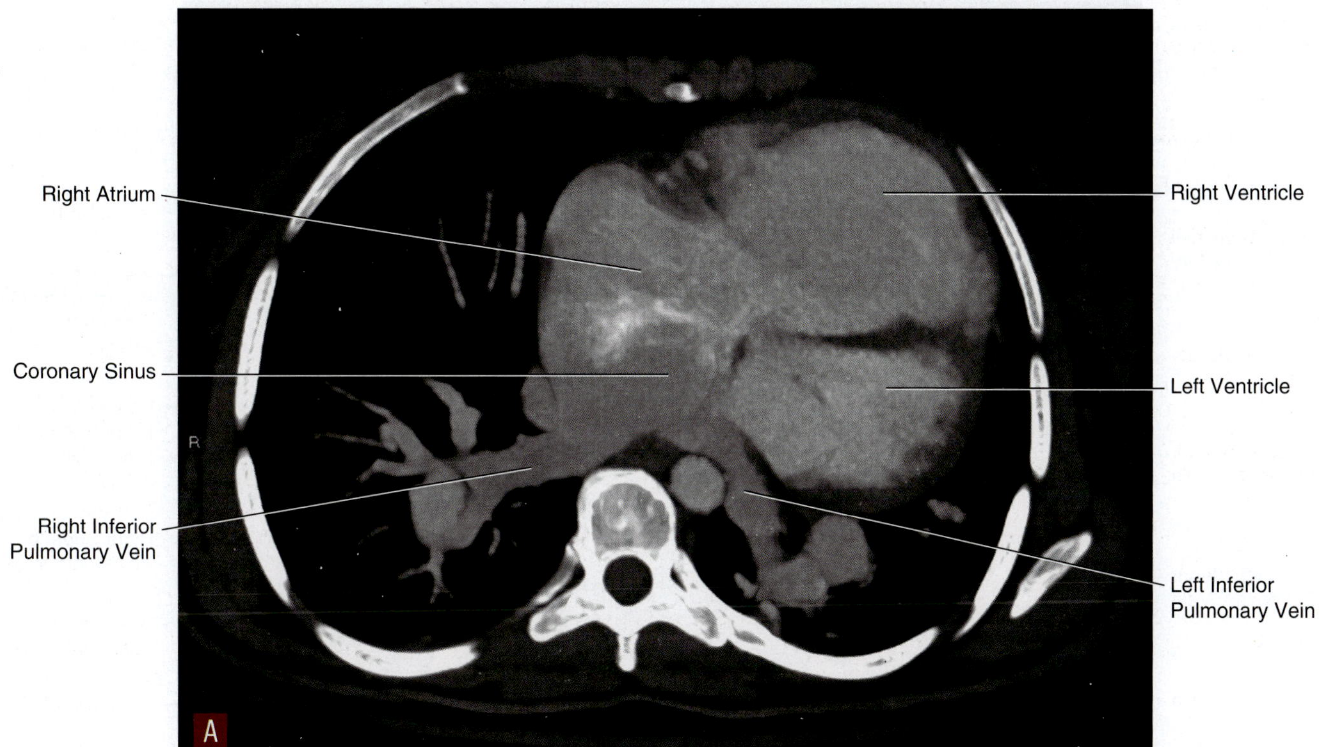

Figure 11.11. Total anomalous pulmonary venous return. A, Maximum intensity projection of a contrast-enhanced **computerized tomography** of the chest showing pulmonary venous drainage into the right atrium of a patient with total anomalous pulmonary venous return. The patient reached adulthood and survived because of a congenital secundum-type atrial septal defect. The left pulmonary veins drain into the coronary sinus. B, Cinematic-rendered reconstruction in a posterior view showing the common confluence of the right and left pulmonary veins. C, Right lateral view showing the right pulmonary veins draining into the right atrium directly. The pulmonary arteries are enlarged.

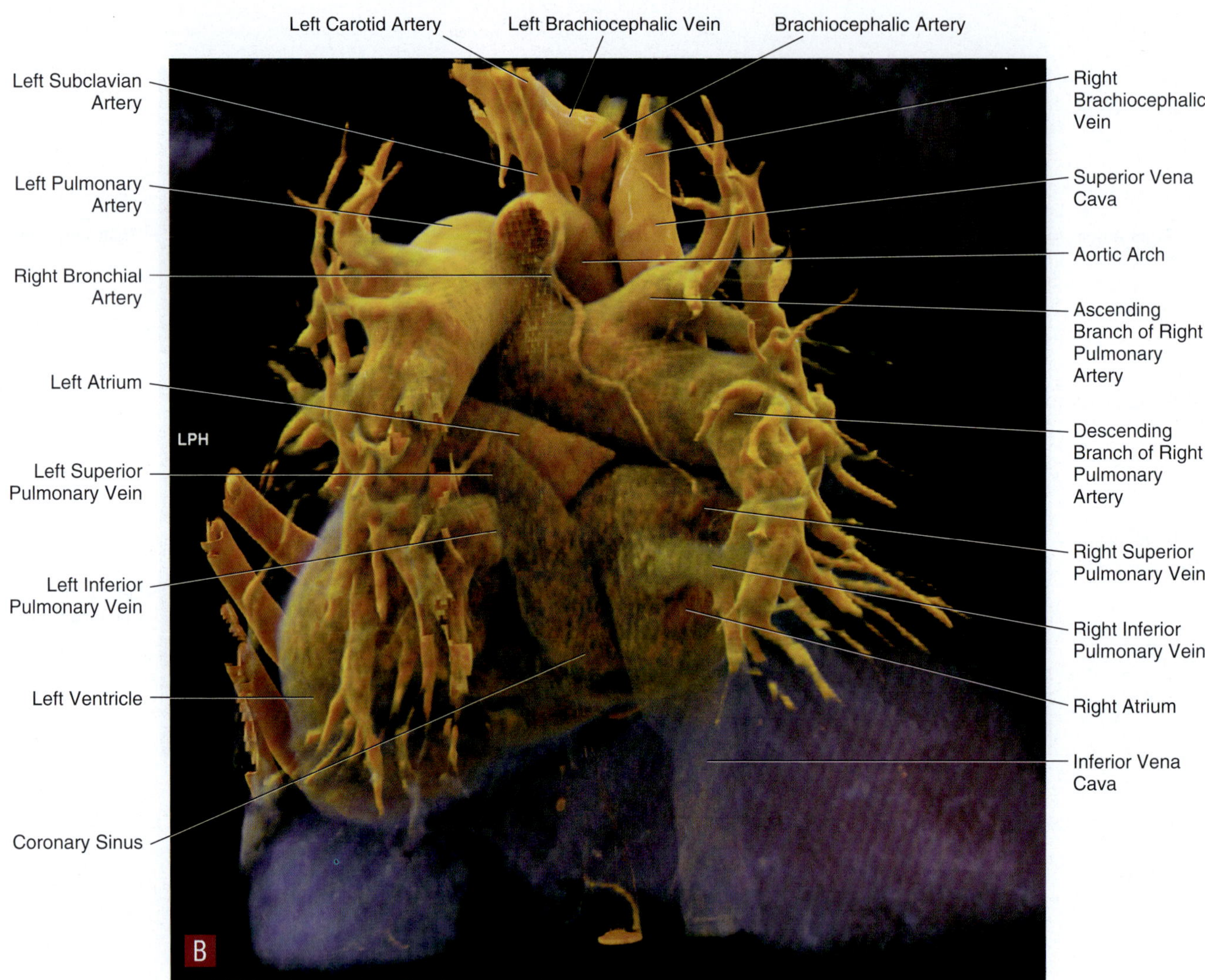

Figure 11.11. *Continued*

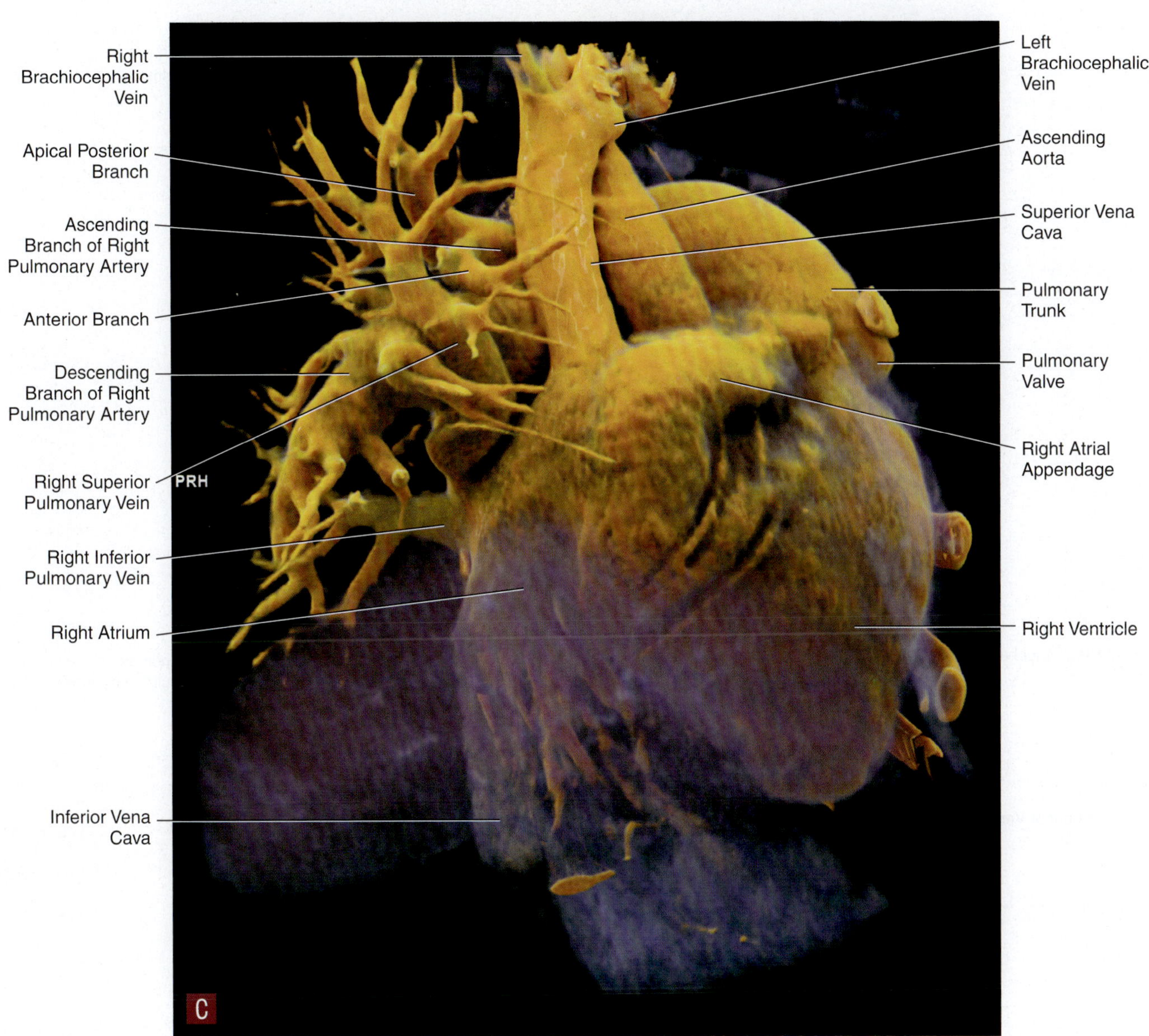

Figure 11.11. *Continued*

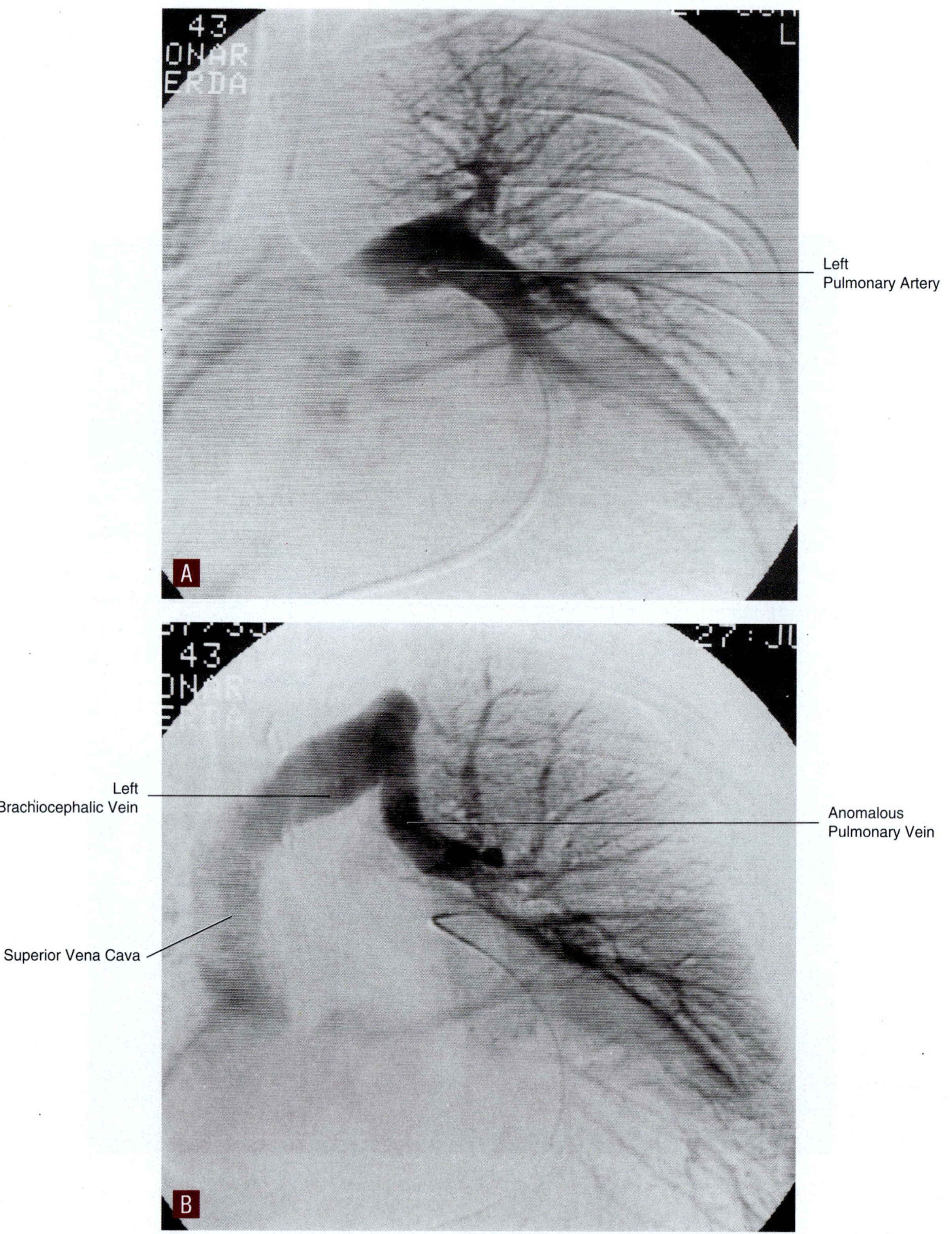

Figure 11.12. Anomalous pulmonary venous drainage. A, Anterior view of the arterial injection. B, Late phase of the pulmonary angiography showing the anomalous pulmonary drainage directly to the left brachiocephalic vein with opacification of the superior vena cava. C, Lateral view of the pulmonary angiography showing posterior displacement of the lung and artery. D, Late phase of the angiography showing the anomalous venous drainage to the left brachiocephalic vein and opacification of the superior vena cava. E, Sagittal view of a different patient from a **computerized tomographic** pulmonary angiogram showing an anomalous superior left pulmonary vein draining into the left brachiocephalic vein. F, 3D volume-rendered reconstruction on the same patient as in (E) showing the anomalous left upper lobe drainage. The intercostal and the vertebral veins are enlarged.

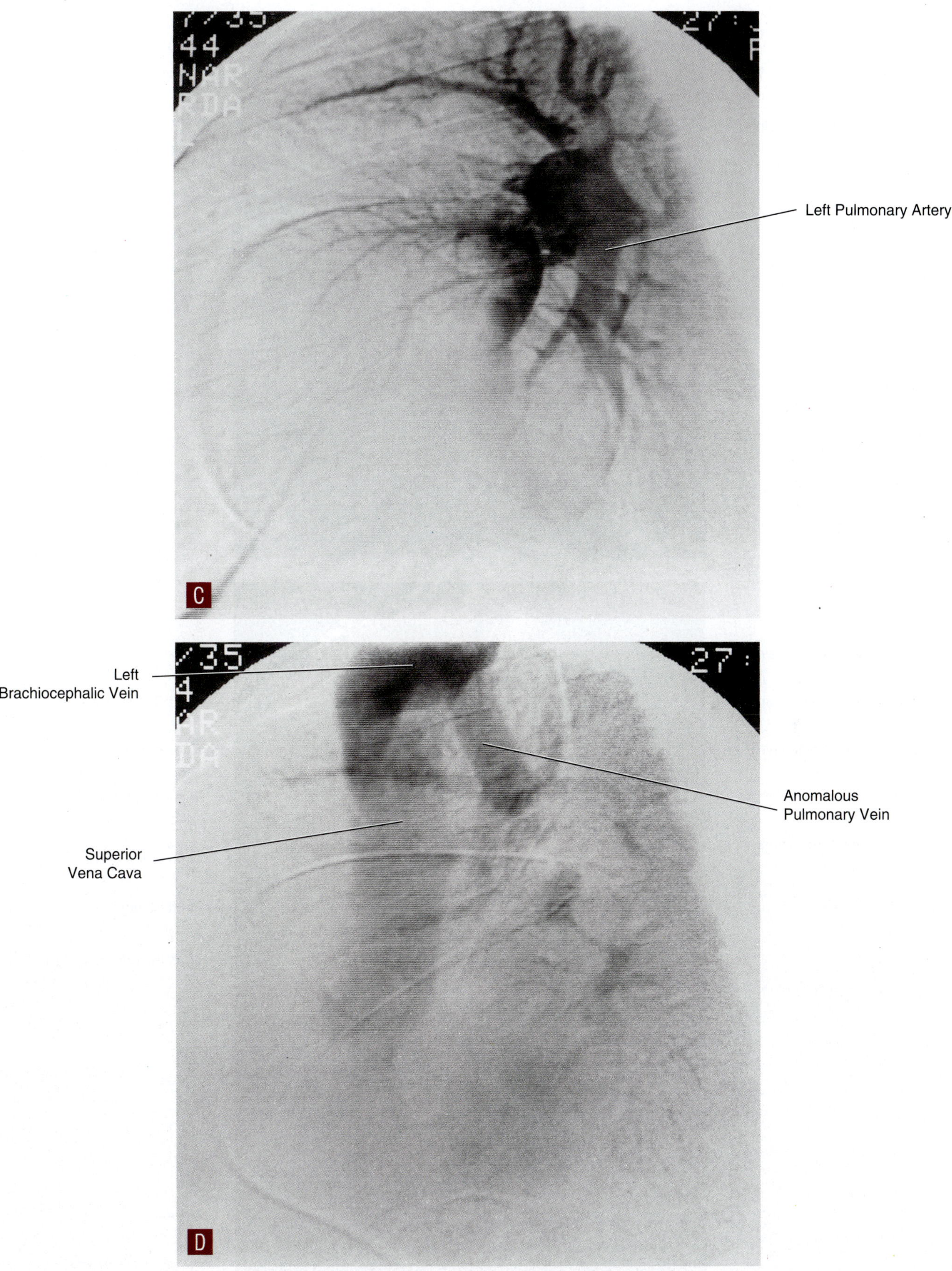

Figure 11.12. *Continued*

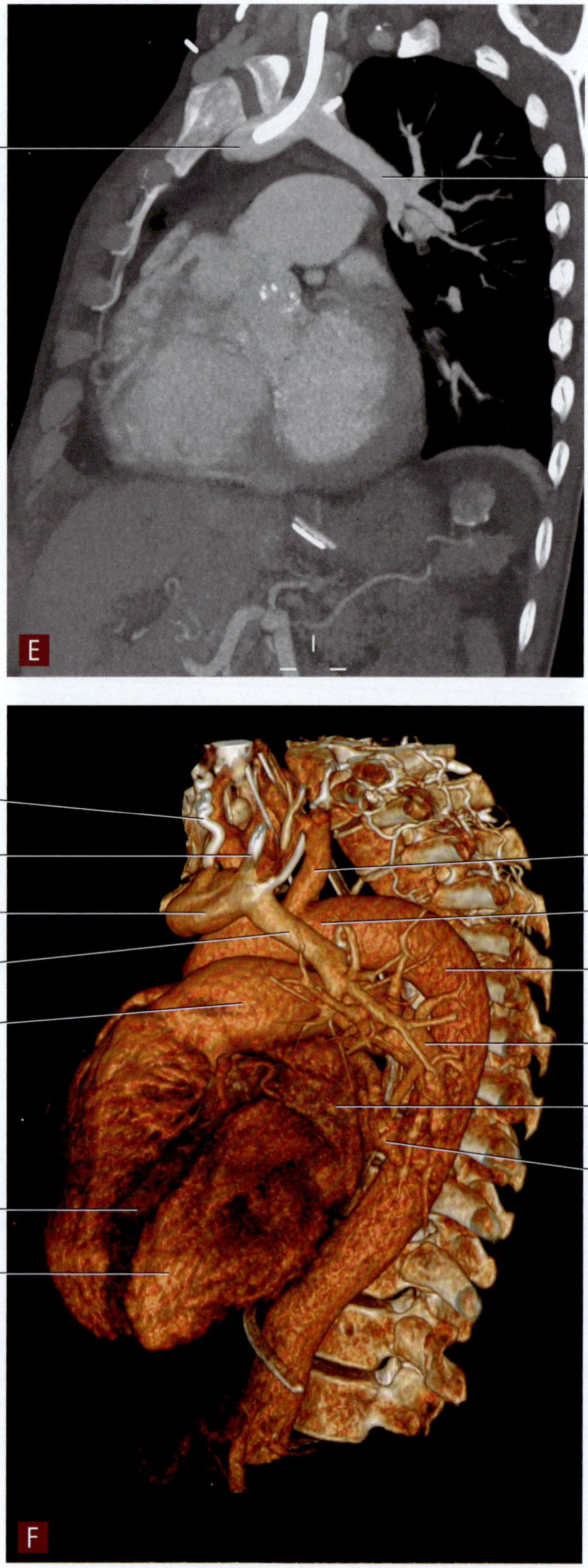

Figure 11.12. *Continued*

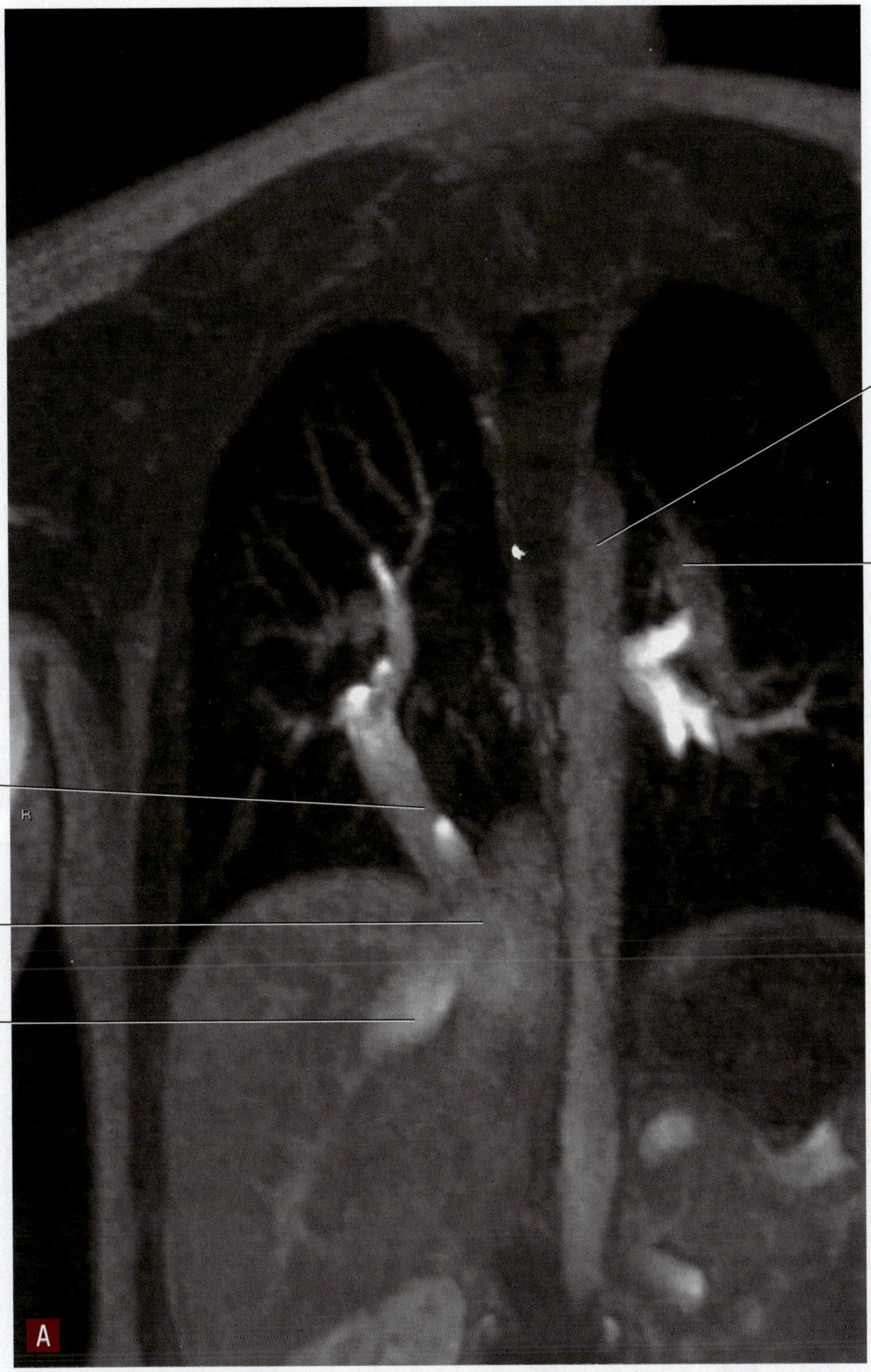

Descending Thoracic Aorta

Left Pulmonary Artery

Right Inferior Pulmonary Vein

R

Inferior Vena Cava

Right Hepatic Vein

A

Figure 11.13. Scimitar-shaped anomalous pulmonary drainage. A, Coronal projection of a magnetic resonance angiogram showing a large right pulmonary vein draining the right upper lobe directly into the inferior vena cava, just central to the intrahepatic segment. B, Left posterolateral view in the same patient on a cinematic-rendered reconstruction from a **computerized tomographic** pulmonary angiogram showing the anomalous pulmonary vein draining into the inferior vena cava (arrow). AAo, ascending thoracic aorta; DAo, descending thoracic aorta; IVC, inferior vena cava. C, Right anterior oblique view of the same patient as above, with the vein draining into the inferior vena cava (arrow). MPA, main pulmonary artery. (Images courtesy of Yoo Jin Lee, MD and Sina Mazaheri, MD.)

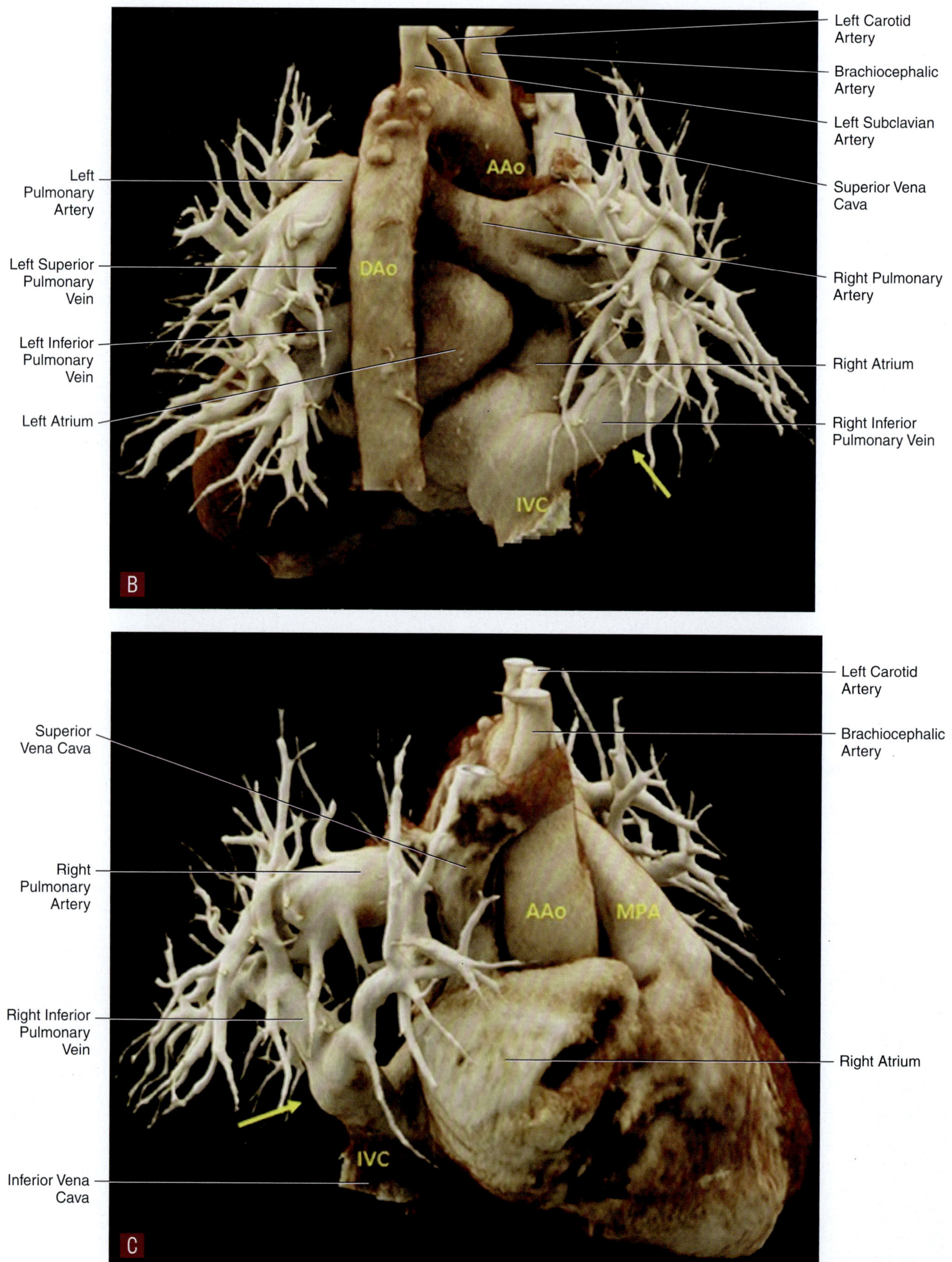

Figure 11.13. *Continued*

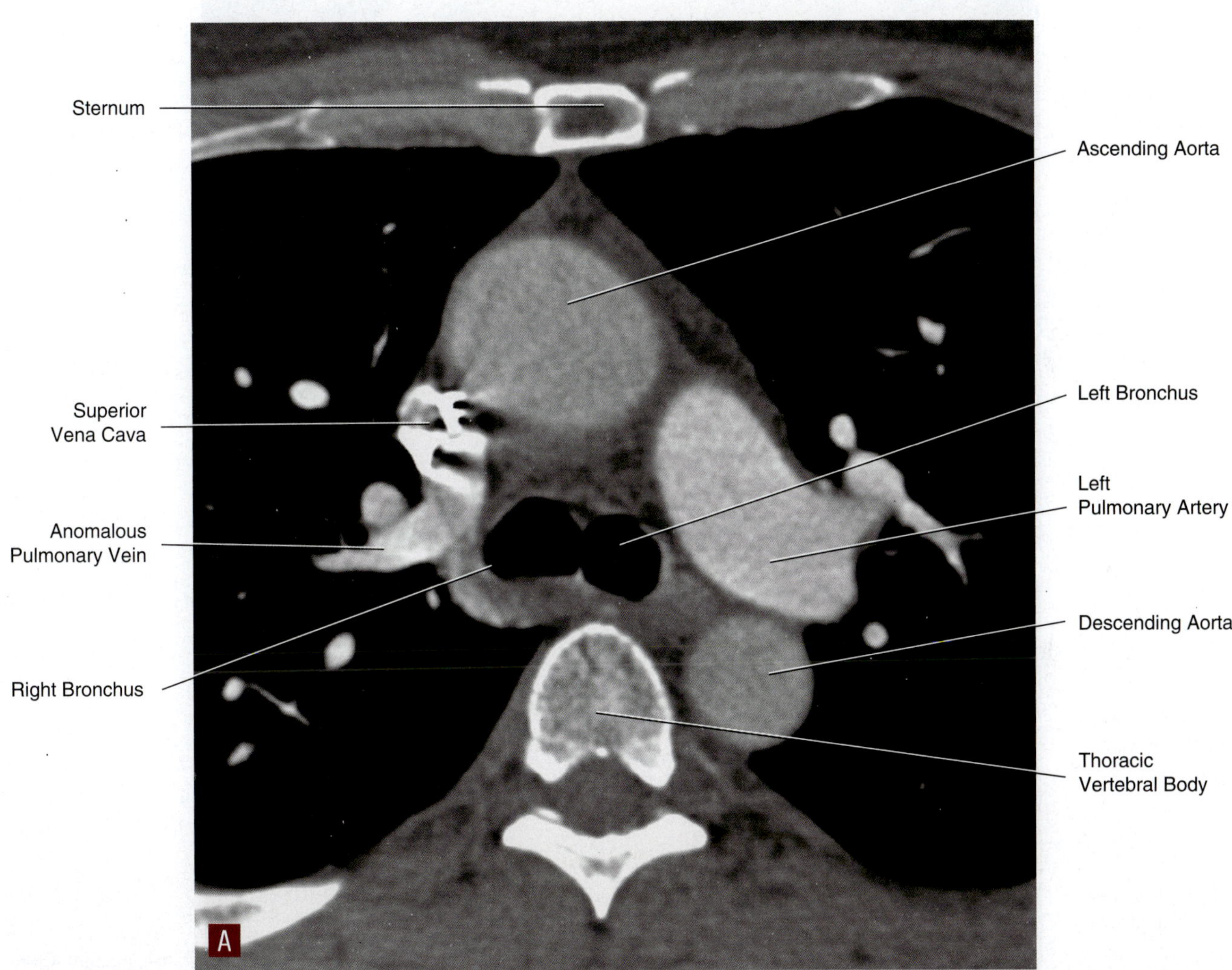

Figure 11.14. Computerized tomographic (CT) image of an asymptomatic patient with partial anomalous pulmonary venous return. A, Axial image shows the vessel draining from the right lung into the superior vena cava. B, 3D CT posterior view. 3D image demonstrates no superior right pulmonary vein in the usual location. The anomalous vessel can be seen near the top of the picture. C, 3D CT anterior view. 3D workstation used to highlight two anomalous right pulmonary veins that were present draining into the superior vena cava.

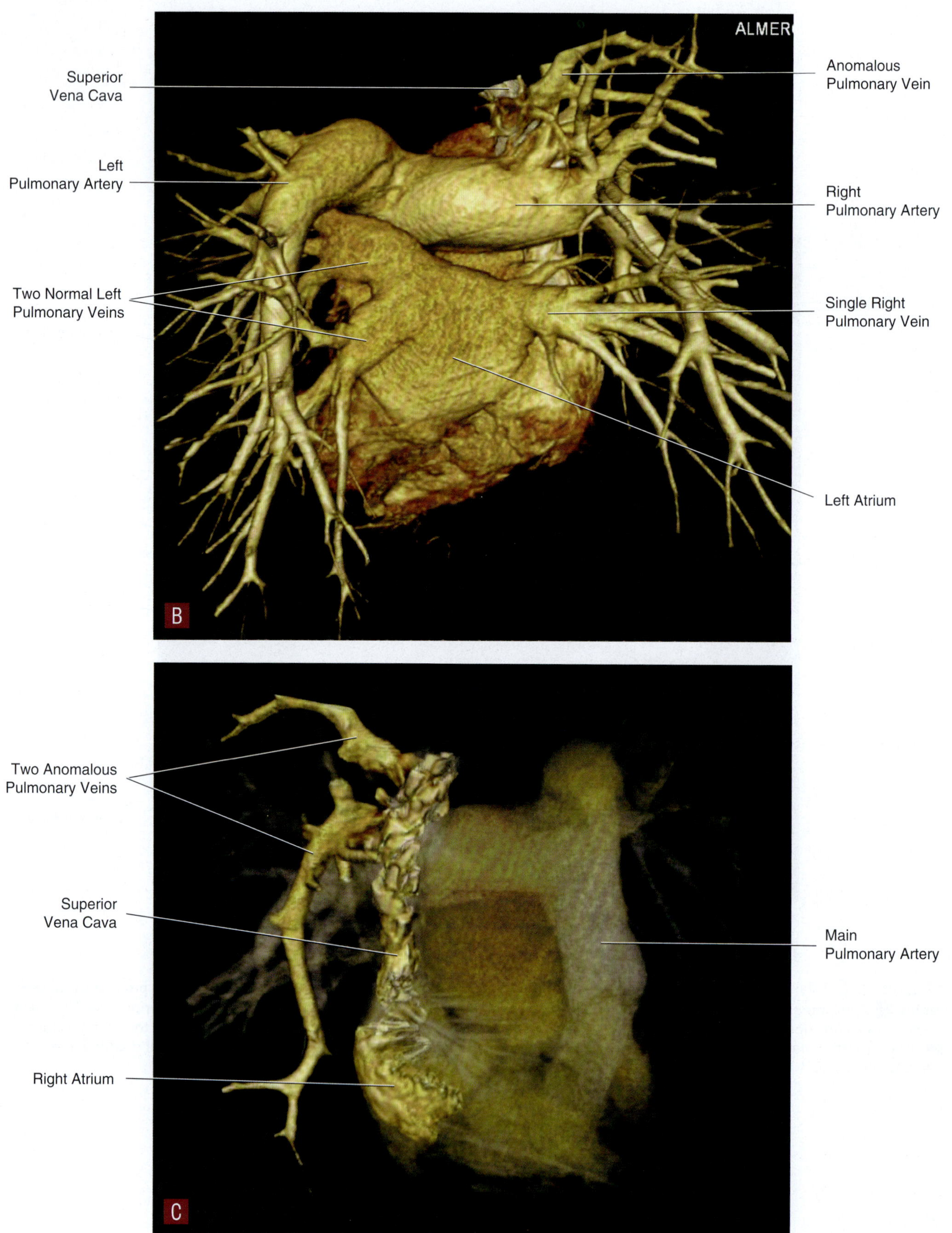

Figure 11.14. *Continued*

12

Pulmonary and Mediastinal Lymphatic System

The pleural lymphatics are variable in size, number, and distribution. They distribute in a plexus with broad channels. There are abundant anastomoses with the pulmonary lymphatics. The lymphatic network is more prominent over the lower than the upper pulmonary lobes. The pleural lymphatics drain to the medial aspect of the lung near the hilum, where there are anastomoses with the lymphatics of the parenchymal plexus (Figs. 12.1 and 12.2).

In the lungs, the lymphatic channels form two major paths: the first in the bronchoarterial and the other in the interlobular septal connective tissue. In both systems, the lymph flows toward the hilum, reaching the bronchial and mediastinal lymph nodes. Multiple anastomoses connect the interlobular perivenous lymphatics with those in the bronchoarterial sheathing. Anastomoses also exist among the bronchoarterial and pleural plexuses. The bronchoarterial lymphatics begin in the region of the distal respiratory bronchioles (Fig. 12.1).

Lymphatics of the Lungs and Pleura

The lungs are subdivided into three main lymphatic drainage areas: superior, middle, and inferior, without correspondence to the pulmonary lobes. On the right lung, the superior area drains directly into the paratracheal and upper bronchopulmonary nodes. The middle zone drains into the paratracheal bifurcation and the central group of bronchopulmonary lymph nodes. The inferior zone drains into the inferior bronchopulmonary and bifurcation nodes and the posterior mediastinal chain. The right lymphatic duct is, therefore, the main drainage system of the right lung. On the left lung, the left superior area drains into the prevascular group of anterior mediastinal nodes and the left paratracheal nodes. The middle zone drains through the bifurcation and the central group of bronchopulmonary nodes and also directly through the paratracheal group. The inferior zone drains into the bifurcation and inferior bronchopulmonary nodes and into the posterior mediastinal group. The left lung, therefore, drains lymph from the superior zone and part of the middle zone to the left paratracheal nodes and into the thoracic duct. The remainder of the lymphatic drainage of the left lung ends up in the right lymphatic duct (Fig. 12.3).

Thoracic Duct and Right Lymphatic Duct

The right lymphatic duct drains the great majority of lymph from both the lungs, whereas the thoracic duct drains the apical portion of the left lung (Fig. 12.3).

The thoracic duct originates at the cisterna chyli on the anterior aspect of the vertebral column at the lever T12 to L2, resulting from the junction of the lumbar lymphatic trunks. The thoracic duct enters the posterior mediastinum through the aortic hiatus of the diaphragm. The thoracic duct ascends cephalad at the right side of the aorta, approximately at the midline or slightly toward the right side. High up in the thorax, the thoracic duct crosses to the left and leaves the thorax between the esophagus and left subclavian artery, joining the left subclavian vein from the posterior aspect. The diameter of the thoracic duct ranges from 1 to 7 mm, and valves are found in the majority of cases.

The right lymphatic duct is poorly documented, but the duct is an inconstant channel and may consist of multiple fine vessels or a network of small ducts rather than a single channel.

Lymph Nodes of the Mediastinum

The intrathoracic lymph nodes are composed of parietal and visceral components. The parietal lymph nodes lie outside the parietal pleura in the extramediastinal tissue, where they drain the thoracic wall and other extrathoracic structures. The visceral lymph nodes are located within the mediastinum between the pleural membranes and are related to the drainage of the intrathoracic content (Chapter 9, Figs. 9.1, 9.8).

Parietal Lymph Nodes

Anterior Parietal Nodes (Internal Mammary Nodes)

The anterior parietal nodes are located bilaterally, either medial or lateral to the internal mammary vessels. They drain the afferent lymph vessels from the upper anterior abdominal wall, anterior thoracic wall, anterior portion of the diaphragm, and medial portion of the breasts. They communicate with the anterior mediastinal nodes and the cervical nodes. The main efferent vessel is the right lymphatic duct or thoracic duct (see Fig. 9.5).

Posterior Parietal Nodes (Intercostal Nodes and Juxtavertebral Nodes)

The posterior parietal nodes drain the intercostal spaces, parietal pleura, and vertebral column. There are communications with other posterior mediastinal lymph nodes. The efferent channels drain superiorly to the thoracic duct and to the cisterna chyli inferiorly (see Fig. 9.1).

Diaphragmatic Lymph Nodes (Anterior Prepericardiac Group, Middle Juxtaphrenic Group, Posterior Retrocrural Nodes)

The diaphragmatic lymph nodes drain the diaphragm and the anterosuperior portion of the liver.

Visceral Lymph Nodes

Anterosuperior Mediastinal Nodes (Prevascular)

The anterosuperior mediastinal nodes are located along the anterior aspect of the superior vena cava, right and left innominate veins, and ascending aorta. They drain most of the structures in the anterior mediastinum, including the pericardium, thymus, thyroid, diaphragmatic and mediastinal pleura, part of the heart, and the anterior portion of the hilum. Efferents drain into the right lymphatic duct or thoracic duct.

Posterior Mediastinal Nodes

Periesophageal Nodes. These nodes are located around the esophagus.

Periaortic Nodes. The periaortic nodes are located anterior and lateral to the descending aorta. They communicate with the tracheobronchial group, particularly with the subcarinal group, and drain mainly to the thoracic duct.

Tracheobronchial Lymph Nodes Group

Paratracheal Lymph Nodes. The paratracheal lymph nodes are located anterior and to the right and left of the trachea. Posterior nodes are occasionally found. The azygos node is one of the large lower paratracheal nodes, medial to the azygos venous arch. The paratracheal nodes receive afferents from the bronchopulmonary and tracheal bifurcation nodes. They also receive afferents from the trachea, esophagus, and right and left lungs. Efferents are the right lymphatic duct and thoracic duct.

Tracheal Bifurcation Nodes (Carinal). These nodes are located in the precarinal and subcarinal fat, as well as around the right and left main bronchi. On the left, the aortopulmonary window nodes are found between the left pulmonary artery and aortic arch. They receive afferents from the bronchopulmonary nodes, anterior and posterior mediastinal nodes, heart, esophagus, pericardium, and lungs. Efferents drain to the paratracheal group.

Bronchopulmonary Nodes (Hilar). The bronchopulmonary nodes are located around the bronchi and vessels, especially at the bifurcation. They receive lymph vessels from the pulmonary lobes. Efferent vessels drain to the carinal and paratracheal nodes (Fig. 12.3).

International Association for the Study of Lung Cancer (IASLC) Lymph Node Map. The IASLC lymph node map was created to encourage the standardized, reproducible labeling of thoracic and mediastinal lymph nodes and was last updated in 2014. This classification system defines 14 different lymph node stations, grouped into seven zones, which can be found in the Table included in the chapter and in a diagrammatic form in Fig. 12.5. The computerized tomographic (CT) appearance of the lymph node zones and certain stations can be seen in Fig. 12.6.

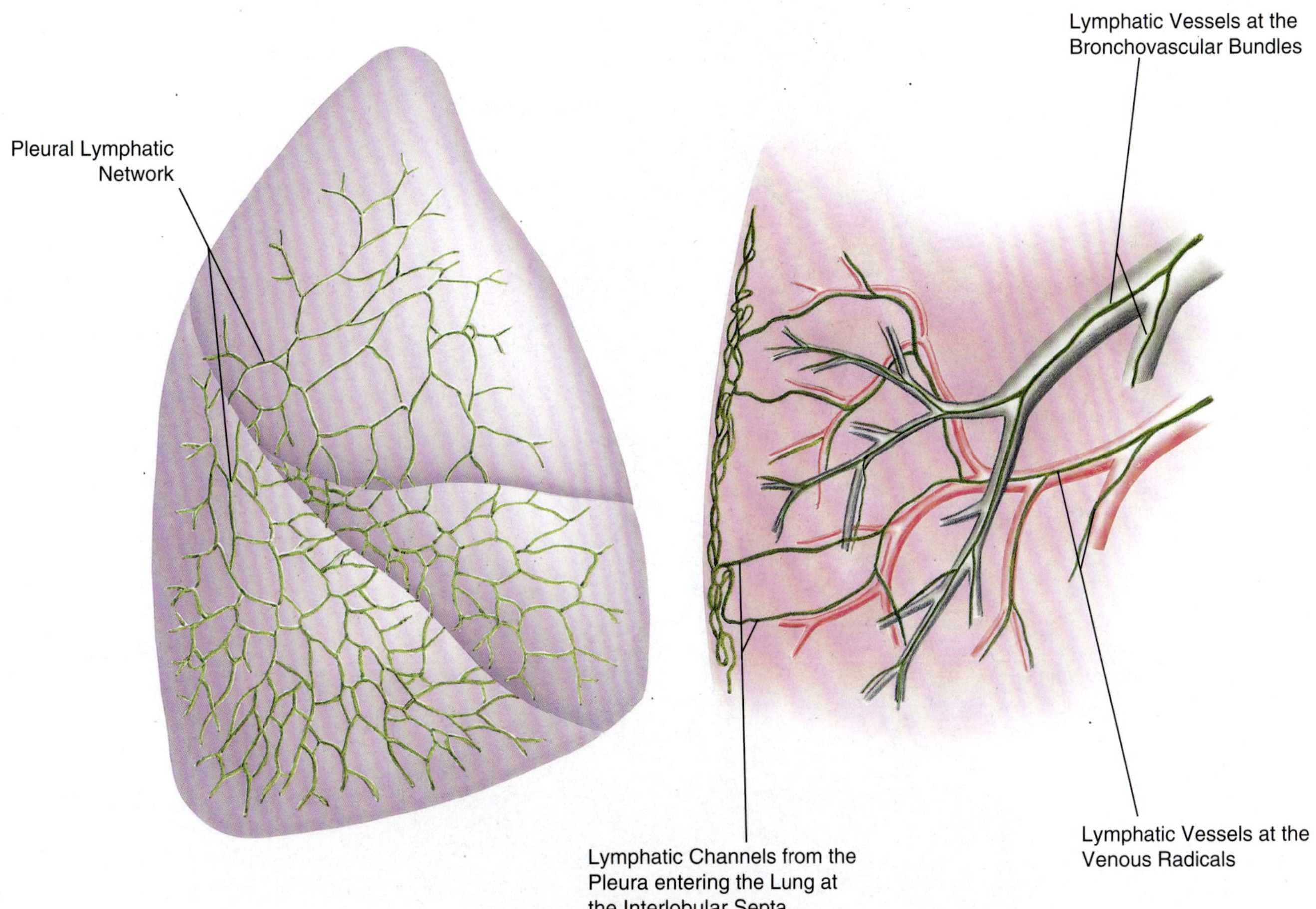

Figure 12.1. Pleural lymphatic drainage. The lateral view of the right lung shows the pleural lymphatic network. The lymphatic network is more prominent over the lower than the upper pulmonary lobes. On close up, the lymphatic channels in the lungs form two major paths, the first in the bronchoarterial bundles and the other in the interlobular septal connective tissue. In both systems, the lymph flows toward the hilum, reaching the bronchopulmonary nodes and mediastinal lymph nodes.

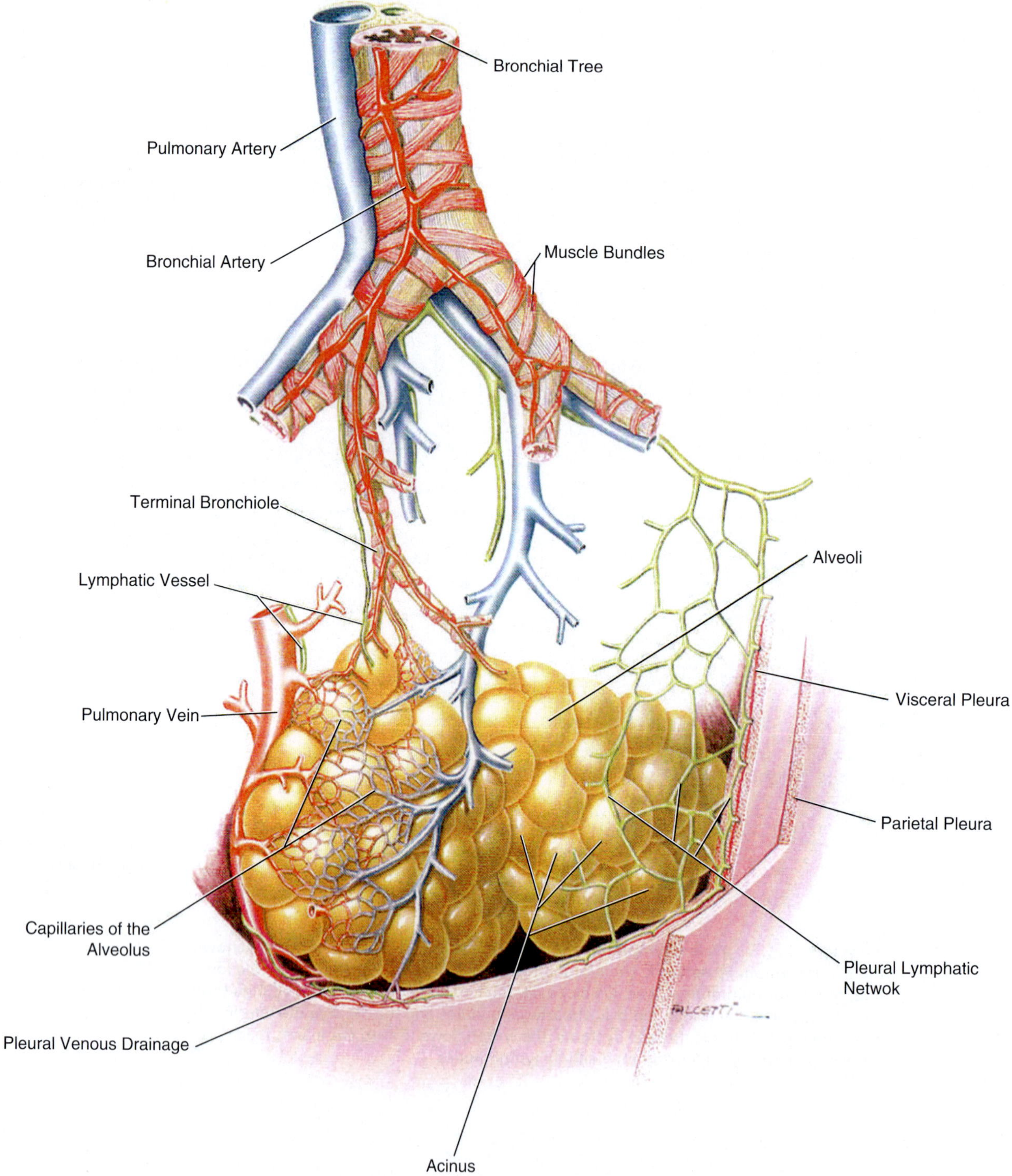

Figure 12.2. Pulmonary microcirculation, showing the relationships of the pulmonary artery, bronchial artery, capillaries of the alveolus, pulmonary vein, and lymphatic network.

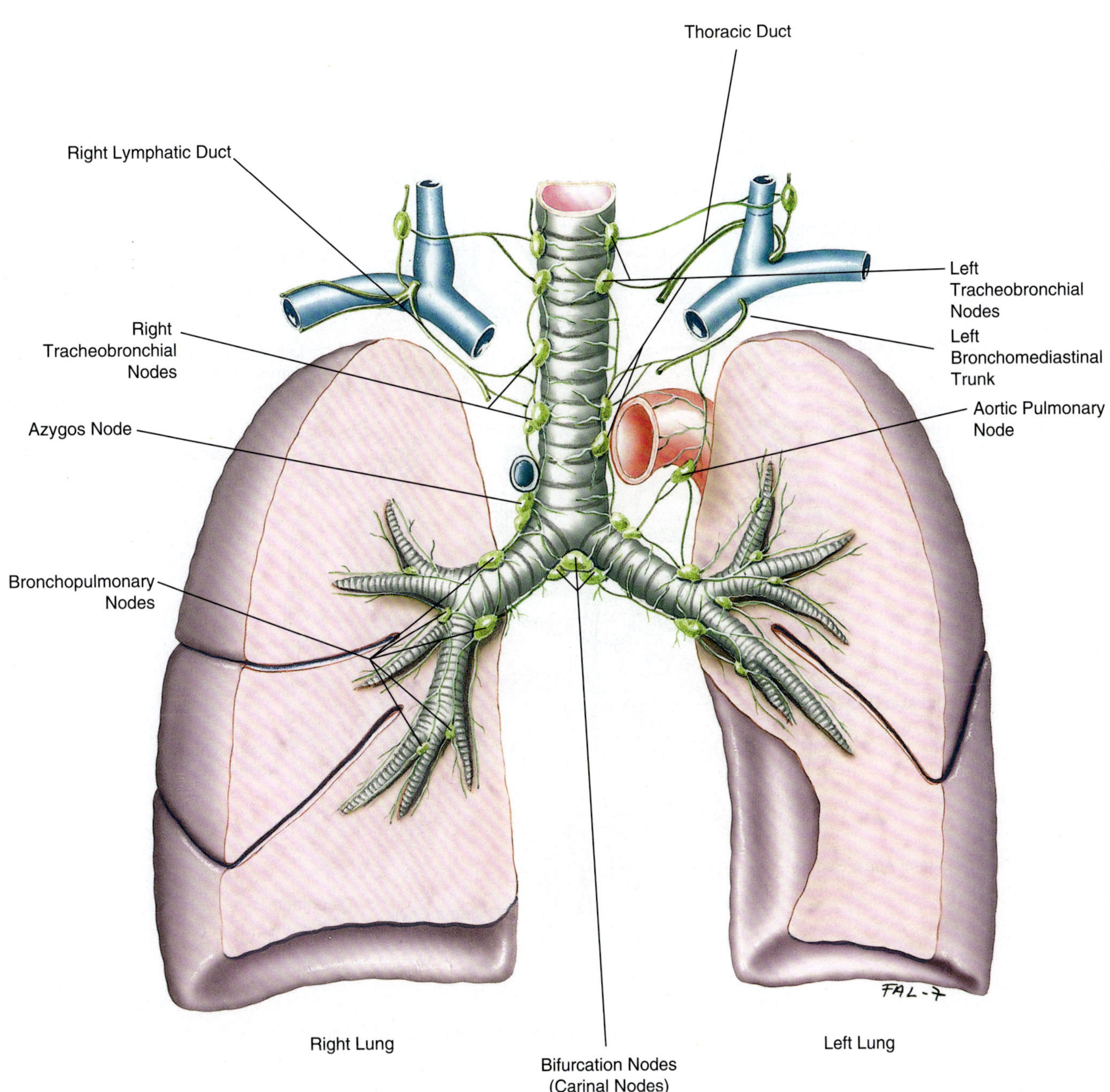

Figure 12.3. Lymphatic pulmonary drainage. The right lymphatic duct drains the great majority of lymph from both the lungs, whereas the apical portion of the left lung drains preferentially to the left system or the thoracic duct.

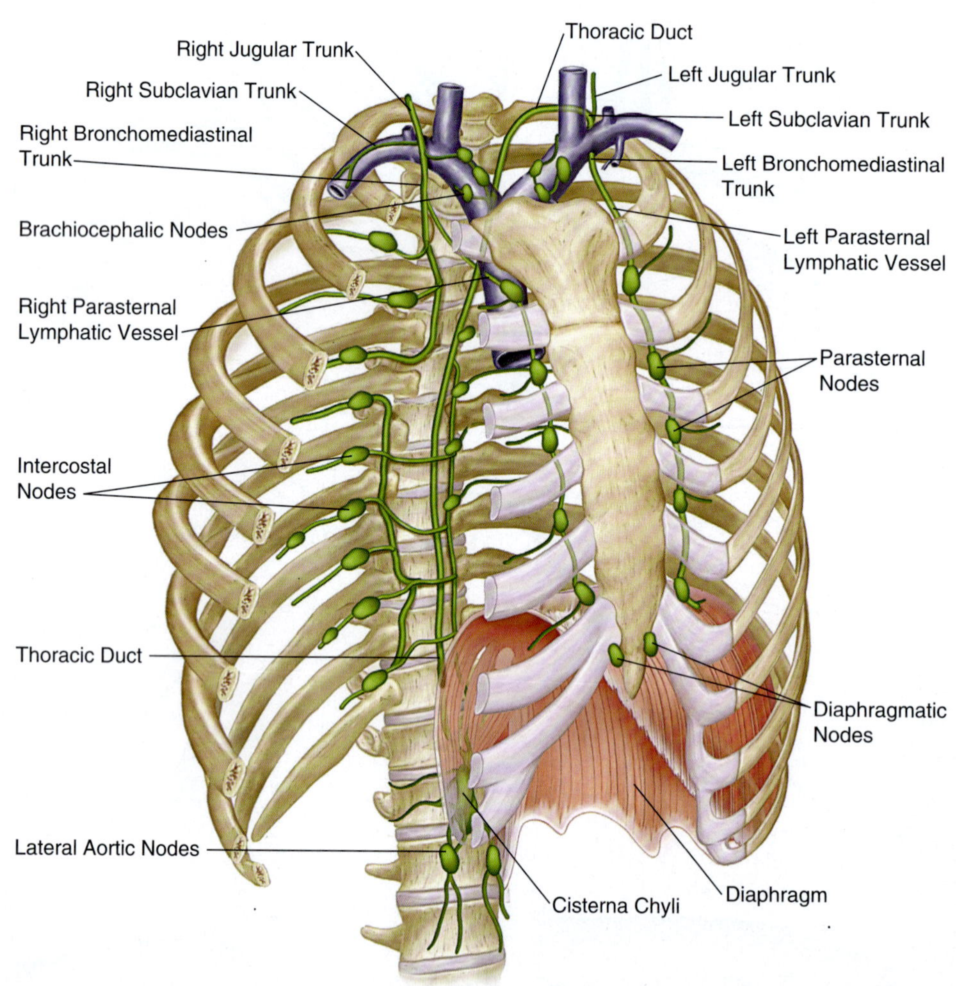

Figure 12.4. Diagram of the lymphatic drainage of the thorax.

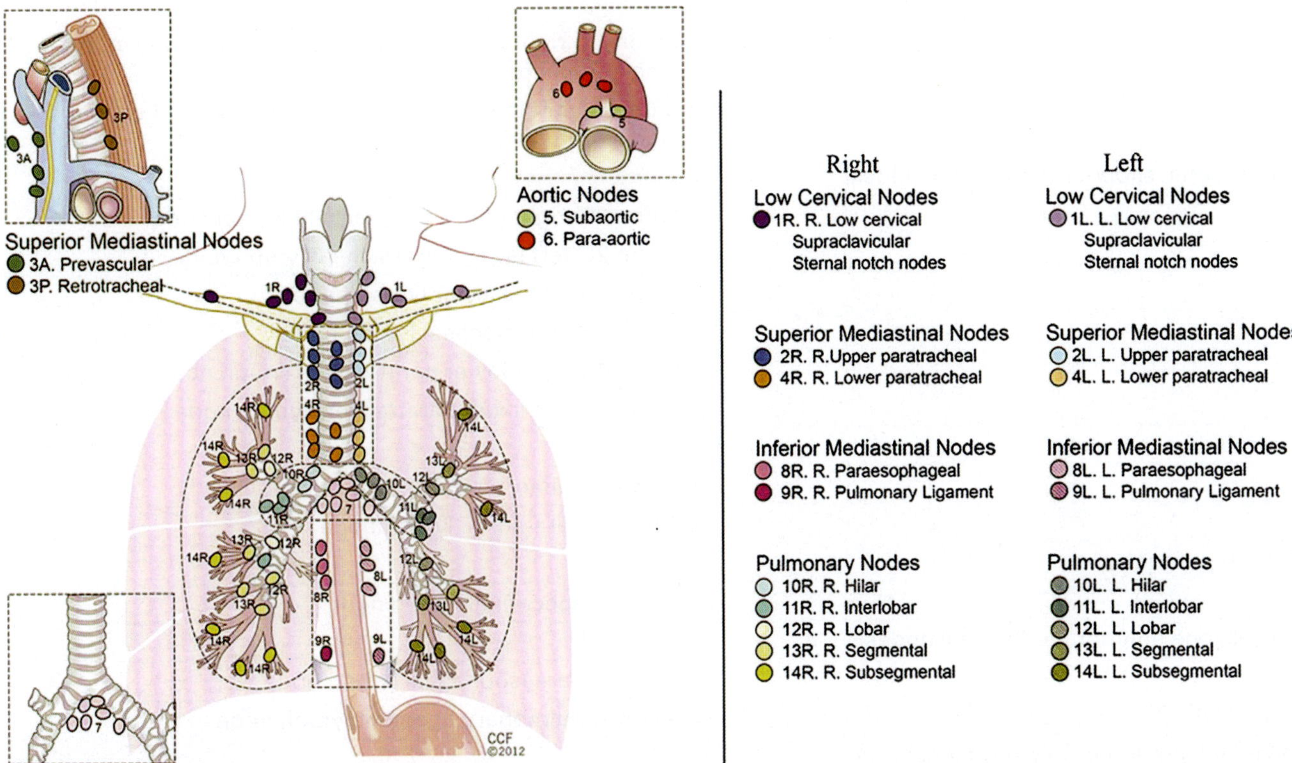

Figure 12.5. Diagram of the International Association for the Study of Lung Cancer lymph node map. (Reprinted from El-Sherief AH, Lau CT, Wu CC, et al. International association for the study of lung cancer (IASLC) lymph node map: radiologic review with CT illustration. *RadioGraphics*. 2014;34:1680-1691 with permission from RSNA.) The reference for each lymph node station can be found in Table 12.1.

TABLE **12.1. Nodal Stations and Zones in the International Association for the Study of Lung Cancer (IASLC) Lymph Node Map**

Supraclavicular Zone	
	Station 1R: right low cervical, supraclavicular, and sternal notch lymph nodes
	Station 1L: left low cervical, supraclavicular, and sternal notch lymph nodes
Upper zone (superior mediastinal nodes)	
	Station 2R: right upper paratracheal lymph node
	Station 2L: left upper paratracheal lymph node
	Station 3A: prevascular lymph node
	Station 3P: retrotracheal lymph node
	Station 4R: right lower paratracheal lymph node
	Station 4L: left lower paratracheal lymph node
Aortopulmonary zone	
	Station 5: subaortic lymph node
	Station 6: para-aortic lymph node
Subcarinal zone	
	Station 7: subcarinal lymph node
Lower zone (inferior mediastinal nodes)	
	Station 8: paraesophageal lymph node
	Station 9: pulmonary ligament lymph node
Hilar and interlobar zone (pulmonary nodes)	
	Station 10: hilar lymph node
	Station 11: interlobar lymph node
	Peripheral zone (pulmonary nodes)
	Station 12: lobar lymph node
	Station 13: segmental lymph node
	Station 14: subsegmental lymph node

Reprinted from Tanoue LT. Staging of non-small cell lung cancer. *Semin Respir Crit Care Med.* 2008;29(3):248-260 with permission.

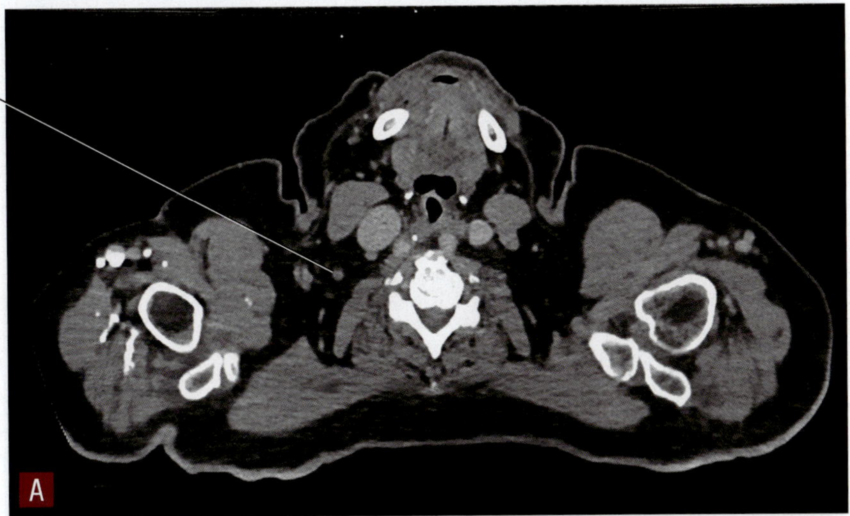

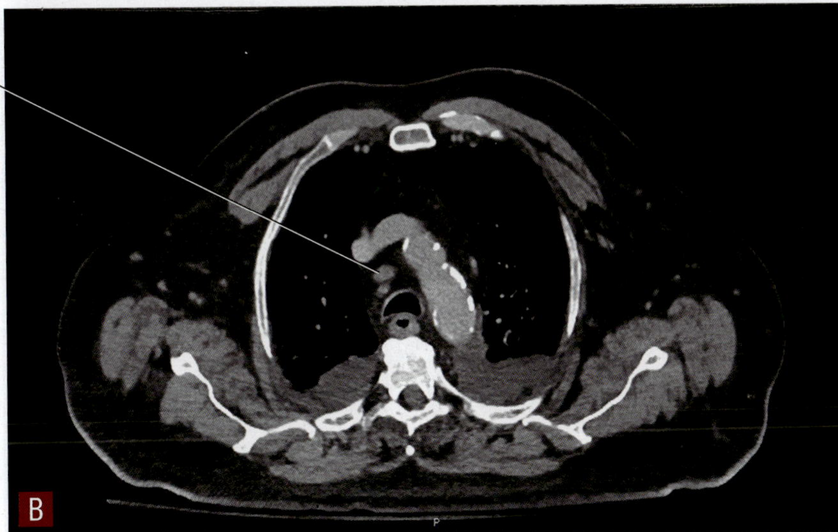

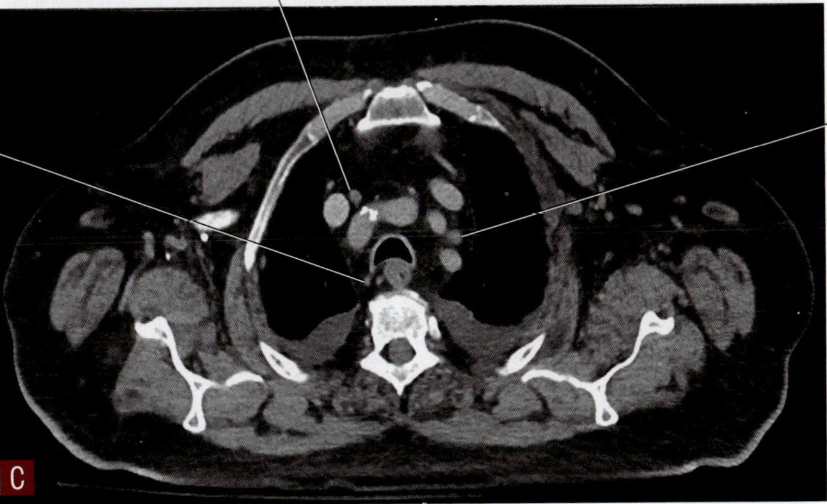

Figure 12.6. **A to I, Computerized tomographic images of the seven lymph node zones and selected stations.**

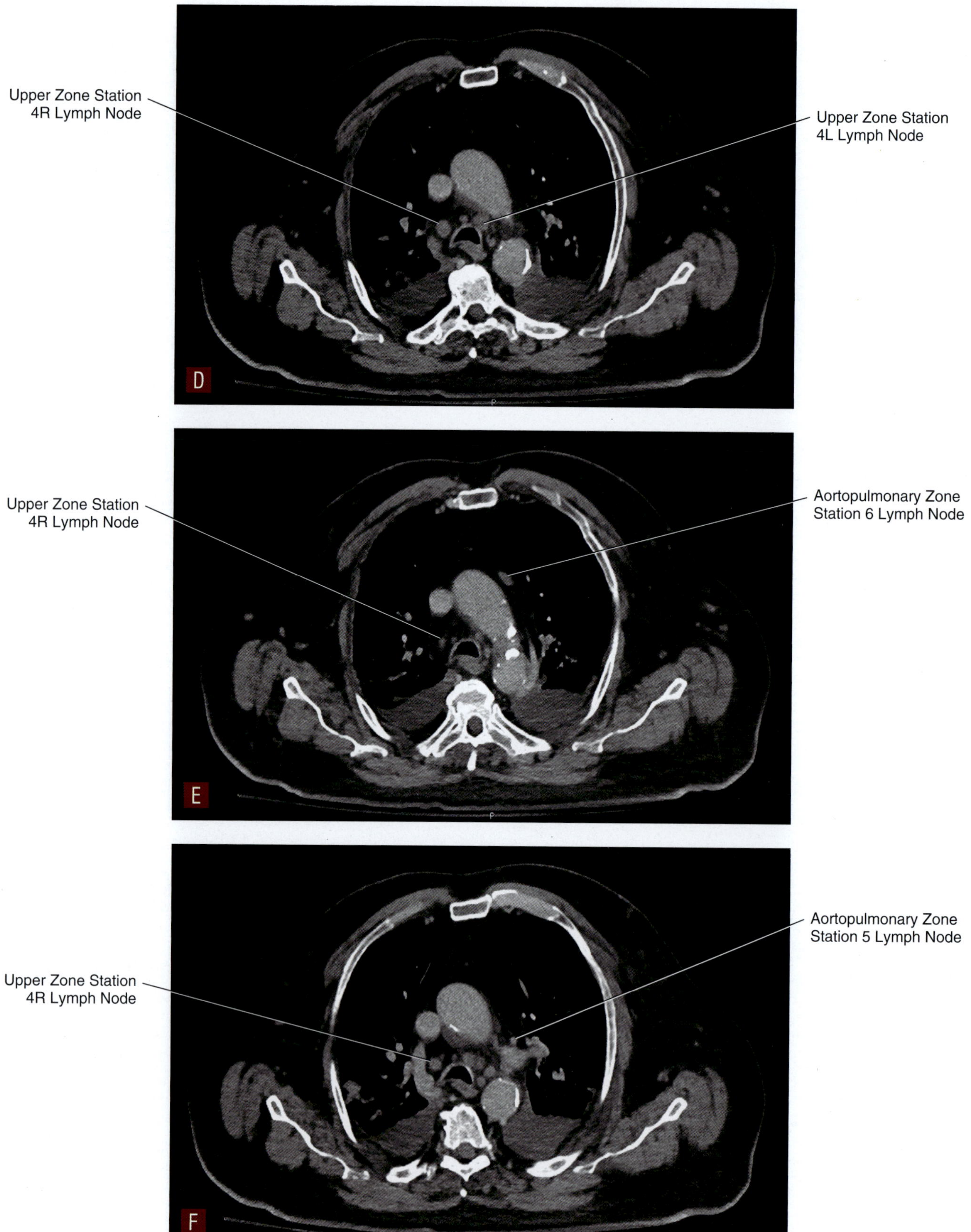

Figure 12.6. *Continued*

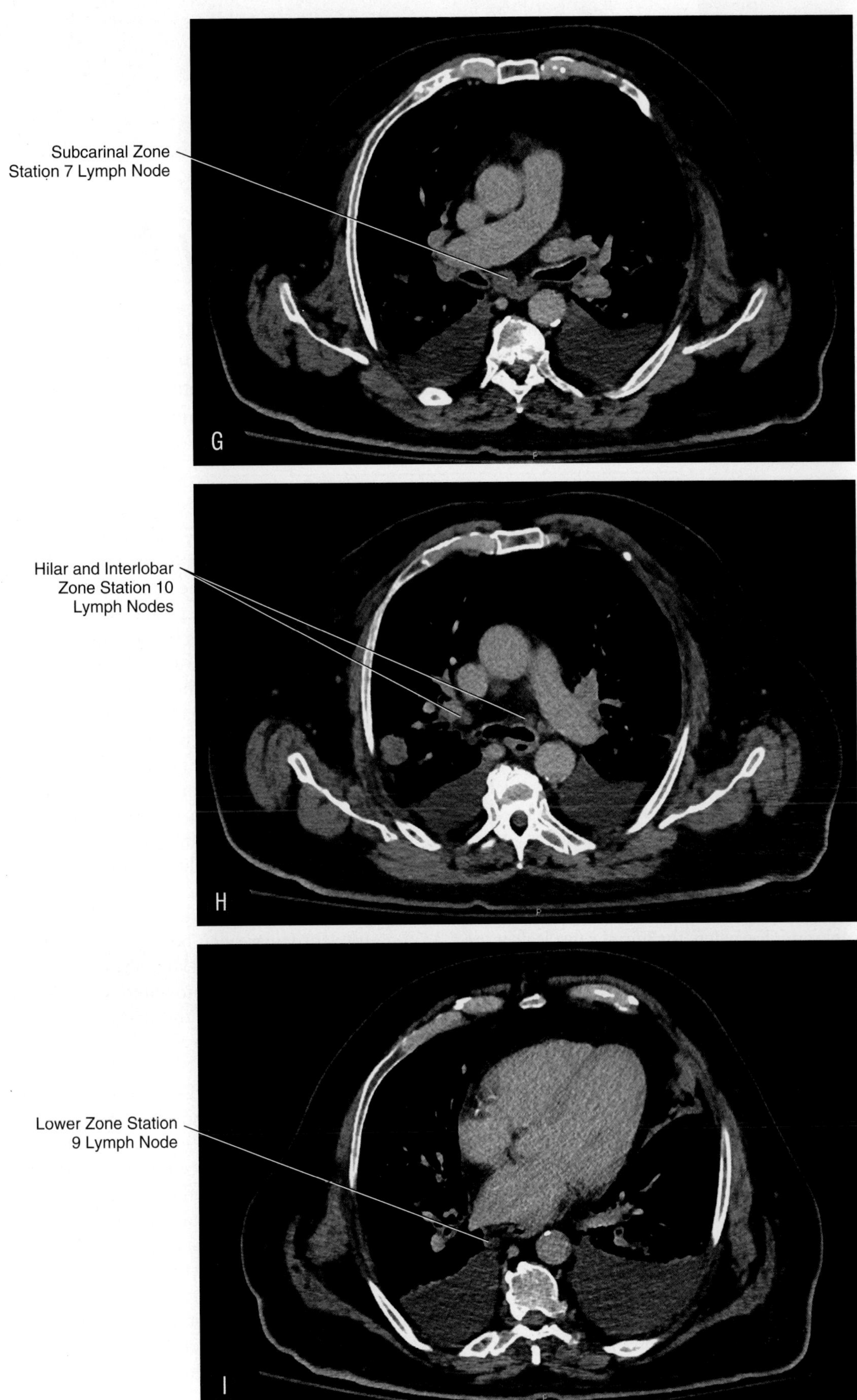

Figure 12.6. *Continued*

13

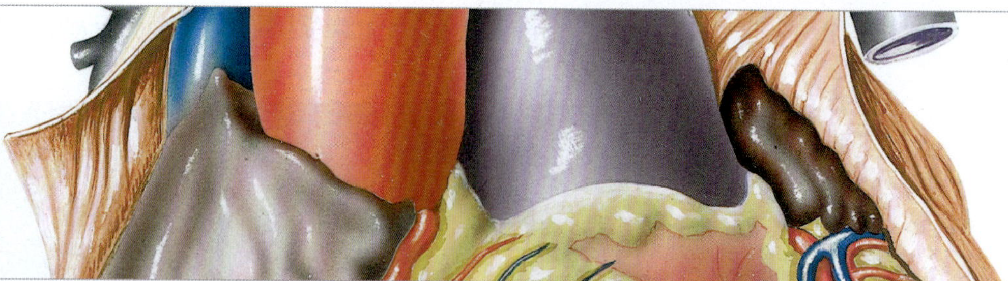

Heart and Coronary Arteries

The heart is an organ asymmetrically situated in the mediastinum. It is protected by a mesodermal-derived structure, the pericardial sac, consisting of two sheets: the external or parietal, which is fibrous, and the internal or visceral, which is a thin serous membrane attached to the heart muscle surface.

The heart is located in the middle portion of the inferior mediastinum bordered laterally by the medial face of the lungs, anteriorly by the chest wall, and posteriorly by the dorsal spine. In the majority of the individuals, a large part of the heart lies in the left hemithorax and is partially covered by the lingula of the left lung (Figs. 13.1-13.3). The right aspect of the heart abuts the right middle lobe of the lung.

In humans, the heart consists of two double-valved pumps that work physiologically in series. The superior and the inferior vena cava (IVC), and the coronary sinus drain the systemic venous blood into the right atrium, which is connected to the right ventricle through the tricuspid valve. The right ventricle pumps the blood to the pulmonary artery across the pulmonic valve. The arterial blood returning from the lungs drains into the left atrium through pulmonary veins, typically two on the left and two on the right. The mitral valve annulus, where the mitral valve leaflets are attached, separates the left atrium from the left ventricle, which ejects the blood into the aorta across the aortic valve (Fig. 13.4).

The longitudinal axis (a.k.a. long axis) of the heart is most frequently oriented anteriorly, inferiorly, and toward the left (Fig. 13.5) (levocardia). The condition where the cardiac apex is pointing toward the right is called dextrocardia. Rarely, the longitudinal axis is almost perfectly in the sagittal plane and the heart occupies the middle mediastinum, which is termed mesocardia.

When the heart is faced in frontal view, the right border is formed by the lateral wall of the right atrium. The left margin is cranially outlined by the left atrial appendage and caudally by the lateral wall of the left ventricle (Figs. 13.1-13.3, 13.6A and B). The right atrium and the right ventricle are both more anterior than their corresponding left-sided chambers (Figs. 13.1, 13.6C and D, 13.7).

The heart has roughly the shape of an inverted pyramid, with the base, formed by the atria and the root of the great vessels, located in the upper mediastinum (Figs. 13.5 and 13.7). The apex of the pyramid corresponds to the apex of the left ventricle and is situated in the left hemithorax toward the diaphragm. The anterior face of the heart or sternocostal face is related to the anterior wall of the chest. The inferior face lies on the diaphragm, and the lateral or pulmonary face is covered by the lingula of the left lung (Figs. 13.3, 13.5, and 13.8). The junction of the sternocostal face with the inferior or diaphragmatic face defines a sharp border called the acute margin. On the left side, the junction of the left face with the diaphragmatic face is the obtuse margin with a rounded and ill-defined border (Fig. 13.9). The divisions of the four cardiac chambers are seen externally as sulci or grooves. Between the atria and ventricles, there are the atrioventricular sulci, both right and left. The ventricle's separation is marked externally by the interventricular sulcus, which is divided into anterior and posterior/inferior portions. The point where the atrioventricular sulcus meets the posterior/inferior interventricular sulcus is termed the crux of the heart.

Although anatomic dissection has been the historical method to define and advance our understanding of human anatomy, medical imaging now plays an invaluable role. In the latter half of the 20th century, angiography was the primary means of visualizing the cardiac structures in a living person. Although this was and is an excellent technique, it suffers from two limitations. First, it is an invasive procedure requiring catheterization of the blood vessels with placement of a catheter into the heart and coronary arteries. Second, only the column of contrast material shows up on the radiographs, so it is the lumen of the arteries and cardiac chambers that is imaged. Angiography gives no direct information about the solid cardiac structures such as myocardium, pericardium, and valves. More recently echocardiography, magnetic resonance imaging (MRI) (Fig. 13.8), and multislice computed tomography (CT) have become advanced to the point where they provide a noninvasive means of evaluating cardiac anatomy. While transthoracic echocardiography may sometimes struggle to visualize certain cardiac structures because of challenging acoustic windows or large body habitus impeding ultrasound penetration, CT and MRI offer unhindered access to visualize all cardiac structures and even extracardiac structures, such as the lungs, airways, and great vessels.

Cardiac Chambers

In invasive angiography, dedicated oblique projections are used to portray cardiac structures. These projections permit the visualization of the septum and the surrounding structures of the heart in more detail than the classical orthogonal frontal and lateral views.

A routine of the angiographic study of the heart consists of three major projections:

Long axial view—30° craniocaudal image intensifier inclination and 60° left anterior oblique patient inclination

Elongated right anterior oblique view—30° craniocaudal inclination of the image intensifier and 30° right anterior oblique patient inclination

Four-chamber view—30° craniocaudal image intensifier inclination and 30° left anterior oblique patient inclination

Additional views may be necessary in special situations. Frontal and lateral views may be the elected projections for adequate visualization of the interventricular septum in some complex cardiac defects. The pulmonary trunk and its bifurcation are better visualized in the sitting-up projection with the patient lying supine and the image intensifier rotating 30° cranially.

On CT, the initial reconstructions are performed in the axial (transverse) plane. With the advent of thin-slice helical scanning modes, isotropic voxels (each voxel is essentially a cube with equal sides) can be obtained, which can subsequently be reformatted into any plane desired. Coronal and sagittal images are usually reconstructed routinely, and 3D postprocessing workstations are then used to create dedicated long- and short-axis views of the heart, similar to those used historically in echocardiography. Even simulated angiographic views can be obtained, which are helpful to predict the appearance of overlapping structures during an invasive catheter-based procedure.

Advancements in MRI technology have also made it possible to obtain high-resolution isotropic 3D datasets of the heart and thoracic vasculature, which can also be reformatted in any desired plane using 3D workstations. When obtaining cine images (movie loops of an entire cardiac cycle), however, dedicated and carefully angulated cardiac views are acquired in the long- and short-axis planes.

Right Atrium

Anatomic Aspects

The right atrium is a somewhat quadrangular chamber that forms the right surface of the heart (Fig. 13.10A). It presents two main portions: the posterior smooth wall called sinus venarum and the anterior with a trabeculated wall called atrium proper and auricle. The crista terminalis is a smooth muscular ridge in the posterolateral wall of the right atrium separating the sinus venarum from the proper atrium. The anterior trabeculated wall of the right atrium extends anteriorly with the auricle or right atrial appendage, which is a conical pouch expanding in front of the root of the ascending aorta. The myocardial trabeculations are called pectinate muscles, from the Latin word "pecten," suggestive of their comblike appearance. The left wall of the right atrium corresponds to the interatrial septum, which separates this chamber from the left atrium. The right face of the interatrial septum presents a central depression called fossa ovalis which is encircled by a prominent margin: the limbus of the fossa ovalis. The most inferior part of the interatrial septum, near the atrioventricular annulus, is formed by the atrioventricular septum (Fig. 13.10B). One more normal structure is sometimes fairly prominent and deserves mentioning, namely, the eustachian valve which is at the junction of the IVC with the right atrium and can be mistaken for a cardiac mass.

Angiographic Aspects

Long Axial View. In this view, the left border of the right atrium corresponds to the anterior portion of the interatrial septum, and the superior border is formed by the free superior wall of the right atrium. The lateral border is represented by a continuous line between the superior and inferior caval veins. The inferior border of the right atrium is the tricuspid valve, and it overlaps the junction of the IVC. The anterior wall and the right auricle are not seen in this projection (Fig. 13.11).

Elongated Right Anterior Oblique View. The superior and inferior vena cavae are separated by a straight line that is the right posterior wall of the right atrium. The tricuspid valve seen in profile is in the inferior and left aspect of the atrial chamber. There is an inferior contour between the IVC and the tricuspid annulus, where the entrance of the coronary sinus is located and is formed partially by the atrioventricular septum. The left and superior aspect of the right atrium corresponds to the right atrial appendage or right auricle (Fig. 13.12).

Four-Chamber View. In this projection, the right atrium has a globular form, very similar to that seen in the long axial view. The left border corresponds to the more posterior portion of the atrial septum, and the right border is related with the anterolateral atrial wall. The atrial appendage and the vena cava are overlapped by the right atrium contour. The tricuspid valve is not well defined in this projection although it forms the left inferior contour (Fig. 13.13).

Right Ventricle

Anatomic Aspects

The right ventricle is a triangular-shaped chamber and is located at the ventral portion of the heart. The base of the right ventricle is more cranial and to the right and the apex is caudal and projected toward the left. The base is formed on the right by the tricuspid valve annulus and the leaflets of the tricuspid valve. On the left, more cranially, is the pulmonary valve (or pulmonic valve). These two valves are separated by a smooth and prominent muscular invagination of the right ventricular wall called ventriculoinfundibular fold. The rest of the right ventricle, including the apex, has coarse trabeculation (Figs. 13.14 and 13.15). The right ventricular chamber is divided into three portions: the inlet, the outlet, and the trabecular zones (Fig. 13.16). The inlet zone includes the tricuspid valve and extends to the implantation line of the papillary muscles. The outlet zone or infundibulum is a tubular muscular formation with the pulmonic valve on its top. The trabeculated zone extends from the papillary muscle's insertion to the apex. The right ventricle is bordered by three walls: the anterior or free wall, the inferior, and the septal wall, which corresponds to the interventricular septum. The interventricular septum is formed by two components: the membranous septum and the muscular septum. The membranous septum is a small fibrous structure divided into two portions by the septal tricuspid leaflet attachment: the superior is the atrioventricular portion and the inferior is the interventricular portion. Of note, the membranous septum superiorly attaches on the aortic valve annulus. The atrioventricular portion is above the tricuspid annulus and separates the left ventricle from the right atrium. The interventricular portion is related to both ventricles. The muscular component, the largest part of the interventricular septum, is divided into three portions: the inlet portion, which divides the inlet of the ventricles; the infundibular portion, which separates the outlet of the ventricles; and the trabeculated portion, situated more apically. The outlet or infundibulum of the right ventricle is bordered anteriorly by the free anterior ventricular wall. Note, the infundibulum can also be called the "conus," since it is a remnant of the embryological conus arteriosus. The posterior wall is the ventriculoinfundibular fold, the muscular formation which separates the tricuspid from the pulmonary valve. The third wall of the infundibulum is the infundibular or outlet portion of the interventricular septum. In normal hearts, the muscular structure, which separates the tricuspid from the pulmonary valve, is called supraventricular crest and is formed in its greater part by the ventriculoinfundibular fold and a small portion of the outlet septum. On the right side of the muscular interventricular septum, there is a well-marked muscular band called septomarginal trabecula (a.k.a. the moderator band), which has two limbs embracing the body of the supraventricular crest. These three structures, the ventriculoinfundibular fold, the outlet septum, and the septomarginal trabecula, are characteristics of the morphologic right ventricle (Fig. 13.17).

The tricuspid valve apparatus consists of an atrioventricular orifice surrounded by a fibrous ring (tricuspid annulus fibrosus), three somewhat triangular cusps or leaflets, various types of chordae tendineae, and three papillary muscles. The cusps are named anterior, septal, and posterior. The anterior cusp is the largest and is interposed between the atrioventricular ring and the infundibulum. The septal cusp is attached to the membranous portion of the interventricular septum. The posterior cusp is attached in the inferior portion of the tricuspid annulus. The papillary muscles in the right ventricle are the anterior with the base arising from the anterolateral ventricular wall, associated with the septomarginal trabecula, and the posterior, smaller than the anterior, arising from the inferior portion of the septum. There may be additional small, papillary muscles arising from the infundibular septal wall.

The pulmonary valve is situated at the summit of the infundibulum. It consists of three semilunar segments or cusps attached to a fibrous annulus. Two of the cusps are anterior (right and left) and the third is posterior.

Angiographic Aspects

Long Axial View. In this view, the right ventricle has a triangular shape with the base at the top. The tricuspid valve is on the right and the pulmonic valve is on the left superiorly. The right contour corresponds to the free anterior wall. The upper left border is formed by the anterior portion of the interventricular septum and the posterior portion is a straight line toward the apex. The right ventricular outflow tract is outlined by the supraventricular crest on the right side and by part of the septomarginal trabecula on the left. It looks like a wide channel (upside-down cone) with the pulmonic valve on top. The negative shadow of the tricuspid valve lies in the right and upper contour of the right ventricle. The anterior leaflet can be visualized superiorly and to the right of the tricuspid annulus. The septal leaflet is seen near and parallel to the interventricular septum. The posterior or mural leaflet is not visualized (Fig. 13.18).

Elongated Right Anterior Oblique View. The tricuspid valve seen on the lateral view is at the posterior border and to the right. The outflow tract is superior and to the left and is demarcated posteriorly by the supraventricular crest and anteriorly by the free wall of the right ventricle (Fig. 13.18).

Four-Chamber View. The morphologic aspect of the right ventricle in this projection is similar to that of the long axial view, but the outflow tract is not well visualized, and the tricuspid valve is localized more medially (Fig. 13.19).

Left Atrium

Anatomic Aspects

Arterial blood returns from the lungs to the left heart—typically—through two pulmonary veins on each side of the left atrium. This is the most dorsal chamber and is localized in front of the lumbar spine and esophagus, under the carina, relatively more superiorly than the other cardiac chambers. It communicates with the left ventricle through the mitral valve. The left atrium has a quadrangular shape and a smooth posterior wall where the four pulmonary veins converge. To the right, there is the interatrial septum, and to the left, the left auricle or left atrial appendage can be found, which is an elongated pouch with a trabeculated wall (pectinate muscles) that encircles the left aspect of the main pulmonary trunk. The left appendage is a fingerlike formation that communicates with the left atrium through a narrow orifice. The right appendage, on the other hand, communicates with the right atrium proper through a wide and triangular orifice. The inferior border of the left atrium is the mitral valve itself (Fig. 13.20).

Angiographic Aspects

Long Axial View. The right contour of the left atrium is formed by the anterior portion of the atrial septum. In the right upper corner, there is the ostium of the right superior pulmonary vein. The left pulmonary veins and the left atrial appendage are not well seen in this view. At the floor of the left atrium is the mitral valve (Fig. 13.21).

Elongated Right Anterior Oblique View. In this view, the most prominent structure is the left atrial appendage which forms the anterior and lateral border of the left atrium. It appears as an irregular and elongated fingerlike protrusion toward the left, between the superior wall and the mitral valve. The entrance of the right superior pulmonary vein is localized on the right in continuation with the roof of the left atrium (Figs. 13.22 and 13.23).

Four-Chamber View. This view shows a similar appearance described in the long axial view but the atrial septum is visualized in its posterior portion (Fig. 13.24).

CT Imaging. CT is particularly useful for visualizing the left atrium and pulmonary veins because of the three-dimensional volume-rendered images that can be generated. This 360-degree visualization of the pulmonary veins can be used to rotate the image to get an overview of the number, location, and size of veins (Fig. 13.25). The most common variation on the left is a single pulmonary vein, whereas on the right, the presence of three veins is the most frequently found variant.

Left Ventricle

Anatomic Aspects

The left ventricle has the thickest chamber wall of the heart and is located to the left and posteriorly to the right ventricle (Fig. 13.26). It has an elongated and conical shape with the base upwards, where the mitral and aortic valves are located. The apex is oriented inferiorly toward the left. The left ventricle is divided into three portions: the inlet tract with the mitral valve complex, the trabeculated zone with less coarse trabeculation than that in the right ventricle, and the outflow tract which supports the aortic valve. Unlike the right ventricle, in the left ventricle, the inlet and outflow tracts are not separated by a well-developed infundibulum and the aortic and mitral annuli are in fibrous contiguity. The left ventricle has a lateral free wall, an inferior or diaphragmatic wall (the anatomical "posterior" wall, which is opposite to the anterior wall), and a septal wall. The left ventricular aspect of the muscular septum is usually nontrabeculated and extends from the membranous septum to the apex (Figs. 13.21, 13.27-13.29).

The mitral valve is formed by two leaflets or cusps attached to a fibrous annulus (can also be spelled just like the original Latin word, "annulus," meaning ring), a number of chordae tendineae, and two papillary muscles: the anterolateral and the posteromedial. The cusps or leaflets are the anterior or septal and the posterior or parietal, separated from each other by two indentations: the anterolateral and the posteromedial commissures. The anterior cusp is longer and narrower than the posterior, but both have about the same overall area.

The aortic valve is located at the top of the left ventricular outflow tract (LVOT), consisting of three cusps attached to the aortic annulus. Two cusps, the right and left coronary cusps, are named after the coronary arteries that originate from their corresponding aortic sinuses of Valsalva. The right coronary cusp is most anterior and is connected to the membranous portion of the ventricular septum inferiorly and is also called "septal" cusp. The left coronary cusp is slightly posterior and to the left. The most posterior cusp is the noncoronary cusp, which straddles the interatrial septum.

Angiographic Aspects

Long Axial View. In this projection, the right contour of the left ventricle corresponds to the trabecular portion of the interventricular septum. A small cranial portion of the septum is formed by the outlet septum located just below the aortic valve. The outlet of the left ventricle (LVOT) is delineated anteriorly and on the right by the outlet portion of the ventricular septum and posteriorly by the anterior leaflet of the mitral valve. The free wall of the left ventricle corresponds to the posterolateral contour and extends from the mitral valve to the apex. The mitral valve is seen as negative shadow in the superior and lateral contour of the left ventricle. The papillary muscles are seen as negative shadows in the middle portion of the left ventricle (Fig. 13.30). This view is similar in projection to the three-chamber parasternal long-axis view, which is typically the first view acquired by sonographers on echocardiography.

Elongated Right Anterior View. In this view, the outflow tract is limited anteriorly, and to the left, by the infundibular septum as a straight vertical line below the right coronary cusp and posteriorly, to the right, by a smooth contour extending from the noncoronary cusp to the crux cordis. It represents the atrioventricular portion of the interventricular septum. The anterior free wall of the left ventricle extends from the infundibular septum toward the apex and the inferior wall corresponds to the contour from the crux cordis to the apex. The mitral valve is not well seen in this view. The aortic valve is localized in the uppermost aspect of the outlet tract and the coronary cusps cover each other on the left. The noncoronary cusp is to the right (Fig. 13.31).

Four-Chamber View. The left ventricle in this view has a semioval shape with a left-rounded contour and a right straight line (Fig. 13.32). The apex is localized inferiorly toward the right. The left contour corresponds to the free anterolateral wall and the right limit is the interventricular septum, whose superior or most basal portion is the atrioventricular portion of the interventricular septum which separates the left ventricle from the right atrium. The leaflets of the mitral valve can be localized near this portion of the septum (corresponding to the crux cordis). The inferior/apical portion of the right contour is formed by the posterior portion of the muscular septum. The aortic valve is visualized above the septal wall. The right coronary and the noncoronary cusps are overlying each other on the right side. The left coronary cusp is on the left side. The mitral orifice is fully exposed, and the mural leaflet implantation is seen in all its length. The septal leaflet is not well visualized, and the papillary muscles appear as two filling defects: anterolateral and posteromedial. They are oriented toward the commissures of the mitral valve. As a rule, the left ventricle shows a relatively smoother, less trabeculated contour on angiography as opposed to the coarse trabeculation of the right ventricle (Figs. 13.14 and 13.27).

Tomographic Anatomy

In the axial view, the relationships between the four chambers are well demonstrated. Moving from a cephalad to caudal direction (Fig. 13.33), the first chamber to come into view is the left atrium (note again, this is the most superior/cranial chamber) at the level of the pulmonic valve. The right atrium begins to appear just above the level of the aortic valve. Immediately below the aortic valve, the right and left ventricles come into view. Although the longitudinal axis of the heart is usually oriented inferiorly, this is variable and will cause some disparity in which structures can be seen at the level of the aortic valve. To get a true "four-chamber" view, an angled reconstruction, called multiplanar reformat (MPR), is necessary (Fig. 13.34A). Using MPRs generated form CT, it is also possible to obtain "short-axis" reconstructions, which allow you to cut the left and right ventricle in cross-section (Fig. 13.34B), as if you were slicing a loaf of bread.

3D volume-rendered images are similar to those seen on angiography (Figs. 13.2 and 13.7). CT better shows the atrial appendages which often hang over the coronary artery origins. From the front, the left and right ventricles, aortic and pulmonary outflow tracts, and a portion of the right atrium are seen. Views at the inferior aspect of the heart show both ventricles with the inferior (or posterior) interventricular groove. It should be noted that the lowermost aspects of the heart are often below the level of the domes of the diaphragm, and thus are more caudal than some intra-abdominal structures such as the dome of the liver and the gastric bubble. A posterior view requires the thoracic spine to be virtually "cut away" to allow better visualization of the descending aorta and the pulmonary veins. If the aorta is also removed, the left atrium is demonstrated to be the most posterior chamber (Fig. 13.25).

Coronary Arteries

The coronary arteries (or coronaries, for short) comprise the vascular network that provides arterial blood to the myocardium. They all stem from the left and right coronary artery (LCA and RCA), which originate from the left (more posterior) and right (anterior) coronary sinuses of Valsalva, ie, from the aortic root (Figs. 13.35-13.39).

The left main coronary artery (LMCA, or "left main" for short) has a variable length, usually 10±4 mm, and shows variable diameter, around 5 mm. In about 1% of the hearts studied in a series, there was no LMCA and two orifices were found in the left coronary sinus with the left anterior descending (LAD) and circumflex arteries originating separately from each one (see anatomic variants at the end of this chapter). The LMCA—in most people—bifurcates into two vessels: the LAD artery, running over the anterior interventricular sulcus and the left circumflex artery (LCX), which follows the left atrioventricular sulcus (Figs. 13.42 and 13.43). The LMCA in a few cases may give rise to a third vessel: the ramus intermedius or intermediary artery (sometimes also referred to as "diagonalis artery," though this is not preferred, as this name can be confused with a diagonal branch off the LAD), which is located between the LAD and LCX and supplies the free anterolateral wall of the left ventricle (Fig. 13. 44).

The LAD artery extends to the cardiac apex or beyond. In fact, in most people, the LAD curves around and courses up in the posterior interventricular sulcus to supply the distal inferior wall. The length of the LAD is thus extremely variable. The main branches of the LAD are the diagonal and septal perforating (or septal perforator) branches. Both diagonals and septal perforators vary in number and size (Figs. 13.42-13.44). Diagonals arise in acute angle from the LAD and supply the anterior and anterolateral walls of the left ventricle. Most frequently, the first diagonal branch is a major artery. The septal branches, usually four to six in number (but sometimes more), originate from the LAD at a right angle, coursing closer to the endocardium on the right side of the interventricular septum and supply the anterior two-thirds of the septal myocardium. They anastomose with the septal branches coming from the posterior descending artery (PDA). In the majority of hearts, the largest septal branch is the first septal artery, originating from the proximal portion of the LAD (Figs. 13.42 and 13.43). In some hearts, the LAD has an unusual configuration: it is short and divided into two parallel vessels called "dual" LAD (Fig. 13.53A and B). One, running over the interventricular sulcus, gives off the septal branches and the other, lying in the anterior left ventricular wall, supplies the diagonal branches (Figs. 13.40-13.44).

The LCX artery is the other principal vessel originating from the LMCA. It commonly emerges at a right or acute angle and is covered by the left atrial appendage in its proximal portion and then takes position in the left atrioventricular sulcus. The circumflex artery may terminate proximal to the obtuse margin of the left ventricle or can extend beyond the crux cordis. The principal branches of the LCX are the obtuse marginal arteries and the left atrial branch. In 40% of hearts, the sinus node artery (or sinoatrial [SA] nodal artery) arises from the circumflex artery. The obtuse marginal arteries are variable in number, but there are usually three. The most prominent marginal artery runs on the obtuse margin of the heart (essentially the true lateral wall) and extends distally approaching the apex. In some cases, the LCX gives rise to posterolateral branches (PLBs) that supply the posterolateral (or inferolateral) and inferior walls of the left ventricle. When the circumflex artery reaches the crux cordis, it may give rise to the posterior descending arteries (PDAs) and atrioventricular nodal arteries (Figs. 13.38-13.44, 13.54). In such an event, the coronary artery system would be termed "left-dominant."

The RCA originates at the right coronary aortic sinus (Figs. 13.45-13.49) (of Valsalva). Often a small branch may arise directly from the aortic sinus with a separate ostium and supply the right ventricle infundibulum or conus. This branch is called the conus artery, which sometimes anastomoses with a left conus branch coming from the LCA to form the arterial ring (arc) or annulus of Vieussens. Shortly after its origin, the RCA gives rise to the SA nodal artery in 60% of the hearts. The RCA courses in the right atrioventricular sulcus and has a variable form of termination. If it is a short artery, it terminates between the acute margin of the right ventricle and the crux cordis as a small branch (left dominance). When there is a dominant RCA, it extends further from the crux supplying the posterolateral wall of the left ventricle with a variable number of PLBs. Near the acute margin of the heart, the RCA gives off (typically several) right marginal or acute marginal arteries that supply the free wall of the right ventricle. The shorter the LCX, the longer the terminal PLBs of the RCA. At the crux cordis, the right coronary gives rise to the PDA, which runs in the posterior interventricular sulcus and supplies the inferior portion (the inferior one-third) of the interventricular septum through a variable number of septal branches. Several of these small septal branches anastomose with the septal branches coming from the anterior descending artery. Just distal to the crux, the RCA appears to make an inverted "U"-turn, giving origin to the atrioventricular node artery (Fig. 13.46).

Coronary arterial anatomy at the inferior aspect of the heart has a greatly variable configuration. The diaphragmatic surface of the heart may be irrigated by vessels (PDA and PLBs) coming from the RCA (right dominant system) or from the left circumflex (left dominant system). Rarely, two PDAs can be seen, one from the LCX and one from the RCA, or the PDA comes from the RCA, while the PLBs originate from the LCX. These variants are called codominant (Figs. 13.45-13.50).

Angiographic Aspects

It is important to visualize all the segments of the main coronary arteries, their branches, anatomic variations, and anastomoses (potential collateral pathways) that occasionally occur. The details of the lesions as well as their locations should be properly defined. To reach these goals, several angiographic projections are used.

Since the anatomic aspects of the coronary arteries are so variable, a number of specific projections with special angles of the X-ray beam are used for each different individual. All major vessels must be visualized in at least two orthogonal projections.

The elongated or cranial left oblique view shows the LMCA, the LAD, and the diagonal branches (Fig. 13.42). The caudal left oblique projection (spider view) shows the LMCA, its bifurcation, and the proximal circumflex artery (Fig. 13.51). To visualize the LAD with its septal and diagonal branches, either the cranial or the caudal right oblique view is obtained. The circumflex artery and its obtuse marginal branches are well defined in the elongated left oblique and in the caudal right anterior oblique projections (Figs. 13.51-13.54).

The anteroposterior view is a good projection to study the LMCA and its bifurcation. In some cases, the caudal anteroposterior or the true lateral views may help visualize the proximal portion of the LAD and LCX.

The RCA is well visualized in the majority of the cases in the conventional right and left oblique projections (Figs. 13.55 and 13.56). The origins of the PDA and the PLBs are best defined in the caudal left anterior oblique view.

Tomographic Anatomy

Coronary arteries run in grooves on the surface of the heart surrounded by epicardial fat. This allows CT to depict the high-density coronary lumen (enhanced by iodinated contrast) vividly against the surrounding low-density fat. Fairly frequently, short segments of the "epicardial" coronaries dive into the myocardium, which is termed "myocardial bridging," referring to the bridge of myocardium overlying the flow of blood in the underlying coronary. 3D volume rendering is useful to get an overview, but for diagnostic purposes, MPRs or curved MPRs are used. Maximum intensity projection images are also useful to evaluate the coronary arteries, but this technique can hide smaller coronary lesions. Current CT technology allows for visualization of all major coronary branches, including diagonals, large septal perforators, obtuse and acute marginals, conus branch, SA nodal branch, PDA, and PLB down to a diameter of 0.5 to 1 mm.

The origin of the coronary arteries can be well seen from a cranial view with the more superior structures removed (Fig. 13.57). In this projection, both the right and left coronary origins are well seen and any anomalies can easily be excluded. Rotating the image to a cranial left anterior oblique defines the LMCA and its bifurcation into the LAD and left circumflex coronary arteries (Fig. 13.58). The LAD runs in the anterior interventricular groove with its diagonal branches serving the anterior wall, and varying degrees of the anterolateral wall, of the left ventricle (Fig. 13.59). The LCX runs in the atrioventricular groove with obtuse marginal branches supplying the lateral wall (and varying degrees of the anterolateral and posterolateral walls) of the left ventricle (Fig. 13.60). As mentioned above, when present, the ramus intermedius will be a third branch arising from the left main, coursing toward the anterolateral wall. This artery may provide flow more for the anterior wall (similar to a diagonal branch) or course more toward the lateral wall (resembling an obtuse marginal branch).

Smaller branches of the RCA (less than 1 mm in diameter) may be difficult to visualize with CT, including the very first branch, the conus branch, which sometimes originates from the aorta directly (Fig. 13.61). The second branch—typically—is the SA nodal branch. Larger branches such as the acute marginal arteries can always be well seen (Figs. 13.61 and 13.62).

After virtual "removal" of the diaphragm, the inferior surface of the heart can be evaluated. About 80% of people have a so-called "right-dominant" system, where the RCA provides flow to the posterior descending coronary artery and the PLBs (Fig. 13.63). The remaining 20% either have a left-dominant (PDA and PLBs from LCX) (Fig. 13.64) or codominant system (dual PDA or PDA from RCA and PLB from LCX) (Fig. 13.50).

Coronary Artery Bypass Grafts

Although these are surgically created vessels, coronary artery bypass grafts have become so common, that basic knowledge of their expected locations and appearances should be part of any anatomic field of study. Bypass grafts, as the name implies, are conduits that are used to bypass severely diseased portions of the native coronary arteries. The material used is always autologous, since man-made grafts have not been found to be effective. Veins or arteries may be used.

If a vein is used, it is used as a "free graft," and the greater saphenous vein in the leg is the donor site of choice. If this is unavailable or not suitable, the lesser saphenous may be used. Less often, veins from other portions of the body may be harvested. These veins are proximally anastomosed to the ascending aorta, and, distally, they are attached just distal to the last coronary stenosis to be bypassed.

Literature has shown that arterial conduits have a slightly higher long-term patency, so they are preferred when possible. The left internal mammary artery (LIMA) is the most common choice, and most commonly it is used as an "in-situ graft," meaning that it is left attached to the left subclavian artery at its origin, but its mid and distal portions are freed up from the chest wall and then anastomosed distally to the vessel to be bypassed (typically the LAD). Of note, the right internal mammary artery (RIMA) can also be used as an in-situ graft. If the in-situ graft does not reach far enough, it can be removed from the chest wall and used as a free arterial graft. Additionally, some institutions utilize the radial artery as a potential donor as well.

The usual nomenclature for coronary artery bypass grafting (CABG) includes the number of bypassed branches, ie, distal anastomoses. Thus, a four-vessel bypass means there are four bypassed coronary artery branches (Fig. 13.65). It is important to examine both proximal and distal anastomoses. Commonly, the LIMA is connected to the LAD or one of the diagonals, while venous grafts are used for other locations (Fig. 13.66A-C). If a second surgery is needed, it is helpful to describe the relationship of the sternum to the grafts (Fig. 13.66D). Some surgeons place metallic rings (bypass markers) around the origins of vein grafts from the ascending aorta. This allows for quicker and easier catheterization if angiography is required (Fig. 13.67).

When evaluating grafts with computed tomography angiography (CTA), it is important to include the origins of the subclavian arteries in the scan field. A stenosis in the proximal left subclavian artery will inhibit flow to an otherwise-good LIMA graft. In these cases, the left subclavian artery can either be treated with a stent or the LIMA can be reattached to the ascending aorta (Fig. 13.68A and B). Surgeons have also begun placing more complex segmental grafts. This requires using the original graft as the origin site for the new segmental communication (Fig. 13.68A and B, 13.69) also known as "Y-grafts." Another form of a sophisticated graft that can have two or more distal anastomoses is the so-called "jump graft" or sequential graft. This graft has a side-to-side anastomosis with a coronary before it attaches end-to-side to a second coronary artery (Figs. 13.70 and 13.71). With these grafts, it is often helpful to use different methods of display to better appreciate the entire course of the graft (Fig. 13.70A and B). Finally, in unusual cases, a surgeon may need to use a more remote site, such as the descending aorta, for the proximal origin of the graft (Fig. 13.72).

Coronary Artery Variants

Although uncommon, anomalies of the coronary arteries can be associated with sudden cardiac death or cardiac disease. Generally, anomalous coronary arteries that course between the ascending aorta and the pulmonary artery (interarterial course) are considered the most significant clinically, as these are most likely to result in serious cardiovascular events (Figs. 13.73 and 13.74). Note also that sometimes the most proximal segment of the coronary artery may run within the layers of the aortic wall, which is called an intramural segment (Fig. 13.74).

There is a wide range of coronary artery anomalies, making an exhaustive discussion of each individual variant outside the scope of this chapter. However, familiarity with the major categories of coronary artery anomalies is useful in identifying clinically significant variants in clinical practice. One can broadly categorize coronary artery anomalies as nonhemodynamically significant and hemodynamically significant groups.

Nonhemodynamically significant anomalies include anomalies typically not associated with symptoms or severe cardiovascular sequelae. These anomalies include duplication of the LAD or RCA, the former being much more frequent. Duplicated LAD arteries often arise from the RCA, taking a prepulmonic, interarterial, or transeptal course. High origins of the coronary arteries are defined as being 1 cm distal to the sinotubular junction. This variant occurs more often in the RCA, and there is an association with bicuspid aortic valve. While not hemodynamically significant, this variant may make catheterization more difficult or complicate surgical aortotomy if not identified. When a major coronary artery courses anterior to the pulmonary outflow tract or pulmonary artery, its course is termed prepulmonic and involves most commonly the LMCA, albeit the RCA may arise from the LAD or LMCA and course anterior to the pulmonary artery. There is an association of prepulmonic course with tetralogy of Fallot.

Additional "benign" anomalies include the retroaortic left circumflex coronary (Fig. 13.75) originating from the RCA or right coronary sinus. Yet another rare finding is having separate origins of the LAD and the LCX from the left coronary sinus of Valsalva (Fig. 13.76), leading to a total of three separate coronary arteries arising from the aortic root. The "flipside" of this is having only a single coronary artery, which is more commonly found with other congenital cardiac malformations (Fig. 13.77). Lastly, a truly unusual form is the Arc of Vieussens (a.k.a. arterial ring or circle of Vieussens), which creates a communication between the left and right coronary systems via a left conus branch from the LAD and a right conus branch from the RCA (Fig. 13.78).

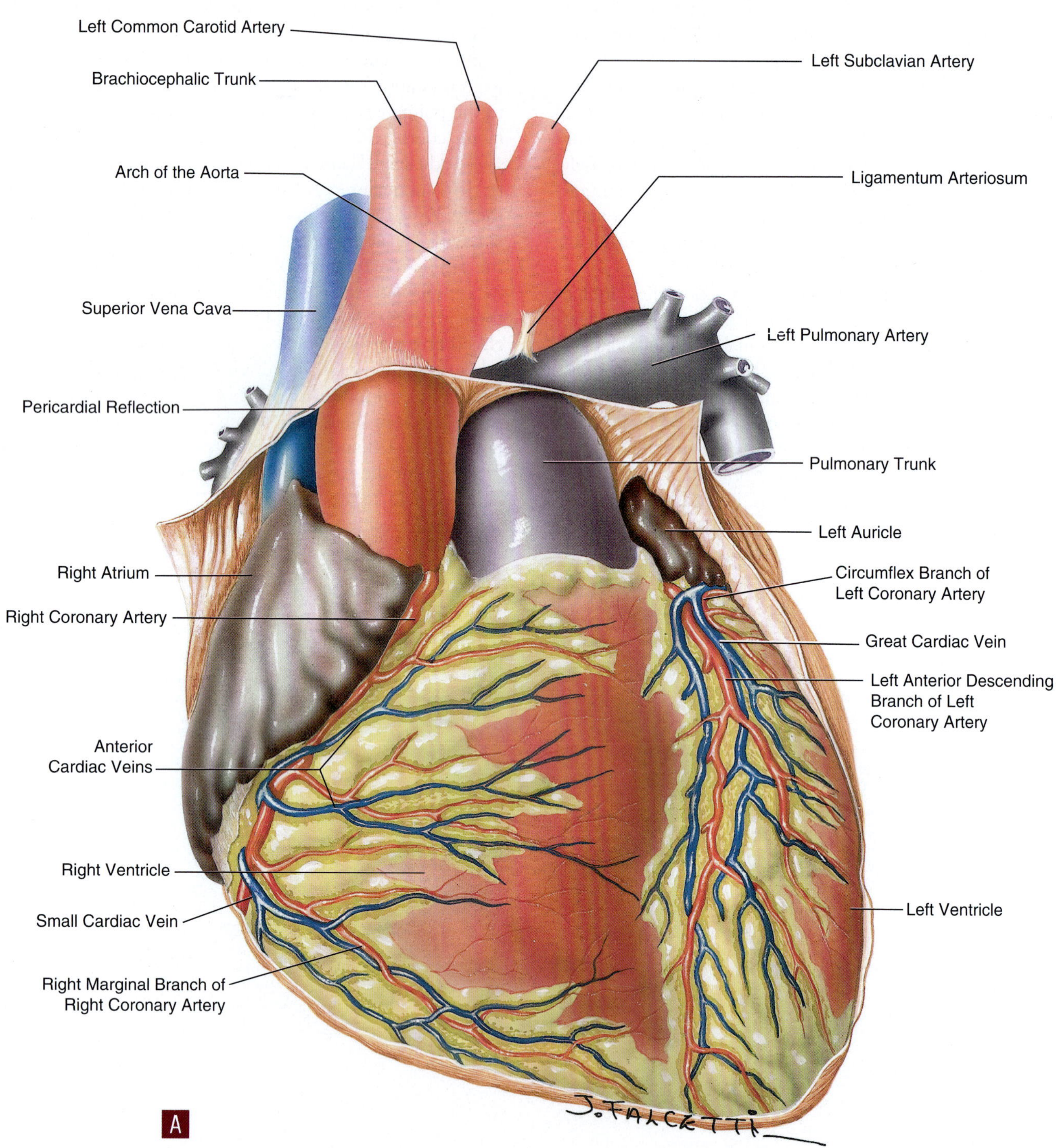

Figure 13.1. A, External aspect of the heart in the frontal view. Note the relationship of the great vessels and the ventricular cavities. B, External aspect of the heart in a posterior view. Note the relationship of the left atrium, pulmonary veins, and the large size of the coronary sinus.

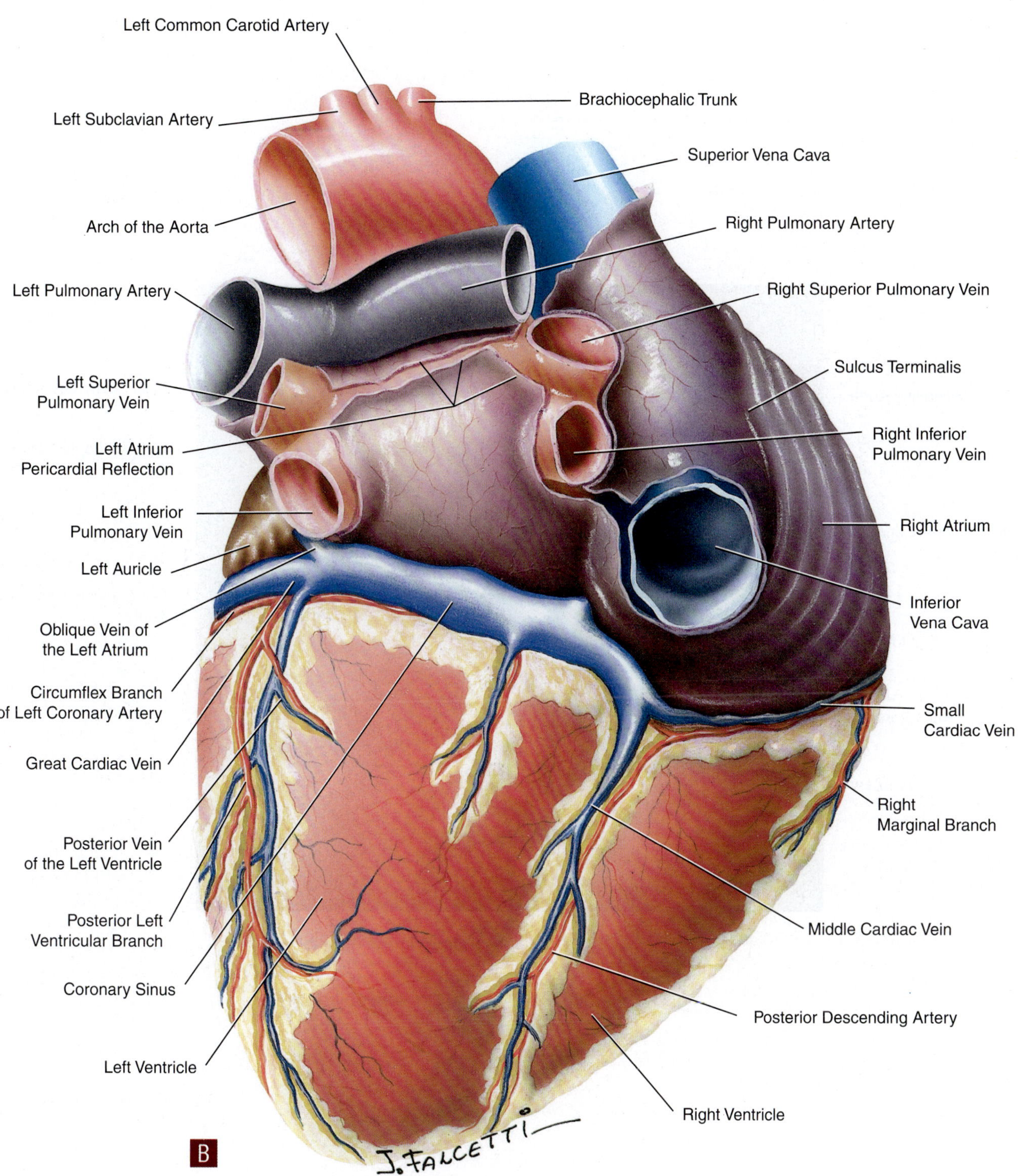

Figure 13.1. *Continued*

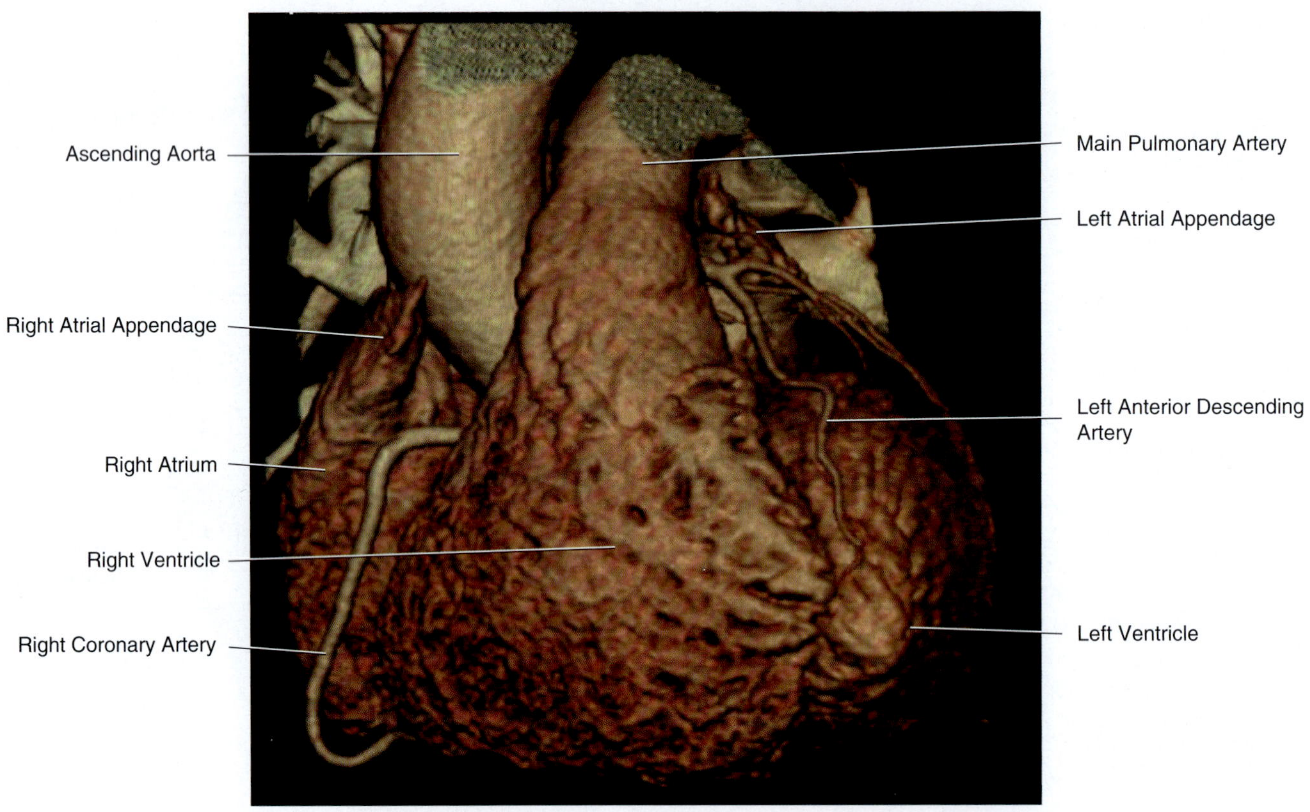

Figure 13.2. CT 3D volume-rendered image—frontal view.

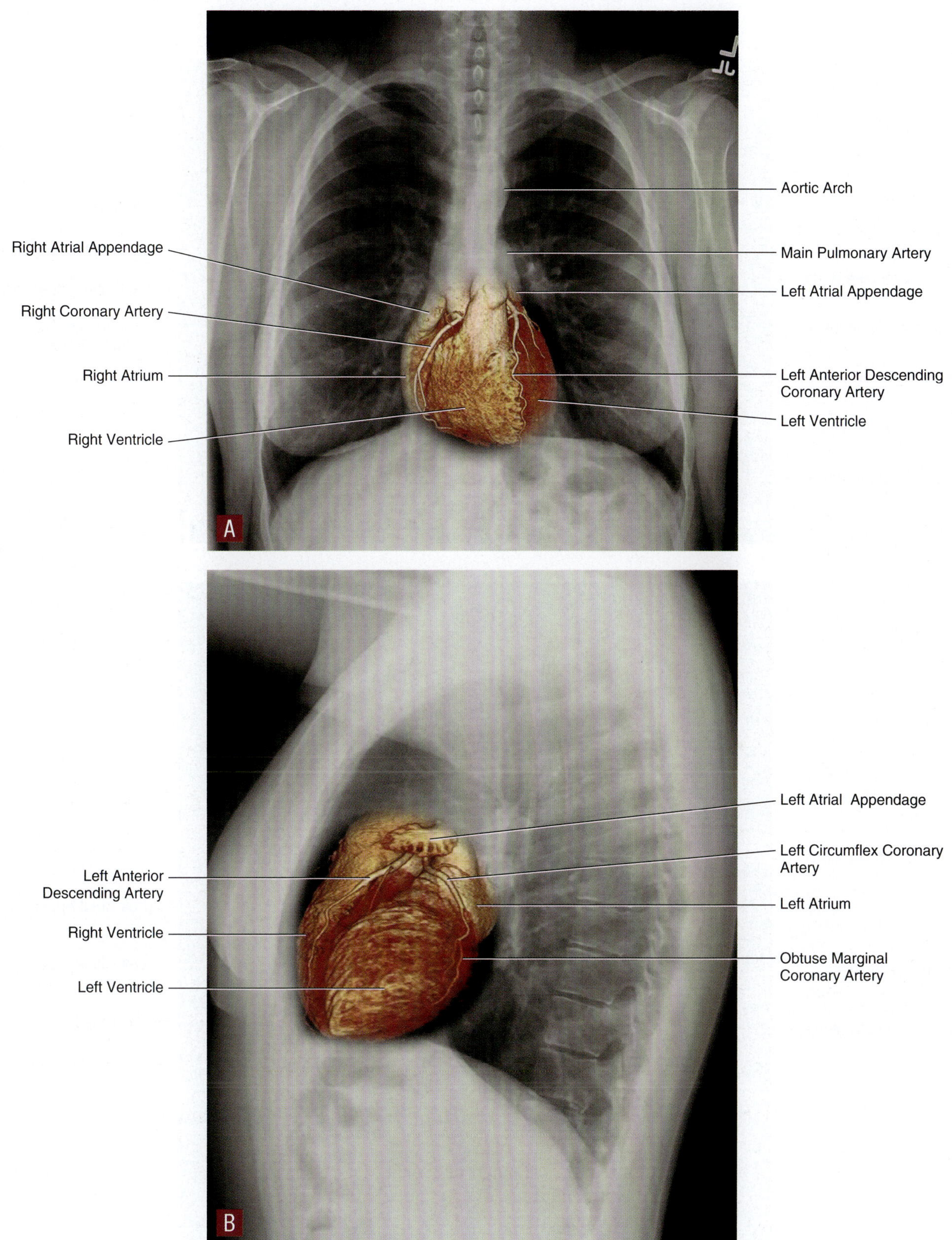

Figure 13.3. **A**, Chest X-ray in posteroanterior projection. A 3D volume-rendered heart is superimposed, located in the middle portion of the inferior mediastinum. The apex of the heart lies in the left hemithorax. **B**, Lateral chest X-ray with superimposed 3D volume-rendered heart. Anteriorly the heart is bordered by the anterior chest wall and posteriorly by the dorsal spine. **C**, Frontal view of volume-rendered CT showing the thoracic cavity and great vessels (semitransparent) and the position of the heart within. **D**, Lateral view of volume-rendered CT showing the thoracic cavity and great vessels (semitransparent) and the position of the heart within.

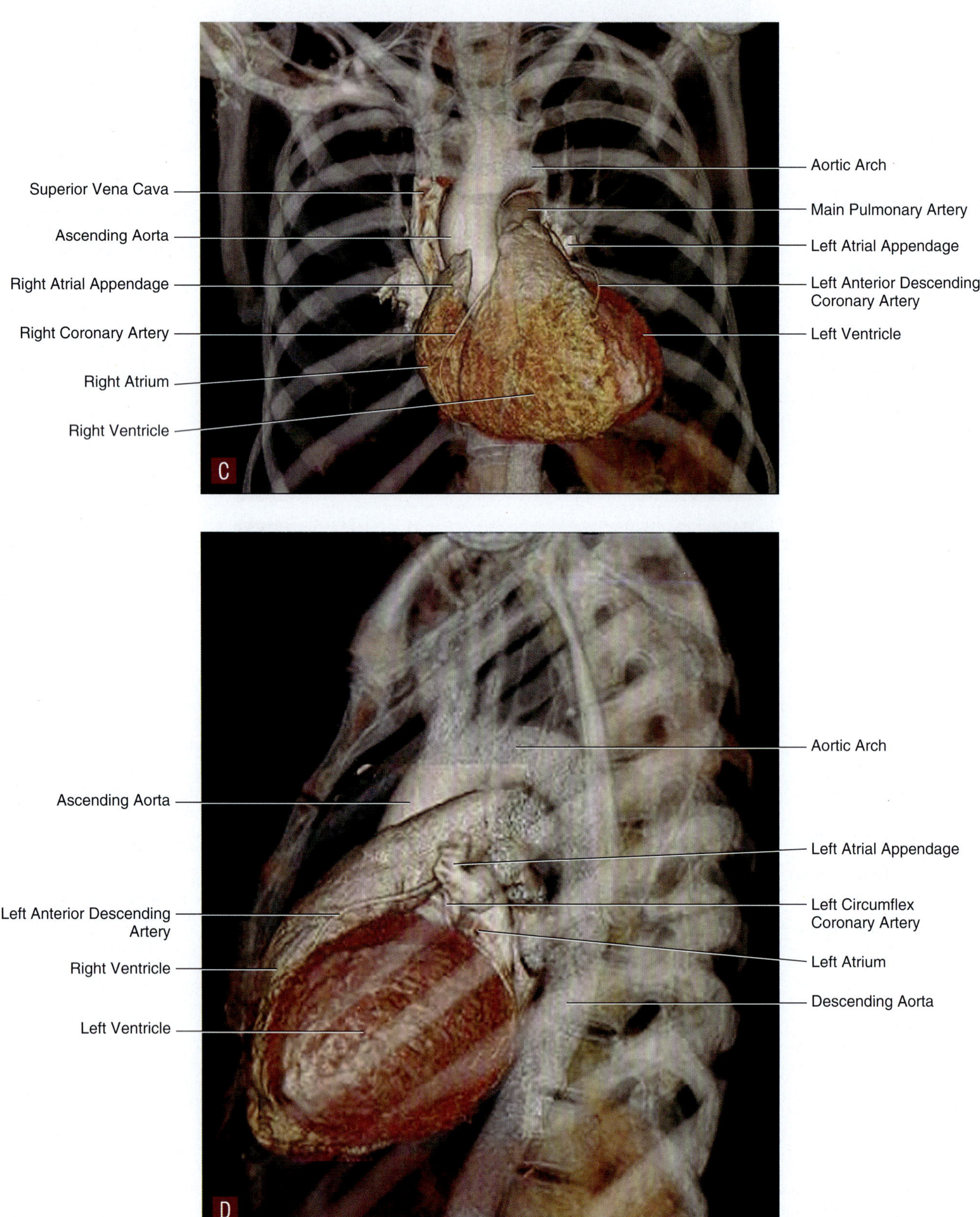

Figure 13.3. *Continued*

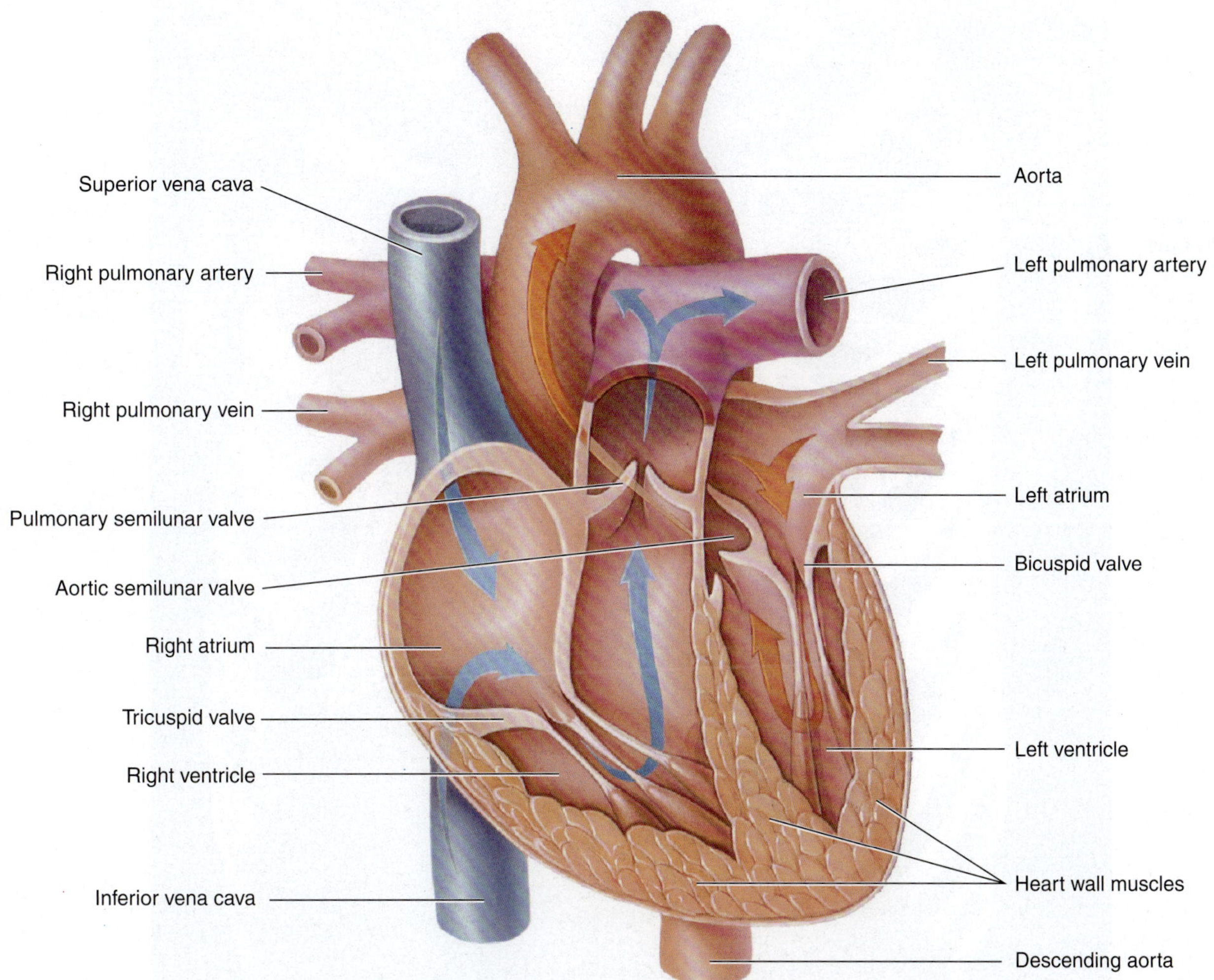

Figure 13.4. Pathways of the blood circulation inside the heart. In blue color is the venous blood and in red is the arterial blood. The pathways are marked by the arrows. (Reprinted from Kraemer WJ, Fleck SJ, Deschenes MR. *Exercise Physiology*. Baltimore: Wolters Kluwer; 2011 with permission.)

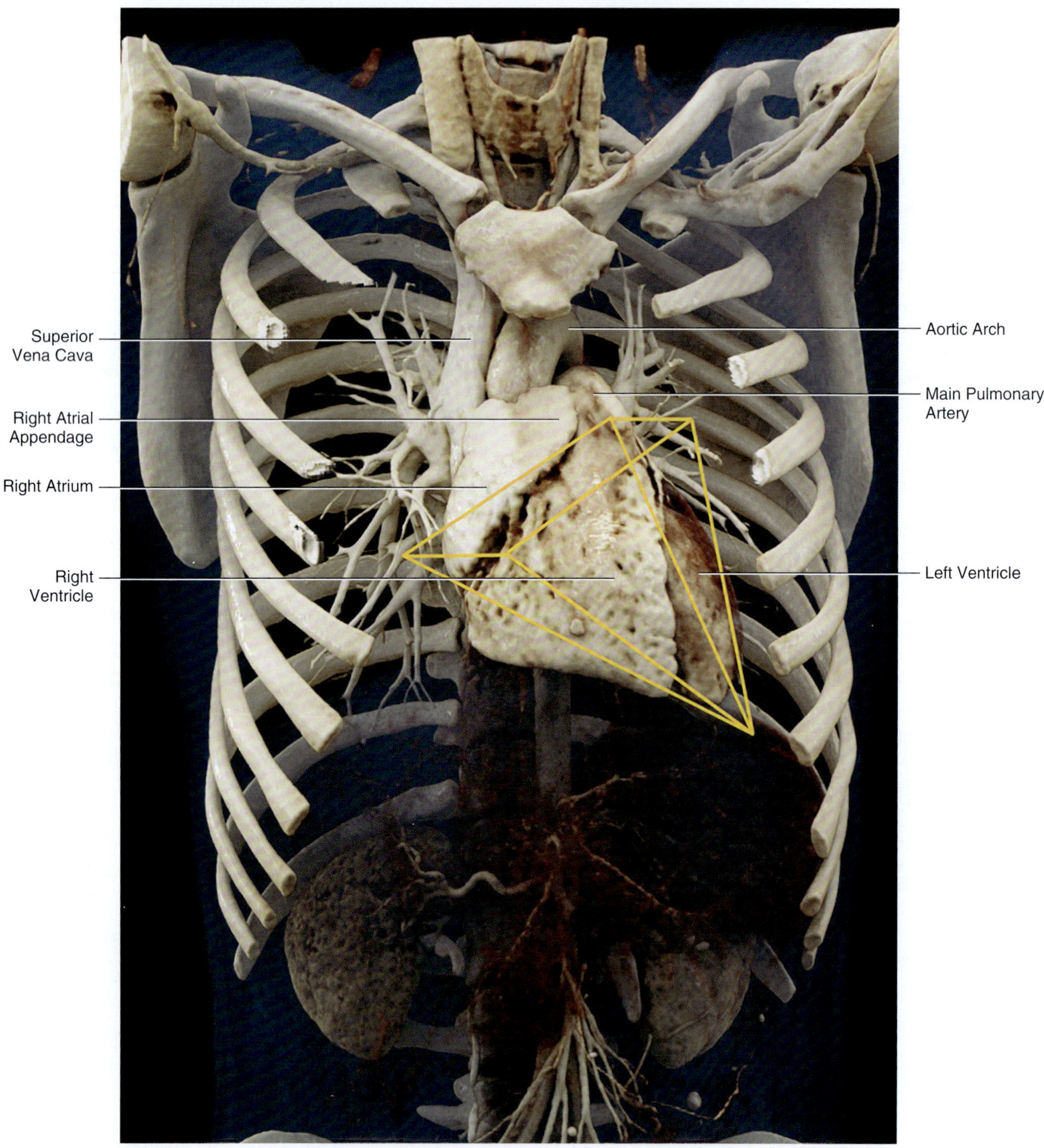

Figure 13.5. Cinematic rendering of CTA of the chest and upper abdomen. The heart looks like an inverted pyramid, with the longitudinal axis oriented anteriorly, inferiorly, and toward the left. CTA, computed tomography angiogram.

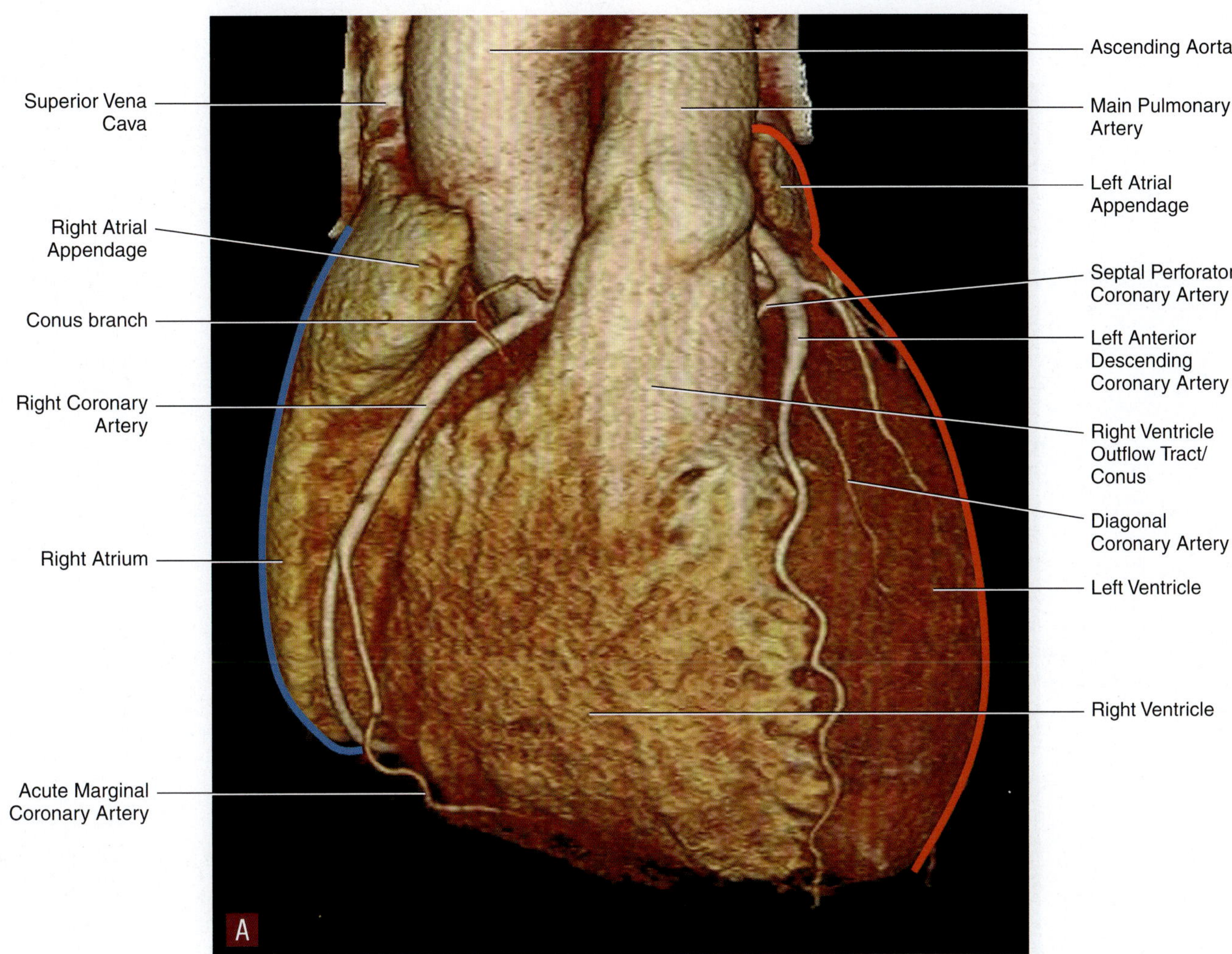

Figure 13.6. **A**, Frontal view of the 3D volume-rendered heart. The right (blue line) and left (red line) heart borders are outlined. **B**, Frontal view with right heart and main pulmonary artery in blue and left heart and aorta in red. **C**, Lateral view of the heart. The anterior border (blue line) corresponds to the anterior wall of the right ventricle and the posterior or dorsal border (red line) to the posterior wall of the left ventricle and left atrium. **D**, Lateral view of the heart with the right heart and main pulmonary artery in blue and the left heart and aorta in red.

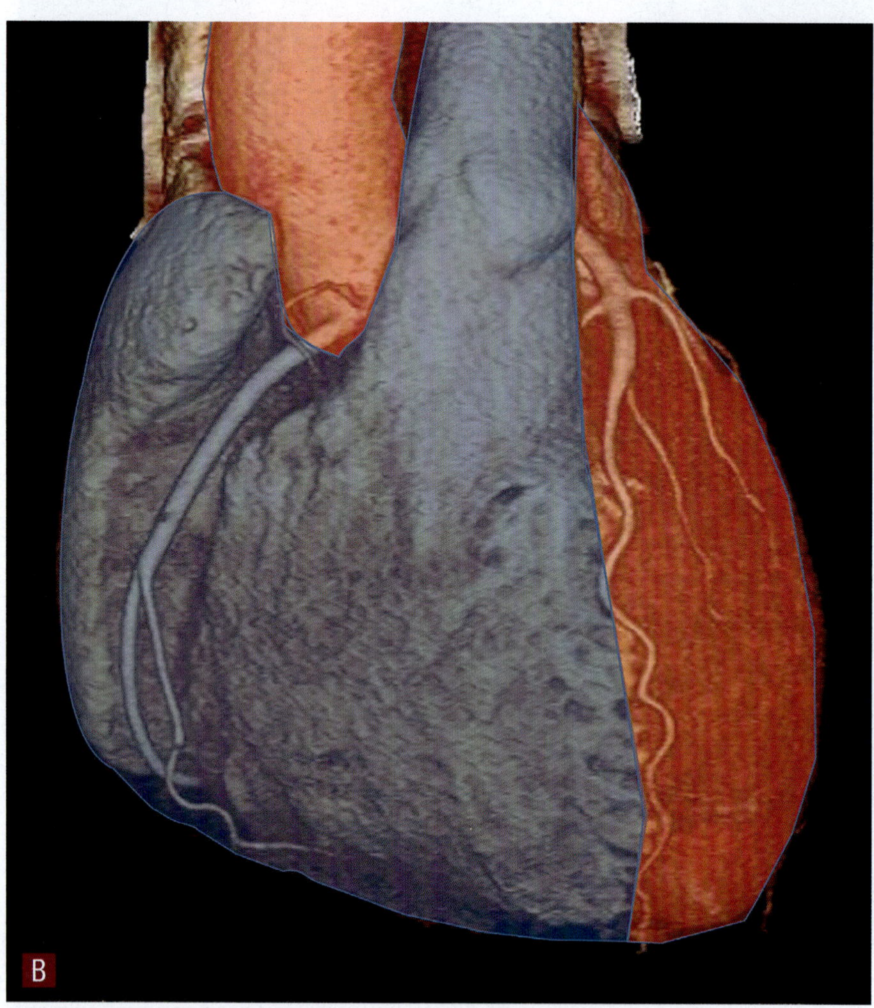

Figure 13.6. *Continued*

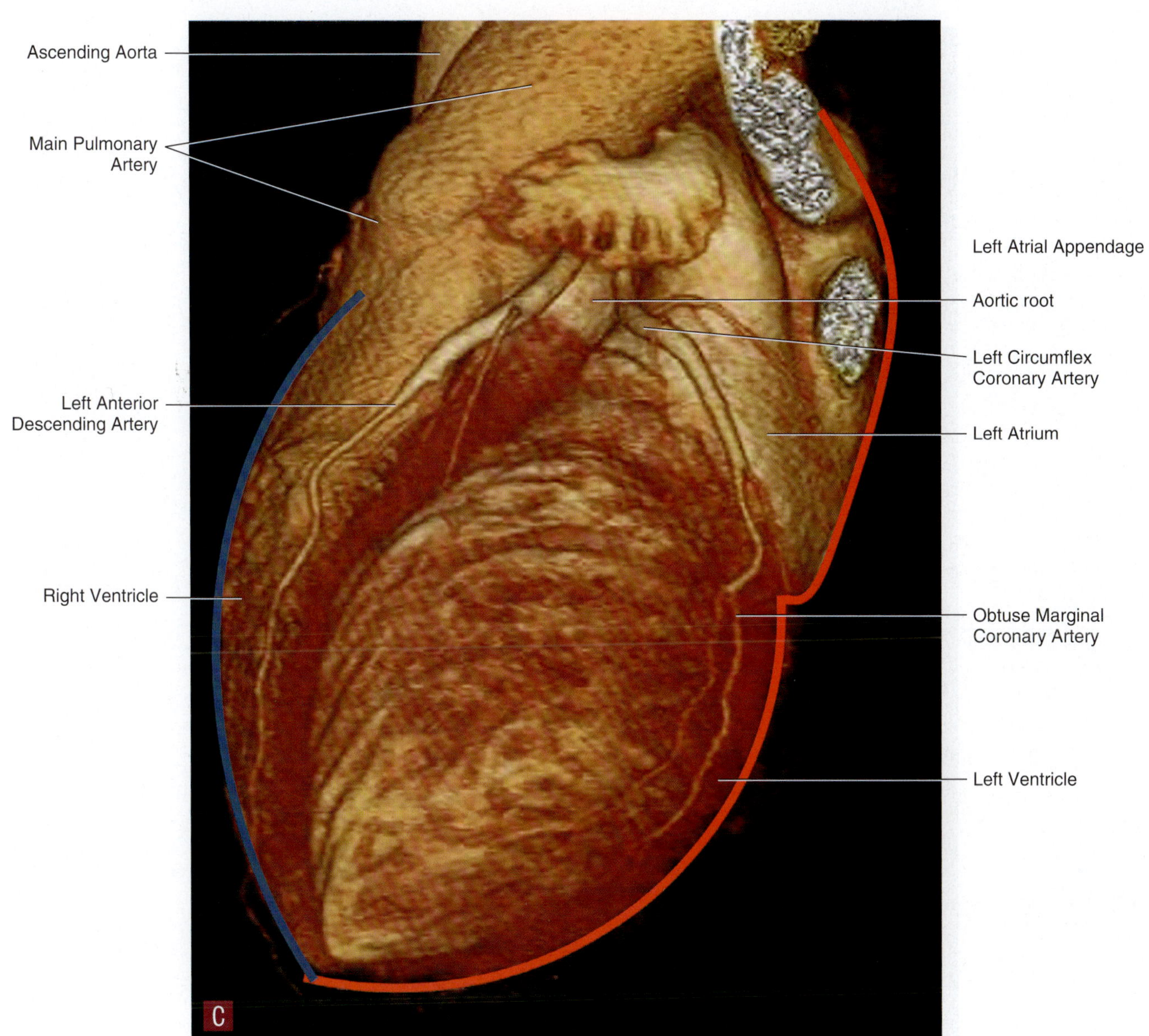

Figure 13.6. *Continued*

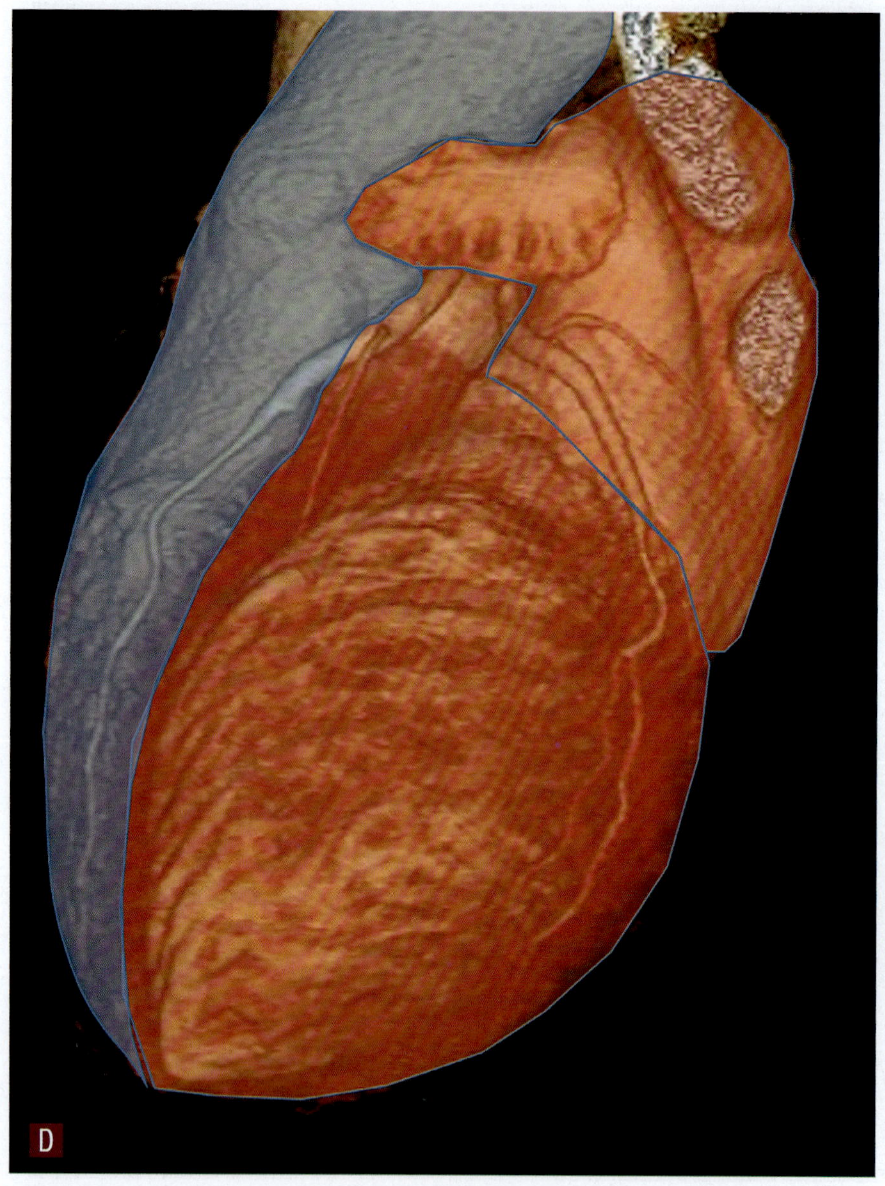

Figure 13.6. *Continued*

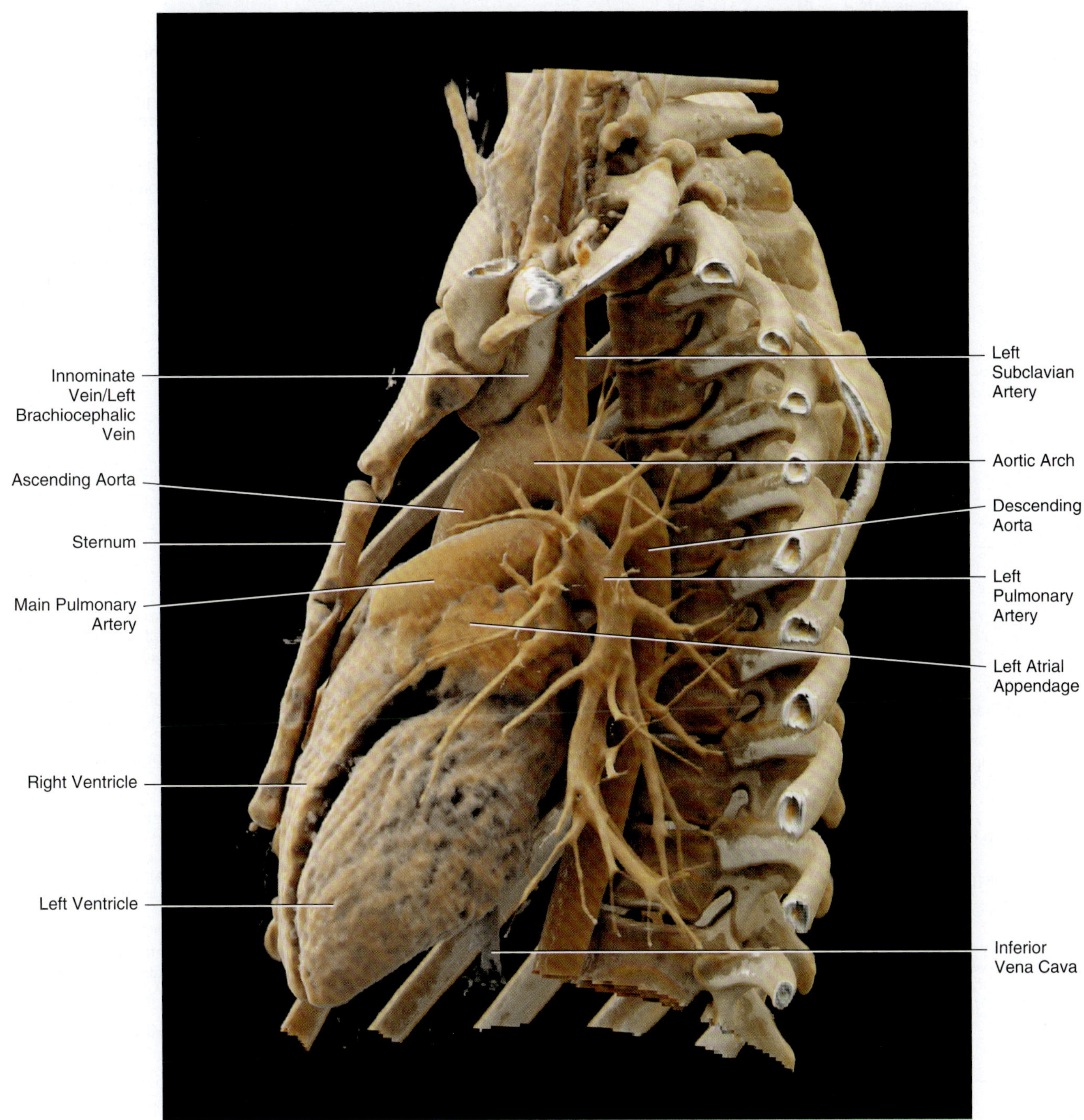

Figure 13.7. CT 3D cinematic volume-rendered image. Left lateral view of the heart with bone overlay.

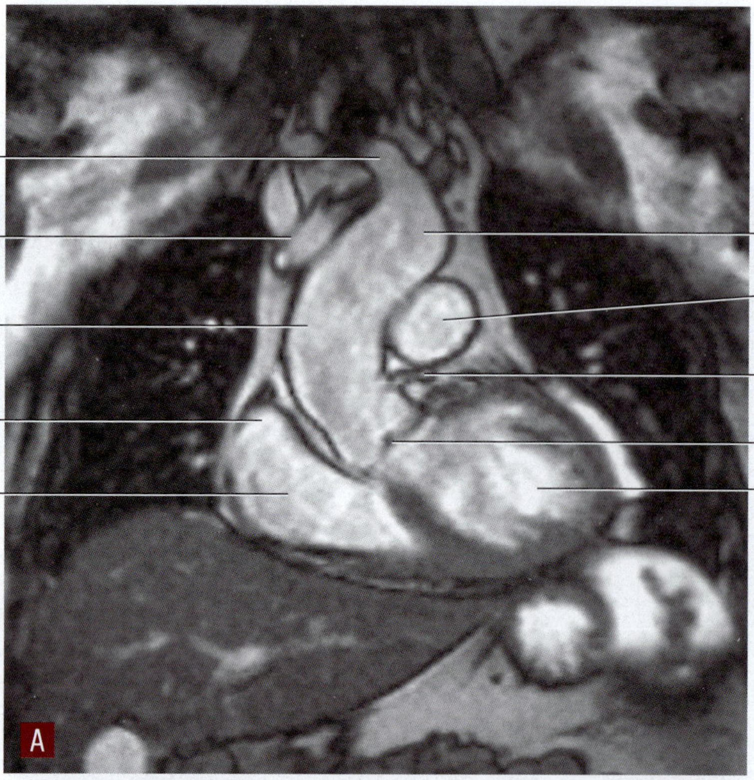

Right Brachiocephalic Artery/ Innominate Artery
Confluence of Brachiocephalic Veins
Ascending Aorta
Right Atrial Appendage
Right Atrium
Aortic Arch
Main Pulmonary Artery
Left Main Coronary Artery
Aortic Valve
Left Ventricle
A

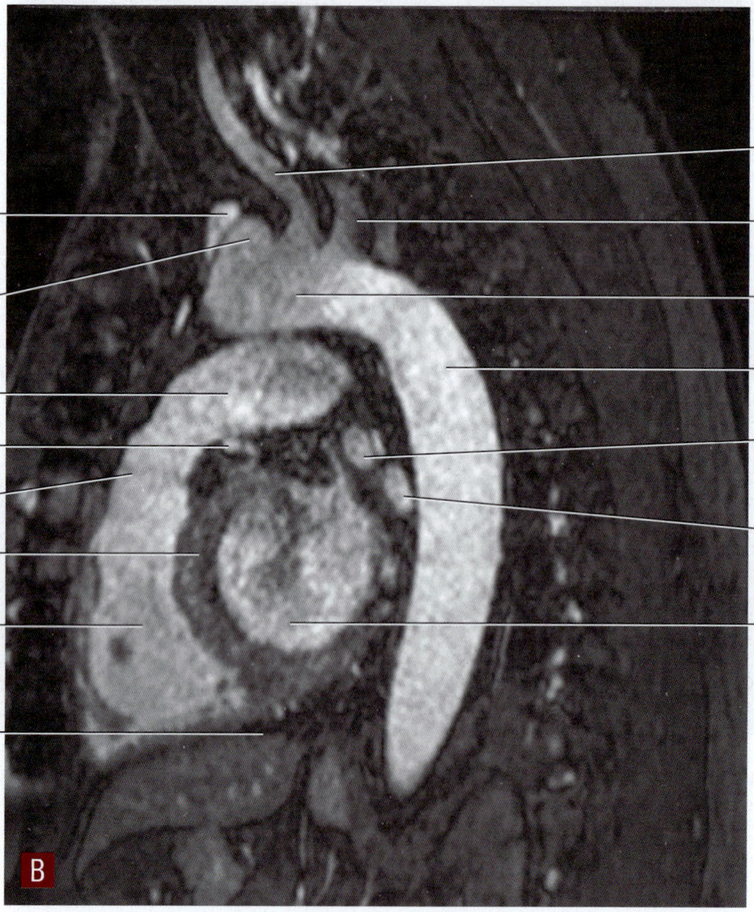

Innominate Vein/ Left Brachiocephalic Vein
Innominate Artery/ Right Brachiocephalic Artery
Main Pulmonary Artery
Left Main Coronary Artery
Pulmonic Valve
Interventricular Septum
Right Ventricle
Left Ventricle
Left Common Carotid Artery
Left Subclavian Artery
Aortic Arch
Descending Aorta
Left Superior Pulmonary Vein
Left Inferior Pulmonary Vein
Left Ventricle
B

Figure 13.8. **A**, Magnetic resonance imaging (MRI) of the heart and mediastinum. Coronal plane. **B**, Magnetic resonance imaging of the heart and mediastinum. Sagittal plane. **C**, Magnetic resonance imaging of the heart and mediastinum. Axial plane.

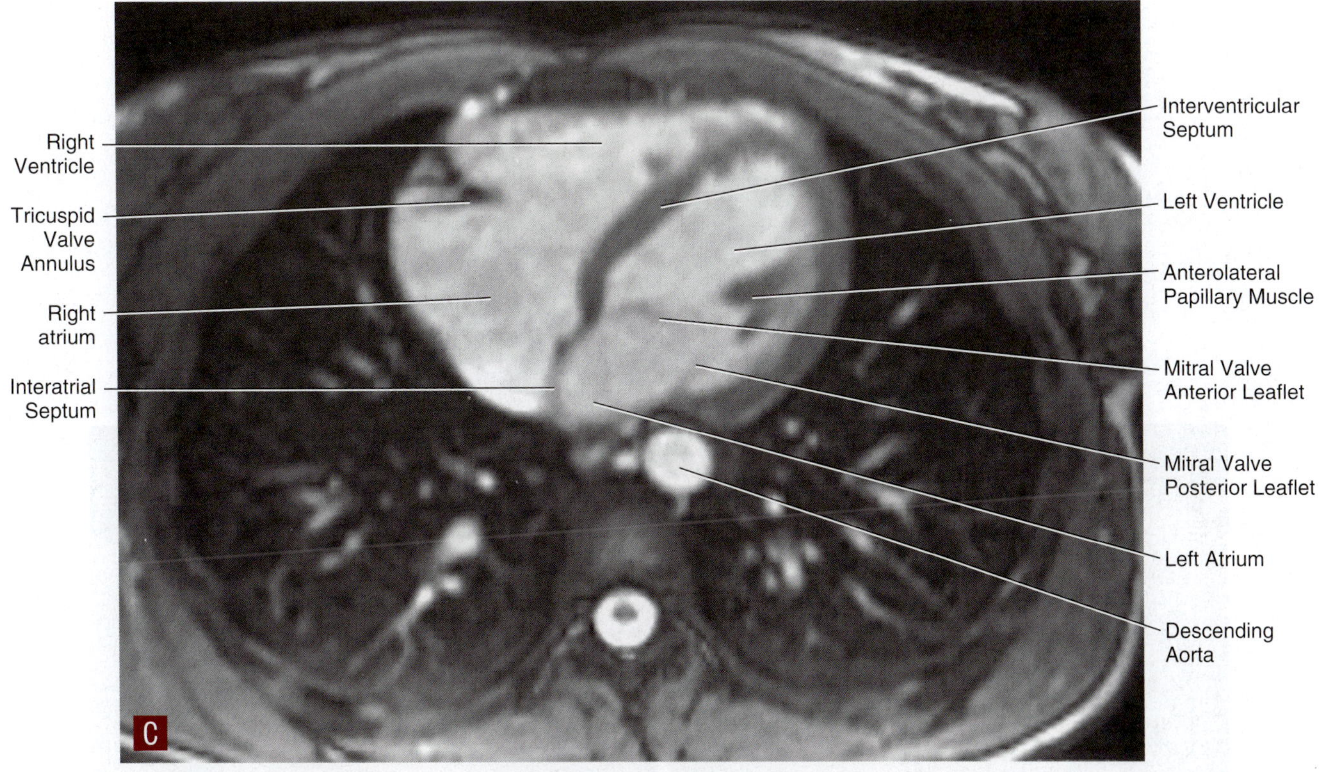

Figure 13.8. *Continued*

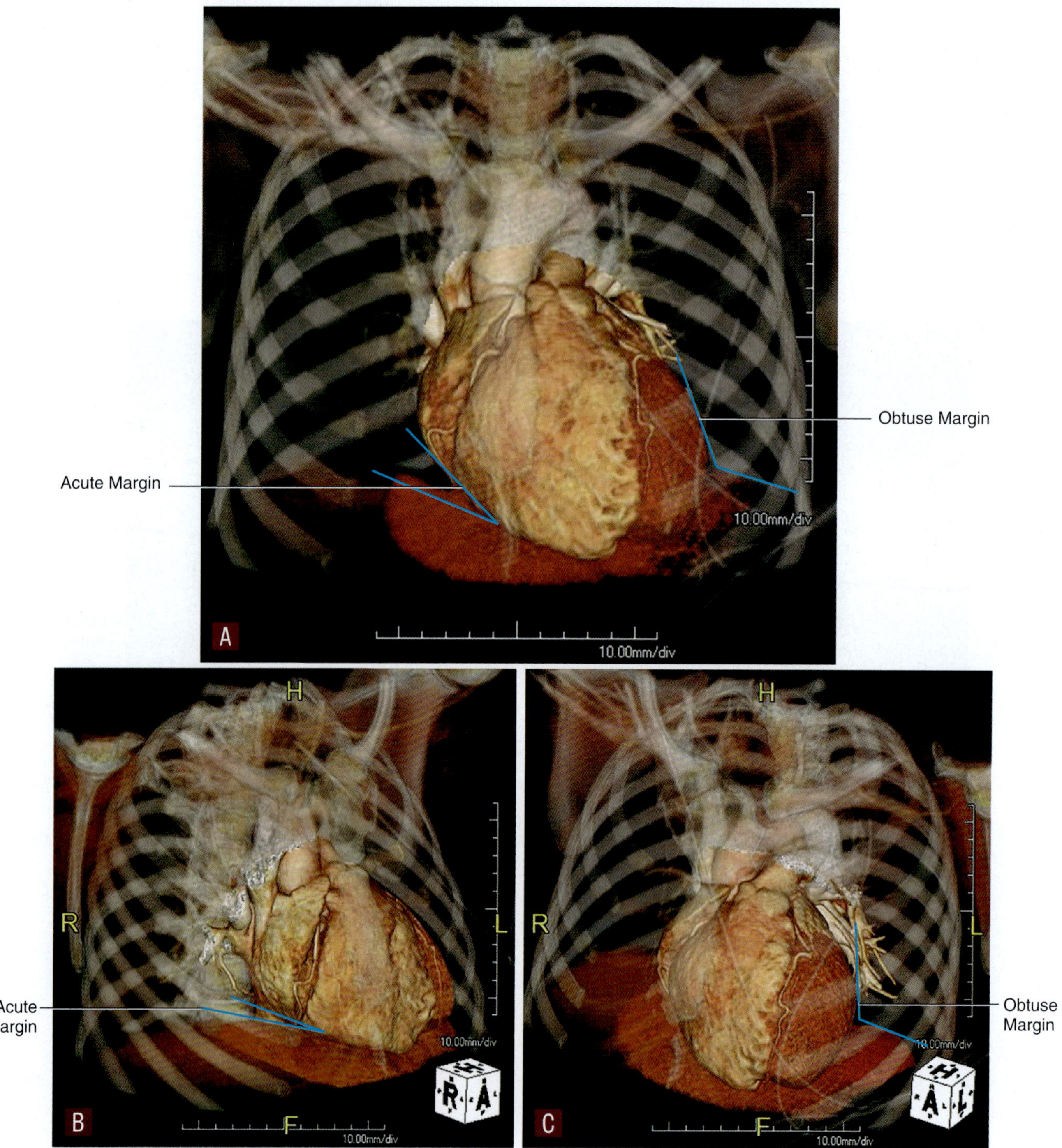

Figure 13.9. **A**, The acute margin of the heart is sharp and is formed mainly by the right ventricle and right atrium. Blue lines denote the acute angle between the heart border and the right diaphragm. The obtuse margin is round and corresponds mainly to the left ventricle. Blue lines denote the obtuse angle between the heart border and the left hemidiaphragm. **B**, Acute margin shown in the RAO view. **C**, Obtuse margin shown in the LAO view. LAO, left anterior oblique; RAO, right anterior oblique.

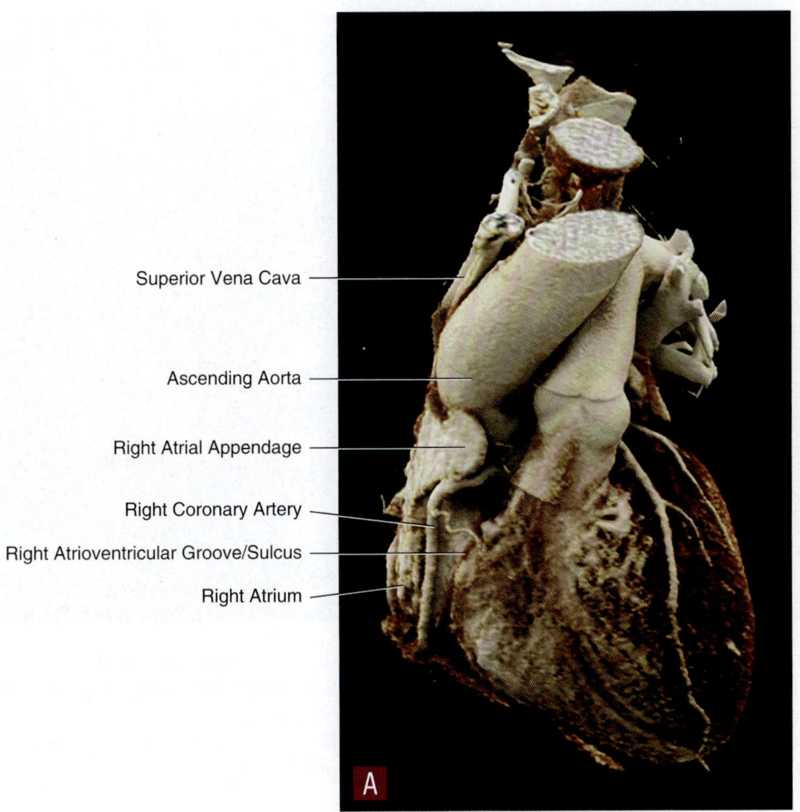

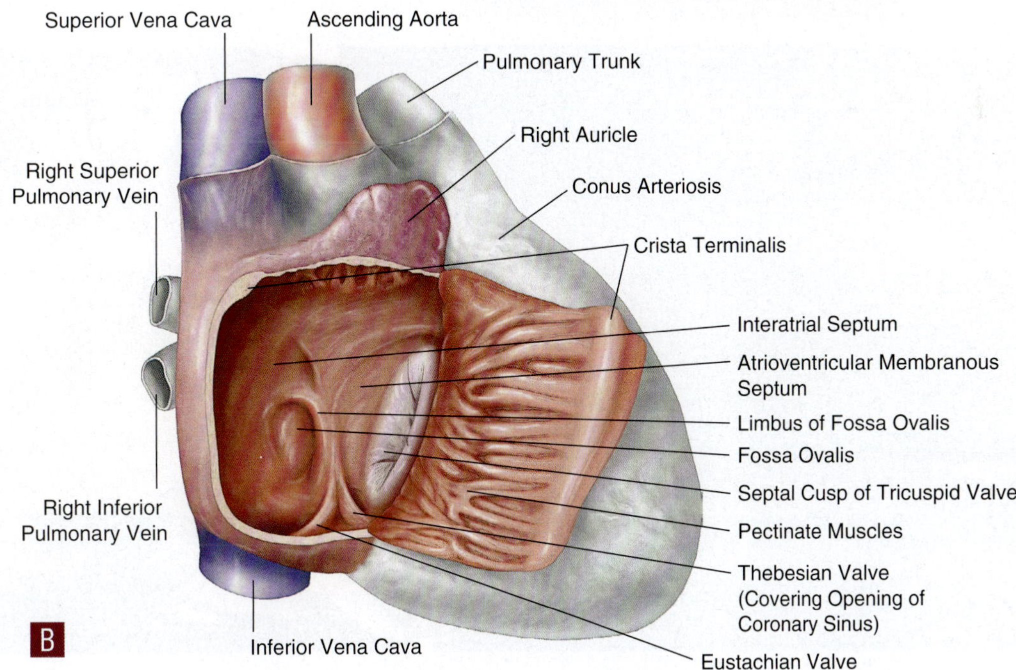

Figure 13.10. **A**, 3D volume-rendered cinematic reconstruction from CTA showing the external features of the right atrium. The lateral wall of the right atrium forms most of the right cardiac border. The right atrial appendage/auricle abuts the ascending aorta. **B**, Internal features of the right atrium. The atrial septum has a central circular depression: the fossa ovalis. CTA, computed tomography angiogram.

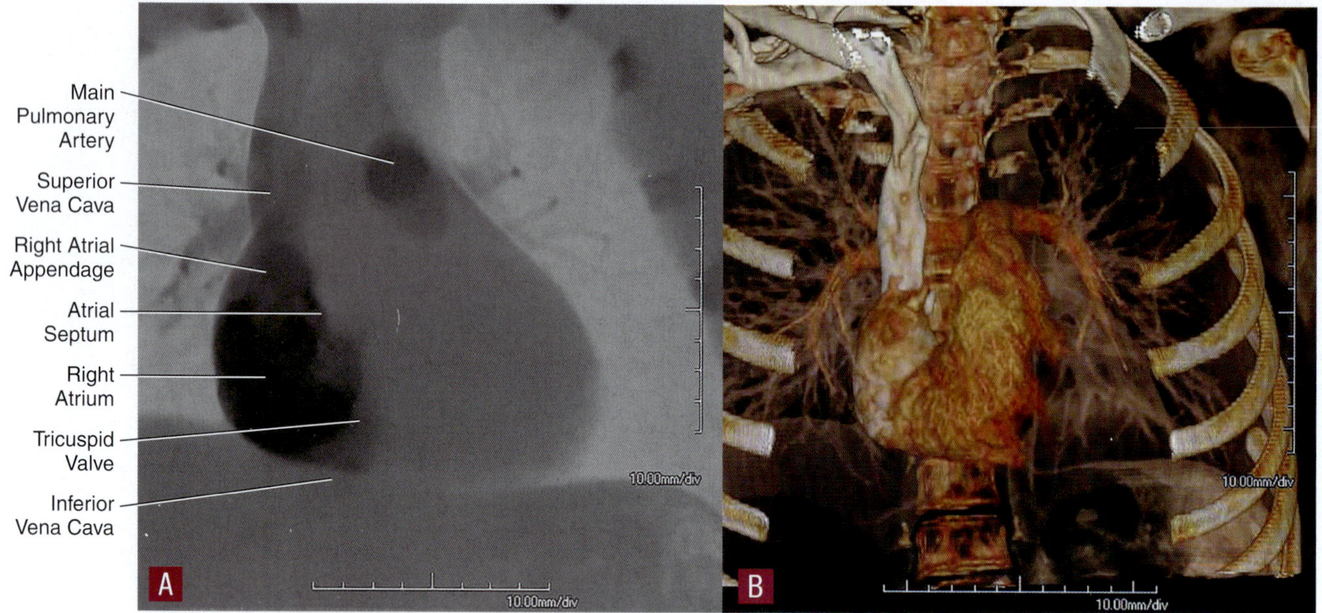

Figure 13.11. Right atrial angiography. **A**, Simulated DSA from CT data. **B**, Corresponding 3D volume-rendered CT in the same patient in the same orientation. The left superior border corresponds to the most anterior portion of the atrial septum. The atrial appendage is not seen clearly in this view. The tricuspid valve is located inferior and to the left. This is a long axial view. DSA, digital subtraction angiogram.

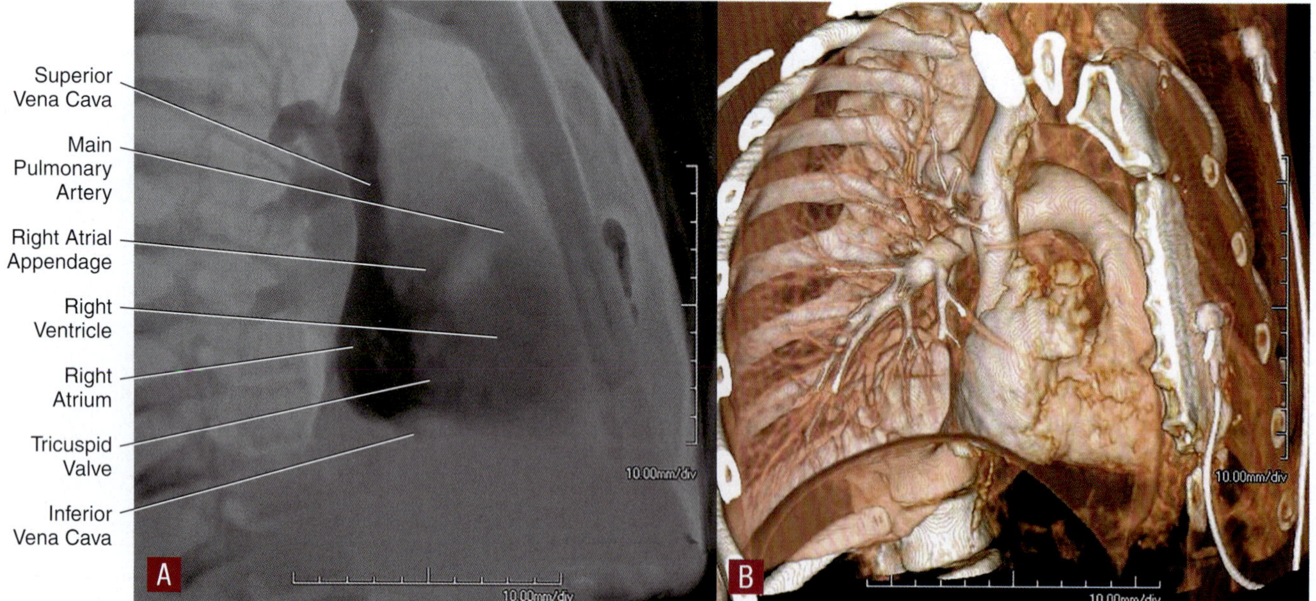

Figure 13.12. Right atrium in elongated right anterior oblique view. **A**, Simulated DSA from CT data. **B**, Corresponding 3D volume-rendered CT in the same patient in the same orientation. The posterior wall is seen as a continuity of the superior and inferior vena cavae in the right border. The right atrial appendage is located superiorly and to the left. Between the inferior vena cava and the tricuspid annulus is the atrioventricular septum. DSA, digital subtraction angiogram.

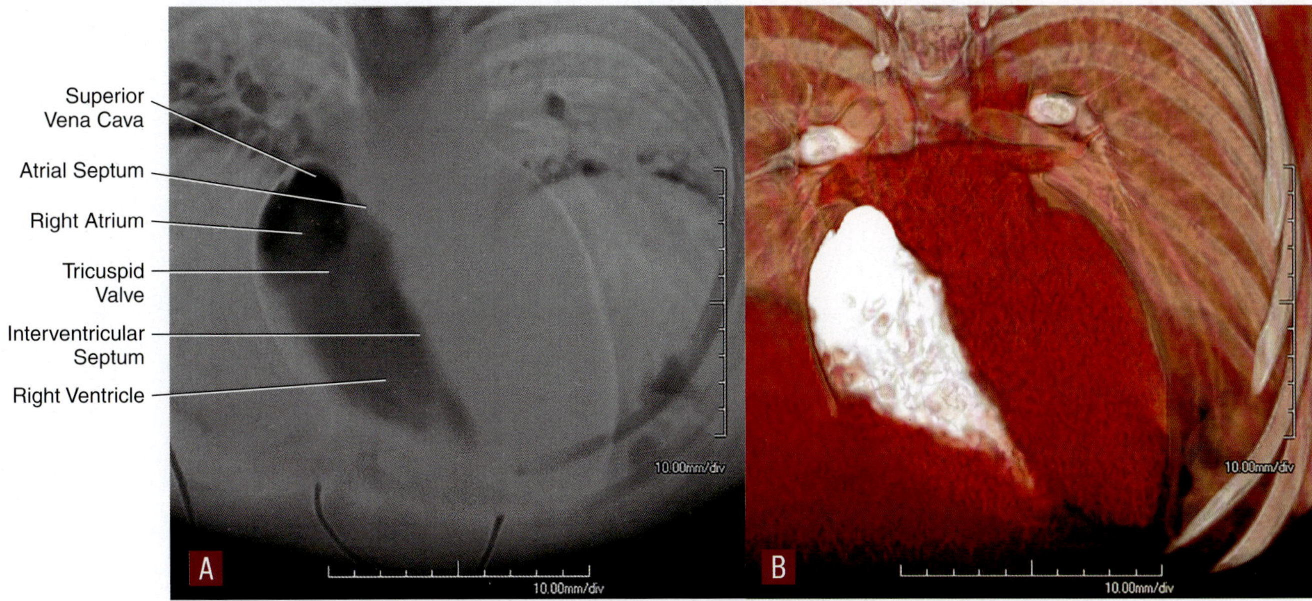

Figure 13.13. Right atrial angiogram in the so-called four-chamber view. A, Simulated DSA from CT data. B, Corresponding 3D volume-rendered CT in the same patient in the same orientation. The atrial appendage is overlapped and therefore not clearly visualized. DSA, digital subtraction angiogram.

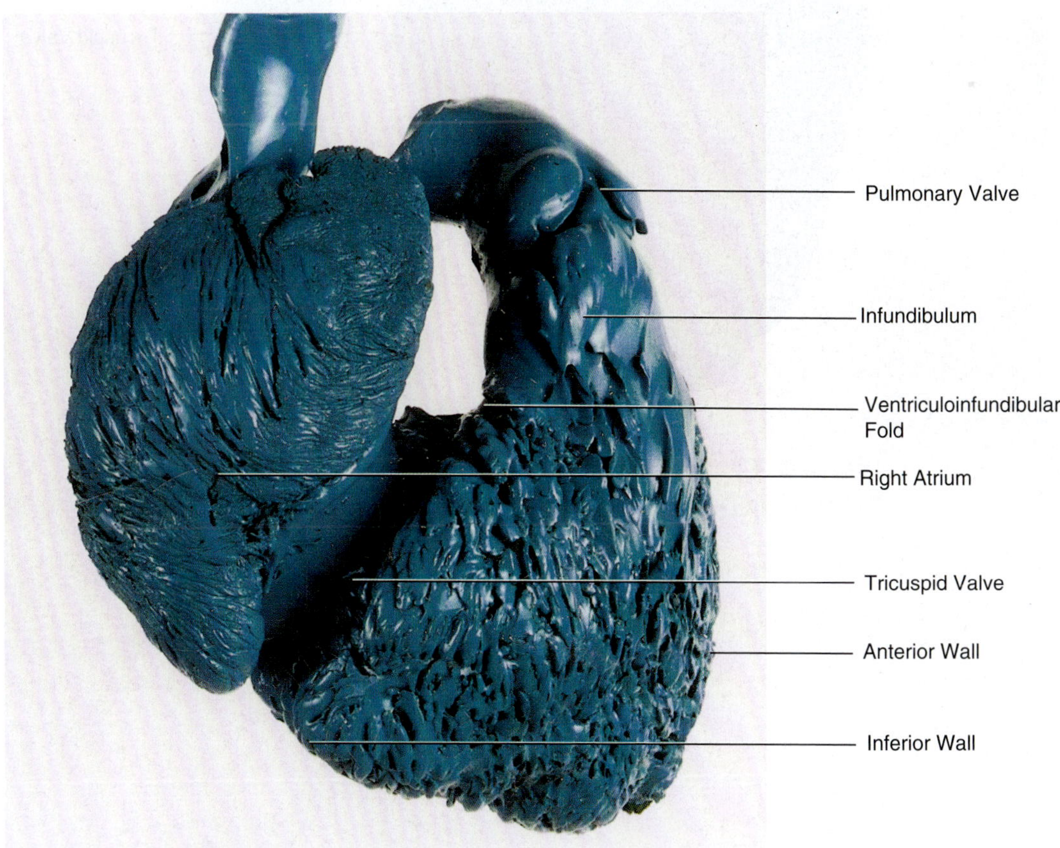

Figure 13.14. Luminal cast of the right atrium and ventricle. Frontal view.

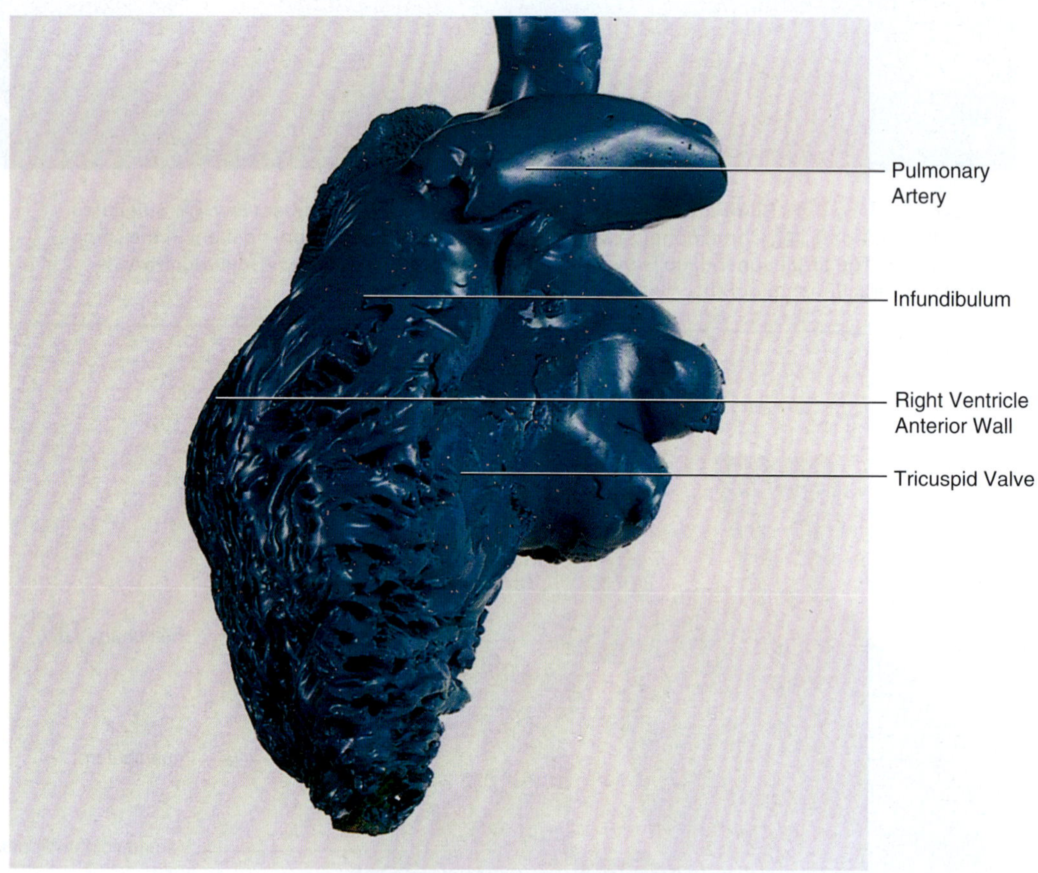

Figure 13.15. **Luminal cast of the right ventricle.** Lateral view.

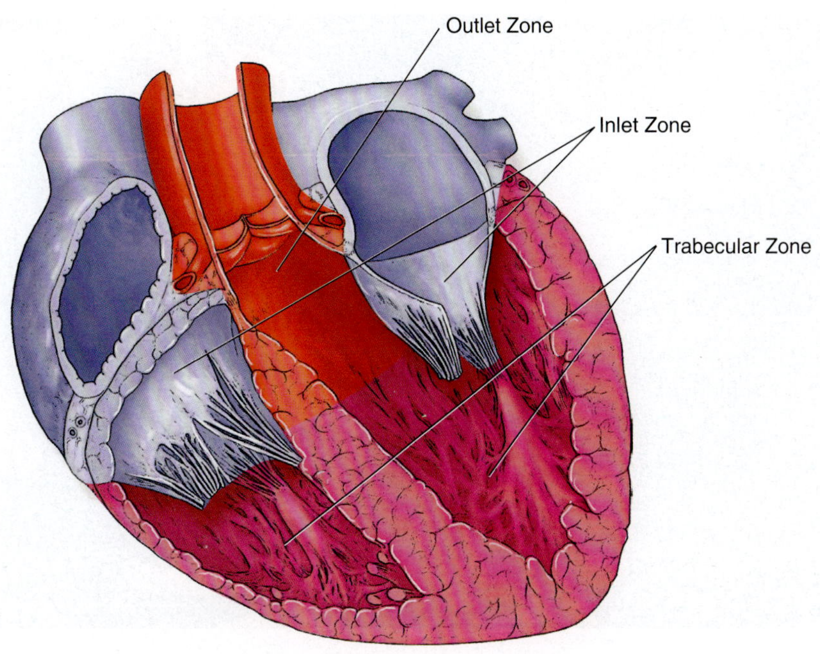

Figure 13.16. The three portions of the right ventricular chamber.

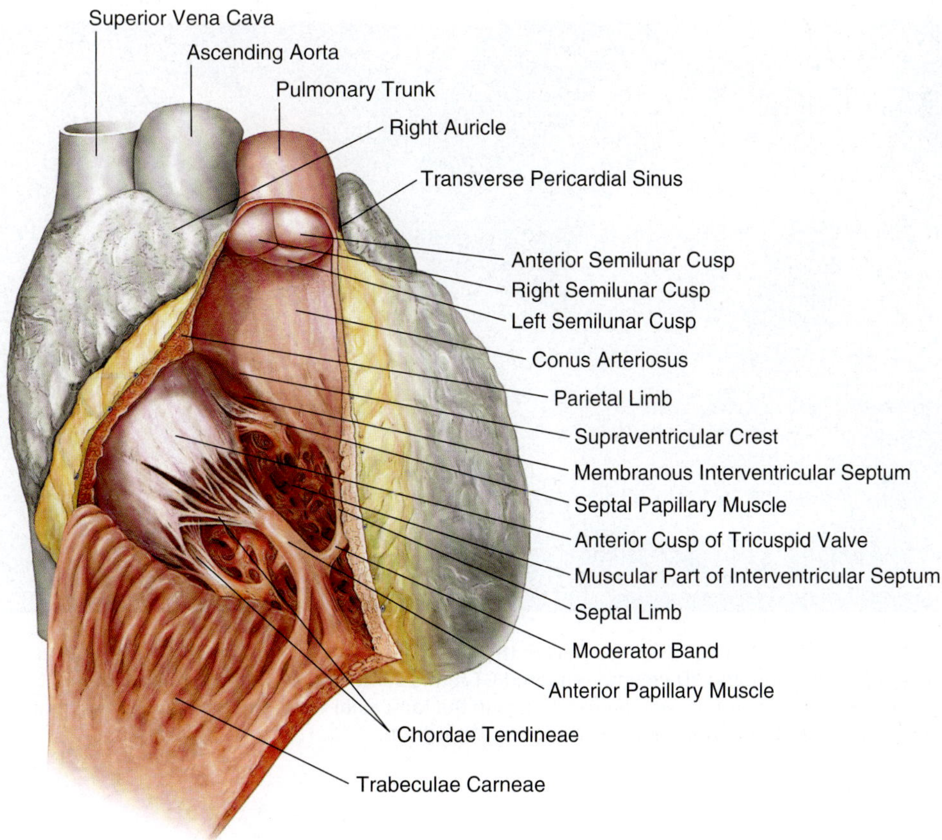

Figure 13.17. Internal features of the right ventricle.

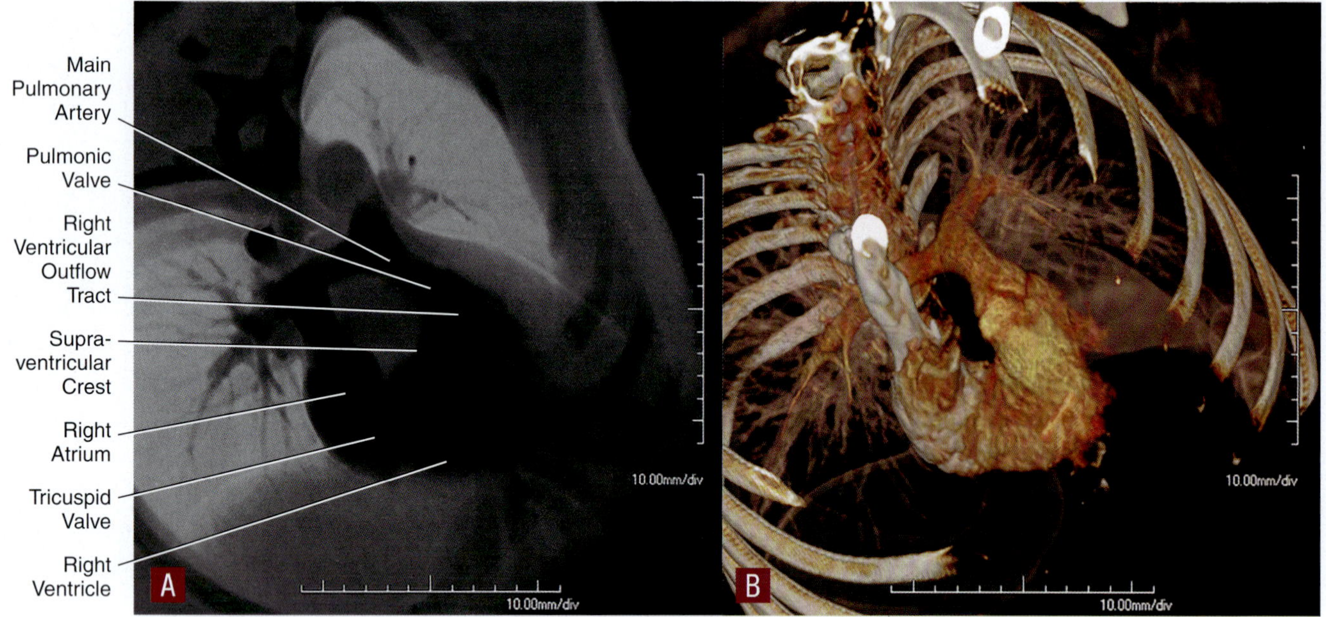

Figure 13.18. Angiographic elongated right anterior oblique view of the right ventricle. **A**, Simulated DSA from CT data. **B**, Corresponding 3D volume-rendered CT in the same patient in the same orientation. DSA, digital subtraction angiogram.

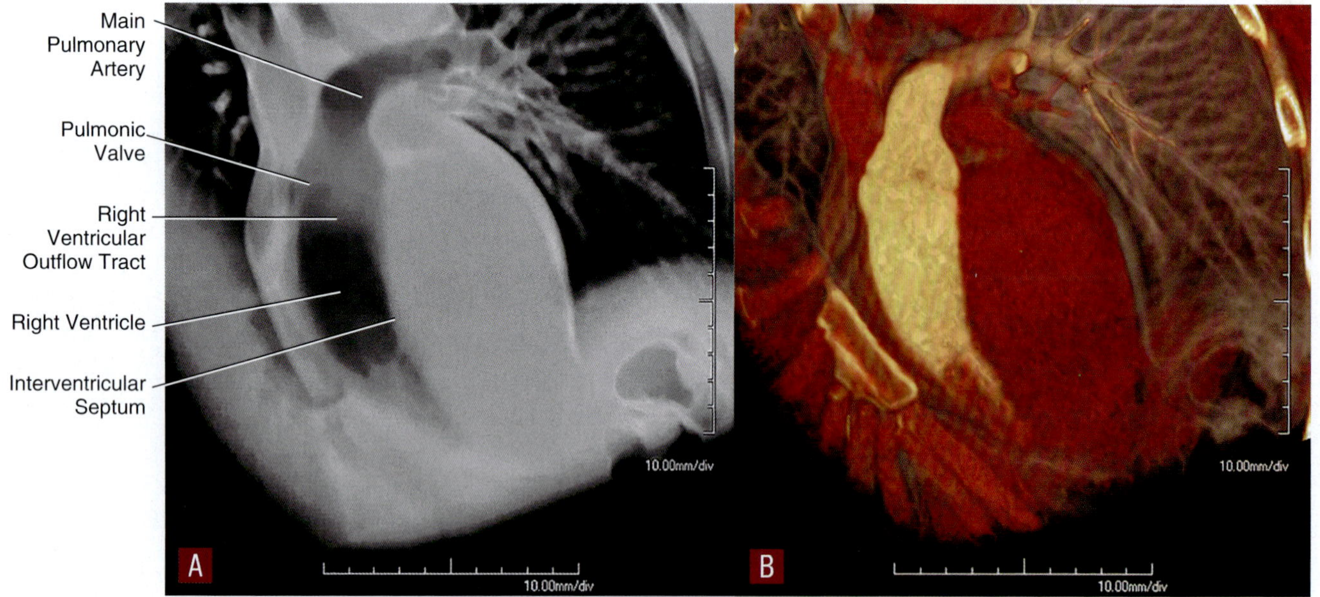

Figure 13.19. Four-chamber view of the right ventricle. **A**, Simulated DSA from CT data. **B**, Corresponding 3D volume-rendered CT in the same patient in the same orientation. The outflow tract is not as well defined as it is in the long axial view, since it overlies the right ventricular inlet zone. DSA, digital subtraction angiogram.

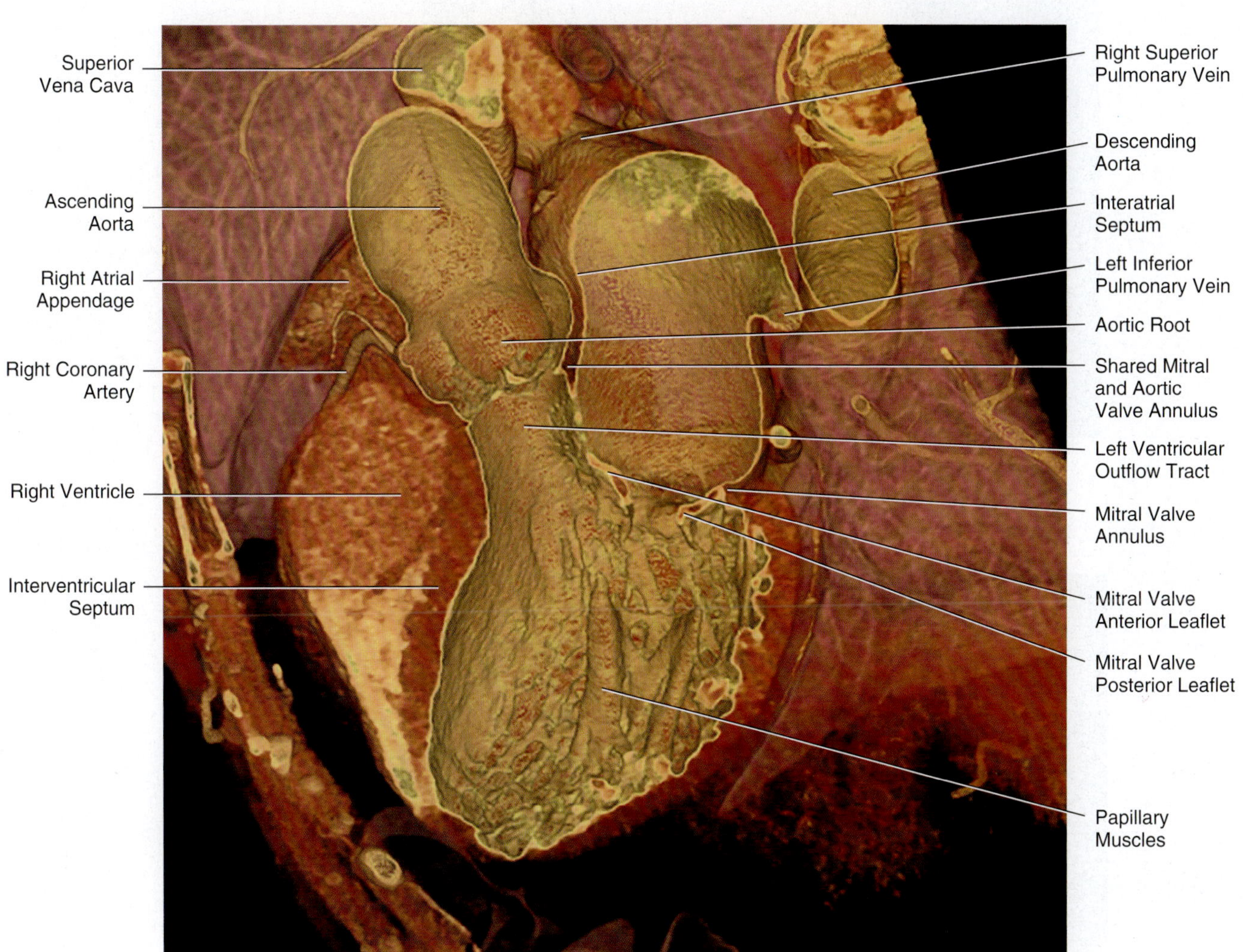

Figure 13.20. Internal features of the left atrium and ventricle. 3D volume-rendered CT.

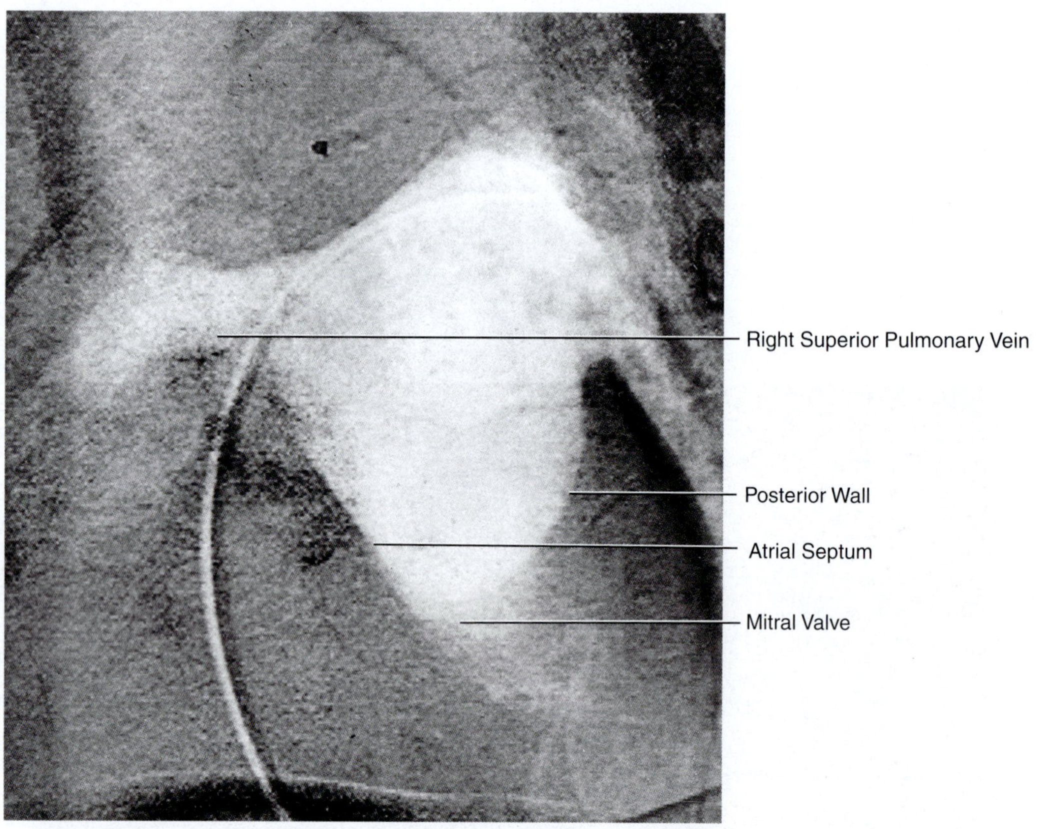

Figure 13.21. **Left atrial angiogram in long axial view.** The left pulmonary veins and the left atrial appendage are not seen clearly in this view.

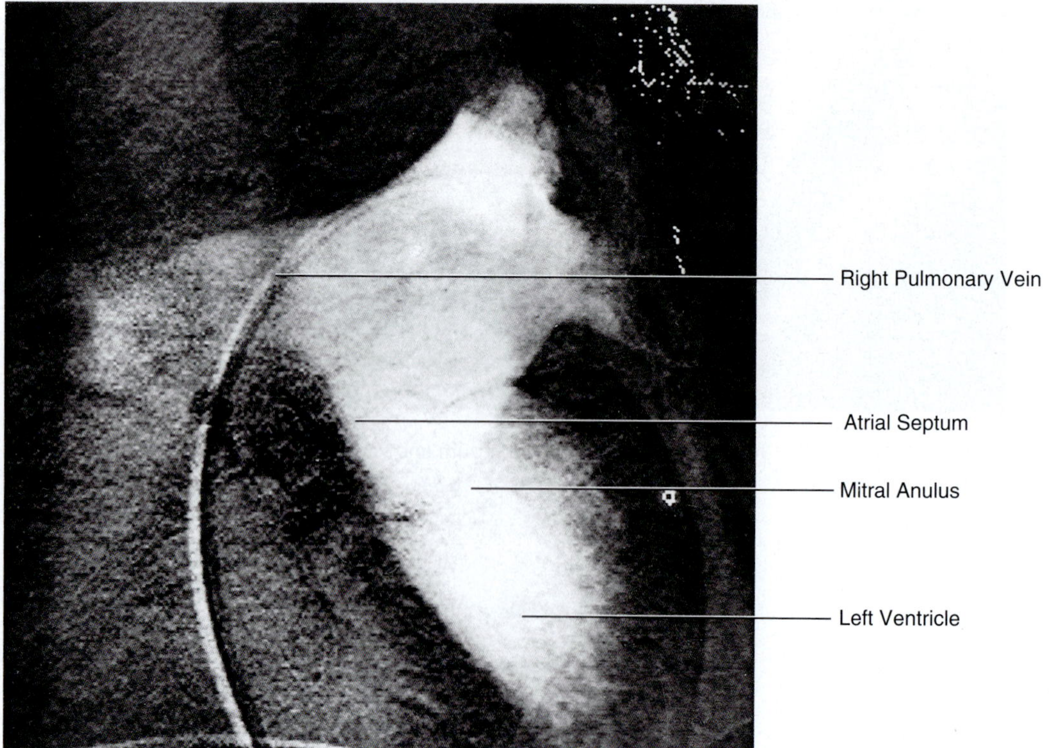

Figure 13.22. **Long axial view of the left atrium.** The anterior portion of the left atrial septum is the right wall of the left atrium. The left atrial appendage is not seen in this projection.

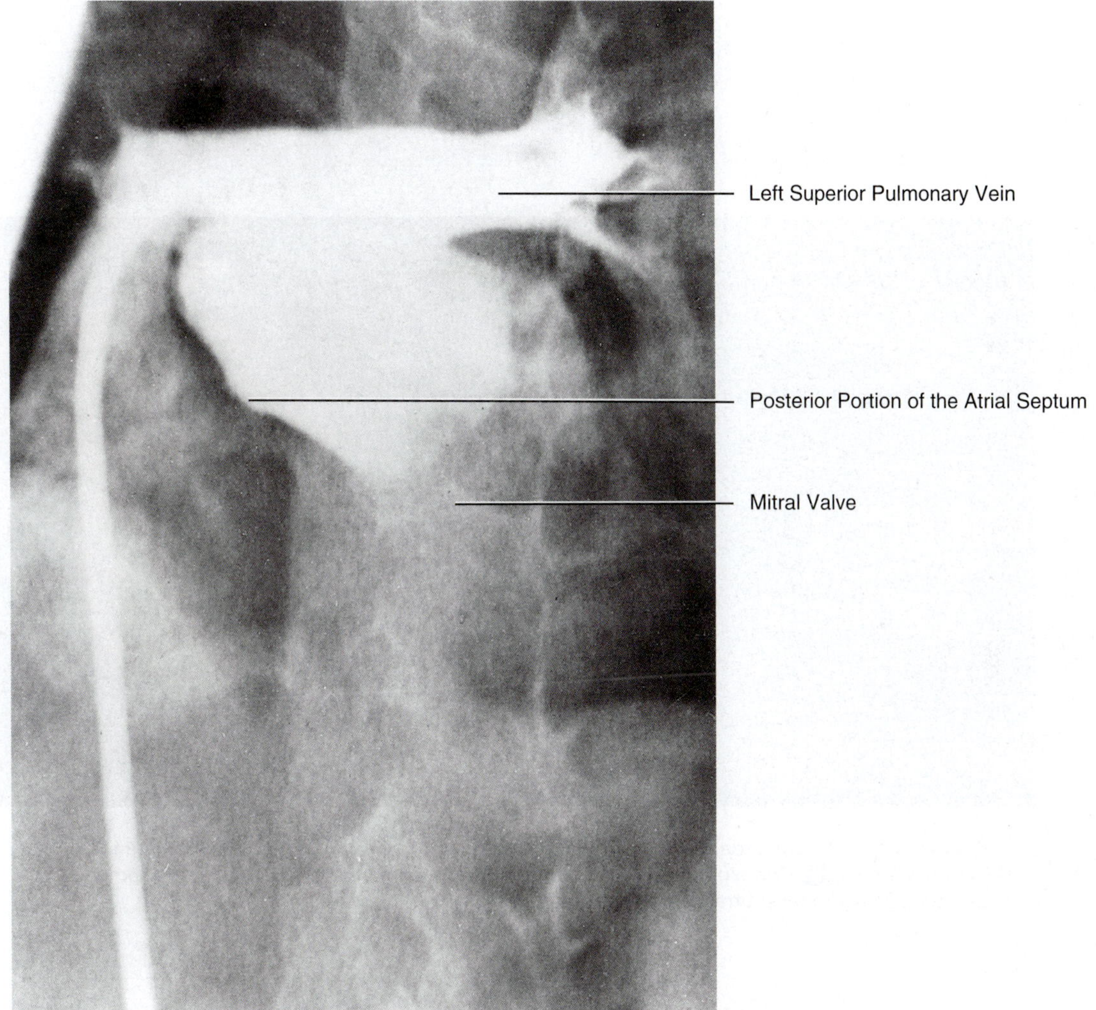

Figure 13.23. Four-chamber view of the left atrium. The posterior portion of the atrial septum is seen as the right border of the left atrium. (Courtesy of Dr. Benigno Soto from University of Alabama, Birmingham.)

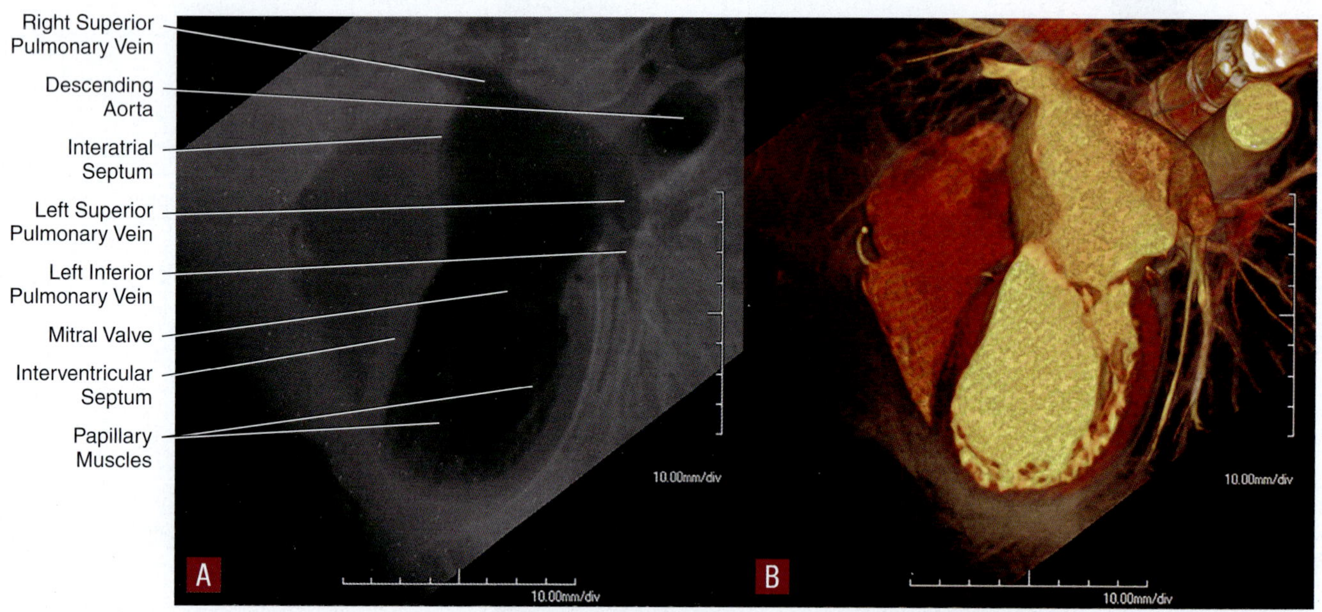

Figure 13.24. Left atrial angiogram in the so-called four-chamber view. **A**, Simulated DSA from CT data. **B**, Corresponding 3D volume-rendered CT in the same patient in the same orientation. DSA, digital subtraction angiogram.

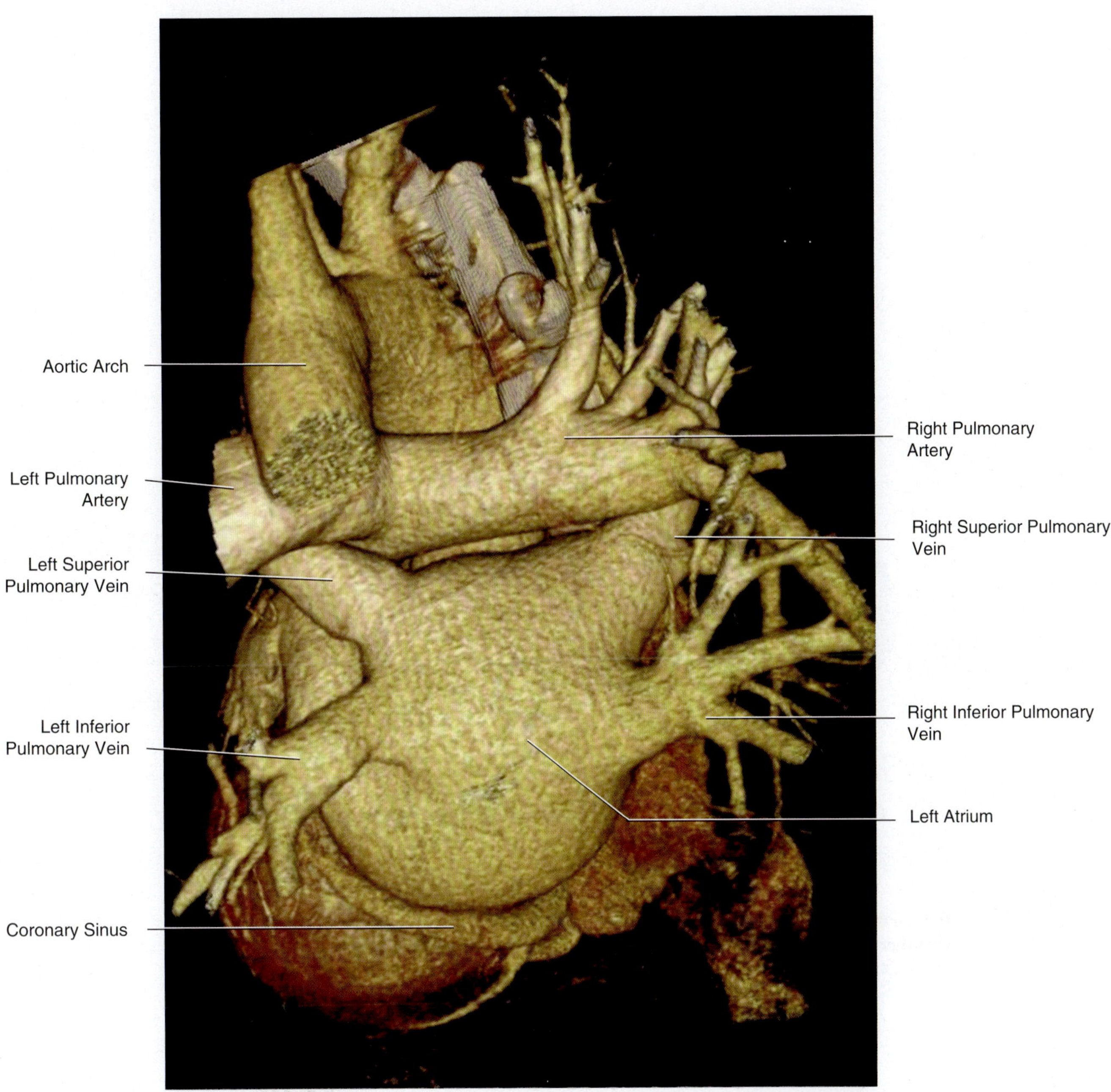

Figure 13.25. CT 3D volume image, left atrium, viewed from posterior.

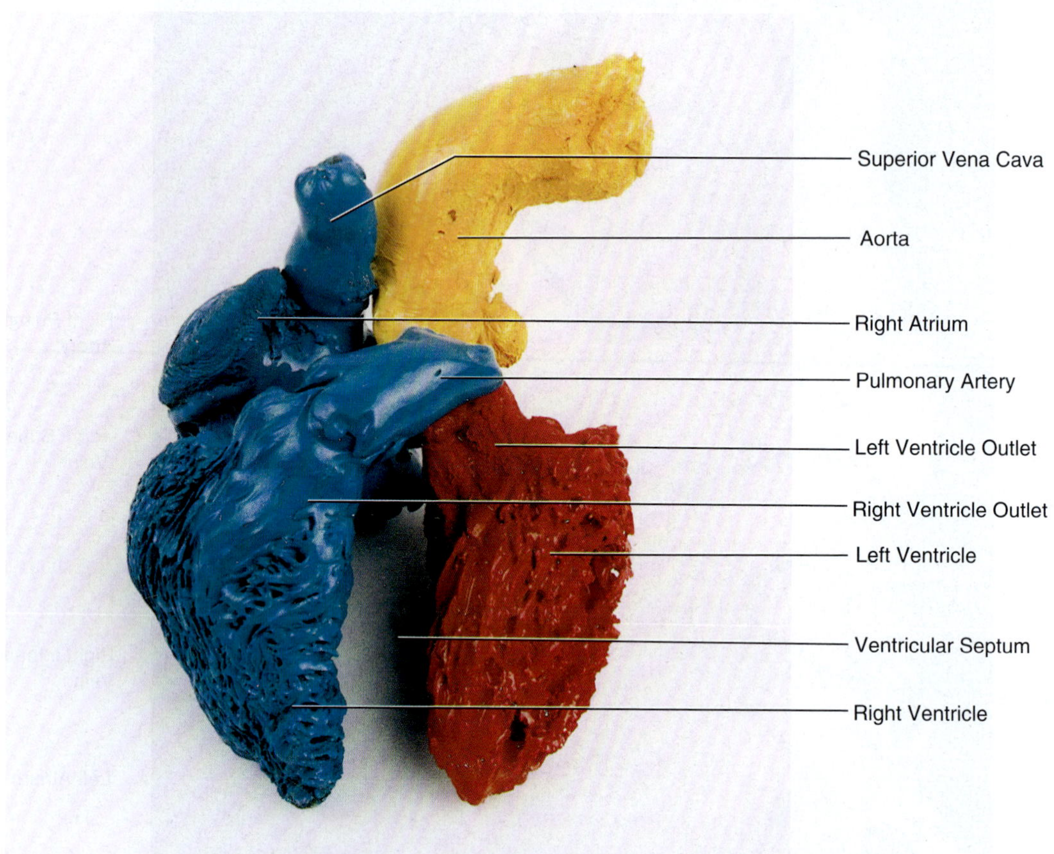

Figure 13.26. Cast of the heart showing the spatial relationships of the ventricular chambers. Note that the left ventricle is red; the aortal is yellow; the right ventricle, right atrium, superior vena cava, and pulmonary artery are blue.

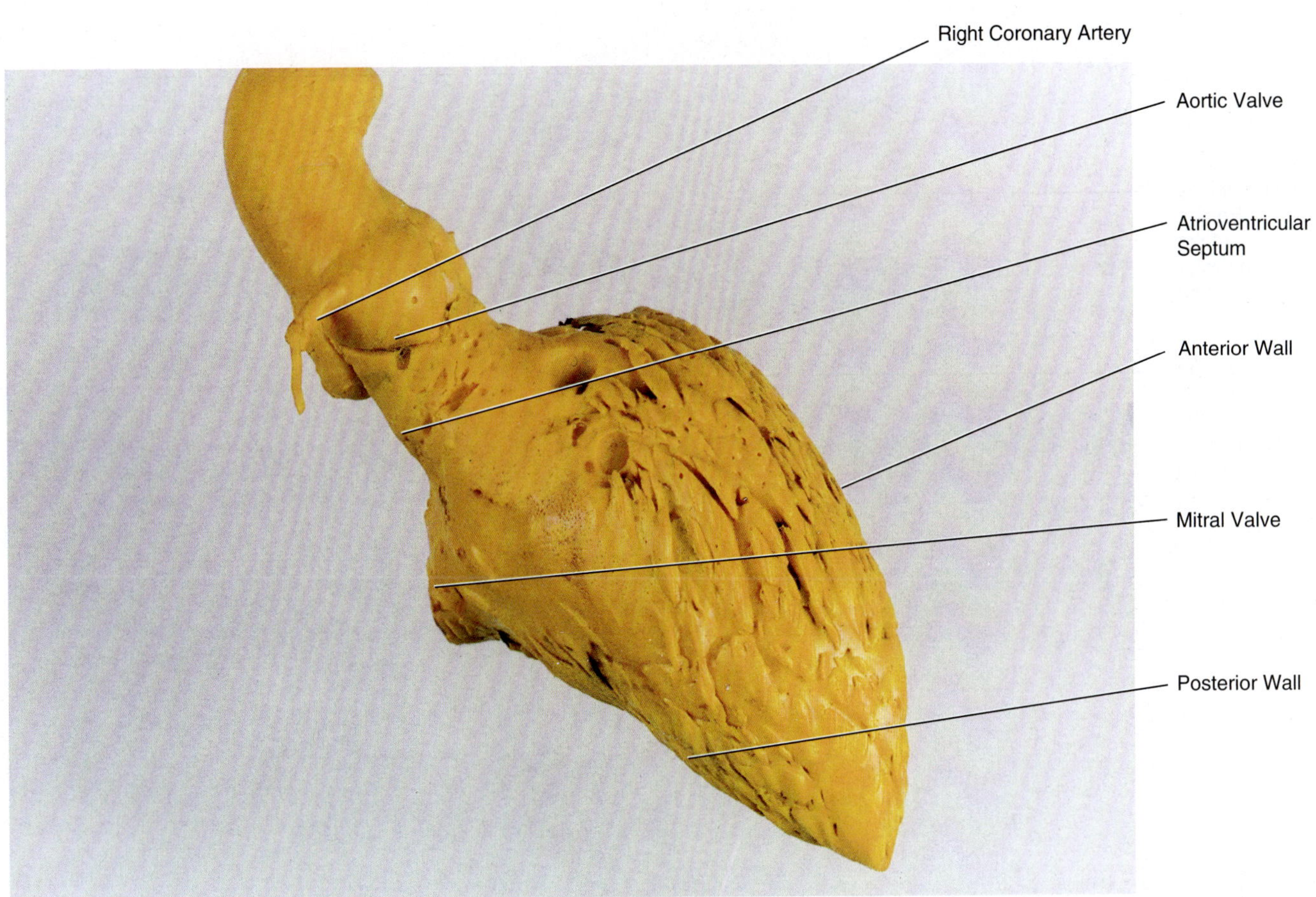

Figure 13.27. Luminal cast of the left ventricle and aorta in a frontal view.

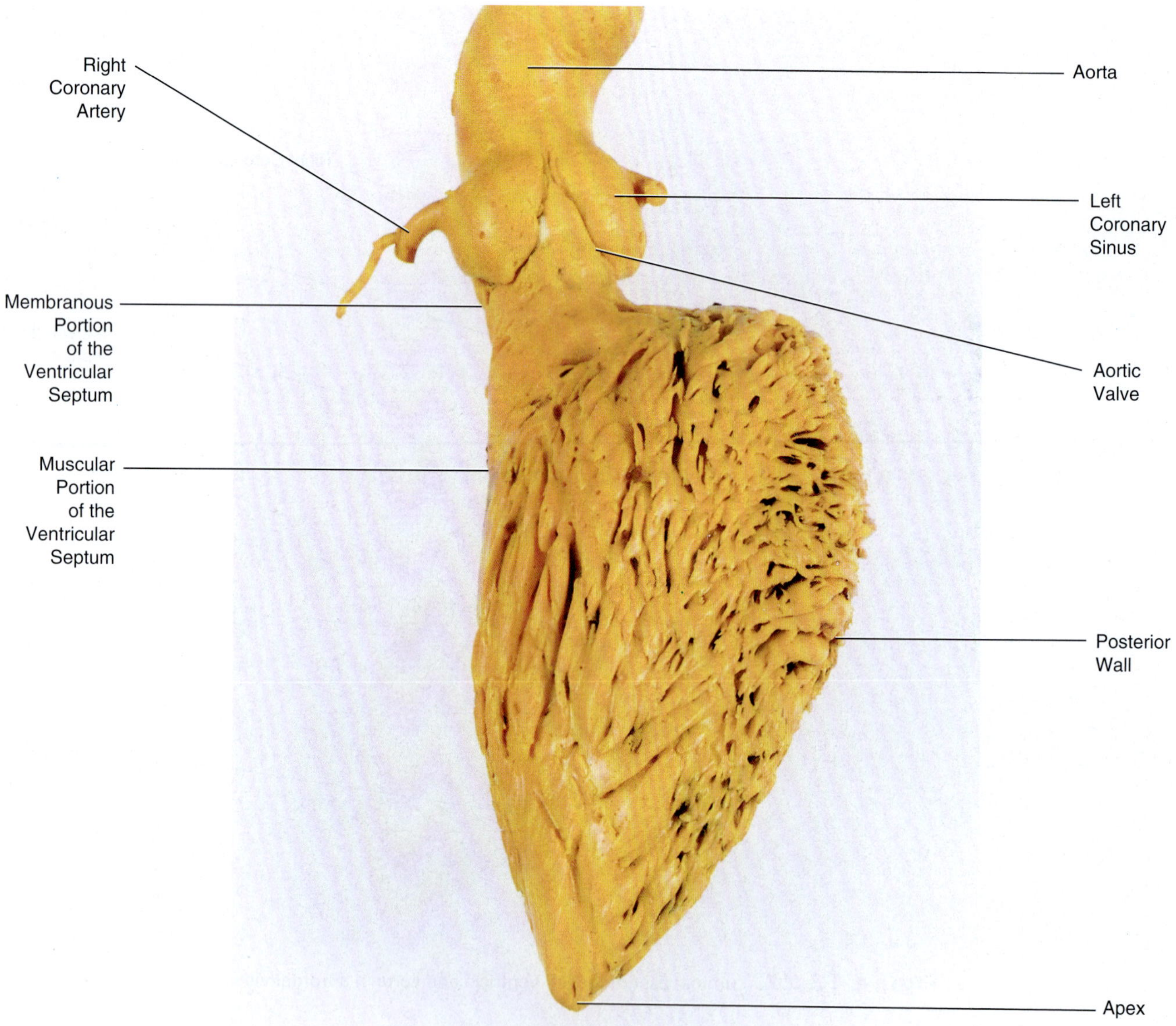

Figure 13.28. Luminal cast of the left ventricle and aorta in a lateral view.

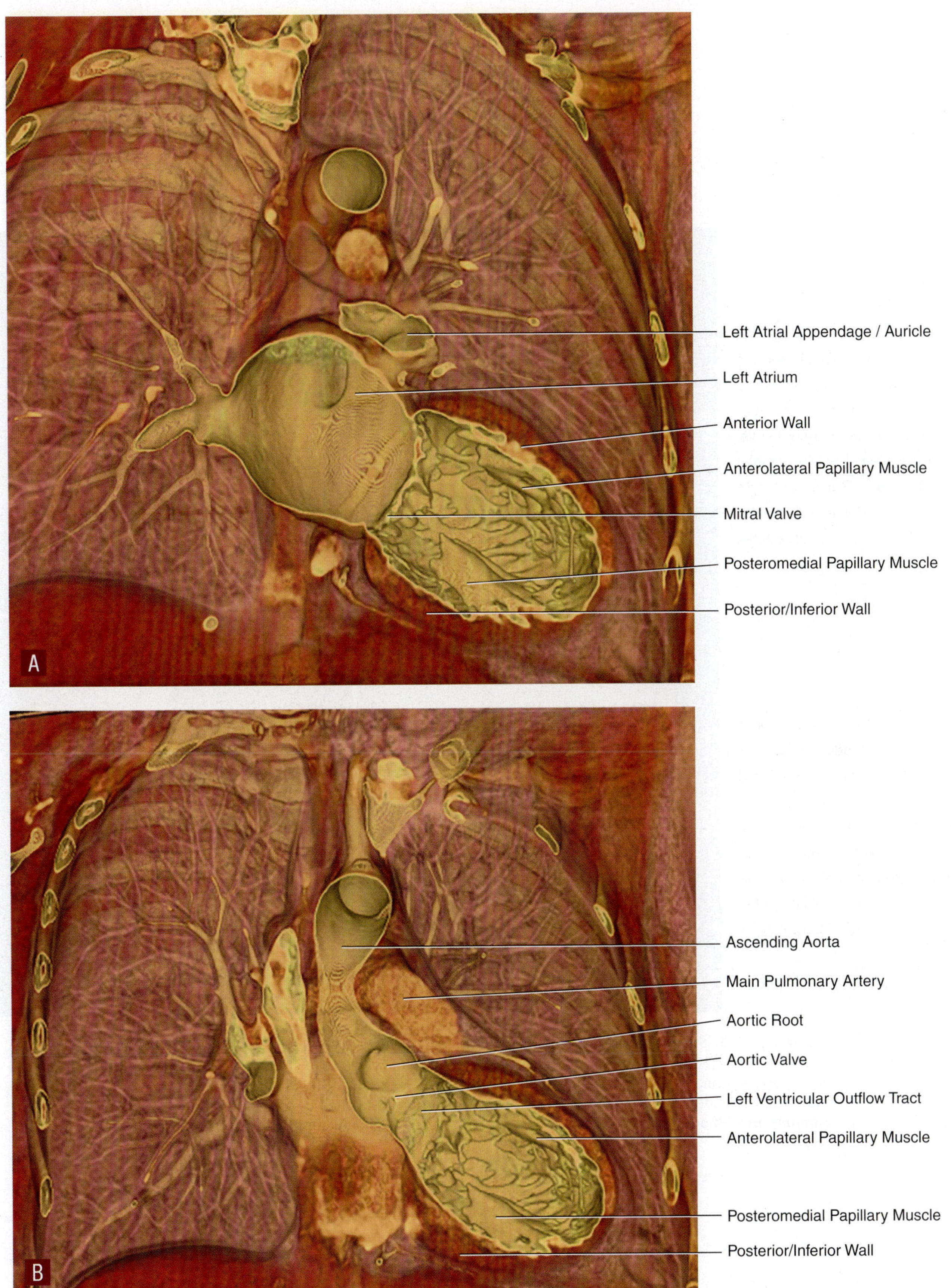

Figure 13.29. Internal features of the left ventricle. 3D volume-rendered CT. **A**, Slightly oblique coronal view, dorsal aspect, showing the left ventricular inflow. **B**, Same orientation, more ventral aspect, showing the LV outflow.

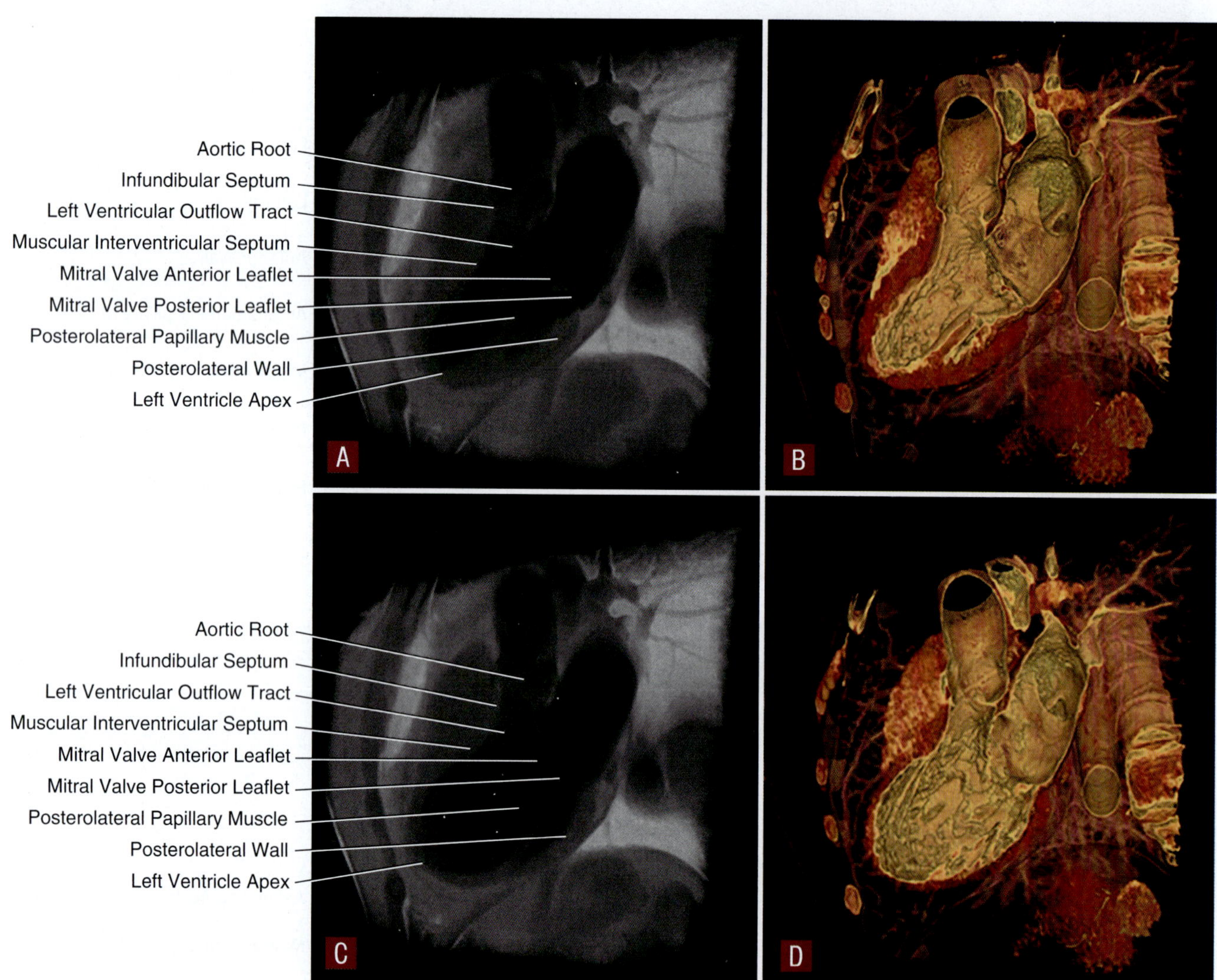

Figure 13.30. Left ventricle angiogram in long axial view. A and C, Simulated DSAs from CT data. B and D, Corresponding 3D volume-rendered CTs in the same patient in the same orientation. A and B, End-systolic phase (on top). C and D, End-diastolic phase (on bottom). The superior portion of the interventricular septum is formed by the infundibular septum (or outflow septum) just below the aortic valve. DSA, digital subtraction angiogram.

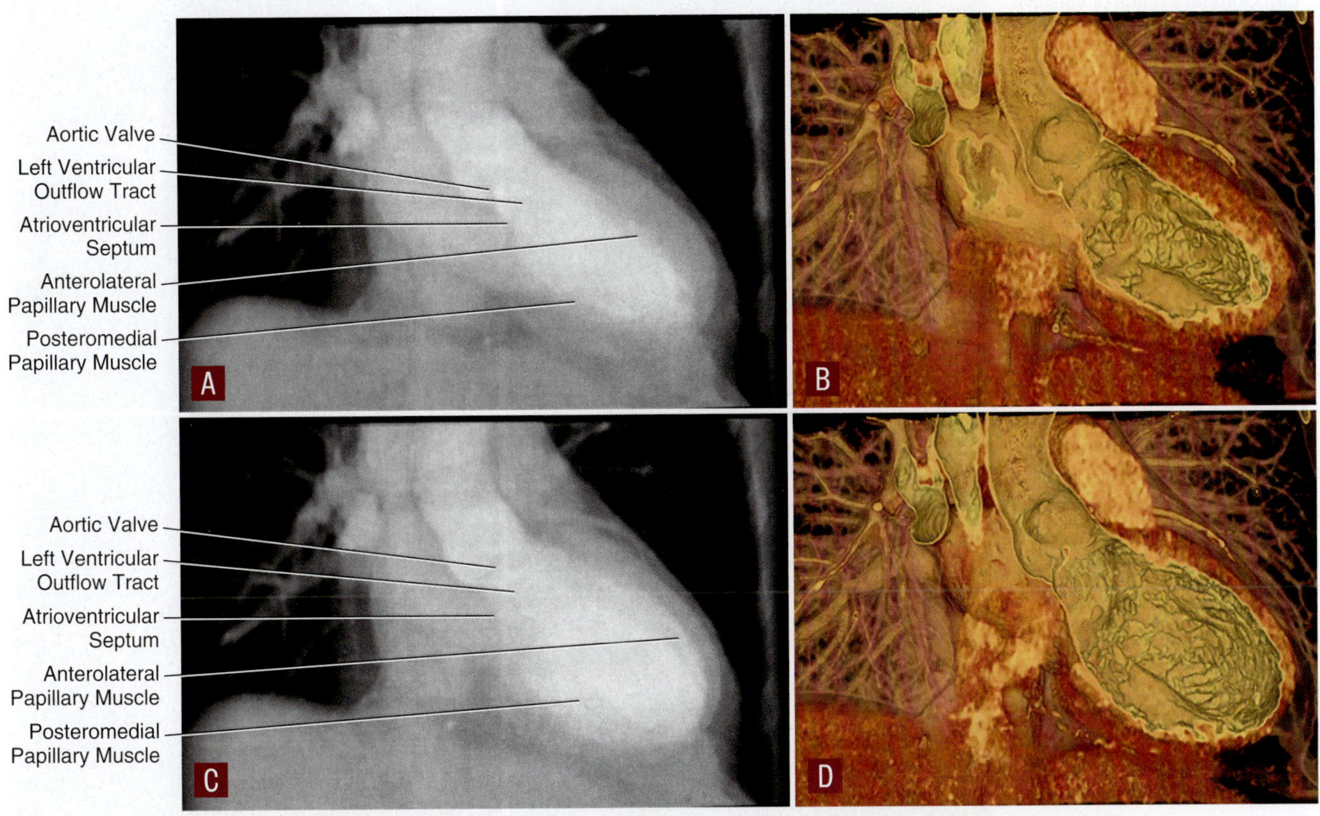

Figure 13.31. **A**, Left ventricular angiogram in elongated right anterior view. **A** and **C**, Simulated X-ray angiograms from CT data. **B** and **D**, Corresponding 3D volume-rendered CTs in the same patient in the same orientation. **A** and **B**, End-systolic phase (on top). **C** and **D**, End-diastolic phase (on bottom). The two papillary muscles appear as two filling defects in the body of the left ventricle.

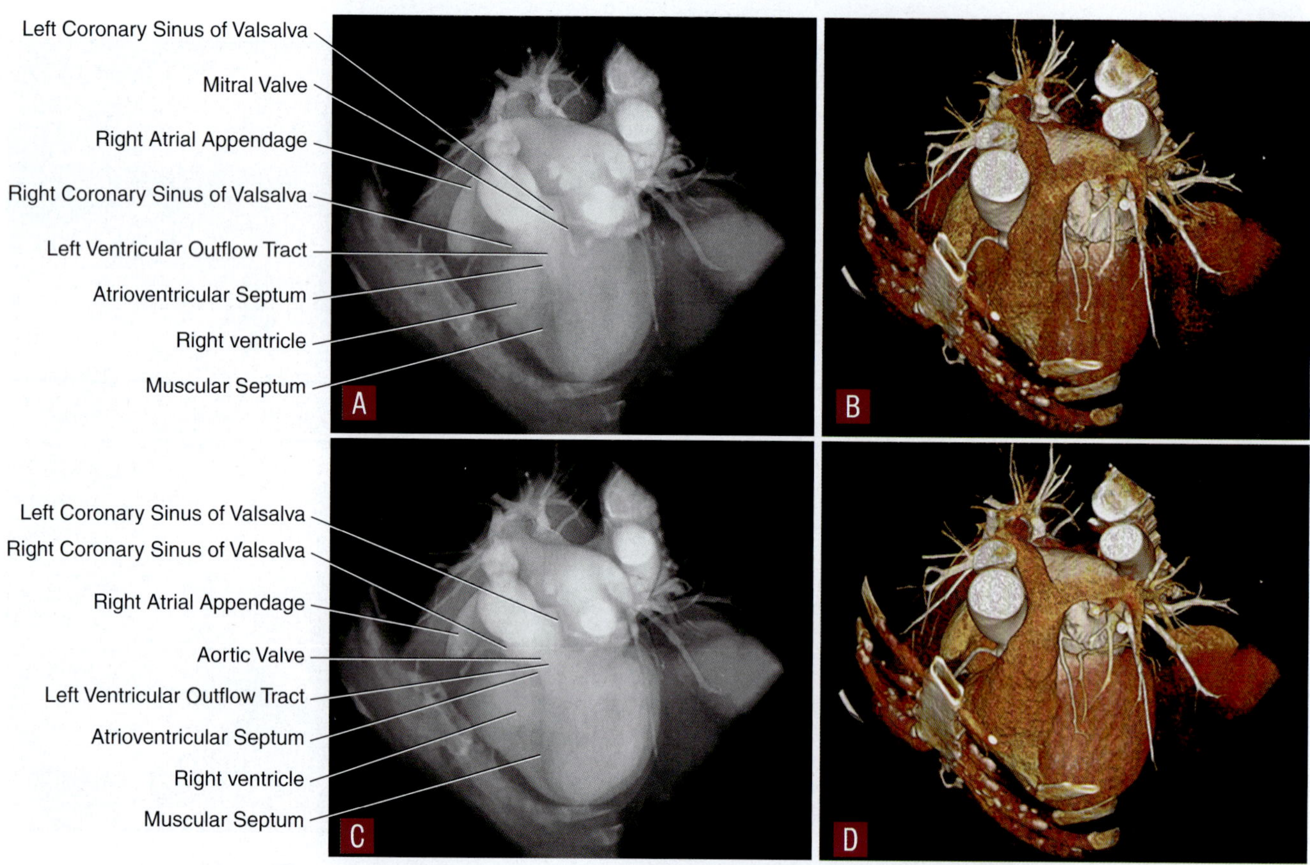

Figure 13.32. A, Left ventricle angiogram in quasi–four-chamber view. A and C, Simulated X-ray angiograms from CT data. B and D, Corresponding 3D volume-rendered CTs in the same patient in the same orientation. A and B, End-systolic phase (on top). C and D, End-diastolic phase (on bottom). The atrioventricular portion of the interventricular septum separates the left ventricle from the right atrium.

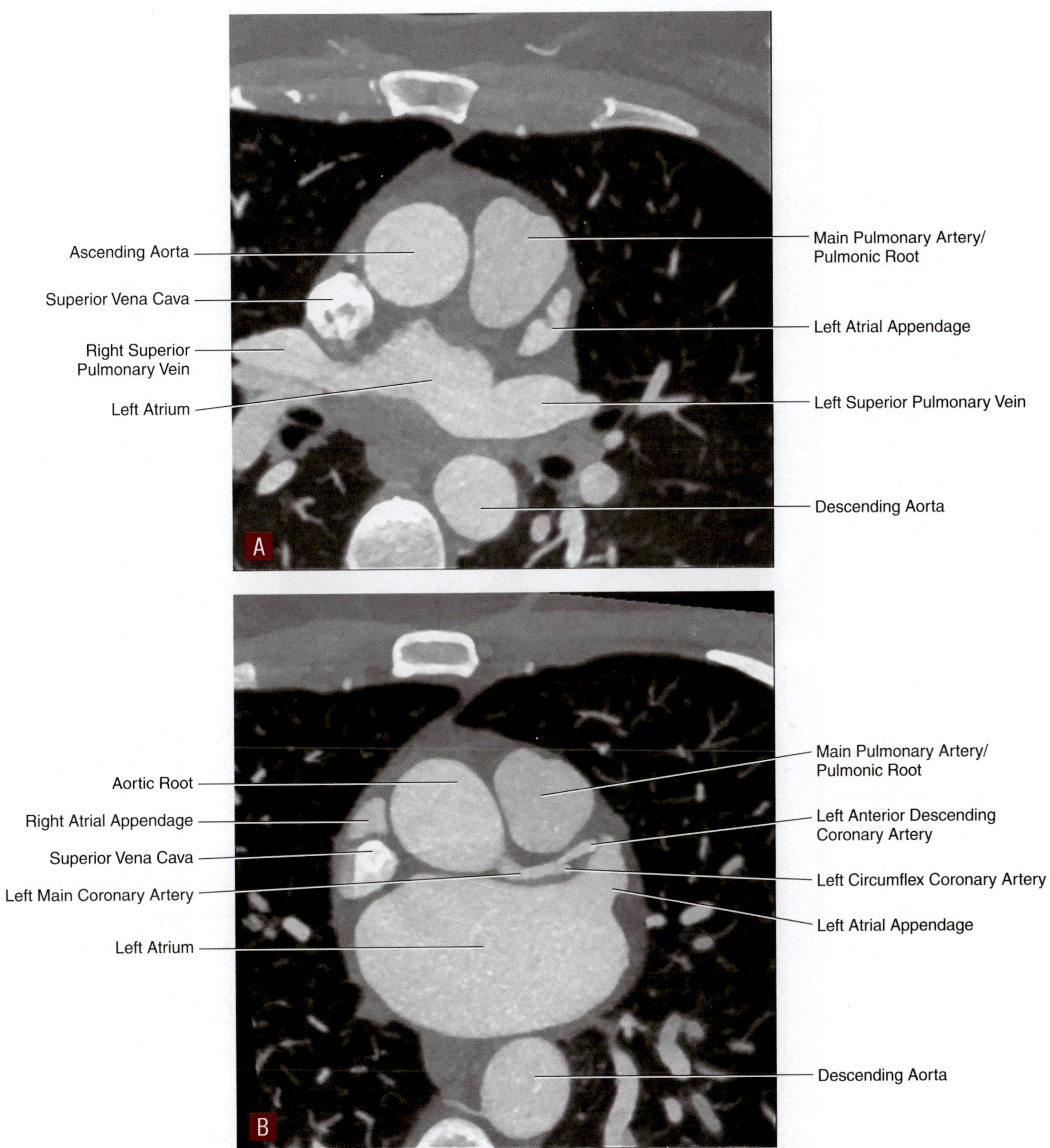

Figure 13.33. Axial CT images from cephalad to caudal border of the heart. **A**, Cephalad extent of the heart with left atrium just coming into view. **B**, Level of the aortic root, left coronary sinus of Valsalva. Right atrium is now beginning to appear. **C**, Level of the aortic root, noncoronary and right coronary sinuses of Valsalva. **D**, At and just below the aortic valve. All four cardiac chambers are partially seen. **E**, Midventricular level. Right atrium is still well visualized, but the section is at the caudal aspect of the left atrium. **F**, Inferior aspect of the heart at the level of the coronary sinus. Note that the lung bases and a portion of the liver are visible at this level. **G**, Caudal most aspect, showing the ventricular apices.

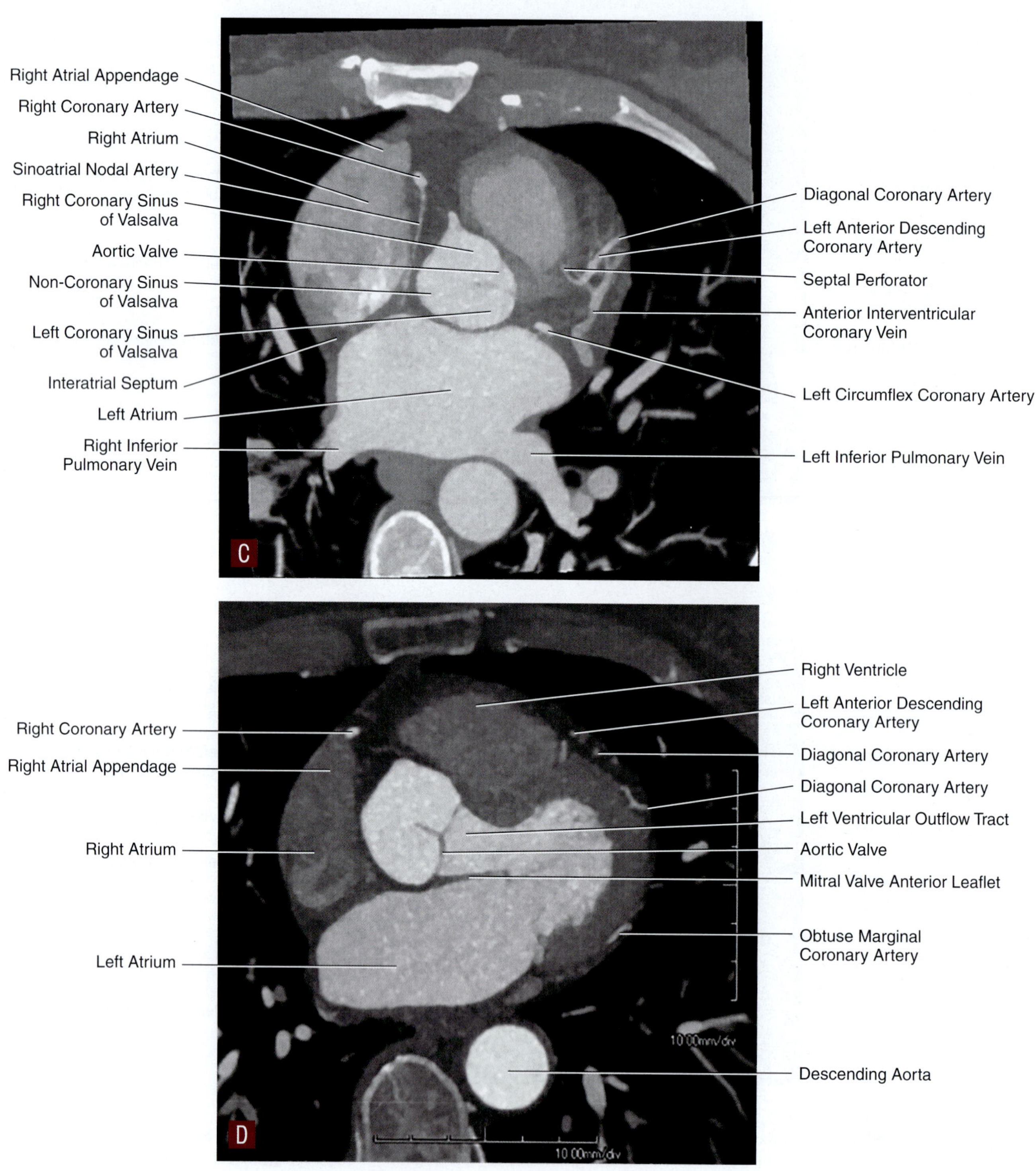

Figure 13.33. *Continued*

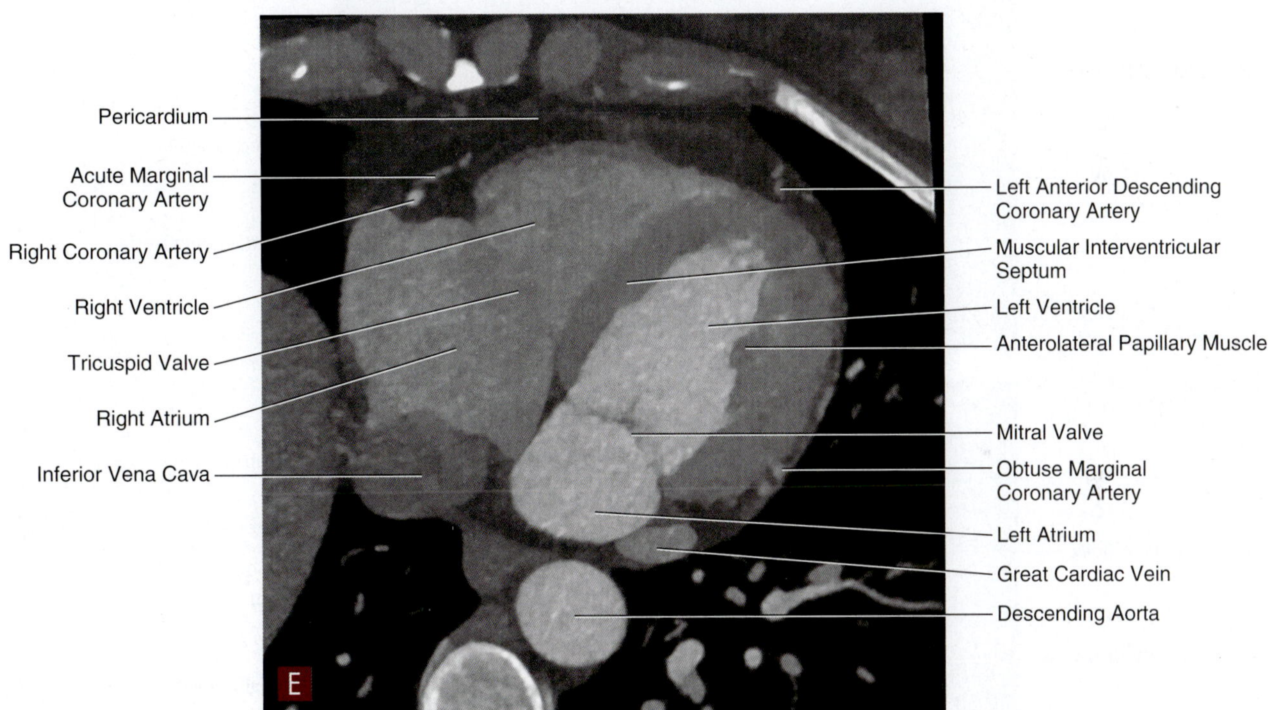

Figure 13.33. *Continued*

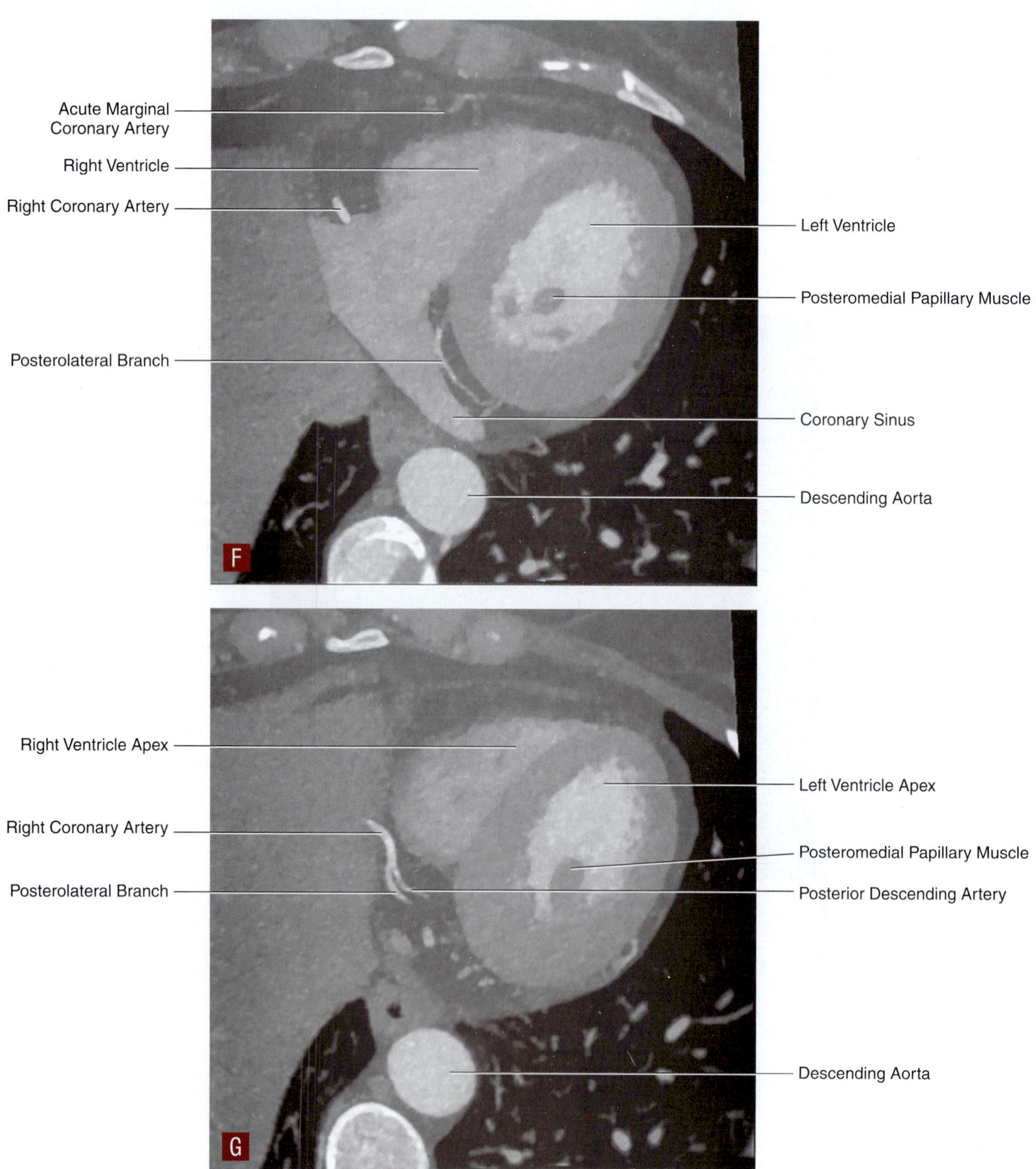

Figure 13.33. *Continued*

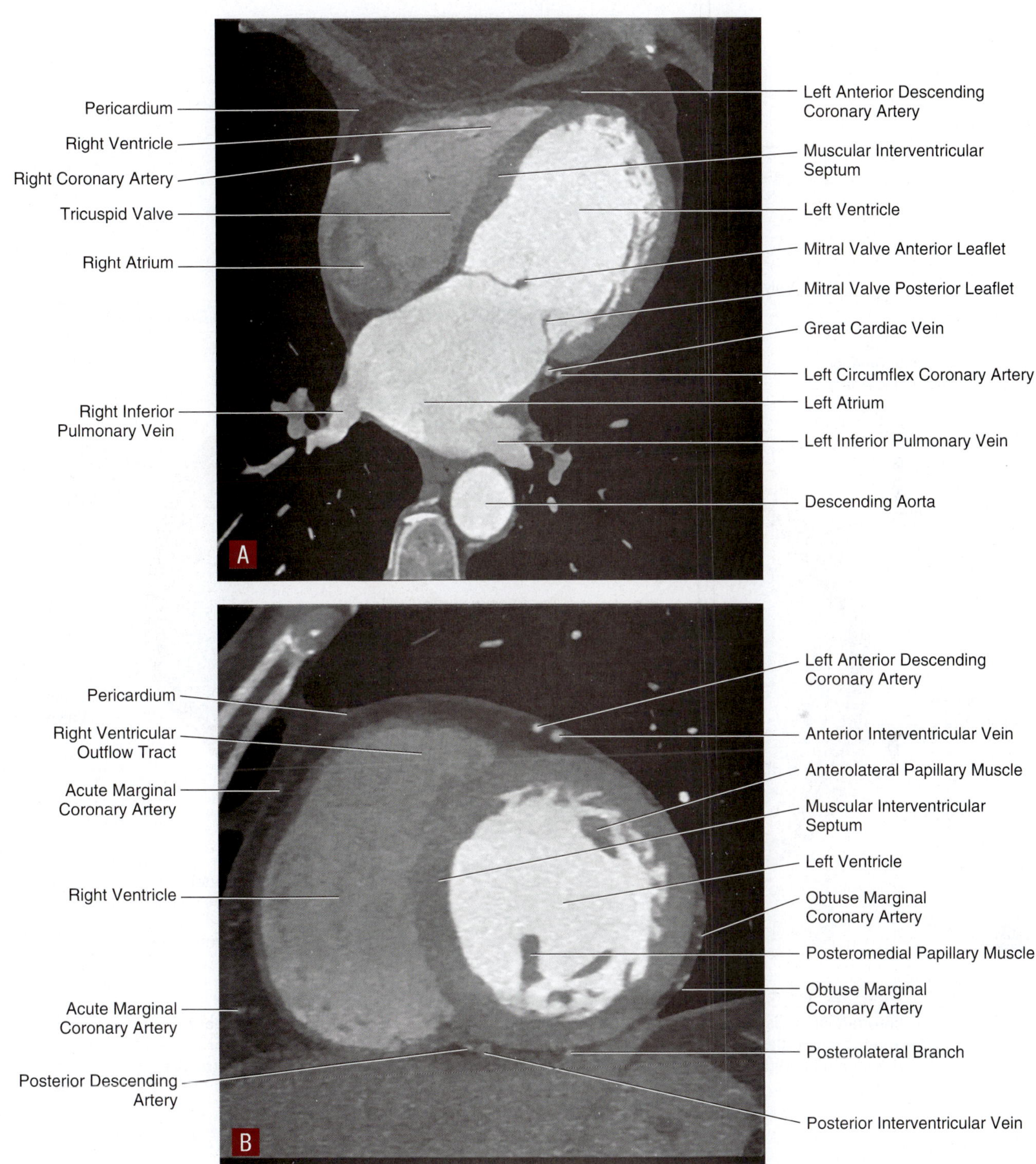

Figure 13.34. **A**, CT multiplanar reformat, oblique four-chamber (long-axis) reconstruction. Note most of the contrast material in the left heart (left atrium, left ventricular) after it has already passed through the right heart (right atrium, right ventricle), which have minimal residual contrast. **B**, CT multiplanar reformat, midventricular short-axis reconstruction (at the level of the papillary muscles). Note thick wall of left ventricle surrounding contrast within the chamber in comparison to the thin wall of the right ventricle.

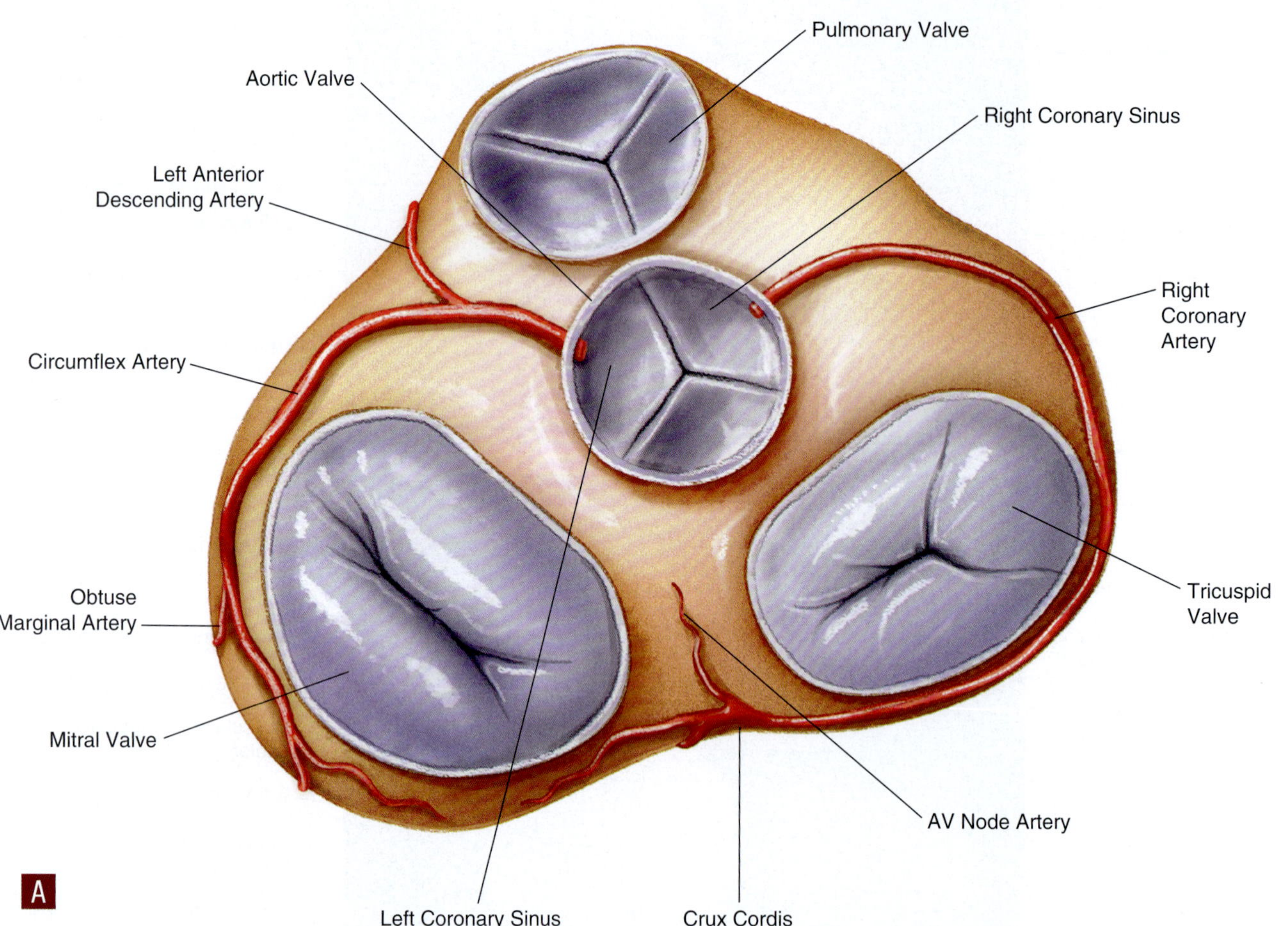

Figure 13.35. **A**, Relationships of the coronary arteries around the heart. The left coronary artery is in red color and the right coronary artery is in blue. **B**, The right coronary and the circumflex arteries form a circle around the atrioventricular sulci. The left anterior descending and the posterior descending arteries form a semicircle around the interventricular sulci.

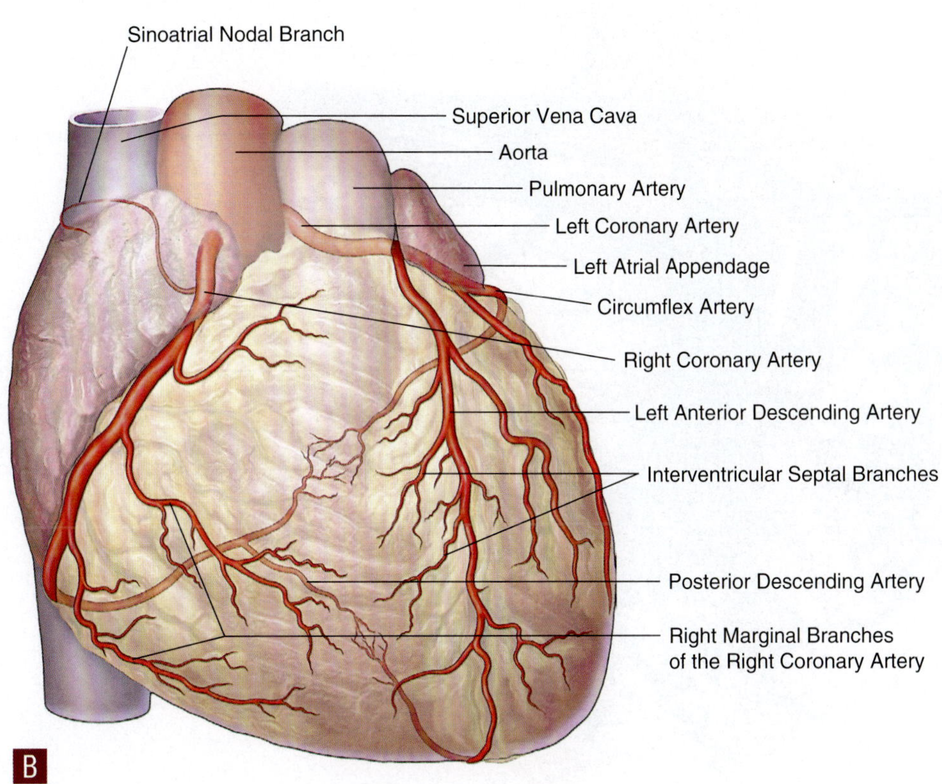

Figure 13.35. *Continued*

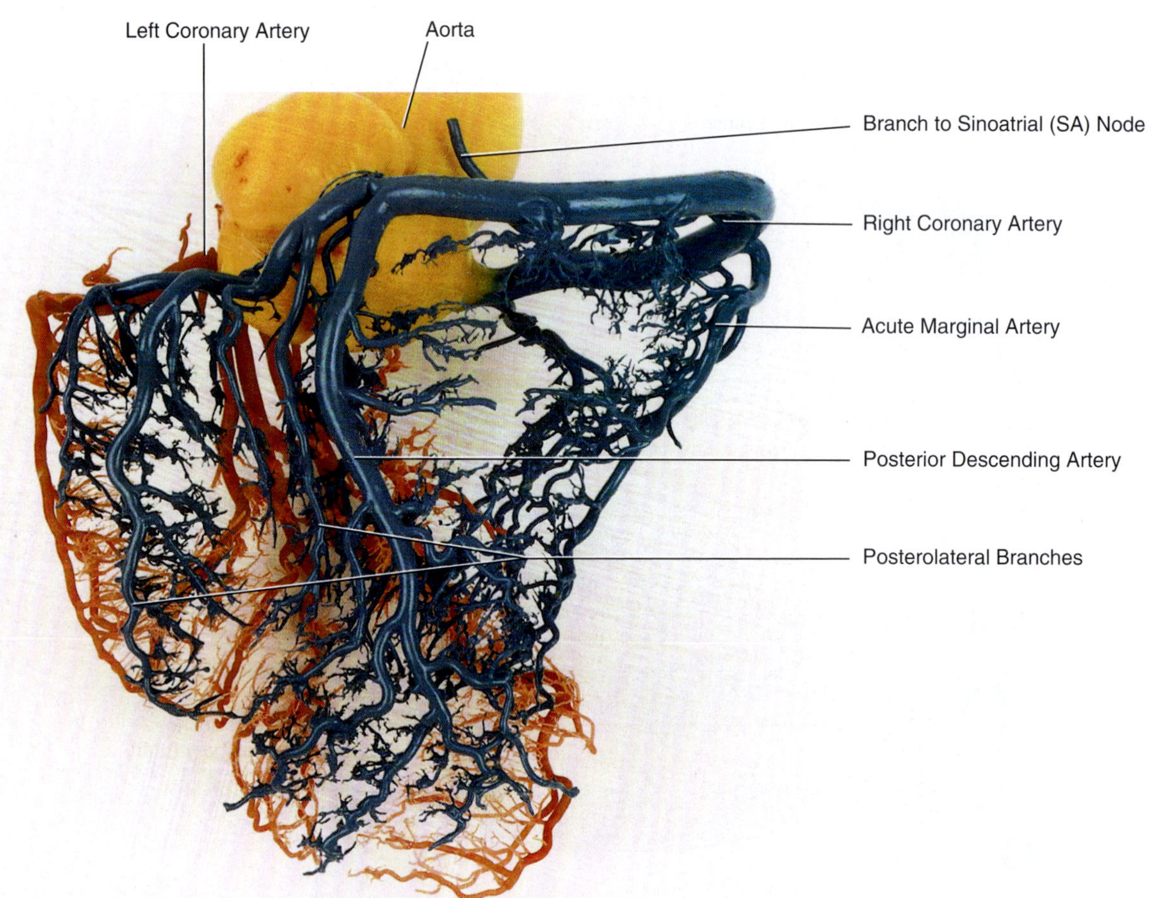

Figure 13.36. Cast of the coronary arteries viewed from the inferior face of the heart. The right coronary artery is blue. It is dominant and supplies the entire inferior wall and part of the left lateral wall of the heart. The aorta is in yellow. The left coronary artery is in red.

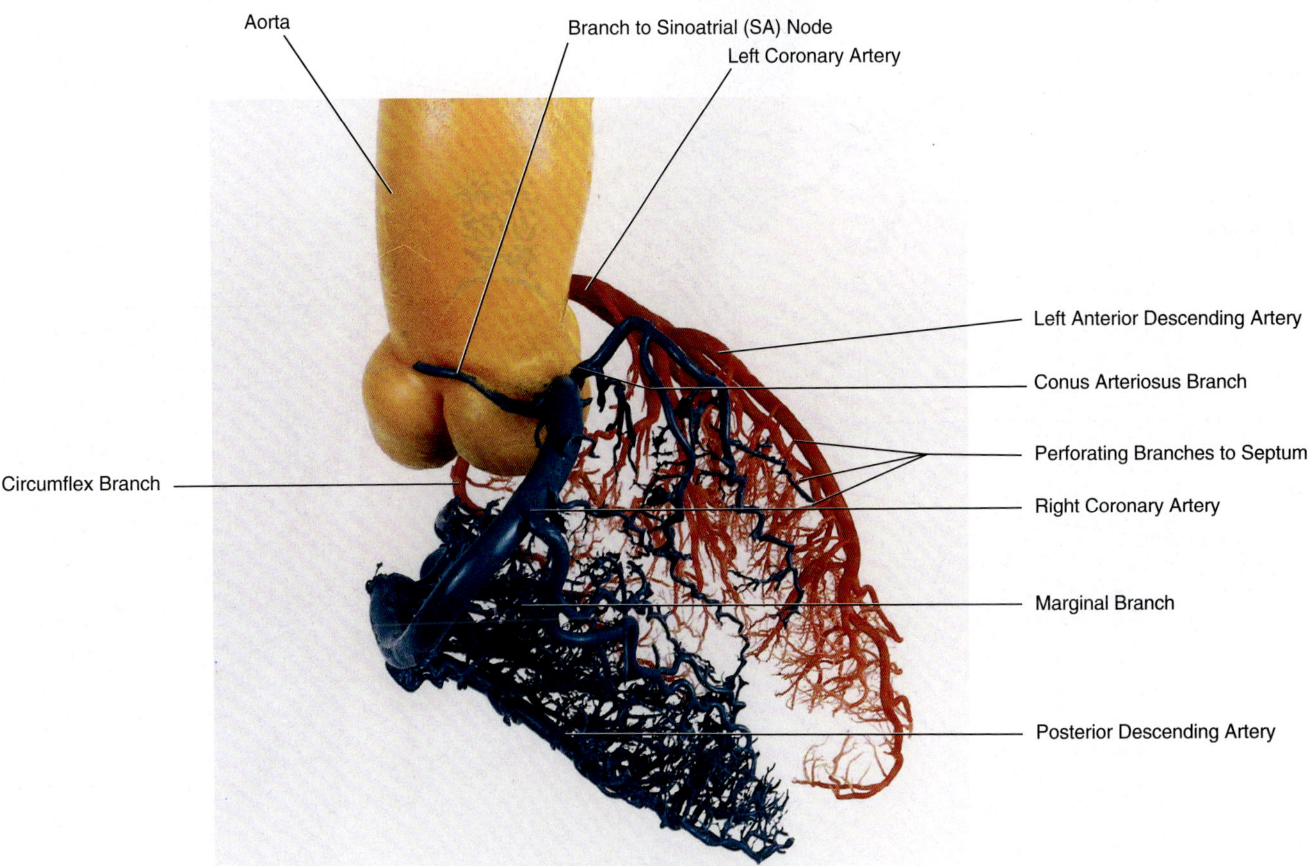

Figure 13.37. Cast of the coronary arteries in lateral view. The right coronary artery is in blue. The left coronary branches are in red and supply the anterior part of the left lateral wall of the heart.

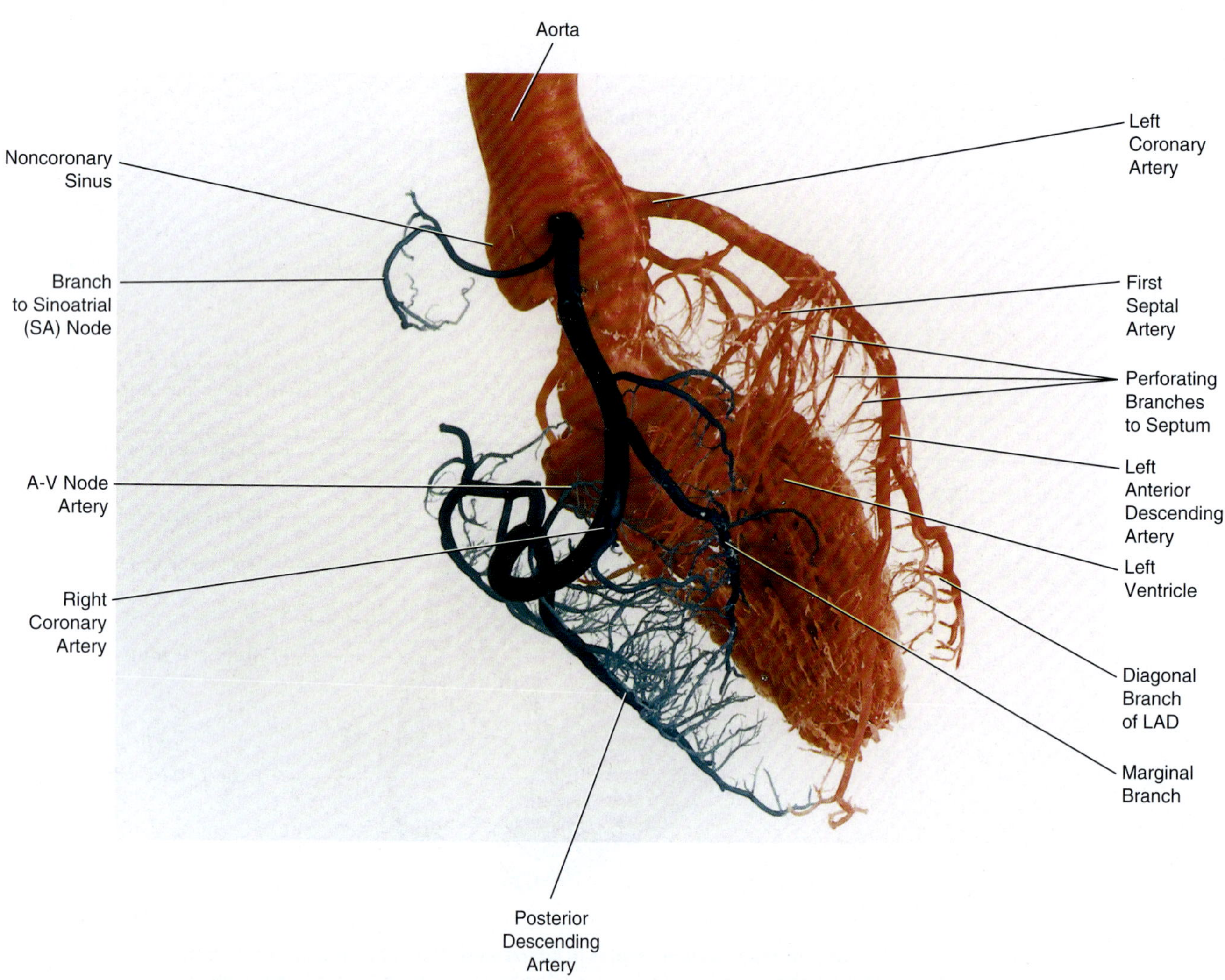

Figure 13.38. Cast of the coronary arteries in right oblique view and their relationships with the left ventricle. The right coronary artery is in blue and gives rise to the posterior descending artery which goes toward the apex of the heart close to the distal portion of the left anterior descending (LAD) artery in red.

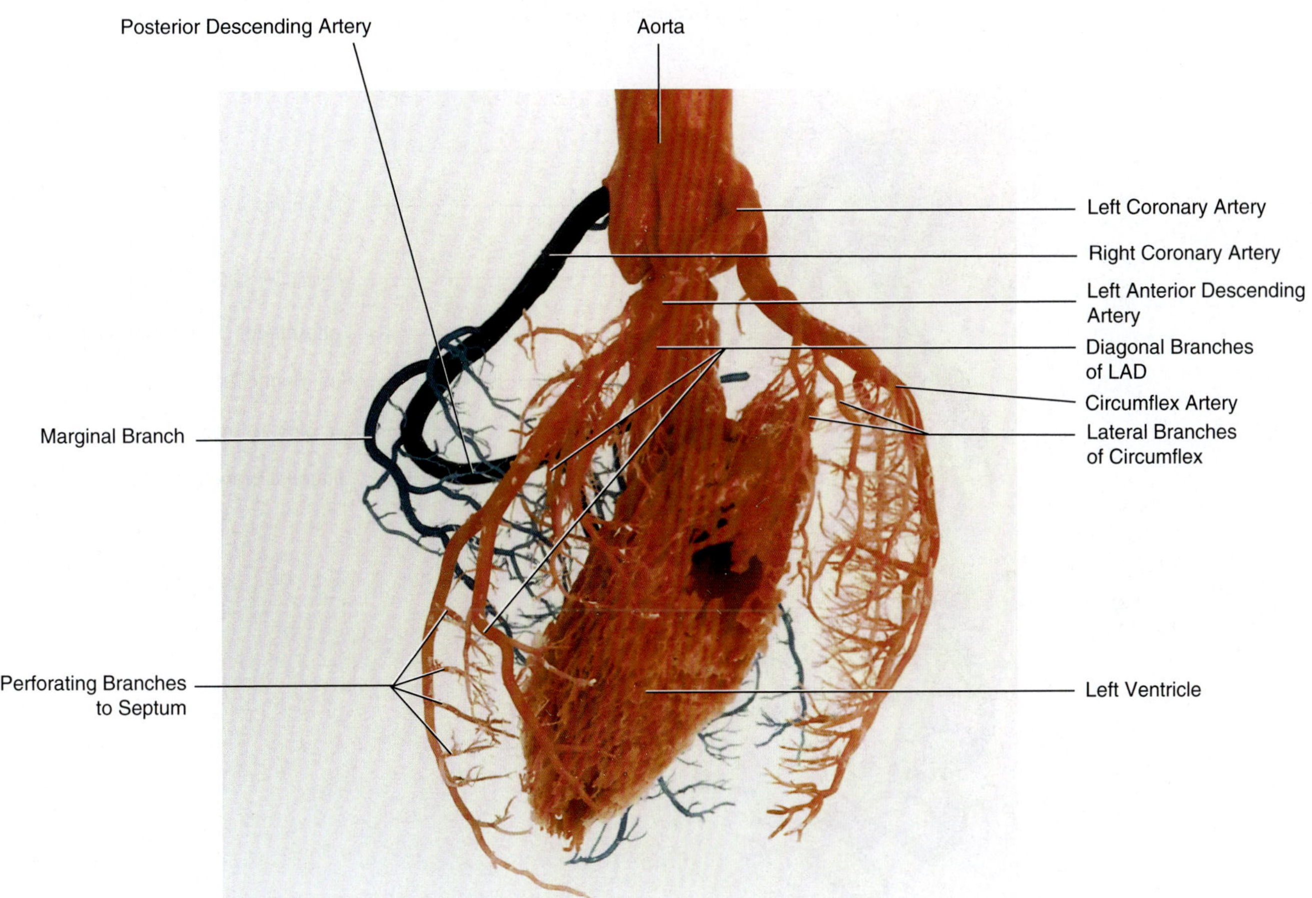

Figure 13.39. Cast of the coronary arteries in a left oblique view and their relations with the left ventricle. The left coronary artery and its branches are in red. The right coronary artery is in blue. LAD, left anterior descending.

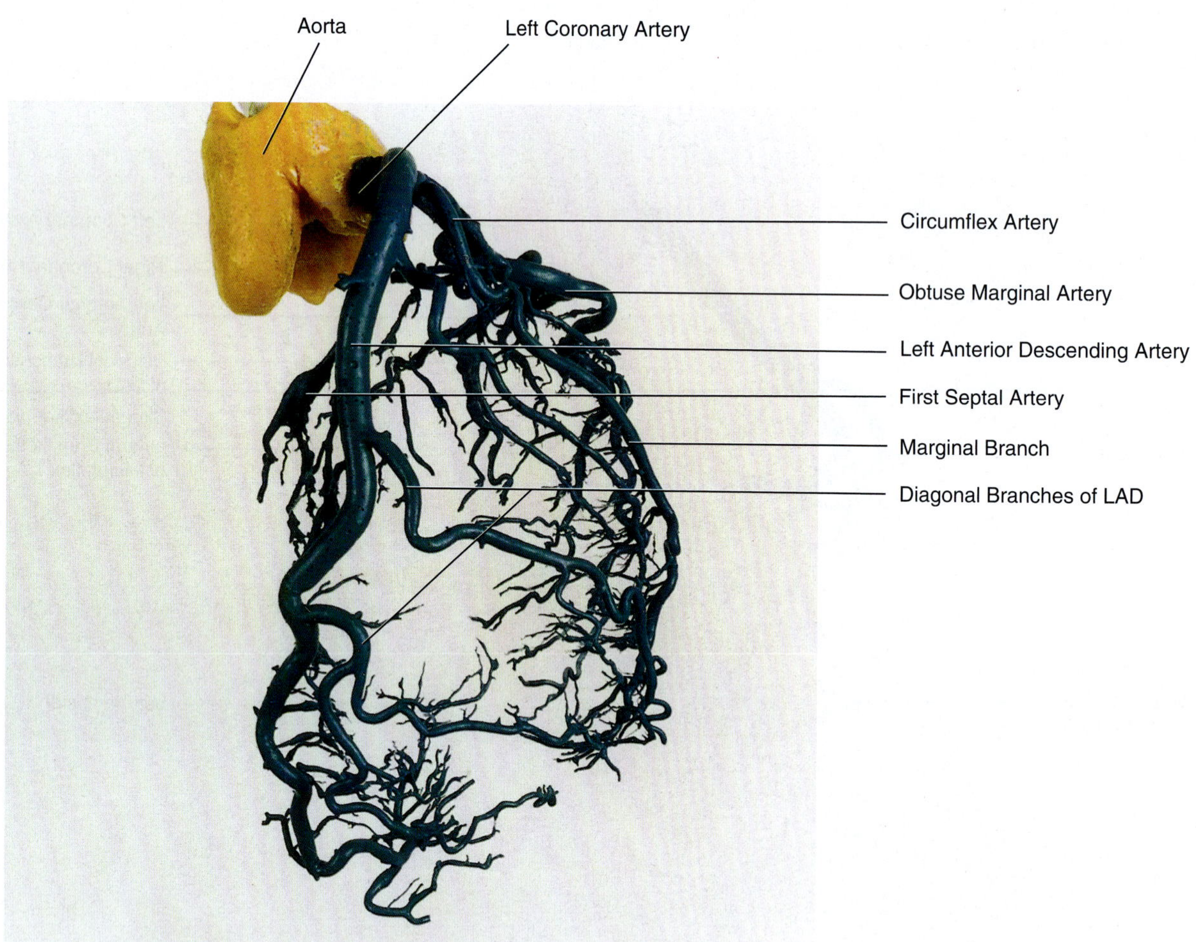

Figure 13.40. Cast of the left coronary artery in a left oblique view. The coronary artery is in blue and the aorta is in yellow. LAD, left anterior descending.

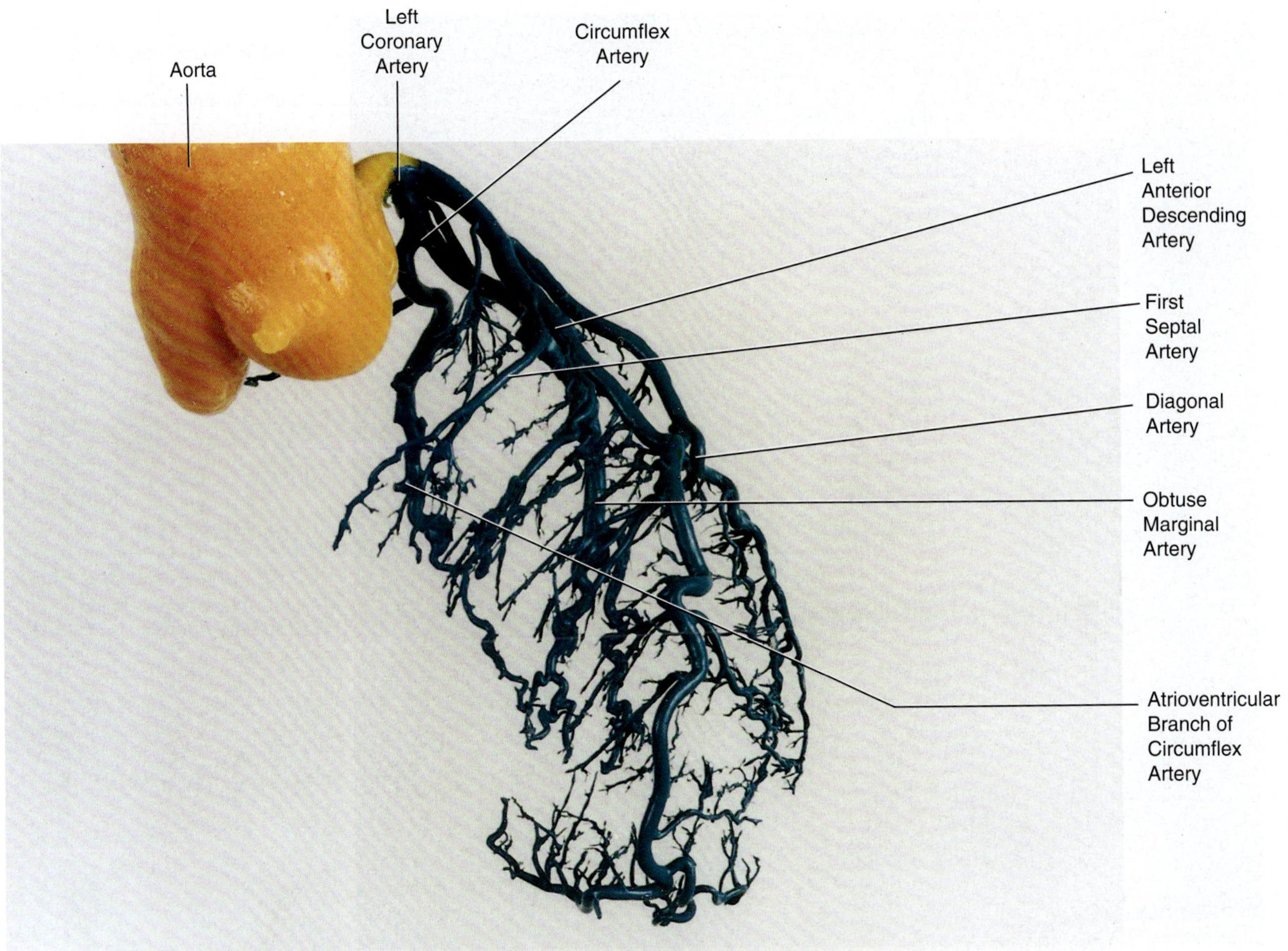

Figure 13.41. Cast of the left coronary artery in a right oblique view. The coronary artery is in blue and the aorta is in yellow.

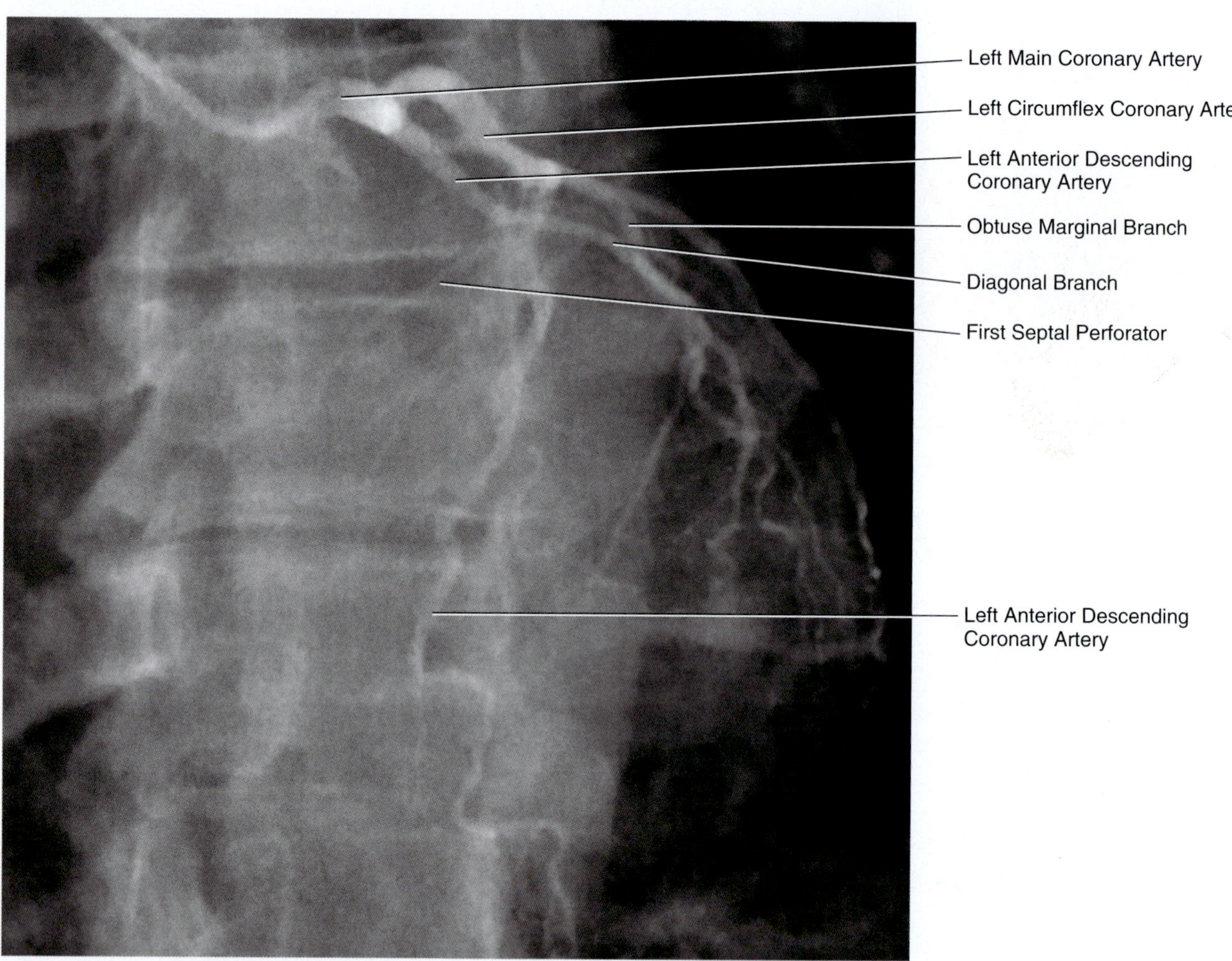

Figure 13.42. Angiogram of the left coronary artery in the cranial left anterior oblique projection.

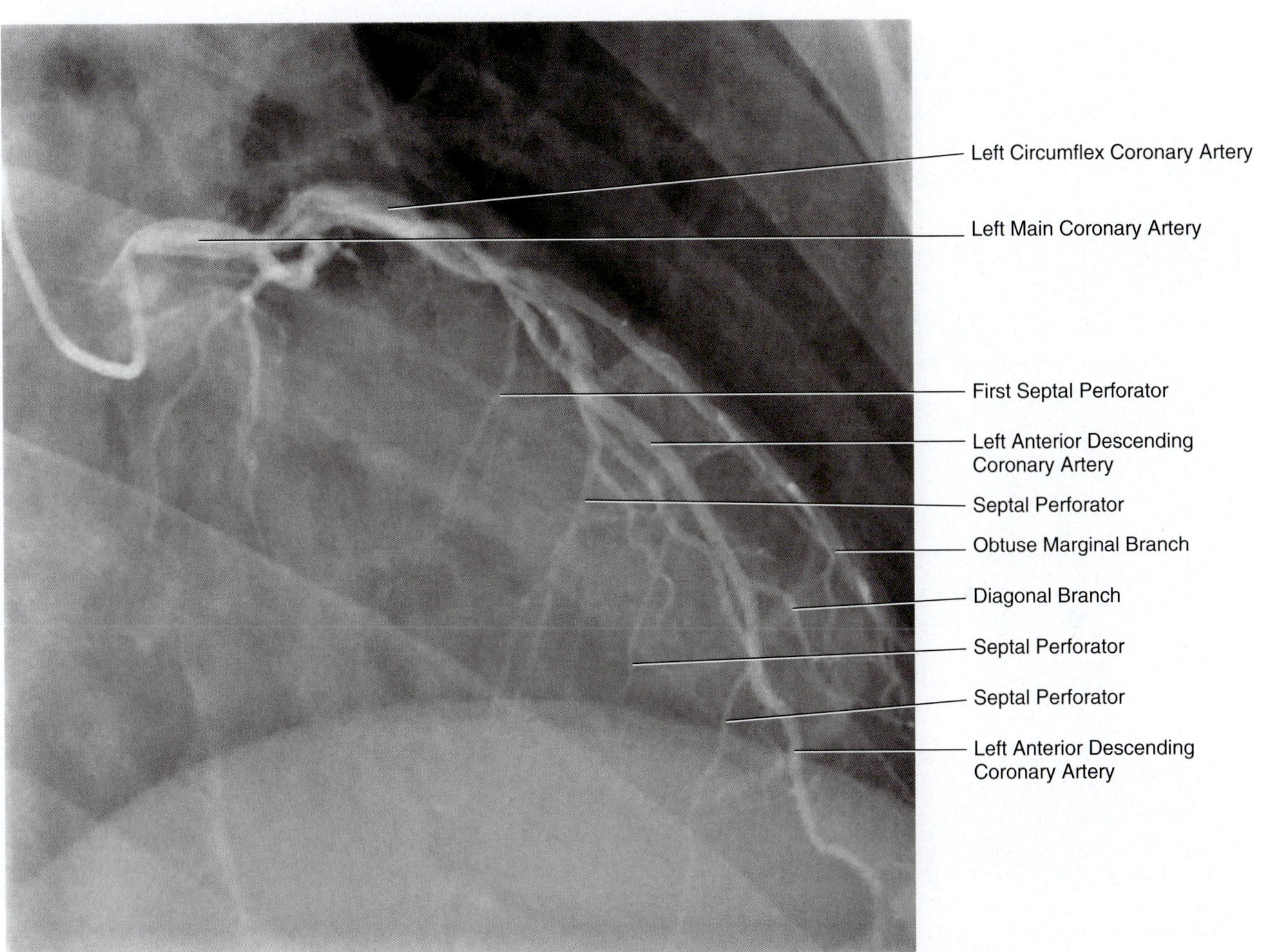

Figure 13.43. Angiogram of the left coronary artery in the cranial right anterior oblique view. The origin of the septal and diagonal arteries is well demonstrated in this projection.

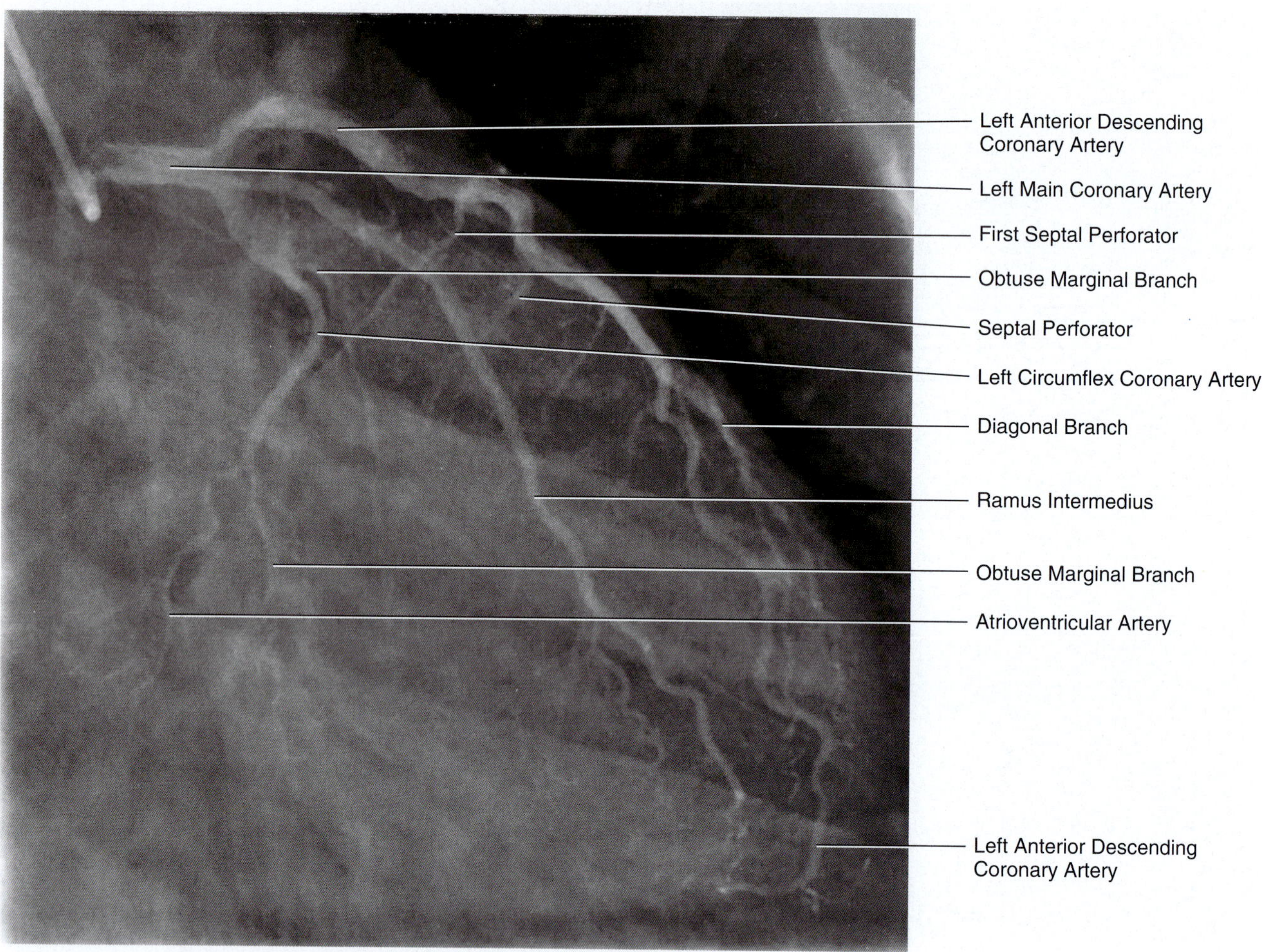

Figure 13.44. Angiogram of the left coronary artery in the right anterior oblique view.

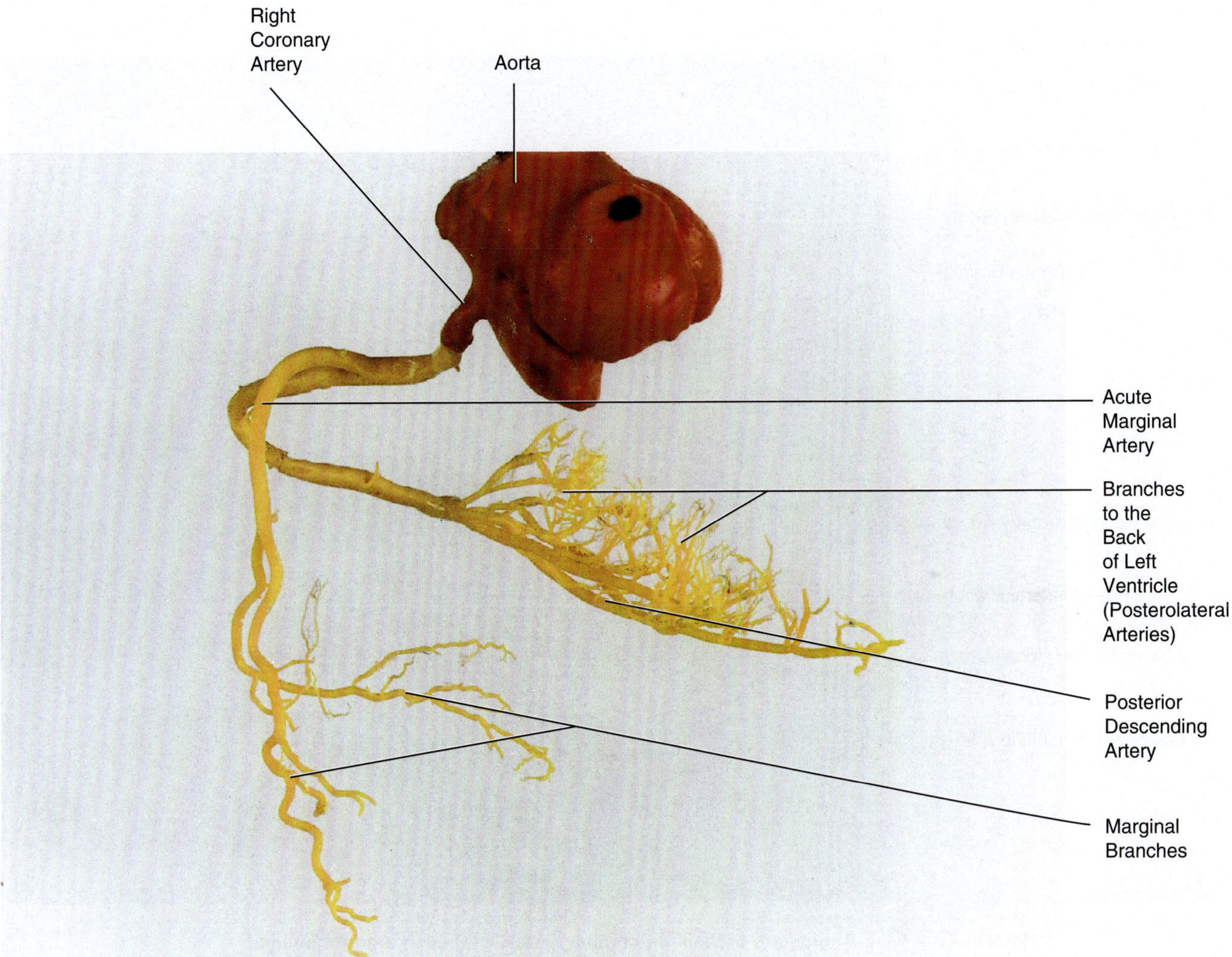

Figure 13.45. Cast of the right coronary artery in a left oblique view.

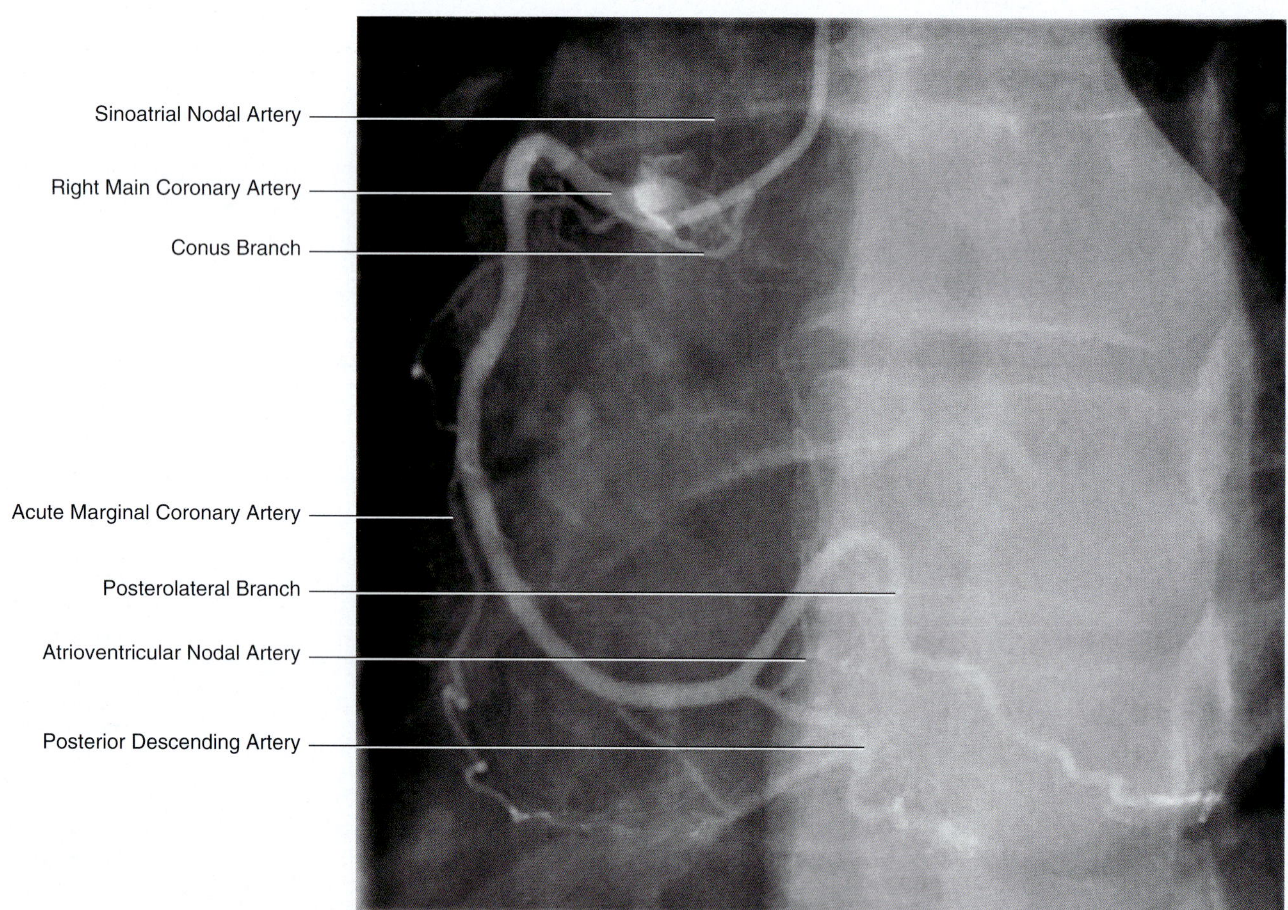

Figure 13.46. Angiogram of the right coronary artery in the left anterior oblique projection. The A-V node artery arises from an inverted U-turn.

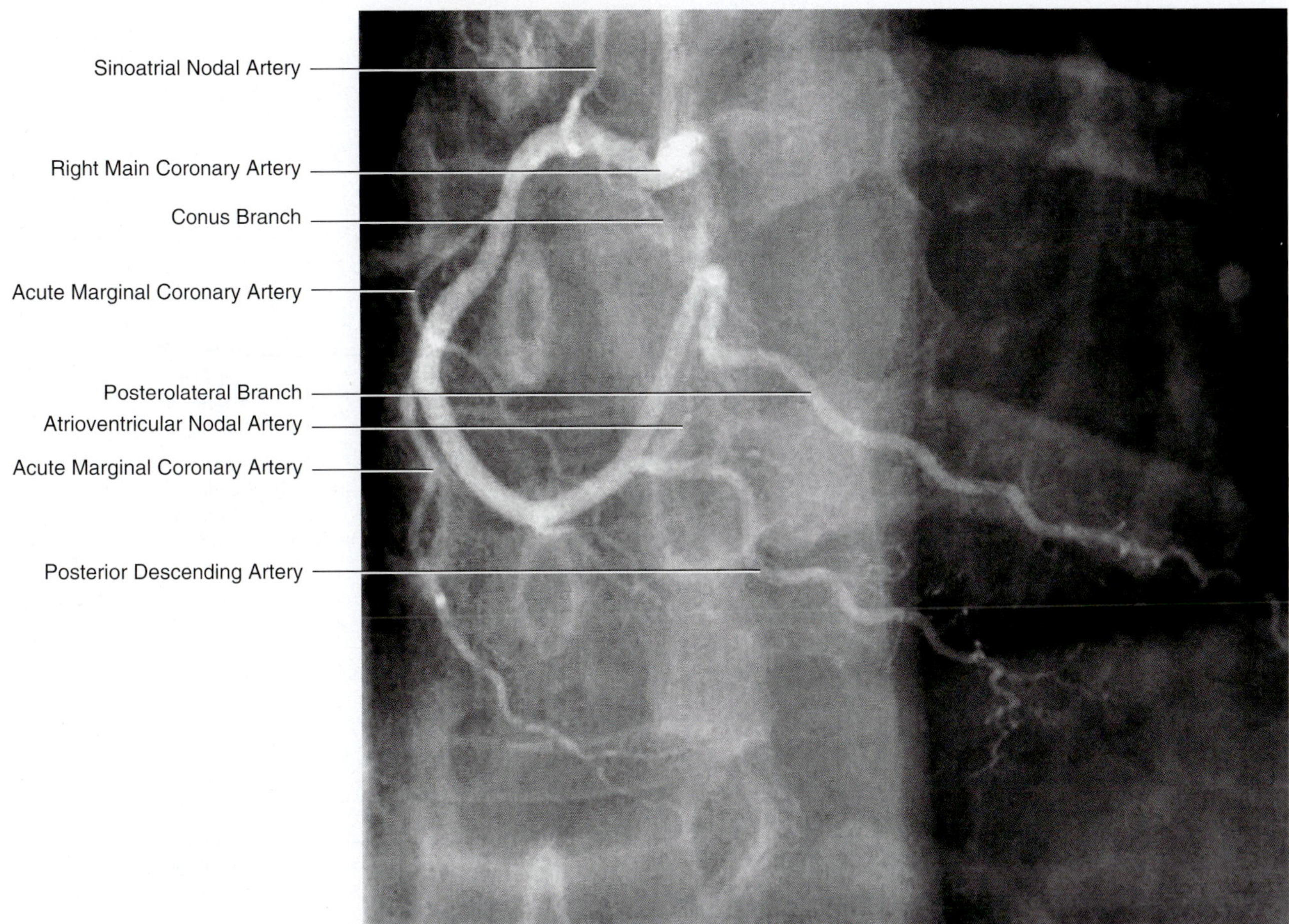

Figure 13.47. Angiogram of the right coronary artery in the left anterior oblique projection. The branches to the A-V node are multiple.

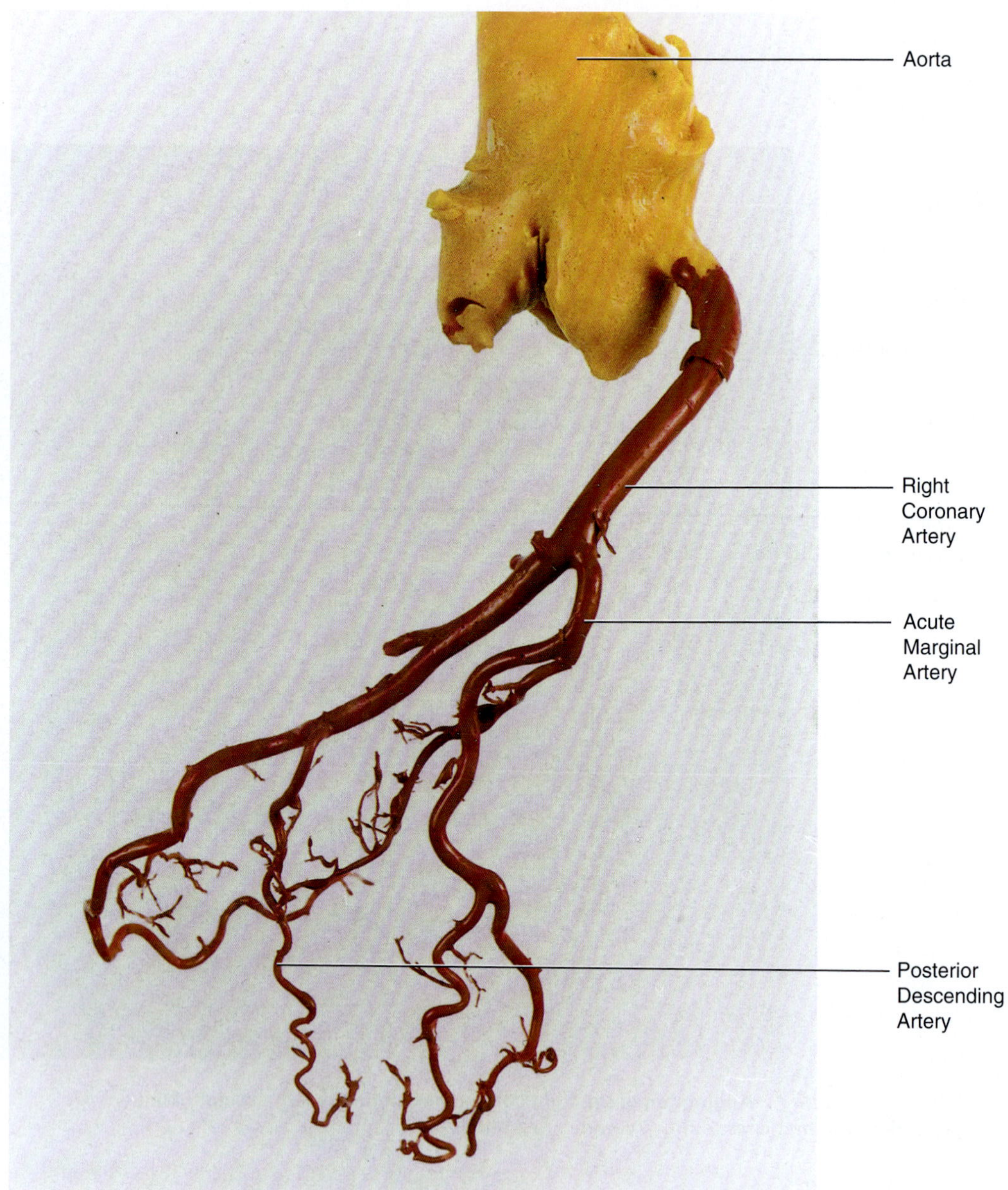

Figure 13.48. Cast of the right coronary artery in a right oblique view. The posterior descending artery is the terminal branch. There are no posterolateral arteries.

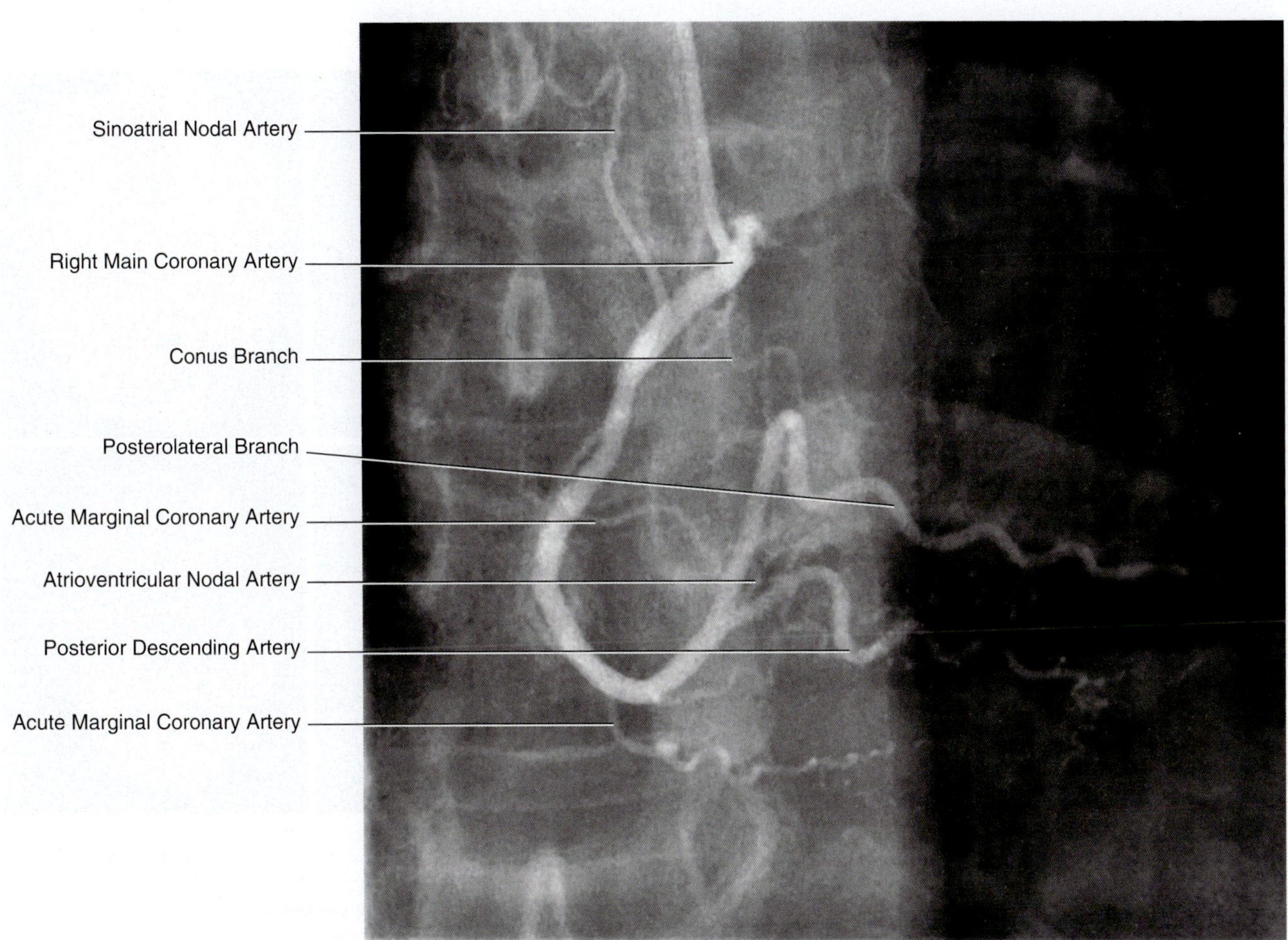

Figure 13.49. **Angiogram of the right coronary artery in the right anterior oblique projection.**

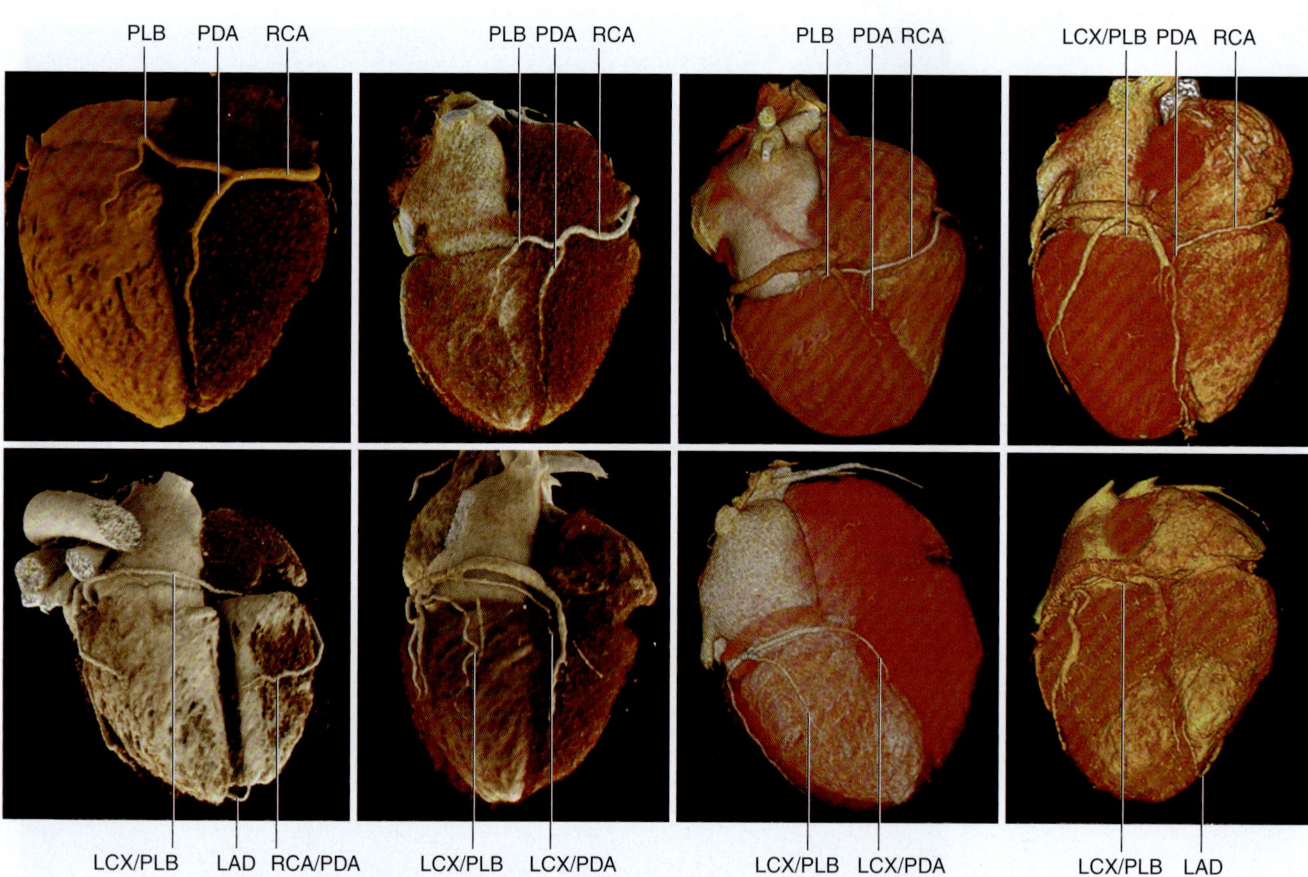

Figure 13.50. Variations of distribution of the coronary branches to the posterior surface of the heart. 3D volume-rendered CTs showing the posterior aspect of the heart in eight different individuals. Note the variability of posterior/inferior wall blood supply. (RCA-right coronary artery, LAD-left anterior descending, LCX-left circumflex, PDA-posterior descending artery, PLB-posterolateral branch.)

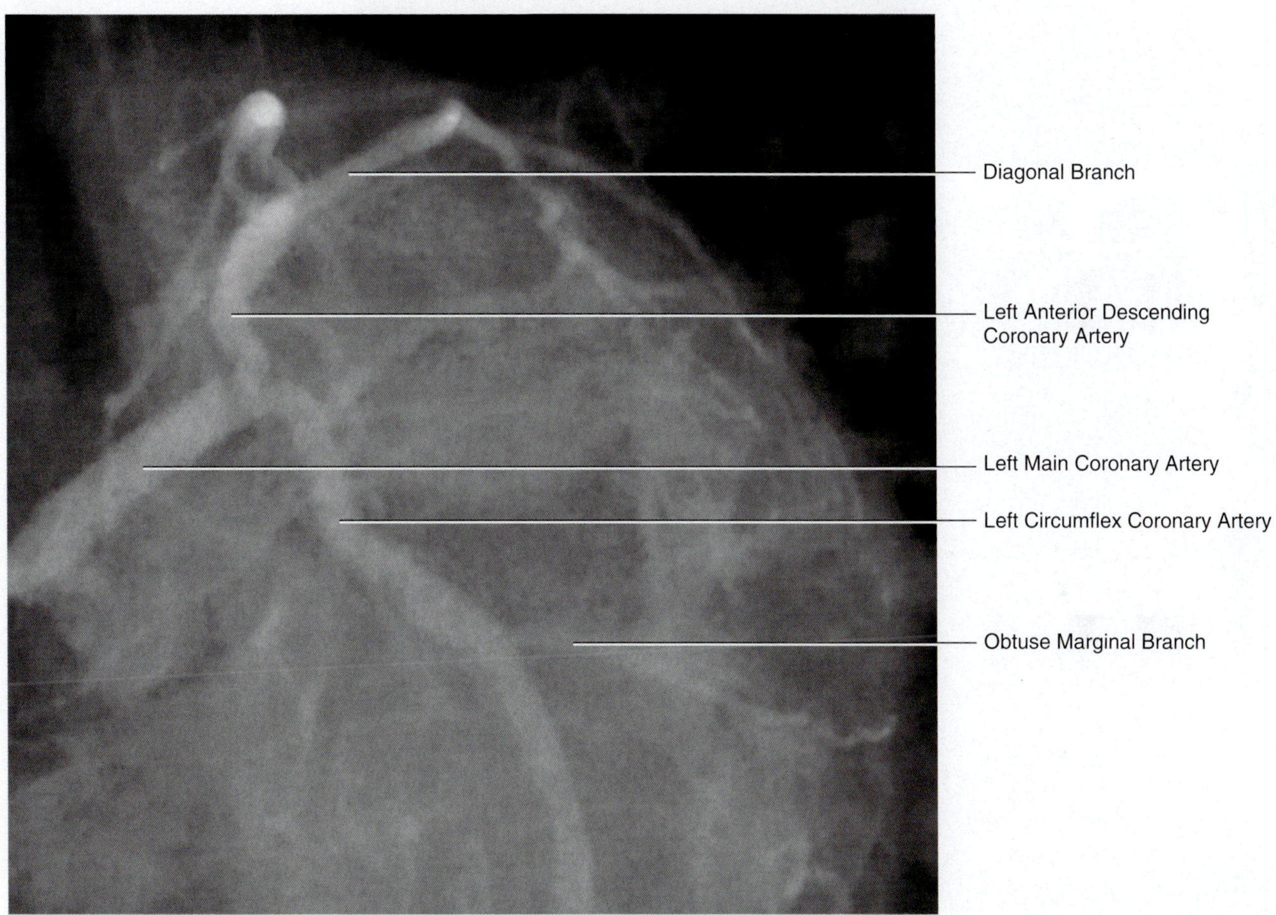

Figure 13.51. Left coronary artery angiogram obtained in the caudal left anterior oblique or spider projection showing the left main coronary and its bifurcation into the left anterior descending artery with its first diagonal branch, and the left circumflex artery with its first obtuse marginal branch.

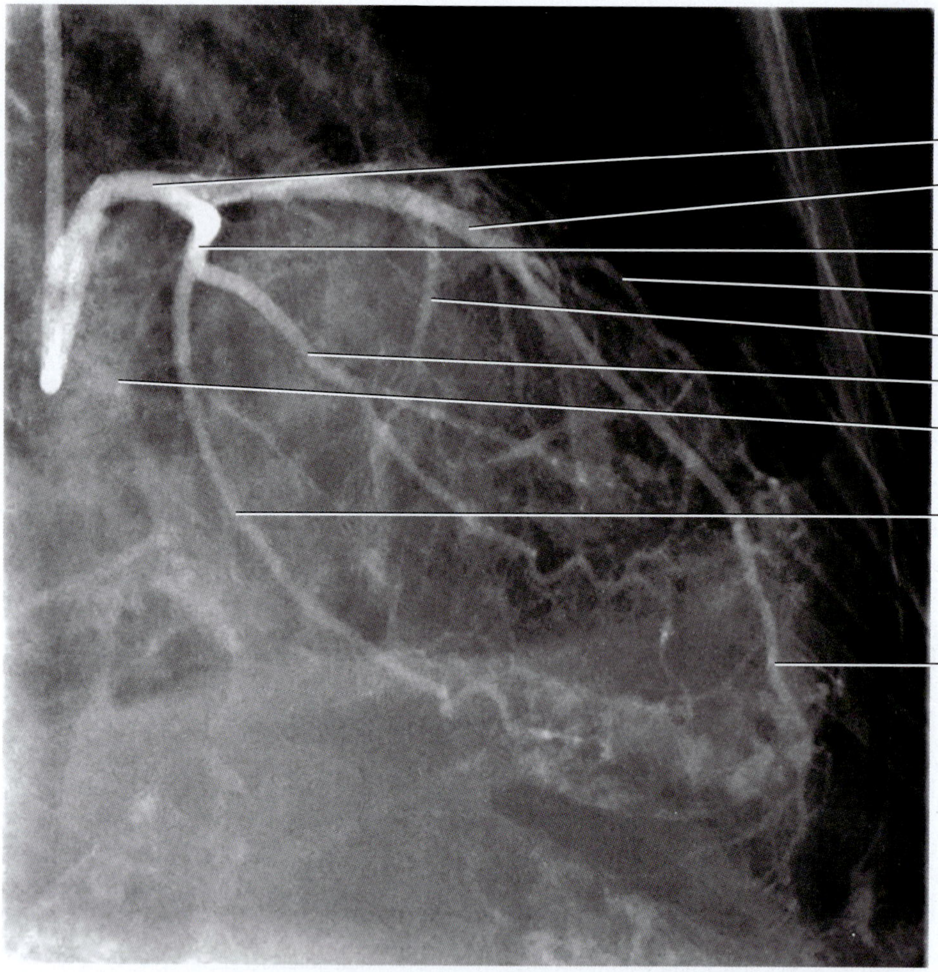

Left Main Coronary Artery
Left Anterior Descending Coronary Artery
Left Circumflex Coronary Artery
Diagonal Coronary Artery
First Septal Perforator
Obtuse Marginal Coronary Artery
Atrioventricular Coronary Artery
Obtuse Marginal Coronary Artery
Left Anterior Descending Coronary Artery

Figure 13.52. Left coronary artery angiogram in the caudal right anterior oblique projection. The circumflex artery is very short and divides into a well-developed obtuse marginal artery and a very diminutive atrioventricular artery.

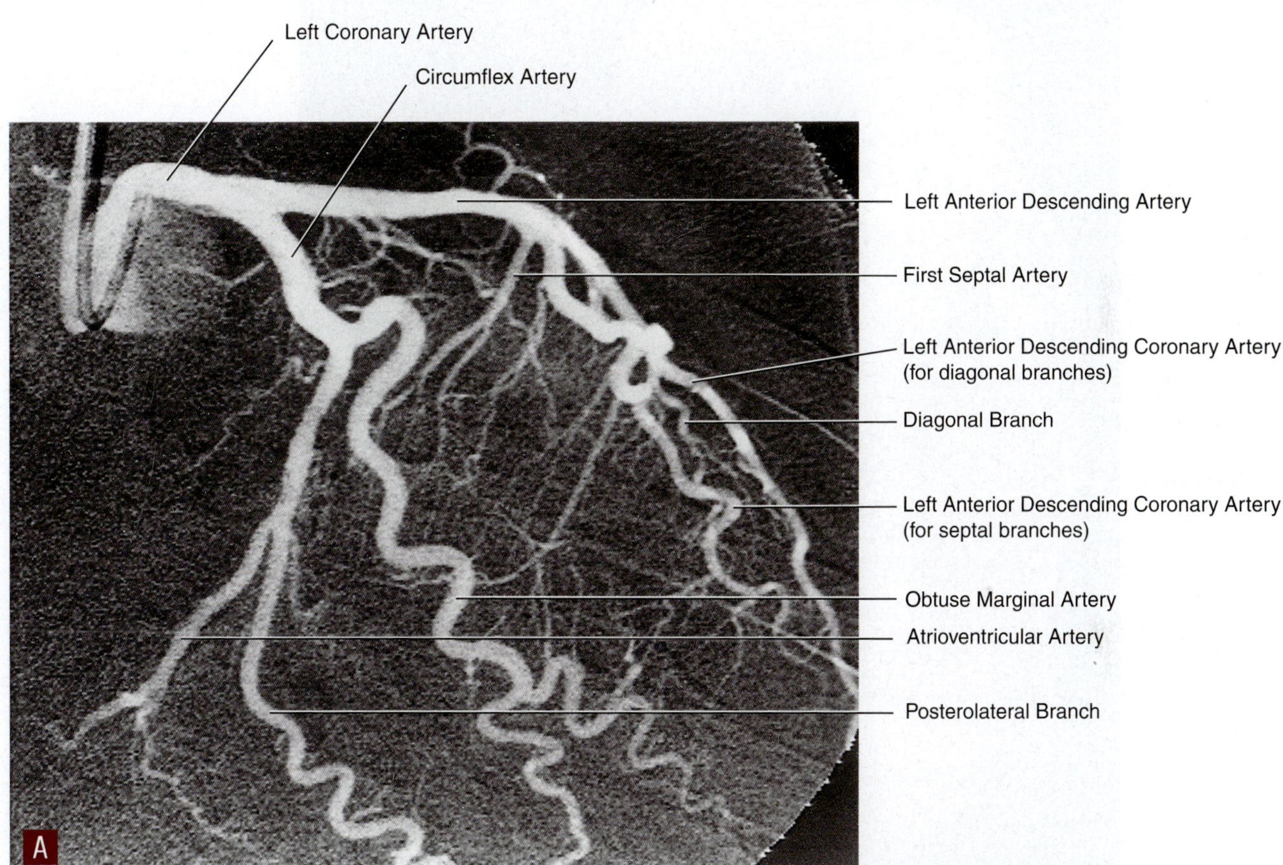

Figure 13.53. **A, Left coronary artery in the caudal right anterior oblique projection.** The left anterior descending (LAD) artery is short and divides into two parallel arteries: one running over the interventricular sulcus supplying the interventricular septum. The other runs along the anterior wall of the left ventricle and gives rise to diagonal branches. This configuration is referred to as "dual left anterior descending artery." B, 3D volume rendering of another patient with "dual LAD."

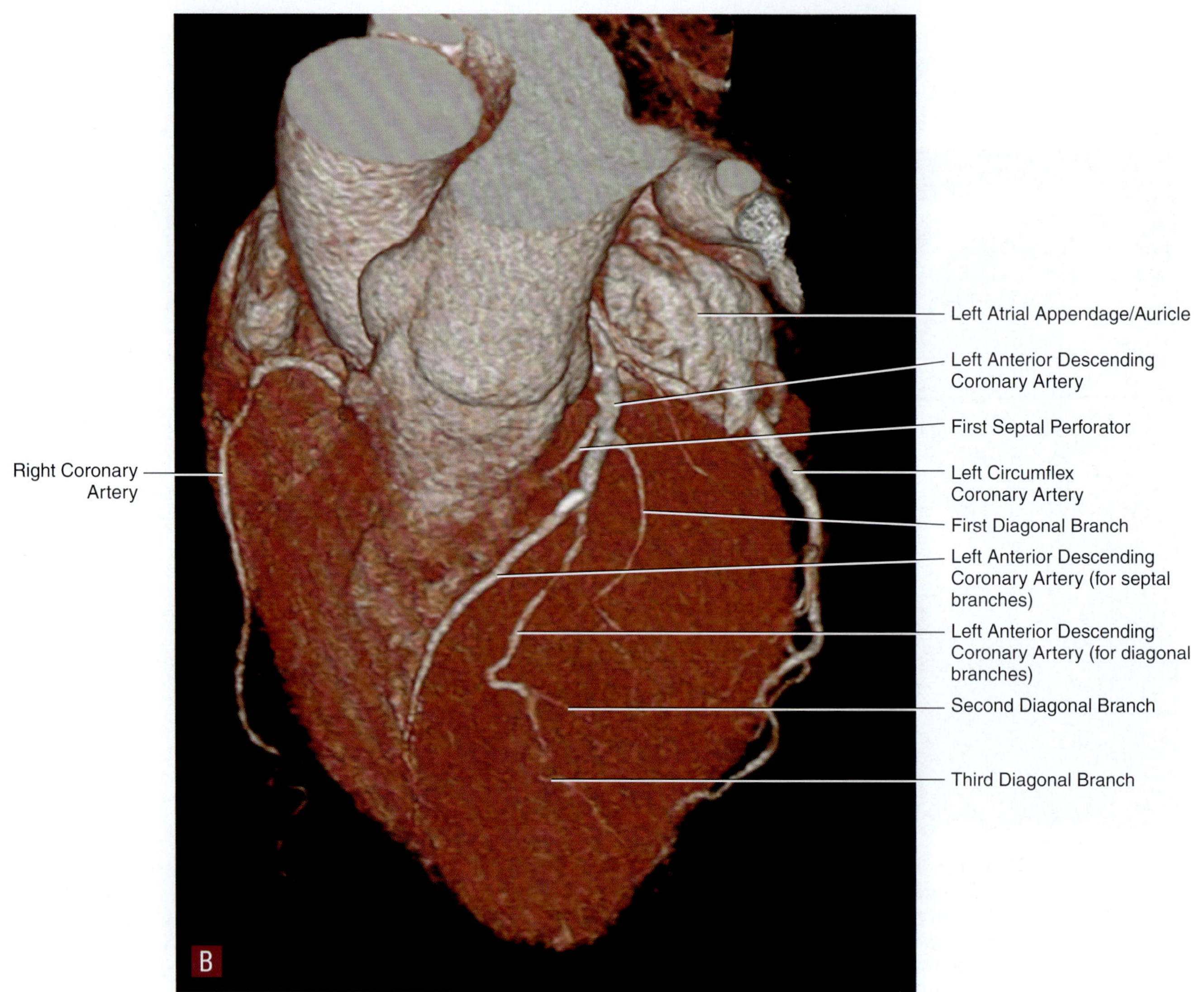

Figure 13.53. *Continued*

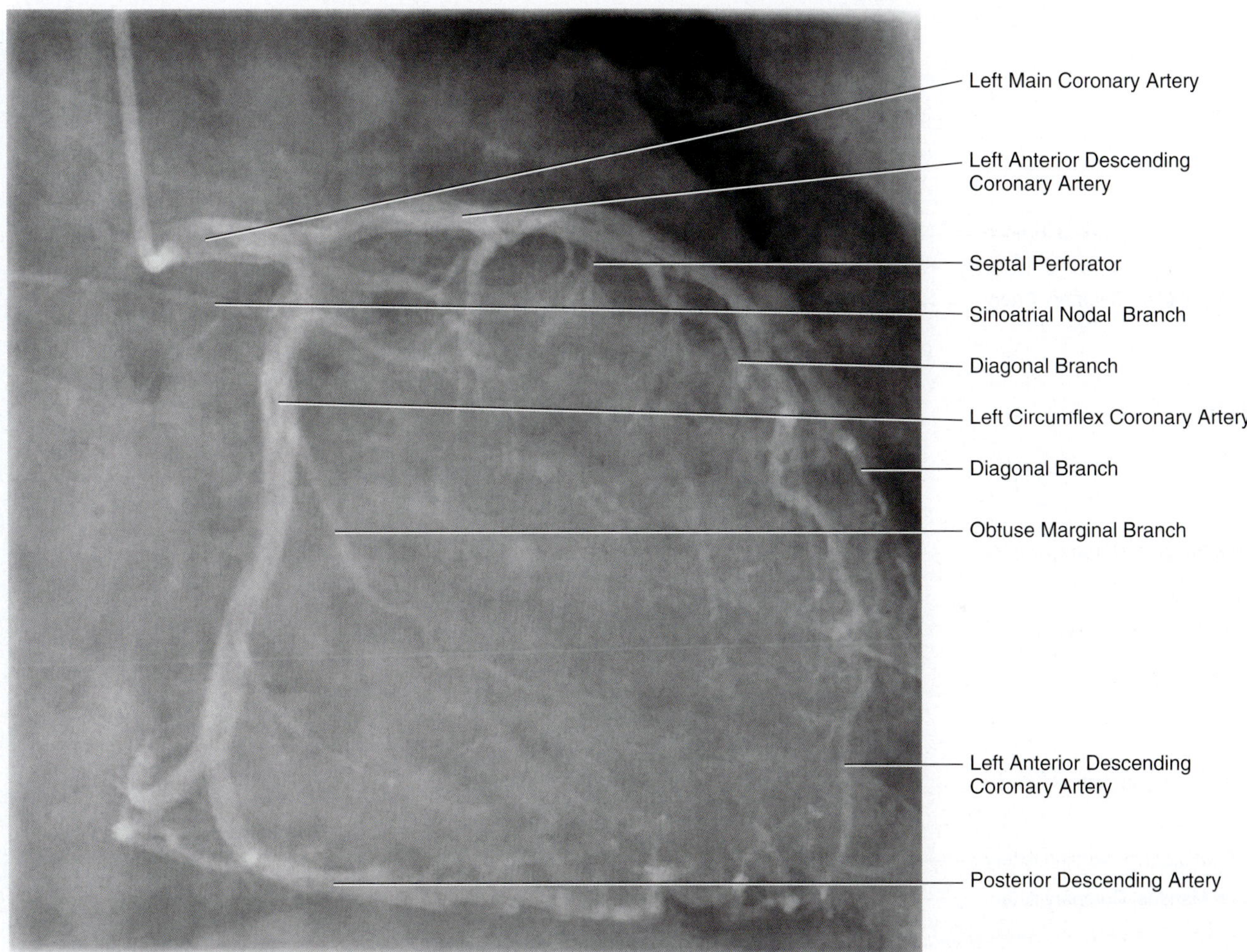

Figure 13.54. Dominant left coronary artery: the posterior descending artery arises distally from the circumflex artery. The sinus node artery (sinoatrial nodal branch) originates from the proximal left circumflex artery. This is an angiogram in the cranial right anterior oblique projection.

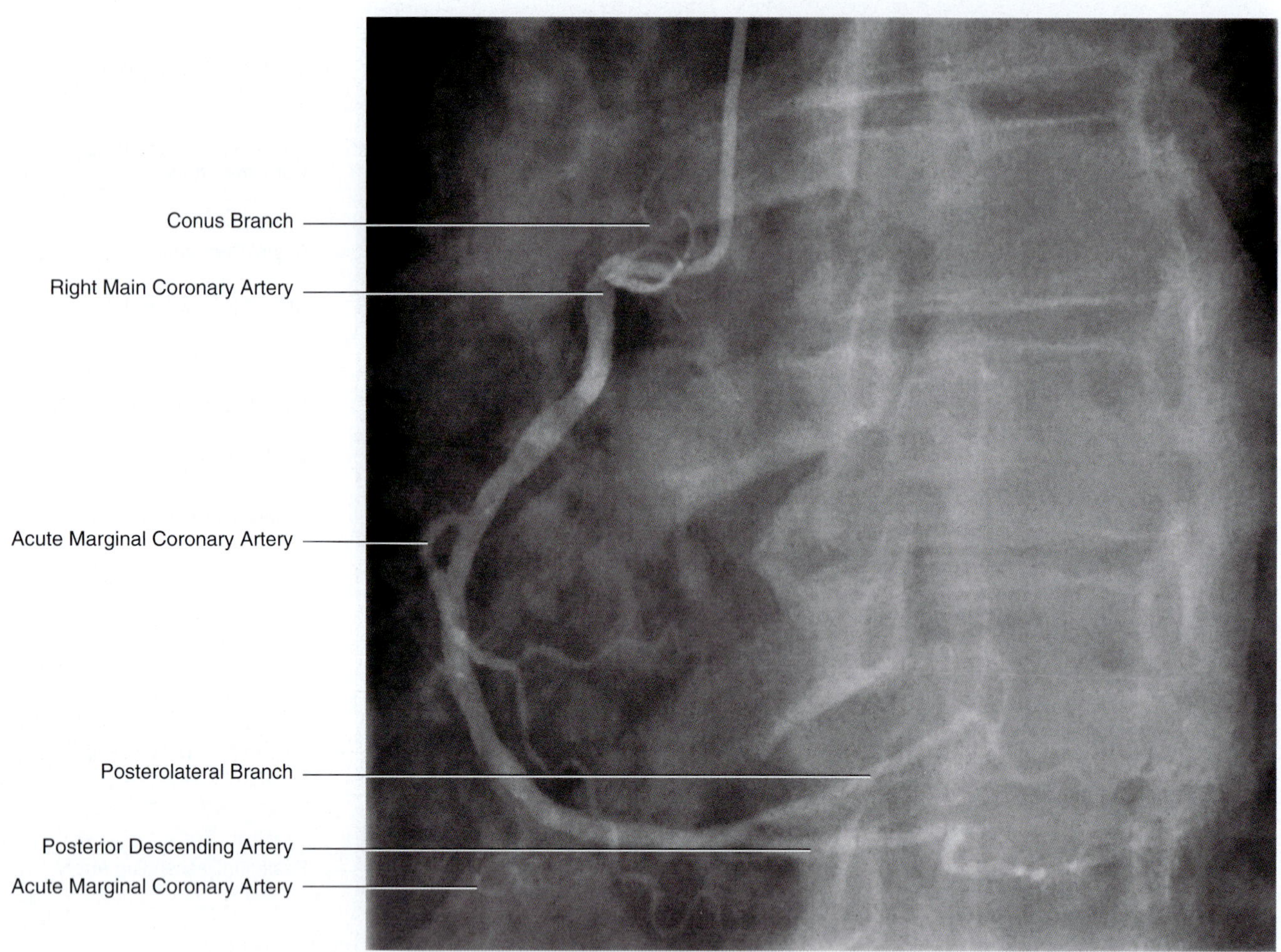

Figure 13.55. Dominant right coronary artery in the left anterior oblique view. The posterior descending artery and posterolateral branch arise from the right coronary artery at the crux cordis.

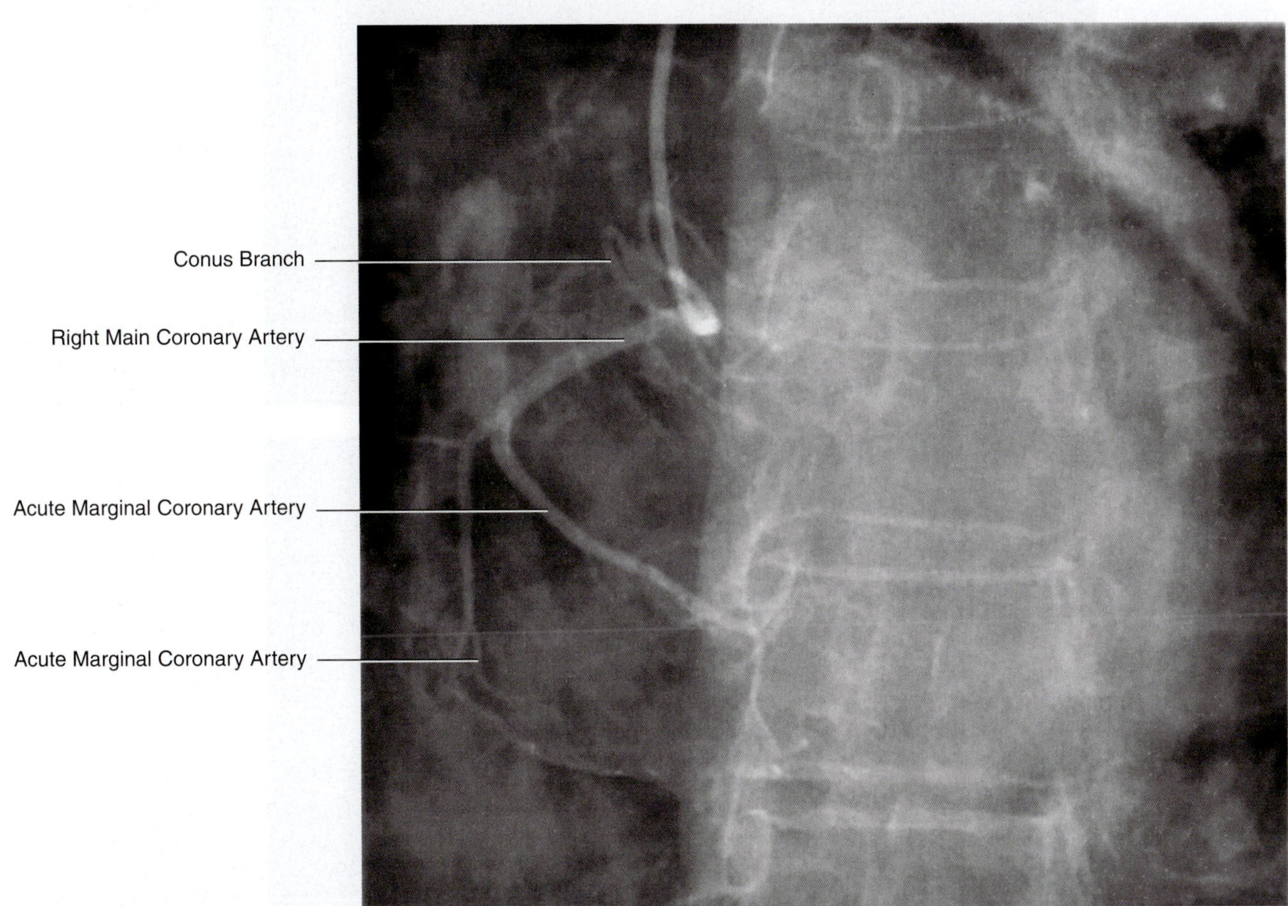

Figure 13.56. Angiogram showing a nondominant right coronary artery (RCA) in the right anterior oblique projection. This RCA becomes diminutive after it gives rise to acute marginal branches.

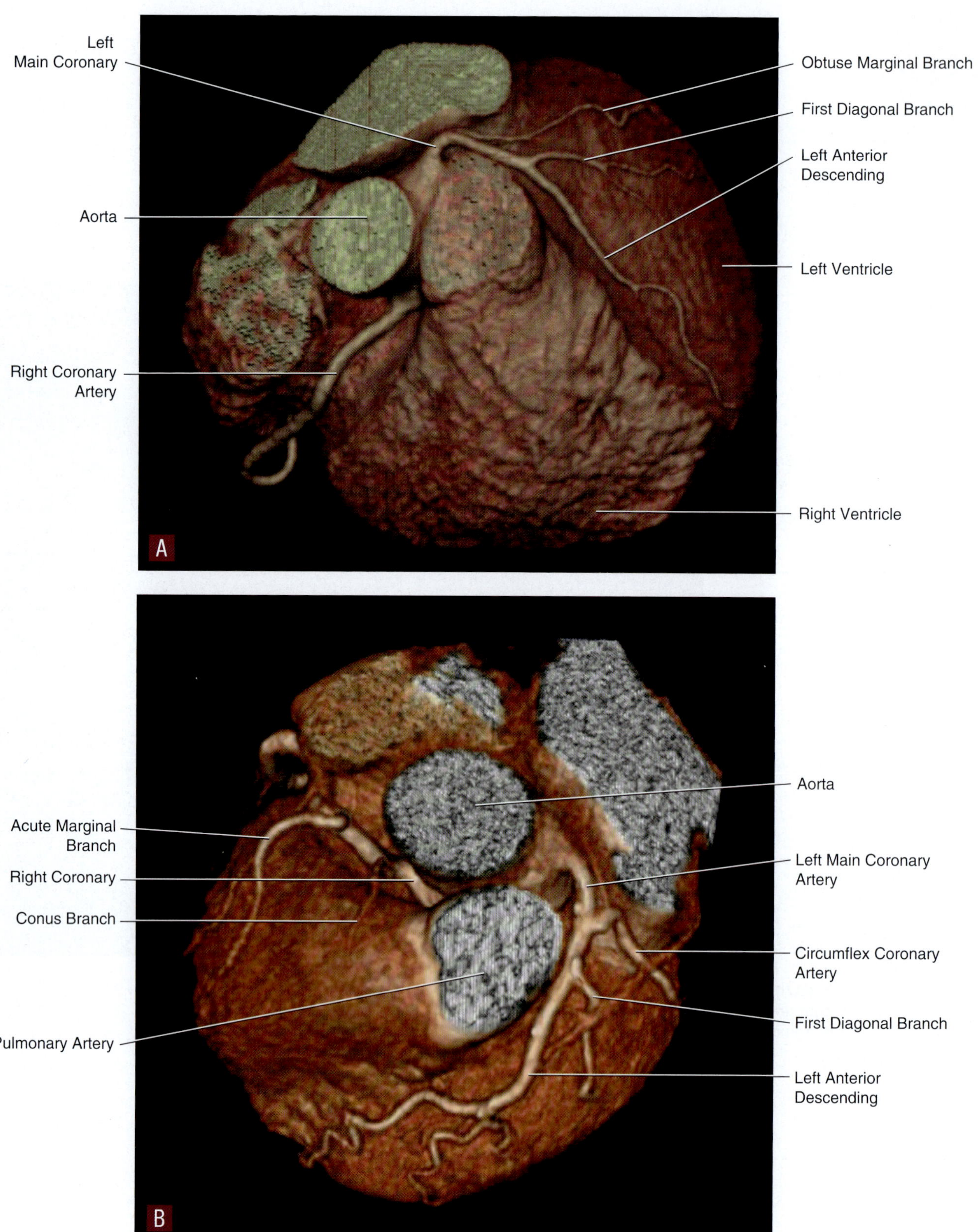

Figure 13.57. **CT 3D volume-rendered image.** A and B, Two examples of normal origins of the right and left coronary arteries.

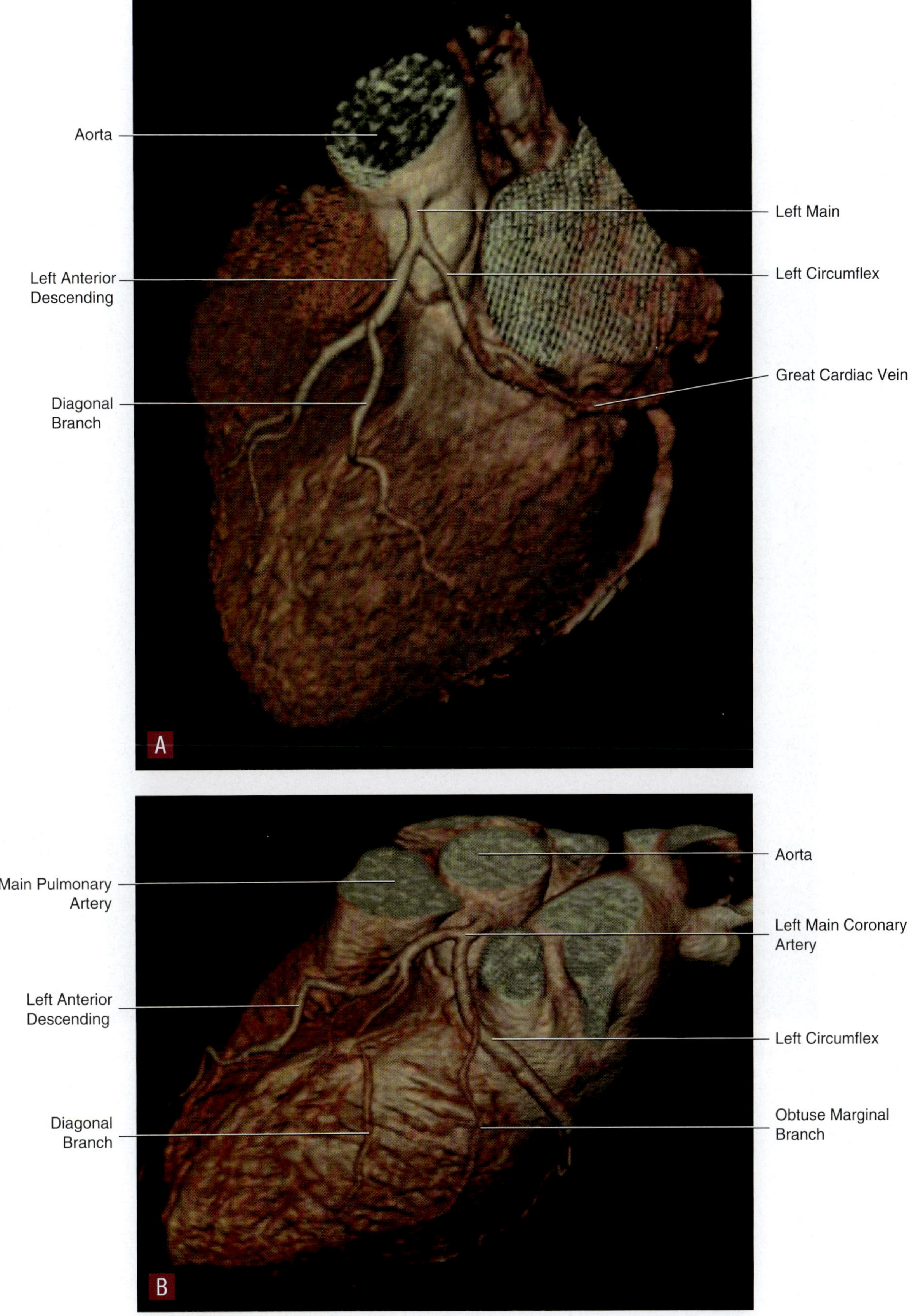

Figure 13.58. CT 3D volume-rendered image. Left main coronary artery bifurcation. A, Note the coronary vein overlapping the left circumflex coronary artery. B, Large left circumflex artery.

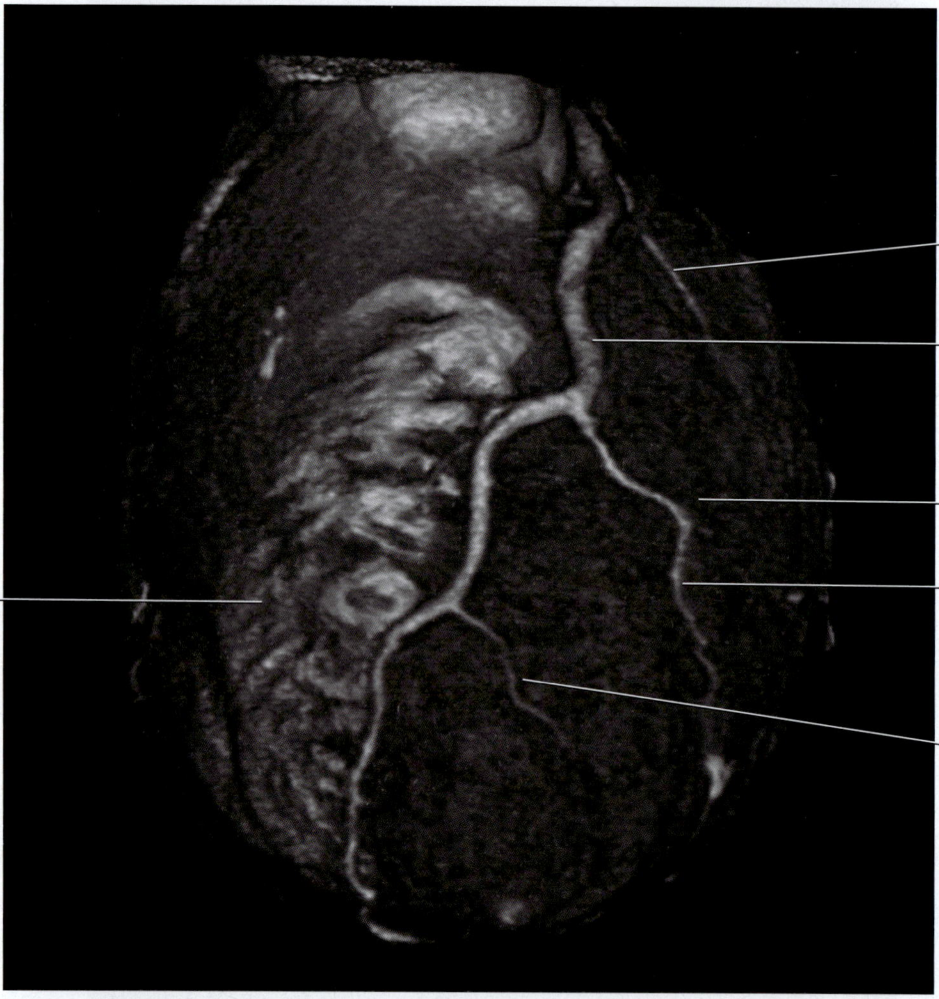

Figure 13.59. **CT 3D volume-rendered image.** Left anterior descending coronary artery in the anterior interventricular groove with multiple diagonal branches.

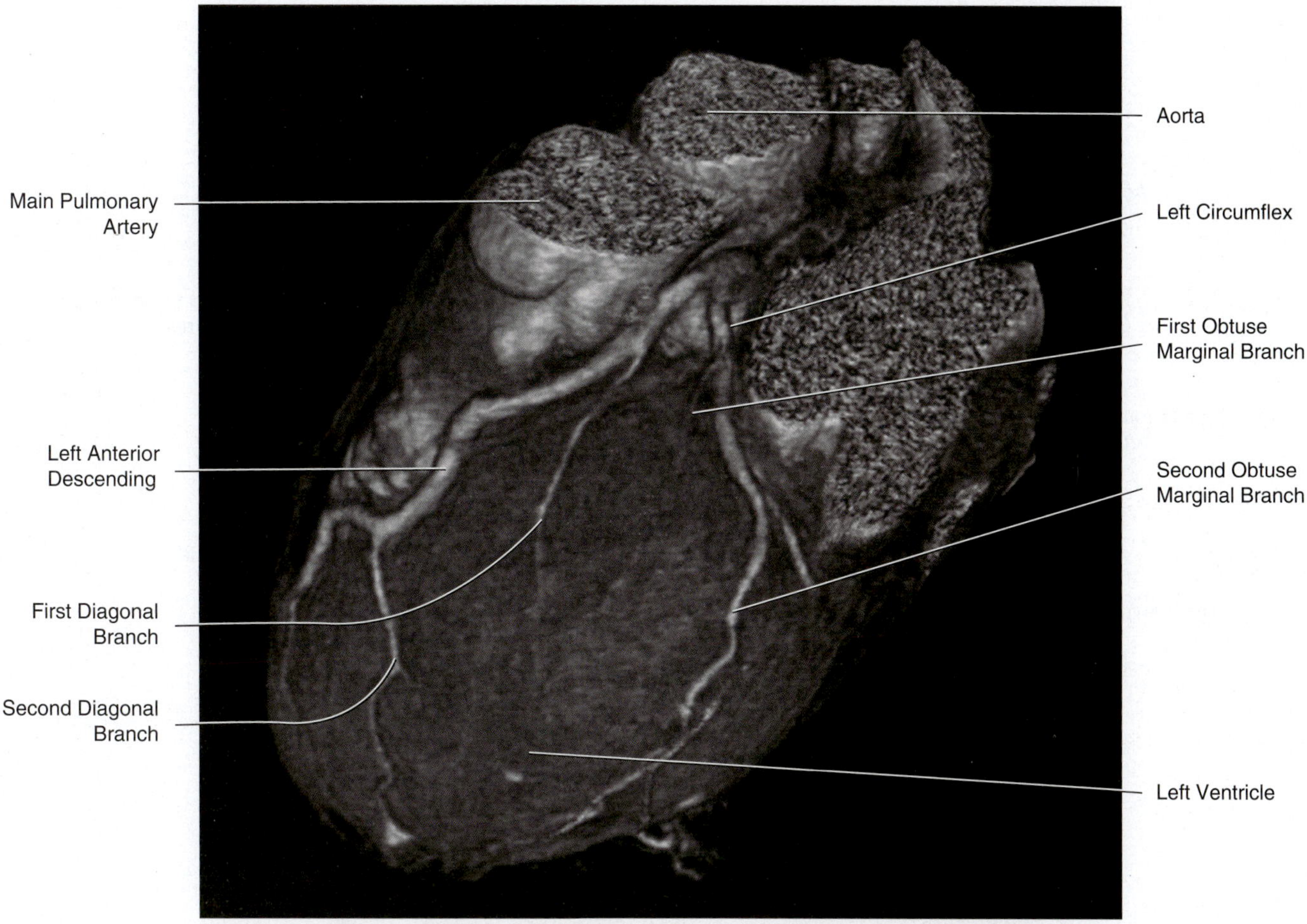

Aorta
Main Pulmonary Artery
Left Circumflex
First Obtuse Marginal Branch
Left Anterior Descending
Second Obtuse Marginal Branch
First Diagonal Branch
Second Diagonal Branch
Left Ventricle

Figure 13.60. CT 3D volume-rendered image. Left anterior descending coronary artery with diagonal branches and left circumflex coronary artery with obtuse marginal branches.

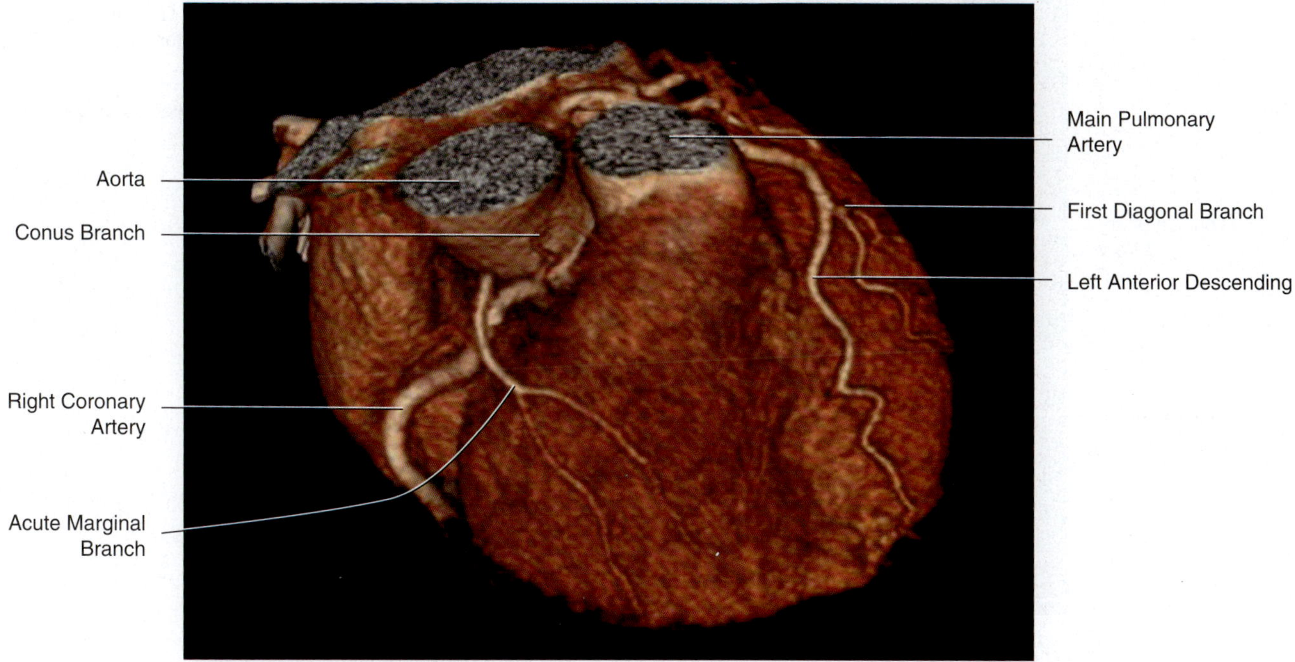

Figure 13.61. CT 3D volume-rendered image. Right coronary artery with an acute marginal branch.

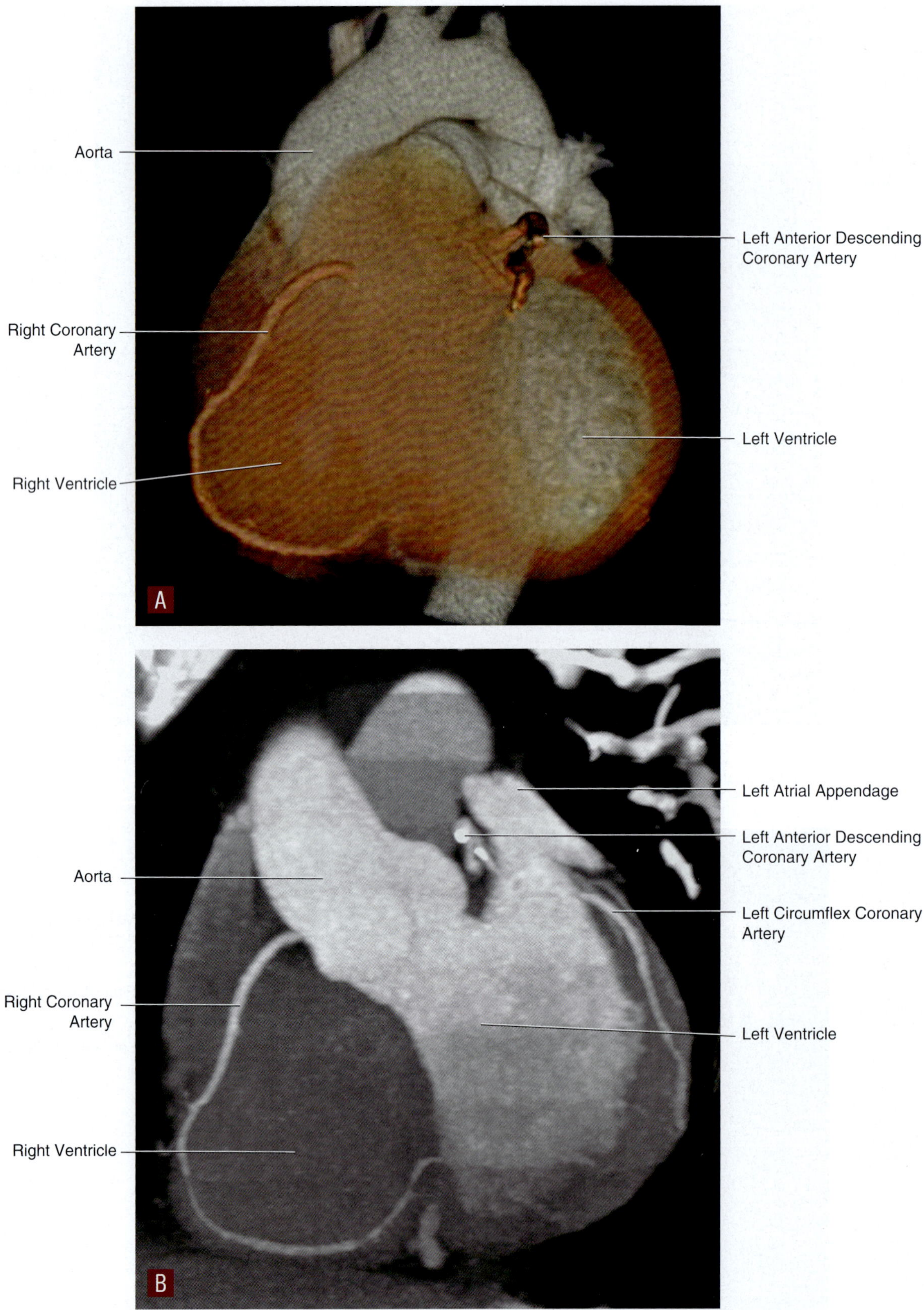

Figure 13.62. **CT 3D volume-rendered image of dominant right coronary artery. Three different methods of representation.** **A**, 3D volume with highlighted coronary artery. **B**, Maximum intensity projection (MIP) image. **C**, Simulated angiographic image.

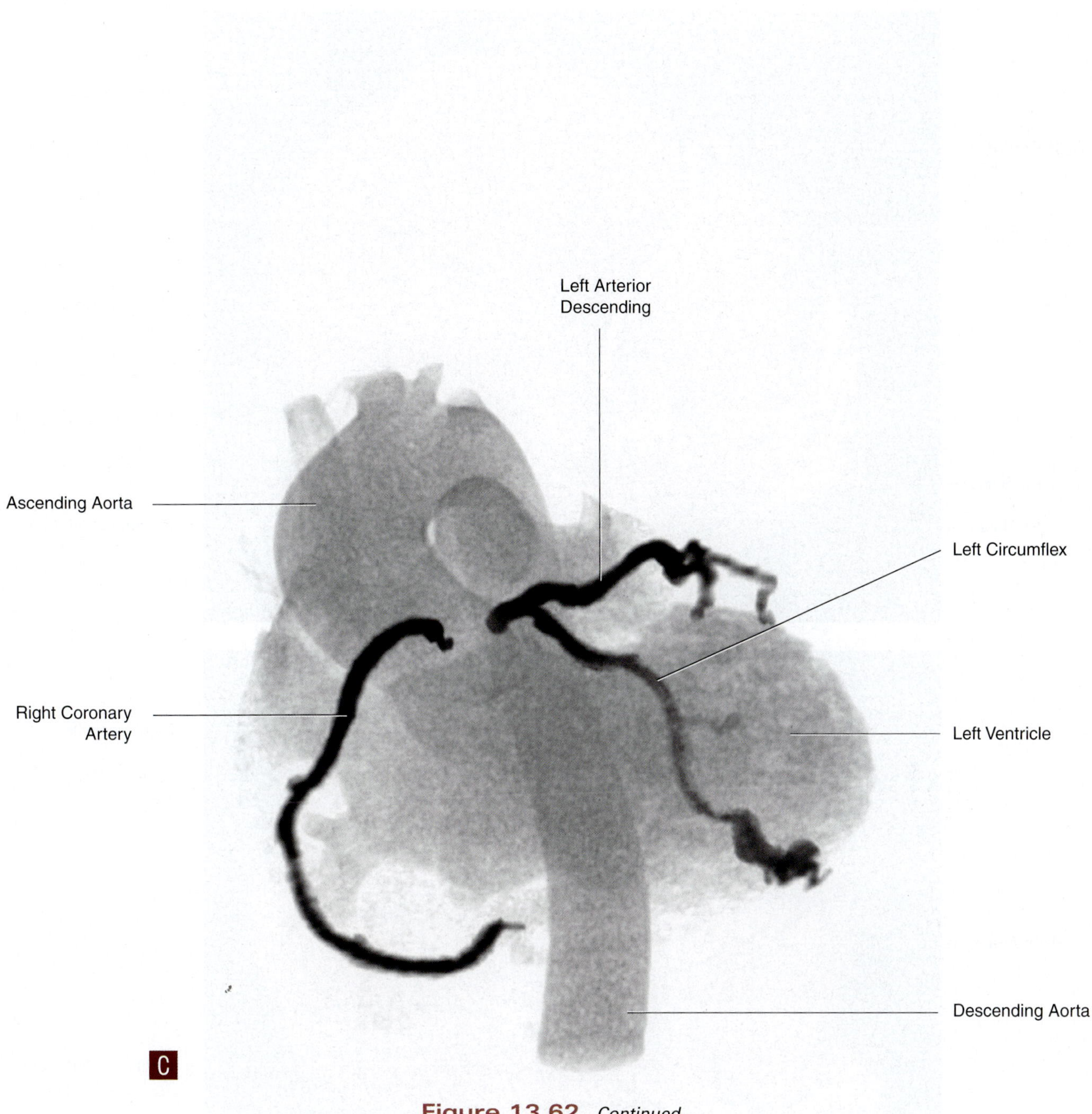

Figure 13.62. *Continued*

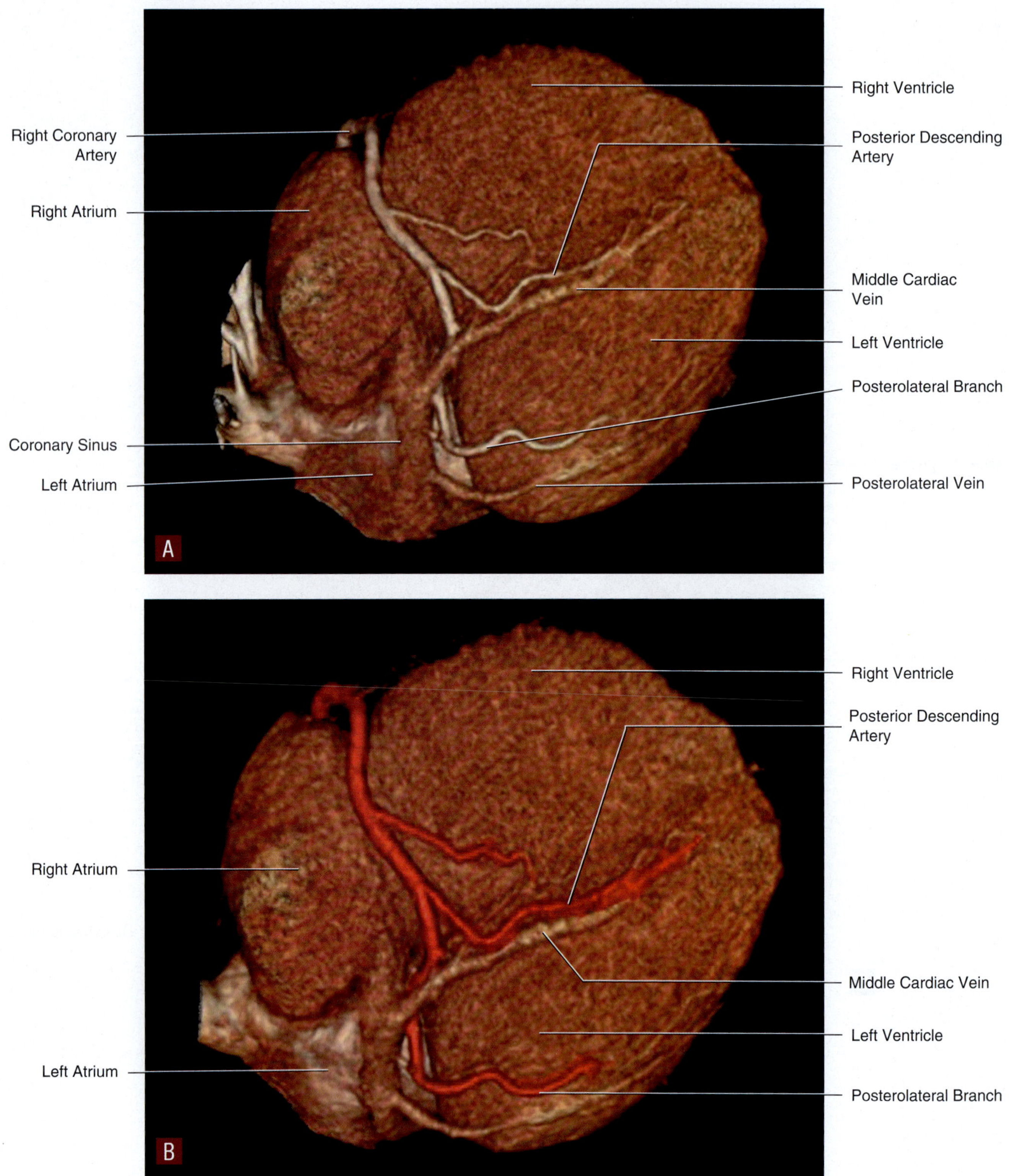

Figure 13.63. CT 3D volume-rendered images with two methods of display. **A**, Inferior surface of the heart with dominant distal right coronary artery giving rise to a posterior descending artery and a posterolateral branch. **B**, CT image with highlighted distal right coronary circulation. Note distinction from venous drainage into coronary sinus.

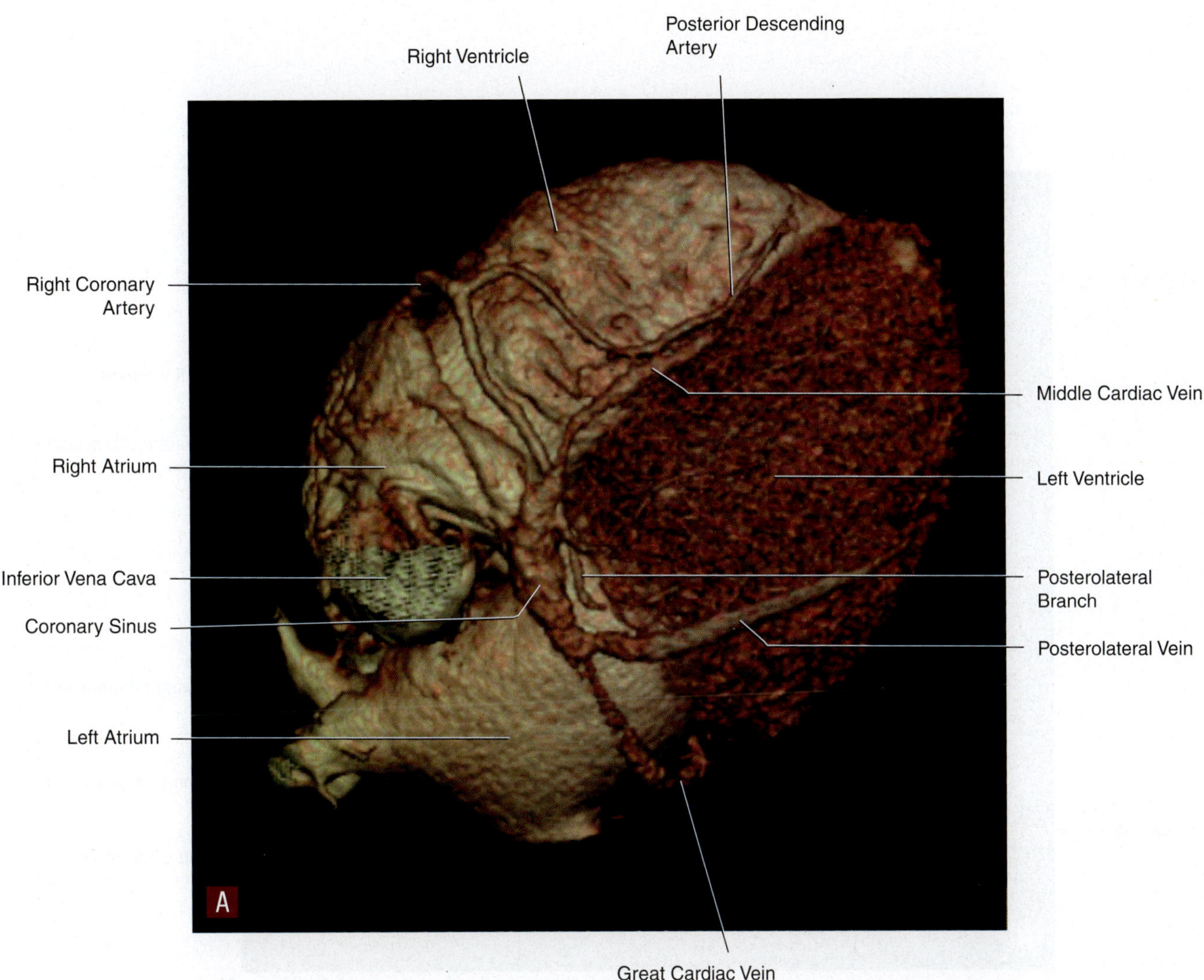

Figure 13.64. **CT 3D volume-rendered image showing the inferior surface of the heart demonstrating right versus left dominance.** A, Right dominant system, with right coronary artery supplying flow to the posterior descending coronary artery and the posterolateral branch. Note slight variant anatomy with early take-off of PDA. B, Left dominant system, with the left circumflex supplying the posterolateral branch and the PDA. Note veins and coronary sinus removed to better demonstrate the distal left circumflex artery. PDA, posterior descending artery.

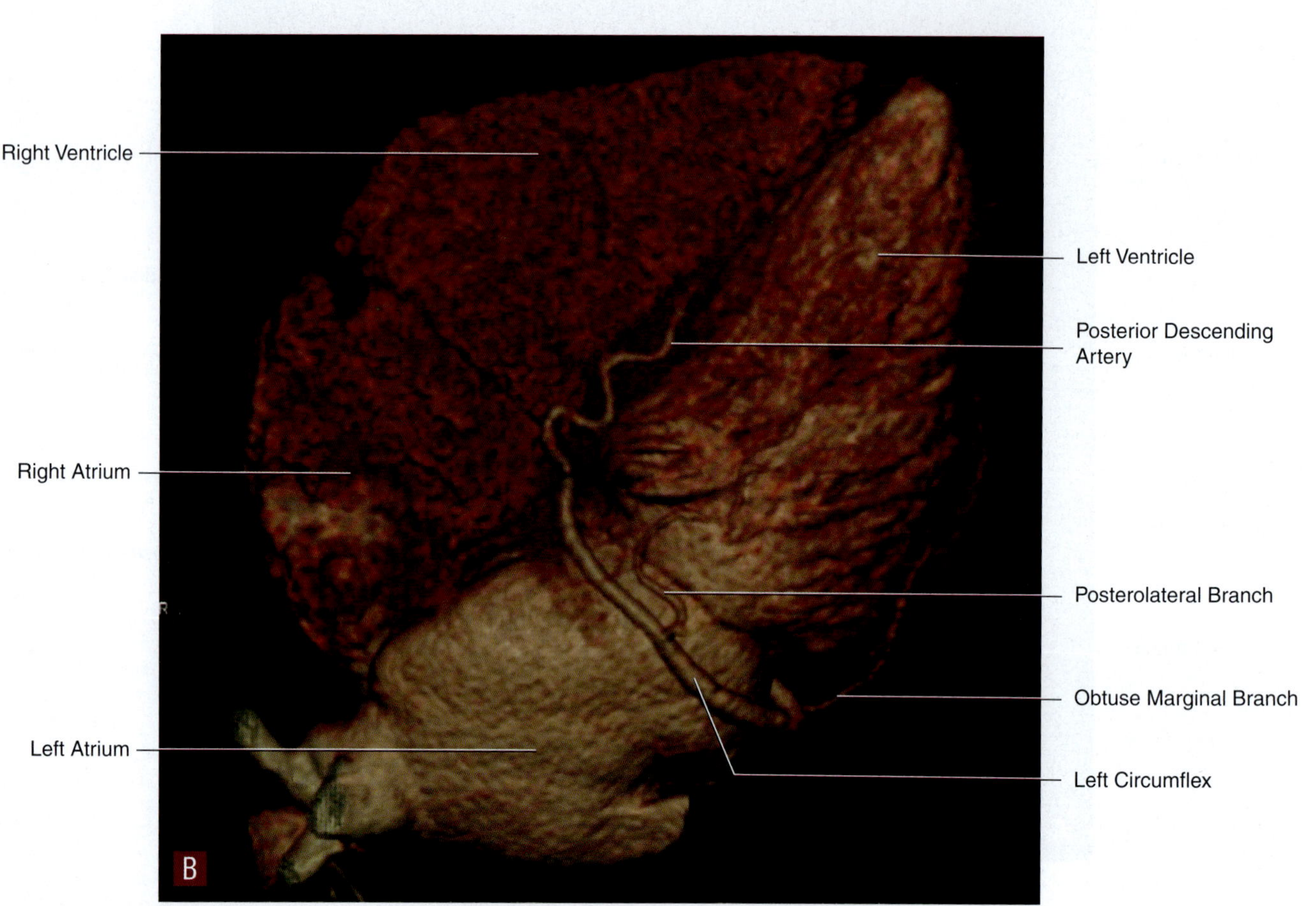

Figure 13.64. *Continued*

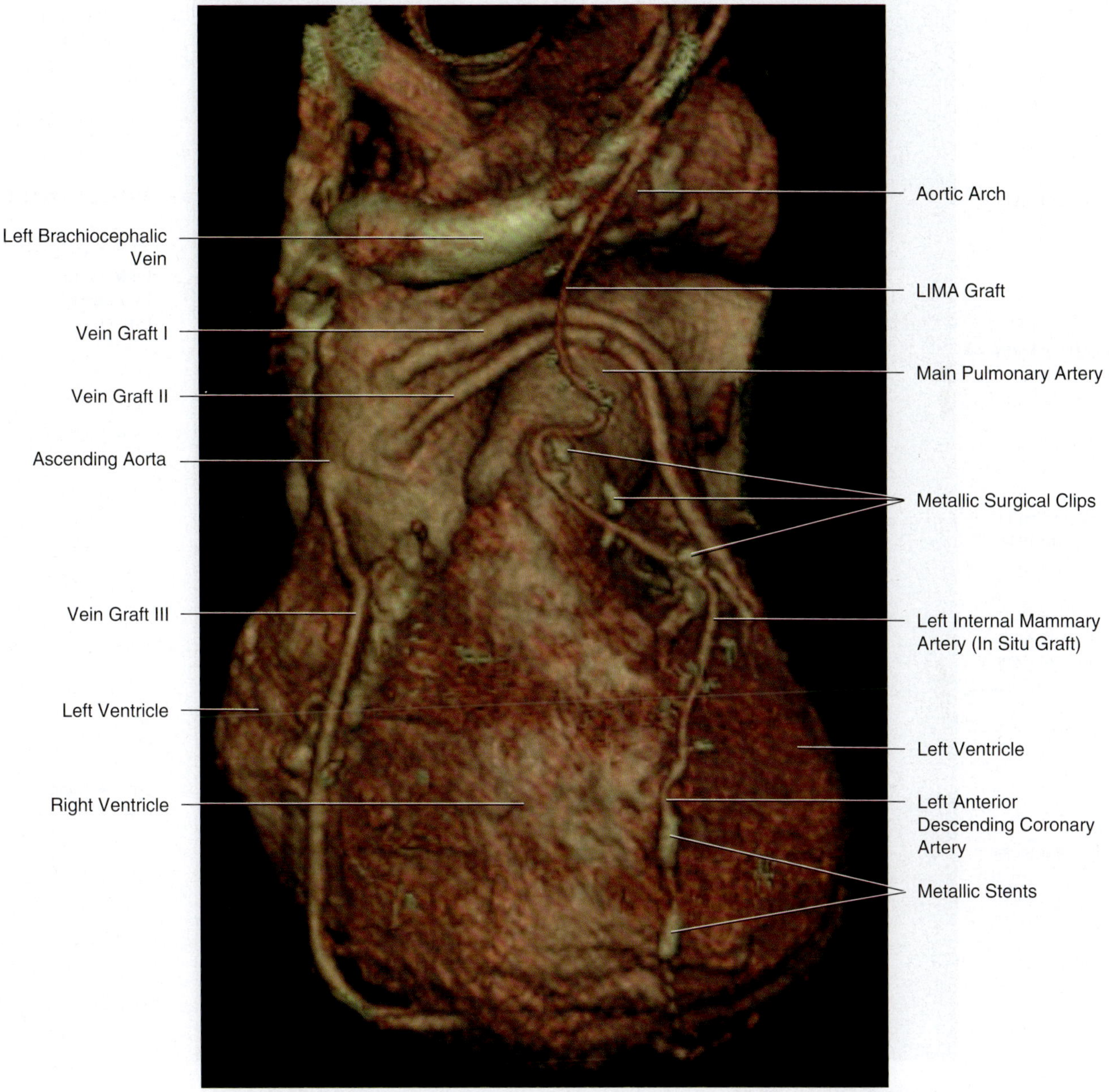

Aortic Arch
Left Brachiocephalic Vein
LIMA Graft
Vein Graft I
Main Pulmonary Artery
Vein Graft II
Ascending Aorta
Metallic Surgical Clips
Vein Graft III
Left Internal Mammary Artery (In Situ Graft)
Left Ventricle
Left Ventricle
Right Ventricle
Left Anterior Descending Coronary Artery
Metallic Stents

Figure 13.65. CT 3D volume-rendered image of four-vessel CABG viewed from the front. Note distal LAD contains previously placed metallic coronary artery stents. CABG, coronary artery bypass grafting; LAD, left anterior descending.

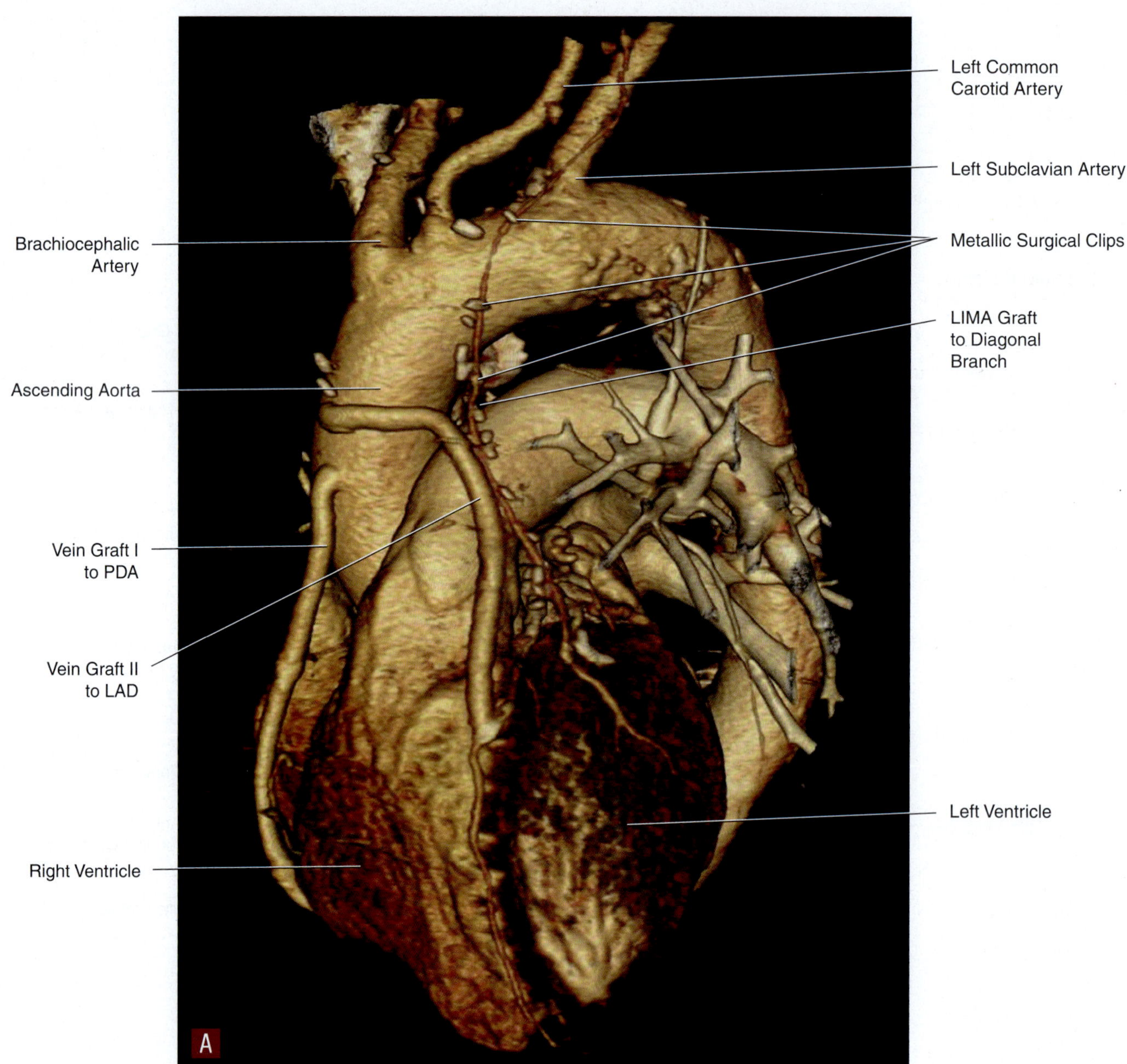

Figure 13.66. CT 3D volume-rendered images of three-vessel CABG. **A**, Two vein grafts arising from the ascending aorta. Left internal mammary artery (LIMA) graft is also present. **B**, Lateral view showing vein graft distal anastamosis with LAD and LIMA graft anastamosis with diagonal branch. **C**, Inferior surface of the heart showing the distal vein graft anastamosis with posterior descending artery. **D**, Lateral view with bones in place to show the relationship of grafts to the chest wall. CABG, coronary artery bypass grafting; LAD, left anterior descending.

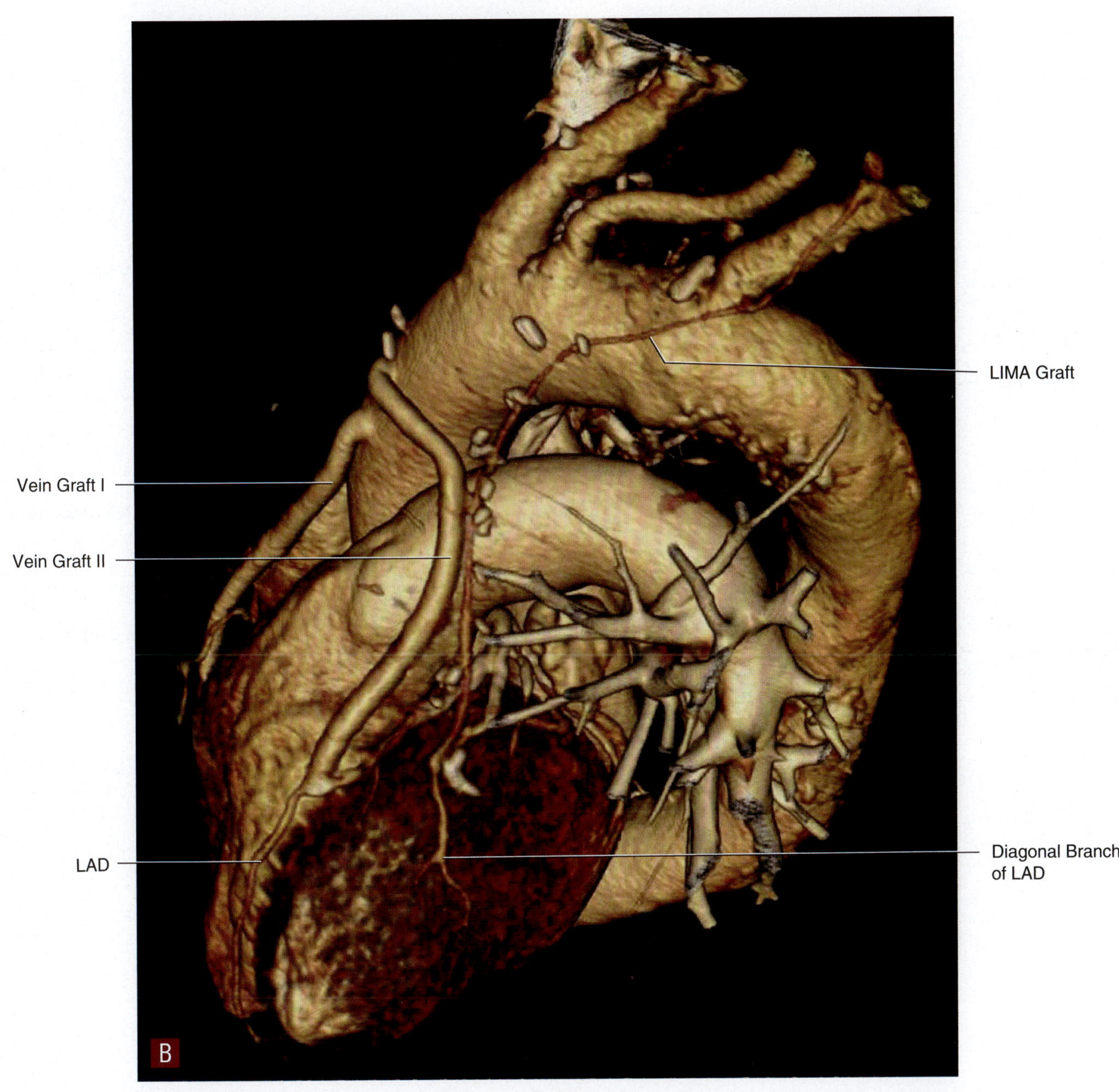

Figure 13.66. *Continued*

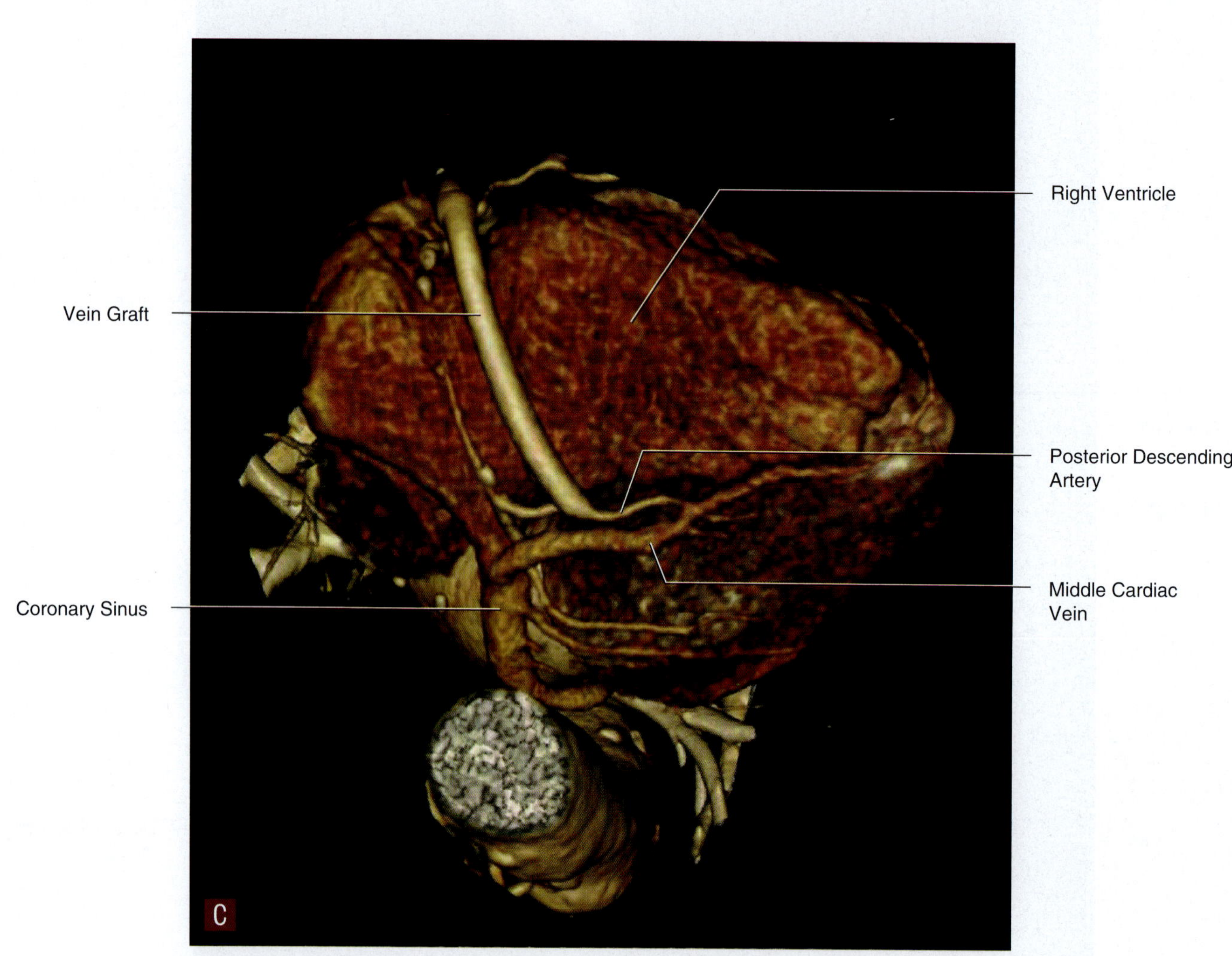

Figure 13.66. *Continued*

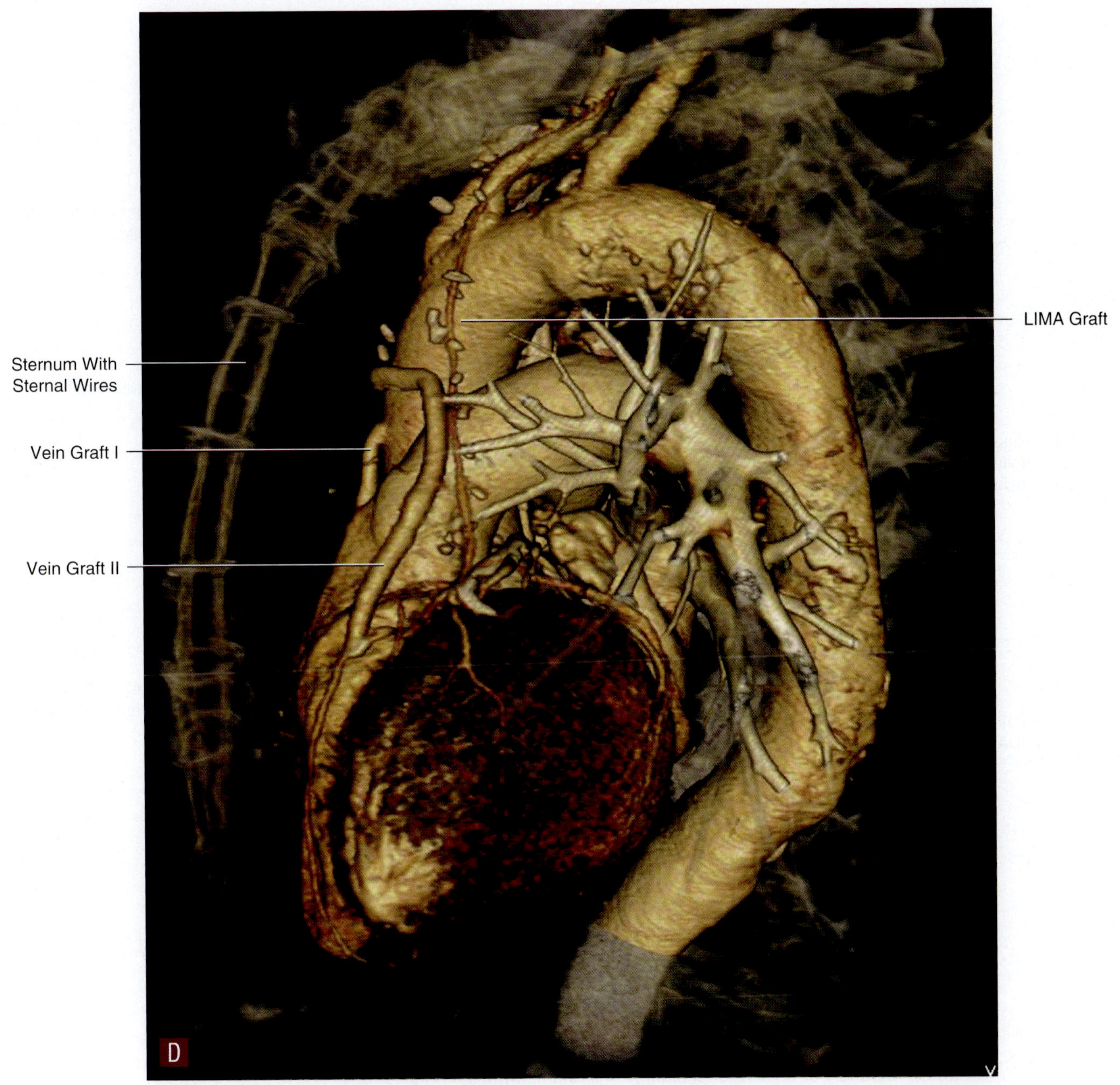

Figure 13.66. *Continued*

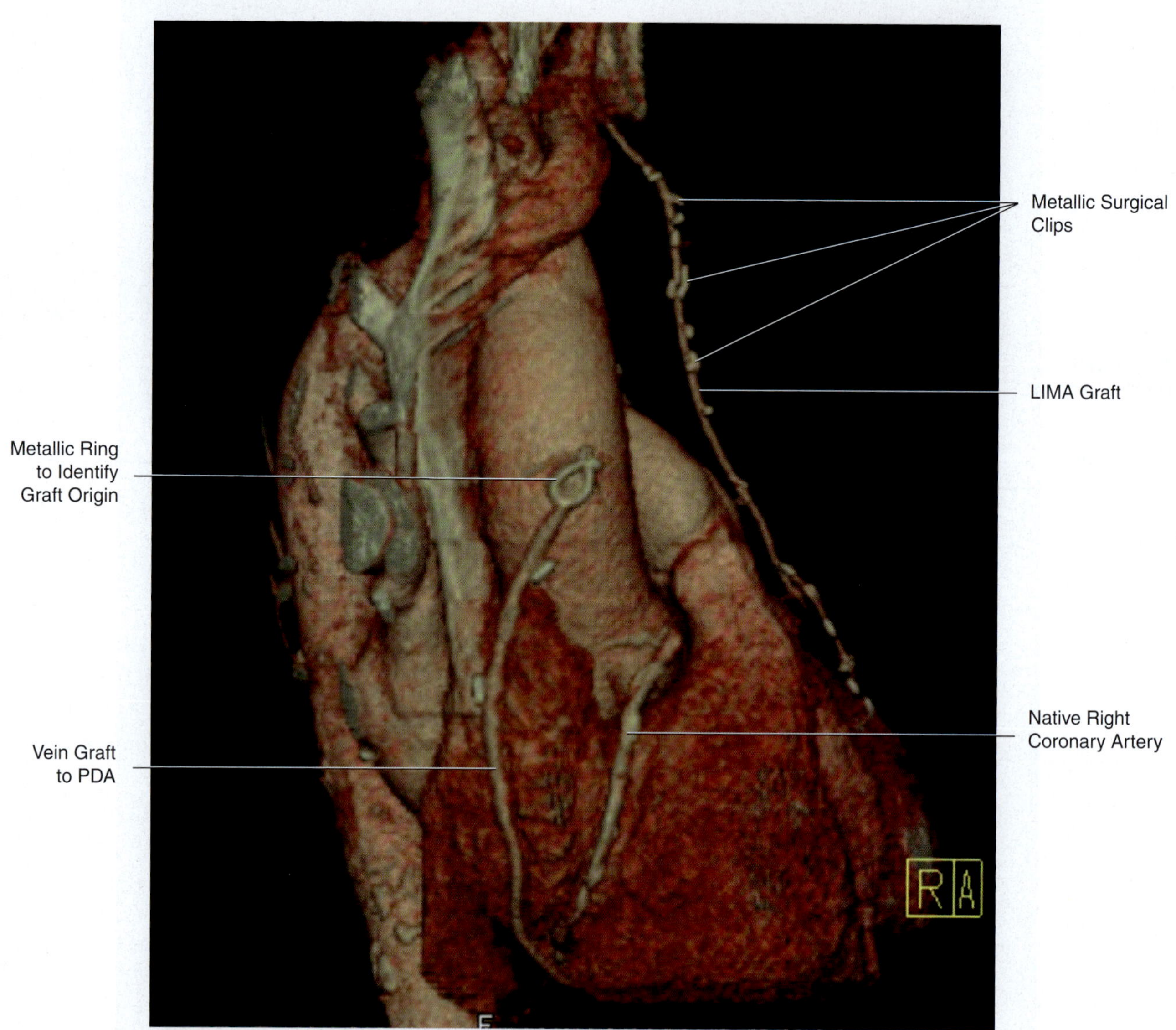

Figure 13.67. CT 3D volume-rendered image of two-vessel CABG. LIMA to left coronary circulation and vein graft to right coronary circulation. Note the metallic ring marker placed at origin of vein graft by surgeons for guidance in subsequent heart catheterizations.
CABG, coronary artery bypass grafting; LIMA, left internal mammary artery.

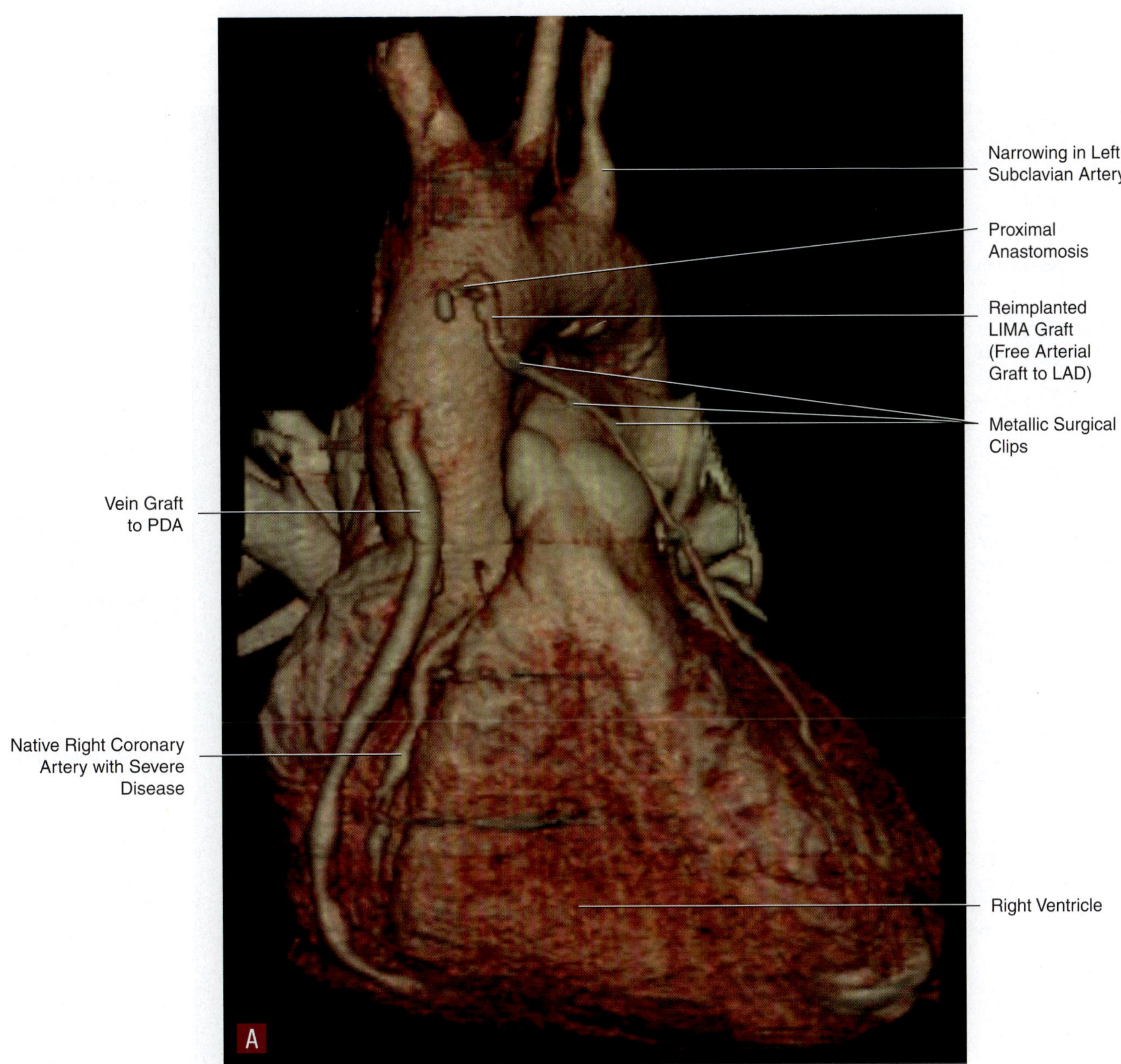

Figure 13.68. CT 3D volume-rendered image. **A**, Narrowing in left subclavian artery led to LIMA being removed and reattached to ascending aorta (free arterial graft). Note severe disease in native right coronary necessitating a vein graft to PDA. **B**, Lateral view again demonstrates narrowing in native left subclavian artery. Note additional graft segment has been anastomosed to LIMA (Y-graft) with supply going to both the LAD and the obtuse marginal branch of the left circumflex. LAD, left anterior descending; LIMA, left internal mammary artery; PDA, posterior descending artery.

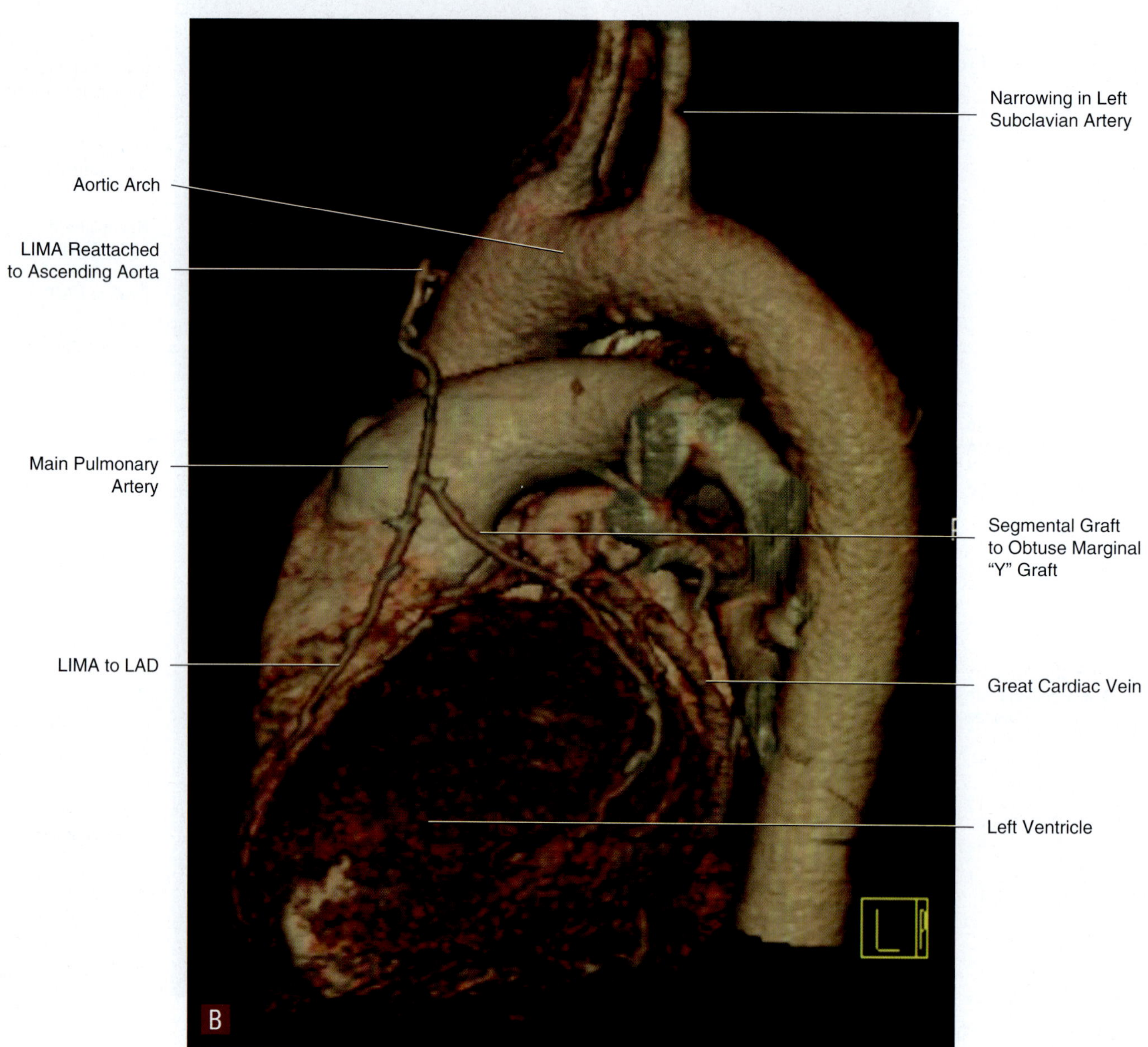

Figure 13.68. *Continued*

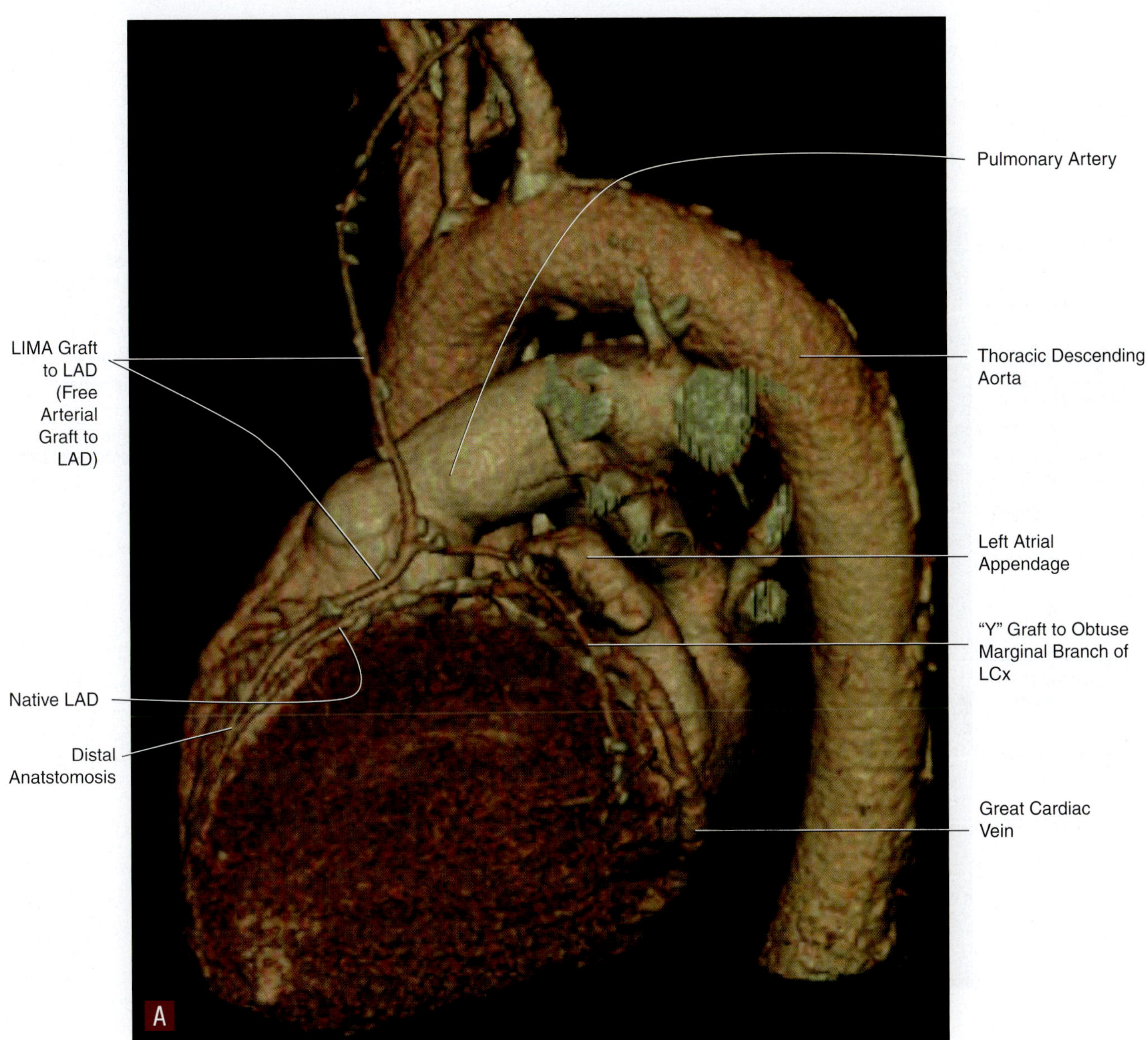

Figure 13.69. **CT 3D volume image.** Additional example of segmental grafts (or Y-grafts). **A**, LIMA goes to native LAD (note disease in proximal LAD) while additional branch goes from the mid portion of the LIMA to the left circumflex distribution obtuse marginal branch. **B**, Different patient, CABGx6, with a venous Y-graft, supplying a diagonal branch and an obtuse marginal branch, note also an occluded vein graft remnant at the anterior aspect of the ascending aorta. CABG, coronary artery bypass grafting; LAD, left anterior descending; LIMA, left internal mammary artery.

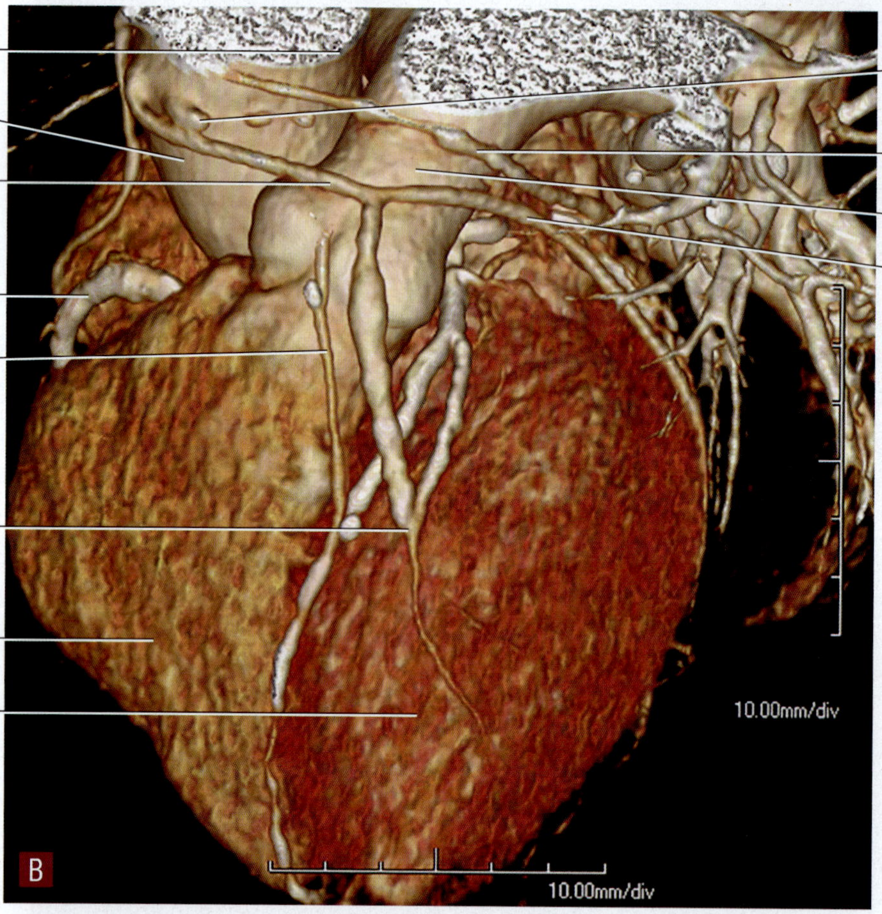

Figure 13.69. *Continued*

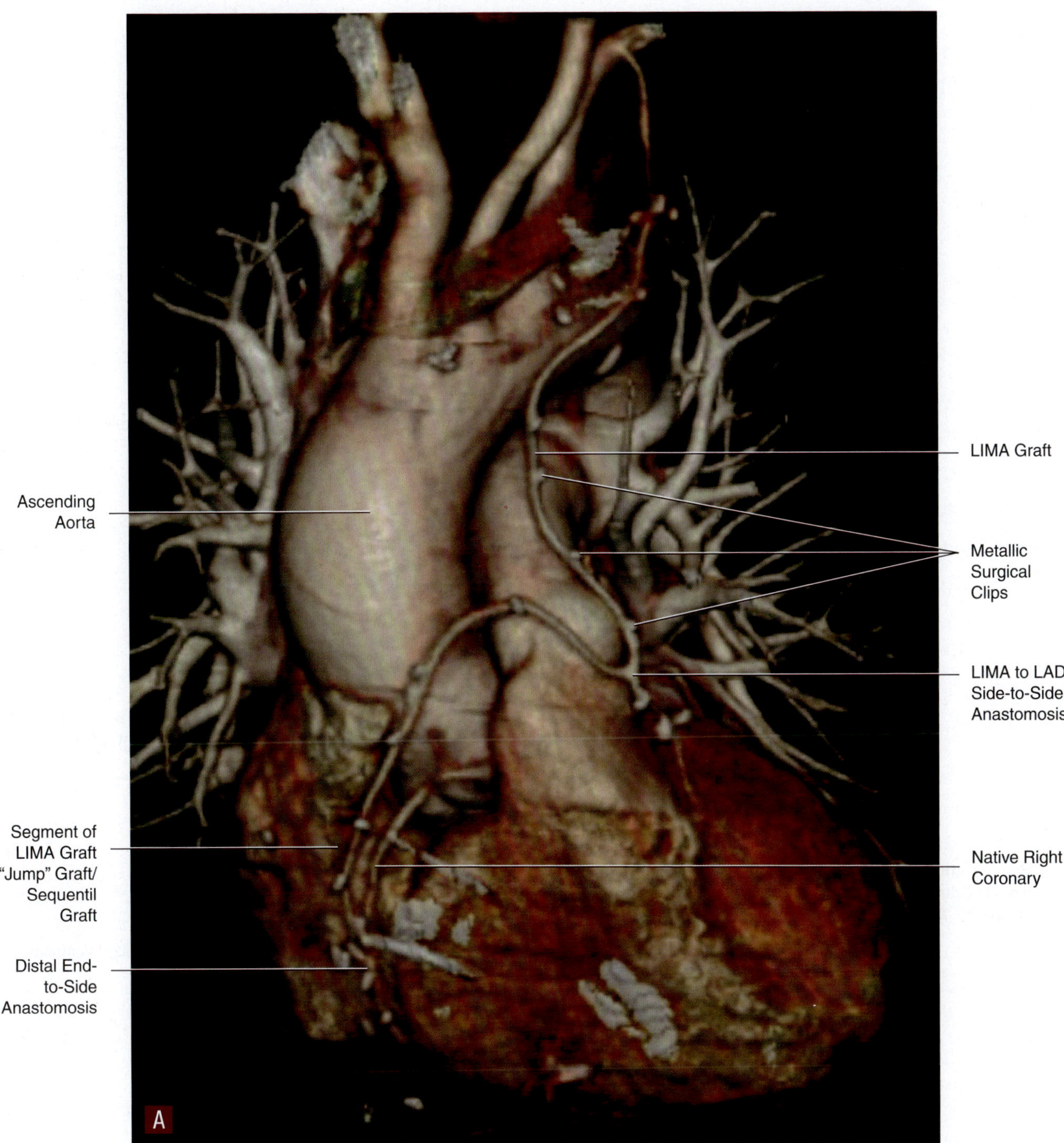

Figure 13.70. CT 3D volume image demonstrating the advantage of alternate methods of display. **A**, Standard 3D view shows LIMA appearing to form a side-to-side anastomosis with the LAD and then continuing to the right coronary. This configuration is sometimes called "sequential graft" or "jump graft." **B**, "Angio" display better delineates graft from its origin at the left subclavian artery to its two anastomoses. LAD, left anterior descending; LIMA, left internal mammary artery.

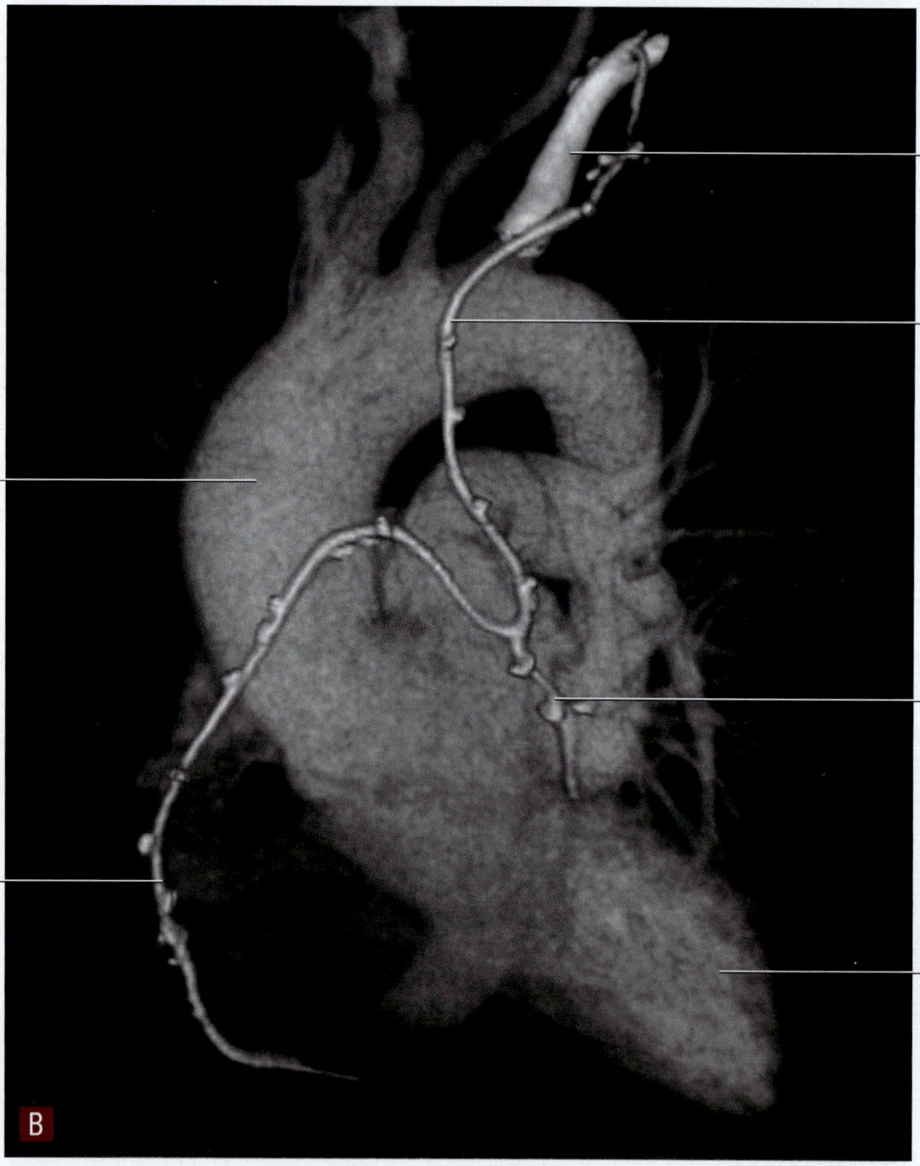

Figure 13.70. *Continued*

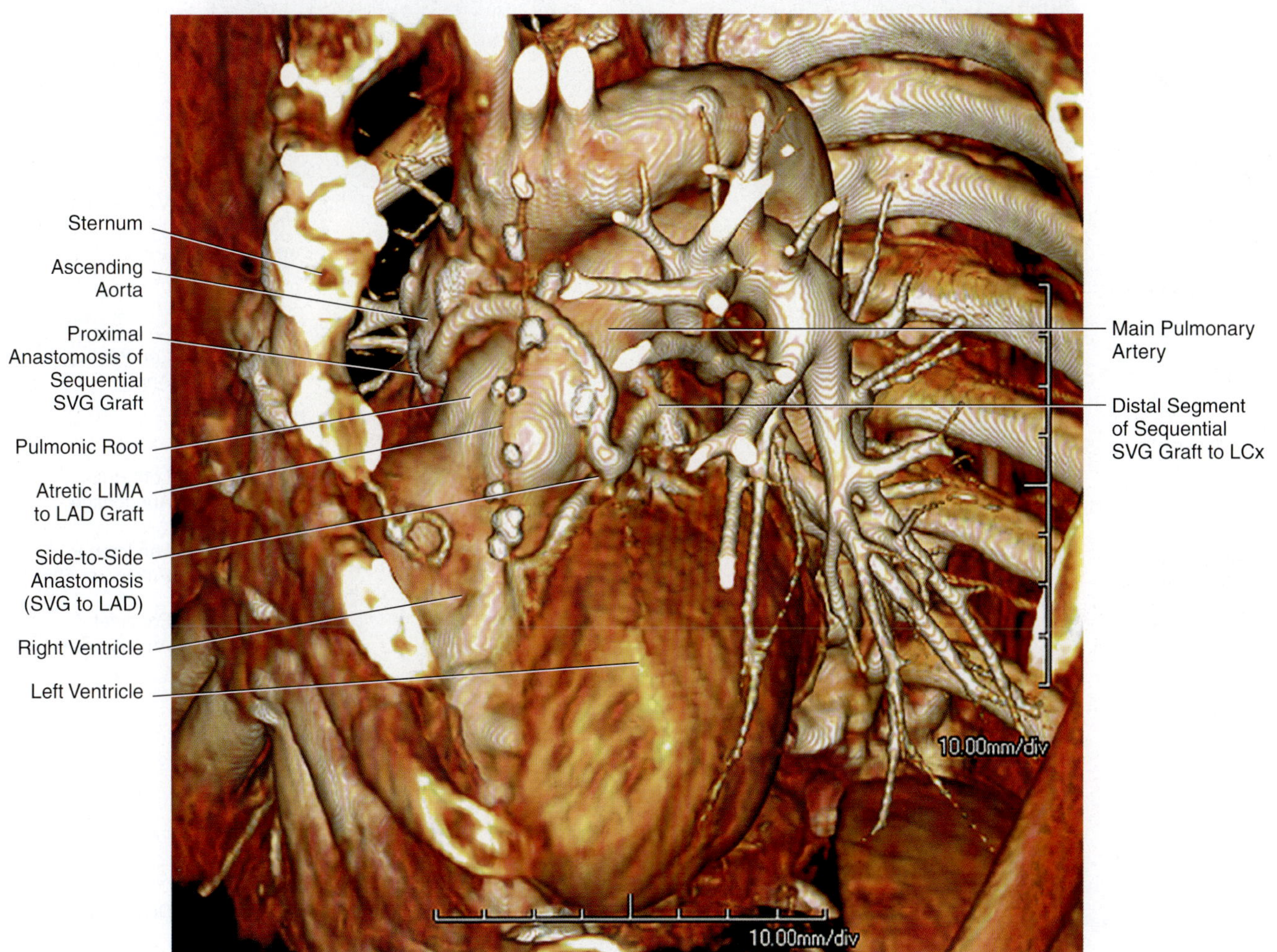

Figure 13.71. CT 3D volume-rendered image. Another example of a jump graft, only this time a vein graft "jumps" from the LAD to the LCX. LAD, left anterior descending; LCX, left circumflex artery.

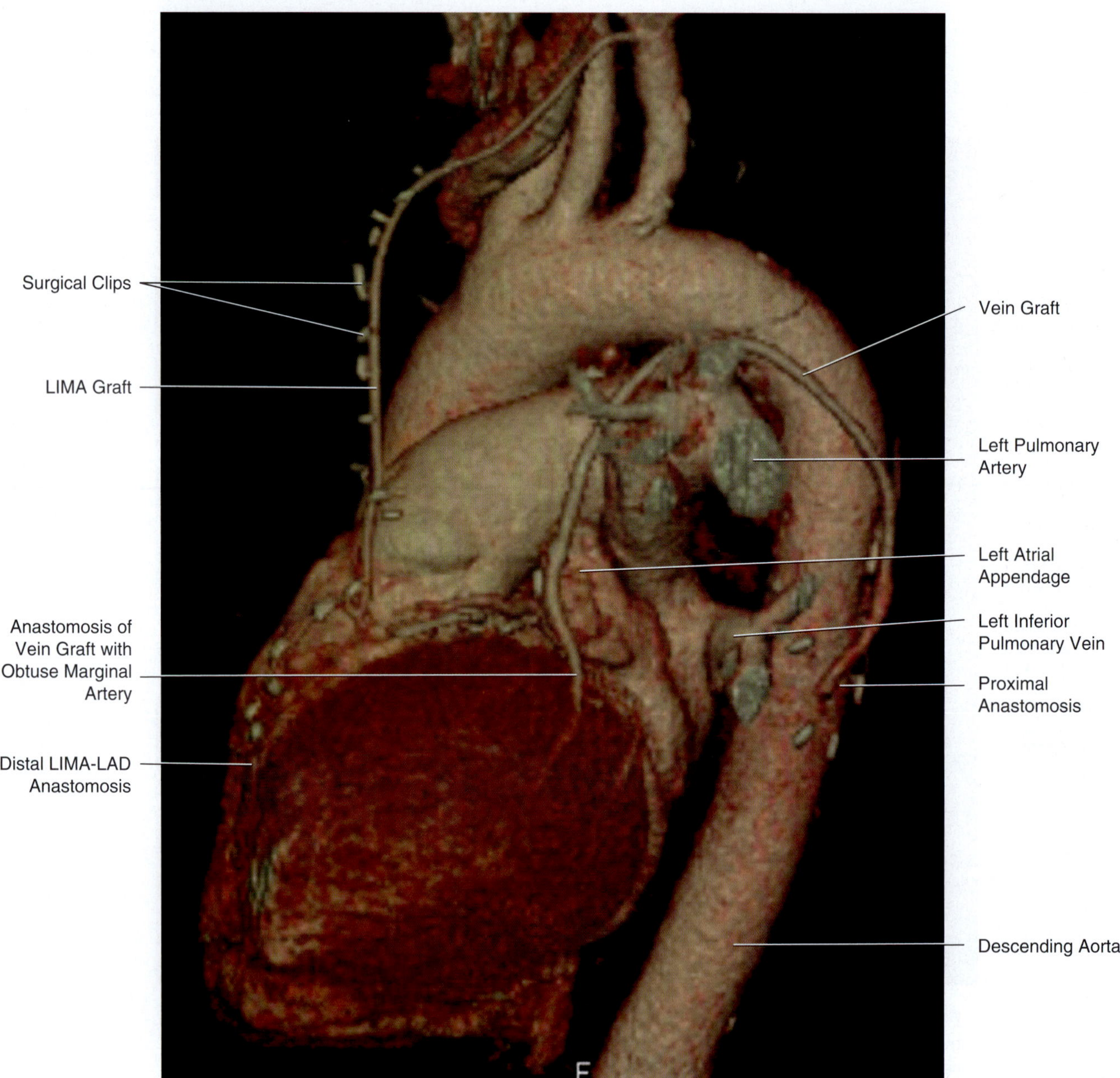

Figure 13.72. CT 3D volume-rendered image. Unusual variation with a vein graft arising from the descending aorta, passing over the left pulmonary artery and then anastomosing with an obtuse marginal branch of the circumflex artery. LIMA graft to LAD is also present. LAD, left anterior descending; LIMA, left internal mammary artery.

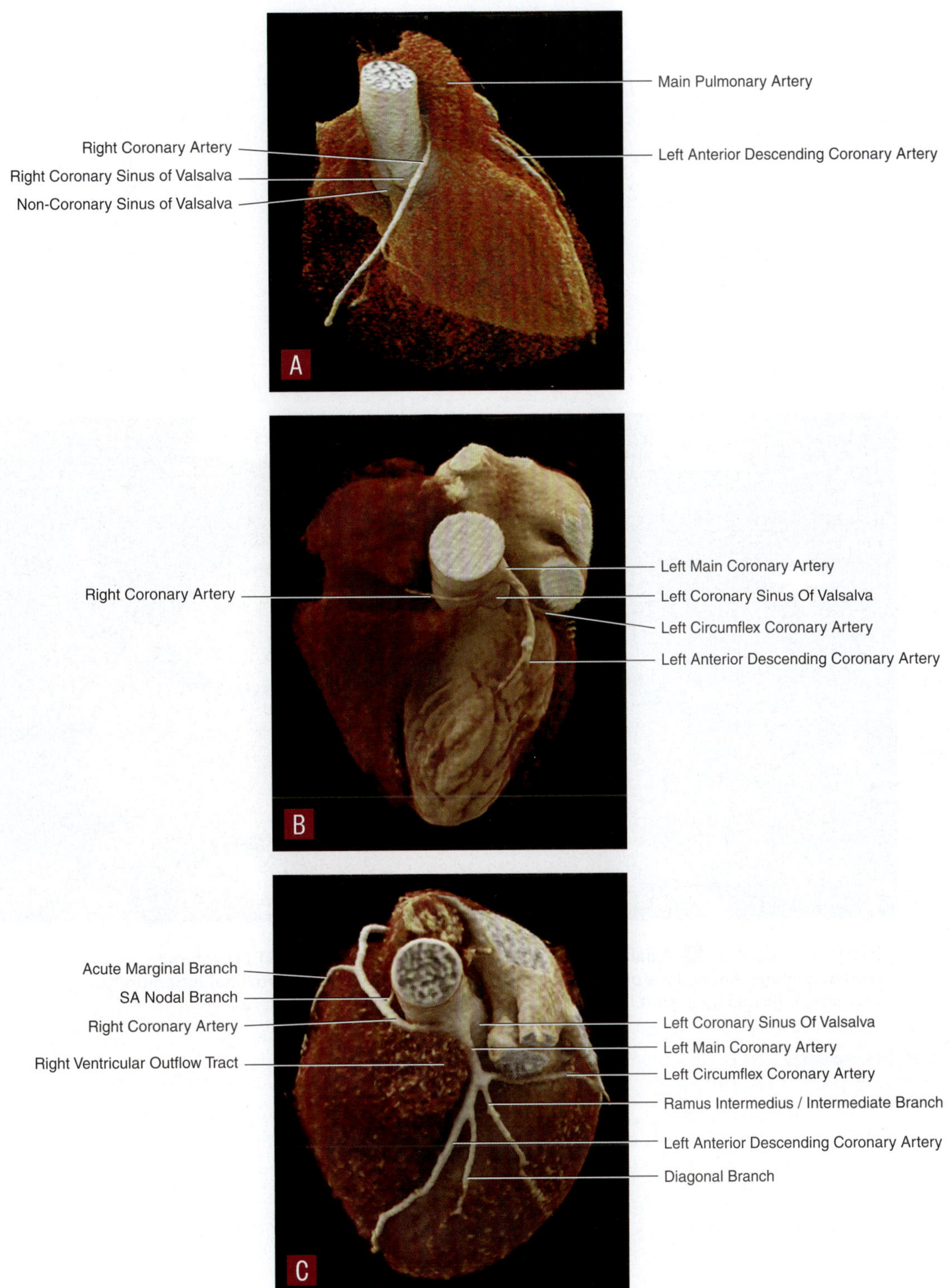

Figure 13.73. CT 3D volume-rendered cinematic images. Potentially "malignant" anomaly of RCA, originating in the left coronary sinus of Valsalva and coursing between the great arteries (interarterial course). A to C, They are different representations and orientations of the same patient's heart. RCA, right coronary artery.

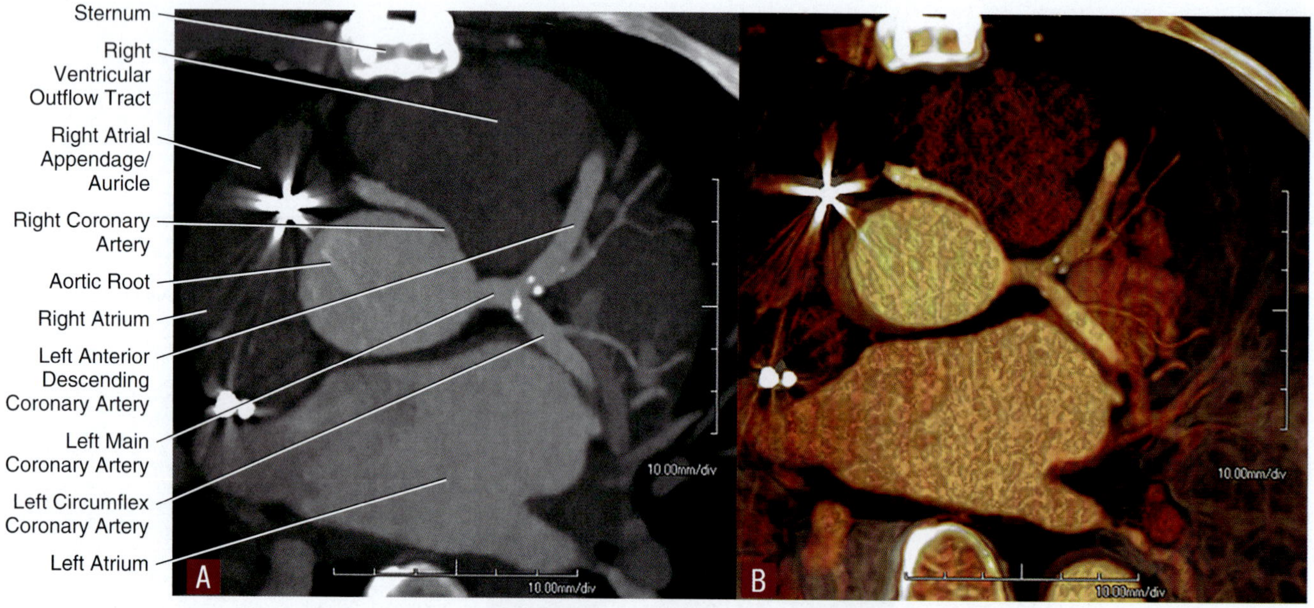

Figure 13.74. **A, Axial MIP (maximum intensity projection). B, CT 3D volume-rendered image.** Anomalous origin of the RCA from the left sinus, with proximal intramural segment, followed by a short interarterial course. RCA, right coronary artery.

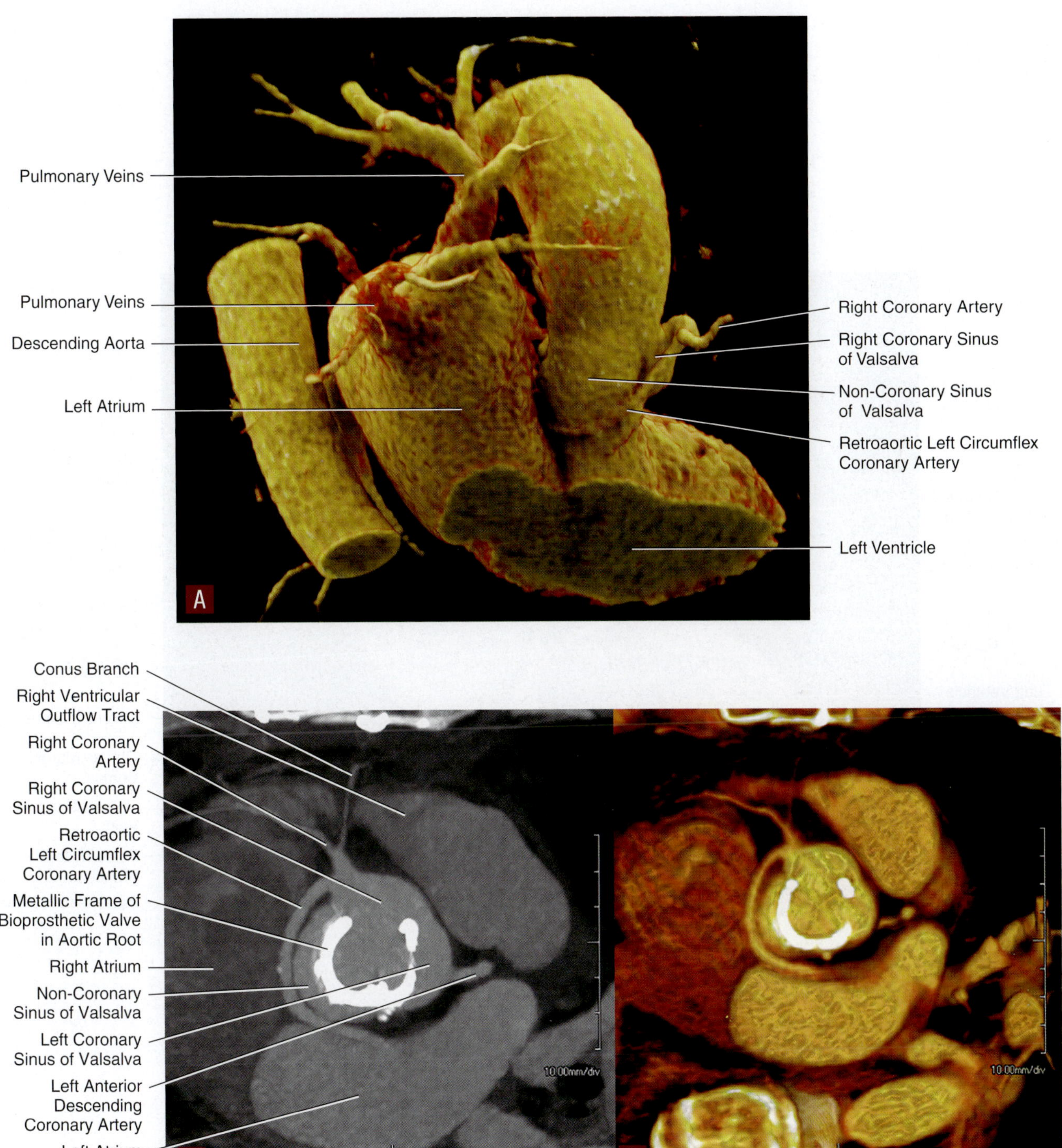

Figure 13.75. **Retroaortic left circumflex coronary artery, a benign anomaly.** **A**, CT 3D volume-rendered cinematic image from an oblique posterior vantage point. **B**, Axial maximum intensity projection (MIP). **C**, 3D volume-rendered axial slab.

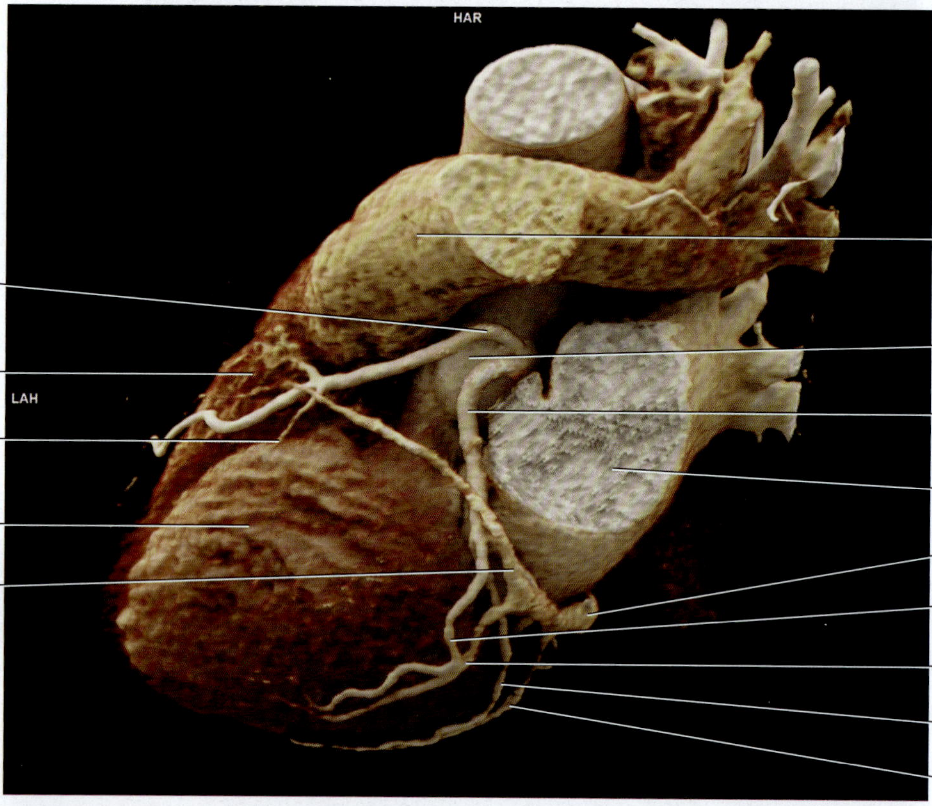

Figure 13.76. **CT 3D volume-rendered cinematic image.** Separate origins of LAD and LCX, both from the left coronary sinus of Valsalva, another benign anomaly. LAD, left anterior descending; LCX, left circumflex artery.

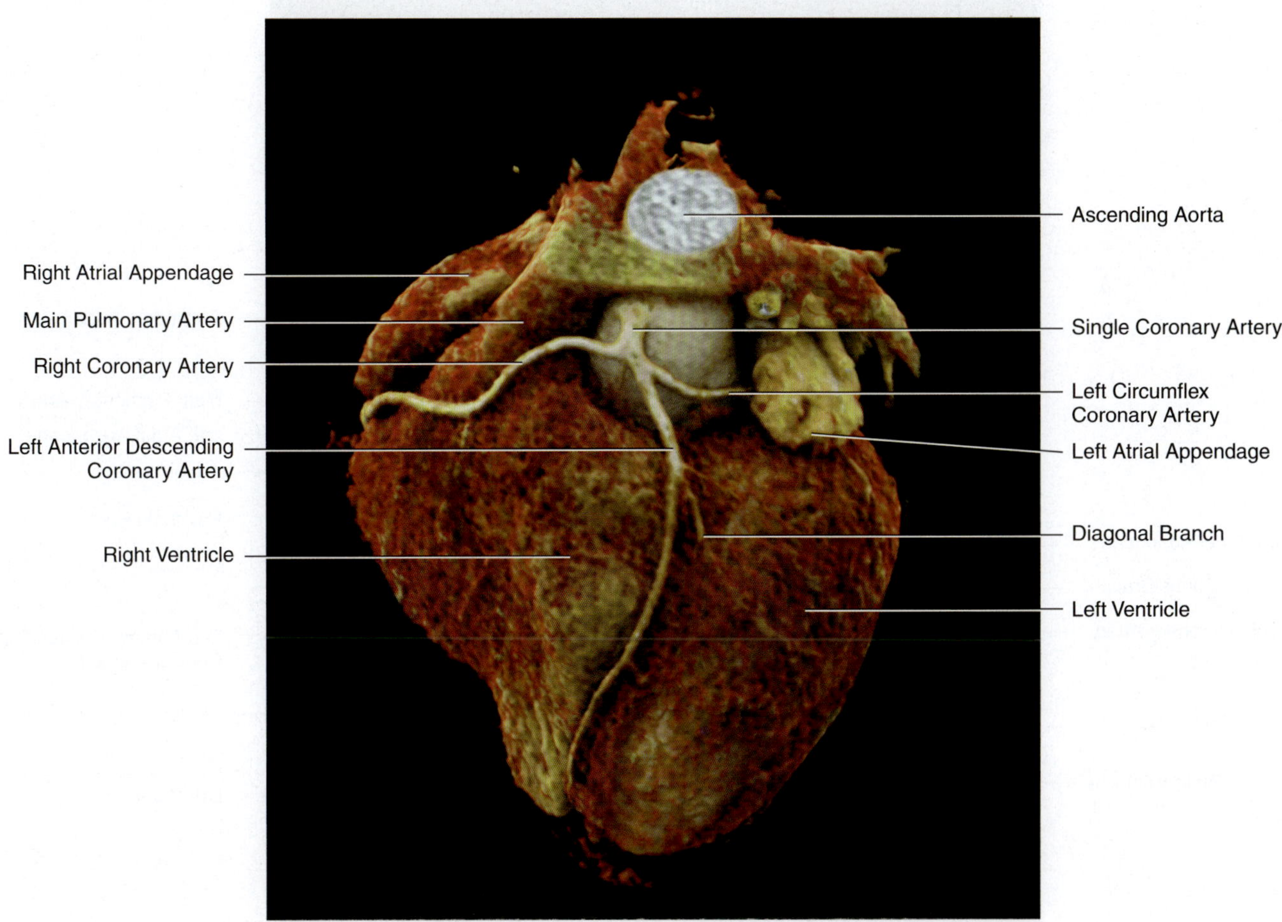

Figure 13.77. CT 3D volume-rendered cinematic image. Patient with history of D-transposition of the great arteries, status post arterial switch with LeCompte maneuver (pulmonary arteries draped over the ascending aorta). A single coronary artery is present, which originates in the ascending aorta.

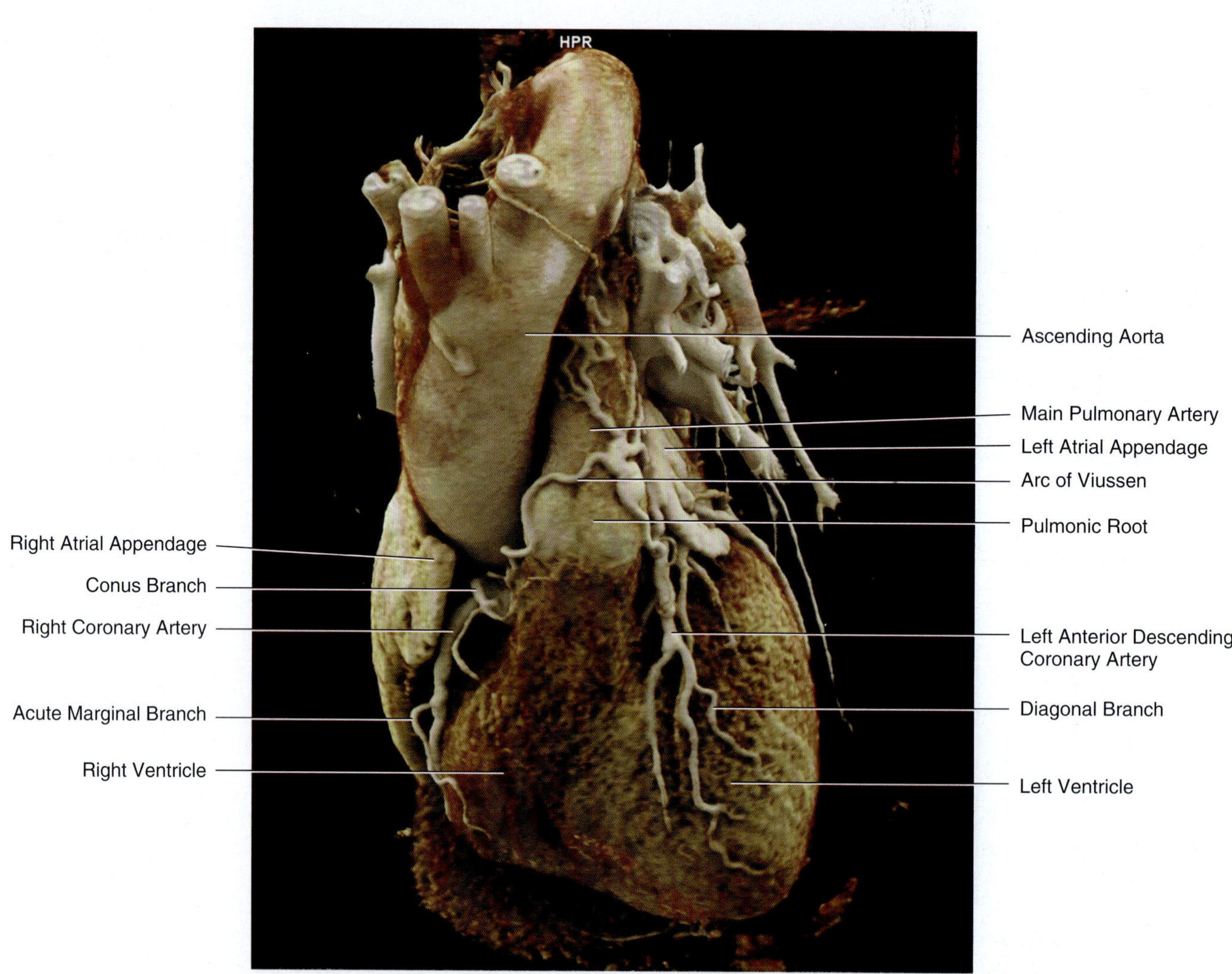

Figure 13.78. **CT 3D volume-rendered cinematic image.** Arc of Vieussens, an unusual communication between the left and right coronary systems.

14

Cardiac Veins

The human heart has three systems of veins: the left ventricular, the right ventricular, and the Thebesian veins. These are separate but intercommunicating systems.

The left ventricular system drains most of the left ventricular venous blood and is formed by the anterior interventricular vein, the great cardiac vein, the left marginal veins (a.k.a. lateral veins), the middle cardiac vein, and the right marginal vein (a.k.a. small cardiac vein) (Fig. 14.1). The anterior interventricular vein ascends parallel to the left anterior descending (LAD) artery (Fig. 14.2) and enters the left atrioventricular sulcus, where it becomes the great cardiac vein (Fig. 14.3) and accompanies the left circumflex coronary artery. The great cardiac vein collects blood from the marginal and lateral veins and continues on to become the coronary sinus that empties into the right atrium (Fig. 14.4). The left marginal veins (also known as obtuse marginal veins or lateral ventricular veins) drain into the great cardiac vein (Fig. 14.5A). Some patients have distinct veins draining the inferolateral wall, called inferolateral or posterolateral veins, which typically empty into the coronary sinus (Fig. 14.5B and C). The posterior interventricular vein, or middle cardiac vein, that runs in the posterior interventricular sulcus, may drain into the right atrium directly or into the coronary sinus. The right marginal vein (or small cardiac vein) drains into the coronary sinus or directly to the right atrium (Fig. 14.6). Note, all the above vessels are highly variable and not all branches are clearly identifiable in all hearts.

The right ventricular veins are known as the anterior cardiac veins and are two to four long veins crossing the anterior surface of the right ventricle and draining directly into the right atrium.

The small Thebesian veins drain directly into the right atrium and right ventricle and are difficult to visualize with clinical imaging.

The coronary sinus is becoming increasingly important in the clinical practice of medicine, as it is a commonly used conduit for the placement of left ventricular pacemaker leads and other electrophysiologic leads. During angiography, a catheter is directed into the right atrium and then into the coronary sinus. The tip of the lead, however, is most commonly placed into a vein on the surface of the left ventricle (eg, marginal or posterolateral vein) or the middle cardiac vein so that the lead tip is in close proximity to the myocardium itself. Lead tips are rarely effective in the coronary sinus or the great cardiac vein itself, as those run in the atrioventricular groove, and may not be in direct contact with myocardium.

Another noteworthy variant is a persistent left-sided superior vena cava, which most commonly empties into the coronary sinus, leading to an unusually large coronary sinus; however, this is considered a normal variant (Fig. 14.7).

A number of structures can be present in the inferior aspect of the right atrium, at the junction of the inferior vena cava and at the ostium of the coronary sinus. There is typically a semilunar valve at the entrance of the inferior vena cava to the right atrium, known as the eustachian valve (Fig. 14.8). In a cadaveric study by Klimek-Piotrowska, the eustachian valve had an average height of 4.9 ± 2.6 mm, with perforations present in 14%. The eustachian valve covers 22.9% ± 14.6% of the caval ostium, on average. The Thebesian valve can be found at the confluence of the coronary sinus with the right atrium (Fig. 14.9).

The Thebesian valve is an embryologic remnant of the right venous sinus valve and was present in 88.2% of cases, originating from the right margin of the coronary sinus ostium. It is on average 4.8 ± 2.9 mm in height, and most commonly appears as an endocardial fold attached to the ostium of the coronary sinus, covering 48% ± 36.6% of the ostium surface area, on average. A meshed or fenestrated Thebesian valve can also be observed, as well as a cord-type valve (Fig. 14.9). The Thebesian valve may be accompanied by a Chiari network, which is also an embryologic remnant of the right venous sinus valve (Fig. 14.10).

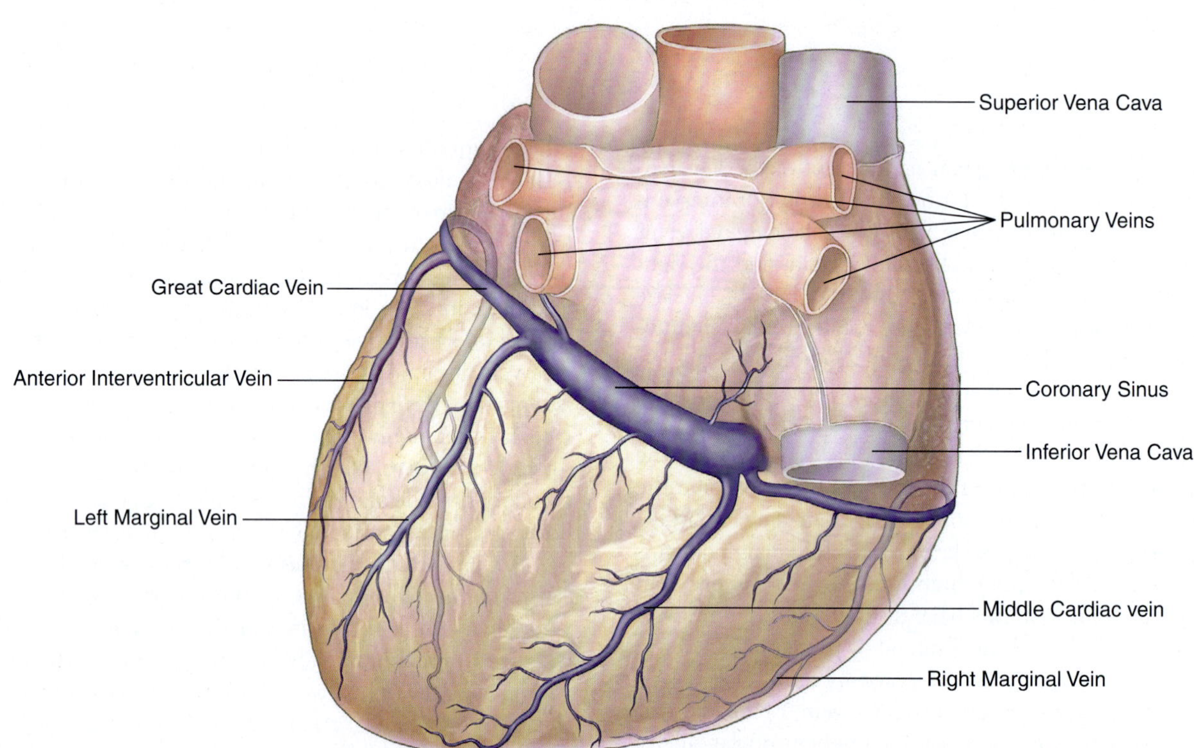

Figure 14.1. Distribution of the cardiac veins.

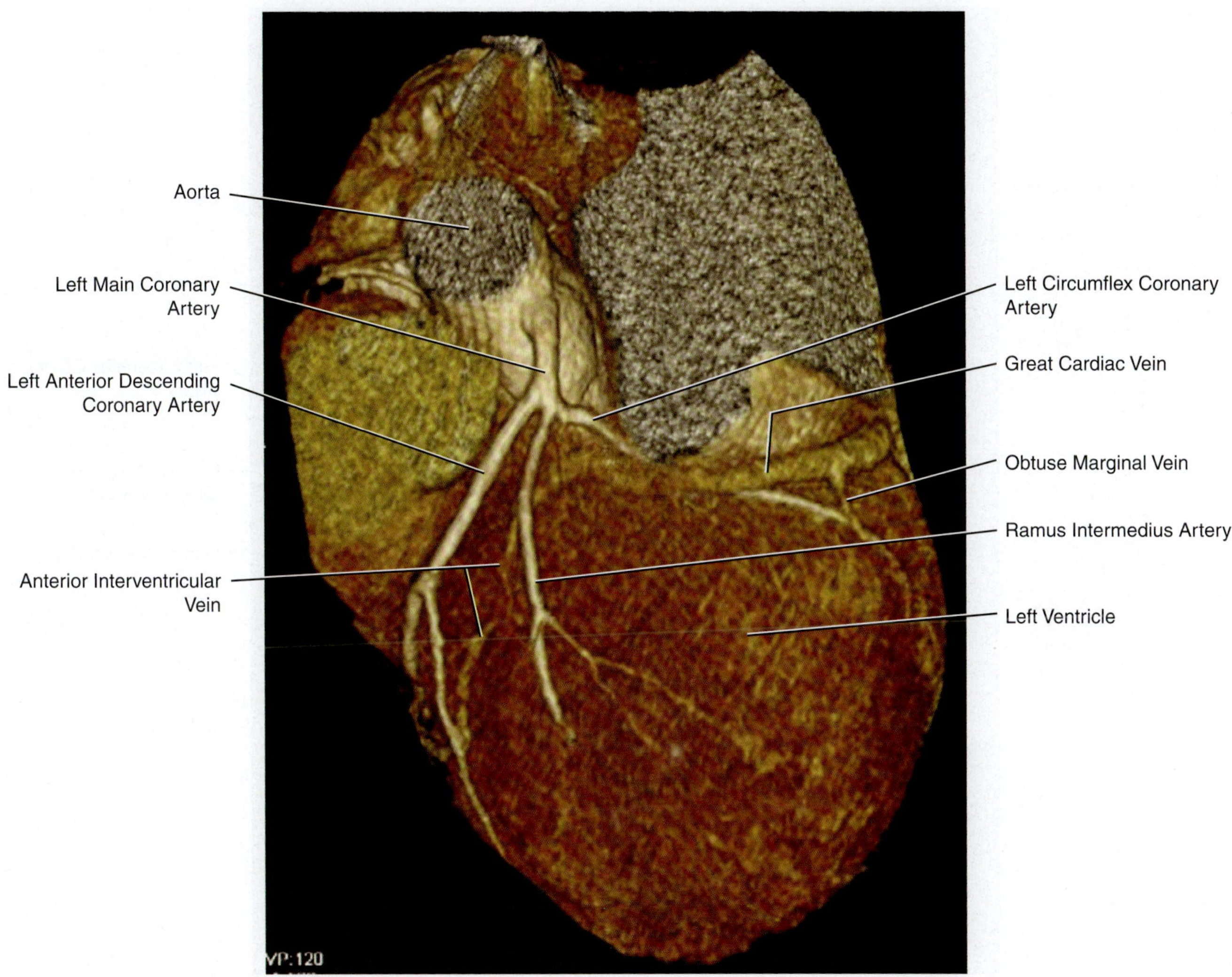

Figure 14.2. Anterior interventricular vein and other small veins emptying into the great cardiac vein. Note veins following the course of the coronary arteries.

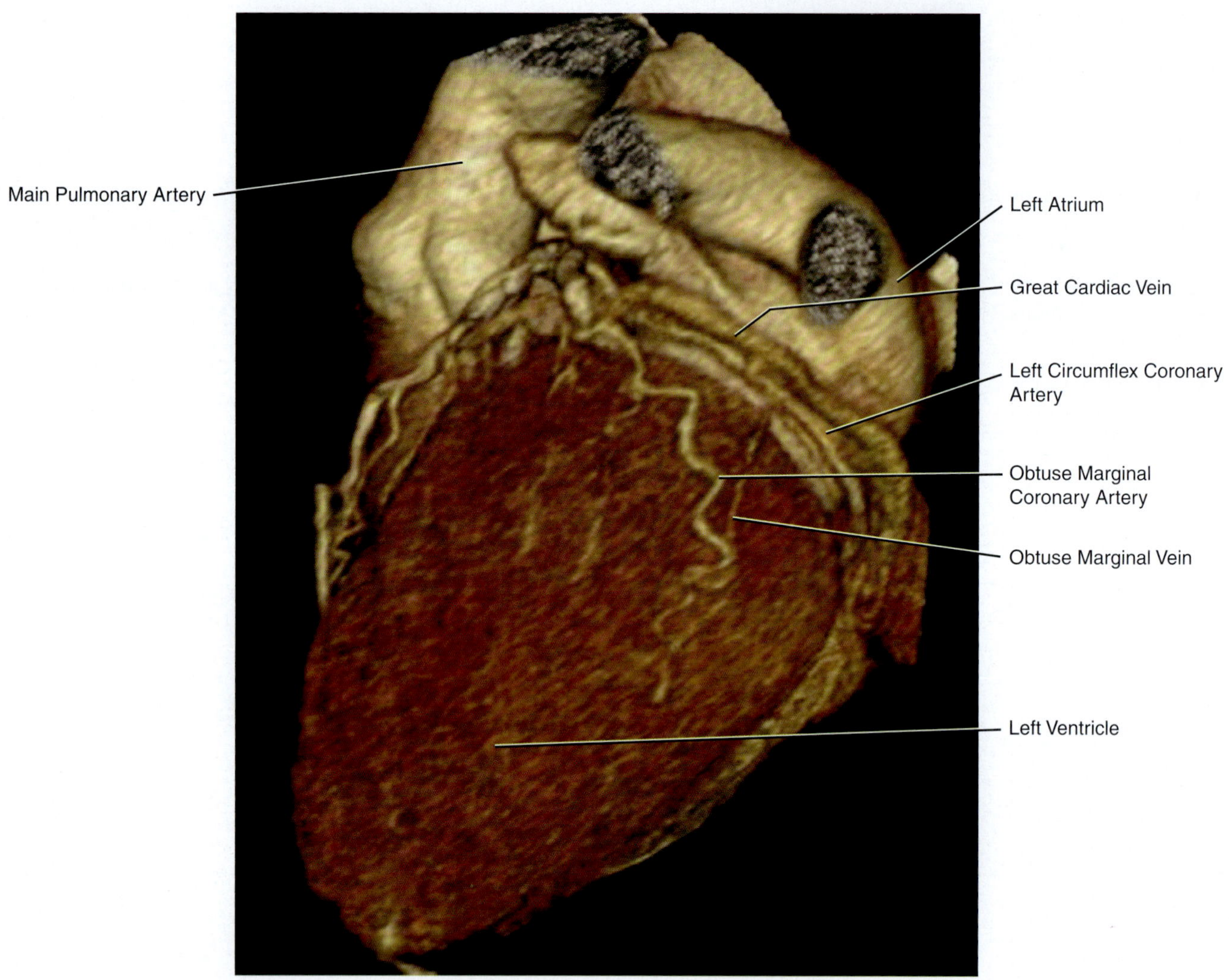

Figure 14.3. The great cardiac vein running in the left atrioventricular groove along with the circumflex coronary artery.

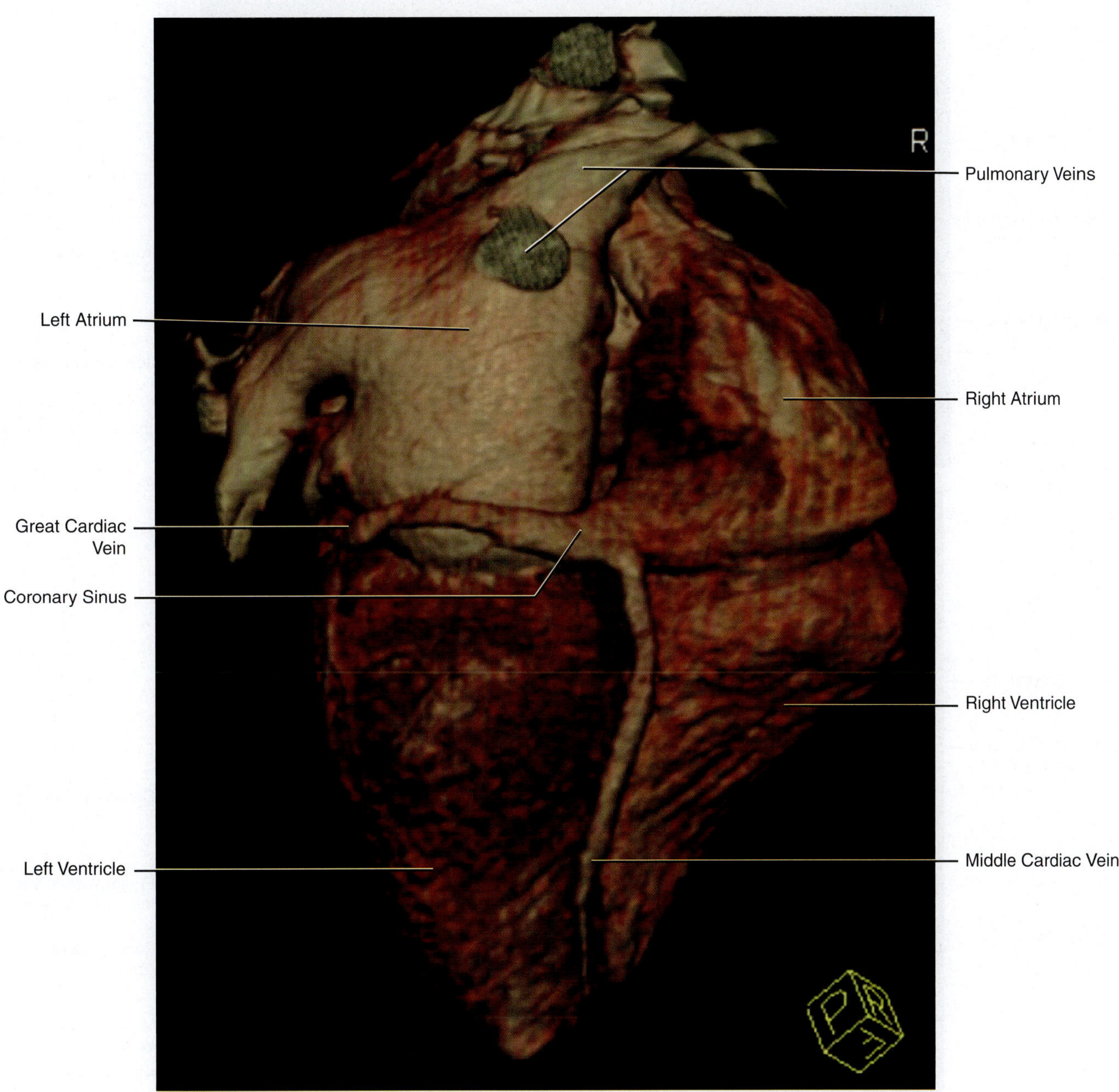

Figure 14.4. The coronary sinus as it enters the right atrium. Typically the sinus widens as it enters the right atrium.

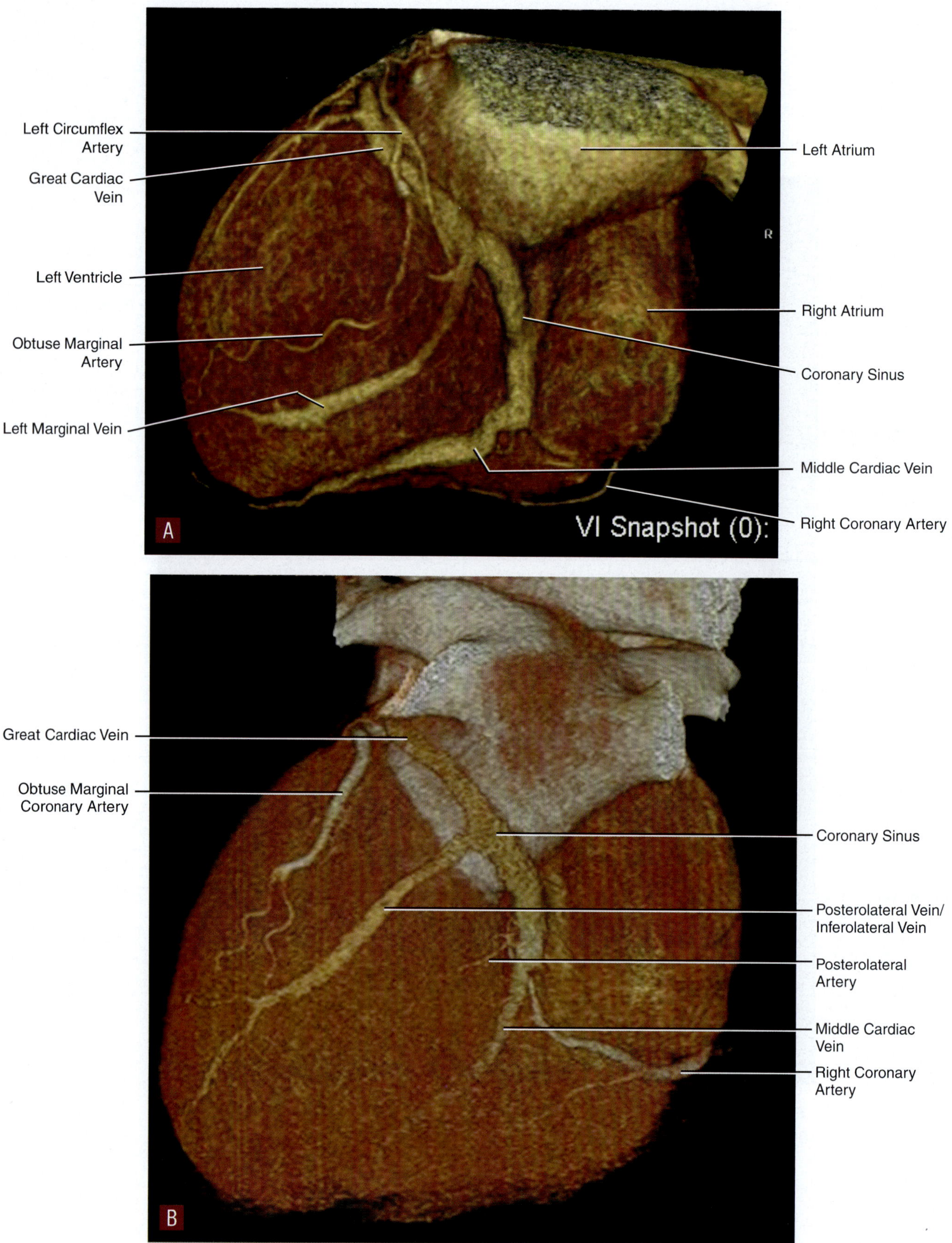

Figure 14.5. The left marginal vein running parallel to a large obtuse marginal branch artery (A). Posterolateral/inferolateral vein draining directly into the coronary sinus (B). Cinematic rendering, lateral view of the left ventricle showing obtuse marginal veins as well as posterolateral veins in the same view (C).

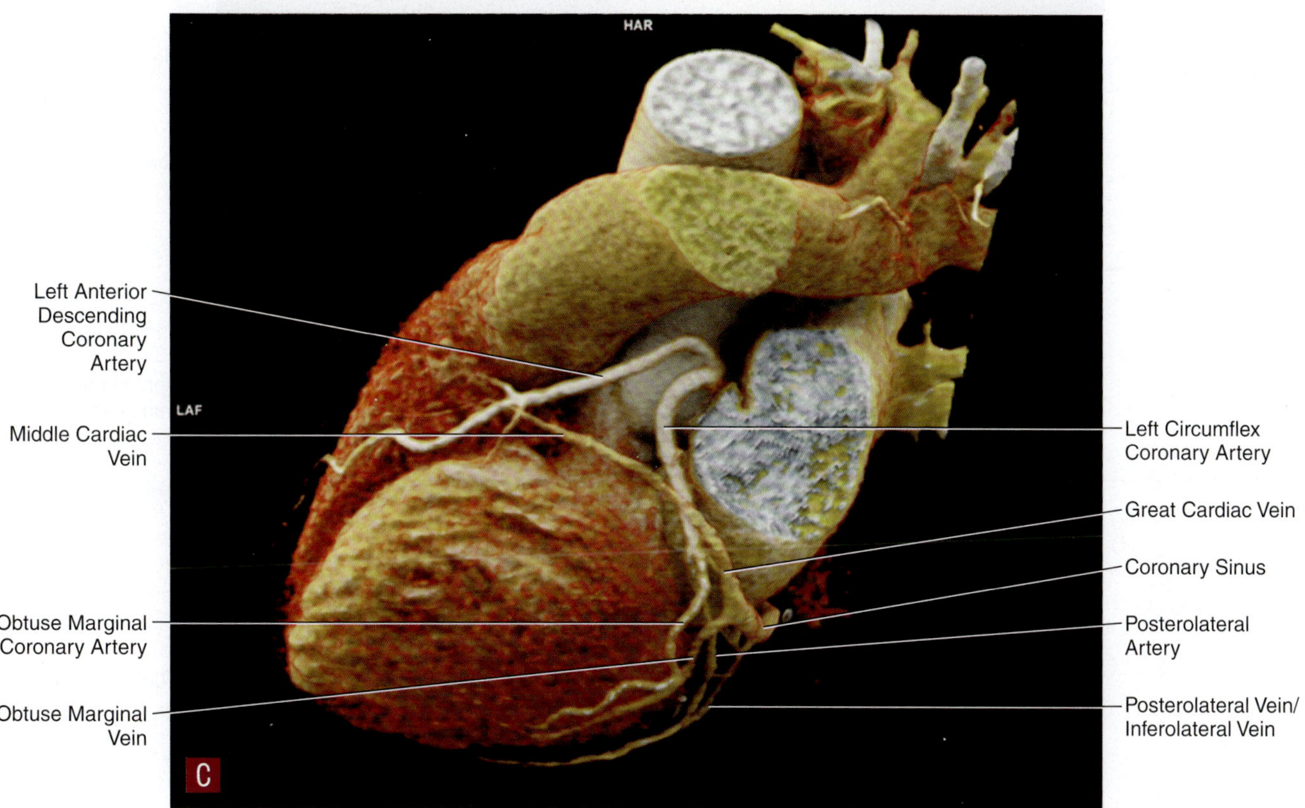

Figure 14.5. *Continued*

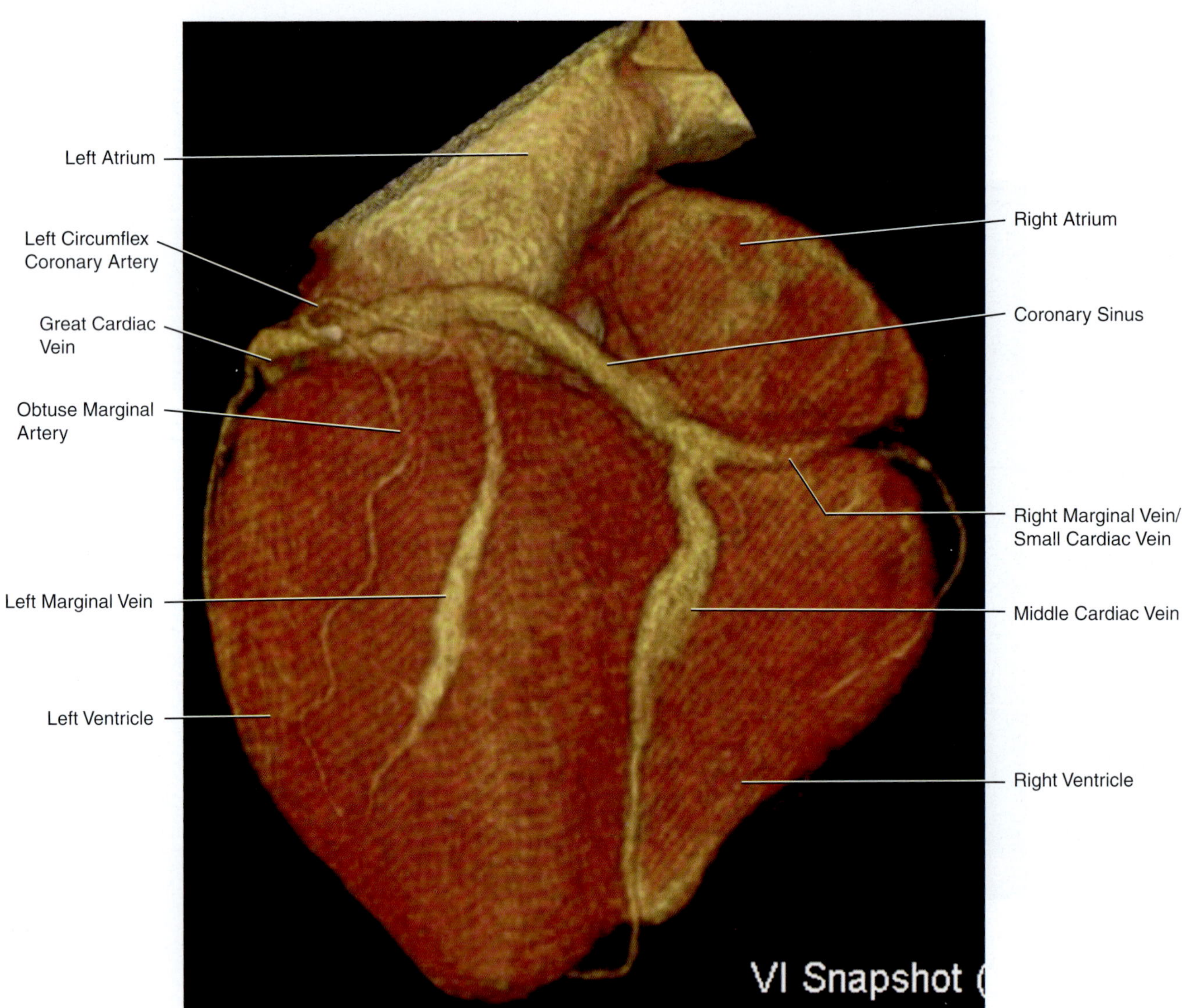

Figure 14.6. View from the bottom of the heart showing drainage of the right marginal (a.k.a. small cardiac vein), middle cardiac vein, left marginal, and great cardiac vein into the coronary sinus.

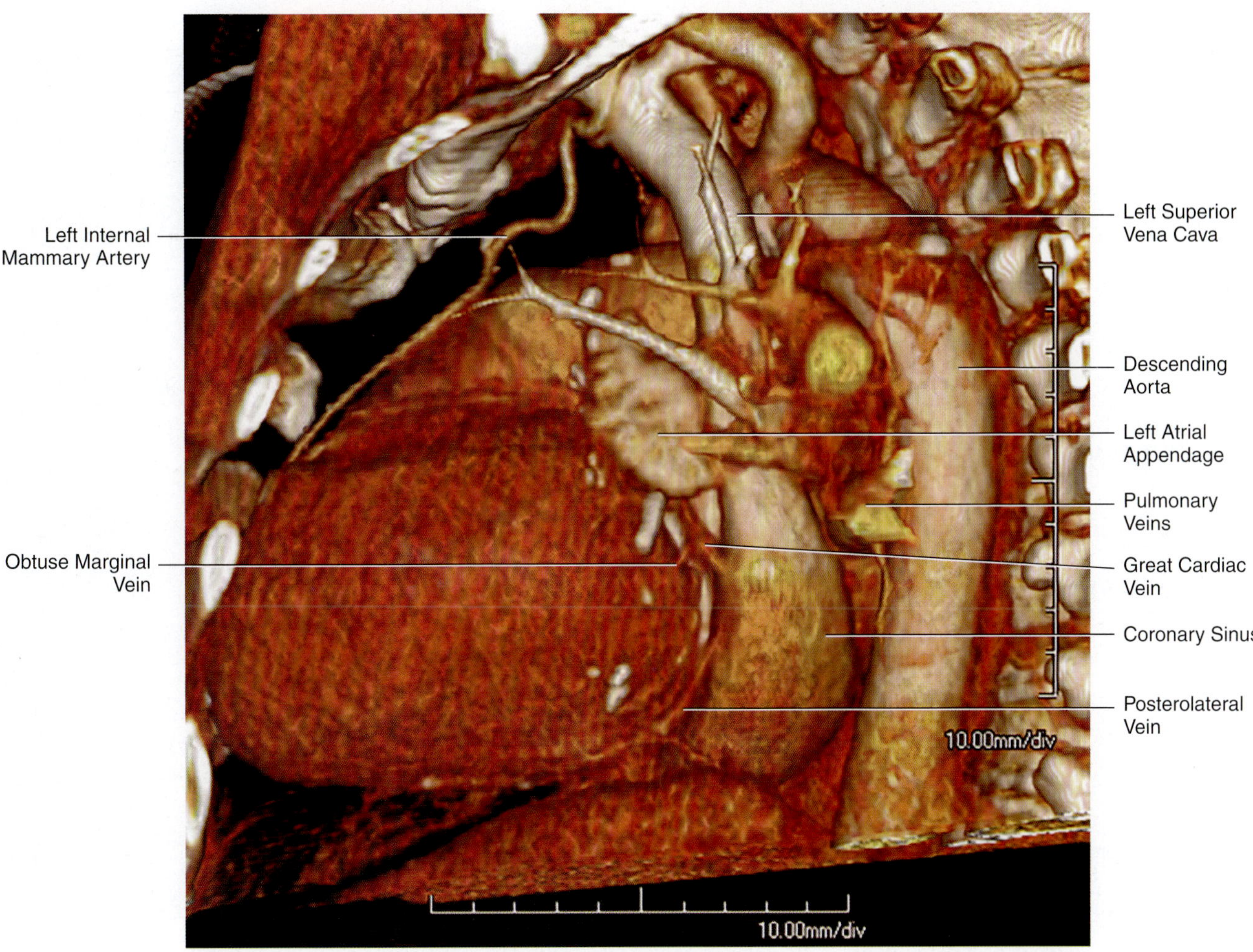

Figure 14.7. Left-sided superior vena cava draining into the coronary sinus. Note marked dilation of the coronary sinus.

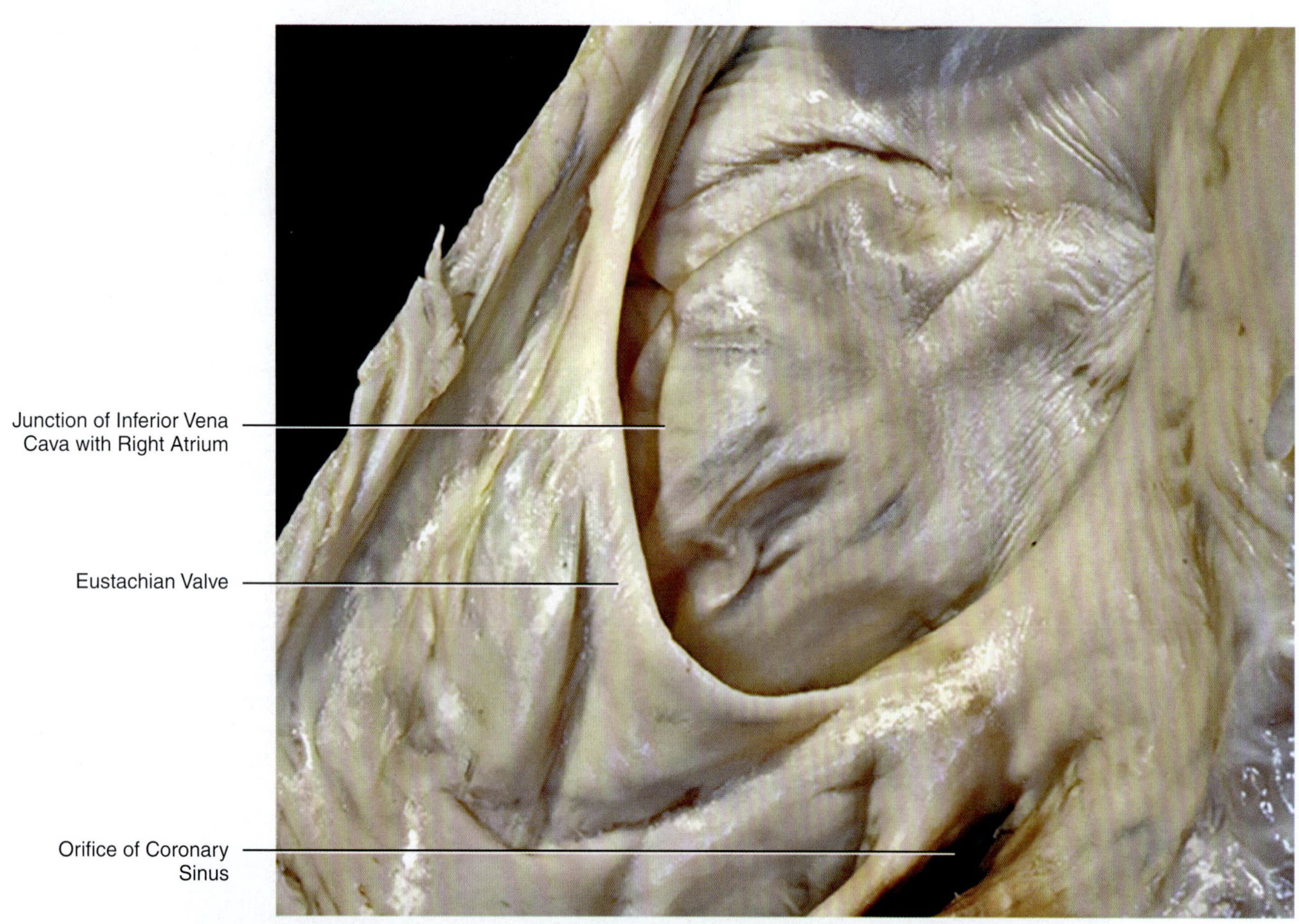

Figure 14.8. Cadaveric hearth specimen of the eustachian valve. (Image courtesy of Matheusz K. Holda, MD, PhD.)

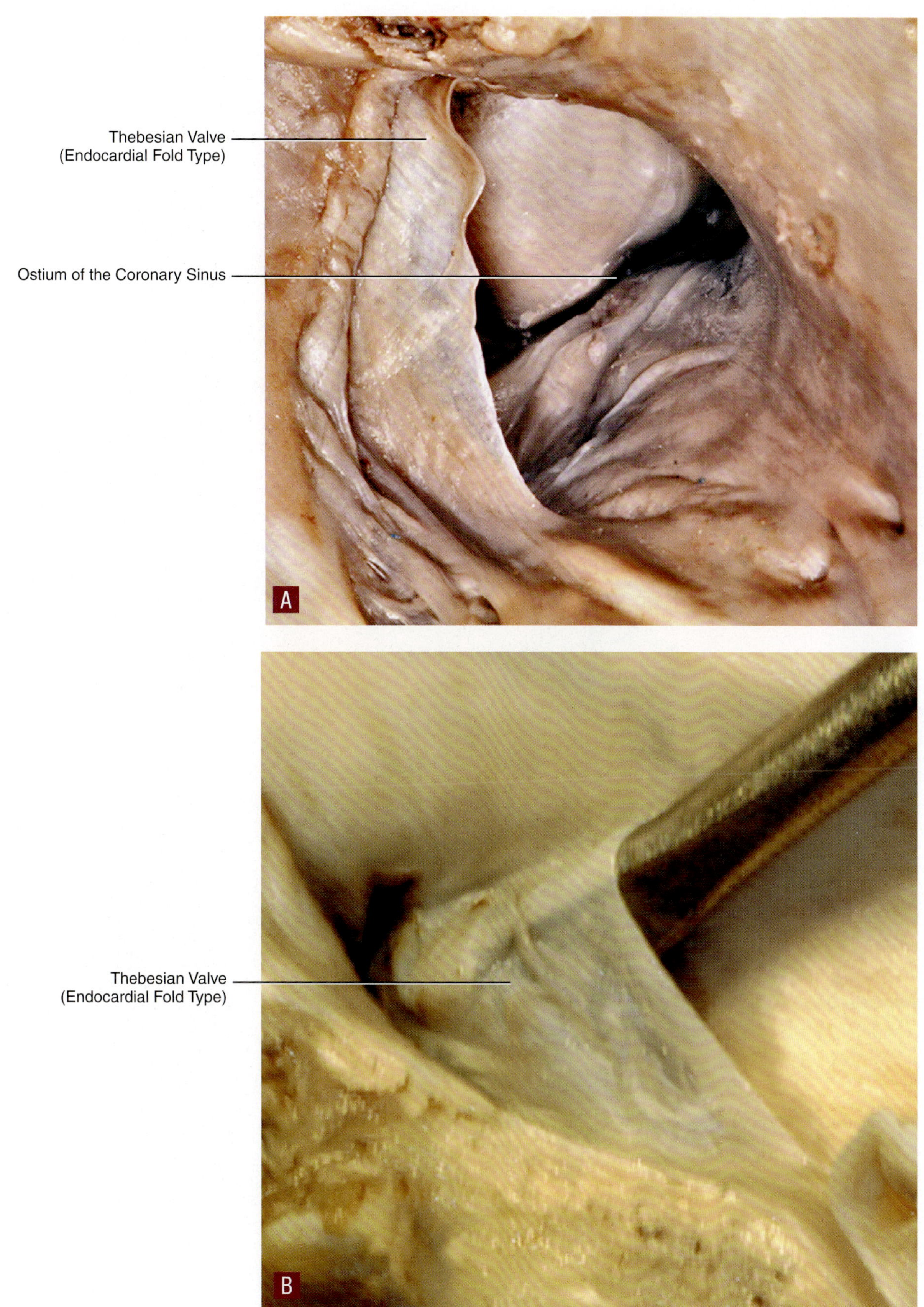

Figure 14.9. Cadaveric heart specimens showing the types of Thebesian valve morphology. The most common form is the endocardial fold (A), which can be very large (B). The mesh or fenestrated type can also be present (C), as well as the cord type (D). (Images courtesy of Matheusz K. Holda, MD, PhD.)

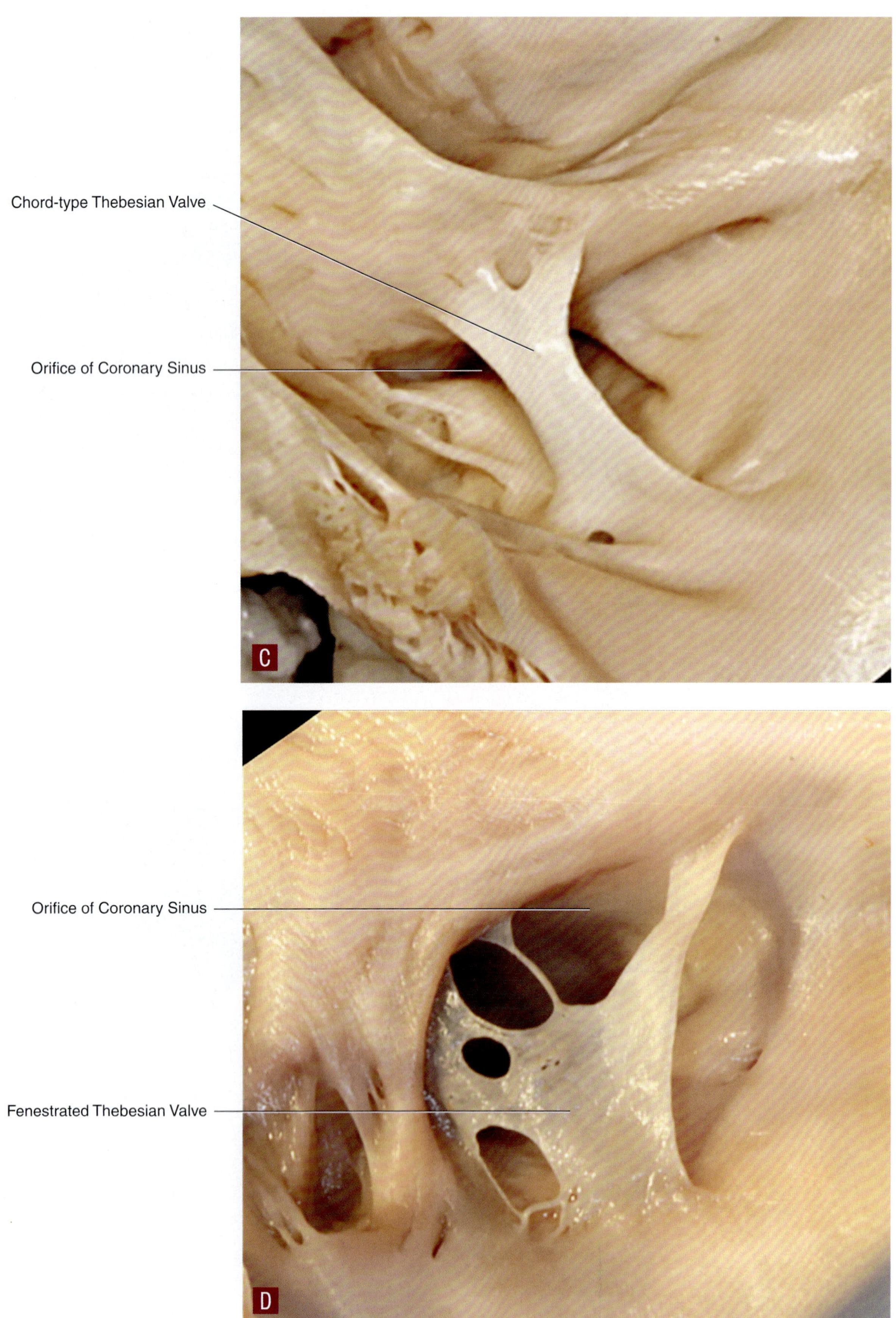

Figure 14.9. *Continued*

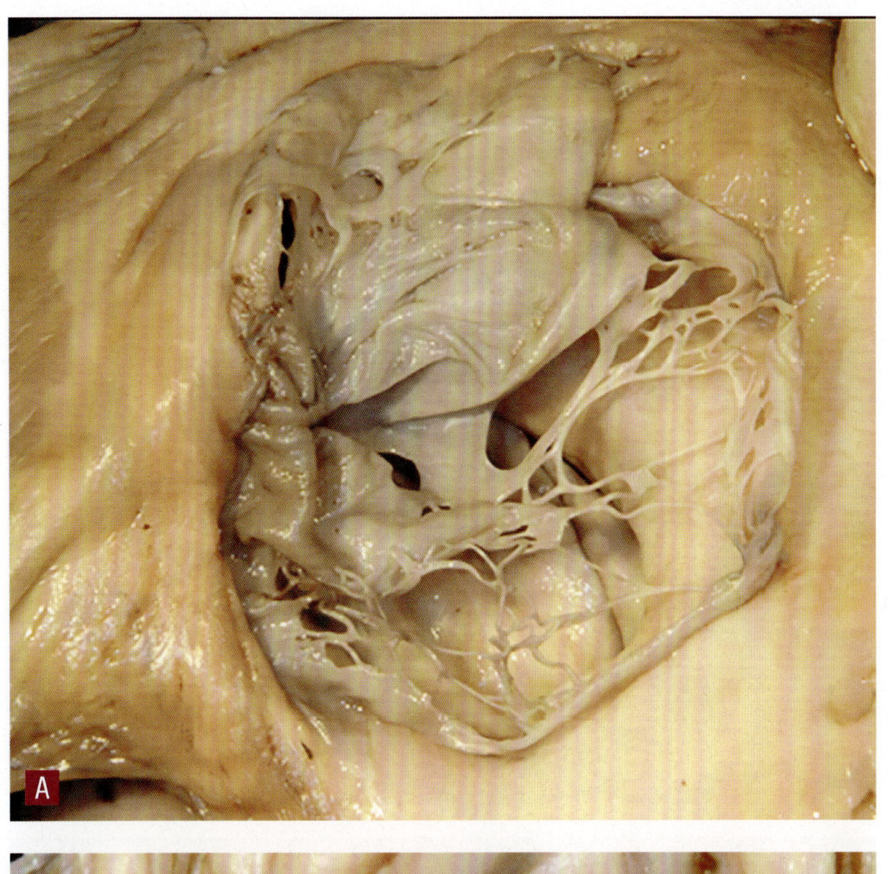

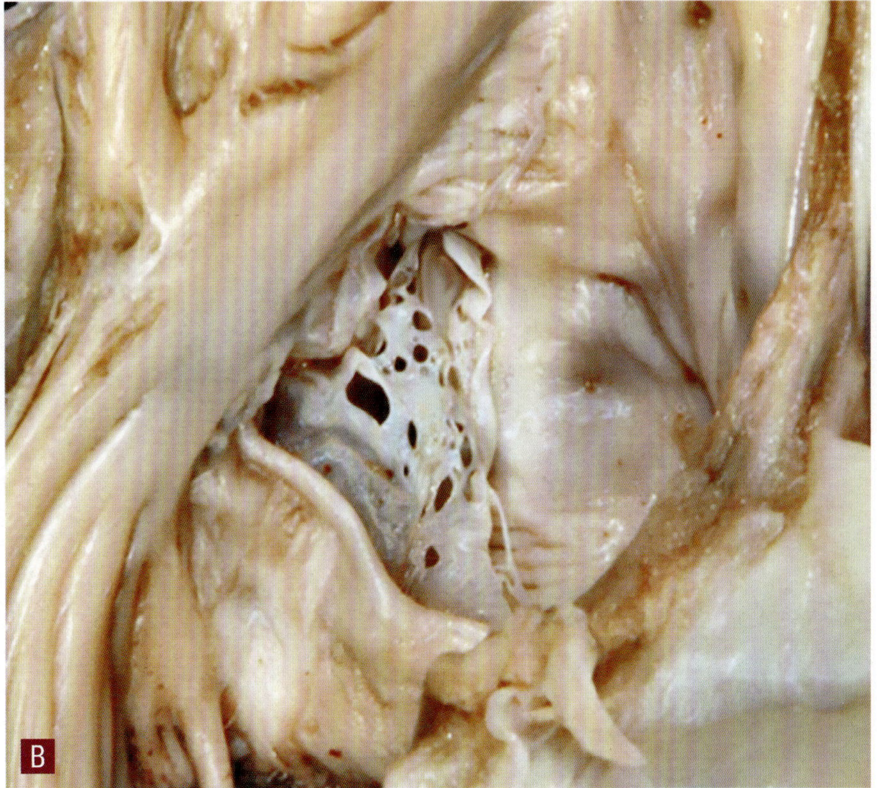

Figure 14.10. A to D. Cadaveric heart specimens showing examples of the Chiari network. (Images courtesy of Matheusz K. Holda, MD, PhD.)

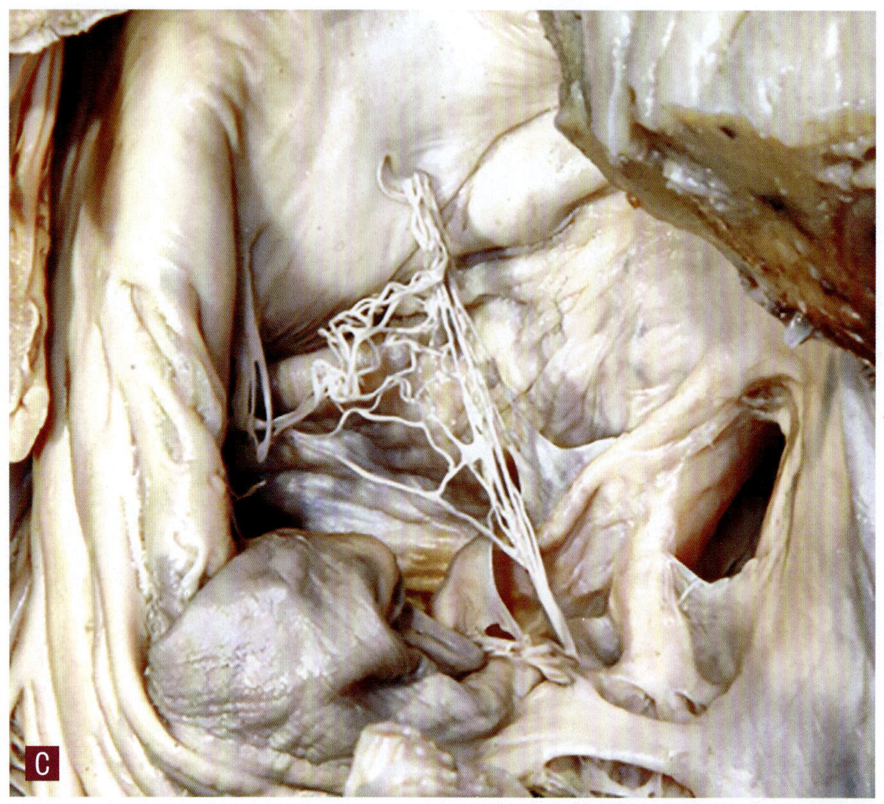

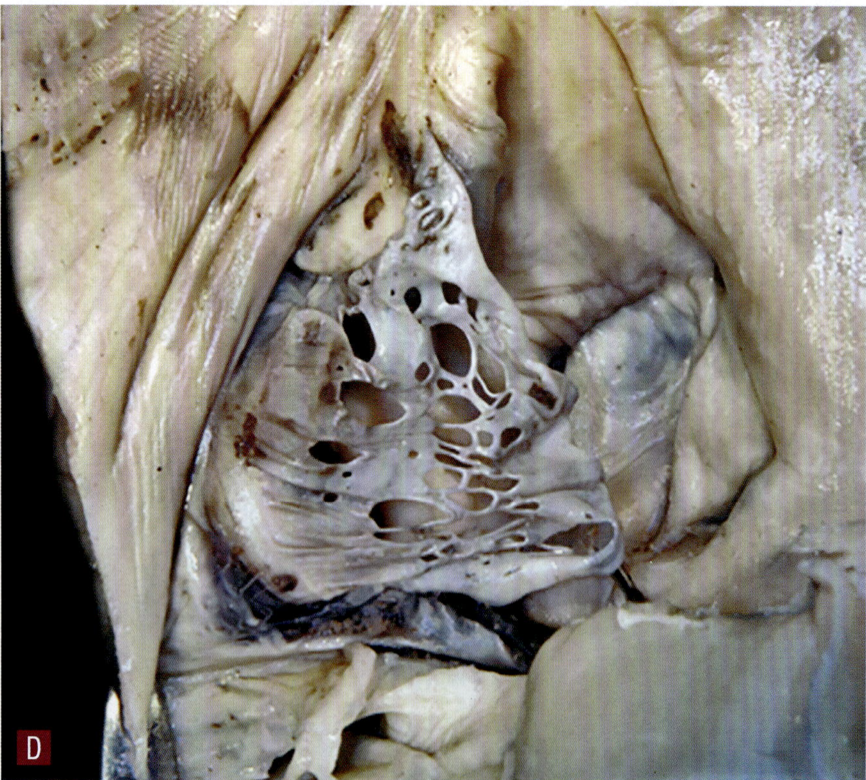

Figure 14.10. *Continued*

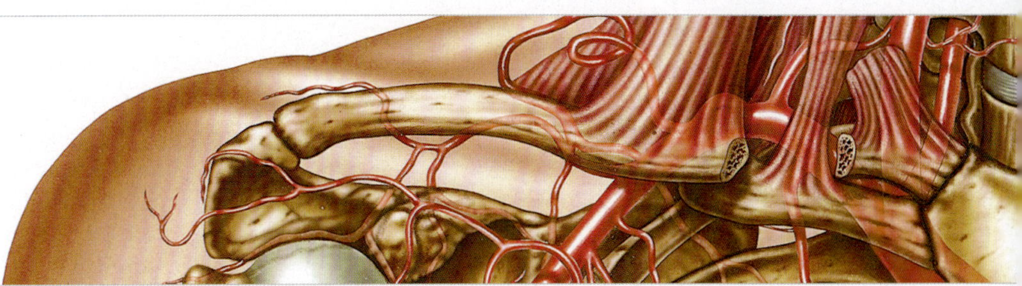

15

Arteries of the Upper Extremity

The right subclavian artery arises from the division of the brachiocephalic trunk (part I), behind the right sternoclavicular joint passing upward behind the scalenus anterior muscle (part II), and coursing horizontally slightly downward to the outer border of the first rib (part III), about the origin of the superior thoracic artery (Figs. 15.1 and 15.2).

The left subclavian artery arises from the aortic arch, after the origin of the left common carotid artery at the level of the third and fourth thoracic vertebra, ascending in the direction of the neck and bending laterally crossing behind the left scalenus anterior muscle (part I), following the same pattern as that of the right subclavian artery on parts II and III.

Subclavian Artery

Branches

- Vertebral artery
- Internal thoracic artery (internal mammary artery)
- Thyrocervical trunk
- Superficial cervical artery
- Costocervical trunk
- Dorsal scapular artery

Vertebral Artery

This artery is described in the head and neck section (Chapter 2).

Internal Thoracic Artery (Internal Mammary Artery)

This artery arises within 2 cm of the origin of the subclavian artery. It courses forward and downward behind the cartilages of the upper ribs and divides into the musculophrenic and superior epigastric arteries at the level of the sixth intercostal space (Figs. 15.3-15.5). The internal thoracic, anterior intercostal, thoracoacromial, and lateral thoracic arteries constitute the main arterial supply to the breast. More recently, authors have described a segmental pattern of blood supply to the breast with the internal thoracic artery nourishing the medial and central breast parenchyma (and the nipple areolar complex) through perforating branches from the upper four intercostal spaces, which anastomose with branches from the lateral thoracic artery, although perforators can also arise from the fifth and sixth anterior intercostal spaces (Fig. 15.6). Cadaveric dissections by van Deventer et al. have shown that this segmental pattern of arterial supply to the breast is variable. The internal thoracic artery supplied the nipple areolar complex in all cases, whereas supply from the lateral thoracic artery was unpredictable. Perforating vessels that supply the nipple-areola complex, while unpredictable, emerge through the thoracic wall on a constant basis at the parasternal border, the submammary fold, and lateral thoracic wall along the pectoralis minor lateral border.

Branches

- Pericardiophrenic artery
- Mediastinal artery
- Pericardial branches
- Intercostal branches
- Perforating branches
- Musculophrenic artery
- Superior epigastric artery

Thyrocervical Trunk

The thyrocervical trunk arises from the first part of the subclavian artery and gives rise to three branches (Fig. 15.2).

Inferior Thyroid Artery (Figs. 15.7 and 15.8)

Branches

- Muscular branches
- Ascending cervical artery
- Inferior laryngeal artery
- Pharyngeal branches
- Tracheal branches
- Esophageal branches
- Large glandular branches
- Ascending (parathyroid)
- Descending (thyroid)

Variation: A bronchial artery may originate from the thyrocervical trunk (Fig. 15.9).

Suprascapular Artery

The suprascapular artery may be a branch of the subclavian or internal thoracic artery (Figs. 15.10-15.12).

Branches

- Suprasternal branch
- Acromial branch
- Articular branches
- Clavicle nutrients
- Scapula nutrients

Superficial Cervical Artery (Fig. 15.13)

This artery anastomoses with the superficial branch of the descending branch of the occipital artery.

Costocervical Trunk

The costocervical trunk arises from the back of the second part of the subclavian artery on the right side, but on the first part on the left side (Fig. 15.14).

Superior Intercostal Artery. The superior intercostal artery anastomoses with the third posterior intercostal artery. It may be supplied by a branch from the aorta.

Deep Cervical Artery. The deep cervical artery arises in most cases from the costocervical trunk but may be a branch of the subclavian artery.

Dorsal Scapular Artery (Figs. 15.15 and 15.16)

This artery arises from the third or second part of the subclavian artery.

Axillary Artery (Figs. 15.1-3, and 17)

The axillary artery is a continuation of the subclavian artery.

Proximal limit—outer border of the first rib.
Distal limit—lower border of the tendon related to the teres major muscle or muscle's tendon.

Branches

- Superior thoracic artery (highest)
- Thoracoacromial (acromiothoracic) artery
  - Pectoral branch
  - Acromial branch
  - Clavicular branch
  - Deltoid branch
- Lateral thoracic (lateral mammary branches)
- Subscapular artery
- Anterior circumflex humeral artery
- Posterior circumflex humeral artery

Superior Thoracic Artery (Highest Thoracic Artery or Arteria Thoracica Suprema)

The superior thoracic artery is a small vessel and arises from the first part of the axillary artery. It may branch from the thoracoacromial artery.

Thoracoacromial Artery (Acromiothoracic Artery) (Figs. 15.18-15.20)

Branches

- Pectoral branch
- Acromial branch
- Clavicular branch
- Deltoid branch (may arise from the acromial branch)

Lateral Thoracic Artery (External Mammary or Inferior Thoracic Artery)

This artery anastomoses with the internal thoracic, subscapular, and intercostal arteries and pectoral branches of the thoracoacromial artery. In females, it is larger and gives off lateral mammary branches reaching the superolateral aspect of the breast parenchyma.

Subscapular Artery (Inferior Scapular Artery)

This artery is the largest branch of the axillary artery. It anastomoses with the lateral thoracic, intercostal arteries and deep branch of the transverse cervical artery and supplies muscles of the chest wall.

Branches

- Circumflex scapular artery
- Infrascapular artery
- Lateral border of the scapula (dorsal thoracic artery)
- Muscular branches

Anterior Circumflex Humeral Artery

This artery is a small branch located anterior to the surgical neck of the humerus. It supplies the head of the humerus and shoulder joint and may have common origin with the posterior circumflex humeral artery.

Posterior Circumflex Humeral Artery (Figs. 15.2, 3, and 17)

This artery is larger than the anterior circumflex humeral artery, arises from the third part of the axillary artery, winds around the surgical neck of the humerus, and distributes branches to the shoulder joint, deltoid, teres major and minor, and long and lateral heads of triceps. The descending branch anastomoses with the deltoid branch of the arteria profunda brachii, the anterior circumflex humeral artery, and the acromial branches of the suprascapular and thoracoacromial arteries.

Alar Thoracic Artery (Variation). The subscapular, circumflex humeral, and profunda brachii arteries may arise as a common trunk (Fig. 15.21). The axillary artery may divide into radial and ulnar arteries or give off the anterior interosseous artery of the forearm. The radial artery may arise from the distal axillary artery (Fig. 15.20). The arteria profunda brachii may originate from the axillary artery (Fig. 15.22A). The subscapular, the lateral thoracic, and pectoral arteries may be part of a common trunk (Fig. 15.22B).

Brachial Artery

The brachial artery is the continuation of the axillary artery. It begins at the lower border of the tendon of the teres major, ending 1 cm below the elbow, dividing into radial and ulnar arteries. It runs down the arm, medially to the humerus and gradually moving to the front of the bone (Figs. 15.22-15.27).

Branches

- Arteria profunda brachii (profunda brachial) (Figs. 15.22 and 15.23)
- Nutrient of the humerus (Fig. 15.25)
- Muscular (Fig. 15.25)
- Superior ulnar collateral (Fig. 15.26)
- Inferior ulnar collateral (Fig. 15.27)
- Radial artery (Fig. 15.27)
- Ulnar artery (Fig. 15.27)

Arteria Profunda Brachii (Brachial Profunda)

Branches

- Nutrient artery of the humerus
- Deltoid artery (ascending anastomoses with posterior humeral artery)
- Middle collateral artery (posterior descending)
- Anastomoses with interosseous recurrent artery
- Radial collateral artery
- Continuation of arteria profunda brachii
- Muscular branches

Main Nutrient Artery

Main nutrient canal—downward.

Muscular Branches

Three or four in number—coracobrachialis, biceps, and brachialis.

Superior Ulnar Collateral Artery

This small artery descends between the medial epicondyle and the olecranon. It anastomoses with the posterior ulnar recurrent and inferior ulnar collaterals.

Inferior Ulnar Collateral Artery (Supratrochlear)

This anastomotic branch forms an arch above the olecranon fossa by a junction with the middle collateral branch. It anastomoses with the anterior ulnar recurrent artery.

Radial Artery (Figs. 15.20, 27, and 28)

The radial artery is the more direct continuation of the brachial artery, arising about 1 cm below the bend of the elbow coursing along the radius bone, reaching the hand. There are three main parts of the radial artery: one in the forearm, one at the wrist, and one in the hand.

Variation. The radial artery may originate at the axillary or upper part of the brachial artery (Fig. 15.20) and run parallel to the brachial artery, reaching the wrist and hand.

Branches at the Forearm and Wrist (Fig. 15.28)

- Radial recurrent artery (anastomoses with the radial collateral branch)
- Muscular branches
- Palmar carpal branch (anastomoses with the palmar carpal branch of the ulnar artery)

Ulnar Artery (Fig. 15.28)

The ulnar artery is the larger of the two distal branches of the brachial artery. It begins at the level of the neck of the radius, passing downward and medially, reaching the ulnar side of the forearm. When it reaches the wrist, it crosses lateral to the pisiform bone and gives off a deep branch, which continues across the palm as the superficial palmar arch.

Branches at the Forearm and Wrist (Figs. 15.23 and 15.29)

- Anterior ulnar recurrent artery
- Posterior ulnar recurrent artery
- Common interosseous artery
- Anterior interosseous artery
- Posterior interosseous artery
- Muscular branches
- Palmar carpal branch

Arteries of the Hand

The arteries of the hand are distal branches of the radial and ulnar arteries, with anastomosis with the posterior and anterior interosseous arteries (Figs. 15.30 and 15.31).

Radial Branches in the Hand

Superficial Palmar Branch

The superficial palmar branch is located at the thenar eminence; it anastomoses with the terminal part of the ulnar artery to complete the superficial palmar arch (arcus volaris superficialis).

Dorsal Carpal Branch

The dorsal carpal branch of the radial artery anastomoses with the dorsal carpal branch of the ulnar artery and anterior and posterior interosseous arteries, forming the dorsal carpal arch (dorsal carpal rete). The dorsal metacarpal arteries descend on the second, third, and fourth dorsal interosseous muscles and bifurcate into dorsal digital branches for the fingers. They anastomose with the palmar digital branches of the superficial palmar arch. The dorsal metacarpal arteries anastomose with the deep palmar arch by the proximal perforating arteries and near their points of bifurcation with the palmar digital vessels of the superficial palmar digital arteries, branches of the superficial palmar arch by the distal perforating arteries.

Arteria Princeps Pollicis (Figs. 15.32-15.34)

The arteria princeps pollicis is the main artery of the thumb. It arises from the radial artery as it turns medially into the palm of the hand. It divides into two branches running along the sides of the thumb.

Arteria Radialis Indicis

The arteria radialis indicis arises from the deep palmar arch and frequently from the arteria princeps pollicis. It runs along the lateral borders of the second finger.

Deep Palmar Arch (Arcus Volaris Profundus) (Figs. 15.30, 32, and 33A, B)

The deep palmar arch is formed by the anastomosis of the terminal part of the radial artery with the deep palmar branch of the ulnar artery.

Branches

- Three palmar metacarpal arteries
- From the convexity of the deep palmar arch (anastomoses with the common digital branches of the superficial palmar arch)
- Three perforating branches
- Anastomoses with the dorsal metacarpal arteries
- Recurrent branches
- Anastomoses with the palmar carpal arch

Ulnar Branches in the Hand

Palmar Carpal Branch

The palmar carpal branch anastomoses with the palmar carpal branch of the radial artery, receiving branches from the anterior interosseous artery, thereby forming the palmar carpal arch at the wrist and carpus.

Dorsal Carpal Branch

The dorsal carpal branch arises above the pisiform bone and anastomoses with the dorsal carpal branch of radial artery.

Deep Palmar Branch

The deep palmar branch is often double and anastomoses with the radial artery to complete the deep palmar arch.

Superficial Palmar Arch (Arcus Volaris Superficialis) (Figs. 15.30 and 15.31)

The superficial palmar arch is the main anastomosis of the ulnar artery. One-third of the superficial palmar arch is formed by the ulnar artery alone. One third is completed by the superficial palmar branch of the radial artery. An additional third is completed by either the arteria radialis indicis, branch of arteria princeps pollicis, or by the median artery.

Three Common Palmar Digital Arteries

These arteries arise from the convexity of the superficial palmar arch and are joined distally by the corresponding palmar metacarpal arteries (from deep palmar arch) and divide into a pair of proper palmar digital arteries, which run along the contiguous sides of the fingers. They are free to anastomose with the dorsal digital arteries by small branches at the level of the joints and at the finger tip vascular tufts (Fig. 15.35).

Variations

The persistent median artery may be the largest artery feeding the hand (Fig. 15.36). The arch is complete in 78.5% of cases (Figs. 15.31 and 15.34) and incomplete in 21.5% of cases (Figs. 15.37 and 15.38).

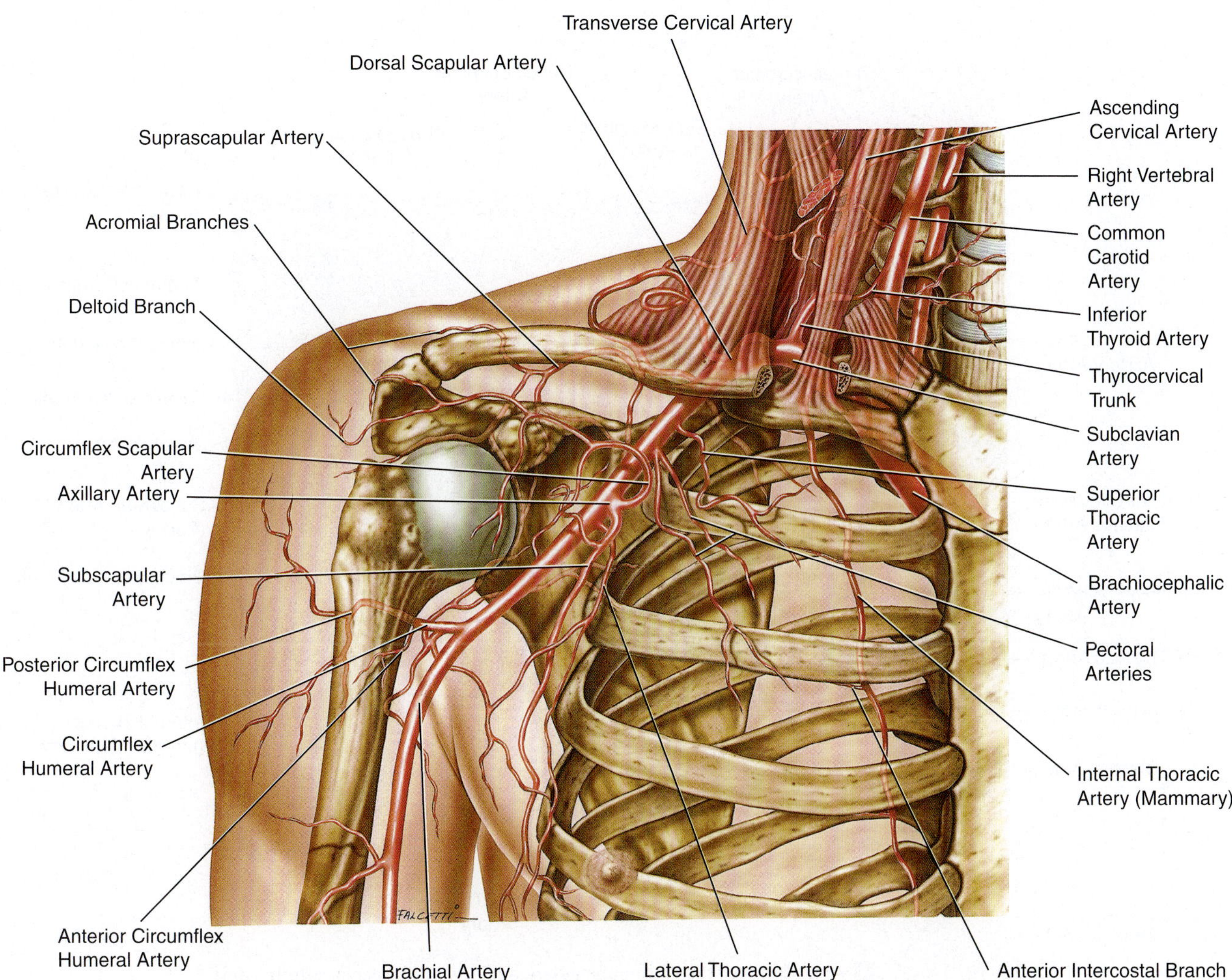

Figure 15.1. Vascular structures of the right shoulder. Note the relationship of the subclavian artery with the clavicle, first rib, and scalenus anterior muscle. The clavicle has been partially removed. (Art based on an actual angiogram.)

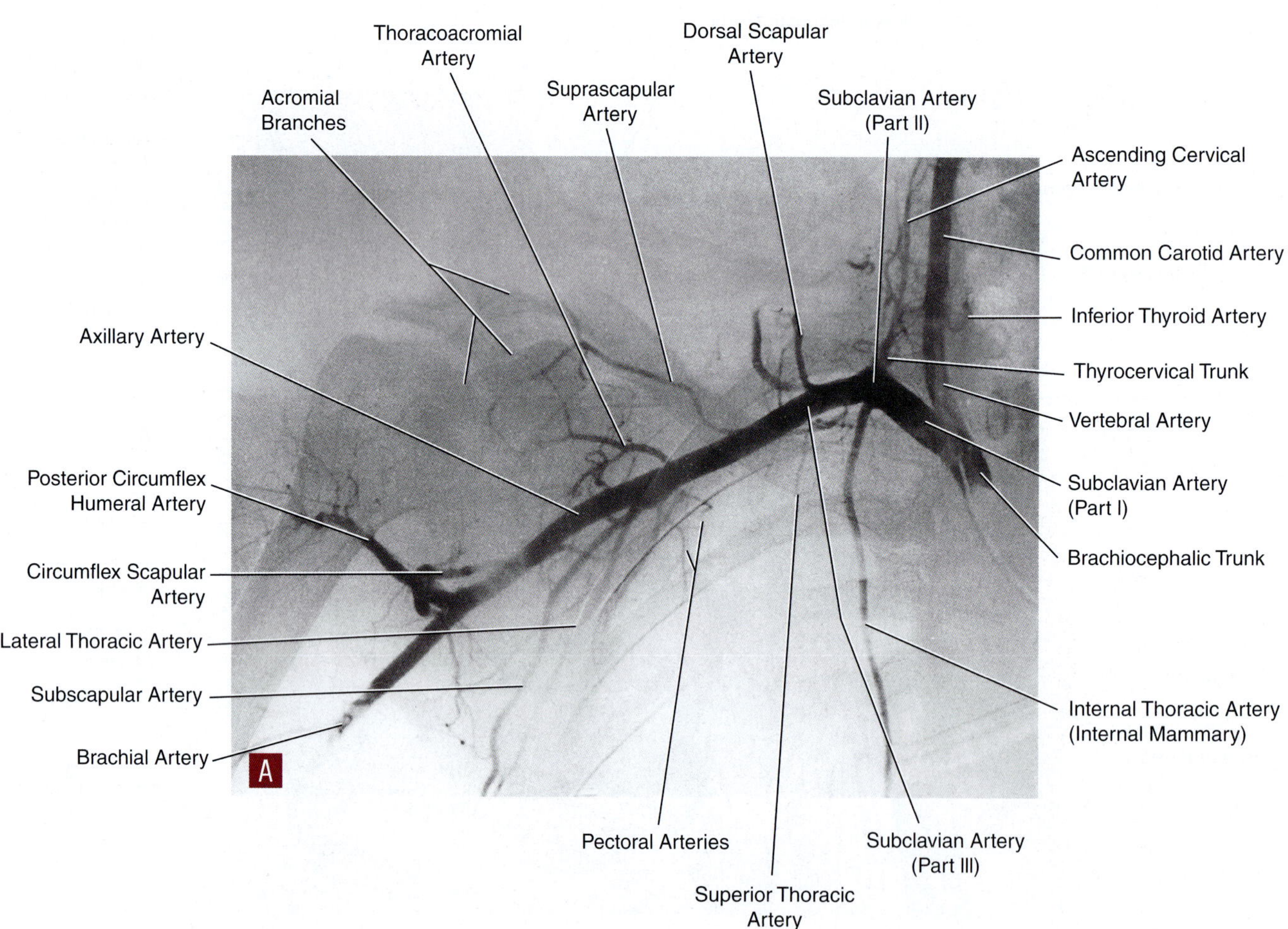

Figure 15.2. A, Angiogram of the right subclavian, axillary, and brachial arteries and branches. B, Angiogram of the left subclavian artery. Note the origin of the vertebral artery arising in the second portion of the subclavian artery.

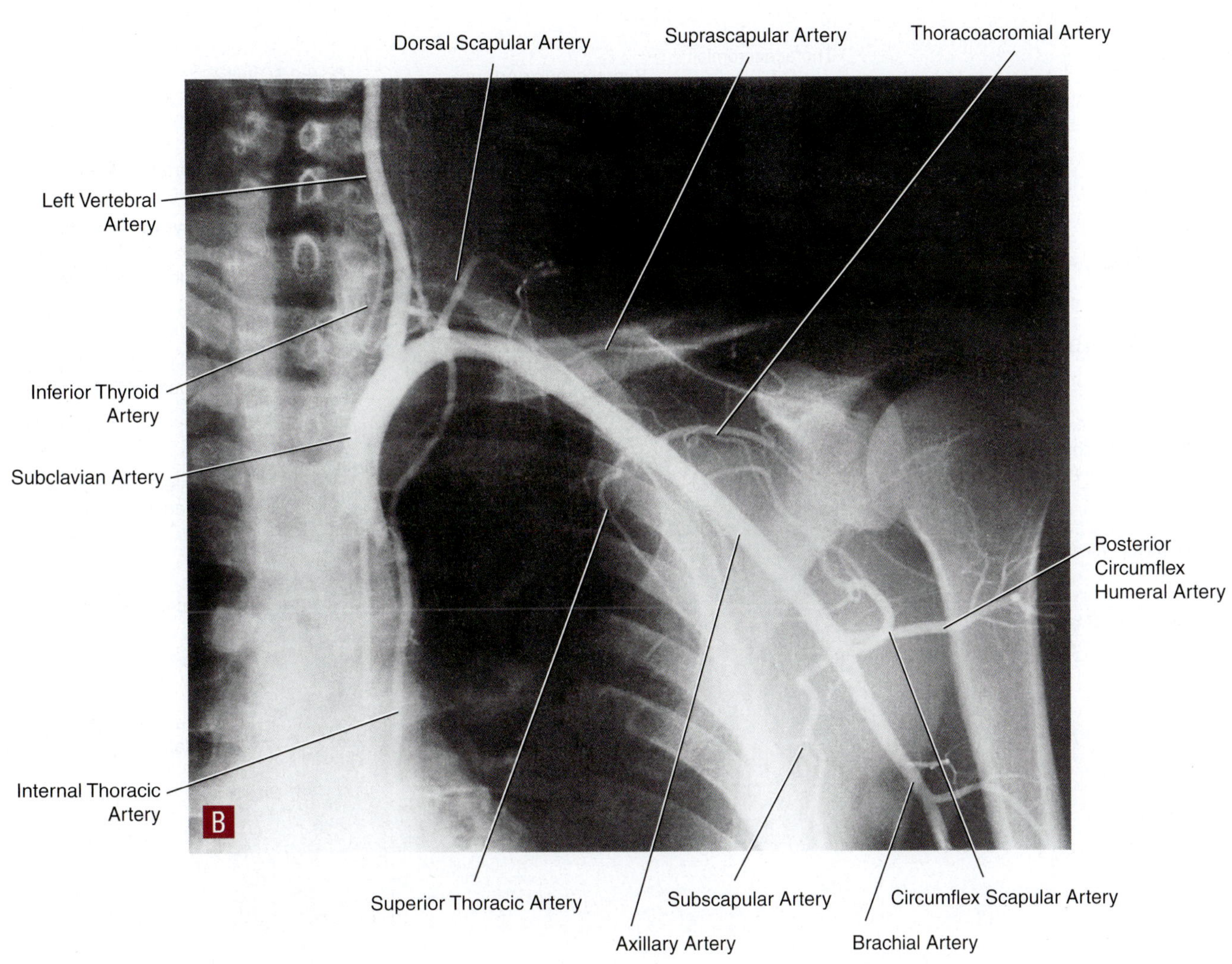

Figure 15.2. *Continued*

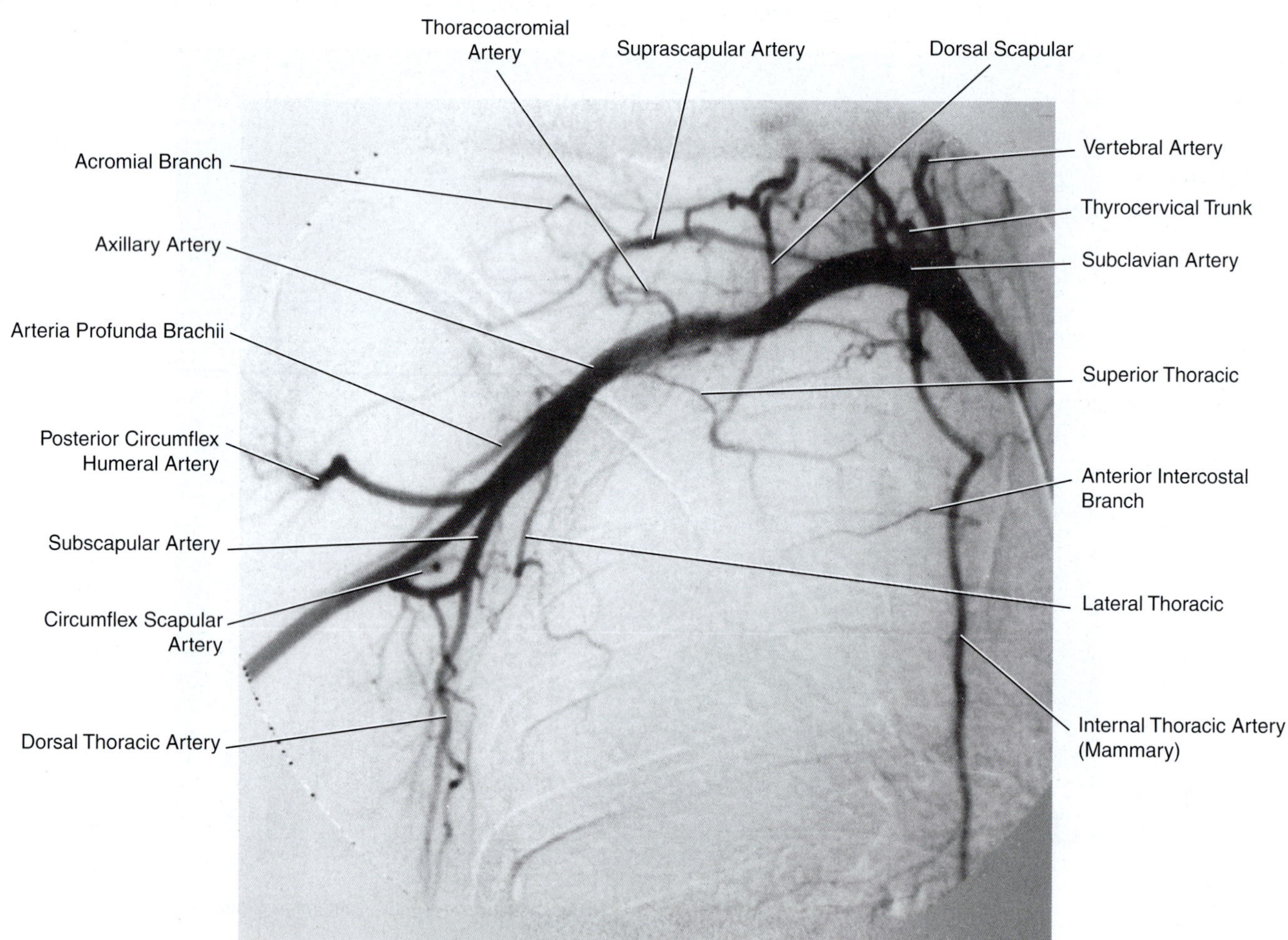

Figure 15.3. **Digital subtraction angiogram of the right subclavian and axillary arteries.**

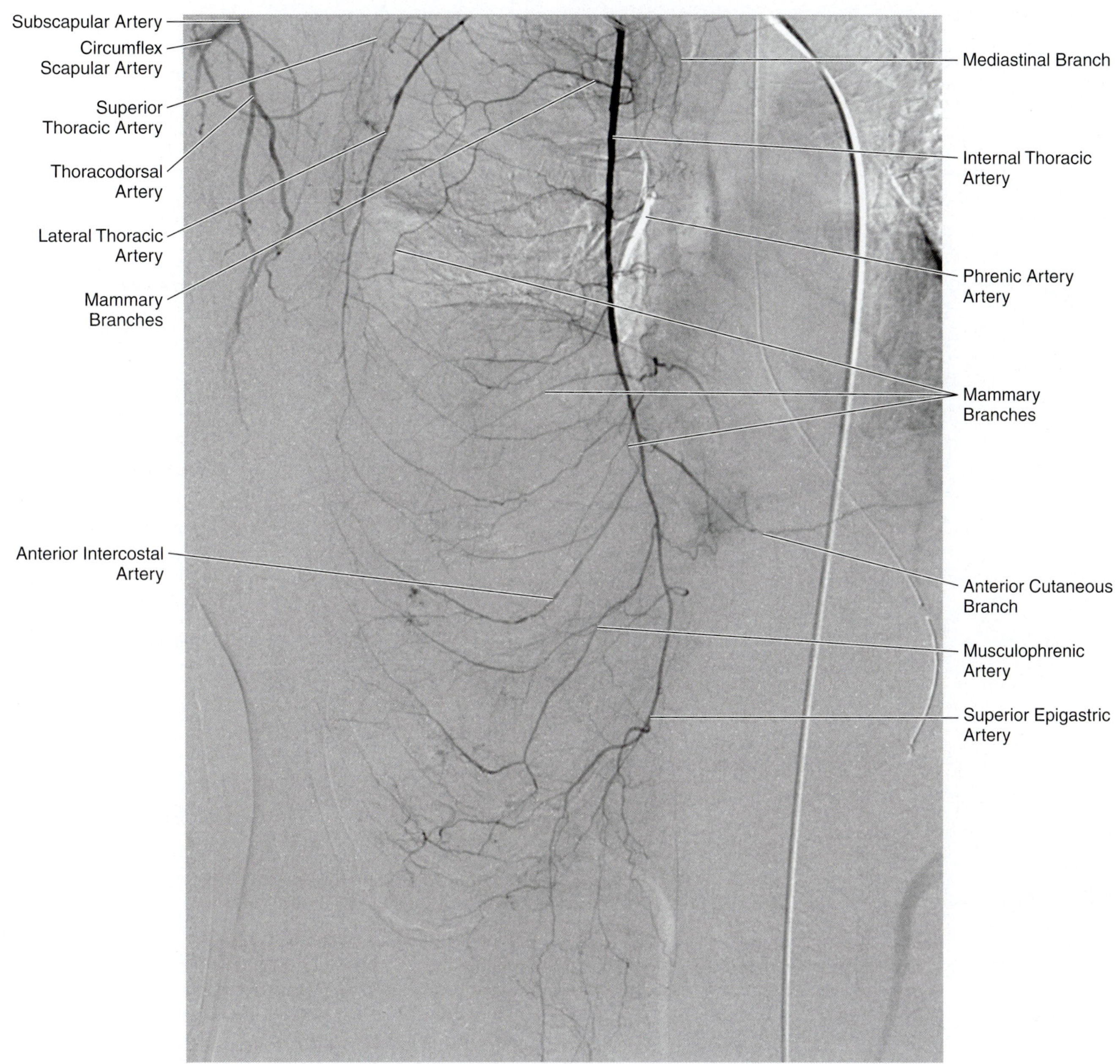

Figure 15.4. **Right internal thoracic (internal mammary) artery and distal branches.**

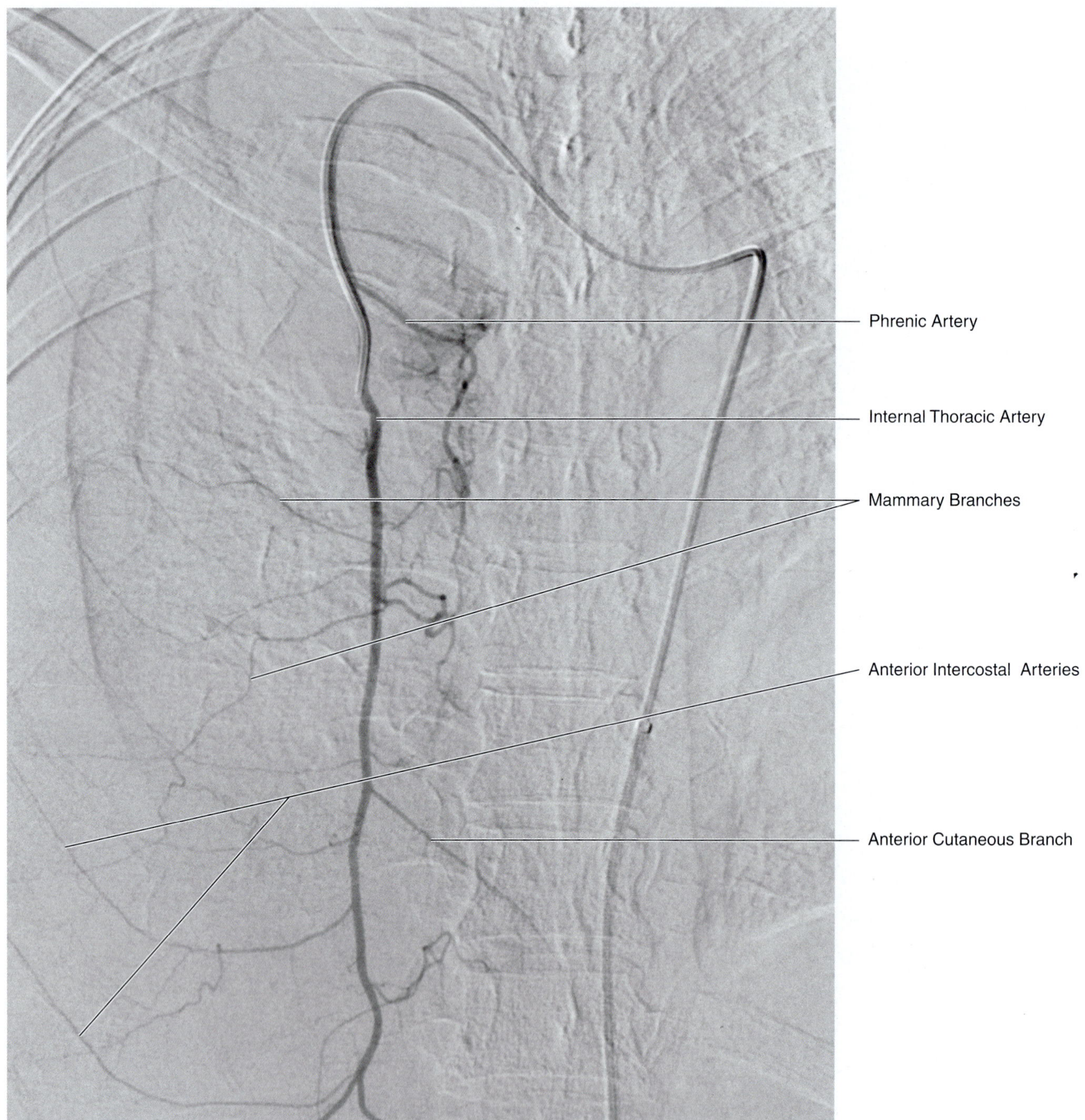

Figure 15.5. **Right internal thoracic artery and the mediastinal and pericardial branches.**

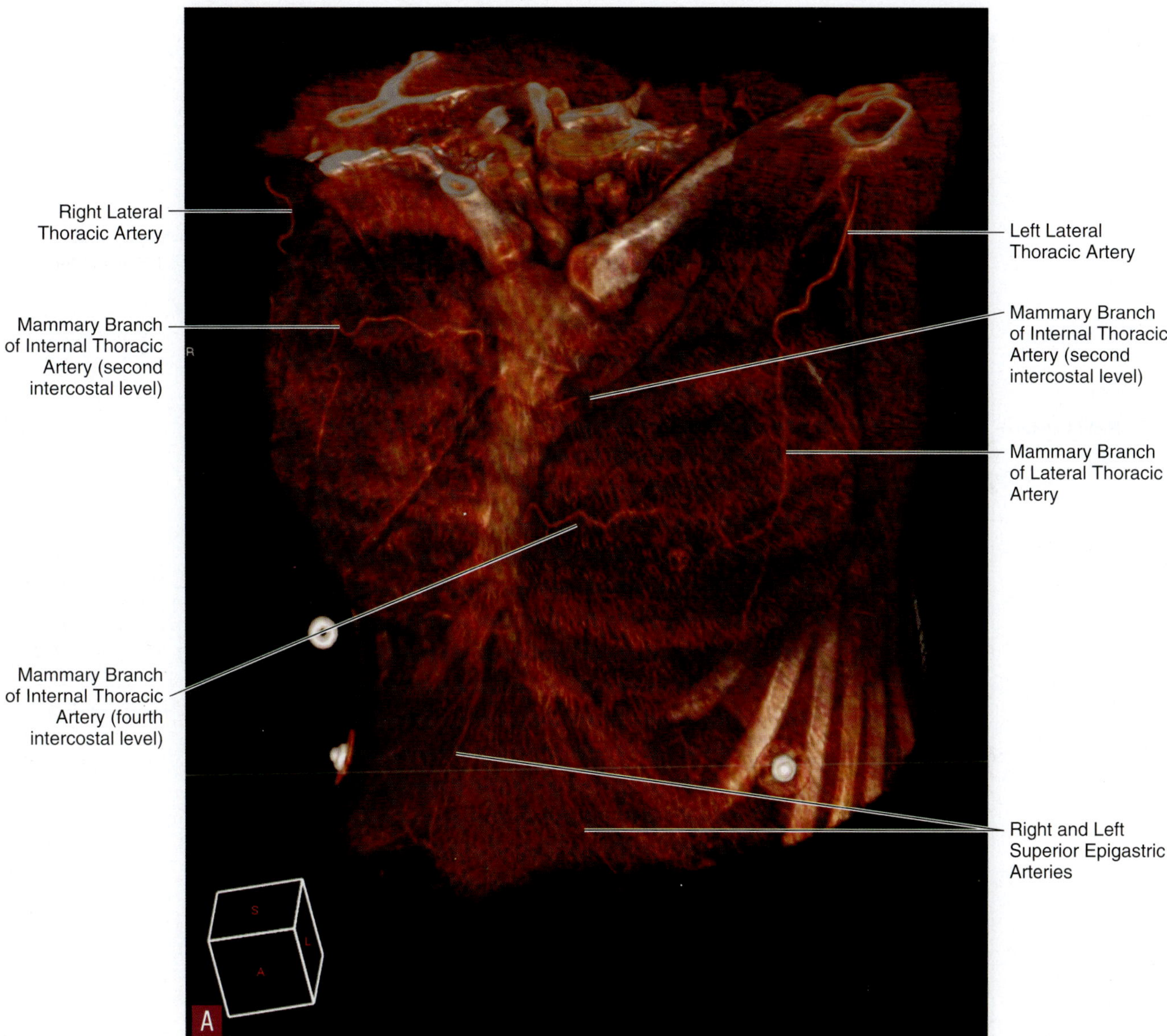

Figure 15.6. **A**, Volume-rendered 3D reconstruction of a thoracic computerized tomographic (CT) angiogram during the arterial phase showing the arterial supply to the breast. There are two branches supplying the medial breast from the first and fourth intercostal spaces on the left, which anastomose with the lateral thoracic artery in the nipple-areola complex. **B**, Volume-rendered 3D reconstruction on the same patient as in (A) showing a single perforating branch from the internal mammary artery on the right, with lateral supply from the ipsilateral lateral thoracic artery. **C**-**E**, Volume-rendered 3D reconstruction on a different patient showing a similar configuration with two medial perforating arteries anastomosing with branches of the lateral thoracic artery in an anterior (**C**), right anterior oblique view (**D**), and left anterior oblique view (**E**). **F**, Maximum intensity projection of a CT angiogram in the arterial phase showing a perforating branch from the left internal mammary artery supplying the medial breast.

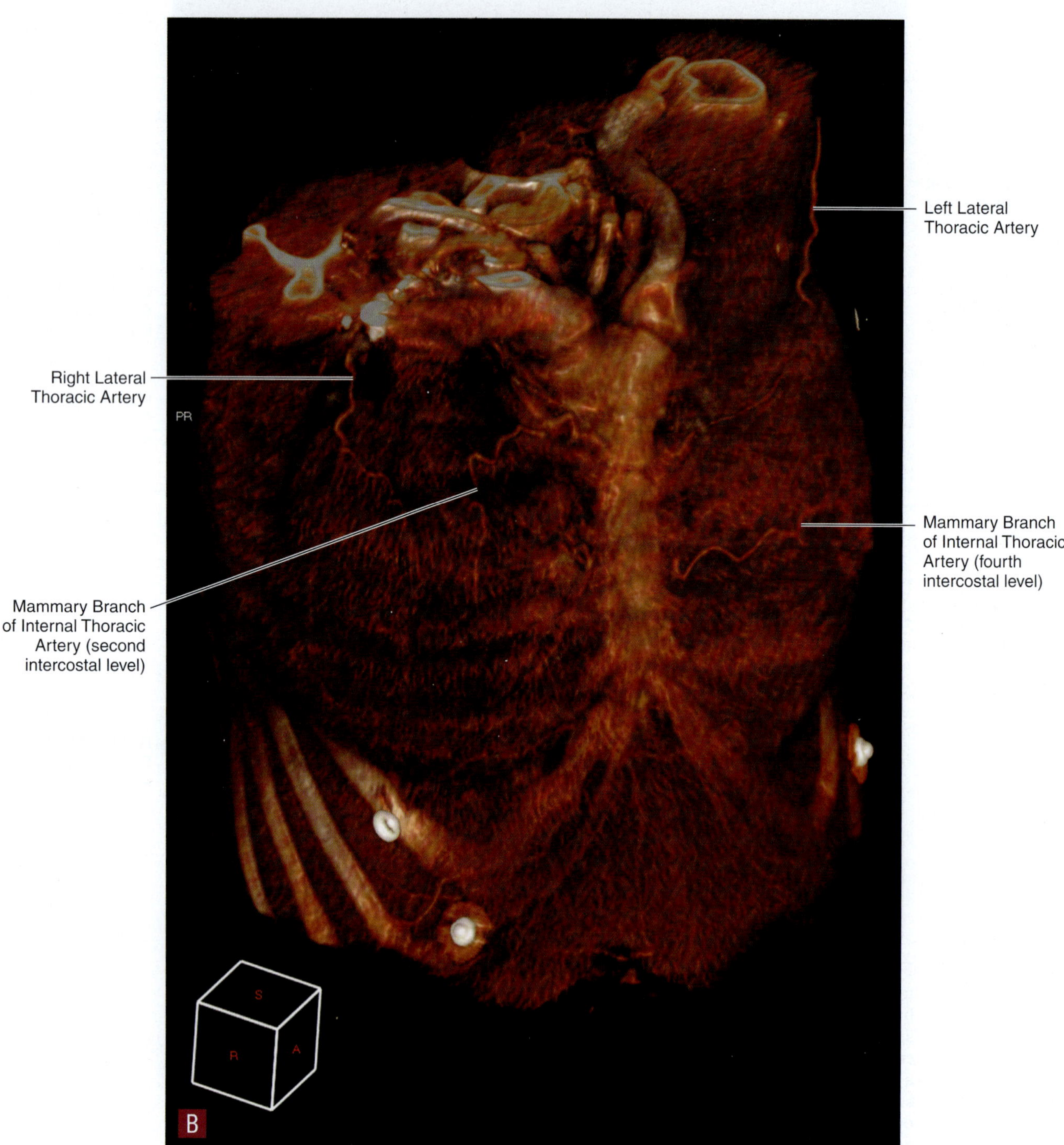

Figure 15.6. *Continued*

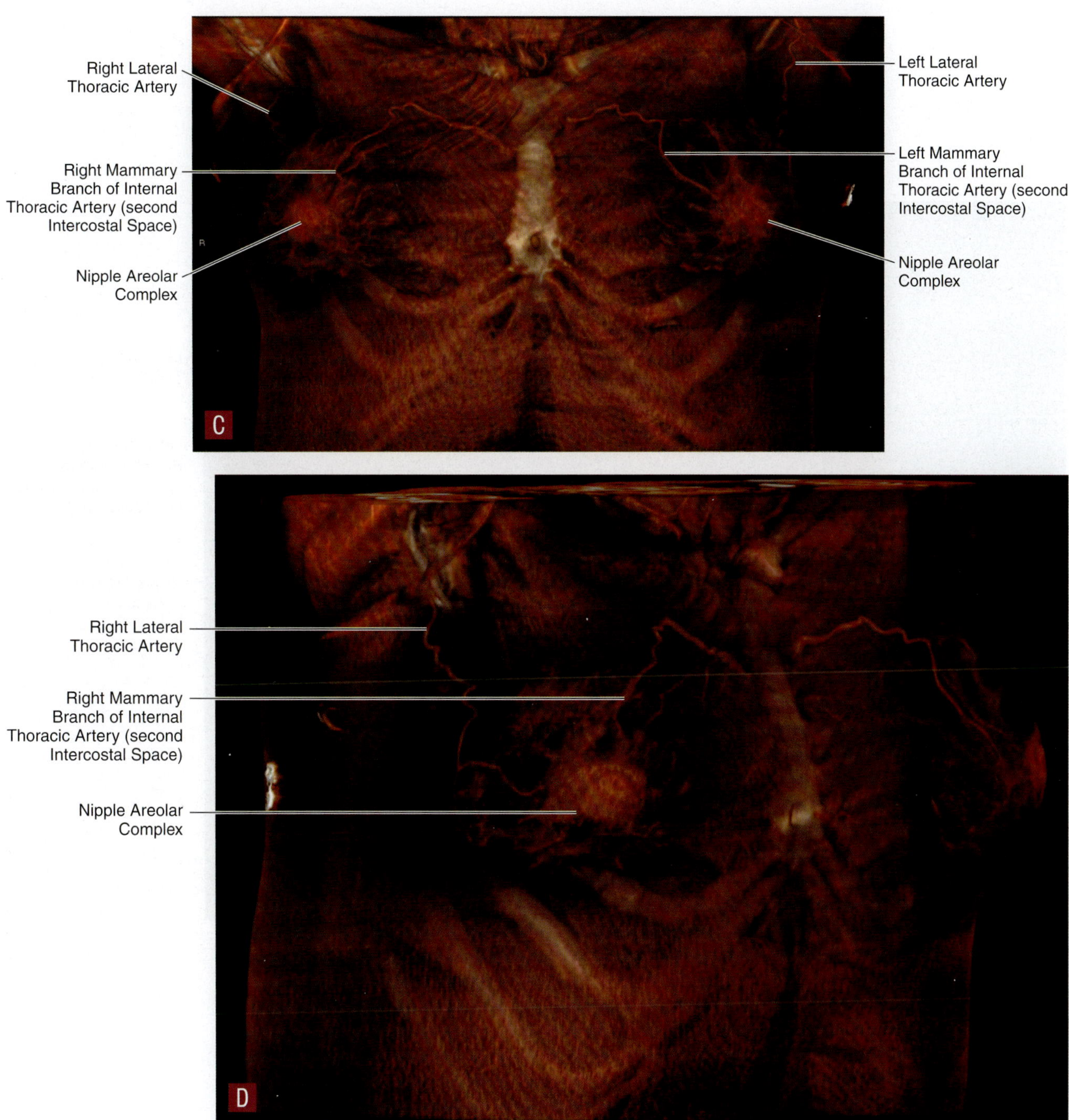

Figure 15.6. *Continued*

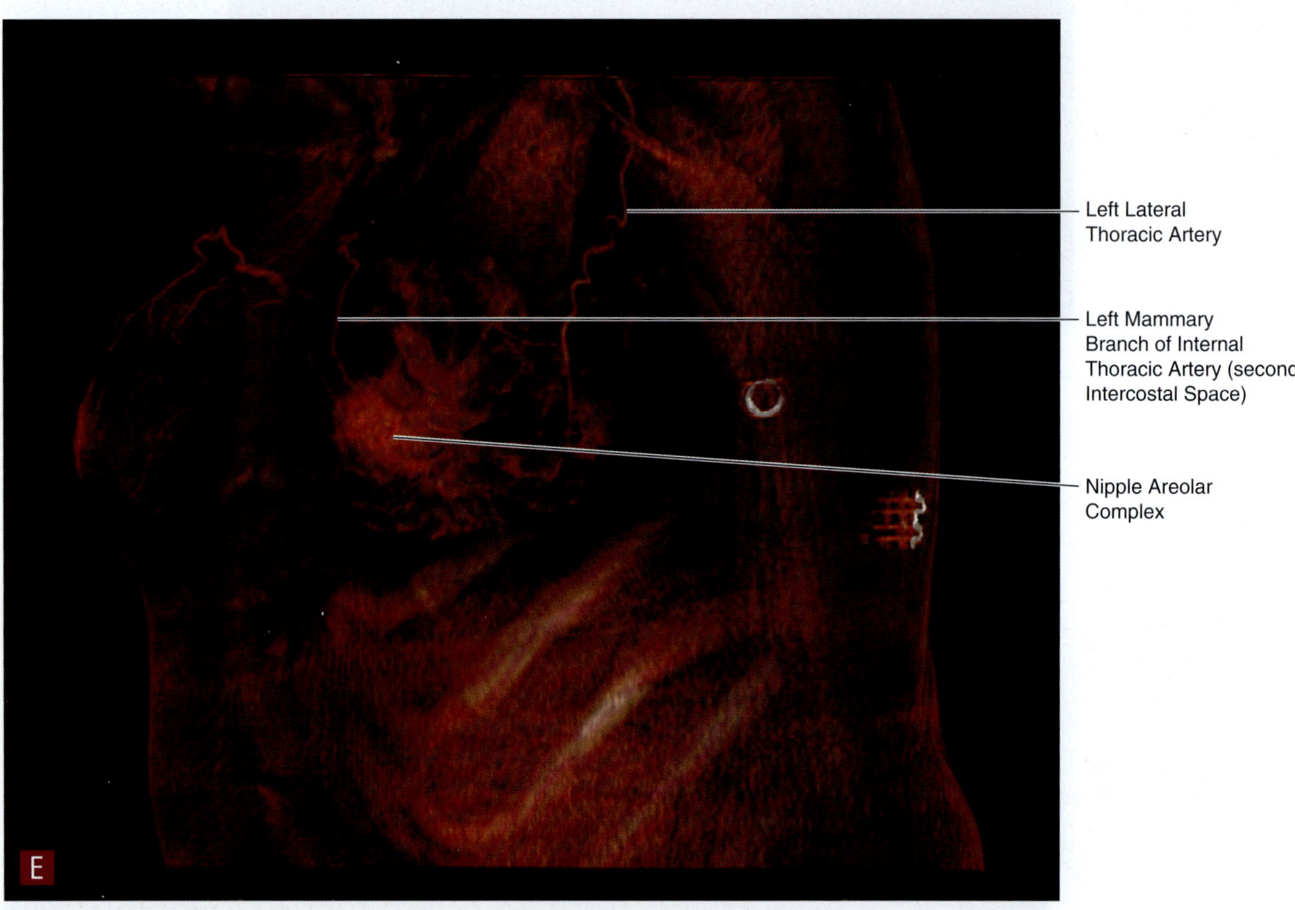

Figure 15.6. *Continued*

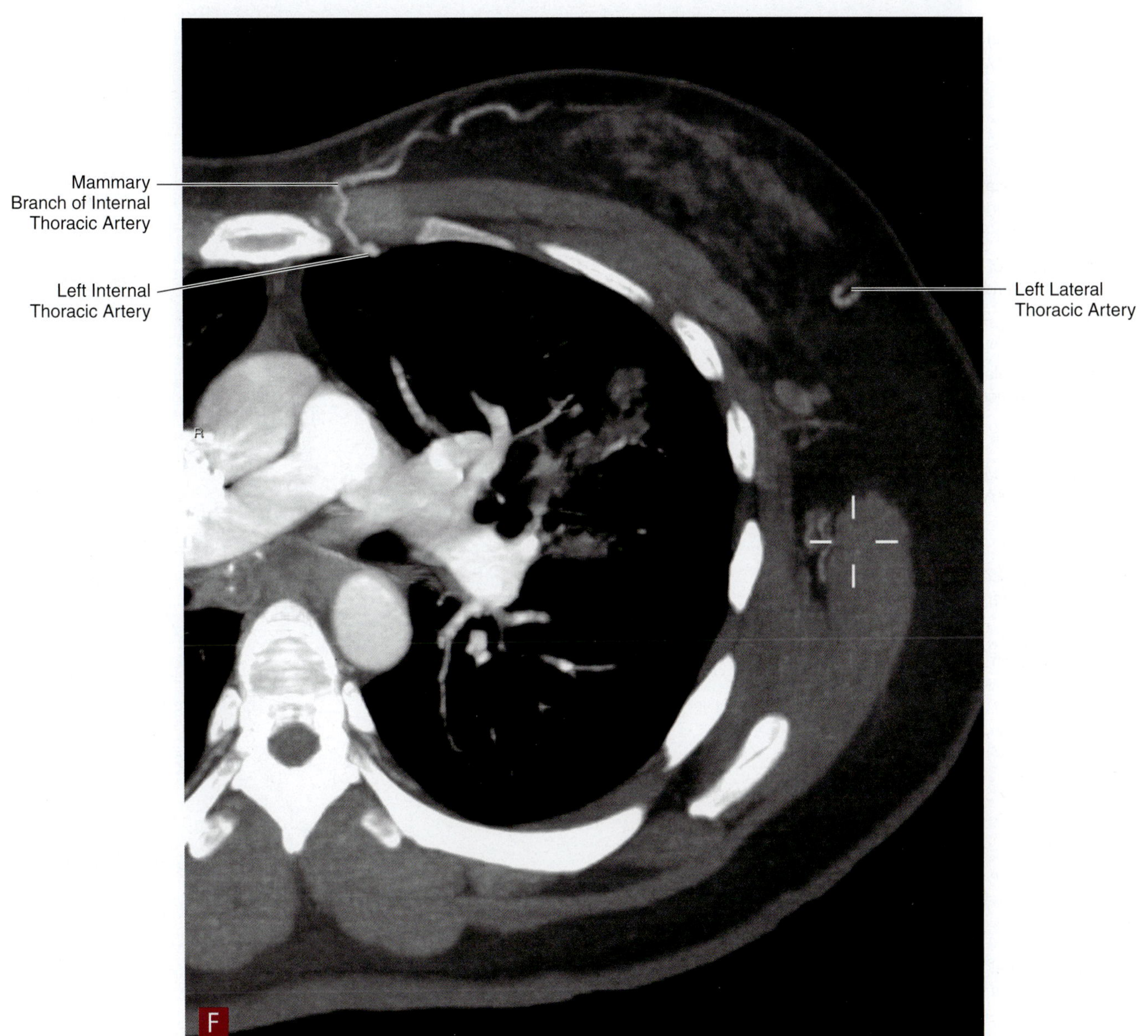

Figure 15.6. *Continued*

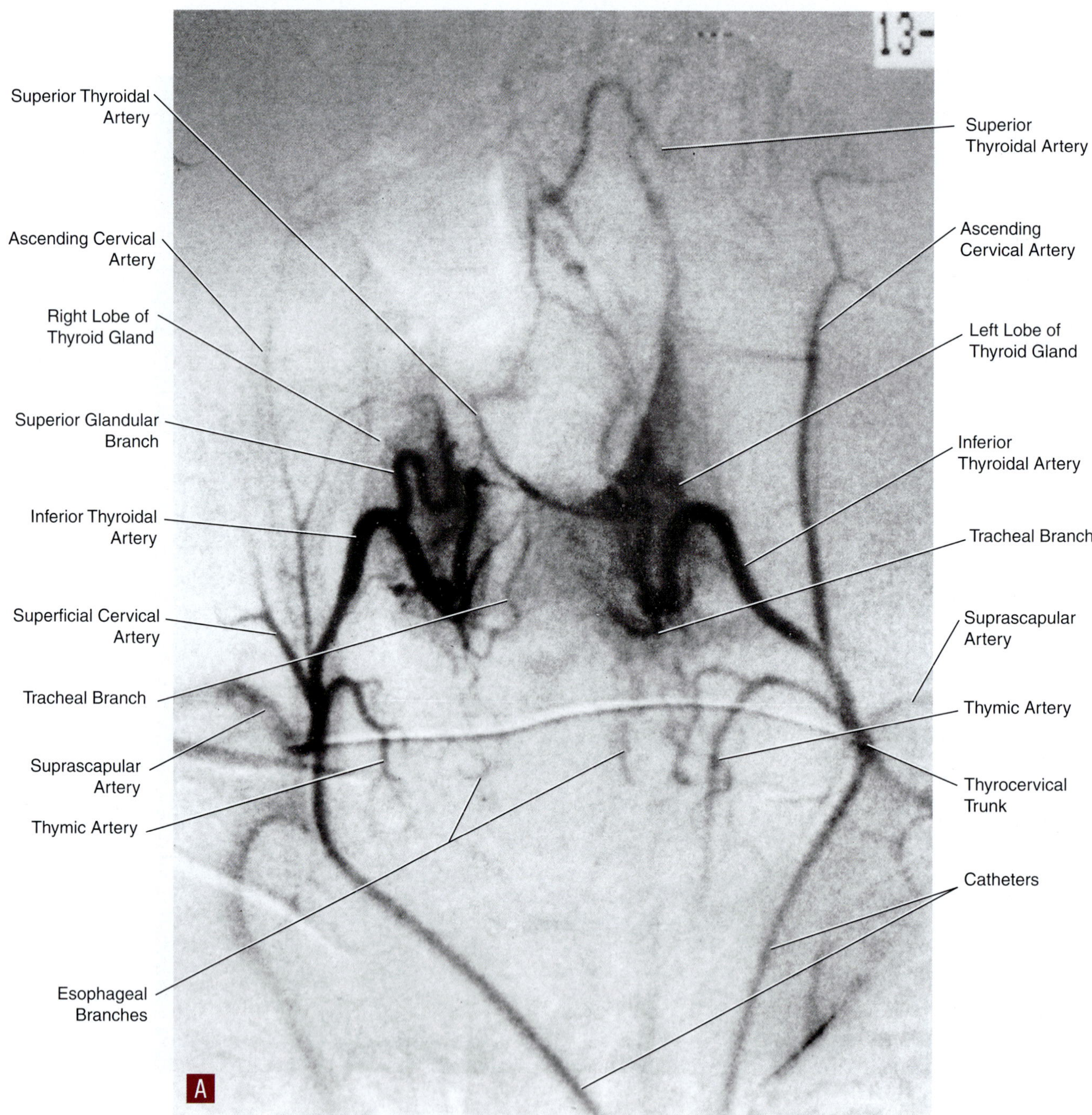

Figure 15.7. A and B, **Simultaneous angiogram of the right and left thyrocervical trunks.** Note the thyroid gland blush and named vessels, as well as the veins in (B).

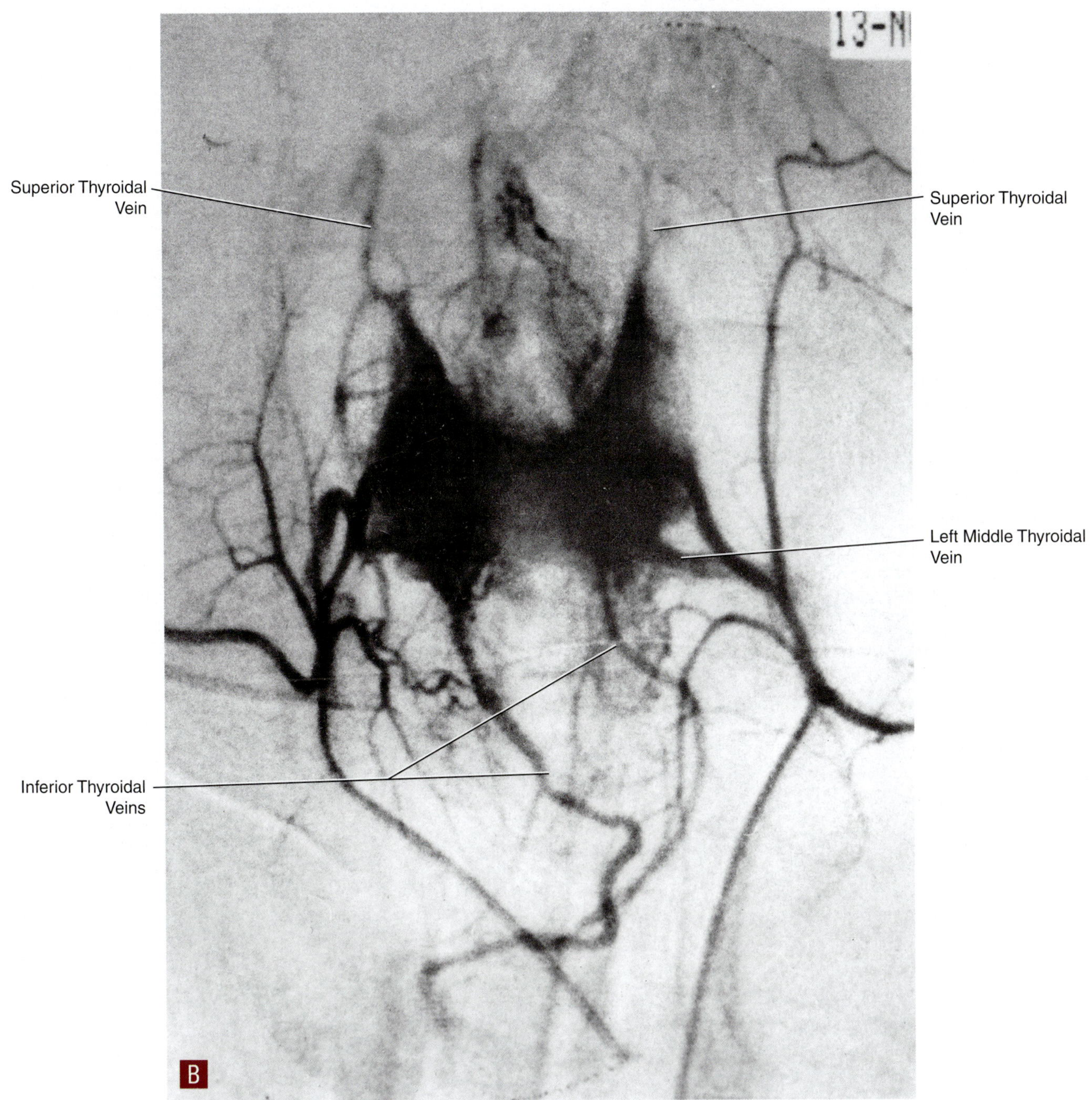

Figure 15.7. *Continued*

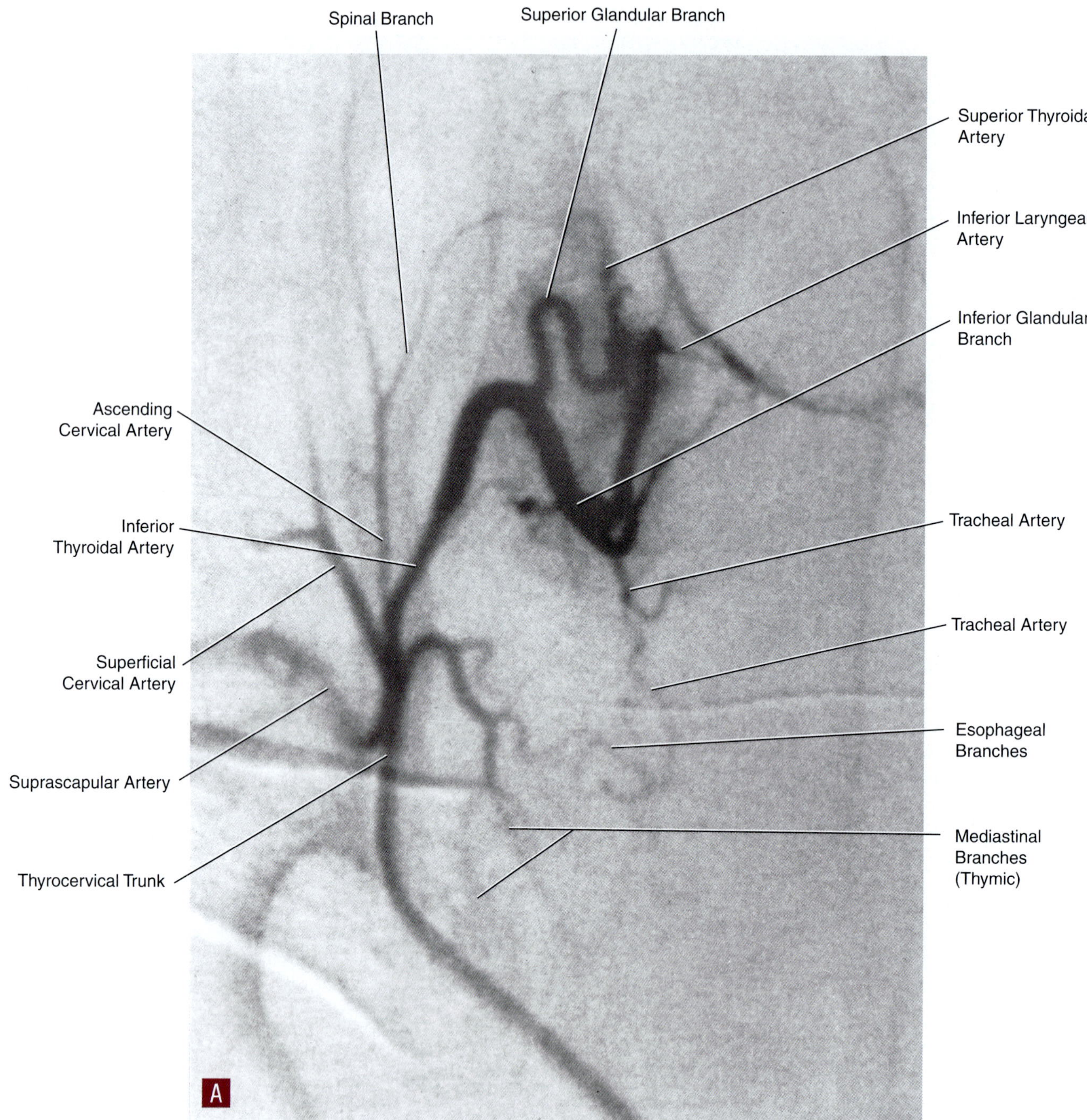

Figure 15.8. A, Closeup view of the right thyroid vessels. B, Closeup view of the left thyroid vessels. C, Selective injection into the right thyrocervical trunk. D, Selective injection into the left thyrocervical trunk.

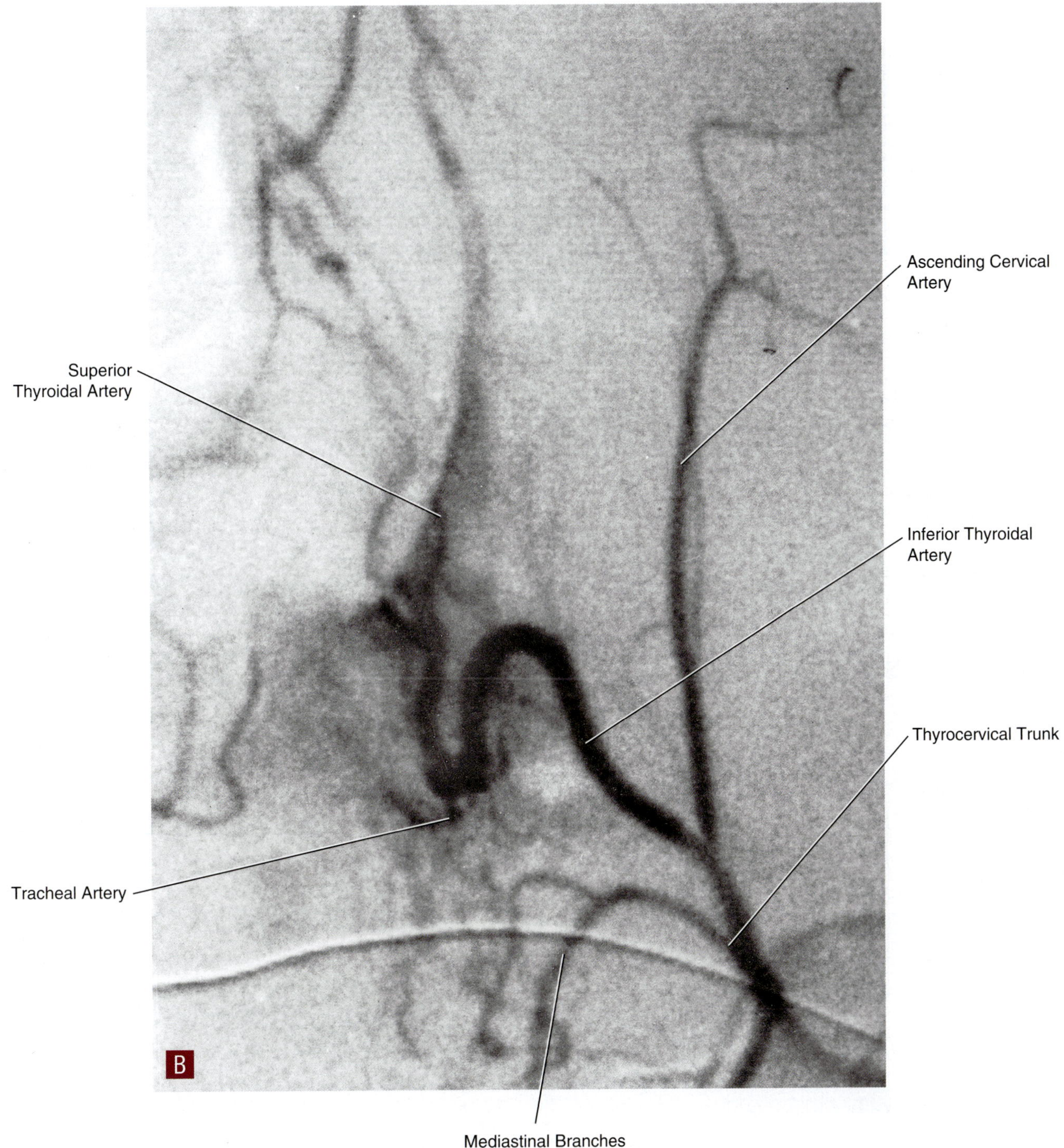

Figure 15.8. *Continued*

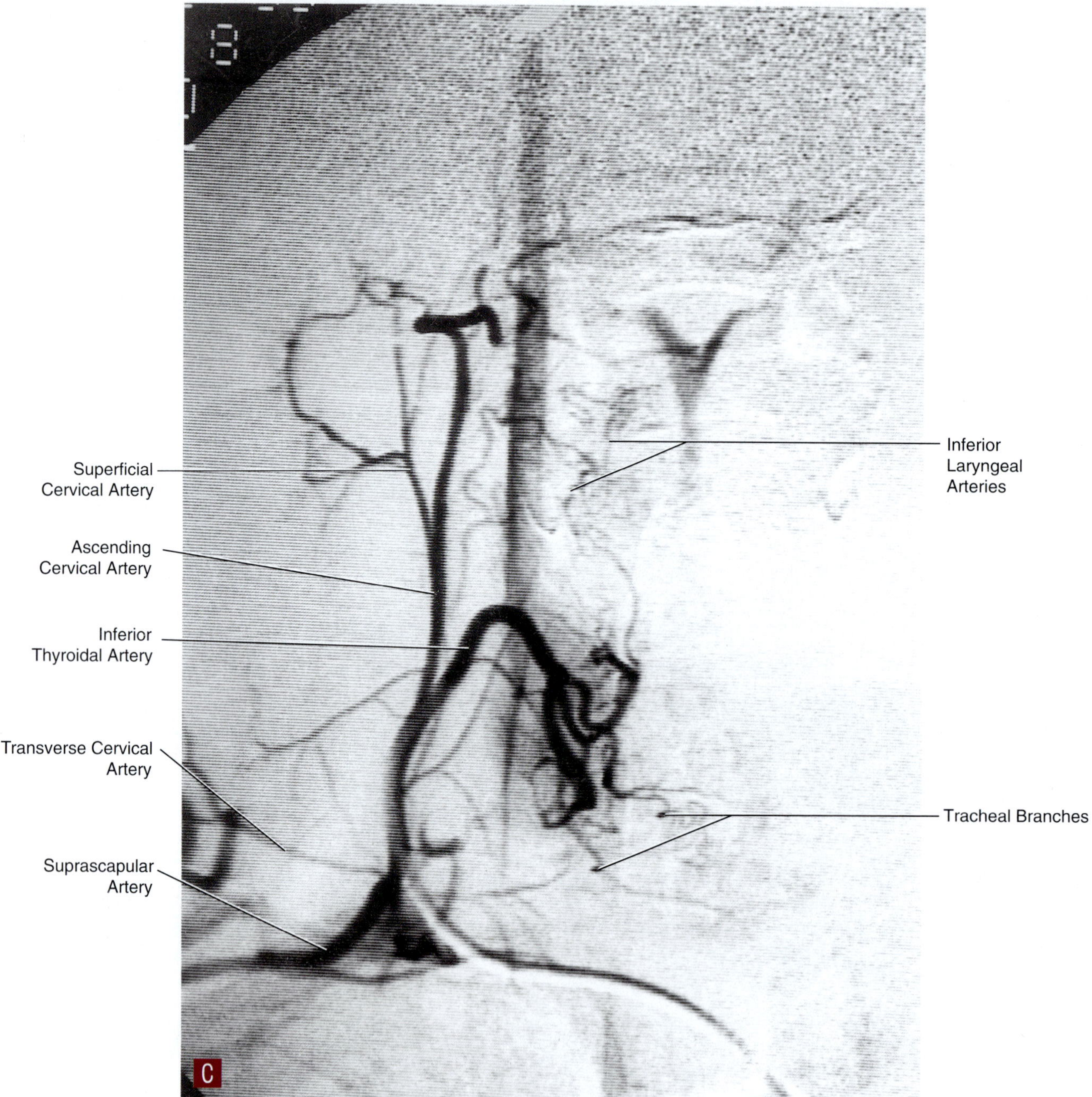

Figure 15.8. *Continued*

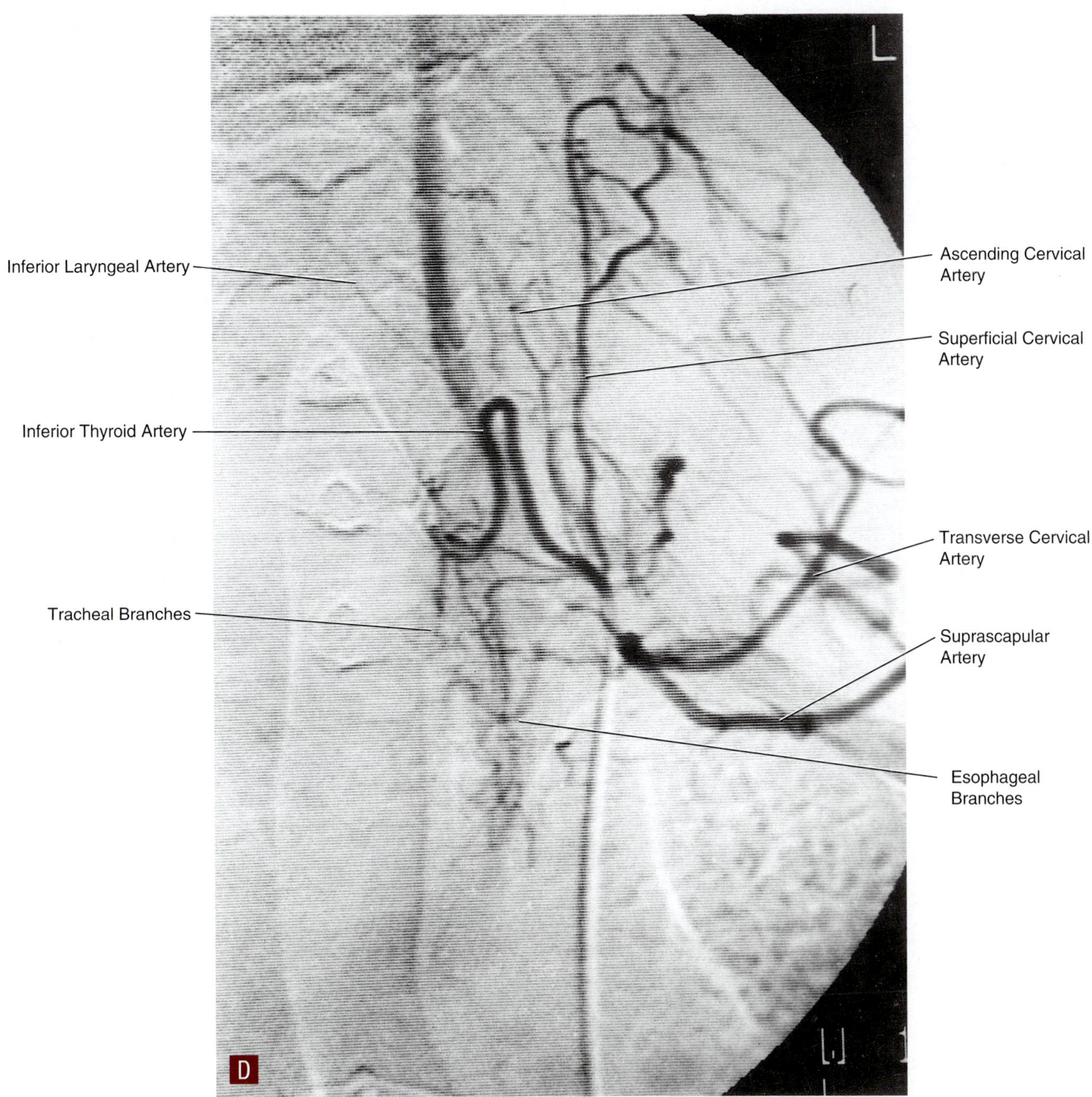

Figure 15.8. *Continued*

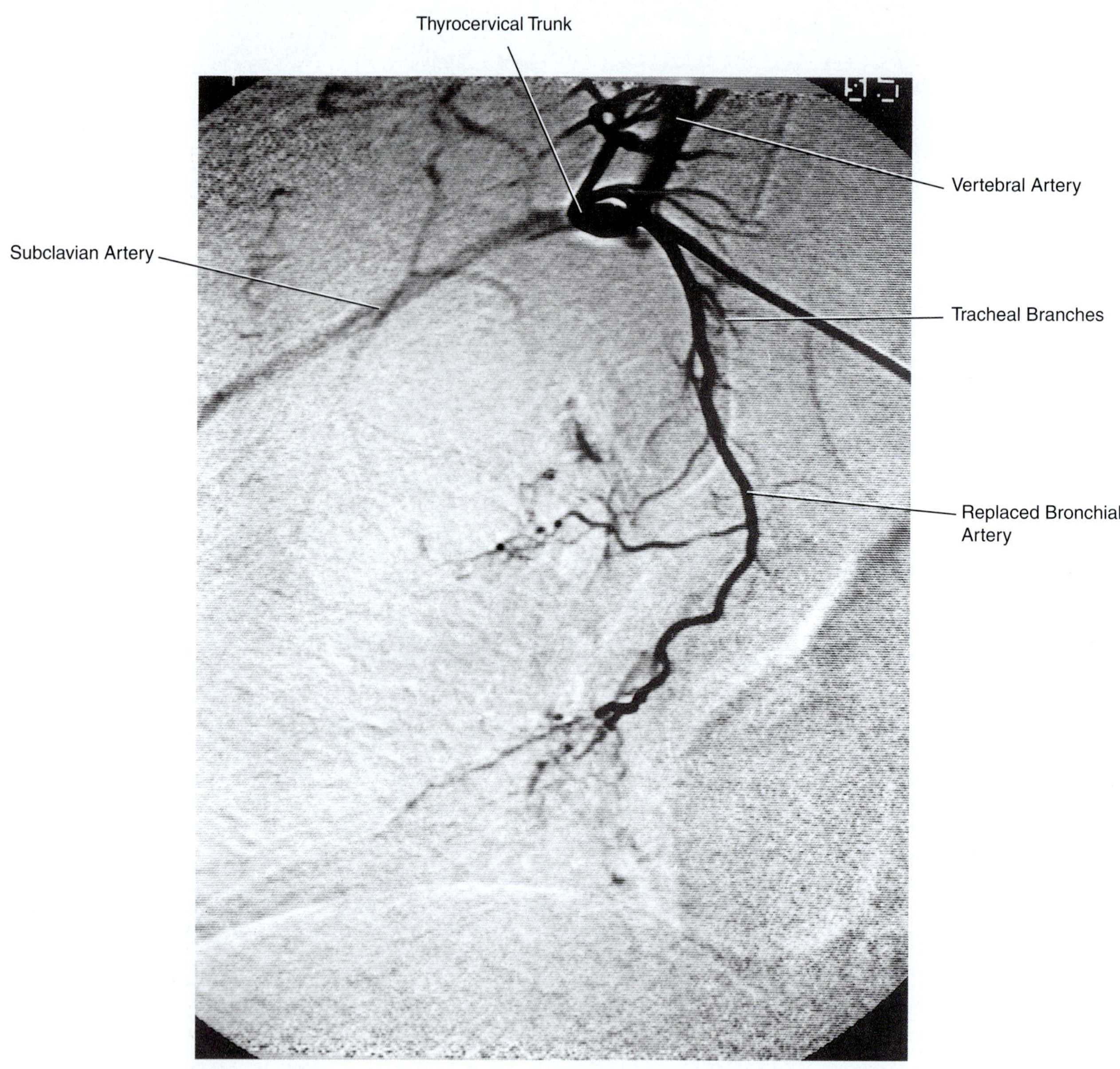

Figure 15.9. Right bronchial artery originating from the right thyrocervical trunk. Variation of the normal anatomy. (See bronchial artery anatomy.)

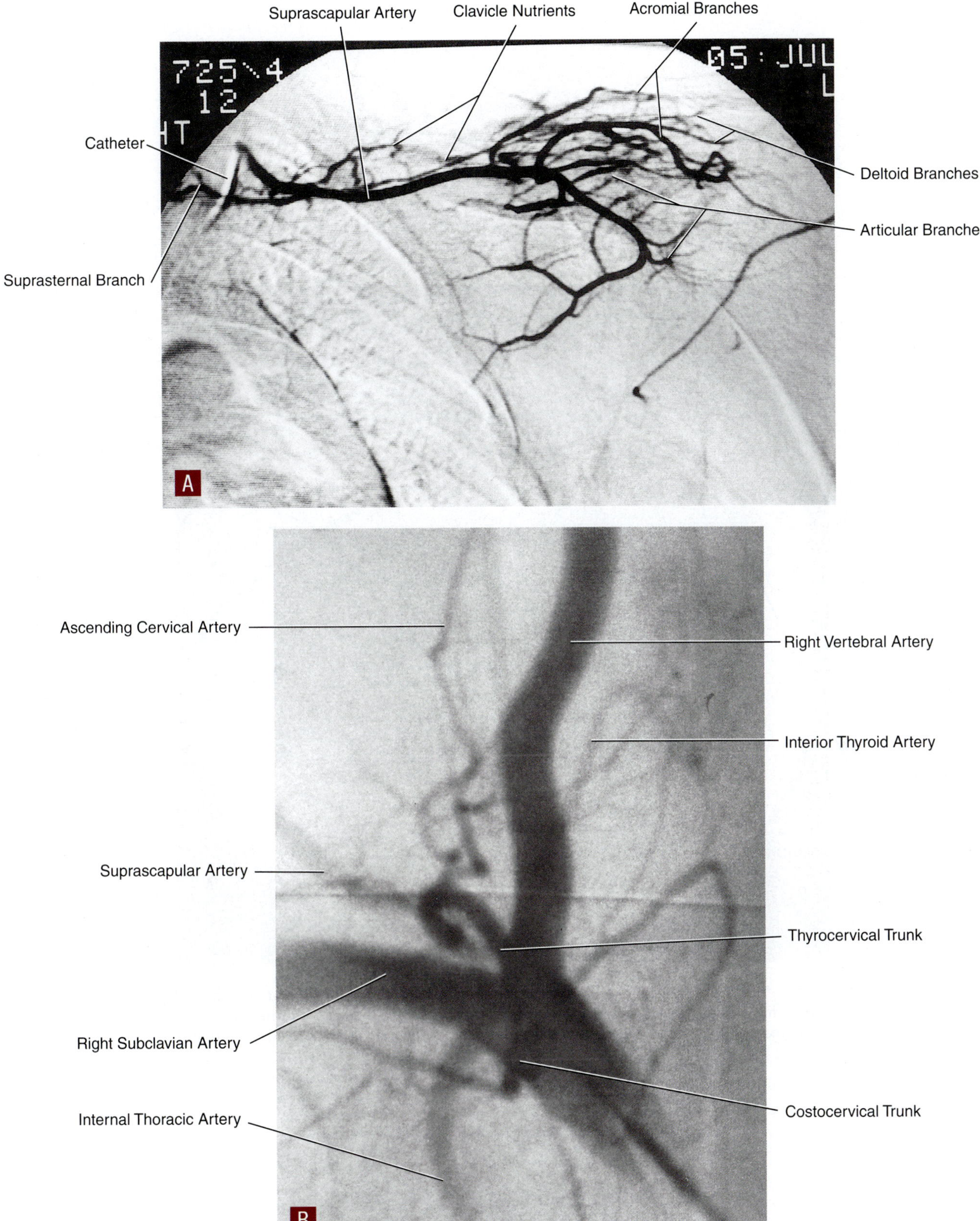

Figure 15.10. A, Selective angiogram of the left suprascapular artery and branches. B, Selective angiogram of the right subclavian artery showing the main branches.

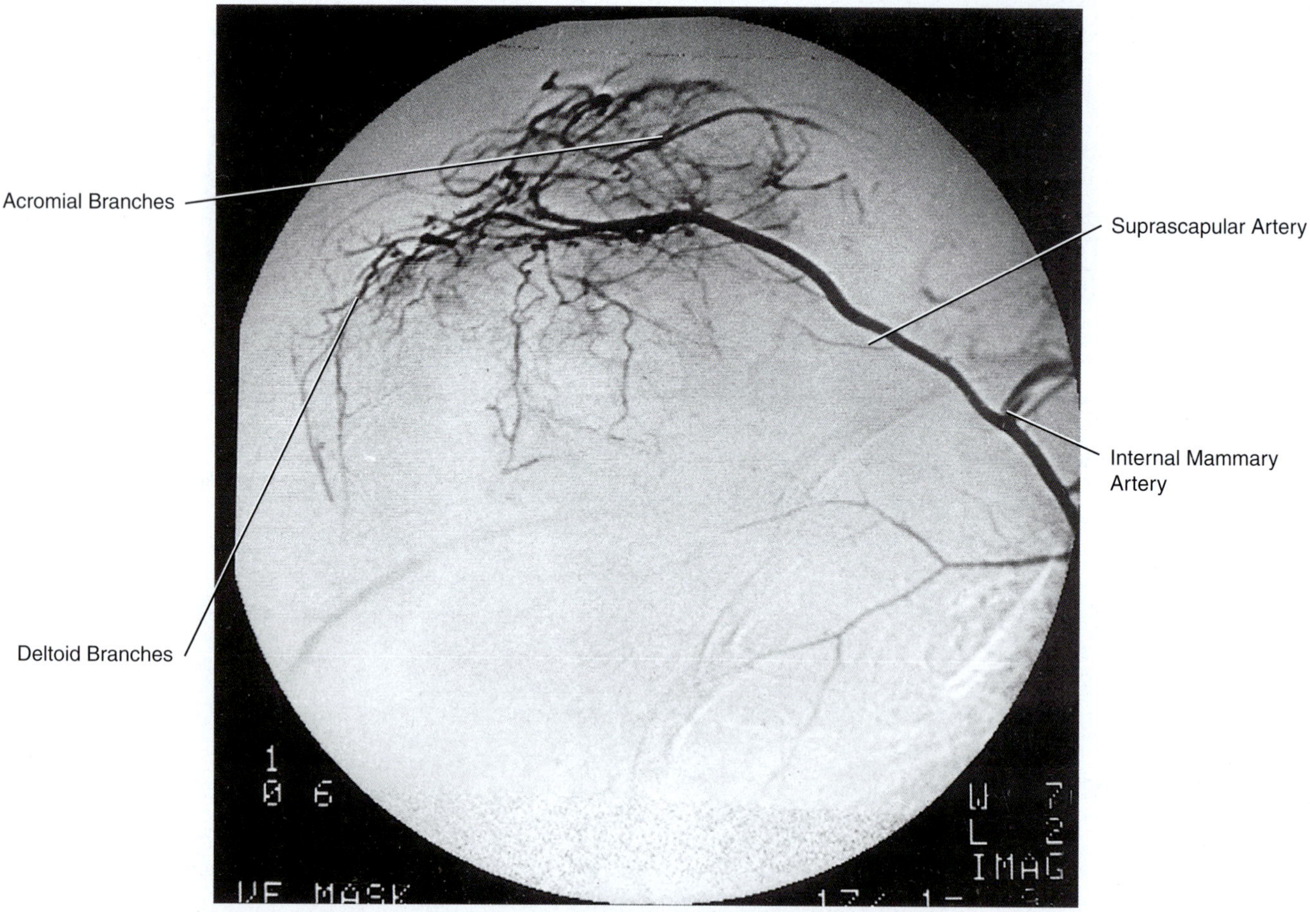

Figure 15.11. Selective angiogram of the right suprascapular artery and branches. Note the anatomic variation. The suprascapular artery originates from the right internal thoracic (internal mammary) artery. The peripheral arteries are displaced by a glenoid aneurysmatic bone cyst.

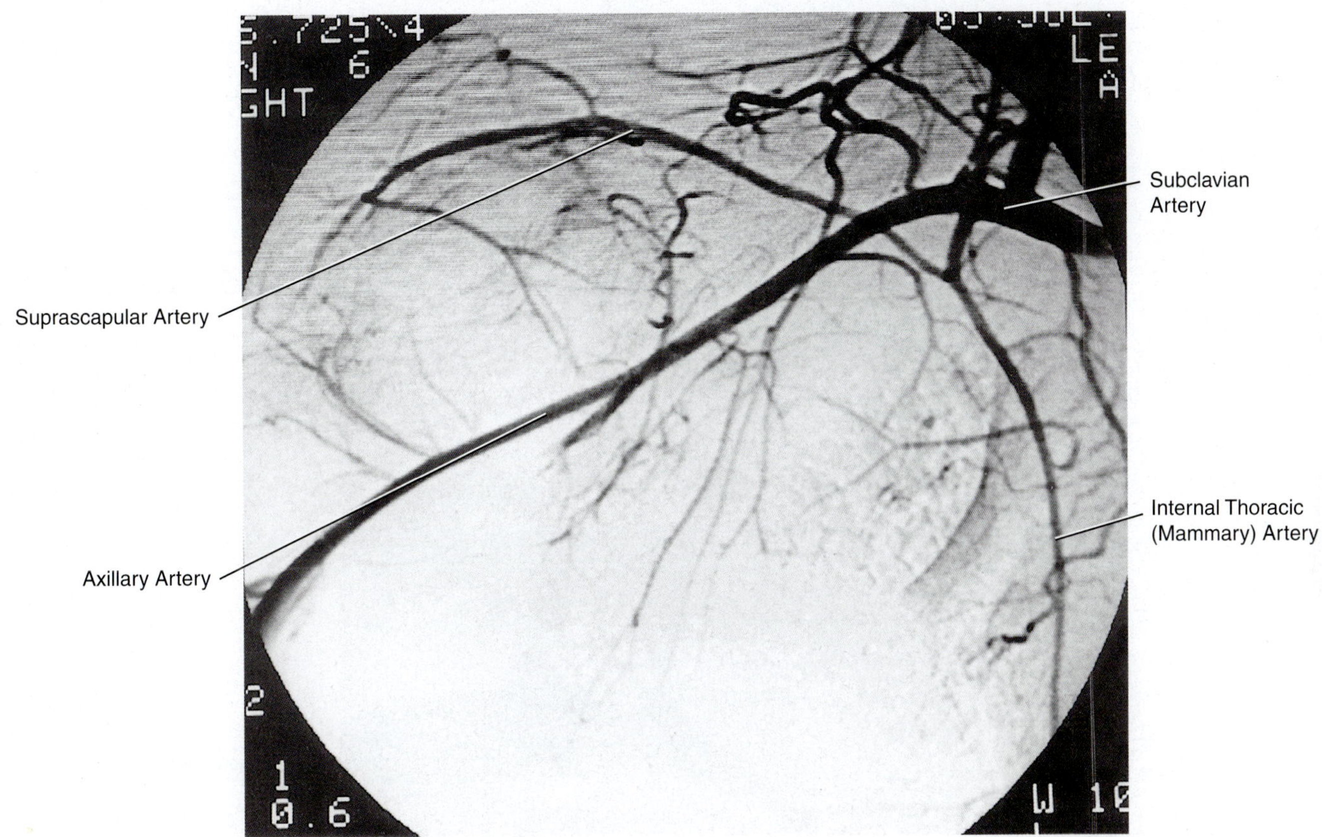

Figure 15.12. **Suprascapular artery arising from the internal thoracic artery.** Note the relationship with the subclavian artery.

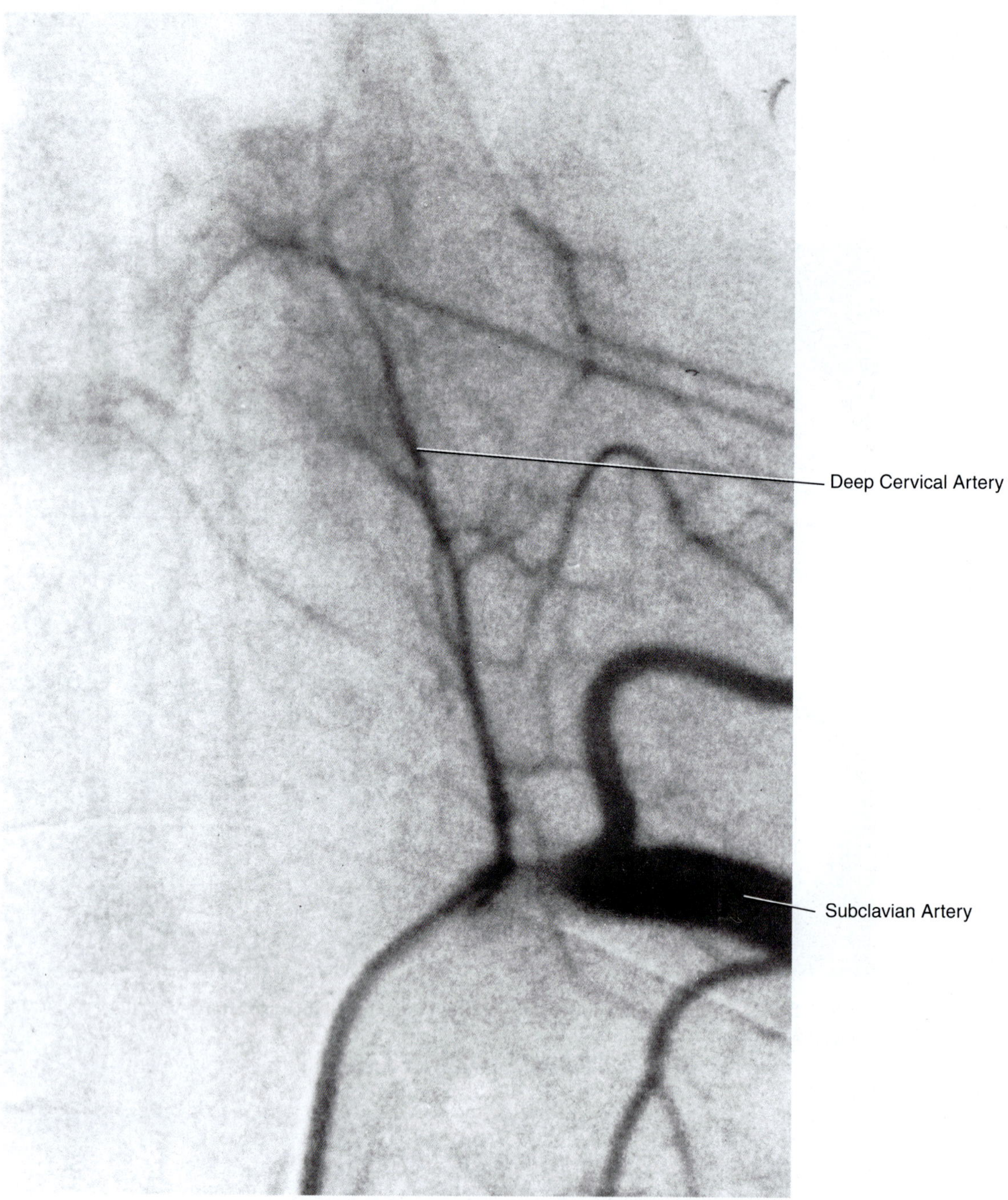

Figure 15.13. Deep cervical artery arising from the internal thoracic artery. Note the relationship with the subclavian artery.

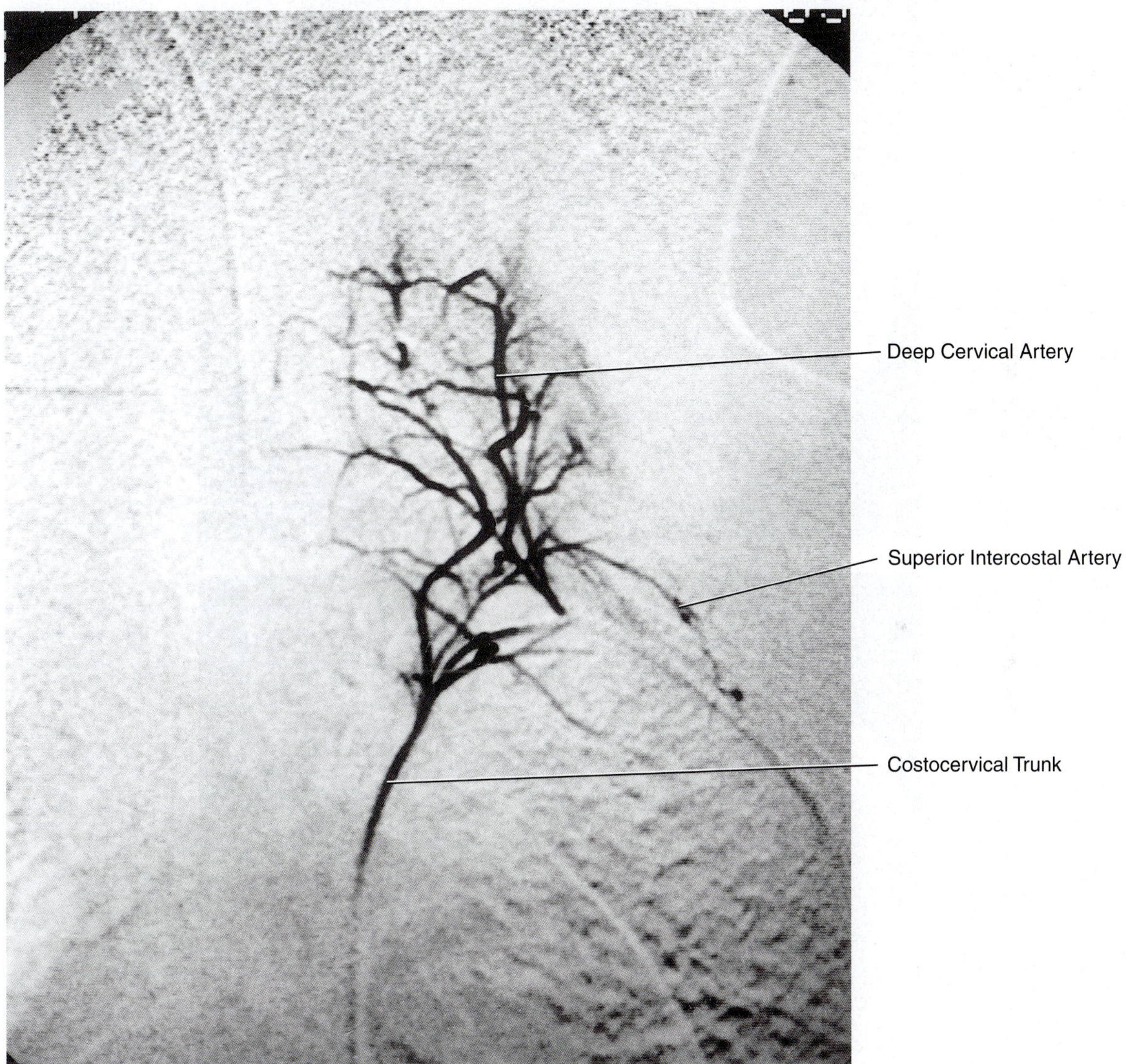

Figure 15.14. **Deep cervical artery, shorter than usual.** Note the muscular arteries and the anastomosis with the intercostal artery. Origin from the costocervical trunk.

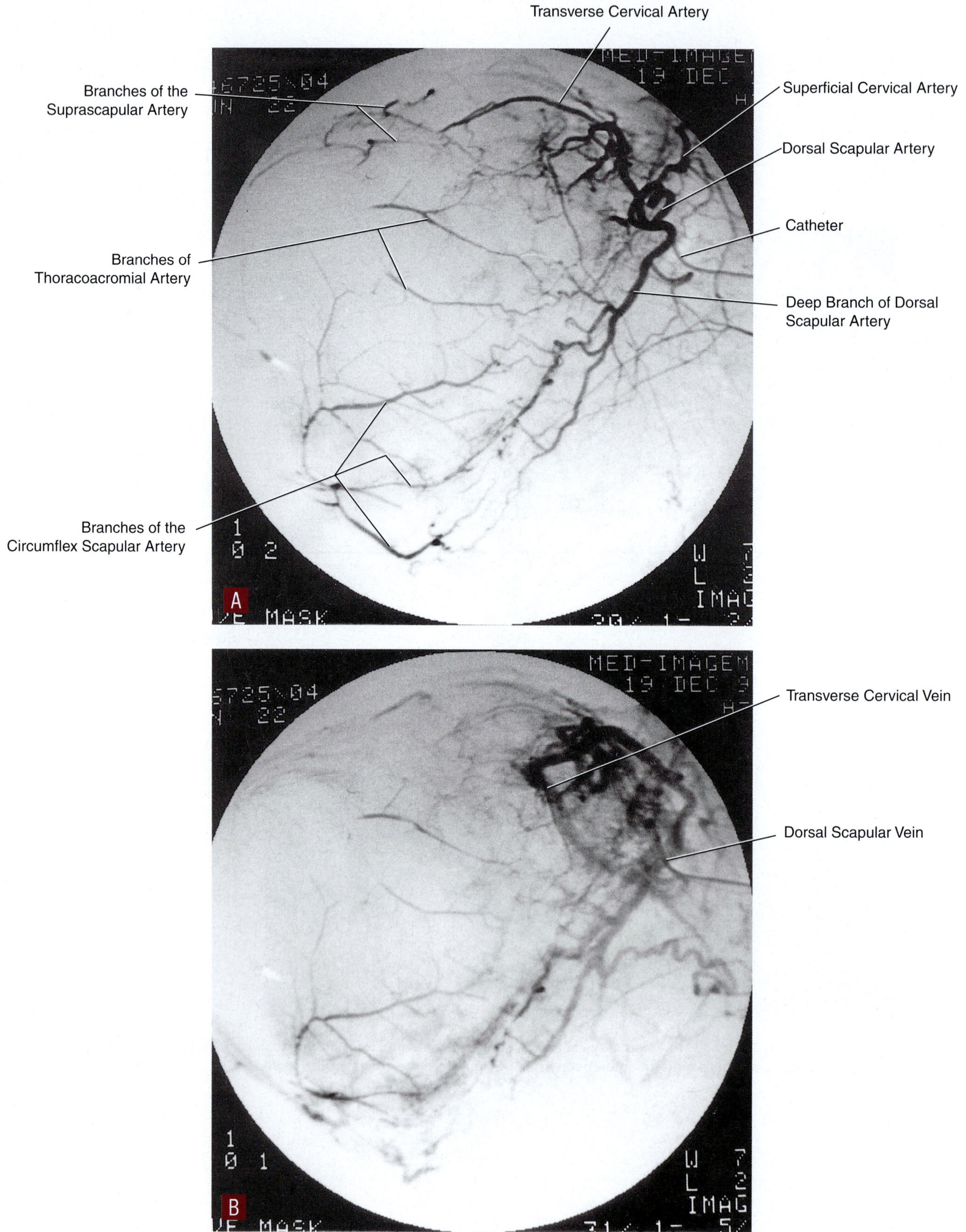

Figure 15.15. **A**, Scapular anastomosis. Angiogram of the dorsal scapular artery and main branches. Distal anastomoses are visible because of embolization of other arteries. **B**, Late phase of the angiogram showing the veins.

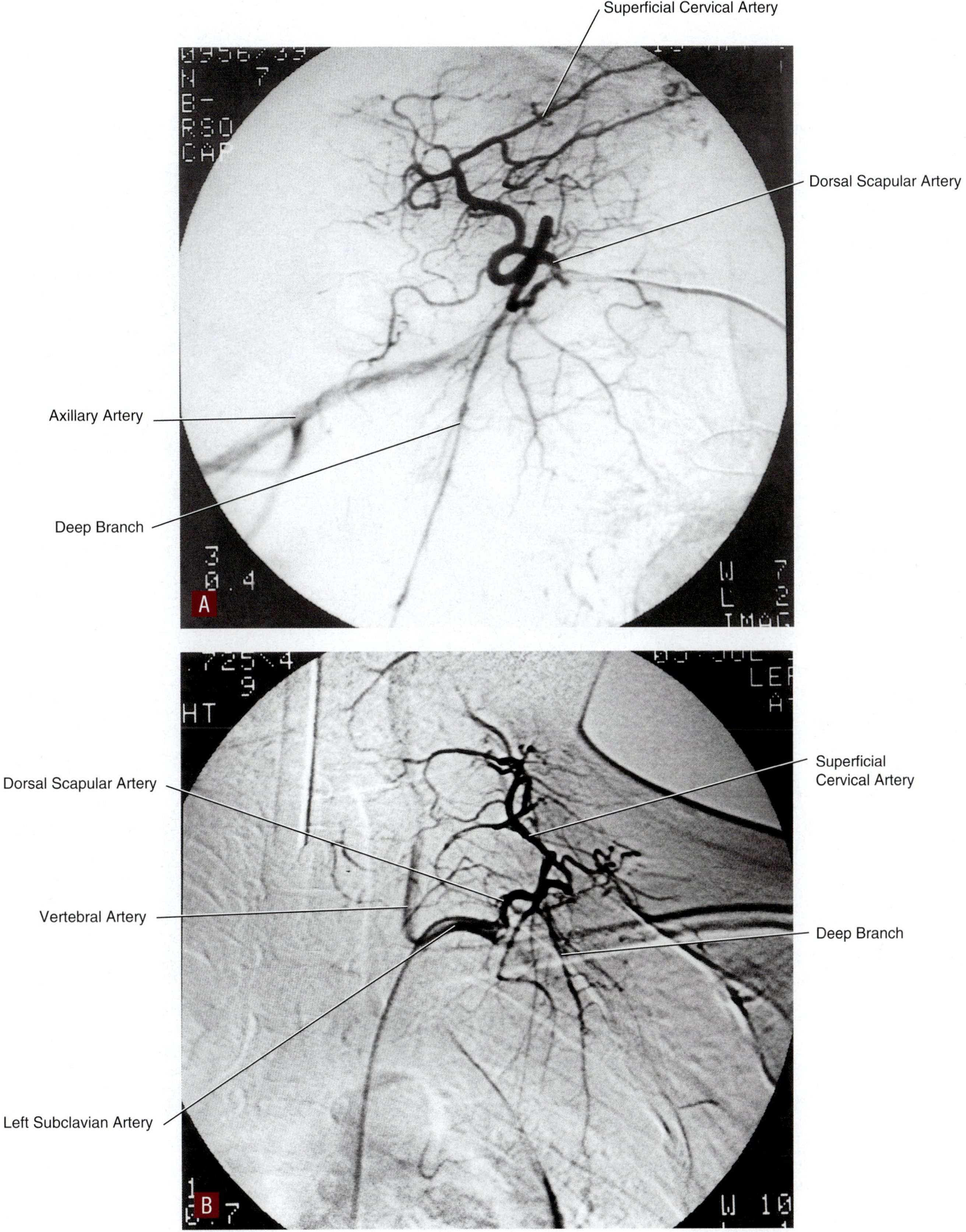

Figure 15.16. A, Angiogram of the dorsal scapular artery on the right side. B, Selective angiography of the left dorsal scapular artery, showing the superficial cervical artery and the deep branch.

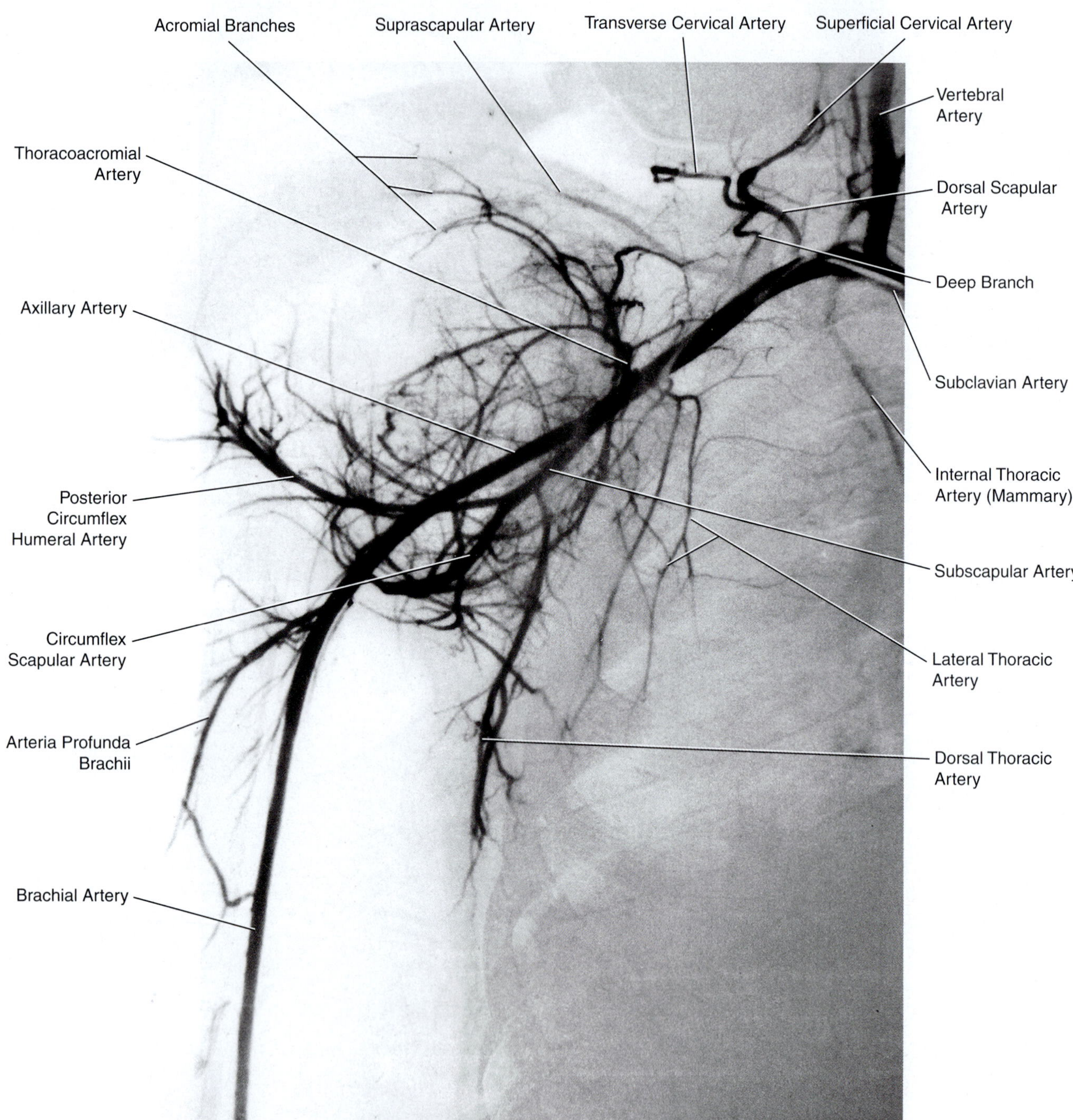

Figure 15.17. Angiogram of the right subclavian, axillary, and brachial arteries. Note the common trunk originating the subscapular, the circumflex scapular, and posterior circumflex scapular arteries.

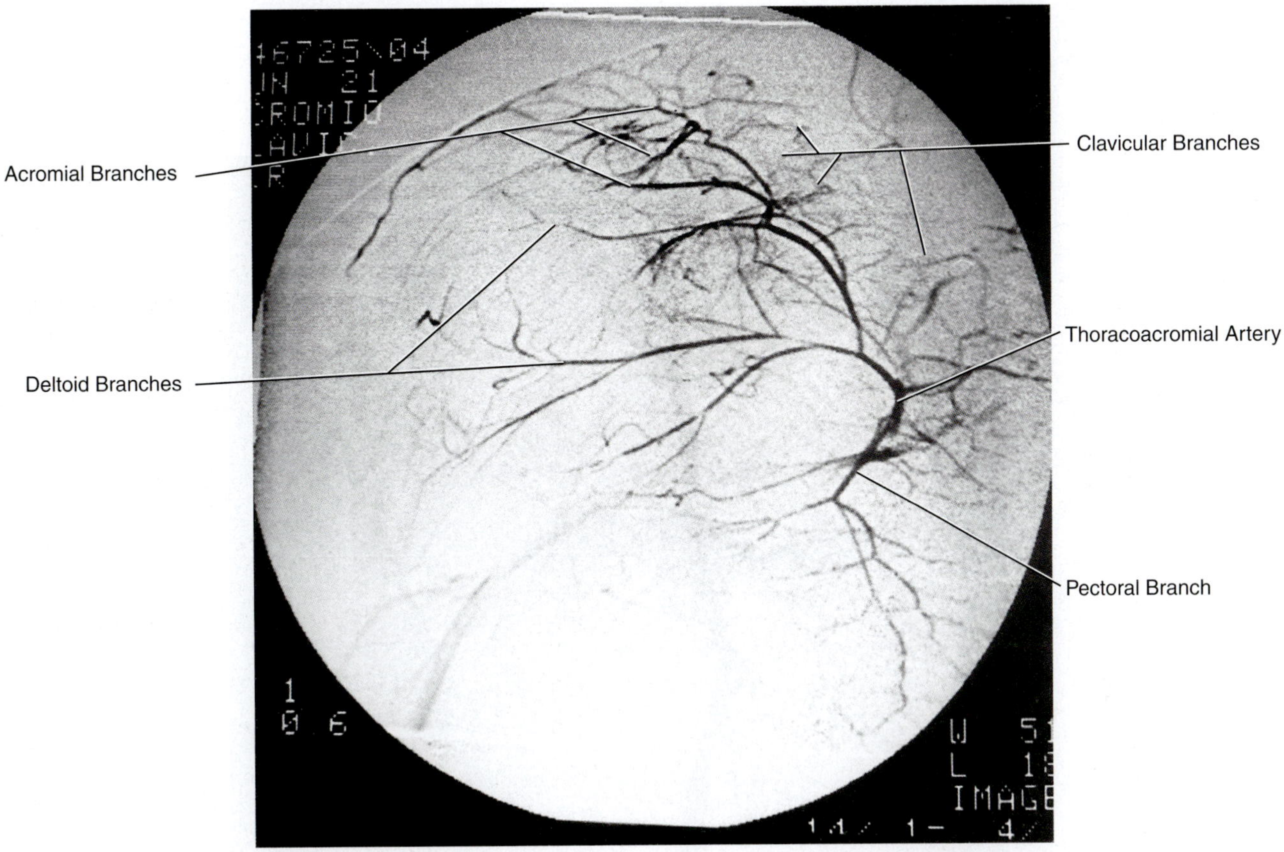

Acromial Branches

Clavicular Branches

Deltoid Branches

Thoracoacromial Artery

Pectoral Branch

Figure 15.18. Right thoracoacromial artery and main branches.

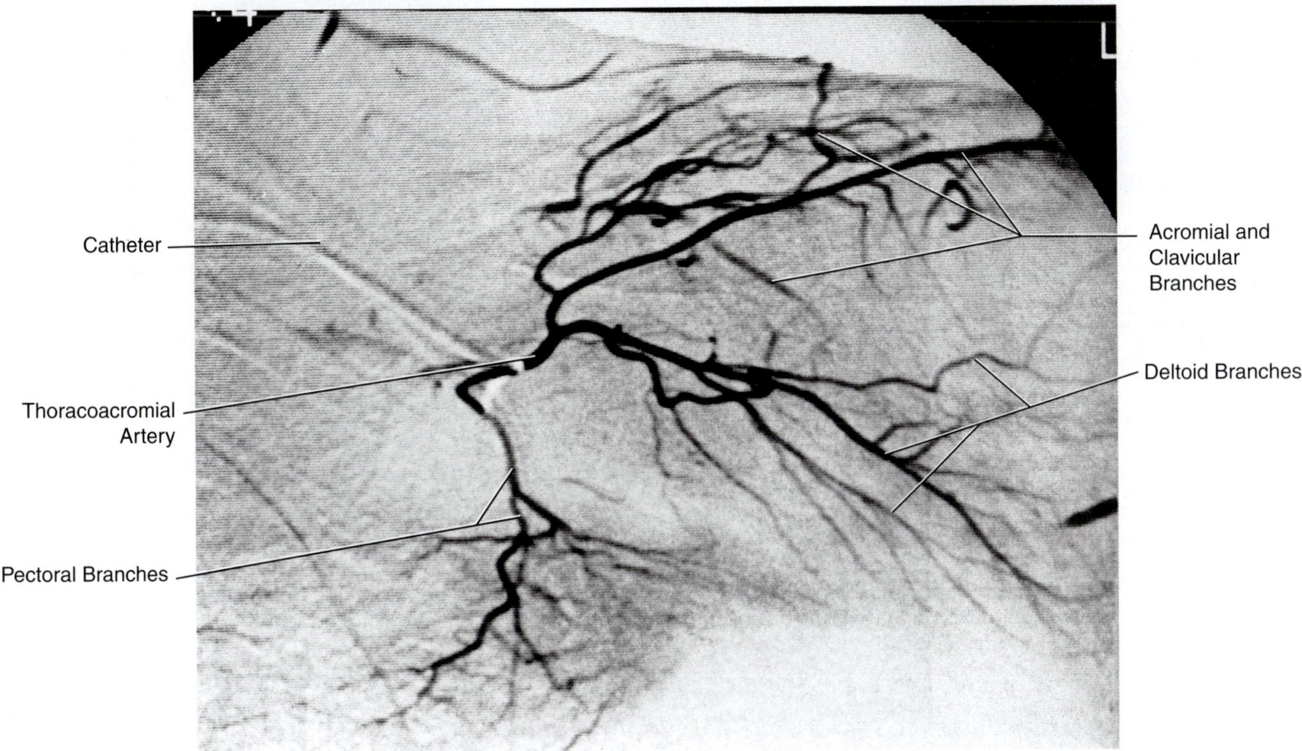

Figure 15.19. Left thoracoacromial artery and main branches.

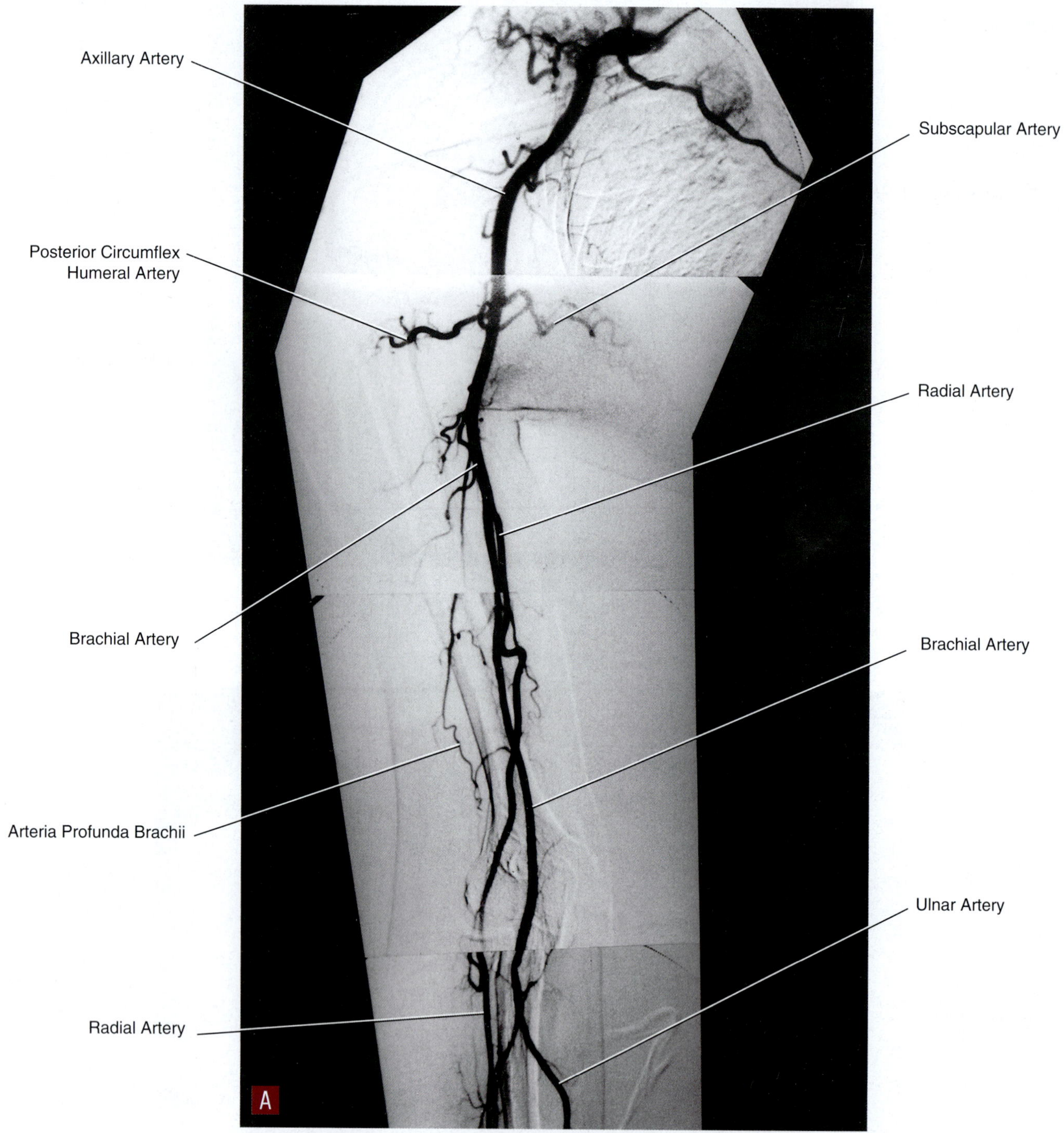

Figure 15.20. **A**, Selective angiogram of the right brachial artery. Note that the radial artery is originated high from the brachial artery. **B**, Distal angiogram showing the radial artery reaching the wrist.

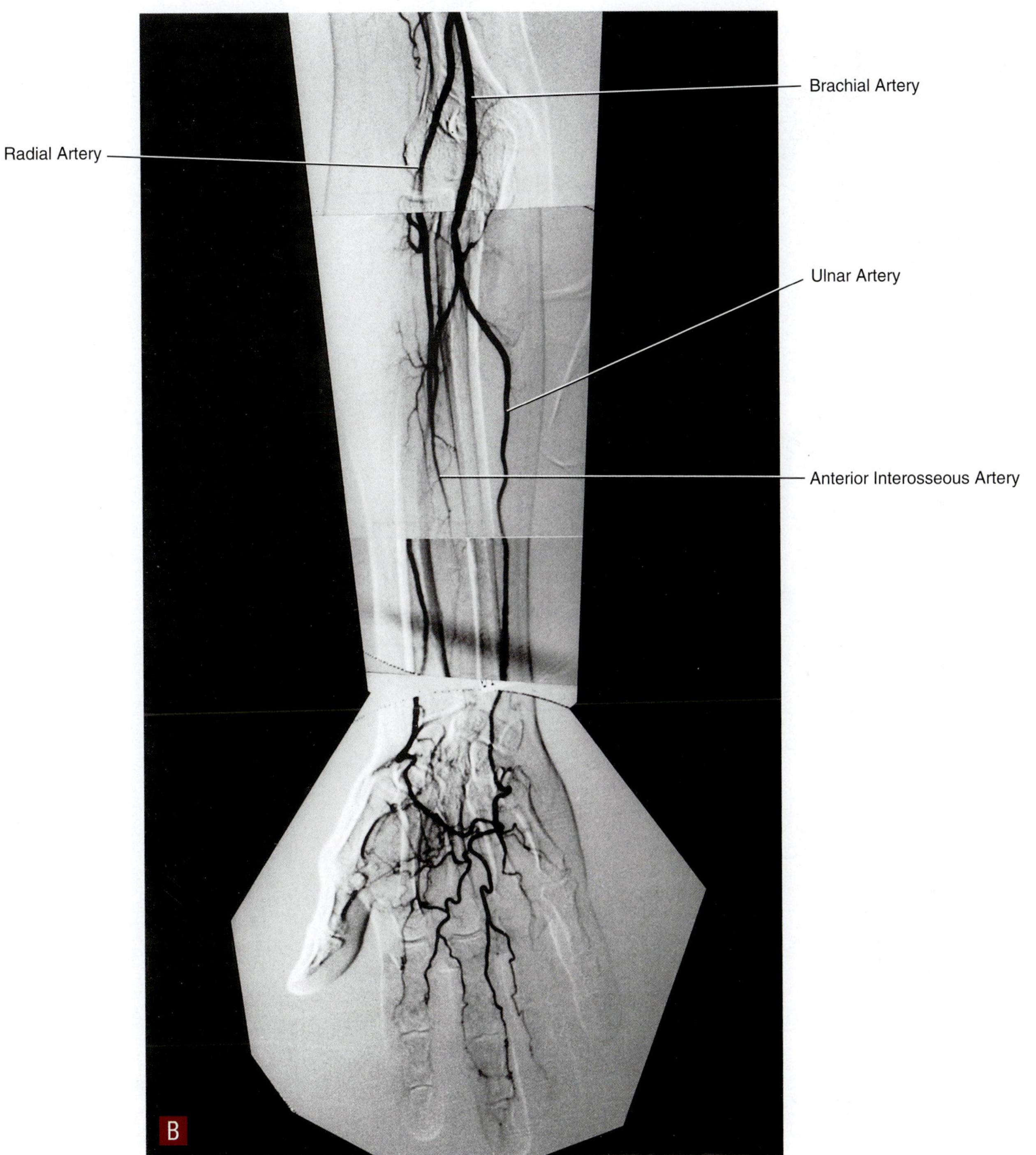

Figure 15.20. *Continued*

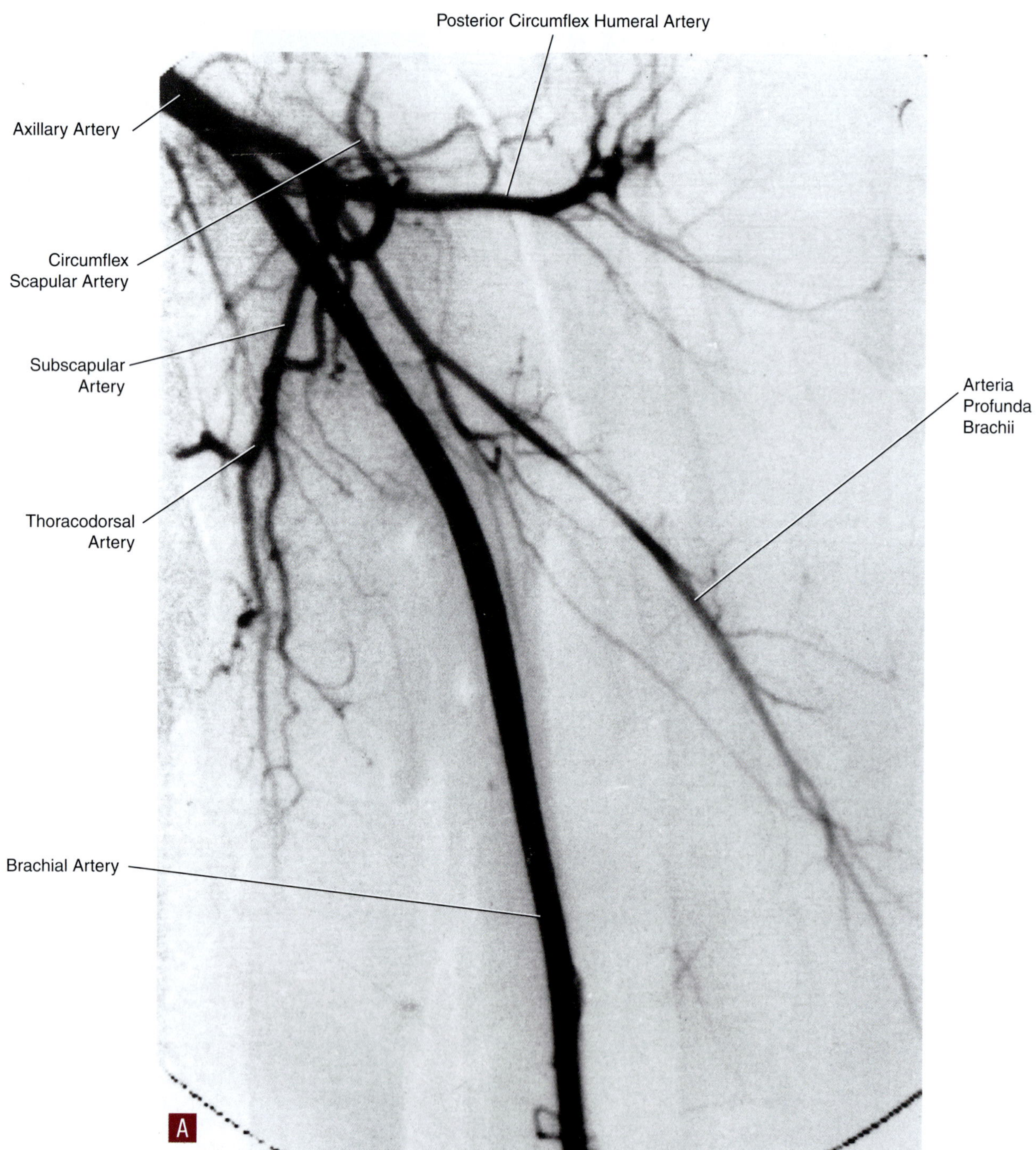

Figure 15.21. The left axillary artery and main branches (A). Note the arteria profunda brachii originating from a common trunk together with the subscapular, posterior circumflex humeral, and circumflex scapular arteries (B).

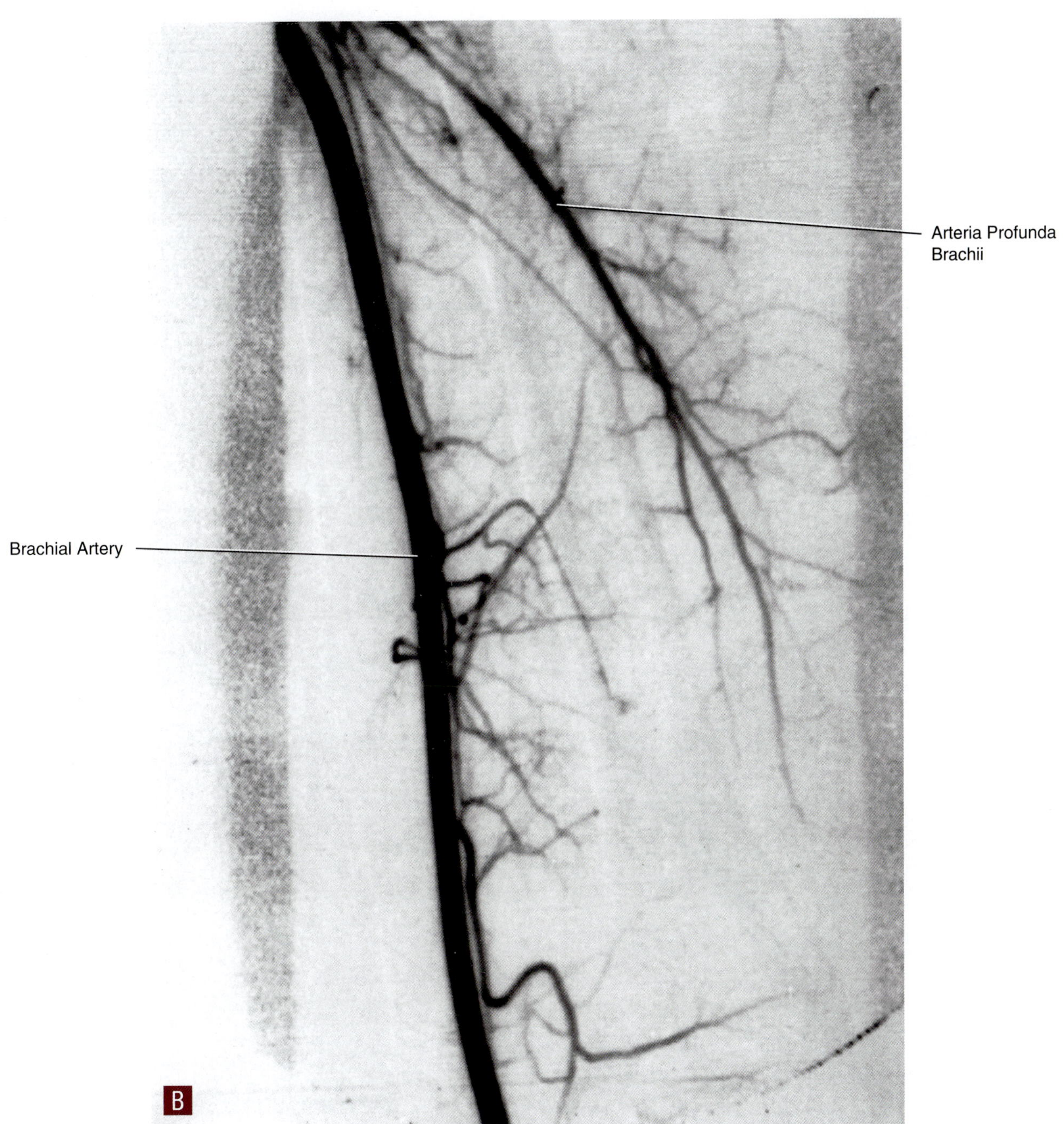

Figure 15.21. *Continued*

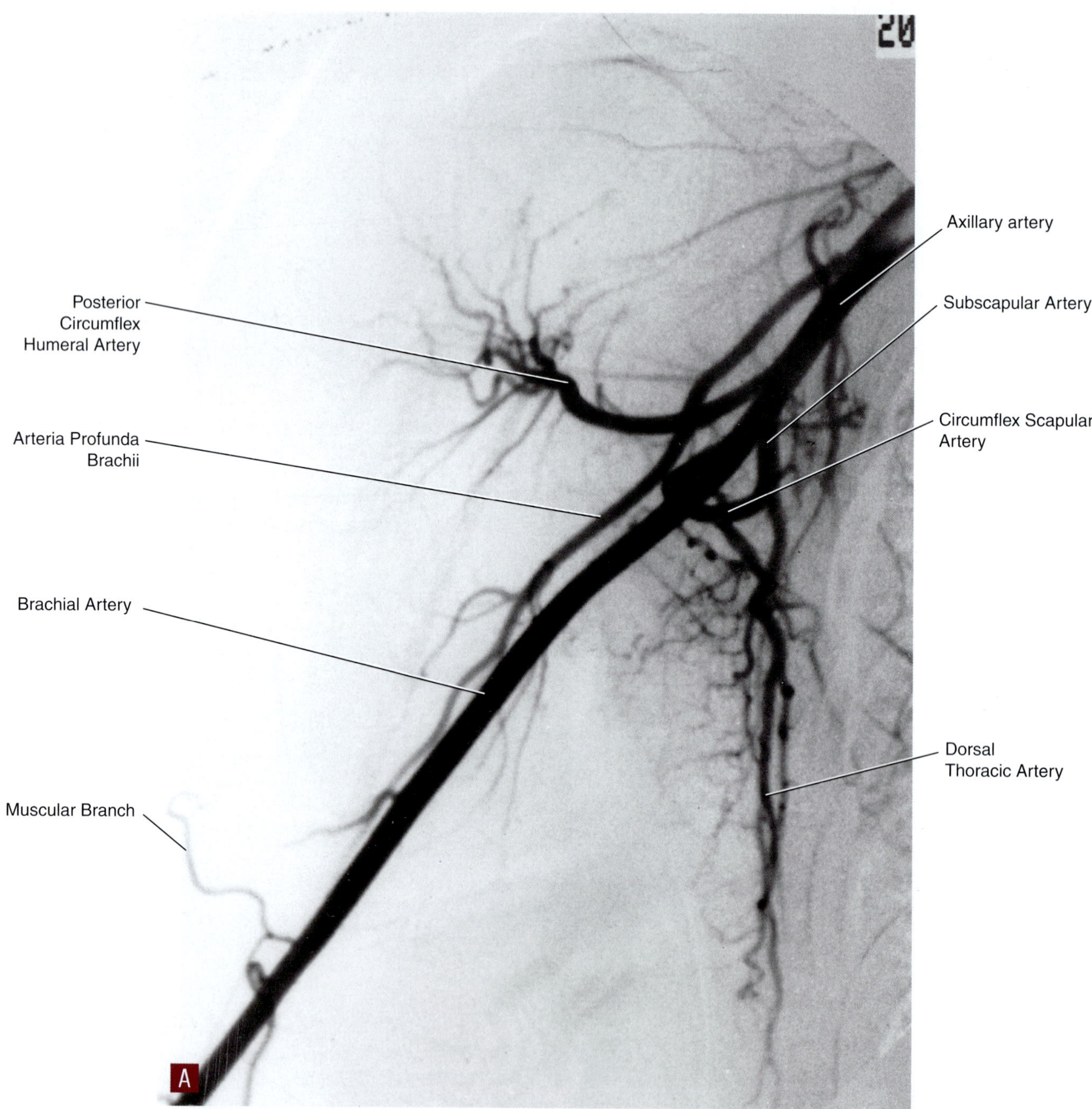

Figure 15.22. **A**, High origin of the arteria profunda brachii from the axillary artery. **B**, Common trunk giving origin to the pectoral, lateral thoracic, and subscapular arteries.

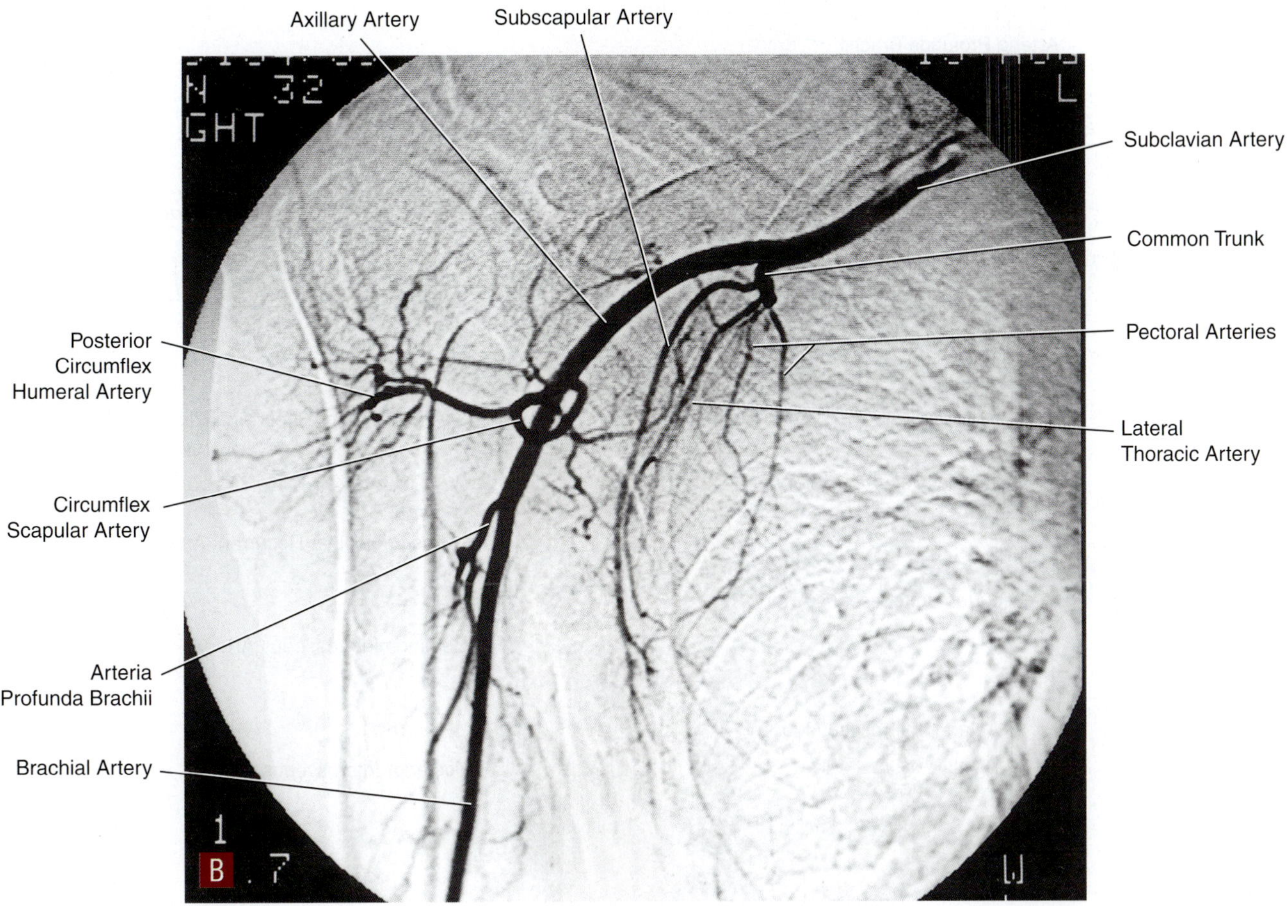

Figure 15.22. *Continued*

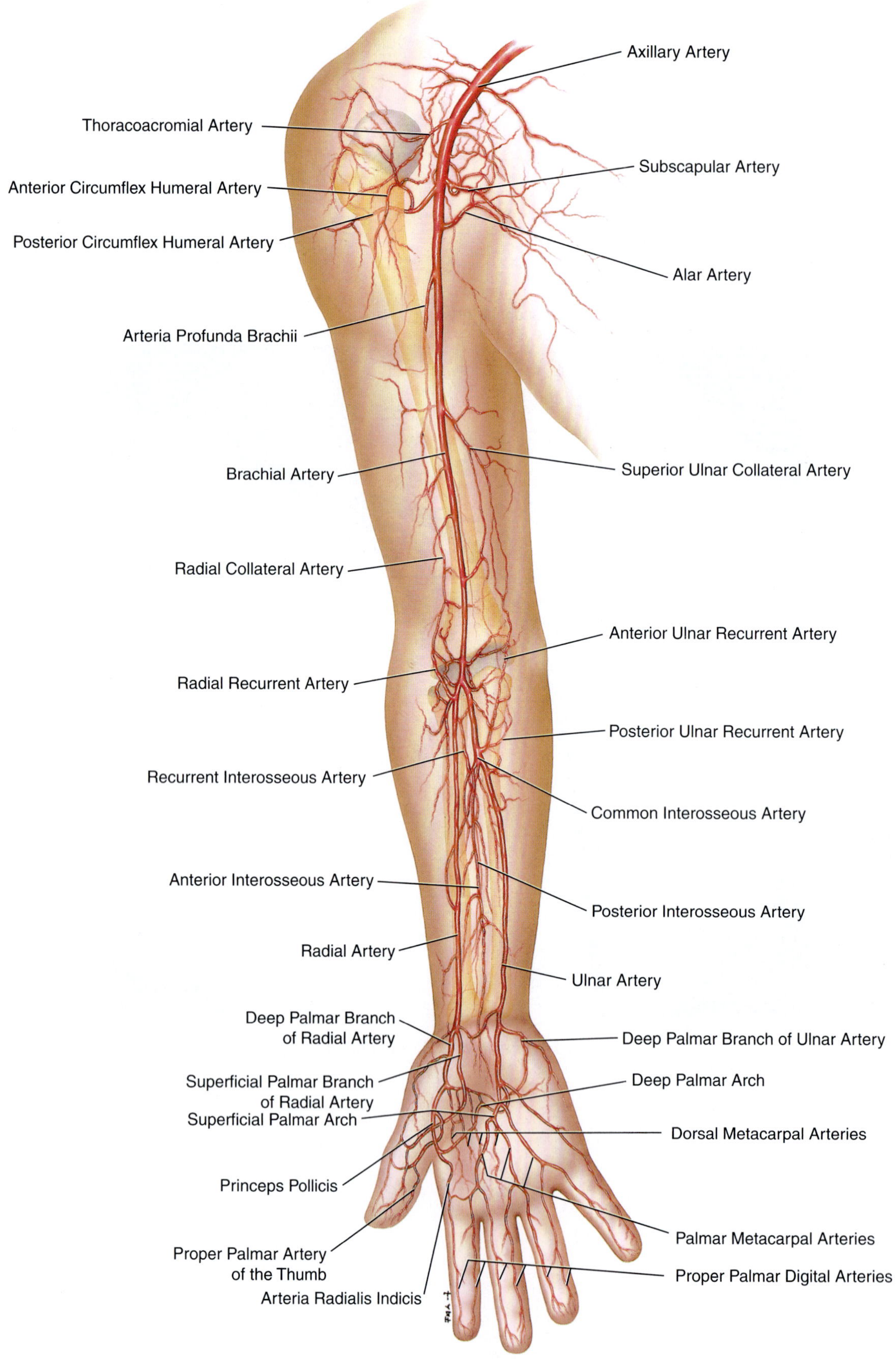

Figure 15.23. The right brachial artery and its branches. Art based on an actual angiogram.

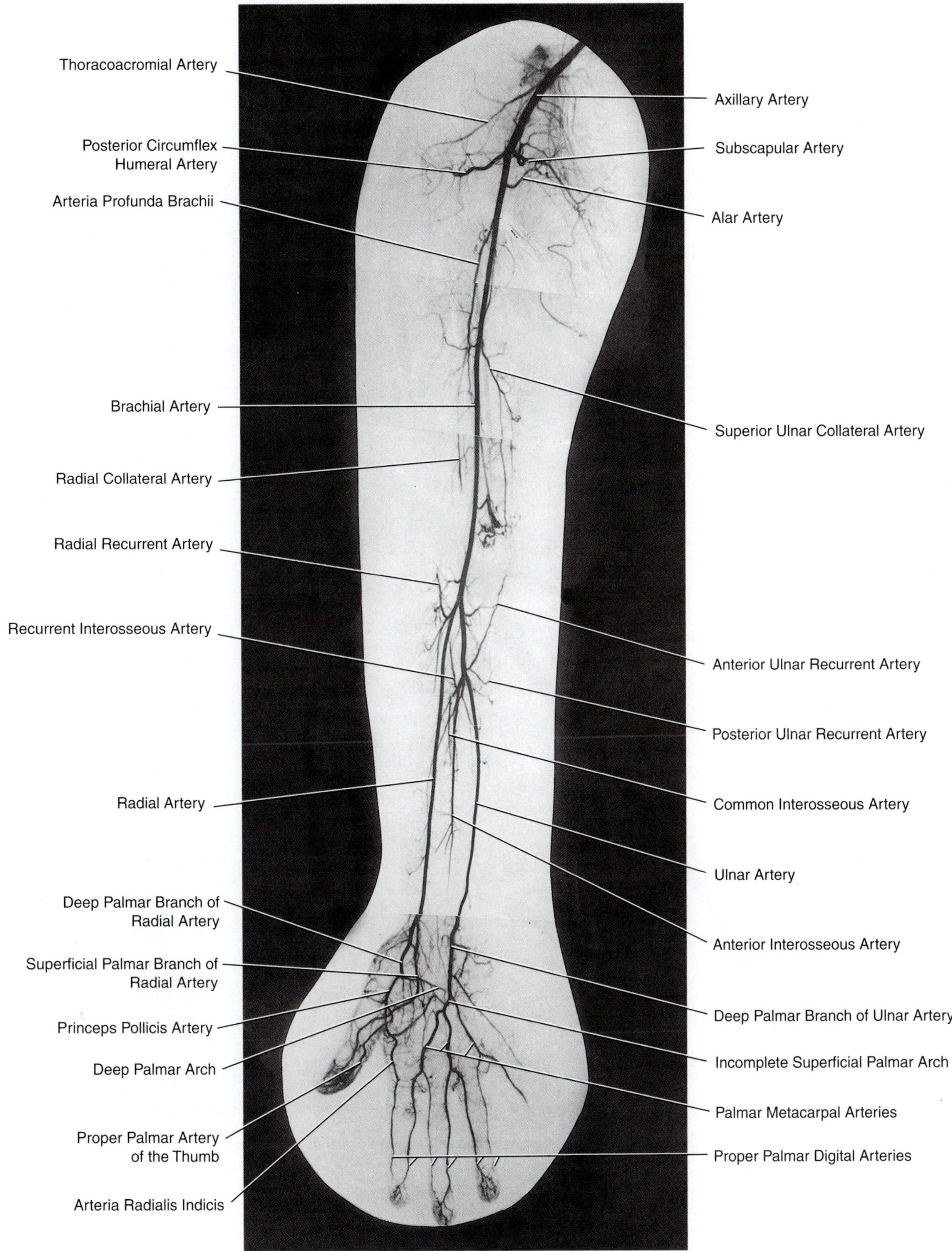

Figure 15.24. Digital subtraction angiogram of the right arm. Brachial artery and main branches.

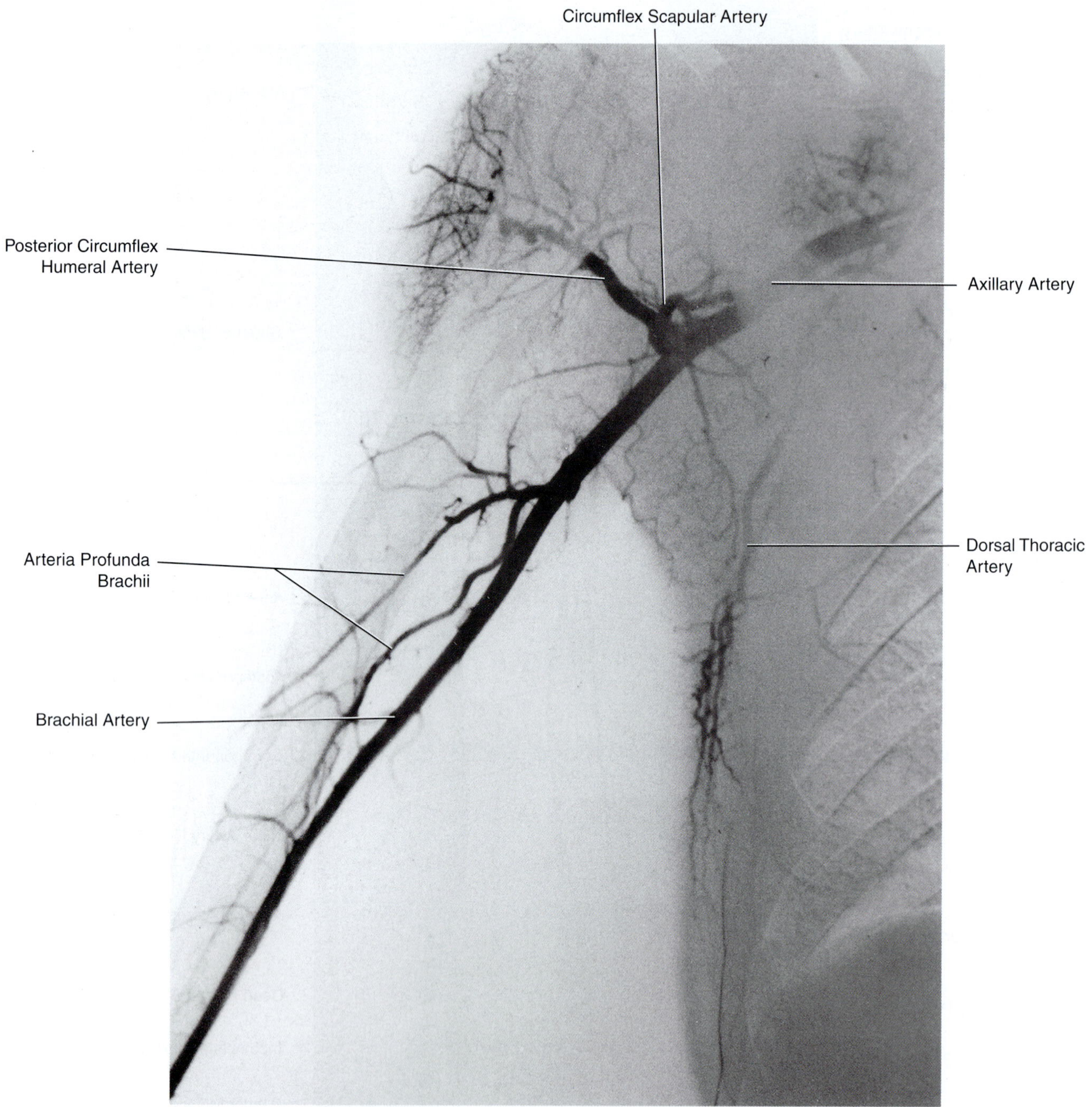

Figure 15.25. **Subtraction angiogram of the axillary and brachial artery and main branches.**

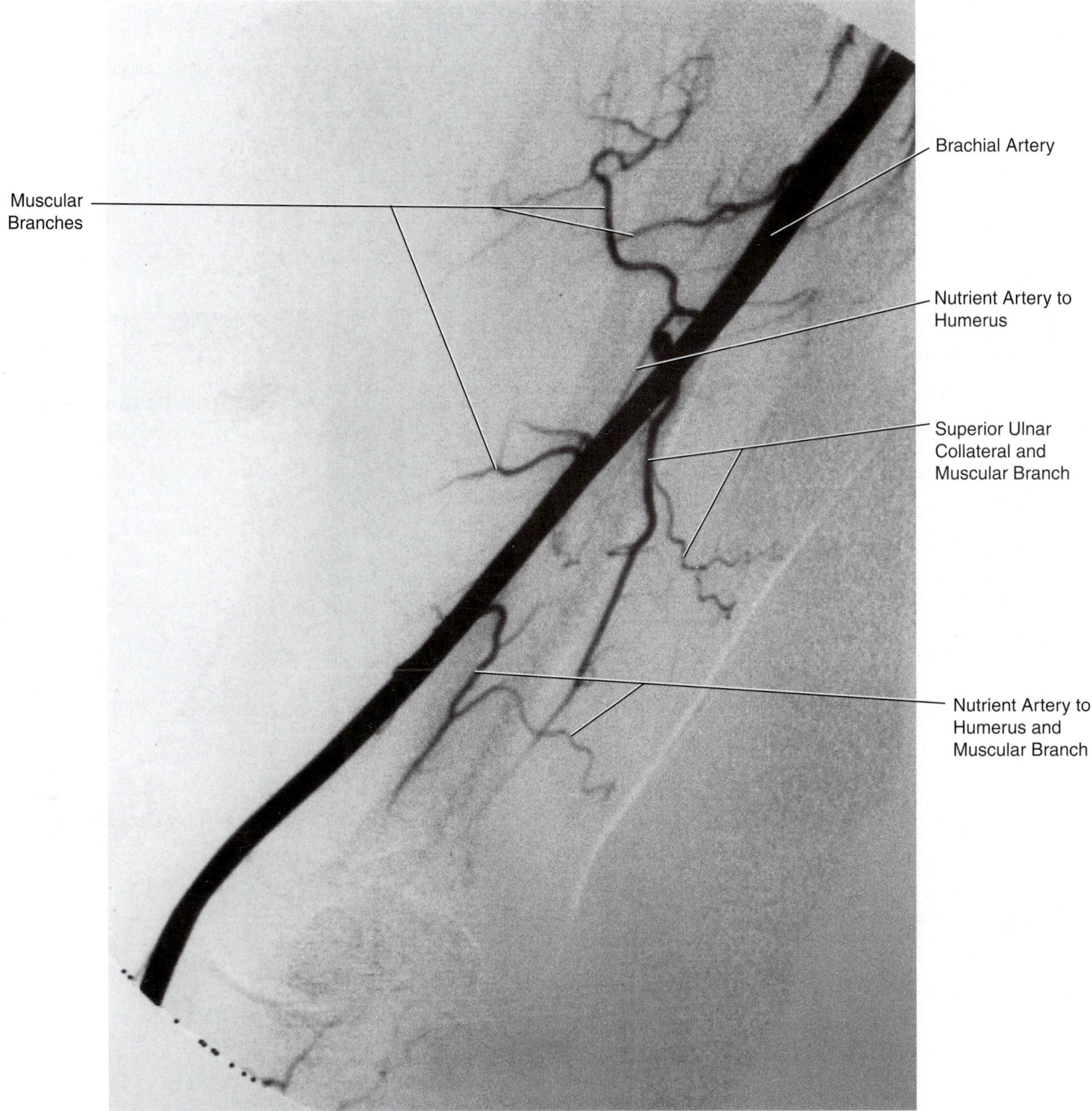

Figure 15.26. **Brachial artery and branches.**

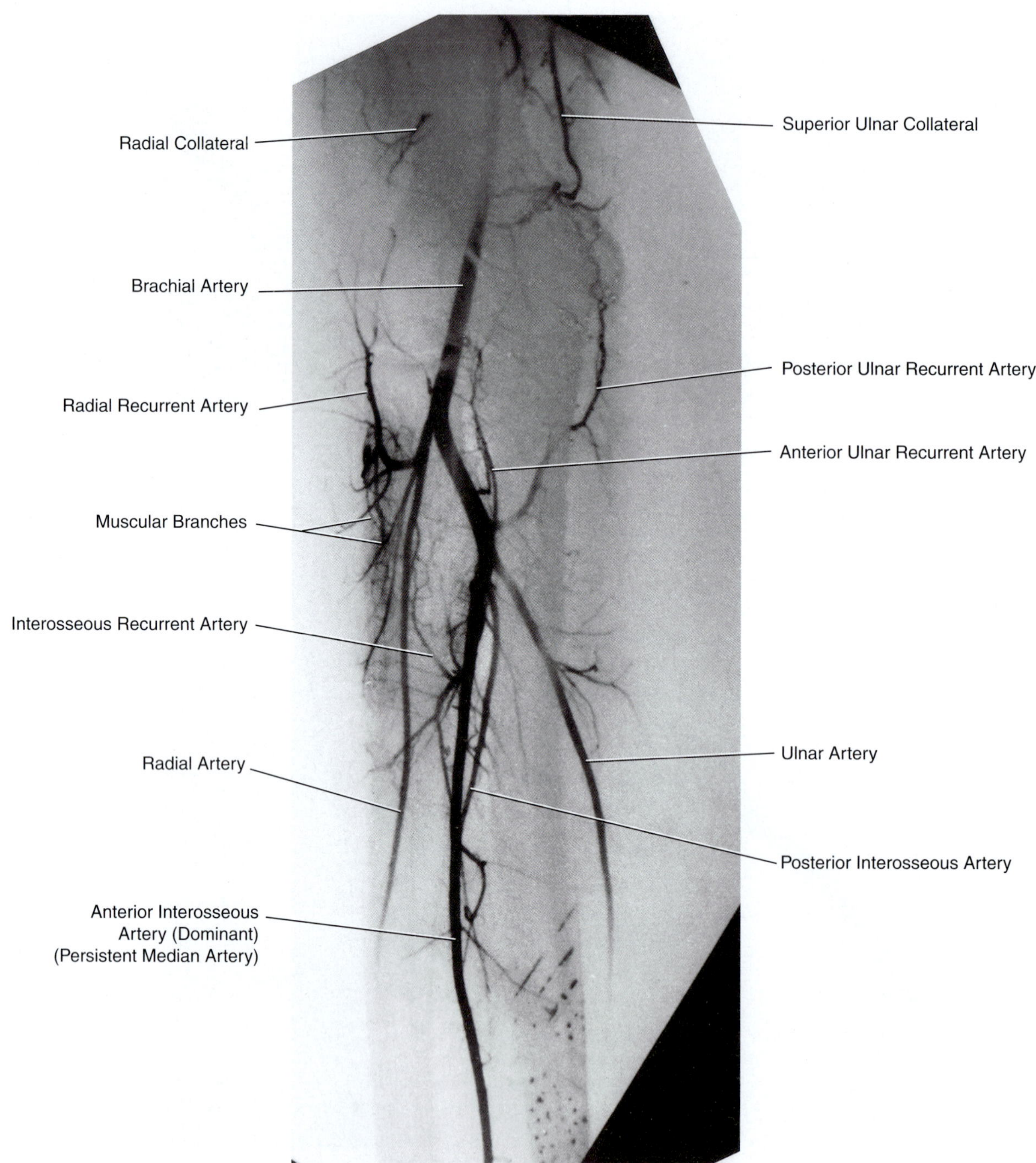

Figure 15.27. Bifurcation of the brachial artery. Note the dominant persistent median artery.

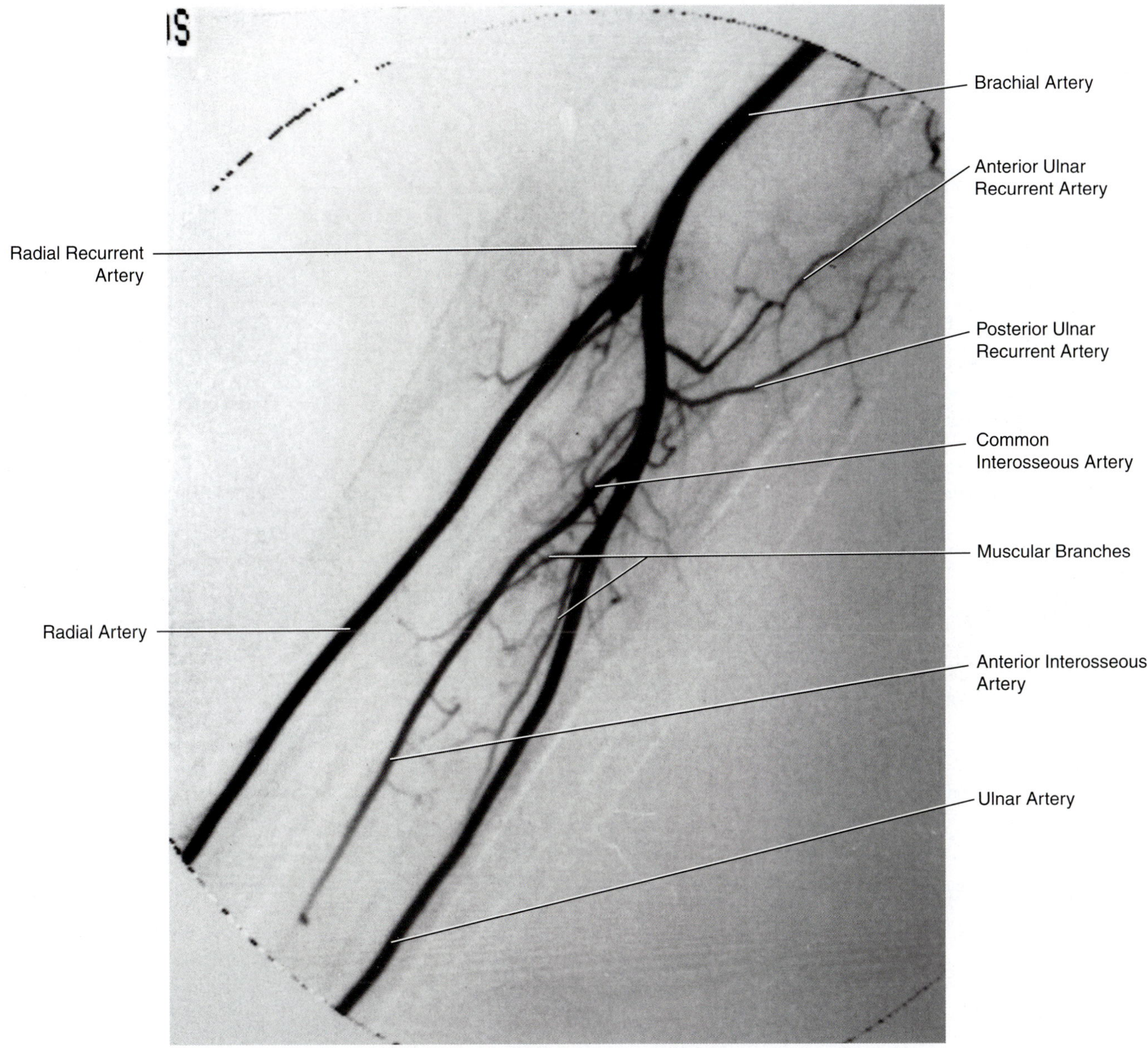

Figure 15.28. **Normal bifurcation of the brachial artery.**

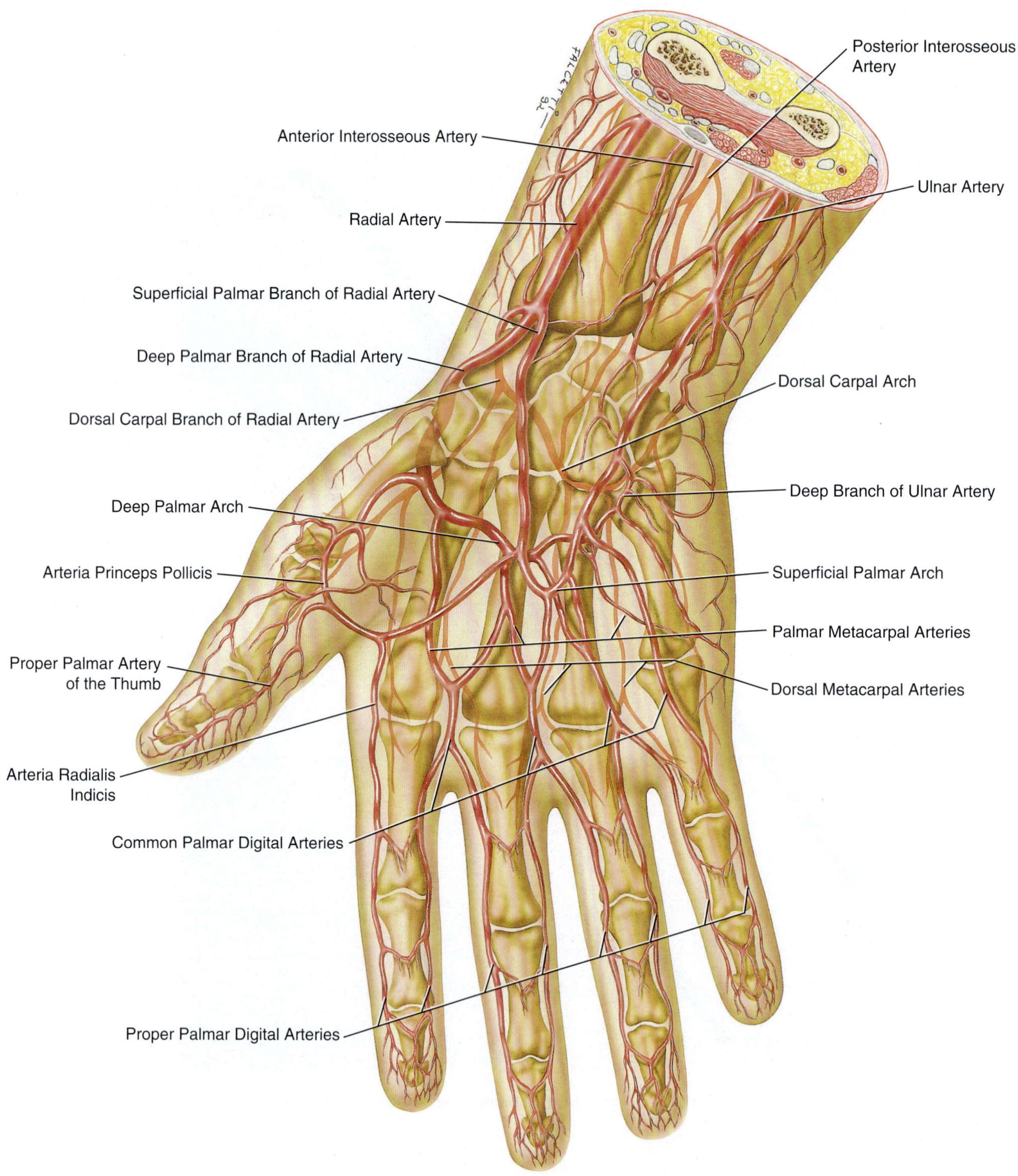

Figure 15.29. **Right hand.** Radial and ulnar branches. The hand is in anatomic position with the palmar aspect showed ventrally. The art is based on an actual angiogram.

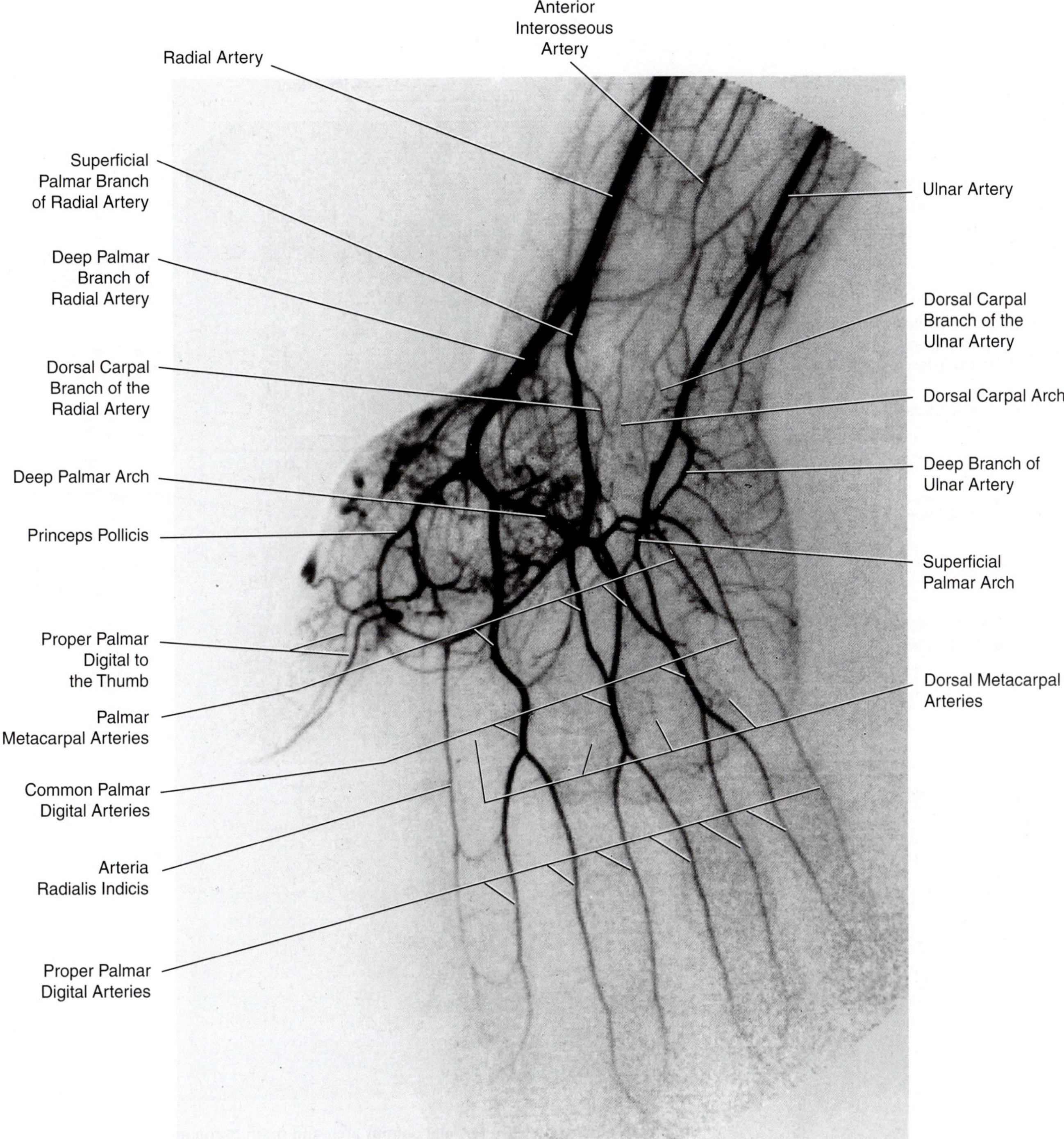

Figure 15.30. Angiogram of the right hand and main arteries. Note the A-V malformation at the tenar region. The deep and superficial palmar arches are complete.

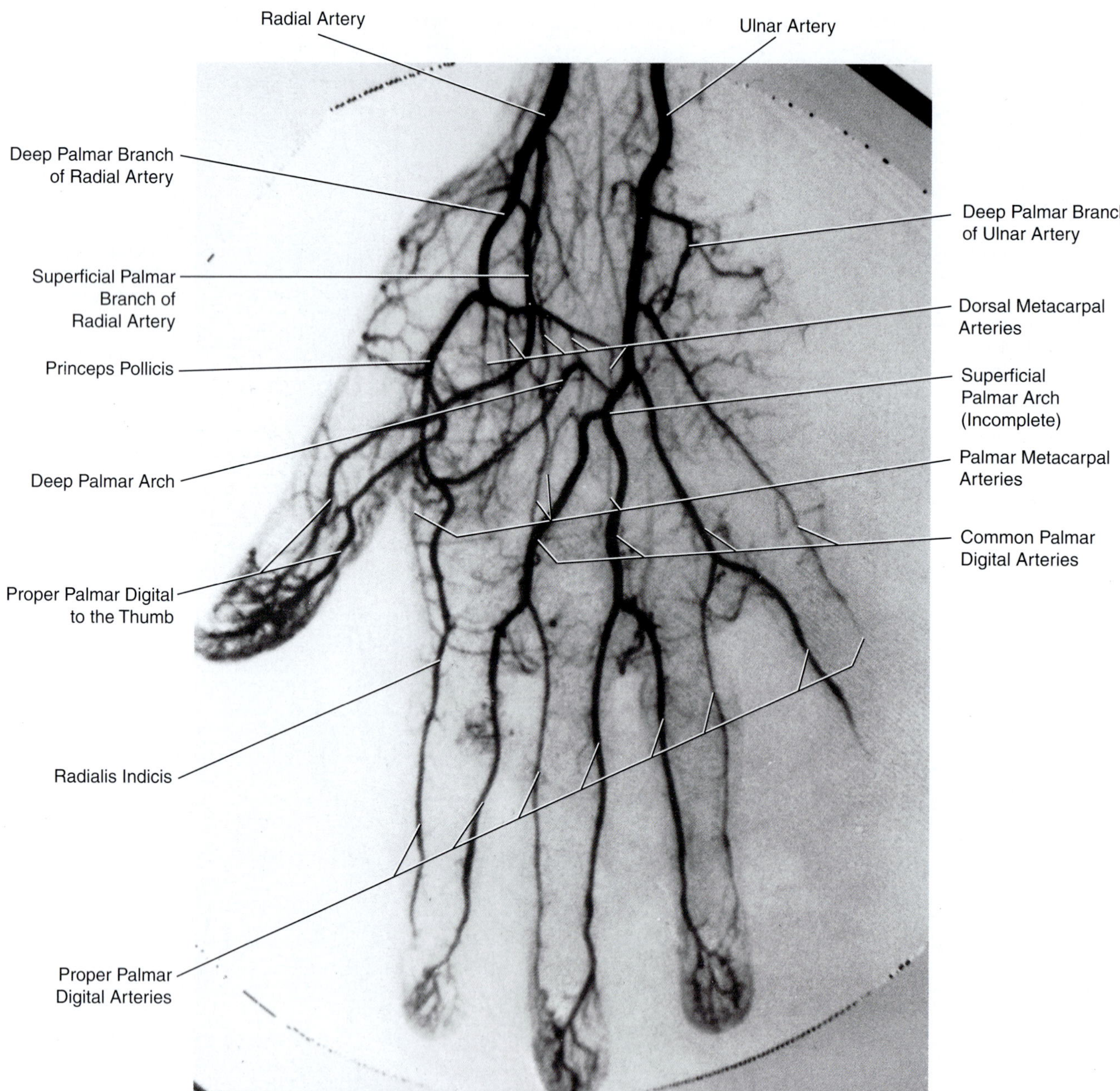

Figure 15.31. Right hand with incomplete superficial palmar arch and main branches.

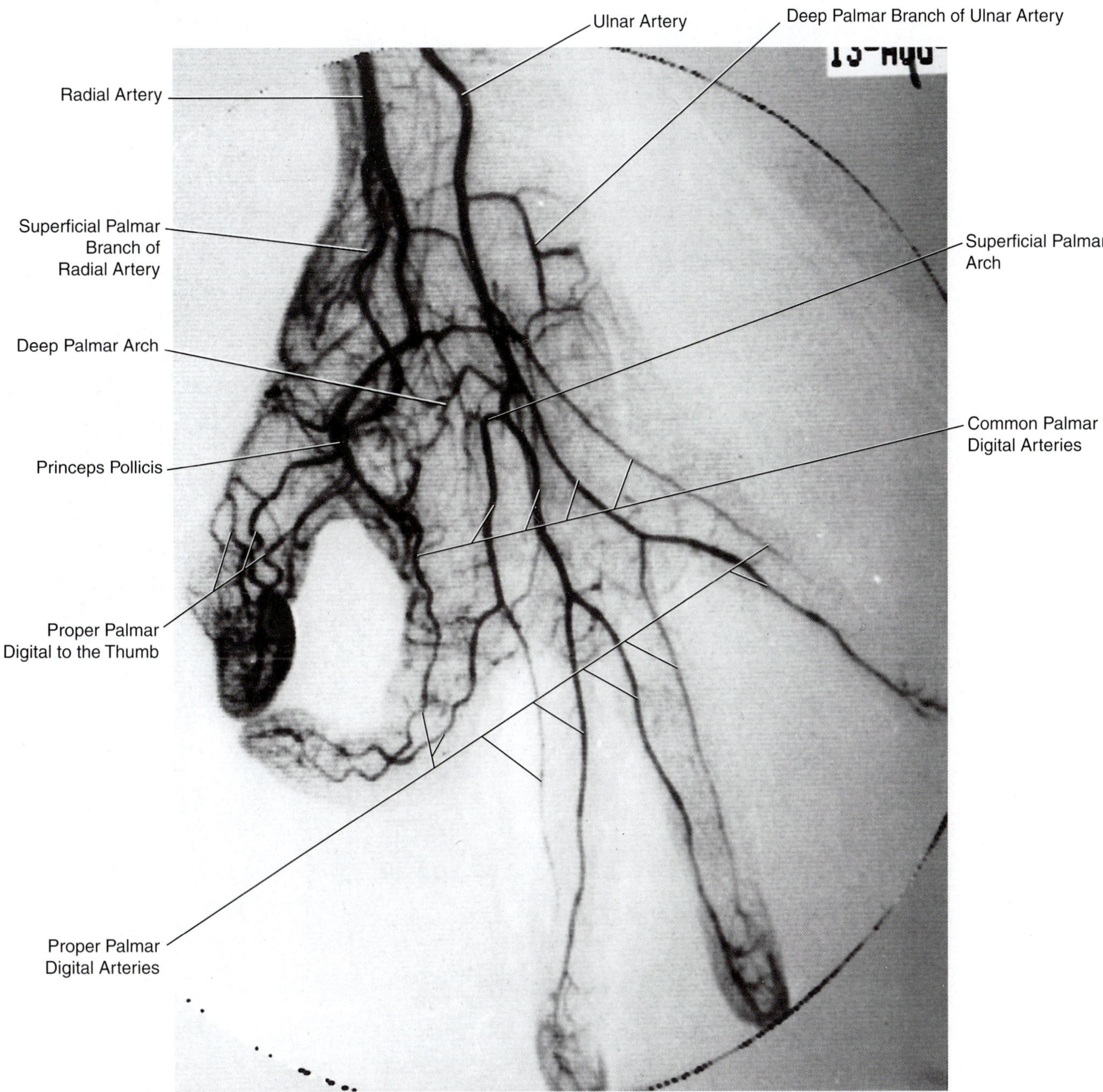

Figure 15.32. **Oblique view of the right hand angiogram.** Same as in Fig. 15.29.

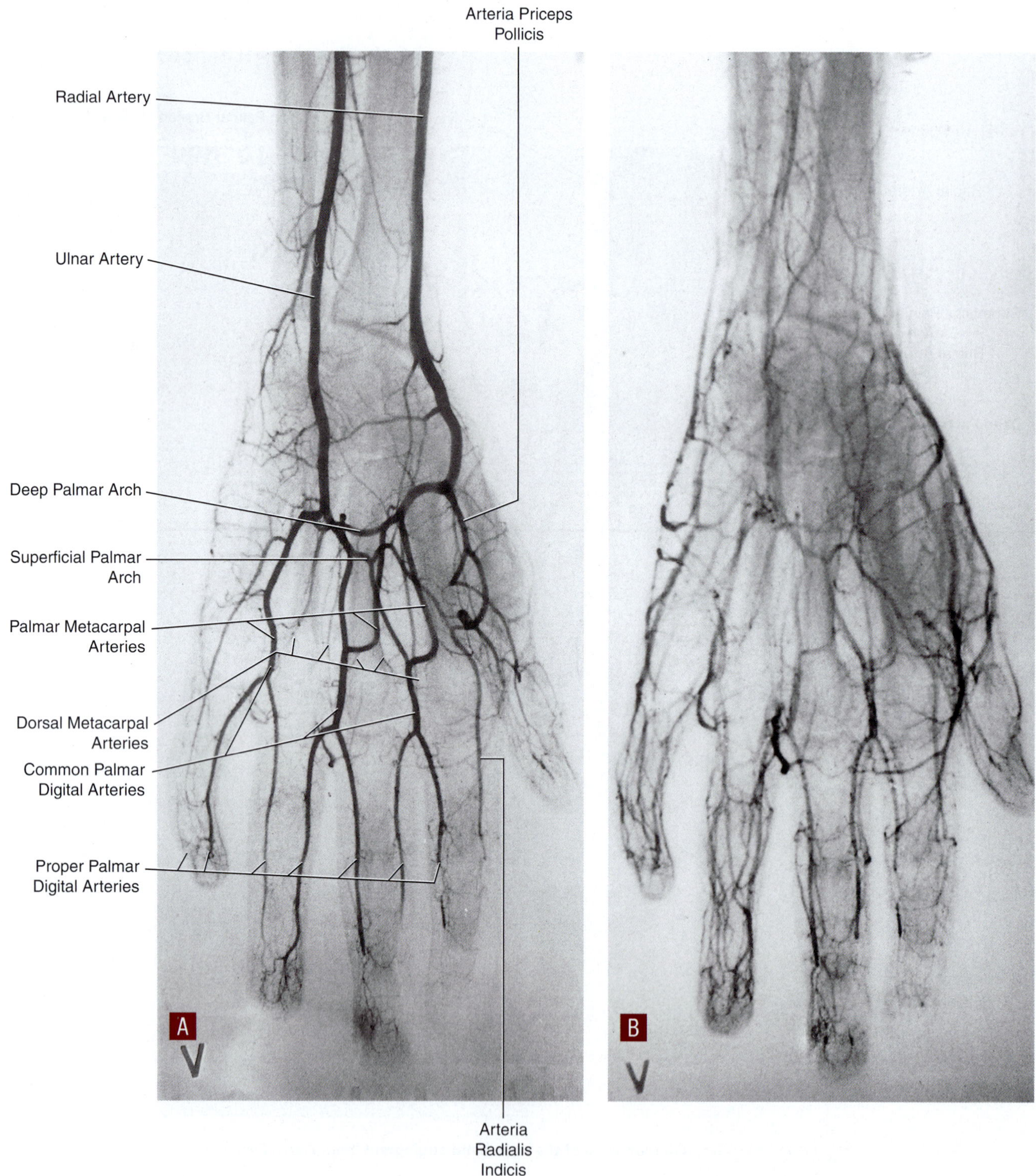

Figure 15.33. **A**, Prone view of the left hand showing a complete superficial palmar arch. **B**, Later phase of the angiogram showing venous drainage. Note distal obstruction of the proper palmar digital arteries.

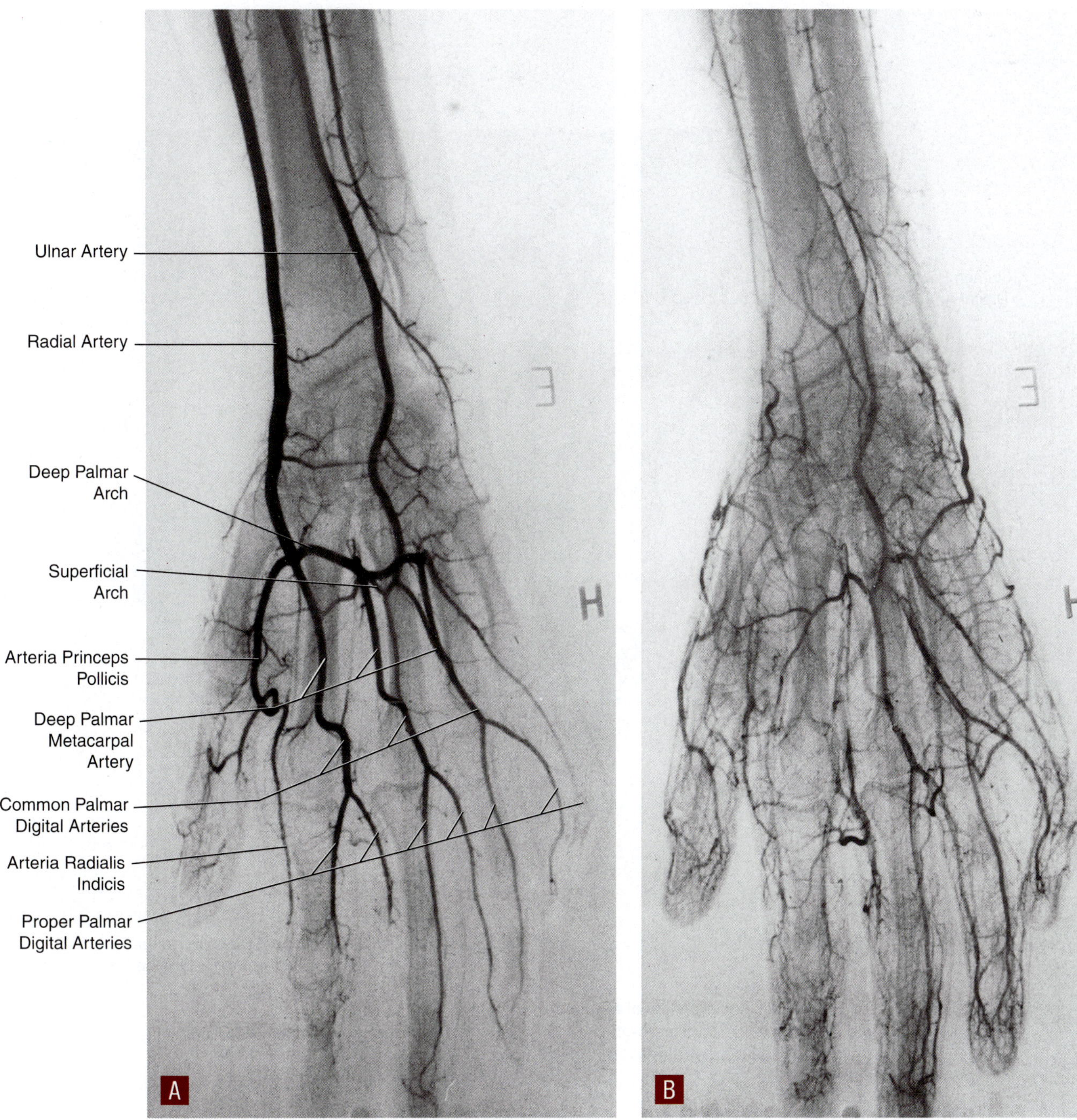

Figure 15.34. A, Prone view of the right hand showing a complete superficial palmar arch. B, Later phase of the angiogram showing the distal arteries and the beginning of the venous drainage. Note distal obstruction of the distal proper palmar digital arteries.

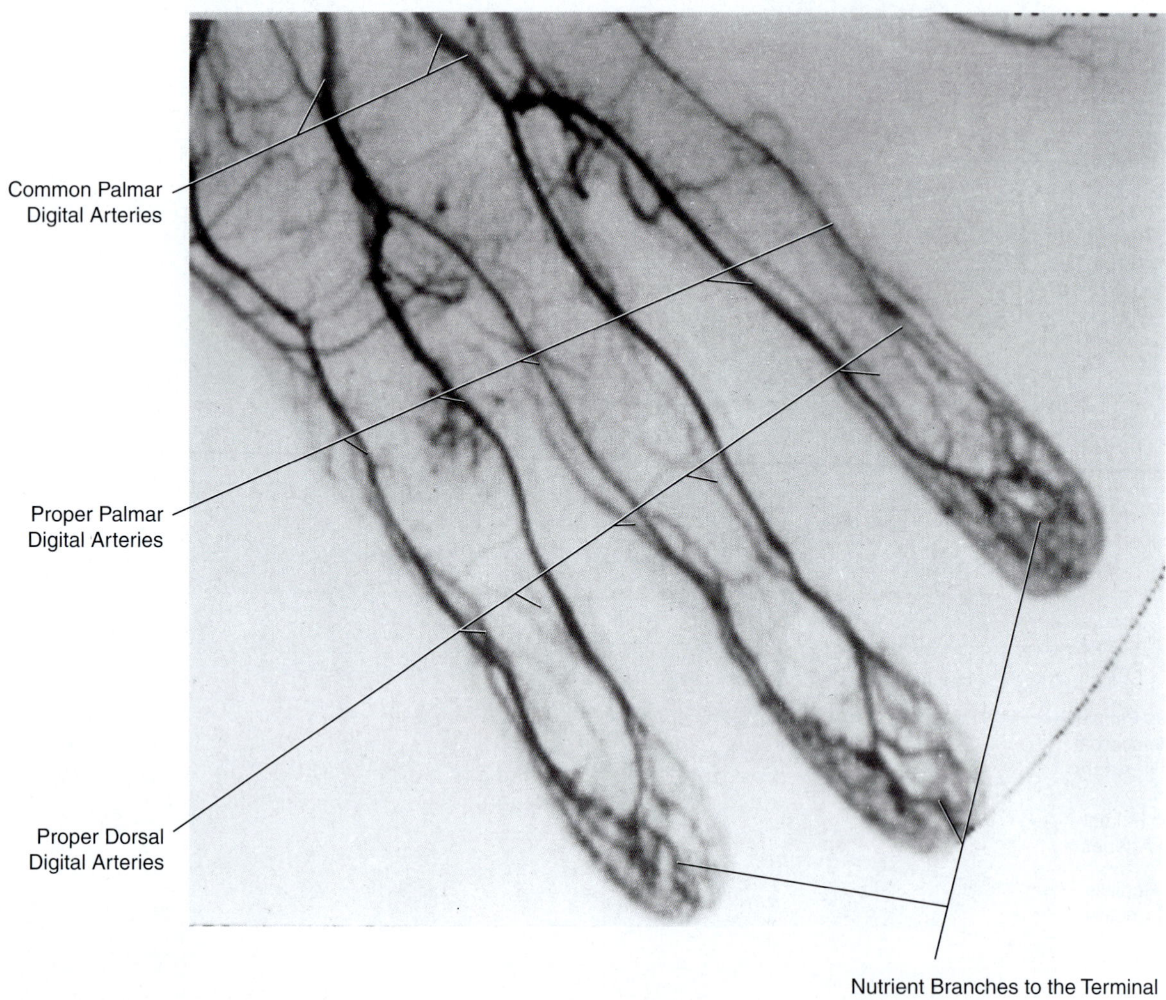

Figure 15.35. Closeup view of the tip of the second, third, and fourth fingers of the right hand showing the rich anastomotic bed of the digital circulation and the digital tufts. The proper dorsal and palmar digital arteries are visible. Note that the dorsal arteries are attenuated.

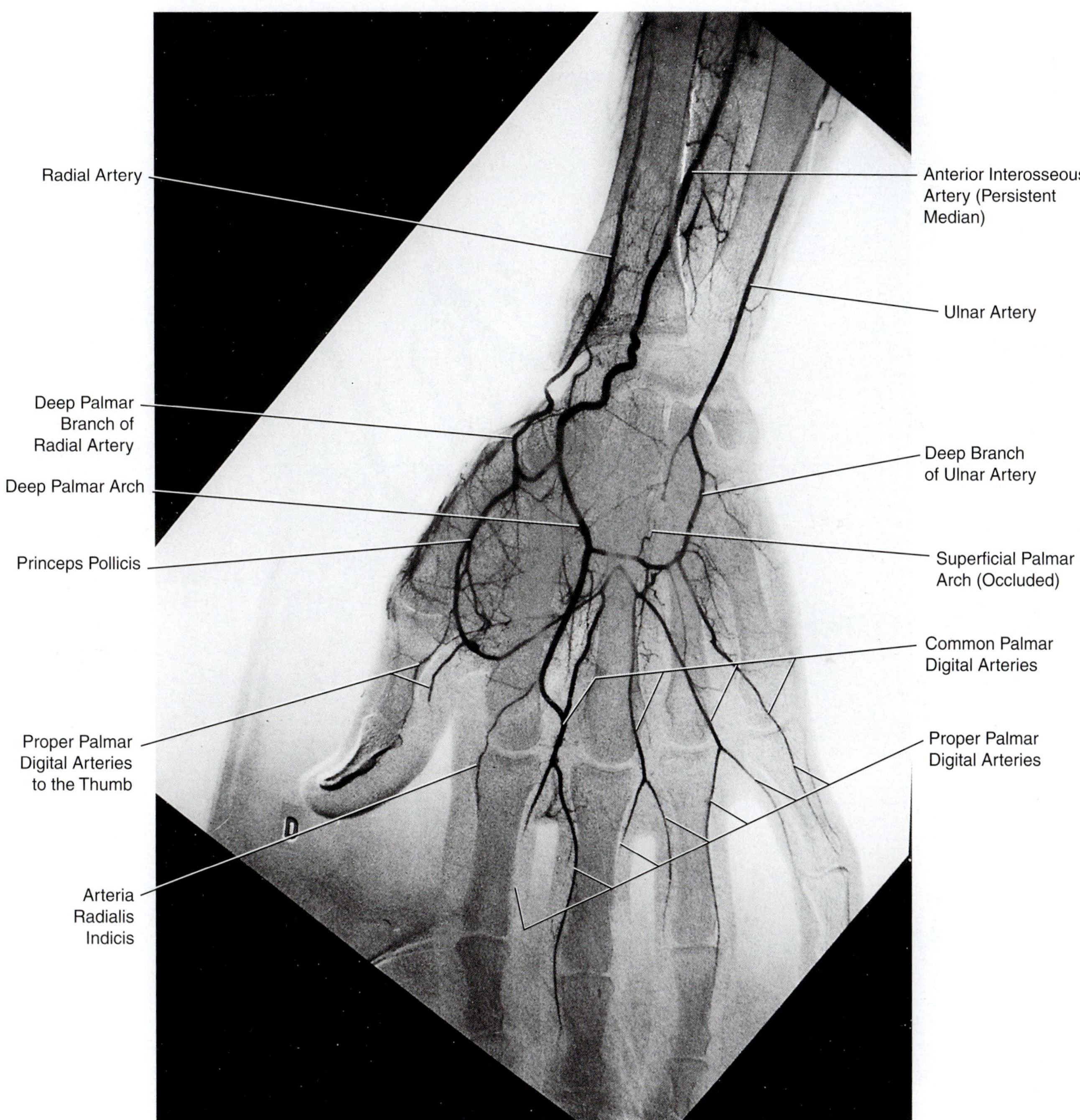

Figure 15.36. Subtraction angiogram showing occluded superficial palmar arch. Note the persistent median artery as part of the deep palmar arch.

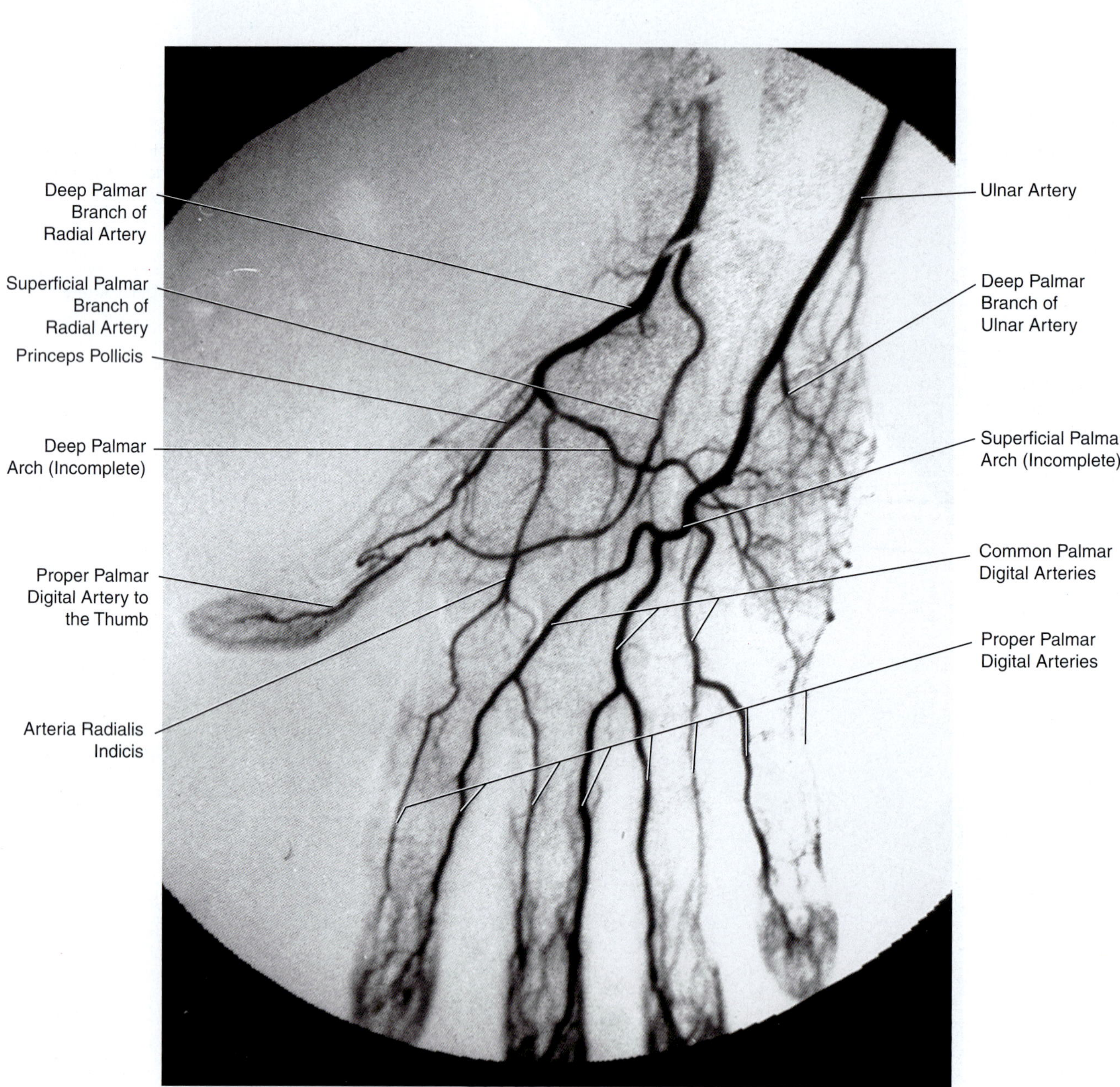

Figure 15.37. Angiogram of the right hand showing the palmar arch and distal arteries.

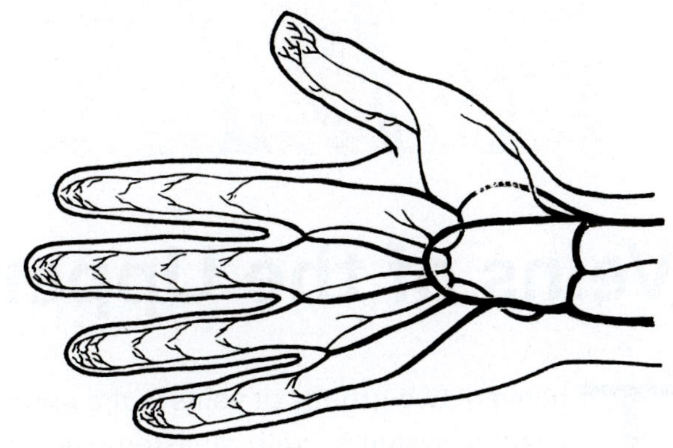

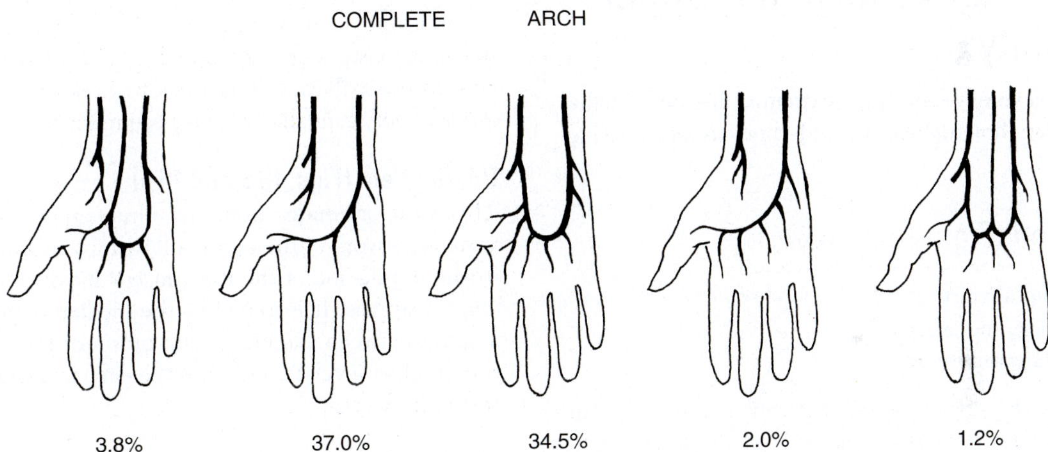

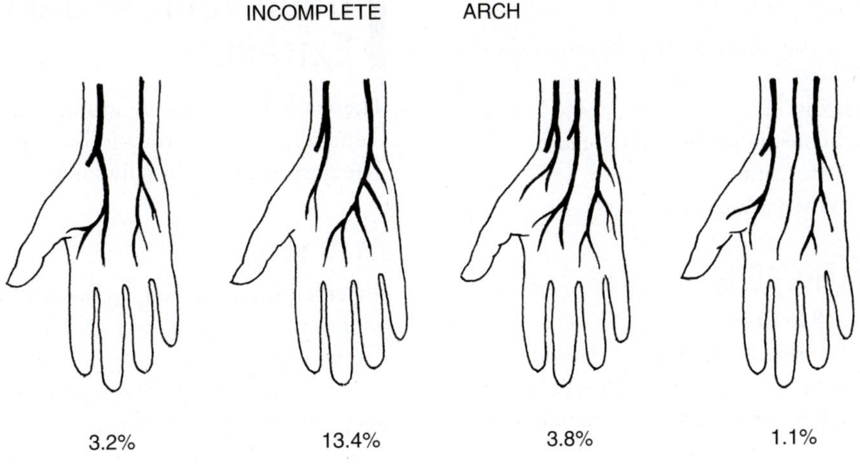

Figure 15.38. Schematic demonstration of the hand with complete arch and variations.

16

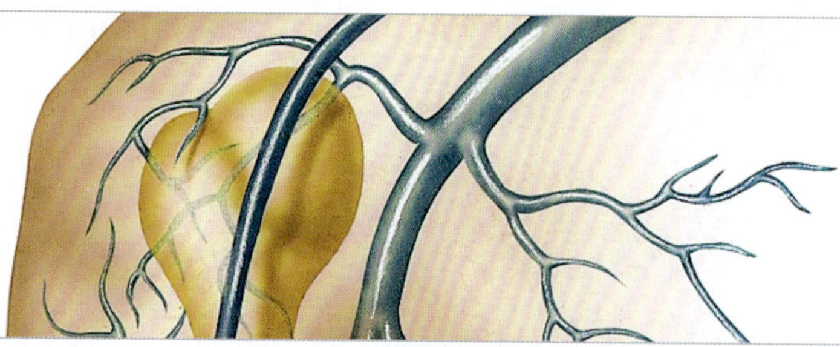

Veins of the Upper Extremity

There are two groups of veins in the upper limb, the superficial and deep venous systems, with anastomoses between them. The superficial veins are in the superficial fascia, immediately under the skin. The deep veins accompany the arteries usually in 2 veins to 1 artery ratio.

Superficial Veins of the Upper Extremity

The superficial veins of the upper extremity are the cephalic, basilic, median brachial veins, and their tributaries (Fig. 16.1).

At the Hand (Figs. 16.2-16.4)

Dorsal digital veins
Three dorsal metacarpal veins
Dorsal venous network

Laterally, the dorsal venous network is joined by the dorsal digital vein from the radial side of the index finger and both dorsal digital veins of the thumb, prolonged proximally as the cephalic vein. Medially, the network receives the dorsal digital vein of the ulnar side of the fifth finger and is continued upwards as the basilic vein.

- Palmar digital veins
  - Connected to the dorsal system by intercapitular veins
- Palmar venous plexus
  - Drains into the median vein of the forearm
- Median vein of the forearm
  - Connected to the basilic vein

At the Forearm (Fig. 16.1)

Cephalic Vein (Figs. 16.5-16.7)

This vein originates from the dorsal venous network and follows the radial border of the forearm. The median cubital vein is given in front of the elbow, which receives a communicating branch from the deep veins of the forearm, passing medially to communicate with the basilic vein. The cephalic vein ascends subcutaneously lateral to the biceps. The infraclavicular fossa ends in the axillary vein just below the level of the clavicle. An accessory cephalic vein may be present.

Basilic Vein (Figs. 16.5 and 16.6)

This vein originates from the ulnar aspect of the dorsal venous network of the hand, following a subcutaneous path in the dorsal side of the forearm but moves forward to the ventral surface. It is joined by the median cubital vein and ascends between the biceps and pronator teres muscles. At the shoulder level, it perforates the deep fascia continuing as the axillary vein.

Median Vein of the Forearm (Fig. 16.5)

This vein is formed by the superficial palmar venous plexus and ends in the basilic or median cubital vein.

Deep Veins of the Upper Extremity

These are the "venae comitans," companions of the arteries. Generally, in pairs, they follow the corresponding arteries. The deep veins are usually small.

At the Hand

Superficial and palmar arches are accompanied by venae comitans, superficial, and deep palmar venous arches. The common palmar digital veins open in the superficial palmar venous arch. The palmar metacarpal veins drain into the deep palmar venous arch.

At the Forearm (Fig. 16.8)

There are companion veins of the radial, interosseous, and ulnar arteries that join at the elbow level as the brachial veins.

Brachial Veins (Fig. 16.1)

These veins follow the brachial artery in pairs and receive tributaries. They join the axillary vein and occasionally the basilic vein.

Axillary Vein (Figs. 16.9-16.17)

This vein begins at the lower border of the teres major, as the continuation of the basilic vein, up to the outer border of the first rib; it lies medially to the axillary artery. Its major tributary is the cephalic vein.

Subclavian Vein (Figs. 16.9-16.11)

The subclavian vein is the continuation of the axillary vein, extending from the outer border of the ribs to the medial border of the scalenus anterior, where it is joined by the internal jugular vein to form the brachiocephalic vein; it lies anterior and inferior to the subclavian artery.

Major venous tributaries are the external jugular and dorsal scapular veins. The left subclavian vein, just before the confluence of the left internal jugular vein, receives the thoracic duct, right at the angle of junction with the internal jugular vein. On the right side, the right lymphatic trunks open independently at the jugular-subclavian junction. In one-fifth of the population, a short right lymphatic trunk is formed and drains directly into the subclavian vein at the junction with the right internal jugular vein.

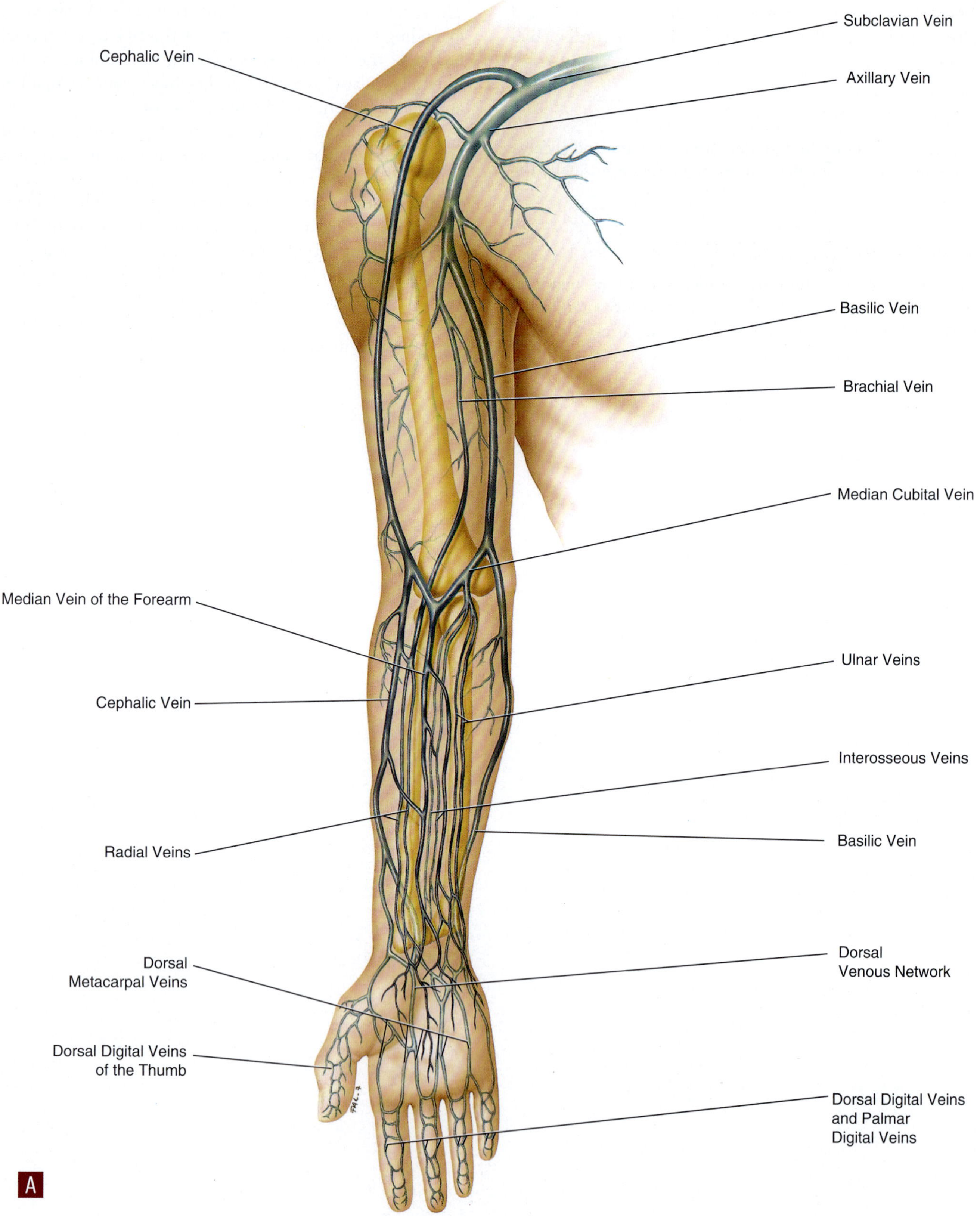

Figure 16.1. **A**, Schematic drawing of the **v**enous anatomy of the right upper extremity. **B**, Venous anatomy of the upper extremity at the axilla.

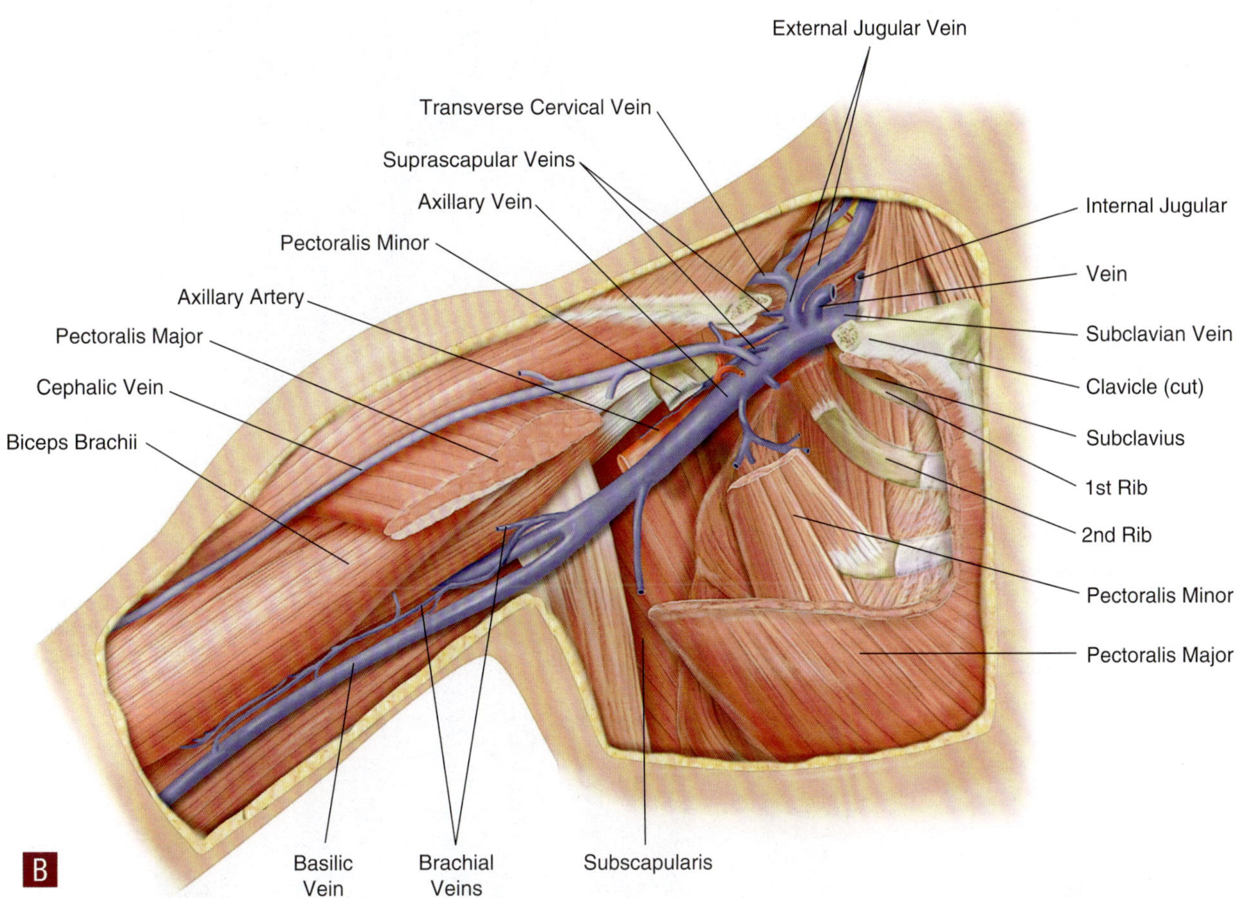

Figure 16.1. *Continued*

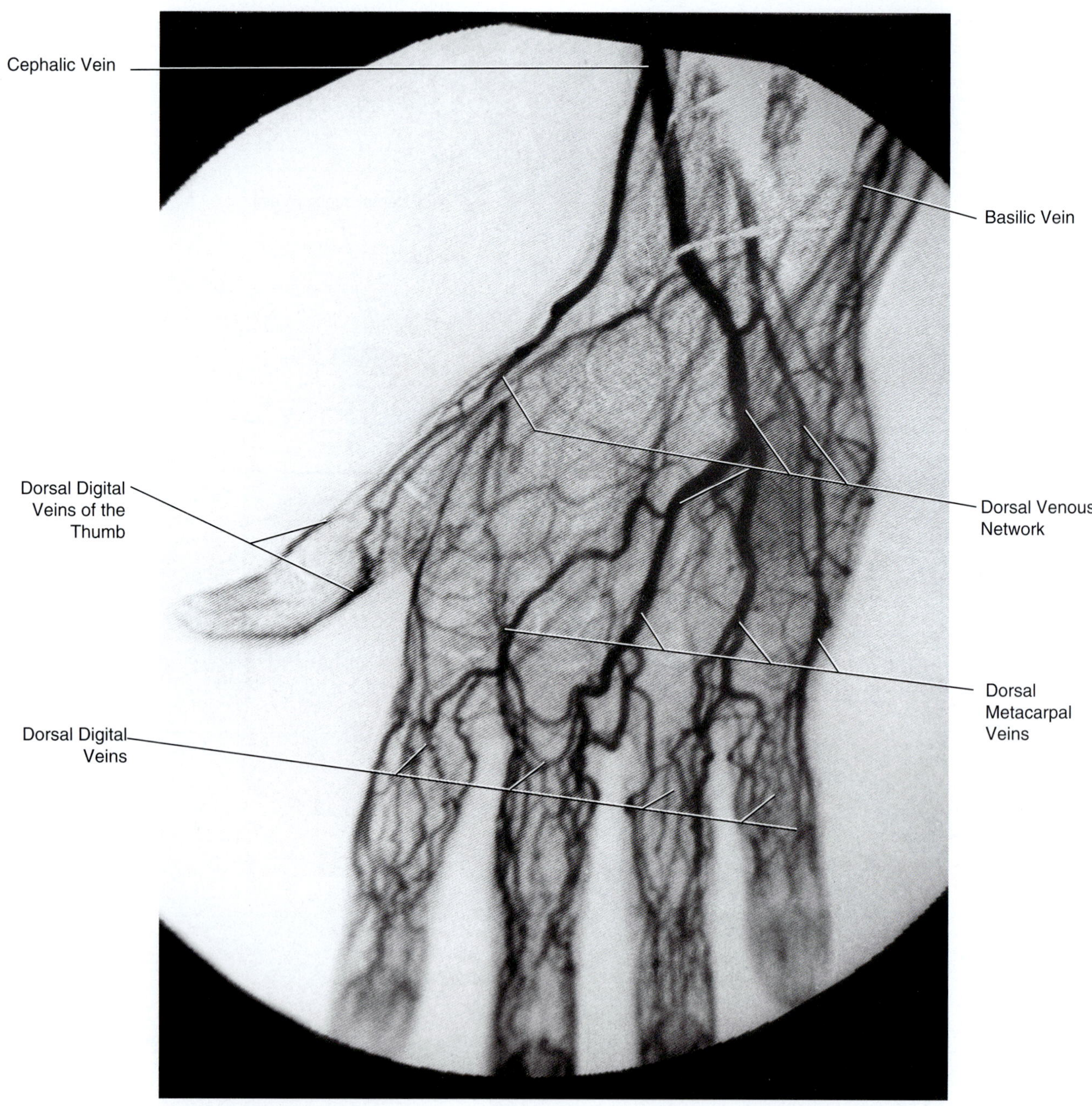

Figure 16.2. Venous phase of a right hand venogram. Note the large dorsal venous network.

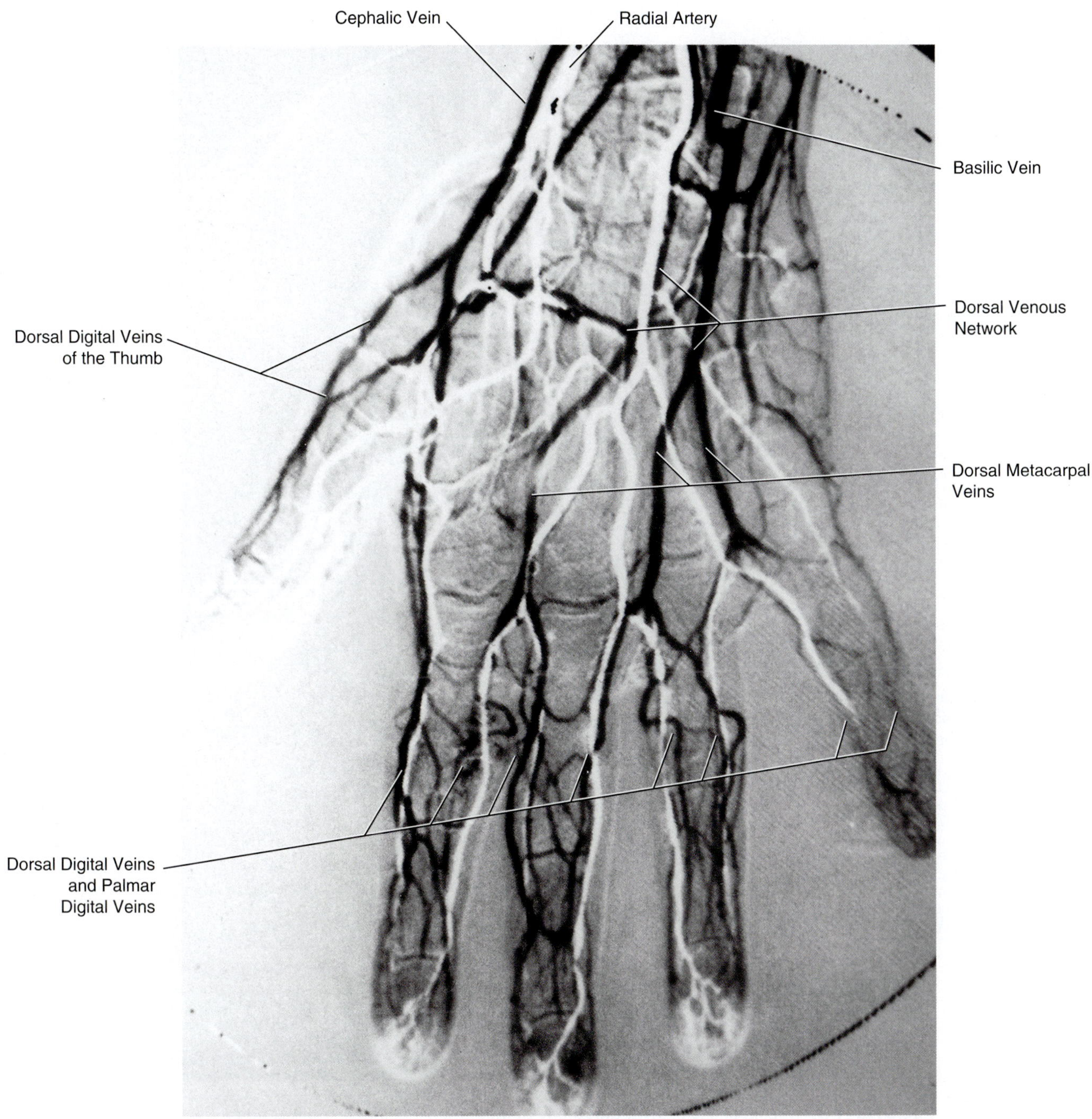

Figure 16.3. Venogram of the right hand overlapping the arteries on a digital subtraction film.

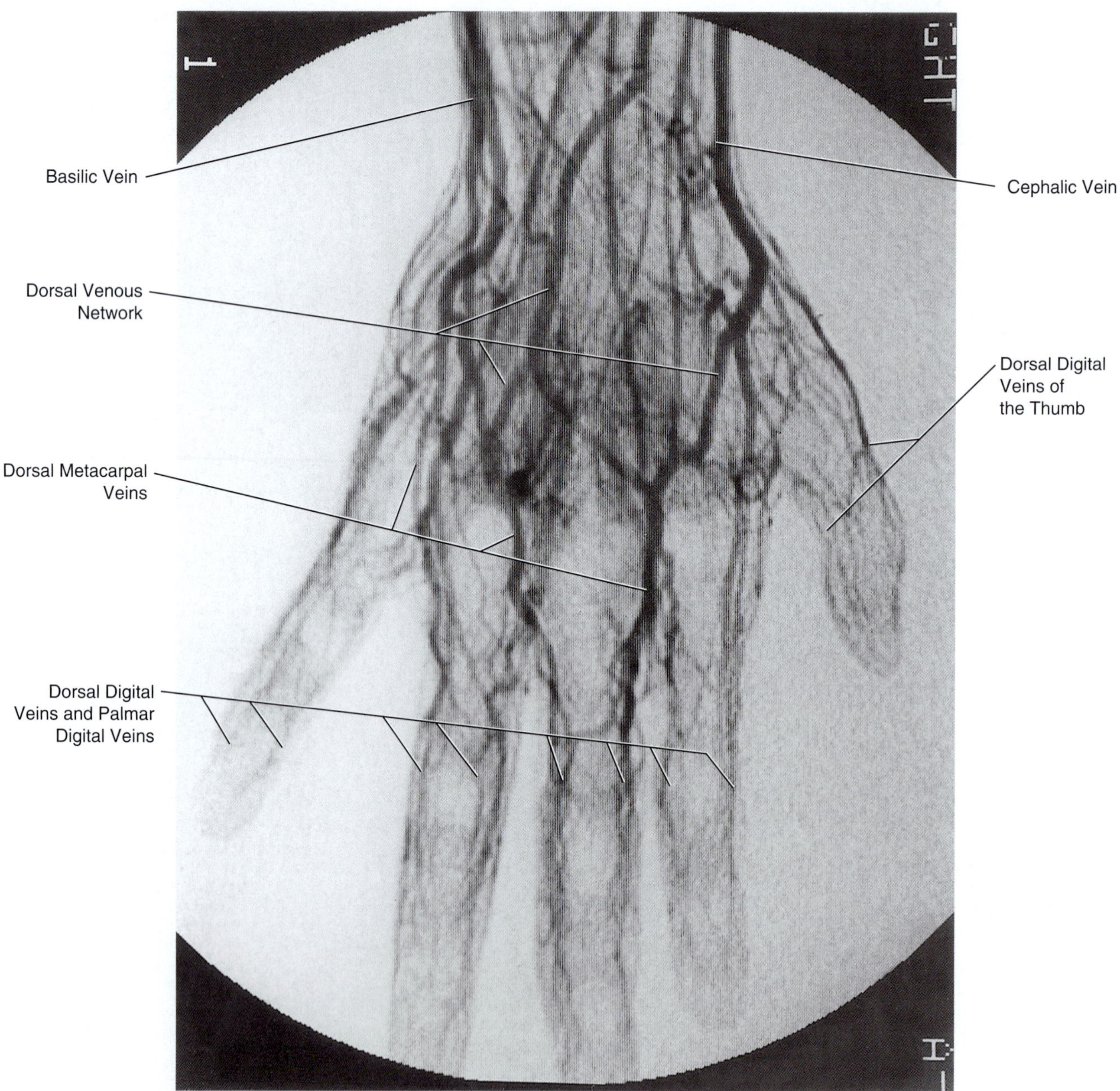

Figure 16.4. Late phase of an angiography of the right hand showing the venous anatomy of the right hand in a prone view.

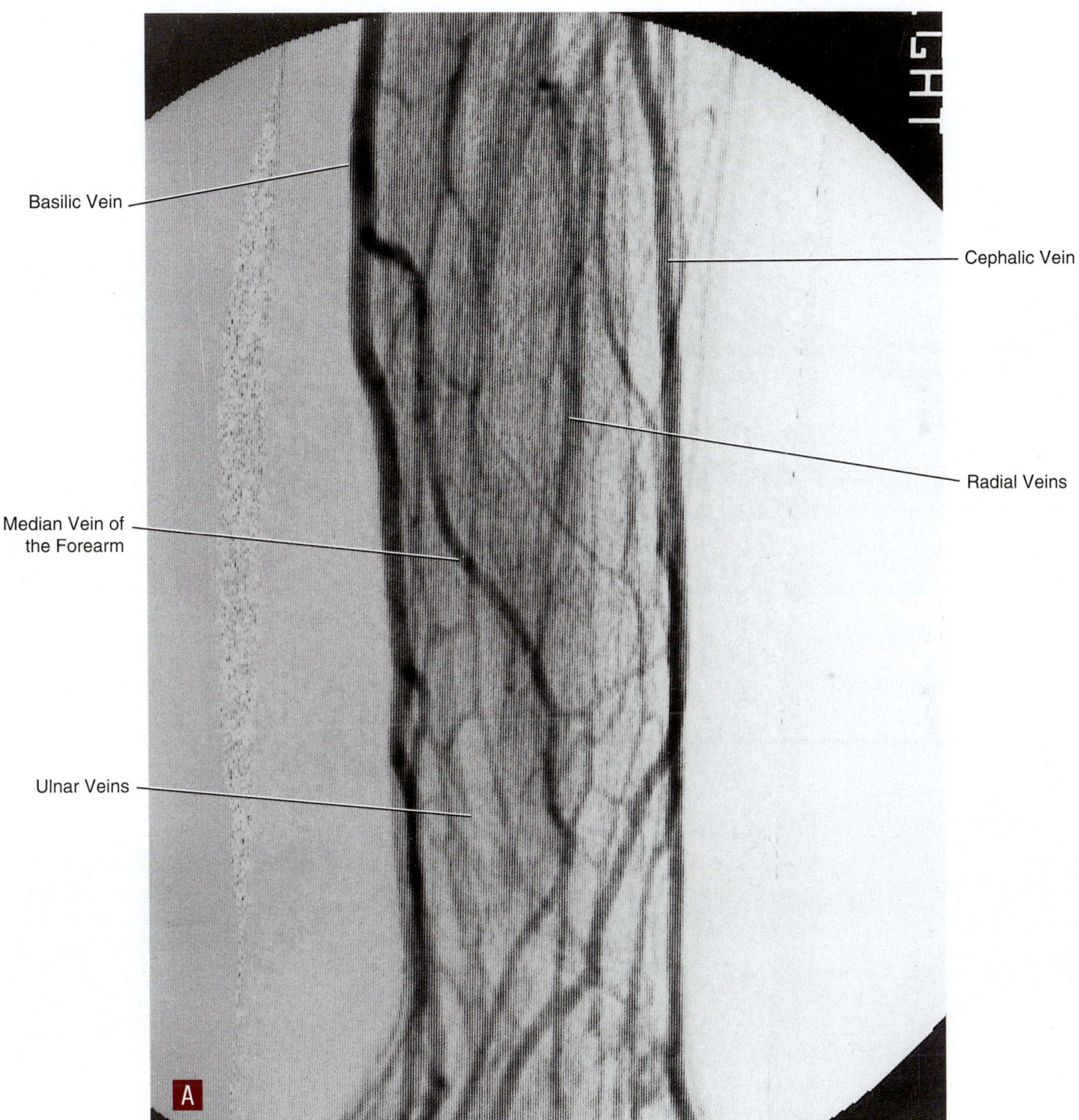

Figure 16.5. A to C, Venous anatomy of the right forearm in anatomical position. The cephalic and basilic veins are part of the superficial venous system. The radial, interosseous, and ulnar veins are part of the deep venous system.

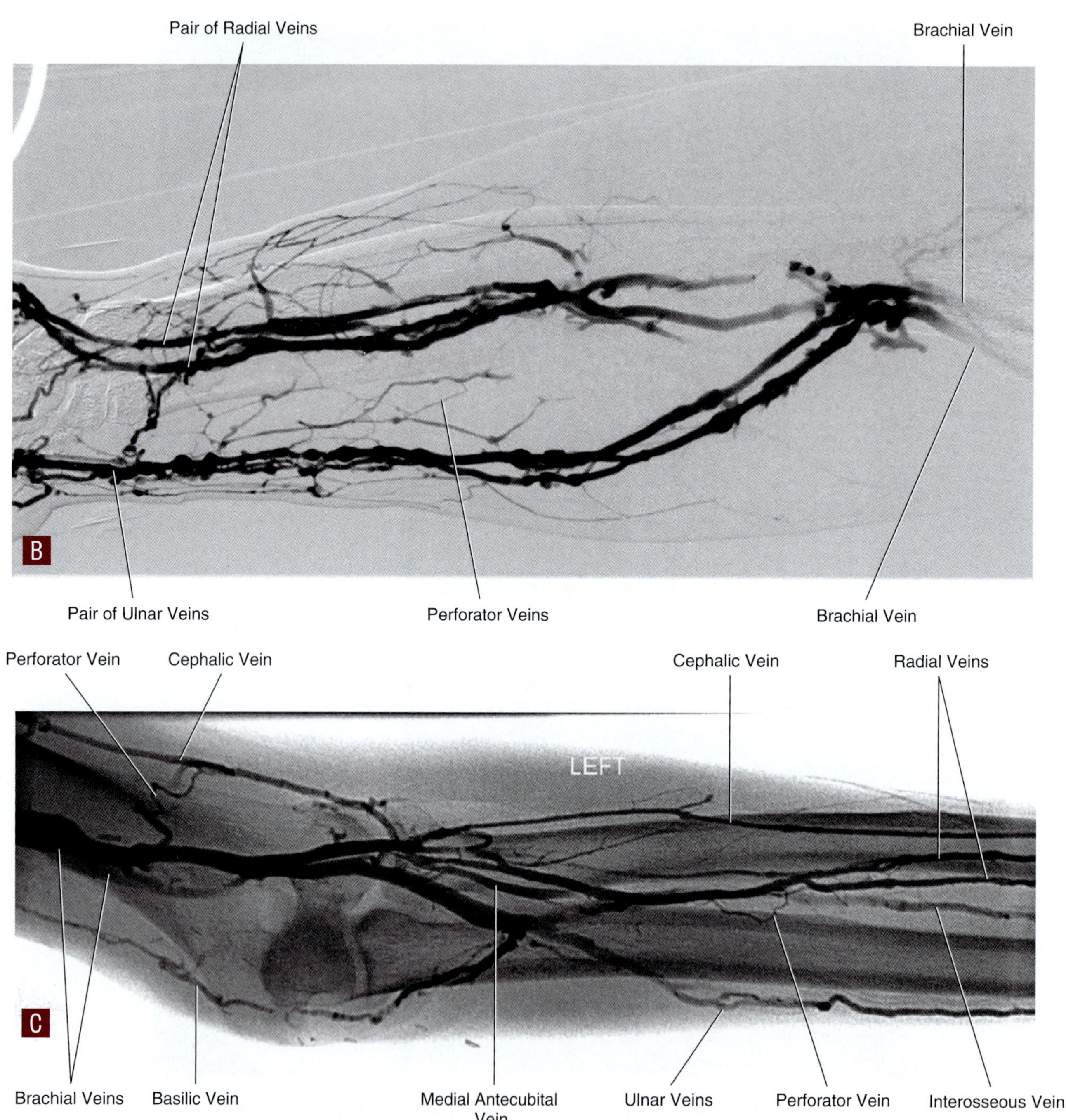

Figure 16.5. *Continued*

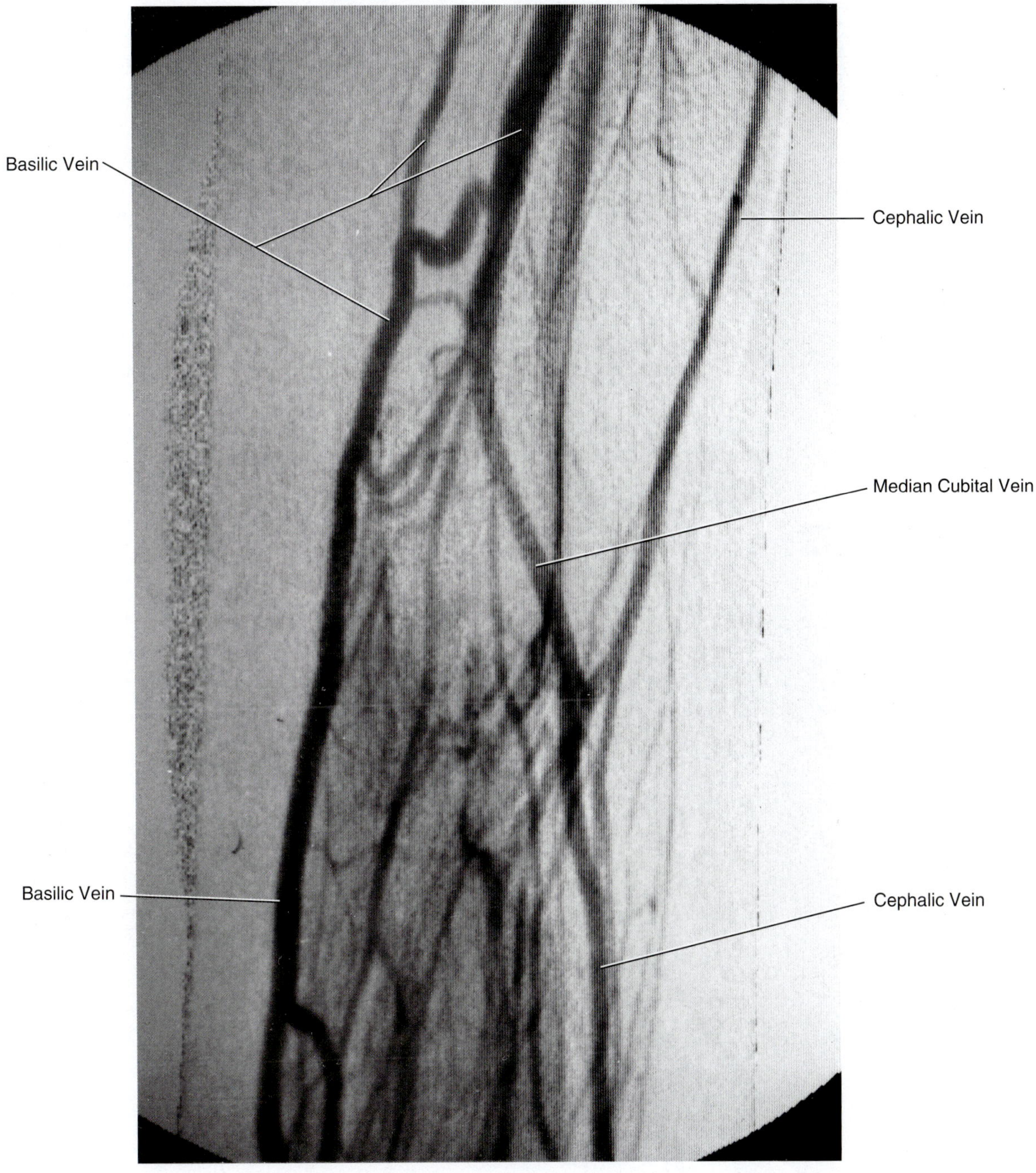

Figure 16.6. Venous anatomy at the right elbow region.

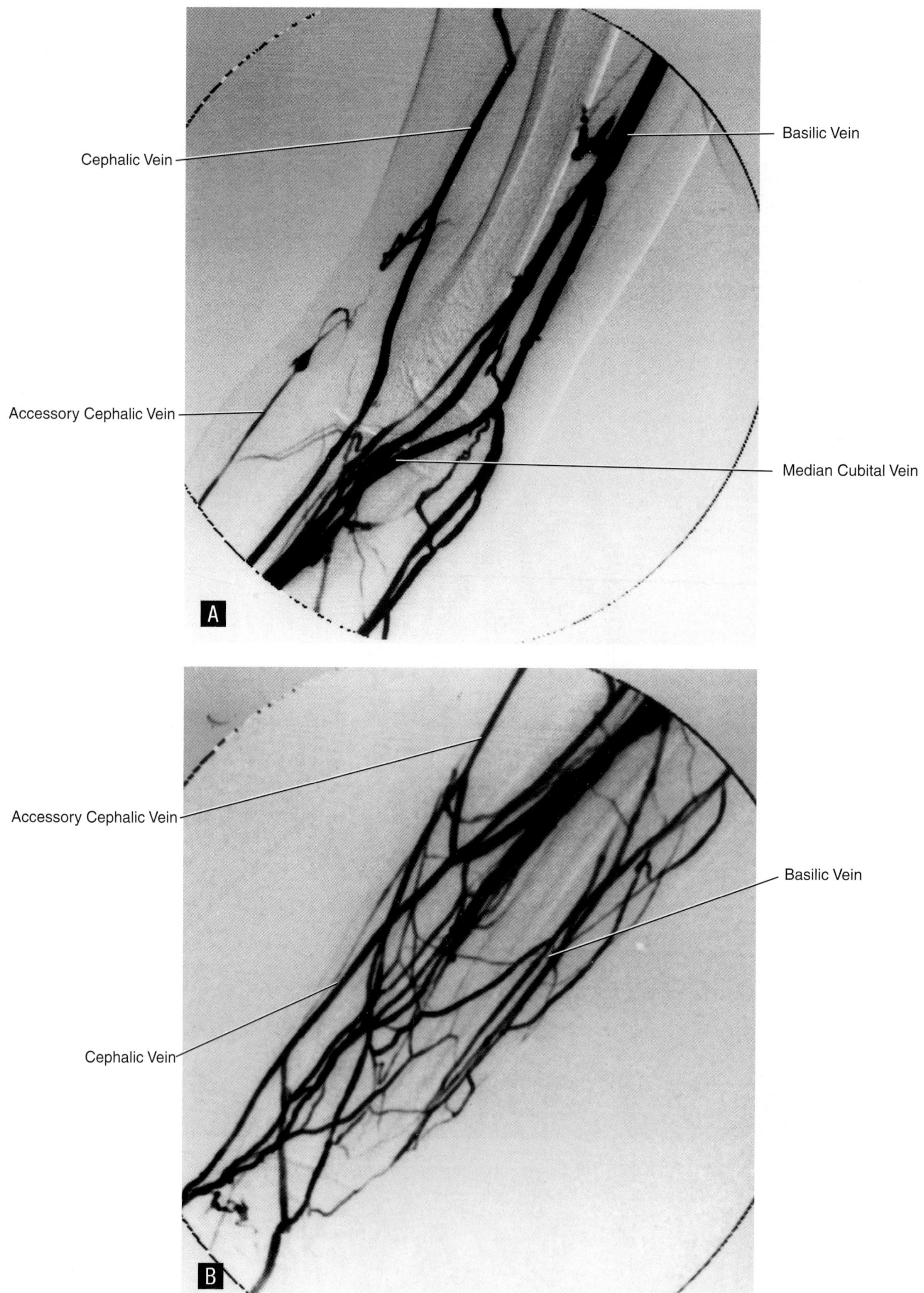

Figure 16.7. Venograms of the right upper extremity. **A**, Forearm. **B**, Antecubital area.

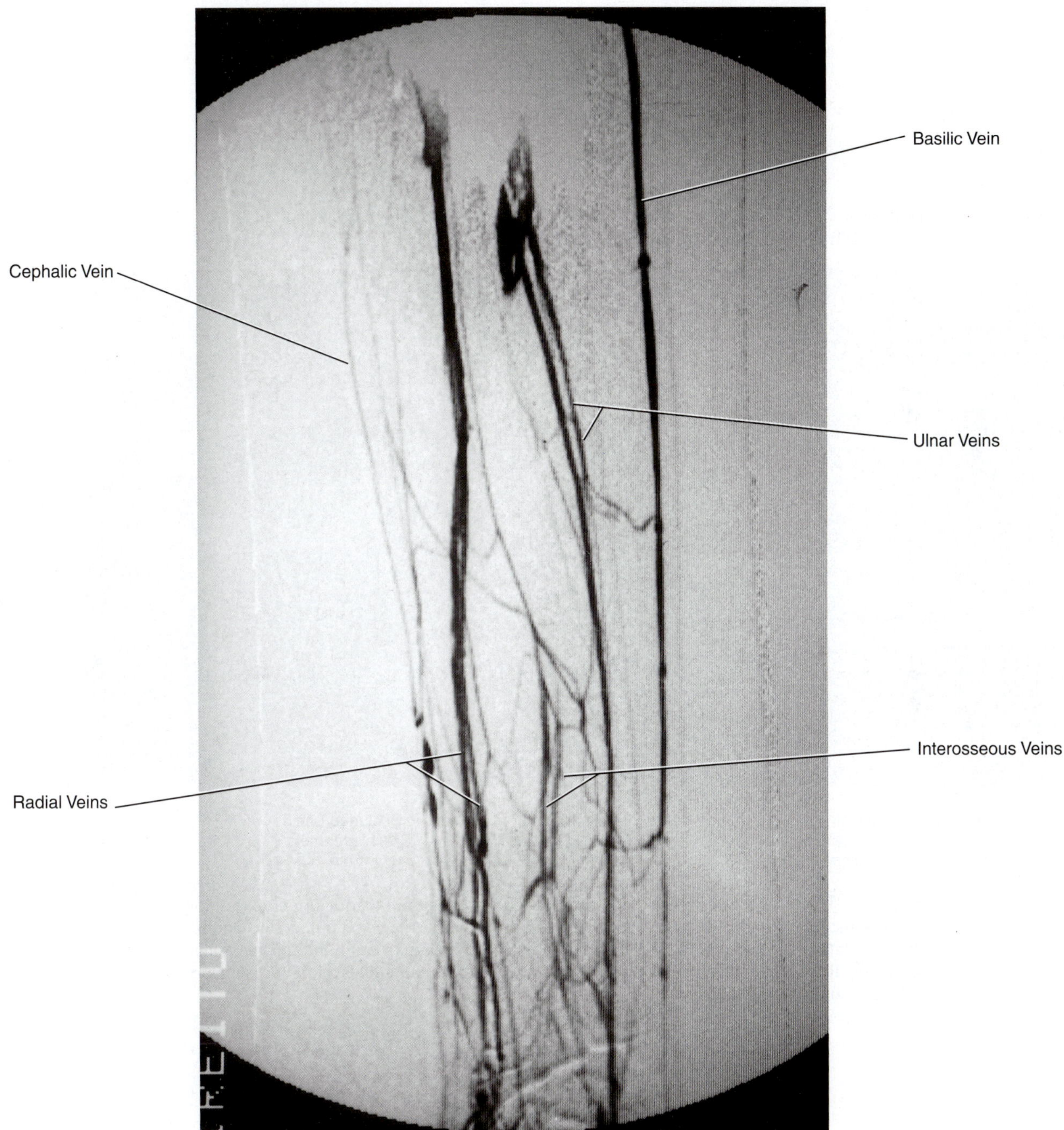

Figure 16.8. Deep venous system at the forearm.

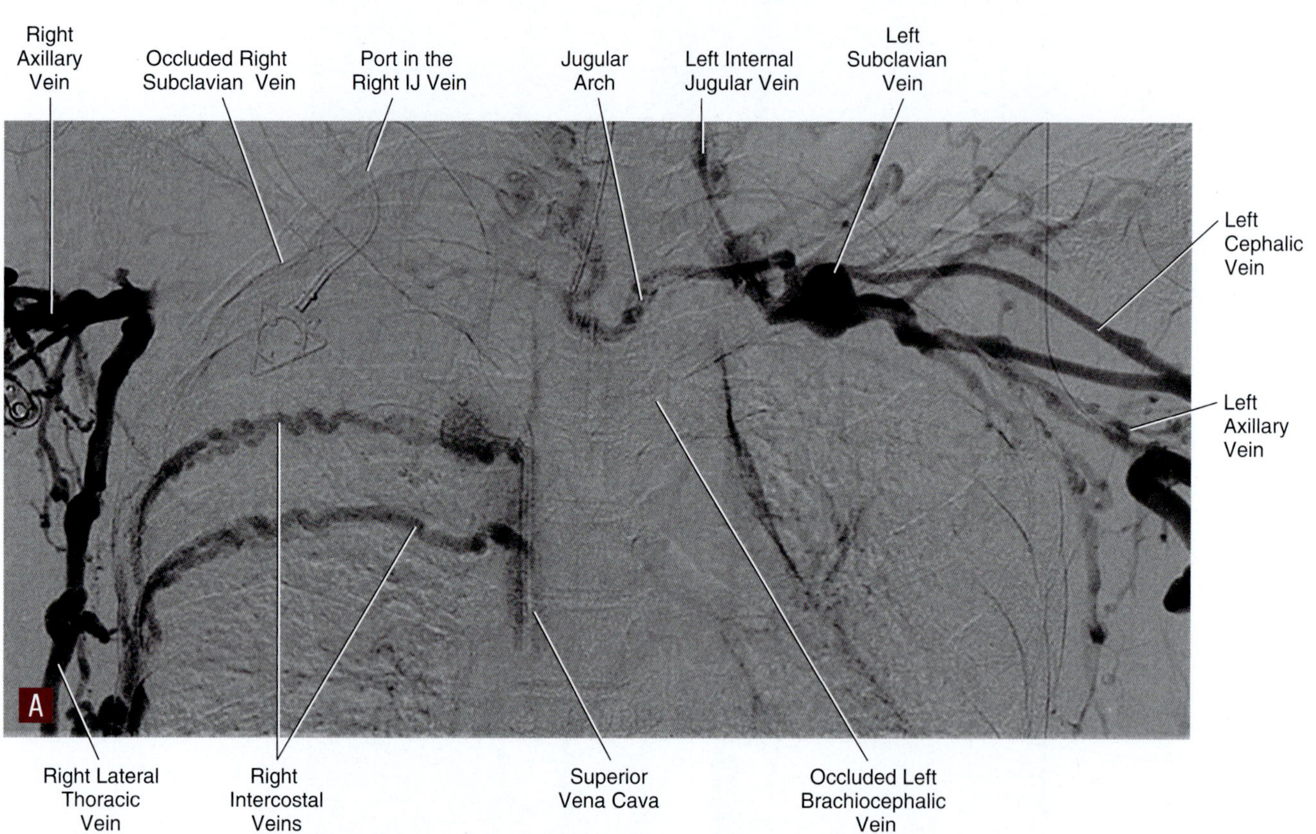

Figure 16.9. **A**, Chest venogram performed through simultaneous upper extremities venograms. Note the occlusion of subclavian and brachiocephalic veins bilaterally. On the right, the lateral thoracic vein drains into the superior vena cava through intercostal veins. **B** and **C**, Right subclavian occlusion. Note presence of different collateral patterns including cervical and chest wall collaterals.

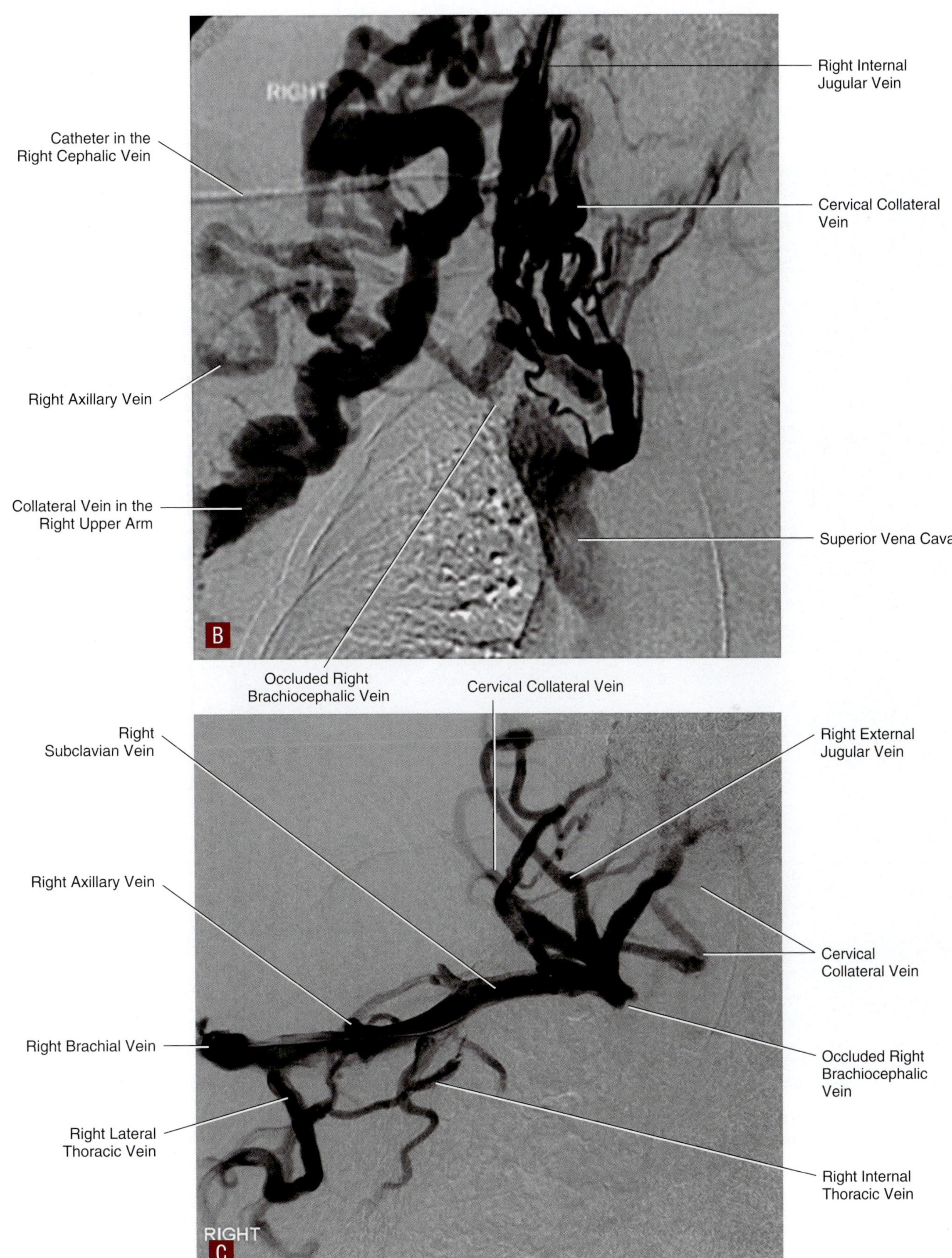

Figure 16.9. *Continued*

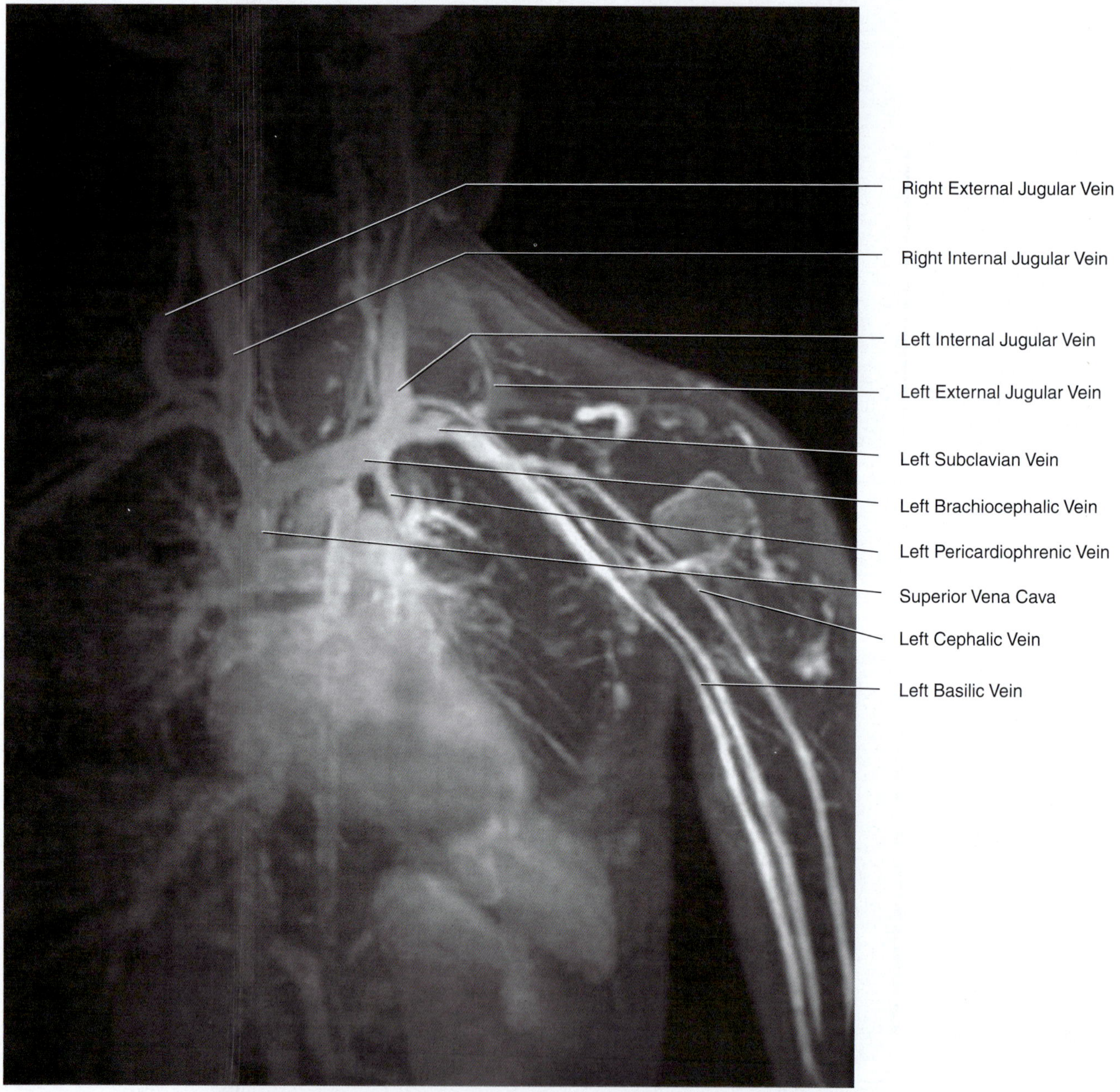

Right External Jugular Vein
Right Internal Jugular Vein
Left Internal Jugular Vein
Left External Jugular Vein
Left Subclavian Vein
Left Brachiocephalic Vein
Left Pericardiophrenic Vein
Superior Vena Cava
Left Cephalic Vein
Left Basilic Vein

Figure 16.10. MRA with 2D reconstruction of the left arm venous system and the internal thoracic veins. This sequence is a late phase, but the artery is still apparent.

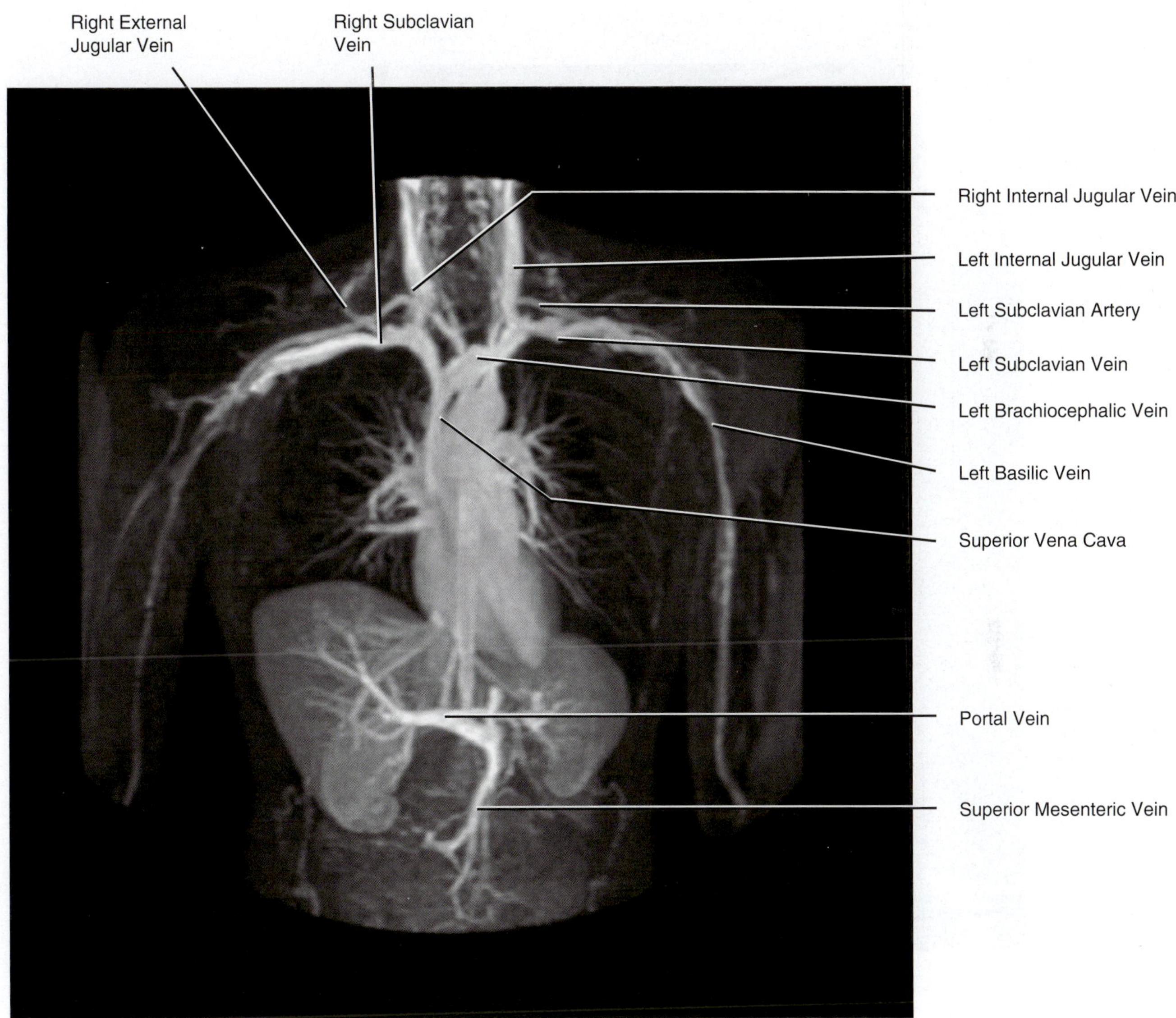

Figure 16.11. MRA with 2D reconstruction of the chest vessels including both arms. Note the late arterial phase still visualized.

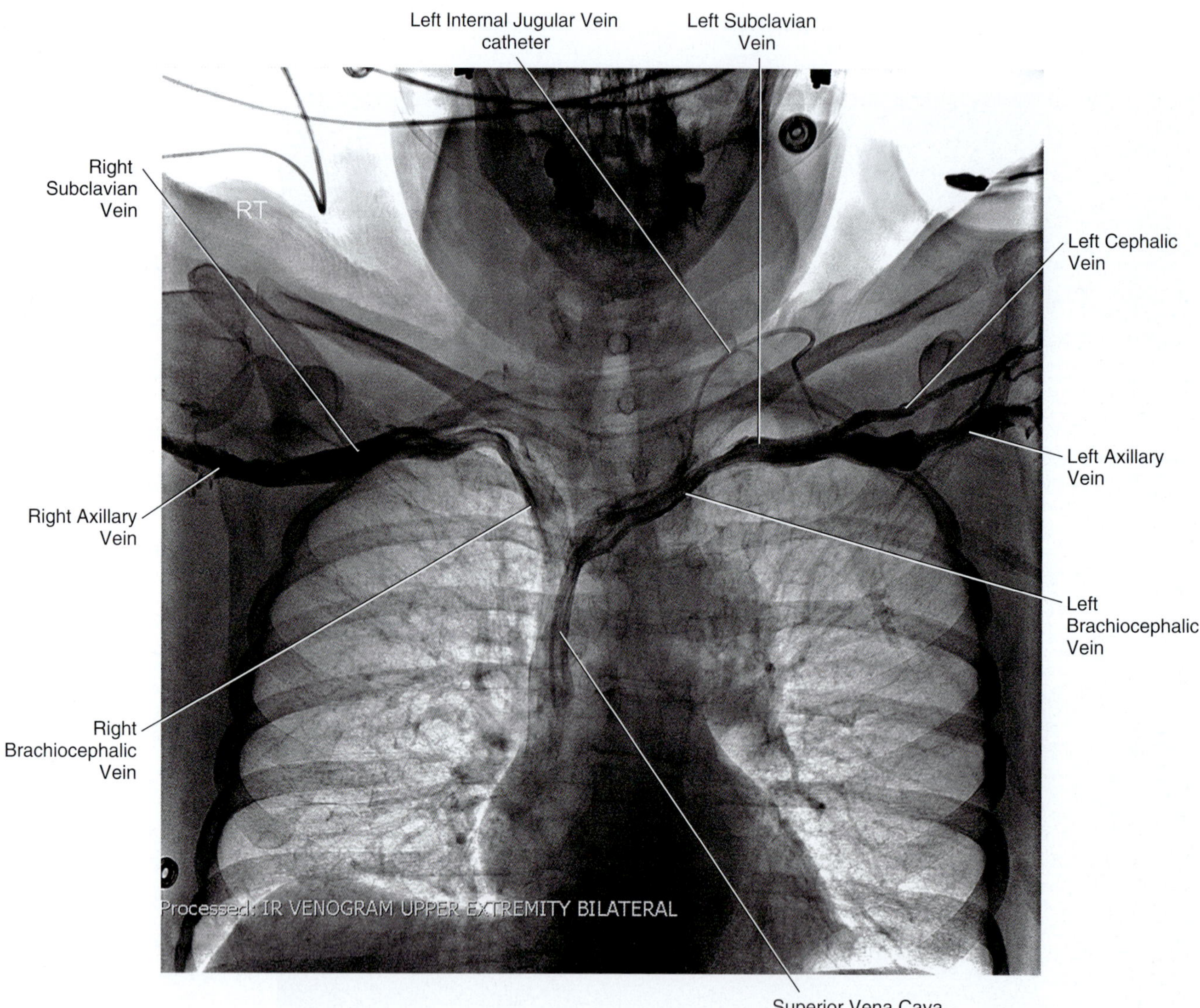

Figure 16.12. Native view of a central venogram. Simultaneous contrast injection was performed through both upper extremities. Central venogram performed through simultaneous injections of contrast.

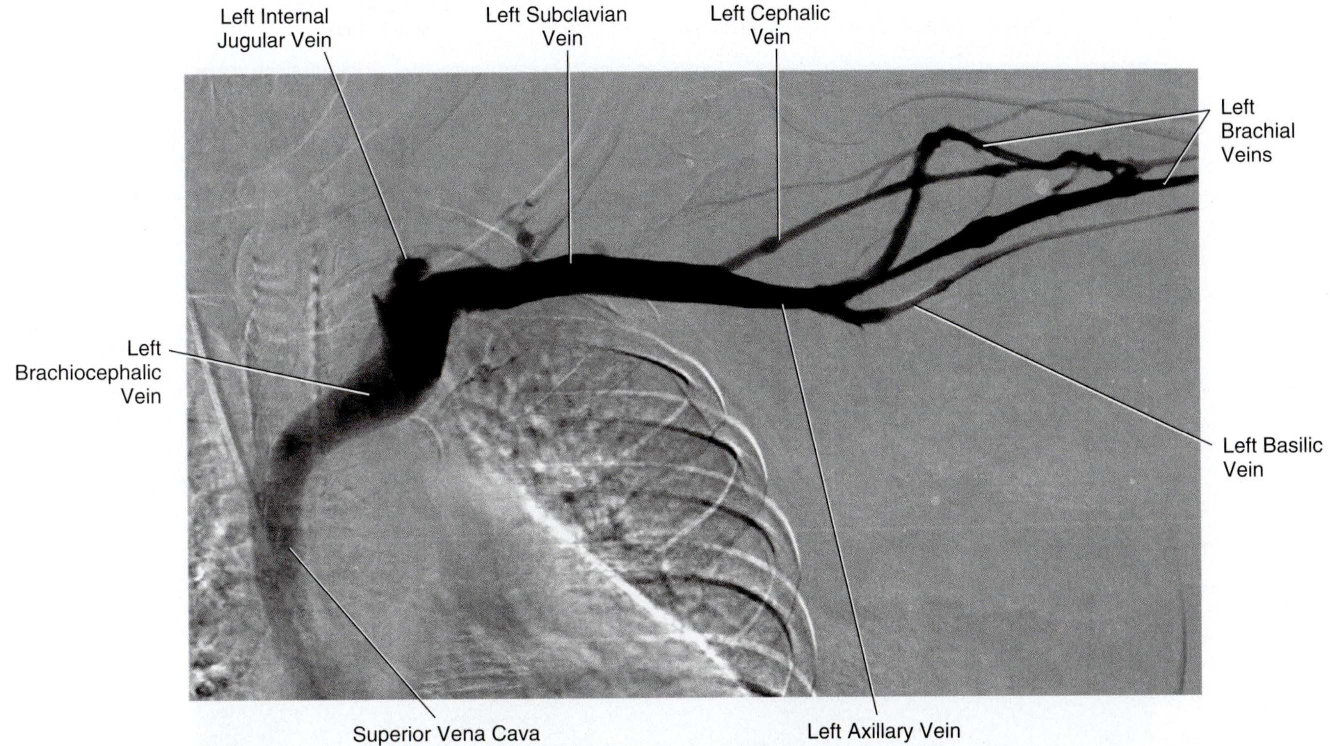

Figure 16.13. Left upper extremity and central venogram. Note patent basilic, a pair of brachial, and the cephalic vein. Note the typical confluence between the left cephalic and the axillary veins.

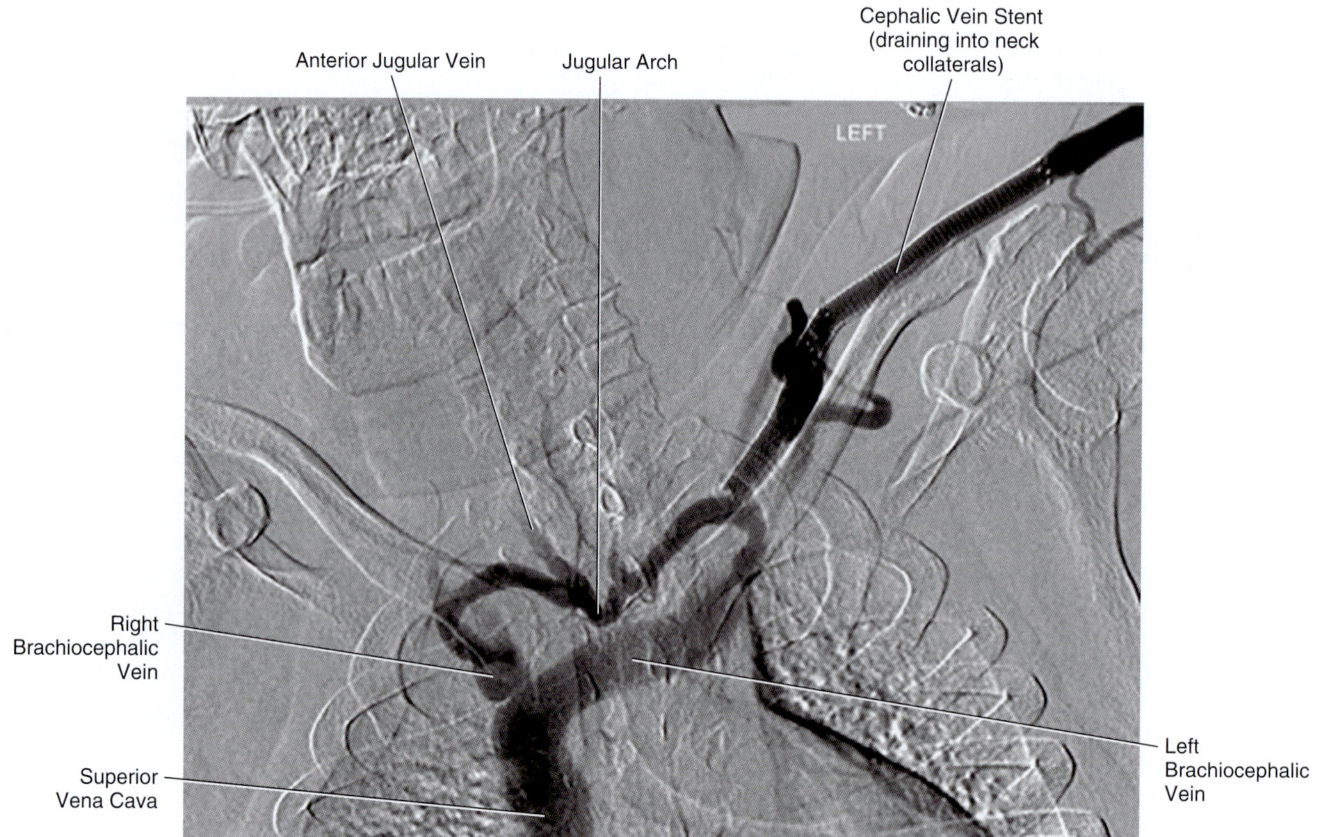

Figure 16.14. Patent cephalic stents associated with high-grade stenosis in between the brachiosubclavian transition. Note the cervical collateral circulation.

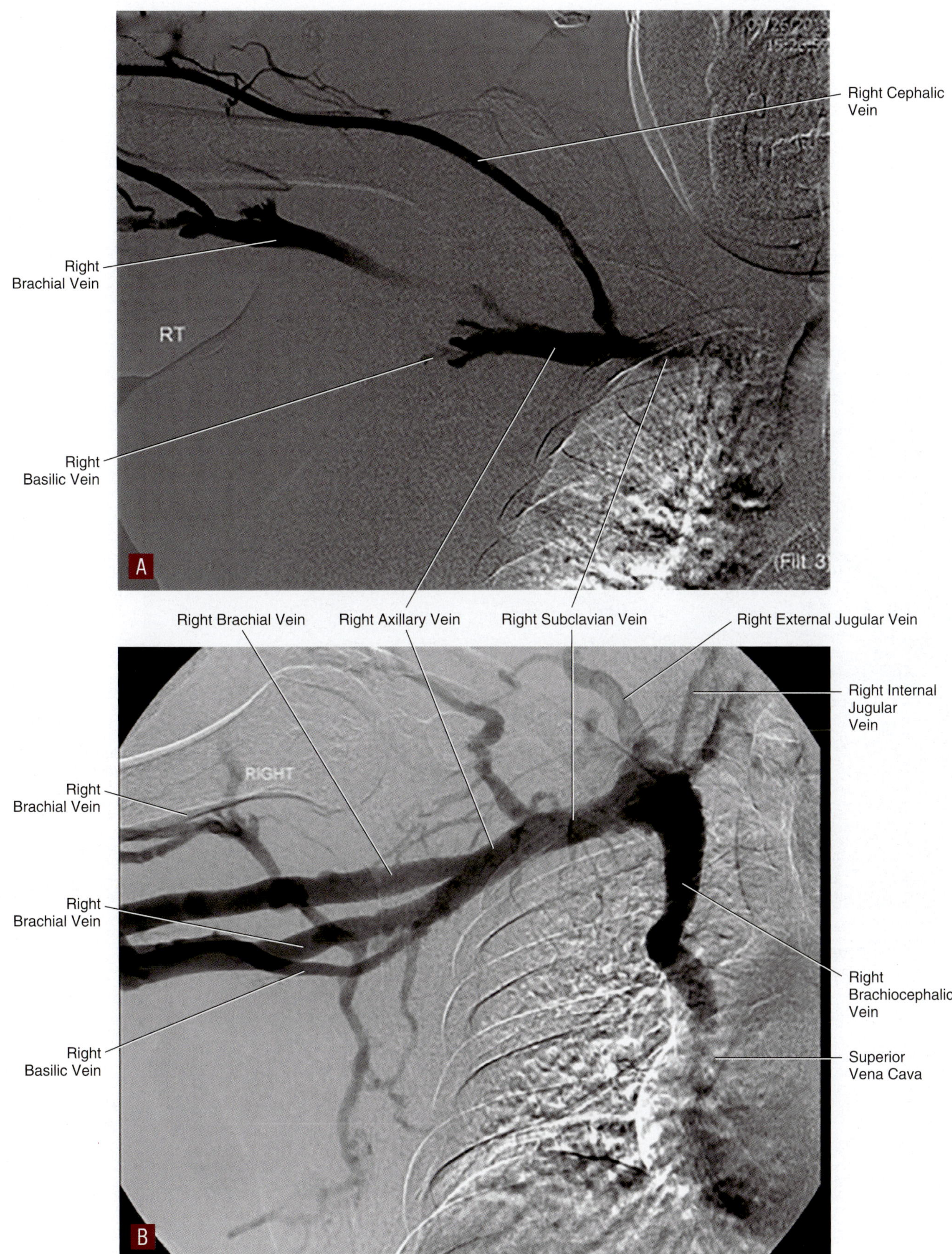

Figure 16.15. A and B, Right upper extremity and central venograms.

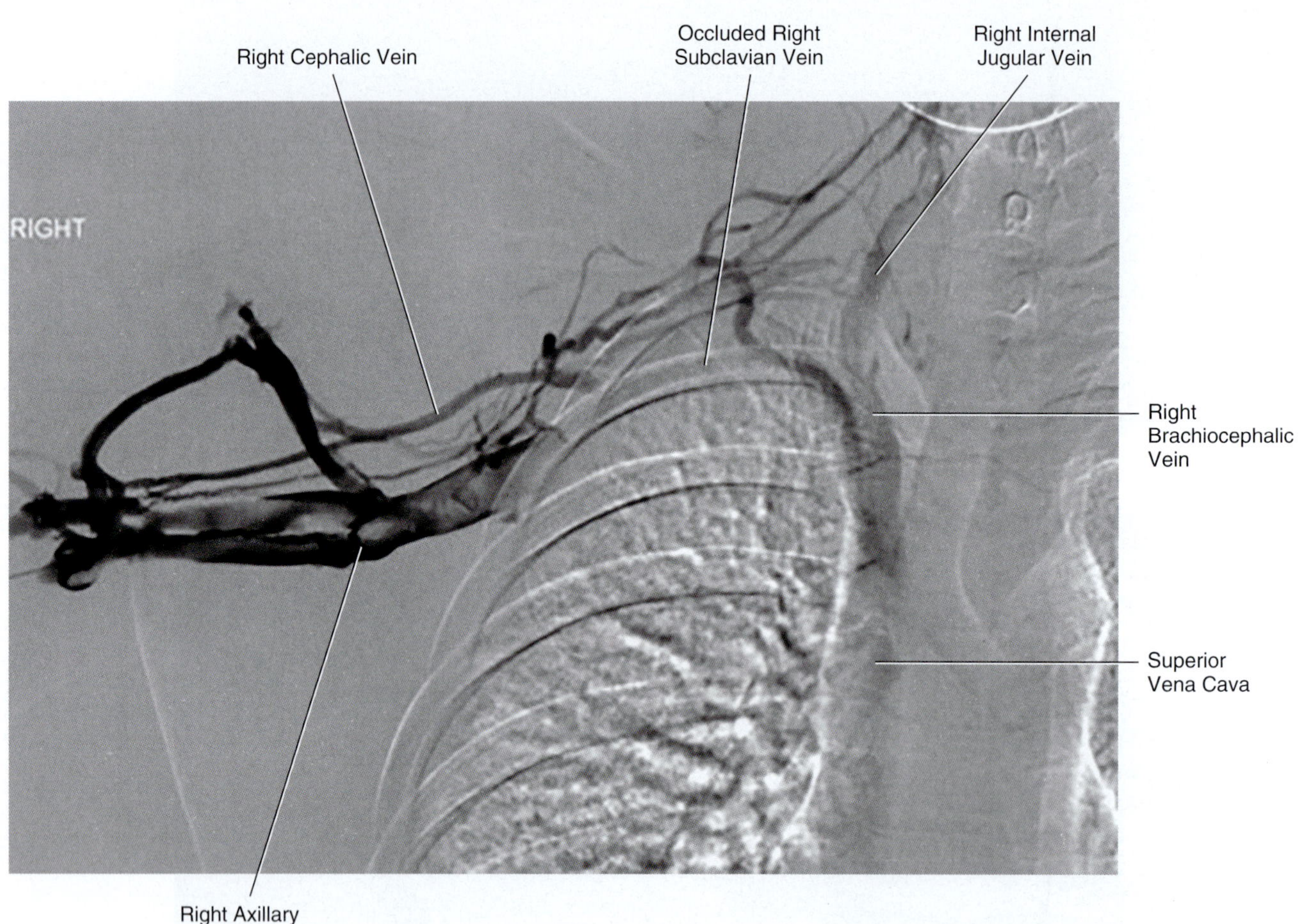

Figure 16.16. Thoracic outlet syndrome. Presence of an occlusion of the right subclavian vein and partial occlusion of the right axillary vein due to acute thrombosis.

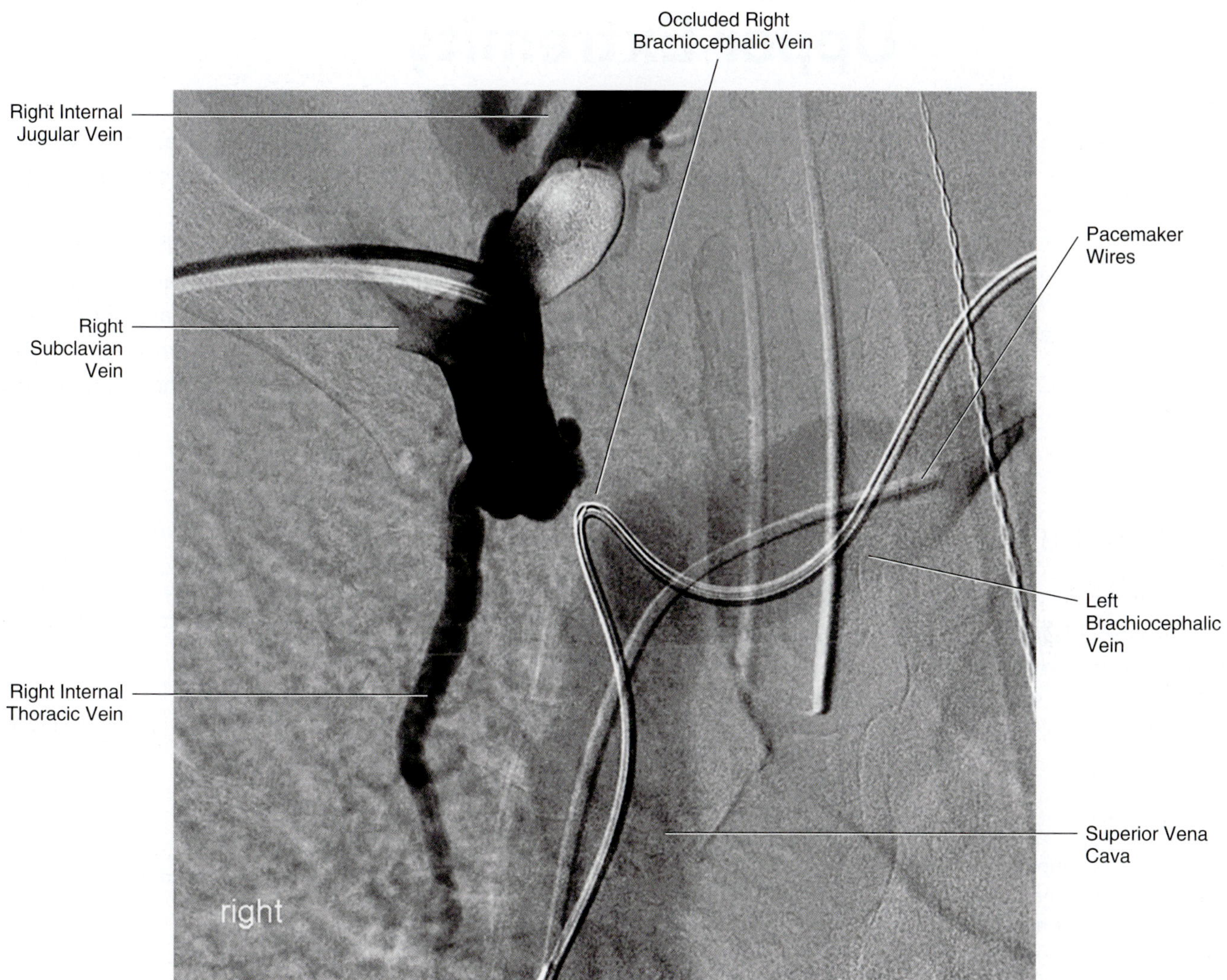

Figure 16.17. Right subclavian venogram showing occlusion of the right brachiocephalic vein with collateralization via the right internal thoracic vein into the superior vena cava and left brachiocephalic vein.

17

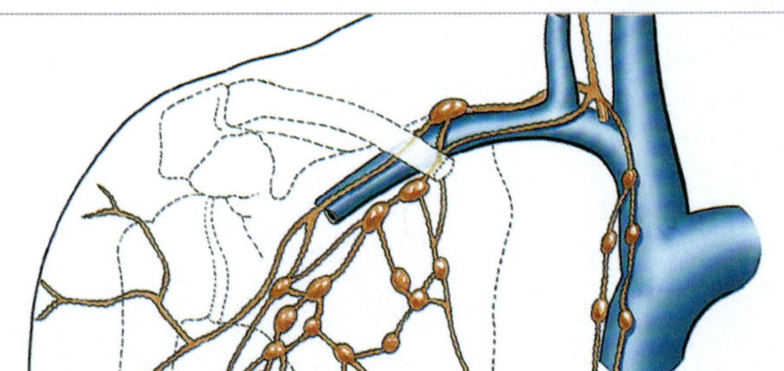

Lymphatic Drainage of the Upper Extremity

The lymphatic drainage of the deep tissues of the upper limb follows the main neurovascular bundles ending in the lateral axillary lymph nodes. Lymphatic vessels draining the deep tissues are internal to the deep fascia (Fig. 17.1). The lymphatic vessels of the arm drain through the lateral group of lymph nodes, the lateral drainage of the subareolar plexus (from the breast), and the pectoral group of lymph nodes drain to the apical group of lymph nodes (Fig. 17.2), which drain through the subclavian lymphatic trunk, joined by the jugular trunk into the subclavian vein or into the thoracic duct (in the left side) (Fig. 17.3).

Lymphatics of the Superficial Tissues

The superficial lymphatic drainage begins at the lymphatic plexuses in the skin and converges in the direction of the superficial veins, following approximately the same direction toward the terminal group of axillary lymph nodes (Fig. 17.1).

At the Hand

The groups of lymphatic plexus are finer on the palmar than on the dorsal surface. The digital vessels run along the border of the fingers and join larger vessels at the palm, passing toward the dorsal aspect of the hand. The main palmar vessels pass toward the wrist, where they join vessels along the ulnar border of the hand and laterally join the draining vessels of the thumb.

At the Forearm and Arm

In the forearm and arm, the lymphatic vessels run together with the superficial veins. The ventral aspect of the forearm and arm contains the largest number of vessels because they pass successively from behind the arm to the front winding around the forearm and joining ventral larger vessels. At the arm level, the vessels above the elbow crowd together and follow the medial aspect of the arm, ending in the lateral group of the axillary lymph nodes (Fig. 17.2). There are small isolated nodes along the radial, ulnar, and interosseous vessels, in the cubital fossa, and in the arm, medial to the brachial vessels.

Lymphatics of the Deep Tissues

Axillary Lymph Nodes

This is the terminal group of nodes for the upper limb, varying from 20 to 30 in number, and is divided into five groups (Figs. 17.1, 17.2, and 17.4).

Lateral Group

The lateral group lies medial and posterior to the axillary vein and drains most of the upper limb. They are connected to the central and apical groups and to the lower deep cervical nodes.

Anterior or Pectoral Group

The anterior group is positioned along the lower border of the pectoralis minor and receives the afferents from the skin and muscles of the lateral and anterior walls of the trunk and central and lateral parts of the mammary gland.

Posterior or Subscapular Group

The posterior (subscapular) group is situated along the lower margin of the posterior wall of the axilla, taking the same course as the subscapular vessels. This group receives afferents that drain the posterior aspect of the trunk and lower part of the neck.

Central Group

The central group is embedded in the axillary fat and receives afferents from all of the above groups.

Apical Group

Situated in the apex of the axilla along the medial side of the axillary vein, the apical group receives afferents from all the other groups. The efferent vessels of this group form the subclavian trunk opening directly into the junction of the internal jugular and subclavian veins. On the left side, this group may end in the thoracic duct.

Other Lymph Nodes of the Upper Limb

Supratrochlear group
Infraclavicular group
Isolated lymph nodes

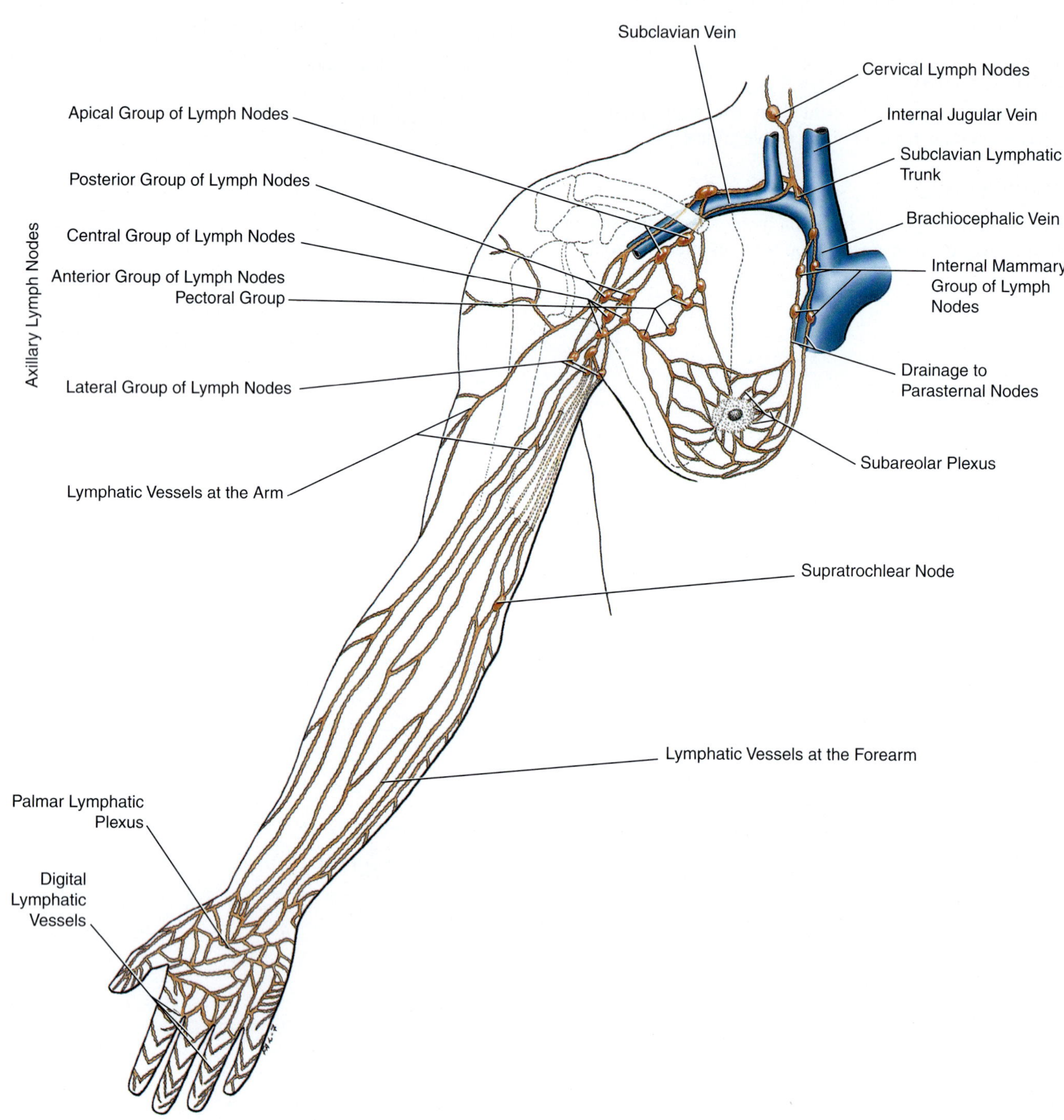

Figure 17.1. Schematic drawing of the lymphatic drainage of the upper extremity.

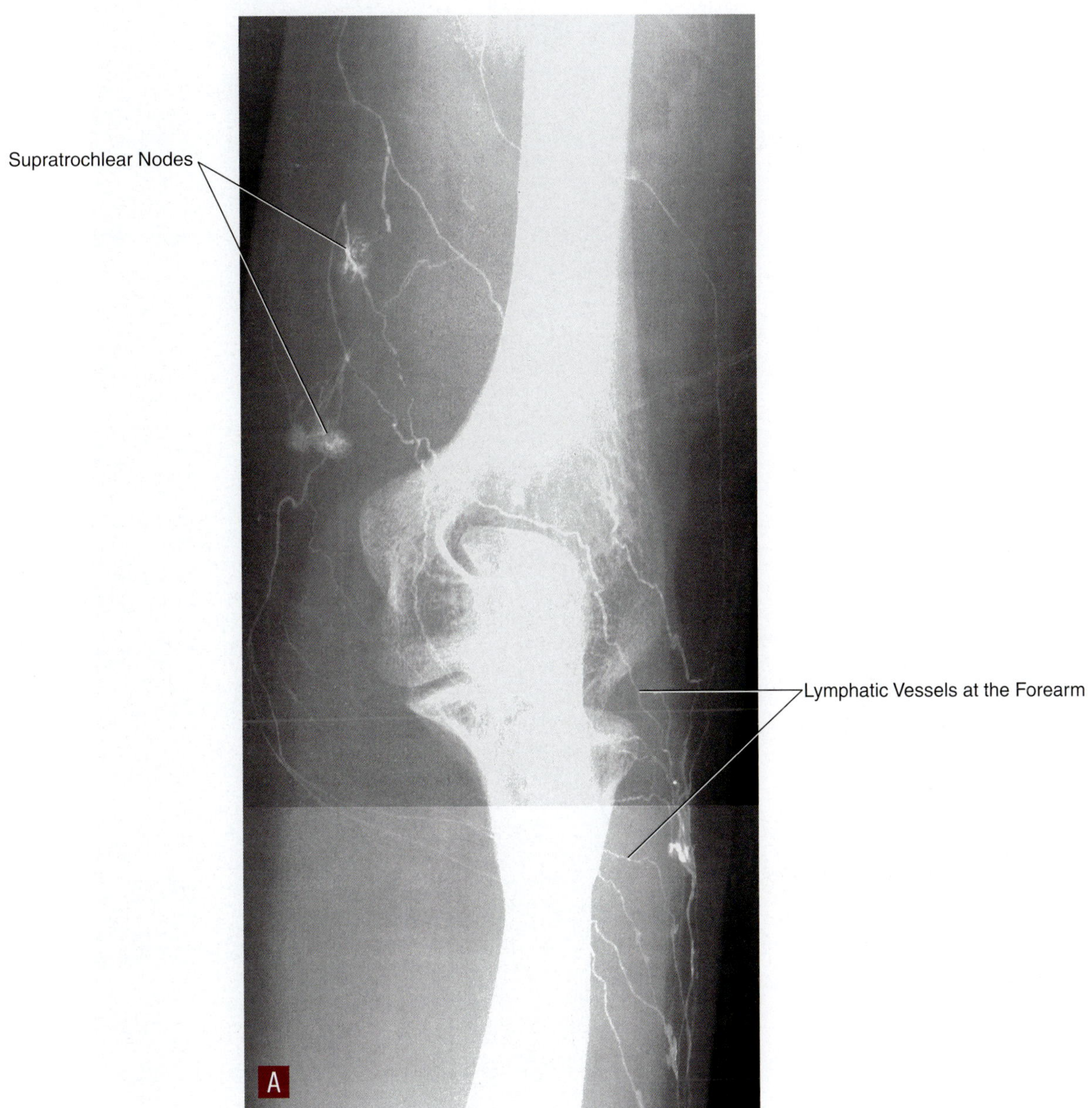

Figure 17.2. A-C. Left upper extremity lymphangiogram showing the forearm, arm, and axillary lymphatic ducts and lymph nodes. (Images 17.2A and 17.2B courtesy of Dr. Fritz Angle, MD.)

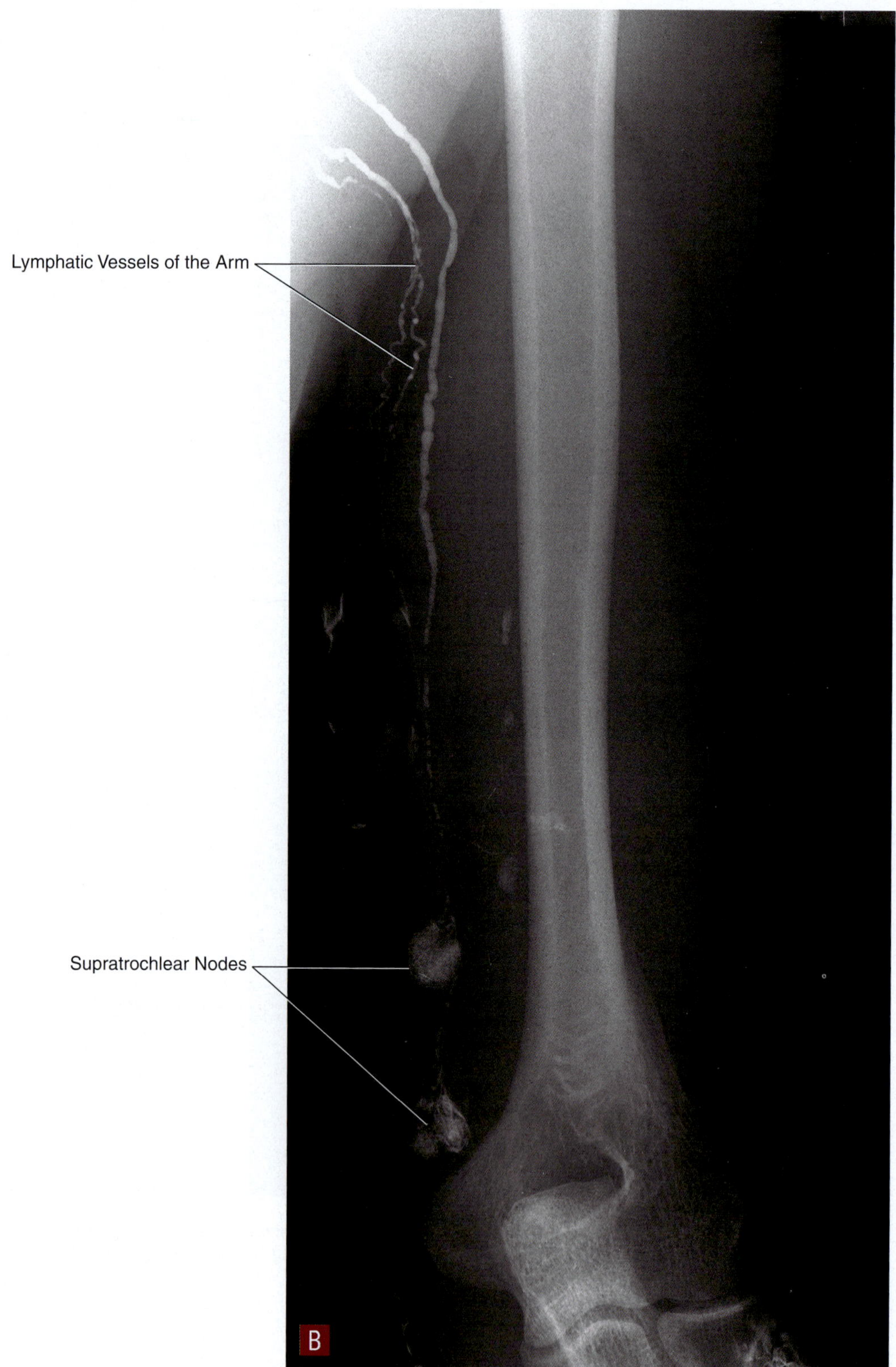

Figure 17.2. *Continued*

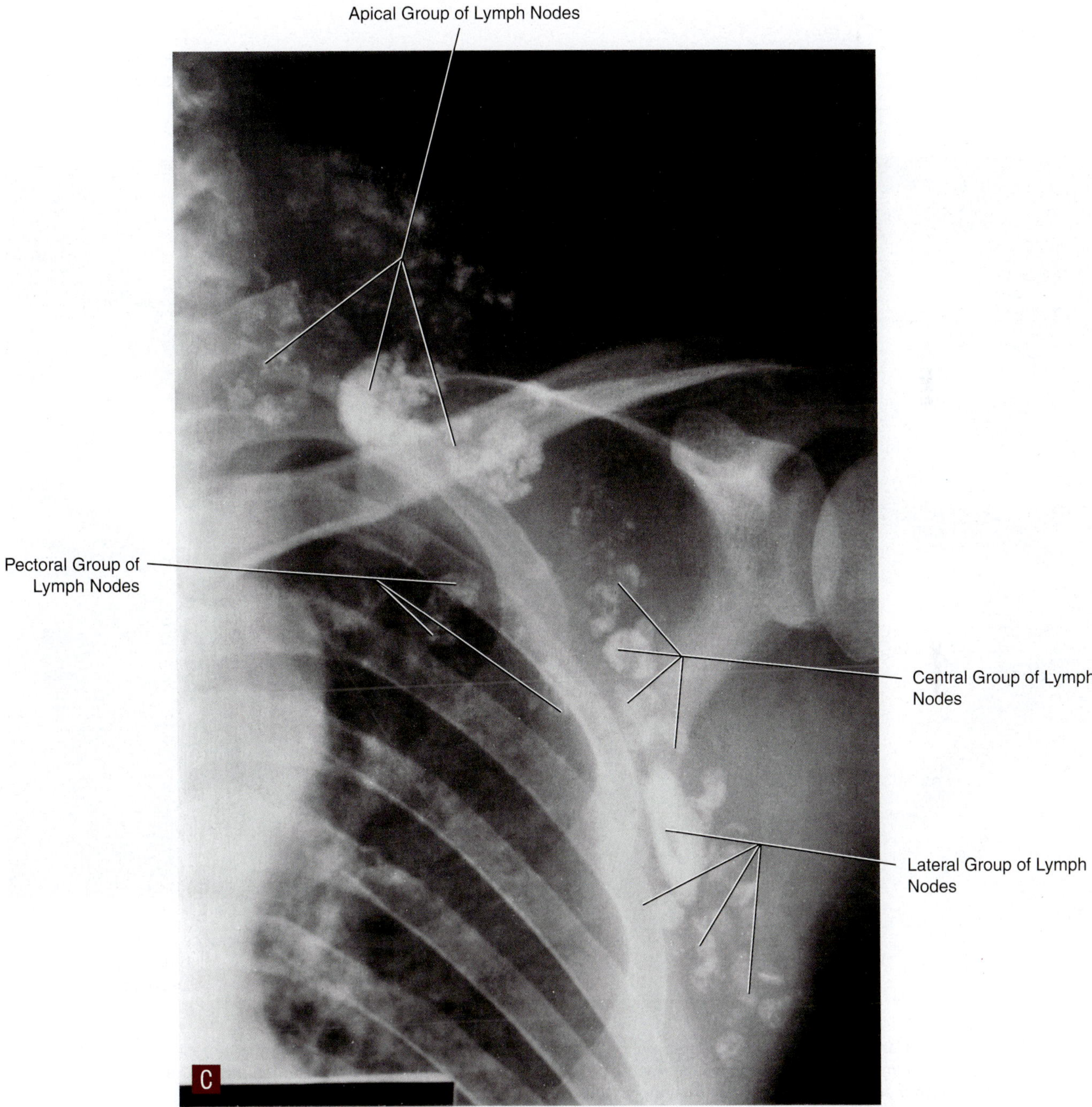

Figure 17.2. *Continued*

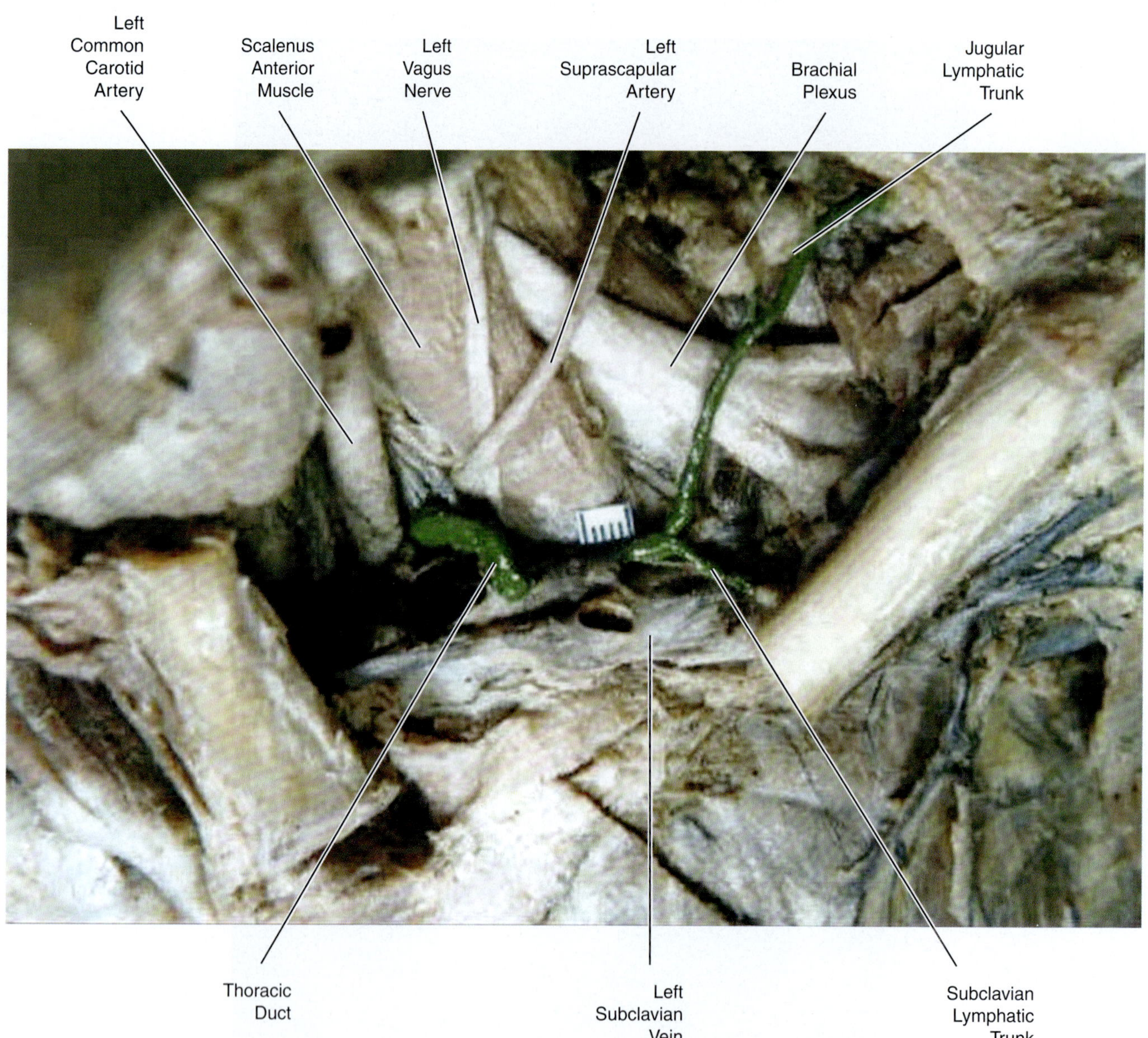

Figure 17.3. Anatomic preparation of the left supraclavicular fossa showing the thoracic duct and jugular and subclavian lymph trunks colorized in green. Note the relationship with the other structures. The subclavian lymph trunk drains the upper extremity through the axillary lymphatic group.

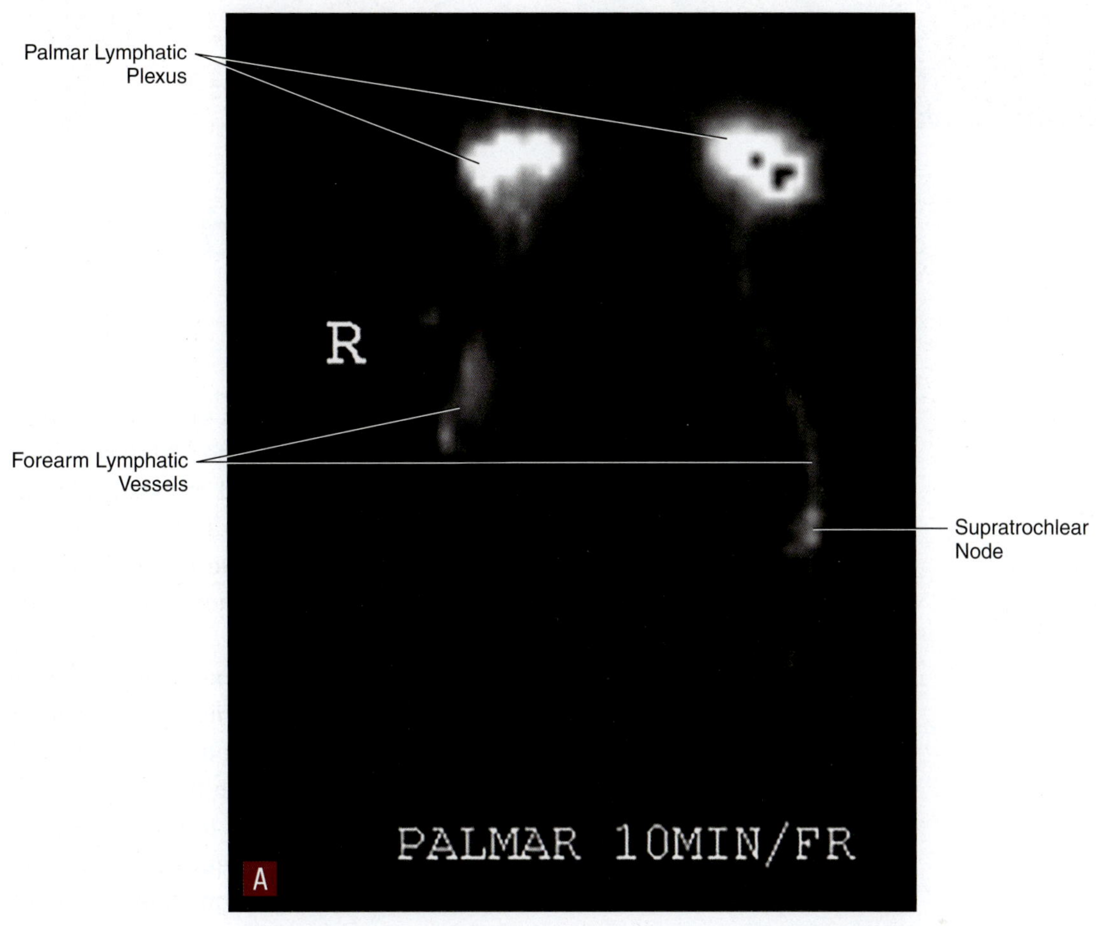

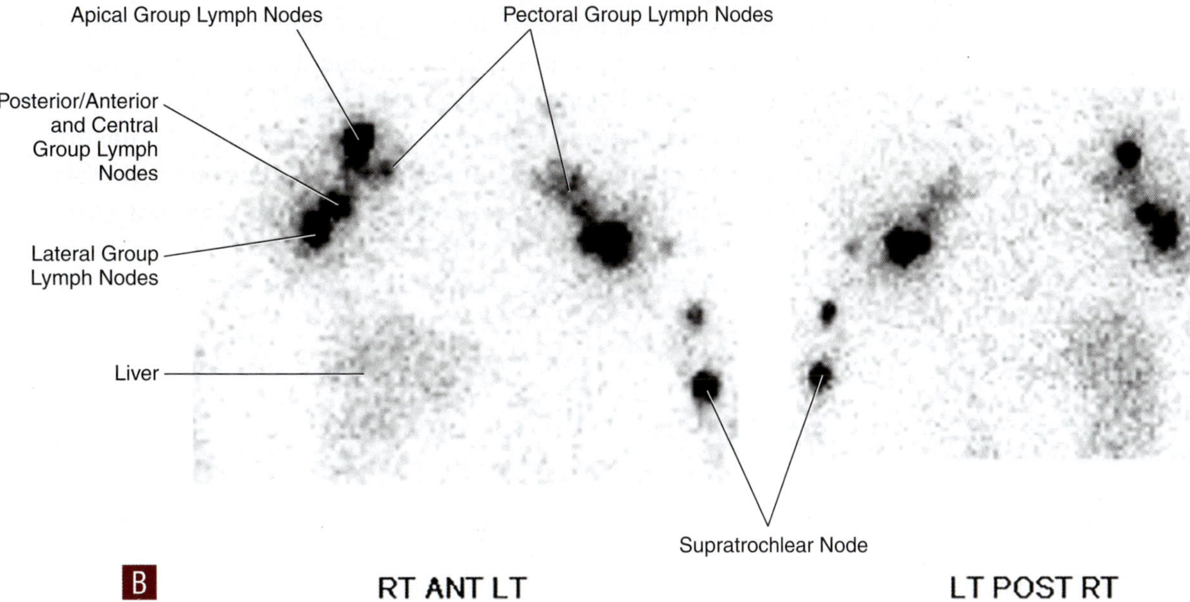

Figure 17.4. A and B. Lymphoscintigram of the upper extremity at the forearm and shoulder.

18

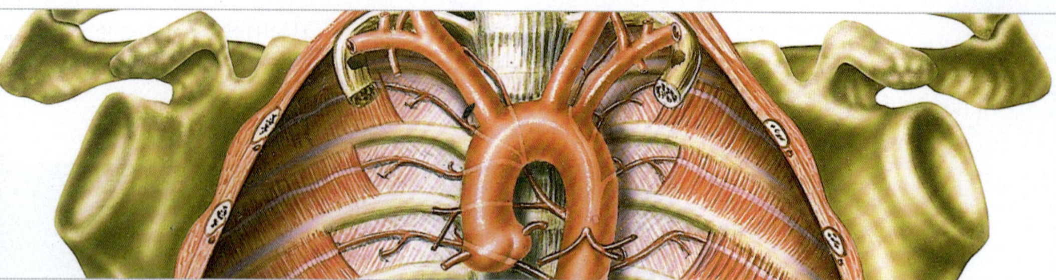

Abdominal Aorta and Branches

The abdominal aorta begins at the aortic hiatus of the diaphragm, anterior to and at the level of the lower portion of the 12th thoracic vertebra, descending slightly lateral to the midline and in close relation to the vertebral bodies, ending at the fourth lumbar vertebra. At that point, it bifurcates into two common iliac arteries forming an angle of 37°. The abdominal aortic diameter diminishes rapidly because the branches are large and numerous (Figs. 18.1 and 18.2).

The aorta is in contact anteriorly with the celiac plexus and the lesser sac or omental bursa, and the pancreatic body with the splenic vein attached posteriorly. Behind the pancreas, between the superior mesenteric artery (SMA) and the aorta, is the left renal vein in close association with the anterior wall of the aorta. Inferior to the pancreas is the horizontal part of the duodenum. Distally, the aorta is covered by the posterior parietal peritoneum and crossed by the oblique parietal attachment of the mesentery. The right lateral aspect of the aorta is in contact with the cisterna chyli, thoracic duct, azygos vein, and right crus of the diaphragm, which separates it from the inferior vena cava. Below the second lumbar vertebra the aorta is in contact with the inferior vena cava until its bifurcation into the iliac arteries. The left lateral aspect of the aorta is in contact with the crus of the diaphragm and celiac ganglion. At the level of the second lumbar vertebra, there is contact with the duodenojejunal flexure and sympathetic trunk, ascending duodenum, and inferior mesenteric vessels. The bifurcation of the abdominal aorta is projected on the abdominal wall surface at the level of the umbilicus (Figs. 18.3-18.8).

Abdominal Aorta

Branches of the Abdominal Aorta

- Ventral
  - Celiac trunk
  - Superior mesenteric artery
  - Inferior mesenteric artery
- Lateral
  - Inferior phrenic artery
  - Middle suprarenal (adrenal) artery
  - Renal artery
  - Testicular or ovarian artery (gonadal)
- Dorsal
  - Lumbar
  - Median sacral
- Terminal
  - Common iliac

Ventral Branches

Celiac Trunk

It is the first wide ventral branch of the aorta, 1.5 cm long, arising just below the aortic diaphragmatic hiatus (Figs. 18.9 and 18.10). It is generally horizontal and oriented anteriorly but may be caudally or cranially oriented (Figs. 18.11-18.15). It may give off the inferior phrenic arteries before the origin of the left gastric artery. In approximately 50% of the population, the celiac trunk follows the standard pattern. A celiac trunk may be absent in 0.4% to 2.5% of the population.

Branches
- Left gastric artery
- Hepatic artery
  - Common hepatic artery
- Gastroduodenal artery
- Pancreaticoduodenal arcades
- Right gastroepiploic artery
- Hepatic artery proper
- Right gastric artery
- Cystic artery
- Arteries of the liver
- Segmental branches
- Microscopic hepatic structure
- Terminal hepatic artery
- Hepatic arterial collaterals
- Variations of the hepatic artery

Splenic Artery

- Arteries of the pancreas
- Pancreaticoduodenal arcades
- Dorsal pancreatic artery
- Arteria pancreatica magna
- Arteria caudae pancreatis
- Short gastric arteries
- Posterior gastric artery
- Left gastroepiploic artery
- Terminal splenic branches
- Segmental splenic branches
- Variations of the celiac trunk

Left Gastric Artery

This is the smallest celiac branch. The origin of the left gastric artery (LGA) may be in the aorta, close to the celiac trunk, or at the cranial aspect of the celiac trunk, all the way, from the ostium to the bifurcation, creating a real trifurcation. It ascends cranially to the left, behind the oriental bursa, to the upper end of the stomach. After giving off distal esophageal branches and branches to the gastric fundus, the artery turns anteroinferiorly into the left gastropancreatic fold, running along the gastric lesser curvature, reaching the pylorus, supplying both gastric walls (anterior and posterior), and ends with an anastomosis with the right gastric artery (Figs. 18.16 and 18.17). The left gastric artery may give origin to the left hepatic artery, or an accessory left gastric artery may arise from the left hepatic artery (Figs. 18.18-18.22). At the gastric fundus, there are anastomoses with the splenic artery through the short gastric arteries (Fig. 18.23).

Hepatic Artery

In the adult, the hepatic artery is smaller than the splenic artery, but larger than the left gastric artery. It originates from the bifurcation of the celiac trunk, directed forward and to the right, toward the porta hepatis, where it divides into the right and left branches to the hepatic lobes (Fig. 18.10). The artery is subdivided into common hepatic artery from the celiac trunk to the origin of the gastroduodenal artery and hepatic artery proper. It is called the proper hepatic artery, from the gastroduodenal artery to the bifurcation into right and left hepatic branches (Fig. 18.12). The common hepatic artery may be extremely short or may not exist at all (Fig. 18.15). The proper hepatic artery may not exist at all (Fig. 18.11) and may be part of a trifurcation of the common hepatic artery. The hepatic artery may arise from the SMA (replaced hepatic artery). The right hepatic branch may arise from the SMA, whereas the left hepatic branch may originate from the left gastric artery. See "Variations of the Hepatic Artery" at the end of this section.

Common Hepatic Artery

Gastroduodenal artery. The gastroduodenal artery arises from the hepatic artery, characterizing the beginning of the proper hepatic artery (Figs. 18.24 and 18.25). It is short and large, descending between the duodenum and neck of the pancreas. It may be located at the left aspect or anteriorly to the bile duct. The gastroduodenal artery has three constant branches: the posterior and anterior pancreaticoduodenal arcades, the terminal branch, and the right gastroepiploic artery (Figs. 18.26 and 18.27). The gastroduodenal artery may be duplicated, or the pancreaticoduodenal arcades may arise from the common hepatic artery (Fig. 18.28).

Posterior pancreaticoduodenal arcade (PPDA). This artery is part of a rich vascular network to the head of the pancreas, uncinate process, and duodenal bulb, together with the anterior pancreaticoduodenal arcade. The PPDA arises 1 to 2 cm from the origin of the gastroduodenal artery in 78% of the cases, but the superior origin may also arise from various branches from the hepatic artery in 15% of the cases, or the SMA in 5% of the cases. It is also called the retroduodenal artery or posterior superior pancreaticoduodenal artery. The retroduodenal artery may become very prominent, tracking along the common hepatic duct (Fig. 18.29). The PPDA gives branches to the duodenum (to the right) and the head of the pancreas (to the left). The pancreatic branches anastomose freely with arteries in the head of the pancreas, anterior pancreaticoduodenal arcade, supraduodenal artery, and dorsal pancreatic artery (Figs. 18.26 and 18.27). The arcades are frequently multiple with two, three, or four branches. The lower part of the bile duct has the main blood supply from the posterior pancreaticoduodenal arcade.

Anterior pancreaticoduodenal arcade. Along with the right gastroepiploic artery, the anterior pancreaticoduodenal arcade is a terminal branch of the gastroduodenal artery. It is also called the superior pancreaticoduodenal or anterior superior pancreaticoduodenal artery and may give a pyloric branch and have distal anastomoses with the SMA or the inferior pancreaticoduodenal artery. The anterior arcade has free communications with the posterior arcade and dorsal pancreatic and transverse pancreatic arteries (Figs. 18.26, 18.27, and 18.30). The middle colic artery may also have anastomoses with the anterior pancreaticoduodenal arcade.

Right gastroepiploic artery. This artery is the terminal branch of the gastroduodenal artery, and the main artery of the stomach (Figs. 18.31 and 18.32). It follows a winding course along the greater curvature of the stomach and gives off an ascending pyloric branch and several ascending gastric branches, which anastomose with descending branches of the right and left gastric arteries. Several omental branches are also originated from the right gastroepiploic artery. The right and left omental branches form an anastomotic arcade at the greater omentum and have anastomoses with the posterior omental branches from the transverse mesocolon. The gastroepiploic artery reaches and anastomoses with the left gastroepiploic artery at its terminus (Figs. 18.33-18.37).

Other branches. Less constant branches are occasionally seen, including the right gastric artery, the transverse pancreatic artery, accessory cystic artery, and supraduodenal artery.

Right gastric artery. This artery arises from any site at the hepatic artery, before or after the gastroduodenal artery. It anastomoses with the left gastric artery (Figs. 18.19 and 18.38).

Cystic artery. This artery usually arises from the right branch of the hepatic artery. It divides into superficial and deep branches. It may originate from the hepatic artery itself at many levels or other arteries such as the gastroduodenal artery. It crosses anteriorly over the common bile duct reaching the gallbladder. An accessory cystic artery may be present and arise from the common hepatic artery or one of its branches. Small branches of the cystic artery may enter the liver parenchyma in the gallbladder bed. The cystic artery arises from the right hepatic artery in 63.9% of the cases, from the hepatic trunk in 26.9% of the cases, from left hepatic artery in 5.5% of the cases, from the gastroduodenal in 2.6% of the cases, from the superior pancreaticoduodenal arcade in 0.3% of cases, and directly from the SMA in 0.8% of cases (Fig. 18.39).

Supraduodenal artery. The supraduodenal artery has been described as a distinctive artery that allows for the surgical mobilization of the horizontal segment of the duodenum. The supraduodenal artery is probably present in more than 90% of the population, but with a high degree of variation in its origin. It provides blood supply to the distal upper two-thirds of the duodenum, with connections to the proximal small bowel (Fig. 18.40). When this artery is absent, it may arise as multiple vessels from the right gastric artery. The supraduodenal artery has been reported to originate from the gastroduodenal artery in 27% of cases, from the common hepatic artery in 20% of the cases, from the left hepatic artery in 20% of cases, the right hepatic artery in 13%, and from the cystic artery in 10% of cases. It may also participate in the blood supply of the extrahepatic bile ducts.

Arteries of the Liver

Hepatic Artery. In the adult individual, the hepatic artery is intermediate in size between the left gastric and splenic arteries. However, in fetal life and early postnatal life it is the largest celiac branch. It has a forward direction and curves to the right, below the epiploic foramen to the upper aspect of the superior part of the duodenum. Crossing anteriorly the portal vein, and roughly parallel, but to the left of the common bile duct, it ascends between layers of the lesser omentum, anterior to the epiploic foramen, to the porta hepatis, where it divides into the right and left branches to the hepatic lobes, accompanying the ramifications of the portal vein and hepatic ducts, within the portal space. The segments of the hepatic artery have been described in the preceding text (Fig. 18.41). Several intra- and extrahepatic branches of the hepatic arteries are identified, including the right gastric artery, the cystic artery, rami to the bile ducts and connections with the supraduodenal artery, and retroduodenal artery.

Interlobar Communicating Arcades

Redman and Reuter first demonstrated the existence of interlobar collateral vessels angiographically and described them as preexisting small arterial communications present in the hilum of most cases. Despite the description of interlobar communications by other authors only recently, Tohma et al. described systematically the presence of communicating arcades (CAs) between the right and left hepatic arteries in more than 85% of cases and proposed a classification (Figs. 18.42-18.44). On the left side, the CAs originated from the segment IV artery (type 1) in 62% of cases. The CAs originated from the left hepatic artery (type 2) in 38% of cases (Fig. 18.44). On the right side, the CAs originated from the right anterior hepatic artery (type 1) in 46% of cases and from the right hepatic artery (type 2) in 15% of cases (Fig. 18.45). In 38% of cases, the CAs originated from both the right hepatic artery and the right anterior hepatic artery (type 3). The CAs bifurcated off two branches to the caudate lobe in 18% of cases and one branch in 45% of cases. No caudate branches were observed in the remaining 36% of cases. The CAs are located extrahepatically cranial to the portal vein bifurcation, close to the hilar bile duct (Fig. 18.46).

Embryologic Aspects

The biliary and hepatic systems have a complex embryologic origin, which causes a significant number of variations and adaptations to the flow patterns. As the embryologic duodenal diverticulum migrates toward the liver hilum carrying the extrahepatic bile ducts, it is supplied by multiple arteries to maintain adequate perfusion for the developing system. These vessels originate from the aorta, celiac trunk, and SMA. The formation of the intrahepatic bile ducts has been suggested, to be dependent upon contact between the developing embryonic liver mass and the preformed extrahepatic duct system, which carries the arteries with it. As the biliary system matures, many of the vessels are resorbed or incorporated into the main arterial bed. However, the resorption and incorporation are variable and multiple arterial patterns develop. Therefore, only 57% to 61% of the population has what is considered the "standard" hepatic arterial perfusion pattern. The presence of significant variations in the hepatic artery anatomic arterial perfusion creates in later life the so-called replaced arteries, which do not correspond to the classical anatomy and perfuse a complete vascular bed. An accessory artery is a secondary artery that contributes to the perfusion of the vascular arterial bed in addition to the conventional anatomic arteries (see "Variations of the Hepatic Artery" in subsequent text).

Other Branches and Connections of the Hepatic Artery

Falciform Artery. The falciform ligament divides the medial and lateral segments of the left lobe of the liver and connects the liver to the diaphragm and the supra-umbilical part of the anterior abdominal wall. Its free edge contains the ligamentum teres and the small para-umbilical veins, and the falciform artery. The falciform artery originates from the middle hepatic artery (when present) and the left hepatic artery. The angiographic incidence of the falciform artery varies from 2% to 25%, but in postmortem dissections, it is identified in as many as 67% of the cases (Fig. 18.47). The terminal branches of the falciform artery are connected to the network of the phrenic arteries, internal mammary artery, and superior epigastric artery (Fig. 18.48).

Middle Hepatic Artery. The middle hepatic artery or segment IV artery is not considered an anatomic variation, although it may serve as an exclusive supplier for the segment IV of the liver. It may also be the origin of the falciform artery, the right gastric artery, and the accessory left gastric artery. It may arise from the proximal right hepatic artery or from the proper hepatic as an independent artery forming a trifurcation.

Hepatic-Phrenic Artery Connections. The hepatic arteries, particularly the left hepatic artery, may develop free communications with the phrenic arterial system. Peripheral hepatic tumors, inflammatory processes of the subphrenic space and base of the lungs, may develop multiple connections, particularly from the bare area of the liver surface. Occasionally a phrenic artery arises directly from the left hepatic artery (Fig. 18.49).

Segmental Anatomy of the Liver

The intrahepatic arteries follow a segmental distribution (Figs. 18.50 and 18.51). The division of the liver into segments is delineated by fissures and the distribution of the vascular and ductal structures. The three main hepatic veins divide the liver into four sectors, each of which receives a portal pedicle, with an alternation between hepatic veins and portal pedicles. Of the four fissures, only one is represented superficially—the portoumbilical fissure. The other three fissures are related to the three large hepatic veins, but not apparent in the liver surface.

Right fissure. This fissure commences at the right margin of the inferior vena cava and follows the attachment of the right superior coronary ligament to about 3 to 4 cm from the junction of the latter with the right inferior layer. The fissure then curves anteriorly to a point on the inferior margin about midway between the gallbladder fossa and the right margin of the liver. Passing posteriorly, the fissure follows a line that runs parallel to the gallbladder fossa and crosses the caudate process to reach the right side of the inferior vena cava. Lying almost in the coronal plane, the fissure contains the right hepatic vein, with branches passing anteriorly to segments V and VIII and posteriorly to segments VI and VII (Figs. 18.50 and 18.51).

Median fissure (main portal fissure, also called Cantlie' line). This fissure passes from the gallbladder fossa to the left margin of the inferior vena cava. Posteroinferiorly, this fissure is represented by a line from the gallbladder fossa to the main bifurcation of the hepatic pedicle (portal triad) to the retrohepatic inferior vena cava (Figs. 18.50 and 18.51).

Left fissure (left portal fissure). This fissure runs from the left side of the inferior vena cava to a point between the dorsal one-third and ventral two-thirds of the left margin of the liver; it divides the left liver into two sectors: anterior and posterior, separating the segments III and II. It is not the umbilical fissure. Inferiorly, the fissure passes to the commencement of the ligamentum venosum (Figs. 18.50 and 18.51).

Portoumbilical fissure (or umbilical fissure). This fissure is marked superficially by the attachment of the falciform ligament, which contains the ligamentum teres hepatis in its inferior border. Angled less generously than the right fissure, it meets the inferior margin of the liver at an angle of about 50°.

The liver is divided into right and left lobes, separated by the main portal fissure or median fissure (projection of the path of the middle hepatic vein upon the liver surface). The portal fissure runs from the medial side of the inferior vena cava to the middle of the gallbladder bed. The right lobe is vascularized by the right hepatic artery and the left lobe is fed by the left hepatic artery. The hepatic lobes are divided in sectors. The right lobe has an anterior and a posterior sector (also called anteromedial and posterolateral), separated by the right portal fissure (projection of the path of the right hepatic vein upon the liver surface). The left lobe has a lateral (left) and a medial sector (right), separated by the falciform ligament and portoumbilical fissure (partial projection of the path of the involuted umbilical vein, called the round ligament) (Figs. 18.50-18.52).

Hepatic Segments

The caudate lobe is an independent segment, supplied by the right and left hepatic artery and portal vein. It is called segment I and has venous drainage directly into the inferior vena cava. It is also called lobule of Spiegel. It is considered part of the left hepatic lobe (segment I of the left lobe) for surgical purposes. The caudate lobe is connected to the right lobe by a narrow bridge called the caudate process, behind the porta hepatis. Below and to the left, there is a small round appendage called the papillary process, which sometimes covers the inferior vena cava completely bridging the caudate lobe to the right liver lobe (Fig. 18.53A-D).

The left hepatic lobe is further subdivided into three segments. The lateral sector is divided into segment II and segment III by the left portal fissure (projection of the path of the left hepatic vein upon the surface of the left lobe of the liver). Segment II is posterior and superior, and segment III is inferior and anterior (Figs. 18.54 and 18.55). The medial sector of the left lobe is segment IV. It has a cuneiform shape, with the base turned anteriorly. It may be subdivided into a cranial and a caudal part, also called segments IVa and IVb. Segment IVa is also called the quadrate lobe of the liver (Fig. 18.56).

The right hepatic lobe is subdivided into four segments. The anterior sector is divided in segment VIII and segment V. Segment VIII is superior and segment V is inferior (Figs. 18.57 and 18.58). The posterior sector is divided in segment VI and segment VII. Segment VI is inferior, and segment VII is superior. The posterior sector is posterior and more lateral than the anterior sector (Figs. 18.59 and 18.60).

The segments of the liver, either at the left or the right hepatic lobes, follow a clockwise distribution. The hepatic artery, the bile ducts, and the portal vein branches run in the center of the hepatic segments, whereas the hepatic veins run within the fissures between the segments. The fissures of the liver cannot be seen at the liver surface, except at the umbilical fissure, due to the presence of the falciform ligament and round ligament (ligamentum teres) (Figs. 18.50-18.52).

Microscopic Hepatic Structure

The classic hepatic lobules are polyhedral structures (hexagonal in histologic sections), about 1 mm in diameter, with a small central vein as a central axis, surrounded by portal triads (Fig. 18.61). Each triad contains a branch of the portal vein, a hepatic artery, a lymphatic vessel, and an interlobular biliary ductule. The portal triad is sheathed by connective tissue, called the portal canal or perivascular fibrous capsule, surrounded by the limiting plate, having in between the space of Mall. In humans, the idea of a functional unit has been proposed instead because the hepatic lobules are not readily perceptible. The functional unit is the portal lobule, consisting of parts of at least three neighboring classic lobules, bile from which drains into a biliary ductule in the portal canal between three such hepatic lobules. Again, the section shows a portal lobule as a polygonal area, centered on a portal triad, with boundaries passing through adjacent central veins. The concept of a portal acinus is more useful considering metabolic organization. The portal acinus is centered on a preterminal branch of a hepatic arteriole and includes the hepatic tissue served by this, and its boundaries are limited by the territory of other acini and by two adjacent central veins (Fig. 18.62). The acinus has been divided into three zones: zone 1 (periportal), zone 2, and zone 3 (close to the central venous drainage). Zone 3 (in the circulatory periphery and close to the central vein) suffers most from injury, developing bridging necrosis. Zone 1, close to the afferent vessels, survives longer and may trigger the regeneration of the liver (Figs. 18.61-18.63).

Portal Space

Portal areas, also called portal triads or portal canals, are located at the corners of the liver lobules. Portal spaces are surrounded by much larger areas with hepatic cords and sinusoids. Each portal space contains three (hence the term portal triad) more-or-less conspicuous tubular structures wrapped together in connective tissue. The tubular structures are branches of the bile duct, the portal vein, and the hepatic artery (Fig. 18.64). There are two less conspicuous structures within the portal space, a nerve and a lymphatic channel, but usually these are not apparent in routine specimens. The portal vein supplies about 70% of the blood flow to the liver, whereas the hepatic artery supplies about 30%; each branch of the portal vein is typically much larger than the associated branch of the hepatic artery. The relative sizes of the paired vessels in a portal area thus differ from those of a typical vein-artery pair in other parts of the body, where the artery delivers the same volume of blood that the vein subsequently returns. The portal vein branches, within the portal space arise at right angles to the main axis of the portal vein in a radial fashion. Direct connections with the sinusoids are provided by the inlet venules (Fig. 18.65). The artery and bile ducts occupy the periphery of the portal space, but the artery and the bile duct may be multiple. Between stroma and hepatocytes, there is a small space, called space of Mall—one of the sites where lymph originates.

Terminal Hepatic Artery

The hepatic artery ramifies parallel with the portal vein branches and bile ducts. Arterioles are released into the lobular parenchyma and terminate at different levels of the lobule, providing arterial blood flow to zone 1 of the acinus through anastomoses with the portal venule inlet

(Fig. 18.66). Much like the bronchial arteries that provide bronchial circulation and pulmonary arterial anastomosis in the lungs, in the liver, the main circulatory arterial flow is provided to the periportal area by arterial branches directly to the peribiliary plexus and to the bile duct. Subsequently and to a much lesser extent, the artery provides nutrition to the acinus and to the liver parenchyma itself through the anastomosis of the arterioles with the portal inlet venule. In fact, due to importance of the hepatic artery to the bile ducts, the hepatic artery should be called biliary artery (Fig. 18.67).

According to Lunderquist, there are four types or levels of arterioportal communications: (1) the peribiliary plexus; (2) the terminal arteriologportal anastomosis connecting to the sinusoids; (3) the vasa vasorum on the wall of the portal vein; and (4) the direct arterioportal communications. The vasa vasorum of the wall of the portal vein is provided by direct small branches from the hepatic artery (Fig. 18.68). There are two concentric vascular layers within the wall of the larger bile duct, constituting the peribiliary plexus. The inner layer is a capillary plexus present in the submucosa, which drains into the outer adventitial venous plexus. The latter opens directly into the hepatic sinusoids via the lobular vein or into the portal vein via the interlobular vein (Figs. 18.69 and 18.70). The intrahepatic bile duct is supplied by the hepatic arterial branches, which form the peribiliary plexus, whereas the extrahepatic bile duct receives its arterial nutrition from various sources, but most commonly from branches of the gastroduodenal artery.

According to Ekataksin, unlike the portal vein which exclusively supplies sinusoids, the hepatic artery supplies five compartments: (1) peribiliary plexus, (2) portal tract interstitium, (3) portal venous vasa vasorum, (4) fibrous capsule of Glisson, and (5) central sublobular-hepatic venous vasa vasorum, which subsequently either secondarily flows through the lobules or directly drains into the hepatic vein.

Within the portal tract, the arterial bed forms distinct collecting vessels, forming a portal system, the so-called hepatic artery-derived portal system, which anastomoses with and/or follows or joins the vein-venule to open at the lobular periphery.

Outside the portal tract, the hepatic artery departs from the tract as an "isolated artery" directed toward the two compartments: the Glisson capsule and the central sublobular-hepatic venous vasa vasorum. The capsular arteriole that eventually drains into the local subcapsular lobules is likely to be misinterpreted as evidence of the hepatic artery being a primary feeder of sinusoids. The hepatic venous vasa vasorum that immediately drains into the respective hepatic vein without passing through lobular sinusoids is a hitherto unrecognized, but occasionally suspected, unusual pathway, a "bypass artery." There are multiple peripheral communications between the hepatic artery and the portal vein radicles, especially in pathologic contexts, such as in liver cirrhosis, when the arterioportal shunts are widely open, contributing therefore to the increase in the portal vein pressure levels and promoting hepatofugal flow in the intrahepatic portal branches (Fig. 18.71). The cirrhotic nodules significantly reduce the number of sinusoids, and perinodular shunts develop. The cirrhotic nodule develops a central feeding artery or group of feeding arteries, visible in a central bundle (Fig. 18.72).

To facilitate description, the biliary duct has been divided into three segments, namely hilar (right and left ducts), supraduodenal (common hepatic duct and upper common bile duct), and retropancreatic (lower common bile duct).

The arterial supply of the hilar bile duct (right and left) is provided by direct numerous small branches from the right and left hepatic arteries that form a rich network on the surface of the ducts in continuity with the plexus around the supraduodenal duct (Fig. 18.73).

The arterial supply of the supraduodenal bile duct is essentially axial, and most arteries arise from named arteries related to its upper and lower ends. The main vessels rim along the lateral aspects of the duct. According to Terblanche, these vessels are named 3 o'clock and 9 o'clock arteries and most commonly originate from the posterior pancreaticoduodenal arcade and gastroduodenal artery. Approximately 60% of the vessels supplying the supraduodenal duct run upward from vessels below, whereas 38% run downward from the right hepatic and other arteries. Only 2% of the supply is nonaxial, arising from the common or proper hepatic artery. The 3 o'clock and 9 o'clock arteries give branches to the duct forming the pericholedocal plexus (Figs. 18.35, 18.73-18.77).

An additional supply to the supraduodenal bile duct may be the retroportal artery, arising from the celiac trunk or SMA close to the origin of these vessels from the aorta. This artery courses to the right, behind the portal vein and to the back of the head of the pancreas, reaching the lower end of the supraduodenal duct. This artery may end, joining the posterior pancreaticoduodenal arcade, close to the distal supraduodenal duct, giving off small branches to the posterior surface of the duct (type I pattern). In one-third of cases, the retroportal artery passes upward on the back of the supraduodenal duct, reaching the right hepatic artery (type II pattern). The retroportal artery along its route gives branches to join the pericholedocal plexus (Fig. 18.74).

The retropancreatic bile duct is supplied by direct small branches from the posterior pancreaticoduodenal artery or gastroduodenal artery, forming a mural plexus (Fig. 18.73). More recently (1999), Vellar described the presence of a 12 o'clock marginal artery in a smaller number of individuals, joining the plexus on the posterior surface of the common hepatic duct, in addition to the previously described 3 o'clock and 9 o'clock arteries.

The hilar plexus: The hilar plate is a condensation of connective tissue, which lines the hilum of the liver and forms a roof over the contents of the hilum, separating these structures from the hepatic substance. The right and left hepatic ducts have an intimate relation to the hilar plate. Bridging between the branches of the left hepatic artery and the right hepatic artery are a number of collateral vessels, which are found on the inferior surface of the hilar plate and which form the hilar plexus. The hilar arterial plexus is not only involved in the blood supply of the confluence of the bile ducts and the right and left hepatic ducts and, therefore, in communication with the arterial plexus over the biliary system, but it is the most important collateral between the right hepatic artery and its branches and the left hepatic artery and its branches, and the same communicating arcade described by Tohma et al. in 2005. Branches from the hilar plexus supply the caudate lobe and process. The caudate lobe is an important bridge for collateral blood flow between the right and left sides of the liver. It is suggested in the literature that the caudate lobe takes its blood supply not only from the segment I artery, but also from the communicating arcade. This may be the reason that transcatheter arterial chemoembolization is often not an especially effective treatment for hepatocellular carcinomas in the caudate lobe. According to that description the arterial branches from the hilar plate ascend posterior to the right and left hepatic ducts (Fig. 18.77). It is supposed that the communicating artery may exist as a marginal artery for the hilar bile duct and connect the parabiliary arteries to form the parabiliary arterial network that supplies the biliary tract, as well as the 3 o'clock and 9 o'clock arteries (from the posterior-superior pancreaticoduodenal arcade), which exist as marginal arteries for the common bile duct.

Hepatic Arterial Collaterals

There are 26 known potential collateral pathways for the arterial supply of the liver. They may be classified as intrahepatic collaterals (Fig. 18.78) and extrahepatic collaterals (Fig. 18.79).

Intrahepatic Collaterals (Fig. 18.78)

- Perivascular
- Interlobar or intersegmental
- Intralobar or intrasegmental
- Vasa vasorum of the portal veins and hepatic veins
- Peribiliary plexus

Extrahepatic Collaterals (Fig. 18.79)

- Pancreaticoduodenal arcades
  - Inferior pancreaticoduodenal artery
  - Dorsal pancreatic artery
  - Arc of Bühler (Fig. 18.80)
- Periportal route
  - Common bile duct collaterals
  - Retroduodenal or supraduodenal artery
  - Cystic artery
  - Right branches of dorsal pancreatic artery
  - Multiple unnamed branches in the porta hepatis
- Left gastric route
  - Left gastric to right gastric anastomosis
  - Left gastric to left hepatic via lesser omentum
- Inferior phrenic route
  - Right inferior phrenic artery
  - Left inferior phrenic artery
- Right paracolic gutter route
  - Branches from middle or right colic artery
  - Direct adhesions to hepatic flexure
- Omental branches
- Internal mammary and superior epigastric artery
- Intercostal and lumbar artery
- Capsular branches of the right renal artery

Variations of the Hepatic Artery

In more than 40% of cases, the origin and course of the hepatic arteries (Fig. 18.81) vary. Two concepts must be defined. The "replaced" artery originates from a different vessel, related to the standard description, and substitutes the typical vessel. The "accessory" artery is an additional vessel to the originated according to the standard description.

Type 1

Type 1 is a replacement of the common hepatic artery, arising from the SMA. The replaced common hepatic artery passes through or behind the head of the pancreas (Figs. 18.81 and 18.82). In 10% of the population, the hepatic artery is replaced; that is, a portion of the hepatic blood supply is from the SMA. The entire hepatic arterial supply is from the SMA in 2.5% of cases and from the aorta in 2% of individuals.

Type 2

Type 2 is early bifurcation of a short common hepatic artery in right and left hepatic arteries. The right and left hepatic arteries may originate separately from the celiac trunk. The gastroduodenal artery arises from the right hepatic artery (Fig. 18.81).

Type 3

Type 3 is a replaced right hepatic artery that originates from the SMA and the left hepatic artery taking origin from the celiac trunk (Figs. 18.81 and 18.83). This is found in 15% of the population.

Type 4

Type 4 is a replaced left hepatic artery, which is a tributary of the left gastric artery, whereas the right hepatic artery originates from the celiac trunk (Figs. 18.20-18.22, 18.81). It runs within the ligamentum venosum and frequently sends smaller branches to the stomach and esophagus. In 12% to 23% of individuals either a branch of the left hepatic artery or the entire left hepatic artery arises from the left gastric artery.

Type 5

The right and left hepatic arteries arise from the celiac trunk, but there is an accessory right hepatic artery from the SMA. The accessory right hepatic artery is in general the first branch of the SMA and almost always originates the main cystic or accessory cystic artery. The accessory passes through or behind the head of the pancreas (Fig. 18.81). It occurs in 10% to 31% of the population, with 96% of cases originating from the SMA and 4% from the pancreaticoduodenal trunk. Rare instances of origin from the phrenic artery or gastroduodenal artery have been encountered.

Type 6

Type 6 is an accessory left hepatic artery arising from the left gastric artery (Fig. 18.81). Found in 8% of the population.

Type 7

Type 7 is an accessory left hepatic artery arising from the right hepatic artery (Fig. 18.81).

Type 8

Right hepatic artery passes anteriorly to the common hepatic bile duct, rather than posteriorly (Fig. 18.81).

Splenic Artery

The splenic artery gives branches to the pancreas, to the stomach, and to the spleen. It originates from the celiac trunk in more than 80% of cases. Normal diameter of the splenic artery is 5.6 mm (±1.3 mm). In situations of hypersplenism the splenic artery may be enlarged three- or fourfold. Most of the arteries feeding the body and tail of the pancreas originate from the splenic artery (Figs. 18.84-18.86).

Arteries of the Pancreas

The pancreas does not have a central hilum like other abdominal organs. It is situated between the celiac trunk and the SMA, receiving the blood supply from several arteries originated from those main trunks (Fig. 18.87). The arteries of the head of the pancreas originate from the gastroduodenal artery, and the arteries of the body and tail originate from the splenic artery, celiac trunk, or common hepatic artery.

Pancreaticoduodenal Arcades

The head of the pancreas is encircled by two arterial arcades: the posterior (retroduodenal artery) and anterior pancreaticoduodenal arcades, branches of the gastroduodenal artery. The posterior arcade is proximal on the gastroduodenal artery, whereas the anterior arcade is a terminal branch of the gastroduodenal artery, together with the right gastroepiploic artery. The anterior pancreaticoduodenal arcade joins the posterior arcade, behind the head of the pancreas, forming a common trunk called inferior pancreaticoduodenal artery (or trunk), and ending in an anastomosis with the SMA or the first jejunal artery. In a number of cases there is an intermediary pancreaticoduodenal arcade, and in some cases it is not a real arcade but a terminal artery to the pancreatic head (Figs. 18.26-18.30).

Dorsal Pancreatic Artery

The main vessel to the neck and proximal body of the pancreas is the dorsal pancreatic artery (Figs. 18.24 and 18.87) (also called superior pancreatic artery, colli, suprema, propria, media, isthmi, or dorsalis, and less correctly the arteria pancreatica magna). The dorsal pancreatic artery arises most commonly from the initial splenic artery but also frequently from the celiac trunk bifurcation (Fig. 18.88) or from the common hepatic artery (Fig. 18.89). Less commonly, it originates from the SMA or from a branch of the SMA (Figs. 18.25, 18.90, and 18.91). The dorsal pancreatic artery is commonly connected, in the right aspect, with the anterior pancreaticoduodenal arcade or other gastroduodenal artery branch by an anastomotic branch (prepancreatic arcade) and originates the transverse pancreatic artery in the left aspect (arteria transversa pancreatis), which crosses all along the pancreatic body and tail (Figs. 18.87 and 18.88). The dorsal pancreatic artery may give rise to omental branches and also an actual or accessory middle colic artery (Fig. 18.92).

Arteria Pancreatica Magna

The body of the pancreas is supplied by the arteria pancreatica magna (arteria corporis pancreatica or great pancreatic artery) (Fig. 18.93). The arteria pancreatica magna may be single, but it is usually a group of comb-shaped branches, perpendicular to the splenic artery, that anastomose with the transverse pancreatic artery.

Arteria Caudae Pancreatis (Caudal Pancreatic Artery)

The tail of the pancreas is supplied by multiple branches originated from the splenic artery, right gastroepiploic artery, or splenic branches (Fig. 18.94). These branches anastomose with the transverse pancreatic artery and branches of the arteria pancreatica magna.

Short Gastric Arteries

The short gastric arteries (rami gastrici breves) arise from the splenic artery, divisional branches, polar arteries for the spleen and splenic parenchyma (Figs. 18.23 and 18.31). They supply the cranial part of the gastric greater curvature (Fig. 18.17). It varies in number from one to four. Up to nine arteries may be found. Anastomoses occur with other gastric branches.

Posterior Gastric Artery

The posterior gastric artery arises from the splenic artery and supplies the posterior fundic portion of the stomach, passing through the gastrosplenic ligament. It may provide splenic branches for the upper pole of the spleen.

Left Gastroepiploic Artery

This artery is also called the left gastro-omental artery. It is most commonly a branch of the splenic artery and arises as a trunk together with the left gastroepiploic artery and the inferior splenic branch. It may, however, arise from the splenic artery isolated. It reaches the greater gastric curvature in the middle and eventually anastomoses with the right gastroepiploic artery (Fig. 18.95). The left omental (epiploic) artery is a major branch of the left gastroepiploic artery and forms the omental arcade in a significant number of cases. Other branches are the omental (or epiploic) arteries and the posterior and anterior short gastric arteries along the gastric body and antrum (Figs. 18.23, 18.31, and 18.86).

Terminal Splenic Branches

The splenic branches enter the hilum after division of the main splenic artery in five or more branches (Figs. 18.96 and 18.97). The splenic arterial circulation consists of multiple separate segments, with adjacent compartments without arterial interconnections. Within the spleen, the finest arteriolar branches pass out of the trabeculae, their adventitia being replaced by a periarteriolar sheath. These sheaths constitute the white pulp with splenic lymphatic follicles. The arterioles divide into a series of straight vessels termed penicillary arterioles. These pass through the marginal zones of the white pulp, developing the ellipsoids by thickening of the sheath by aggregation of macrophages and fibroblasts. Beyond the ellipsoids, each vessel continues as a fine arteriole or divides into two. Eventually the blood passes into the red pulp and the venous sinusoids, venules, and small veins. The small veins form the larger veins and exit through the hilum.

Segmental Splenic Branches

In more than 80% of cases, there are only two segments, the superior and the inferior. The superior segment is larger and heavier than the inferior segment in more than 65% of cases. In fewer cases, there are three or four splenic segments (superior, intermediate, and inferior).

Variations of the Celiac Trunk

In 55% to 65% of cases, the celiac trunk divides into three branches: the left gastric artery, the splenic artery, and common hepatic artery. In more than 55% of cases, the inferior phrenic arteries also arise from the celiac trunk either as a single trunk or separately. The rest of the population presents one or more replaced arteries in origin. The celiac trunk may be absent, and the three arteries arise independently from the aorta (Fig. 18.98).

Couinaud described the following eight different types of variations of the celiac trunk.

Type 1. Classic Celiac Trunk: Hepato-Gastro-Splenic Trunk

This is the classic configuration of the celiac trunk, with the hepatic, left gastric, and splenic artery arising as a trunk from the abdominal aorta (Fig. 18.99). Three subtypes are described: (1) hepatosplenic trunk with the left gastric artery arising from the trunk (Fig. 18.96); (2) hepatogastrosplenic trunk, with the three arteries arising at the same time in a trifurcation (Fig. 18.99); and (3) gastrosplenic trunk, the splenic is dominant and the hepatic artery arises from the splenic (Figs. 18.20 and 18.100).

Type 2. Hepatosplenic Trunk

The hepatic and splenic arteries form a trunk, and the left gastric artery arises from the aorta (Fig. 18.16).

Type 3. Hepatogastric Trunk

The hepatic and left gastric arteries arise from a common trunk, and the splenic artery arises directly from the aorta (Fig. 18.85) or from the SMA, called splenic-mesenteric trunk.

Type 4. Hepato-Splenic-Mesenteric Trunk

The left gastric artery arises directly from the aorta and the hepatic, the splenic, and the mesenteric arteries form a single trunk (Figs. 18.101 and 18.102).

Type 5. Gastrosplenic Trunk

This is the most complex configuration. The left gastric artery and the splenic artery form a common trunk. The middle hepatic artery, when present, may arise from the aorta or from the SMA. When the middle hepatic artery does not exist, it is replaced by the right or left or both at the same time.

Type 6. Celiac-Mesenteric Trunk (Celiacomesenteric Trunk)

The SMA arises from the celiac trunk; this type is found in less than 1% of the population (Fig. 18.102).

Type 7. Celiac-Colic Trunk

The left colic artery or the middle colic artery arises from the celiac trunk.

Type 8. Absent Celiac Trunk

The three main arteries arise directly from the abdominal aorta.

Superior Mesenteric Artery

This is the second ventral branch of the abdominal aorta. This artery supplies all of the small intestine, the right colon, and most of the transverse colon (Figs. 18.103 and 18.104). The origin of the SMA is about 1 cm below the origin of the celiac trunk, behind the pancreas, and is crossed anteriorly by the splenic vein. The left renal vein crosses posteriorly to the most proximal centimeters of the SMA, followed by the uncinate process of the pancreas and the horizontal part of the duodenum.

Branches

- Inferior pancreaticoduodenal artery
  - Anterior branch
  - Posterior branch
- Jejunal and ileal branches
  - Straight vessels (vasa recta)
- Ileocolic artery
  - Superior branch
  - Inferior branch
  - Ascending colic artery

Anterior and posterior cecal artery
Appendicular artery
Ileal branch
Right colic artery
Ascending branch
Descending branch
Middle colic artery
Right branch
Left branch
Other replaced and accessory branches
Different origins of the SMA
Terminal arteries and intestinal villi

Inferior Pancreaticoduodenal Artery

This is the first branch of the SMA on the right. It may originate from the first jejunal branch. It divides into an anterior and a posterior branch. The anterior branch crosses anteriorly to the head of the pancreas joining the anterior pancreaticoduodenal arcade. The posterior branch crosses posteriorly to the head of the pancreas anastomosing with the posterior pancreaticoduodenal arcade (Fig. 18.105).

Jejunal and Ileal Branches

The jejunal and ileal branches arise from the left aspect of the SMA, varying in number from 12 to 15. These branches vascularize the jejunum and ileum, except for the terminal ileum, forming a series of arches and anastomoses in three or four levels. The straight arteries (vasa recta) and the short arteries (vasa brevia) arise from the fourth- or fifth-level arches and supply the intestinal wall and mucosa (Fig. 18.106).

Ileocolic Artery

This artery is the last branch on the right side of the SMA. It is oriented to the right underneath the retroperitoneal layer and vascularizes the terminal ileum, the right colon, the cecum, and the appendix (Figs. 18.107 and 18.108). Four major branches are identified: the ascending branch, to the right colon (with anastomoses to the right colic artery); the cecal branches (anterior and posterior) to the cecum; the ileal branch to the ileum, with anastomoses to the terminal SMA; and the appendicular artery of the appendix.

Right Colic Artery

This artery originates at the middle of the SMA, but may share a common origin with the ileocolic artery. It courses behind the parietal peritoneum, reaching the right ascending colon. It presents two main branches: the descending and the ascending branches. The descending anastomoses with the ileocolic artery and the ascending with the middle colic artery (Figs. 18.109-18.113).

Middle Colic Artery

This artery arises from the SMA just after passing the pancreas, following a path at the transverse mesocolon. It has a right branch and a left branch. The right branch anastomoses with the right colic artery, and the left branch with the left colic artery, a branch of the inferior mesenteric artery through the marginal arteries. It may be replaced and arises from the dorsal pancreatic artery or from the celiac trunk (Figs. 18.114-18.119).

Other Replaced and Accessory Branches

The common hepatic artery, the gastroduodenal artery, an accessory right hepatic artery, and an accessory pancreatic artery or splenic artery, may arise from the SMA. The dorsal pancreatic artery arises from the SMA in 14% of cases (Figs. 18.25 and 18.90). The replaced hepatic artery or accessory hepatic artery follows a path behind the head of the pancreas, in intimate contact with the pancreas tissue, sometimes actually encircled by pancreatic parenchyma (Fig. 18.120). The arc of Bühler is an uncommon direct pathway between the celiac and superior mesenteric arteries, due to the remaining embryologic ventral anastomosis (Fig. 18.80).

Different Origins of the Superior Mesenteric Artery

The SMA most commonly arises from the abdominal aorta; it may, however, originate as a celiac-mesenteric trunk. It may also originate together with the splenic artery (Fig. 18.98).

Terminal Arteries and Intestinal Villi

The intramural vessels of the bowel arise from both vasa recta and the vasa brevia forming the external muscular plexus (Fig. 18.121). After crossing the muscle, a rich submucosal plexus is formed from which a few recurrent branches course backward into the muscle and may join the external muscular plexus. The submucosal plexus is found over the length of the bowel and is arranged in a coarse rectangular pattern. The vertical arterioles arise from the submucosal plexus, reaching the villi and mucous membrane. A mucosal plexus is also found in the small bowel (Fig. 18.122).

The circulation to the villus is supplied from a single arteriole, about 20 μm in diameter, which originates from the submucosal plexus and runs up to the villi stroma and becomes capillarized, losing its smooth muscle coat. At the tip of the villus, the arteriole is arborescent and divides into a fine subepithelial channel system, which eventually drains into a central venule. There is also a central lymphatic channel. The arterial and venous loops in the villi are so close that there is evidence of a countercurrent exchange of oxygen and nutrients in the intestinal villus, aggravated in low flow states as in intestinal ischemia (Fig. 18.123).

There is evidence of arteriovenous anastomoses in the submucosal plexus of the gut wall, better demonstrated in the stomach and colon rather than the small bowel. The regulation of the blood flow reaching the intestine is complex and interdependent, playing an important role in the theory of vascular circuits running in parallel, with resistance in series (Fig. 18.124) among several other central and regional mechanisms.

Inferior Mesenteric Artery

The inferior mesenteric artery (IMA) supplies the left third of the transverse colon, the descending colon, the sigmoid colon, and part of the rectum. It arises a few centimeters from the aortic bifurcation and is much smaller in diameter compared with the SMA. It follows a retroperitoneal path in the left colonic branches and enters the sigmoid mesocolon with the rectal arteries (Figs. 18.125 and 18.126).

Branches

- Left colic artery
  - Ascending branch
  - Descending branch
- Sigmoid arteries (inferior left colic artery)
- Superior rectal artery (superior hemorrhoidal artery)
  - Right branch
  - Left branch

Left Colic Artery

This artery courses a retroperitoneal route and divides into ascending and descending branches. The ascending branch reaches the transverse mesocolon where it anastomoses with the middle colic artery (Fig. 18.127). Arches that originate from this ascending branch provide the blood supply of the distal transverse colon and descending left colon. The descending branch anastomoses with the highest sigmoid artery. From the anastomosis between these arteries, the continuous marginal artery near the colon wall originates; this artery is called the marginal artery of Drummond (Figs. 18.128 and 18.129). The anastomosis of the marginal artery with the ascending branch of the left colic artery and the distal left middle colic artery is frequently made through an additional arcade, the arc of Riolan. When the arc of Riolan is not well developed, there will be a critical area of anastomosis, called Griffith's point, at the splenic flexure of the colon, which is important in the etiology of ischemia of the left colon when occlusion of one of the mesenteric arteries develops.

Sigmoid Arteries

There are two or three sigmoid arteries within the sigmoid mesocolon. Branches supply the left descending colon and the sigmoid colon. There is an upper anastomosis with the descending branch of the left colic artery and a lower anastomosis with the superior rectal artery (Figs. 18.129 and 18.130).

Superior Rectal Artery

This artery descends into the pelvis in the sigmoid mesocolon and when it reaches the rectum divides into two lateral branches, right and left, dividing further into smaller branches reaching the sphincter ani internus, forming loops around the lower rectum (Fig. 18.131). There are communications with the middle rectal artery (branch of the internal iliac artery) and with the inferior rectal artery (branch from the internal pudendal artery) (Fig. 18.132).

Lateral Branches of the Abdominal Aorta

Inferior Phrenic Artery

The inferior phrenic arteries may arise together as a trunk or separately as independent vessels, just above or at the origin of the celiac trunk (Figs. 18.1 and 18.4). These arteries ascend along the diaphragmatic crura (Fig. 18.133). Each artery divides into a medial and a lateral branch (Fig. 18.134). The medial curves forward and the lateral reaches the thoracic wall, having anastomosis with the posterior intercostal and musculophrenic arteries (Fig. 18.135). Each artery gives the small superior suprarenal branches to the upper portion of the adrenal glands (Figs. 18.136-18.138). The inferior phrenic artery supplies the Glisson capsule of the liver through anastomoses at the bare area of the liver within the triangular ligaments (Fig. 18.139).

Middle Suprarenal Artery

These are small arteries that arise laterally to the aorta, at about the same level of the origin of the SMA, reaching the adrenal glands, and with anastomoses with the superior phrenic artery, and inferior suprarenal artery originated from the renal artery (Figs. 18.1 and 18.4). The right middle suprarenal artery passes behind the inferior vena cava.

Arteries of the Adrenal Glands

The adrenal glands are vascular organs and are supplied by three groups of arteries (Fig. 18.140): the superior adrenal artery (Fig. 18.138), the middle adrenal artery (Fig. 18.141), and the inferior adrenal artery, originated from the inferior phrenic artery, the aorta, and the renal artery, respectively.

The capsular arteries ramify extensively before entering the gland to form a subcapsular plexus, which extends into the zona glomerulosa as sinusoids. The sinusoids continue into the zona fasciculata as straight cortical sinusoids between columns of cells. These are followed by a deep plexus of sinusoids at the zona reticularis. At the internal aspect of the zona reticularis, there are muscle fibers which modulate the adrenal arterial flow, and act as a dam at the corticomedullary junction. Some larger arterioles bypass the described route and connect the capsular artery with the medullary capillaries (Fig. 18.142). There is a medullary plexus that connects with the medullary vein, which emerges from the hilum to form the suprarenal vein, draining to the inferior vena cava on the right and to the renal vein on the left side.

Renal Arteries

Extrarenal Arteries

Each renal artery is described as a single vessel, emerging on each side of the vertebral column between the first and the second lumbar vertebra, immediately below (1 to 2 cm) of the SMA. The renal artery usually has a slightly oblique cranial-caudal course, and close to the renal sinus, after giving off the inferior suprarenal artery, it divides into an anterior and a posterior branch. The aortic origin of the left renal artery is higher than the right renal artery origin; nevertheless, it is not a definitive rule.

Anatomic variations of the renal blood supply occur frequently. Multiplicity of renal arteries is more common than multiple veins and is more prevalent than any other arteries of the same size in other organs.

Material of investigation. Renal pedicles (266) were analyzed that were dissected from 133 formalin-fixed cadavers of adult patients, of both sexes, who died of causes not related to the urinary tract.

Findings. Figs. 18.143-18.145 show schematic drawings with the frequency of each type of renal arterial supply that we have found. The current nomenclature used and that must be adopted to denominate the renal arteries is the following.

Hilar artery. Aortic branch that penetrates the kidney in the hilar region (Fig. 18.143A).

Extrahilar artery. Renal artery branch that has an extrahilar penetration (superior pole) in the kidney (Fig. 18.143B).

Superior polar artery. Aortic branch that penetrates the kidney in the superior pole (Fig. 18.143D).

Inferior polar artery. Aortic or common iliac artery branch that penetrates the kidney in the inferior pole (Fig. 18.144A).

Precocious bifurcation. Renal artery in which the main trunk has less than 1 cm in length before branching off (Fig. 18.144C). When variations in the renal arteries exist, these vessels shall be named multiple arteries; the words "extra," "aberrant," and "accessory" should be avoided because these vessels are normal segmental end arteries, without anastomoses between them. Even the term "supernumerary" should not be used because it might imply that these vessels are superfluous.

The presence of the superior pole extrahilar branch (Fig. 18.143B) should not be considered an anatomic variation because this vessel is a ramification of the main trunk of the renal artery. Variations in the kidney arterial supply in 81 of the 266 pedicles analyzed (30.5%) were found. There was no significant statistical difference in arterial variations between right and left kidneys. In 12 cases (4.5%), an individual presented bilateral variation; among these, in five cases (1.9%), the variation was the same on both sides (Fig. 18.145).

A low incidence of multiple renal arteries (0.17%) has been reported in patients of African ancestry. In individual cases, the number of multiple arteries (when present) tends to be greater in patients of African ancestry than in Caucasian subjects.

Angle of the Origins of the Renal Arteries

In the transverse plane, the location of the origin of the right renal artery tends to be anterolateral, with an angle ranging from 0° to 70°, and the average angle is 30° to 35°. The left renal artery tends to be posterolateral or lateral, with an angle ranging from −50° to 35°, and the average angle is −11° to 15°. The variation in location and distribution width of the renal arteries, however, is great (Fig. 18.146).

Renal Ectopy

Ectopic kidneys are rare, occurring in about 0.1% of the population. It is assumed that caudal ectopic kidneys have multiple arteries, but it is not always the case. The most common type of fused kidney is the horseshoe kidney, but a variety of ectopic kidneys exist, including crossed ectopia, fused presacral kidney, and pelvic kidney. The vascular supply of these malformations is unpredictable. Multiple arteries originating from the lower aorta or pelvic arteries are usually present to supply the ectopic kidney (Figs. 18.147 and 18.148).

Intrarenal Arteries

The main renal artery divides into an anterior and a posterior branch after giving off the inferior suprarenal artery. Whereas the posterior branch (retropelvic artery) proceeds as the posterior segmental artery to supply the homonymous segment without further significant branching, the anterior branch of the renal artery provides three or four segmental arteries. The renal artery branches are terminal vessels, and there is no anastomosis between the segmental arteries. These segmental arteries divide before entering the renal parenchyma into interlobular arteries (infundibular arteries), which progress adjacent to the caliceal infundibula and the minor calices, entering the renal columns between the renal pyramids (Figs. 18.149-18.151).

As the interlobar arteries progress, they give origin (usually by dichotomous division) to the arcuate arteries (Figs. 18.149-18.151). The arcuate arteries give off the interlobular arteries, which run to the periphery, thereby giving off the afferent arterioles of the glomeruli (Fig. 18.150). The afferent arteriole invaginates into the glomerular capsule (Bowman), forming the glomerulus, from which an efferent arteriole leaves (Fig. 18.152). The complex formed by the glomerulus invaginated into the capsule is called the renal corpuscle (Malpighi). In the renal corpuscle, one may identify a vascular pole (site where the afferent and efferent arterioles are located) and, in a diametrically opposite position, a urinary pole (site where the glomerular capsule narrows into a tube) (Fig. 18.152).

Because the division branches of the renal artery and the intrarenal distribution of these vessels vary, study of the isolated vessels has a limited practical value. An analysis considering the anatomic relationship between the intrarenal arteries and the kidney collecting system, and considering these relationships in the specific kidney regions, is useful. Moreover, the anatomic relationships between the arteries and the collecting system have a fairly constant pattern in the different kidney regions. Also, these relationships are independent of both the number and the arrangement of the arterial segments.

Material of investigation. Eighty-two three-dimensional endocasts of the renal collecting system together with the intrarenal arteries, obtained from 41 male and female fresh cadavers from patients who died of causes not related to the urinary tract, were studied.

A yellow polyester resin was injected into the ureter to fill the kidney collecting system, and a red resin was injected into the main trunk of the renal artery to fill the renal arterial tree, according to the proportions and technique described previously. For this research, only the kidneys presenting a single main renal were used.

To study the intrarenal arteries and their anatomic relationships to the collecting system, the arterial tree was injected to its full capacity to preserve the same spatial associations as existed in vivo. Because the polyester resin has low viscosity and consequently high penetration power, the injection reached the interlobular arteries, the afferent arterioles, the glomerular tufts, the efferent arterioles, and even the vasa recta. Therefore, after organic matter corrosion and washing of the injected specimen, the cast looks like a sponge (Fig. 18.153). The aspect of a sponge corresponds to glomeruli filled with resin. If one examines the cast under magnification, it is easy to identify the microcirculation of the kidney (Figs. 18.154 and 18.155). The fine vessels and glomerular tufts were removed by needle handpicking, allowing clear visualization of the targeted arteries and the underlying collecting system (Fig. 18.156).

Findings. The findings were presented in relation to the pelvicaliceal system and considering the specific kidney regions.

Superior Pole

The superior segmental artery (apical) can have different origins, but it usually arises from the anterosuperior segmental artery, being positioned in the medial midline and progressing to the uppermost region of the superior pole. This artery often has a proximal origin, passes far from the upper infundibulum to reach the superior segment (apical) (Figs. 18.157A and 18.158) and is not related to the collecting system.

In 86.6% of cases (71 of 82 casts), the arterial supply related to the upper caliceal group arose from two arteries: one originated from the anterior division and the other from the posterior division of the renal artery. The upper caliceal group was involved by these two arterial trunks, which coursed alongside the anterior and posterior surfaces of the caliceal infundibulum (Fig. 18.157A and B). In the remaining 13.4% of cases (11 casts), these two arteries originated only from the anterior division or only from the posterior division of the renal artery.

Midzone (Hilar)

In all cases, the arterial supply to the anterior surface of the kidney midzone arose from the anterior division of the renal artery. Two possibilities may be found: in 64.6% (53 of 82 casts) there was one artery that coursed horizontally in the mid-renal pelvis (Figs. 18.159A and 18.160); the mid-kidney receives secondary division branches from arteries of other regions (Figs. 18.159B and 18.161). The relationship between the calices and the anterior artery varied amply and followed the caliceal variations, which are typical and large in the mid-kidney. One may predict the mid-kidney arterial vascularization through an intravenous pyelogram: if the mid-kidney caliceal drainage is independent of the superior and inferior caliceal groups, the mid-kidney usually has an individualized artery; conversely, when the caliceal drainage is dependent on the superior and the inferior caliceal groups, the mid-kidney usually receives secondary division branches from arteries of other regions (Fig. 18.14 referring to veins).

Inferior Pole

In the inferior pole, two possibilities of arterial distribution may be found. In 62.2% of the cases (51 of 82 casts) the arterial supply to the inferior pole, both front and back, arose from the inferior segmental artery (Figs. 18.162 and 18.163). This vessel, which originates from the anterior division of the main renal artery, passes in front of the ureteropelvic junction, and, after entering the inferior pole, divides into an anterior and a posterior branch. The anterior branch is related to the anterior surface of the lower infundibulum (Fig. 18.162A). The posterior branch progresses under the neck of the lower calyx to reach the posterior aspect of the kidney (Fig. 18.162A and B). In these cases, the posterior segmental artery does not reach the lower infundibulum, leaving its posterior surface free from arteries (Fig. 18.162B). In this situation, both anterior and posterior aspects of the inferior pole are supplied by a single anterior artery (inferior segmental artery).

In the other 37.8% of cases (31 of 82 casts), the anterior branch arose from the inferior segmental artery and the posterior branch was an extension of the posterior segmental artery (retropelvic artery) (Figs. 18.164A and B, 18.165). In these cases, the anterior aspect of the inferior pole is supplied by the anterior branch and its posterior aspect is supplied by the posterior branch.

Dorsal Kidney

The dorsal kidney is supplied by the posterior segmental artery (retropelvic artery), which is a direct extension of the posterior division of the main renal artery. Within the kidney substance, the retropelvic artery usually describes an arc and from its convexity three constant subdivision branches emerge and may be identified (superior, middle, and inferior; Figs. 18.166 and 18.167). The superior branch is close to the posterior surface of the upper caliceal infundibulum. In some instances, the posterior segmental artery may give off two, or even three, superior branches related to the dorsal aspect of the superior pole (Fig. 18.166). The middle branch supplies the middle portion of the posterior segment and may interdigitate with the anterior branches of the mid-kidney. The inferior branch is an extension of the retropelvic artery itself (Fig. 18.166). Its course and arrangement is dependent on the inferior vascularization, as described previously (Figs. 18.162 and 18.164).

The posterior segmental artery itself was in close relationship to the upper infundibulum or to the junction of the pelvis with the upper calix in 57.3% of the cases (Fig. 18.168A). In this situation, this artery usually described an arc that contacted the upper infundibulum (Fig. 18.168B). In the other 42.7% of cases, the posterior segmental artery coursed in the middle posterior surface of the renal pelvis (Fig. 18.168C).

Relationships to the Ureteropelvic Junction

In 53.7% of cases (44 of 82 casts), a close relationship between the inferior segmental artery and the anterior surface of the ureteropelvic junction (UPJ) was found when this vessel passed this region to enter the inferior pole (Fig. 18.169A). Among these cases, there was one artery anterior and another artery posterior to the UPJ, simultaneously (Fig. 18.170). In the remaining 46.3% of cases (38 of 82 casts), the UPJ was not related to the arteries, either anteriorly or posteriorly (Figs. 18.169B-18.172).

Arterial Segmental Analysis

The independence between portions of an organ (segments) may be based on different structures, according to their specifically functional importance. Concerning the kidney, no branch of the renal artery anastomoses with another. Some of the primary and secondary branches of the renal artery have been called segmental arteries, and the zones supplied by these arteries are named renal segments. Because the intrarenal veins have no segmental organization and anastomoses freely, the segmentation of the kidney is mainly based on the arterial supply.

In addition to a study of the arterial segmental arrangement, it is presented an analysis of the surface proportional area of each segment as measured on polyester resin endocasts of the kidney arterial vasculature.

Material of investigation. Forty-nine three-dimensional endocasts of the intrarenal arterial tree were analyzed, which were obtained from 33 fresh cadavers of both sexes (cause of death not related to the urinary tract). In 16 subjects, the kidneys were studied bilaterally, and in 17 subjects, only one side was studied. For this study, only kidneys with a single renal artery were considered.

A segmental artery is defined as a primary or a secondary branch of the main renal artery that can be identified and isolated outside the renal hilum. The posterior segmental artery (retropelvic artery) is considered the posterior branch of the renal artery, not considering the subdivisions (branches) inside the renal parenchyma or segmental arteries.

A polyester resin (volume ranging from 2.0 to 6.0 mL) was injected into each segmental branch as defined previously. The segments were injected with resins of different colors, corresponding to the following:

Posterior segment: red
Superior (apical) segment: brown
Anterosuperior segment: blue
Anteroinferior segment: white
Inferior segment: yellow

Two other possibilities existed: First, when the main artery to the apex of the kidney (superior segment) was a branch of the posterior segmental artery (retropelvic artery), the superior segment was injected with the same color as the posterior segment (red), because in these cases, both anatomically and functionally, the arterial supply of the kidney apex is dependent on the posterior segmental artery. Second, when the mid-kidney has only one segmental artery, the anterosuperior and the anteroinferior segments were fused in the anterior segment (blue resin).

The possibilities of segmental arrangement are shown in Figs. 18.173 and 18.174.

After the endocasts were obtained, they were positioned horizontally, and their anterior and posterior sides were photographed (Fig. 18.175). A B-100 translucent Weibel grid 11 was placed over the photographs to evaluate the surface area of each segment by using the "point-counting planimetry method" (Fig. 18.175). The B-100 grid presents 100 points, and each point is the geometric center of a square (Fig. 18.175C). If a B-100 translucent grid is superimposed on a photograph of a cast, one may evaluate the number of points that correspond to one surface of the cast (Fig. 18.175D). Because individual segments are injected with different colors, it is also possible to evaluate the number of points that correspond to each segment. By performing this technique for both sides and adding the results, one may achieve an estimated evaluation concerning the proportional area that each arterial segment represents in the whole kidney.

Just the absolute values in percentage were used; that is, the number of points on each side of the cast (anterior and posterior) was evaluated. After adding these results, the number of points that represents the whole kidney (100.0%) was obtained. Afterward, the number of points for each segment on both sides was evaluated by using a single rule of three. The proportional area of each segment was determined.

For example: The whole kidney (anterior and posterior surfaces) corresponds to 85 points. The inferior segment (anterior and posterior surfaces) corresponds to 27 points.

Thus:

85 points (whole kidney) = 100.0%
27 points (inferior segment) = X

$$X = \frac{100 \times 27}{85} = 31.8\% \text{ (inferior segment)}$$

Findings. The bifurcation of the main renal artery into an anterior and a posterior branch was found in all cases of kidneys with a single artery. The anterior branch usually had greater caliber than the posterior branch.

In 61.2% of cases (30 of 49 casts), kidneys with five arterial segments (Fig. 18.176A and B) were found; in 38.8% of cases (19 of 49 casts), we found kidneys with four arterial segments (Fig. 18.176C and D).

Superior segment (apical). The superior segmental artery usually has an extrahilar origin. In 73.5% of cases (36 of 49 casts), this artery arose from the anterior division of the main renal artery and in 26.5% of the cases (13 of 49 casts) from its anterior division (posterior segmental artery). When the main artery to the apex of the kidney (superior segment) was a branch of the posterior segmental artery (retropelvic artery), we did not consider the superior segment as independent and it was included with the posterior segment. When the superior segment existed independently (Fig. 18.176), its area varied from 1.84% to 27.02% of the total kidney area (mean: 13.02%).

Anterosuperior segment. In 61.2% of cases (30 of 49 casts), an anterosuperior segment (Fig. 18.176A and B) was found. Its area varied from 5.17% to 34.22% of the total kidney area (mean: 21.36%).

Anteroinferior segment. The anteroinferior segment (Fig. 18.176A and B) was also found in 61.2% of cases (30 of 49 casts), and its area varied from 1.29% to 25.8% of the total kidney area (mean 17.18%).

Anterior segment. In 38.8% of cases (19 of 49 casts), there was only one segmental artery to the mid-kidney, the anterosuperior and the anteroinferior segments being fused as the anterior segment (Fig. 18.176C and D). When the anterior segment existed, its area varied from 16.57% to 42.95% of the total kidney area (mean: 28.44%).

Inferior segment. The inferior segment was found in 100.0% of the cases (Fig. 18.176). Its area varied from 7.42% to 38.18% of the total kidney area (mean: 22.65%).

Posterior segment. Just as with the inferior segment, the posterior segment was found in 100.0% of the specimens studied (Fig. 18.177). Its area varied from 14.57% to 52.93% of the total kidney area (mean: 33.76%).

The posterior segment, supplied by the posterior segmental artery (called retropelvic artery), presented the greatest median value of proportional area (33.76%) and also the greatest maximum value of proportional area, consisting of up to 52.93% of the total kidney area (Fig. 18.177B). This knowledge is important because it demonstrates the significance of the posterior segmental artery.

Capsular and Perirenal Collateral Circulation

The renal capsular arterial system is composed of three basic pathways: superior, medial, and inferior capsular arteries (Figs. 18.178 and 18.179). These vessels usually arise from or together with the adrenal arteries. The system may also originate from the main renal artery or from the gonadal artery.

The superior capsular artery usually arises from the inferior adrenal artery, or from the main renal artery or a branch. It may also originate from the inferior phrenic artery, from the aorta or a superior polar artery.

The middle capsular artery arises from the renal artery or its main branches at the renal hilum.

The inferior capsular artery is uncommonly observed, but usually arises from the gonadal artery or from an inferior polar artery.

There is a number of perforating capsular arteries arising from arcuate and interlobular arteries, connecting the intrarenal circulation with the larger capsular arteries. The perforating capsular arteries are usually small and enlarge only when advanced nephropathy or arterial occlusion is encountered.

The pelvic arteries are small and difficult to observe either angiographically or at dissection. When there is renal artery occlusive disease, they may enlarge and may be observed as tortuous small vessels. The ureteric and pelvicoureteric arteries are also small and originate from the main renal artery (or its main branches), or from the gonadal artery.

Testicular and Ovarian Artery

The testicular and ovarian arteries arise anterolaterally from the abdominal aorta, a few centimeters below the renal arteries in 80% to 90% of the population (Fig. 18.1). The ovarian or testicular arteries follow a descending path, anterior to the inferior vena cava and parallel to the gonadal vein, anteriorly to the ureter in the right side, and posterior to the left gonadal vein at the beginning, but anterior to the left ureter (Figs. 18.178 and 18.180). The gonadal artery may arise from an inferior polar renal artery (Fig. 18.181) and may send branches to the ureter. Rarely the ovarian or testicular arteries arise from lumbar, adrenal, or iliac arteries. Both testicular arteries pass the deep inguinal ring to enter the spermatic cord, traversing the inguinal canal into the scrotum. At the posterosuperior aspect of the testis, two branches are found on its medial and lateral surfaces, which form the tunica vasculosa after ramifying (Fig. 18.182). The ureter, the perirenal fat and iliac lymph nodes, and the cremaster muscle are arterialized by the testicular artery. The ovarian arteries correspond to the testicular arteries, but follow a different path in the pelvis, to supply the ovaries, reaching the uterine broad ligament. Some branches of the gonadal artery supply the ureters, the uterine tubes, and have anastomoses with the uterine artery. The ovaries are supplied by ovarian arteries in 40% of the cases, by both uterine and ovarian arteries in 56% of cases, and by uterine arteries alone in about 4% of the cases.

Dorsal Branches of the Aorta

Lumbar Arteries

There are usually four lumbar arteries in each side, arising from the posterior aspect of the abdominal aorta. A smaller fifth pair of lumbar arteries may arise from the middle sacral artery, but lumbar branches of the iliolumbar arteries are usually in their place. These arteries follow a posterior path over the lumbar vertebral bodies, continuing in the posterior abdominal wall (Fig. 18.1). They anastomose with one another (Fig. 18.183) and with the lower posterior intercostal, subcostal, iliolumbar, deep circumflex iliac, and inferior epigastric arteries (Figs. 18.184-18.186).

Branches

Dorsal ramus
Spinal branches
Muscular branches

The dorsal ramus of the lumbar arteries supplies the dorsal muscles, joints, and skin (Figs. 18.184 and 18.185).

The spinal branches of the dorsal ramus enter the spinal canal to supply its structures and adjacent vertebra. They anastomose with arteries from above and from below, crossing the midline. The spinal branch of the first lumbar artery supplies the terminal spinal cord, and the others the cauda equina, meninges, and the vertebral canal.

Muscular branches of the dorsal rami supply the adjacent muscles, fascia, bones, red marrow, ligaments, and joints (Fig. 18.186).

Median Sacral Artery

This is a small posterior branch of the abdominal aorta, arising from the aorta above its bifurcation that descends in the middle line, anterior to the fourth and fifth lumbar vertebra, sacrum, and coccyx. There are anastomoses with the rectum, lumbar branches of the iliolumbar artery, and the lateral sacral arteries (Fig. 18.185).

Terminal Branches

Common Iliac Arteries

The abdominal aorta bifurcates at the level of the fourth lumbar vertebra, into two arteries, called right and left common iliac arteries, which supply the pelvis and lower extremities. The common iliac arteries divide into the external iliac artery, which courses parallel to the axis of the common iliac artery, and the internal iliac artery, which is a posteromedial branch.

In addition to the terminal branches, the common iliac arteries give branches to the surrounding tissues, peritoneum, psoas muscle, ureter, and nerves. Occasional branches are the iliolumbar and accessory renal arteries for topic or ectopic kidneys.

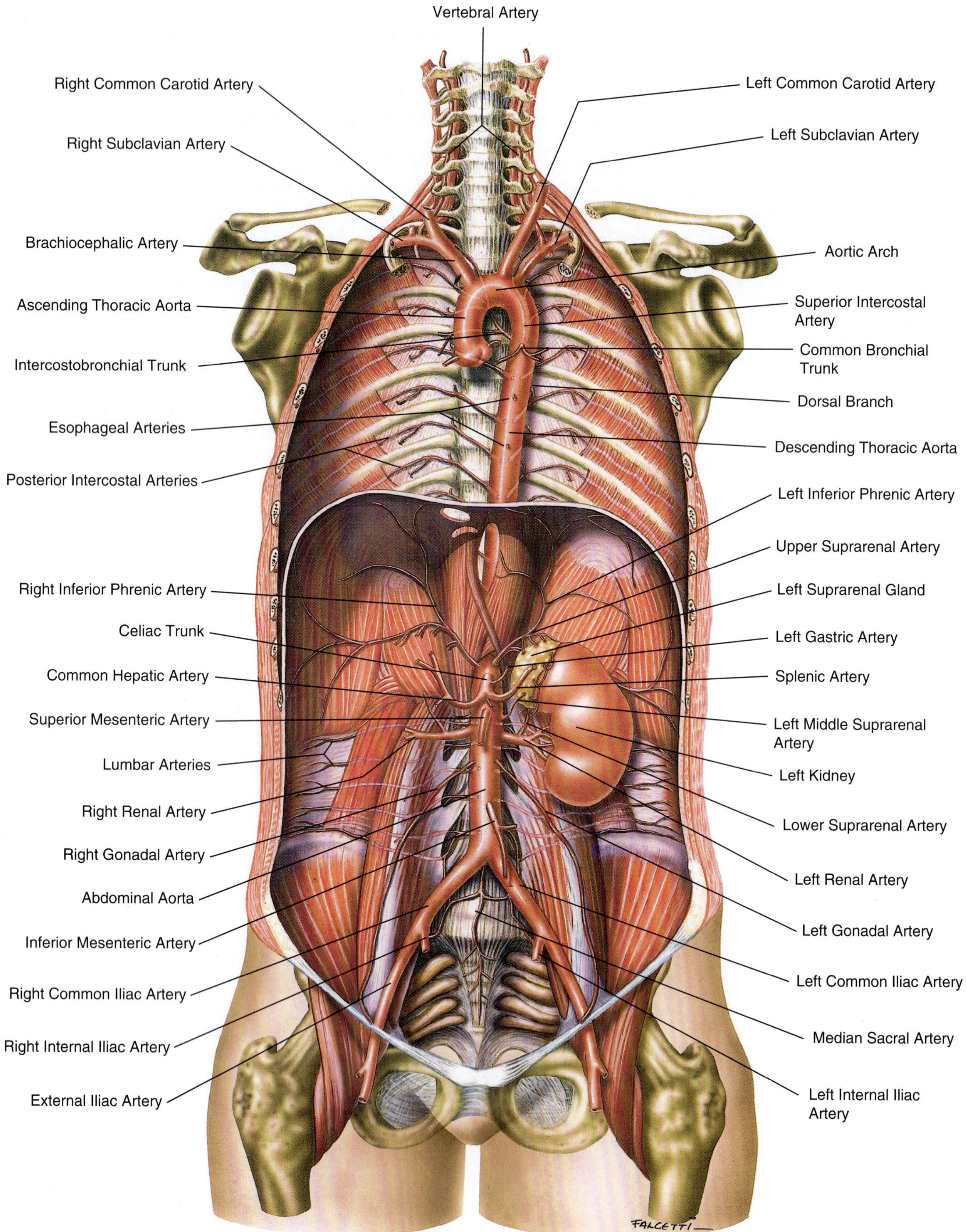

Figure 18.1. Schematic drawing of the thoracic and abdominal aorta and branches.

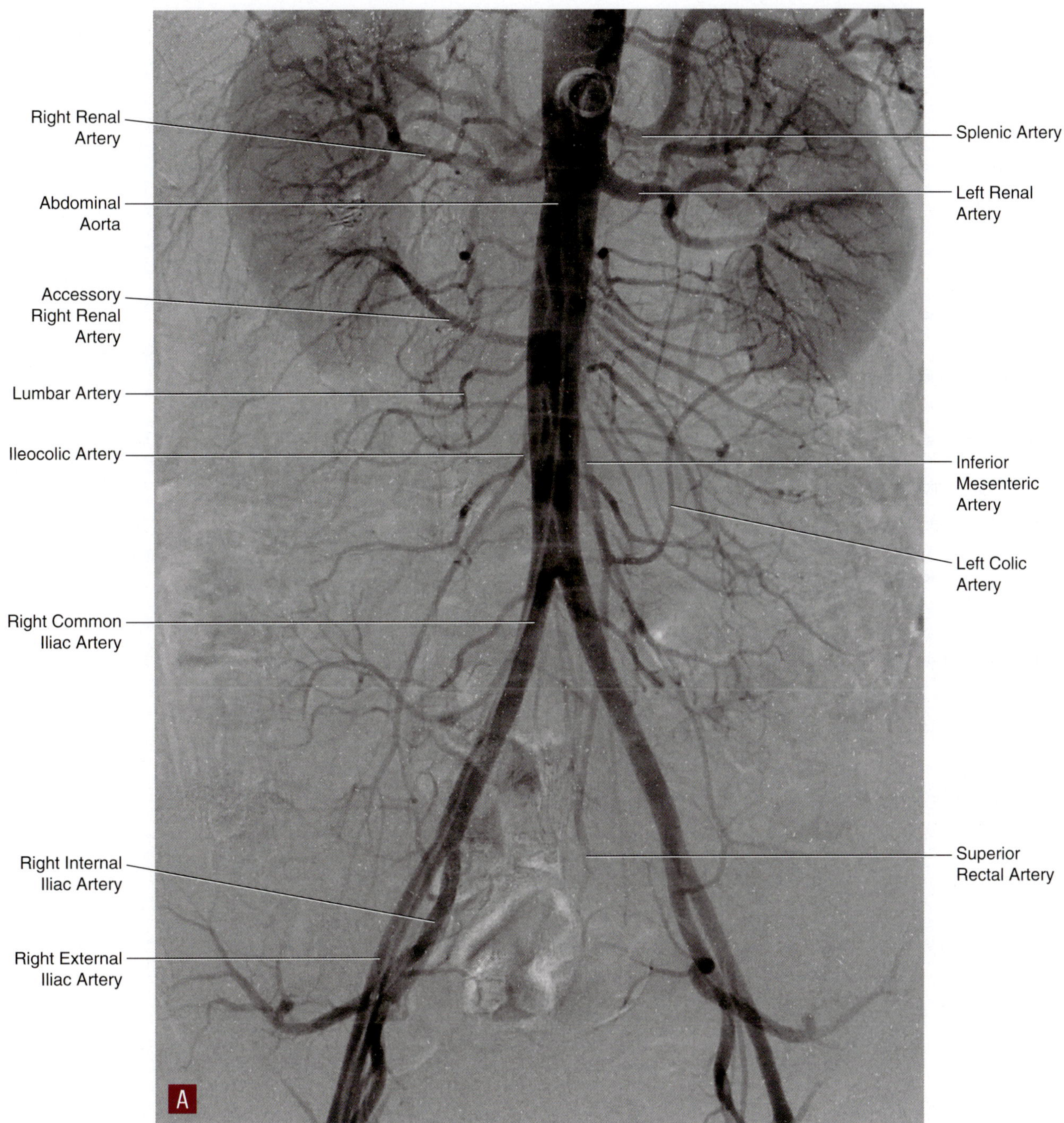

Figure 18.2. A, Angiography of the thoracoabdominal aorta and the main branches. B, Cinematic reconstruction of the abdominal aorta and main branches.

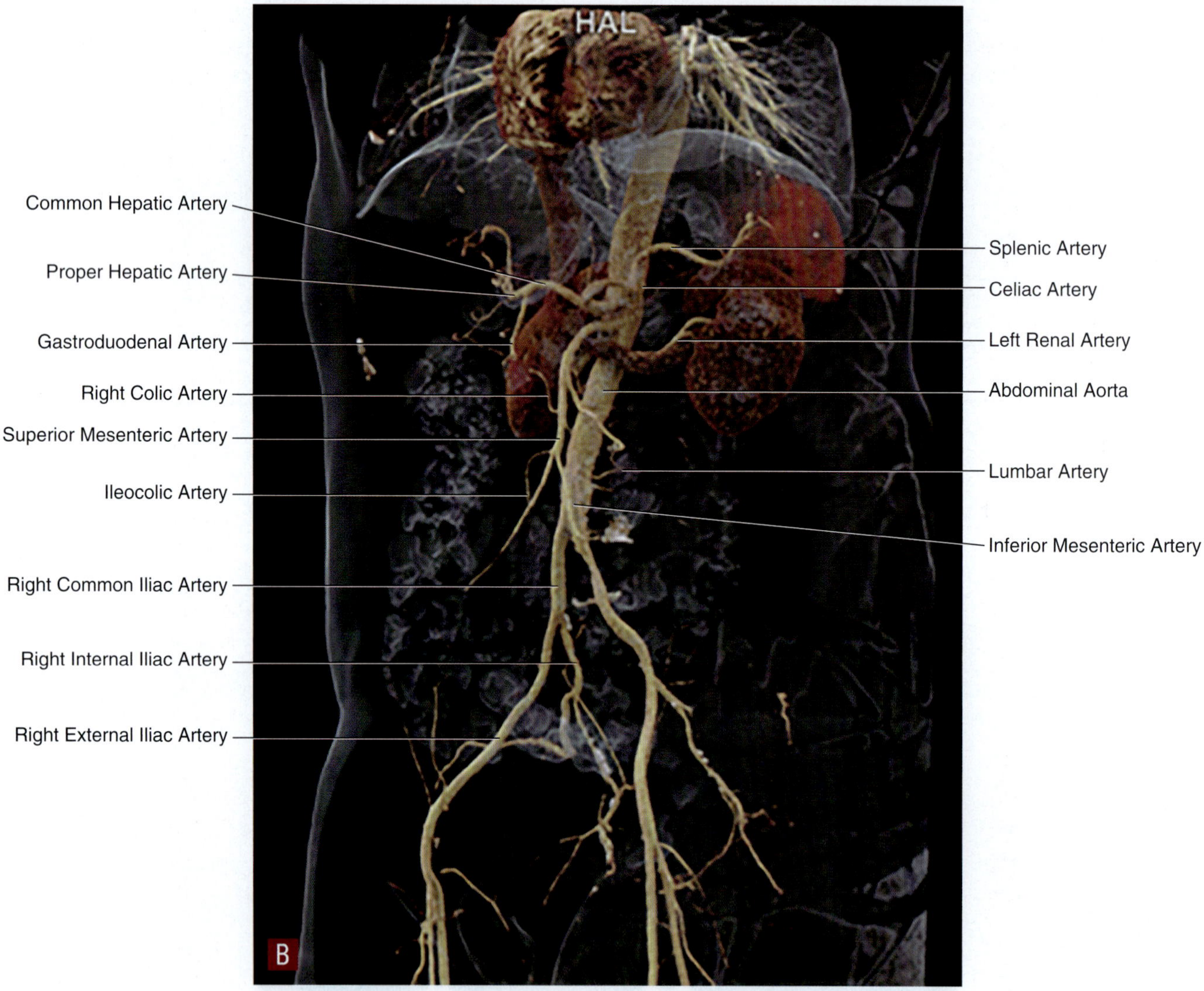

Figure 18.2. *Continued*

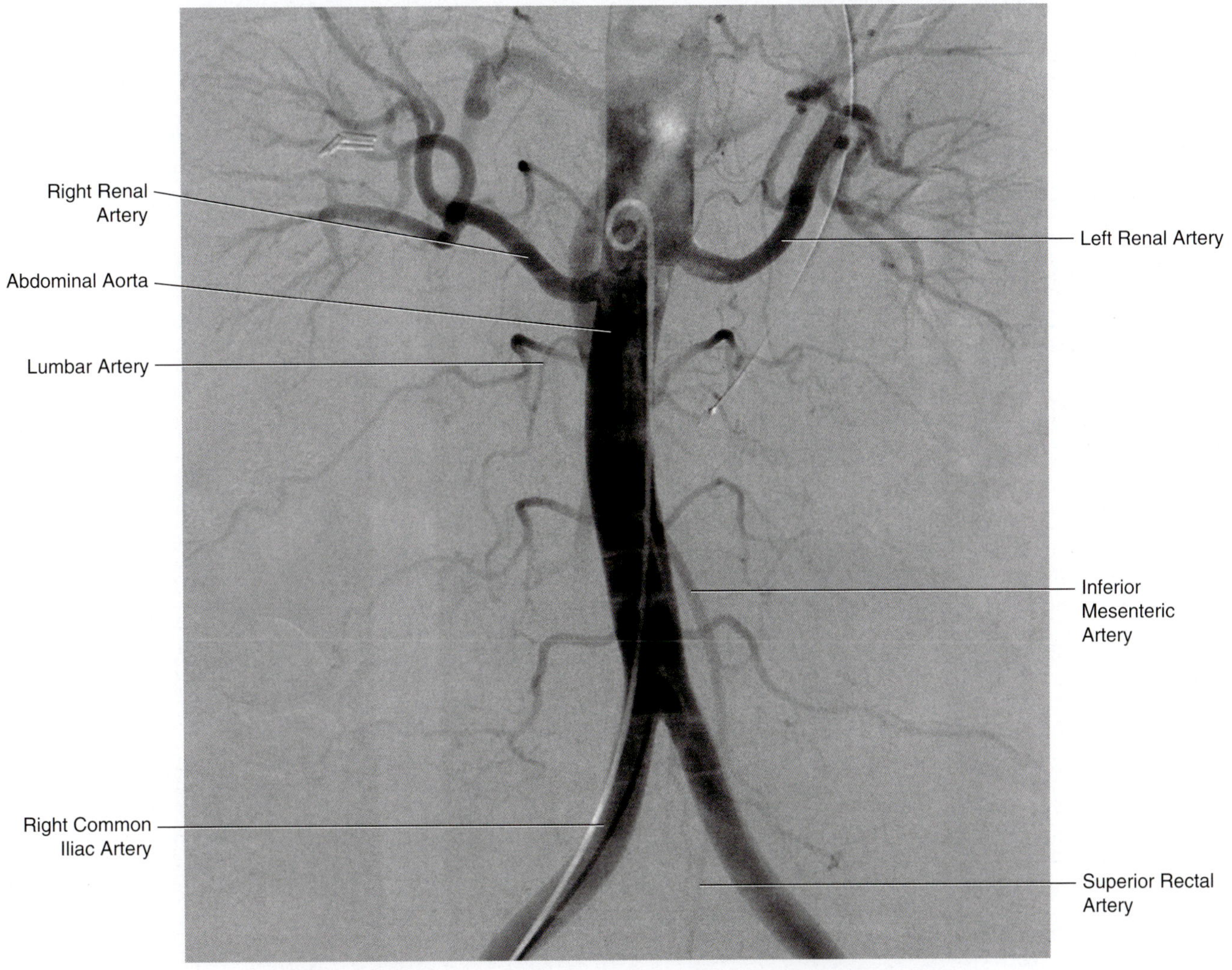

Figure 18.3. Angiography of the abdominal aorta and main branches.

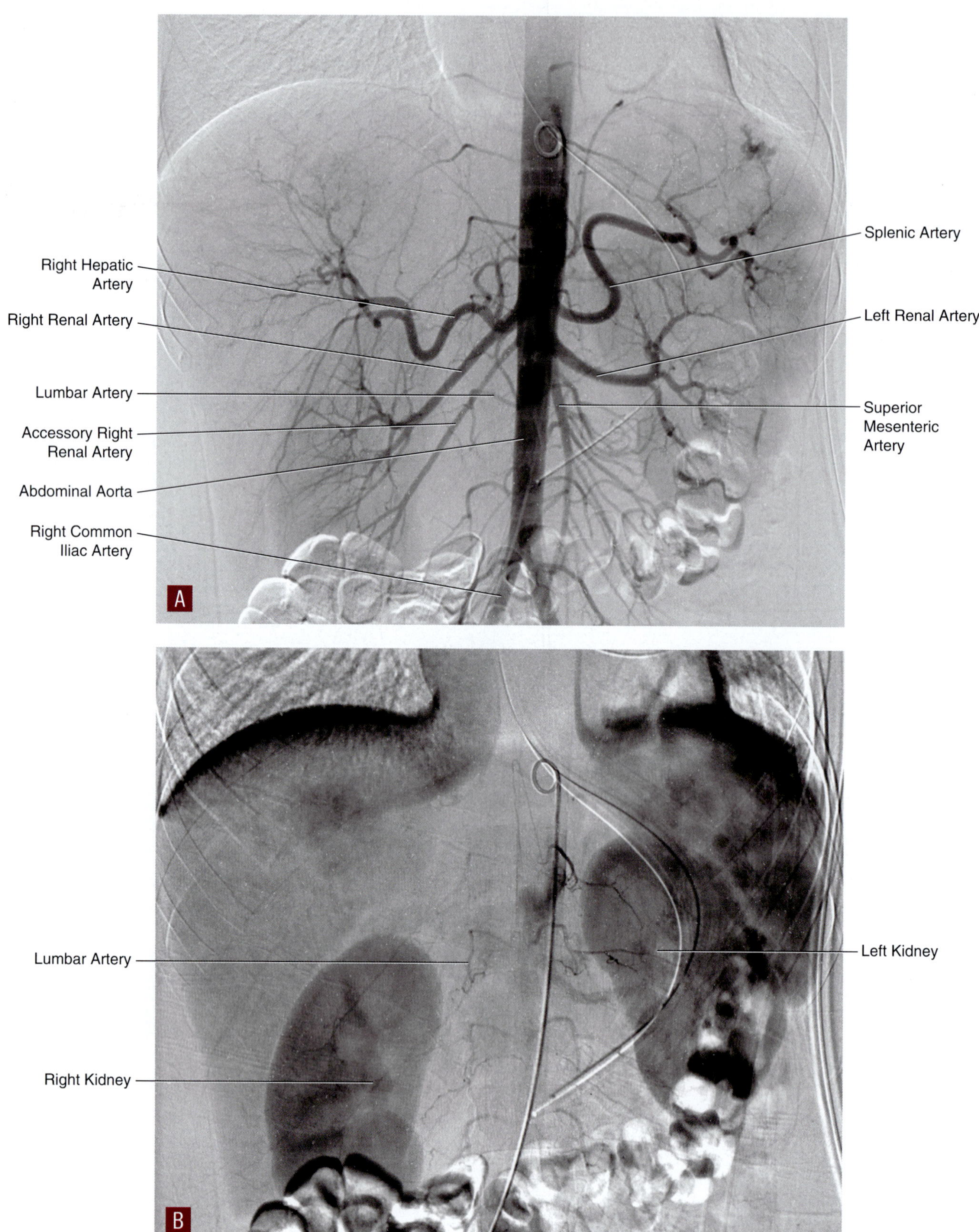

Figure 18.4. **A**, Angiography of the abdominal aorta on digital subtraction. Note the relationship of the renal arteries and the origin of the celiac trunk and SMA. **B**, Late phase of the aortography showing bilateral nephrogram.

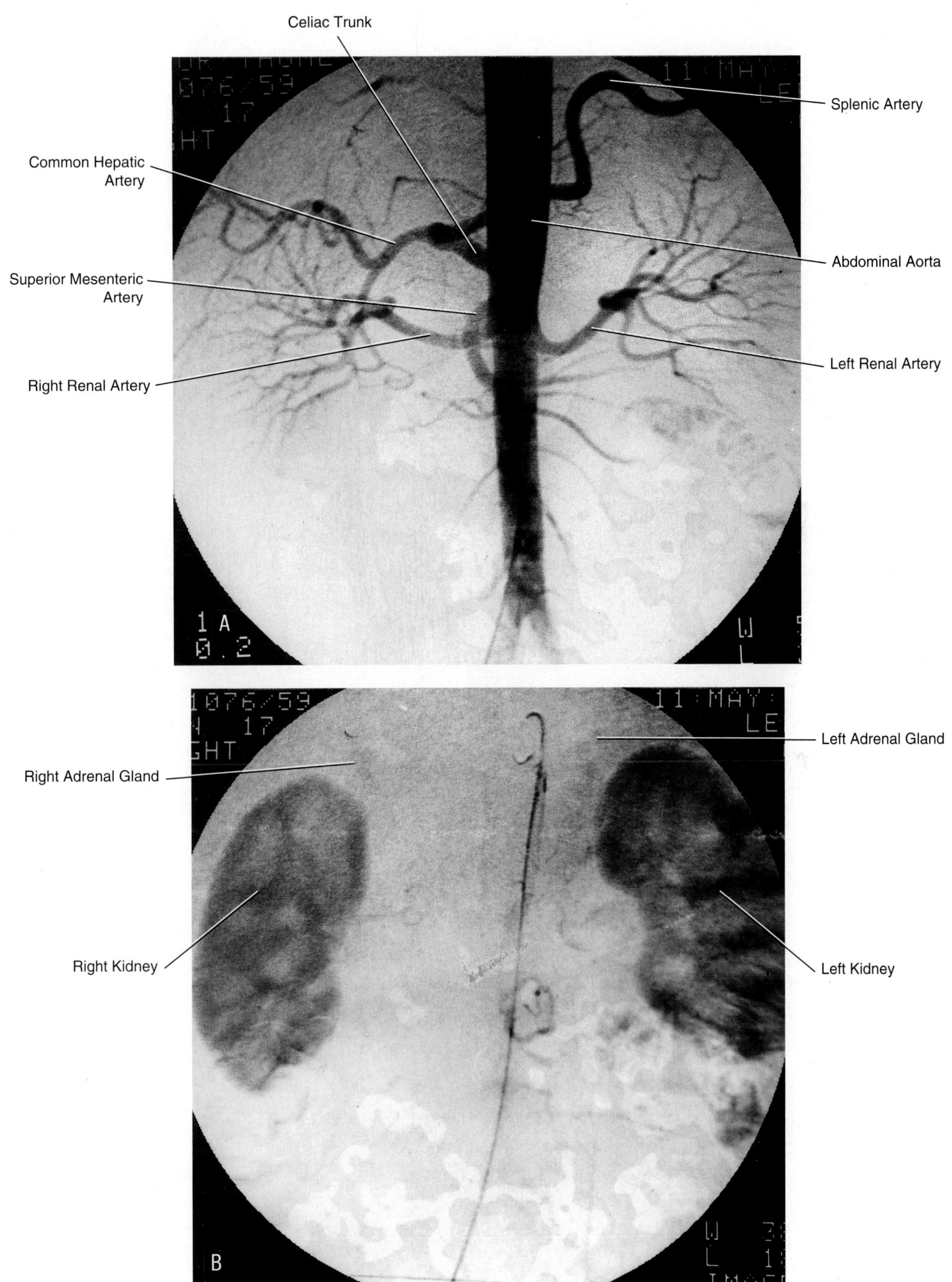

Figure 18.5. A, Abdominal aortography on digital subtraction. B, Late phase aortography showing the bilateral nephrogram.

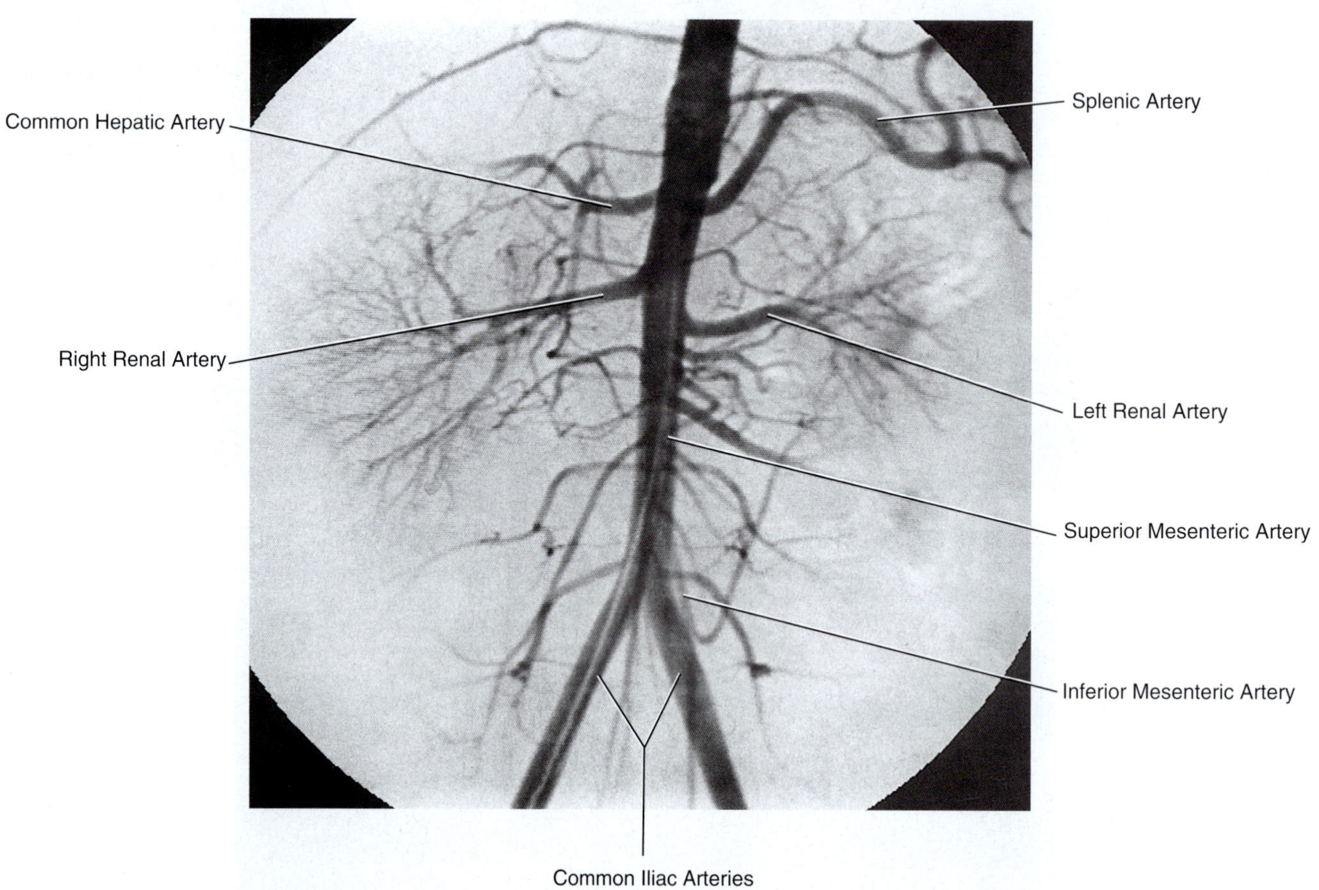

Figure 18.6. **Abdominal aortography.**

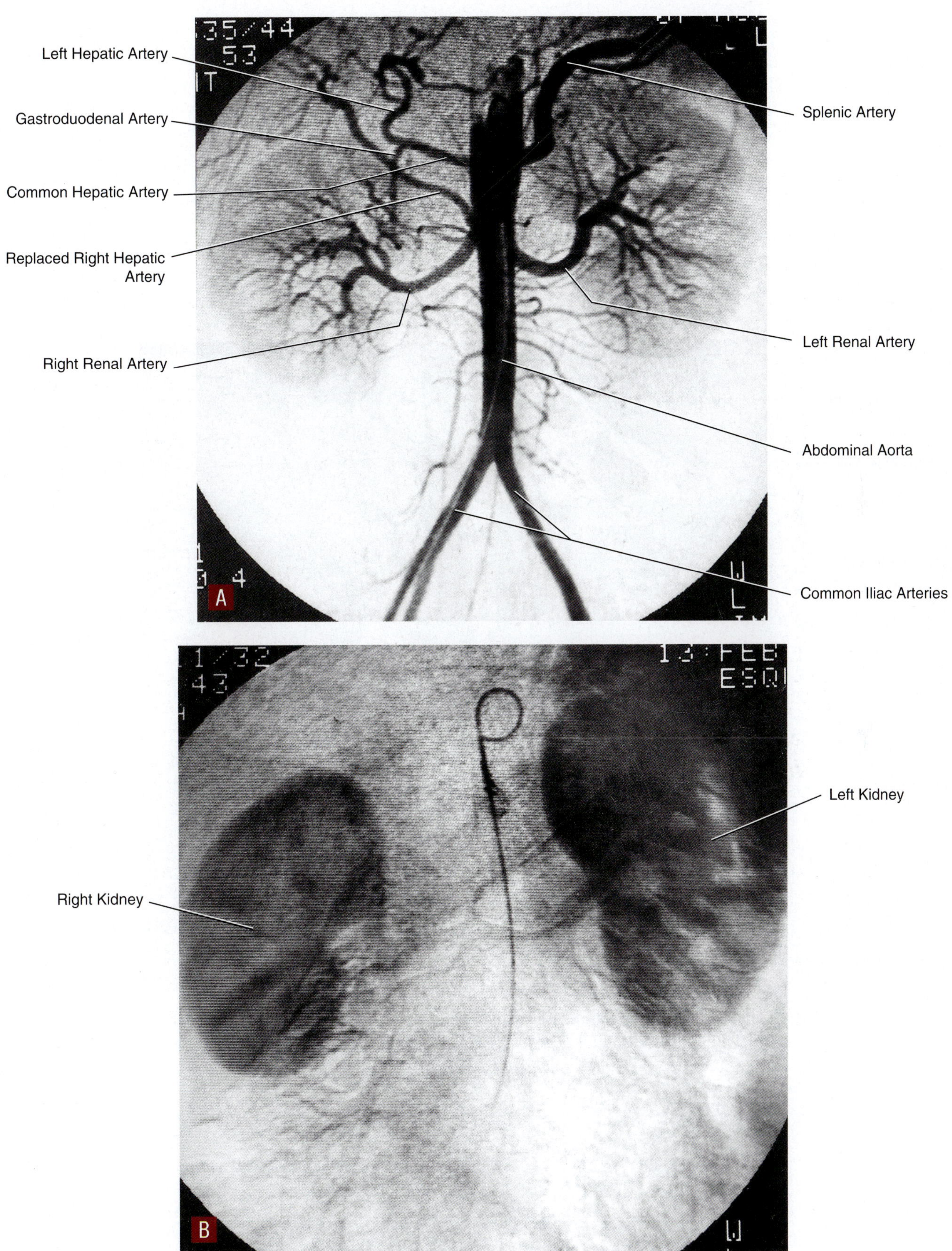

Figure 18.7. **A**, Abdominal aortography. **B**, Late phase showing the bilateral nephrogram.

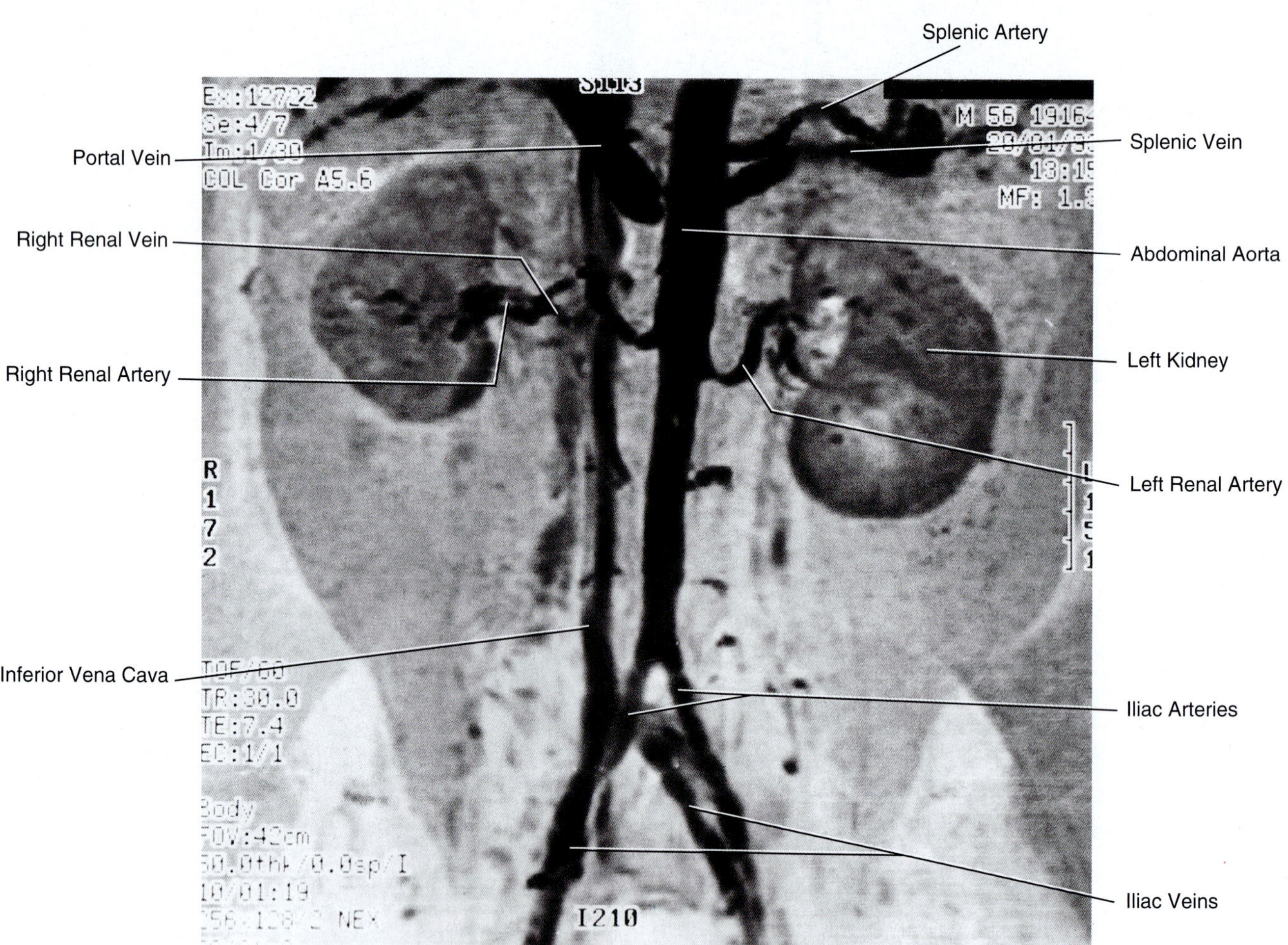

Figure 18.8. Magnetic resonance imaging showing the abdominal aorta, the inferior vena cava (partially), and the portal and splenic veins.

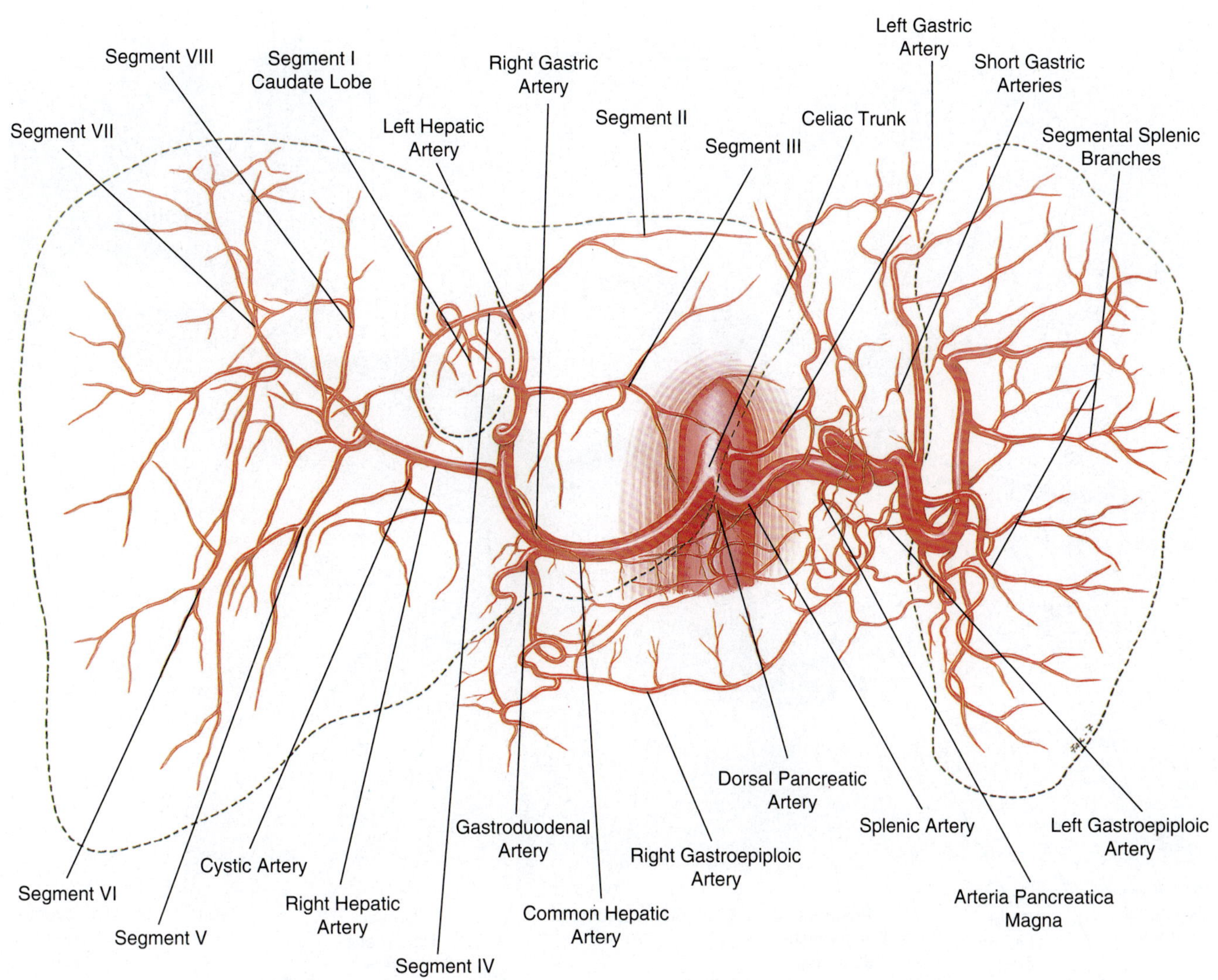

Figure 18.9. Schematic drawing of the celiac trunk, showing the hepatic arteries, segments (Couinaud), and the gastric and splenic circulation. Based on a real angiogram.

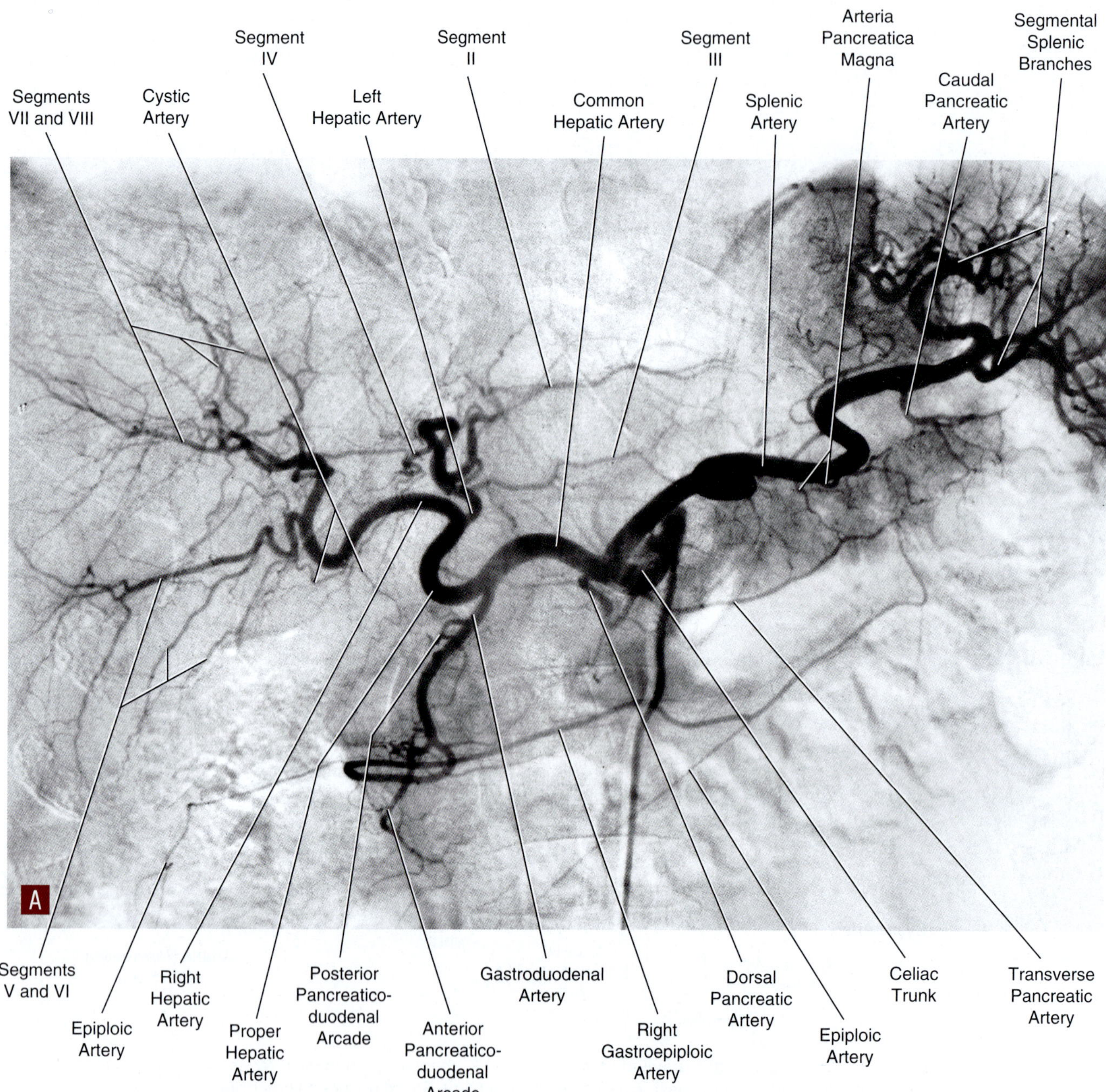

Figure 18.10. A, Selective angiogram of the celiac trunk, showing the hepatic circulation, and the gastric, pancreatic, and splenic circulation. The pattern presented here is the most common and present in about 40% to 50% of the population. B, Late phase of the angiogram showing the splenic and portal veins, as well as the splenic blush and the hepatic blush.

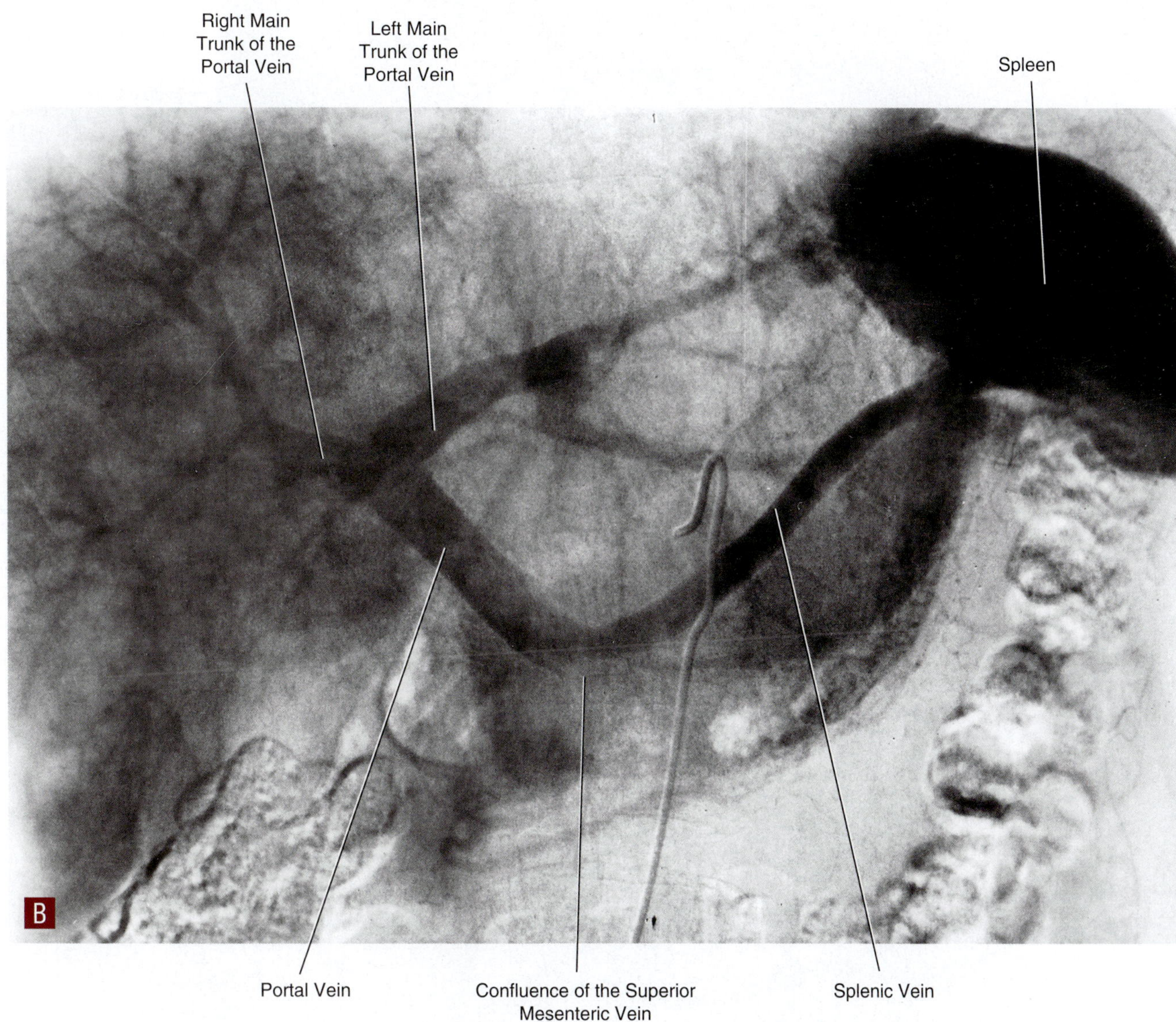

Figure 18.10. *Continued*

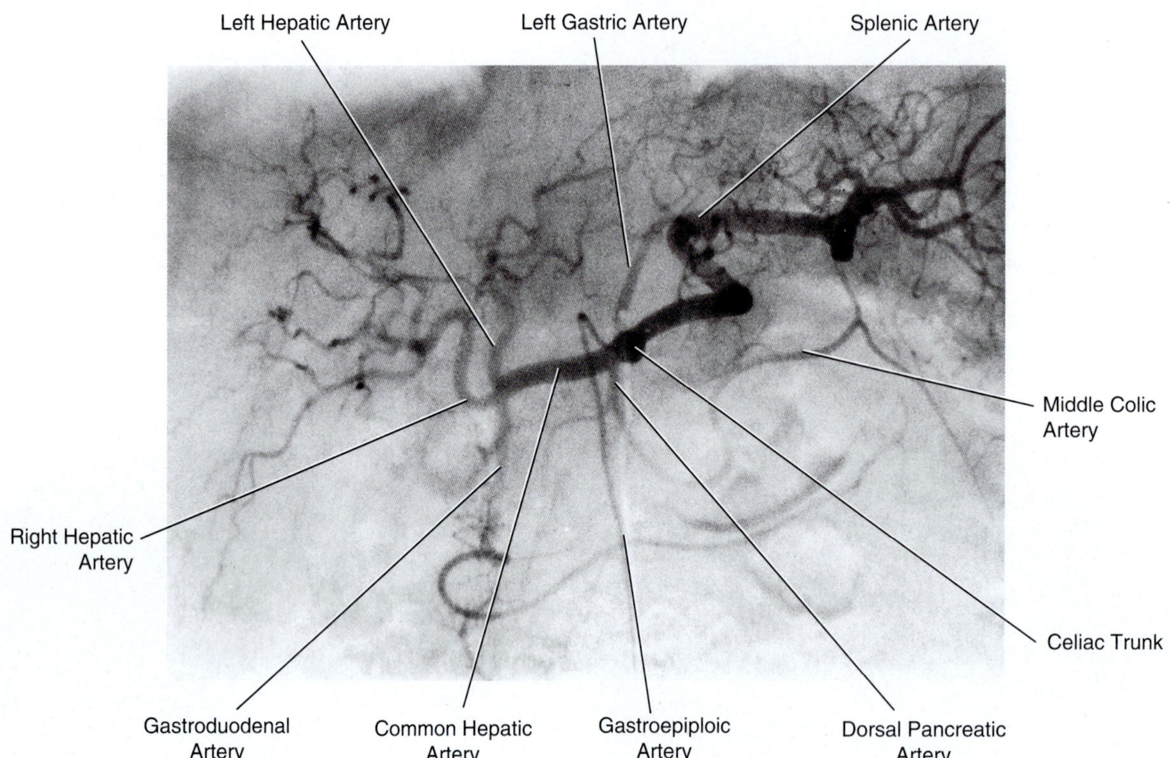

Figure 18.11. Selective angiogram of the celiac trunk, showing absence of the proper hepatic artery due to the trifurcation of the common hepatic artery into the right and left hepatic arteries and the gastroduodenal artery. Note that the dorsal pancreatic artery gives rise to the middle colic artery.

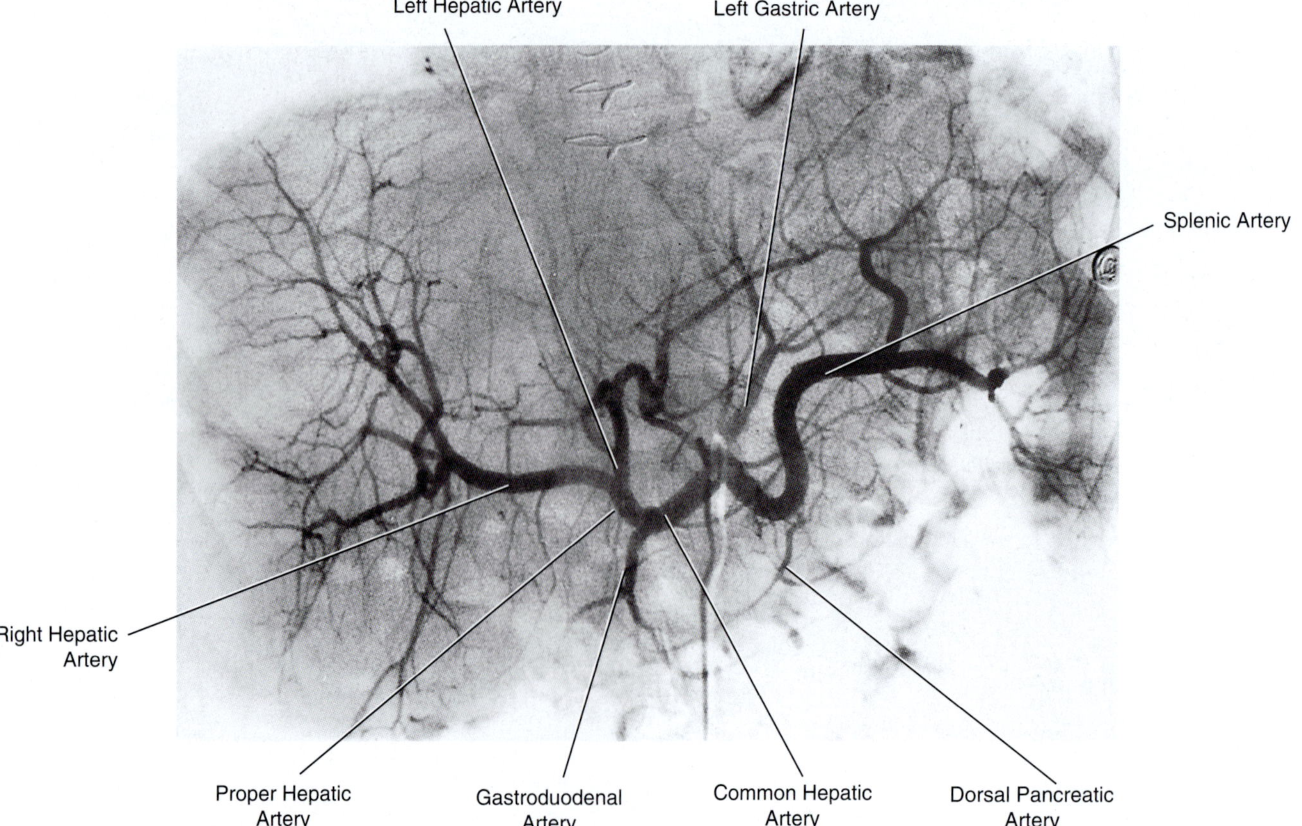

Figure 18.12. Selective angiogram of the celiac trunk, showing normal distribution of the hepatic and splenic arteries. This is an example of a horizontal celiac trunk.

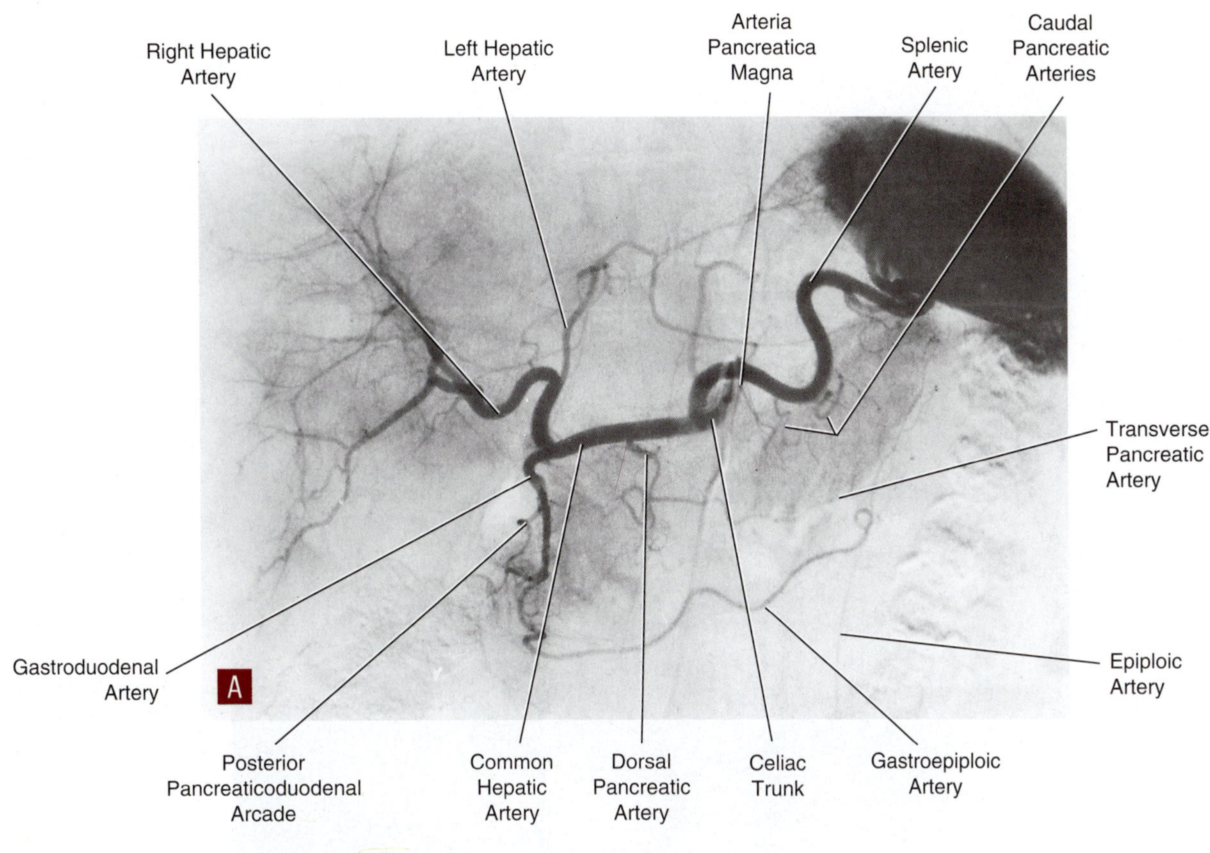

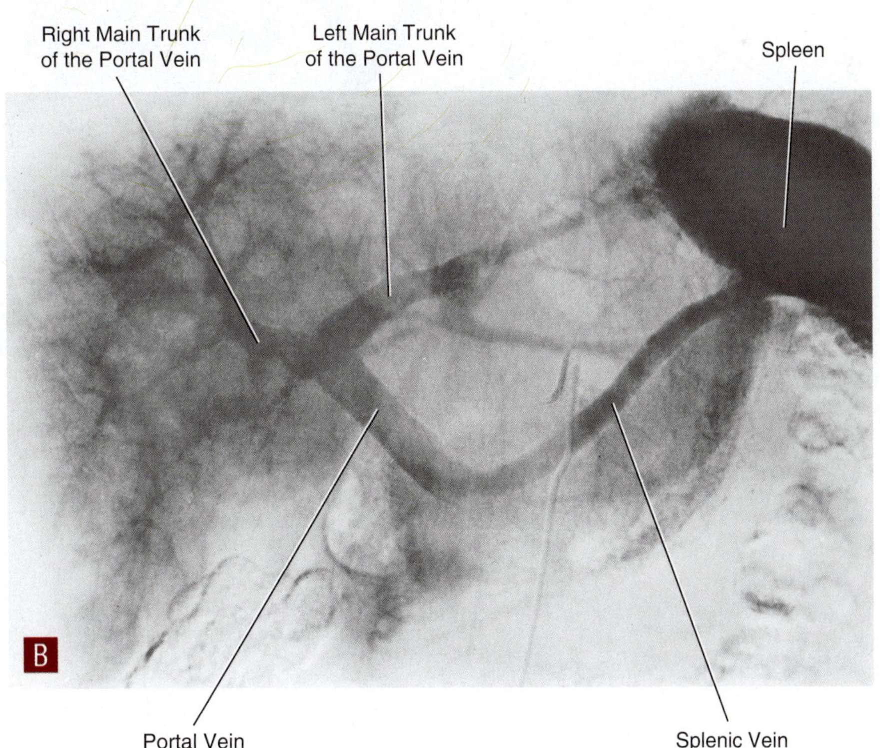

Figure 18.13. A, Selective angiogram of the celiac trunk, showing normal distribution of the arteries. The celiac artery is caudally oriented. B, Normal splenic and portal veins.

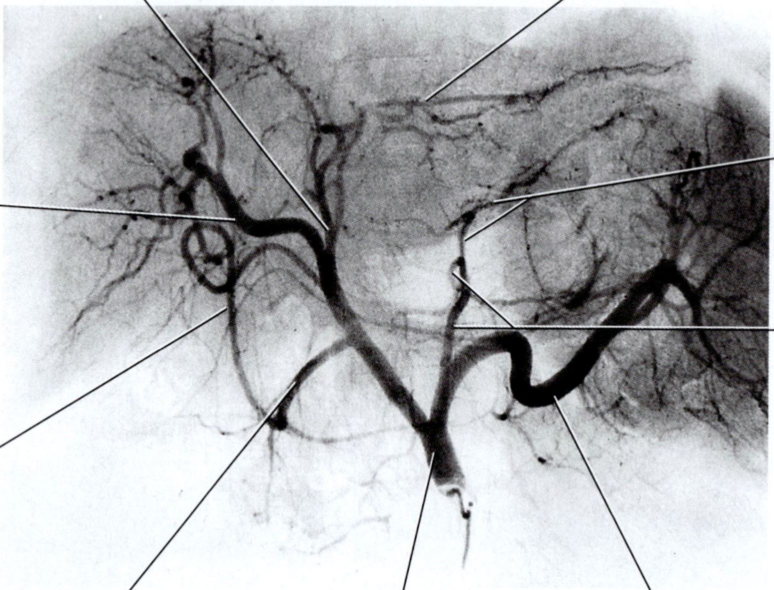

Figure 18.14. Selective angiogram of the celiac trunk, showing a cranial orientation. The distribution of the arteries is of the most common pattern.

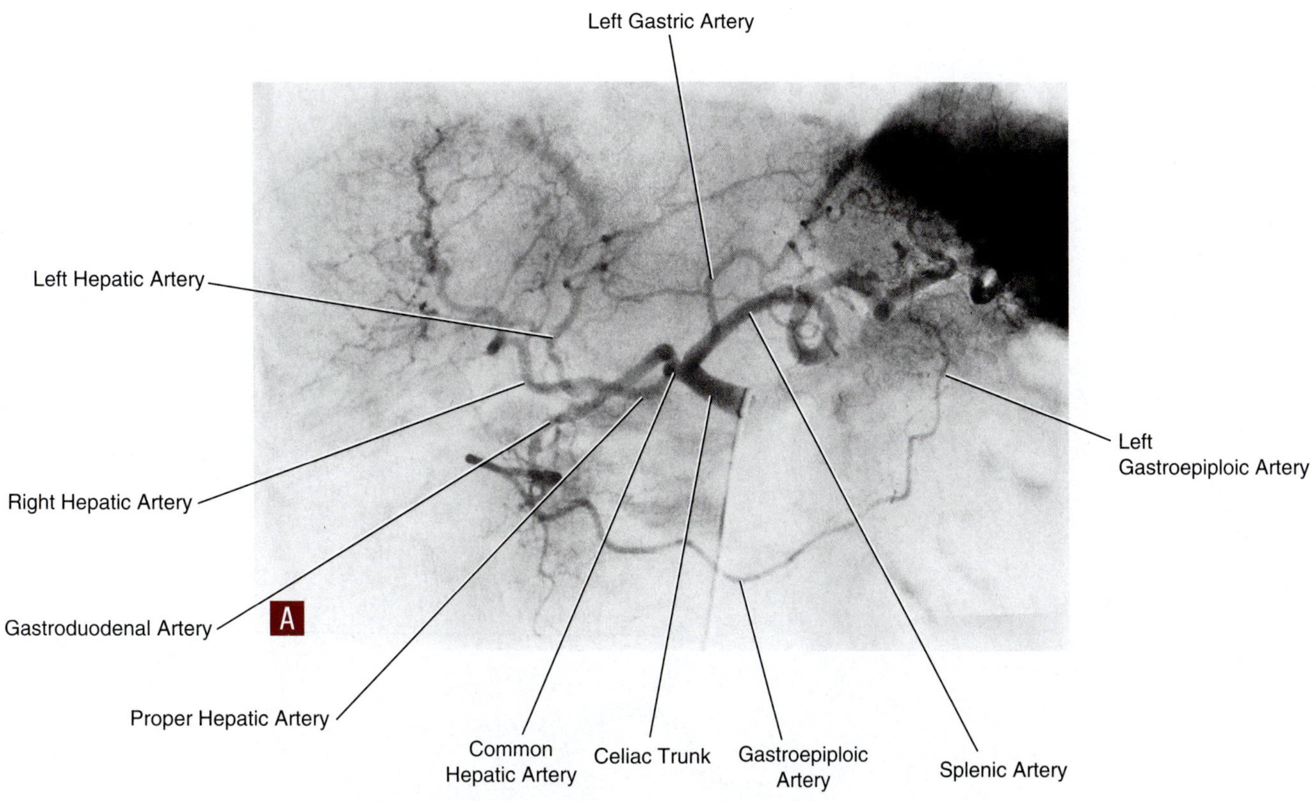

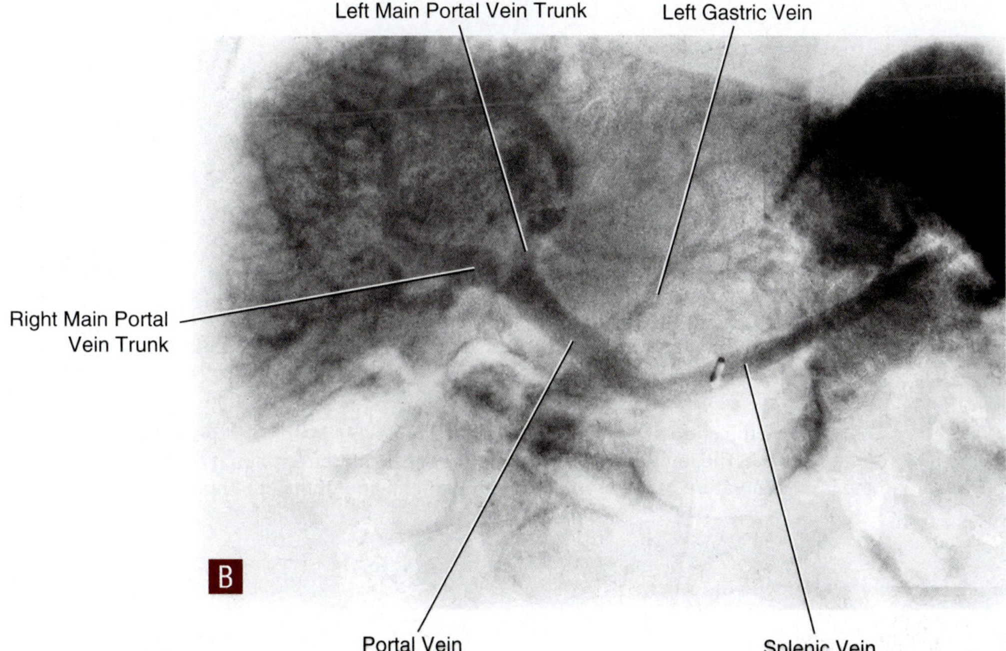

Figure 18.15. A, Angiogram of the celiac trunk, showing absence of the common hepatic artery. The gastroduodenal artery arises directly from the bifurcation of the celiac trunk. The proper hepatic artery divides into the right and left hepatic arteries. B, Late phase of the angiogram showing the normal splenic and hepatic veins.

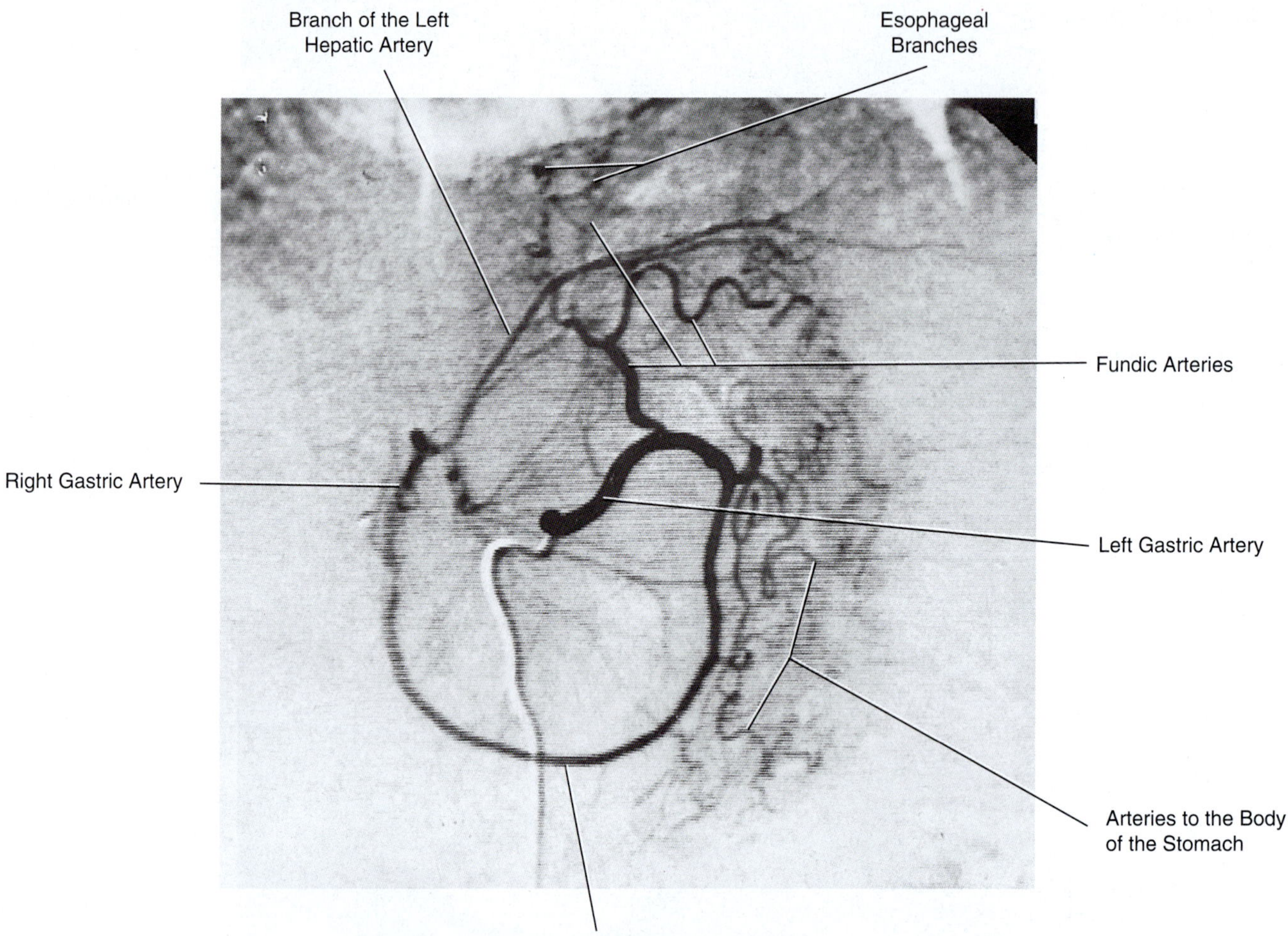

Figure 18.16. Selective injection at the left gastric artery. Note the gastric arteries at the fundus and body of the stomach. The left gastric artery anastomoses with the left hepatic artery and courses along the lesser curvature of the stomach. Note partial filling of the left hepatic artery.

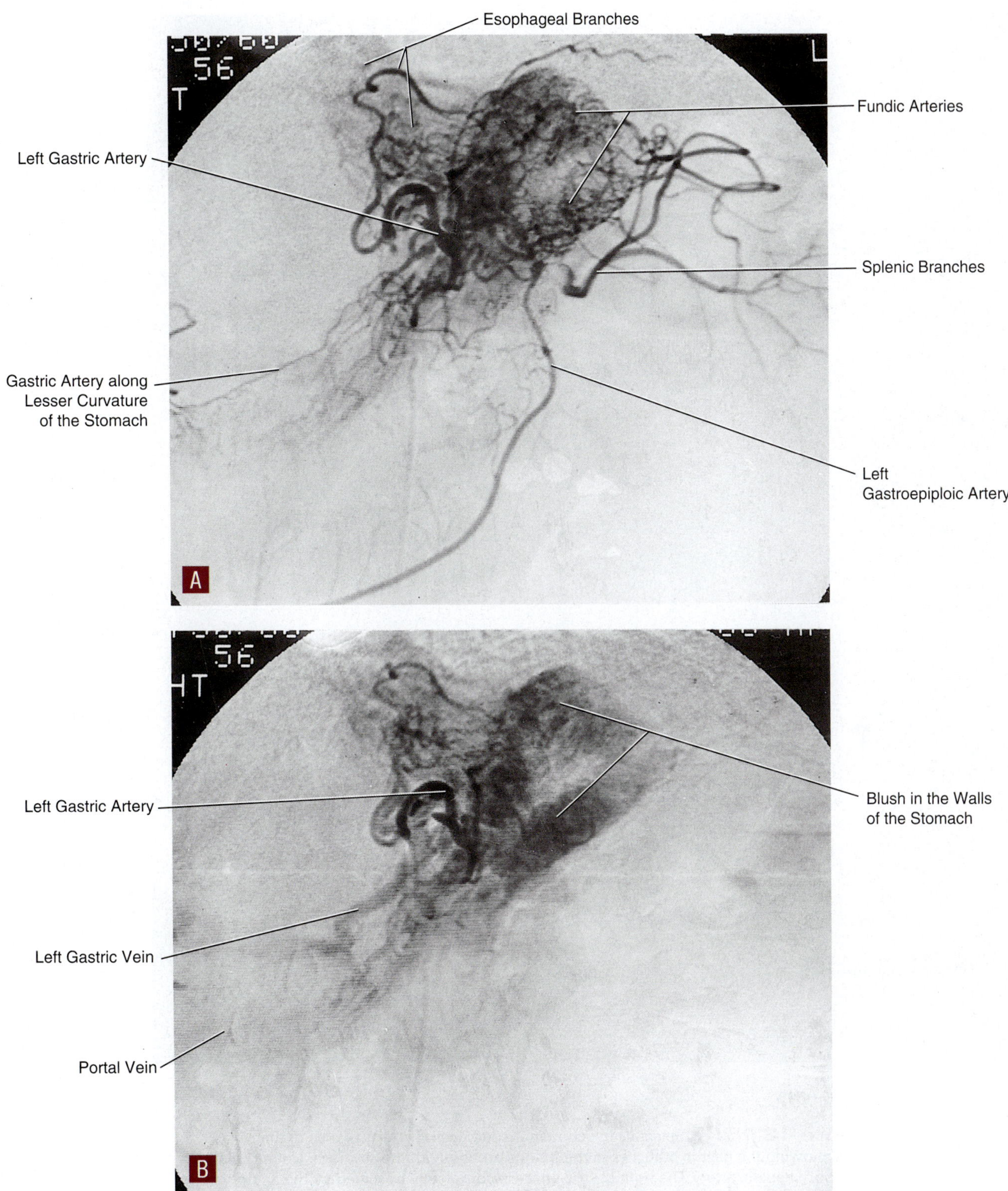

Figure 18.17. A, Selective angiography of the left gastric artery. Note the filling of the arteries of the fundus of the stomach and the anastomoses with the splenic arteries, as well as filling of the left gastroepiploic artery. B, Later phase of the left gastric artery injection, showing blush at the gastric wall and filling of the drainage veins, especially the left gastric vein.

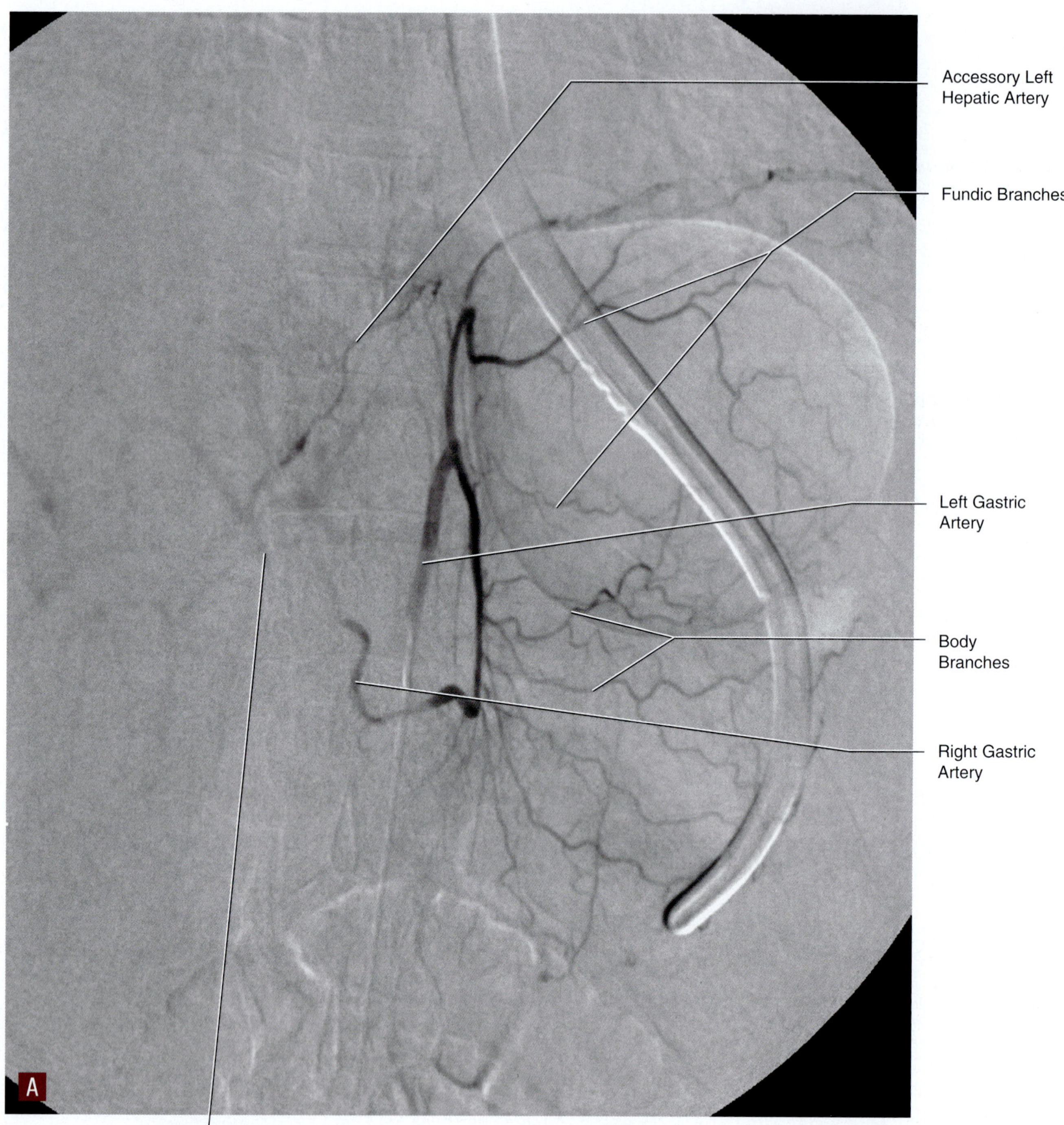

Figure 18.18. **A**, Selective injection in the left gastric artery, branch of the celiac trunk showing the gastric branches in the fundus and body of the stomach. Note a small left accessory hepatic artery. The right gastric artery is completely opacified by the angiographic injection and the anastomosis with the hepatic artery is visible. The gastric branches of the right hepatic artery are smaller than the fundic and body branches. There is a Blakemore tube with the gastric balloon inflated. **B**, Late phase of the left gastric artery angiography showing the venous return of the fundic and body veins draining into the left gastric vein and into the portal vein (faintly opacified). There is also filling of distal esophageal veins with a varicose aspect.

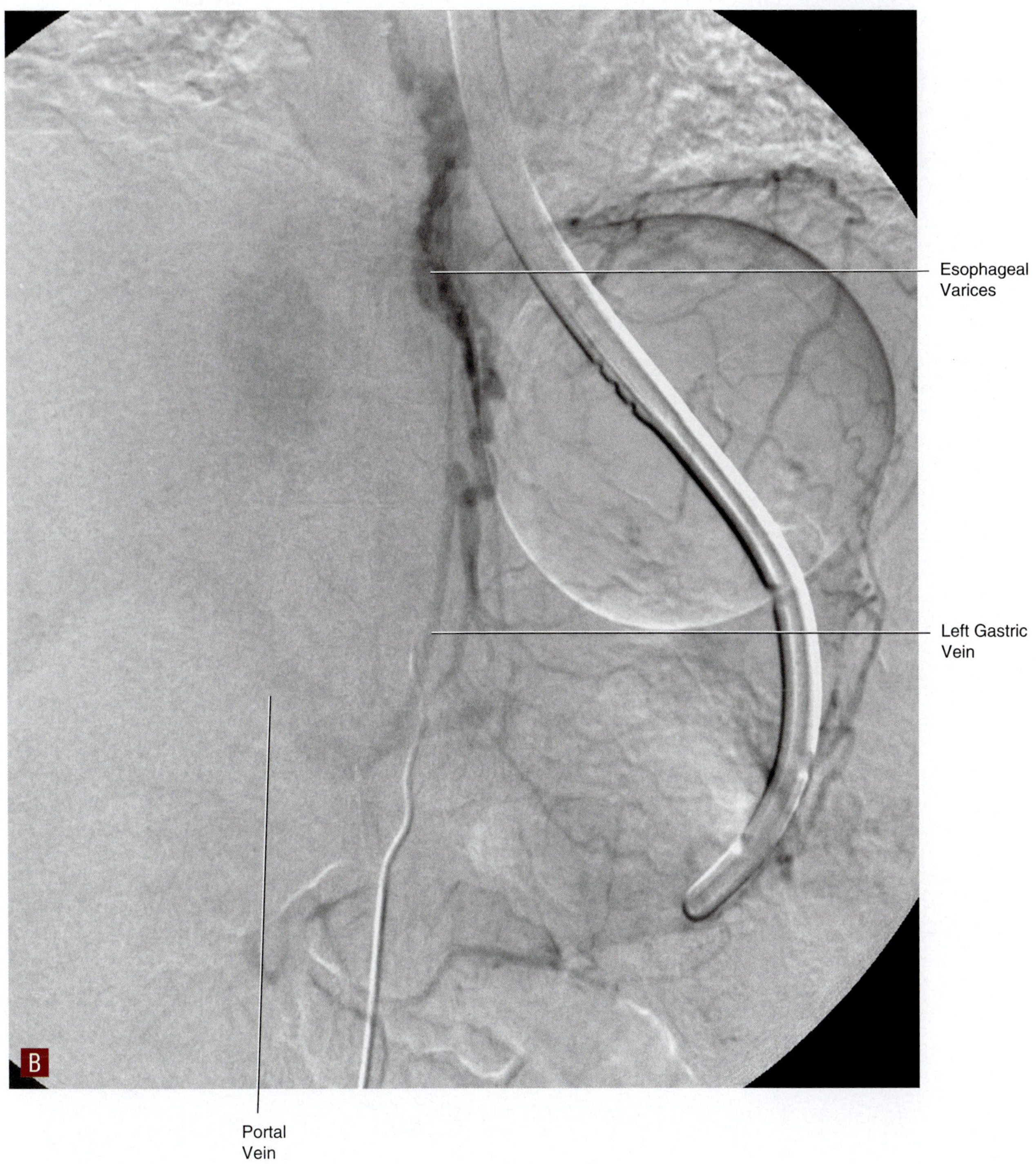

Figure 18.18. *Continued*

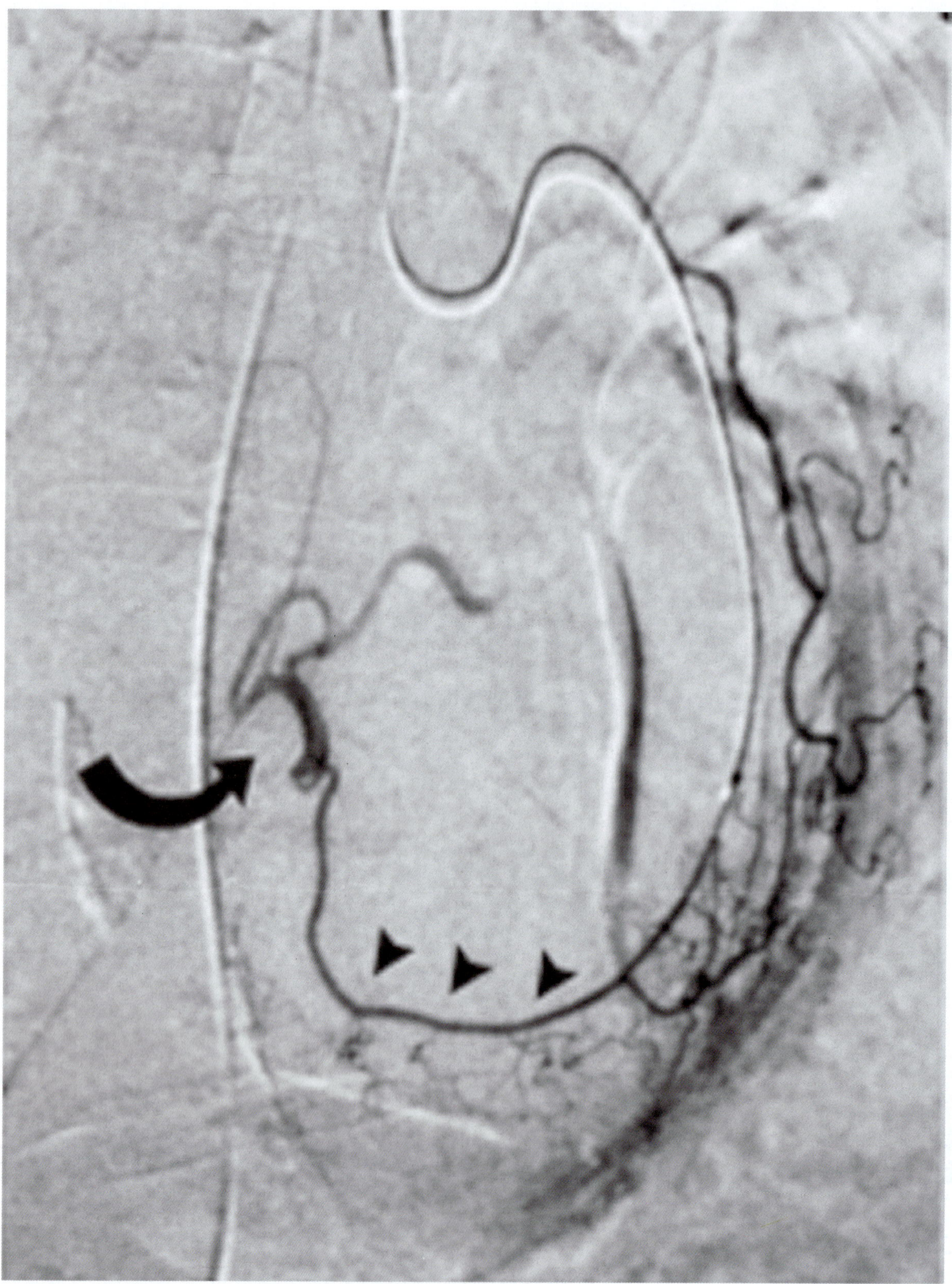

Figure 18.19. Left and right gastric artery arcade, opacified by superselective catheterization and angiography of the left gastric artery. The right gastric artery is densely opacified (arrow heads) and connects with the left hepatic artery (curved arrow). (Reprinted from Liu DM, et al. Angiographic considerations in patients undergoing liver-direct therapy. *J Vasc Interv Radiol.* 2005;16:911-935 with permission from Elsevier.)

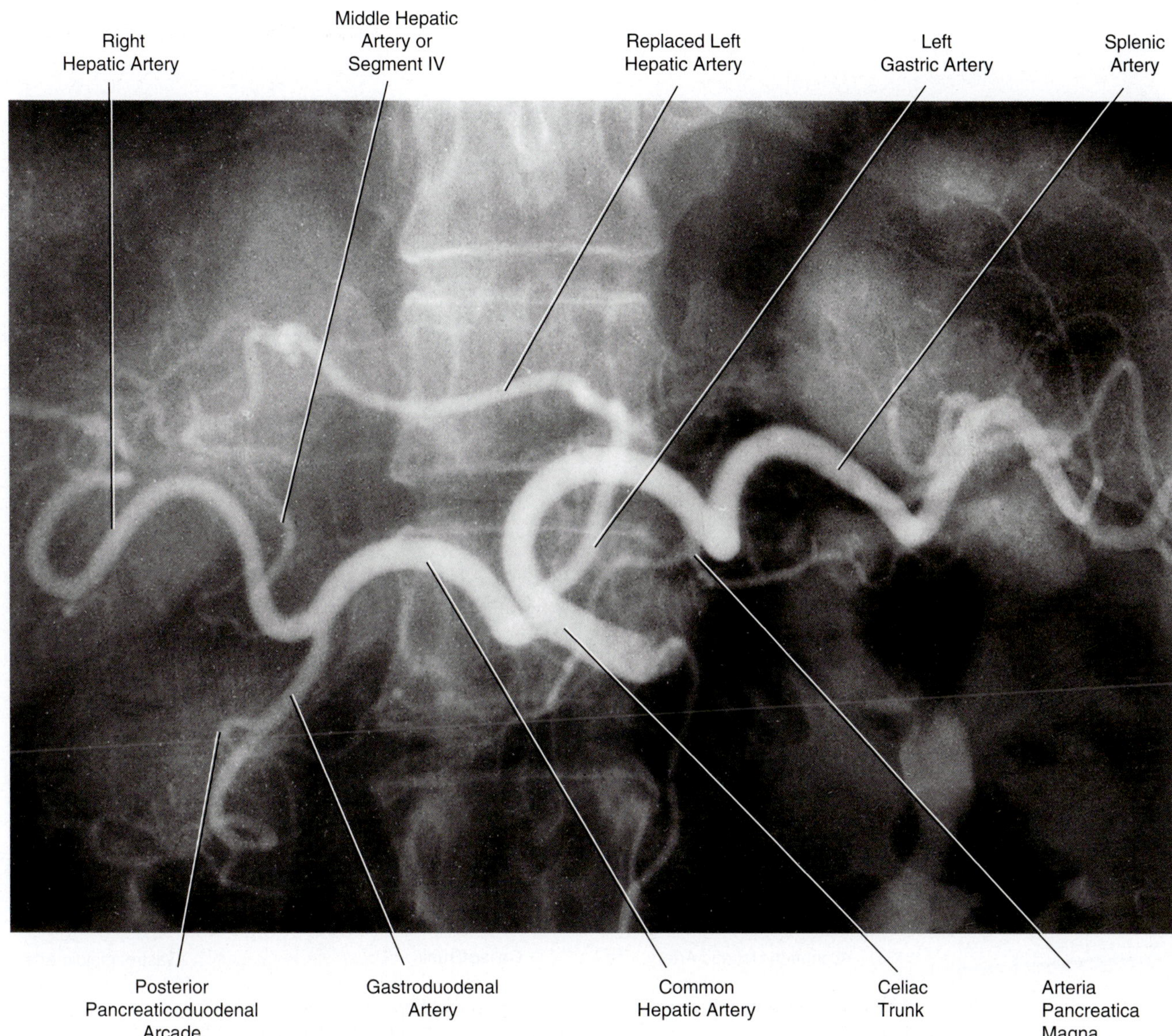

Figure 18.20. Selective injection at the celiac trunk showing the normal bifurcation, with distal origin of the left gastric artery giving rise to the left hepatic artery. There is a "middle hepatic artery" or the artery to segment IV arising from the proximal right hepatic artery. The splenic artery is long and tortuous. There is no visible dorsal pancreatic artery and the circulation of the body and tail of the pancreas is supplied mainly by the arteria pancreatica magna.

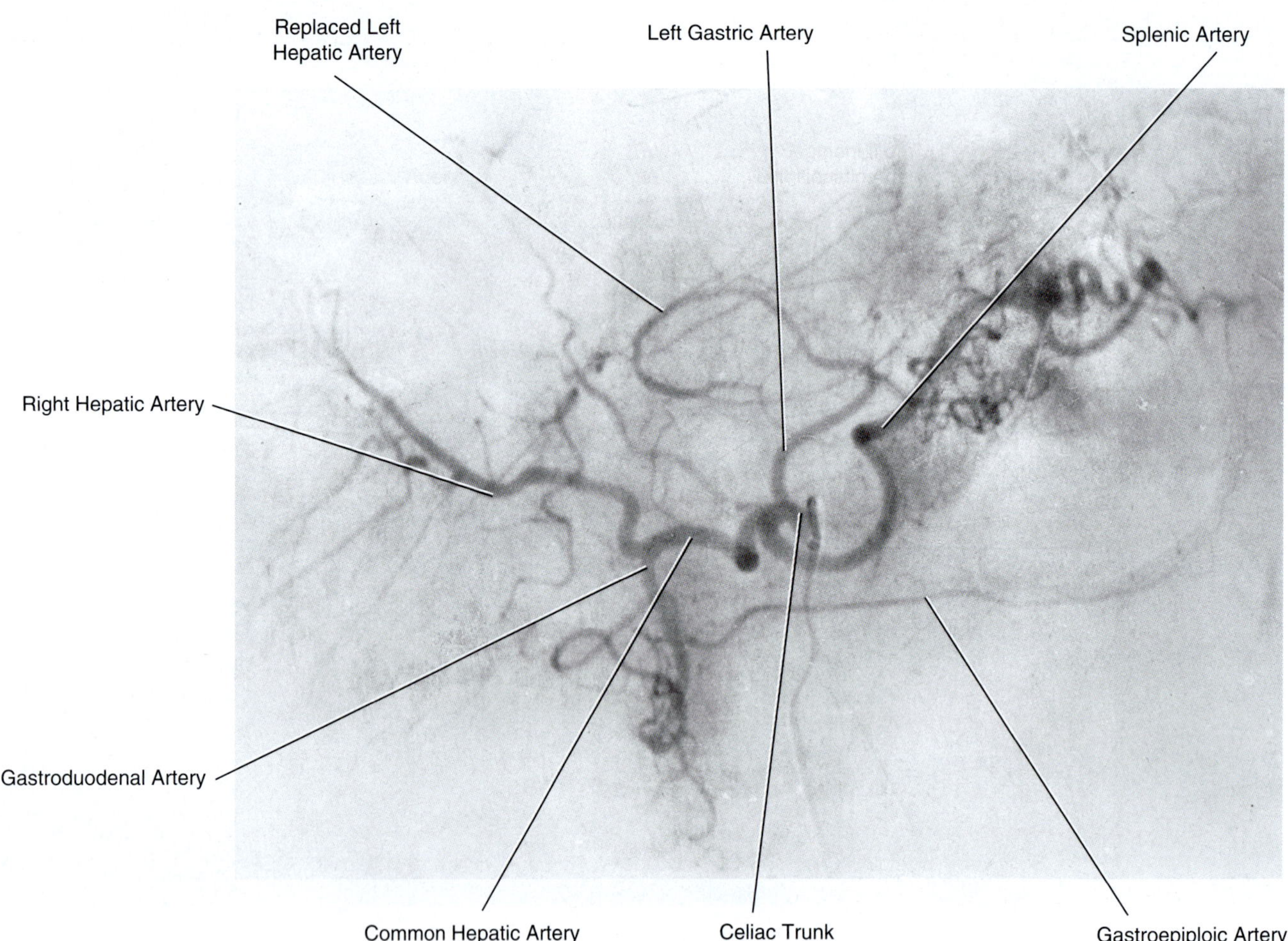

Figure 18.21. Injection at the celiac trunk, showing normal bifurcation, but with an enlarged left gastric artery giving origin to the left hepatic artery. The artery to the segment IV originates from the right hepatic artery. The splenic artery is long and tortuous. The pancreatic tail is partially stained by the contrast.

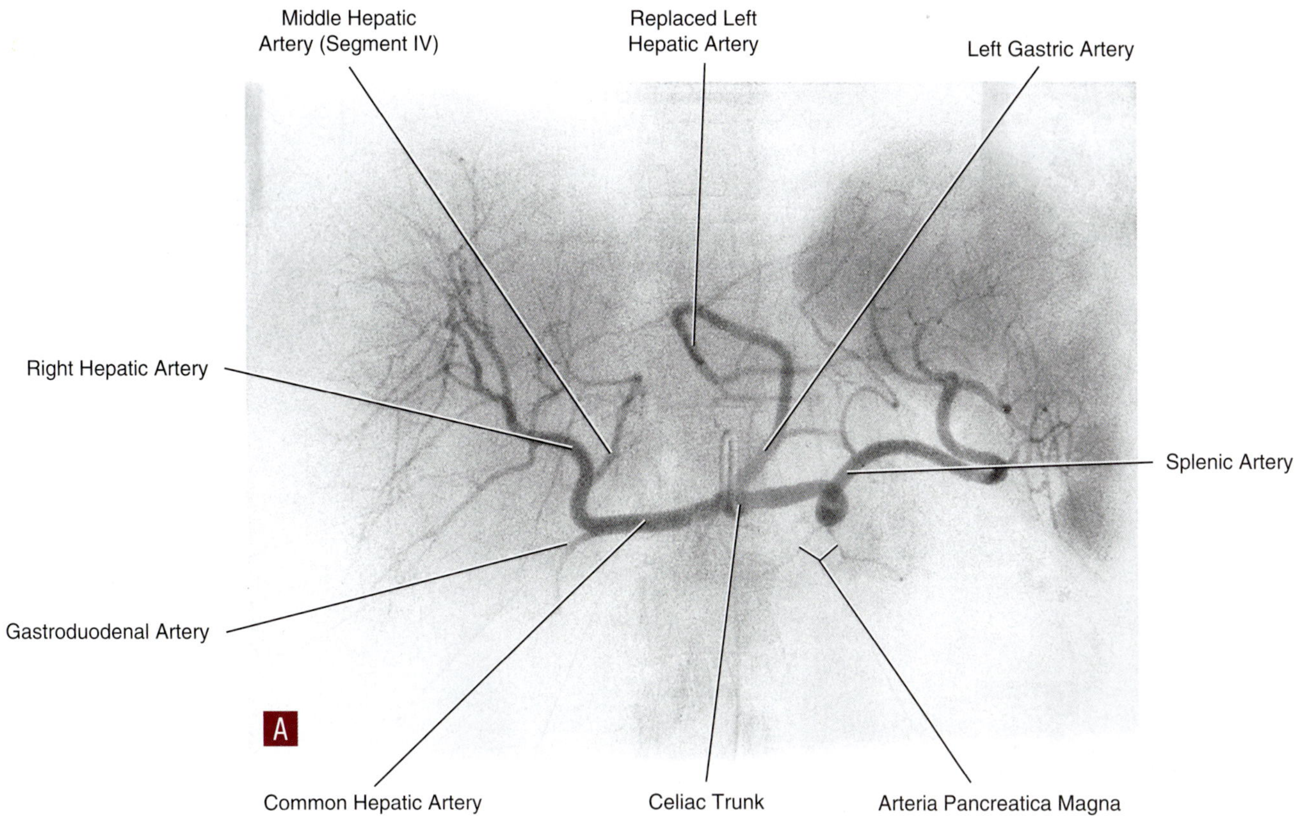

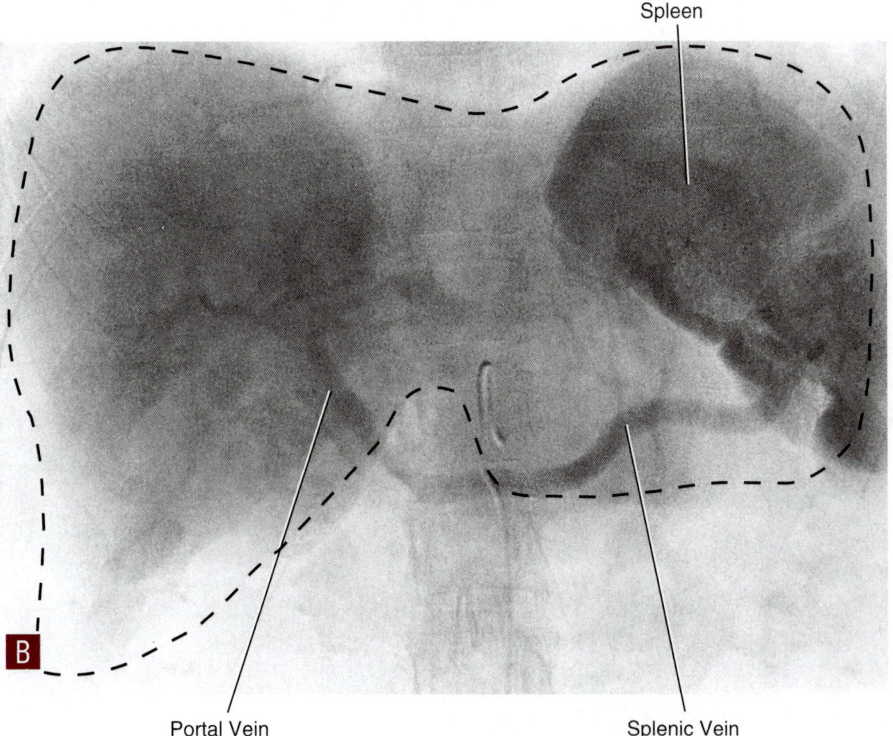

Figure 18.22. **A**, Selective injection at the celiac trunk showing a horizontal celiac trunk, with the replaced left hepatic artery arising from the left gastric artery. The artery to segment IV is a branch of the right hepatic artery. **B**, Late phase of the celiac injection showing the patent splenic and portal veins. Note the laminar flow into the portal vein. **C**, Late phase of a superior mesenteric artery (SMA) injection showing the superior mesenteric vein and the intrahepatic portal vein. The segments can be individualized. Segment V has a specific branch originating from the main portal vein.

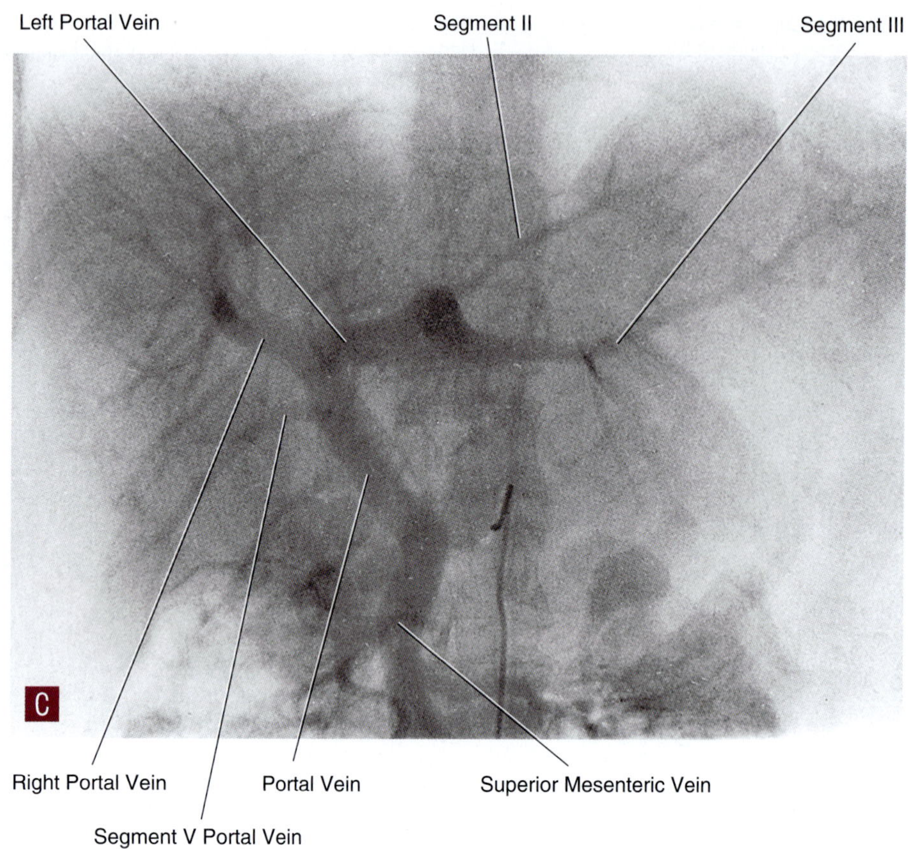

Figure 18.22. *Continued*

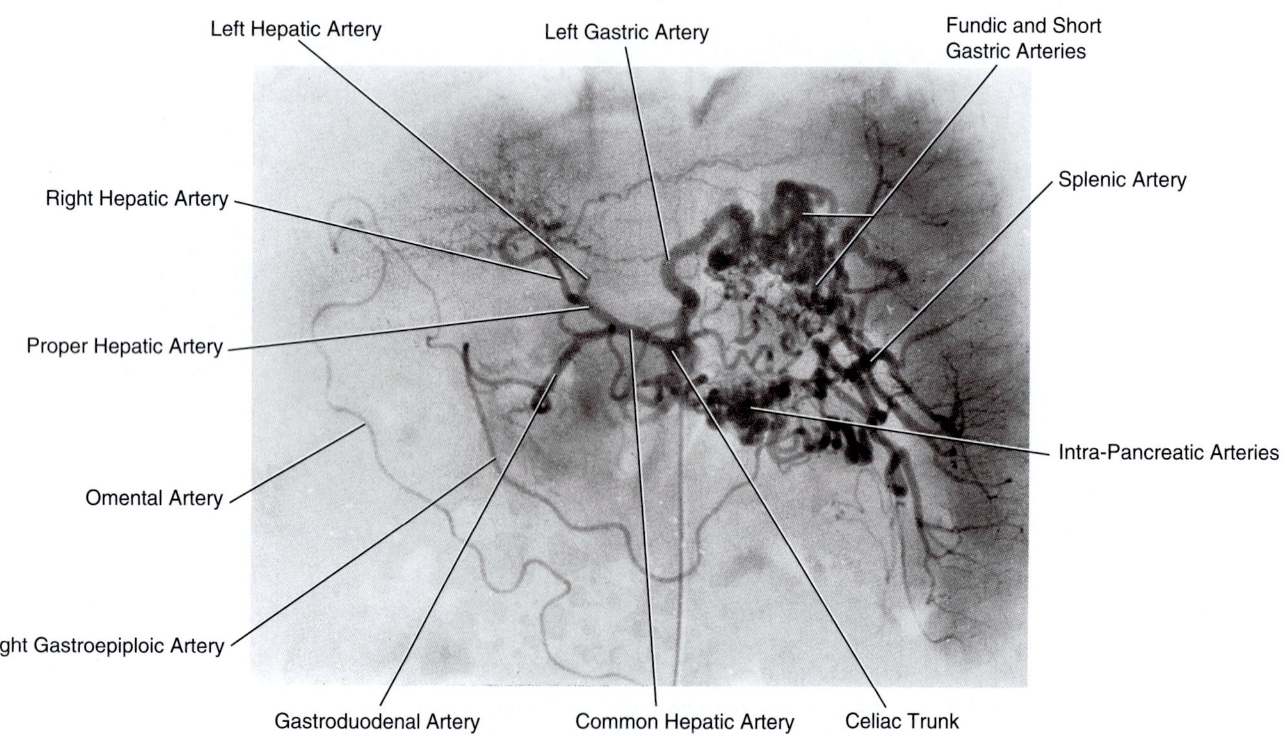

Figure 18.23. Celiac injection showing occlusion of the splenic artery and development of the collateral circulation through the left gastric artery, gastric fundus arteries, short gastric arteries and with filling of the splenic artery at the hilum. There is some collateralization through pancreatic arteries on the tail and body of the pancreas, through the dorsal pancreatic artery.

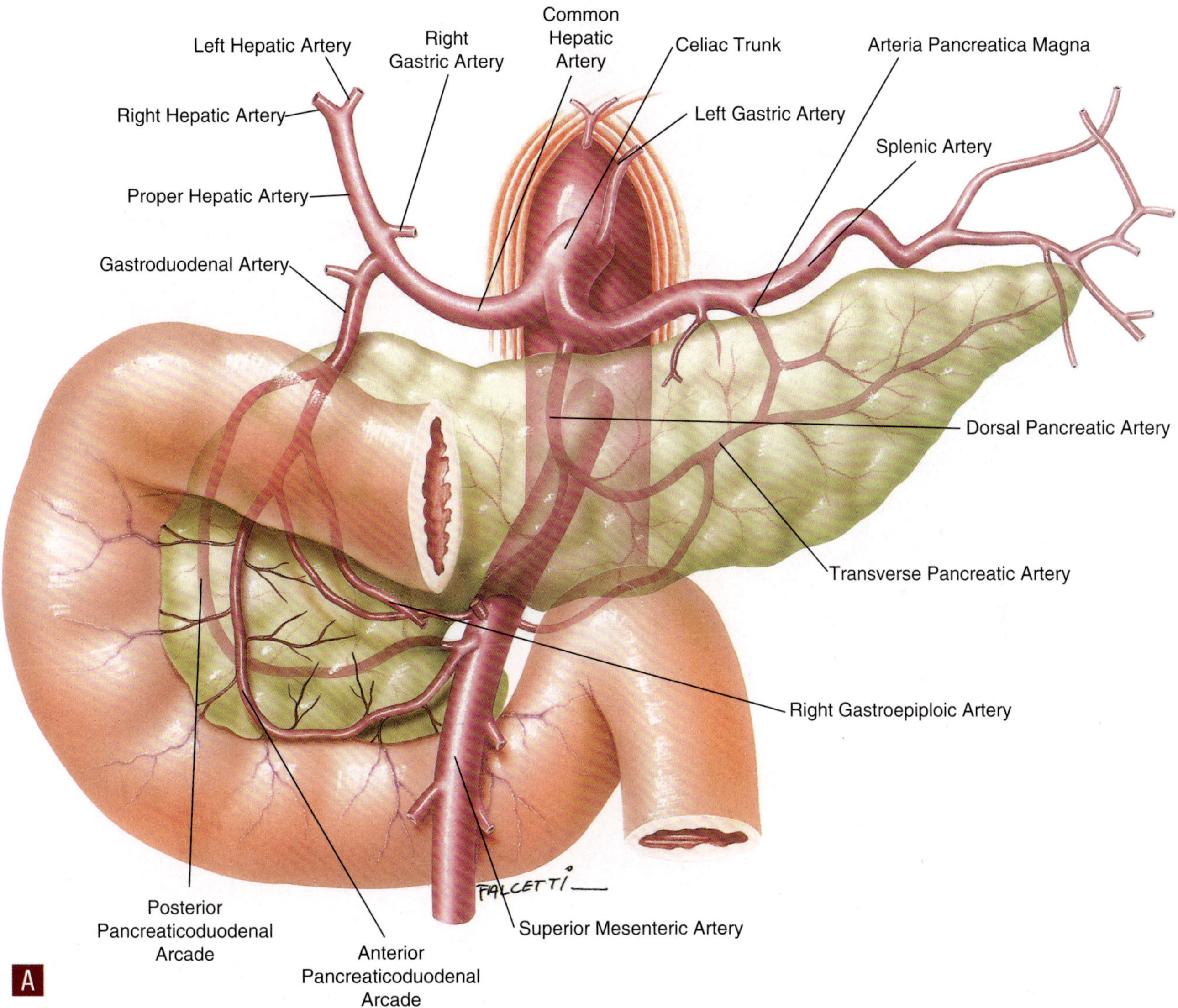

Figure 18.24. Schematic drawings of the celiac artery and variant branches of the left gastric artery. **A**, Schematic drawing of the celiac artery and branches to the duodenum, pancreas, and connections with the SMA. **B**, Origin of the left gastric artery from the superior mesenteric artery. **C**, Left gastric artery originating directly from the aorta. **D**. Duplicated left gastric artery arising from the celiac artery. **E**, Trifurcation of the celiac artery with a common origin of the common hepatic, splenic, and left gastric arteries.

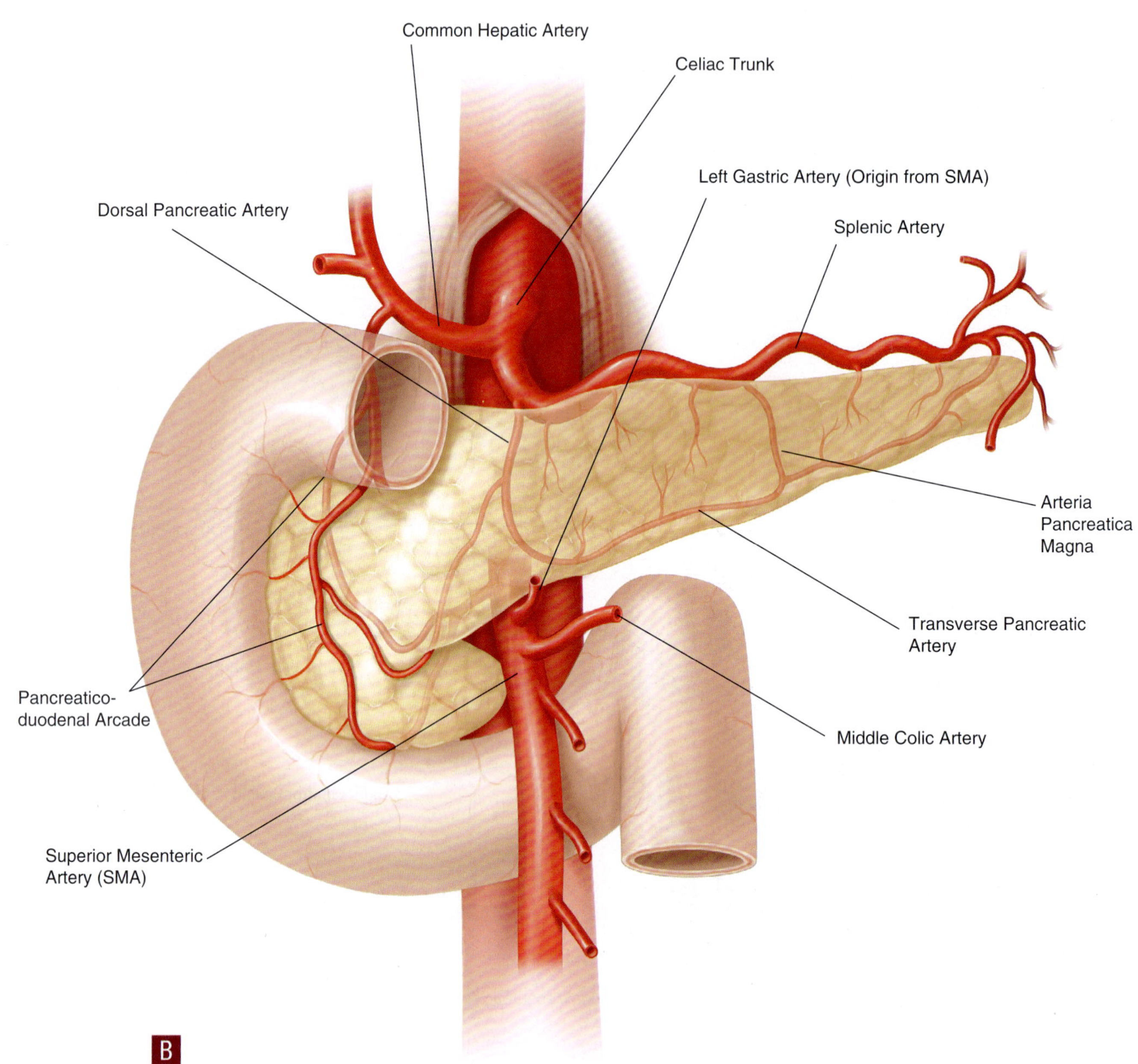

Figure 18.24. *Continued*

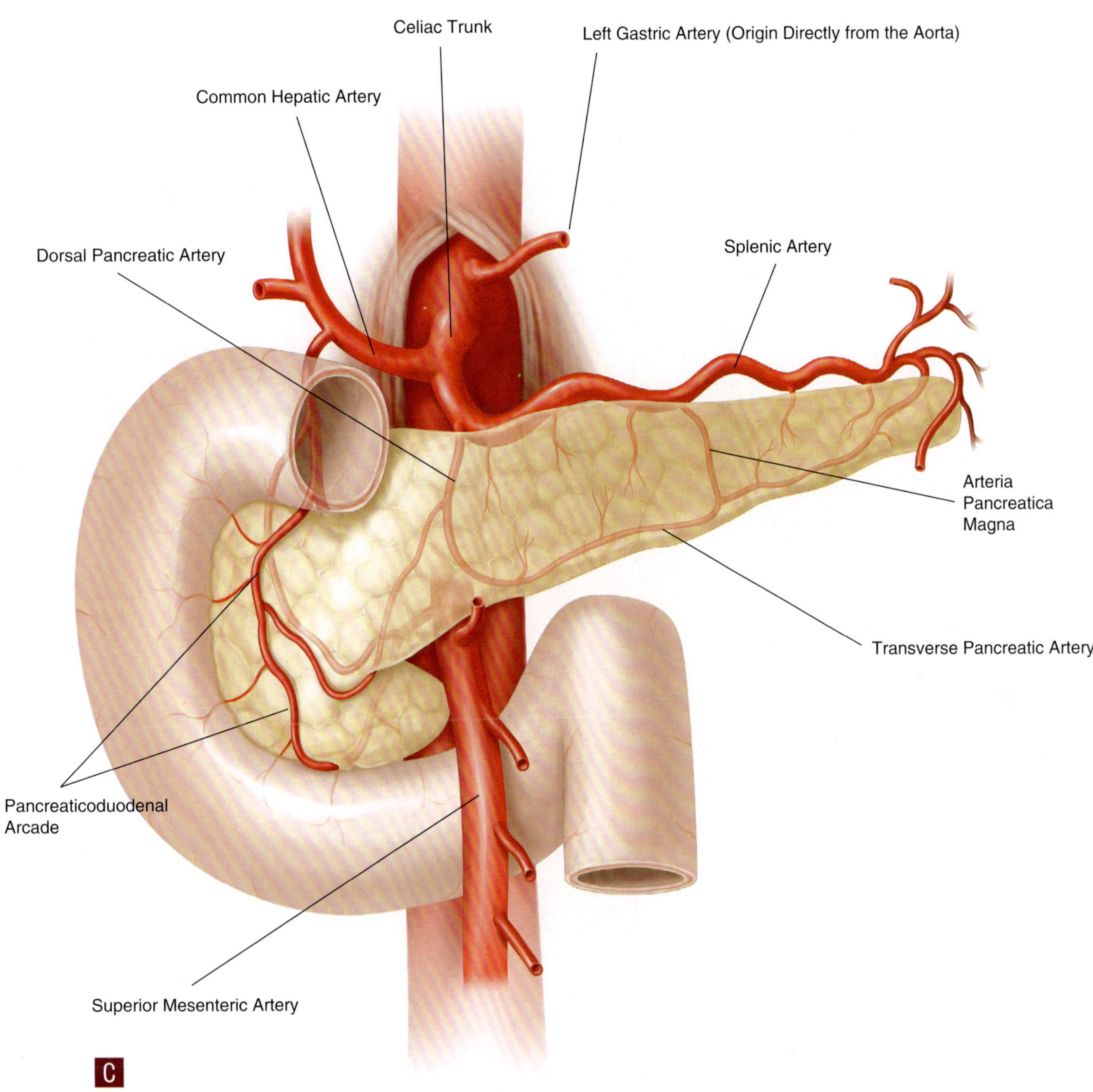

Figure 18.24. *Continued*

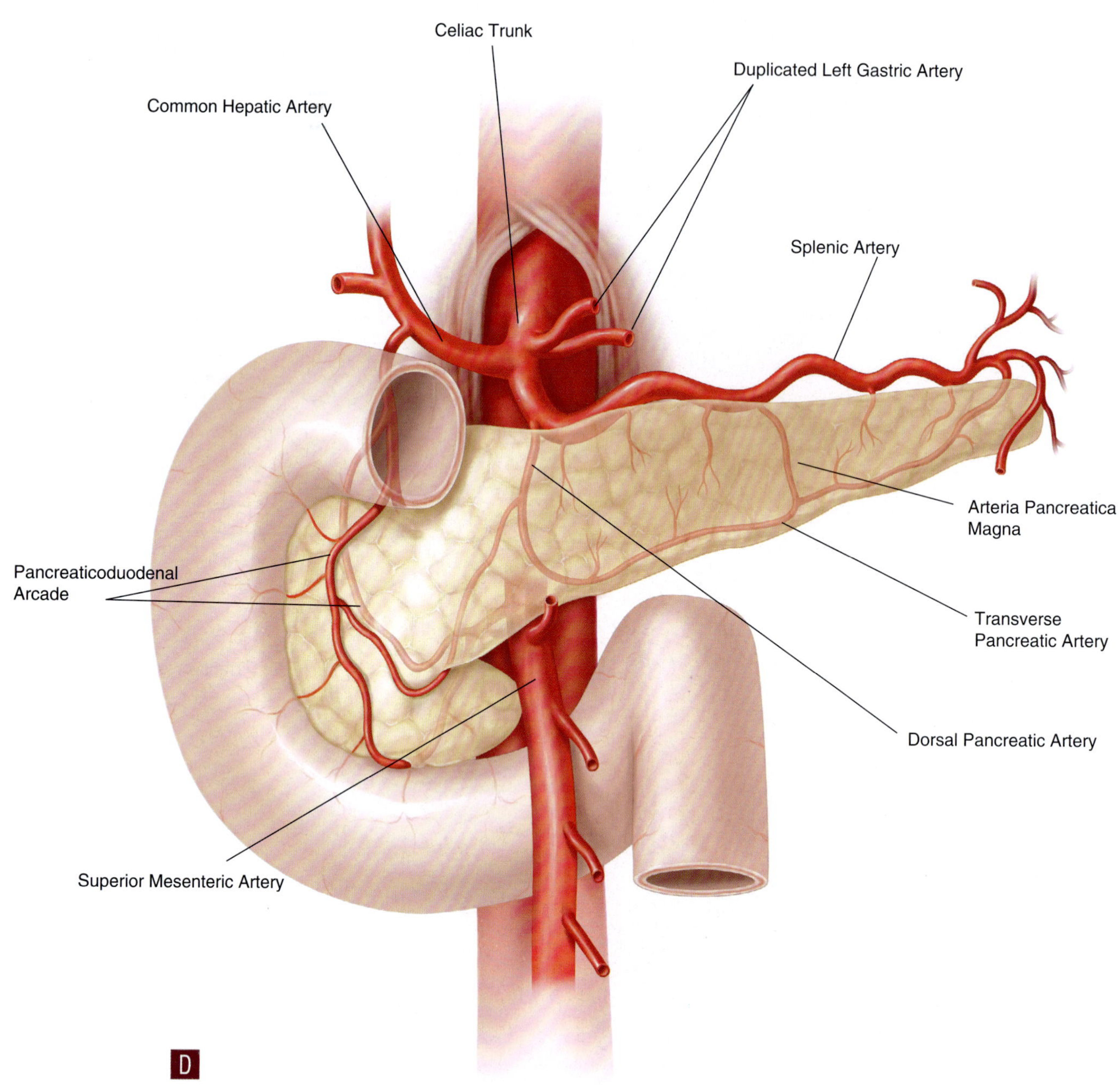

Figure 18.24. *Continued*

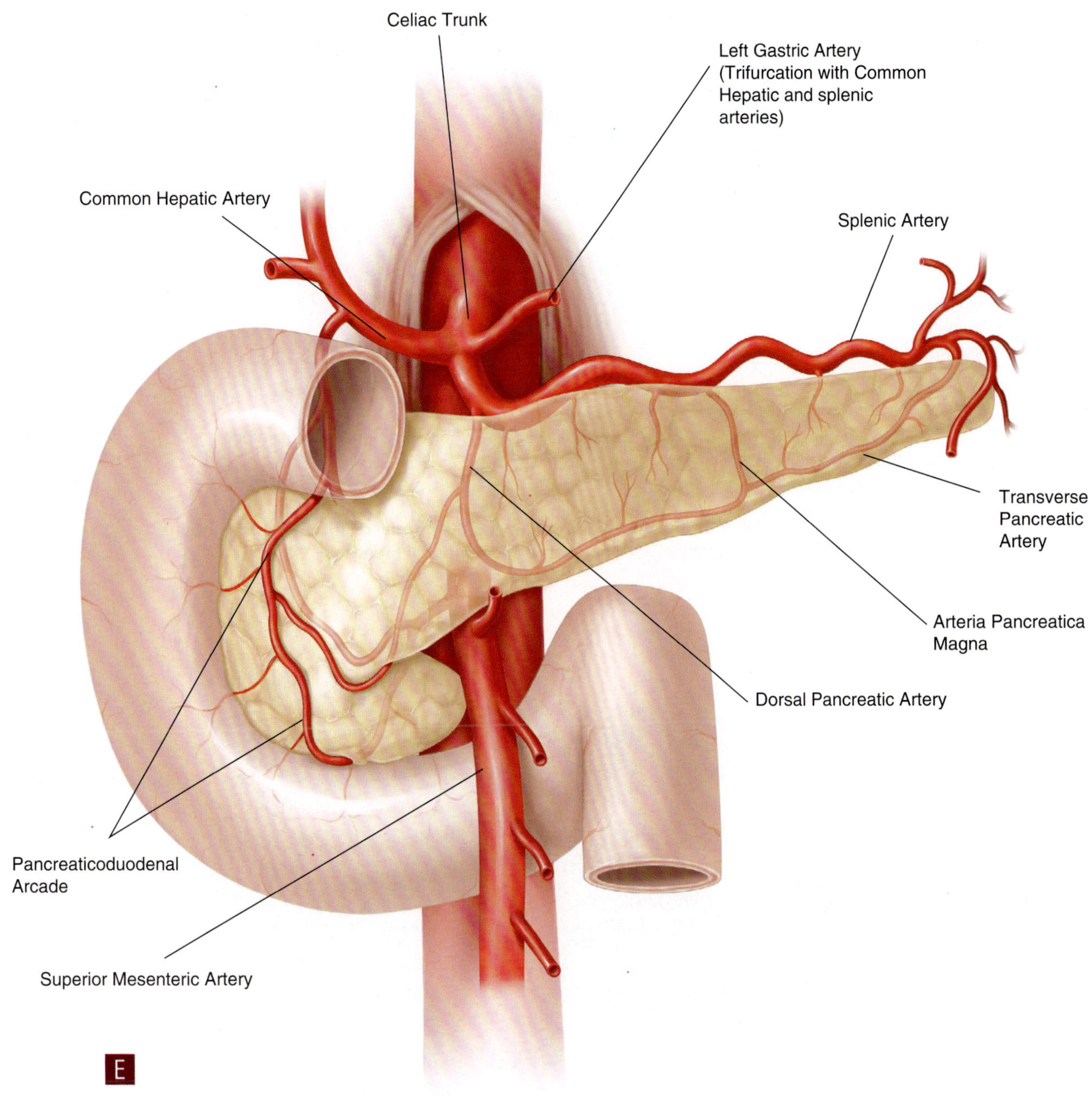

Figure 18.24. *Continued*

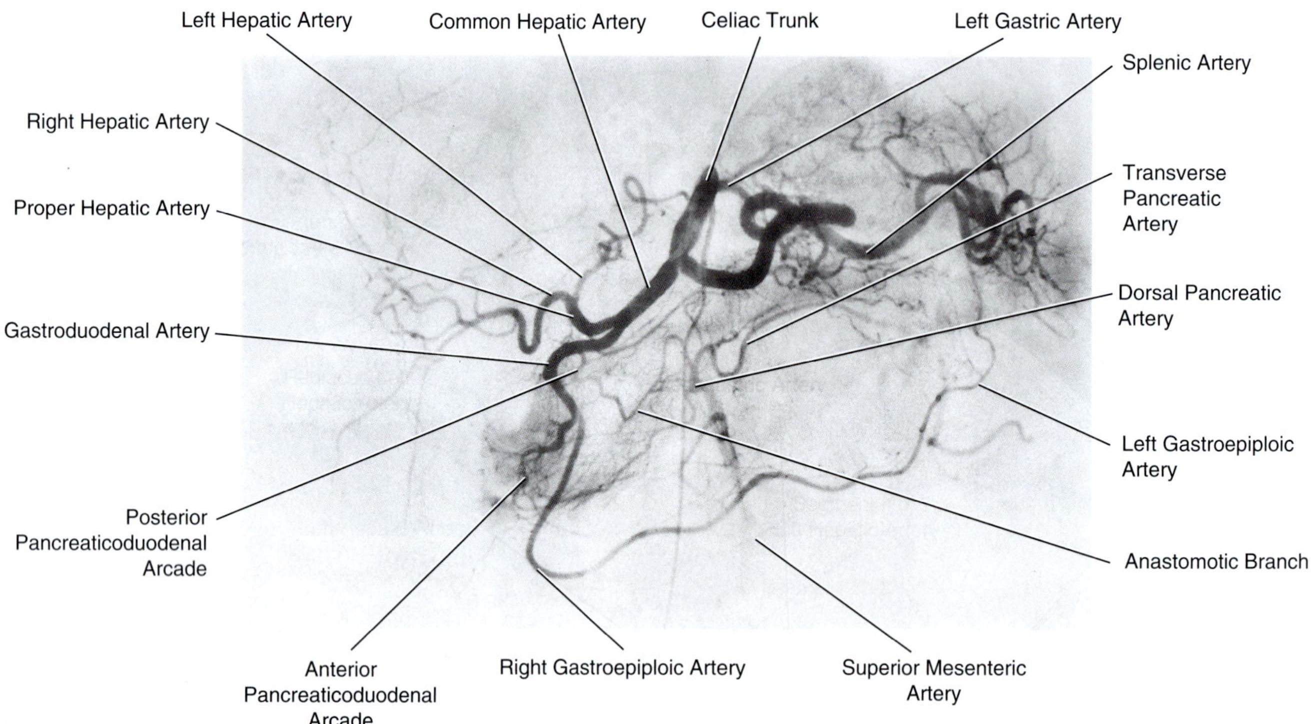

Figure 18.25. Celiac artery angiography showing the normal distribution of the main branches, the pancreatic branches, and the gastric and duodenal branches.

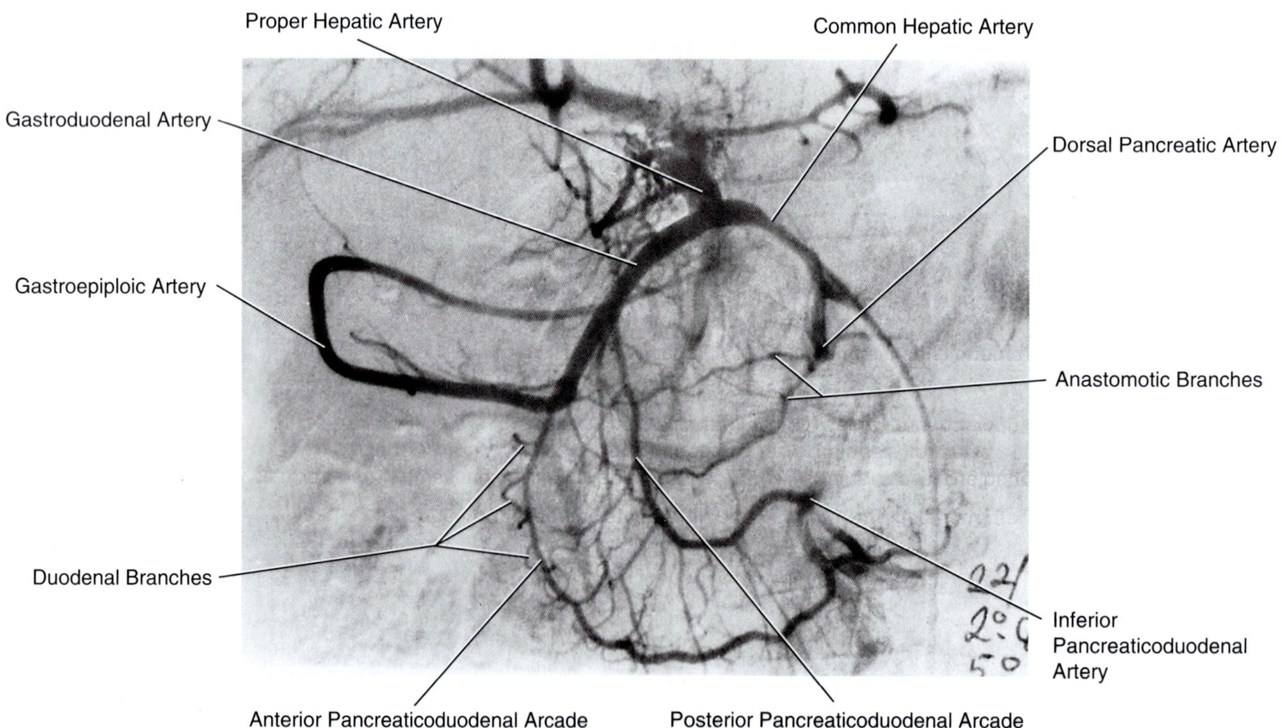

Figure 18.26. Selective injection at the gastroduodenal artery, showing the duodenal and pancreatic head branches. The proper hepatic artery is occluded. The dorsal pancreatic artery is a branch of the common hepatic artery and is retrograde filled.

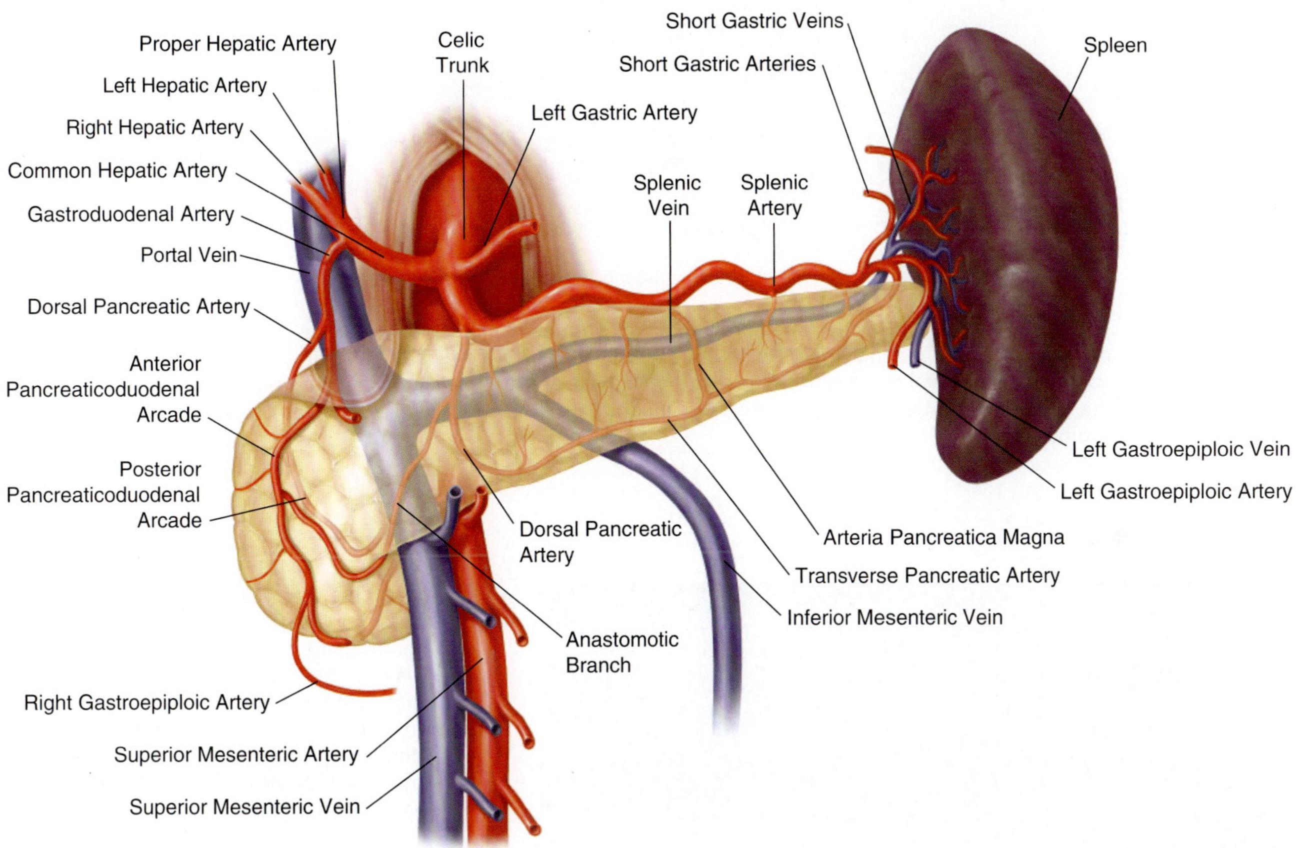

Figure 18.27. **Schematic drawing of the pancreatic and celiac branches.**

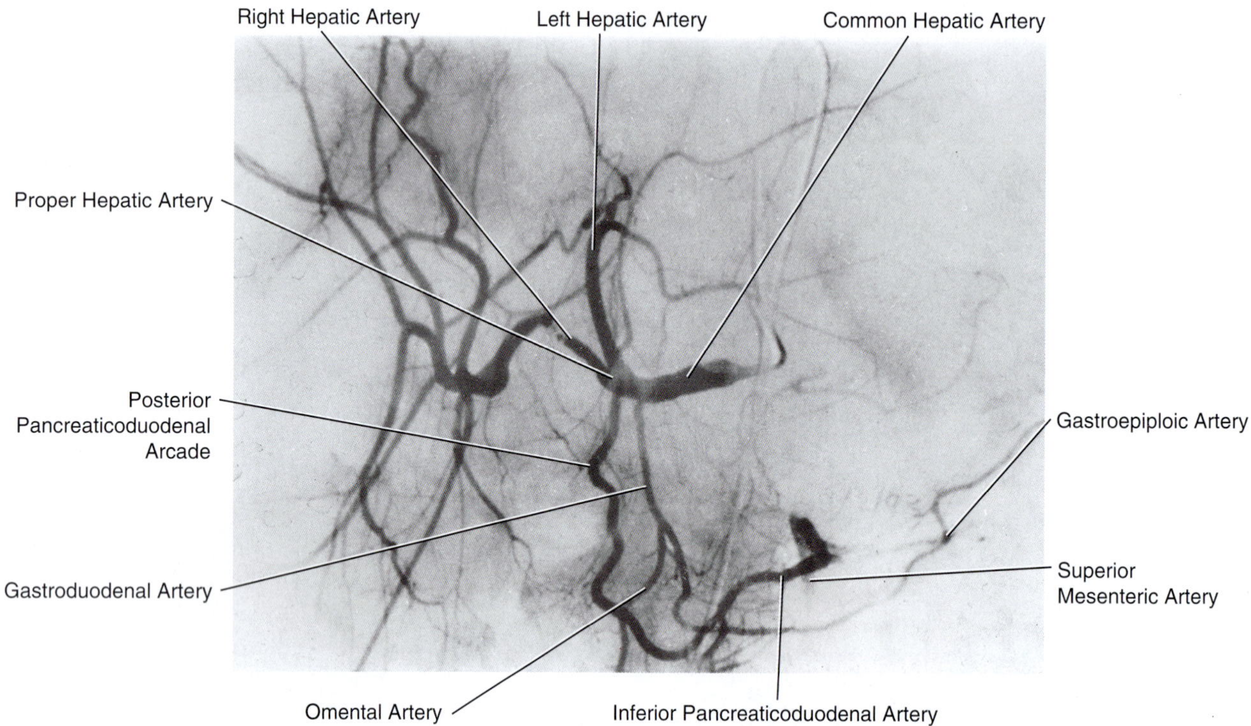

Figure 18.28. Selective angiography of the common hepatic artery showing the duplicated gastroduodenal artery (GDA) or absence thereof, with direct origin of the pancreaticoduodenal arcades from the common hepatic artery. Note significant spasm of the right hepatic artery. There is filling of the inferior pancreatic artery and a small proximal segment of the SMA.

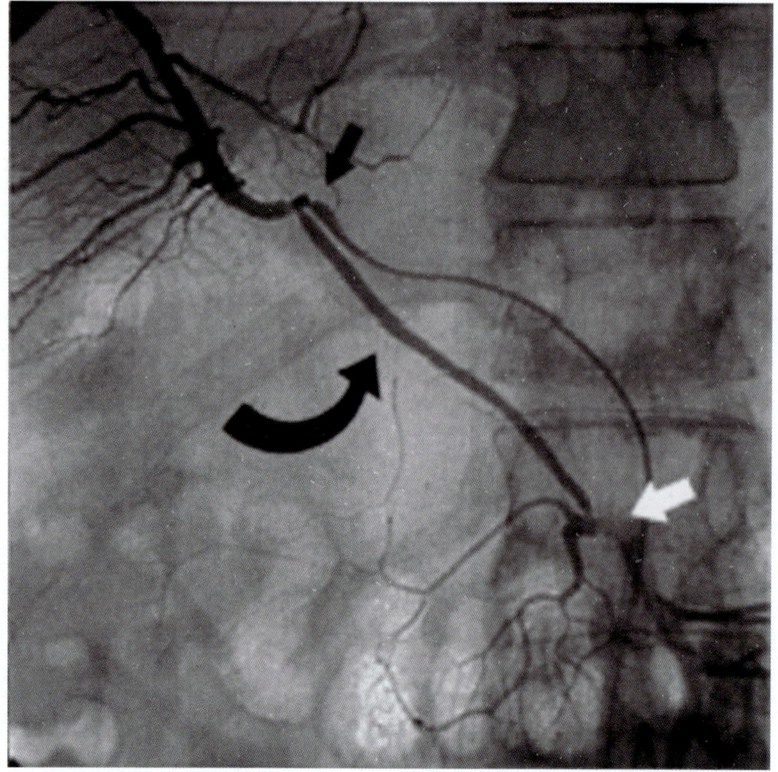

Figure 18.29. Selective angiogram of the proper hepatic artery with spasm at the catheter tip (black arrow). A large retroduodenal artery is depicted (curved arrow) with reflux and opacification of the SMA (white arrow). (Reprinted from Liu DM, et al. Angiographic considerations in patients undergoing liver-direct therapy. *J Vasc Interv Radiol.* 2005;16:911-935 with permission from Elsevier.)

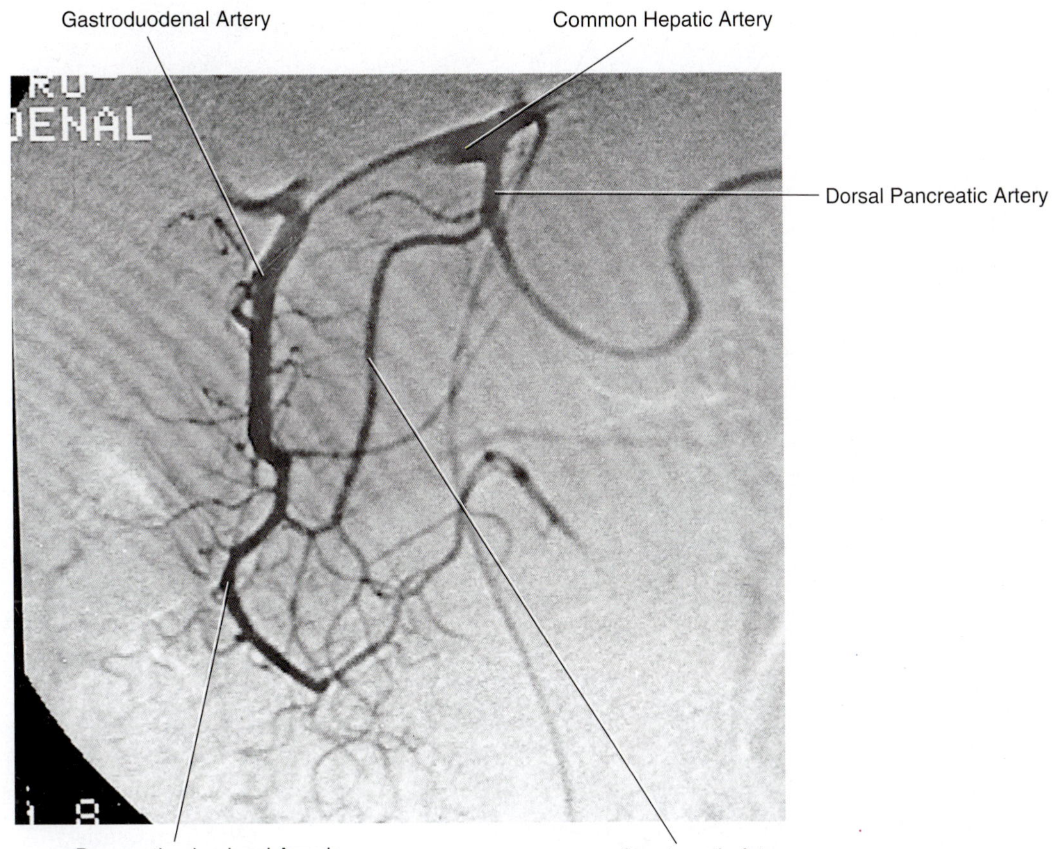

Figure 18.30. Selective angiography at the gastroduodenal artery, showing the pancreaticoduodenal arcades and the anastomosis with the dorsal pancreatic artery and filling of the inferior pancreatic artery.

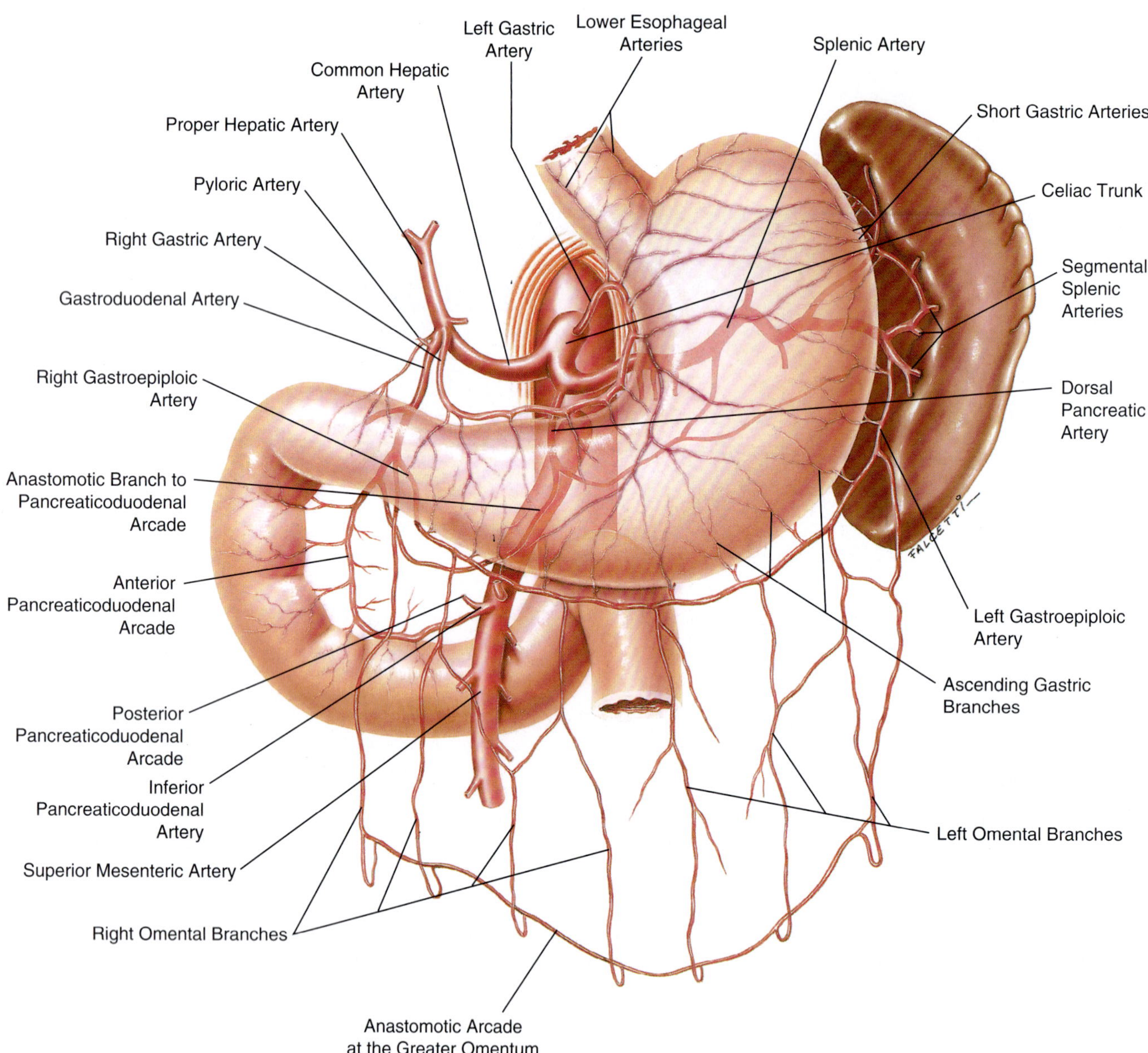

Figure 18.31. Schematic drawing showing the arterial circulation of the duodenum, stomach, spleen, and greater omentum, as well as the anastomotic collaterals.

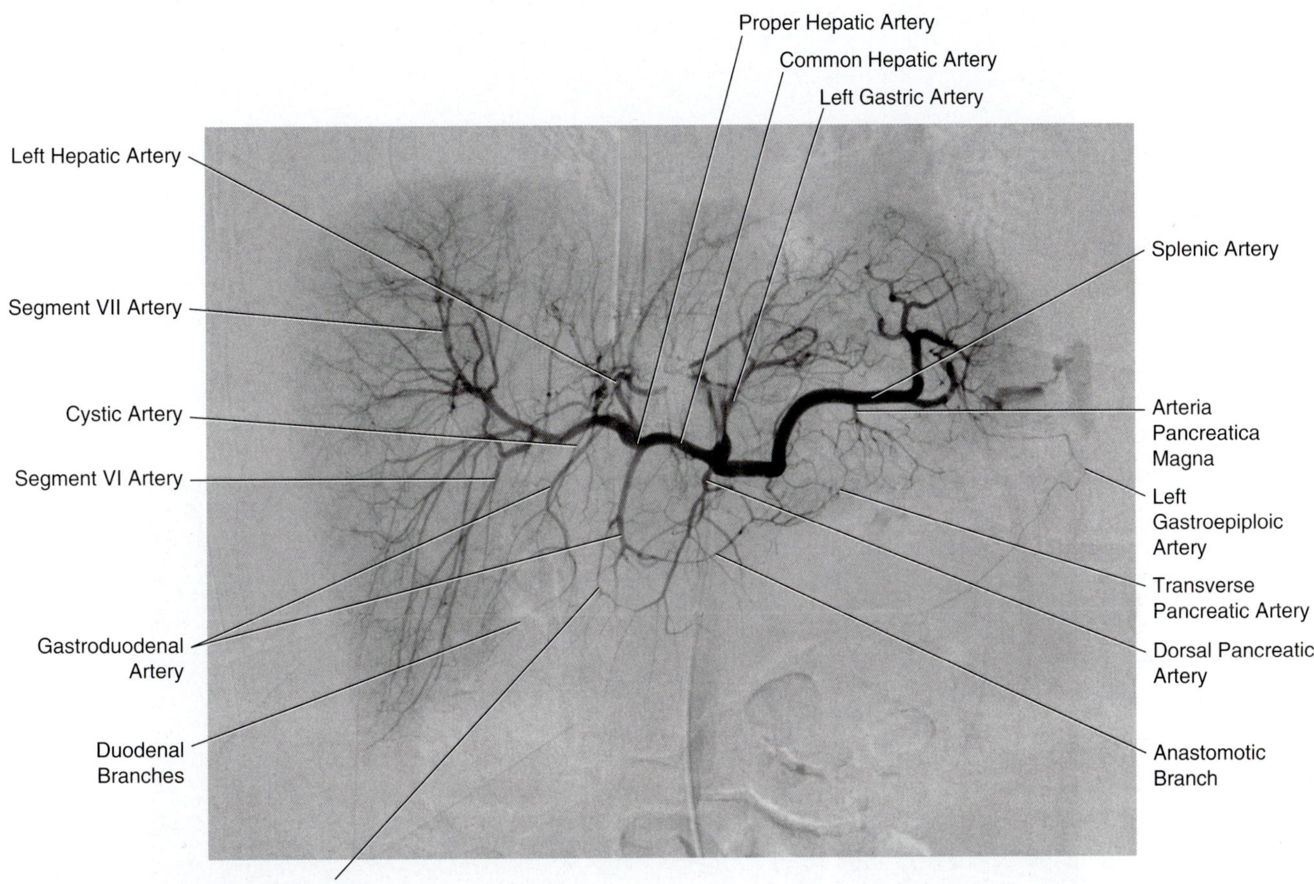

Figure 18.32. Selective injection at the celiac trunk with a normal distribution of the branches. Note the dorsal pancreatic artery arising from the bifurcation of the celiac artery and that most of the arterial circulation of the pancreas arises from the dorsal pancreatic artery. The transverse pancreatic artery is diminutive.

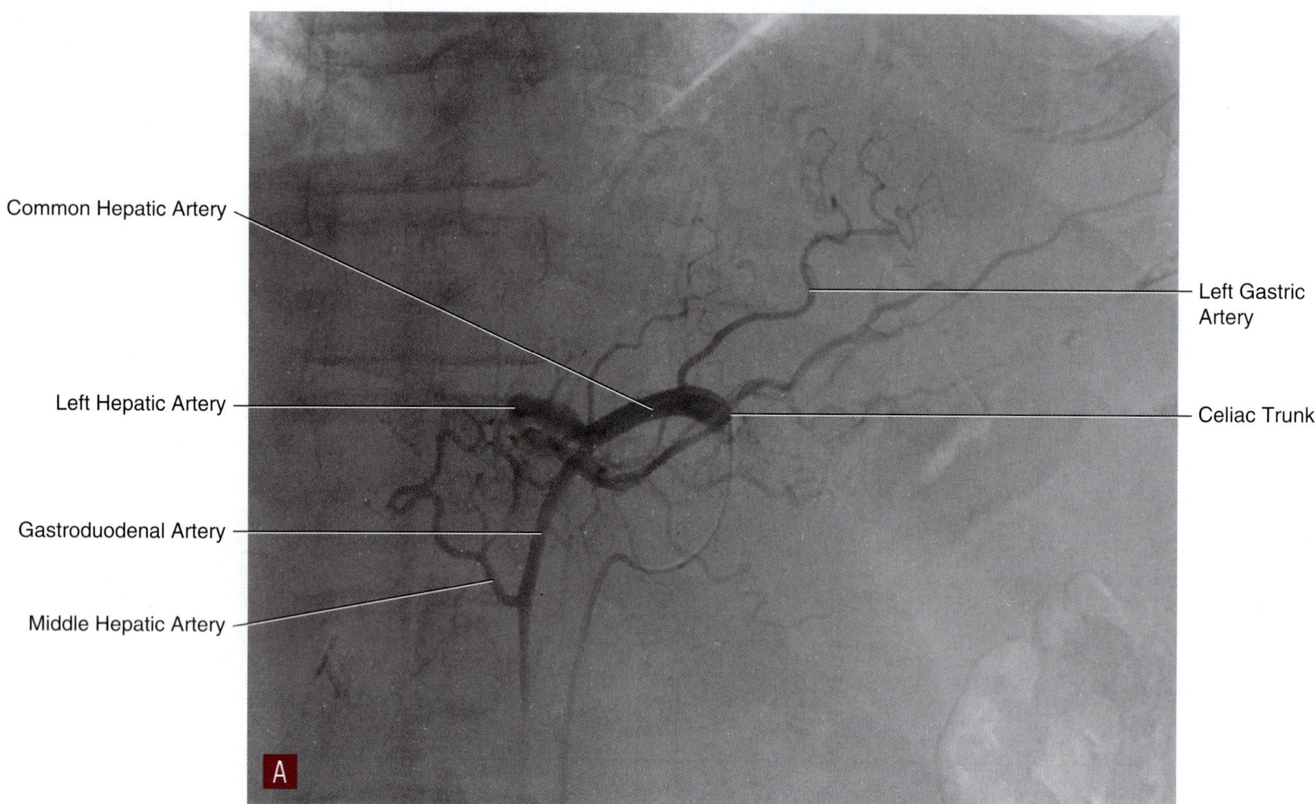

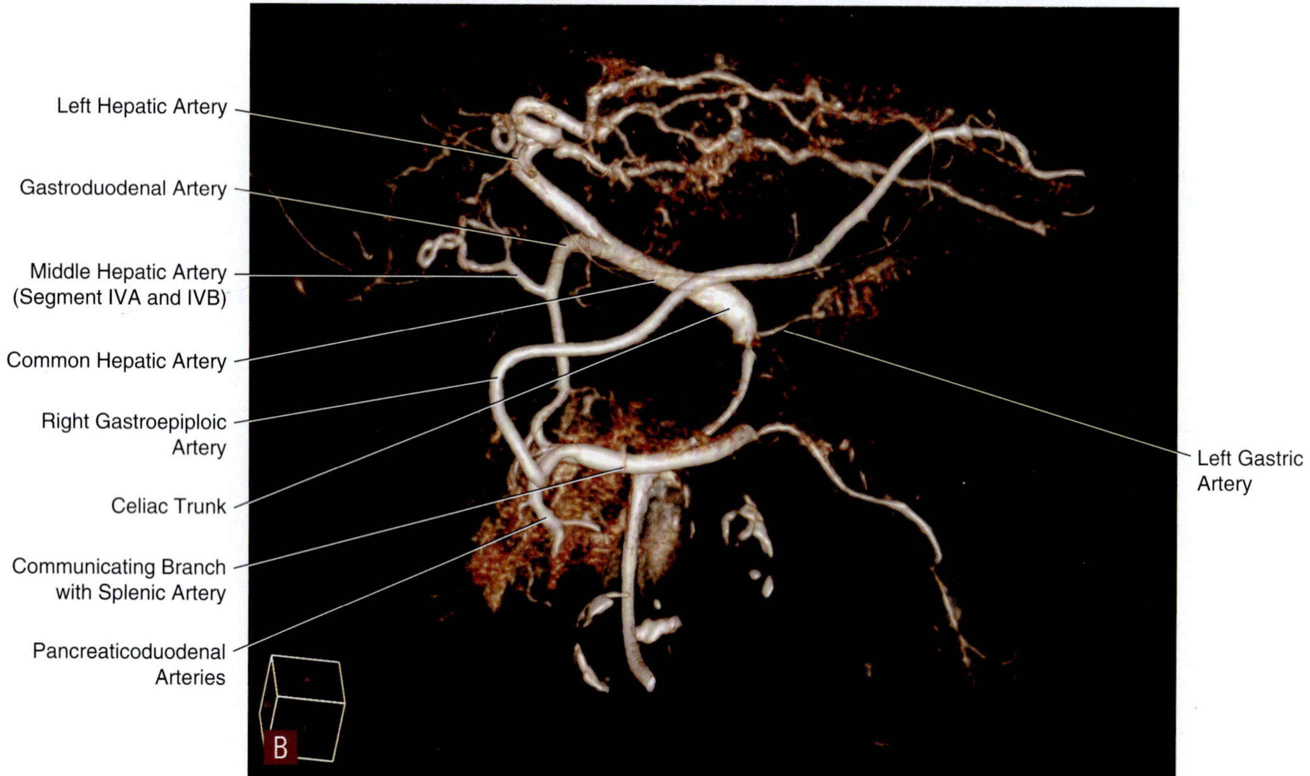

Figure 18.33. **A**, Selective angiogram of the celiac trunk with the left hepatic artery arising from the proper hepatic artery. The middle hepatic artery supplying segment IVA and IVB arises directly from the gastroduodenal artery. The right hepatic artery is replaced from the superior mesenteric artery. **B** and **C**, 3D reconstruction of the celiac artery injection during cone beam CT showing the variant middle hepatic artery without an anastomosis with the superior mesenteric artery through the pancreaticoduodenal arcade. **D**, Selective splenic angiogram demonstrating a large communicating branch with the gastroduodenal artery and no anastomosis to the superior mesenteric artery.

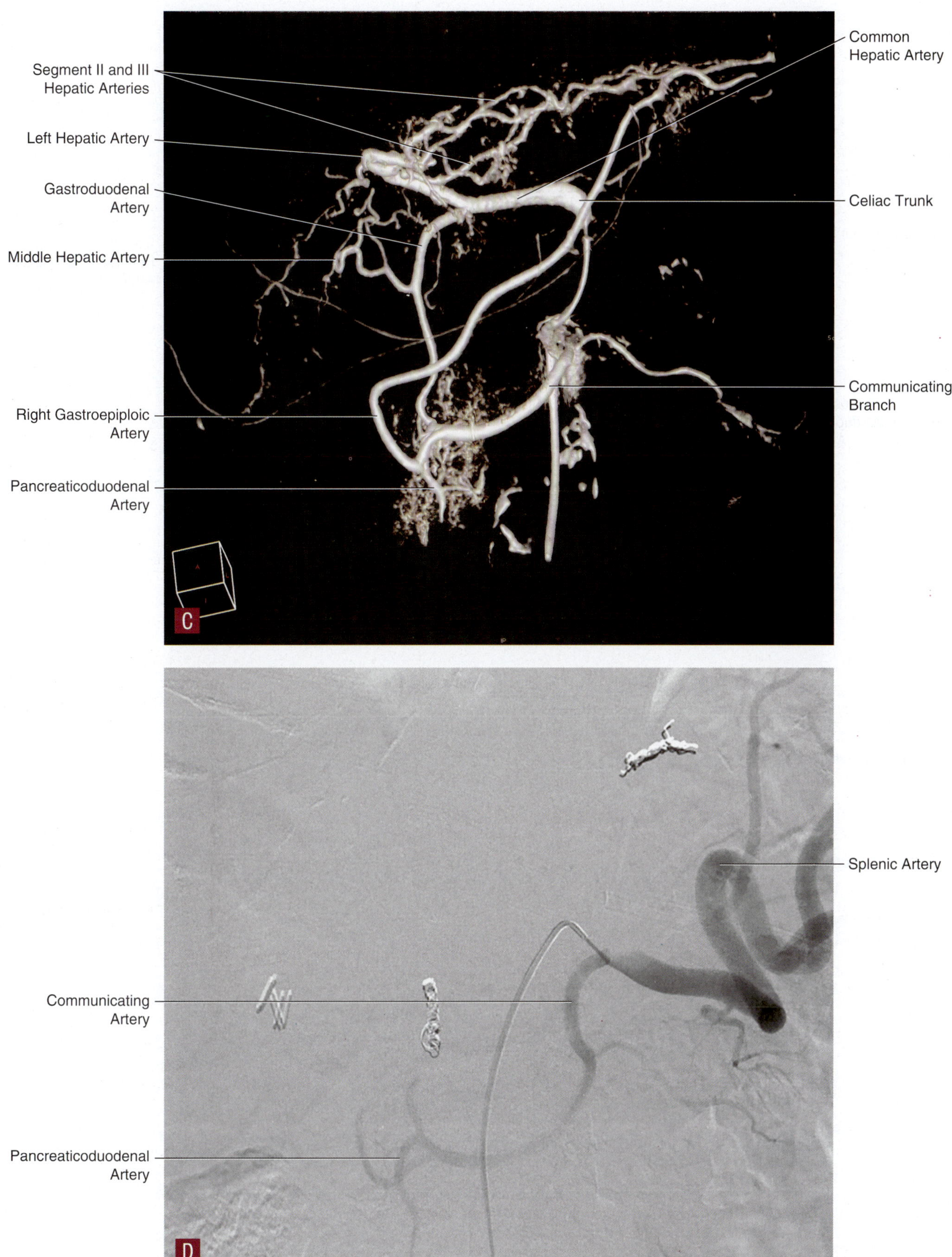

Figure 18.33. *Continued*

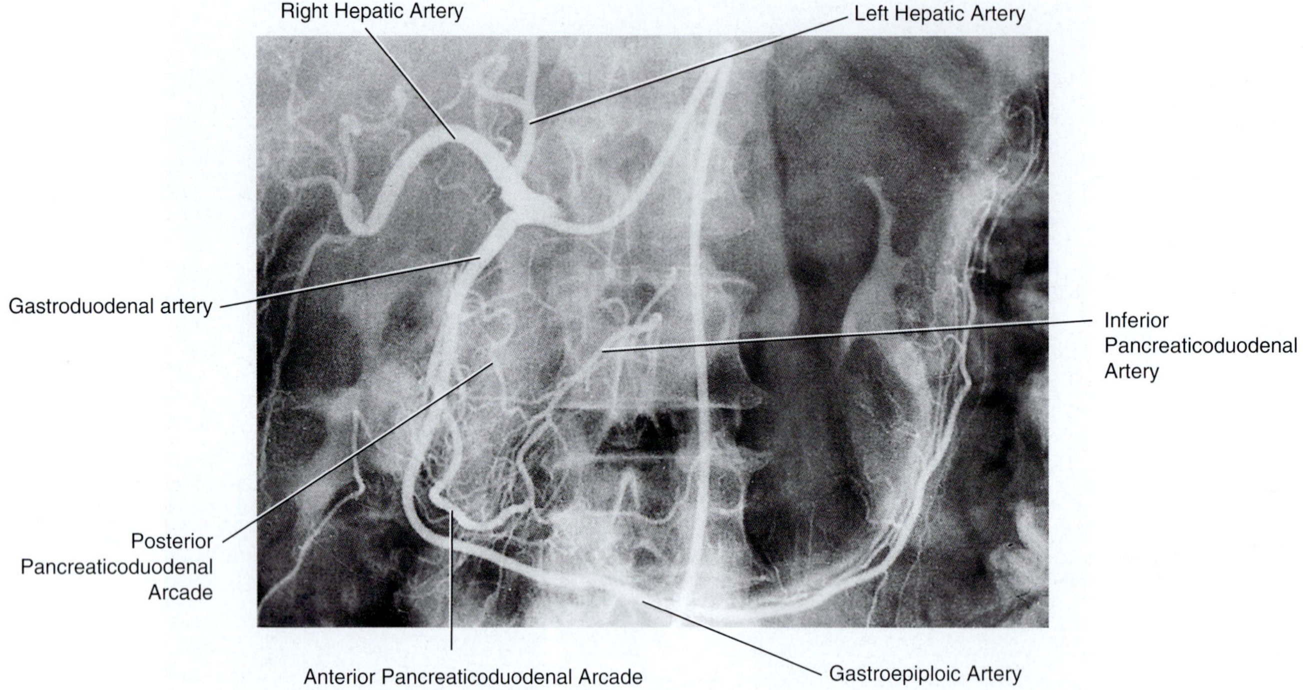

Figure 18.34. Selective angiography of the gastroduodenal artery showing the pancreaticoduodenal arcades and the gastroepiploic arteries. There is dominance of one of the pancreaticoduodenal arcades.

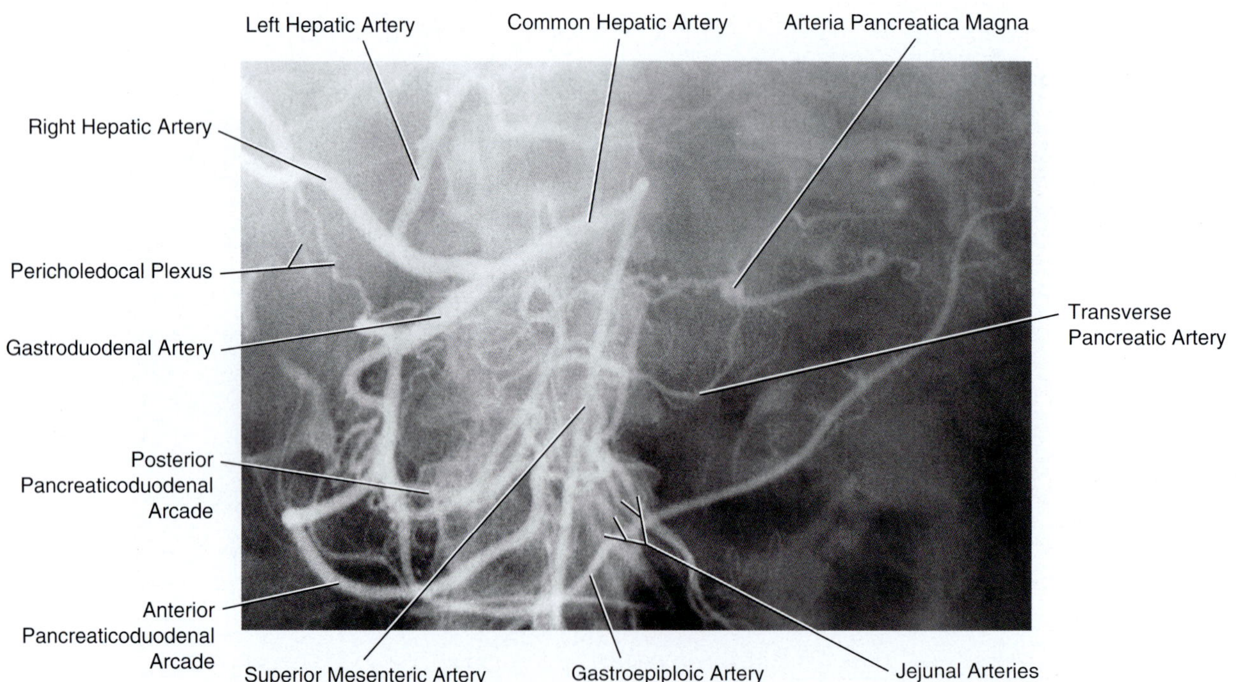

Figure 18.35. Selective angiography of the gastroduodenal artery showing the arteries supplying the pancreatic head and the anastomoses within the pancreas. Note filling of the arteria pancreatica magna and opacification of the gastroepiploic artery.

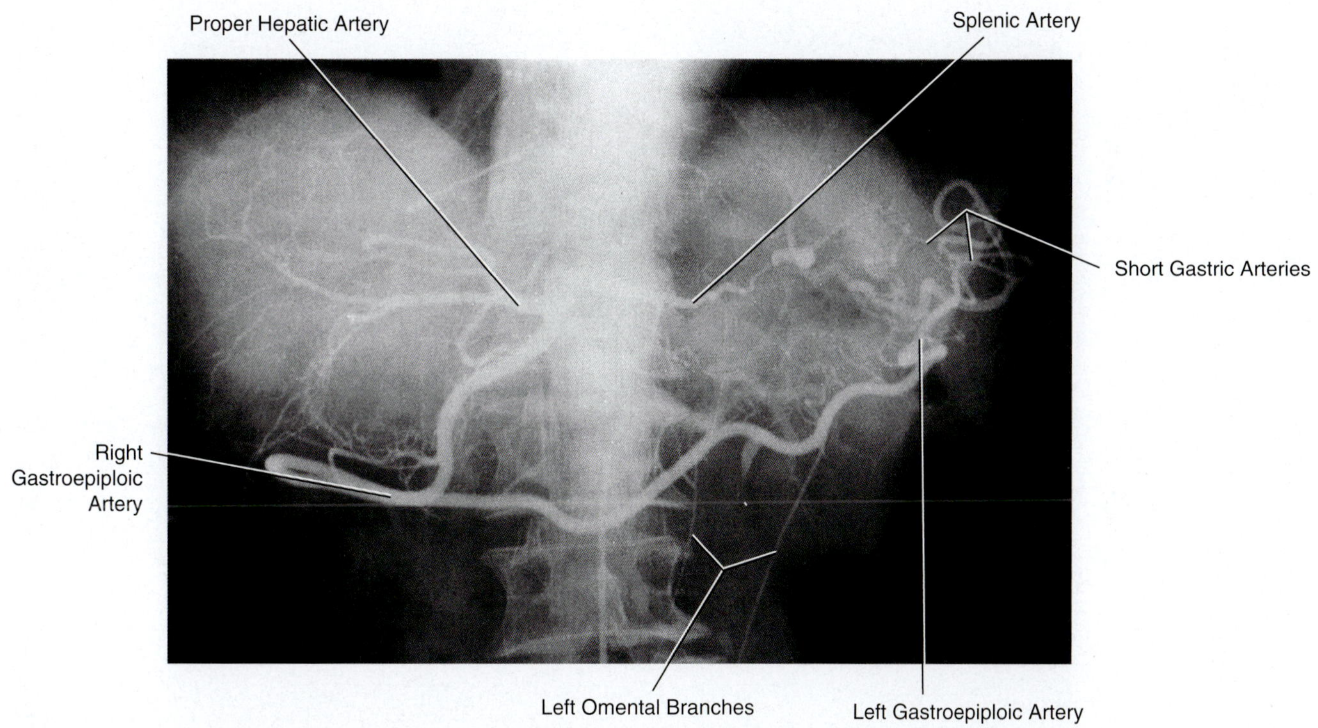

Figure 18.36. Selective angiography of the celiac trunk. Note the enlargement of the gastroepiploic artery and the anastomosis with the splenic circulation, due to the partial occlusion of the splenic artery by a pancreatic tumor.

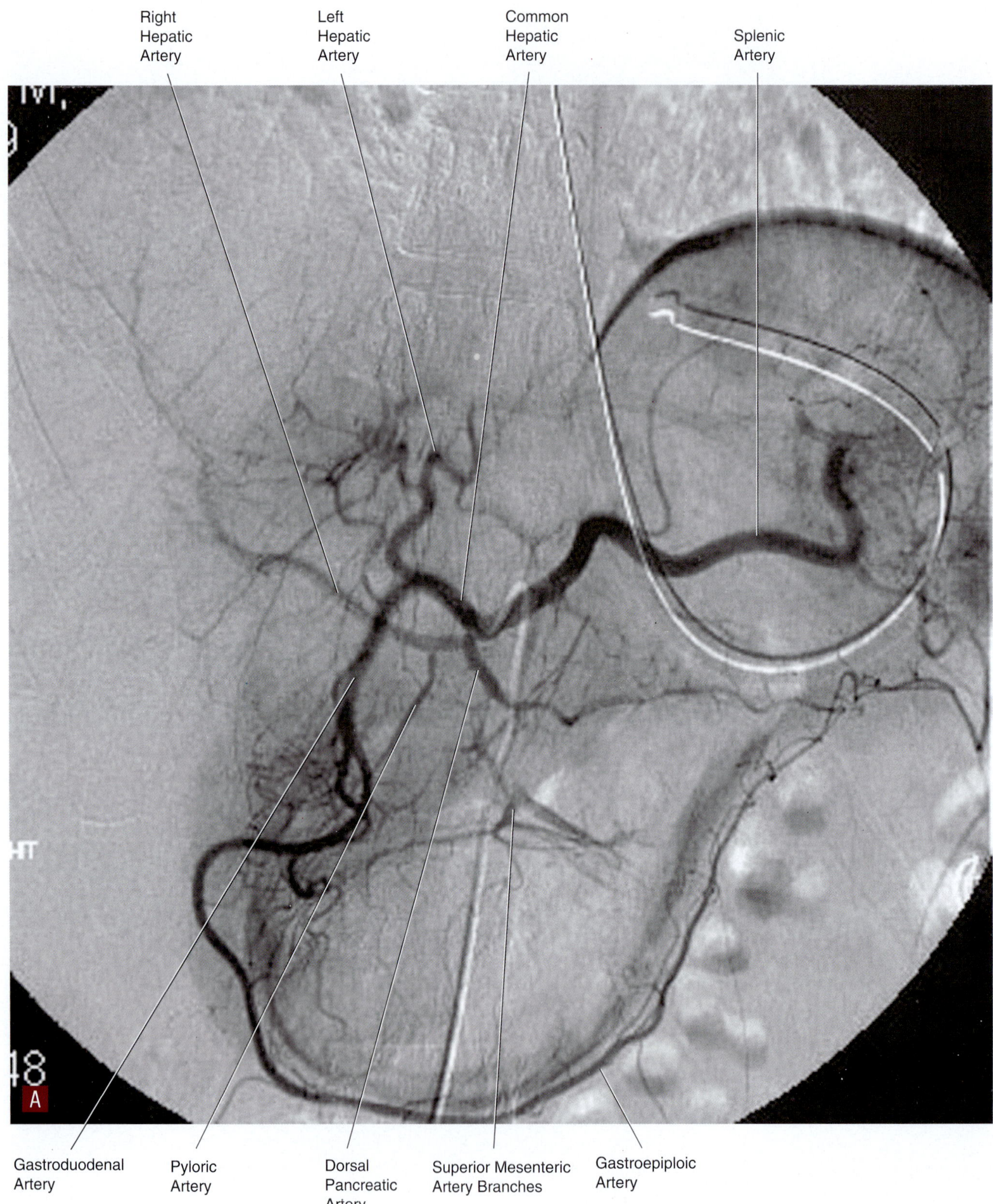

Figure 18.37. **A**, Selective angiography of the celiac trunk. Note the early bifurcation of the hepatic artery, without a proper hepatic artery. The left hepatic artery arises from the common hepatic artery and the dorsal pancreatic artery originates from the proximal right hepatic artery. The pyloric artery is also a branch of the right hepatic artery. The gastroduodenal artery is a branch of the common hepatic artery and the middle hepatic artery is a branch of the proximal gastroduodenal artery. Note the long gastroepiploic artery along the great curvature of the stomach, with the gastric body branches visible and enhancement of the stomach wall. Note also filling of proximal branches of the SMA from connections with the dorsal pancreatic artery. **B**, Late phase of the celiac angiogram showed the venous phase, with filling of the gastroepiploic vein, draining into the superior mesenteric vein and the portal vein. Note the thickness of the gastric wall.

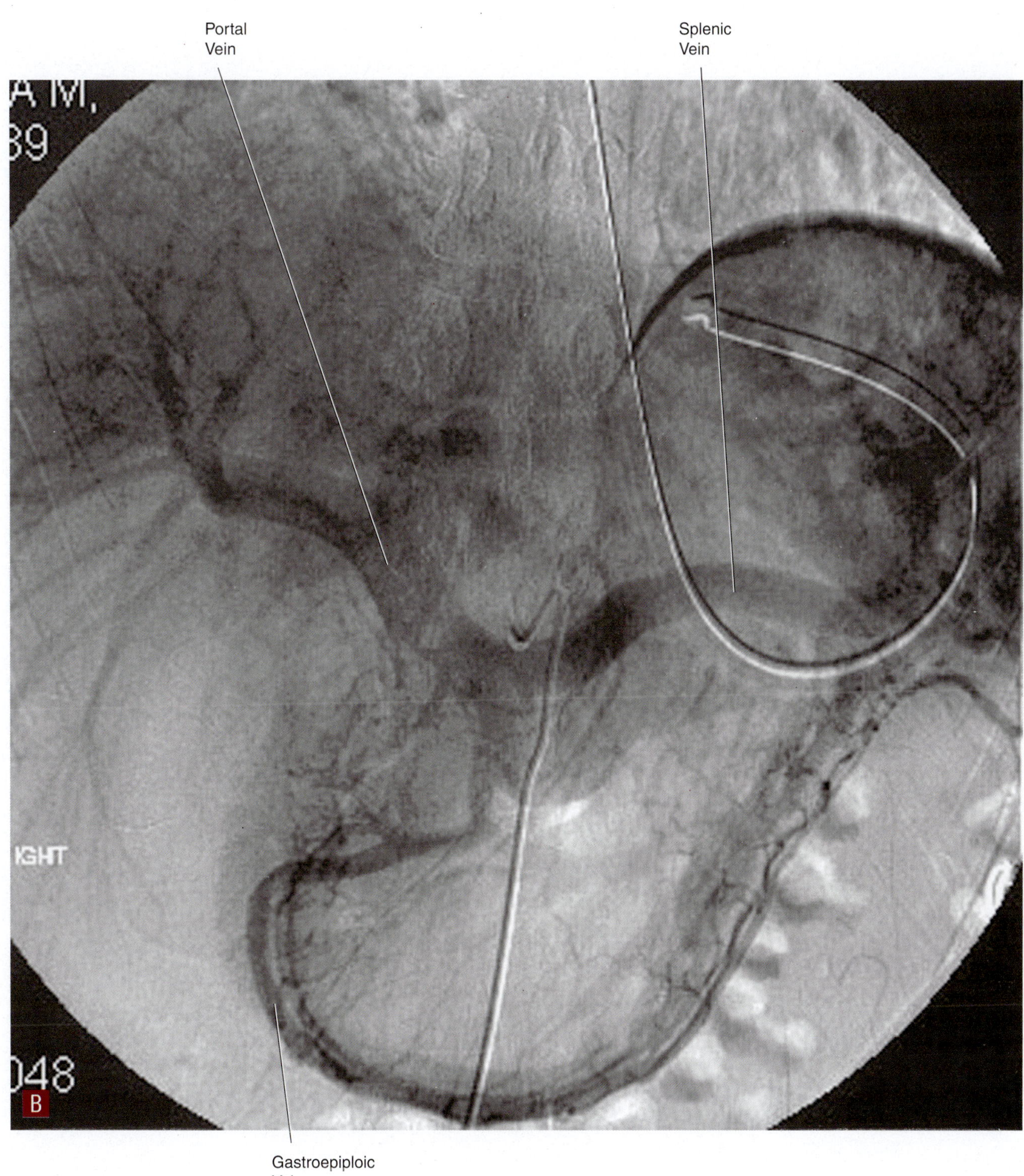

Figure 18.37. *Continued*

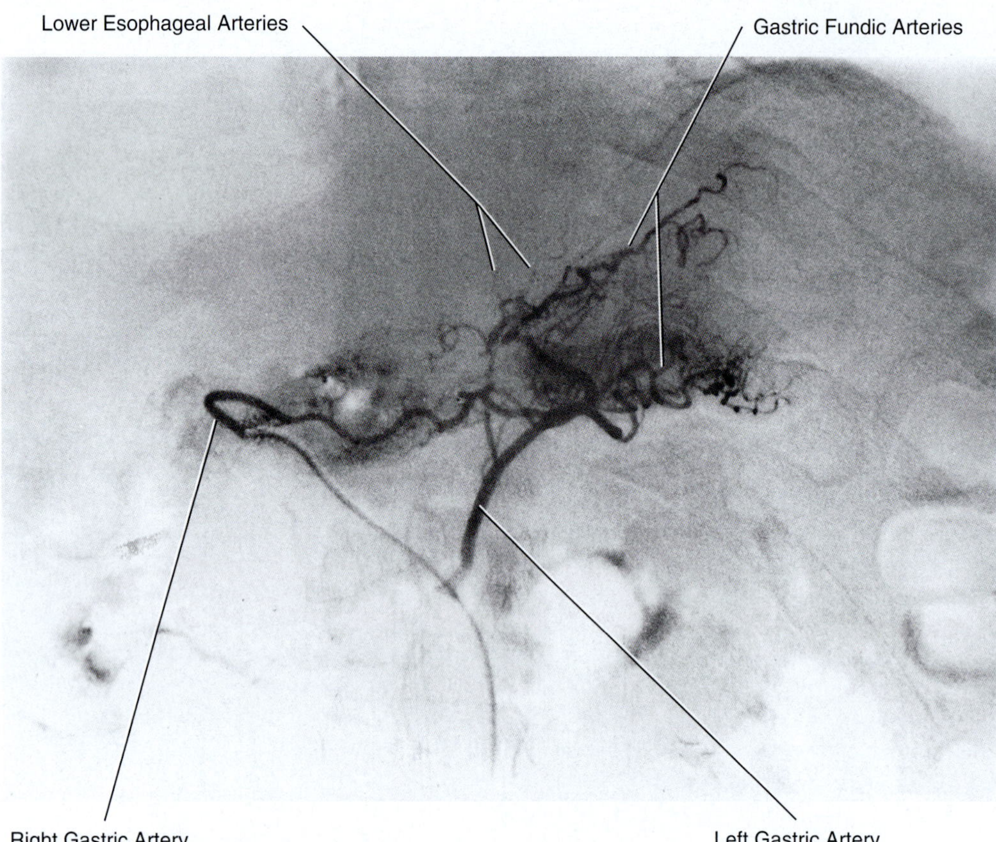

Figure 18.38. Selective angiography of the right gastric artery showing the anastomosis with the left gastric artery and the filling of the gastric wall circulation at the fundus.

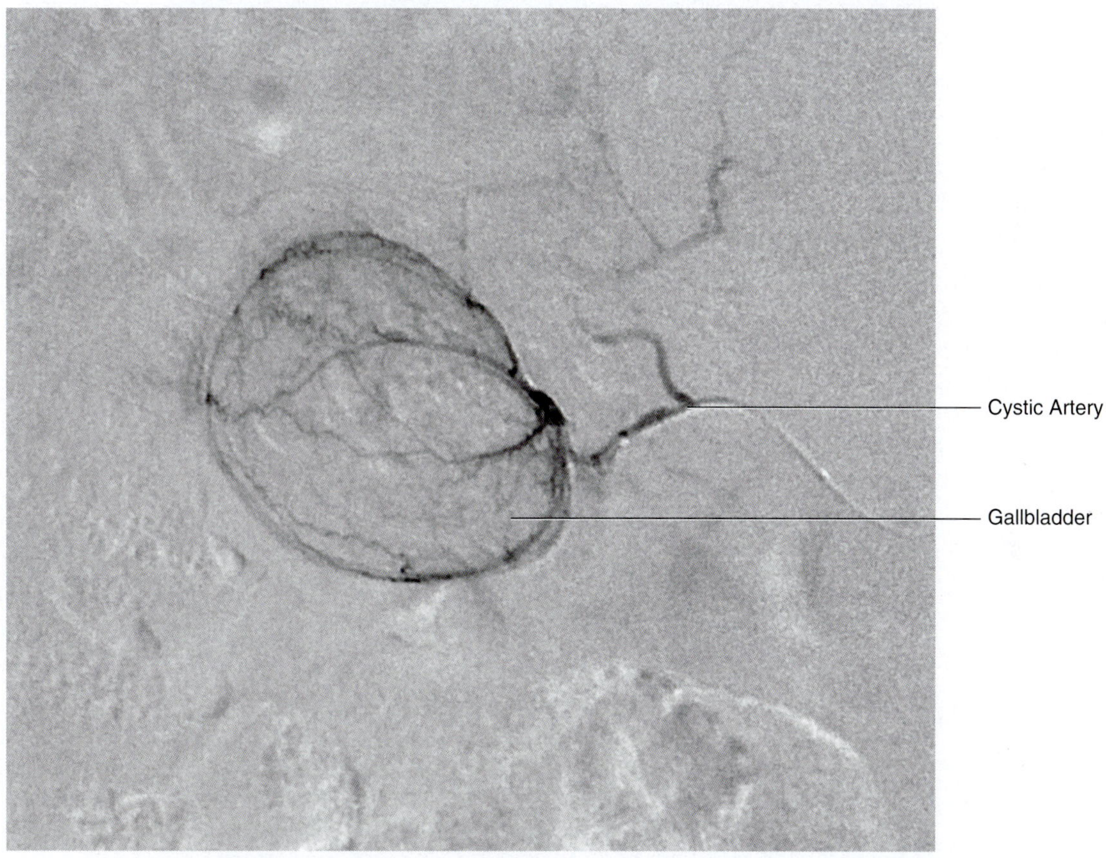

Figure 18.39. **Selective injection at the cystic artery.** Note the small size of the arteries and the bulging of the arteries around the gallbladder.

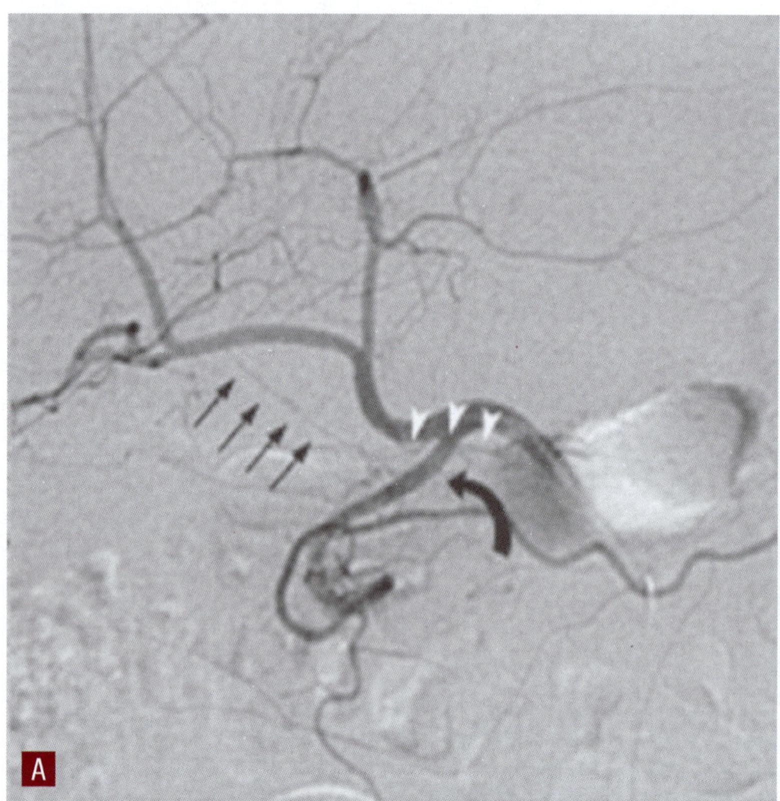

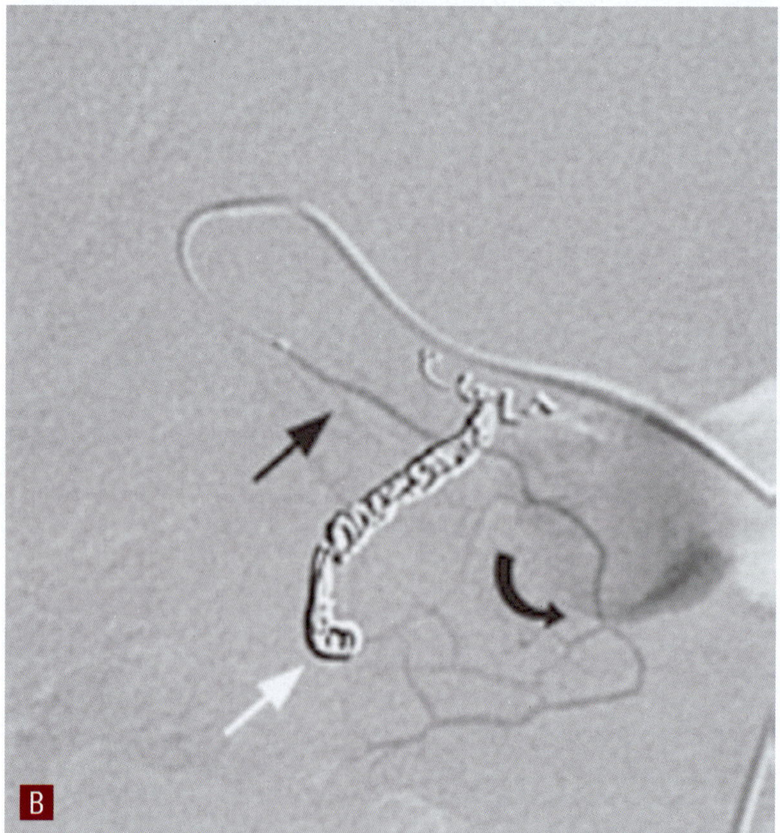

Figure 18.40. A, Hepatic arteriography showing a small supraduodenal artery, arising from the right hepatic artery (straight arrows). The gastroduodenal artery is indicated by the curved arrow. The right gastric artery arises from the proper hepatic artery (white arrowheads). B, Superselective catheterization of the supraduodenal artery (straight arrow) demonstrates the connection with duodenal branches (curved arrow). The gastroduodenal artery and right gastric artery were embolized (white arrow). (Reprinted from Liu DM, et al. Angiographic considerations in patients undergoing liver-direct therapy. *J Vasc Interv Radiol.* 2005;16:911-935 with permission from Elsevier.)

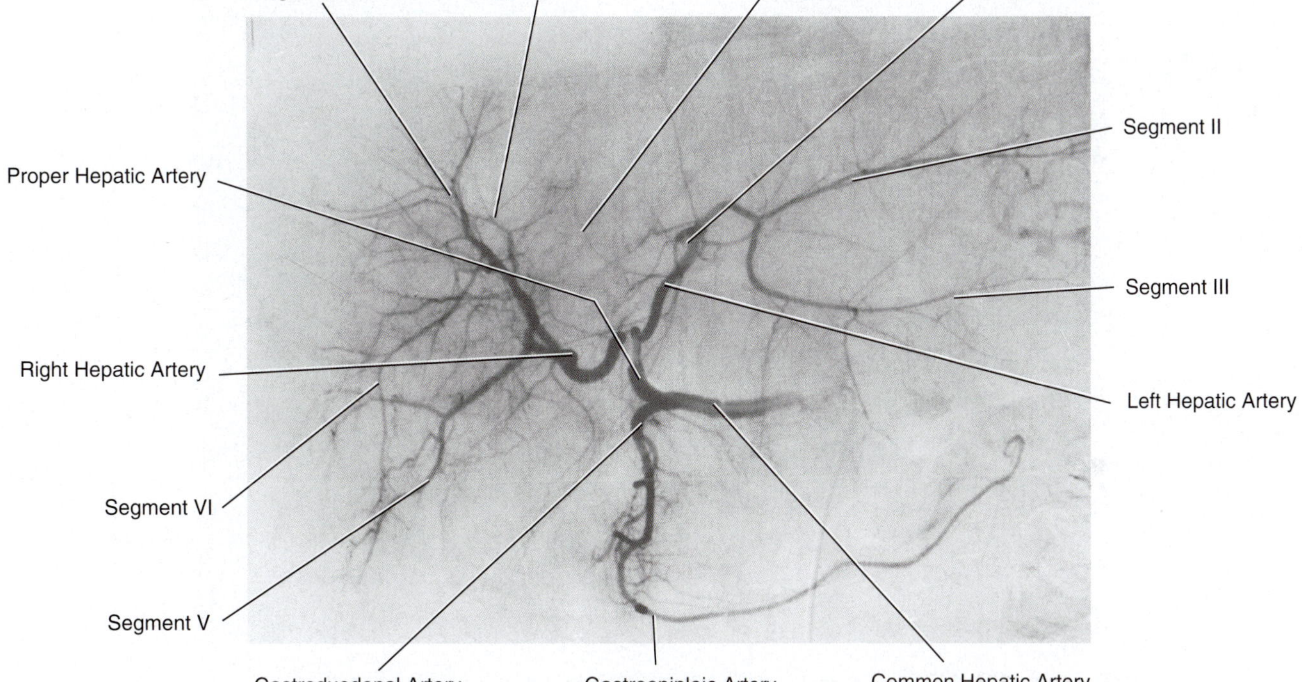

Figure 18.41. Selective injection of the proper hepatic artery showing the intrahepatic circulation, the gastroduodenal artery, and the gastroepiploic artery. The left lobe of the liver is enlarged. There is spasm of the hepatic arteries at the bifurcation.

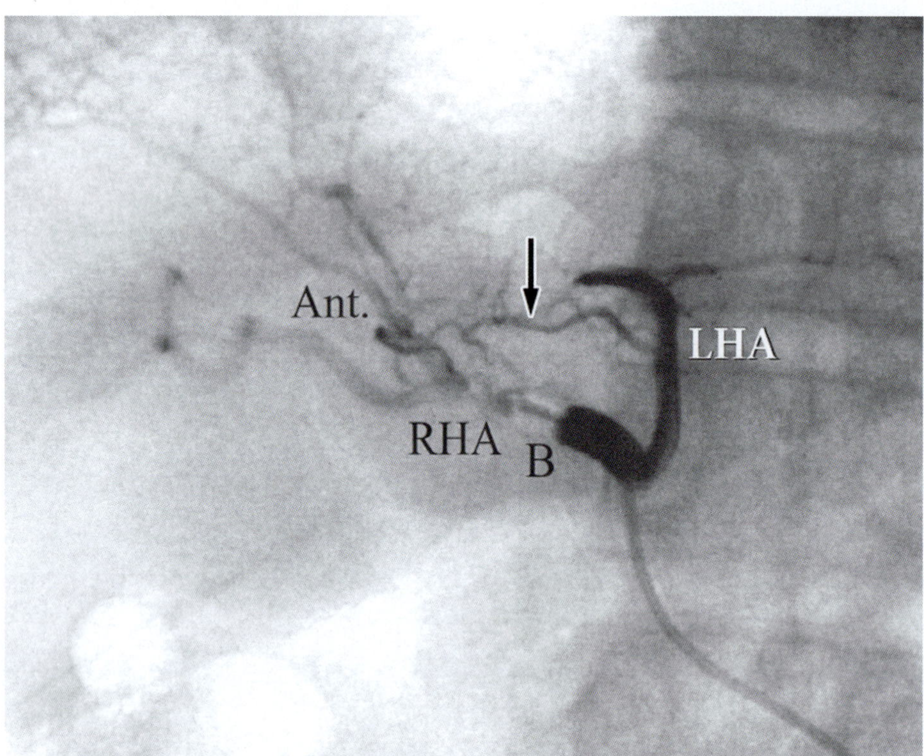

Figure 18.42. Angiography of the left hepatic artery during temporary balloon occlusion of the right hepatic artery. The communicating arcade is seen as a thin artery (arrow) in the hepatic hilum and originates from the left hepatic artery and joins both the right hepatic artery and right anterior hepatic artery. Ant, right anterior hepatic artery; B, balloon; LHA, left hepatic artery; RHA, right hepatic artery. (Reprinted from Tohma T, et al. Communicating arcade between the right and left hepatic arteries: evaluation with CT and angiography during temporary balloon occlusion of the right or left hepatic artery. *Radiology*. 2005;237:361-365 with permission from RSNA.)

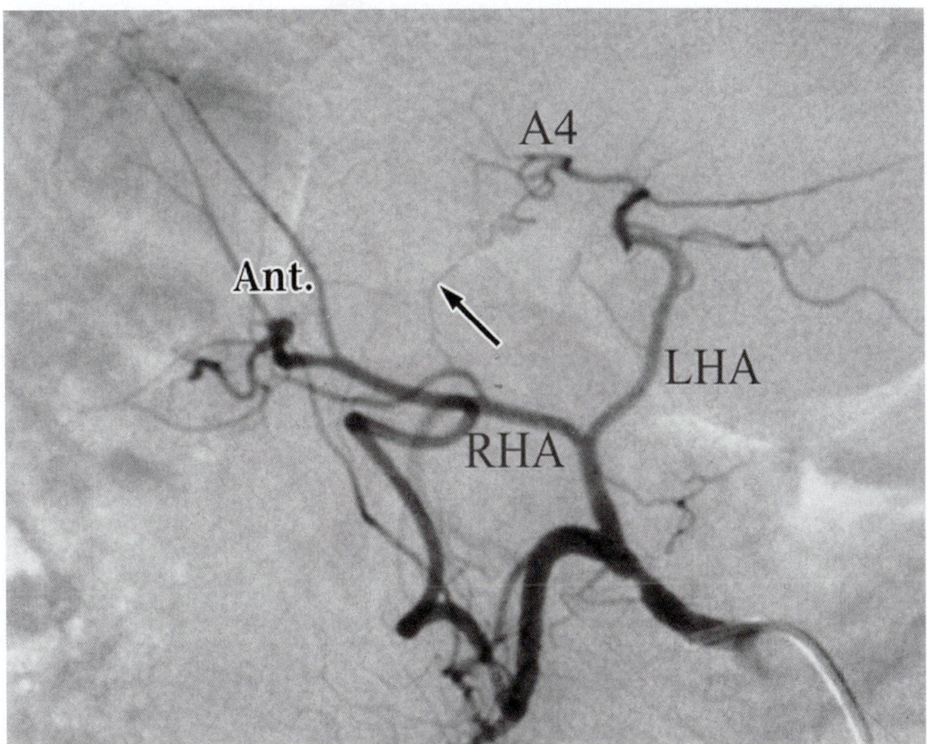

Figure 18.43. Angiography of the proper hepatic artery showing the communicating arcade (arrow) in the hepatic hilum, originating from the segment IV artery (branch of the left hepatic artery), reaching both the right hepatic artery and the arcade right anterior hepatic artery. A4, segment IV artery; Ant, right anterior hepatic artery; LHA, left hepatic artery; RHA, right hepatic artery. (Reprinted from Tohma T, et al. Communicating arcade between the right and left hepatic arteries: evaluation with CT and angiography during temporary balloon occlusion of the right or left hepatic artery. *Radiology*. 2005;237:361-365 with permission from RSNA.)

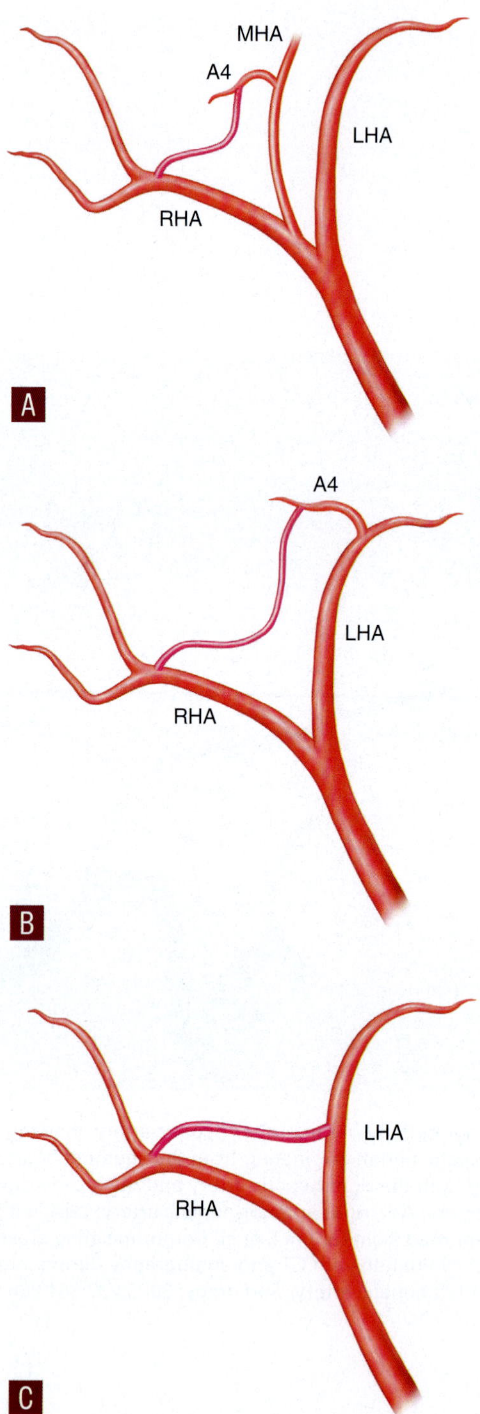

Figure 18.44. Diagram showing the branching patterns of the communicating arcade (CA) (solid black line) on the left side. **A**, Diagram of the CA originating from the segment IV artery from the middle hepatic artery (type 1a). **B**, Diagram of CA originating from the segment IV artery, from the left hepatic artery (type 1b). **C**, Diagram of CA originating from the left hepatic artery (type 2). A4, segment IV artery; LHA, left hepatic artery; RHA, right hepatic artery. (Reprinted from Tohma T, et al. Communicating arcade between the right and left hepatic arteries: evaluation with CT and angiography during temporary balloon occlusion of the right or left hepatic artery. *Radiology*. 2005;237:361-365 with permission from RSNA.)

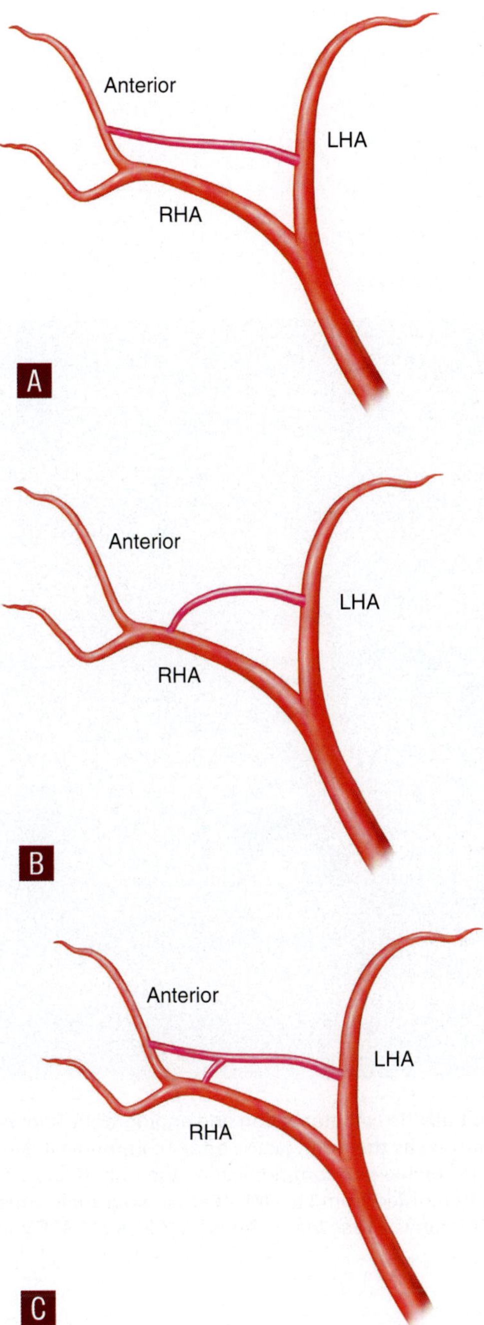

Figure 18.45. Diagram showing the branching point of the communicating arcade (CA) (solid black line) on the right side. **A**, Diagram of CA originating from the right anterior hepatic artery (type 1). **B**, diagram of CA originating from the right hepatic artery (type 2). **C**, Diagram of CA originating from both the right anterior hepatic artery and the right hepatic artery (type 3). A4, segment IV artery; LHA, left hepatic artery; RHA, right hepatic artery. (Reprinted from Tohma T, et al. Communicating arcade between the right and left hepatic arteries: evaluation with CT and angiography during temporary balloon occlusion of the right or left hepatic artery. *Radiology*. 2005;237:361-365 with permission from RSNA.)

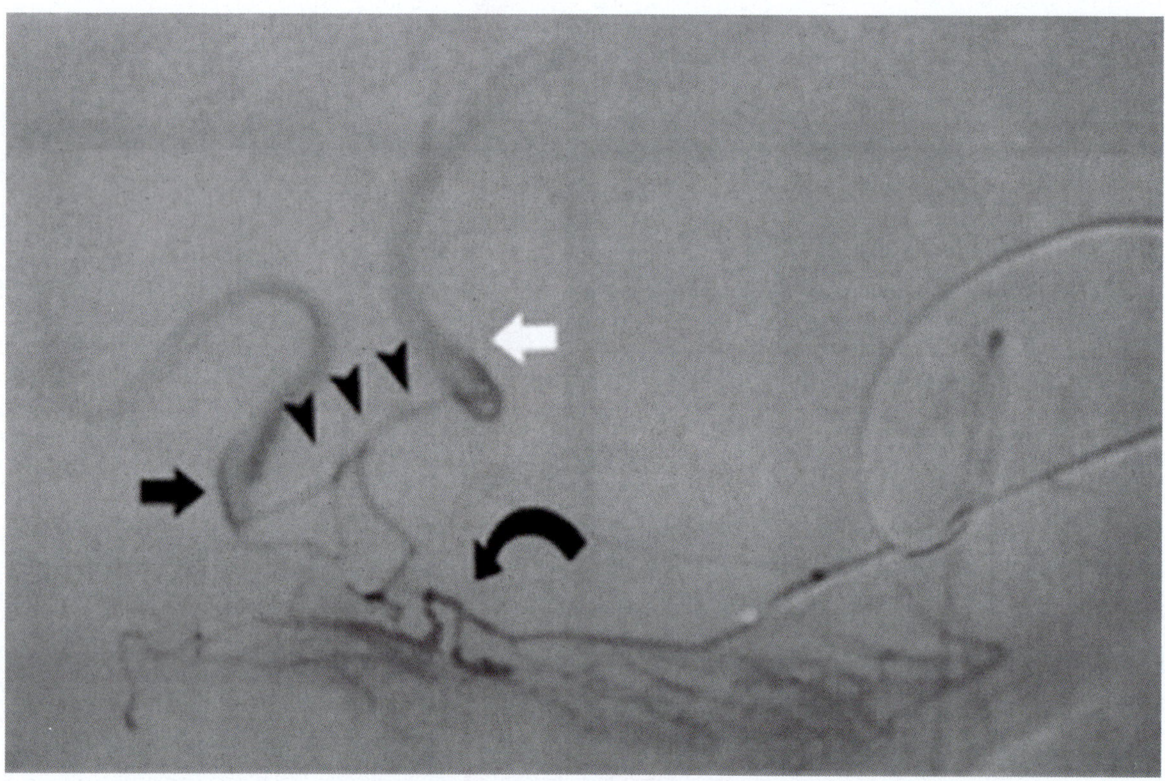

Figure 18.46. Left gastric catheterization and angiography shows the square-shaped vessel (curved arrow) as the right gastric artery communicates with an intrahepatic communicating arcade (arrowheads), communicating the right (black arrow) and left (white arrow) hepatic arteries. (Reprinted from Liu DM, et al. Angiographic considerations in patients undergoing liver-direct therapy. *J Vasc Interv Radiol.* 2005;16:911-935 with permission from Elsevier.)

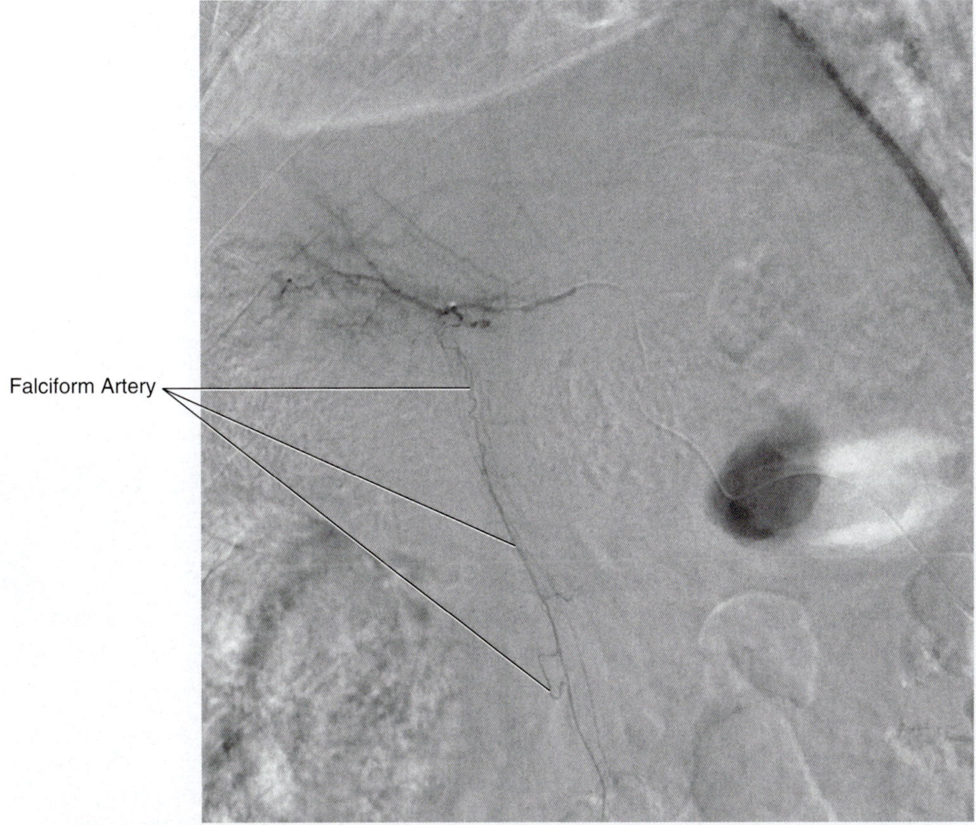

Figure 18.47. Left hepatic arteriogram demonstrates the falciform artery as it travels through the falciform ligament, terminating in the anterior abdominal wall, and anastomoses with the superior epigastric vessels.

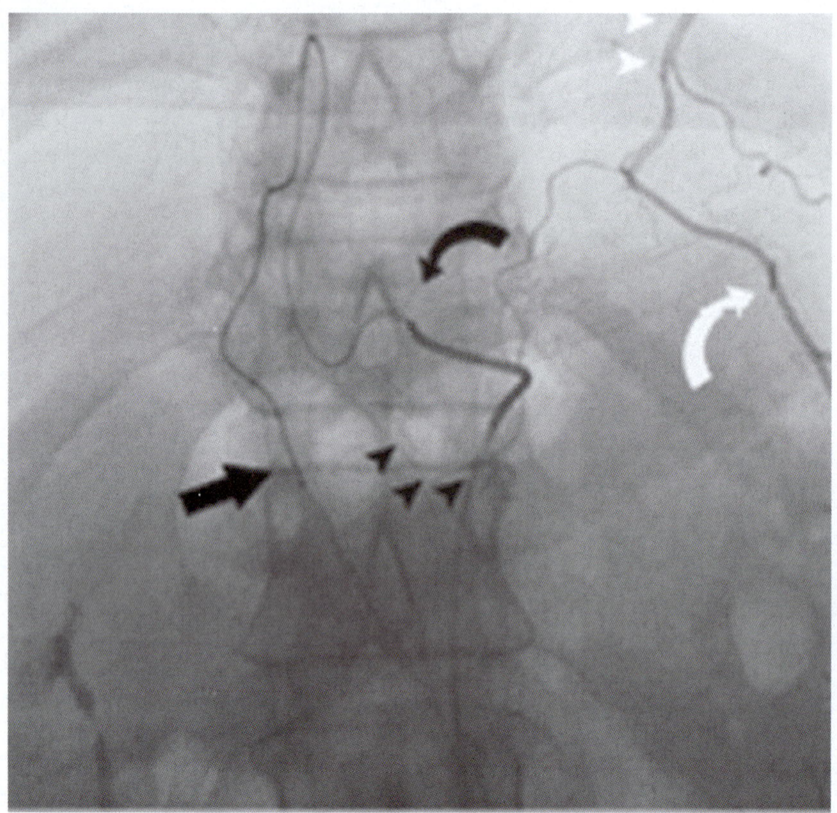

Figure 18.48. Angiogram of the falciform artery (straight arrow) in a different patient demonstrates the communication (black arrowheads) with the superior artery (white curved arrow) and musculophrenic artery (white arrowheads). The catheter is shown (curved arrow). (Reprinted from Liu DM, et al. Angiographic considerations in patients undergoing liver-direct therapy. *J Vasc Interv Radiol.* 2005;16:911-935 with permission from Elsevier.)

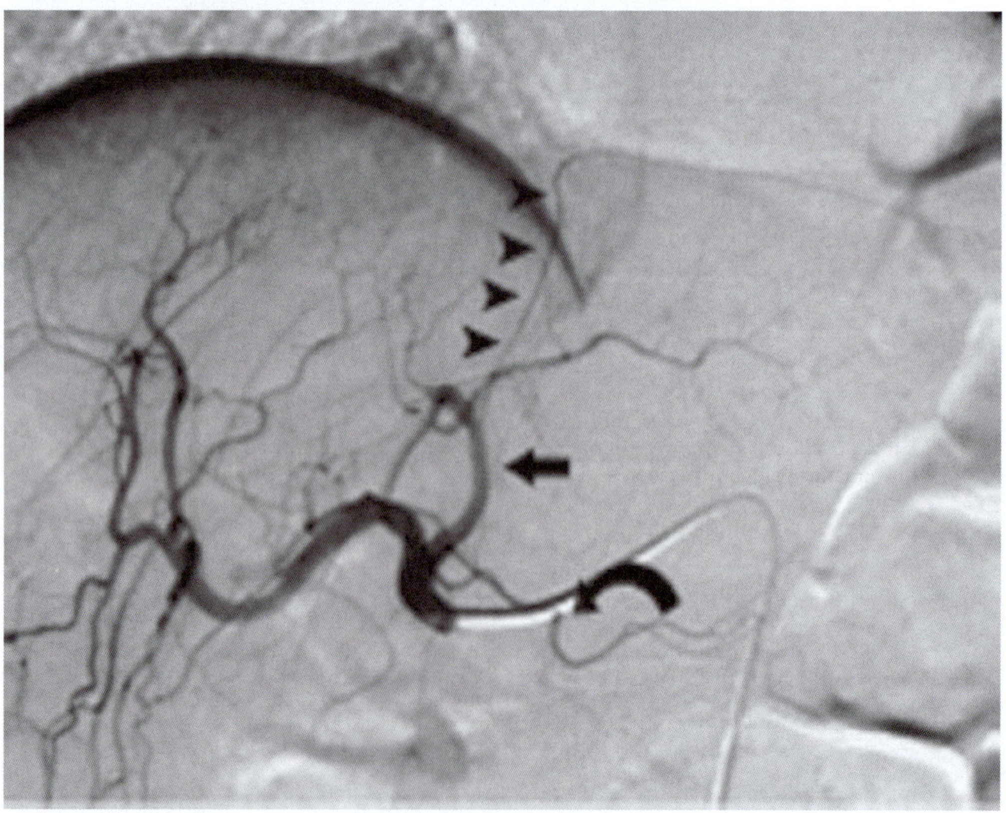

Figure 18.49. Common hepatic arteriogram with phrenic-esophageal branch (arrowheads) arising from the left hepatic artery (arrow) and right gastric artery (curved arrow). (Reprinted from Liu DM, et al. Angiographic considerations in patients undergoing liver-direct therapy. *J Vasc Interv Radiol.* 2005;16:911-935 with permission from Elsevier.)

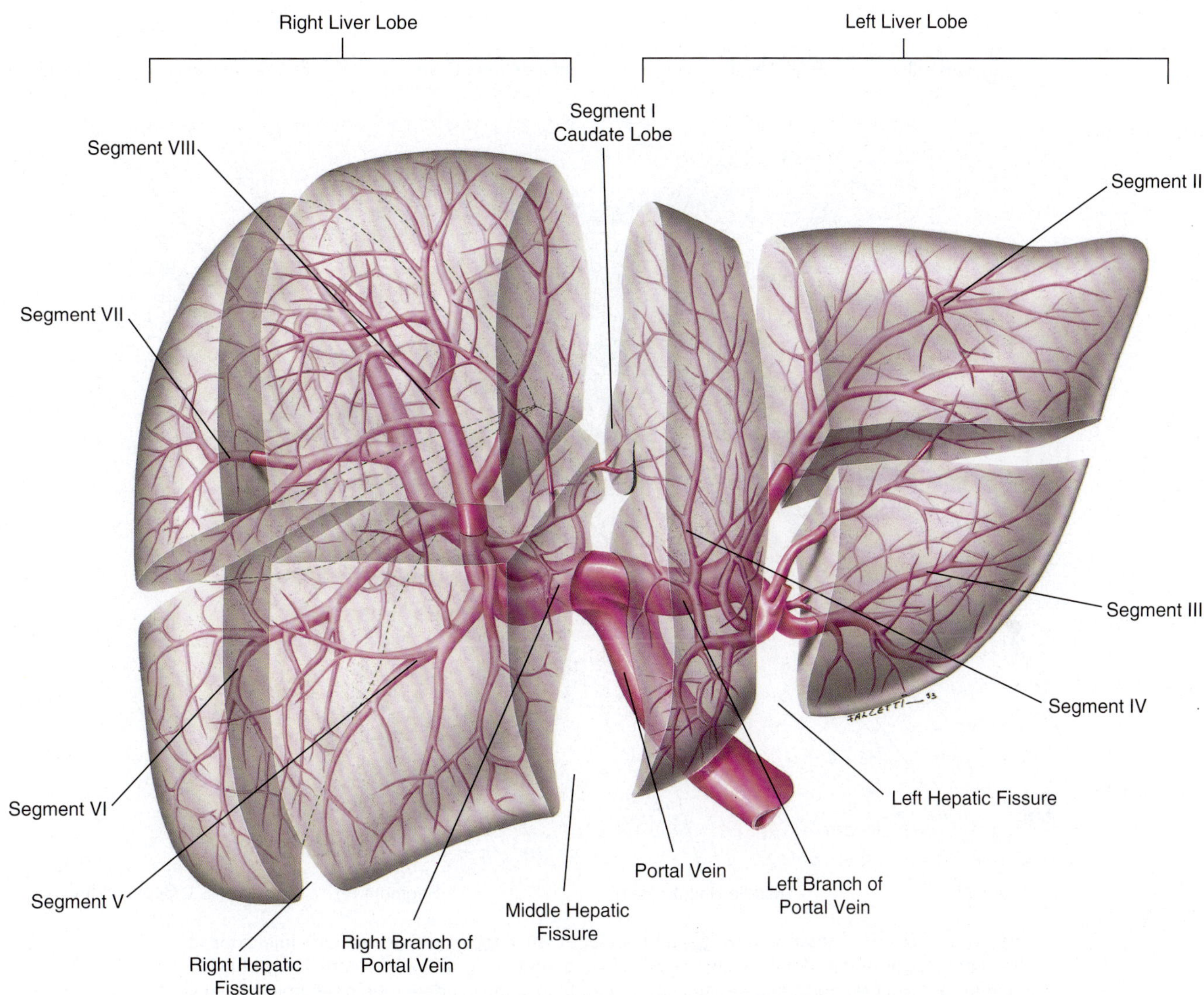

Figure 18.50. Schematic drawing of the hepatic segments according to the Couinaud description, showing the portal vein distribution, the hepatic lobar division, and hepatic fissures.

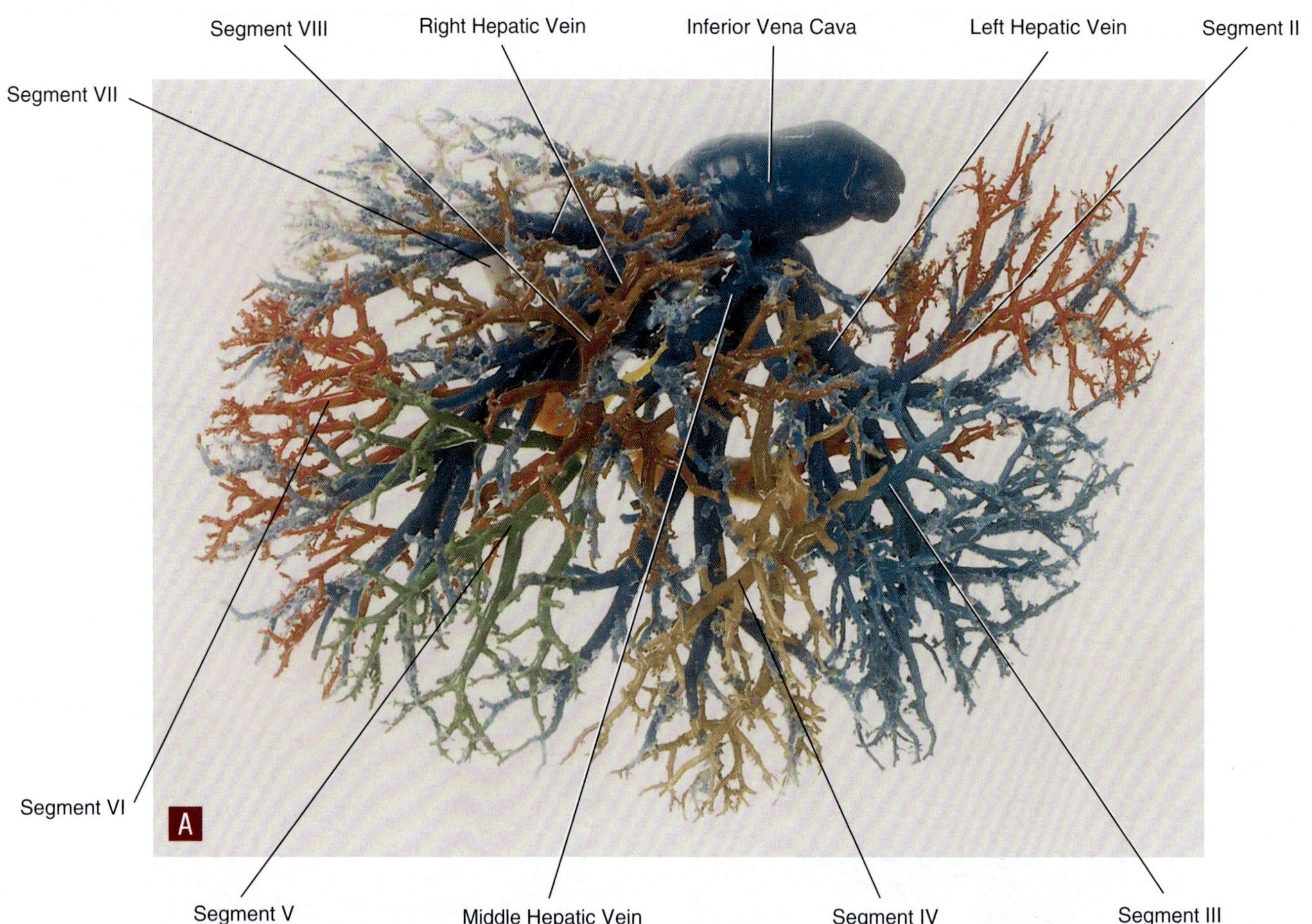

Figure 18.51. Anterior view (A) and posterior view (B) of a liver cast with injections in the hepatic veins and portal vein, showing the liver segments in different colors. Navy blue is the inferior vena cava (IVC) and hepatic veins, light blue is the caudate lobe or segment I, red is segment II, darker blue is segment III, light brown is segment IV, green is segment V, light red is segment VI, white is segment VII, and brown is segment VIII.

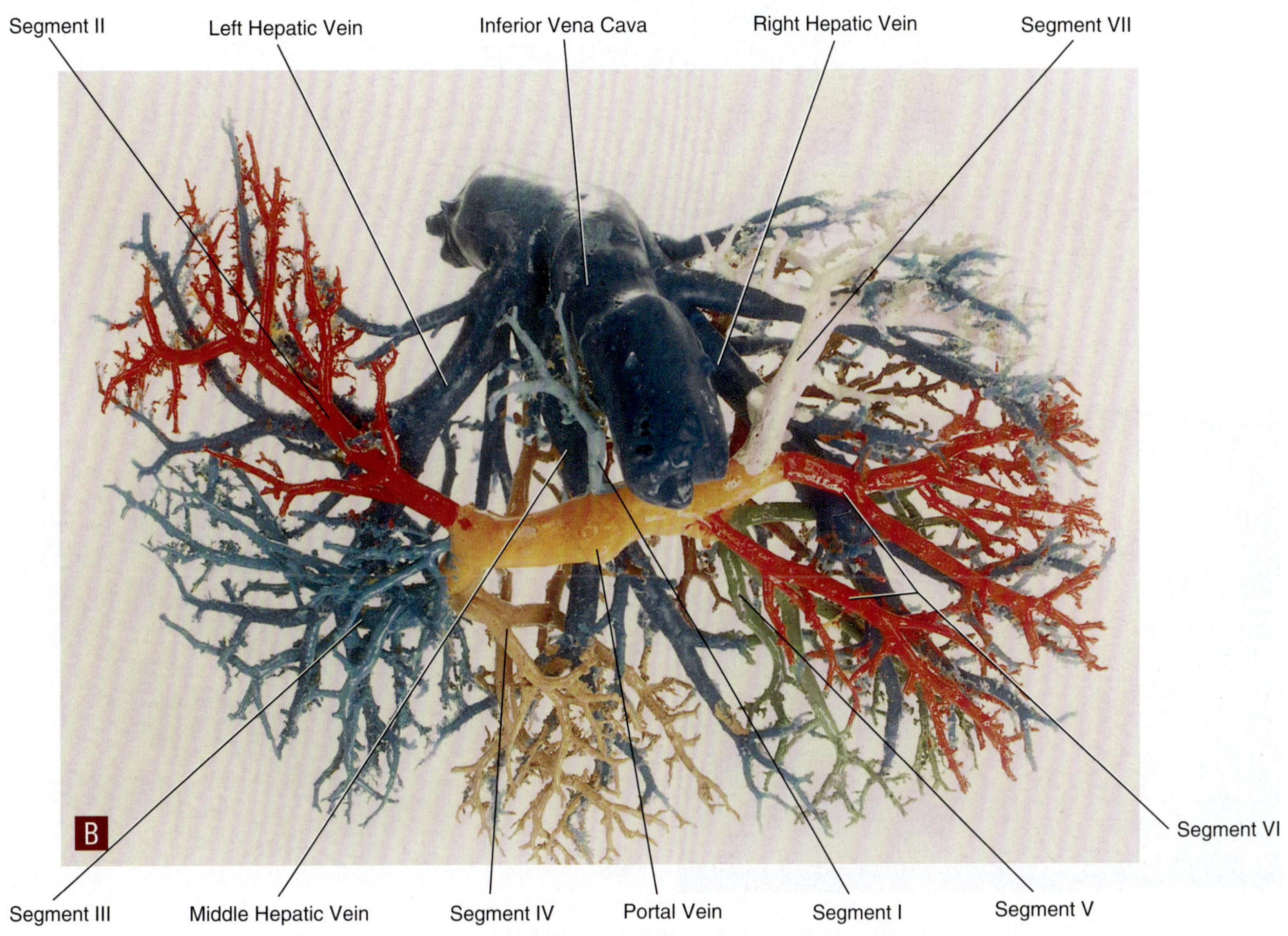

Figure 18.51. *Continued*

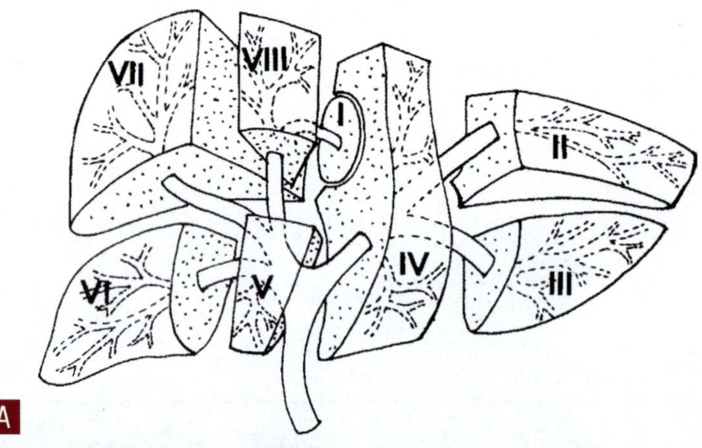

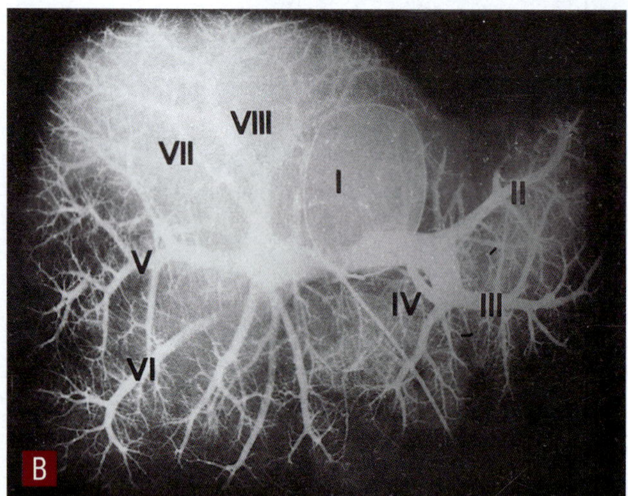

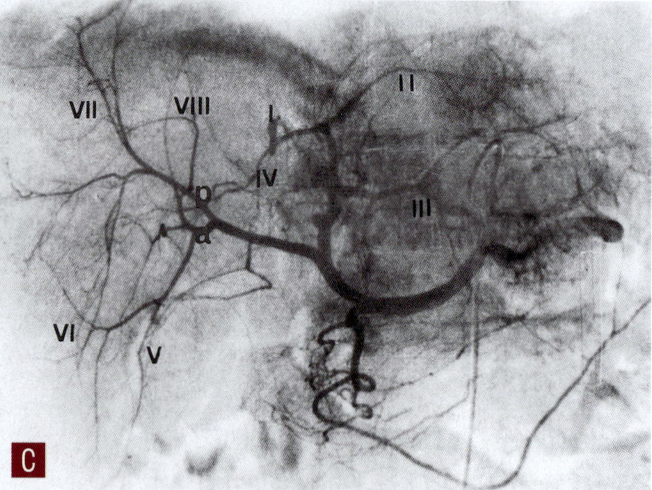

Figure 18.52. **A**, Schematic drawing of the liver segments according to Couinaud description. **B**, Specimen injection in the portal vein depicting the liver segments I through VIII. **C**, Arterial angiogram of the liver showing the hepatic segments in the hepatic artery branches. Note the presence of a large tumoral mass in the left lobe of the liver.

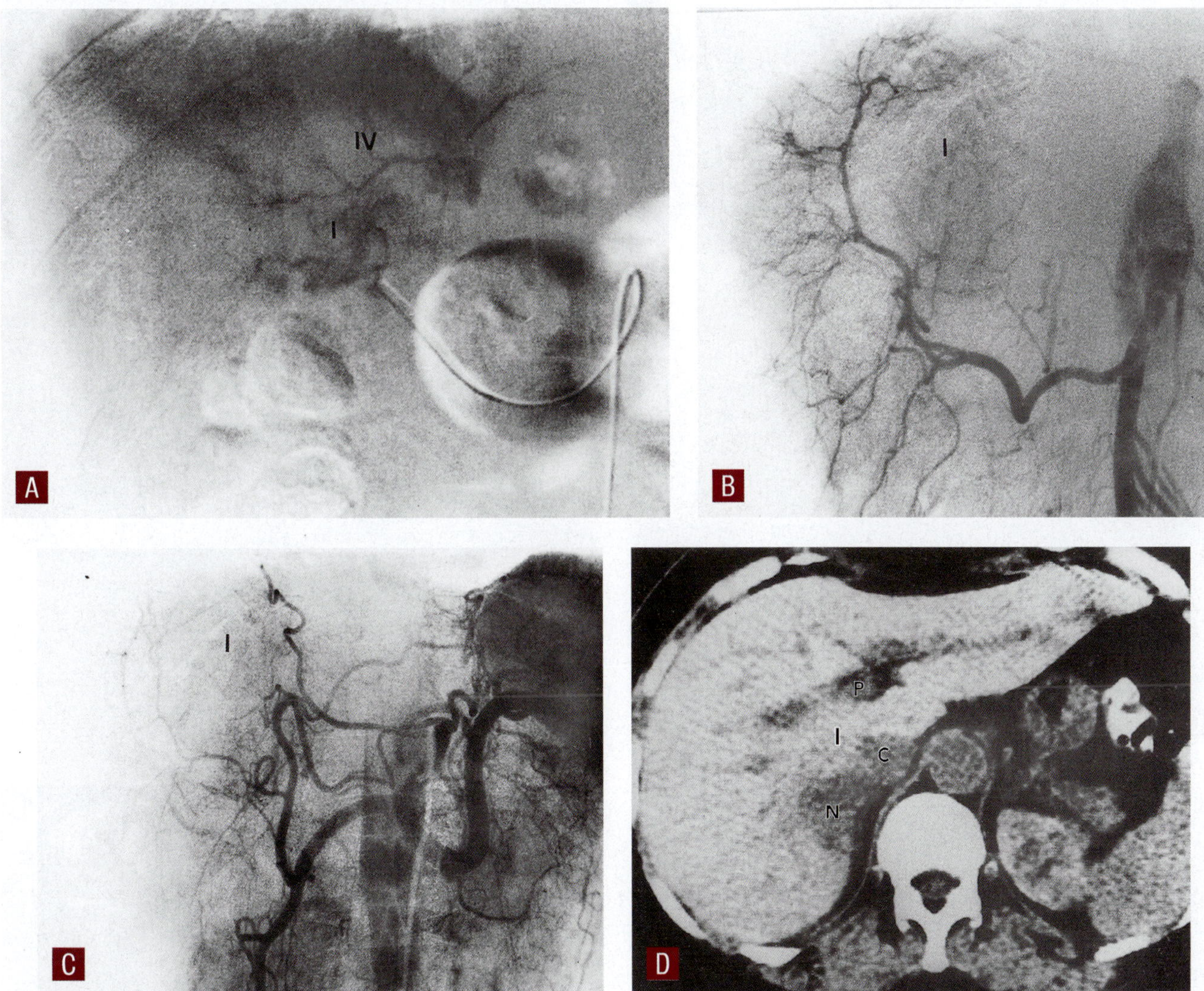

Figure 18.53. Hepatic arteriography. A, Selective injection at the segment I (caudate lobe). Note that segment IV is also opacified. B, Replaced right hepatic artery showing some contrast stain at segment I with arterial feeders from the right hepatic artery. C, Same patient as in B, showing feeders from the left hepatic artery to segment I. Note the liver stain at the same place due to the tumoral lesion observed in the computerized tomographic (CT) scan of the liver. D, CT scan of the liver showing the metastatic tumoral lesion at the segment I, adjacent to the IVC.

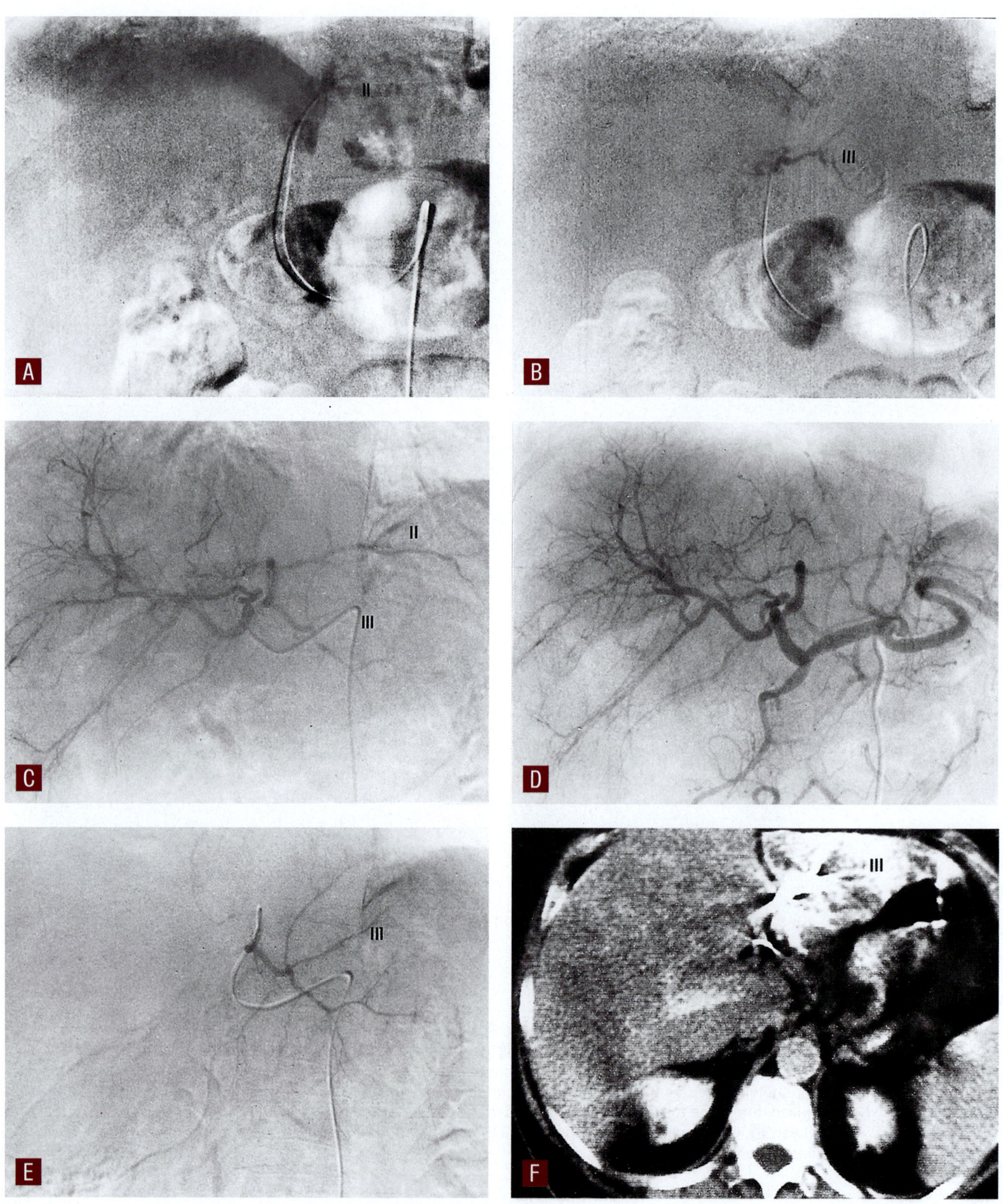

Figure 18.54. A, Superselective angiography of the hepatic segment II. B, Superselective angiography of hepatic segment III. C, Celiac angiography showing the liver arterial segments. D, Superselective hepatic angiography showing the segments II and III well opacified. E, Superselective injection at the hepatic segment III. F, CT scan of the liver showing selective stain of the hepatic segment III. Note the medial limit of segment III by the falciform ligament.

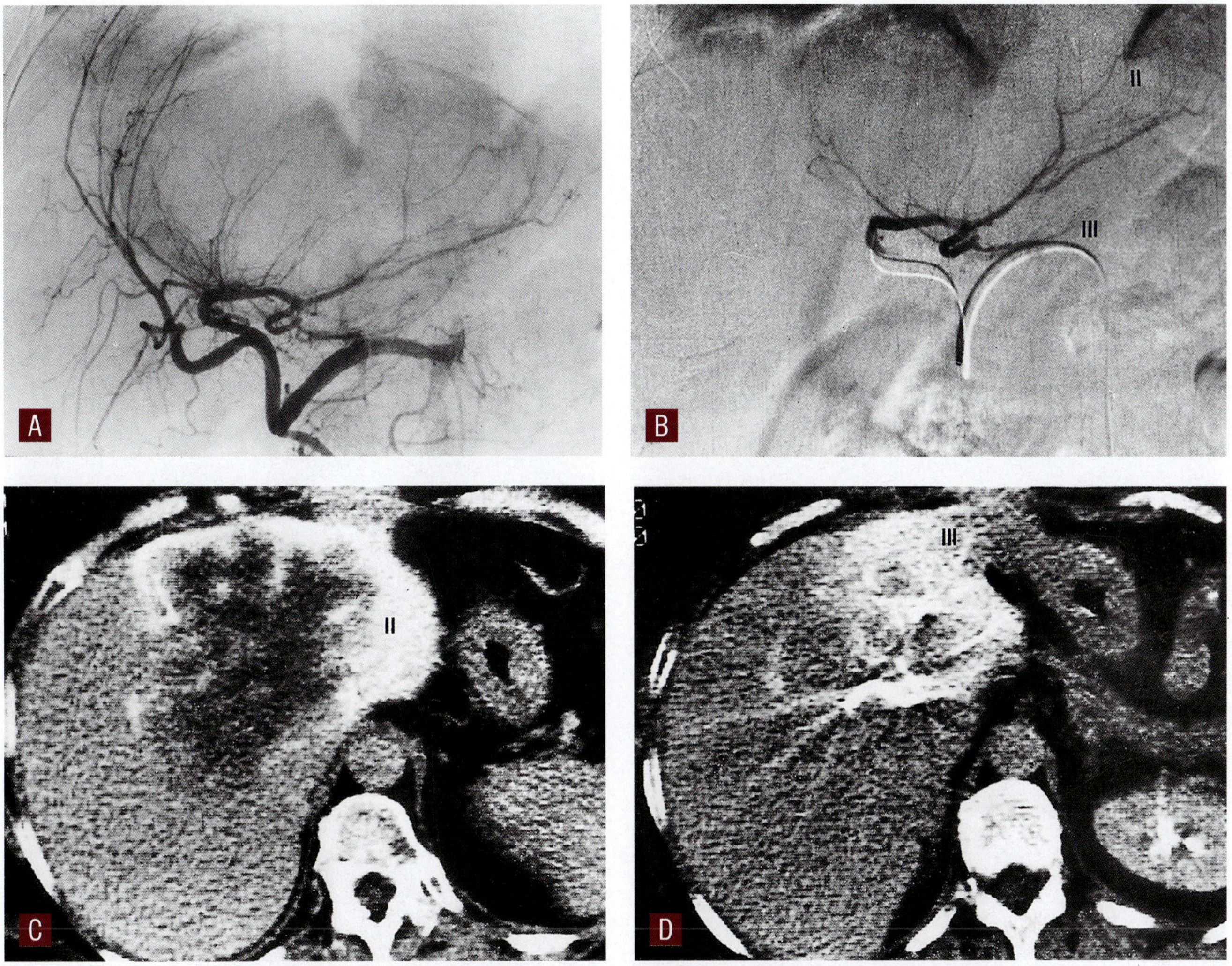

Figure 18.55. A, Hepatic angiography showing the left lobe of the liver enlarged and with the arteries displaced by a metastatic lesion but showing the segments II and III. B, Selective injection in the left hepatic artery showing segments II and III. C, CT scan of the liver showing selective stain of the segment II. D, CT scan of the liver showing selective stain of the segment III.

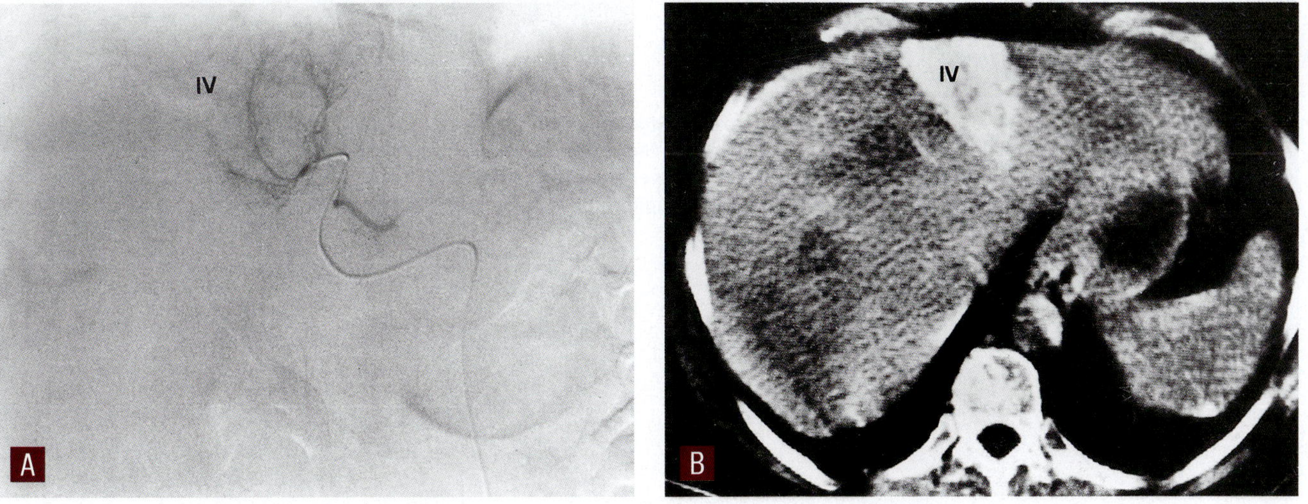

Figure 18.56. A, Superselective angiography of the segment IV. B, CT scan of the liver showing the segment IV with the typical appearance of a wedge with the base turned ventrally.

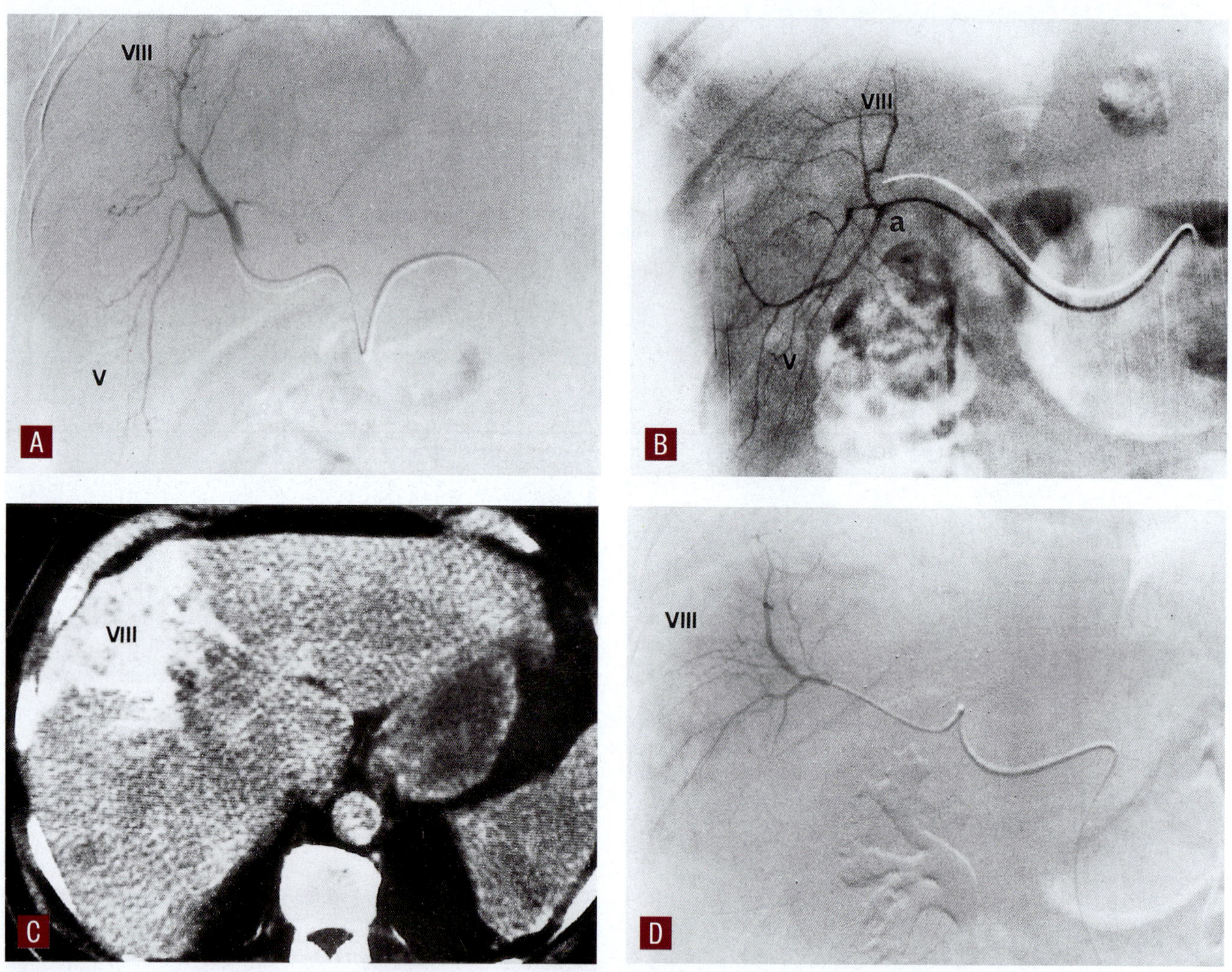

Figure 18.57. **A**, Superselective angiography of the segments V and VIII (sector anteromedial of the right lobe of the liver). **B**, Superselective angiography of the segments V and VIII in another patient. **C**, CT scan of the liver showing segment VIII with a dense stain due to the selective injection. **D**, Superselective angiography of the segment VIII of the liver used to perform the CT shown in part C of the figure.

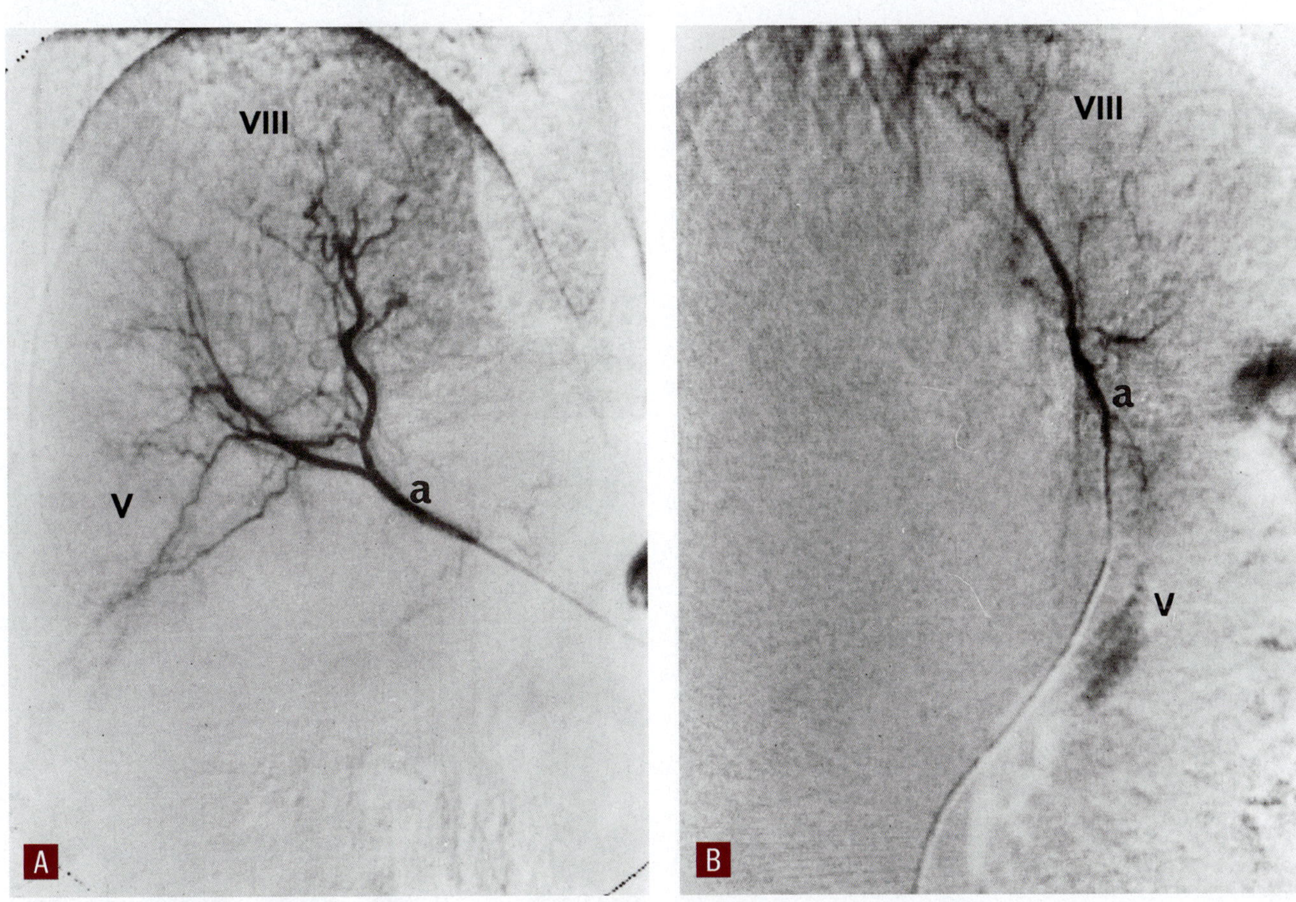

Figure 18.58. A, Anterior view of a selective injection of the anterior branch of the right hepatic artery showing segments V and VIII. B, Lateral view of the selective injection of the anterior branch of the right hepatic artery depicting segments V and VIII.

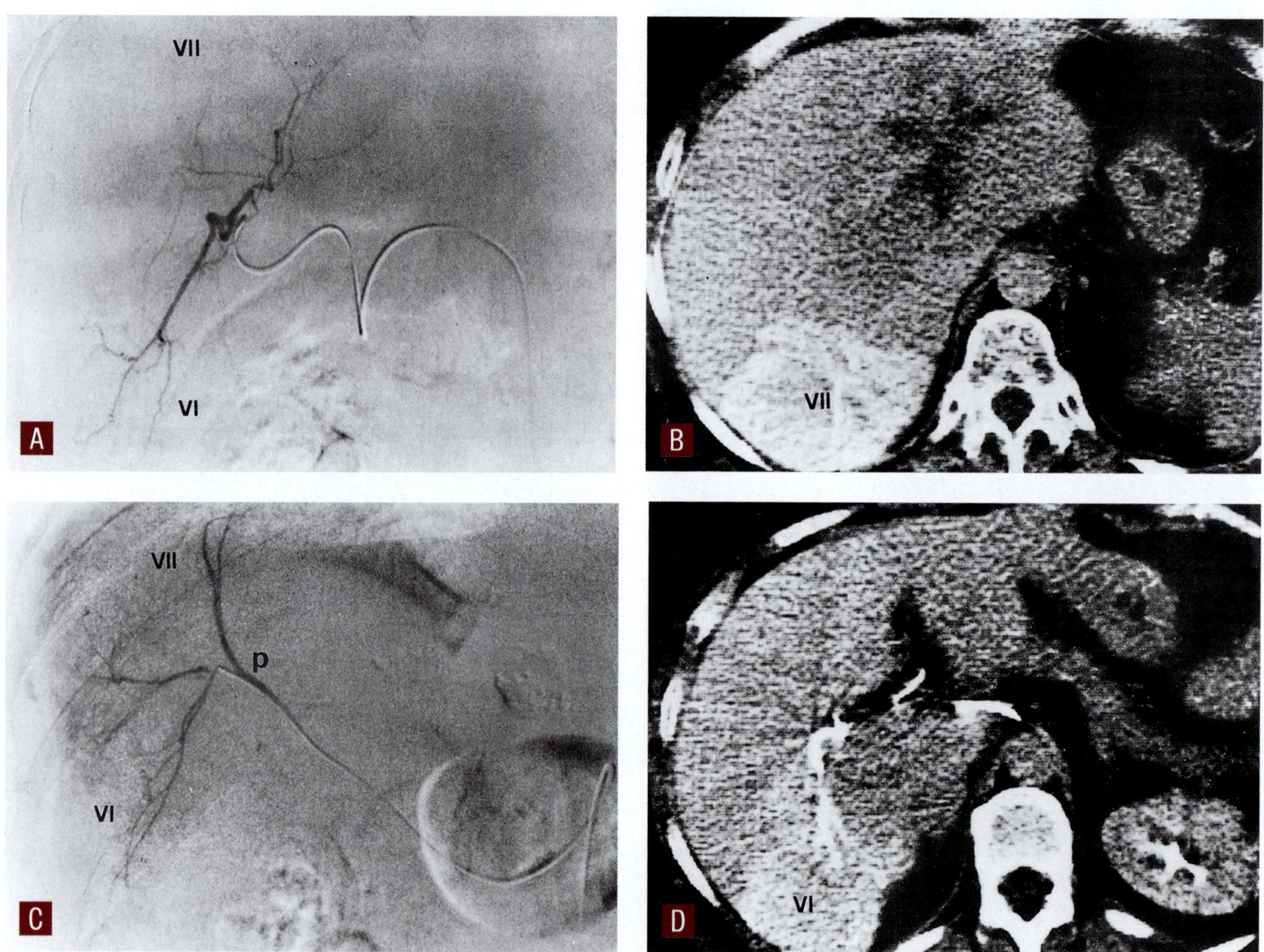

Figure 18.59. **A**, Anterior view of a selective injection of the posterior branch of the right hepatic artery showing segments VI and VII (sector posterolateral of the right lobe of the liver). **B**, CT scan of the liver showing the stain at the segment VII. **C**, Selective angiography at the posterior branch of the right hepatic artery, showing segments VI and VII. **D**, CT scan of the liver showing the stain at the segment VI.

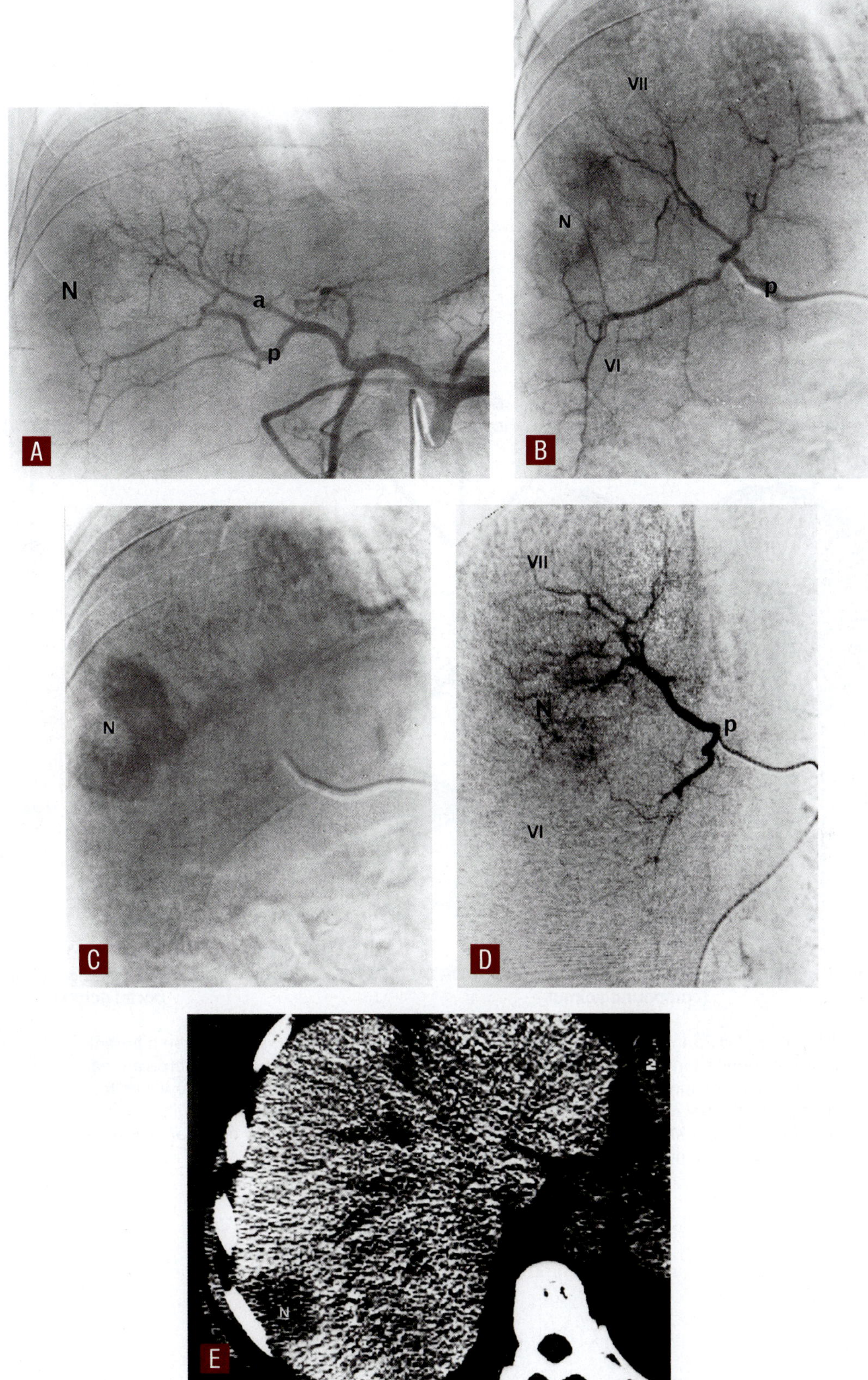

Figure 18.60. A, Celiac artery injection showing the bifurcation of the right hepatic artery in anterior and posterior branches. N denotes a tumoral nodule. B, Superselective angiography of the right posterior branch of the hepatic artery. Segments VI and VII are clearly visualized. N denotes the tumoral lesion with nutrient arteries from both segments. C, Later phase of the angiogram showing the tumoral nodule (N). D, Lateral view of the injection at the posterior branch of the right hepatic artery, showing the segments VI and VII. Note the tumor nodule stain. The selective injection at the anterior branch of the right hepatic artery of the same patient is seen on Fig. 18.45A and B, E, CT scan of the liver showing the lesion (N) between the segments VI and VII, at the posterolateral sector of the right lobe of the liver.

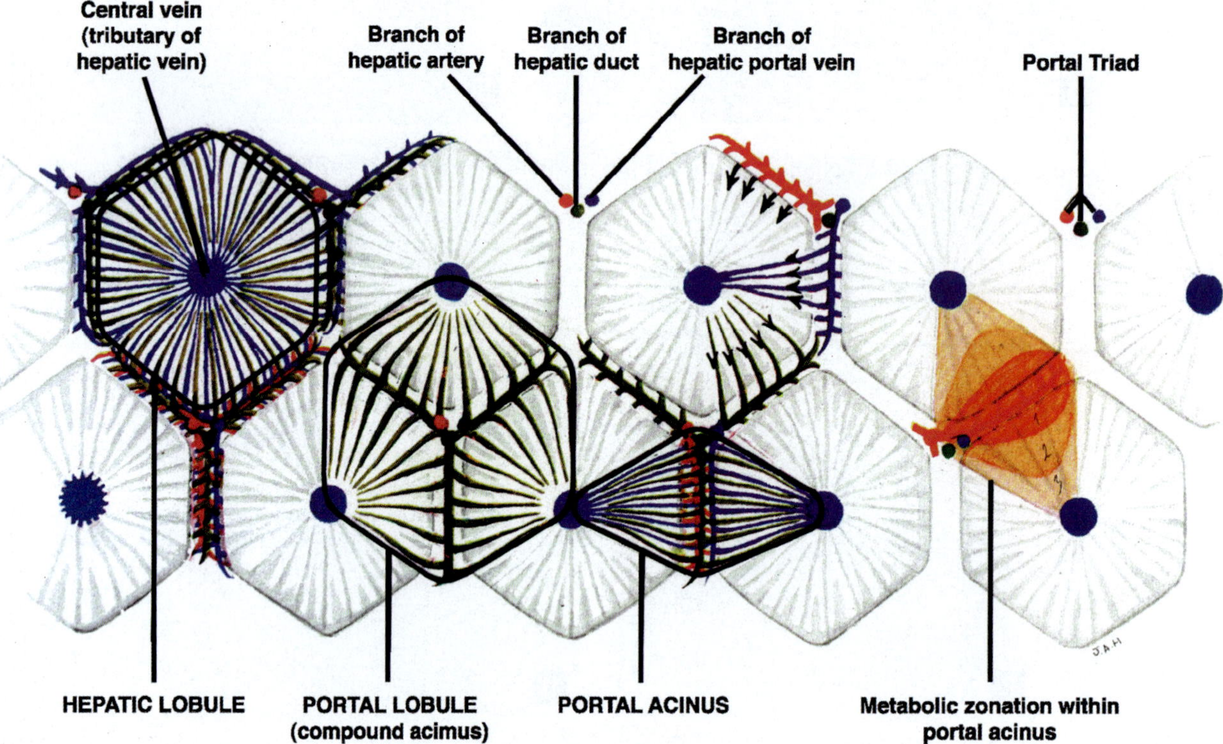

Figure 18.61. Diagram of the histologic structure of the liver, showing the different types of subdivisions proposed. The hexagonal structure depicted is based in some animal species, and not applicable to humans, for which structure is highly variable; however, for purposes of clarity it is showed in the highly schematic way. (Reprinted from Williams PL, Warwick R, Dyson M, Bannister LH. Angiology. In: *Gray's Anatomy.* 37th ed, Chap 6. Edinburgh: Churchill Livingstone; 1989:661-858 with permission.)

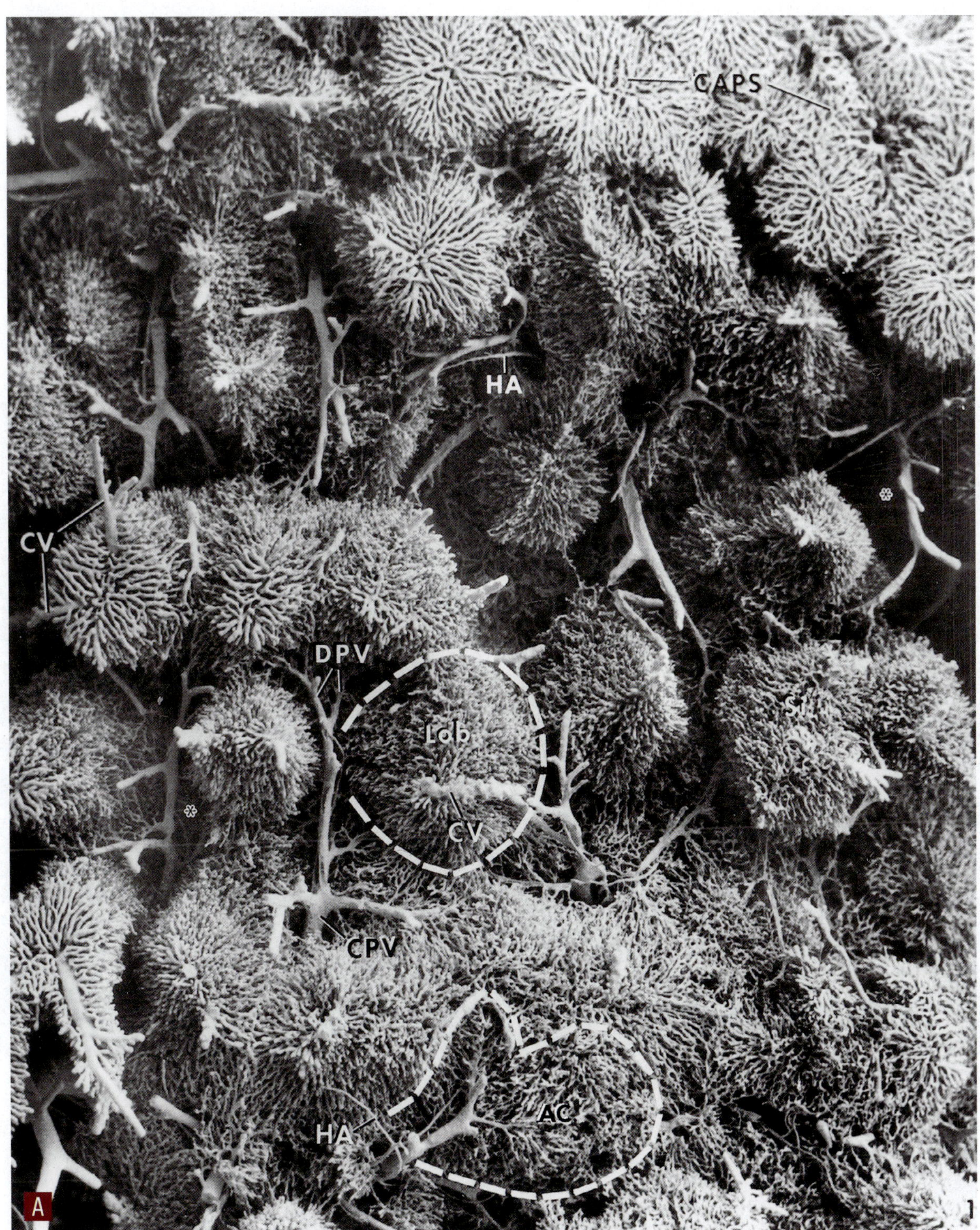

Figure 18.62. **A**, **Scanning electron microscopy** (SEM) of casted hepatic microcirculation in both capsular (CAPS) and subcapsular regions. The capsular surface is shown in upper right of figure, and the adjacent regions of the cast are from areas underlying this plane. Zone one (1), two (2), and three (3) of the liver acinus are denoted at the bottom of the figure. Adjacent areas also contain sinusoids (Si), the arrangement of which corresponds to a lobular (Lob) parenchymal organization; conducting portal vein (CPV); distributing portal vein (DPV), collecting venule (CV); hepatic arteriole (HA); and noncasted areas in portal tracts (*) (×65). **B**, The left side of Fig. 18.48B, is an enlargement of the lower portion of Fig. 18.48A (×75), and the right side is an enlargement of the area enclosed by the rectangle (×200). The approximate boundary of zone 1 of the liver acinus is denoted by broken lines in the figure on the right. Conducting portal vein (CPV), terminal divisions of the distributing portal vein (DPV), hepatic arteriole (HA), collecting venule (CV), blind-ends of portal vein (*), and anastomoses of sinusoids (arrows). The hepatic arteriole in Fig. 18.62B on the right extends into acinar zones 2 and 3. (Reprinted from Kardon RH, Kessel RG. Three-dimensional organization of the hepatic microcirculation in the rodent as observed by scanning electron microscopy of corrosion casts. *Gastroenterology*. 1980;79:72-81 with permission.)

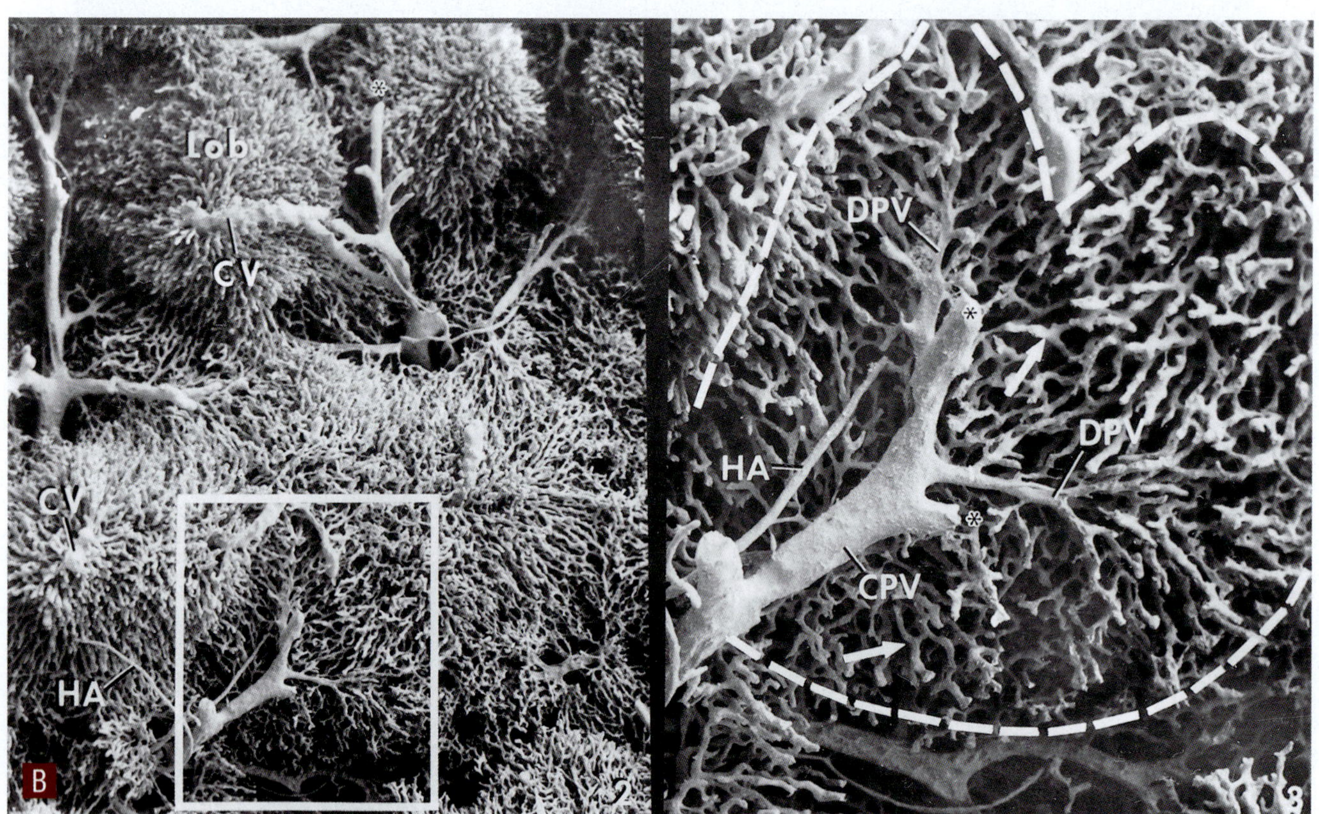

Figure 18.62. *Continued*

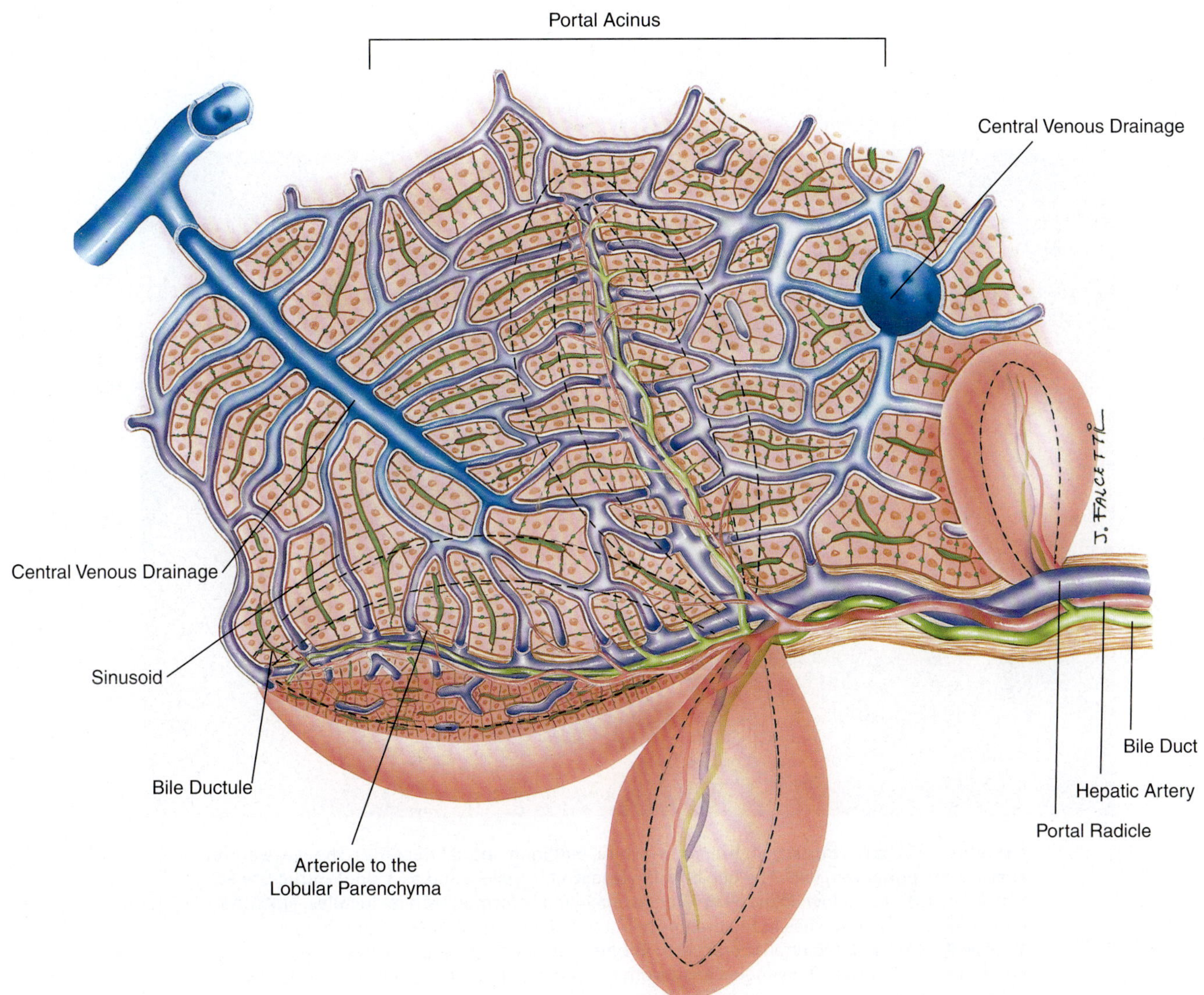

Figure 18.63. Schematic drawing of the microcirculation of the liver. The functional liver acinus zone 1, zone 2, and zone 3 are denoted by the broken line. The acinar three-dimensional (3D) nature is showed by the pearlike structures. Zone 3 represents everything on the liver parenchyma around zone 2 until the draining vein. The artery, the portal radicle, and the bile duct are in the center of the acinus surrounded by sinusoids.

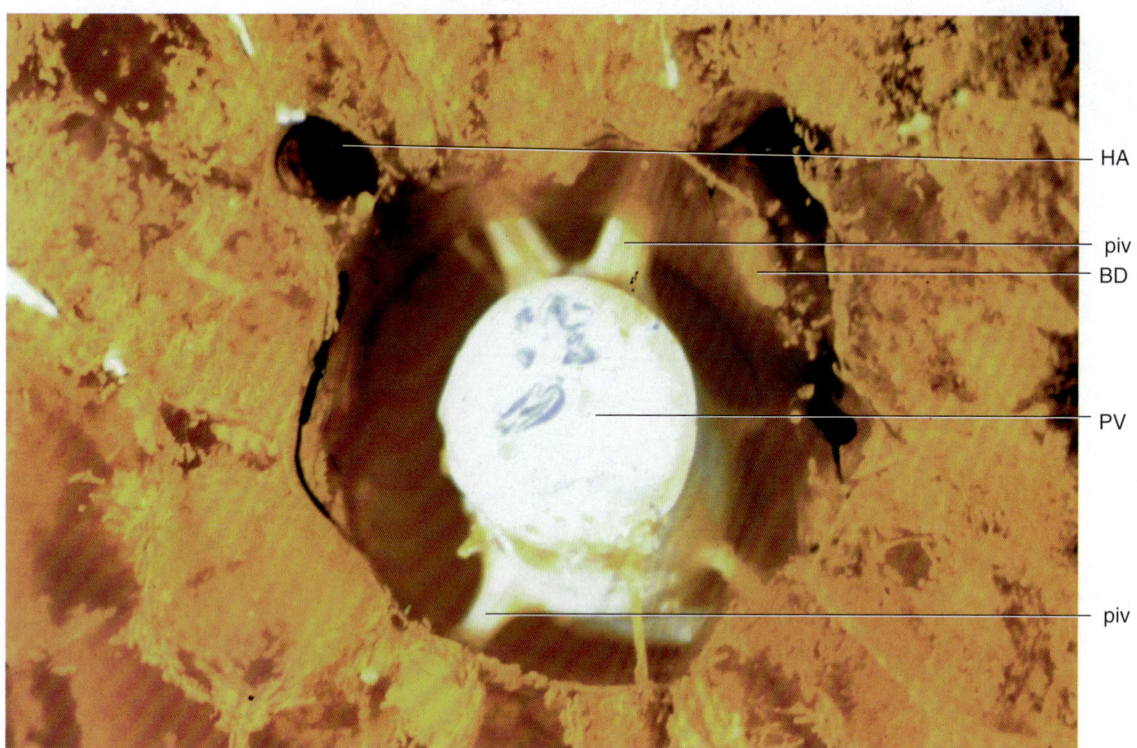

Figure 18.64. Portal vein branch, in white, within the portal tract (PV). The large empty space is the portal vein wall. The bile duct is visualized in yellow and as a single structure at 2 o'clock (BD). The yellow color in the liver parenchyma is formed by bile ductules. Note the two hepatic artery branches in the proximity of the bile duct (HA). There is another artery at 10 o'clock (HA). Note the arterial branches, in blue, surrounding the portal vein within the portal tract. The portal inlet venules arise from the portal vein in right angles entering the liver substance (piv).

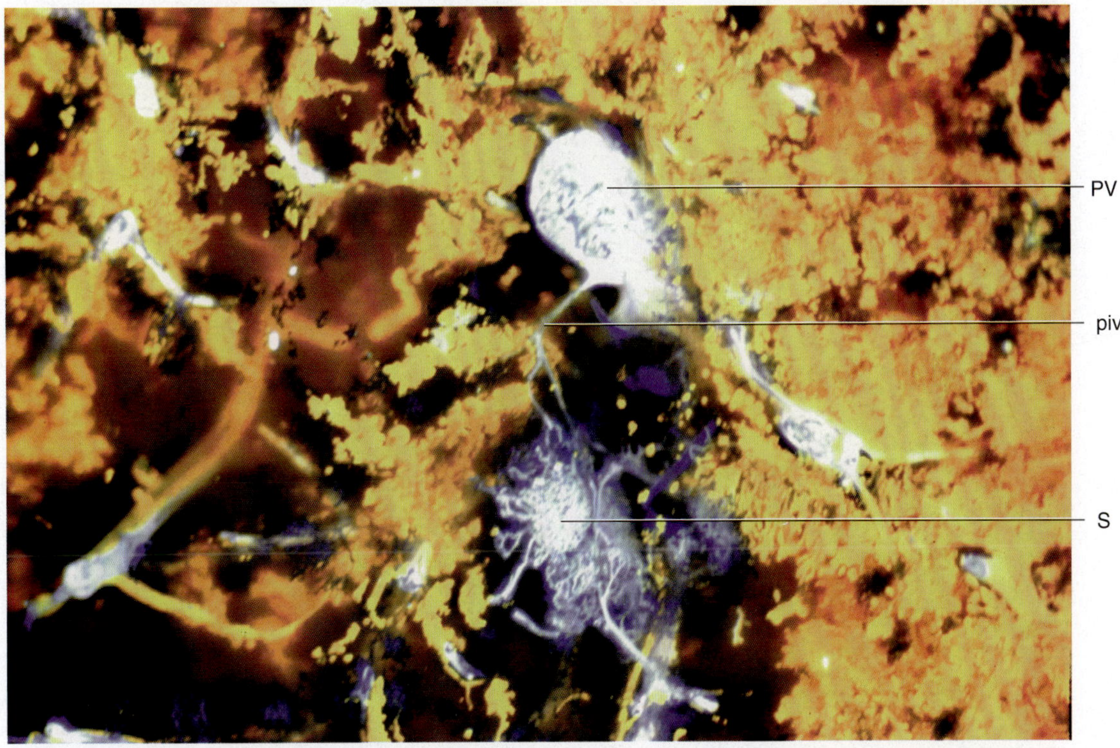

Figure 18.65. Pig liver. Demonstration of direct communication from the portal vein, in white (PV) through a portal inlet venule (piv) into a group of sinusoids (S) at 6 o'clock, with some blue color from the arterial injection. The artery, injected in blue, was not immediately identified in this section of the liver. The dominant color is yellow, which results from the filling of the bile ductules within the hepatic lobules.

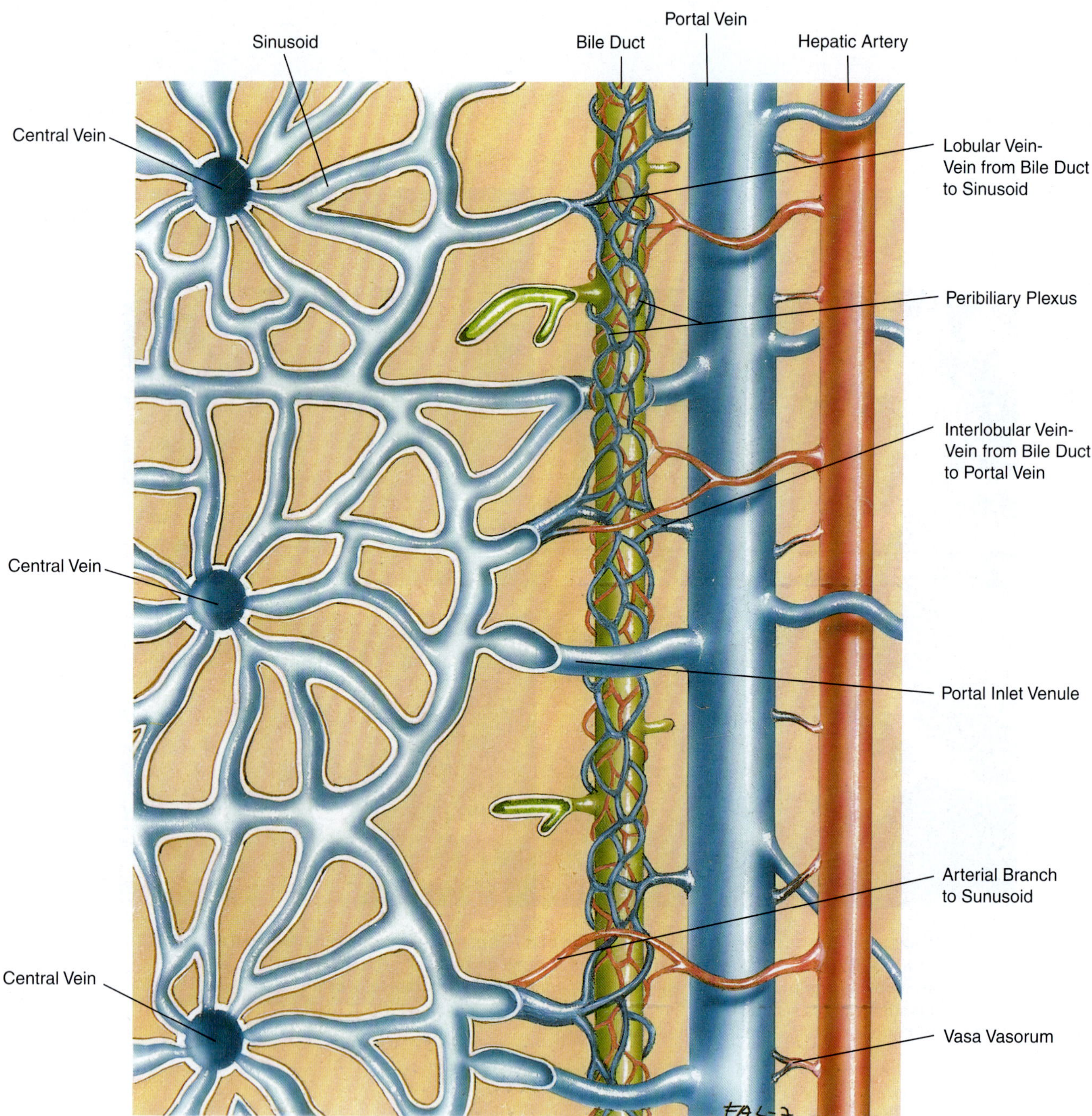

Figure 18.66. Schematic diagram showing the vascular plexus and venous drainage of the bile duct (peribiliary plexus). The hepatic artery gives off its branches to the sinusoid, the bile duct, and the portal vein (vasa vasorum). The venous plexus of the bile duct (blue vessels around the bile duct) is drained into the portal vein via the interlobular vein and into the sinusoids via the lobular vein. Note that there are four types of arterioportal communications: (1) the peribiliary plexus, (2) the terminal arterioportal anastomosis, (3) the vasa vasorum on the wall of the portal vein, (4) and direct arterioportal connections. (Modified from Cho YJ, et al. *Radiology*. 1983;147:357-364.)

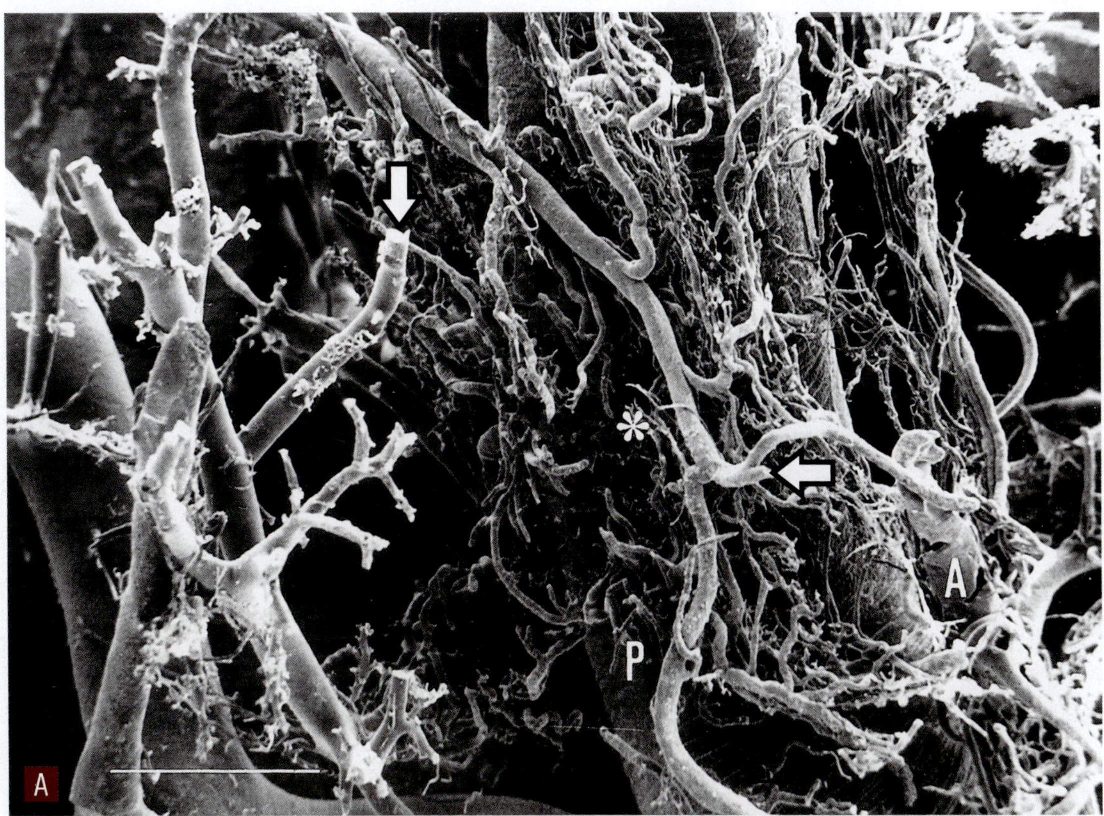

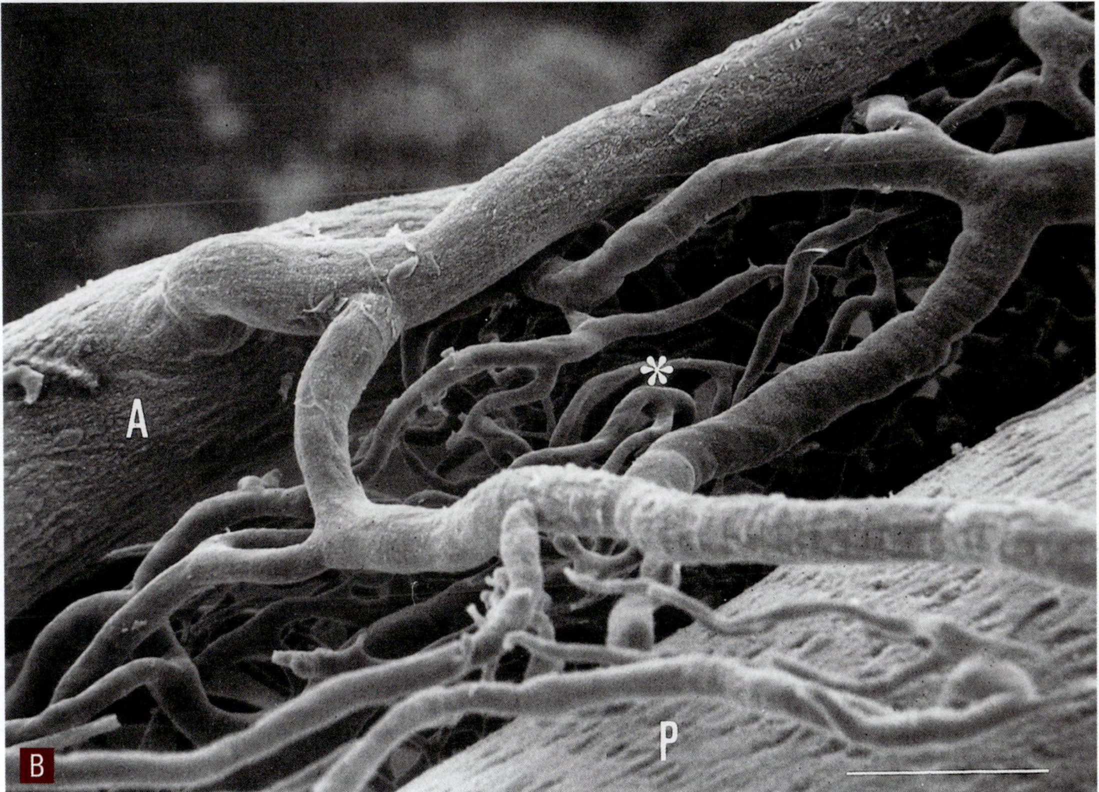

Figure 18.67. A, SEM of the intrahepatic microvasculature, 3 hours after hepatic artery embolization with Gel foam particles. The hepatic artery (A) measures about 290 mm in diameter and is occluded (arrow). The peribiliary plexus around the occluded artery (*) is well filled with the casting medium. Portal vein (P). Bar = 1000 mm. B, SEM of the intrahepatic vasculature in a normal rat. The peribiliary plexus (*) consists of two layers. The hepatic artery (A) supplies the peribiliary plexus (*). Portal vein (P). Bar = 100 mm.

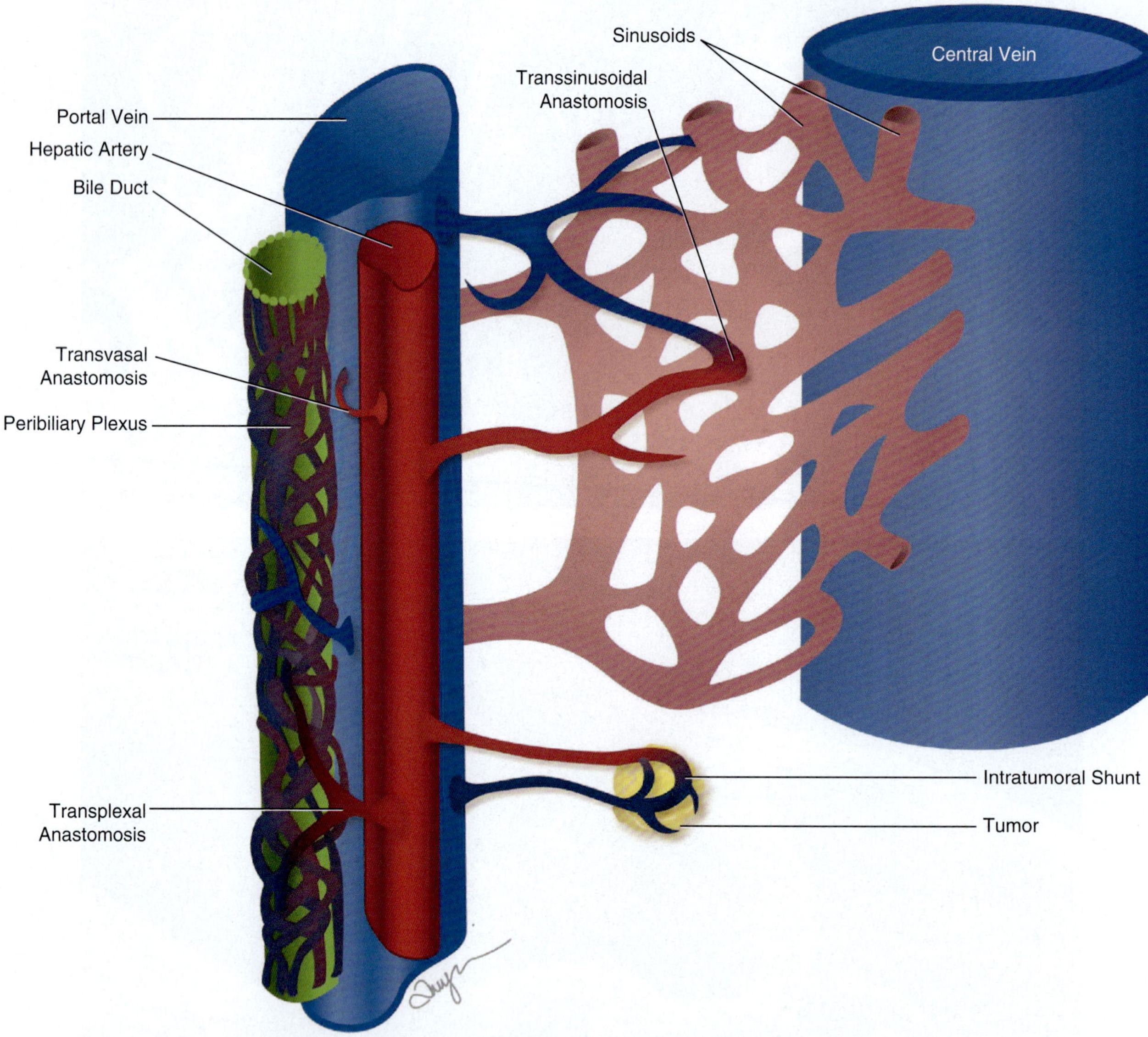

Figure 18.68. The hepatic microcirculation. Arterioportal communication occurs via the peri-biliary venous plexus, via the sinusoid itself, and via the vasa vas ora of the portal venules. In addition, transtumoral shunting may occur if the neoplasm drains to portal venules. (Reprinted from Desser TS. Understanding transient hepatic attenuation differences. *Semin Ultrasound CT MRI.* 2009;30:408-417, with permission from Elsevier.)

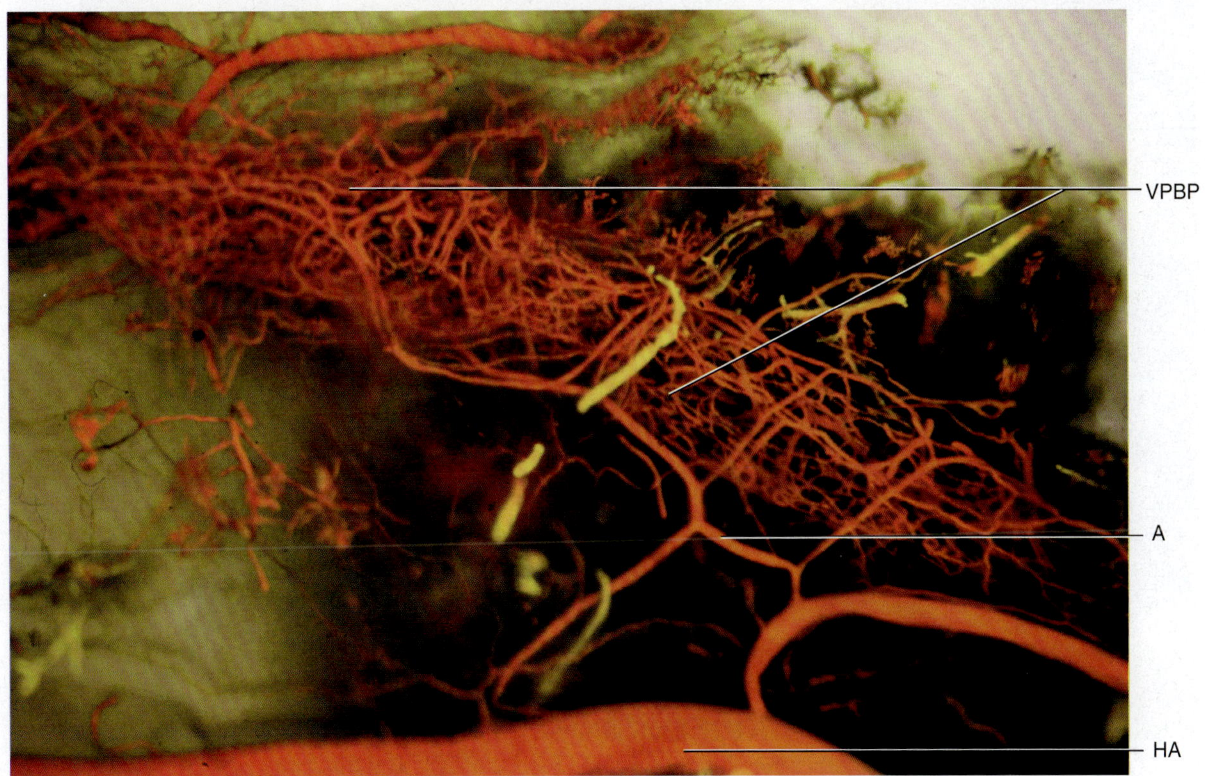

Figure 18.69. Demonstration of the vascular peribiliary plexus (VPBP). Note the hepatic artery (HA) at the bottom of the figure and two smaller branches (A) supplying the dense peribiliary plexus in orange.

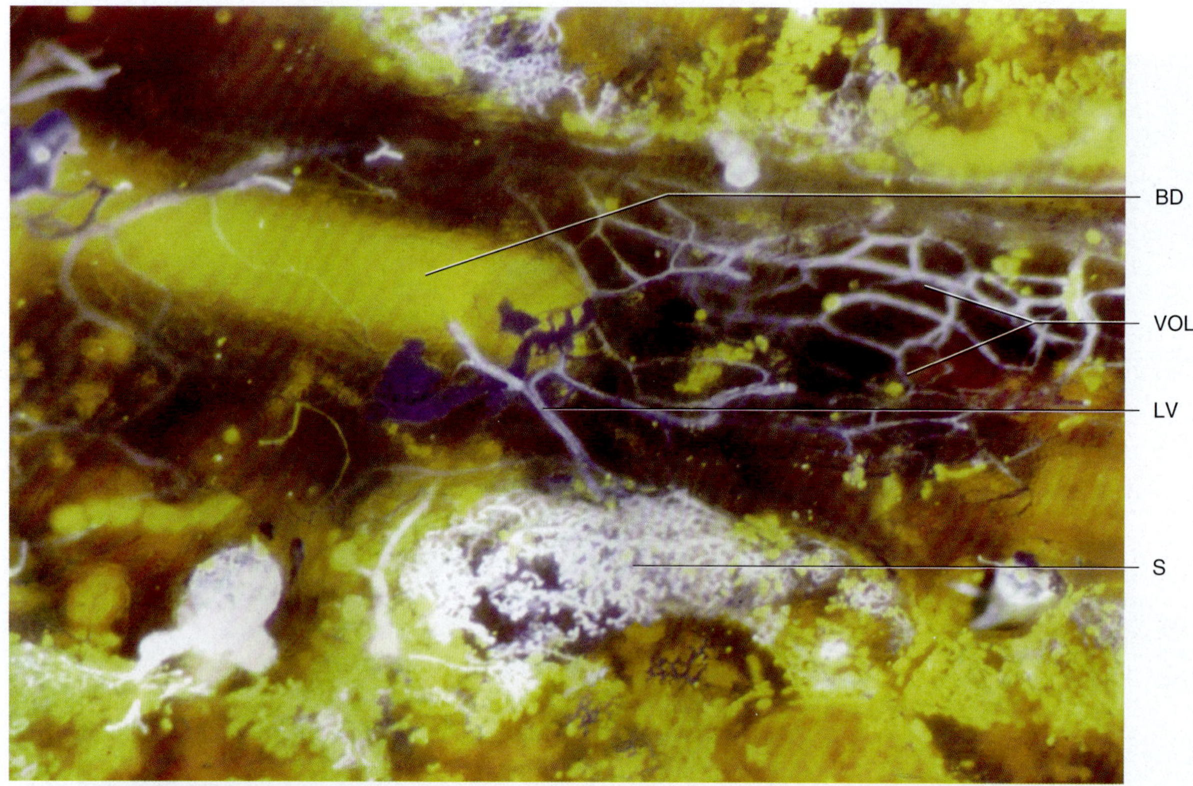

Figure 18.70. Demonstration of the venous outer layer (VOL) of the vascular peribiliary plexus, in light blue (mixture of the dark blue from the artery and the white from the portal vein), and draining through a lobular vein (LV) into the nearby group of sinusoids at 6 o'clock (S). Note the lumen of the bile duct within the peribiliary plexus in yellow (BD). The bile duct is visible in the middle of the vascular peribiliary plexus in yellow (BD) and out of focus. The artery is not readily visible, and only some segments in dark blue are observed.

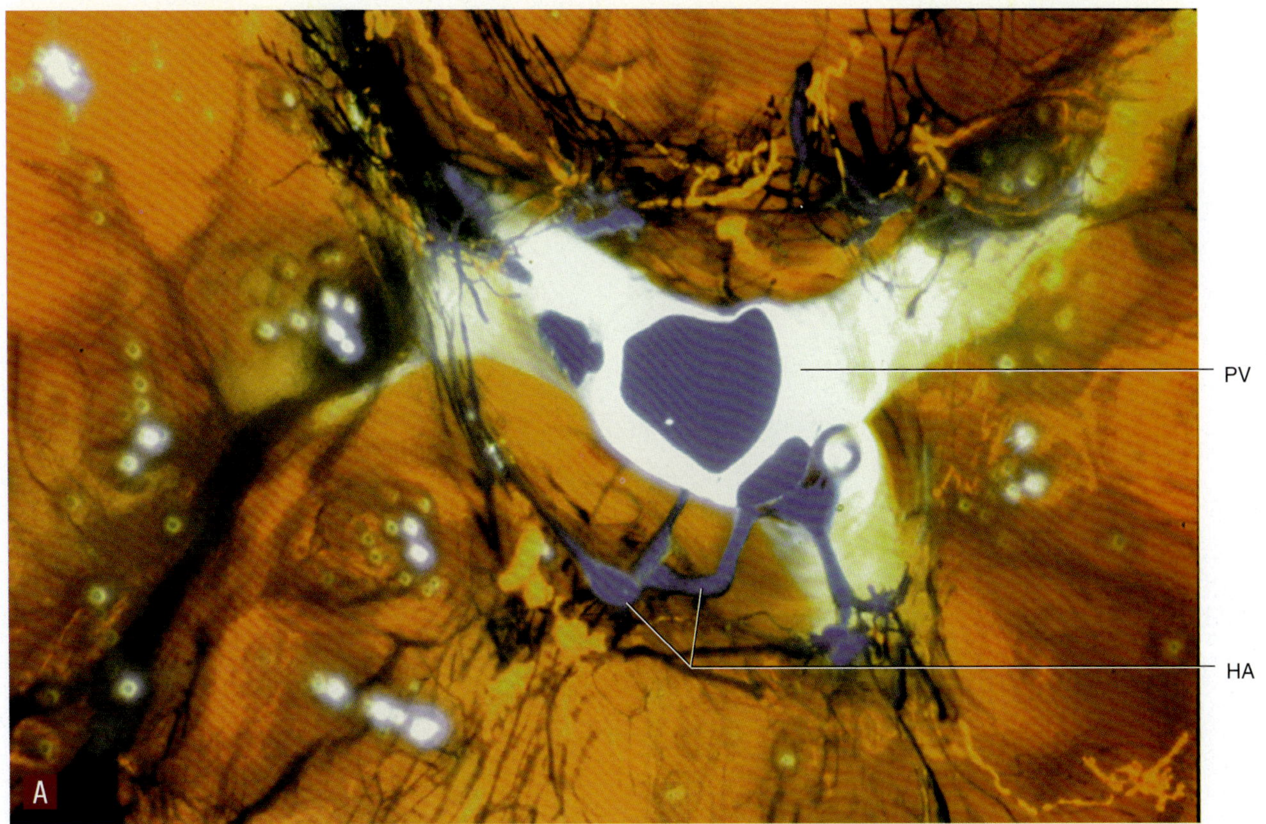

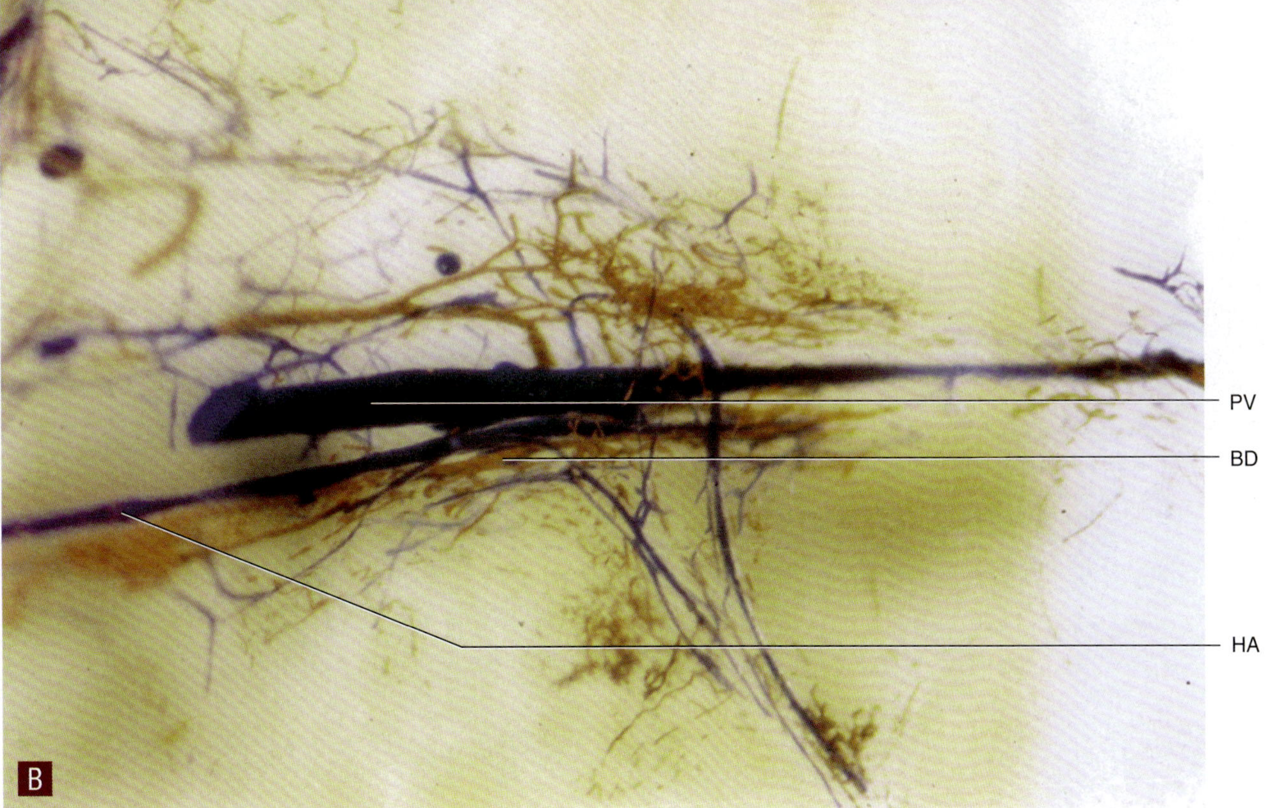

Figure 18.71. Direct arterioportal communications are observed in central and peripheral branches of portal vein. **A**, Portal vein injection showing the portal vein in white (PV) with spots of dark blue inside. Note a dark blue artery entering directly though the wall of the portal vein (HA). The bile duct is filled with orange. **B**, Peripheral smaller portal radicle (PV) showing an arterioportal communication before entering the nodules. Note the smaller straight artery in dark blue (HA) communicating with the peripheral portal radicle also in dark blue (PV). The surrounding bile ducts are orange (BD).

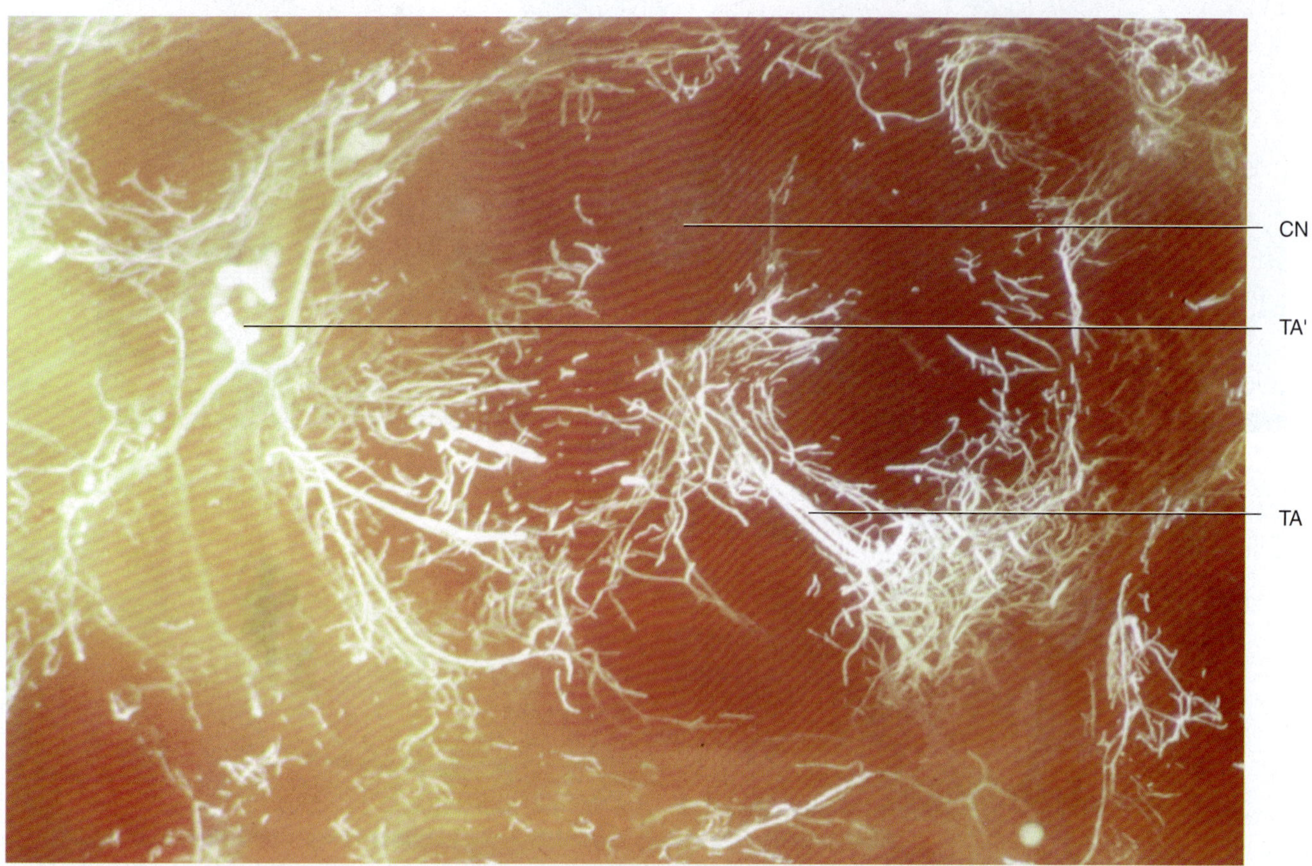

Figure 18.72. A terminal hepatic arteriole (TA) is observed entering the cirrhotic nodule; a terminal portal venule should also enter the nodule at the same level but is observed less frequently as in this case. Another terminal hepatic arteriole (TA′) is visible at the periphery of the cirrhotic nodule (CN) displaced by the nodule and with bowed branches around the nodule.

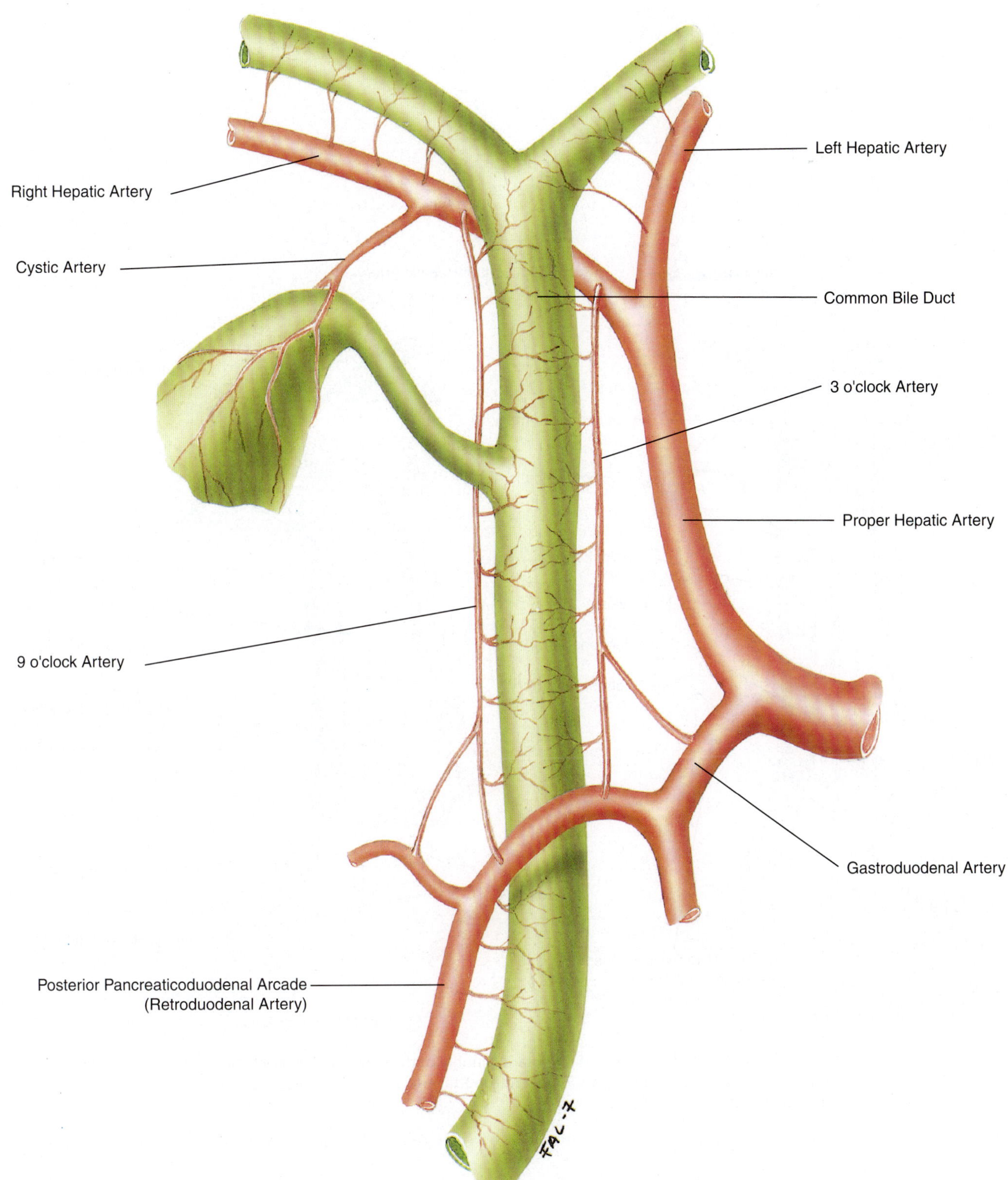

Figure 18.73. Schematic diagram showing the arterial supply of the main bile ducts. The right hepatic duct is supplied by small branches from the right hepatic artery, whereas the left duct is supplied by small branches from the left hepatic artery. The common bile duct (supraduodenal segment) is supplied by the 9 o'clock and 3 o'clock arteries. The common bile duct (infraduodenal segment) is supplied by direct small branches of the pancreaticoduodenal arcade.

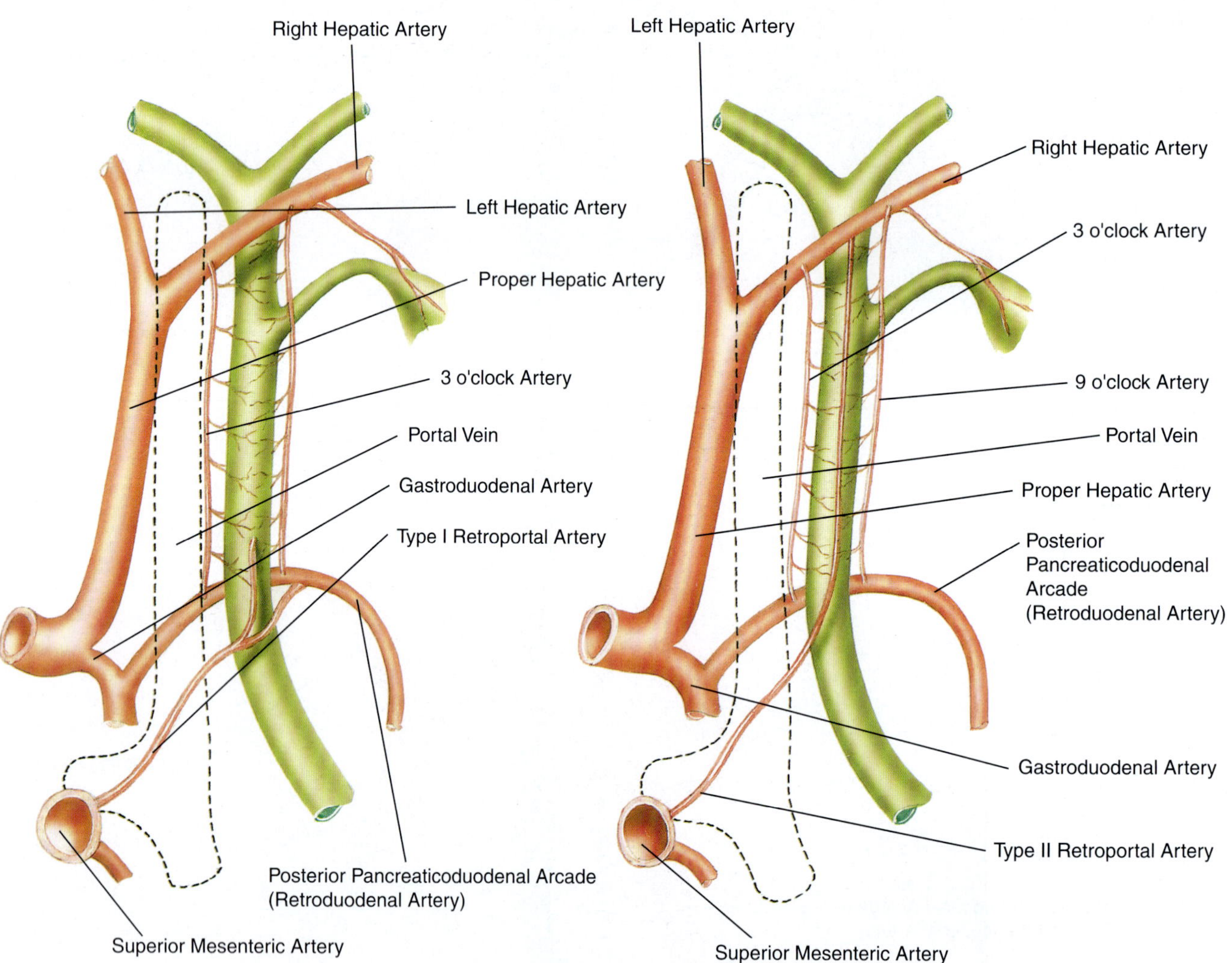

Figure 18.74. Posterior view of the arterial supply of the common bile duct showing the retroportal artery, type I and type II. Type II retroportal artery increases the supply of the common bile duct.

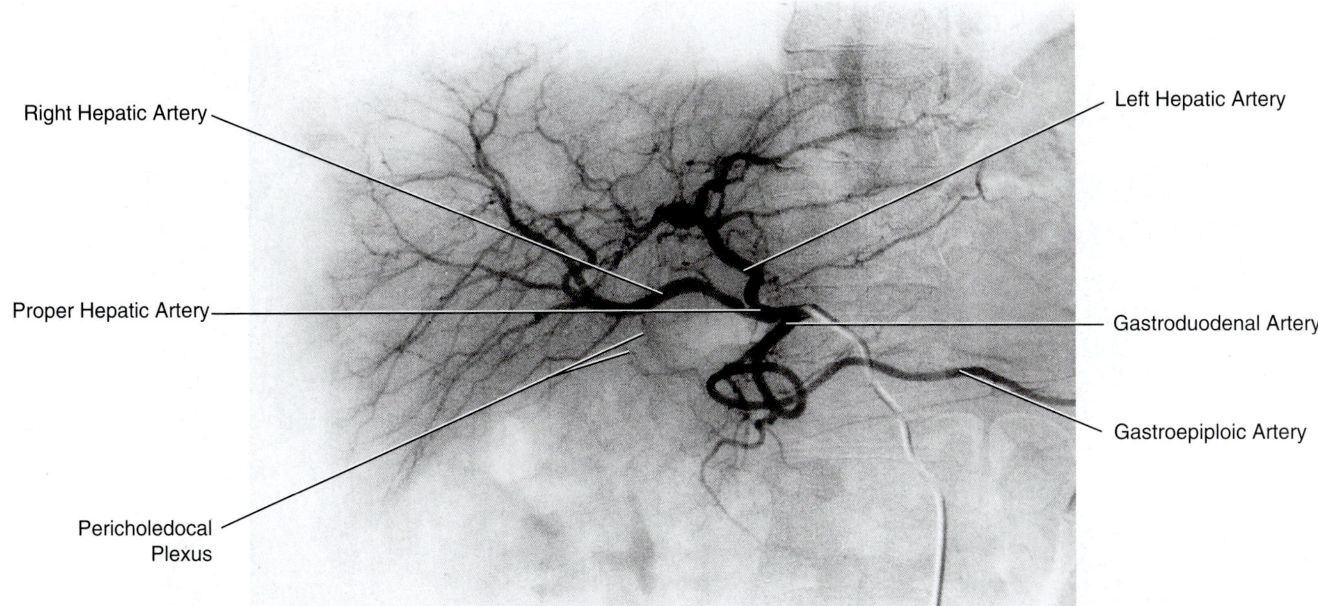

Figure 18.75. Common hepatic arteriography, arterial phase. The peribiliary arteries are filled from the pancreatic arcade and reach the hepatic arterial branches at the hilum. The 3 o'clock and 9 o'clock arteries are seen. There is an early bifurcation of the proper hepatic artery.

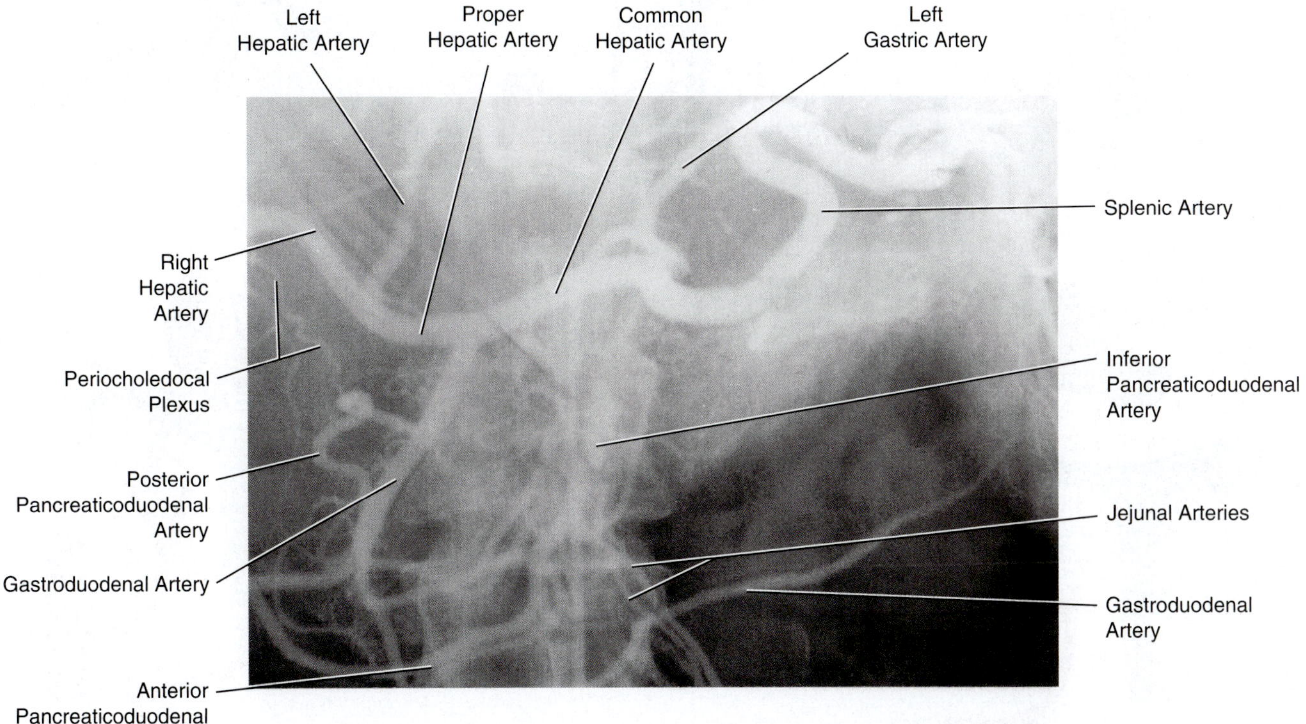

Figure 18.76. Celiac artery injection showing the peribiliary arteries parallel to the main bile duct, arising from the pancreatic arcade.

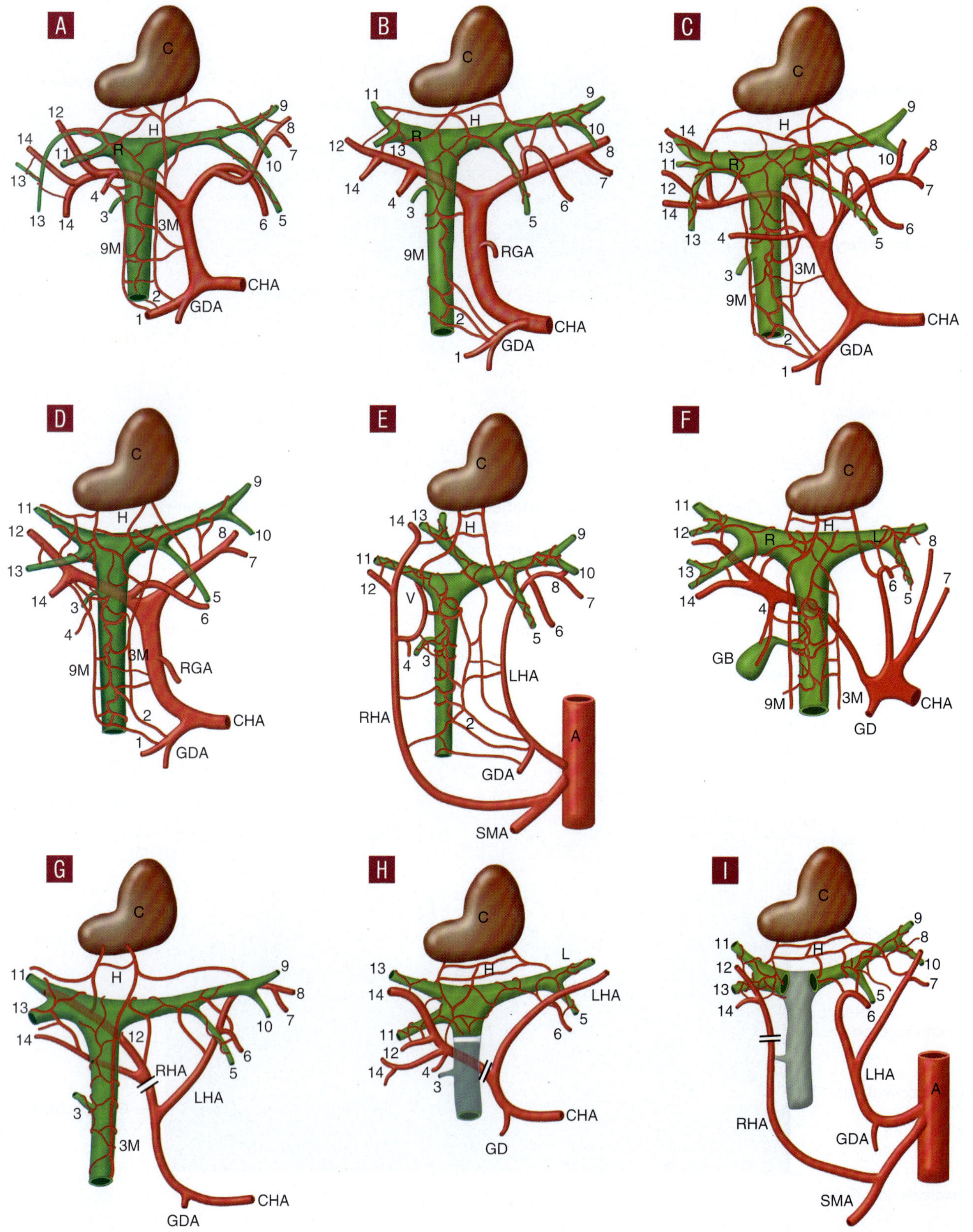

Figure 18.77. A to E, Diagrams based in dissected specimens showing the arterial supply of the bile ducts. F to I, Diagrams based on dissected specimens representing vasculobiliary injuries caused by cholecystectomy. A, aorta; C, caudate lobe; CHA, common hepatic artery; GB, gallbladder; GDA, gastroduodenal artery; H, hilar plate arterial plexus; L, left hepatic duct; LHA, left hepatic artery; R, right hepatic bile duct; RGA, right gastric artery; RHA, right hepatic artery; SMA, superior mesenteric artery; 3M, 3 o'clock marginal artery; 9M, 9 o'clock marginal artery. 1, posterosuperior pancreaticoduodenal artery; 2, marginal arteries; 3, cystic duct; 4, cystic artery; 5, duct to segment IV; 6, artery to segment IV; 7, artery to segment III; 8, artery to segment II; 9, duct to segment II; 10, duct to segment III; 11, right anterior sectoral duct; 12, right anterior sectoral artery; 13, right posterior sectoral duct; 14, right posterior sectoral artery.

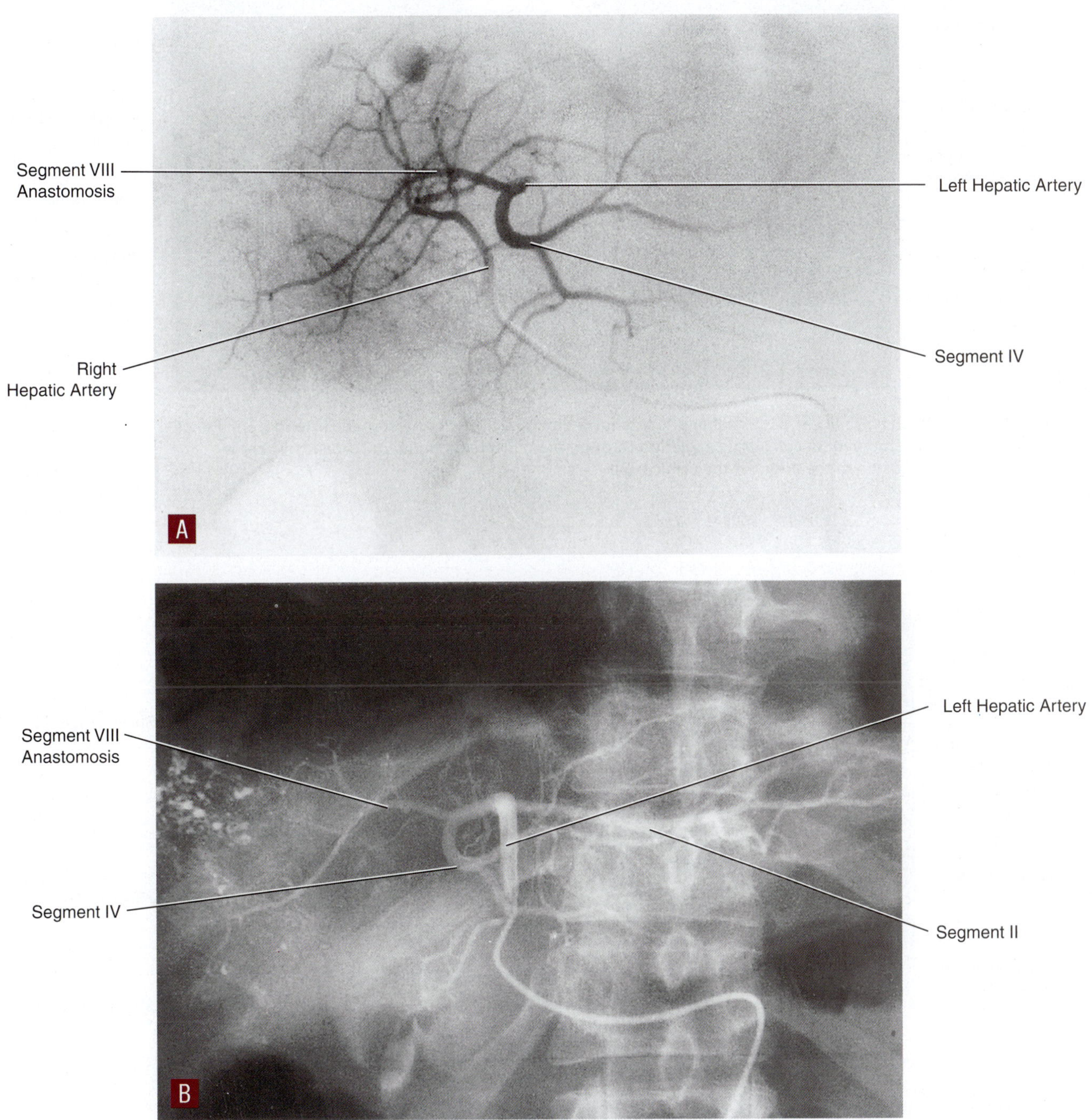

Figure 18.78. Interlobar intrahepatic arterial collaterals. A, Selective injection in the right hepatic artery shows simultaneous filling of the left hepatic artery, segments IV and III. B, Selective injection in the left hepatic artery shows no filling of the right hepatic artery.

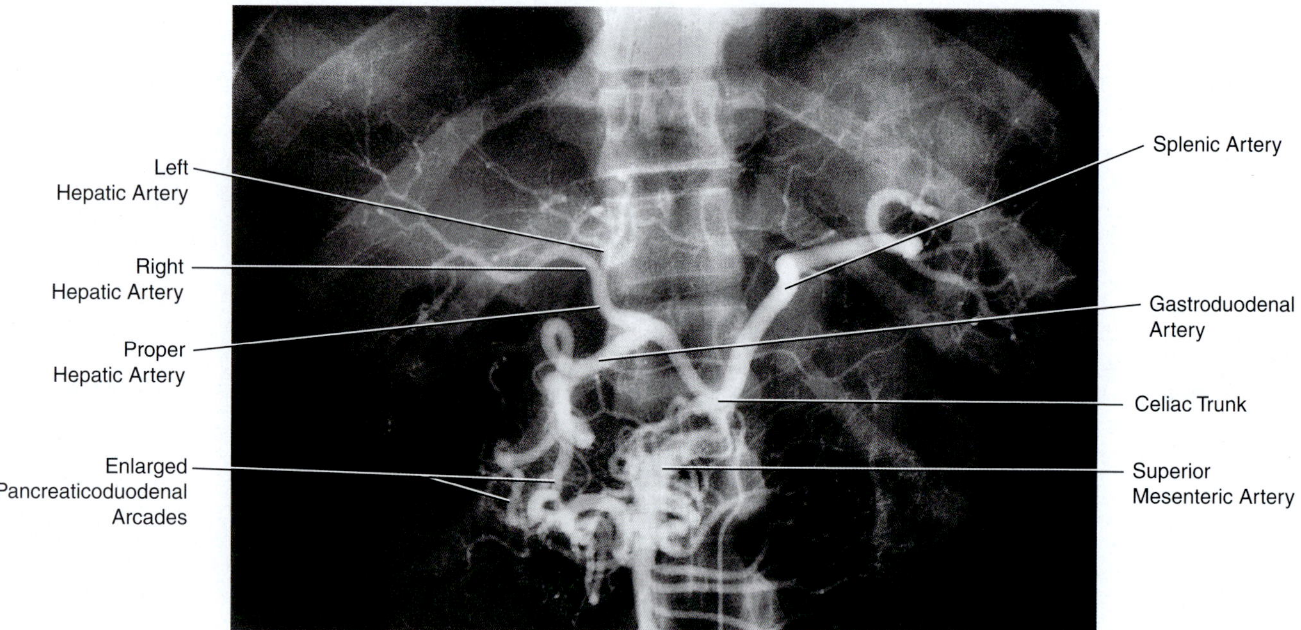

Figure 18.79. **Extrahepatic arterial collaterals.** Superior mesenteric arteriogram shows development of collateral circulation through the pancreaticoduodenal arcades. There is occlusion of the origin of the celiac trunk.

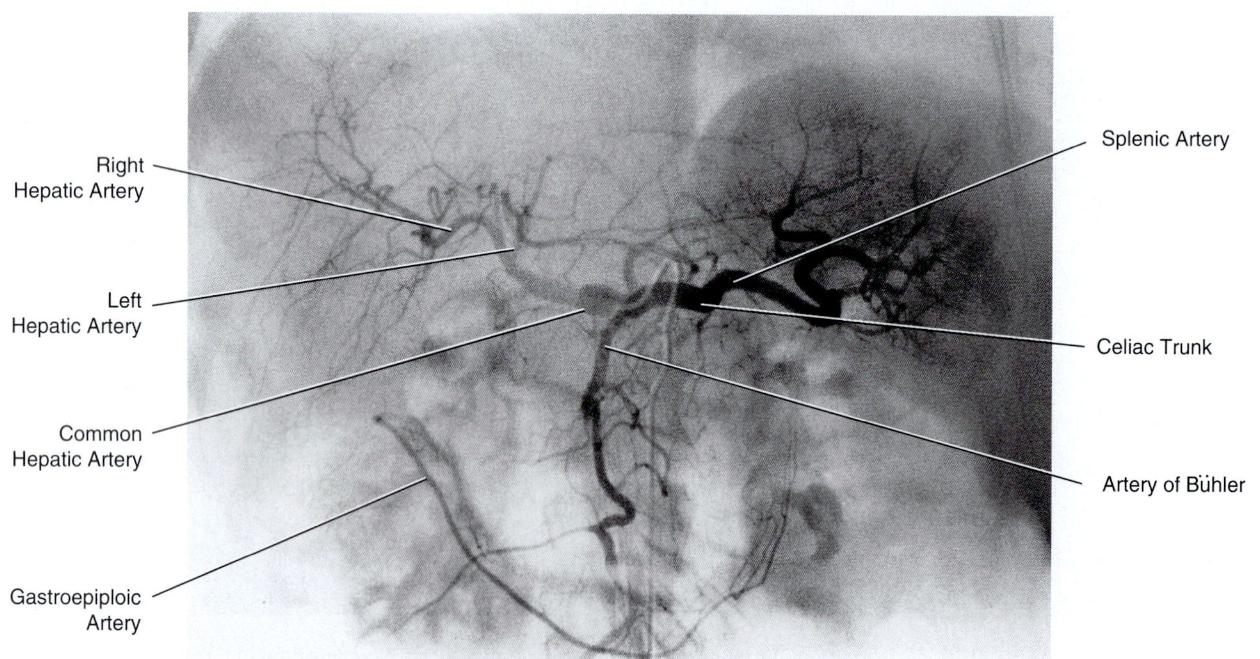

Figure 18.80. **Extrahepatic arterial collaterals.** Celiac artery angiogram showing opacification of the Arc of Bühler, connecting to the superior mesenteric artery.

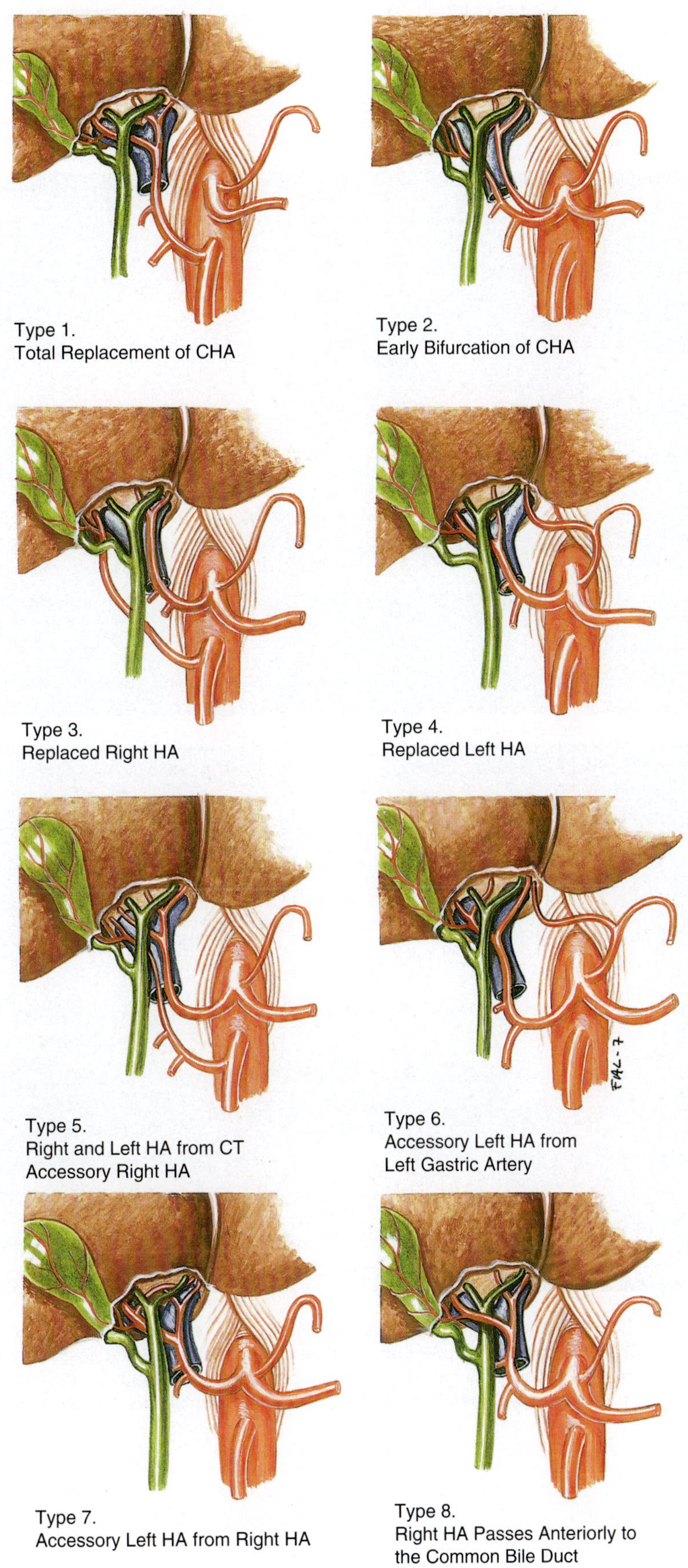

Figure 18.81. **Variations of the hepatic artery.** Types 1 through 8. The most frequent variation is replacement of the hepatic artery. There are variations in about 40% of the population.

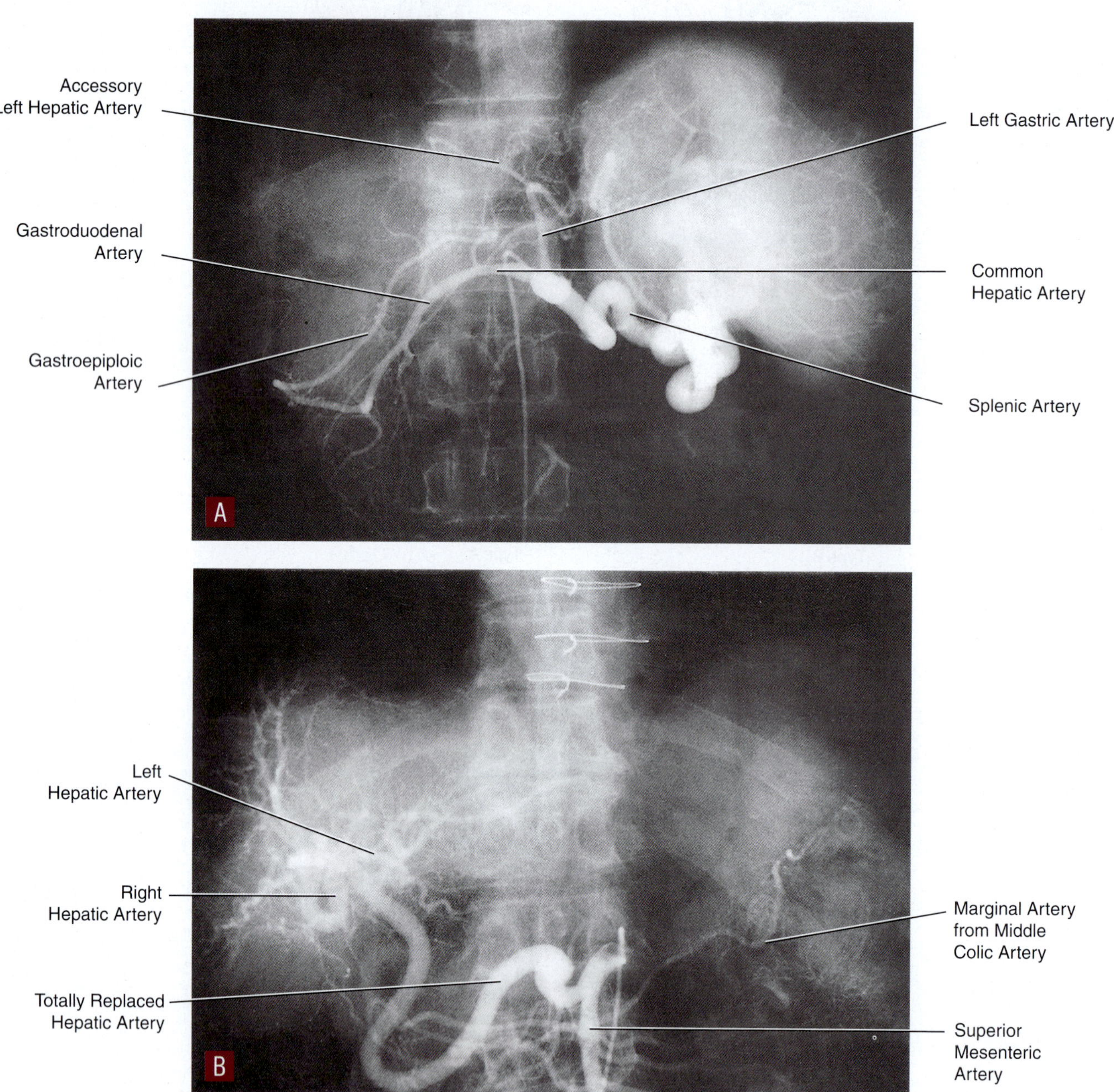

Figure 18.82. Variation of the hepatic artery. Type 1. Total replacement of the common hepatic artery. **A**, Celiac injection shows only the gastroduodenal artery, left gastric artery, and splenic artery. This patient may have a very small accessory left hepatic artery, originated from the left gastric artery. **B**, Superior mesenteric artery injection shows the totally replaced hepatic artery.

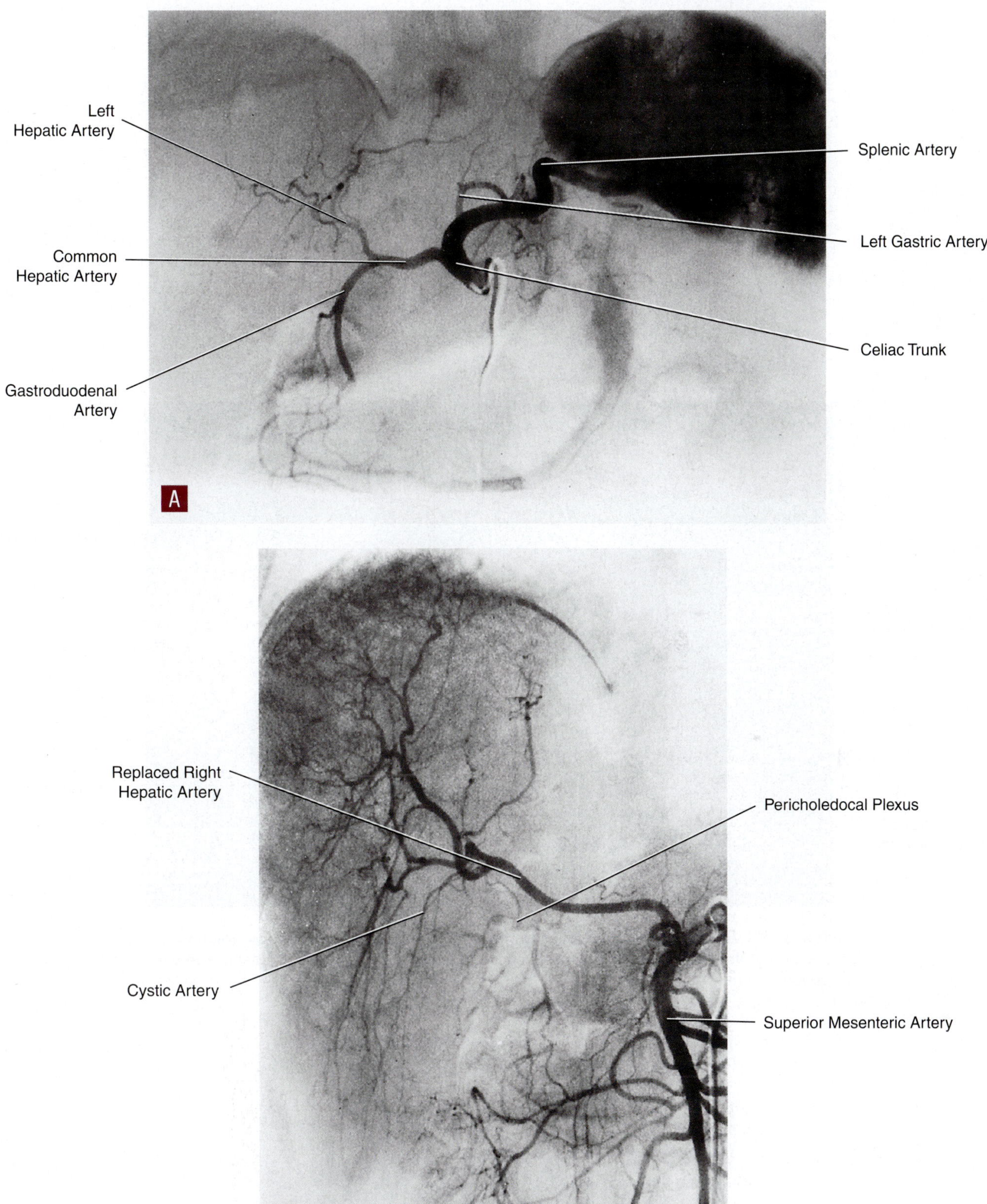

Figure 18.83. Variation of the hepatic artery. Type 3. Replaced right hepatic artery. **A**, Celiac trunk injection shows the left gastric artery originated from the common hepatic artery. **B**, SMA injection giving origin to the right replaced hepatic artery.

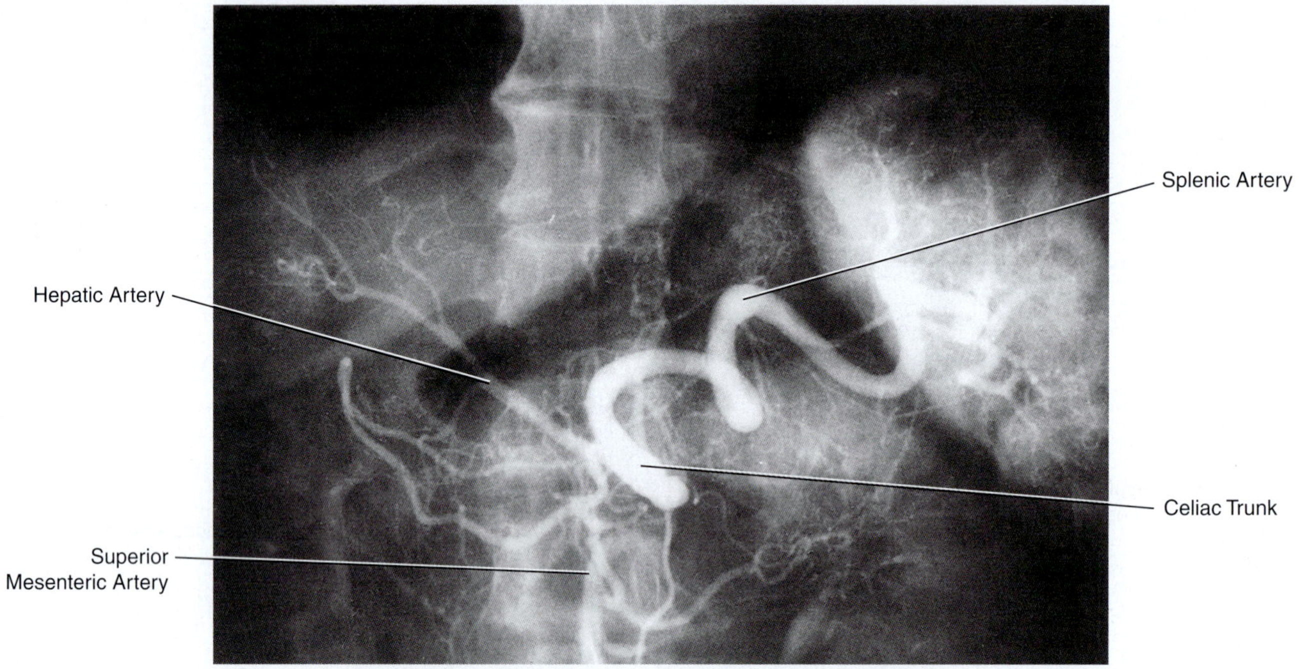

Figure 18.84. **Splenic artery.** Celiac trunk injection shows the large and convoluted splenic artery. Note the several pancreatic branches and the bifurcation of the splenic artery in the splenic hilum.

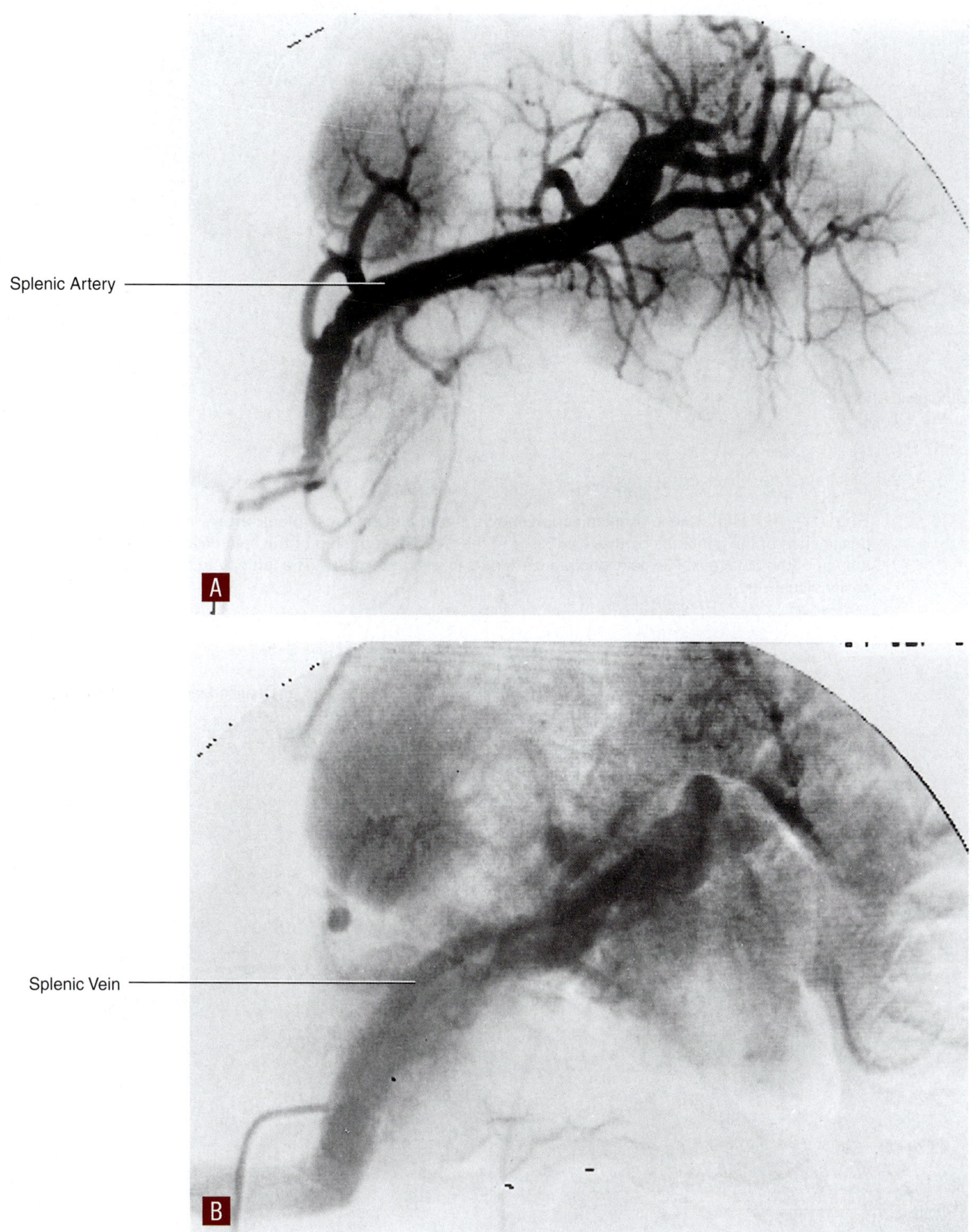

Figure 18.85. A, Selective splenic artery injection shows the intrasplenic circulation as well as the pancreatic arteries originated from the splenic artery. B, Late angiographic phase shows the splenic venous drainage, with dense opacification of the splenic vein.

Common Hepatic Artery
Pancreatic Blush
Gastroduodenal Artery
Gastroepiploic Artery
Splenic Artery
Celiac Trunk
Omental Branch

Figure 18.86. **Celiac trunk injection shows a long and sinuous splenic artery.** Note the dense stain of the pancreas by the injection and the close relationship of the splenic artery and the tail of the pancreas. The gastroepiploic artery is long and tortuous. The left epiploic artery is easily visualized.

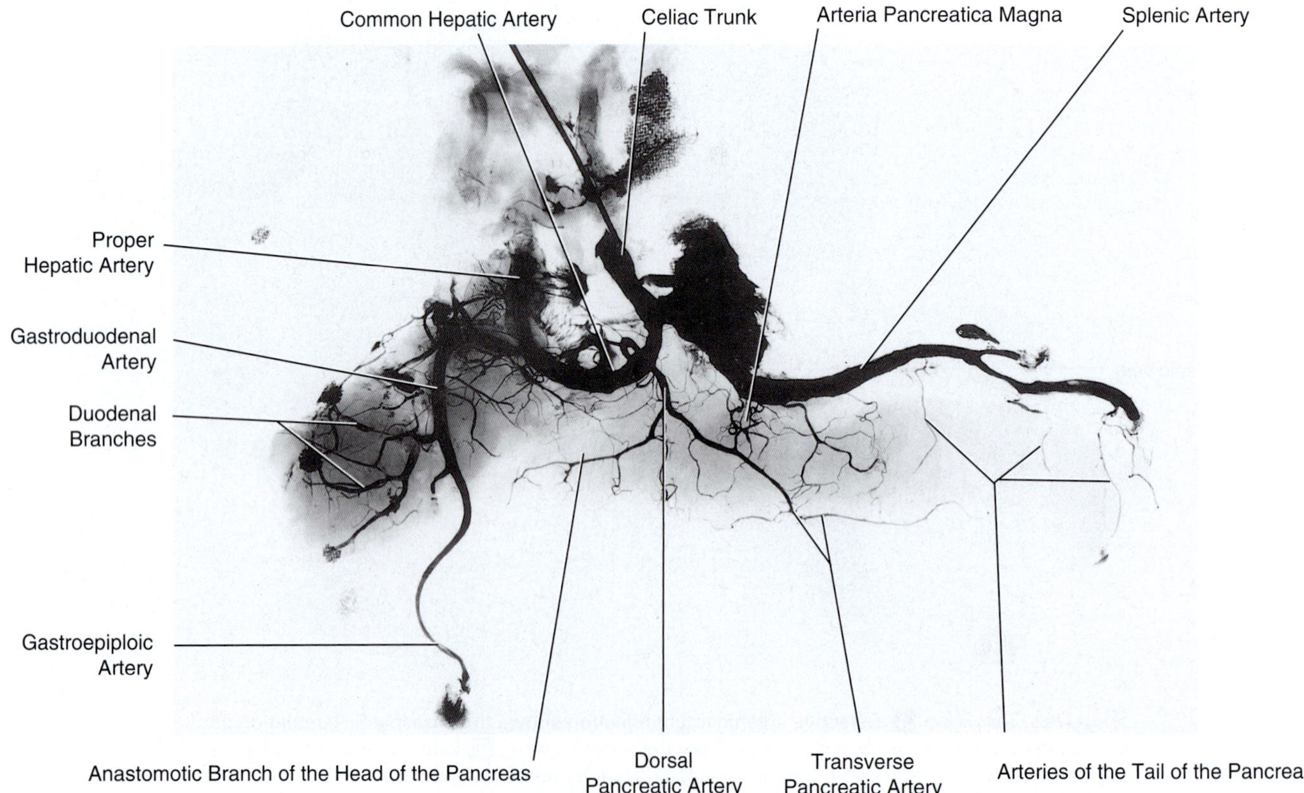

Figure 18.87. **Necropsy specimen injection of contrast media showing the pancreatic arteries.** There are artifacts due to extravasation of contrast.

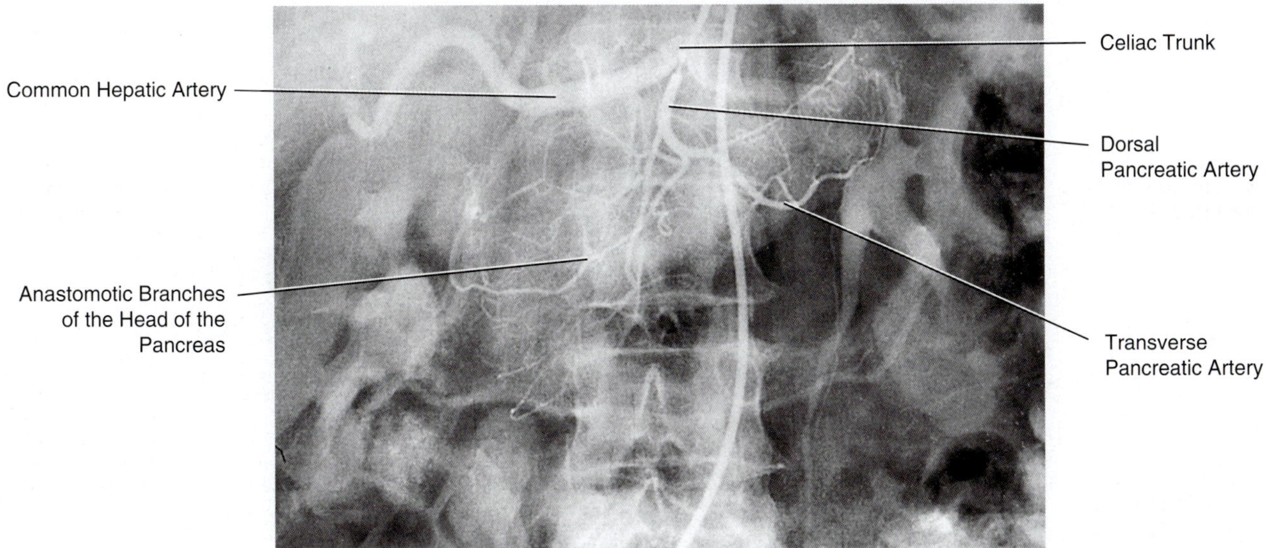

Figure 18.88. Selective angiography of the dorsal pancreatic artery arising from the bifurcation of the celiac trunk. Note the communications with the pancreaticoduodenal arcades and with the transverse pancreatic artery.

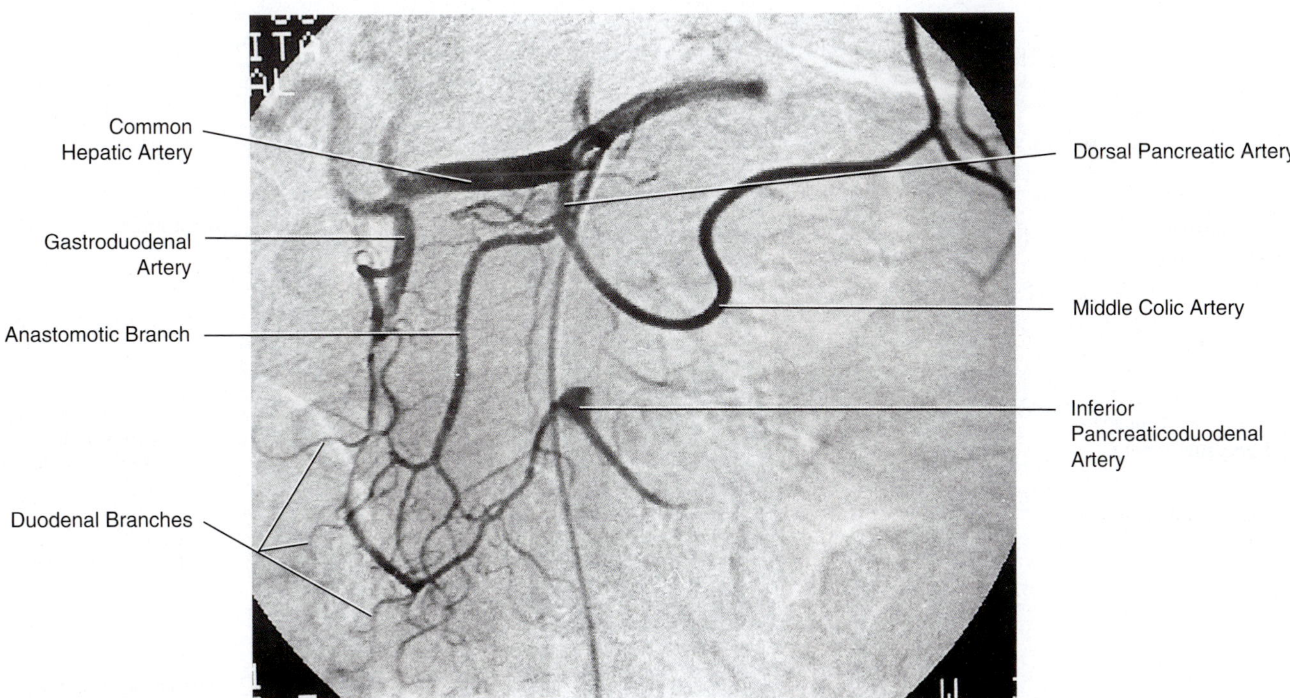

Figure 18.89. Selective angiography of the common hepatic artery shows the origin of the dorsal pancreatic artery from the common hepatic artery; in this case, it anastomoses with the pancreaticoduodenal arcade. Note that the middle colic artery originates from the dorsal pancreatic artery.

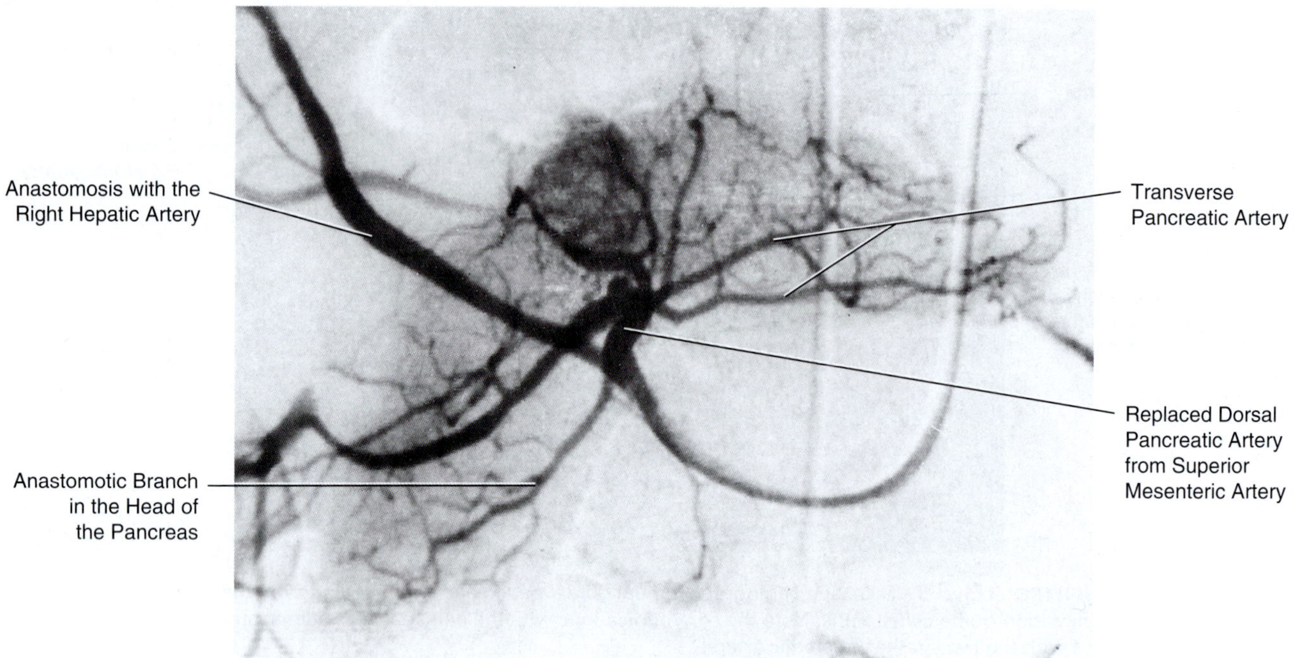

Figure 18.90. Variation of the origin of the dorsal pancreatic artery. Selective angiography of the dorsal pancreatic artery, in this case originated from the SMA. Incidentally a hypervascular lesion (insulinoma) is observed. Note that there is an anastomose with the right hepatic artery, directly from the dorsal pancreatic artery.

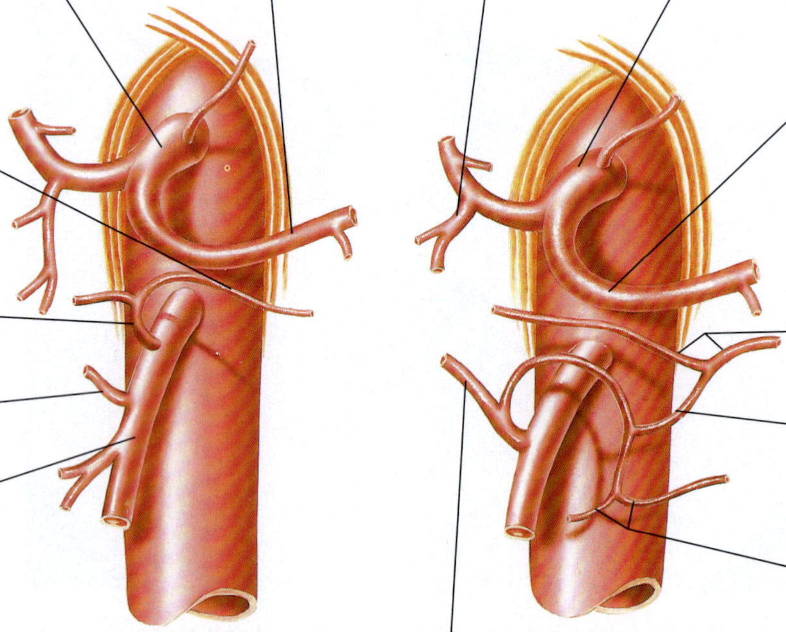

Figure 18.91. Schematic diagram showing variations in origin of the dorsal pancreatic artery. Note that the middle colic artery and the dorsal pancreatic artery may have a common origin.

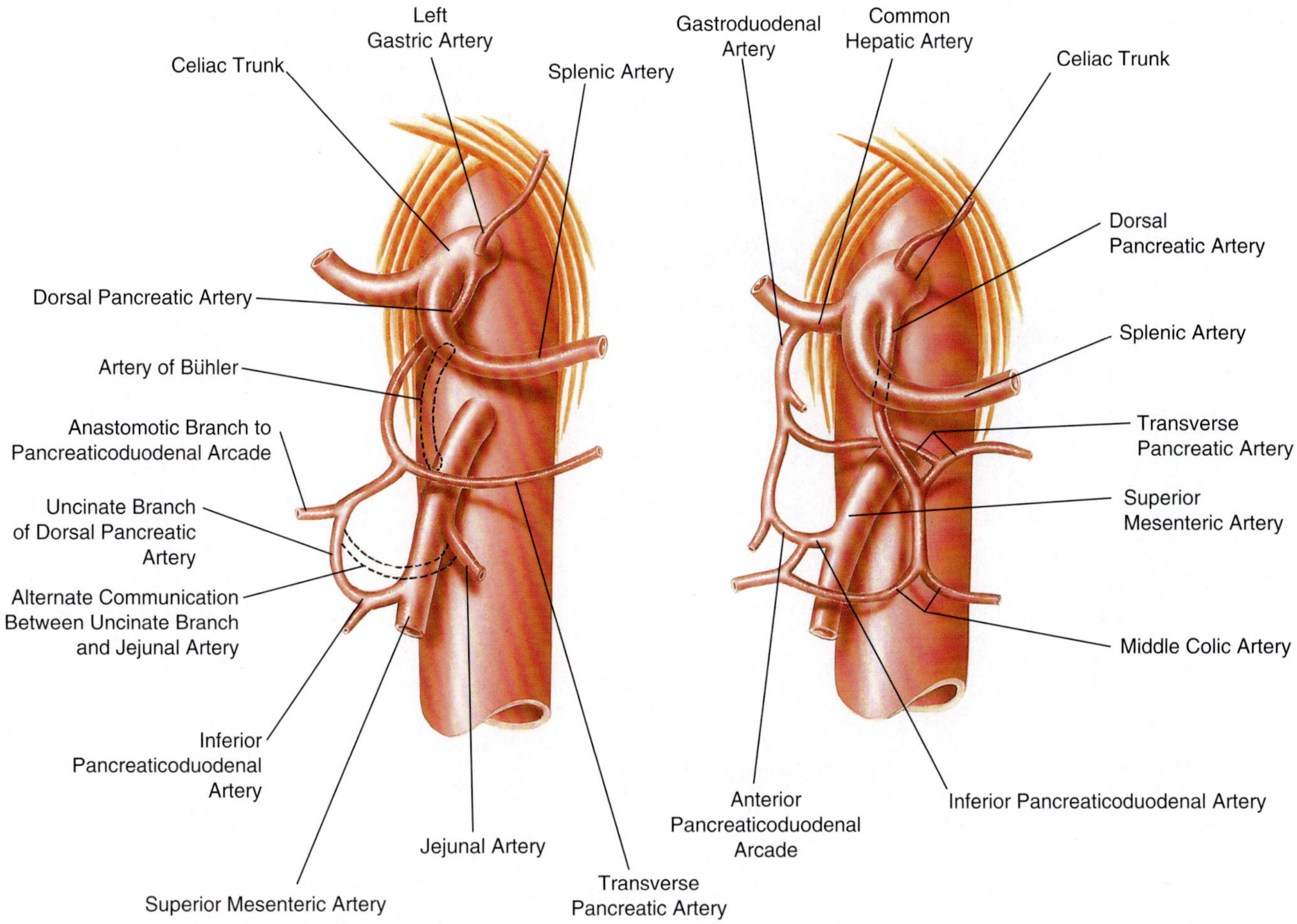

Celiac Trunk
Left Gastric Artery
Splenic Artery
Dorsal Pancreatic Artery
Artery of Bühler
Anastomotic Branch to Pancreaticoduodenal Arcade
Uncinate Branch of Dorsal Pancreatic Artery
Alternate Communication Between Uncinate Branch and Jejunal Artery
Inferior Pancreaticoduodenal Artery
Superior Mesenteric Artery
Jejunal Artery
Transverse Pancreatic Artery
Gastroduodenal Artery
Common Hepatic Artery
Celiac Trunk
Dorsal Pancreatic Artery
Splenic Artery
Transverse Pancreatic Artery
Superior Mesenteric Artery
Middle Colic Artery
Inferior Pancreaticoduodenal Artery
Anterior Pancreaticoduodenal Arcade

Figure 18.92. Schematic diagram shows possible connections between the celiac trunk and superior mesenteric artery through the dorsal pancreatic artery and the artery of Bühler.

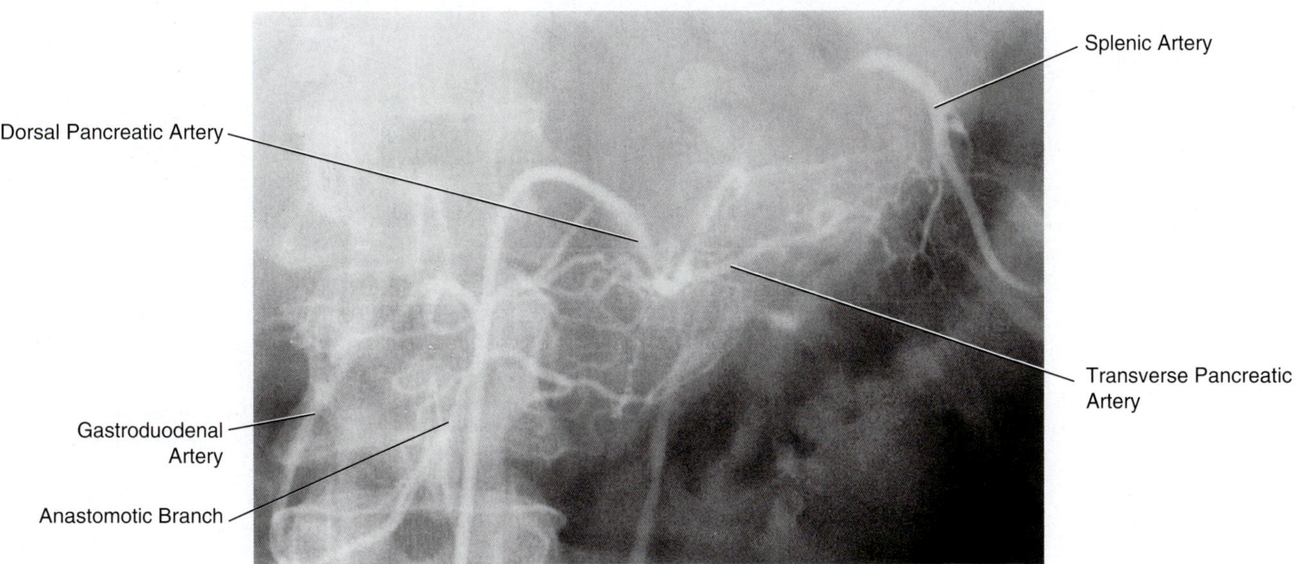

Figure 18.93. Selective arteriography injection at the arteria pancreatica magna (great pancreatic artery) branch of the splenic artery. Note the connections with the arteries in the neck and head of the pancreas and the arteries in the tail of the pancreas with filling of the transverse pancreatic artery and smaller branches.

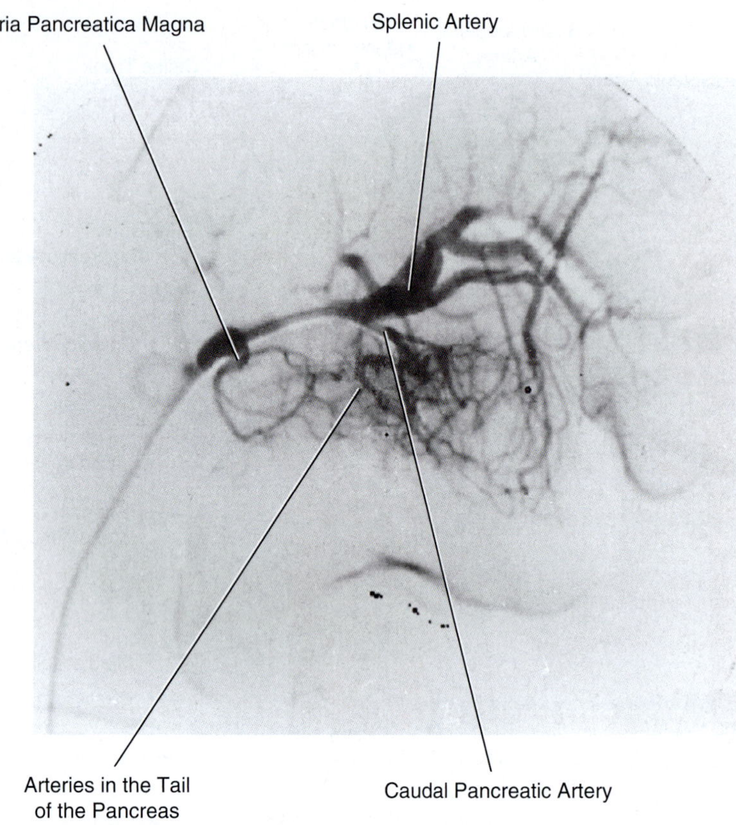

Figure 18.94. Selective arteriography of the caudal pancreatic artery, branch of the splenic artery. Note partial filling of the splenic arteries and smaller branches in the distal tail of the pancreas.

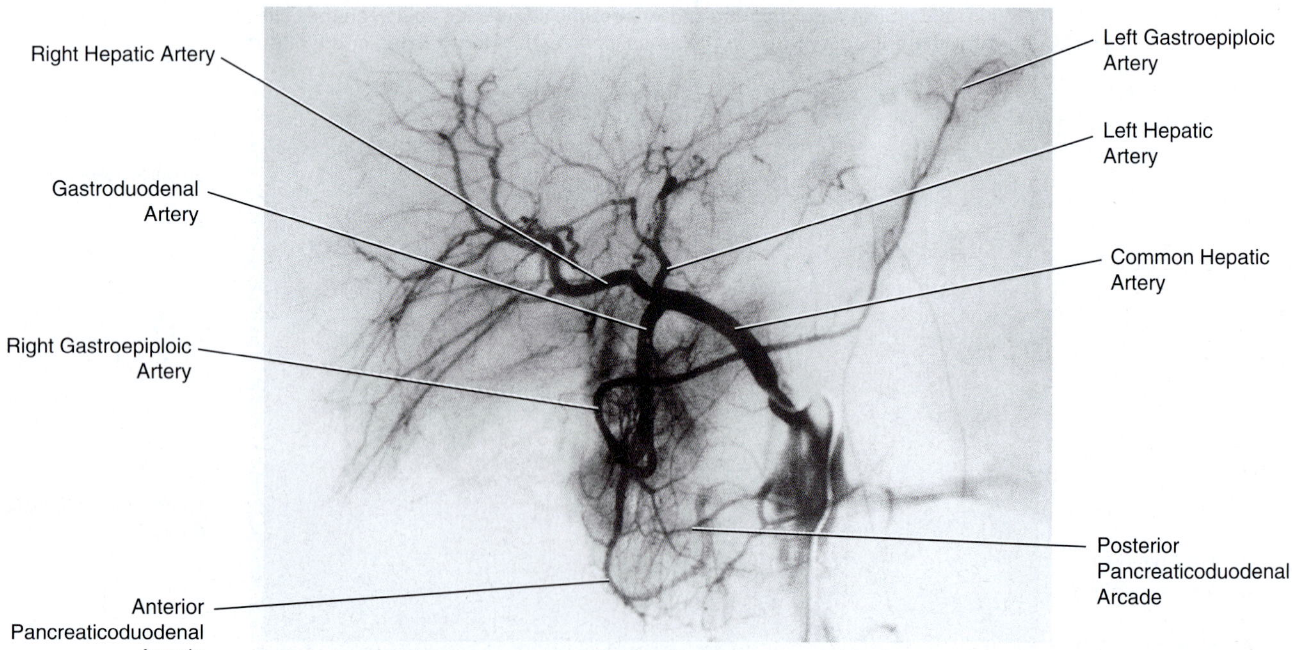

Figure 18.95. Selective injection in the common hepatic artery showing filling of the gastroduodenal artery, as well as the pancreaticoduodenal arcades, intrahepatic arteries, and the right gastroepiploic artery. The right gastroepiploic artery is a continuation of the gastroduodenal artery, vascularizes the stomach wall, and originates the omental branches (epiploic arteries).

Segment IV
Left Hepatic Artery
Left Gastric Artery
Splenic Artery
Splenic Branches
Right Hepatic Artery
Great Pancreatic Artery
(Pancreatica Magna)
Gastroduodenal Artery
Common Hepatic Artery
Gastroepiploic Artery

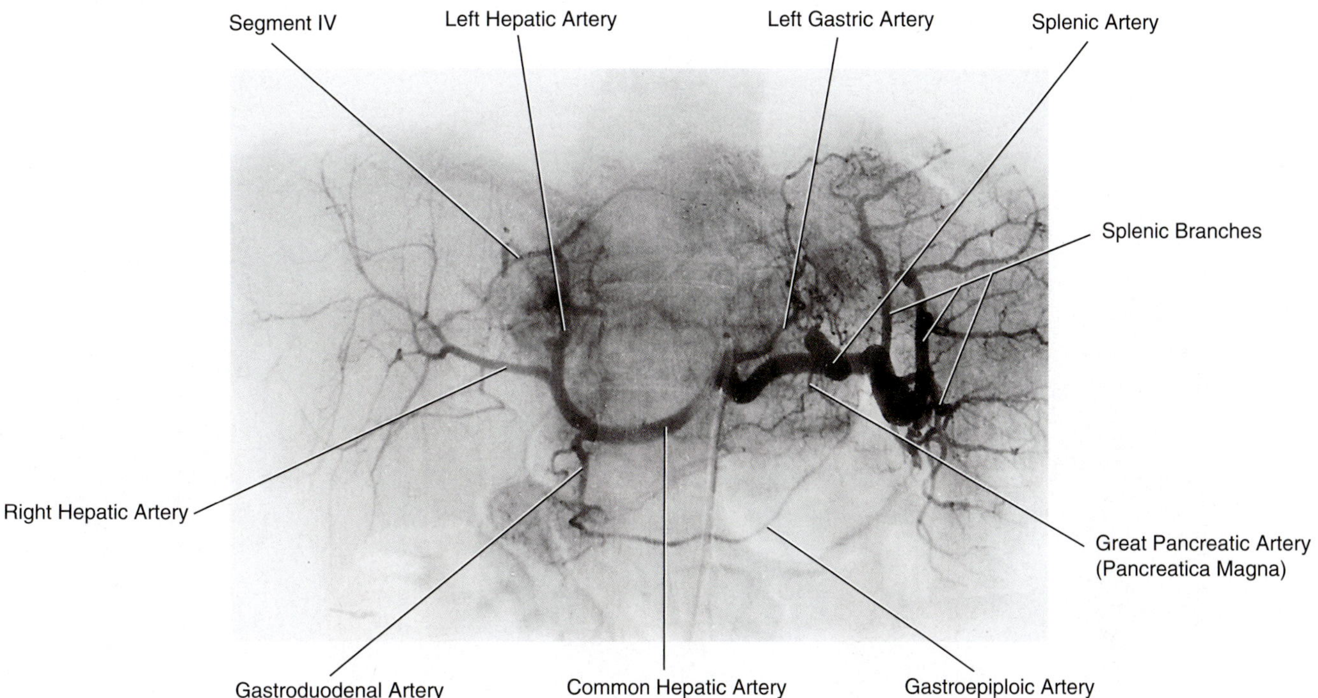

Figure 18.96. Celiac trunk injection showing the large splenic artery and the intrasplenic circulation. Note the presence of an arterial bifurcation at the hilus making at least three independent segments in the spleen. In this specific case the spleen is enlarged.

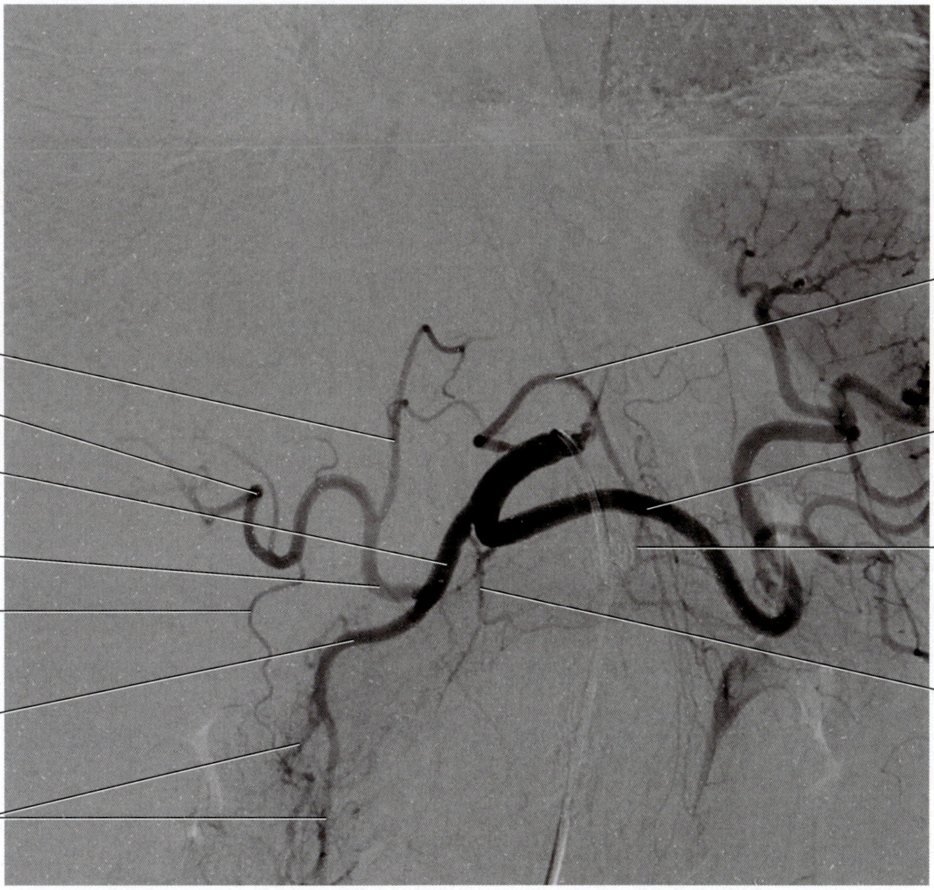

Left Hepatic Artery
Right Hepatic Artery
Common Hepatic
Artery
Proper Hepatic Artery
Pericholedochal
Plexus Artery
Gastroduodenal
Artery
Pancreaticoduodenal
Arcades
Left Gastric
Artery
Splenic Artery
Arteria
Pancreatica
Magna
Dorsal
Pancreatic
Artery

Figure 18.97. Splenic artery angiography shows a tortuous splenic artery with bifurcation in at least three segments in the spleen.

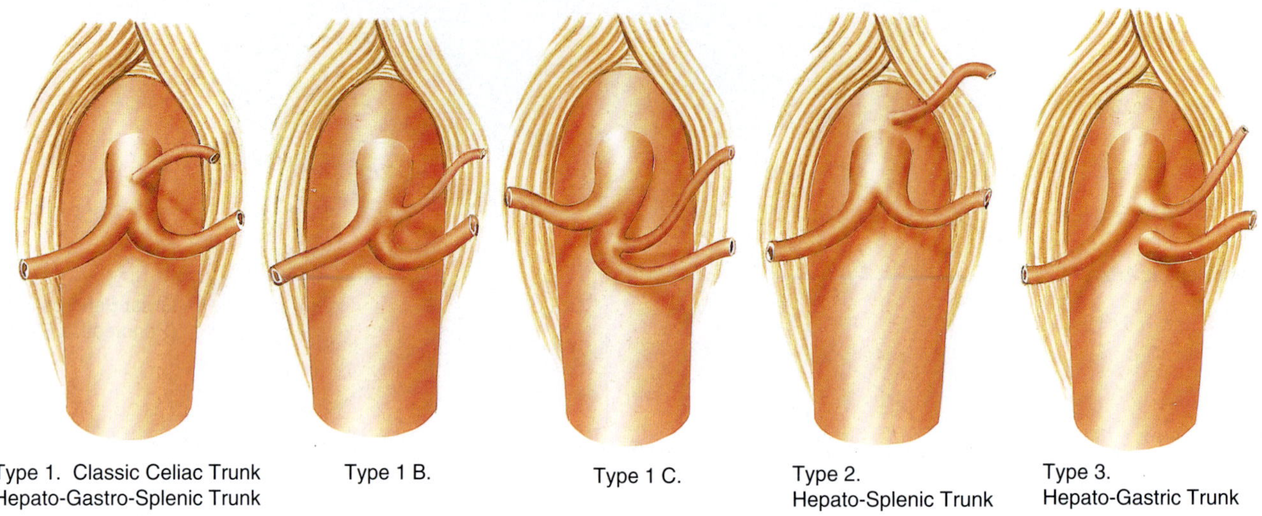

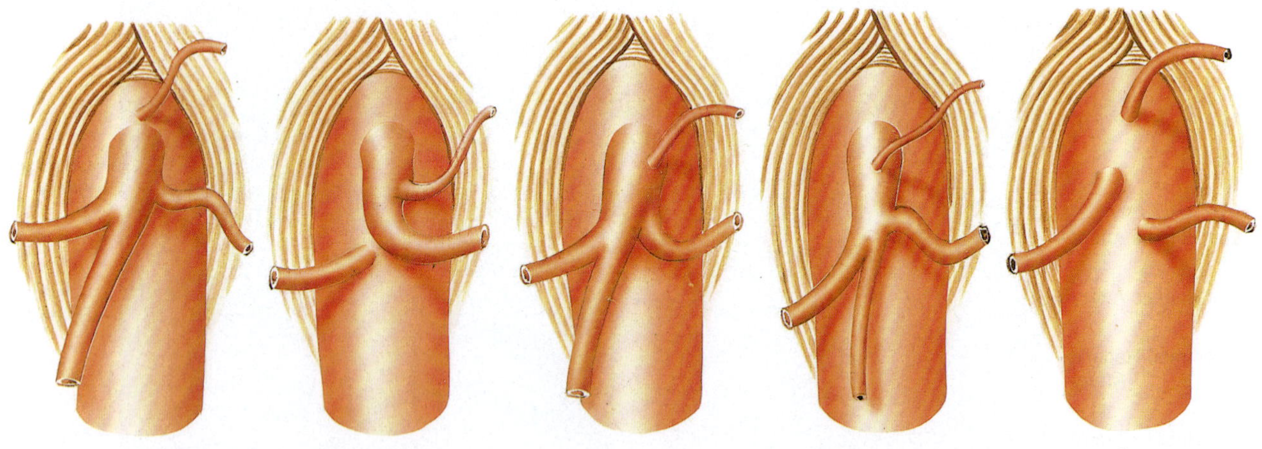

Figure 18.98. Schematic drawing showing the variations in the configuration of the celiac trunk.

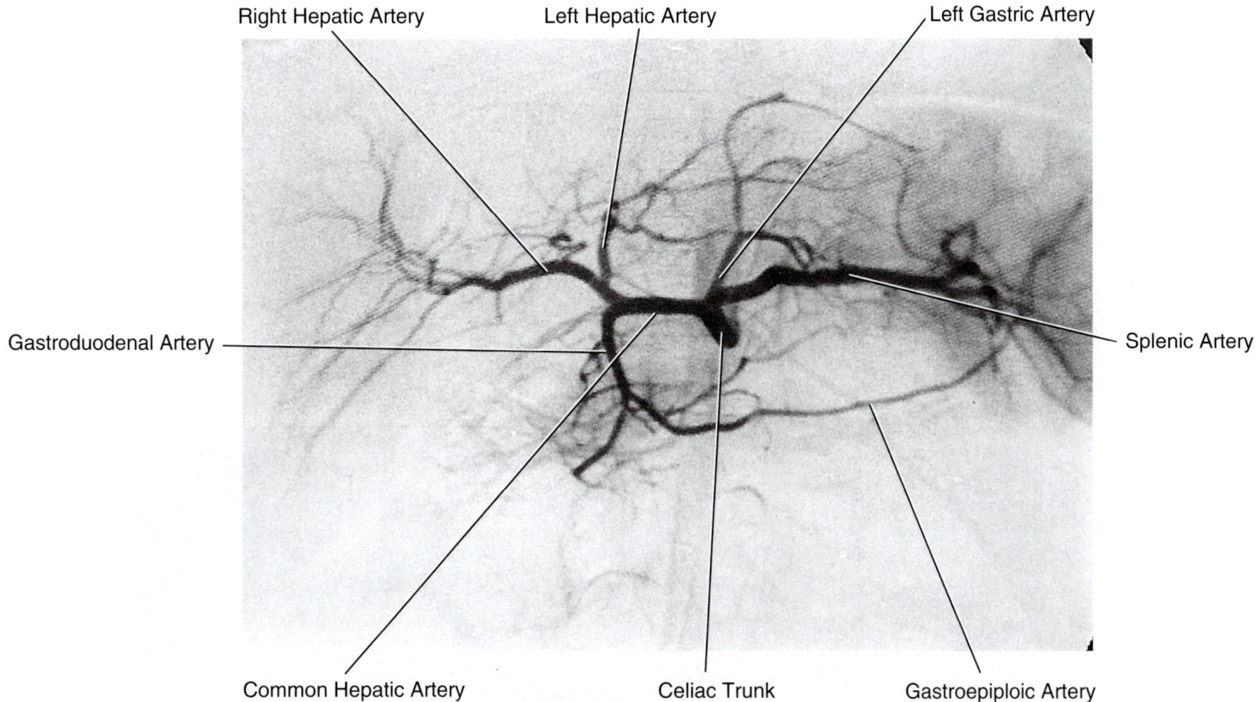

Figure 18.99. Celiac angiography shows the classical configuration of the celiac trunk also called type 1, hepatogastrosplenic trunk.

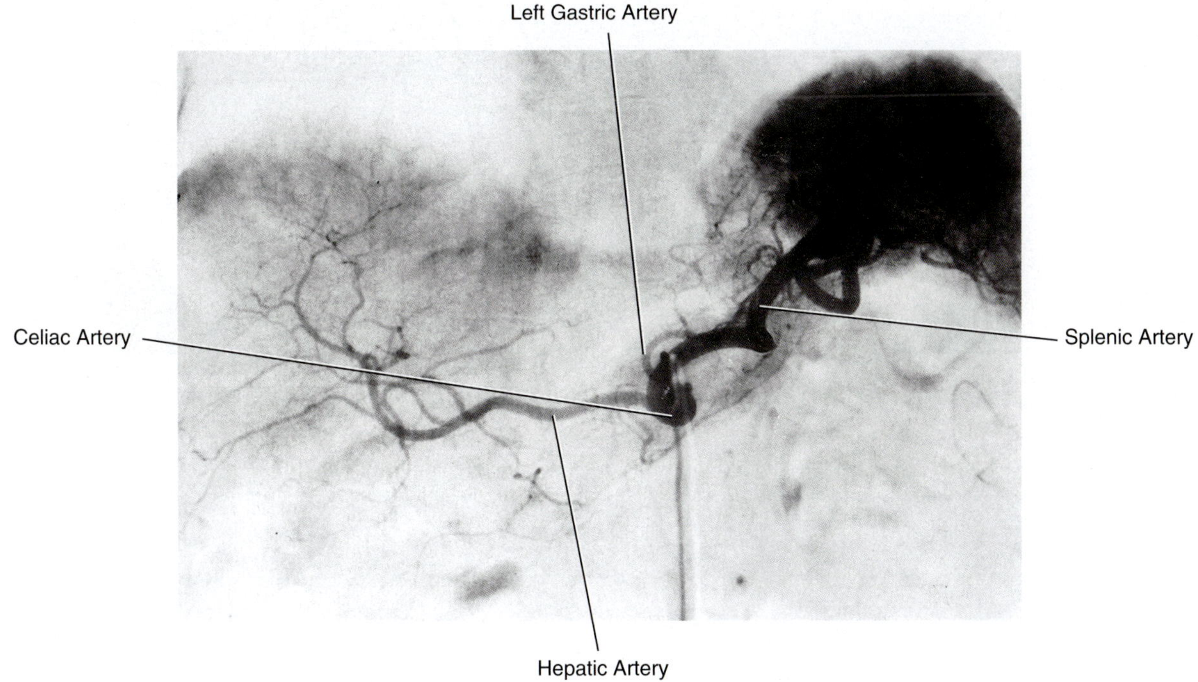

Figure 18.100. Celiac angiography shows the type 7c celiac trunk, also called gastrosplenic trunk. The splenic artery is dominant, and the hepatic artery arises from the splenic artery.

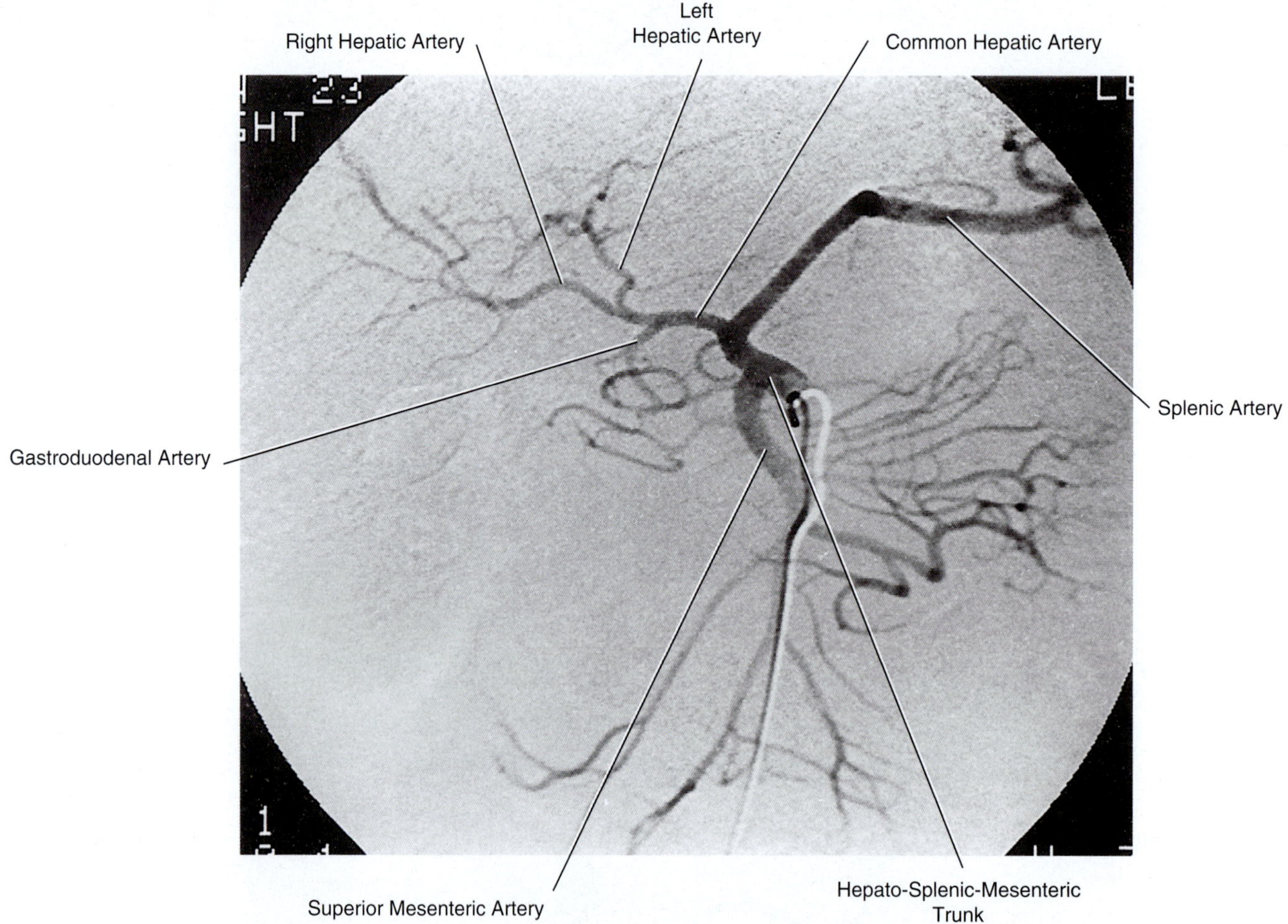

Figure 18.101. Celiac angiography shows a hepatosplenicmesenteric trunk. The left gastric artery arises directly from the aorta. The hepatic, splenic, and mesenteric arteries form a single trunk.

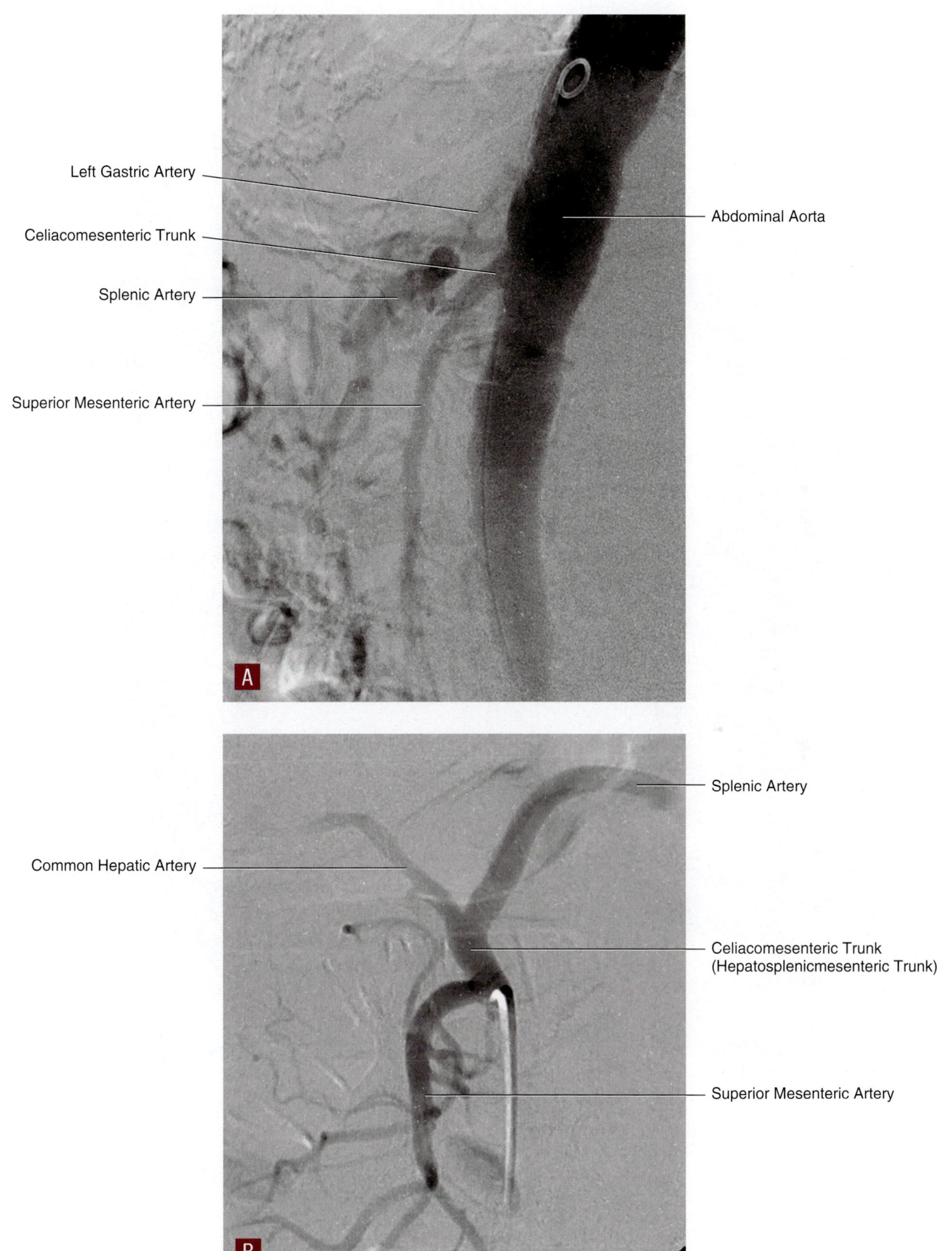

Figure 18.102. A and B, **Celiac angiography showing a hepatosplenicmesenteric (celiacomesenteric) trunk.** The hepatic, splenic, and mesenteric arteries have common origin from a single trunk.

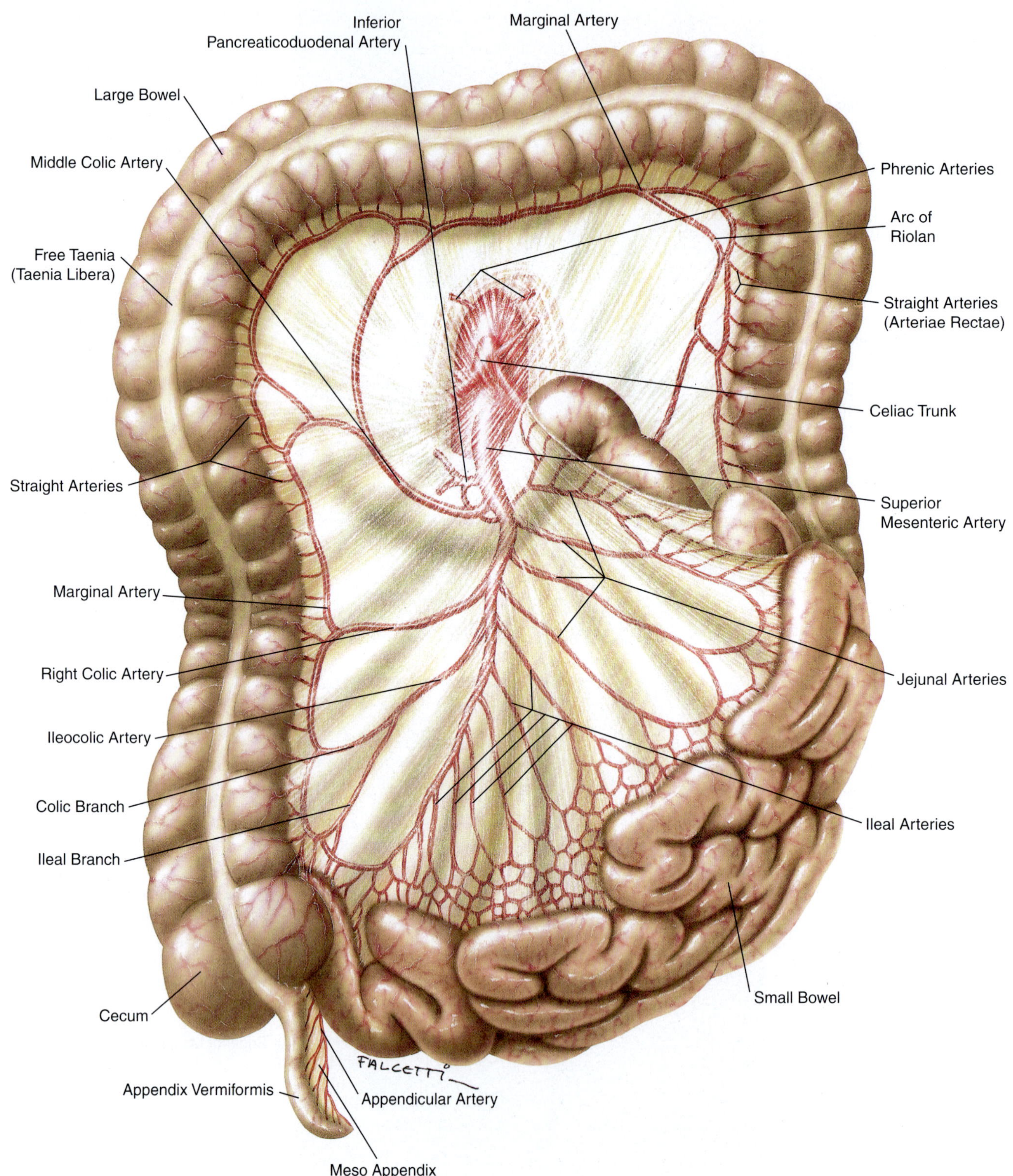

Figure 18.103. Schematic drawing of the SMA and main branches to the large bowel and to the small bowel.

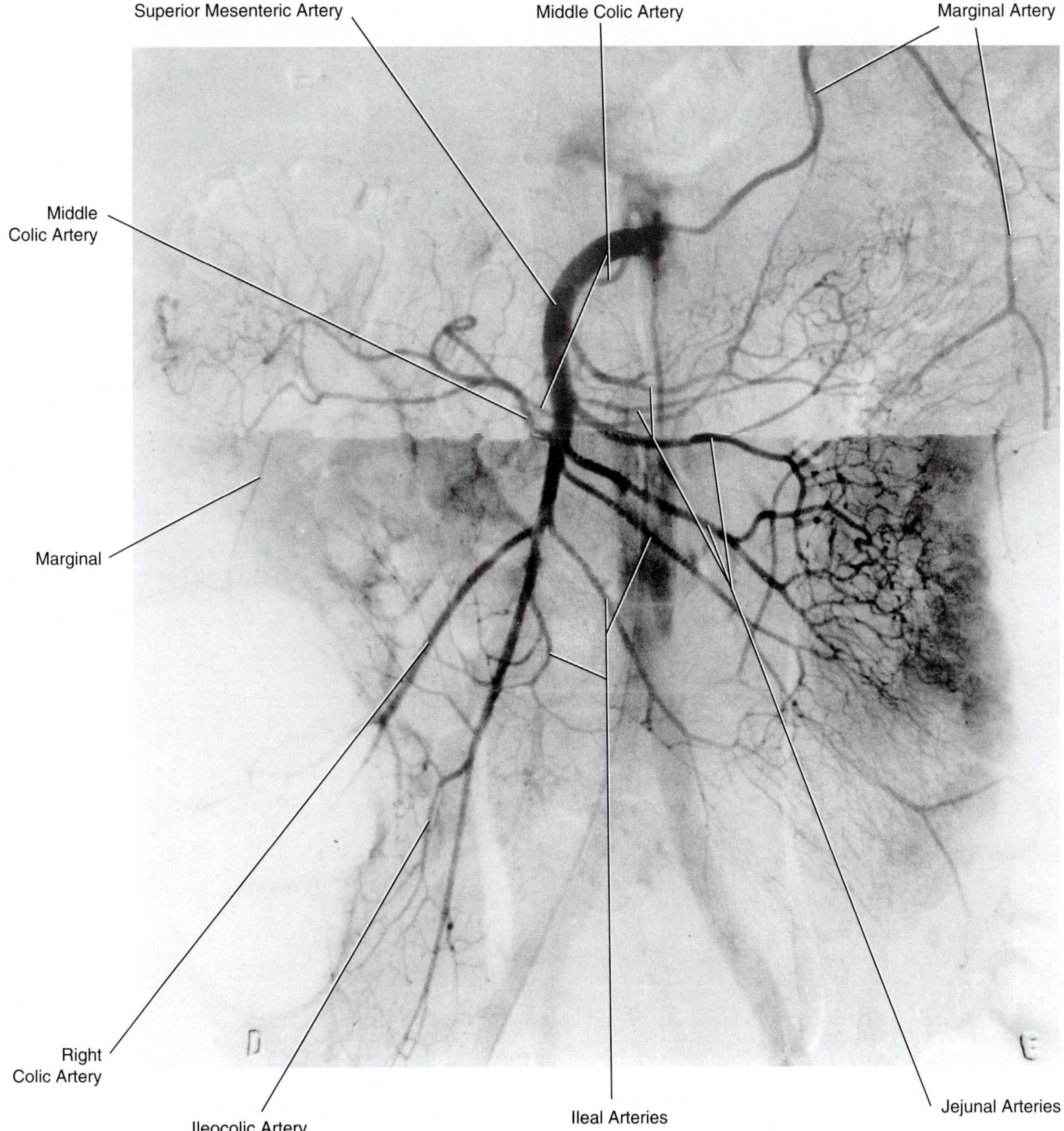

Figure 18.104. Superior mesenteric angiography showing the main branches to the large bowel and to the small bowel. The middle colic artery has two separate origins from the SMA.

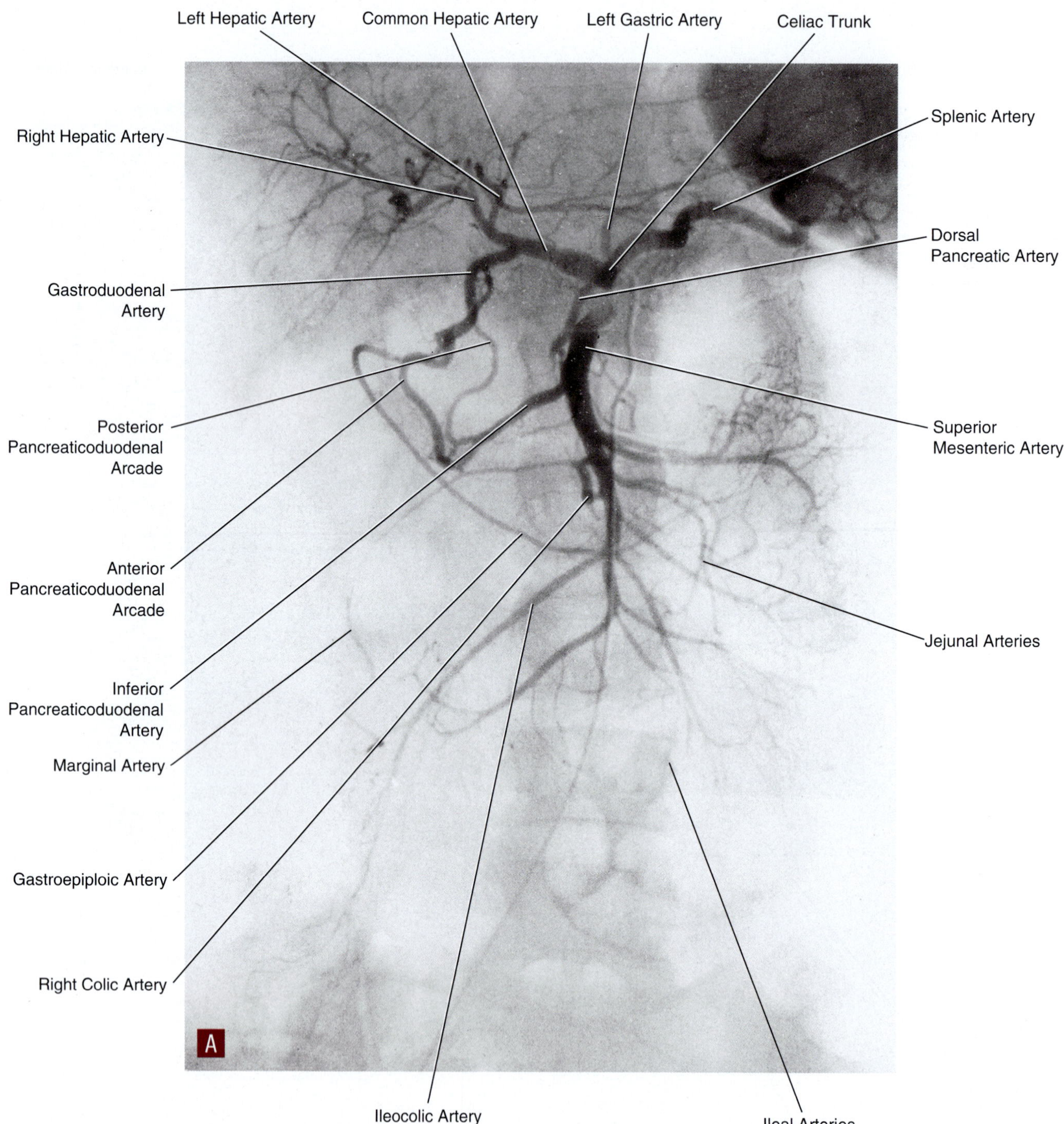

Figure 18.105. **A**, Superior mesenteric angiography shows the enlarged pancreaticoduodenal arcades communicating the SMA with the common hepatic artery through the inferior pancreaticoduodenal artery and gastroduodenal artery. There is severe stenosis of the celiac trunk. **B**, Late phase of the SMA angiogram showing the superior mesenteric vein, the colic veins, and the jejunal and ileal veins, as well as the portal and splenic veins.

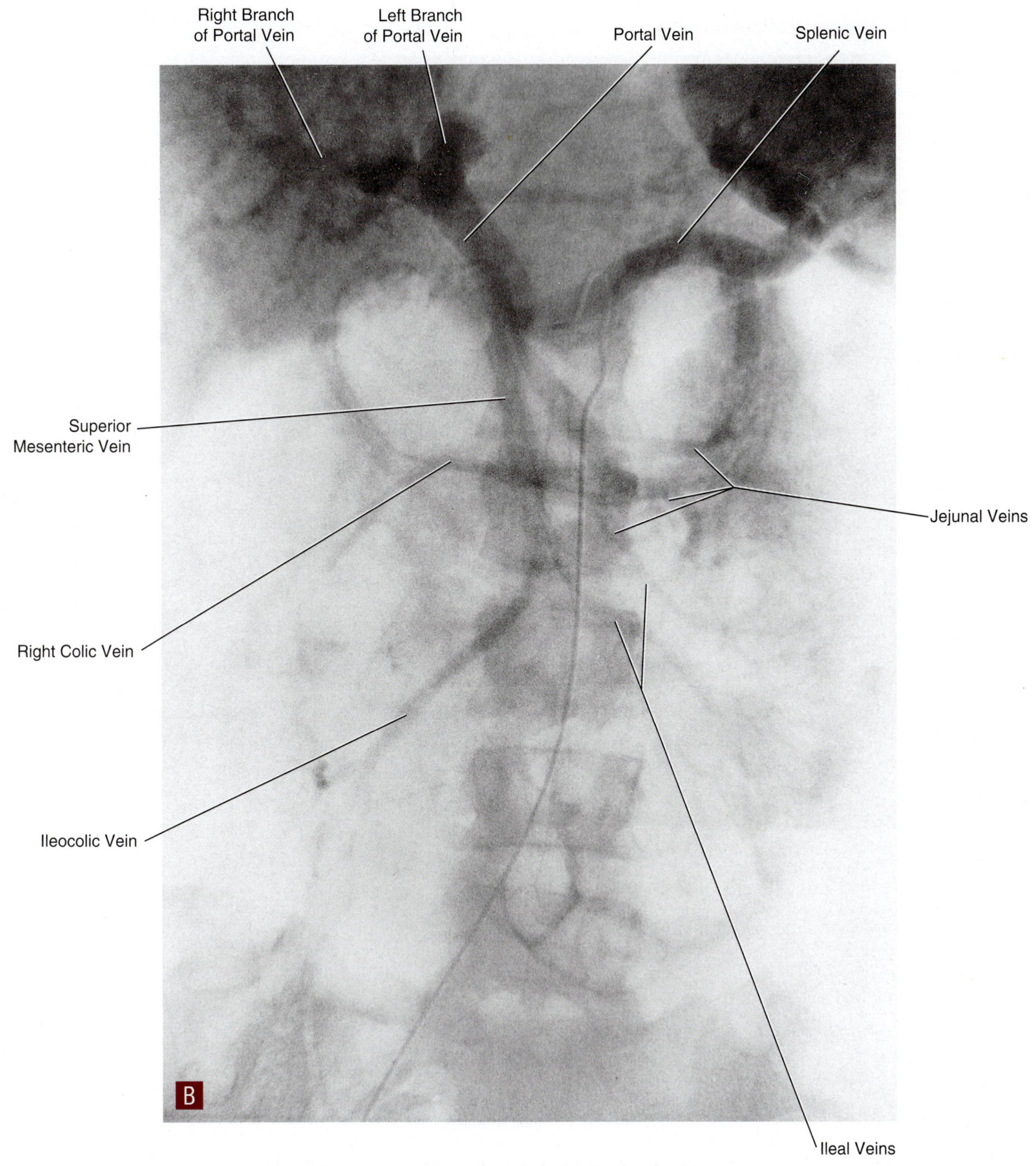

Figure 18.105. *Continued*

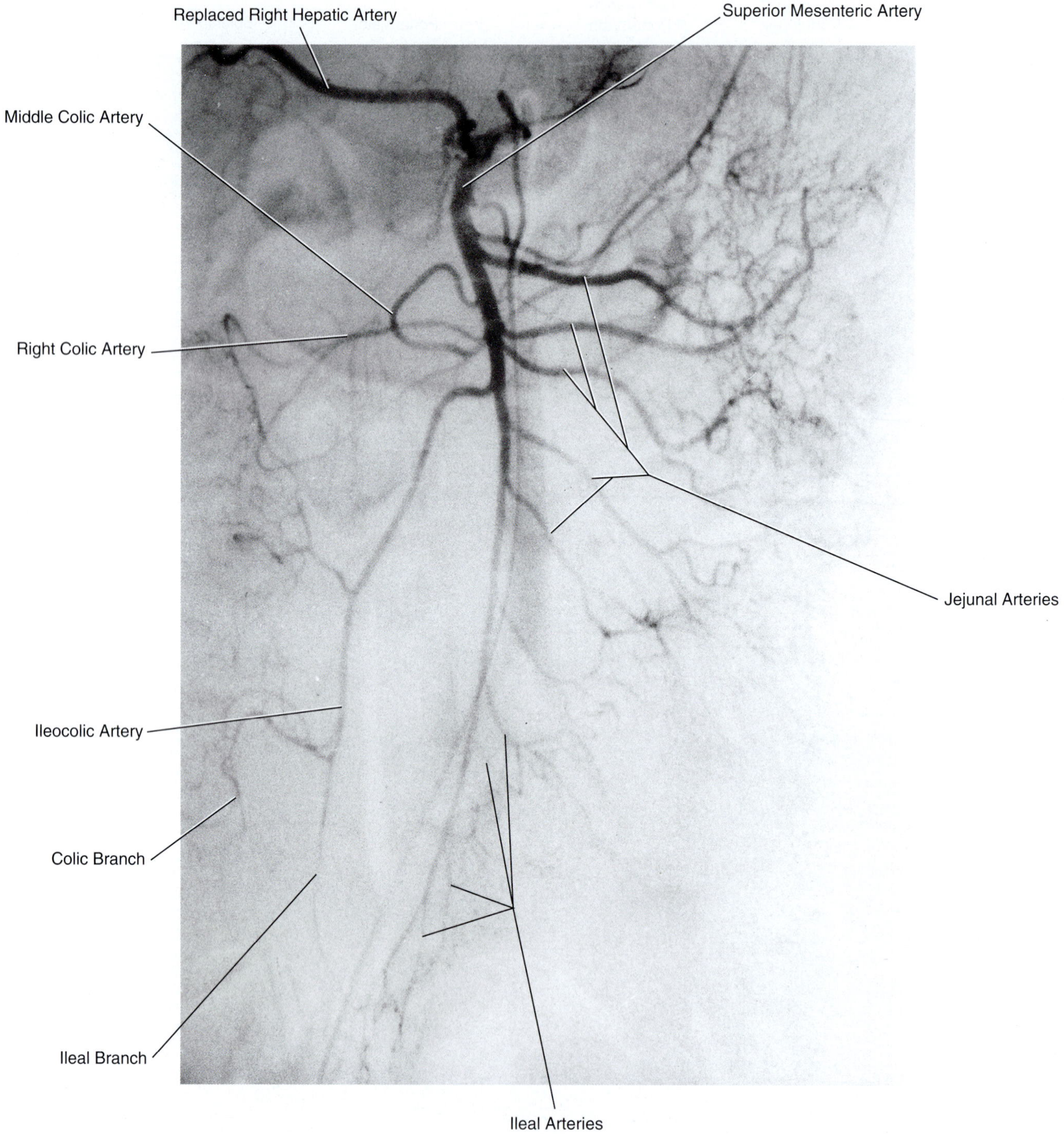

Figure 18.106. Superior mesenteric angiography showing the main branches to the large bowel and small bowel. Note the replaced right hepatic artery.

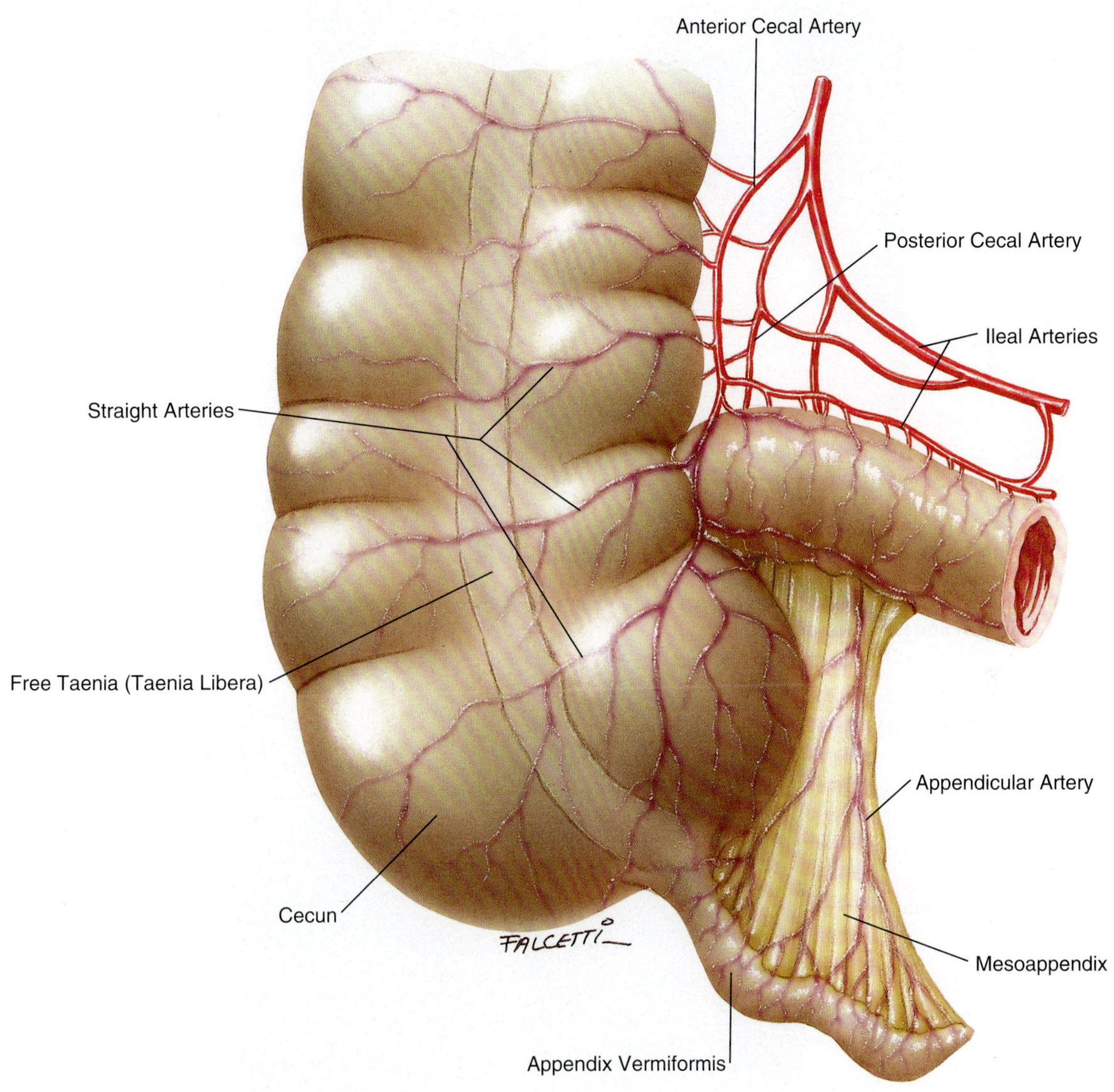

Figure 18.107. Schematic drawing showing closeup of the distal ileal arteries and the cecal arteries, as well as the appendicular artery.

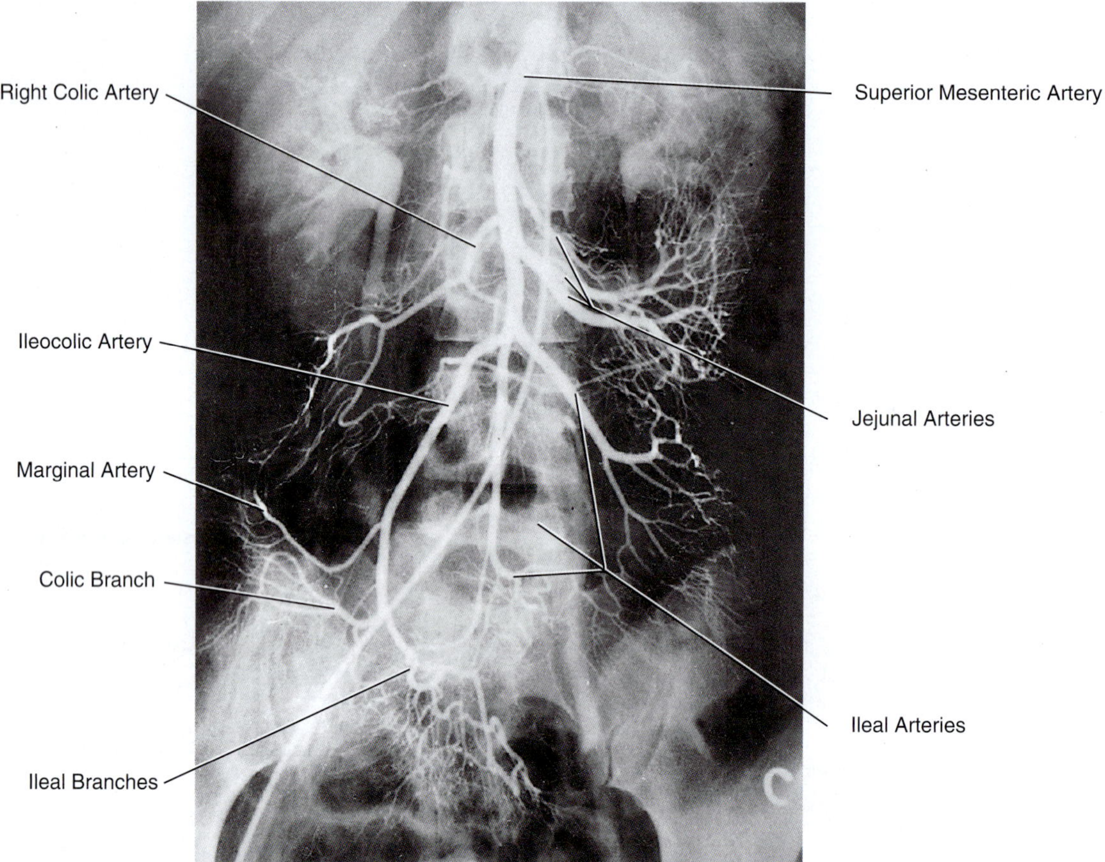

Figure 18.108. **Superior mesenteric angiography showing the branches to the small bowel and large bowel.**

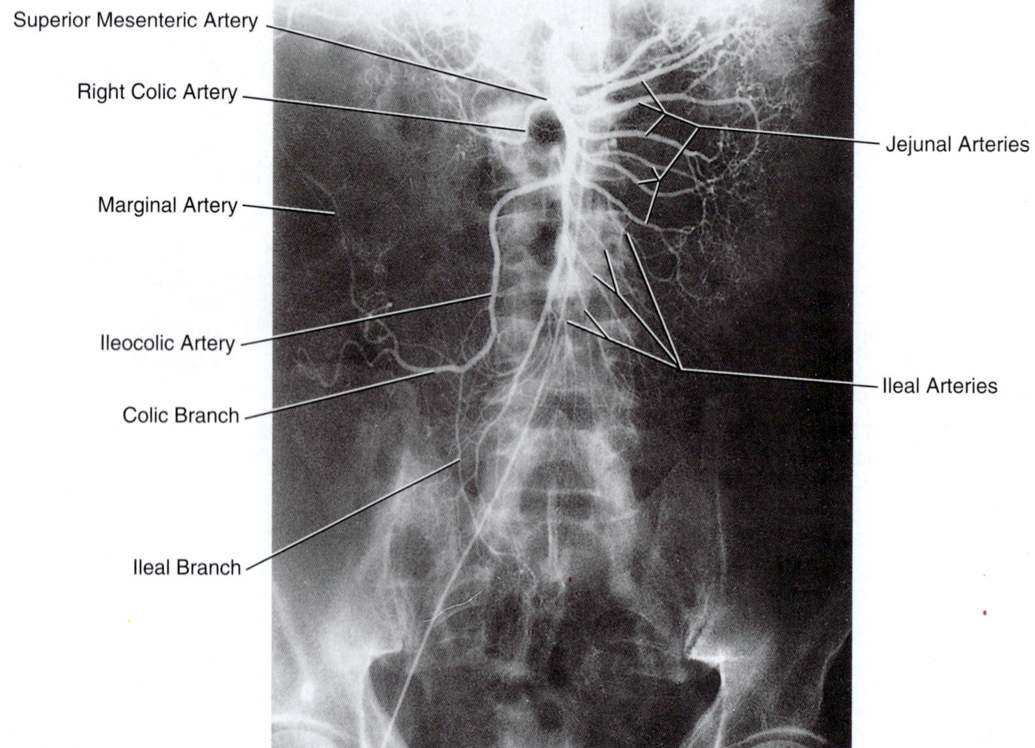

Figure 18.109. **Superior mesenteric angiography showing the branches to the small bowel and large bowel.**

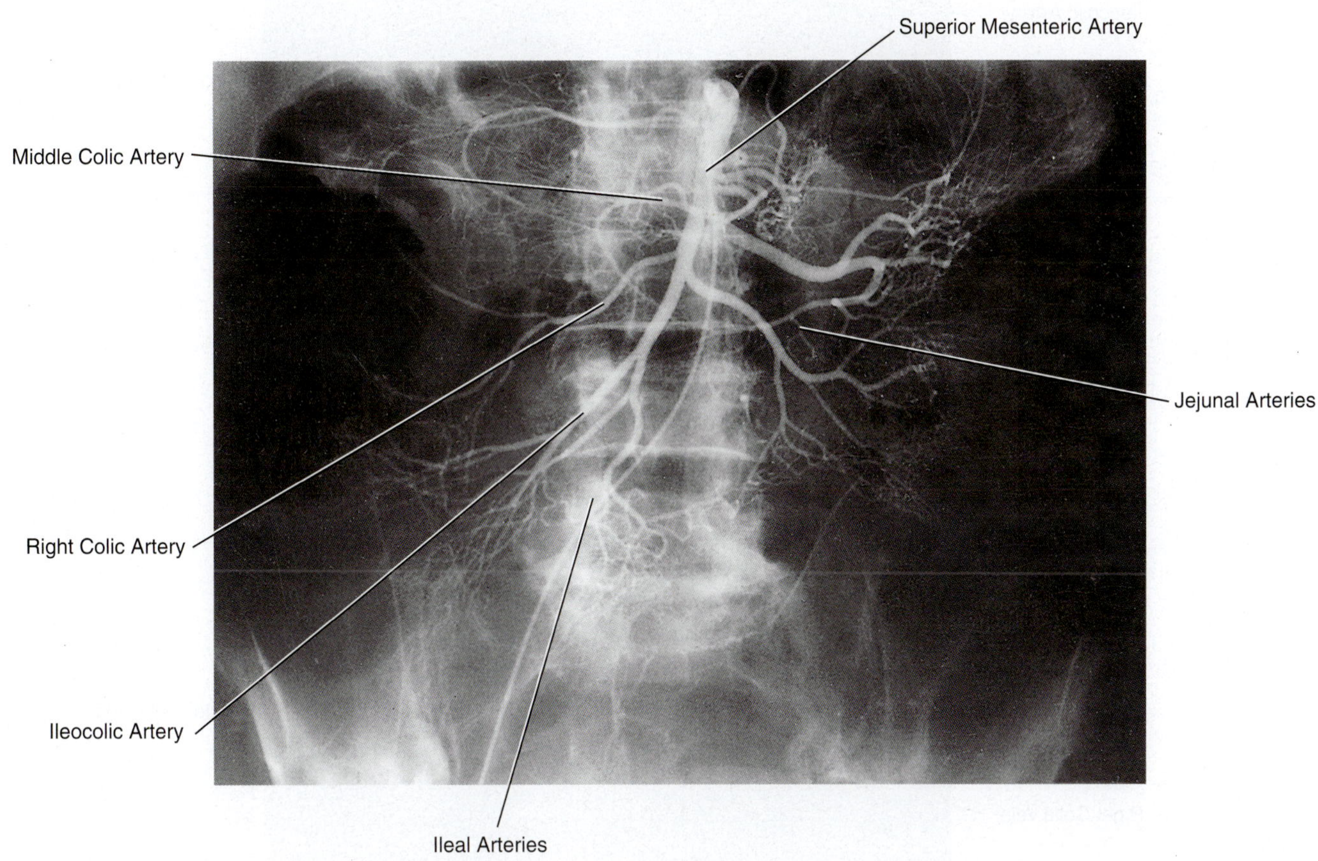

Figure 18.110. **Magnification view of superior mesenteric angiography showing the branches to the small bowel and large bowel.**

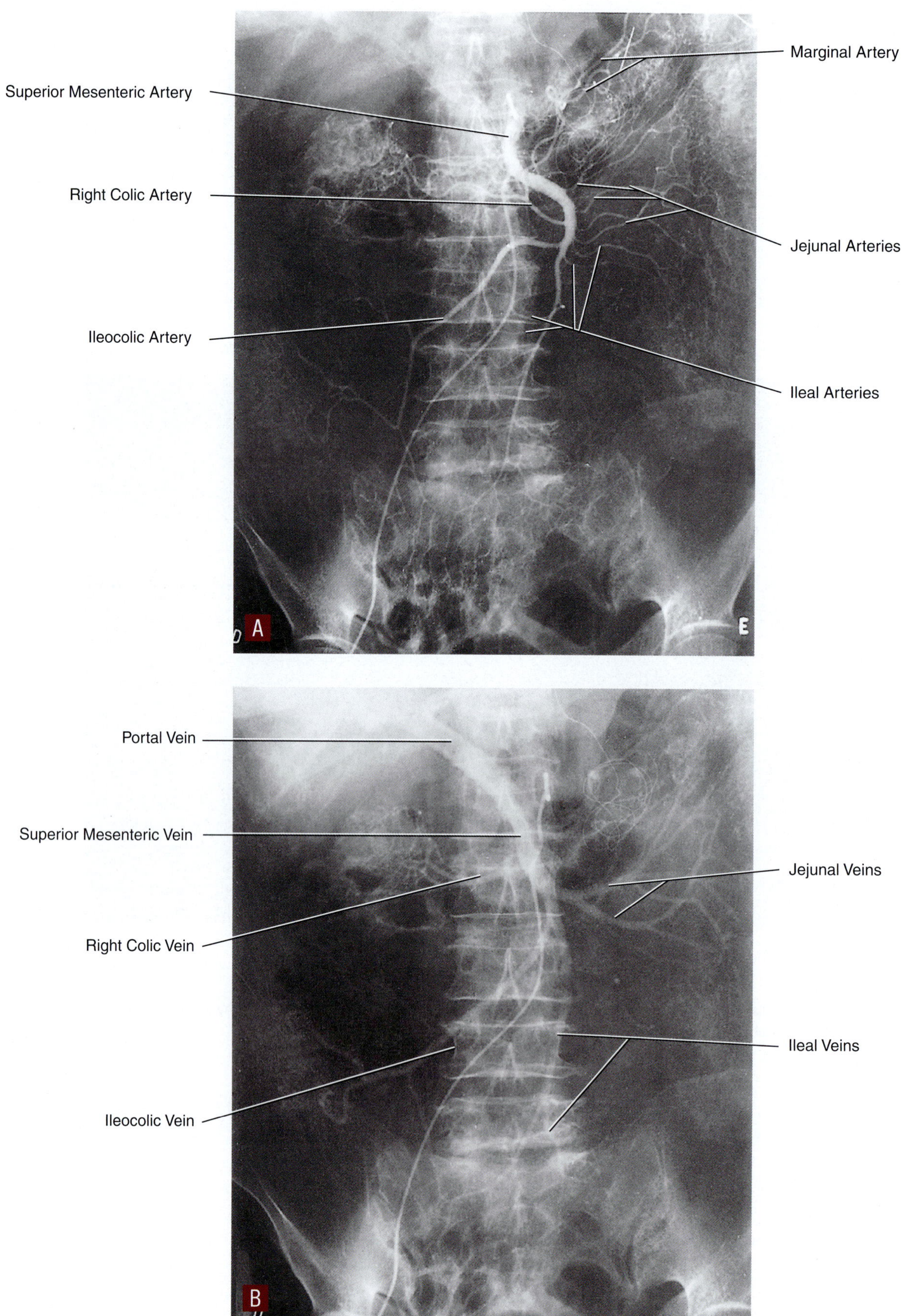

Figure 18.111. **A**, Early phase of the superior mesenteric angiography showing the branches to the small bowel and large bowel. **B**, Late phase of the SMA angiography showing the superior mesenteric vein, and the colic, jejunal, and ileal veins.

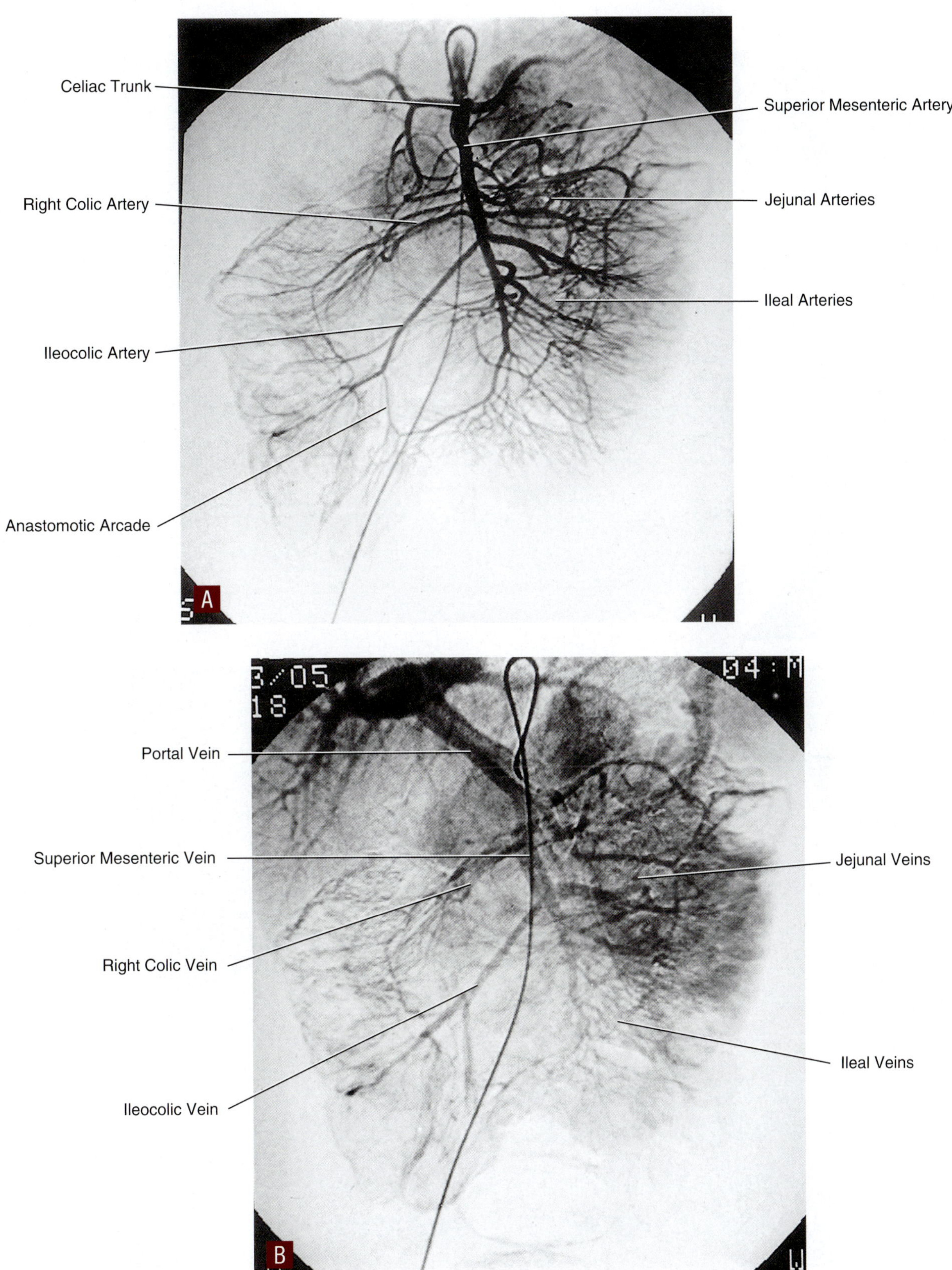

Figure 18.112. **A**, Superior mesenteric angiography showing the branches to the small bowel and large bowel. **B**, Later phase of the SMA angiography showing the superior mesenteric, jejunal and ileal veins, as well as the portal vein.

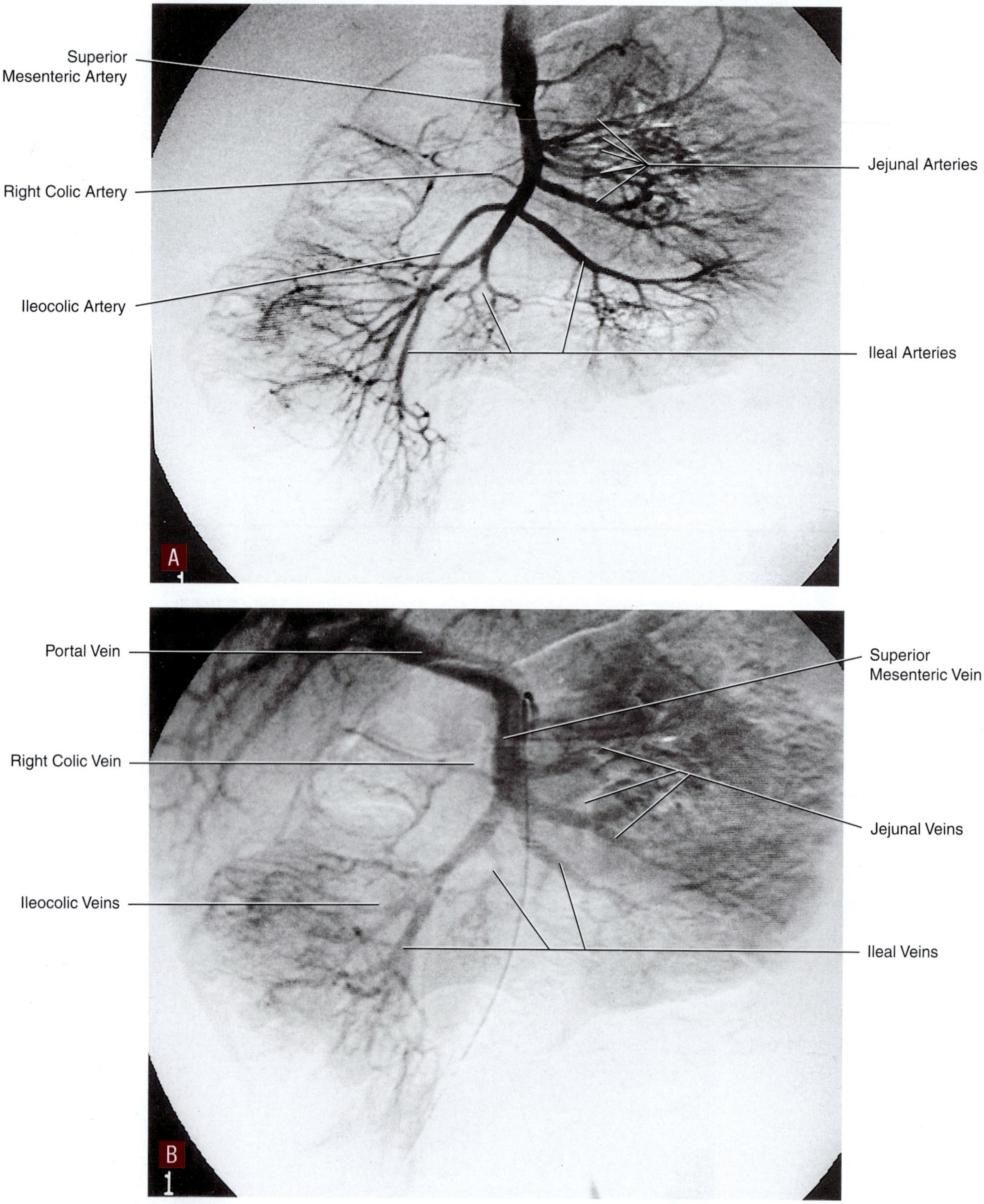

Figure 18.113. **A**, SMA angiography showing the arteries to the small bowel and large bowel. **B**, Later phase of the SMA angiography showing the bowel veins and the portal vein.

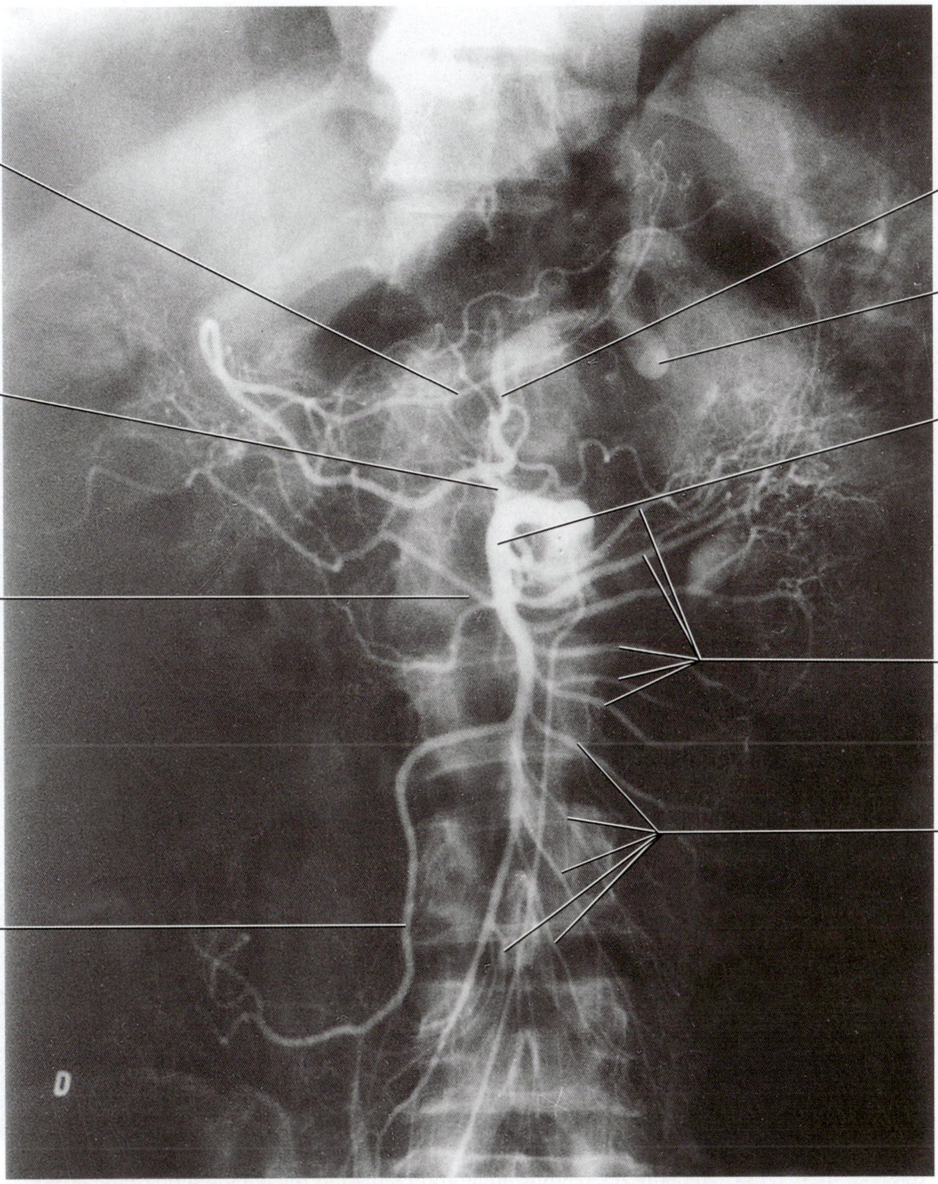

Marginal Artery
Artery of Bühler
Splenic Artery
Middle Colic Artery
Superior Mesenteric Artery
Right Colic Artery
Jejunal Arteries
Ileal Arteries
Ileocolic Artery

Figure 18.114. Superior mesenteric arteriogram shows the branches to the small and large bowel. Note the artery of Bühler connecting the middle colic artery to the celiac trunk. The splenic artery is faintly seen.

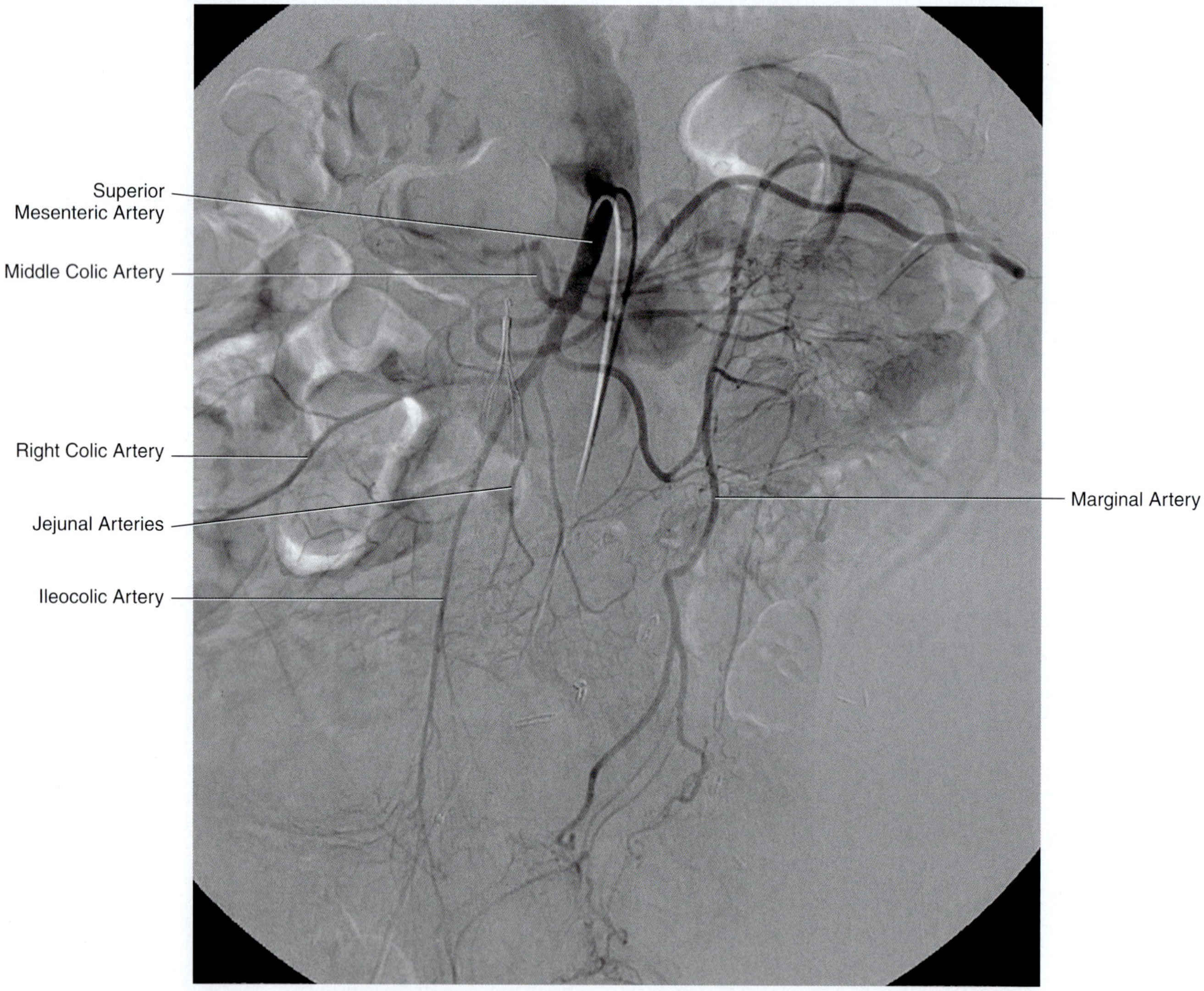

Figure 18.115. Superior mesenteric angiogram showing the enlarged marginal artery, branch of the middle colic artery.

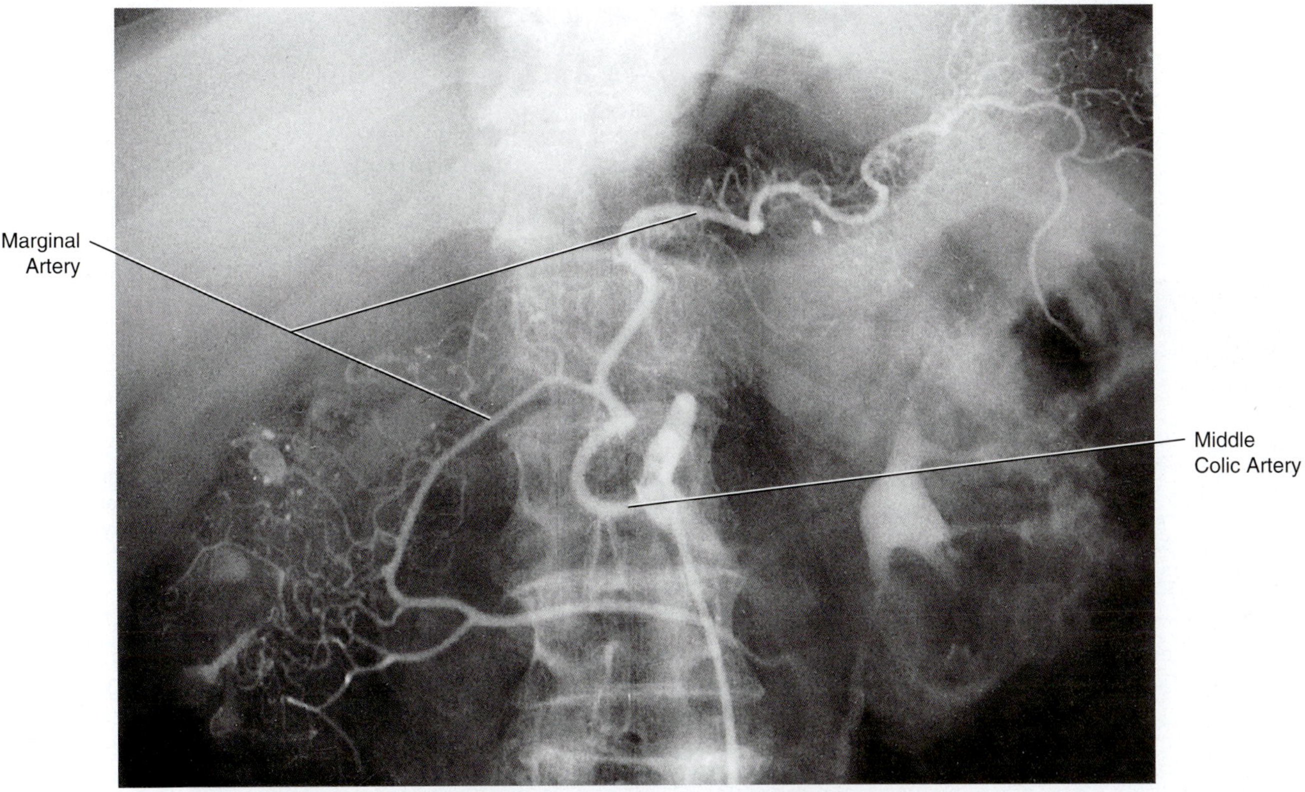

Figure 18.116. Selective injection at the middle colic artery. Note the marginal artery at the transverse colon.

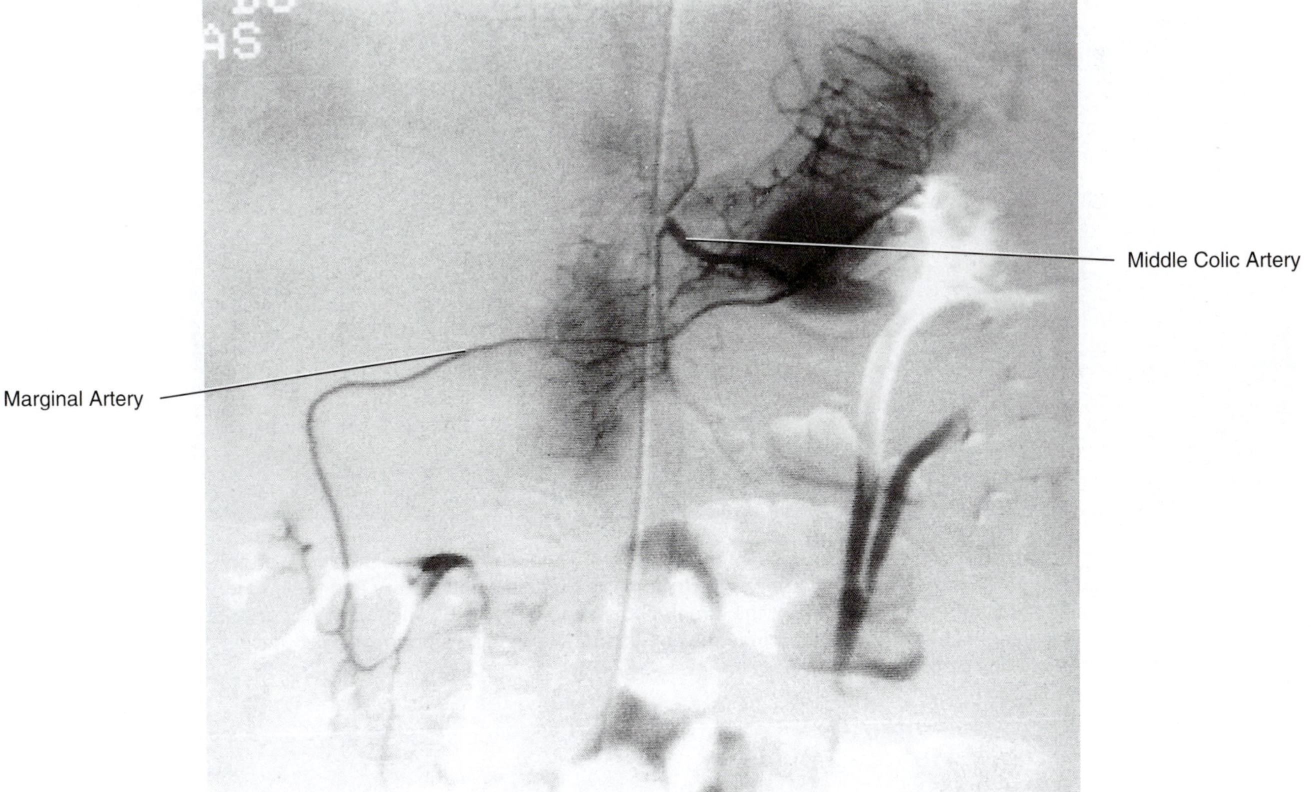

Figure 18.117. Selective injection at the middle colic artery.

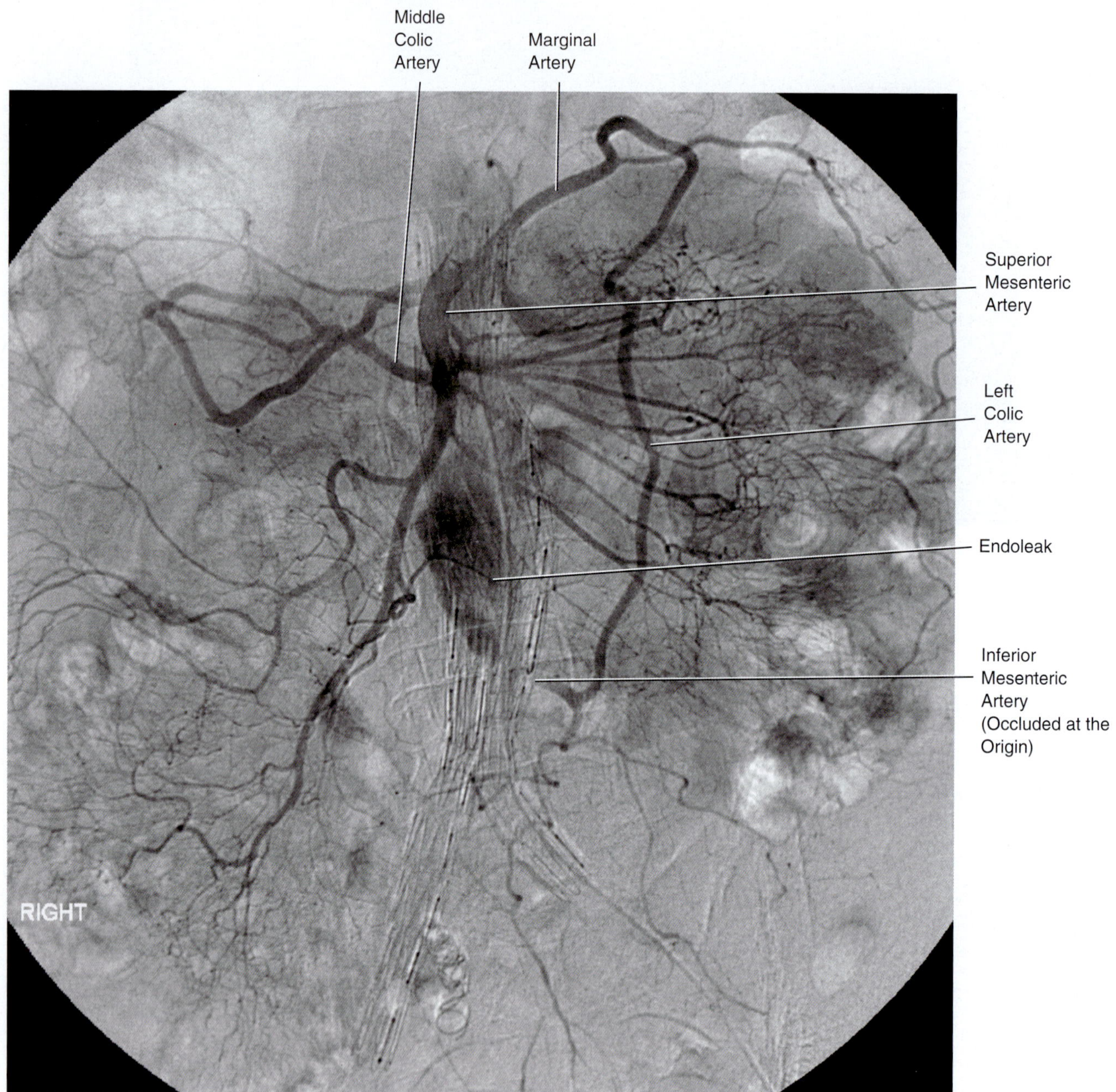

Figure 18.118. Superior mesenteric arteriogram showing a large middle colic artery supplying an enlarged marginal artery, which connects to the left colic artery and the inferior mesenteric artery. Note the filling of the lumen of the abdominal aortic aneurysm sac, despite the placement of a stent-graft to exclude the aneurysm. A large type II endoleak was present and treated by embolization.

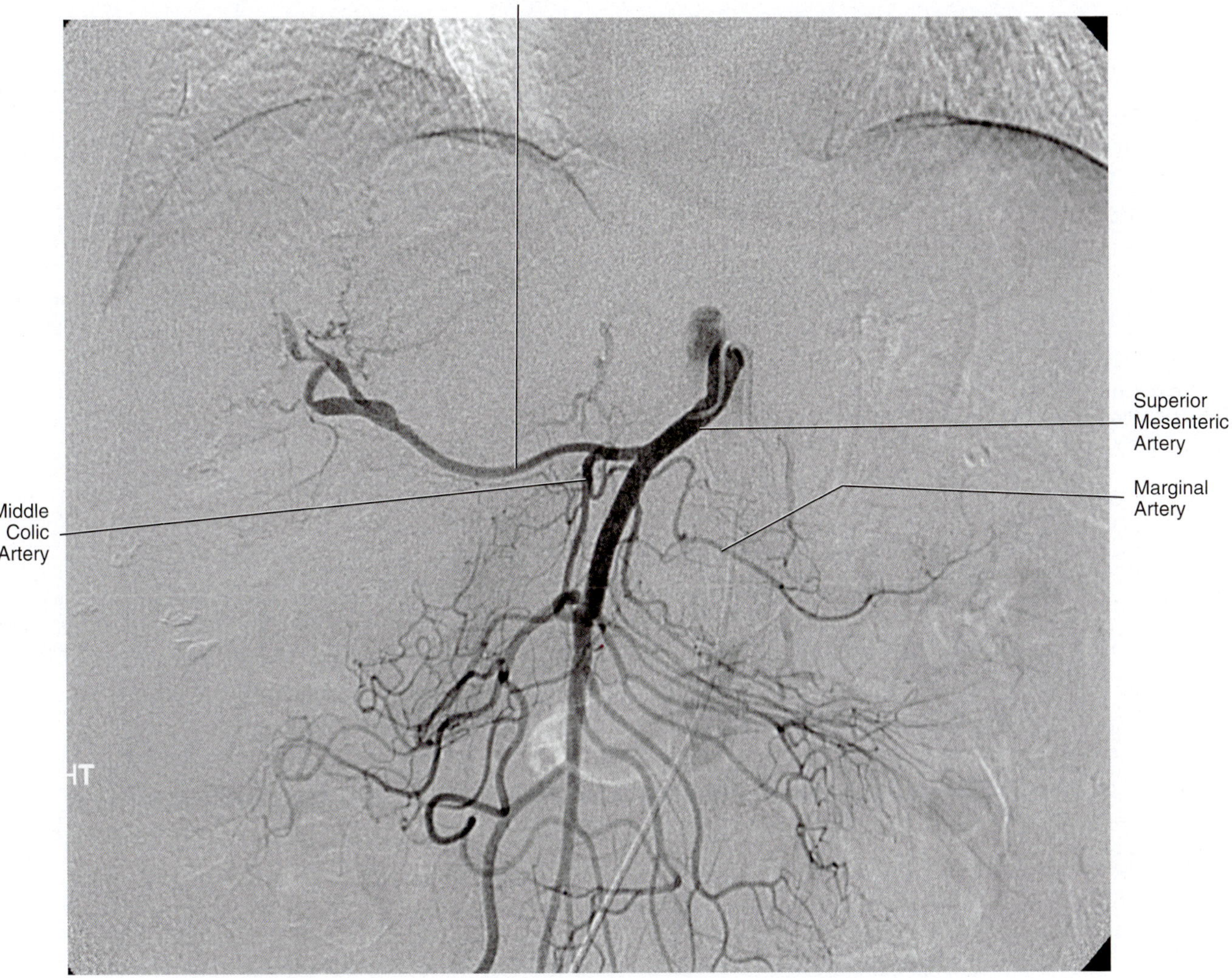

Figure 18.119. Superior mesenteric arteriogram showing a replaced right hepatic artery with an abnormal middle colic artery arising from the proximal hepatic artery. The gastroduodenal artery was a branch of the common hepatic artery from the celiac trunk.

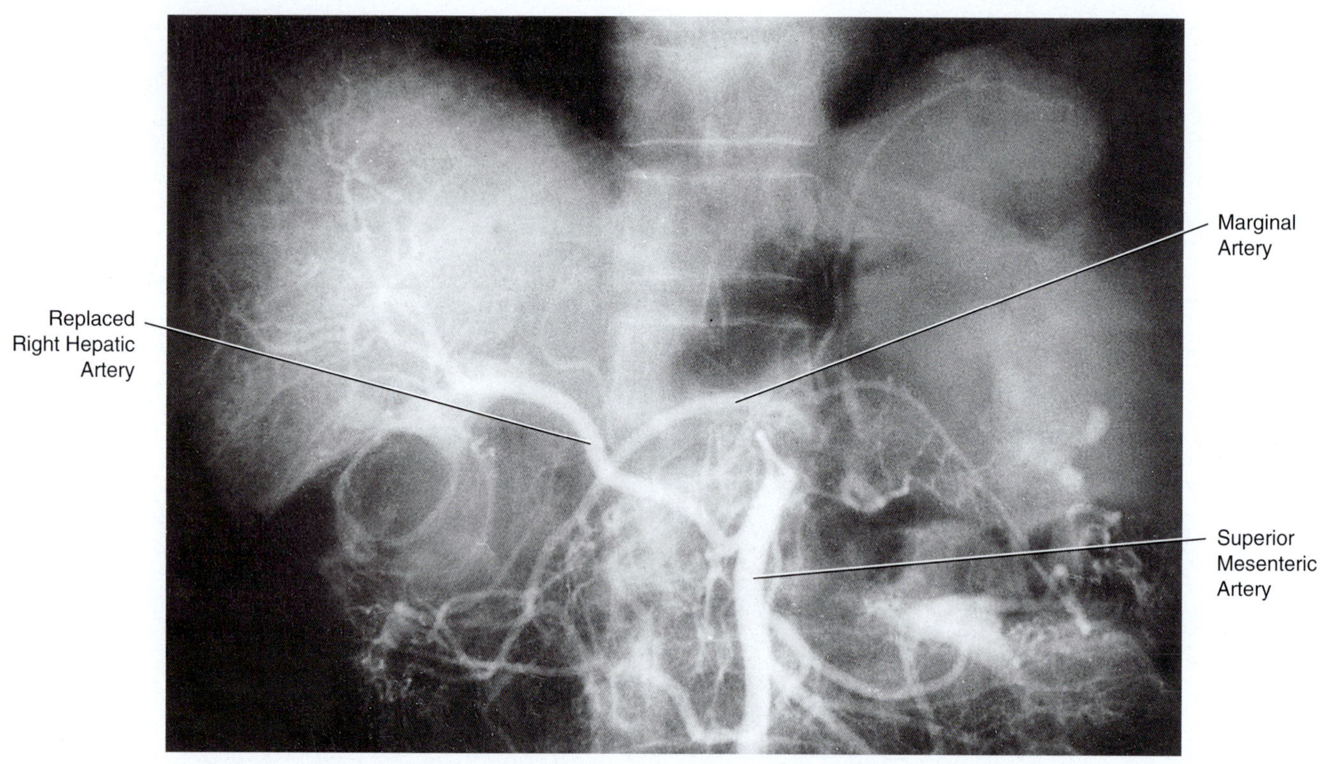

Figure 18.120. Selective angiogram of the superior mesenteric artery. Note the replaced right hepatic artery.

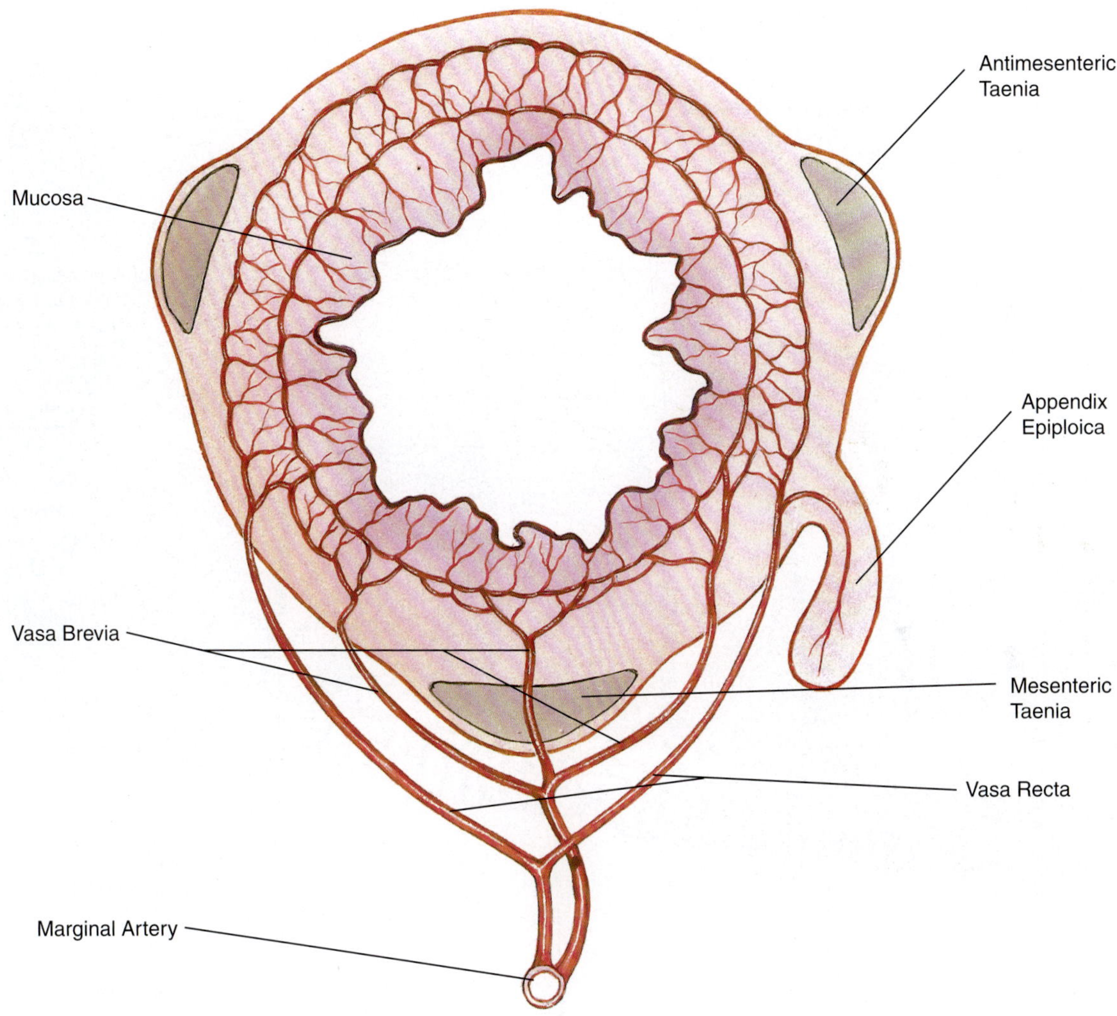

Figure 18.121. Schematic drawing showing a transverse cut of the large bowel with demonstration of the mucosal arteries, from the vasa brevia, and the muscular arteries, from the vasa recta.

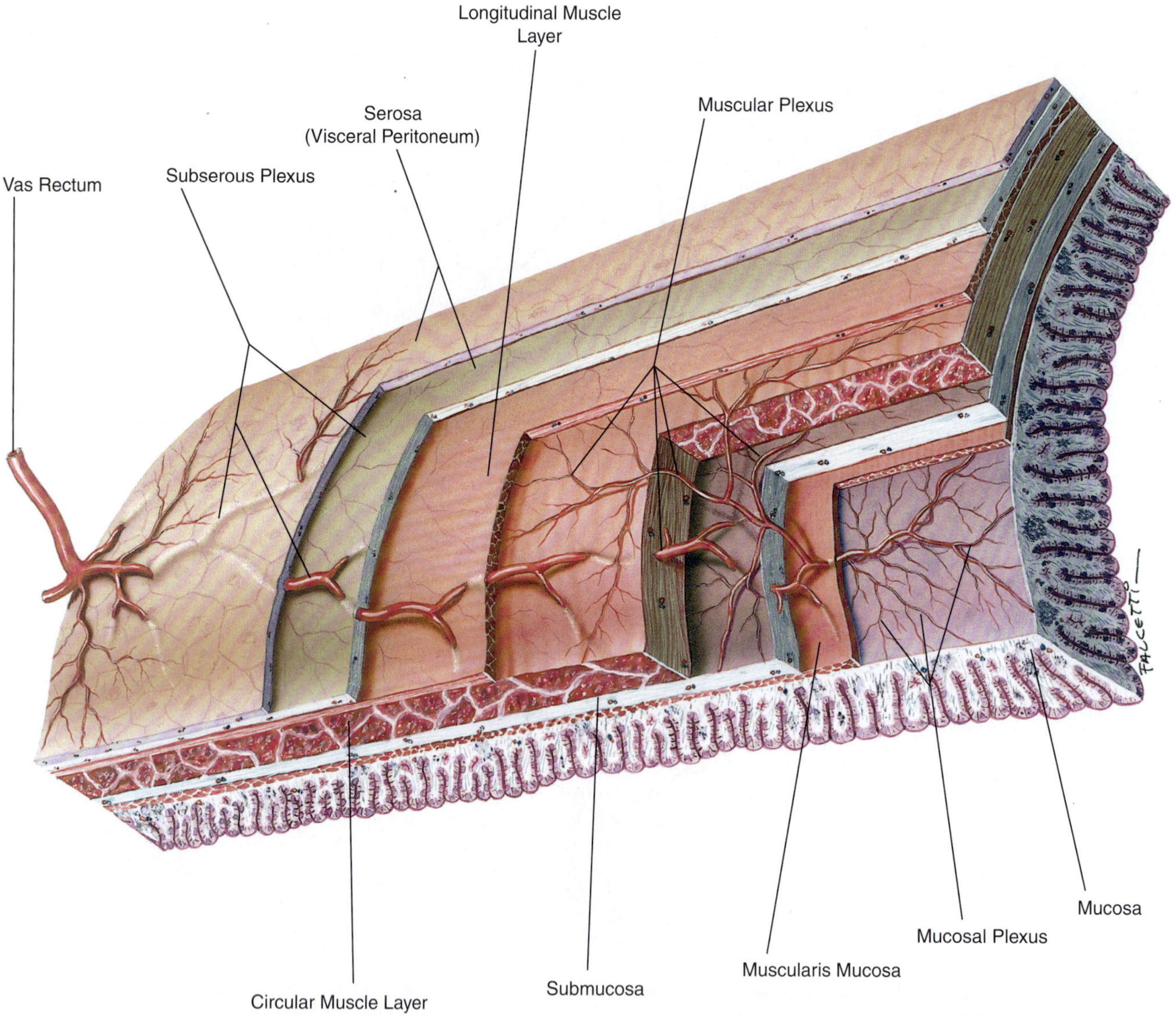

Figure 18.122. Schematic drawing showing the multiple layers of the wall of the small bowel with the vascular distribution from the peritoneum to the mucosa.

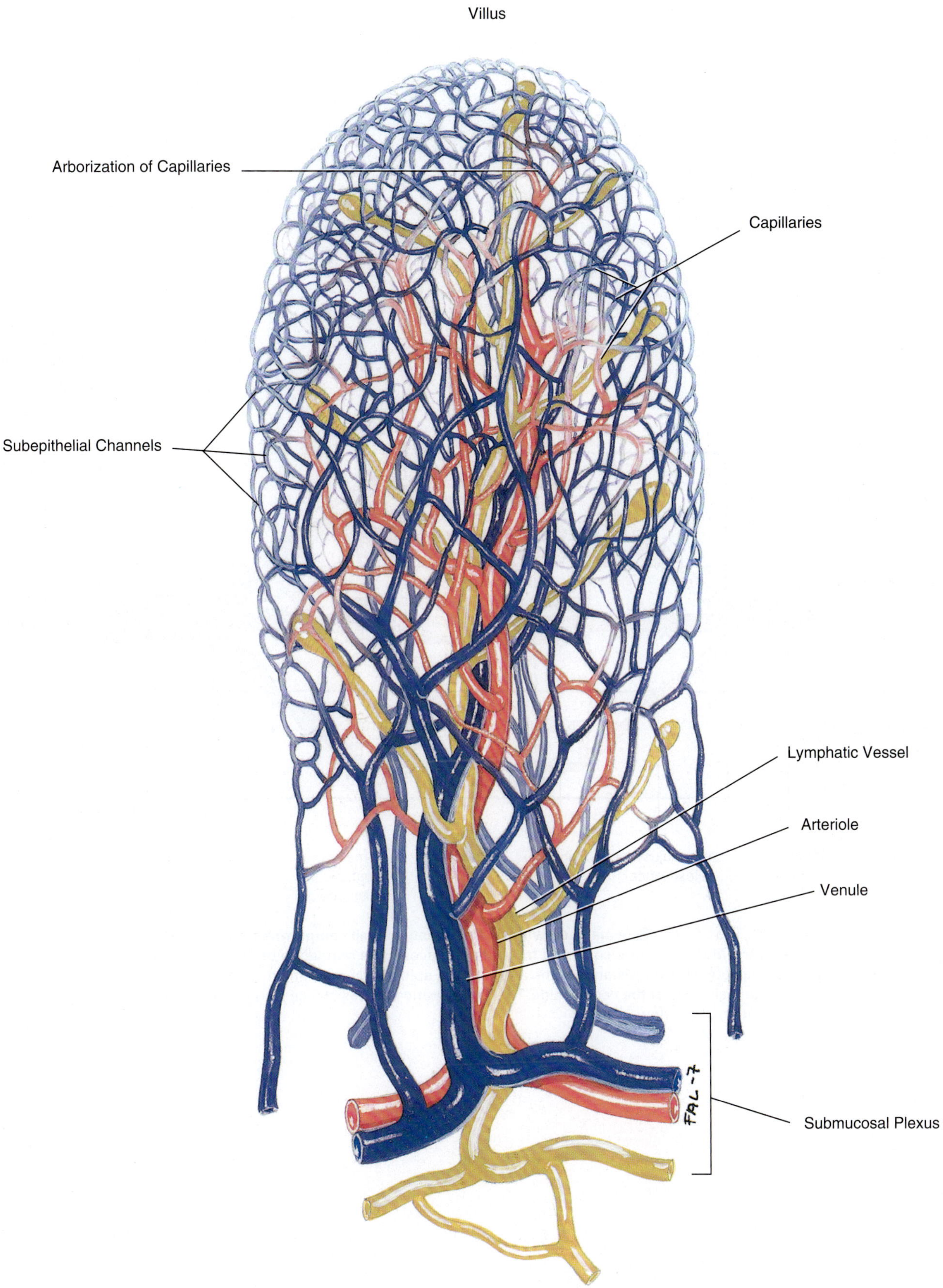

Figure 18.123. Schematic drawing of an intestinal villus showing the venules in blue, the arterioles in red, and the lymphatic vessels in brown. Note the close relationship of the vessels in the center of the villus, being responsible for the countercurrent mechanism of O_2 exchange between the arteriole and venule.

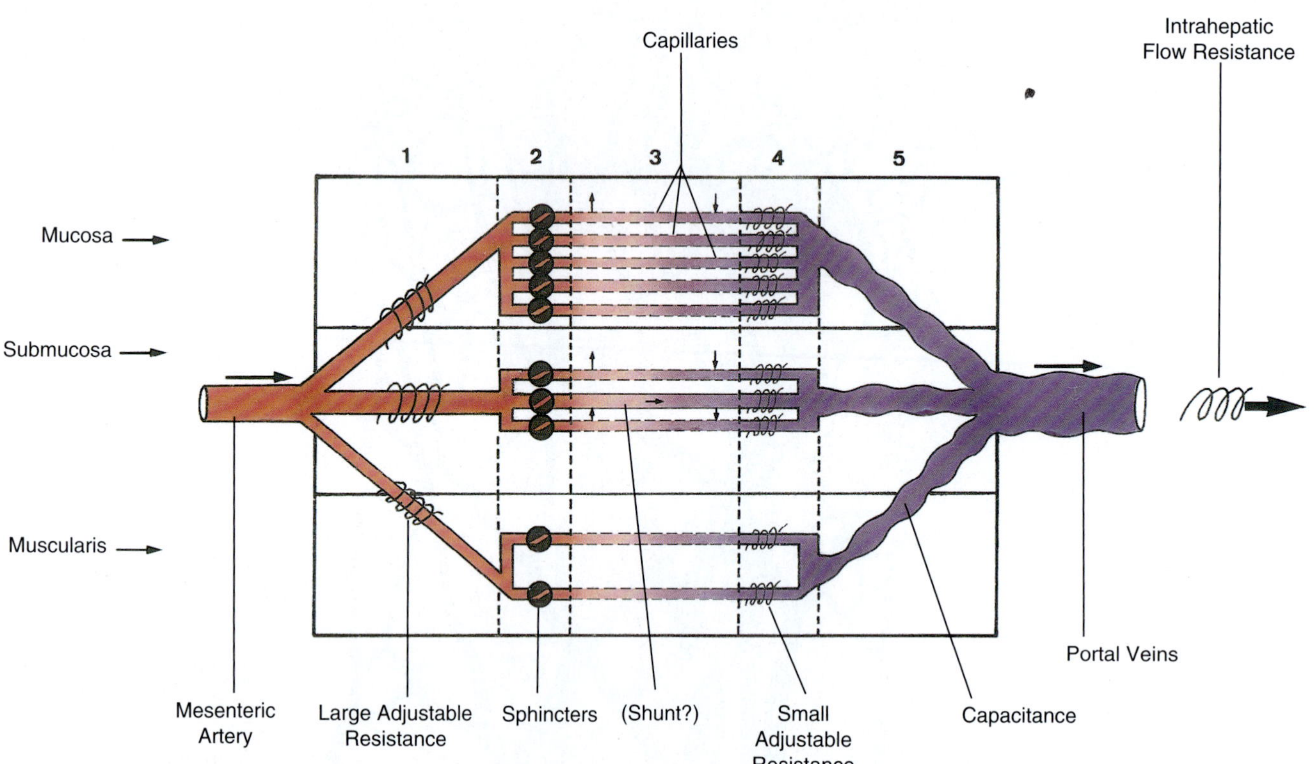

Figure 18.124. Schematic drawing of the intestinal wall compartments with the three layers. Mucosa, submucosa, and muscularis mucosa. The regulation of the flow is done by the large adjustable resistance at the arterial side, sphincteric mechanisms, and small adjustable resistance at the venous side. The intrahepatic flow resistance also plays a role in the regulation of the flow.

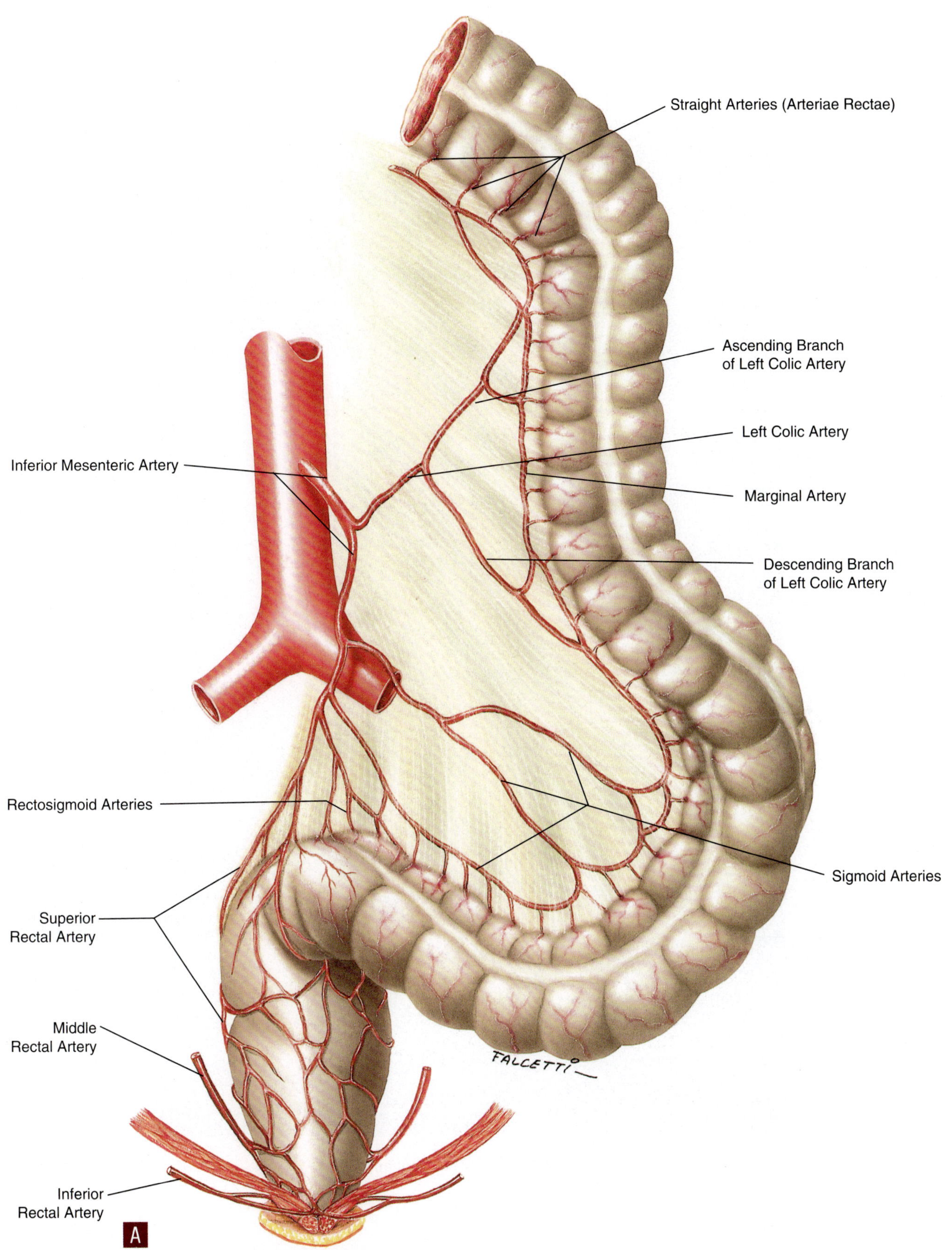

Figure 18.125. A, Schematic drawing of the inferior mesenteric artery circulation. B, Selective angiogram of the middle rectal artery showing anastomotic communications with the superior rectal artery and the bilateral inferior rectal arteries.

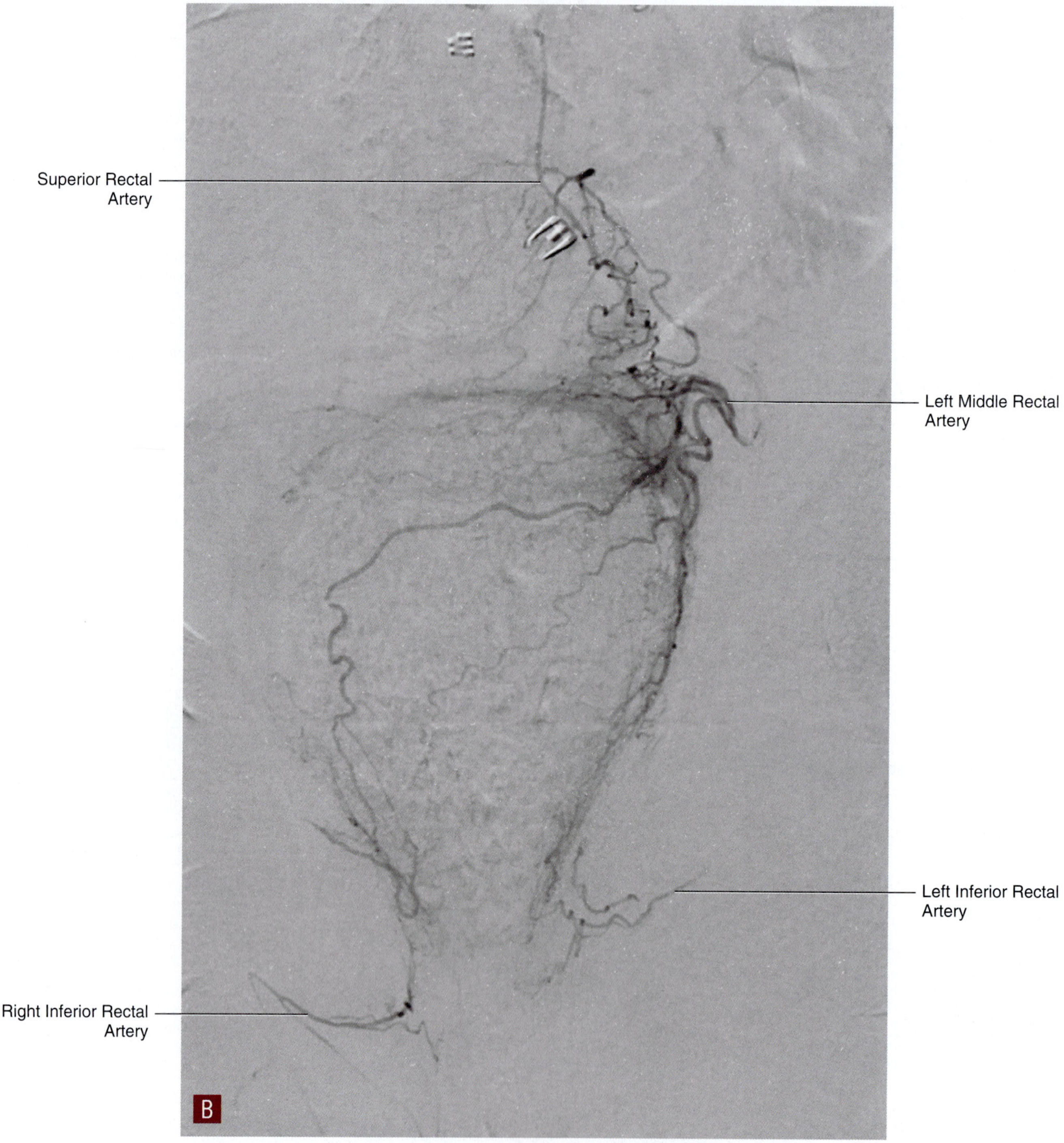

Figure 18.125. *Continued*

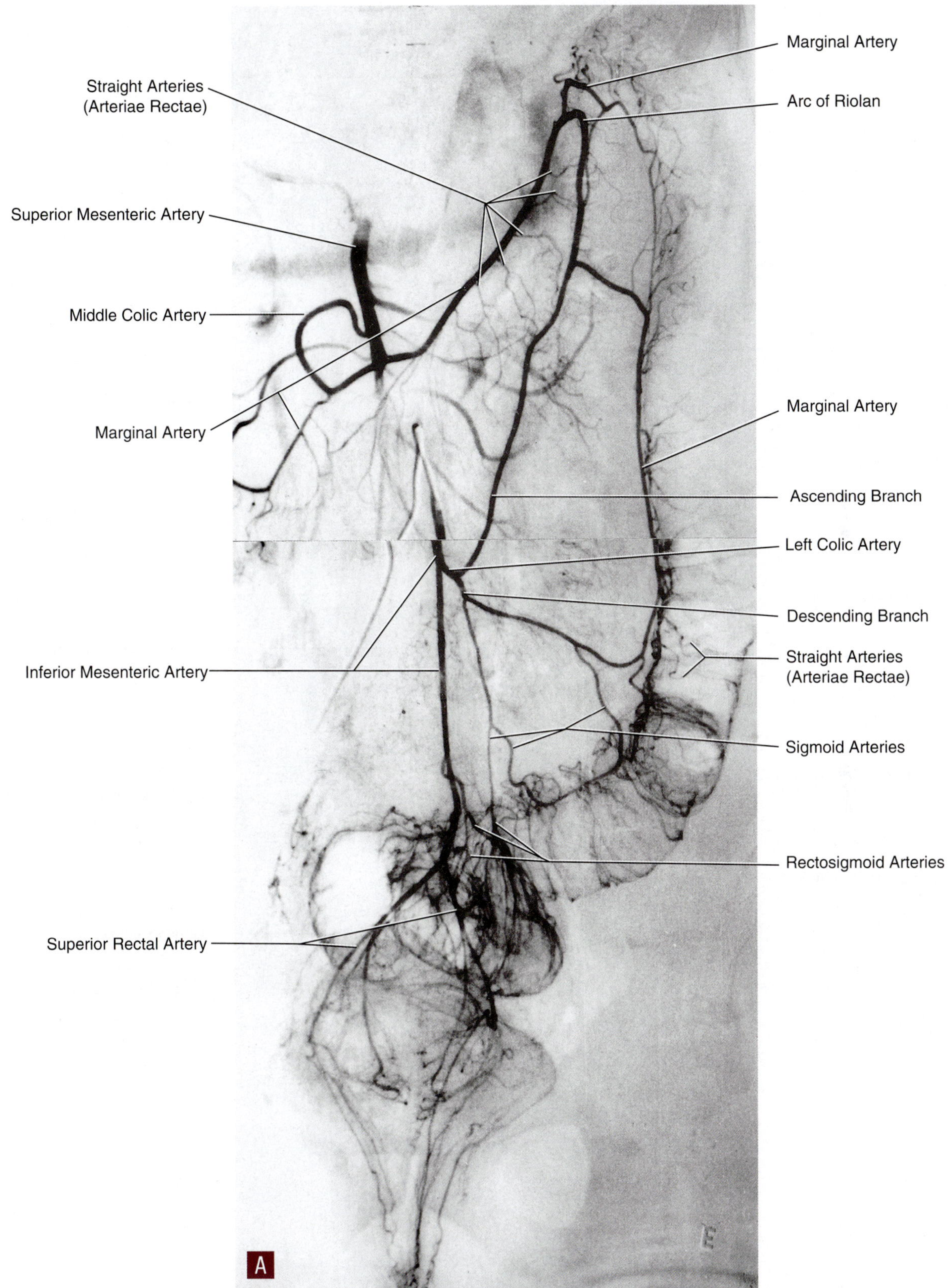

Figure 18.126. **A**, Selective angiogram of the inferior mesenteric artery. Note the filling of the superior mesenteric artery through the middle colic artery. The arc of Riolan is the main connection of the ascending branch of the left colic artery and the marginal artery of the middle colic artery in this case. **B**, Late phase of the inferior mesenteric angiography showing the hypoplastic inferior mesenteric vein. The marginal vein along the left colon is the main via of drainage of the inferior mesenteric arterial venous system directly into the middle colic vein. The venous companion of the arc of Riolan is also depicted.

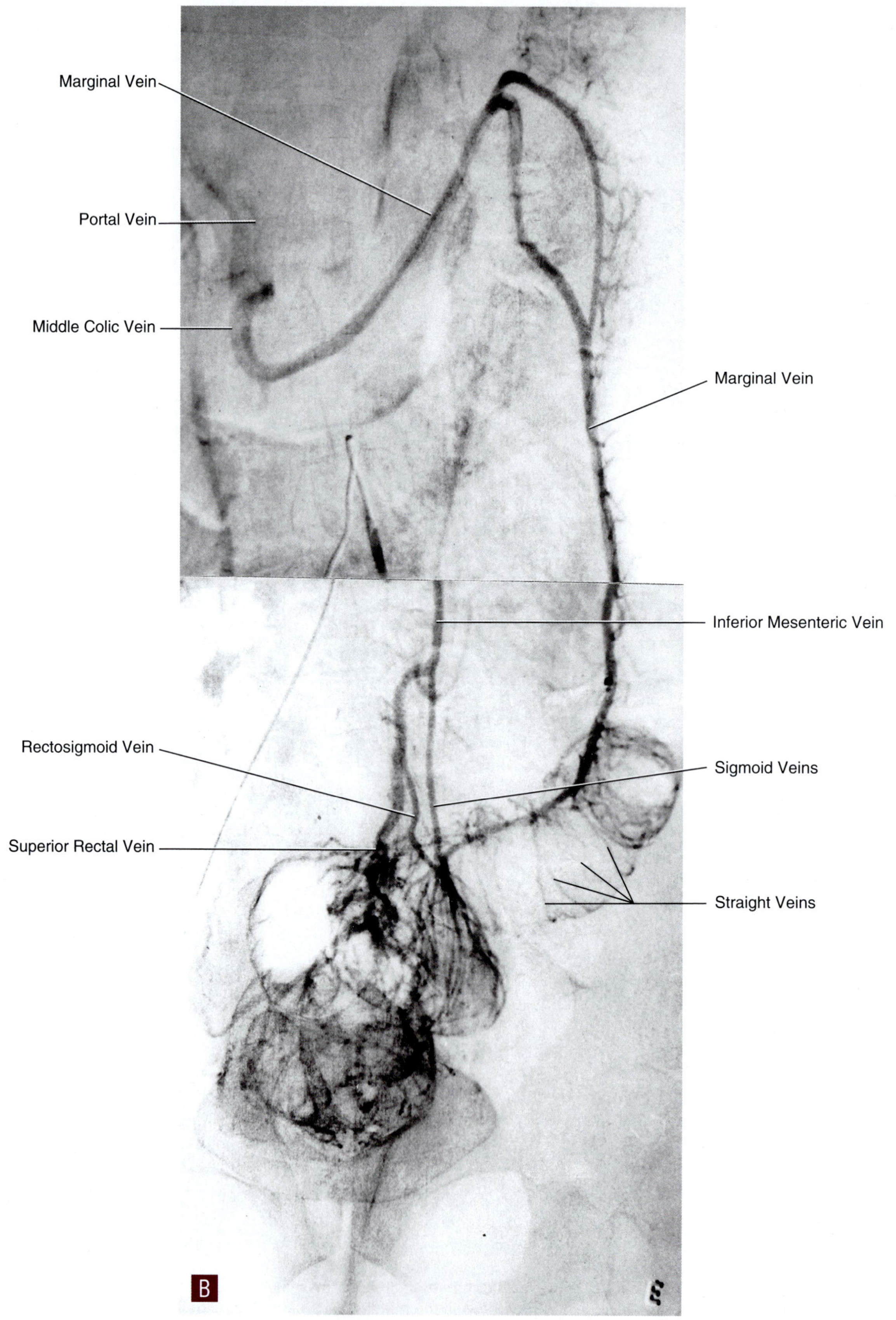

Figure 18.126. *Continued*

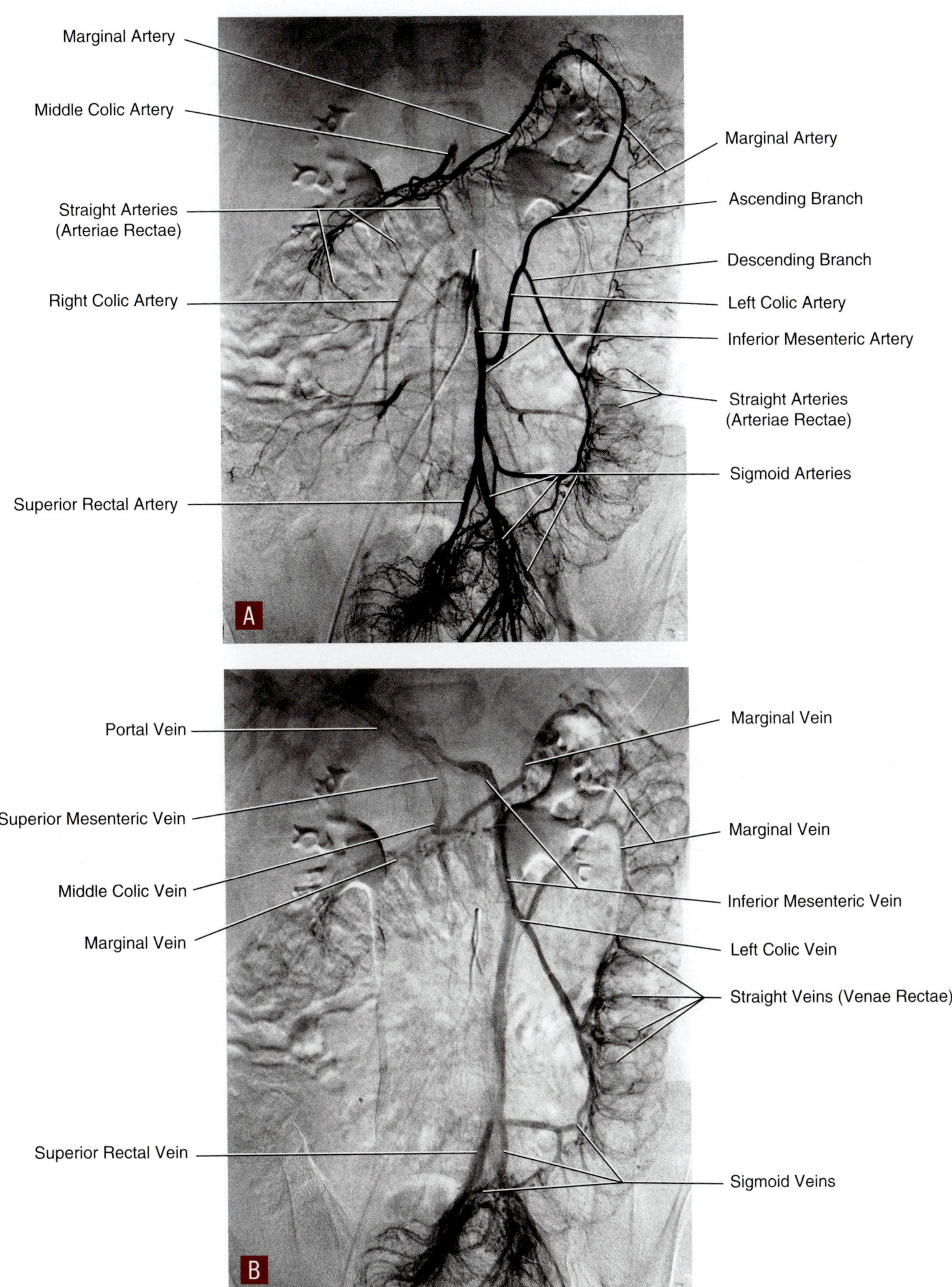

Figure 18.127. **A, Selective inferior mesenteric angiogram showing the superior rectal, the sigmoid, the left colic, and marginal arteries.** Note the communication between the left colic and the middle colic artery. **B**, Late phase of the angiogram showing the venous drainage of the left and transverse colon through the inferior mesenteric vein into the portal vein.

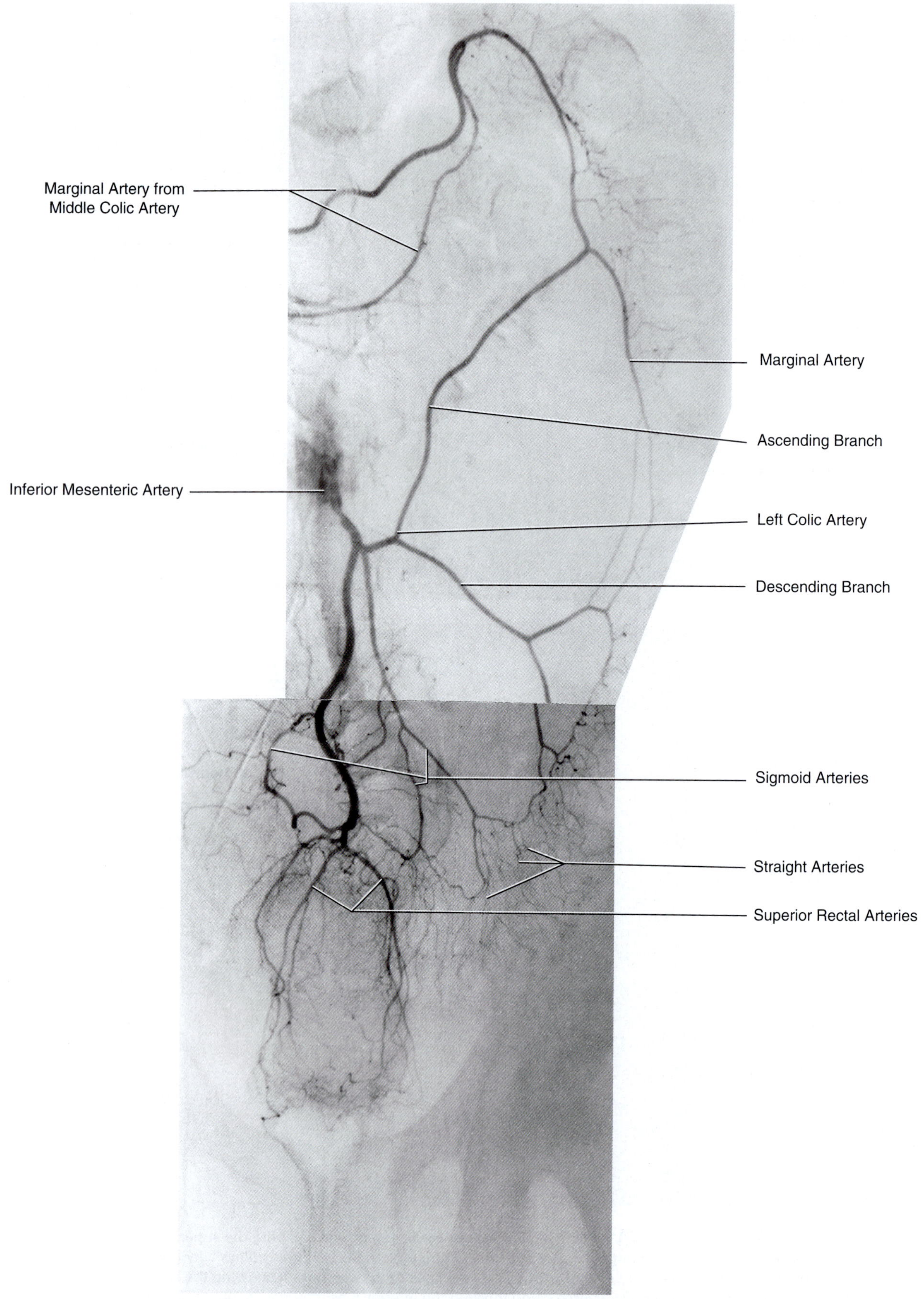

Figure 18.128. Selective angiogram of the inferior mesenteric artery, showing the circulation to the sigmoid, the rectum, the left colon, and the transverse colon.

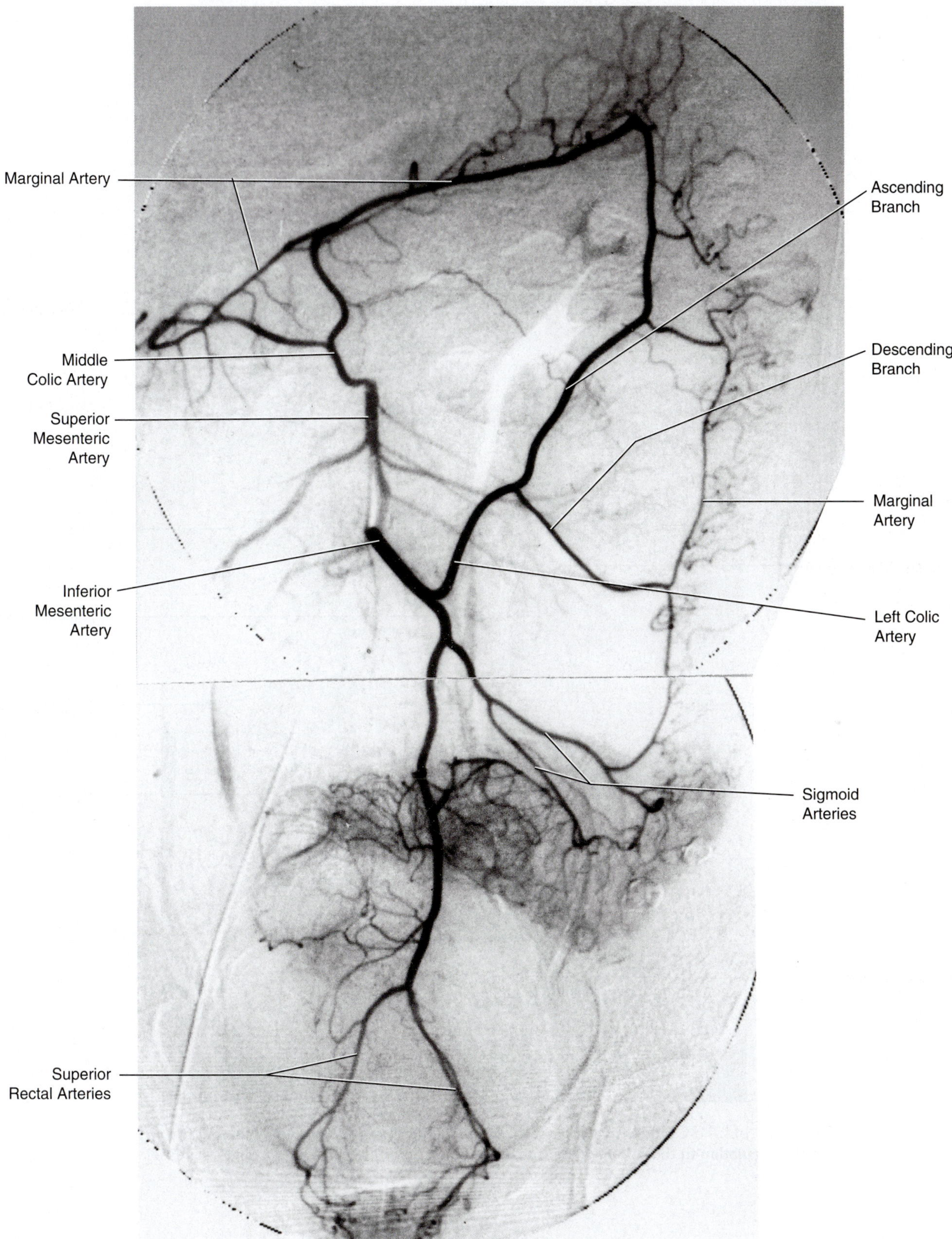

Figure 18.129. Selective angiogram of the inferior mesenteric artery showing the arterial circulation to the colon and rectum. Note filling of the superior mesenteric artery through the connections through the middle colic artery.

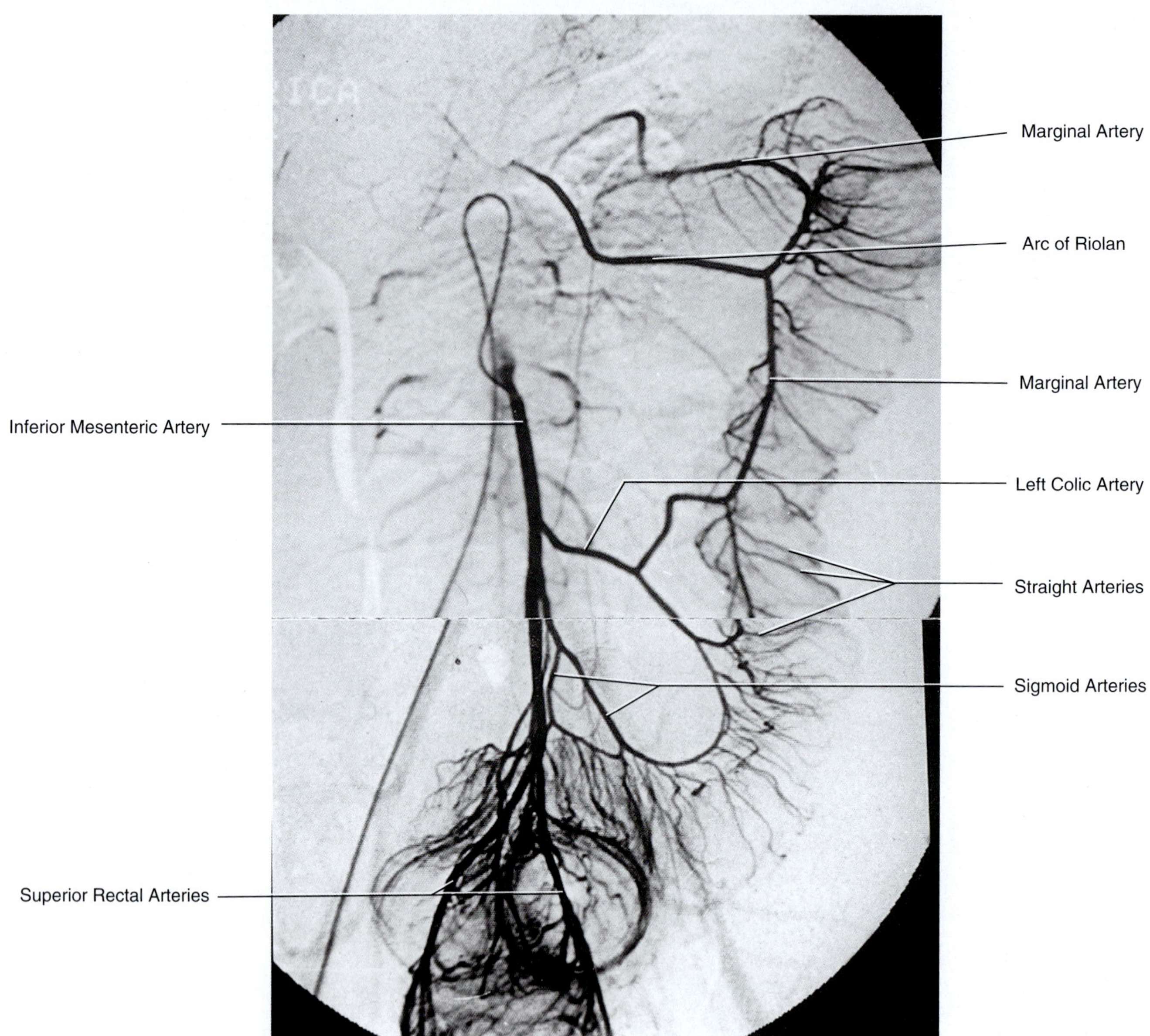

Figure 18.130. Selective angiogram of the inferior mesenteric artery showing the arterial circulation to the colon and rectum. Note the arc of Riolan as a large collateral vessel.

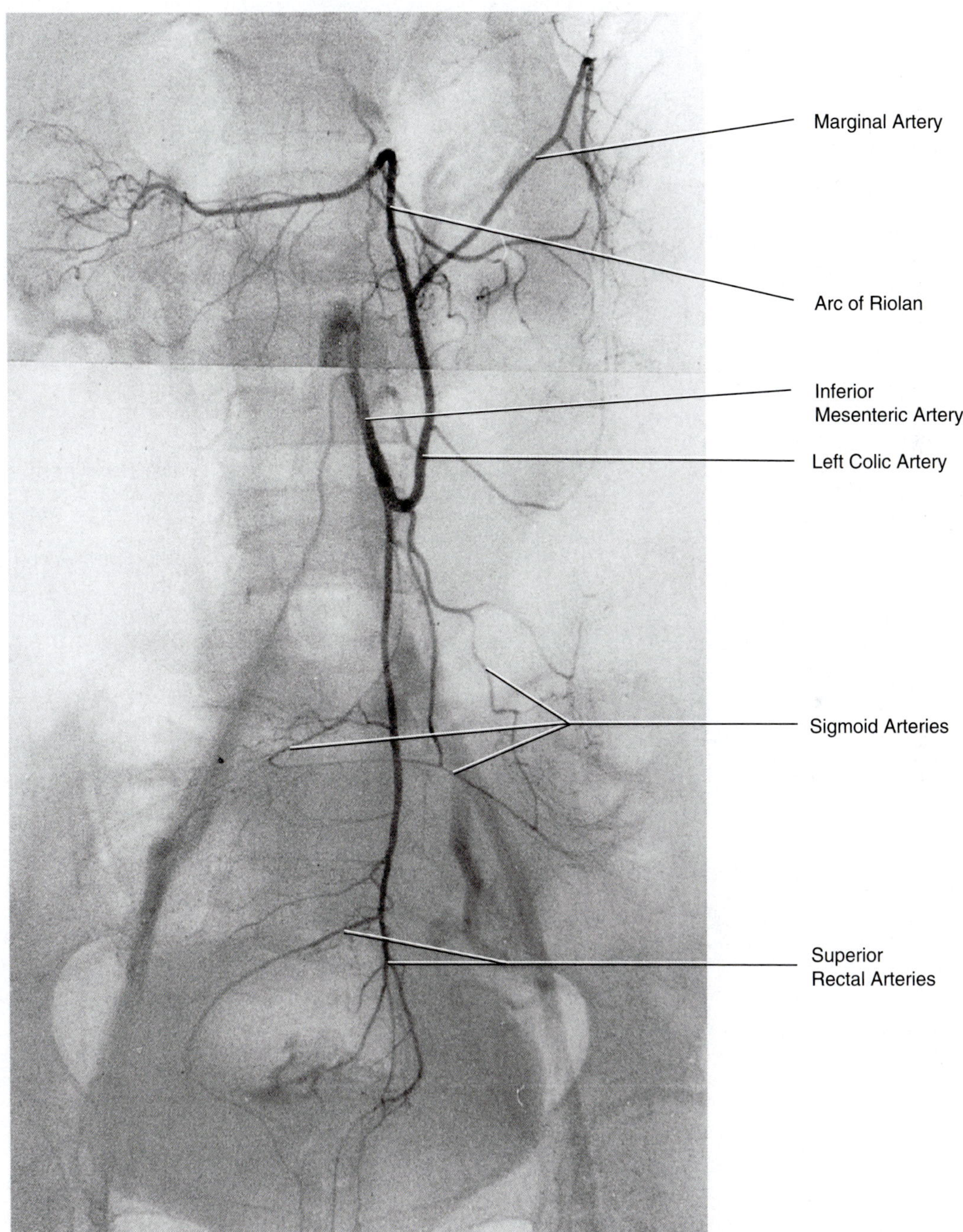

Figure 18.131. **Selective angiogram of the inferior mesenteric artery.**

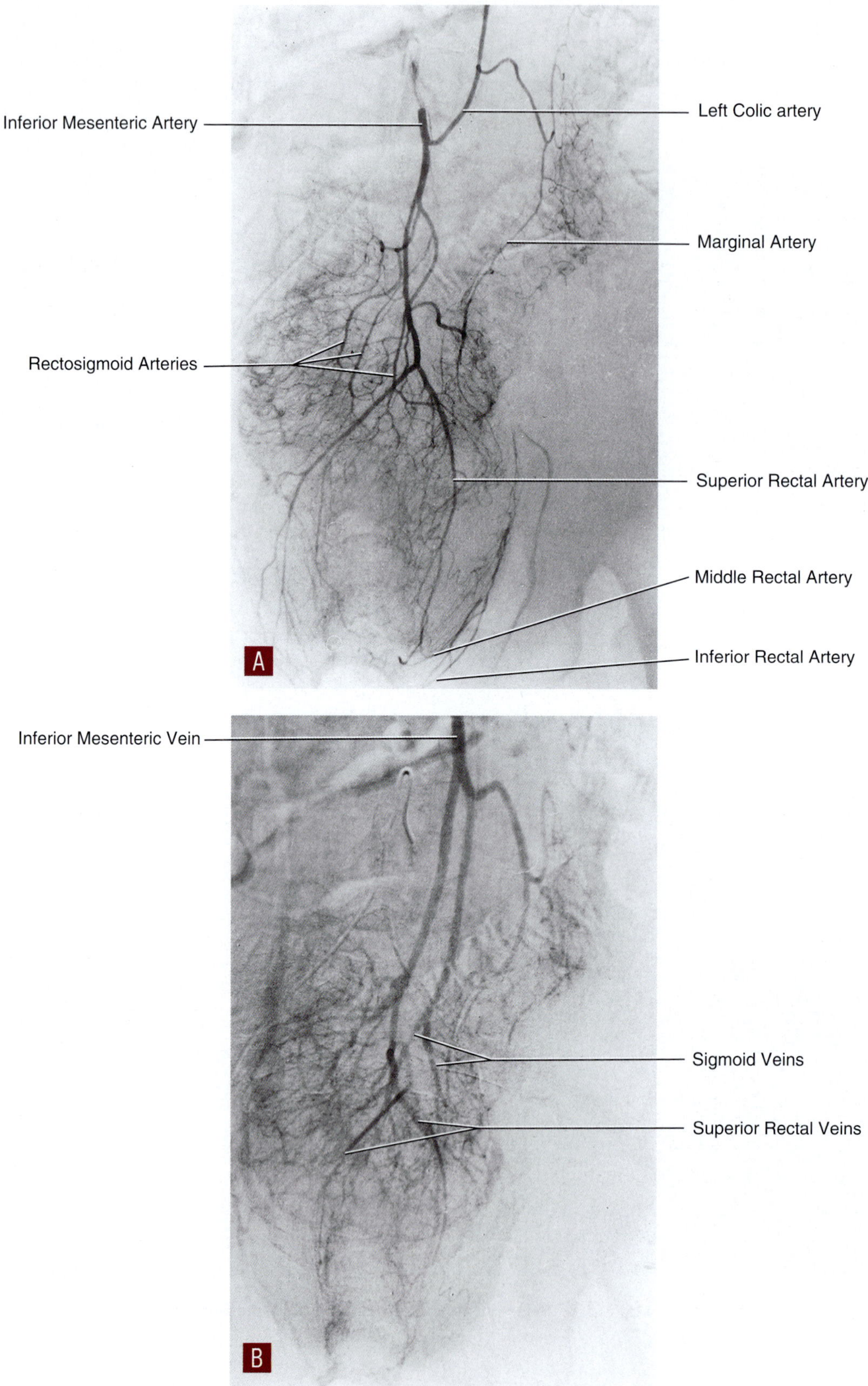

Figure 18.132. A, Selective angiogram of the inferior mesenteric artery showing the anastomosis of the superior rectal arteries with the middle rectal and inferior rectal arteries. B, Late phase of the angiogram showing the venous drainage of the rectum.

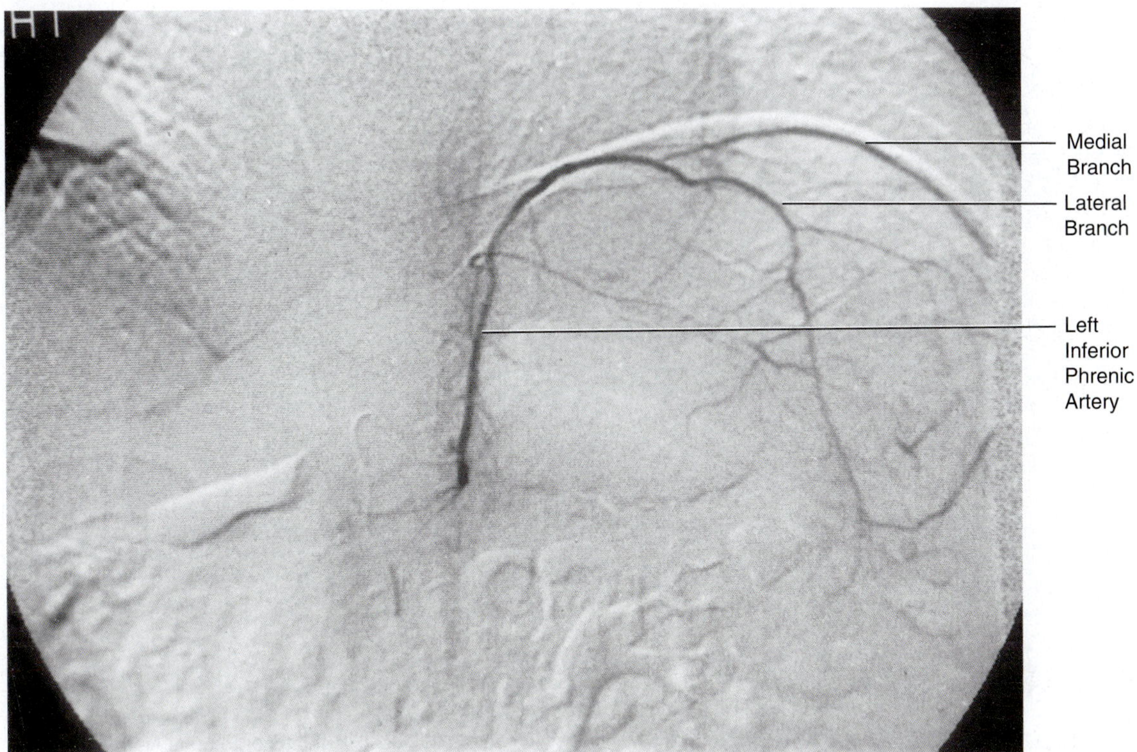

Figure 18.133. Selective angiogram of the left inferior phrenic artery. Note the lateral and medial branches.

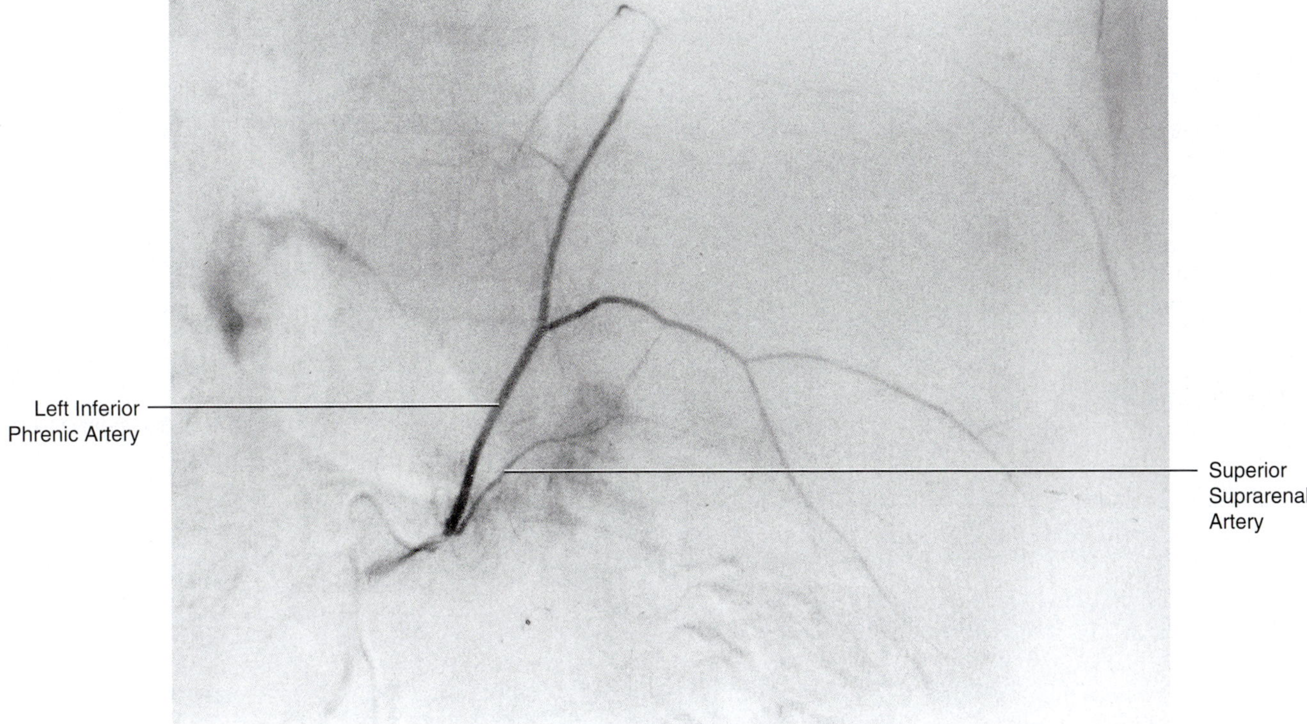

Figure 18.134. Selective angiogram of the left inferior phrenic artery. The superior suprarenal artery is the first branch. Note the adrenal blush.

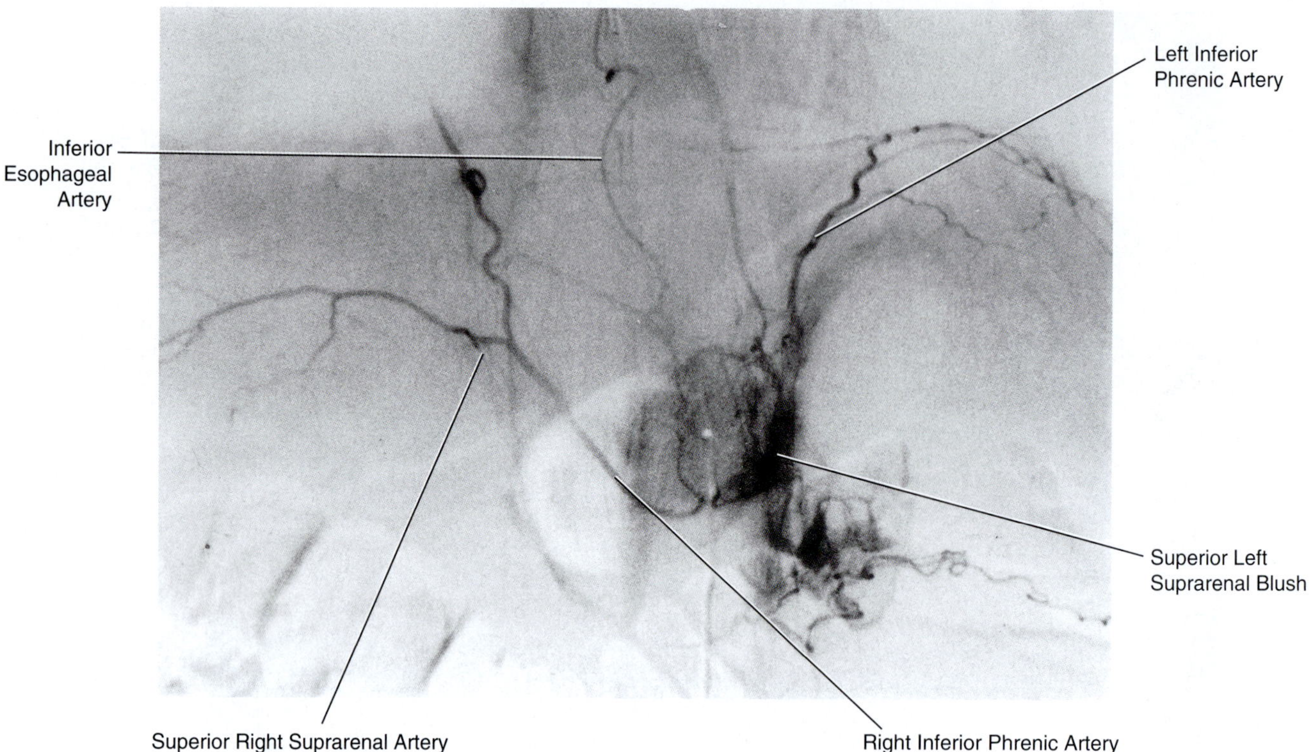

Figure 18.135. Selective angiogram of the inferior phrenic artery, presented as a common trunk with branches to the left and right side. The superior suprarenal arteries are filled. Note the adrenal blush on the left. Some inferior esophageal arteries are also noted.

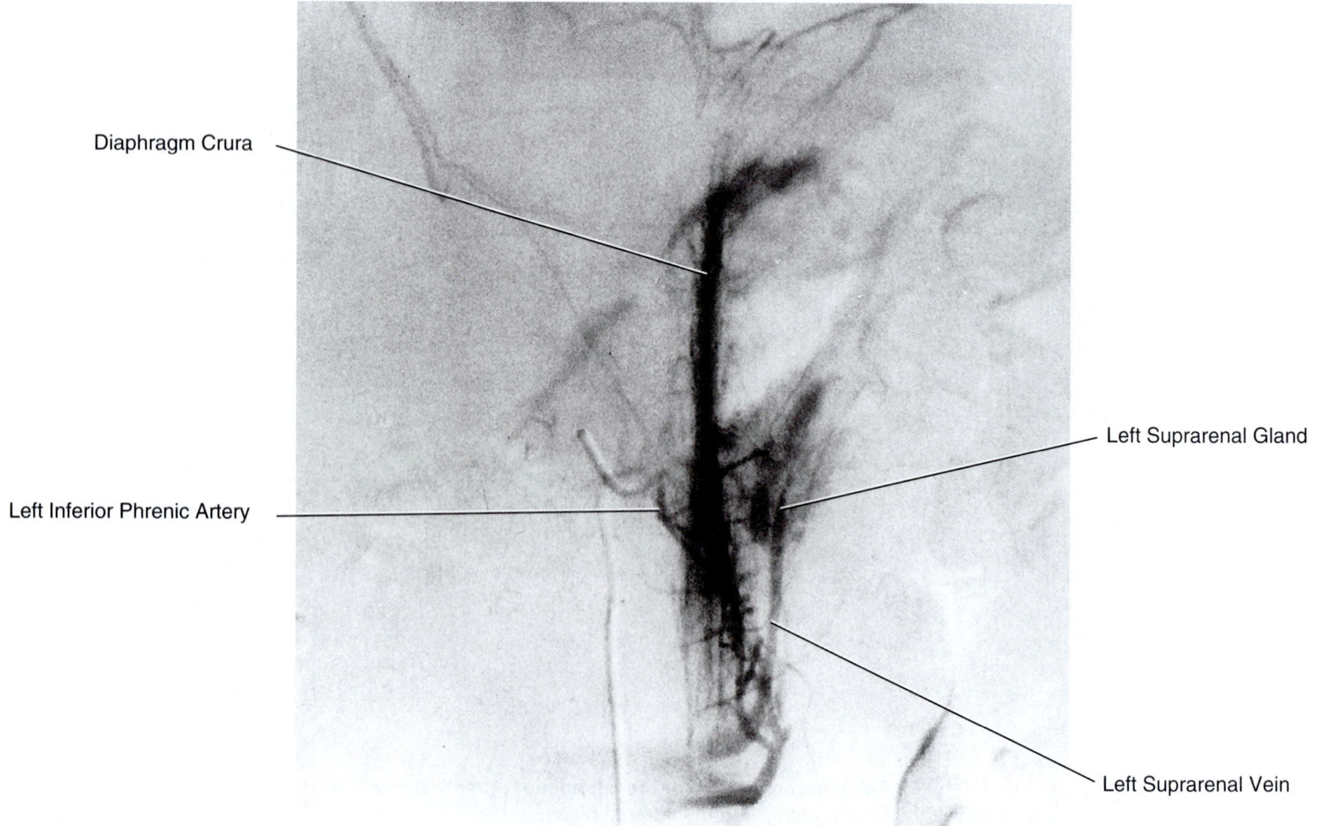

Figure 18.136. Selective angiogram of the left inferior phrenic artery. Note the diaphragmatic crura stain. The left adrenal blush is observed as well as the left suprarenal vein draining into the left renal vein.

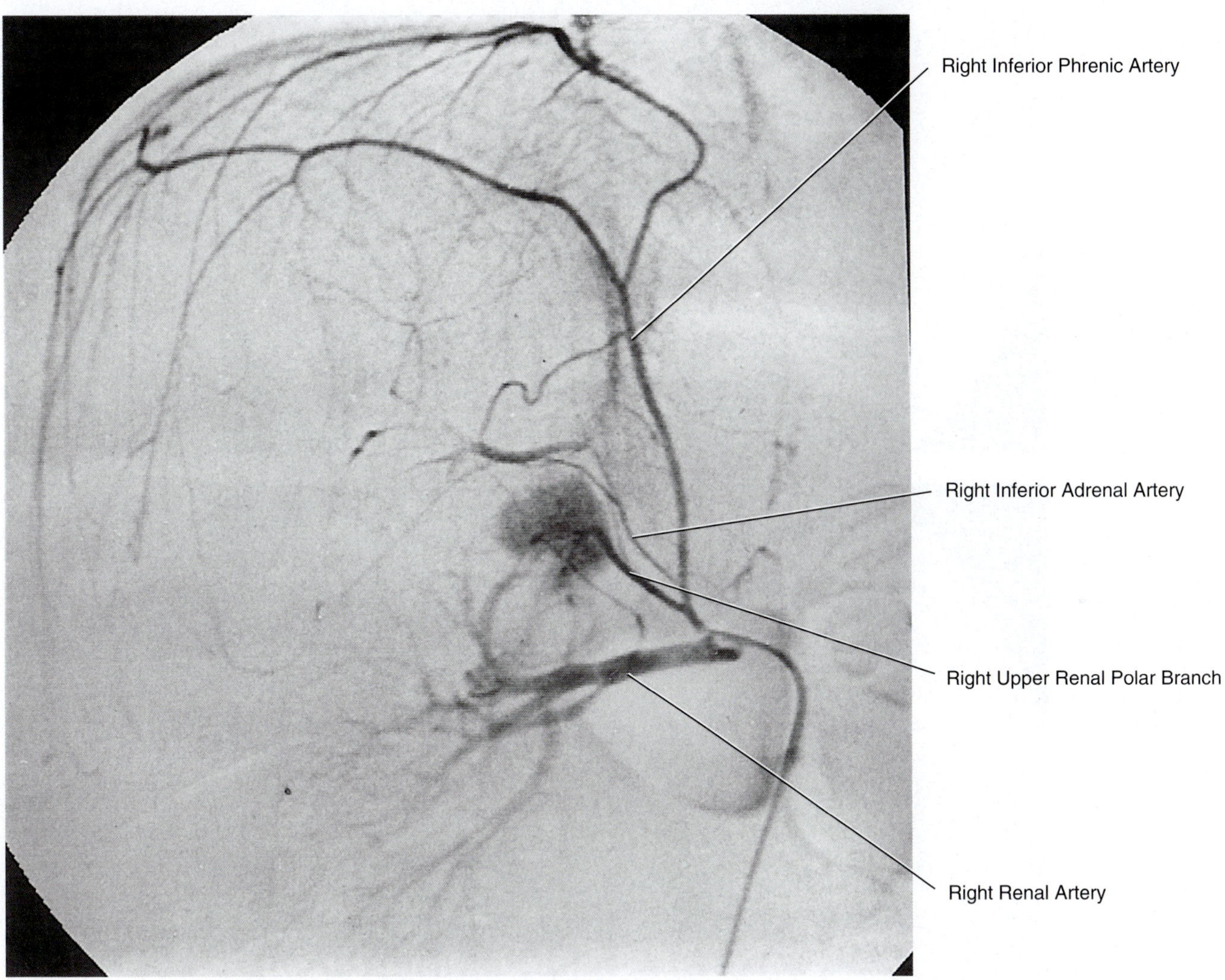

Figure 18.137. Selective injection at the right inferior phrenic artery arising as a common trunk with the right inferior adrenal artery as well as an upper renal polar branch. The right main renal artery is partially filled. Note an ill-defined right adrenal blush.

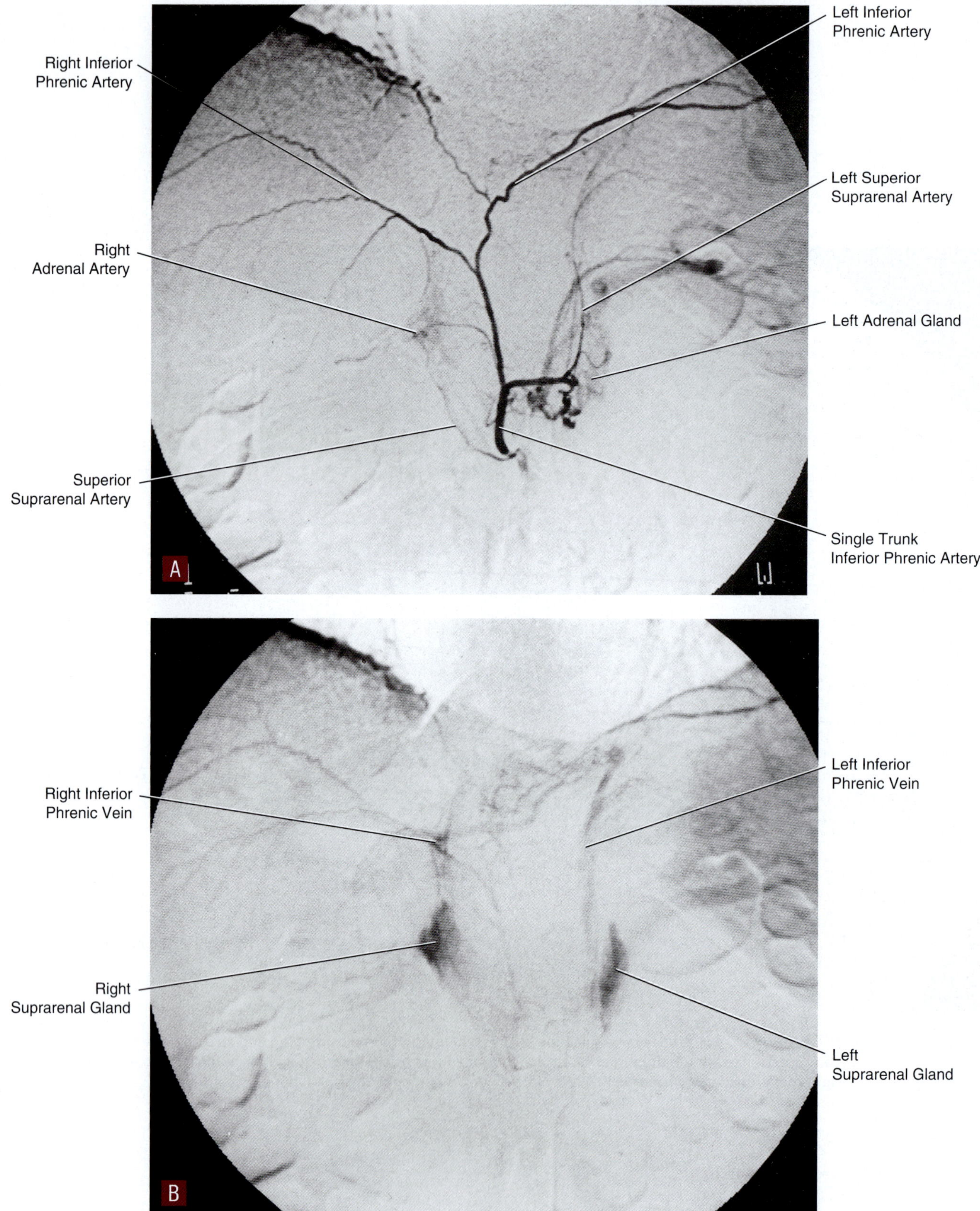

Figure 18.138. **A**, Selective angiogram of the inferior phrenic arteries observed as a trunk giving origin to the right and left inferior phrenic arteries. Note the origin of the right and left superior suprarenal arteries. The adrenal blush is ill-defined on both sides. The right superior suprarenal artery is hardly visible. **B**, Late phase angiogram shows the right and left adrenal blush and the right and left inferior phrenic veins.

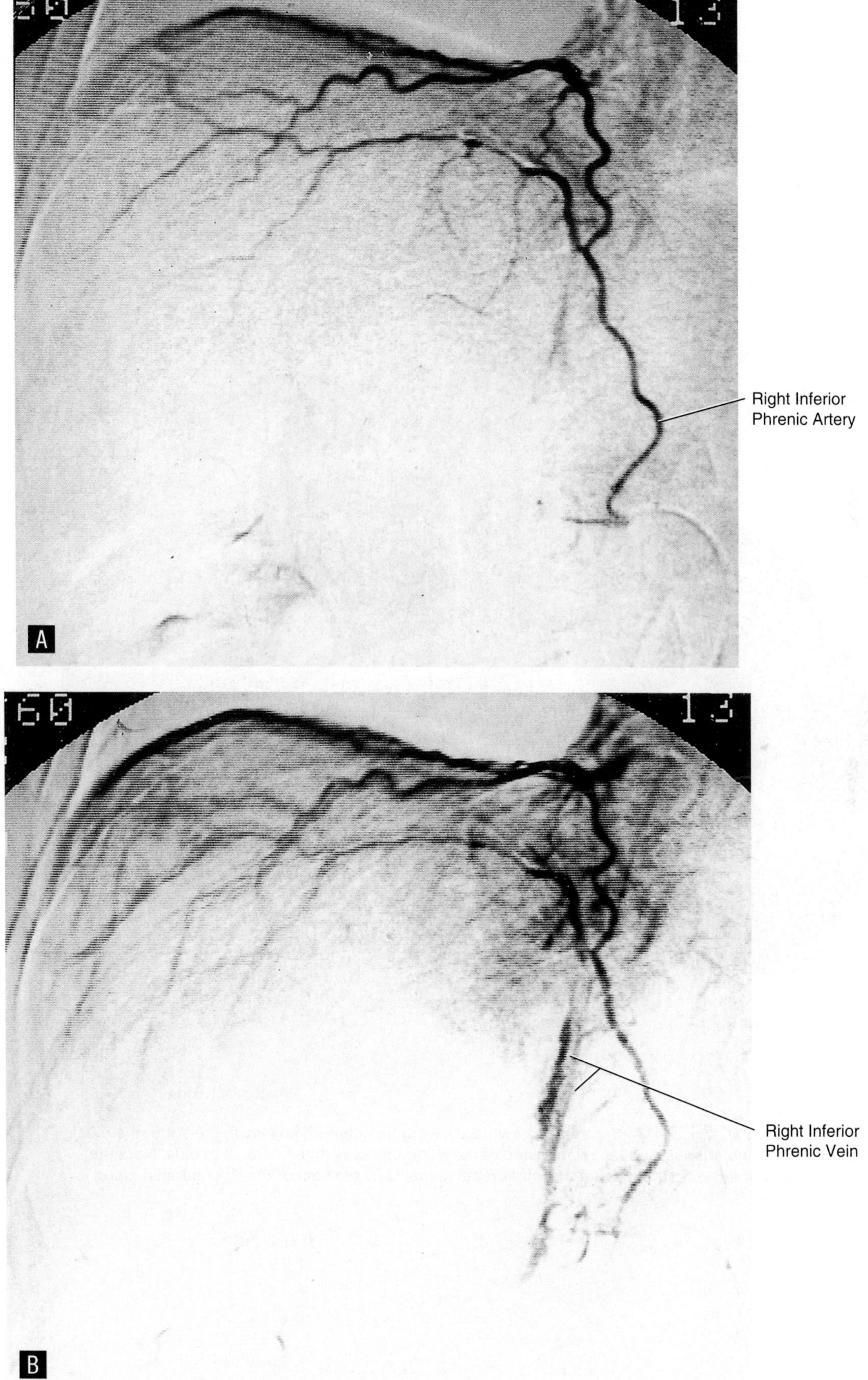

Figure 18.139. **A**, Right inferior phrenic artery angiogram. **B**, Late phase of the angiogram shows the venous drainage parallel to the arteries and the right inferior phrenic vein.

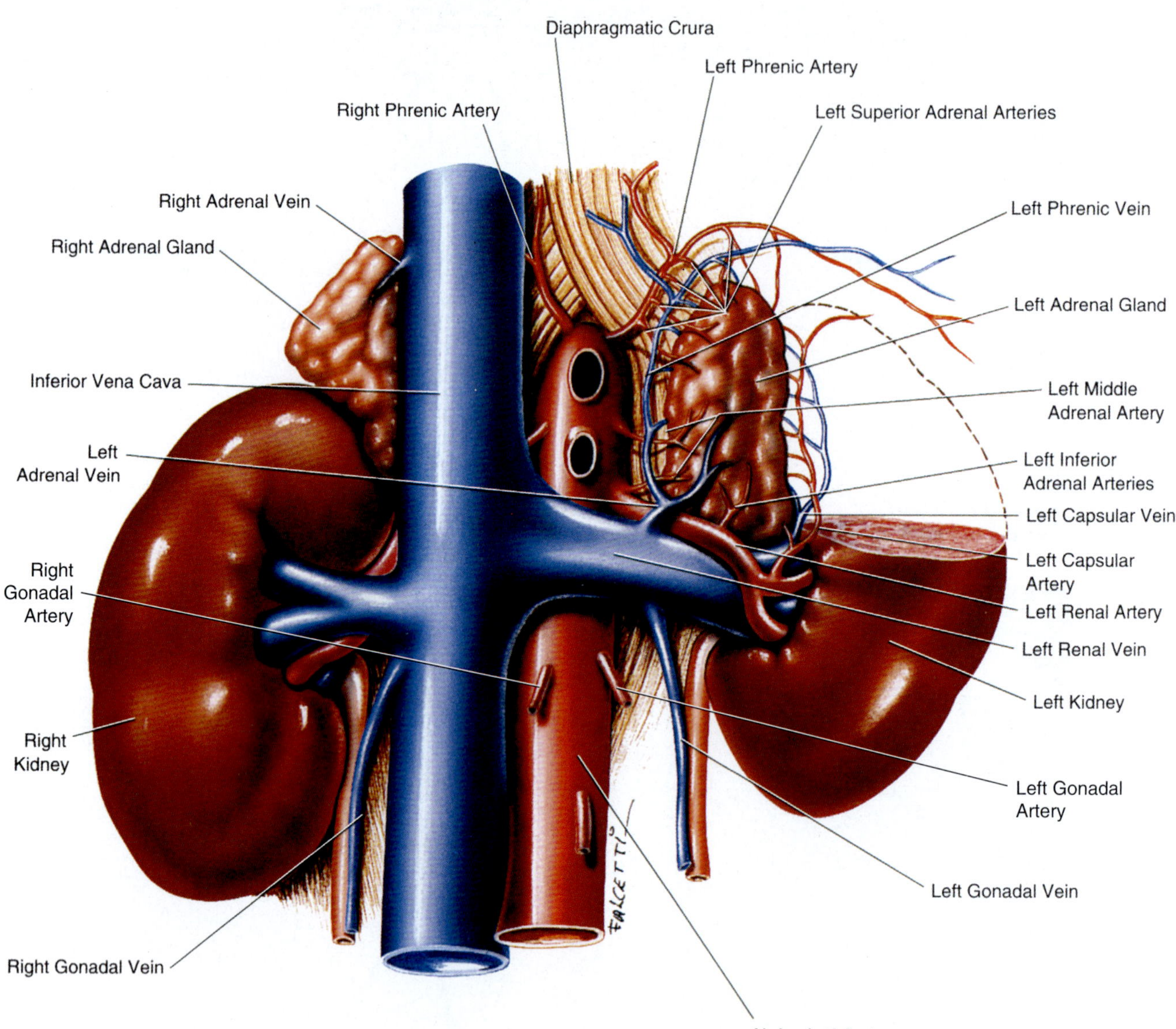

Figure 18.140. Schematic drawing showing the inferior vena cava, the aorta, the renal veins and arteries, and the relationship of these structures with the adrenal glands. Note the arterial and venous supply of the left adrenal gland. Only the vein of the right adrenal gland is shown.

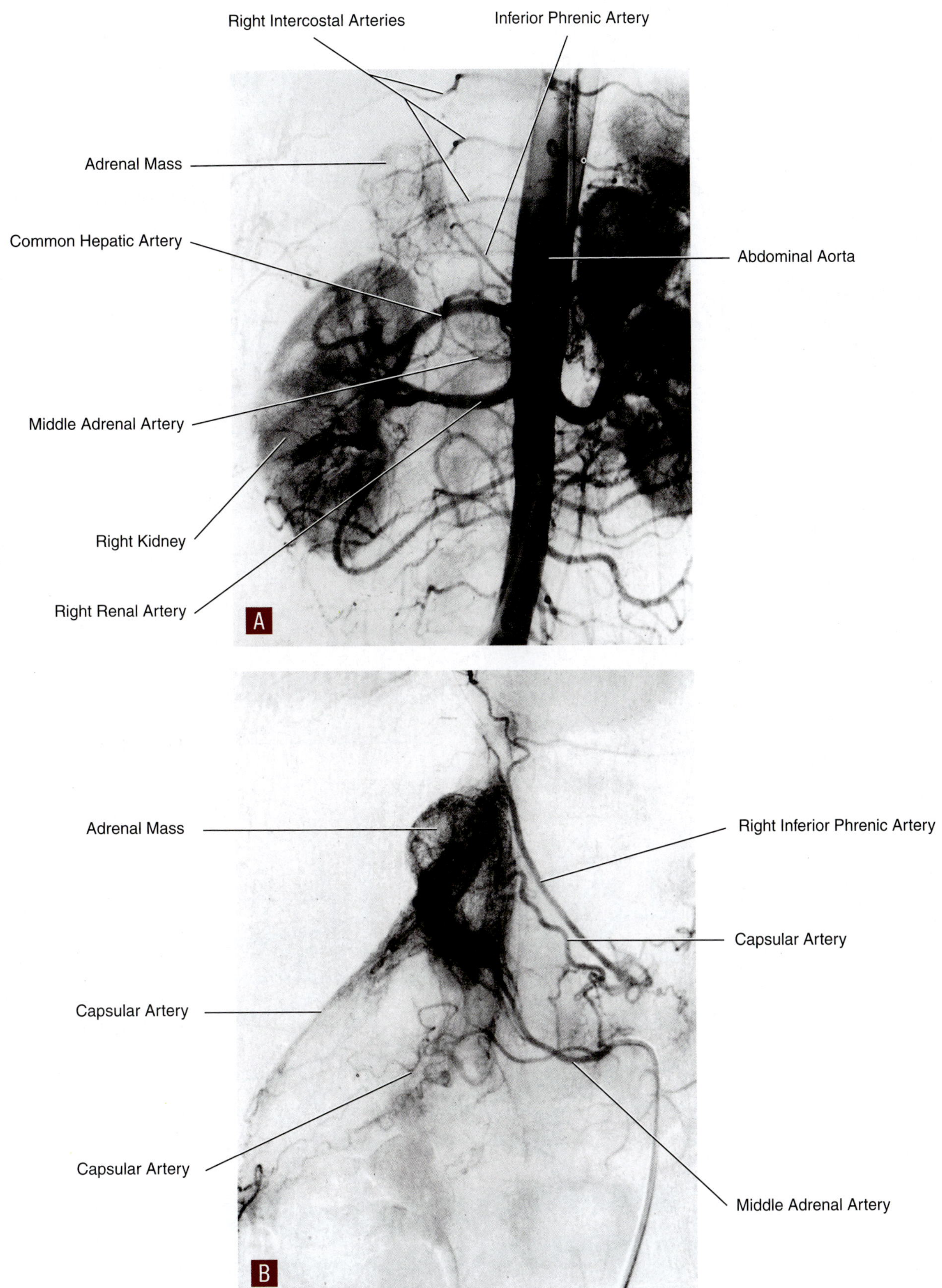

Figure 18.141. **A**, Aortogram of the abdomen, showing the arteries to the right kidney and to the right adrenal gland. A vascular mass (pheochromocytoma) is demonstrated replacing the right adrenal gland. **B**, Selective injection into the middle adrenal artery shows retrograde filling of the inferior phrenic artery via the superior adrenal artery.

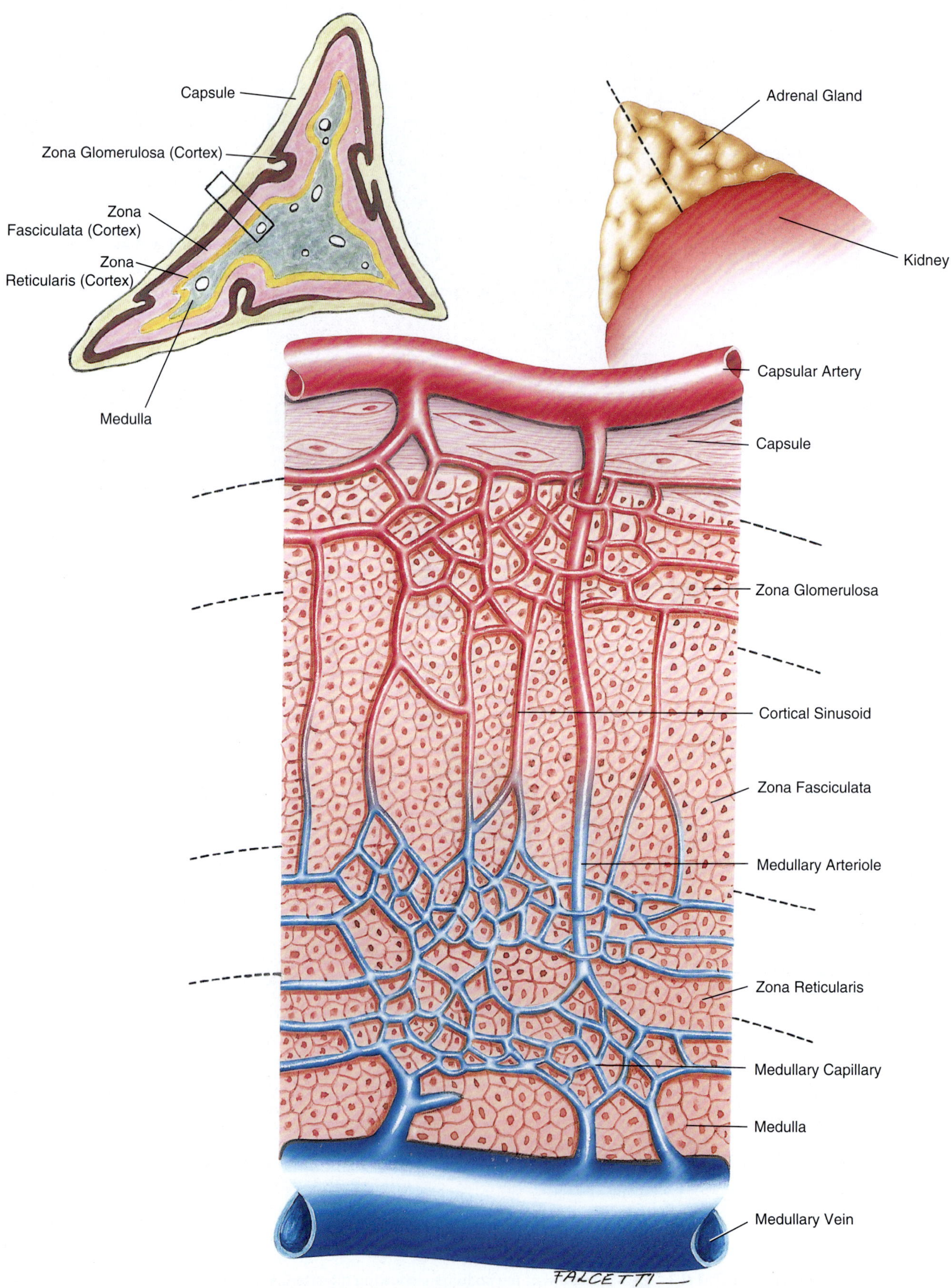

Figure 18.142. Schematic drawing of the left adrenal gland showing the microstructure of the gland on a transverse cut. Note the capsular circulation and the connections through the sinusoids to the medullary vein.

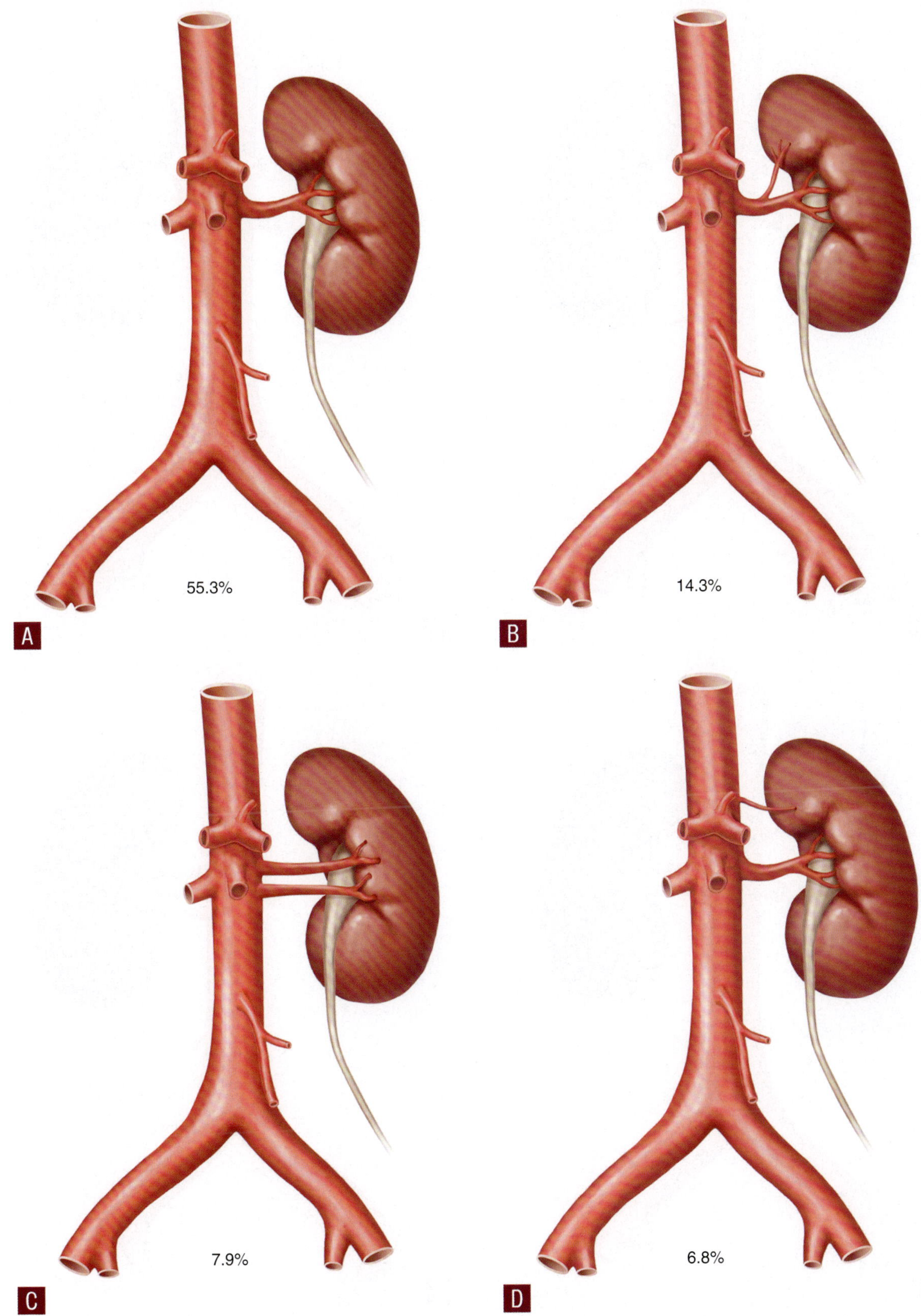

Figure 18.143. Types and incidence of renal arterial supply. A, One hilar artery, 55.3% (147 of 266 pedicles). B, One hilar artery with one superior pole extrahilar branch, 14.3% (38 of 266 pedicles). C, Two hilar arteries, 7.9% (21 of 266 pedicles). D, One hilar artery with one superior polar artery, 6.8% (18 of 266 pedicles).

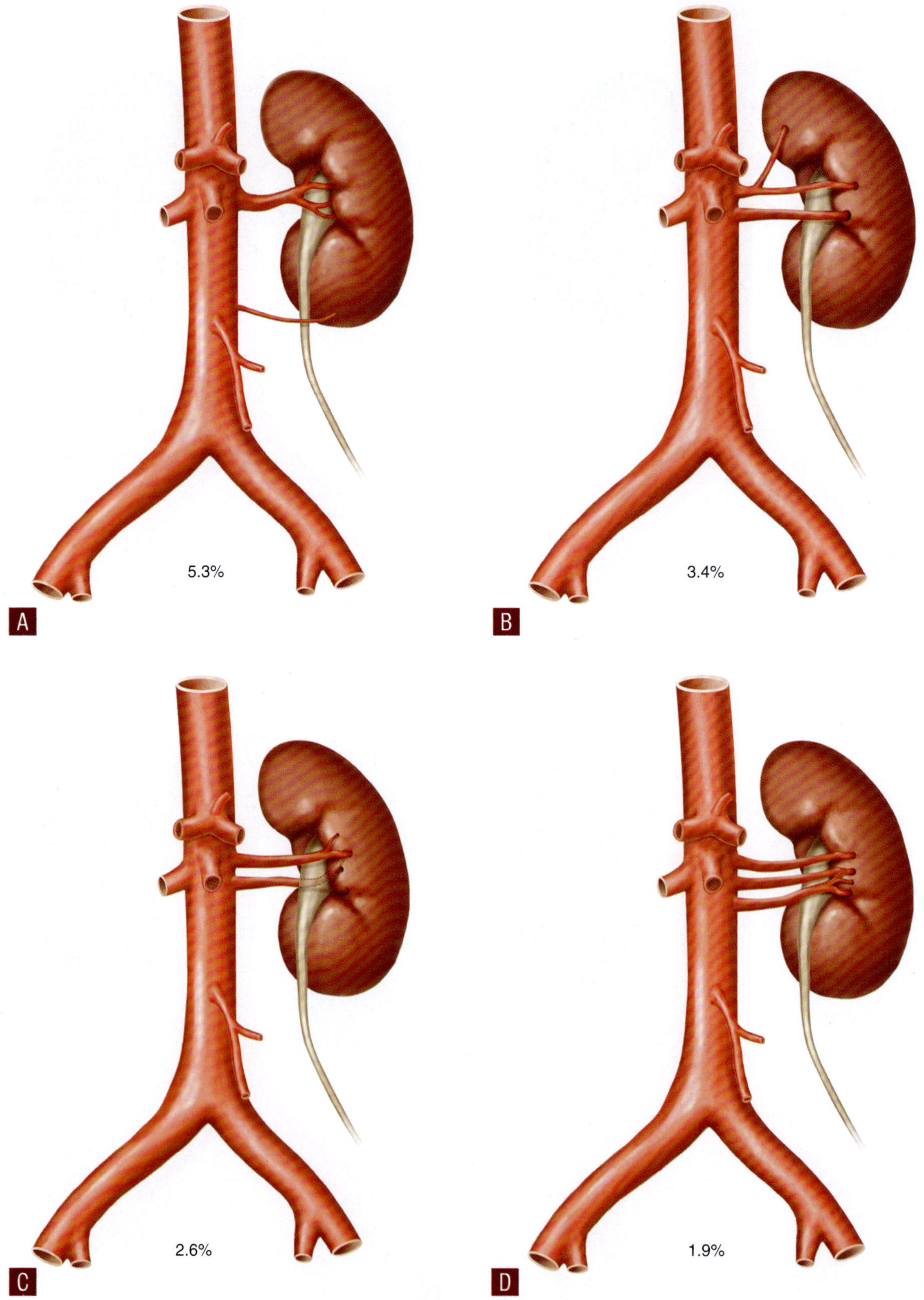

Figure 18.144. **Types and incidence of renal arterial supply.** A, One hilar artery with one inferior polar artery, 5.3% (14 of 266 pedicles). B, Two hilar arteries with one superior pole extrahilar branch, 3.4% (9 of 266 pedicles). C, One hilar artery with a precocious bifurcation, 2.6% (7 of 266 pedicles). D, Three hilar arteries, 1.9% (5 of 266 pedicles).

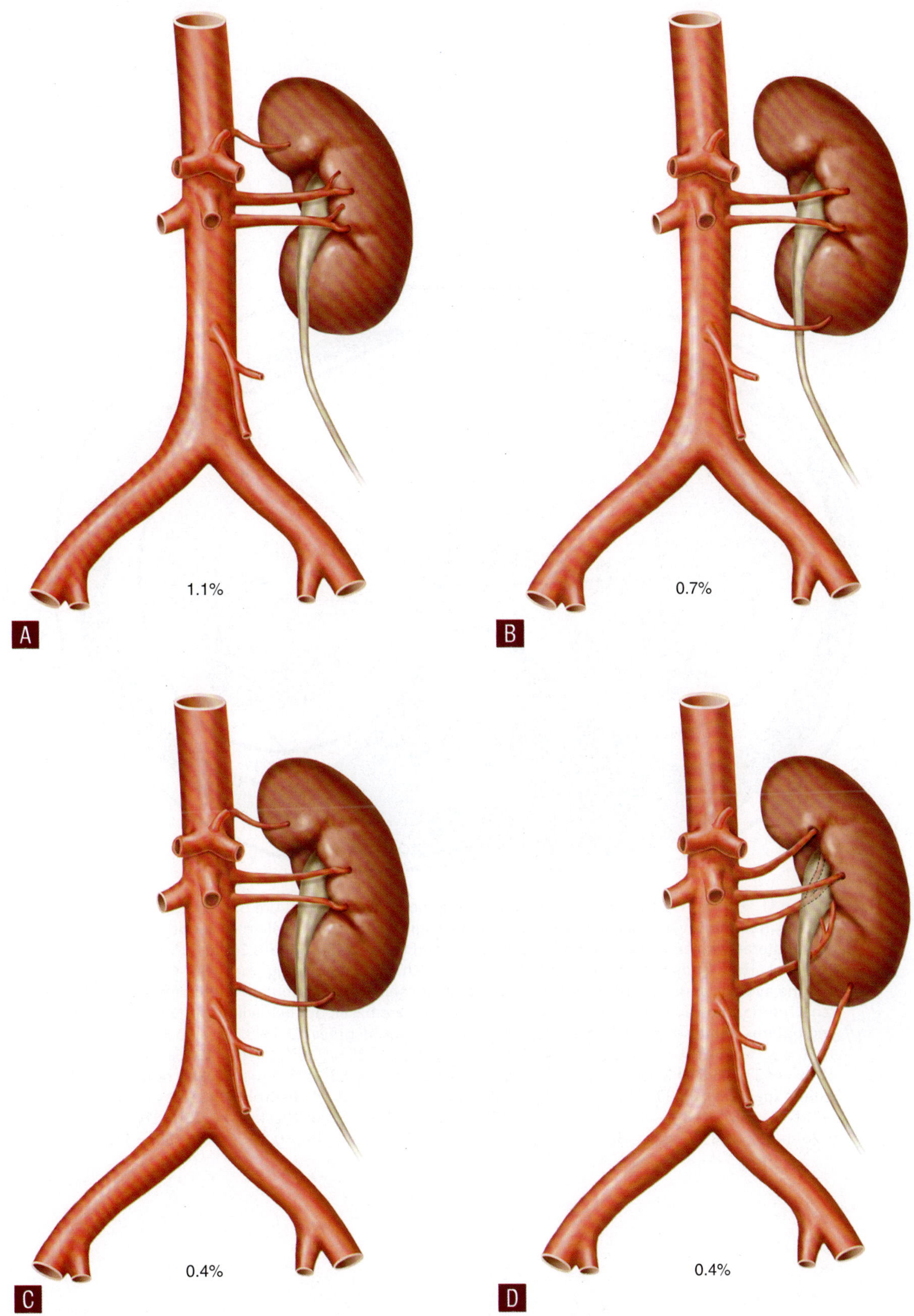

Figure 18.145. **Types and incidence of renal arterial supply.** **A**, Two hilar arteries with one superior polar artery, 1.1% (3 of 266 pedicles). **B**, Two hilar arteries with one inferior polar artery, 0.7% (2 of 266 pedicles). **C**, Two hilar arteries with one superior polar artery and one inferior polar artery, 0.4% (1 of 266 pedicles). **D**, Three hilar arteries with one superior polar artery and one inferior polar artery, 0.4% (1 of 266 pedicles).

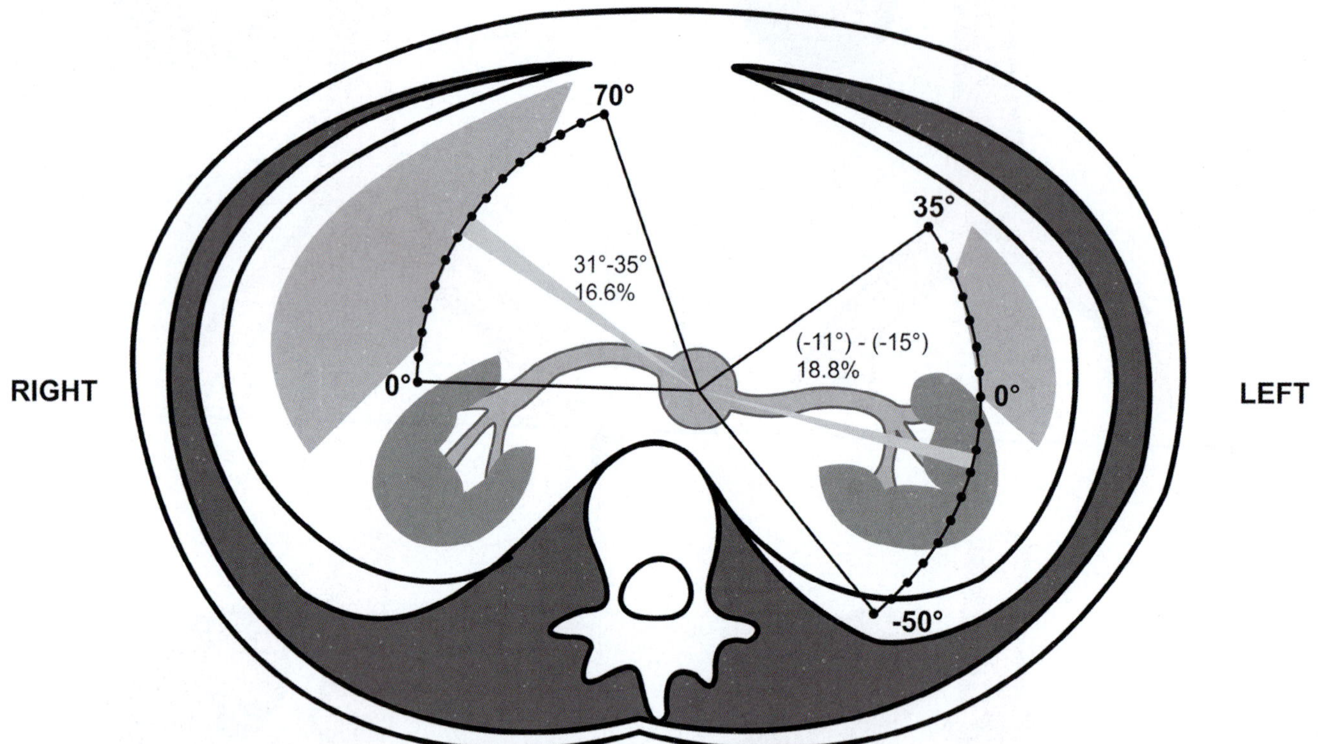

Figure 18.146. Schematic drawing showing the angle of the ostium of the renal arteries in the transverse plane, the location of the origin of the right renal artery tends to be anterolateral, with an angle ranging from 0° to 70°, and the average angle is 30° to 35°. The left renal artery tends to be posterolateral or lateral, with an angle ranging from −50° to 35°, and the average angle is −11° to 15°. The variation in location and distribution width of the renal arteries, however, is great. The following numbers are based on the review of the CT angiograms of the aorta in 400 patients. Right renal ostium (degrees), 0-5 = 3.3%, 6-10 = 2.8%, 11-15 = 5.7%, 16-20 = 13.2%, 21-25 = 14.3%, 26-30 = 16.0%, 31-35 = 16.6%, 36-40 = 13.5%, 41-45 = 8.3%, 46-50 = 2.8%, 51-55 = 2.0%, 56-60 = 0.8%, 61-65 = 0.2%, 66-70 = 0.50. Left renal ostium (degrees), 35-30 = 0.2%, 29-25 = 1%, 24-20 = 2%, 19-15 = 3.7%, 14-10 = 5.3%, 9-5 = 7.3%, (−1)-(−5) = 7.5%, (−6)-(−10) = 8.3%, (−11)-(−15) = 18.8%, (−16)-(−20) = 18%, (−21)-(−25) = 11%, (−26)-(−30) = 3.8%, (−31)-(−35) = 2.8%, (−36)-(−40) = 1.2%, (−41)-(−45) = 0.8%, (−46)-(−50) = 1%.

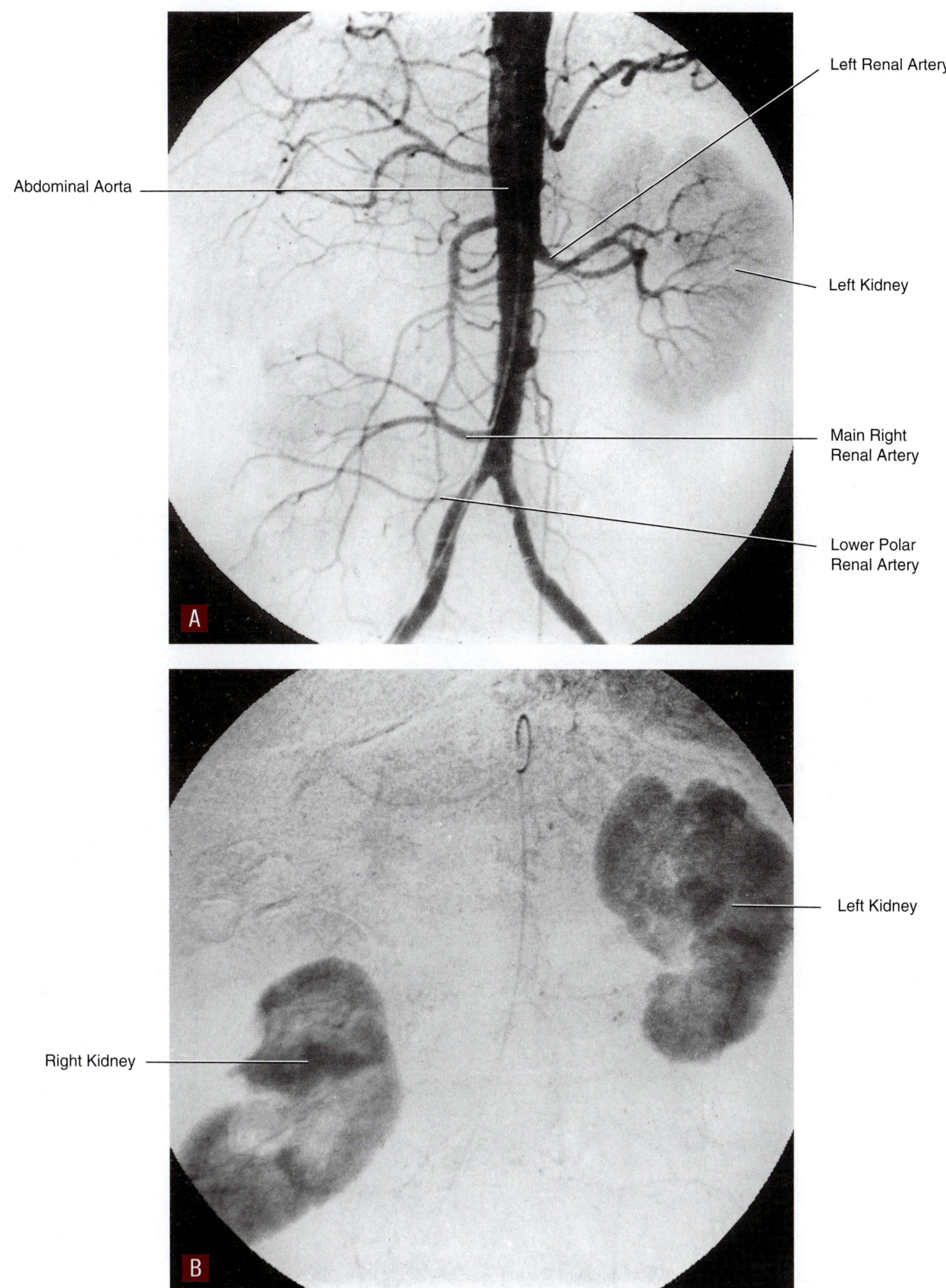

Figure 18.147. A, Abdominal aortogram. Normal positioned left kidney. The main renal artery on the right side originates from the distal aorta, close to the bifurcation. Note the smaller renal branch arising from the right common iliac artery. B, Late phase of the aortogram showing the bilateral nephrogram. Note the caudal position of the right kidney.

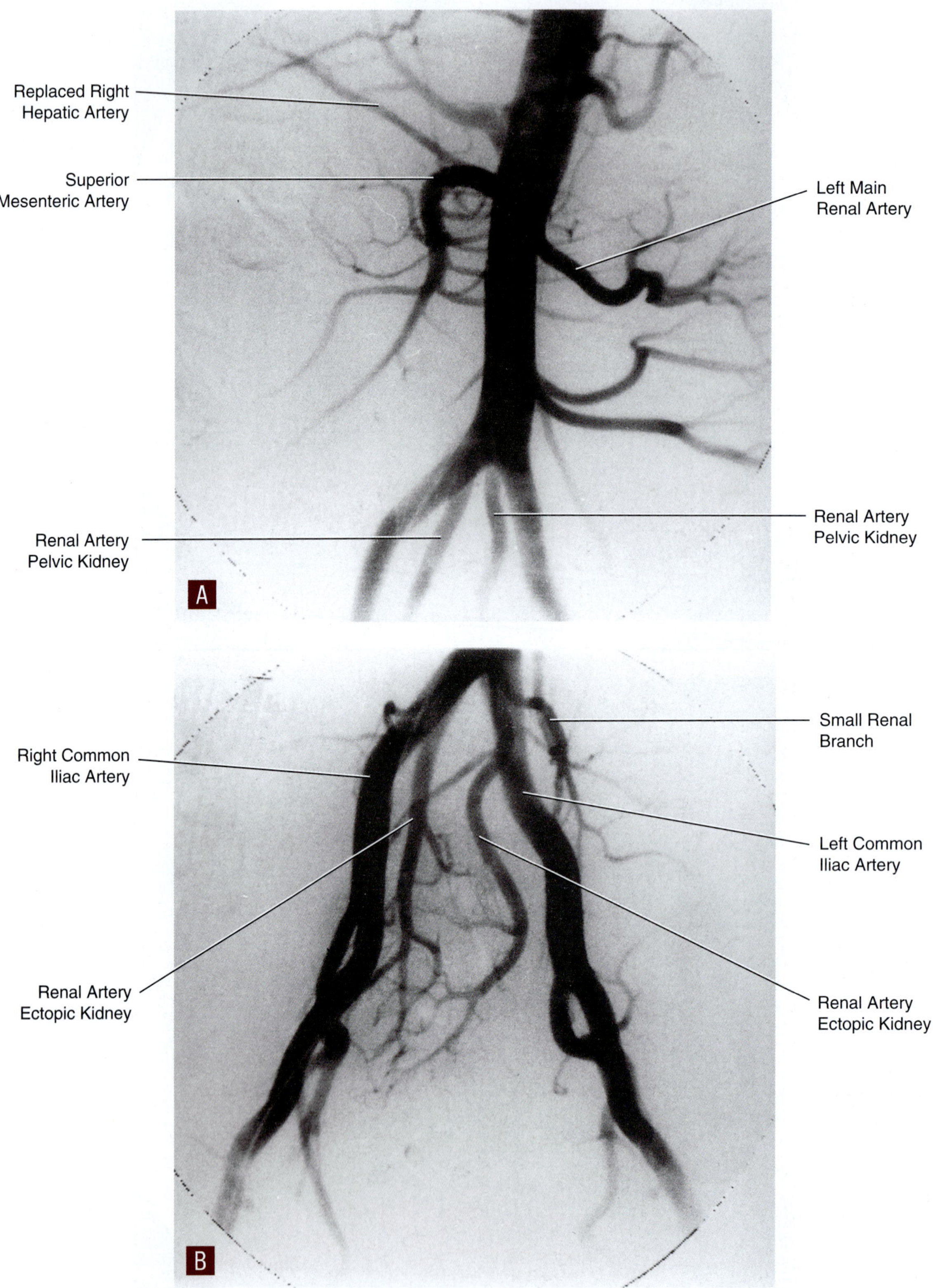

Figure 18.148. A, Abdominal aortogram showing an ectopic left kidney with the origin of the left main renal artery in the abdominal aorta. Note the vessels arising from the bifurcation of the aorta and common iliac arteries. B, Angiography of the iliac vessels shows the three renal arteries supplying the intrapelvic kidney. Two of the main arteries arise from the common iliac arteries while a small artery arises from the distal aorta.

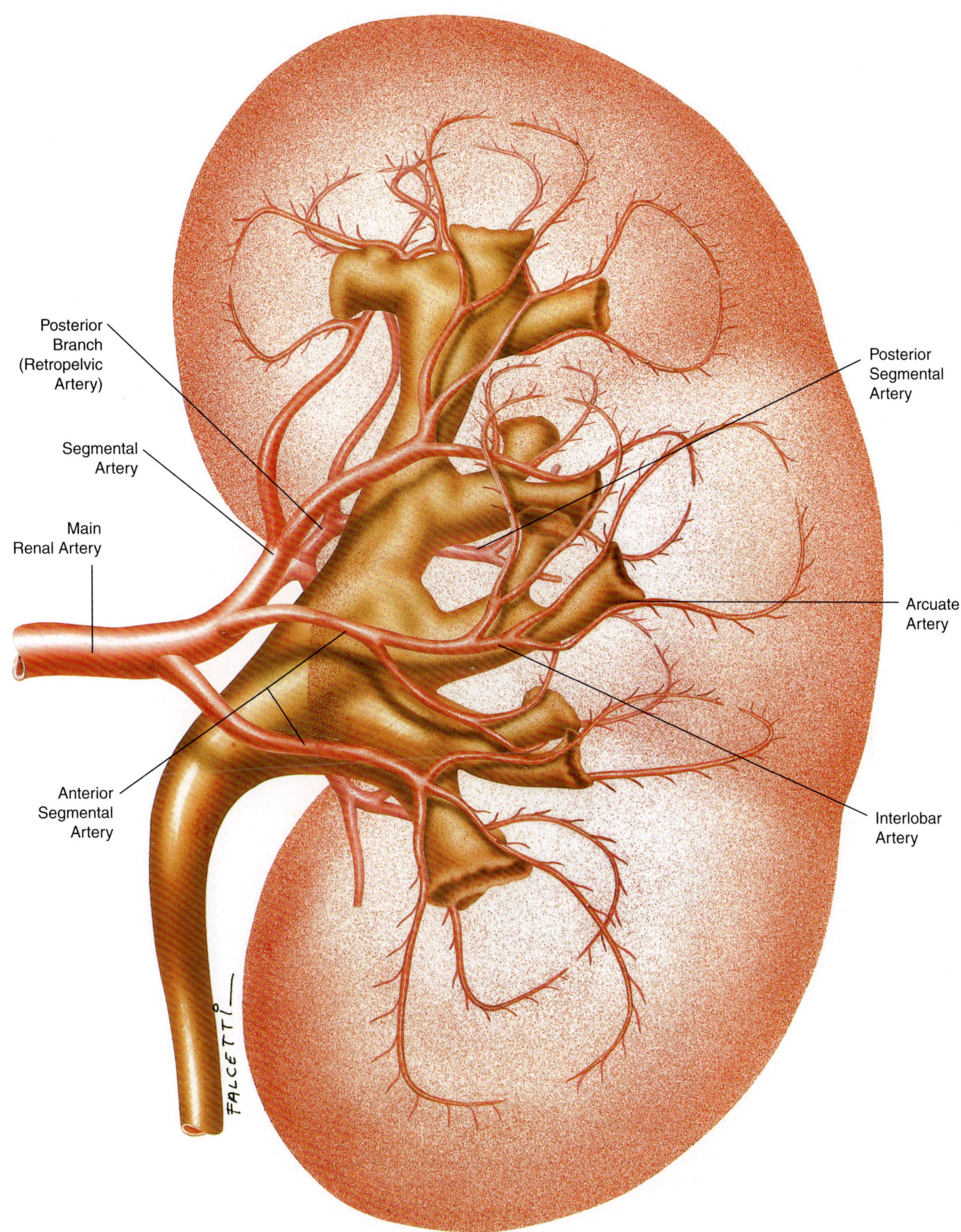

Figure 18.149. Schematic drawing of an anterior view from a left kidney shows the branching of the renal arteries and their official nomenclature according to kidney regions. Renal artery; segmental artery; interlobar artery (infundibular), and arcuate artery.

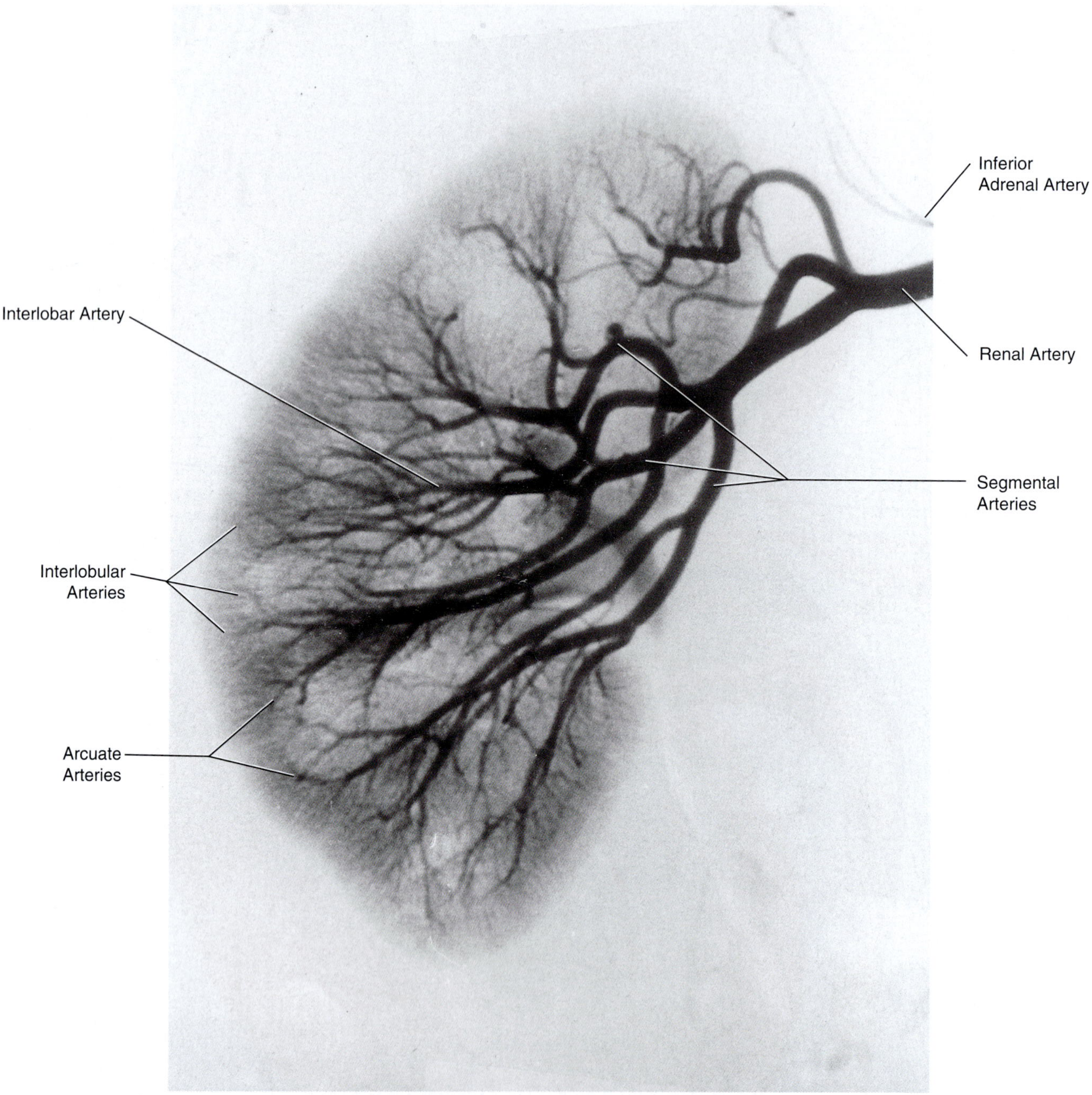

Figure 18.150. Right kidney angiogram shows the normal branching of the renal artery and the official nomenclature according to the kidney regions.

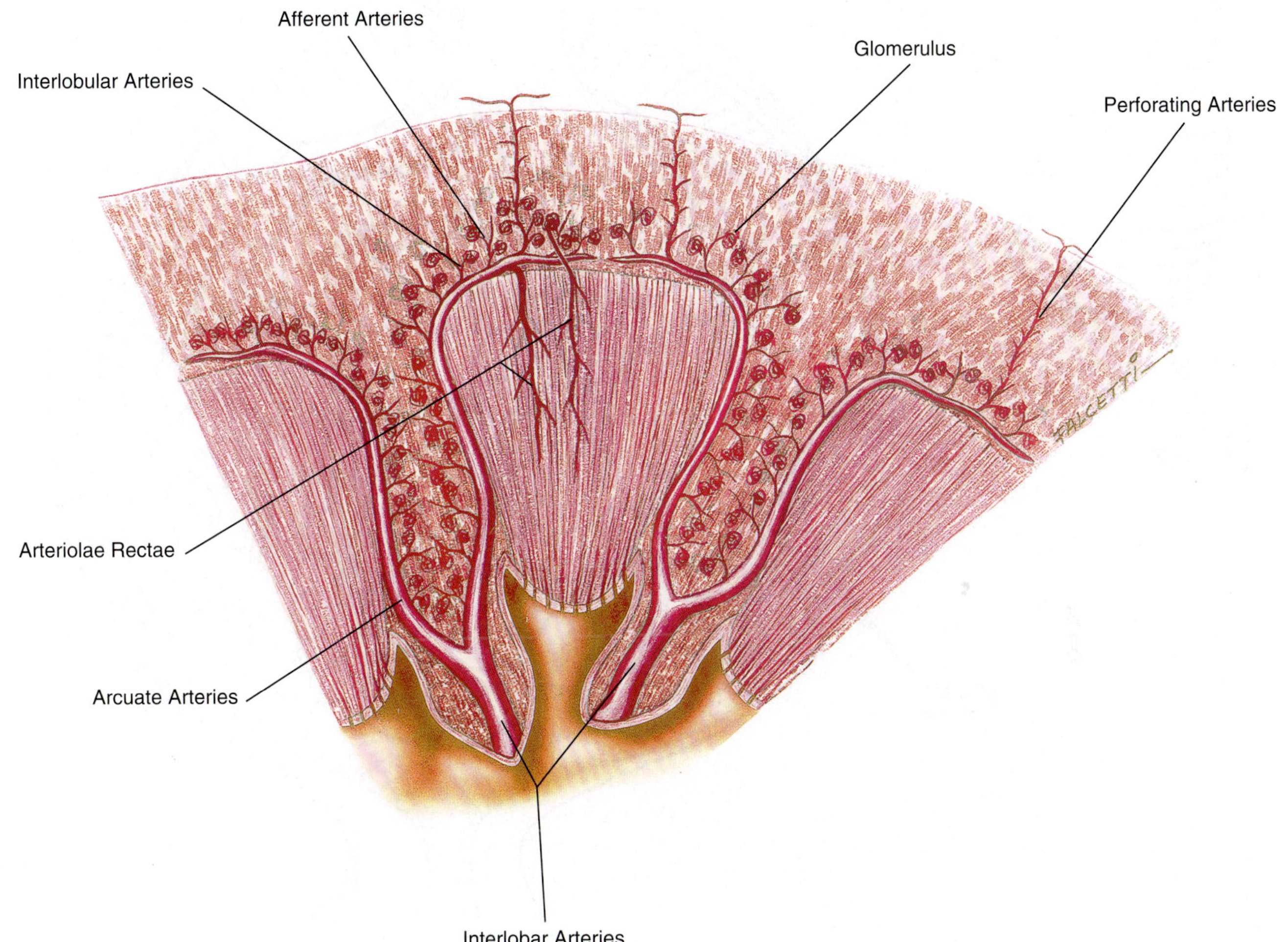

Figure 18.151. Schematic diagram of two adjacent pyramids and minor calices depicts the vasculature of the renal parenchyma from the level of the interlobar arteries to the glomerular level.

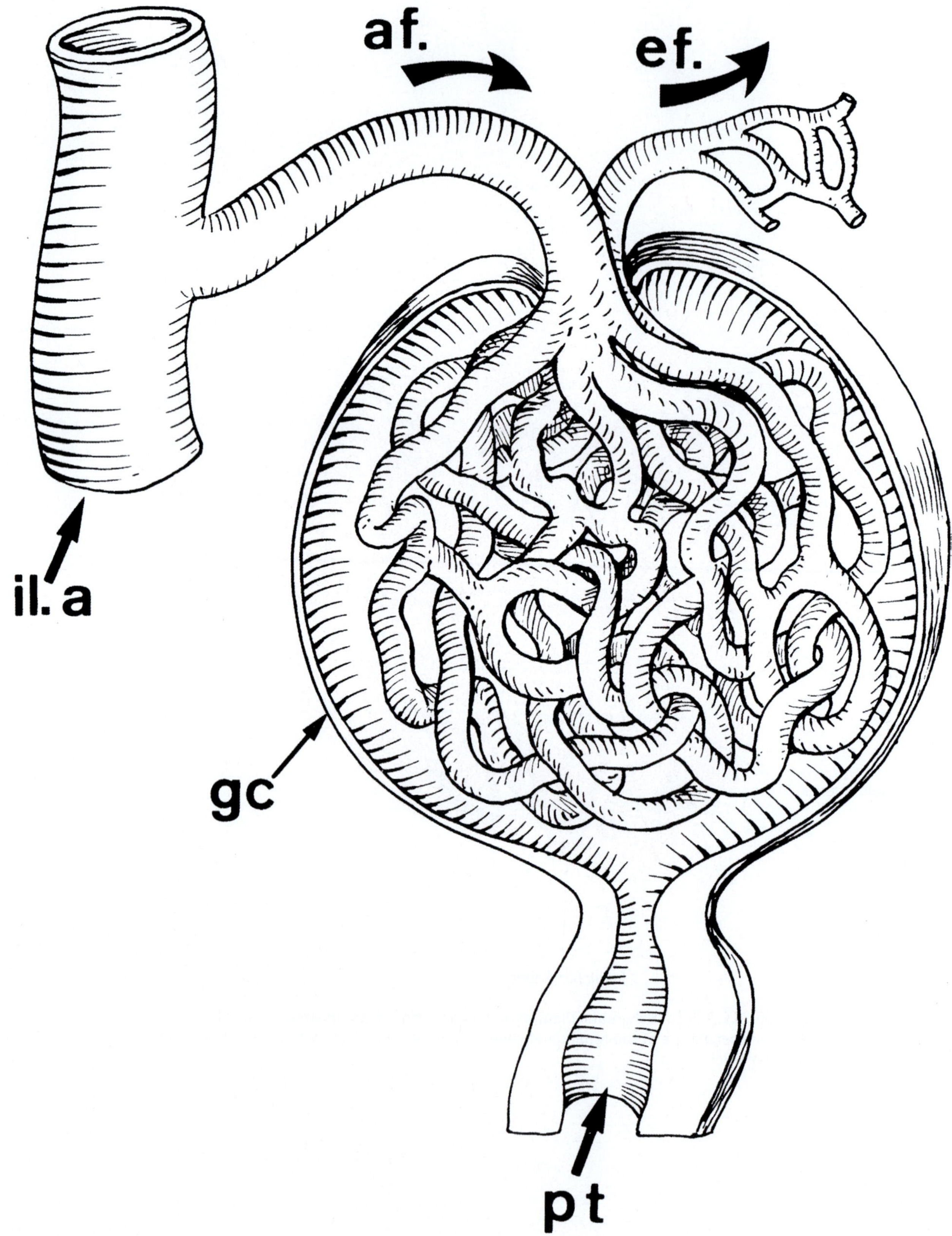

Figure 18.152. Schematic drawing representing the renal corpuscle (of Malpighi). il.a, interlobular artery; af., afferent arterioles; ef., efferent arterioles; gc, glomerular capsule (Bowman); pt., proximal tubule.

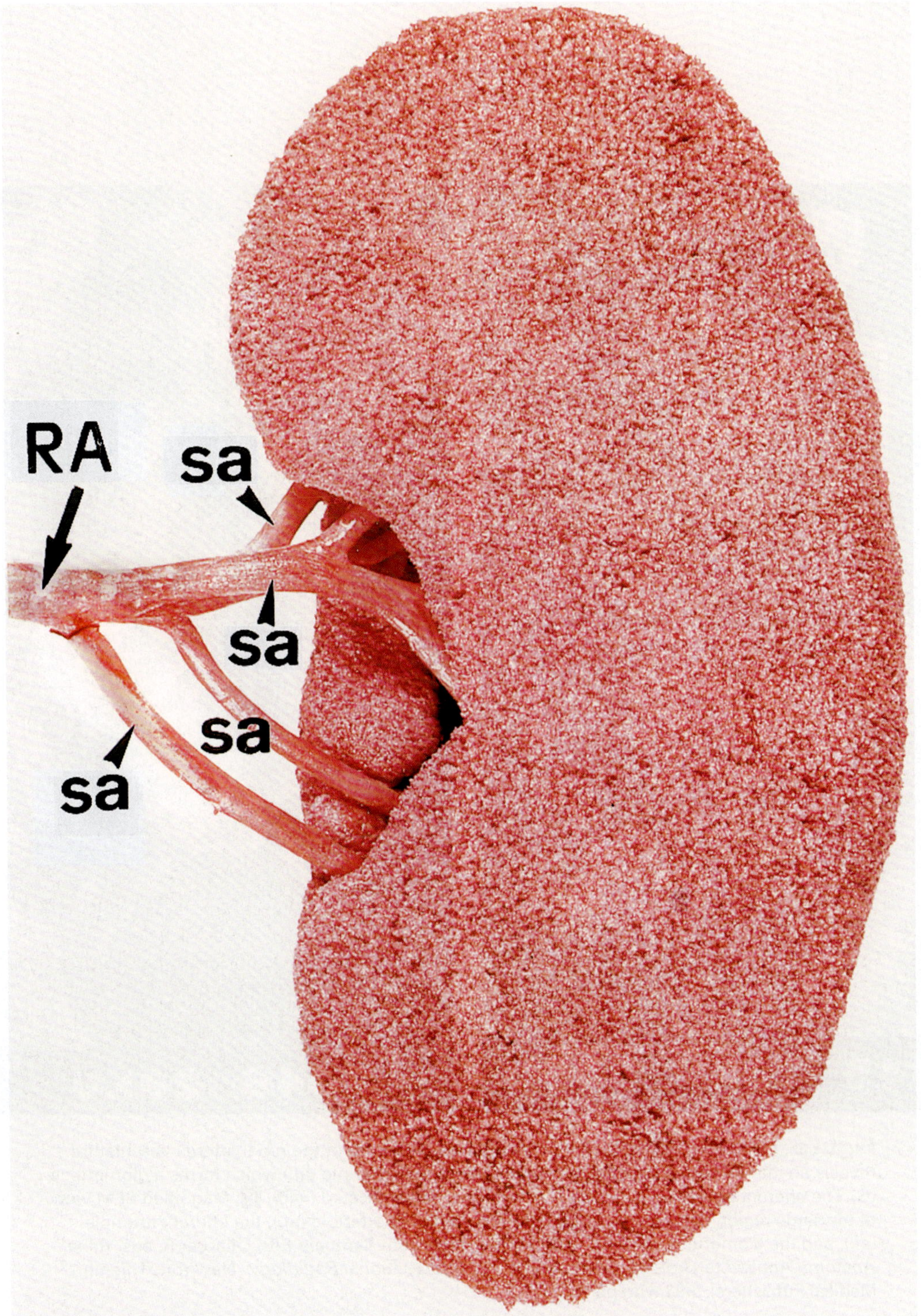

Figure 18.153. Anterior view of a left kidney polyester resin endocast of the renal arterial vasculature. Note the "spongelike" appearance of the endocast, which represents the glomeruli filled with the polyester resin. RA, main trunk of the renal artery; sa, anterior segmental arteries.

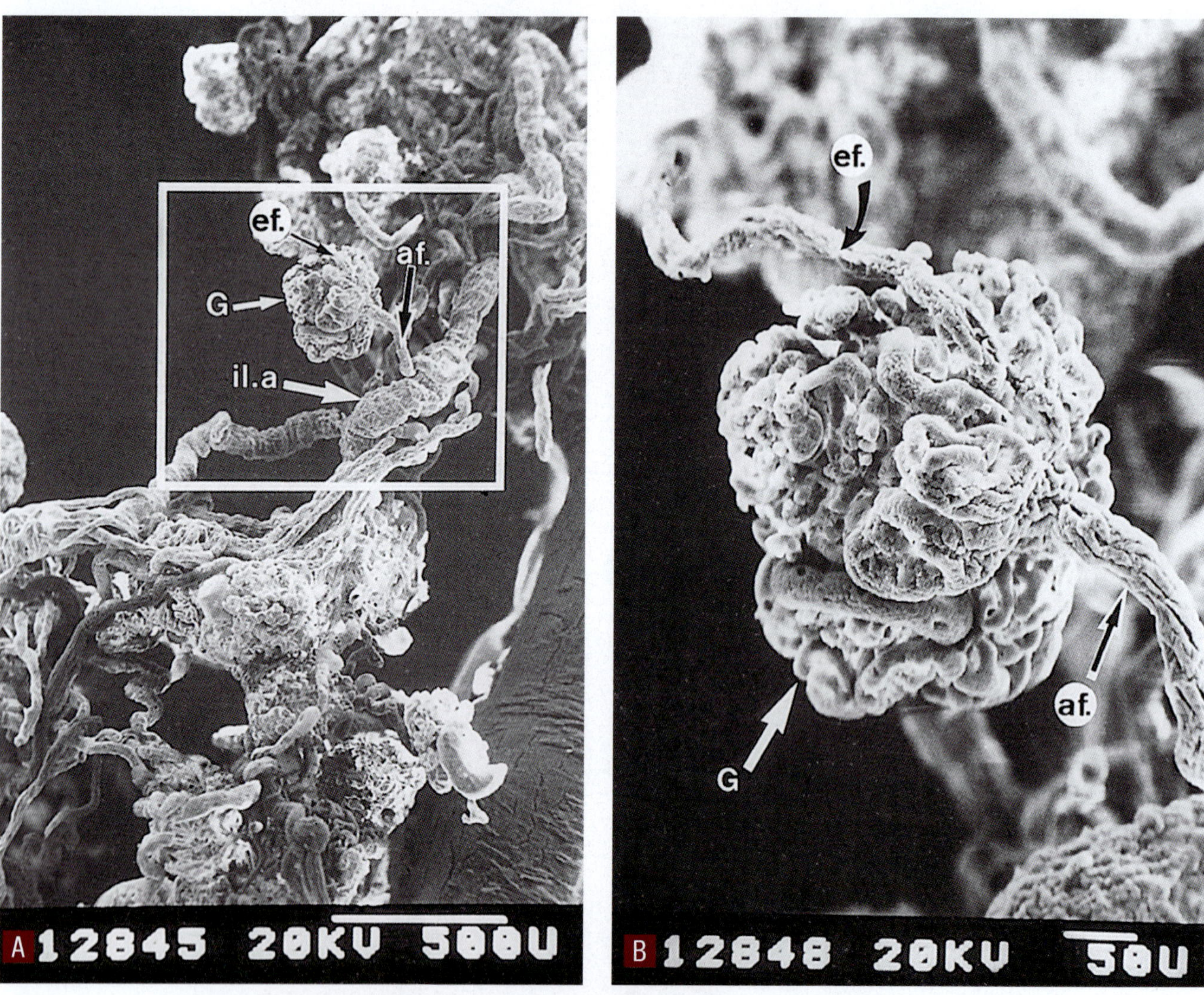

Figure 18.154. A, SEM of a polyester resin endocast of the renal arterial vasculature reveals an interlobular artery (il.a) giving off an afferent arteriole (af.) which forms a glomerulus (G). The efferent arteriole (ef.) of the glomerulus is also indicated (×40). B, Magnified SEM view of the same region demarcated in A, details the afferent arteriole (af.), the efferent arteriole (ef.), and the glomerulus itself (G) (×300). (Reprinted from Sampaio FJB, Uflacker R, eds. *Renal Anatomy Applied to Urology, Endourology and Interventional Radiology.* New York: Thieme Medical Publishers; 1993 with permission.)

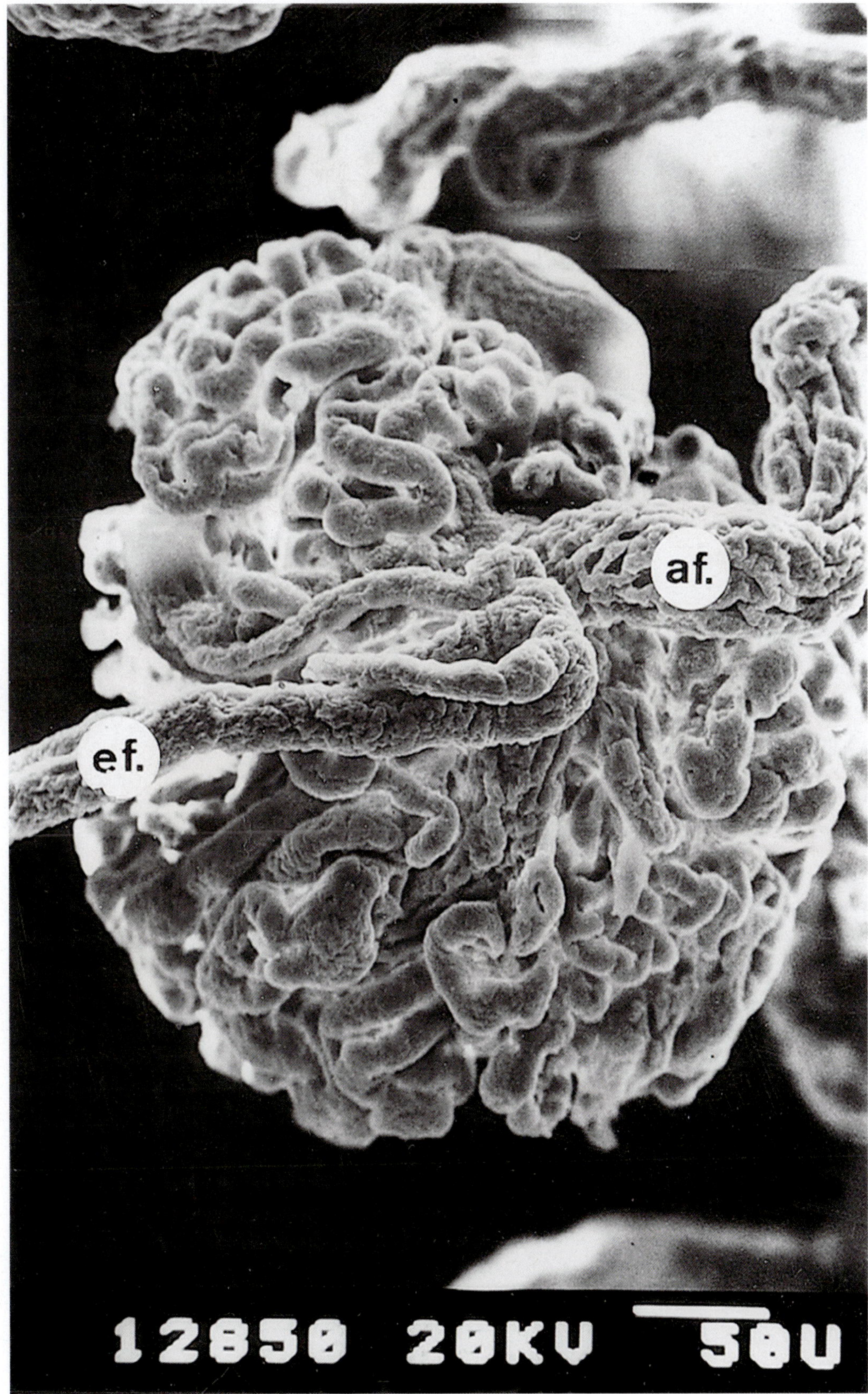

Figure 18.155. Scanning electron microscopy close-up view of a glomerular endocast reveals the vascular pole with the afferent (af.) and efferent (ef.) arterioles. This figure demonstrates that the afferent arteriole has a greater caliber than the efferent arteriole (×300). (Reprinted from Sampaio FJB, Uflacker R, eds. *Renal Anatomy Applied to Urology, Endourology and Interventional Radiology.* New York: Thieme Medical Publishers; 1993 with permission.)

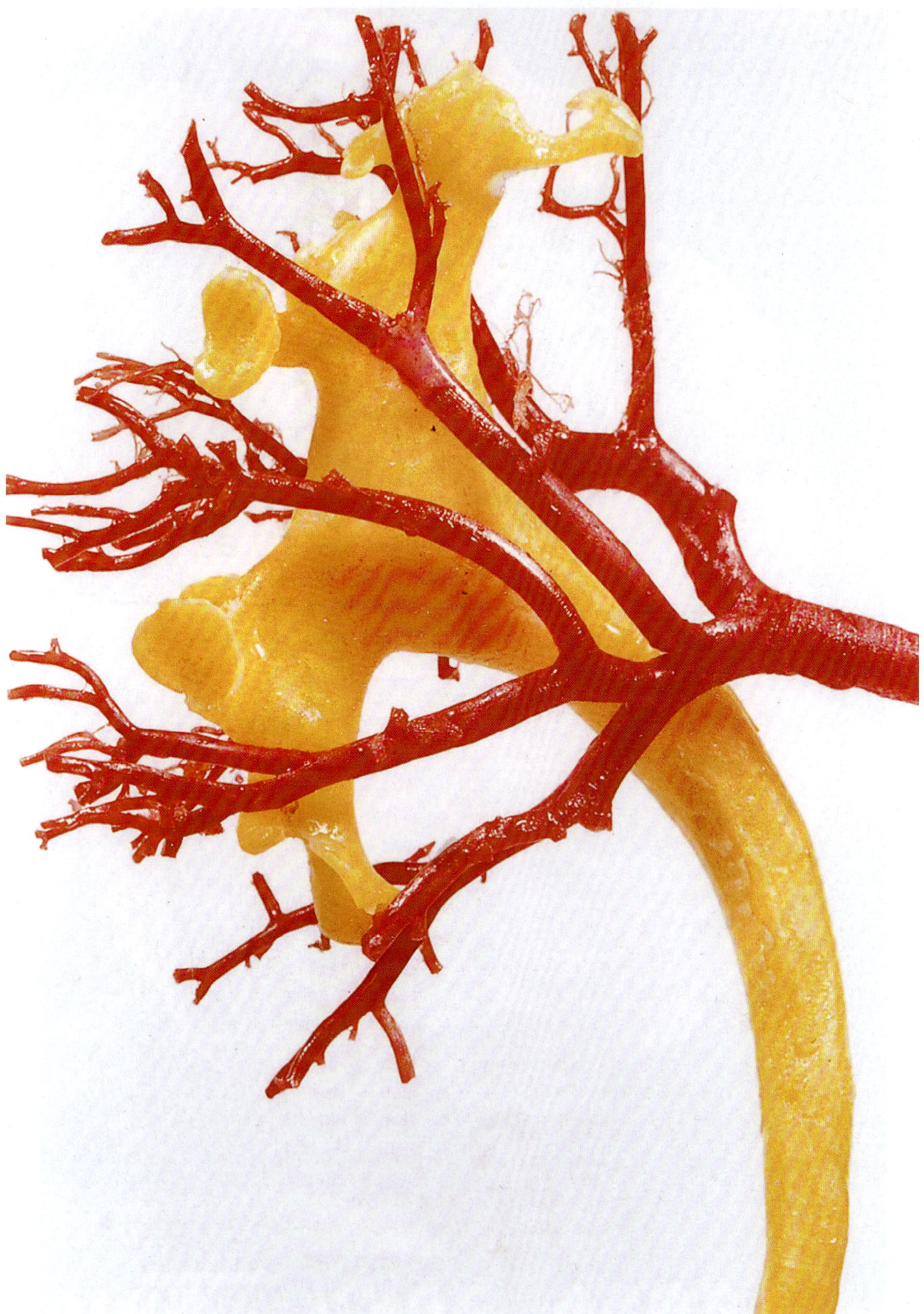

Figure 18.156. Anterior view of endocast (pelvicaliceal system and arteries) from a right kidney. This cast shows that the fine arterial vessels and the glomerular tufts were removed by needle handpicking, allowing a clear visualization of the major intrarenal arteries and the underlying collecting system.

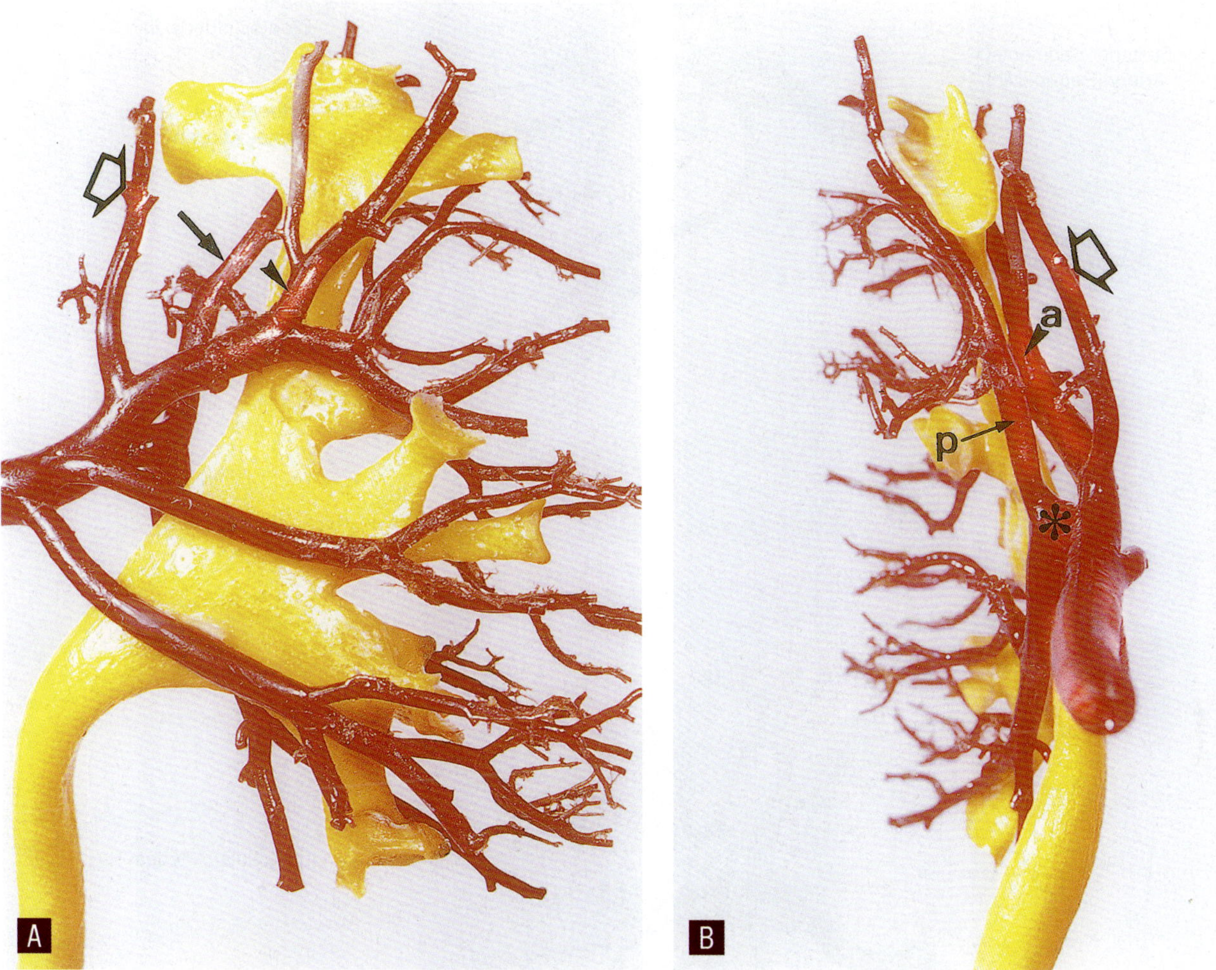

Figure 18.157. A, Anterior view of an endocast (pelvicaliceal system and arteries) from a left kidney shows arterial supply related to the superior pole: the superior (apical) segmental artery (open arrow), the artery related to the anterior surface of the upper infundibulum (arrowhead), and the branch of the posterior segmental artery related to the posterior surface of the upper infundibulum (arrow). B, Oblique posterior view of the same endocast shown in A reveals the artery related to the anterior surface (a) and the artery related to the posterior surface (p) of the upper infundibulum. The open arrow points to the superior (apical) segmental artery, which is not related to the upper infundibulum. The asterisk marks the posterior segmental artery (retropelvic artery). (Reprinted from Sampaio FJB, Uflacker R, eds. *Renal Anatomy Applied to Urology, Endourology and Interventional Radiology.* New York: Thieme Medical Publishers; 1993 with permission.)

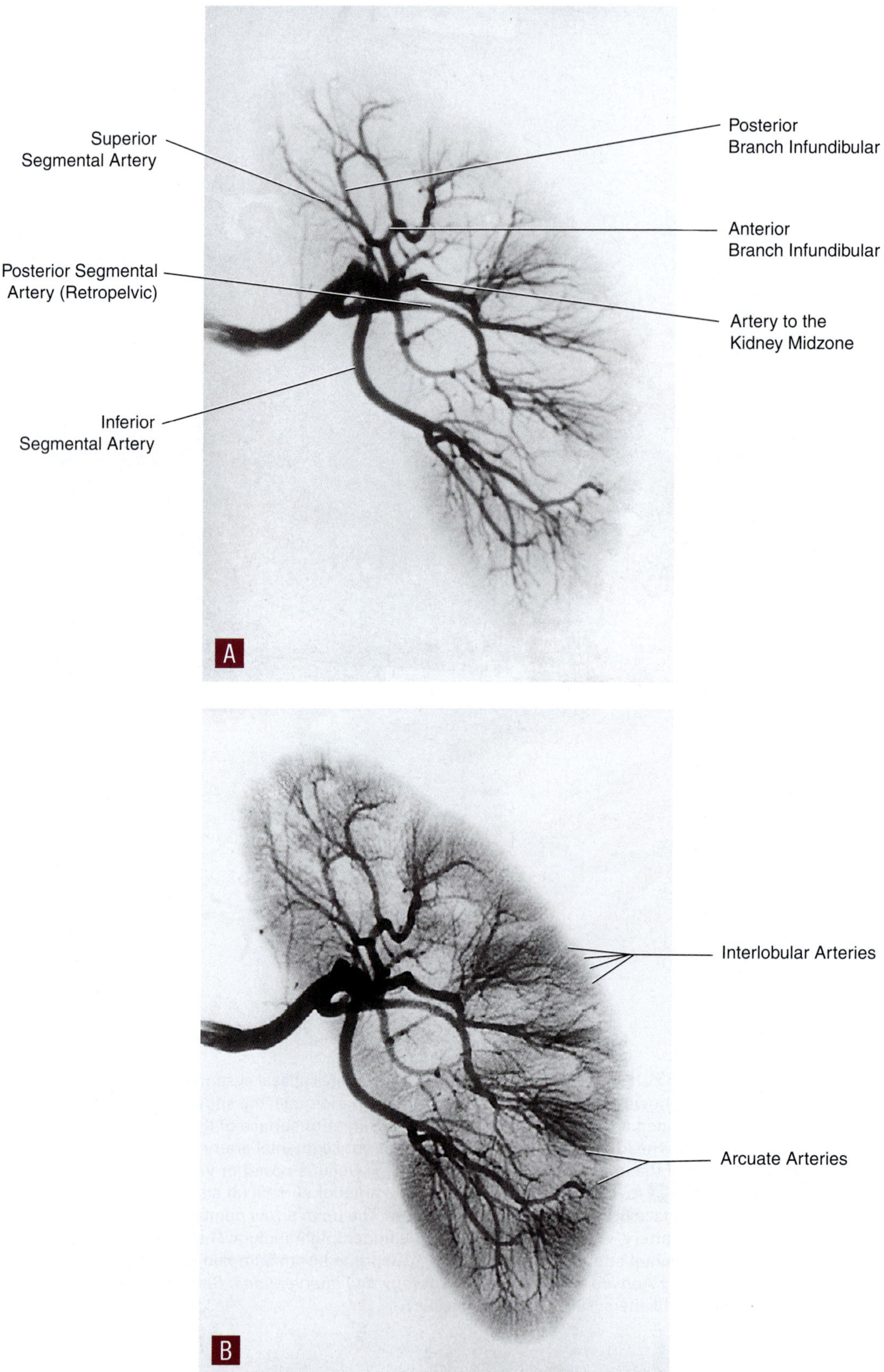

Figure 18.158. A, Anterior view of a left renal angiogram shows the arterial supply related to the superior pole: the superior segmental artery, the artery related to the anterior surface of the upper infundibulum, and the branch of the posterior segmental artery related to the posterior surface of the upper infundibulum. B to D, Later phase of the renal angiogram showing the progressive filling of the peripheral vessels, including the interlobar arteries, the arcuate arteries and the interlobular arteries. In D, the nephrogram is more prominent.

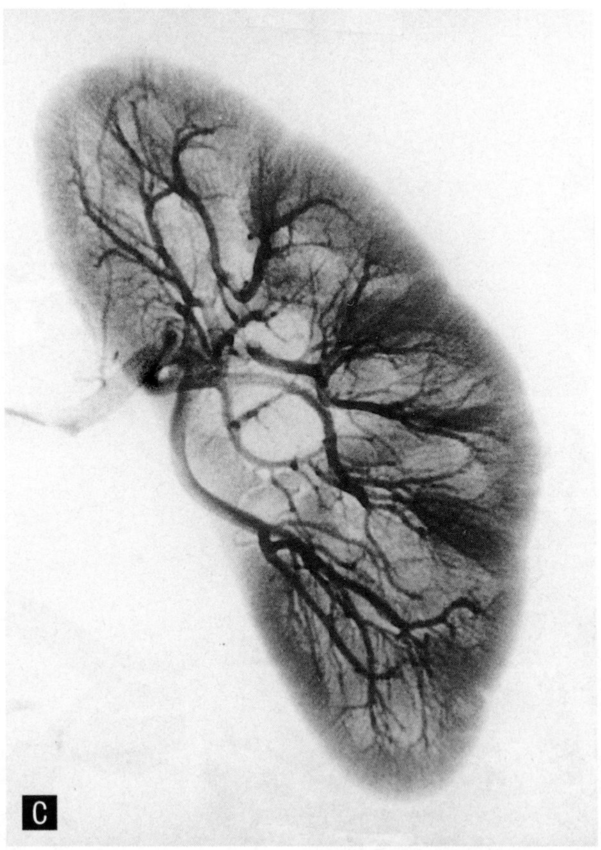

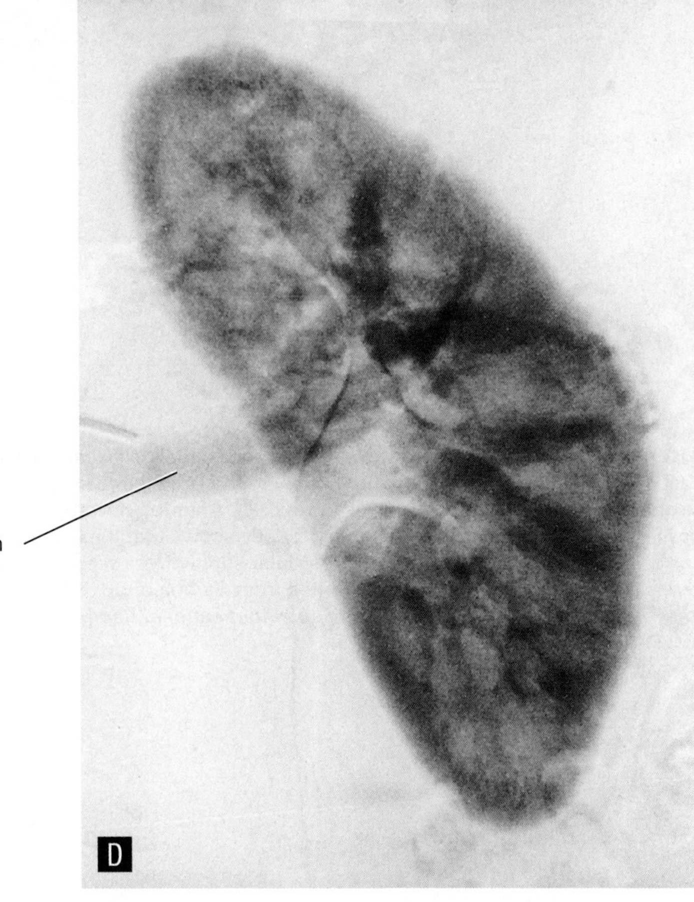

Figure 18.158. *Continued*

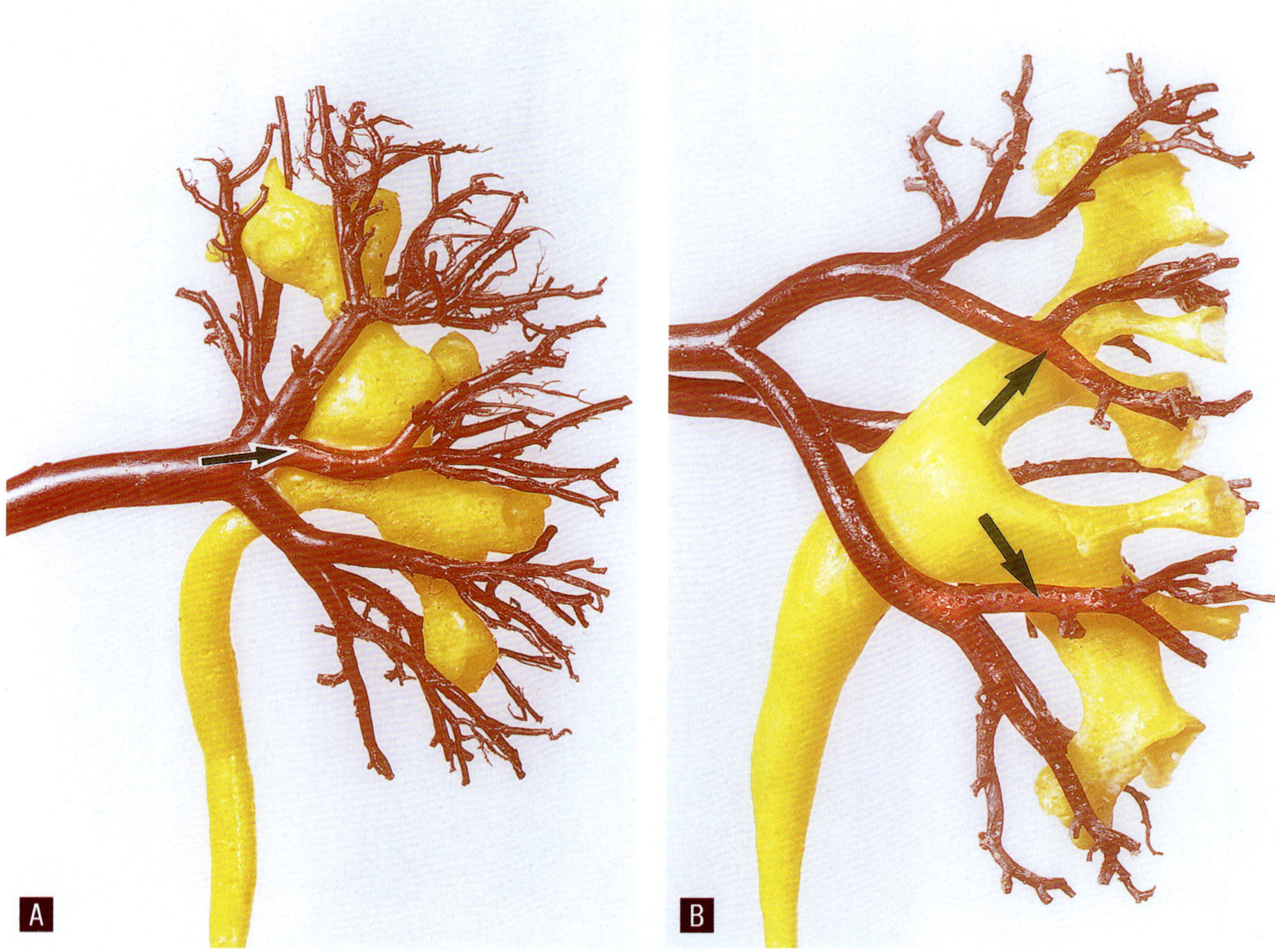

Figure 18.159. **A**, Anterior view of an endocast (pelvicaliceal system and arteries) from a left kidney shows an individualized artery to the kidney midzone coursing horizontally on the anterior surface of the renal pelvis (arrow). **B**, Anterior view of an endocast (pelvicaliceal system and arteries) from a left kidney shows that the kidney midzone does not have an individualized artery and receives vascular supply from secondary division branches of arteries of other regions (arrows). (Reprinted from Sampaio FJB, Uflacker R, eds. *Renal Anatomy Applied to Urology, Endourology and Interventional Radiology.* New York: Thieme Medical Publishers; 1993 with permission.)

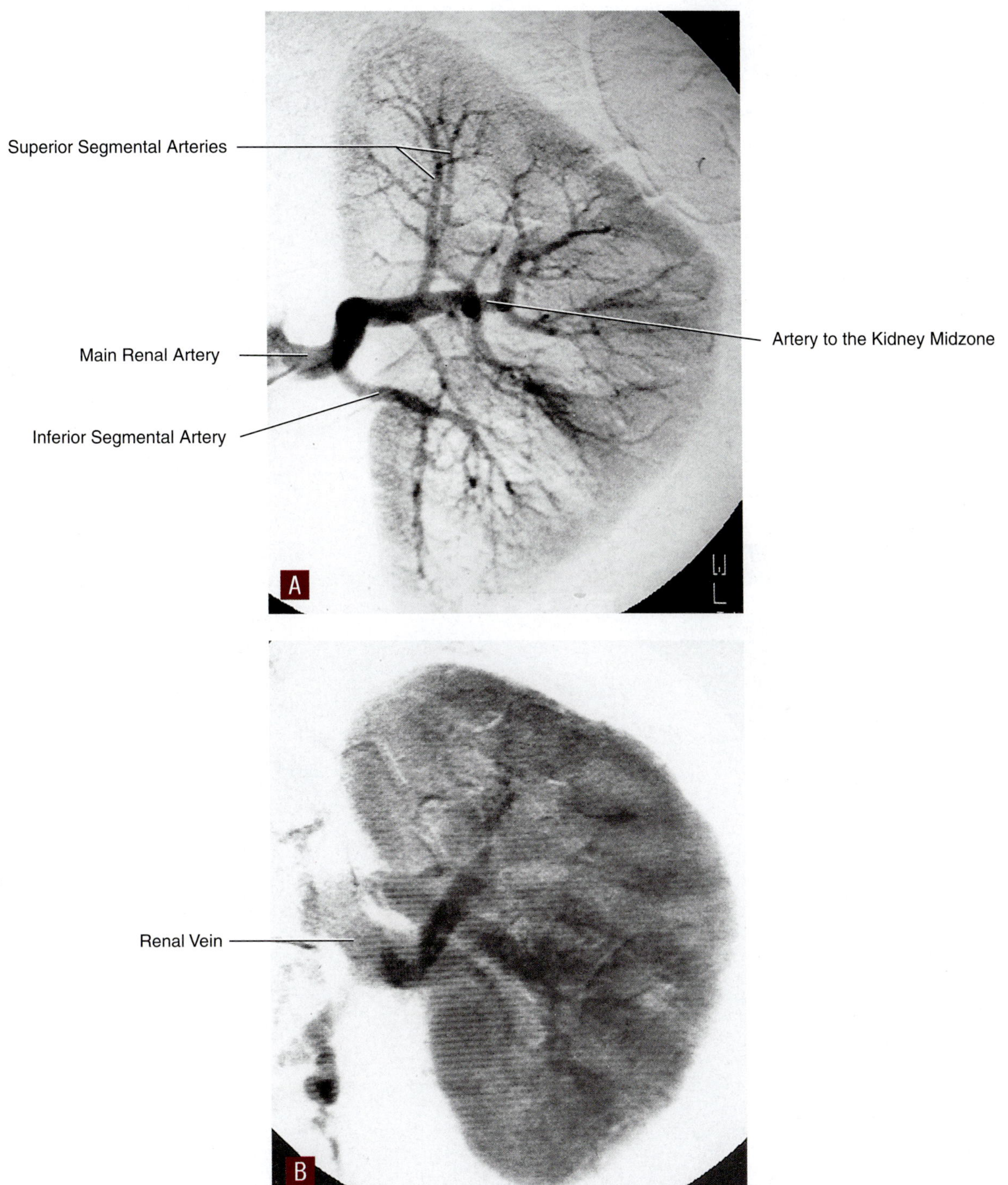

Figure 18.160. **A**, Anterior view of a left renal angiogram showing the artery to the kidney midzone, as well as the superior and inferior segmental arteries. **B**, Late angiographic phase shows the renal nephrogram and the drainage vein.

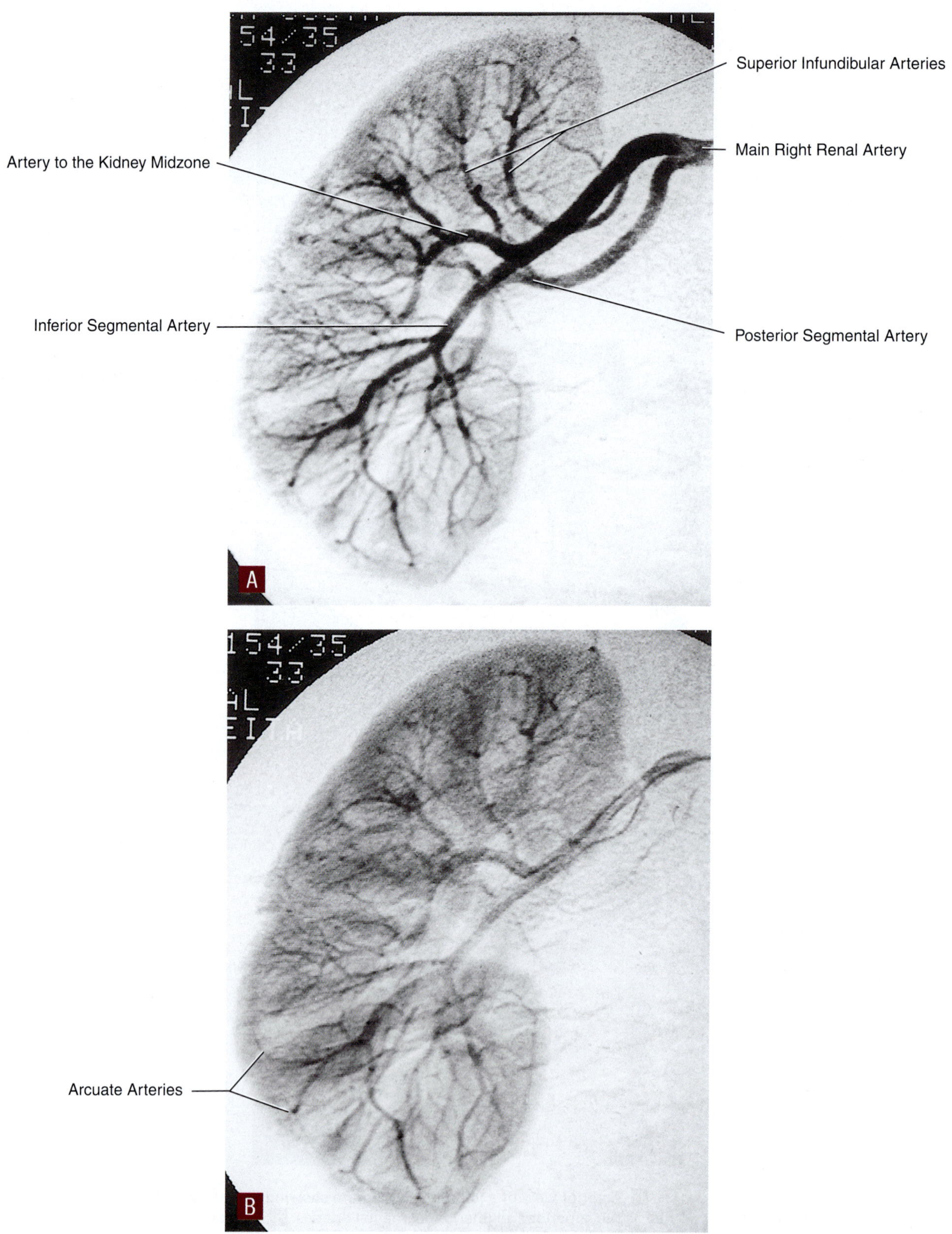

Figure 18.161. **A**, Anterior view of a right renal angiogram showing the artery to the kidney midzone, the posterior segmental artery, and the superior and inferior segmental arteries. **B**, Later phase of the angiogram shows more peripheral arteries.

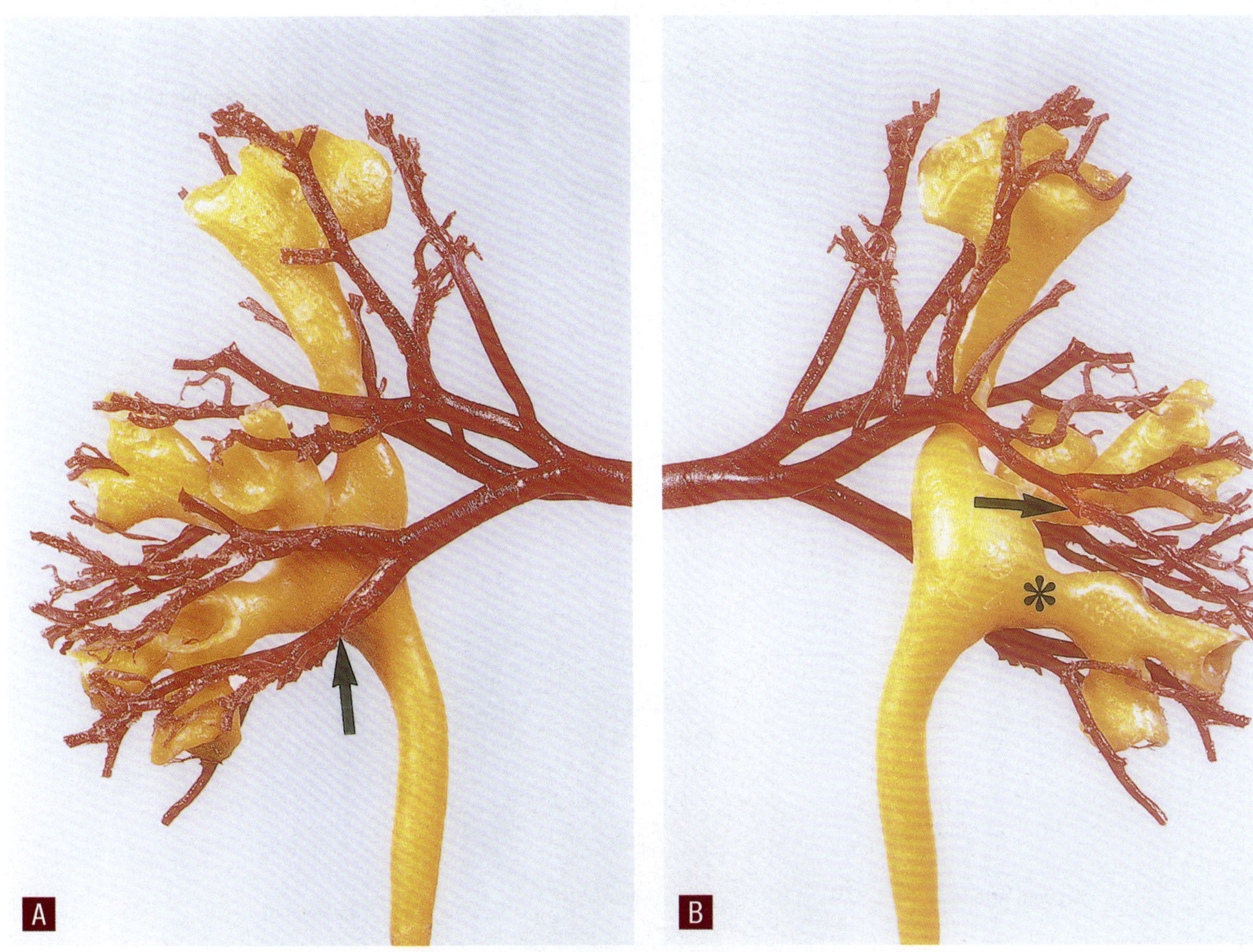

Figure 18.162. A, Anterior view of an endocast (pelvicaliceal system and arteries) from a right kidney demonstrates front and back arterial supply to inferior pole (arrow) arising from the anterior division of the renal artery (inferior segmental artery). B, Posterior view of the same cast shown in A demonstrates that the posterior segmental artery (retropelvic artery) does not reach the lower infundibulum (arrow). The posterior aspect of the lower infundibulum is free of arteries (asterisk). (Reprinted from Sampaio FJB, Uflacker R, eds. *Renal Anatomy Applied to Urology, Endourology and Interventional Radiology.* New York: Thieme Medical Publishers; 1993 with permission.)

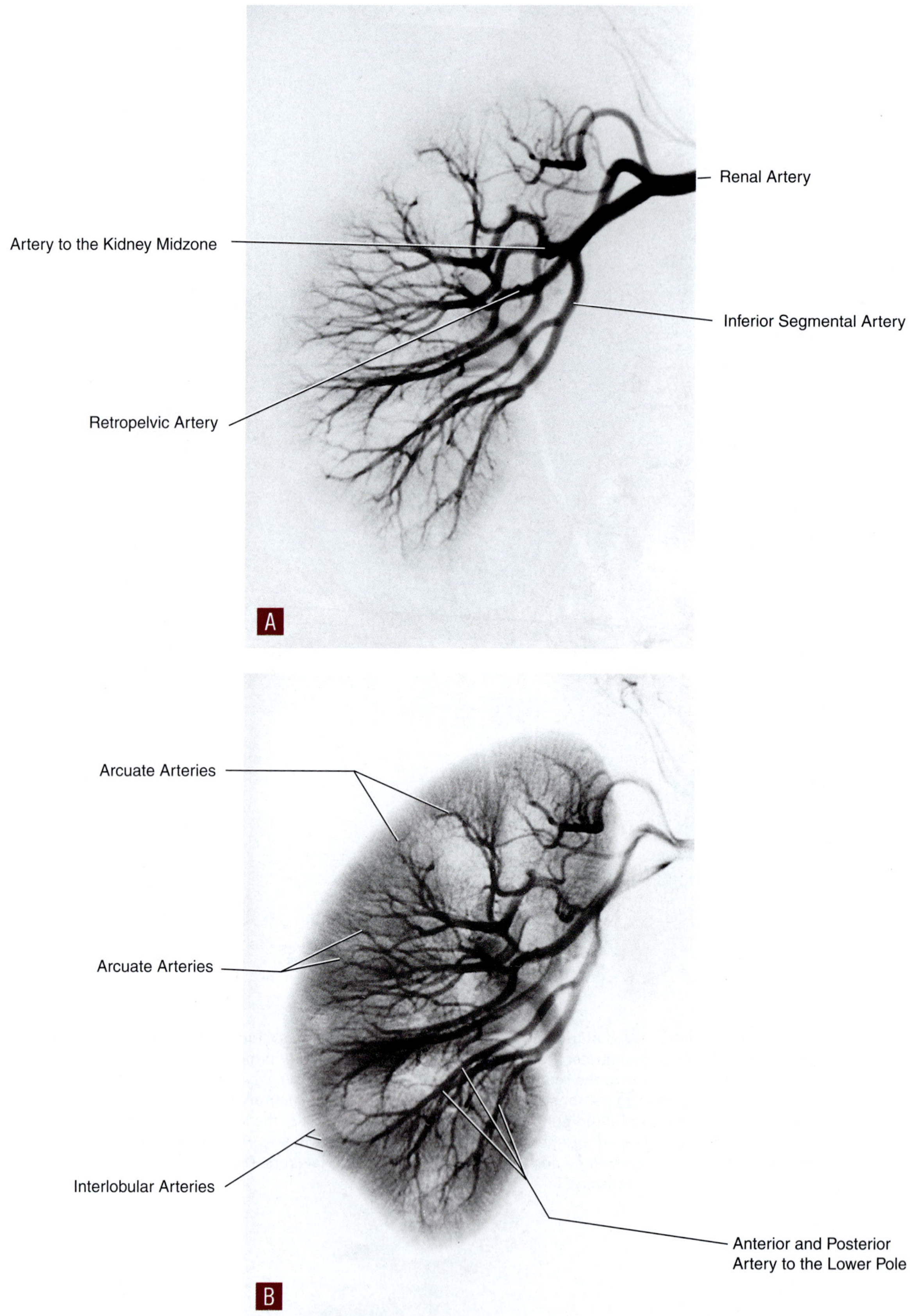

Figure 18.163. A, Selective right kidney angiogram shows the arteries to the lower infundibulum arising from the inferior segmental artery. The artery to the midzone of the kidney is also seen. The retropelvic artery is also observed. B, Later arterial phase shows the interlobar and interlobular arteries. C, Nephrographic phase shows the renal cortex and the drainage vein.

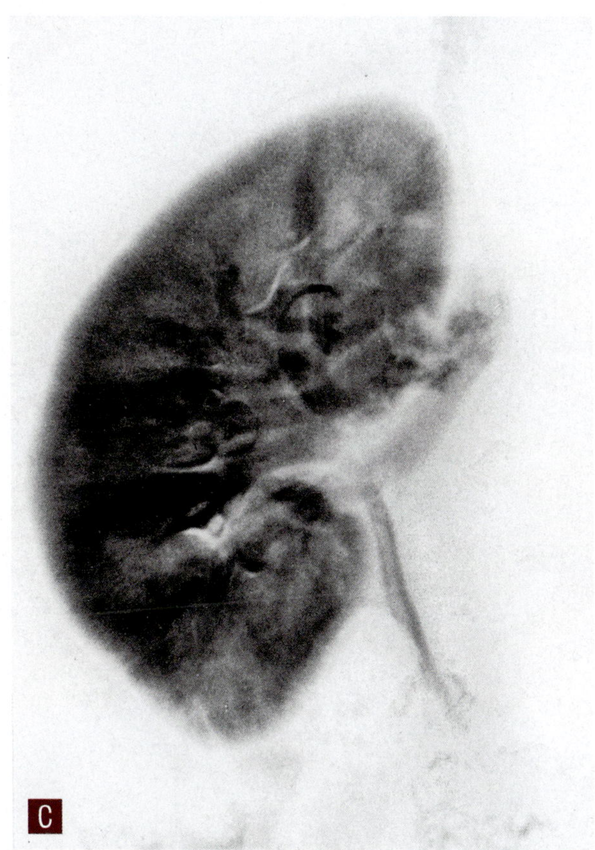

Figure 18.163. *Continued*

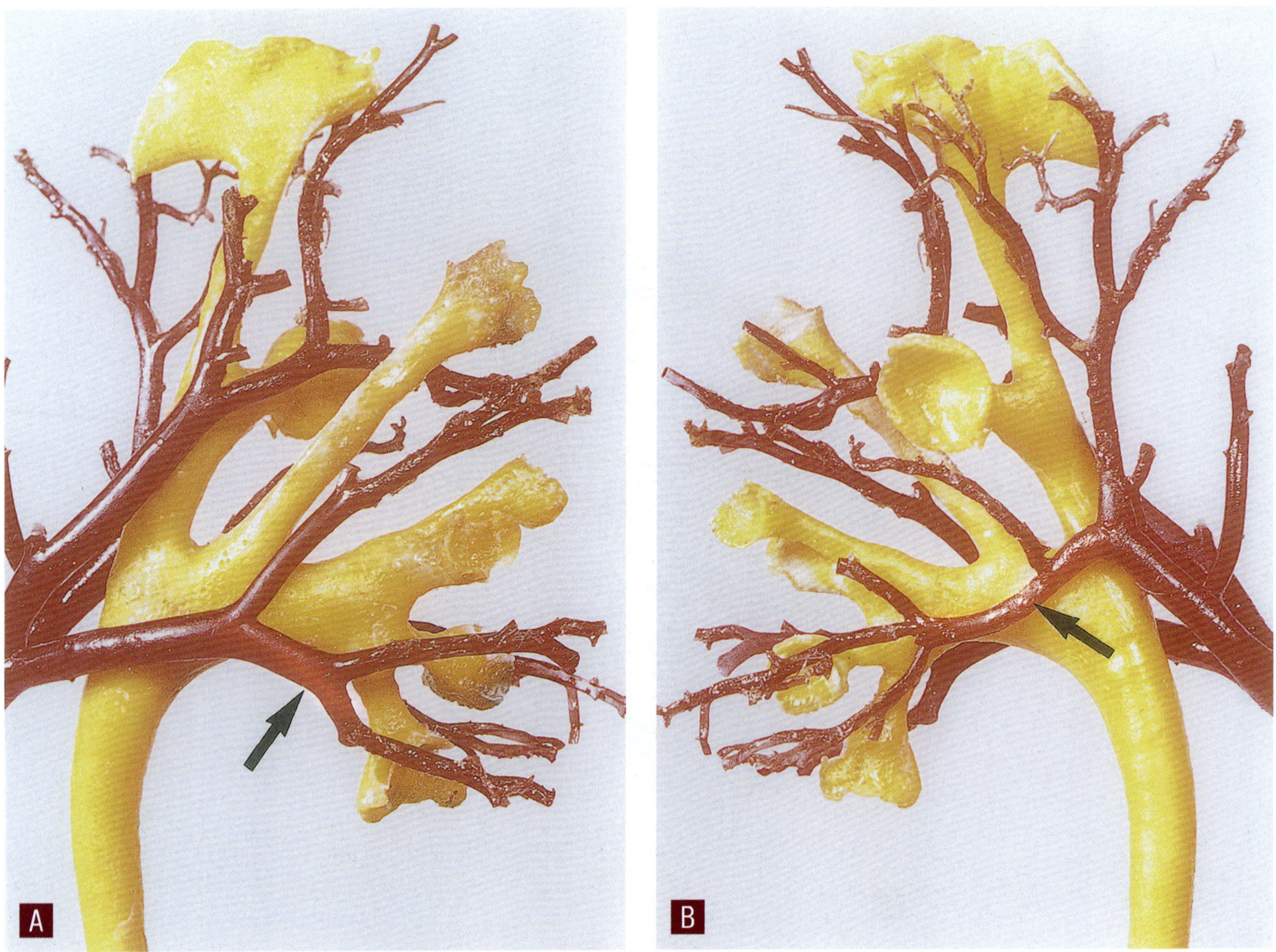

Figure 18.164. A, Anterior view of an endocast (pelvicaliceal system and arteries) from a left kidney shows the artery to the anterior surface of the lower infundibulum arising from the inferior segmental artery (arrow). B, Posterior view of the same cast shown in A reveals the posterior aspect of the lower infundibulum supplied by the inferior branch of the posterior segmental artery (arrow). (Reprinted from Sampaio FJB, Uflacker R, eds. *Renal Anatomy Applied to Urology, Endourology and Interventional Radiology.* New York: Thieme Medical Publishers; 1993 with permission.)

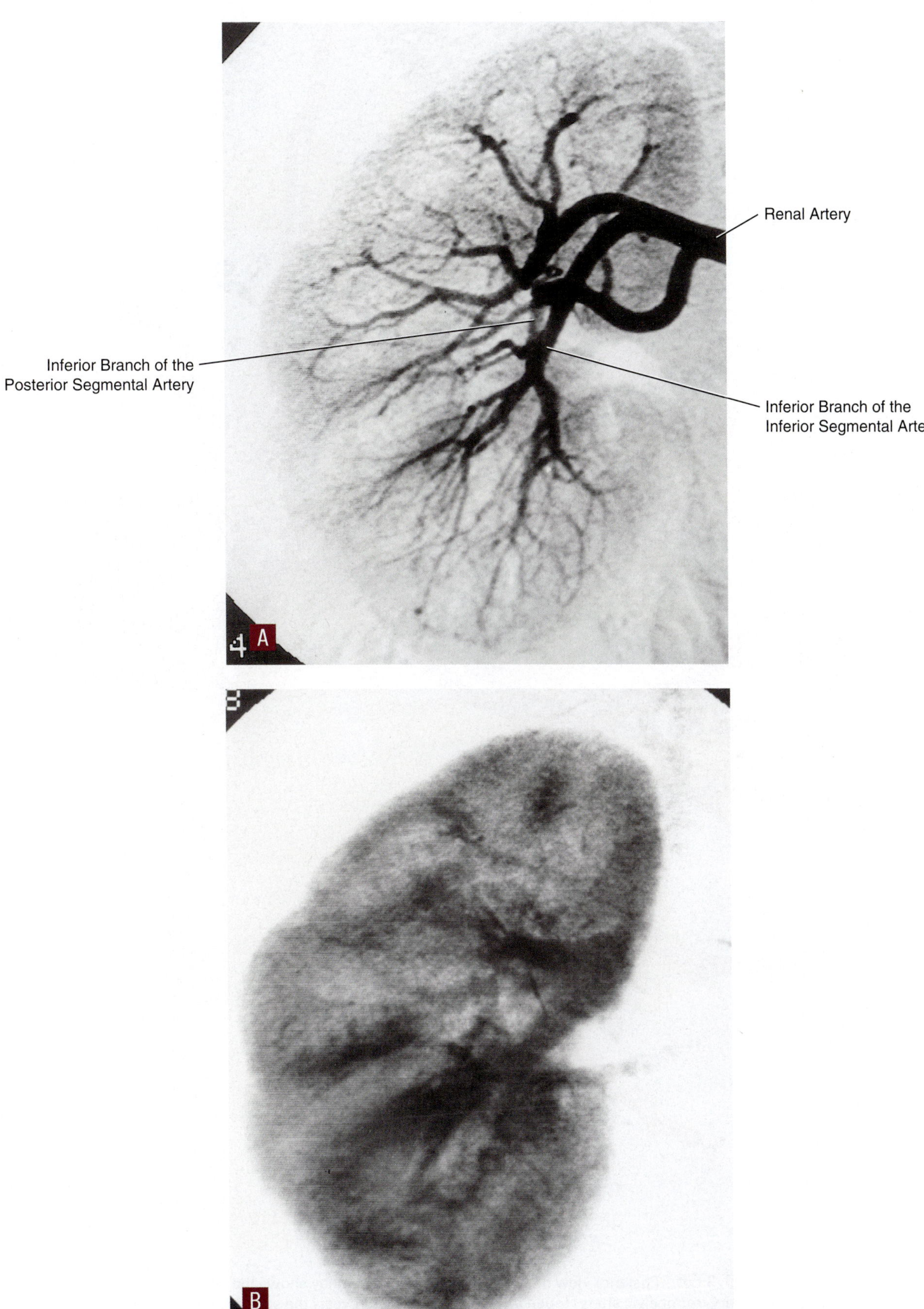

Figure 18.165. A, Anterior view of a right renal angiogram. The artery to the anterior surface of the lower infundibulum arises from the inferior segmental artery. The inferior branch of the lower infundibulum arises from the posterior segmental artery. B, Nephrographic phase of the kidney. The vein is ill-defined.

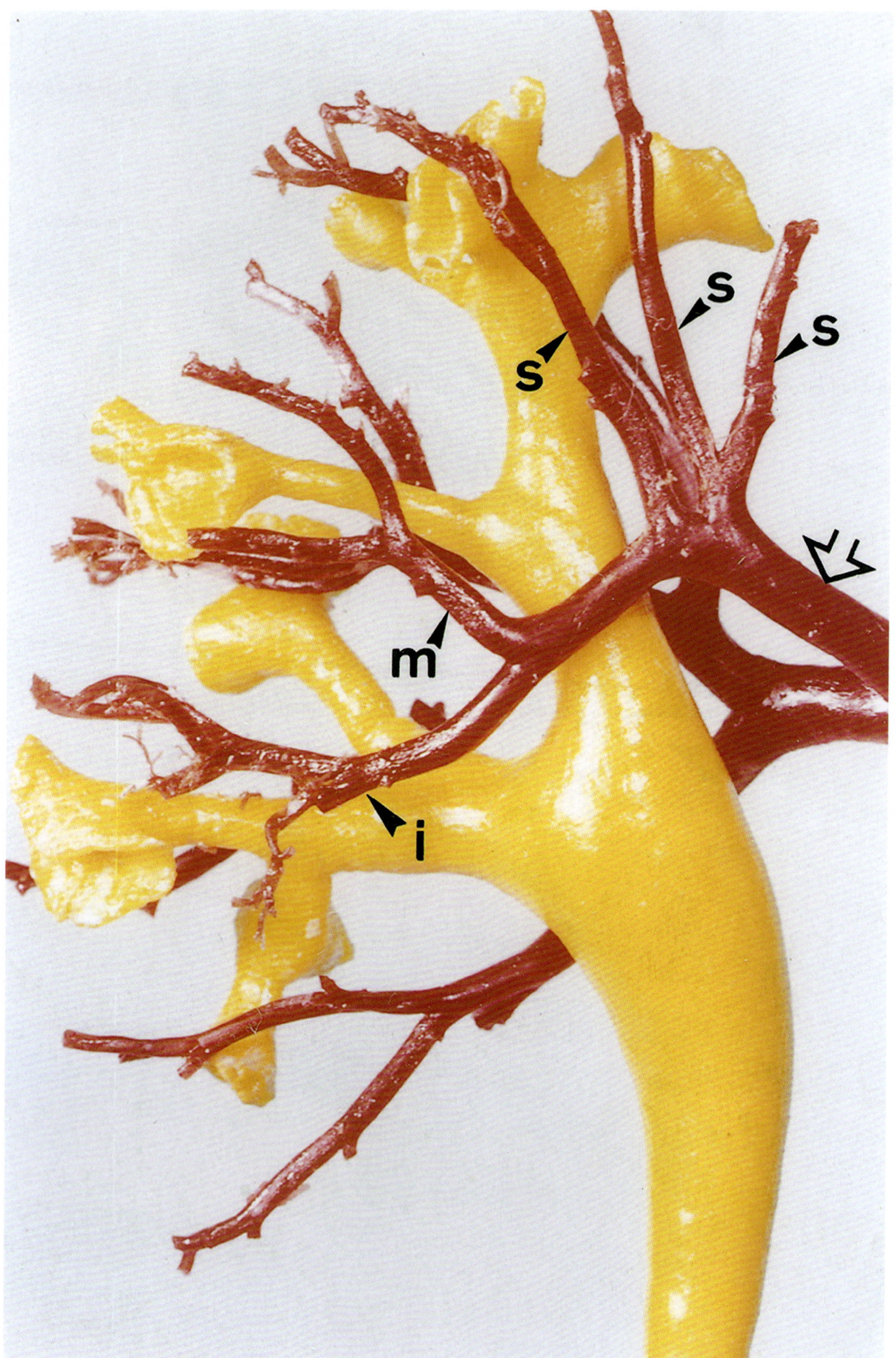

Figure 18.166. Posterior view of an endocast from a left kidney shows the posterior segmental artery (retropelvic artery) (open arrow). This cast also reveals the subdivision branches of the posterior segmental artery. In this case, there are three superior branches related to the posterior aspect of the upper infundibulum. s, superior subdivision branches; m, middle subdivision branch; i, inferior subdivision branch. (Reprinted from Sampaio FJB, Uflacker R, eds. *Renal Anatomy Applied to Urology, Endourology and Interventional Radiology.* New York: Thieme Medical Publishers; 1993 with permission.)

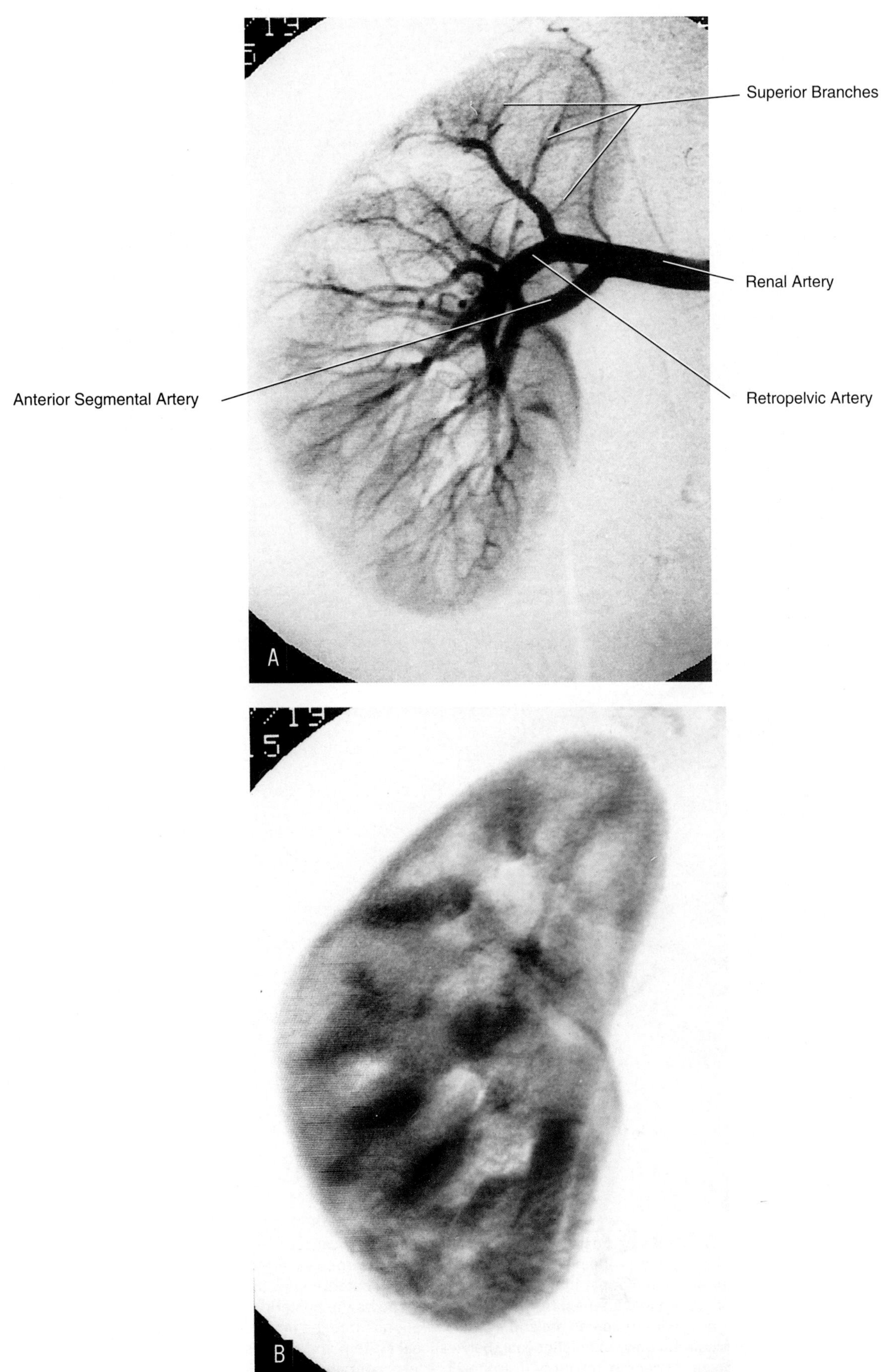

Figure 18.167. **A**, Anterior view of a right renal angiogram showing subdivision branches of the retropelvic artery. **B**, Nephrographic phase. No vein is visible at that phase.

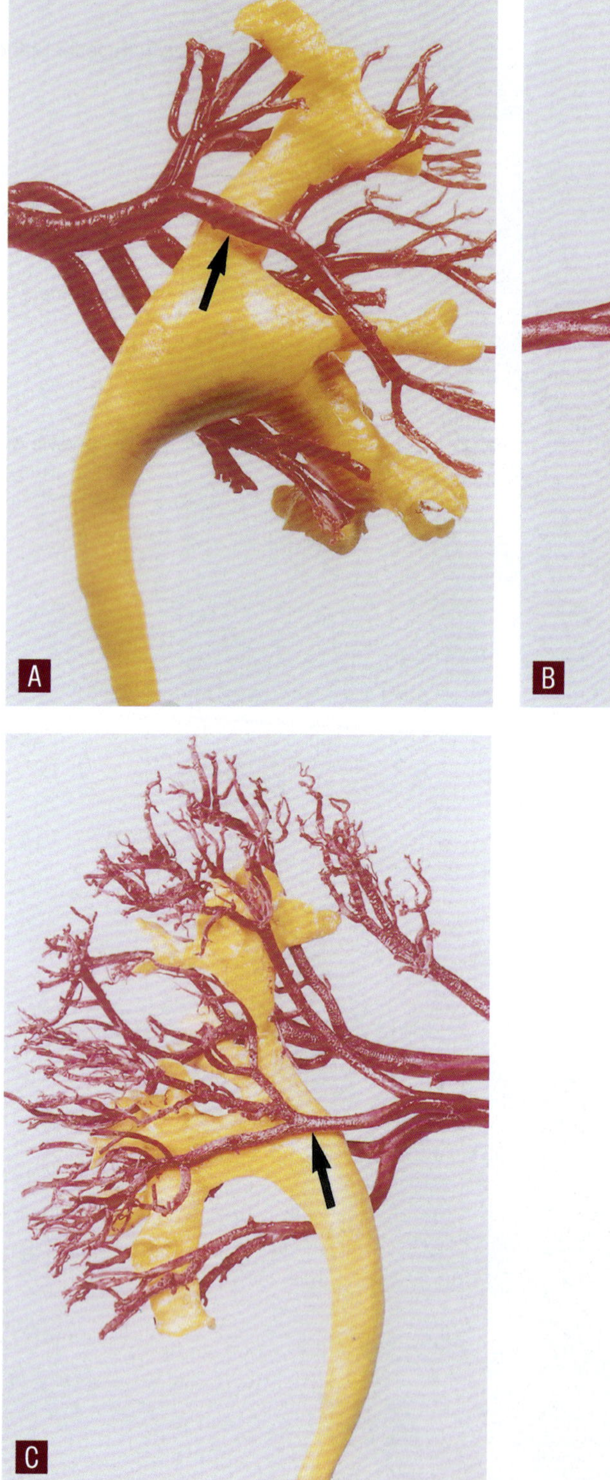

Figure 18.168. **A**, Posterior view of an endocast (pelvicaliceal system and arteries) from a right kidney shows the posterior segmental artery (retropelvic artery) crossing the dorsal surface of the upper infundibulum (arrow). **B**, Posterior view of an endocast (pelvicaliceal system and arteries) from a right kidney shows the posterior segmental artery (retropelvic artery) describing an arc and in close relationship to the upper infundibulum (arrow). **C**, Posterior view of an endocast (pelvicaliceal system and arteries) from a left kidney shows the posterior segmental artery (retropelvic artery) coursing in the middle posterior surface of the renal pelvis (arrow). (Reprinted from Sampaio FJB, Uflacker R, eds. *Renal Anatomy Applied to Urology, Endourology and Interventional Radiology.* New York: Thieme Medical Publishers; 1993 with permission.)

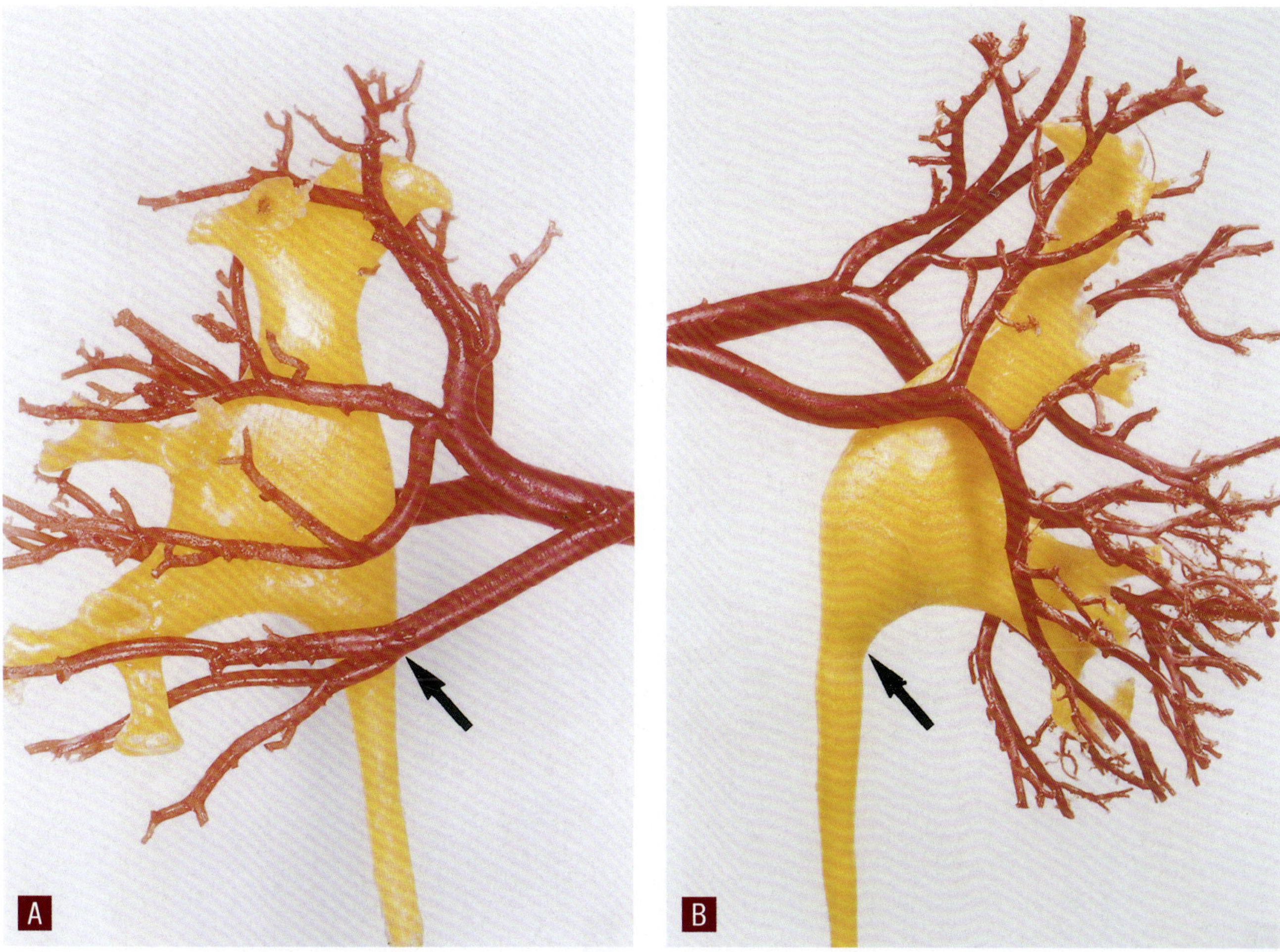

Figure 18.169. Anatomic relationships between ureteropelvic junction (UPJ) and renal arteries. A, Anterior view of an endocast from a right kidney shows a close relationship between the inferior segmental artery and the anterior aspect of the UPJ (arrow). B, Posterior view of an endocast from a right kidney shows the UPJ free of arteries (nonvascular area), (arrow). (Reprinted from Sampaio FJB, Uflacker R, eds. *Renal Anatomy Applied to Urology, Endourology and Interventional Radiology.* New York: Thieme Medical Publishers; 1993 with permission.)

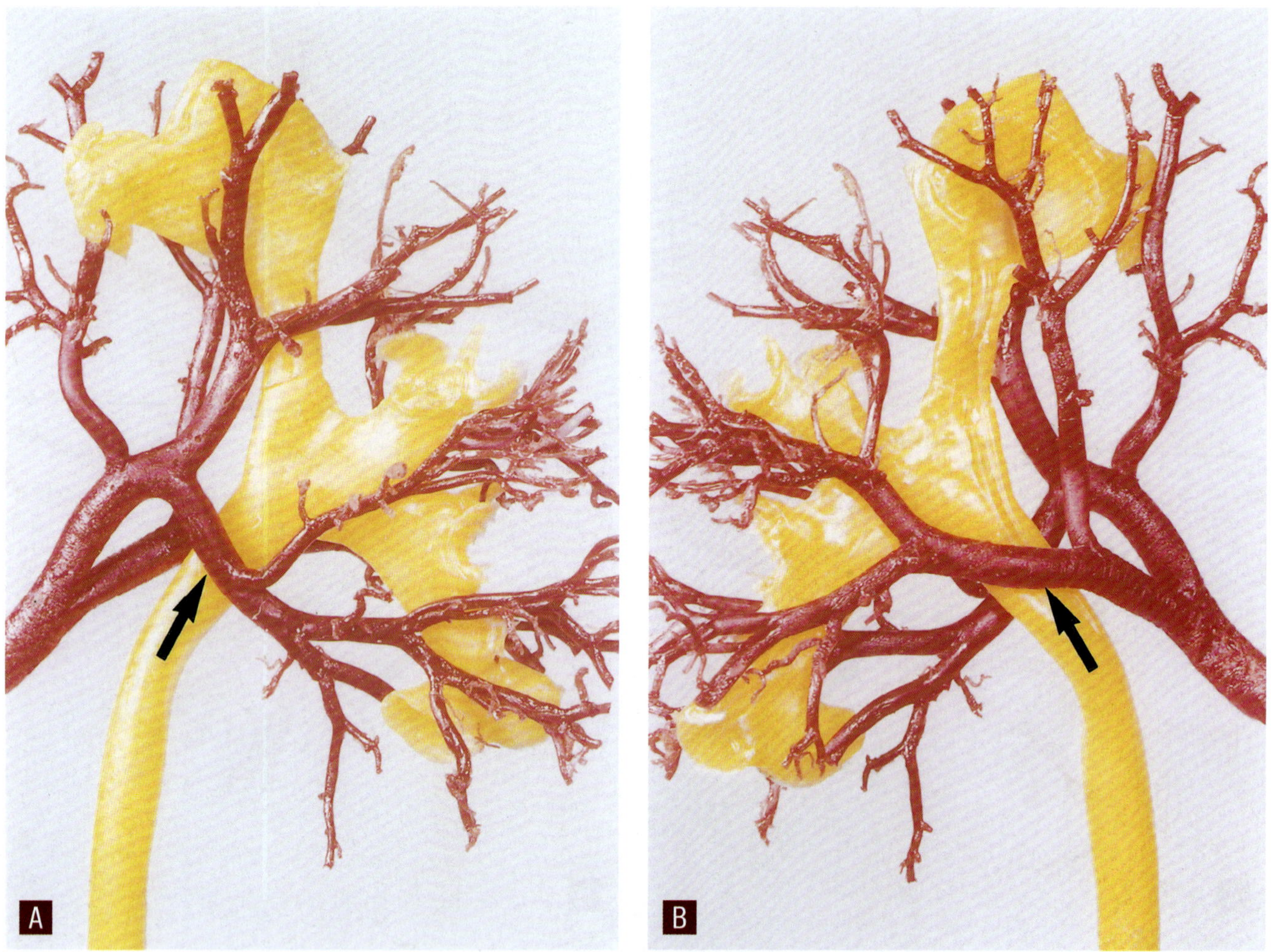

Figure 18.170. Anatomic relationships between ureteropelvic junction (UPJ) and renal arteries. A, Anterior view of an endocast from a left kidney shows a close relationship between an anterior segmental artery and the UPJ (arrow). B, Posterior view of the endocast shown in A reveals the UPJ in close relationship to a retropelvic artery (arrow).

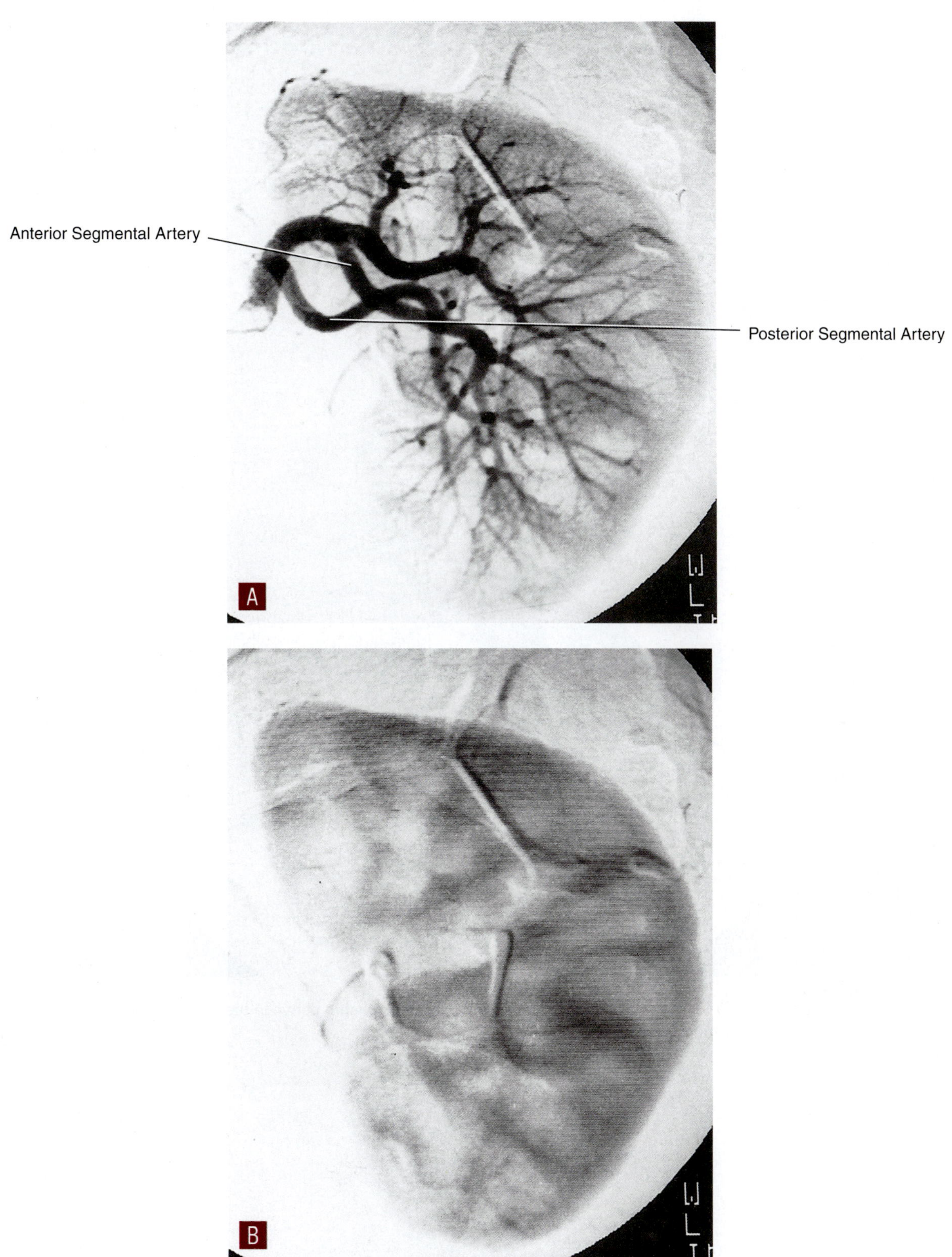

Figure 18.171. A, Left renal angiogram shows the relationship of the anterior segmental artery with the UPJ. B, Late nephrographic phase.

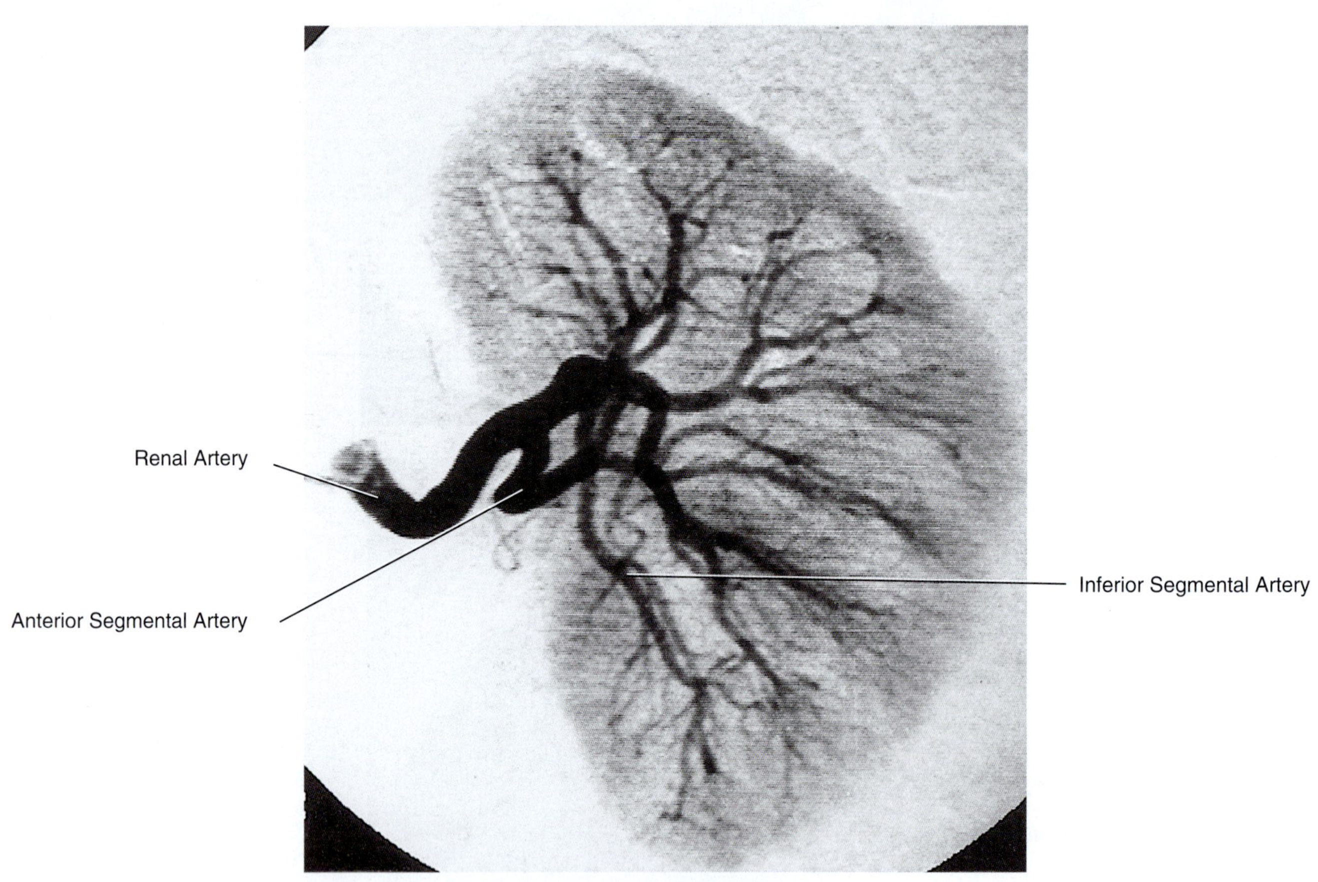

Figure 18.172. Left renal angiogram shows the relationship between the ureteropelvic junction and the renal arteries.

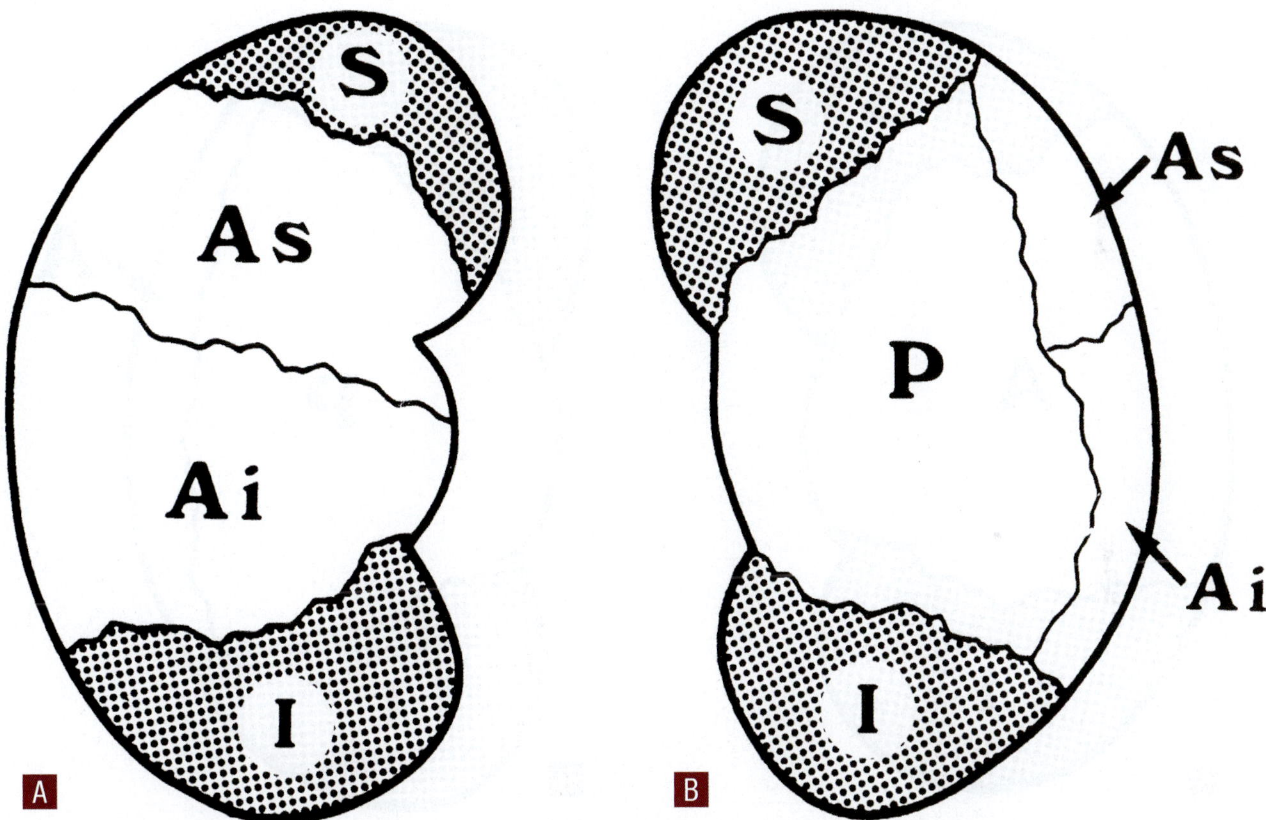

Figure 18.173. **Schematic drawing depicts the more frequent kind of renal arterial segments distribution (five segments).** A, Anterior view. B, Posterior view. S, superior segment; As, anterosuperior segment; Ai, anteroinferior segment; P, posterior segment.

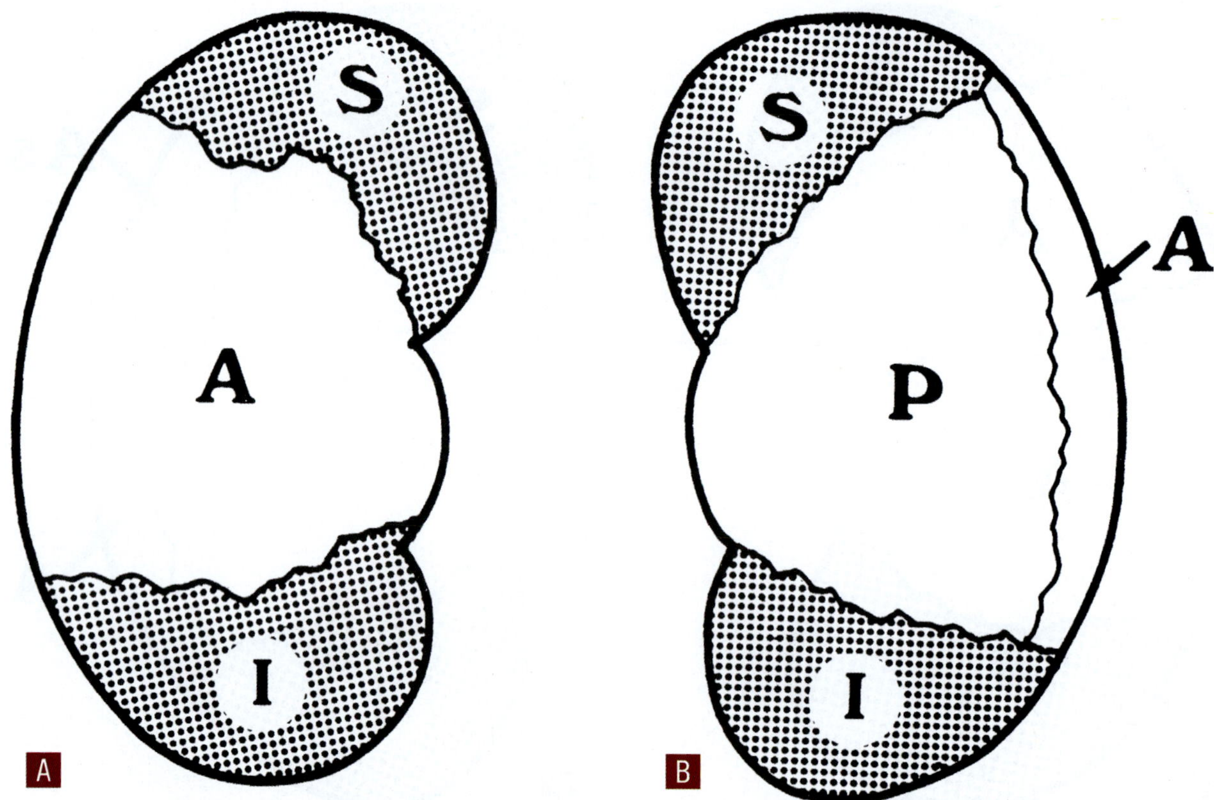

Figure 18.174. **Schematic drawing depicts a kidney with four arterial segments.** A, Anterior view. B, Posterior view. S, superior segment; A, anterior segment; I, inferior segment; P, posterior segment.

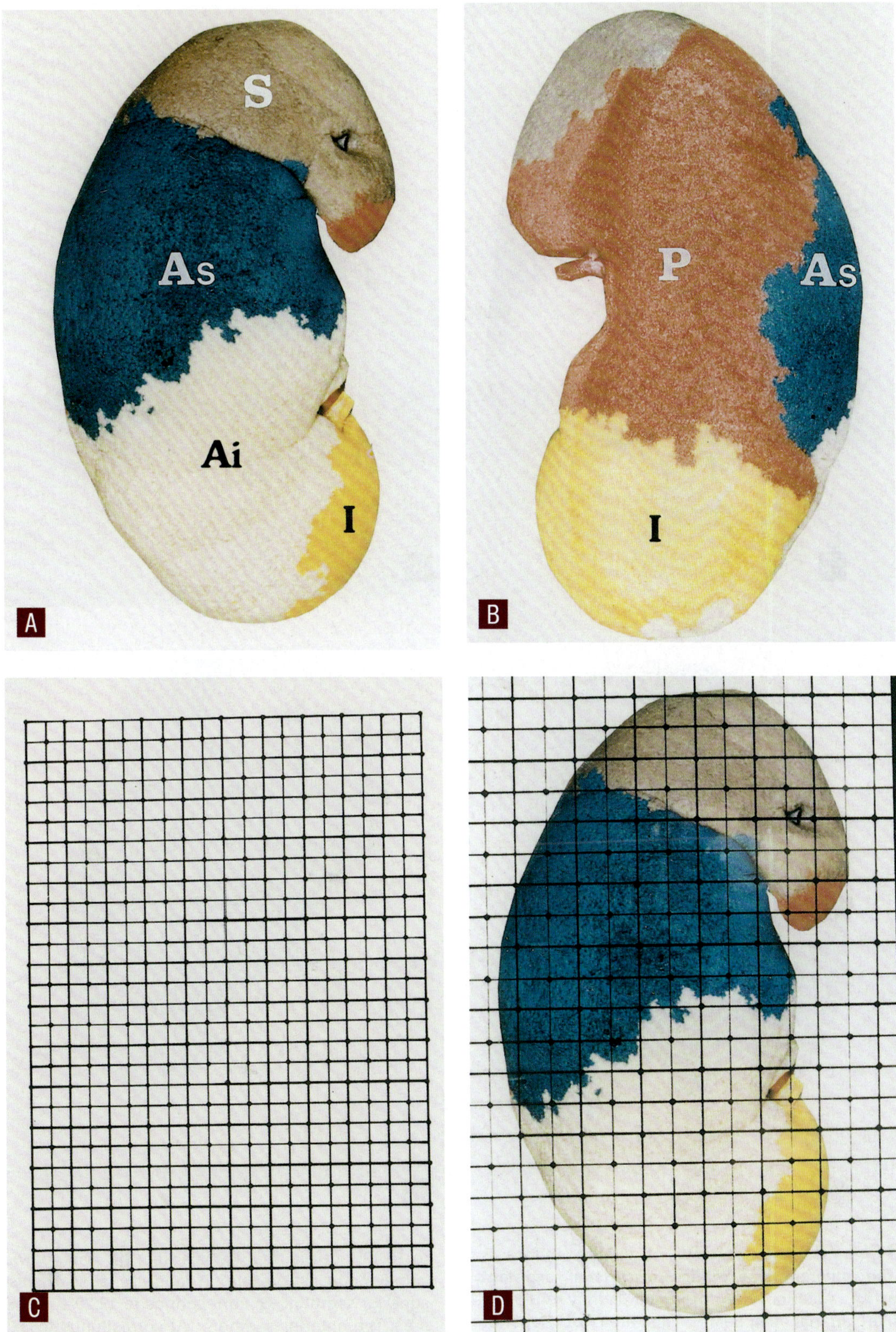

Figure 18.175. This figure shows an example of a polyester resin endocast obtained from a right kidney and illustrates the evaluation of the surface segmental area by using the "point-counting planimetry method." **A**, Anterior view of a right kidney endocast presenting five arterial segments that were injected with different colors. **B**, Posterior view of the same endocast shown in A. S, superior segment (brown); As, anterosuperior segment (blue); Ai, anteroinferior segment (white); I, inferior segment (yellow); P, posterior segment (red). **C**, The B-100 grid of planimetry used in the "point-counting method." **D**, The B-100 grid of planimetry placed over a photograph of the endocast shown in A depicts the evaluation of the surface segmental area by using the "point-counting method." (Reprinted from Sampaio FJB, Uflacker R, eds. *Renal Anatomy Applied to Urology, Endourology and Interventional Radiology.* New York: Thieme Medical Publishers; 1993 with permission.)

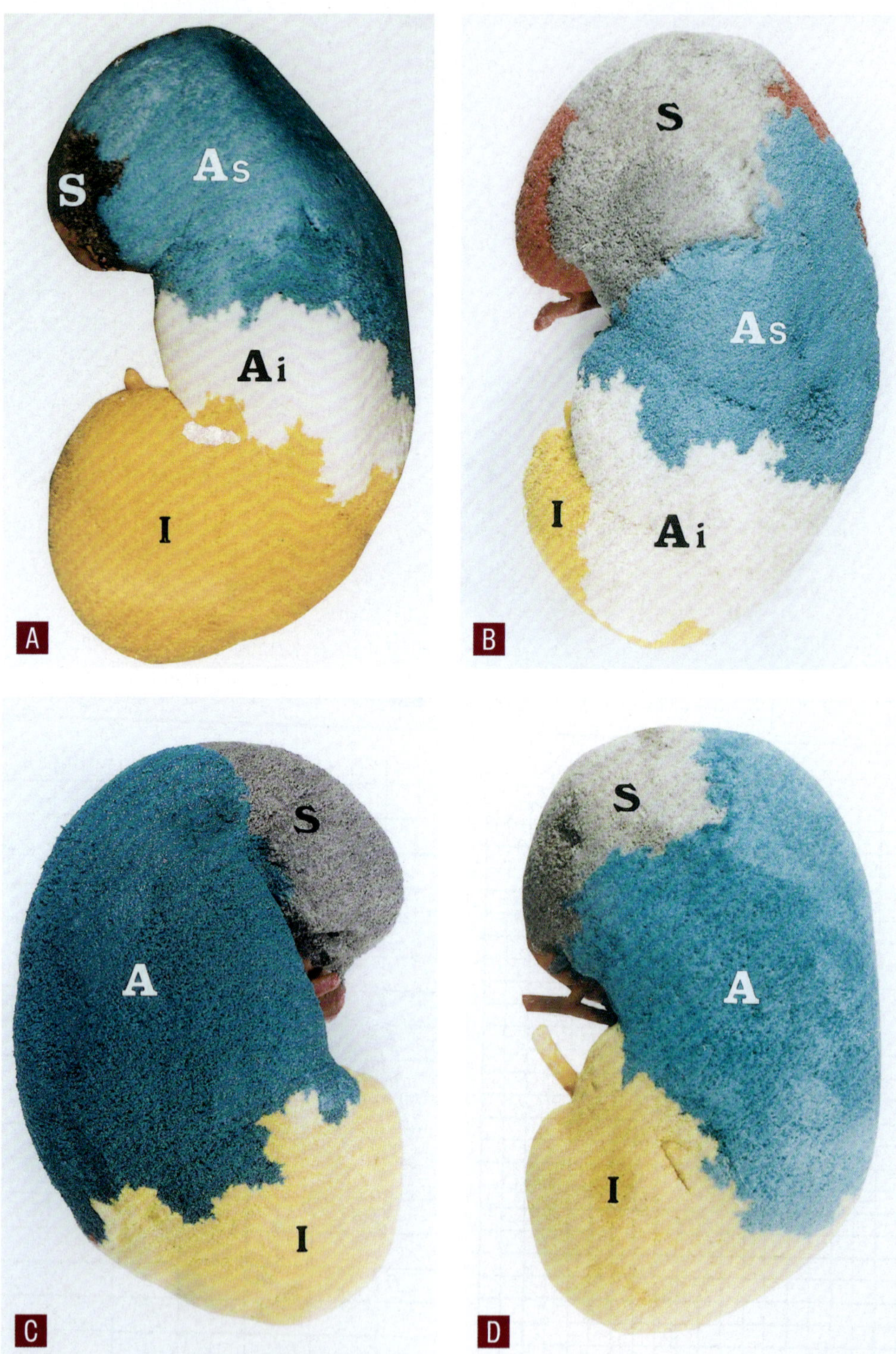

Figure 18.176. Anterior view of kidney endocasts exemplifies the different possibilities of arterial segment arrangements. **A**, Anterior view of a left kidney endocast presenting five arterial segments. The area of superior segment (S) corresponds to 1.84% of the total kidney area. The anterosuperior segment (As) corresponds to 28.16%, the anteroinferior segment (Ai) corresponds to 18.95%, and the inferior segment (I) corresponds to 30.0% of the total kidney area. **B**, Anterior view of a left kidney endocast presenting five segments. The area of the superior segment (S) corresponds to 16.59% of the total kidney area. The anterosuperior segment (As) corresponds to 19.75%, the anteroinferior segment (Ai) corresponds to 16.04%, the inferior segment (I) corresponds to 16.49% of the total kidney area. **C**, Anterior view of a right kidney endocast presenting four arterial segments. The area of superior segment (S) corresponds to 12.20% of the total kidney area. The anterior segment (A) corresponds to 37.28% and the inferior segment (I) corresponds to 23.21% of the total kidney area. **D**, Anterior view of a left kidney endocast presenting four arterial segments. The area of the superior segment (S) corresponds to 19.71% of the total kidney area. The anterior segment (A) corresponds to 34.90% and the inferior segment (I) corresponds to 27.39% of the total kidney area. (Reprinted from Sampaio FJB, Uflacker R, eds. *Renal Anatomy Applied to Urology, Endourology and Interventional Radiology.* New York: Thieme Medical Publishers; 1993 with permission.)

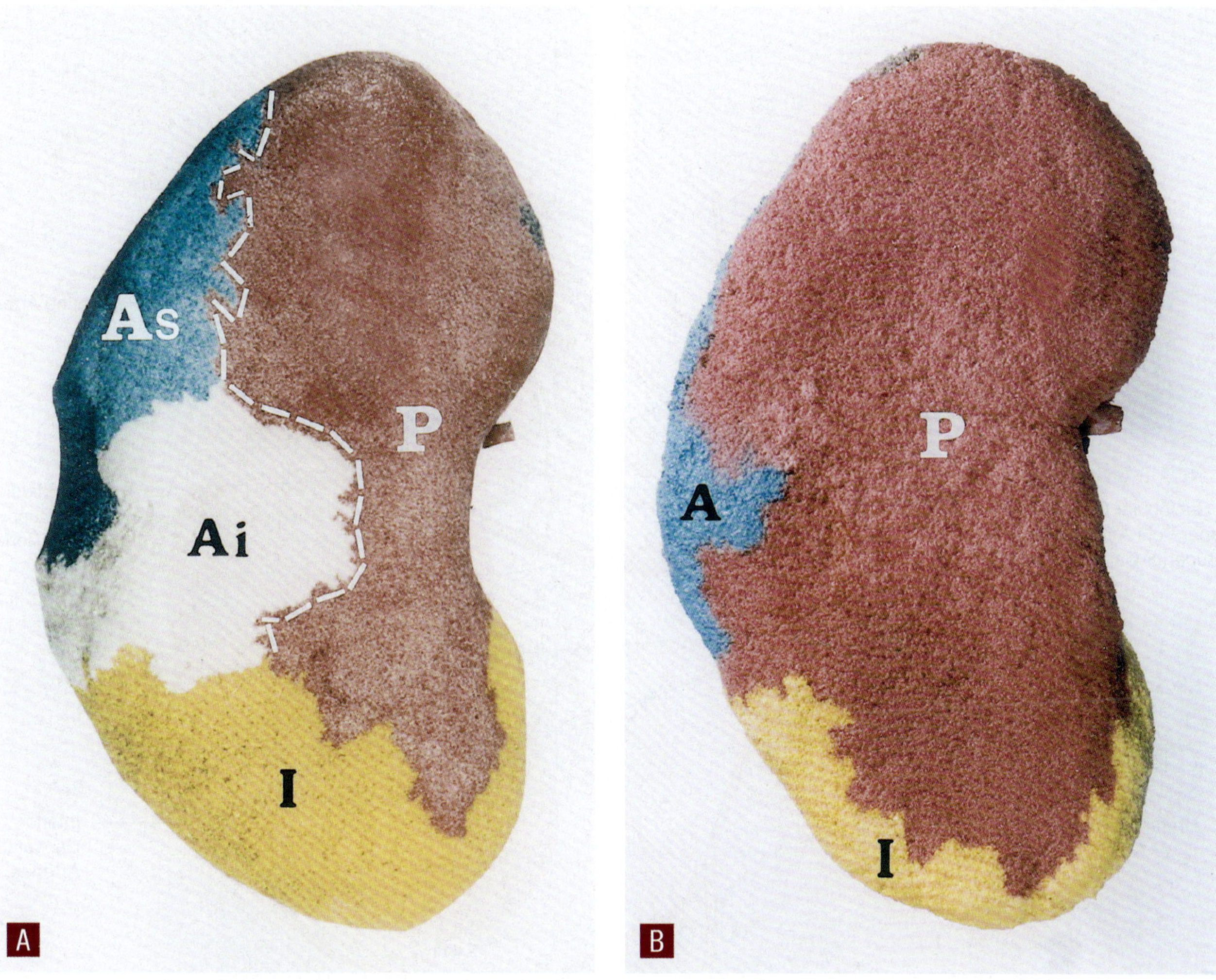

Figure 18.177. Posterior view of endocasts shows different types of posterior arterial segment arrangements. A, Posterior view of a left kidney endocast shows the limit between posterior (P) and anterior segments (Brodel' line) far from the lateral kidney margin (dashed white line). B, Posterior view of a left kidney endocast reveals a posterior segment (P) in red, corresponding to 49.36% of the total kidney area. In this case, the limit between posterior and anterior segments is located close to the lateral kidney margin. As, anterosuperior segment; Ai, anteroinferior segment; A, anterior segment; I, inferior segment. (Reprinted from Sampaio FJB, Uflacker R, eds. *Renal Anatomy Applied to Urology, Endourology and Interventional Radiology.* New York: Thieme Medical Publishers; 1993 with permission.)

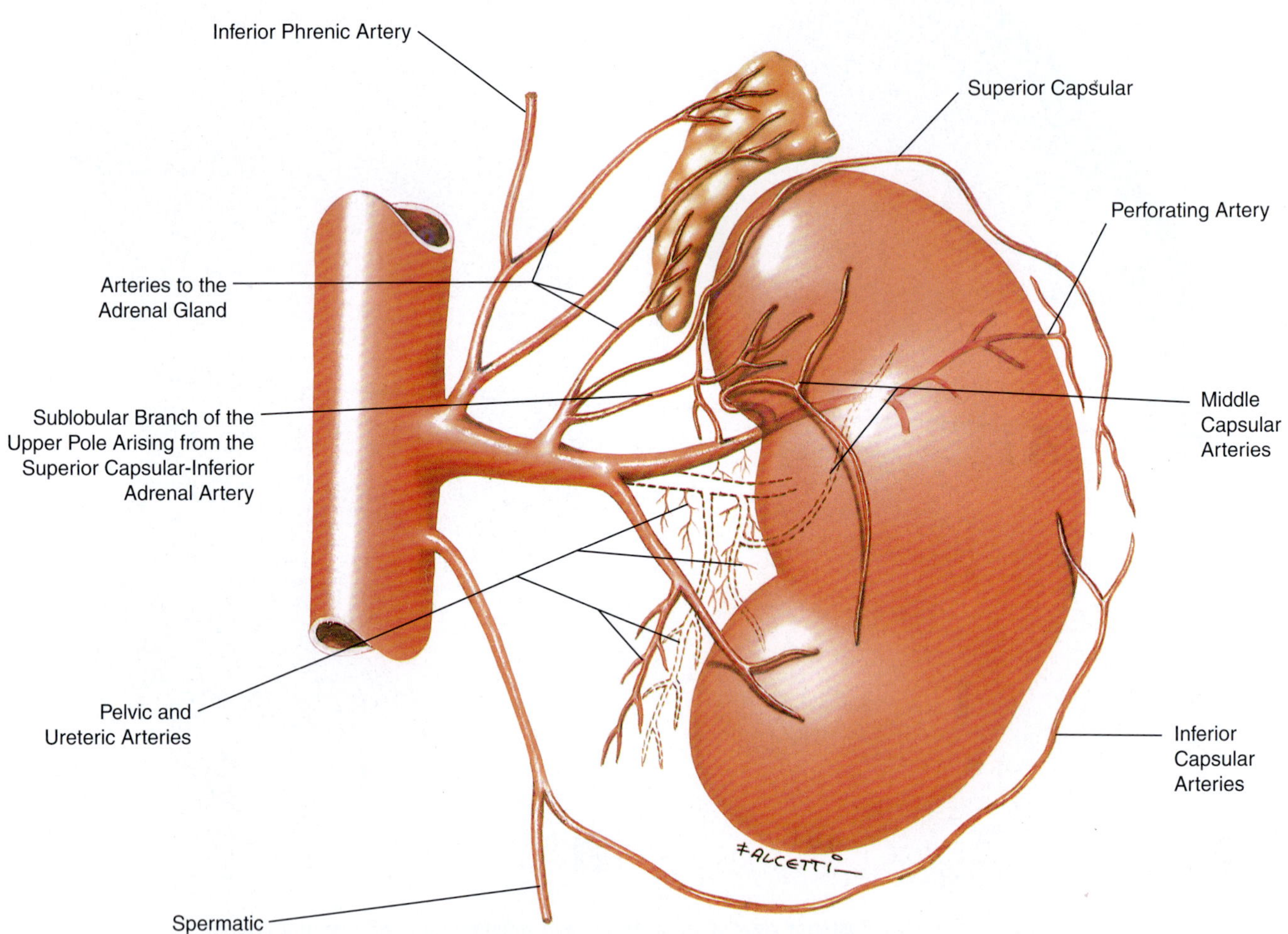

Figure 18.178. Schematic diagram showing the potential adrenal capsular and pelvic collateral arteries around and inside the kidney, most frequently observed in angiograms.

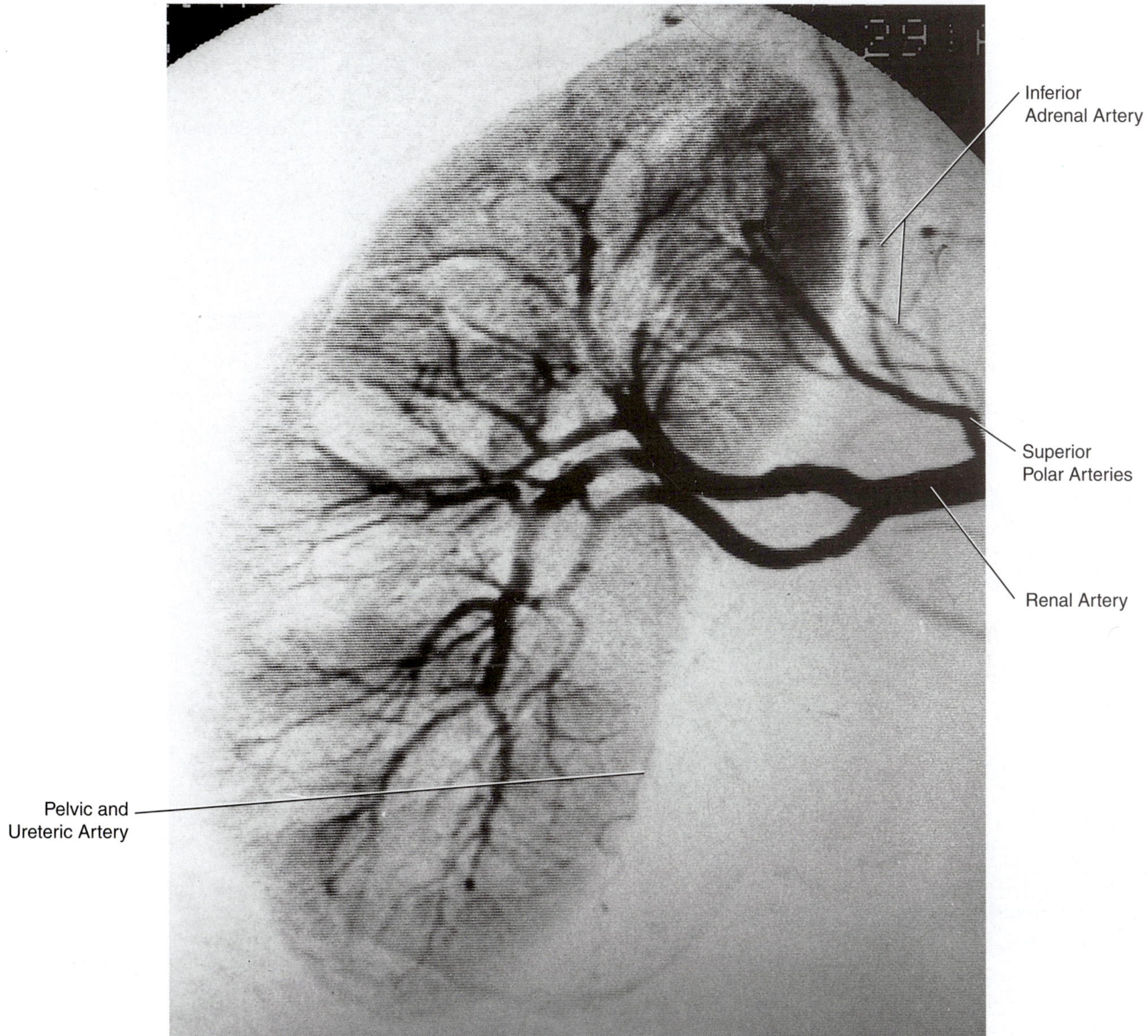

Figure 18.179. Right renal angiogram showing the inferior adrenal artery as the origin of the superior capsular arteries. Note the pelvic and ureteric artery.

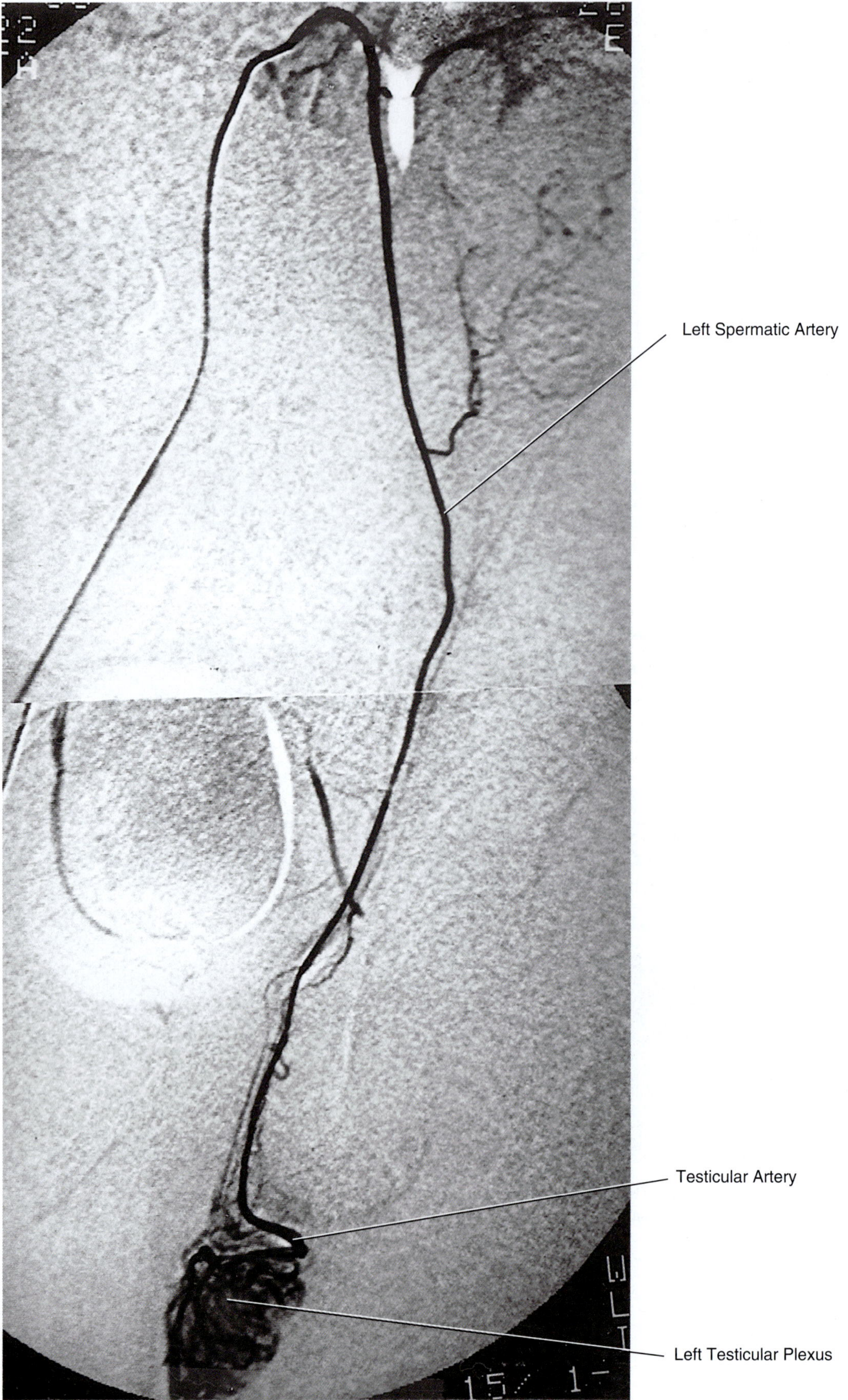

Figure 18.180. Selective angiogram of the left spermatic artery, arising from the abdominal aorta, and descending to the testis. Note the collaterals and the plexus at the testis.

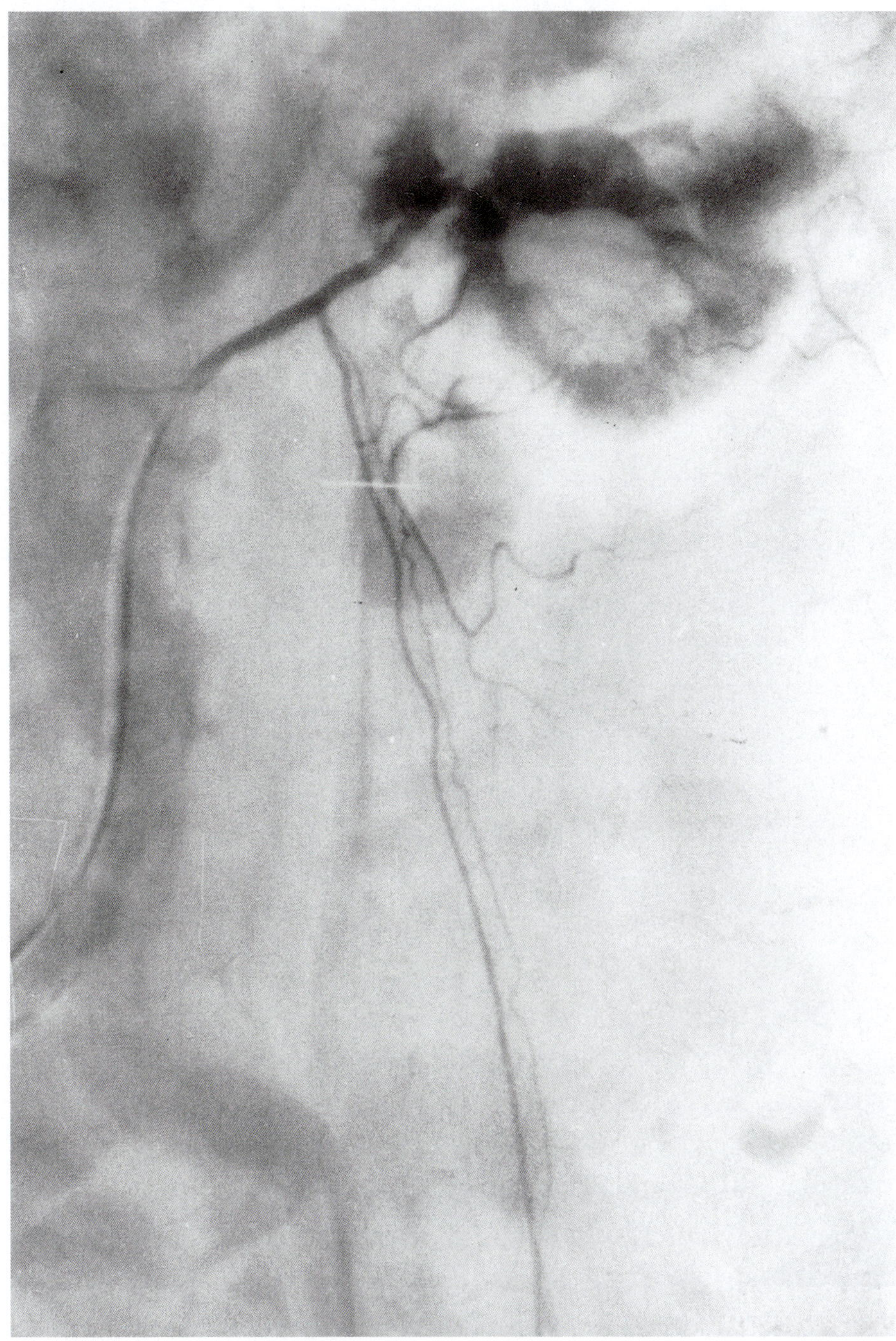

Figure 18.181. Selective angiogram of a lower polar artery of the kidney, giving origin to the left spermatic artery. Note the collaterals and anastomosis with the capsular arteries.

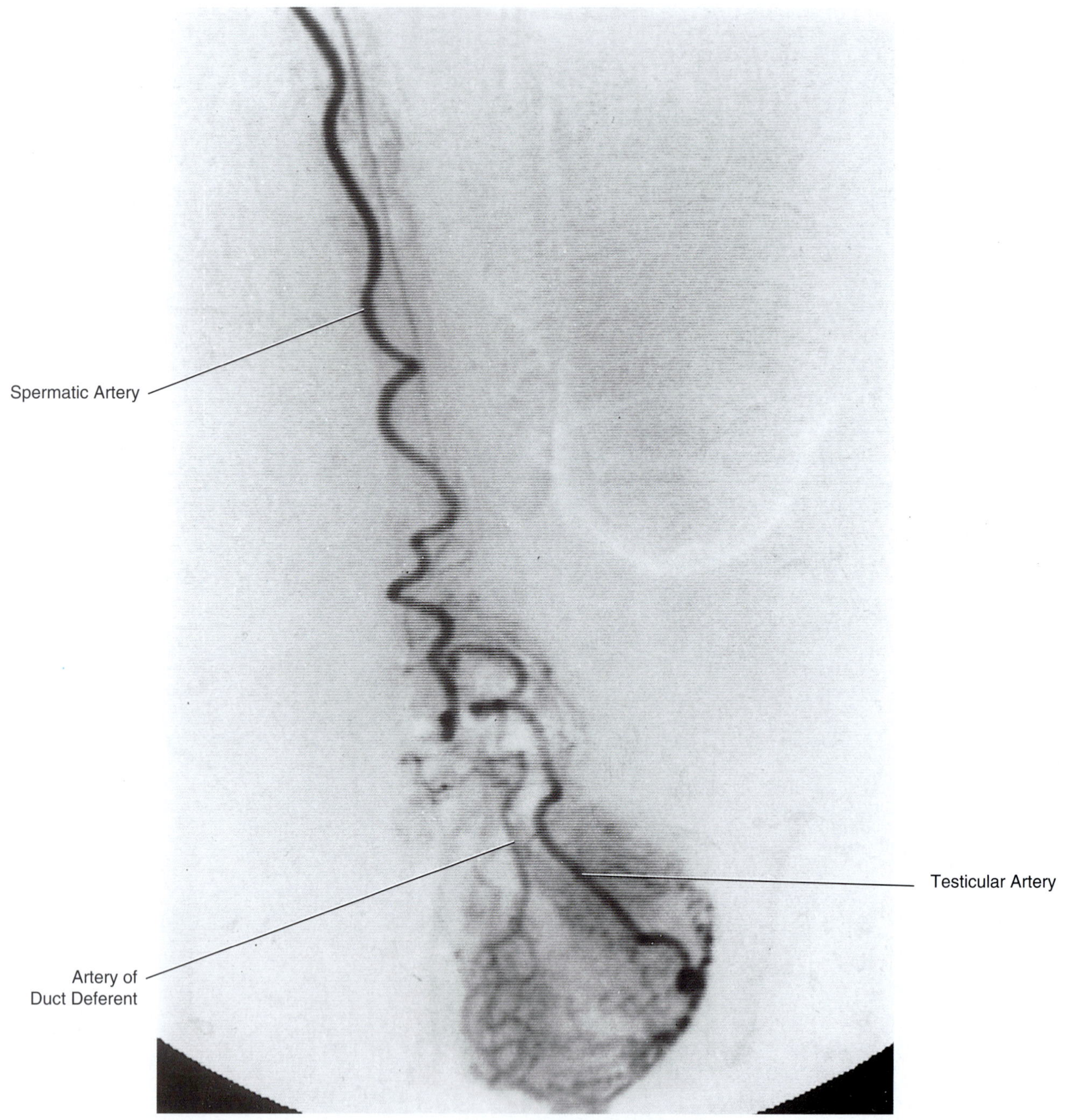

Figure 18.182. Close-up view of the left testis, showing the spermatic artery and the plexus at the testis.

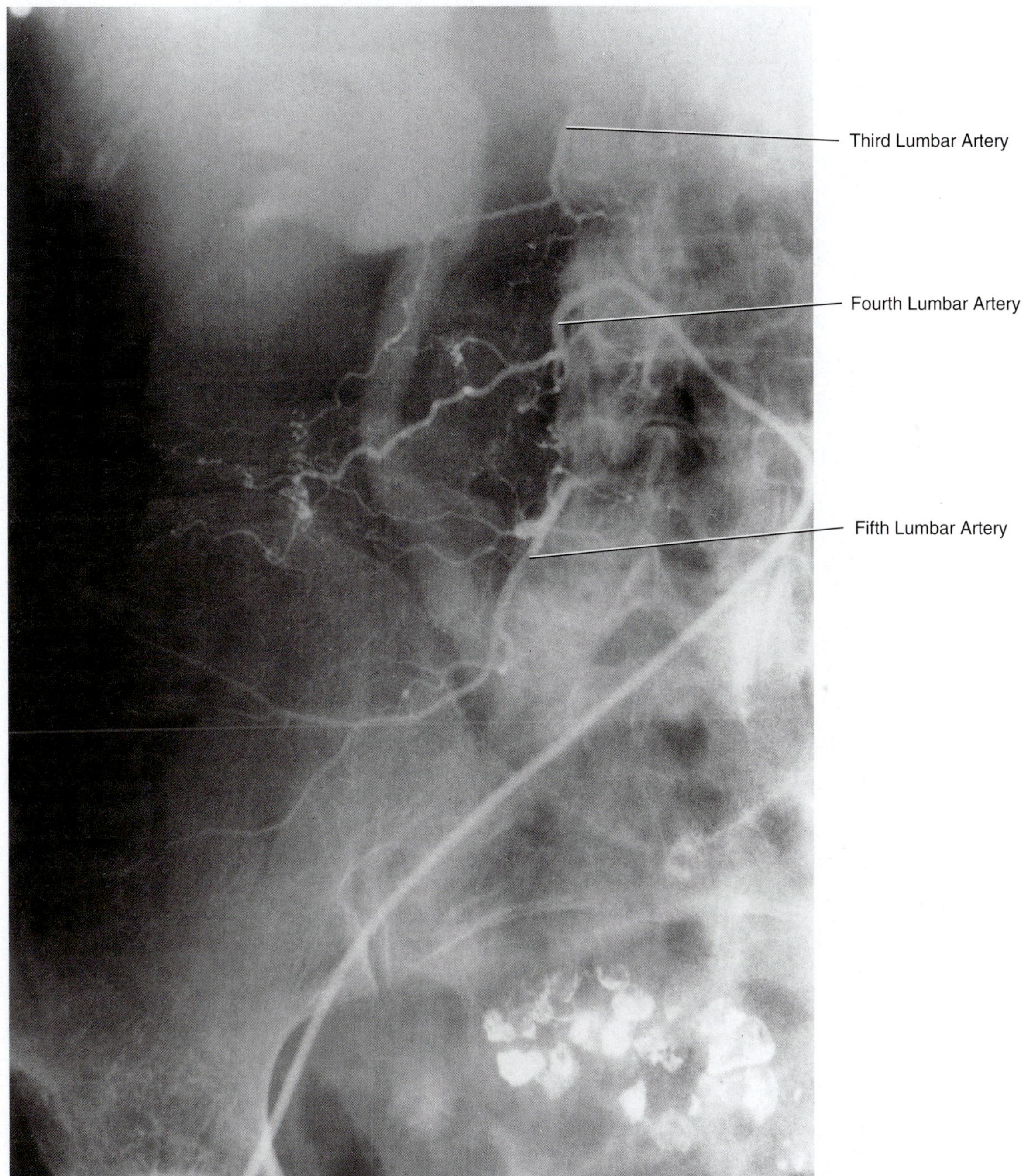

Figure 18.183. Selective angiogram of the fourth right lumbar artery. Note the anastomosis and retrograde filling of the third and fifth right lumbar arteries.

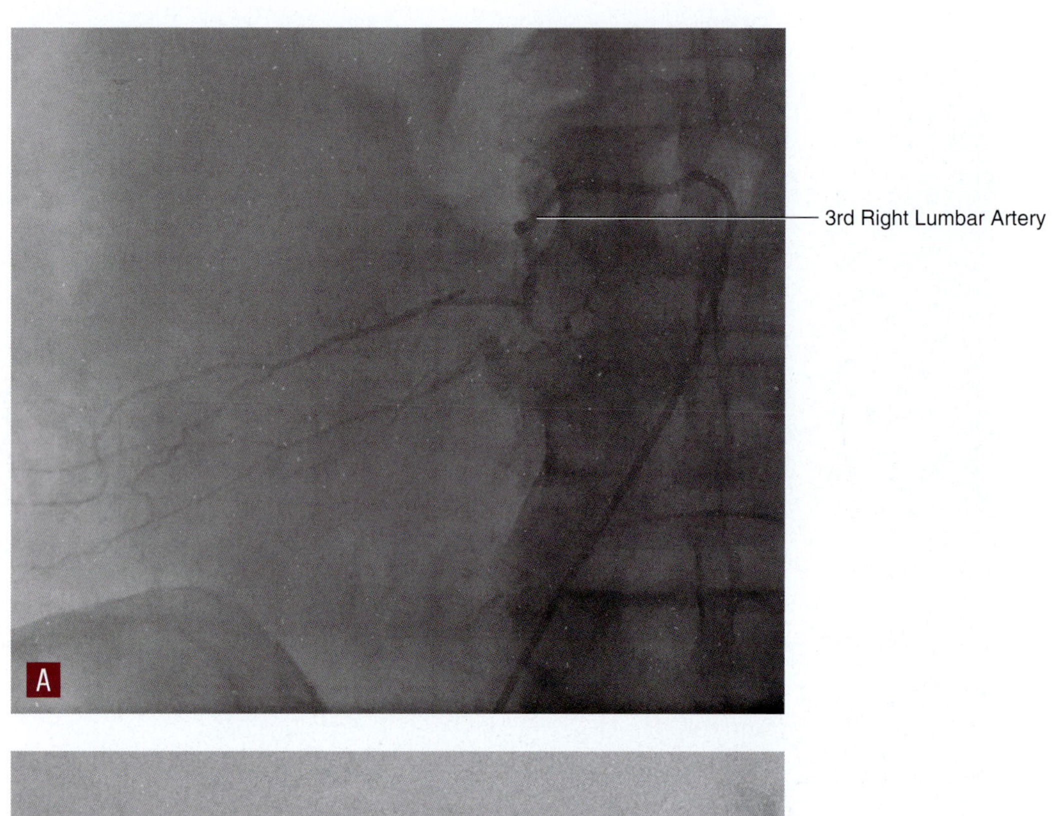

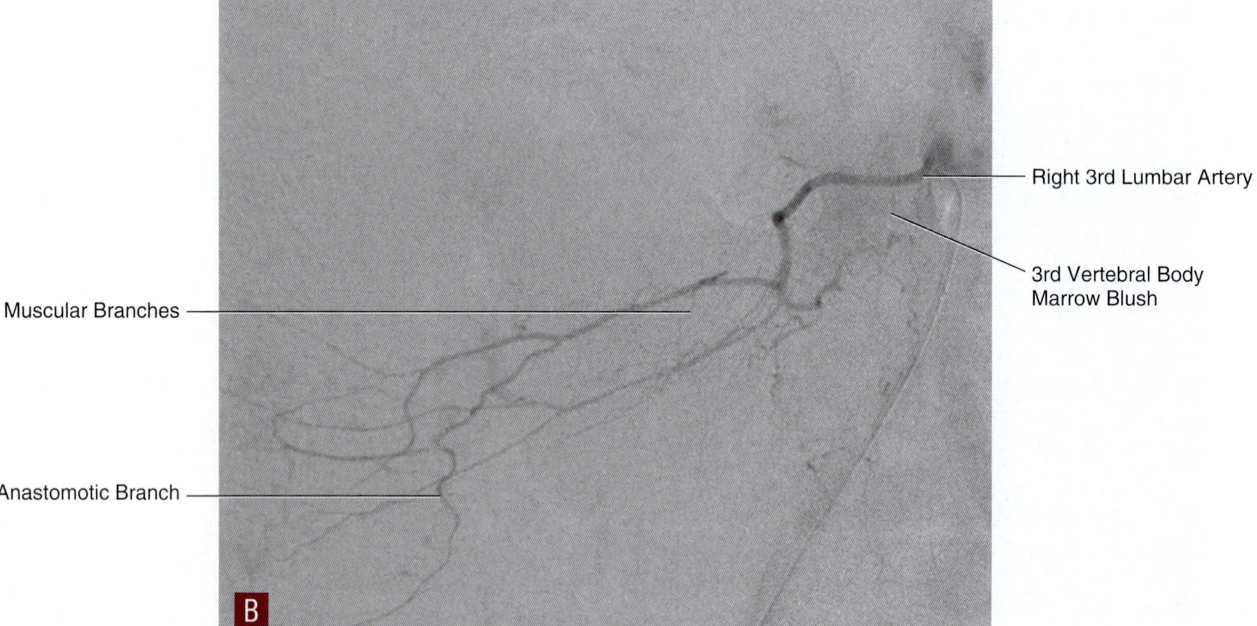

Figure 18.184. A and B, Selective angiogram of the third right lumbar artery and the muscular and vertebral branches with enhancement of the right side of the third vertebral body marrow cavity on the subtracted angiogram.

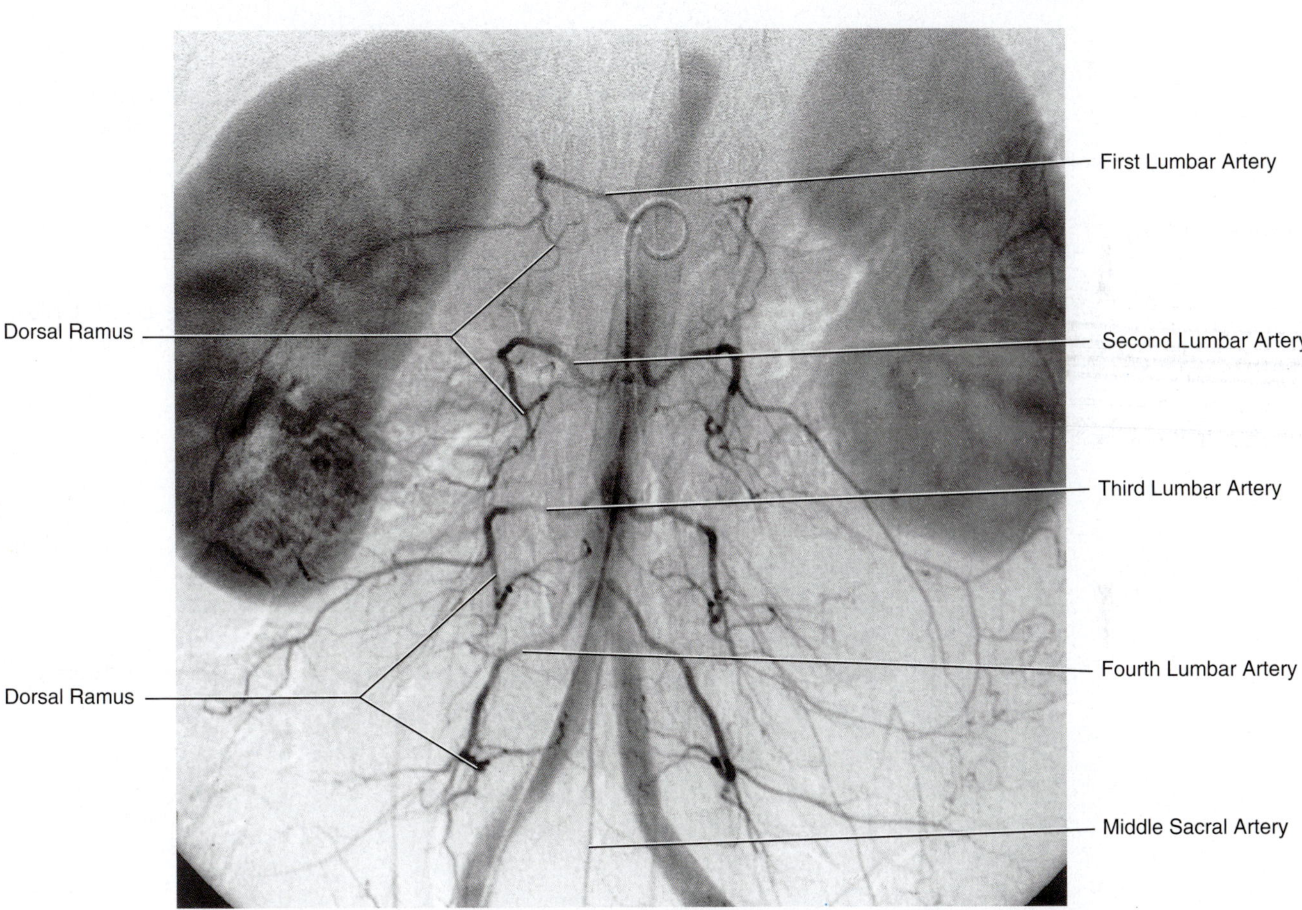

Figure 18.185. Late phase angiogram of the abdominal aorta, showing the lumbar arteries and normal branches.

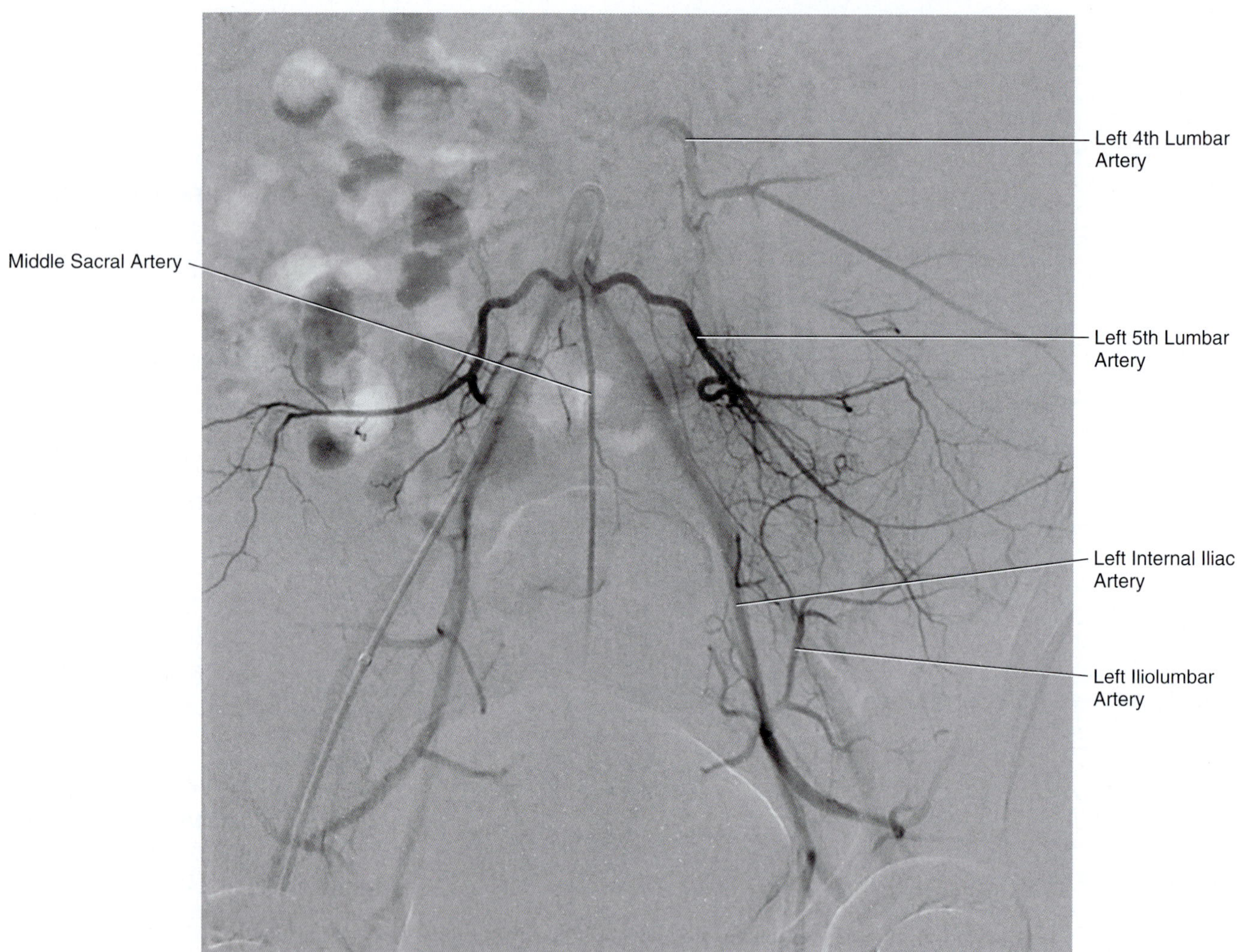

Figure 18.186. Selective angiogram of the common trunk of the fifth bilateral lumbar arteries. Note the anastomosis with the iliolumbar artery and with the fourth left lumbar artery.

19

Arteries of the Pelvis

Common Iliac Arteries

The right and left iliac arteries have been described as the terminal branches of the abdominal aorta (Fig. 19.1). The abdominal aorta bifurcates at the level of the fourth lumbar vertebra, into two large arteries, the right and left common iliac arteries, supplying the pelvis and the lower extremities. The right common iliac artery crosses to the right over the left common iliac vein, often causing compression of that vein with occlusion or severe stenosis. Compression of the left iliac vein may cause hypertension in the venous circulation of the left lower extremity and deep venous thrombosis, known as iliac compression syndrome, May-Thurner syndrome or Cockett syndrome. The anatomical abnormality is present in 15% to 20% of the population. The wall of the common iliac vein thickens and progressive occlusion develops. Adhesion of the iliac vein wall is observed in some cases causing obstruction (Fig. 19.2). The common iliac arteries usually do not have branches above the bifurcation into the external iliac artery and internal iliac artery. Occasional branches of the common iliac arteries are inferior renal polar arteries with an abnormal origin from the common iliac, usually in a situation of multiple renal arteries. Ectopic pelvic kidneys are rare, found in about 0.1% of the population, and single or multiple renal arteries may also originate from the iliac arteries, most commonly from the common iliac arteries. The common iliac artery may give small branches to the surrounding tissues, peritoneum, psoas muscle, ureter, and pelvic nerves. The common iliac arteries divide into the external iliac artery, which is normally in a straight line with the axis of the common iliac artery, and the internal iliac artery, which is a posteromedial branch.

Internal Iliac Arteries (Hypogastric Arteries)

The internal iliac arteries are typically 4 cm long, arising from the bifurcation of the common iliac arteries (Figs. 19.1-19.3). There are four distinct branching patterns of the internal iliac artery, according to Yamaki (Fig. 19.4A-D), termed group A through D. The group A branching pattern is the most common, consisting of 60% to 80% of pelvic halves, followed by group B, which is present in 15% to 30% of pelvic halves. Groups C and D are the least common, being present in 5% to 7% and less than 1% of pelvic halves, respectively. Group A consists of an anterior division that gives rise to the internal pudendal artery and the inferior gluteal artery, also called a gluteal-pudendal trunk (or anterior trunk), with the posterior division giving rise to the superior gluteal artery. Group B branching patterns have the internal pudendal artery being the major branch of the anterior division, with the posterior division giving rise to the superior and inferior gluteal arteries. When the internal iliac artery trifurcates into the internal pudendal, superior gluteal, and inferior gluteal arteries, the pattern is termed group C. The rarest pattern, group D, consists of an anterior division giving rise to the superior gluteal and internal pudendal arteries, and the posterior division consisting of the inferior gluteal artery.

The anterior division branches typically supply the bladder, the uterus, the rectum, and the vagina, and through the obturator artery supplies pelvic bone and muscles, inside and outside the pelvis, including the femoral head via the foveal artery via the ligamentum teres. The posterior division branches usually supply the bones, muscle, and nerves, including proximal lumbar and sacral nerves, which will form the sciatic nerve. Absence of the internal iliac artery is rarely observed.

In the fetus, the internal iliac artery is larger than the external iliac artery and is a direct continuation of the common iliac artery. As the superior vesical artery ascends on the anterior abdominal wall to the umbilicus, it converges with the contralateral superior vesical artery. After passing the umbilicus opening, the artery is named umbilical and enters the umbilical cord, coiling around the umbilical vein reaching the placenta. At birth, when the placental circulation ceases, the artery closes down and only the pelvic segment of the internal iliac artery remains, and the remainder turns into a fibrous cord termed the medial umbilical ligament.

Branches of the Internal Iliac Artery (Figs. 19.6 and 19.7)

Internal Pudendal Artery (Figs. 19.1, 19.7, 19.12, and 19.13)

The internal pudendal artery is the smaller branch of the anterior trunk of the internal iliac artery.

Supplies the external genitalia.

Branches

Inferior rectal artery (anastomoses with the contralateral inferior rectal artery and with the superior and middle rectal arteries)

- Perineal artery (Figs. 19.17 and 19.20)
  - Transverse branch
  - Scrotal arteries
  - Muscular branches
- Artery of the penis (Figs. 19.16-19.19)
  - Name of the internal pudendal artery beyond the perineal artery
- Artery to the bulb of the penis (Figs. 19.16-19.18)
  - Corpus spongiosum
  - Bulb urethral gland
- Urethral artery (Figs. 19.16-19.18)
  - Urethra and erectile tissue (corpus spongiosum)
- Deep penile artery (cavernosal artery) (Figs. 19.16 and 19.17)
  - One of the two terminal branches of the internal pudendal artery, the deep penile artery enters the crus penis and transverses the corpus cavernosum longitudinally, supplying the erectile tissue on each side
- Dorsal penile artery (Figs. 19.16-19.20)
  - The terminal branch of the internal pudendal artery, ascends between the crus of the penis and the pubis, running along the dorsum reaching the glans; anastomoses with the deep artery of the penis and supplies the skin and fascia of the penis
- Erectile tissue (Fig. 19.21)
  - The penis contains the corpus spongiosum, corpora cavernosa, and glans penis, made of erectile tissue. Erection results from parasympathetic stimulation via the pudendal nerves, with contraction of the smooth muscles enlarging the sinusoids and the intersinusoidal connections, with simultaneous closure of the venous outflow and increase of the arterial inflow
- Transverse root communication (Figs. 19.20 and 19.23)
  - There are constant anastomoses between the right and left arterial circulation through transverse root communication at the pubic area, either from branches of the obturator artery or from the internal pudendal

Accessory Pudendal Arteries (Fig. 19.22)

Accessory pudendal arteries have been defined as an artery in the periprostatic region, superior to the pelvic diaphragm, posterior to the pubic bone, which enters the penile hilum. The prevalence is not well known because of inconsistent definition, which varies among studies, and depending on the series, can range from 4% to 75% of men, with 20% to 30% being likely closer to the true prevalence. The origin is variable and has been observed to arise from the obturator, inferior vesical, superior vesical, or internal pudendal arteries. The term aberrant pudendal artery has been used to describe an accessory pudendal artery which is solely responsible for the arterial supply to the corpora cavernosa in a pelvic half and occurs in about 3% of men. Accessory pudendal arteries have been classified by Secin et al. as lateral or apical. Lateral accessory pudendal arteries course along the pelvic fascial tendinous arch, within the groove of the prostate, bladder, and pelvic wall. Apical accessory pudendal arteries course laterally and inferior to the puboprostatic ligament along the anterolateral surface of the prostatic apex before entering the dorsal vascular complex. Accessory pudendal arteries anastomose with the internal pudendal arteries, when present, in about 70% of cases, and can put a patient at risk of erectile dysfunction or penile ischemic injury during embolization if not recognized.

Inferior Gluteal Artery

Usually the largest terminal branch of the anterior trunk of the internal iliac artery, the inferior gluteal artery supplies the muscles of the buttock and thigh (Figs. 19.5 and 19.7). It passes the lower part of the greater sciatic foramen to reach the gluteal region. The inferior gluteal and internal pudendal arteries are often a common stem from the internal iliac, sometimes including the superior gluteal artery. It continues down the thigh with the sciatic and posterior femoral cutaneous nerves, supplying these nerves as well, and anastomoses distally with branches of the perforating arteries in the thigh. Internal iliac and inferior gluteal artery embolization may cause nerve ischemia and paralysis of segments of the lower extremity. The artery profunda femoris is also important blood supplier to the sciatic nerve, and embolization of this artery may cause nerve damage by ischemia.

Branches

- Inside the pelvis
  - Muscular (piriformis, coccygeus, and levator ani)
  - Perirectal fat
  - Vesical fundus, seminal vesicles, and prostate
- Outside the pelvis
- Muscular branches
  - Anastomoses with superior gluteal, internal pudendal, obturator, and medial circumflex femoral arteries
- Coccygeal branches
- Artery of the sciatic nerve
- Anastomotic branch
  - Join the cruciate anastomosis (perforating arteries)
- Articular branch
  - Cutaneous branch

Superior Gluteal Artery (Figs. 19.1, 19.4, and 19.7)

The superior gluteal artery is the largest branch of the internal iliac artery and, in most cases, the continuation of the posterior trunk. It leaves the pelvis through the greater sciatic foramen above the piriformis and dividing in superficial and deep branches.

Branches

- Superficial branch
  - Supplies the gluteus maximus; anastomoses with the inferior gluteal artery and posterior branches of the lateral sacral arteries
- Deep branch
  - Divides into superior and inferior rami. The superior ramus anastomoses with the deep circumflex iliac artery and the ascending branch of the lateral circumflex femoral artery. The inferior ramus anastomoses with the lateral circumflex femoral, inferior gluteal, and ascending branch of the medial circumflex femoral artery.

Superior Vesical Artery (Fetal Umbilical Artery)

- Supplies
  - Vesical fundus
  - Ductus deferens
  - Ureteral arteries

Inferior Vesical Artery (May Arise With the Middle Rectal Artery)

- Supplies
  - Vesical fundus
  - Prostate (prostatic branches communicate across the midline)
  - Seminal vesicle
  - Lower ureter
  - Ductus deferens

Middle Rectal Artery

The middle rectal artery is present in about one-third of patients, being typically unilateral and arising as a prostatorectal trunk in a majority of cases. The middle rectal artery anastomoses with the superior and inferior rectal arteries.

- Supplies
  - Lower rectum
  - Seminal vesicle
  - Prostate
  - Vesical walls

Prostatic Artery

The prostatic artery is typically described as a branch of the inferior vesical artery, although its origin is highly variable. Up to three prostatic arteries can be observed in a pelvic half. In up to a third of cases, the prostatic artery arises as a single branch directly from the internal pudendal artery as a prostatovesical trunk, which supplies the inferior aspect of the bladder. Other common origins of the prostatic artery include the anterior division of the internal iliac artery, where it usually arises as a common trunk with the superior vesical artery, or from the anterior division proper without an association with the superior vesical branch. Other origins include the obturator artery, the middle rectal artery, the inferior and superior gluteal arteries, and accessory pudendal arteries. The prostatic arterial supply is also rich in anastomotic connections to other pelvic branches, most commonly the internal pudendal arteries. Common connections also occur with ipsilateral and contralateral prostatic arteries, rectal arteries, vesical arteries, and accessory pudendal arteries. Table 19.1 shows the origins of the prostatic artery and types of anastomosis as well as the incidence of these findings from a study of 214 pelvic halves by Bilhim et al. Table 19.2 provides a suggested anatomical classification according to de Assis et al.

The prostatic artery can provide branches to the ductus deferens and seminal vesicles. When a branch is identified supplying seminal vesicles and ductus deferens is encountered, it is termed a vesiculodeferential artery. When more than one prostatic artery is present, the branches supply either the central gland or the periphery. An artery supplying the central gland can be termed the anterolateral prostatic artery, and an artery supplying the peripheral gland, the posterolateral prostatic artery.

Uterine Artery (Figs. 19.9 and 19.11)

The uterine artery is a branch from the anterior division of the internal iliac artery. The artery penetrates the anterior or posterior wall of the uterus itself. At the level of the internal os, the arteries course at right angles to the long axis of the uterus. Below the internal os, the arteries are inclined downwards: above this level, the inclination is upwards. The terminal branch of the uterine artery is the intramural branch, also described as the arcuate artery. The arcuate arteries lie between the outer and the middle third of the uterine wall, either anterior or posterior. The arcuate arteries terminate in medial peripheral and radial branches. Free anastomoses between the arcuate arteries on either side of the uterus can be seen. The blood supply of the tube and the ovary is derived from both the uterine and the ovarian arteries. In general, the uterine supplies the medial half of the ovary and the medial two-thirds of the tube, whereas the rest of the blood supply arises from the ovarian artery. The ovarian artery alone may supply the entire tube and the ovary.

The uterine artery crosses above the ureter and there is a ureteric branch. It anastomoses with the vaginal arteries, forming the azygos artery of the vagina. The cervicovaginal branch arises directly from the uterine artery in 91% of cases, whereas in 9% of its origin is directly from the internal iliac artery (Figs. 19.11-19.14). The origin of the uterine artery is extremely variable, but four different patterns were identified. Type I is defined as the uterine artery arising as the first branch of the inferior gluteal artery (45%). Type II is defined as the uterine artery arising as the second or third branch of the inferior gluteal artery (6%). Type III is a true trifurcation, where the origins of the superior gluteal, inferior gluteal, and uterine arteries are at the same level (43%). In type IV, the uterine artery origin is proximal to the bifurcation of the anterior and posterior division (6%). Rarely, one may encounter an artery of the round ligament as the predominant supply to the uterine half in question (Fig. 19.15C). The artery of the round ligament is normally diminutive and arises from the inferior epigastric artery.

Uterine artery supplies
- Ureter
- Vagina
- Uterus
- Broad ligament of uterus
- Round ligament of uterus
- Uterine tube and part of the ovary
- The tortuous terminal branches in the uterus are called helicine arteries.

Ovarian Artery

Knowledge of the ovarian artery anatomy is important for the success of certain procedures of embolization on pelvic organs such in uterine fibroids. An important implication of the ovarian artery-to-uterine artery communications is the possibility of ovarian failure and premature menopause after uterine artery embolization. There are three main patterns of anastomoses between the ovarian artery and the uterine artery following a physiologic point of view. Type Ia—The ovarian artery is the major source of blood supply to the fibroid in the uterus by means of anastomosis with the intramural uterine artery. In this case, the flow in the tubal artery is toward the uterus, without evidence of retrograde reflux in the direction of the ovary (13.2%). Type Ib—The ovarian artery supplies the fibroid in the uterus in a similar manner as that of type Ia. Flow in the tubal artery was toward the uterus; however, reflux into the ovarian artery is seen on the preembolization-selective uterine artery angiogram (8.6%). Type II—The ovarian artery supplies the fibroids directly. Some anastomoses to the intramural uterine artery may exist; the flow to the fibroid is independent from the uterine artery (3.9%). Type III—Flow in the tubal artery is toward the ovary on selective uterine angiograms with washout of contrast toward the ovary (6.6%). The three types of uterine-ovarian anastomoses are shown in Fig. 19.10.

Vaginal Artery

The vaginal artery may be two or three arteries and corresponds to the inferior vesical artery in males.

Supplies
- Vagina
- Vesical fundus
- Rectum

Obturator Artery

This artery leaves the pelvis through the obturator canal and has an anterior and a posterior branch (Figs. 19.1, 19.7, 19.12, and 19.23C).

Branches

- Inside the pelvis
  - Iliac branches
  - Vesical branch
  - Pubic branch
- Outside the pelvis
  - Anterior and posterior branches encircle the foramen
  - Anterior branches supply various muscles and anastomoses with the medial circumflex femoral artery
  - Posterior branches supply various muscles and anastomoses with the inferior gluteal artery; give an acetabular branch that supplies the acetabular fossa and the femoral head through the ligament teres (foveal artery)

A pubic branch of the inferior epigastric artery may replace the obturator artery. It may be a branch either of the anterior or posterior trunks of the internal iliac artery and may be a branch of the superior or inferior gluteal artery. When present, this variant is termed the aberrant obturator artery, also known as the "corona mortis."

Iliolumbar Artery (Figs. 19.1 and 19.26)

This artery ascends laterally anterior to the sacroiliac joint and lumbosacral trunk, posterior to the obturator nerve and external iliac vessels, dividing into the lumbar and iliac branches.

Branches

- Lumbar branch (psoas and quadratus lumborum)
  - Anastomoses with the fourth lumbar artery and sends a small spinal branch to the cauda equina between the fifth lumbar and first sacral vertebrae. The ventral rami of the L5, S1, and S2 from the sacral and coccygeal plexus have supply from the iliolumbar artery. Embolization of this artery can cause paresthesia and paralysis of the lower extremity.
- Iliac branch (iliac bone through a nutrient branch)
  - Anastomoses with the superior gluteal, circumflex iliac, and lateral circumflex femoral arteries

Lateral Sacral Arteries (Figs. 19.1, 19.12, and 19.27)

Branches

Superior lateral sacral branch (first and second sacral foramen) supplies the sacral vertebrae, sacral canal, and the skin and muscles dorsal to the sacrum

- Inferior lateral sacral branch
  - Anastomoses with the median sacral artery, anterior to the coccyx and enters the sacral canal through the anterior sacral foramina

Persistent Sciatic Artery (Figs. 19.28-19.30)

Persistent sciatic artery is a rare embryologic anomaly, seen in approximately 0.05% of individuals, affecting both sexes equally. The sciatic artery is the axial artery of the lower extremity, providing blood supply during the early stages of embryonic development. It normally regresses to form the proximal part of the inferior gluteal artery after the third month of embryologic life after the development of the femoral artery from the external iliac artery. If the femoral system fails to develop, the sciatic artery becomes the dominant supply to the leg and the superficial femoral artery remains hypoplastic. Conversely, failure of complete involution of the sciatic artery may result in a hypoplastic sciatic artery with a normal femoral system. Aneurysm formation in the persistent sciatic artery occurs in as many as 46% of cases and may be the first evidence of the presence of the anomaly, causing buttock pain and sometimes sciatic nerve compression with sciatic pain in the affected leg. The sciatic vein usually follows the same path of the artery but is less perceptible on imaging.

External Iliac Arteries (Figs. 19.1, 19.3, and 19.8)

These arteries are the natural continuation of the common iliac artery. Larger than the internal iliac arteries, they descend laterally along the medial border of the psoas major, entering the thigh posteriorly to the inguinal ligament, becoming the femoral artery.

Branches

Inferior Epigastric Artery (Figs. 19.1 and 19.3)

The inferior epigastric artery arises medially from the distal external iliac artery just above the inguinal ligament, ascending behind the rectus abdominis muscle. It anastomoses with the superior epigastric and lower posterior intercostal arteries. The branching pattern of the inferior epigastric artery has been classified into three distinct types (types 1 to 3) based on the number of branching trunks from which perforating branches arise (up to three).

Branches

Cremasteric artery
Pubic branch
Muscular branches
Cutaneous branches

Deep Circumflex Iliac Artery (Fig. 19.1)

This artery arises laterally from the external iliac artery, opposite of the inferior epigastric artery. It anastomoses with the ascending branch of the lateral circumflex femoral artery and the iliolumbar and superior gluteal arteries and has a large ascending branch.

Collateral Pathways (Fig. 19.31)

There are large number of potential pathways of collateral circulation, connecting the abdominal aorta and thoracic aorta with the pelvic arteries that may be developed in the case of aortoiliac femoral occlusive disease. The potential collateral circulation connectors are the superior epigastric (Fig. 19.32), intercostal, subcostal, lumbar, middle sacral, common iliac, external iliac, iliolumbar, superior gluteal, lateral sacral, obturator, internal pudendal, external pudendal, deep iliac circumflex, superficial iliac circumflex, medial femoral circumflex, lateral femoral circumflex, lateral ascending branch, lateral descending branch, profunda femoris, superficial femoral, and inferior epigastric arteries (Figs. 19.33 and 19.34).

It is important to be aware of the terminology employed in discussing collateral circulation. An affluent vessel is a collateral branch that arises from a patent main vessel above the obstruction or from a patent contralateral mate. An effluent vessel is a branch below the obstruction that receives blood from the affluent vessel and allows it to flow retrogradely to reconstitute the occluded artery.

The affluent vessel may pass blood into the effluent vessel as a continuous line in a phenomenon called inosculation or may be connected to the effluent vessel by a network of fine vessels forming what is called retiform anastomosis. Inosculation usually maintains adequate flow with a heavy pressure head through the anastomosis, leading to refilling of the main vessels distal to the occlusion. Retiform anastomosis allows passage of blood with decrease inflow and pressure. An example of retiform anastomosis is the communication between the lumbar and iliolumbar arteries or the Winslow's pathway (ie, from the intercostal and internal mammary arteries to the external iliac arteries via the epigastric arteries) (Figs. 19.1 and 19.32). An example of inosculation would be between the lateral ascending branch of the arteria profunda femoris and lateral branches of the superior gluteal artery (Figs. 19.33 and 19.34).

TABLE **19.1.** **Origins of the Prostatic Artery and Anastomoses**

Origin	Incidence (%)
Internal pudendal artery	34.1
Common trunk with superior vesical artery	20.1
Anterior division (gluteopudendal trunk)	17.8
Obturator artery	12.6
Middle rectal artery (prostatorectal trunk)	8.4
Inferior gluteal artery	3.7
Accessory pudendal artery	1.9
Superior gluteal artery	1.4
Anastomoses*	
Internal pudendal artery	43.3
Lateral accessory pudendal artery	20
Contralateral prostatic artery	17.6
Rectal arteries	14.4
Ipsilateral prostatic artery	13.4
Vesical arteries	11.3

*Percentages for anastomoses are not cumulative

TABLE **19.2.** **Angiographic Classification of the Prostatic Artery (de Assis)**

	Description	Incidence (%)
Type I	Prostatovesical trunk arising as a common trunk with the superior vesical artery	28.7
Type II	Prostatovesical trunk arising from the anterior division	14.7
Type III	Prostatovesical trunk arising from the obturator artery	18.9
Type IV	Prostatovesical trunk arising from the inferior vesical artery	31.1
Type V	Other origins	5.6

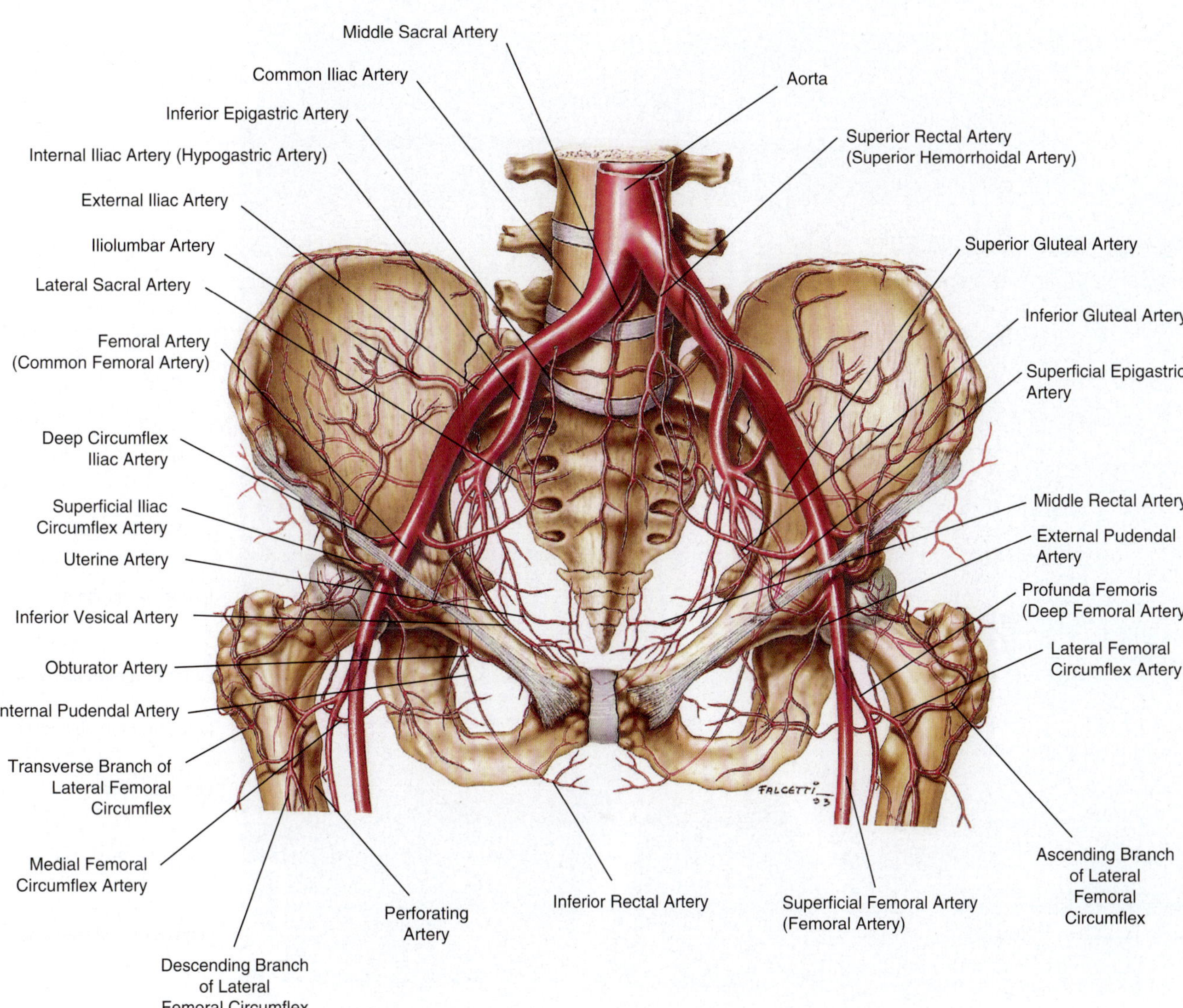

Figure 19.1. Schematic diagram of the pelvic circulation.

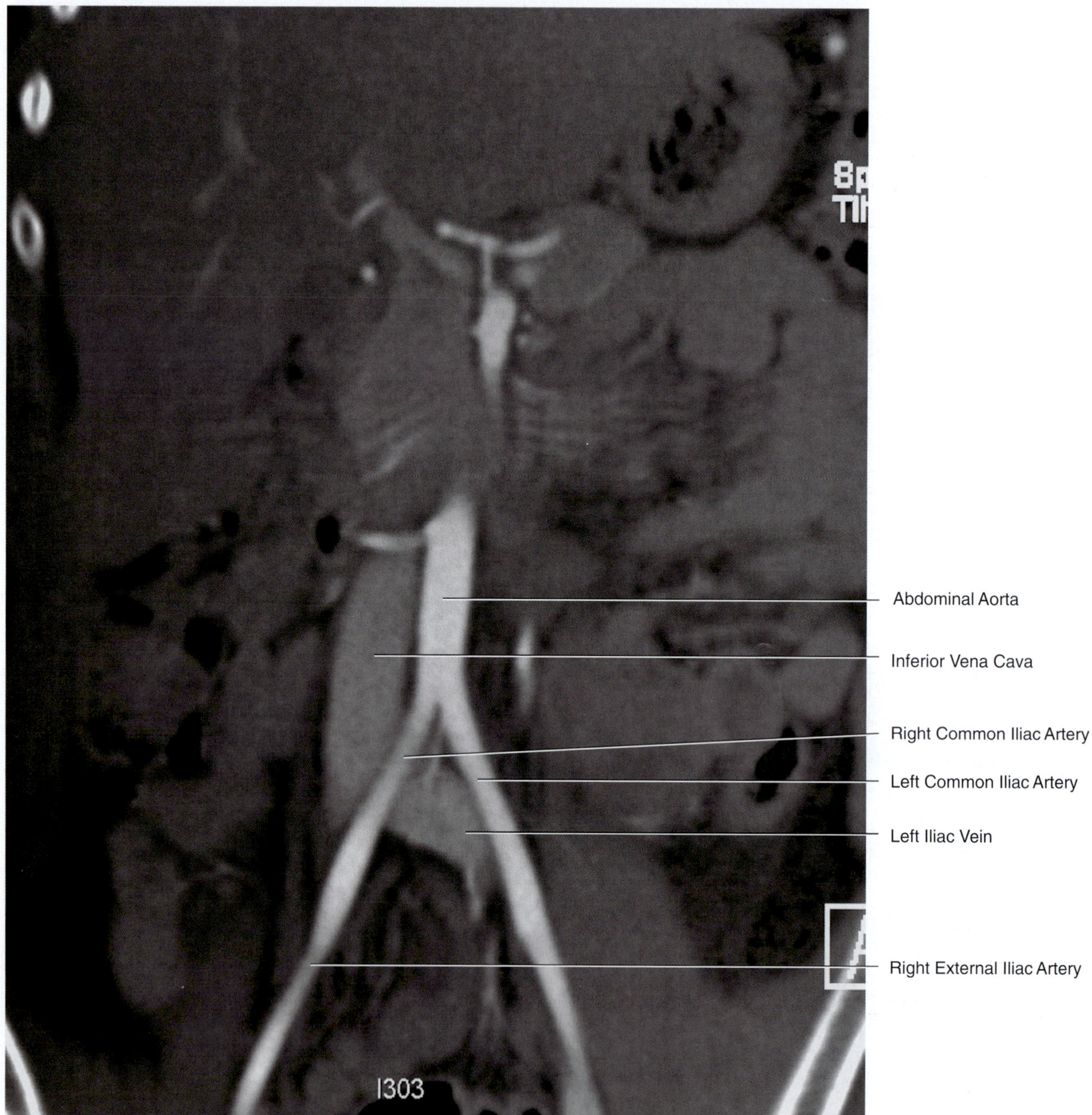

Figure 19.2. Pelvic computerized tomographic angiography (CTA) showing the relationship between the right common iliac artery crossing over the left common iliac vein, causing compression.

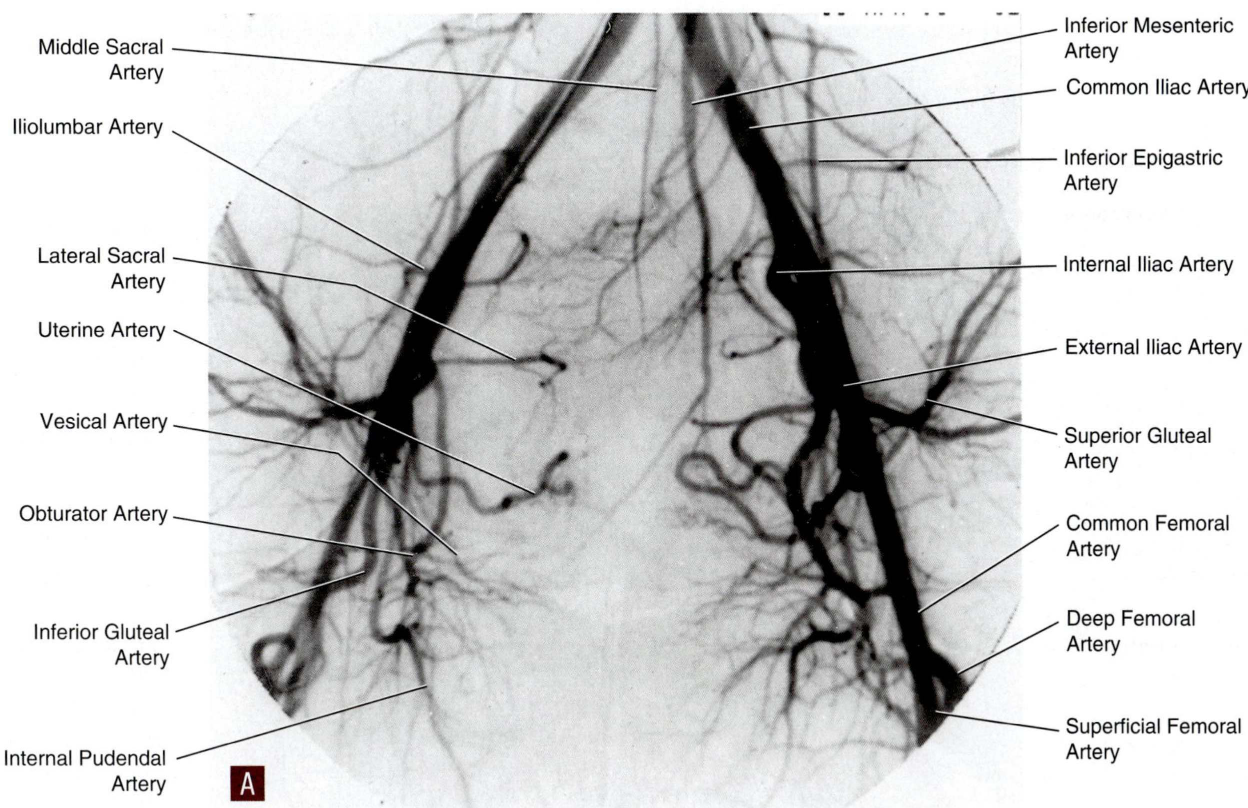

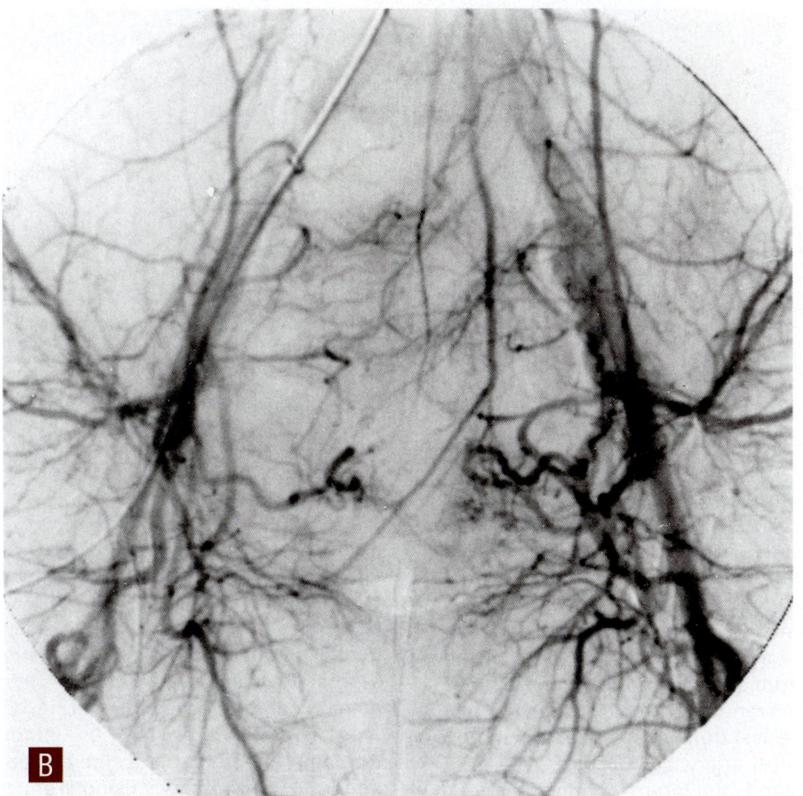

Figure 19.3. A, Early pelvic angiography in a female patient. B, Late phase of the same pelvic angiography.

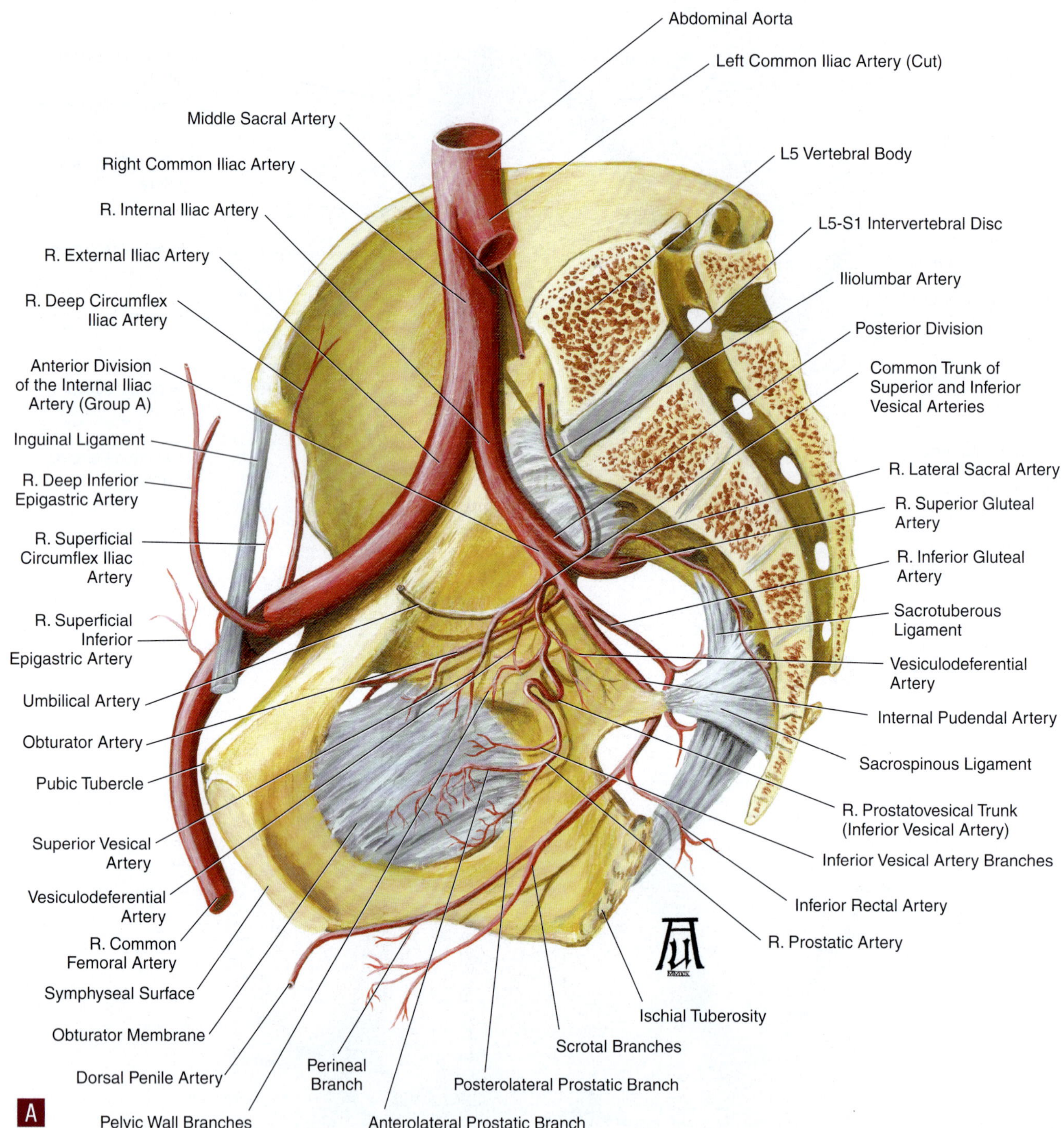

Figure 19.4. Schematic diagram of the four Yamaki internal iliac branching types and several pelvic arterial variants. Note that there is no association between the branching types and the pelvic arterial variants, which are shown as illustrative examples. **A**, Group A: the anterior division consists of the internal pudendal and inferior gluteal arteries with superior gluteal artery being the main branch of the posterior division. In this example, the prostatovesical trunk arises from a common trunk with the superior vesical artery. **B**, Group B: the main branch of the anterior division is the internal pudendal artery, with the posterior division consisting of a common trunk that gives rise to the superior and inferior gluteal arteries. This example shows a prostatovesical trunk arising from the internal pudendal artery, an aberrant obturator artery, and an anastomosis between the prostatic artery and ipsilateral internal pudendal artery. **C**, Group C: consists of a trifurcation of the internal iliac artery into the superior gluteal, the inferior gluteal, and the internal pudendal arteries. This example shows a prostatovesical trunk arising from the obturator artery with a middle rectal artery. **D**, Group D: the rarest of the four types, group D consists of an anterior division giving rise to the superior gluteal and internal pudendal arteries with the inferior gluteal artery arising from the posterior division. In this example, an accessory pudendal artery gives rise to the anterolateral prostatic branch, with a posterolateral branch arising from the internal pudendal artery.

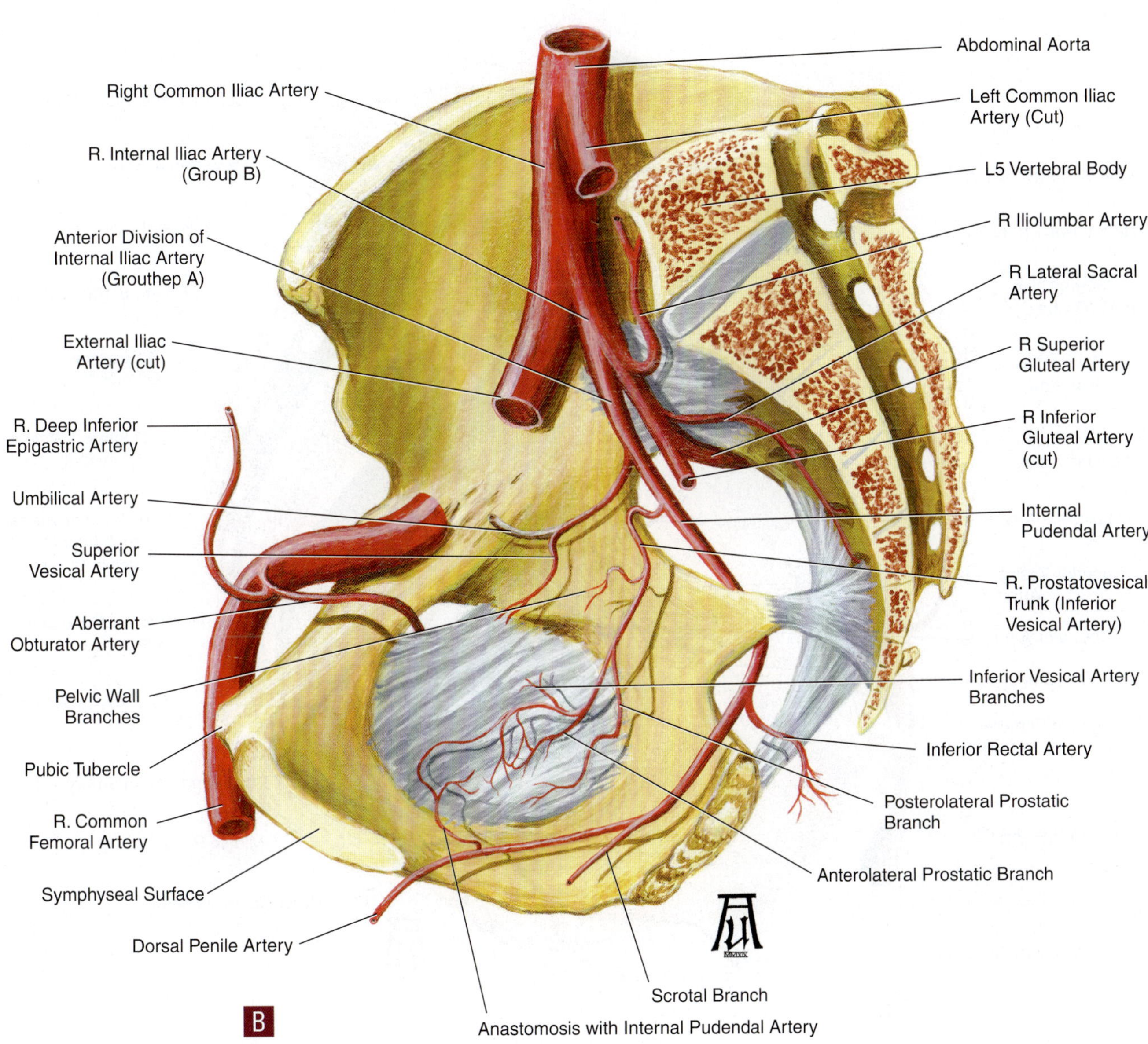

Figure 19.4. *Continued*

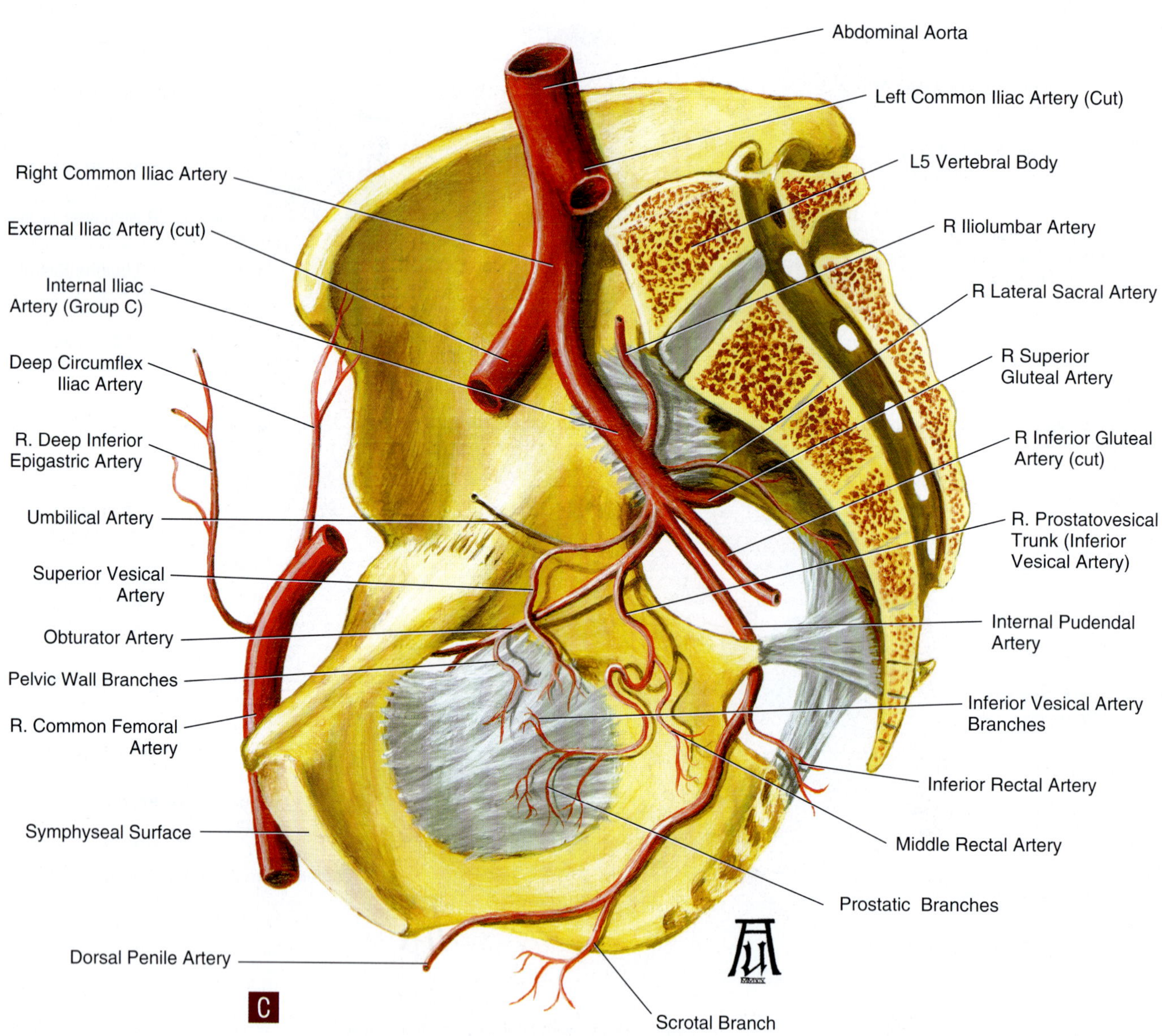

Figure 19.4. *Continued*

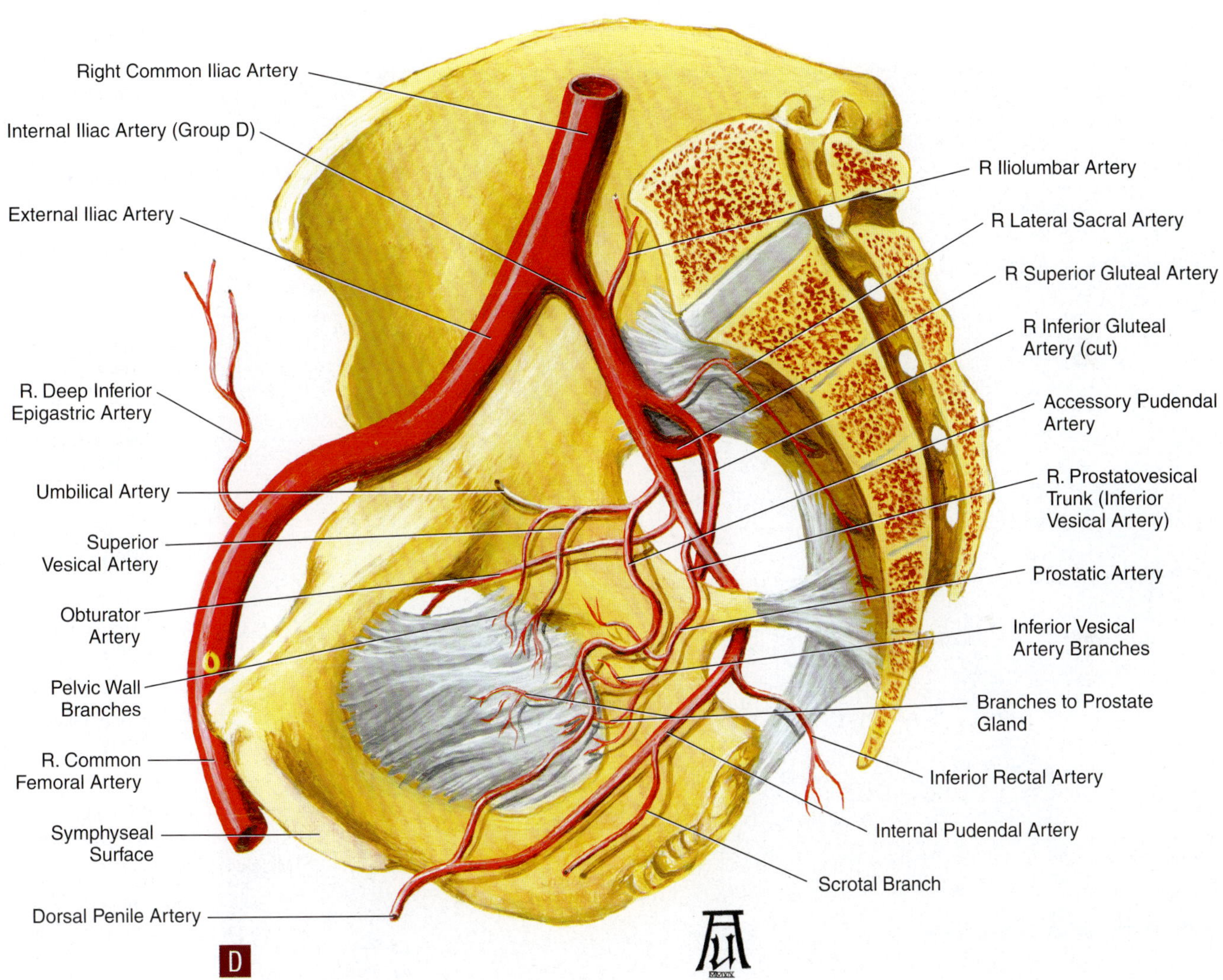

Figure 19.4. *Continued*

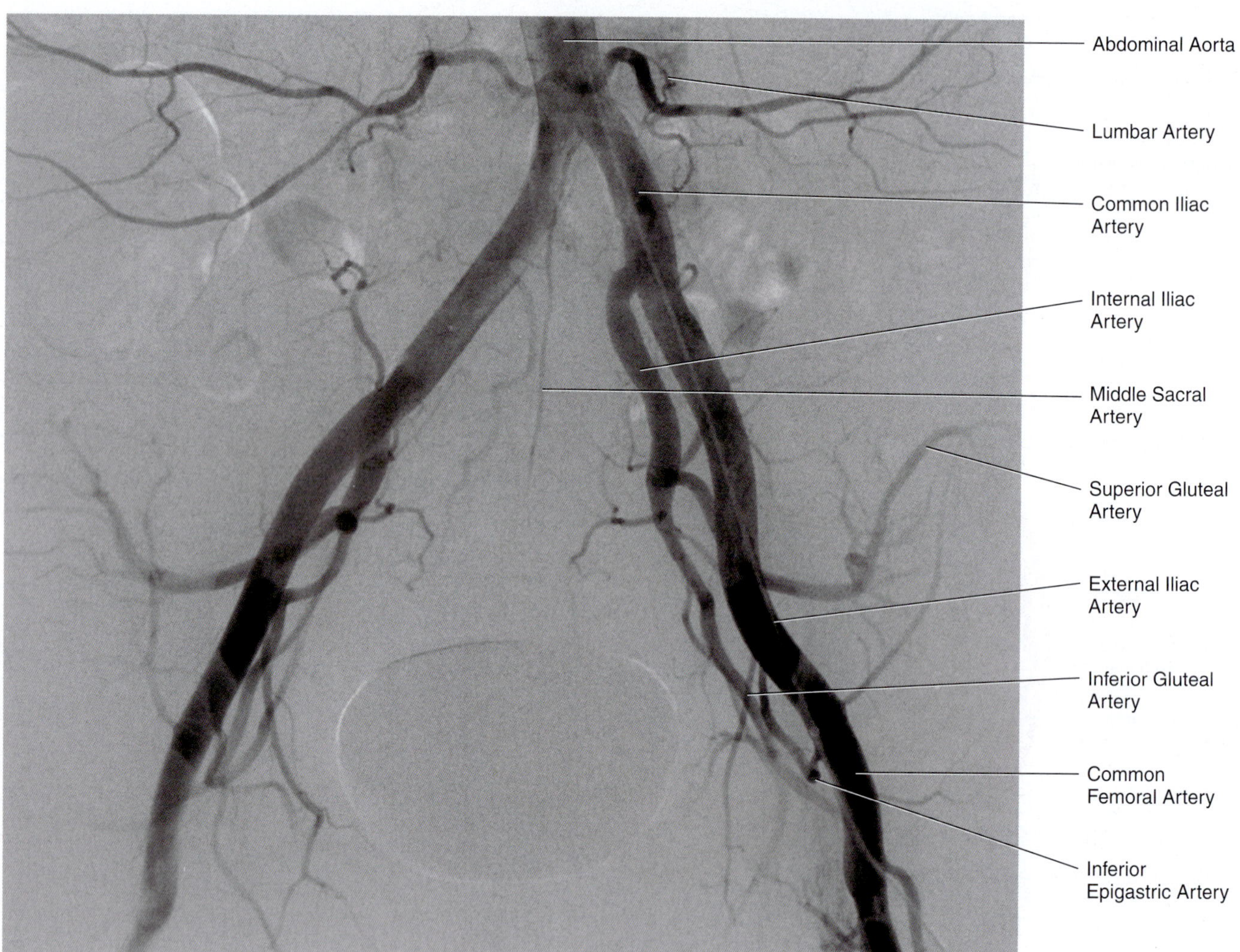

Figure 19.5. Pelvic angiography in a male patient.

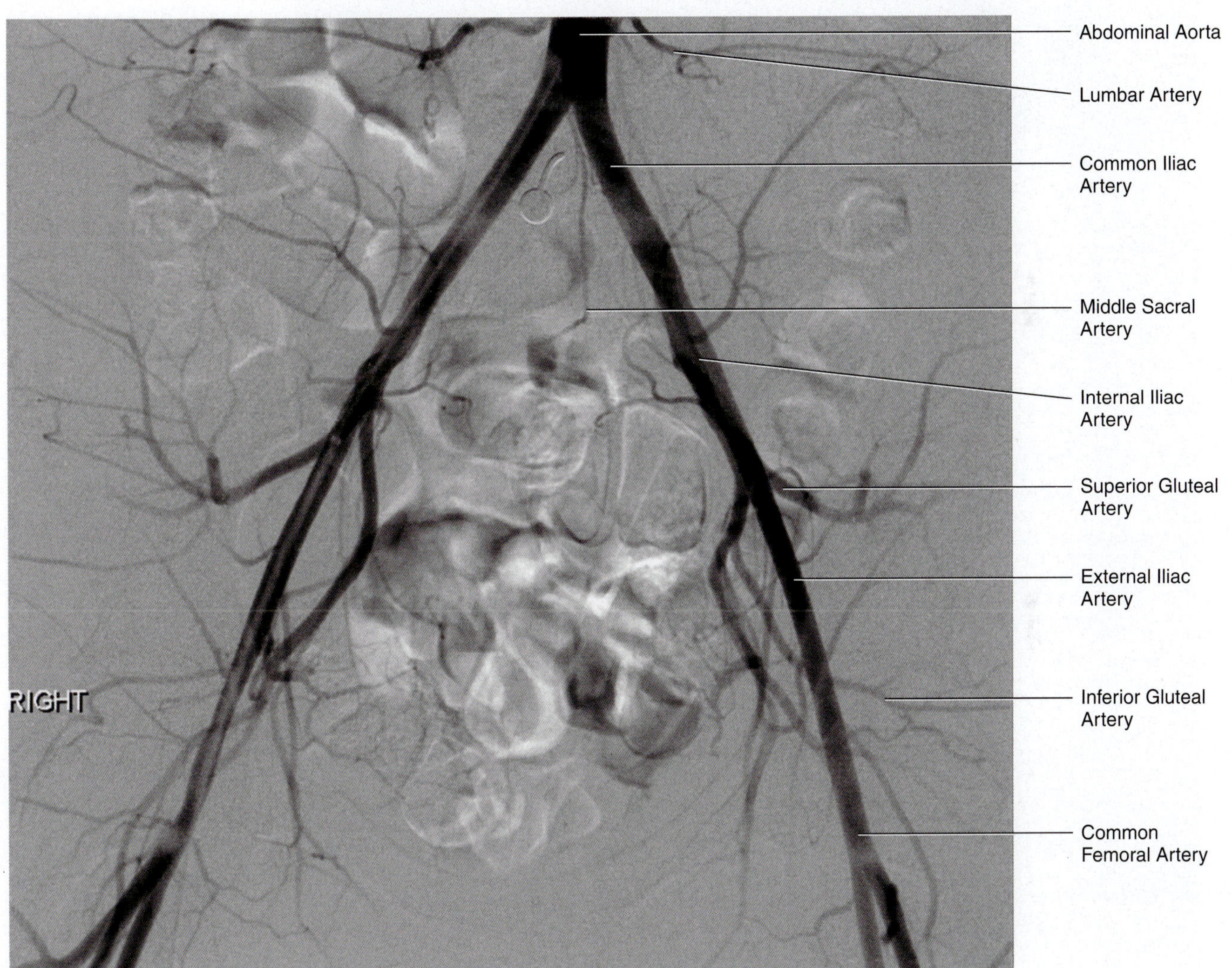

Figure 19.6. Pelvic angiography in a normal female patient.

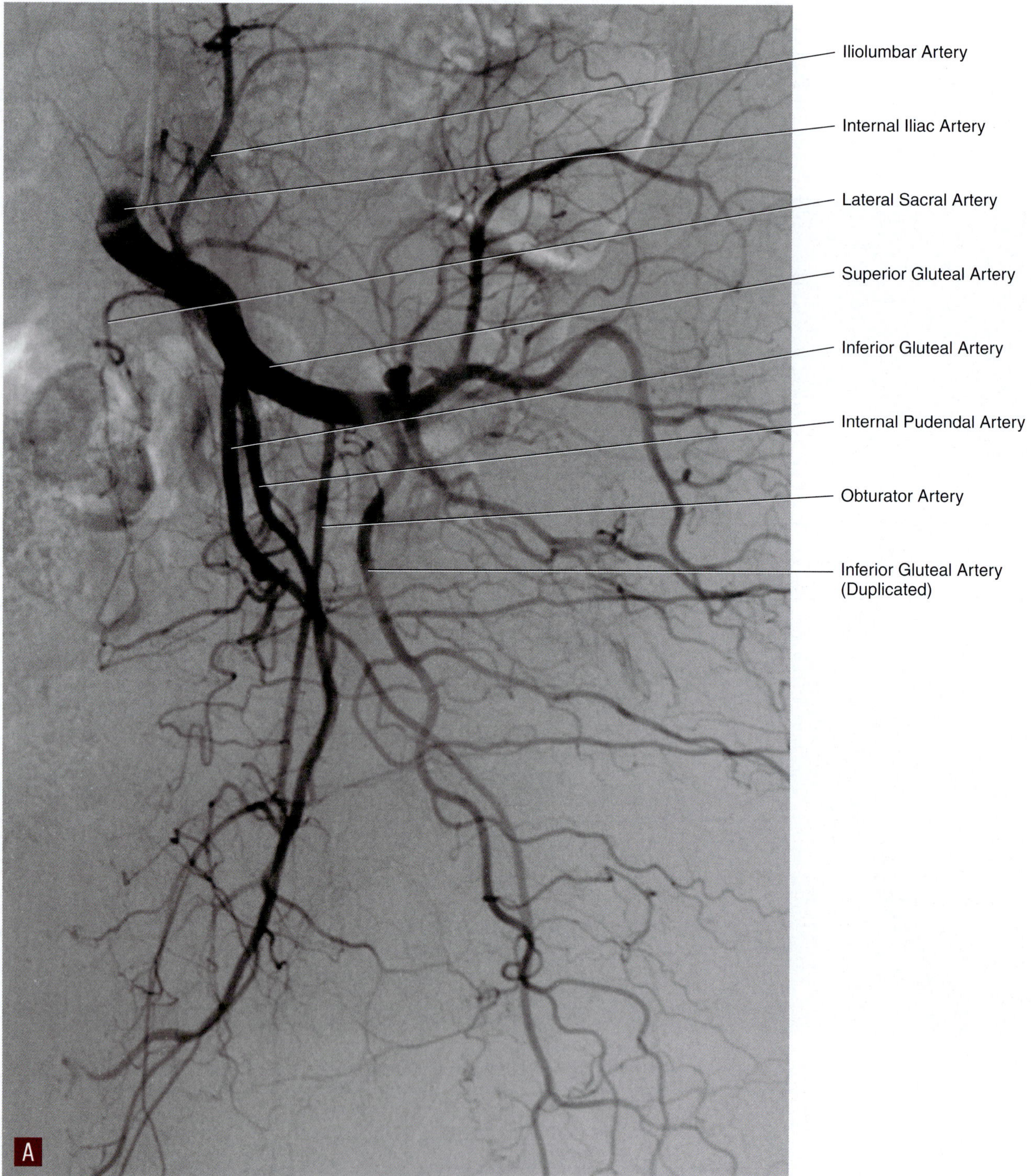

Figure 19.7. A, Selective arteriography of the left internal iliac artery showing the gluteal arteries and branches. B, Selective angiogram of the right internal iliac artery showing an example of the Yamaki group A configuration.

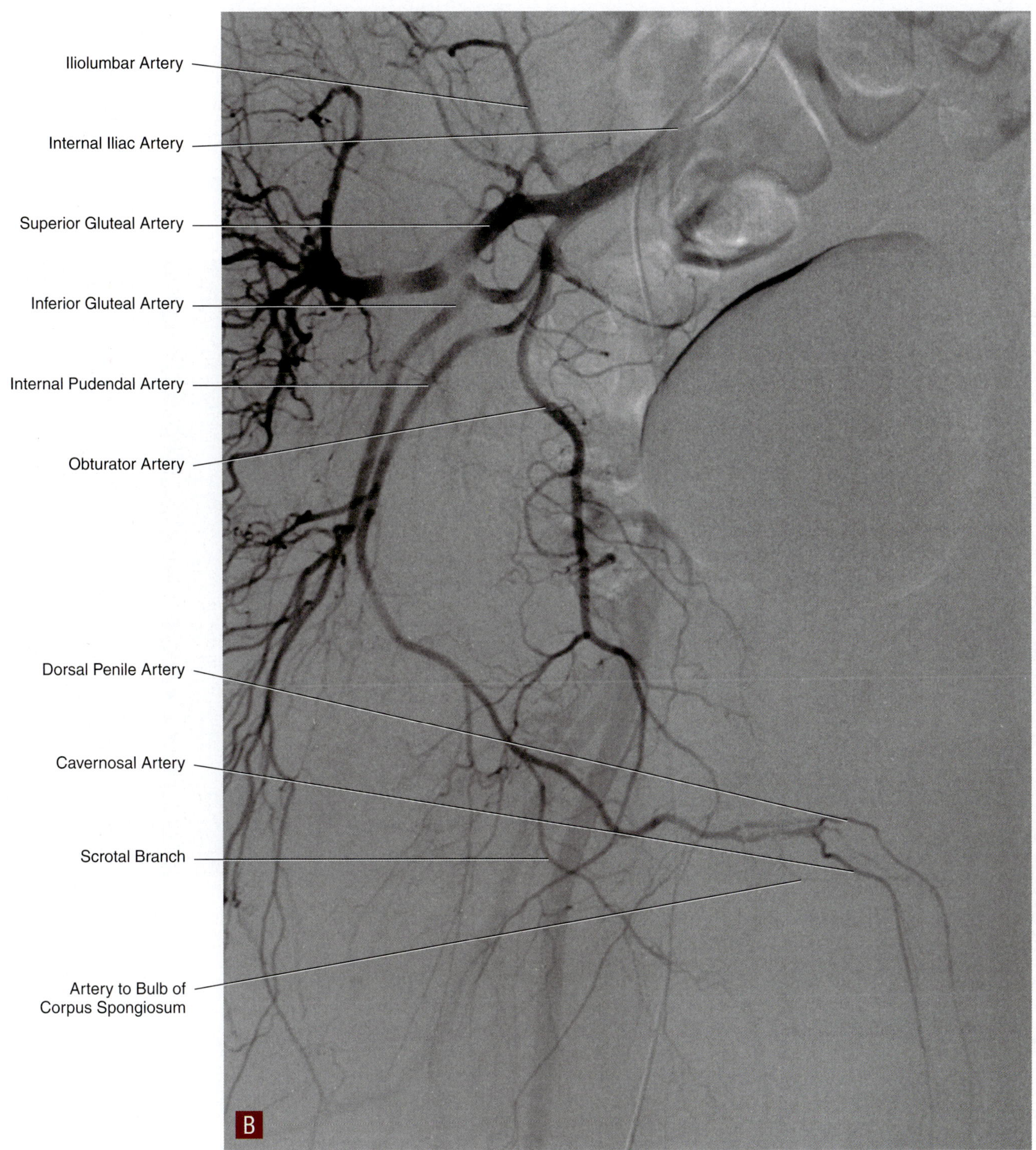

Figure 19.7. *Continued*

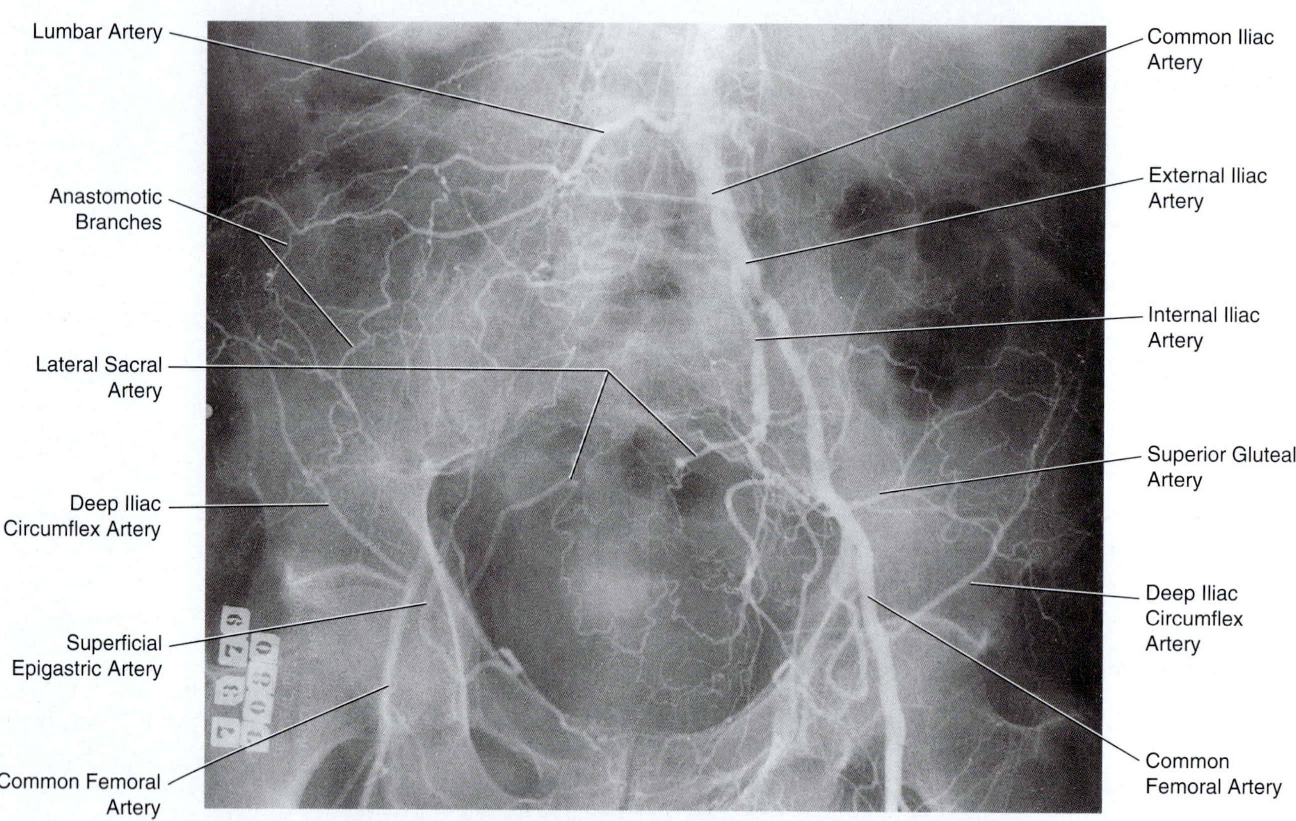

Figure 19.8. Pelvic angiography in a patient with occlusive disease, showing the development of the collateralization in the pelvis.

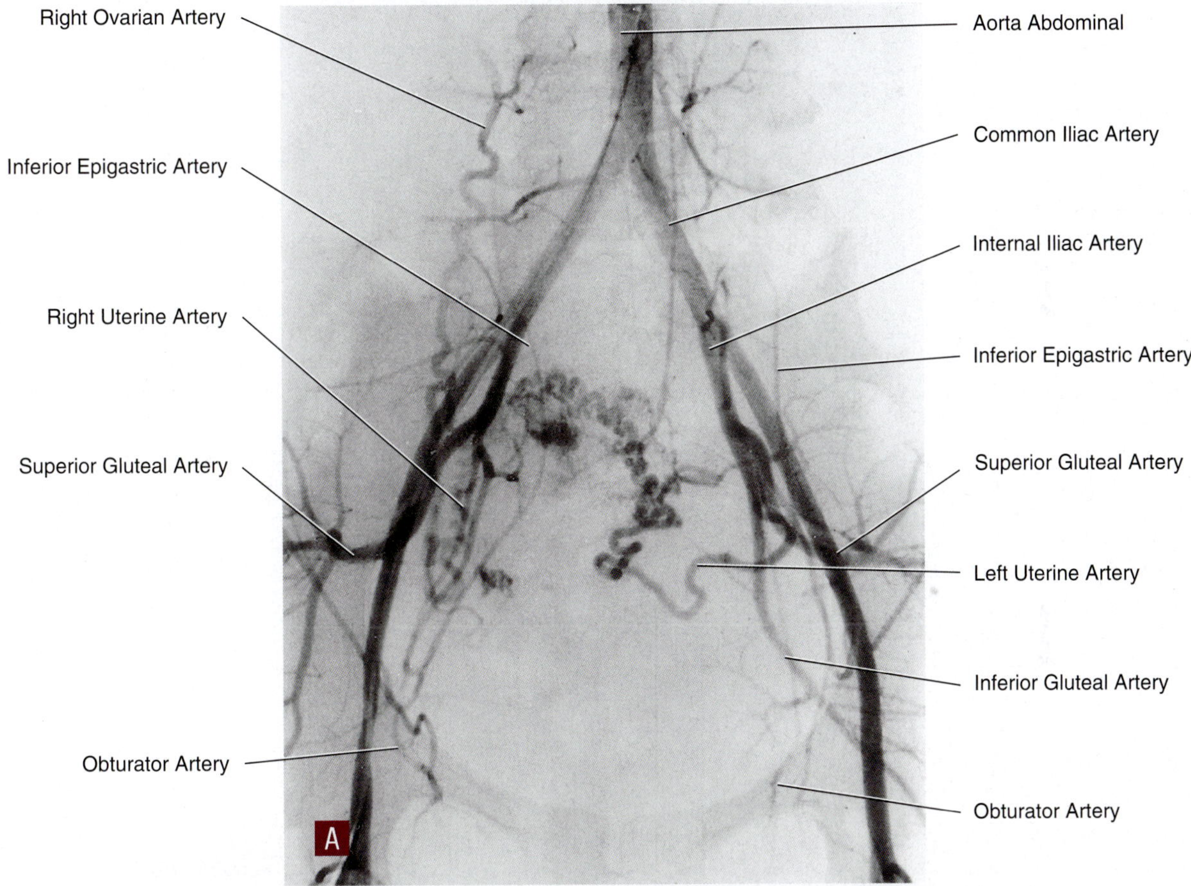

Figure 19.9. A, Pelvic angiography in a female patient with a uterine leiomyoma showing the enlargement of the uterine arteries. B and C, Later phase of the angiogram shows contrast stain in the uterus. D, Selective angiography of the right internal iliac artery shows the pelvic circulation, mainly the uterine artery. E, Selective injection at the left uterine artery shows the typical vascular pattern of the enlarged uterus.

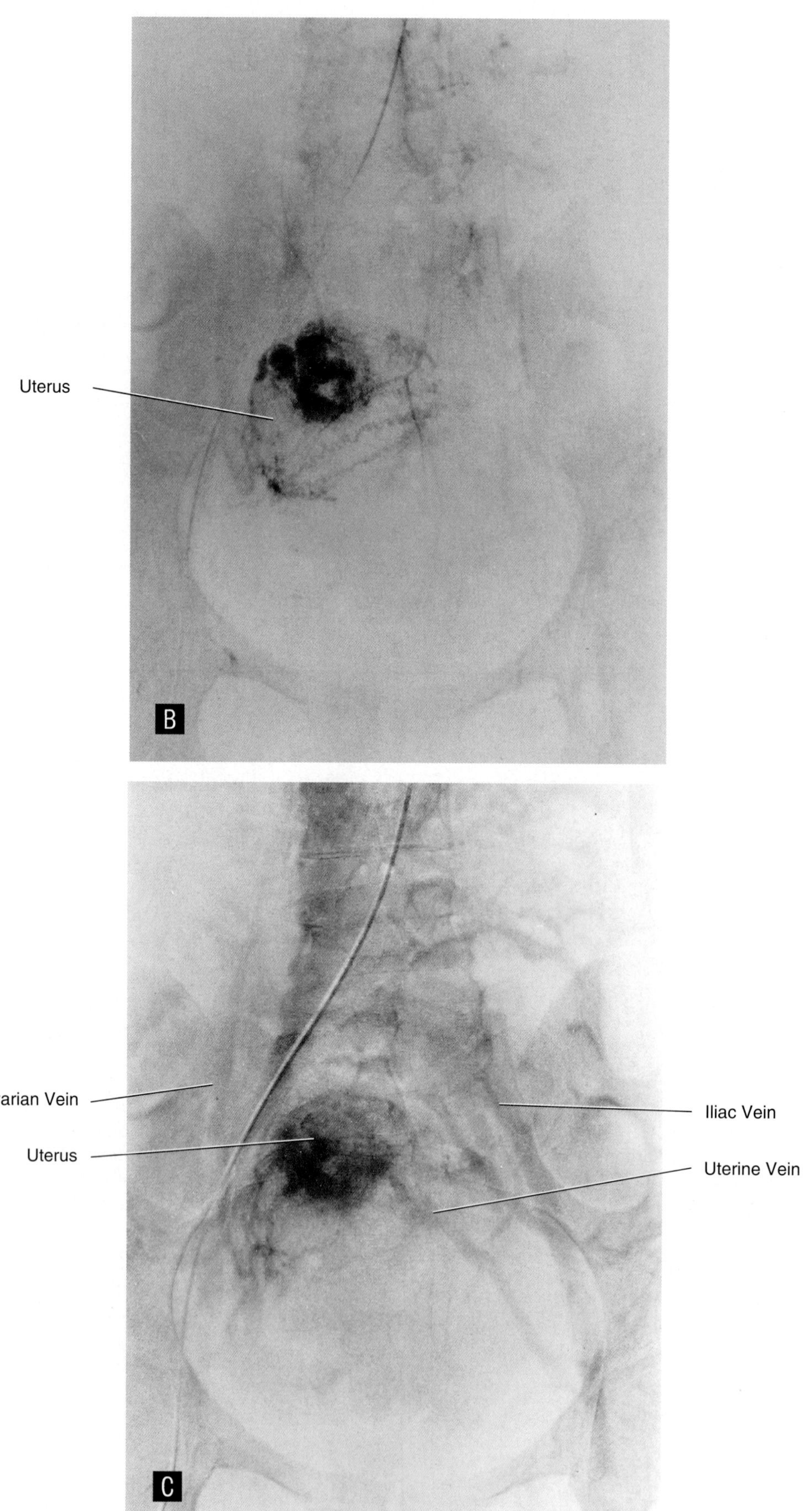

Figure 19.9. *Continued*

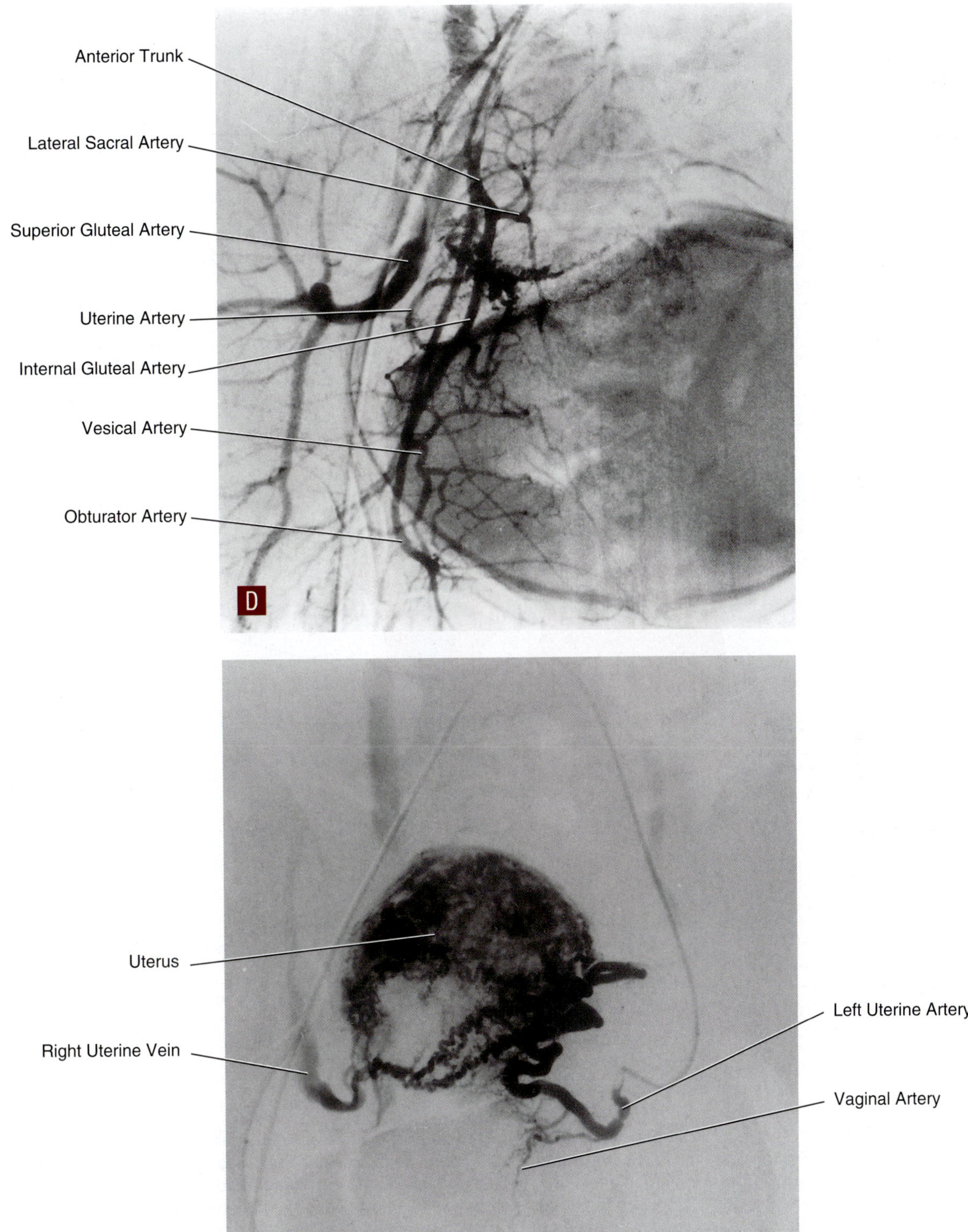

Figure 19.9. *Continued*

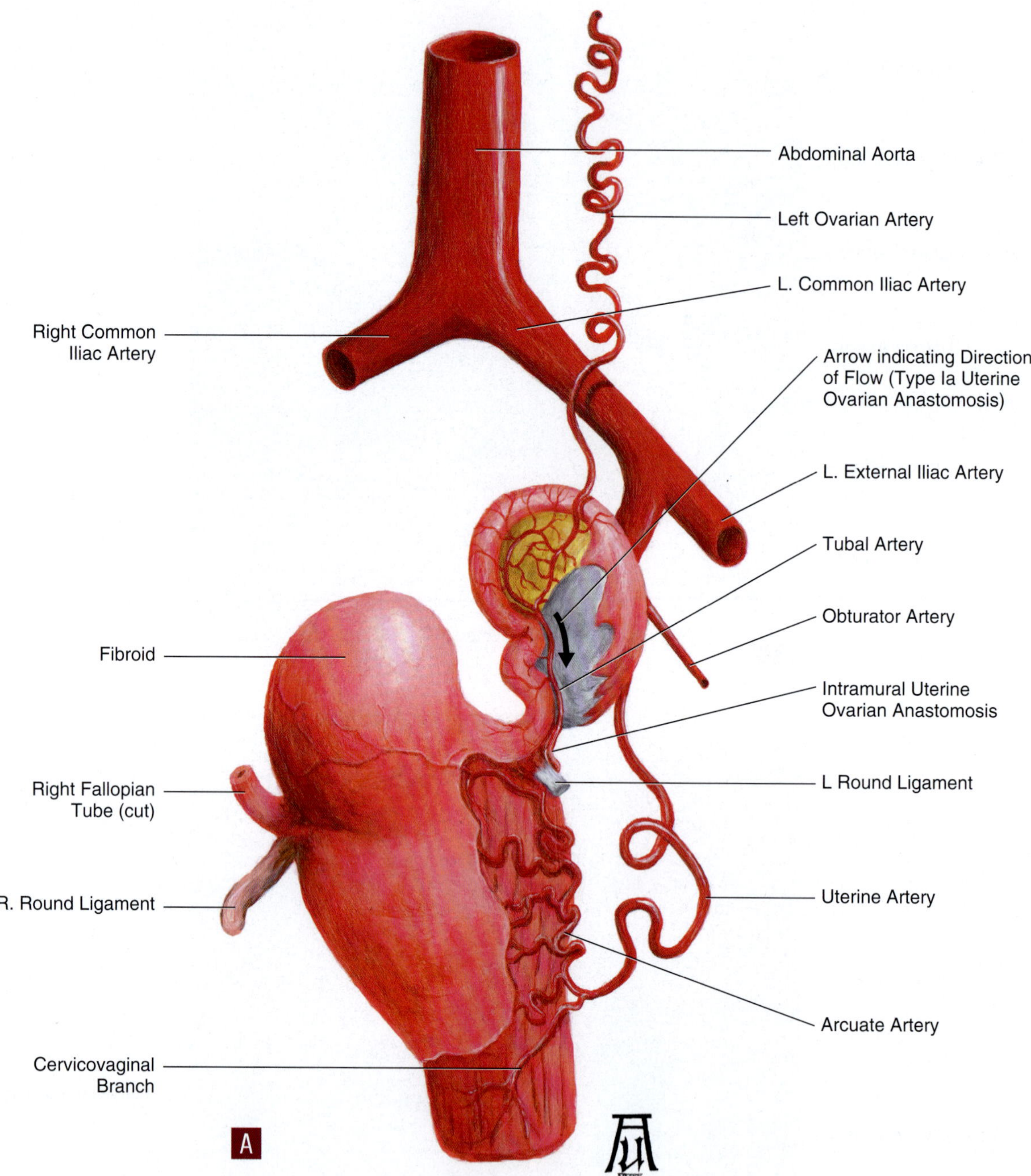

Figure 19.10. **Schematic diagram of the uterine-ovarian anastomotic types.** **A**, Uterine-ovarian anastomosis type Ia (13.2%) and type 1b (8.6%)—the fibroid derives blood supply predominantly from the ovarian artery with an anastomosis in the intramural uterine artery. Flow in the tubal artery is toward the uterus, without reflux into the ovary. In the type 1b pattern, the anatomical configuration is similar to type 1a, except that the type Ib flow pattern shows reflux into the ovarian artery on the preembolization selective uterine artery angiogram. **B**, Type II (3.9%)—the ovarian artery supplies the fibroids directly with anastomoses to the intramural uterine artery, although flow to the fibroid is independent of the uterine artery. **C**, Type III (6.6%)—flow in the tubal artery is toward the ovary, with the anastomosis being through the tubal artery.

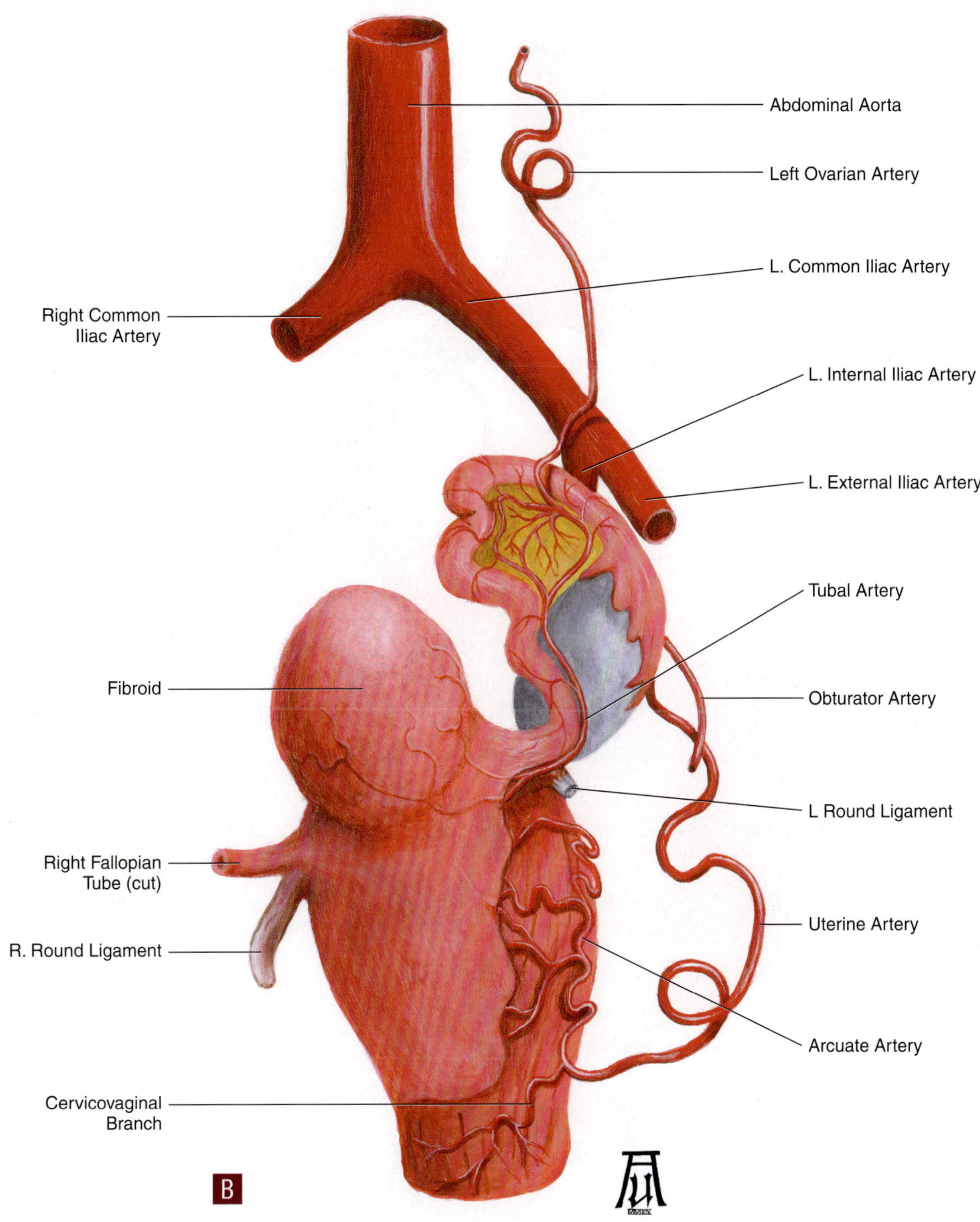

Figure 19.10. *Continued*

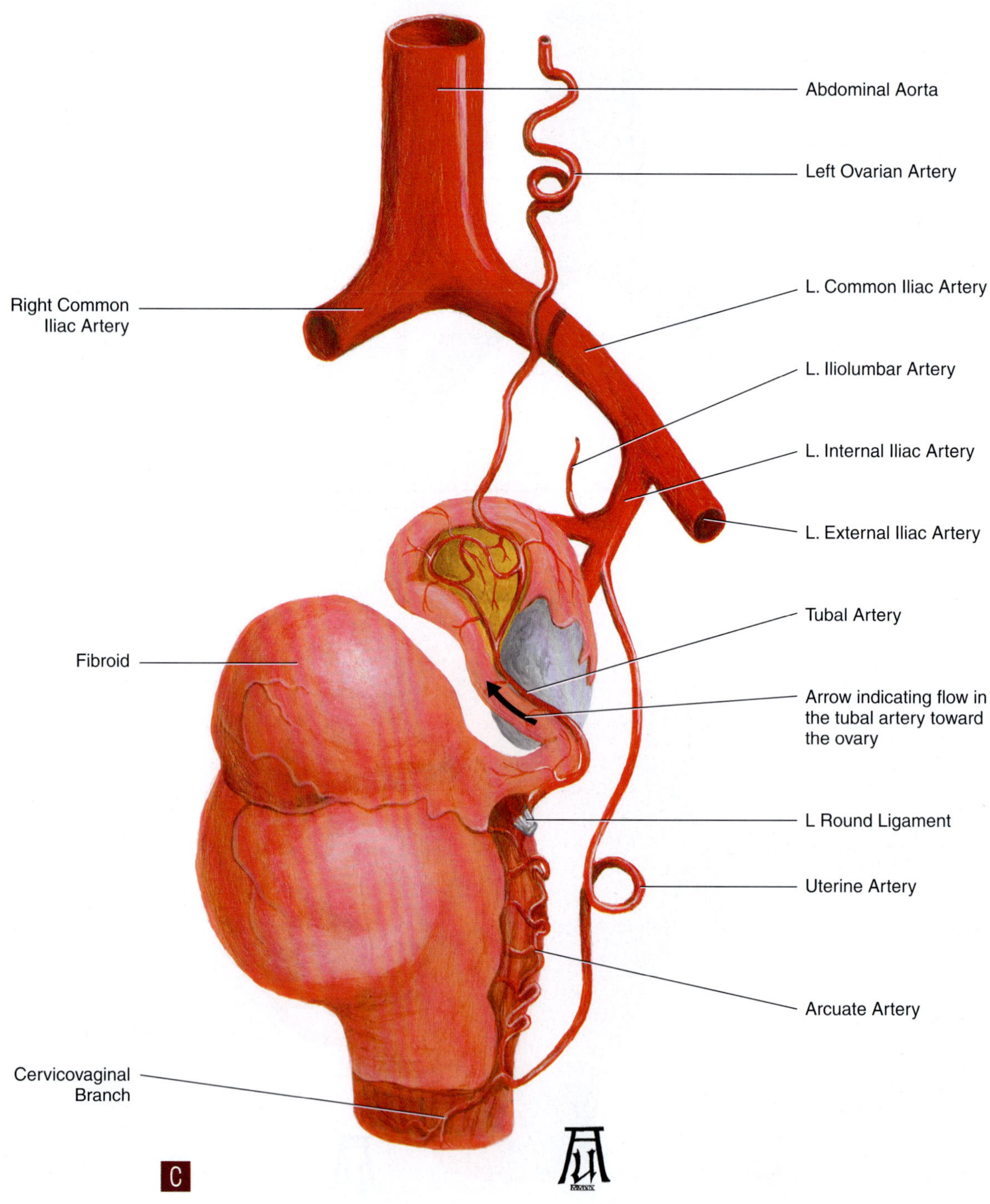

Figure 19.10. *Continued*

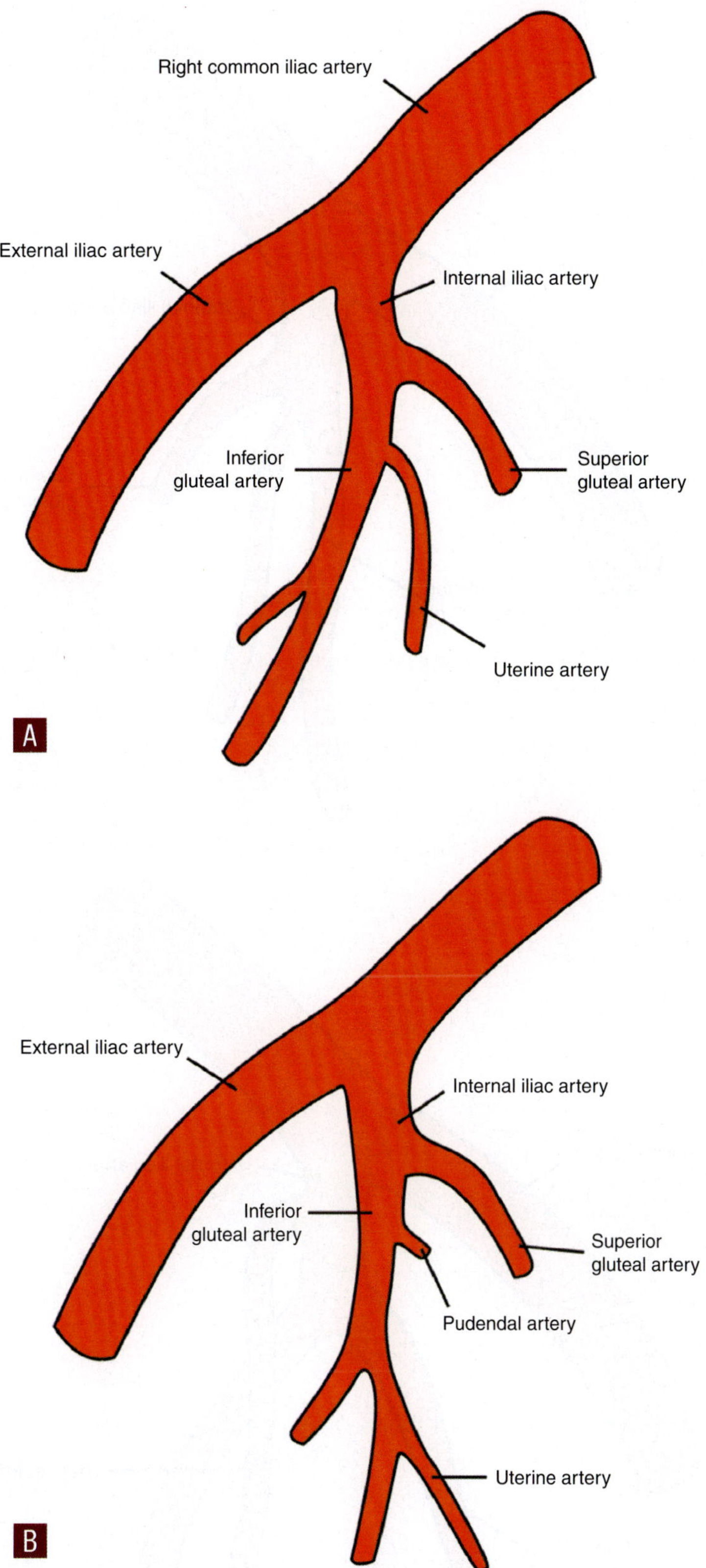

Figure 19.11. **A**, Type I uterine artery arising as the first branch of the inferior gluteal artery or anterior trunk. This is the most common origin of the uterine artery, representing about 65% of cases. **B**, Type II uterine artery arising as the second or third branch of the inferior gluteal artery (6%). Other branches such as the internal pudendal artery may be the first branch of the inferior gluteal artery. **C**, Type III uterine artery, the inferior gluteal artery, and the superior gluteal artery arise at the same level as a trifurcation in about 43% of cases. **D**, Type IV uterine artery arising proximally to the origin of the inferior gluteal artery and superior gluteal arteries (6%).

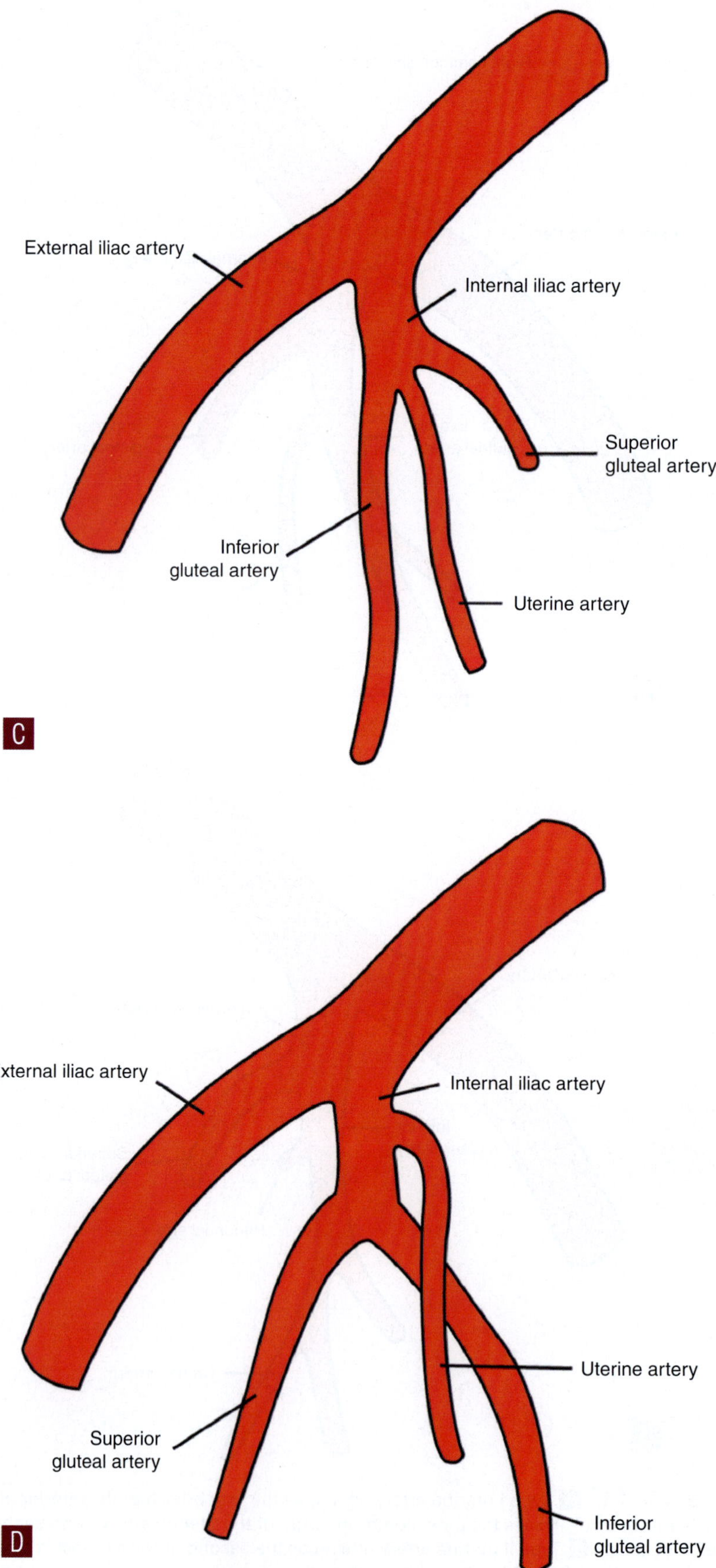

Figure 19.11. *Continued*

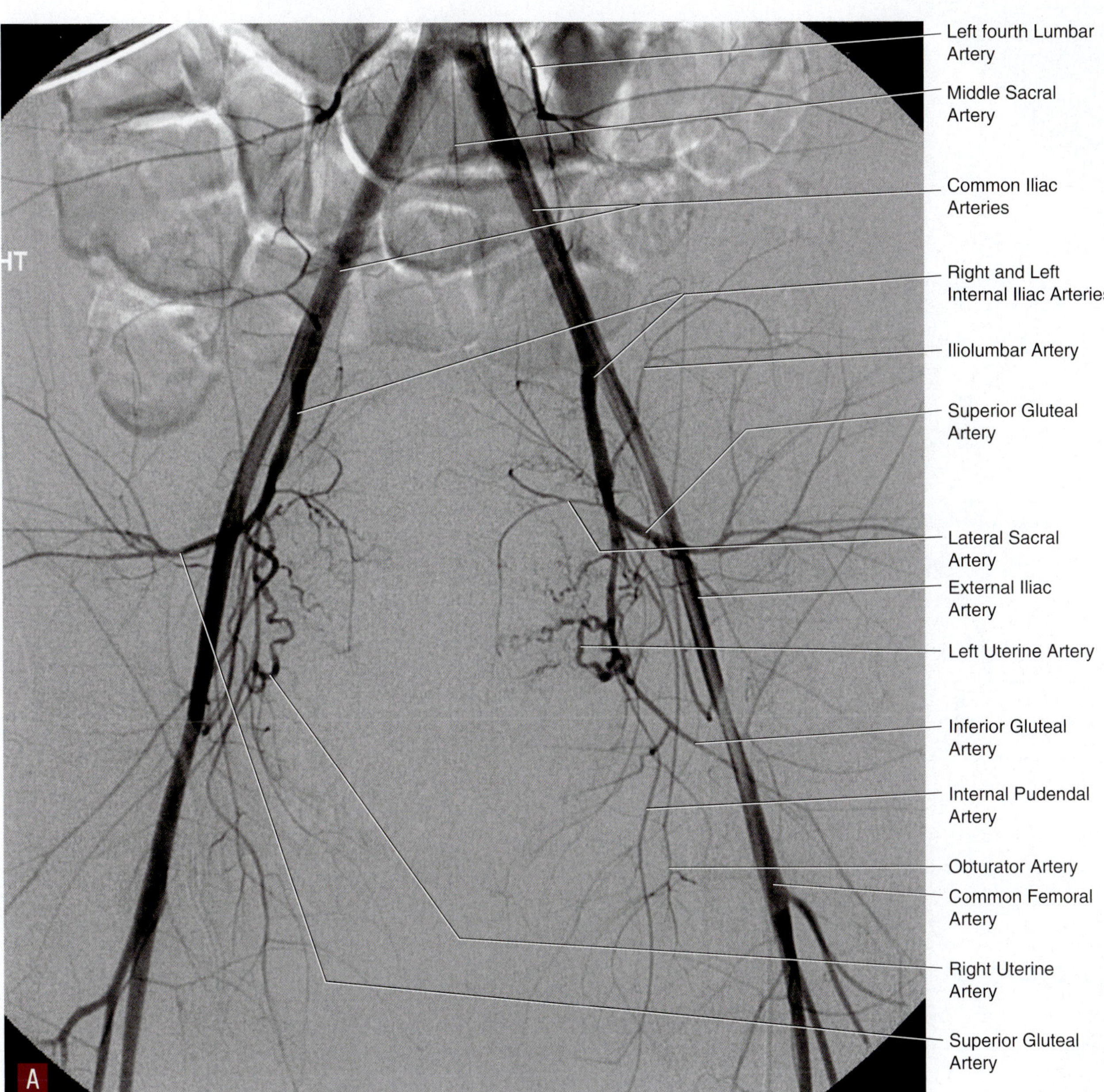

Figure 19.12. **A**, Pelvic arteriogram in a female patient with uterine fibroids. Note the prominent right and left uterine arteries. **B**, Selective angiogram of the right internal iliac artery. The right uterine artery is the first branch of the anterior trunk, inferior gluteal artery (type I). **C**, Selective angiogram of the left internal iliac artery. The left uterine artery is the first branch of the inferior gluteal artery but not as evident (type I).

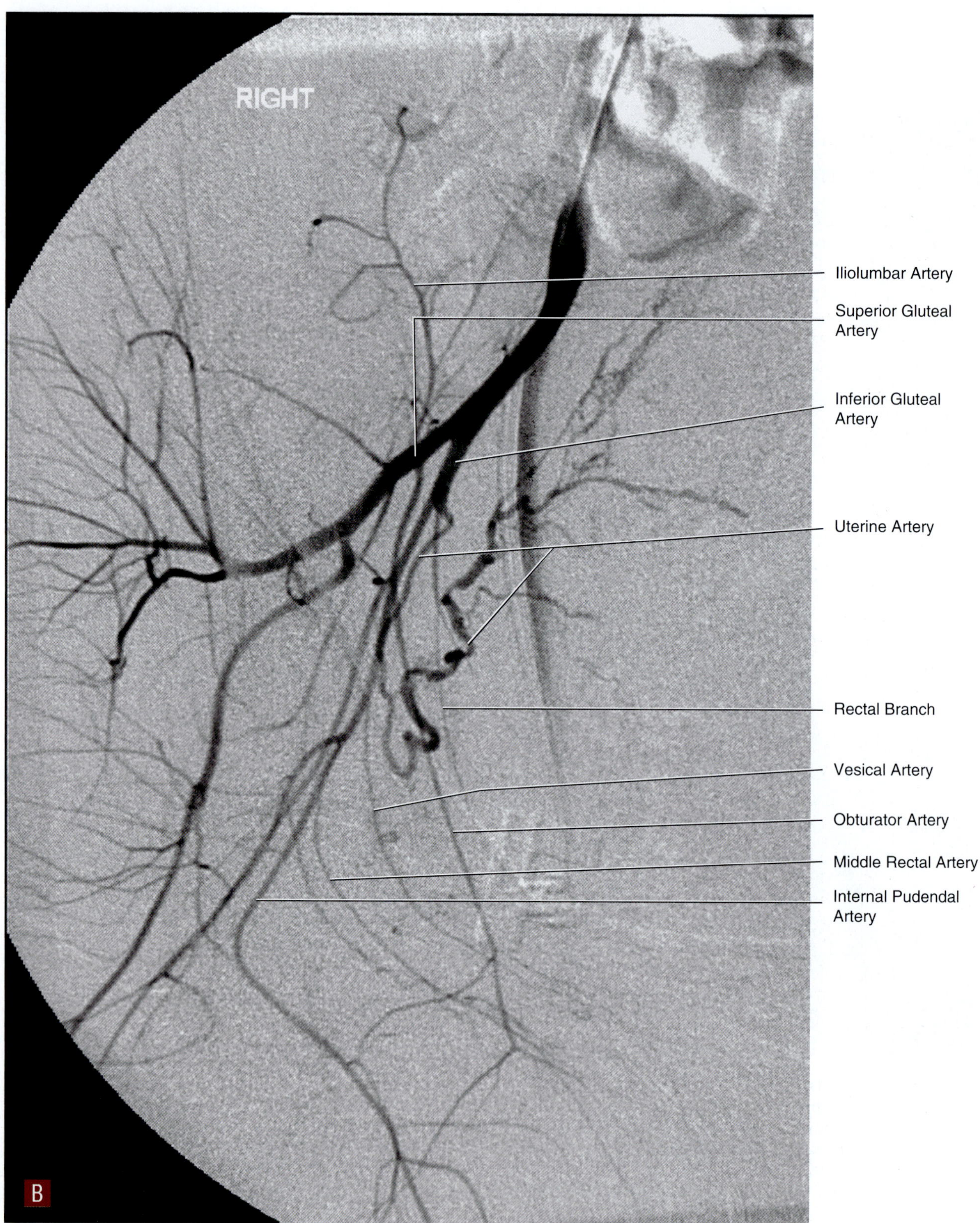

Figure 19.12. *Continued*

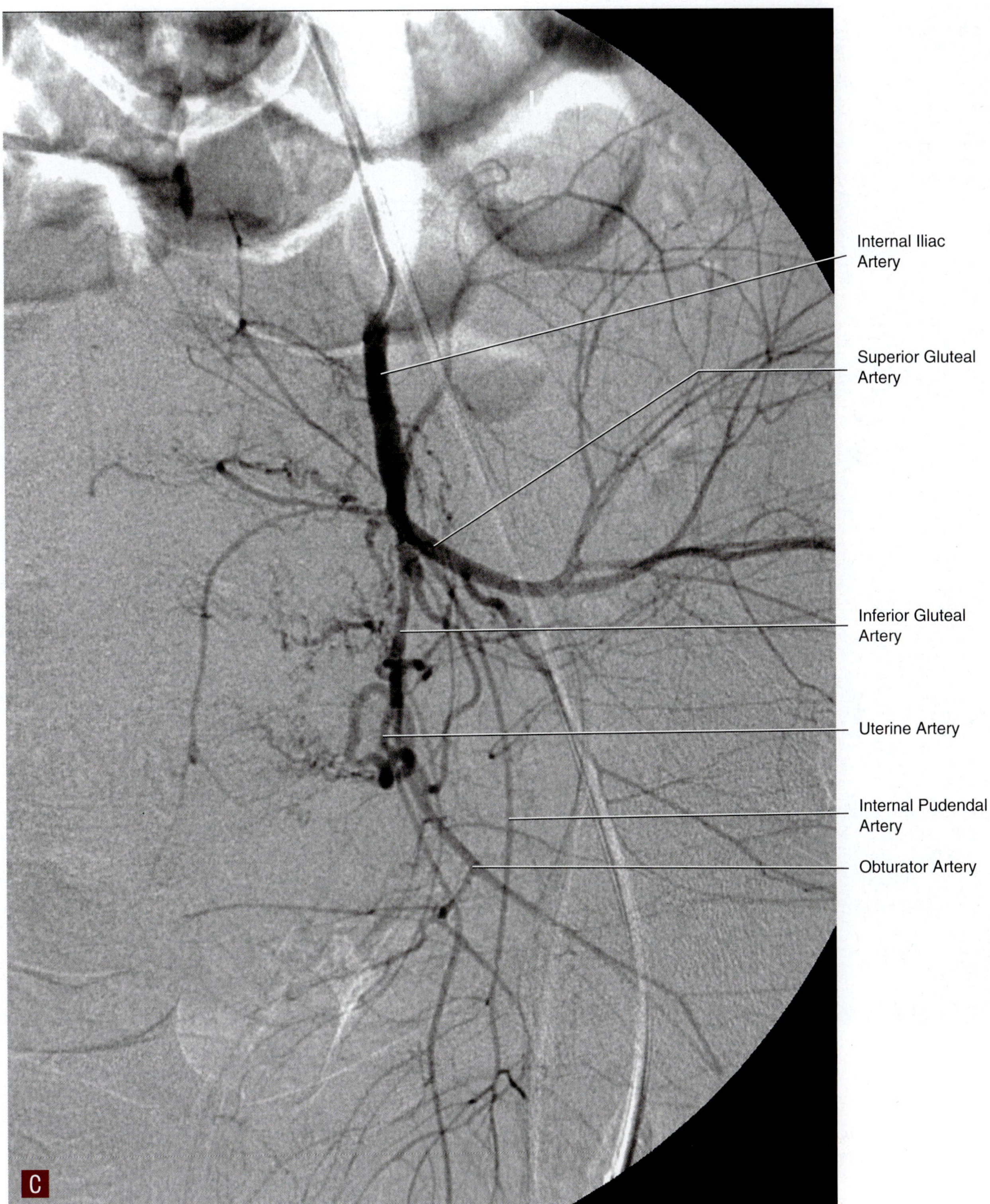

Figure 19.12. *Continued*

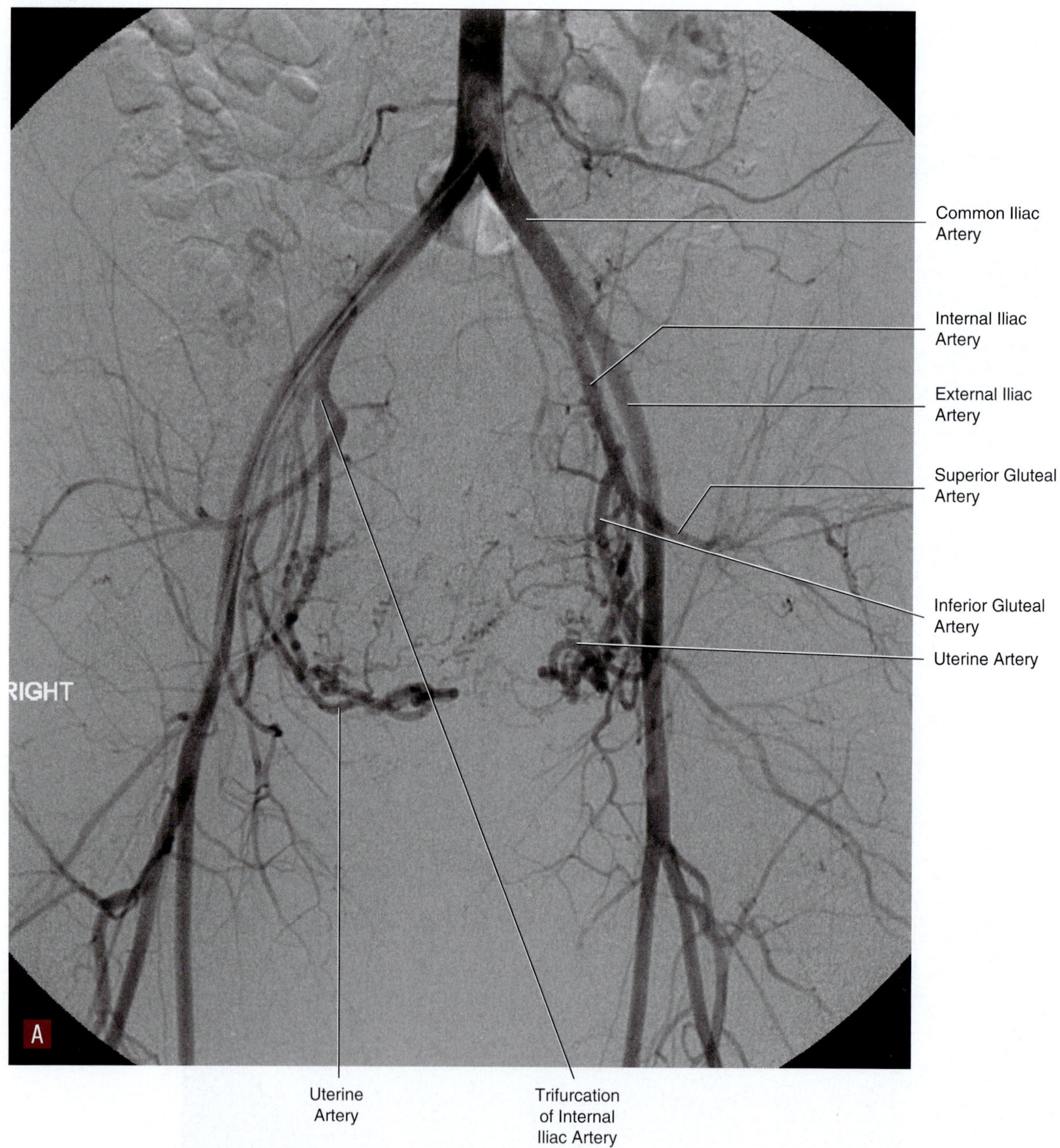

Figure 19.13. **A**, Pelvic arteriogram in a female patient with uterine fibroid. The uterine arteries are enlarged and tortuous. **B**, Selective angiogram of the right internal iliac artery. The uterine artery origin arises together with the superior gluteal artery and the inferior gluteal artery (type III). **C**, Selective angiogram of the left internal iliac artery. The uterine artery origin arises together with the superior gluteal artery and the inferior gluteal artery in a trifurcation (type III).

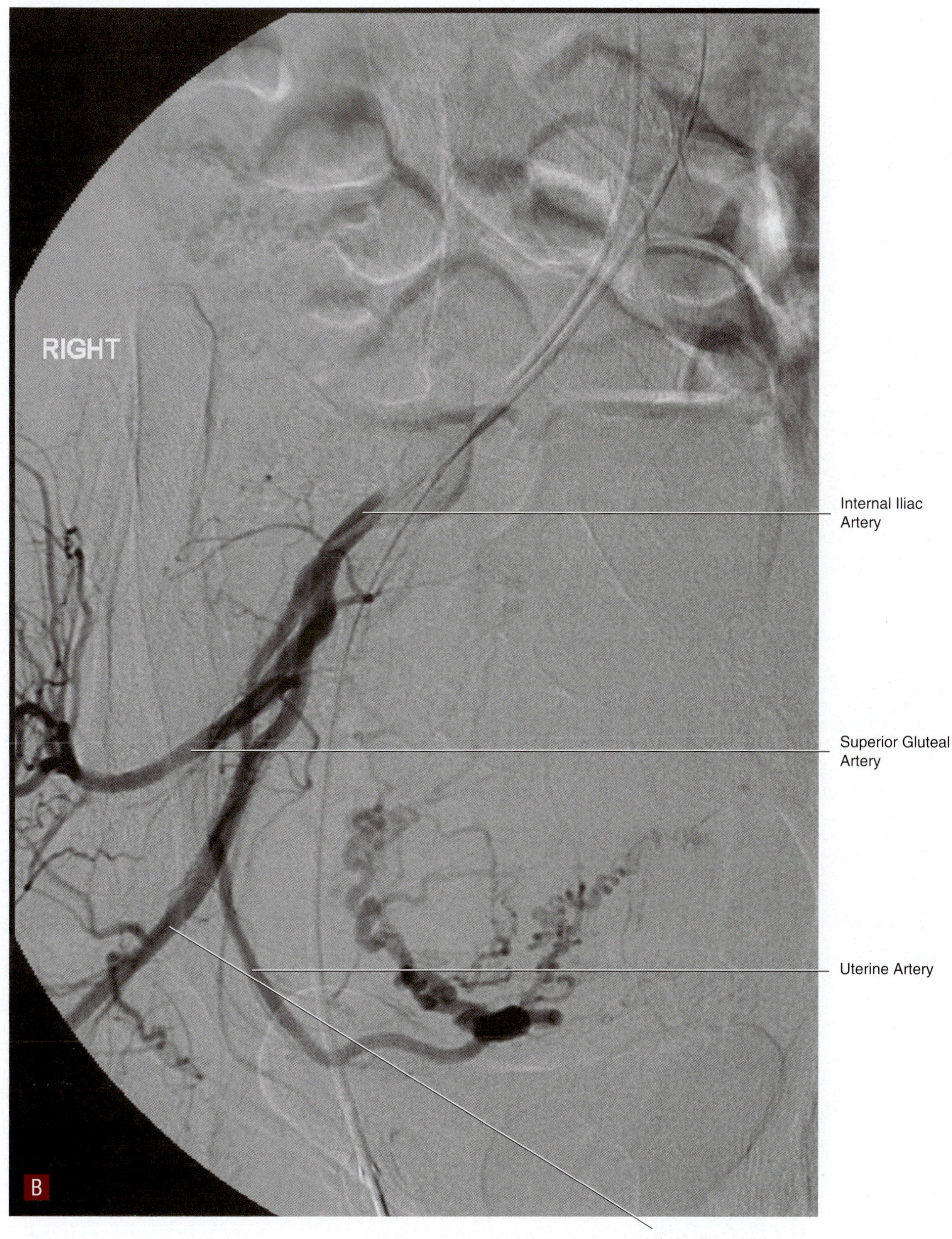

Figure 19.13. *Continued*

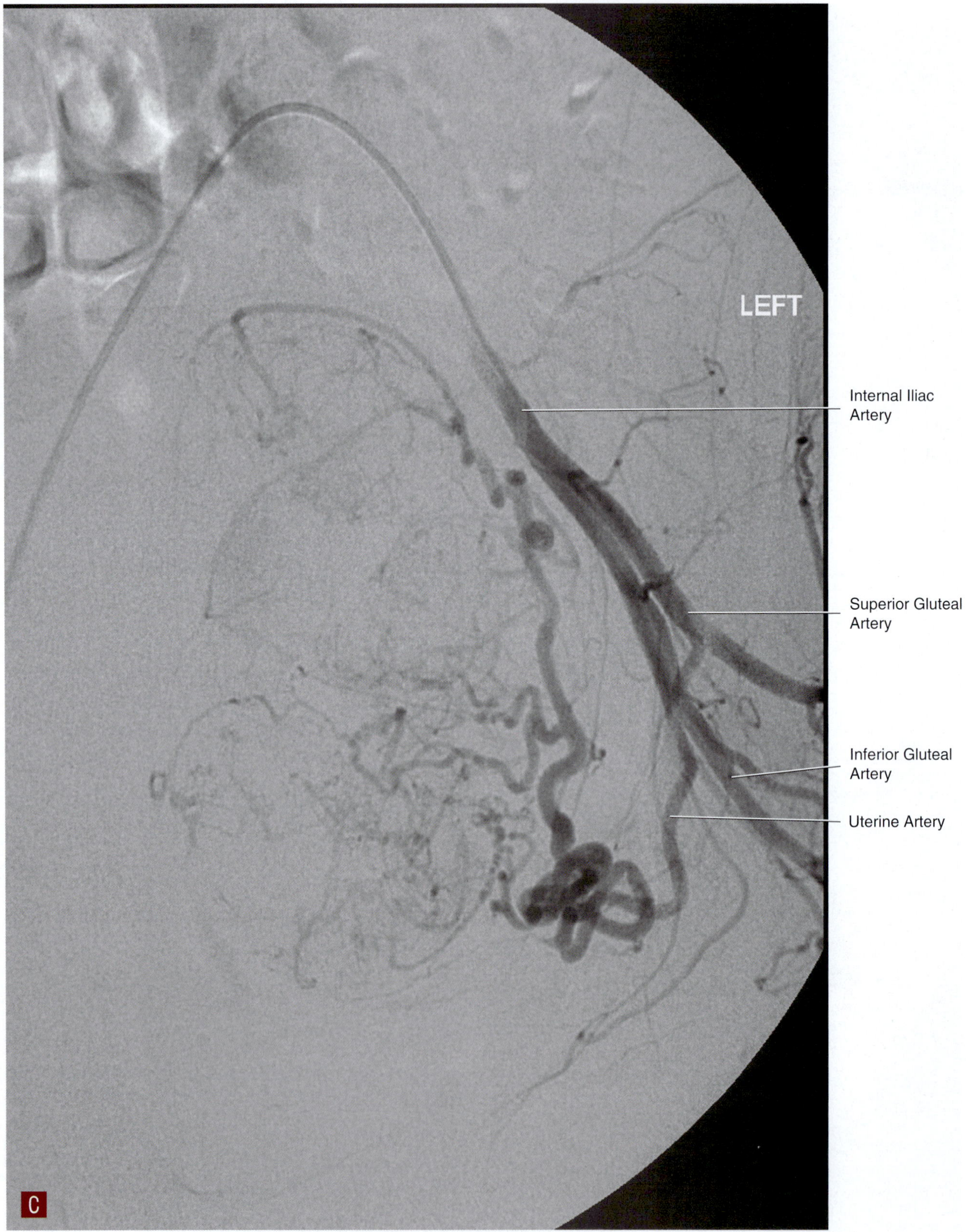

Figure 19.13. *Continued*

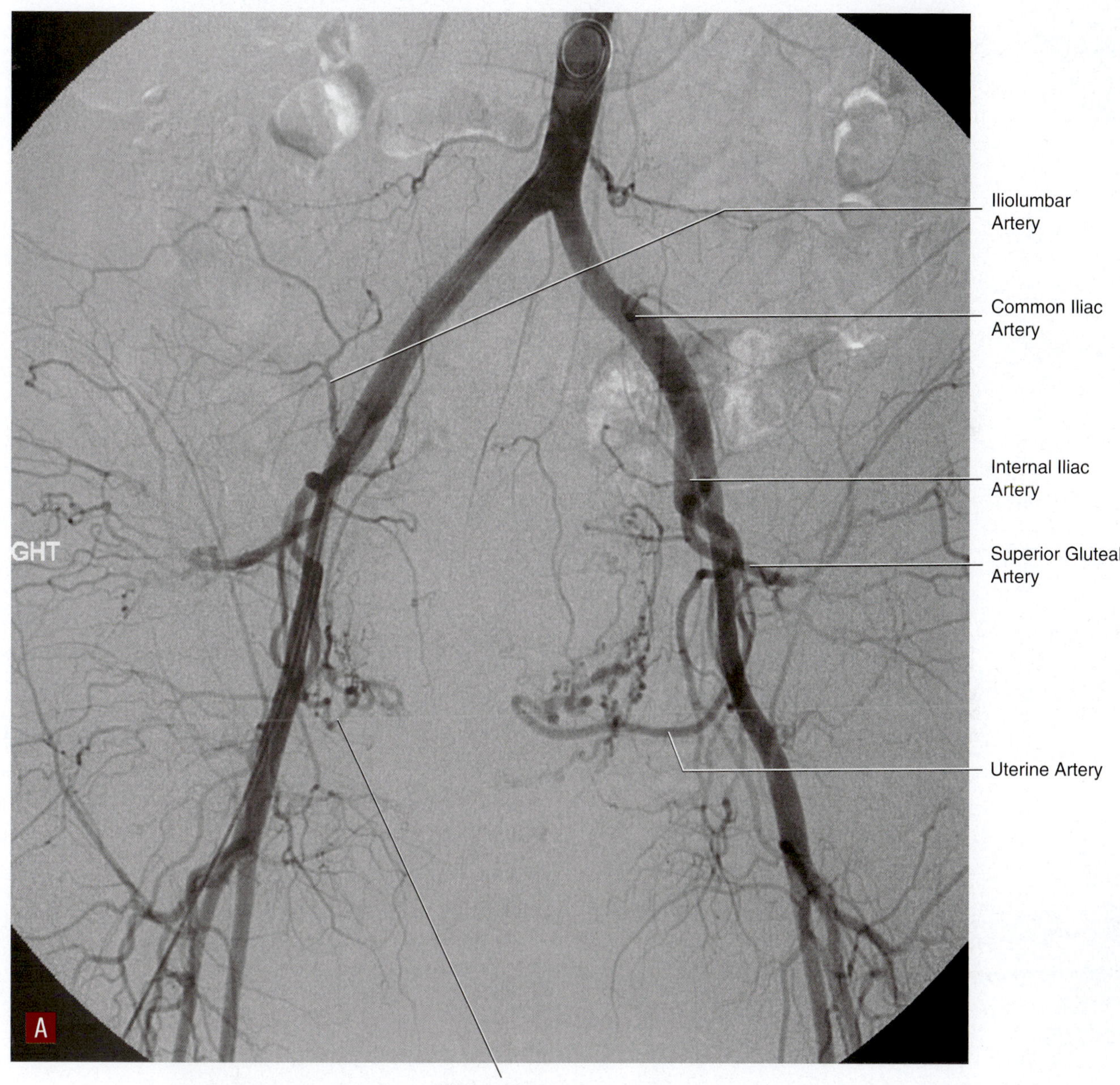

Figure 19.14. **A**, Pelvic arteriogram in a female patient with uterine fibroid. The uterine arteries are enlarged and tortuous, but the left is more prominent. **B**, Selective angiogram of the right internal iliac artery. The uterine artery origin is below the origin of the pudendal artery (type II). **C**, Selective angiogram of the left internal iliac artery. The uterine artery origin is the first branch of the inferior gluteal artery (type I).

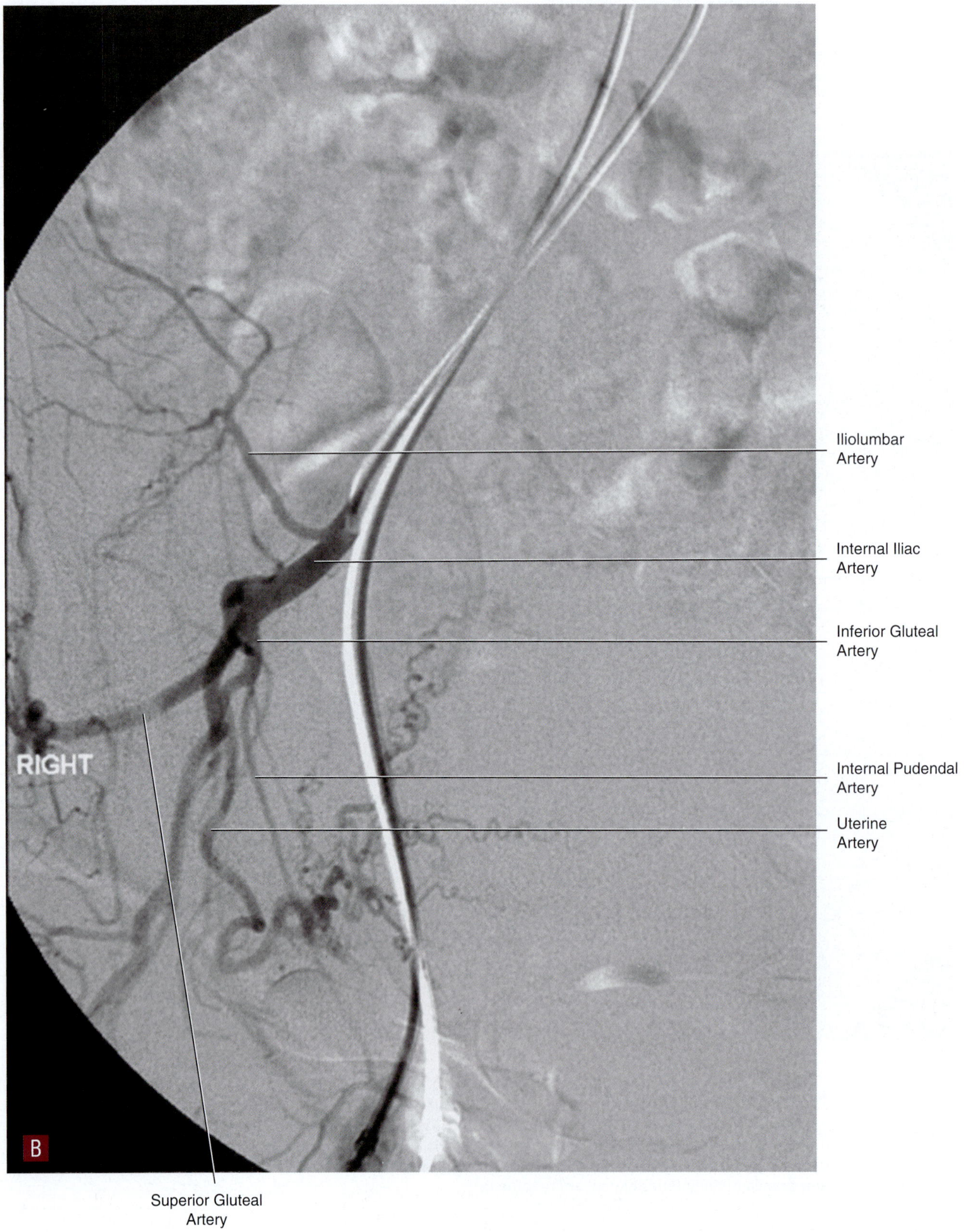

Figure 19.14. *Continued*

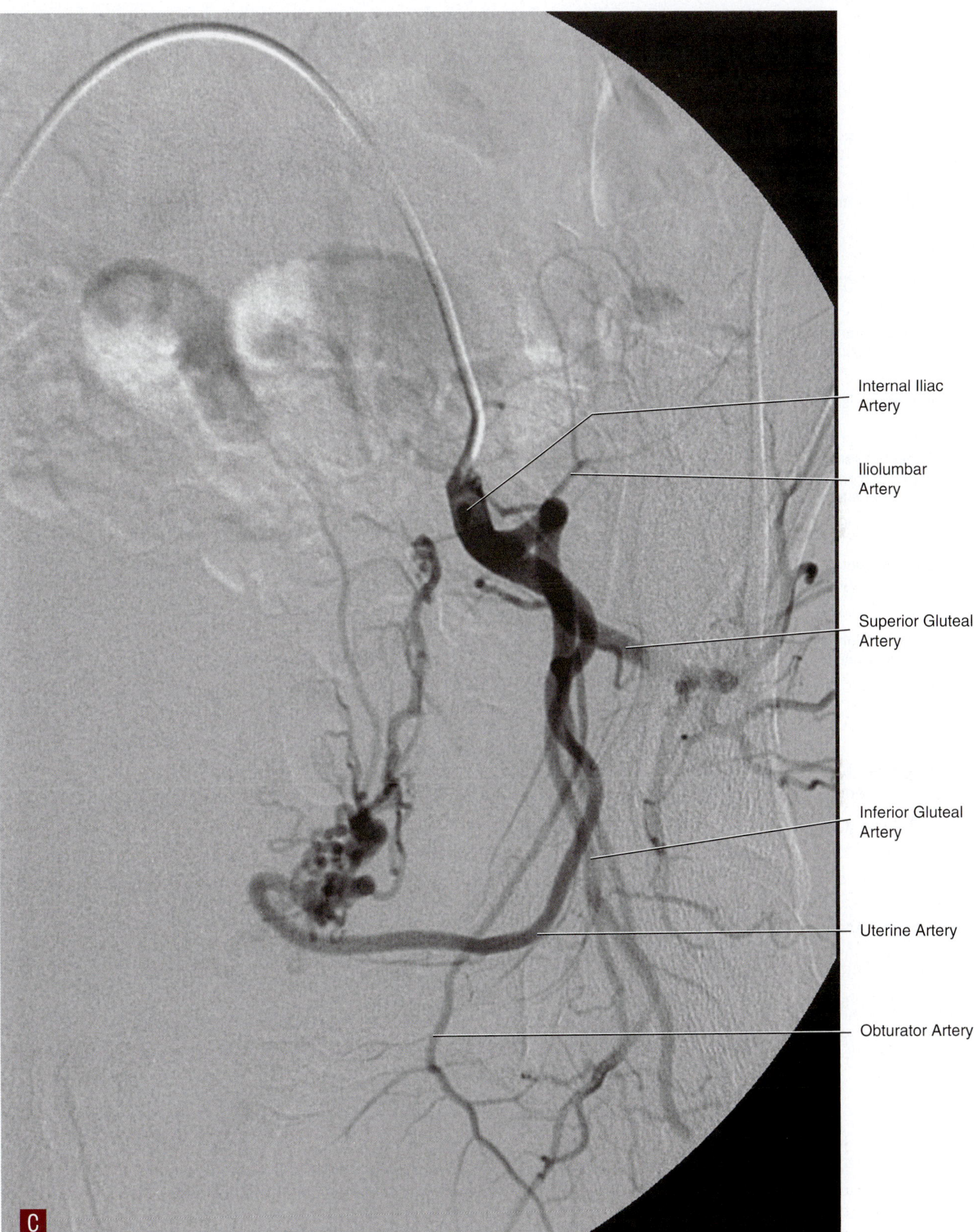

Figure 19.14. *Continued*

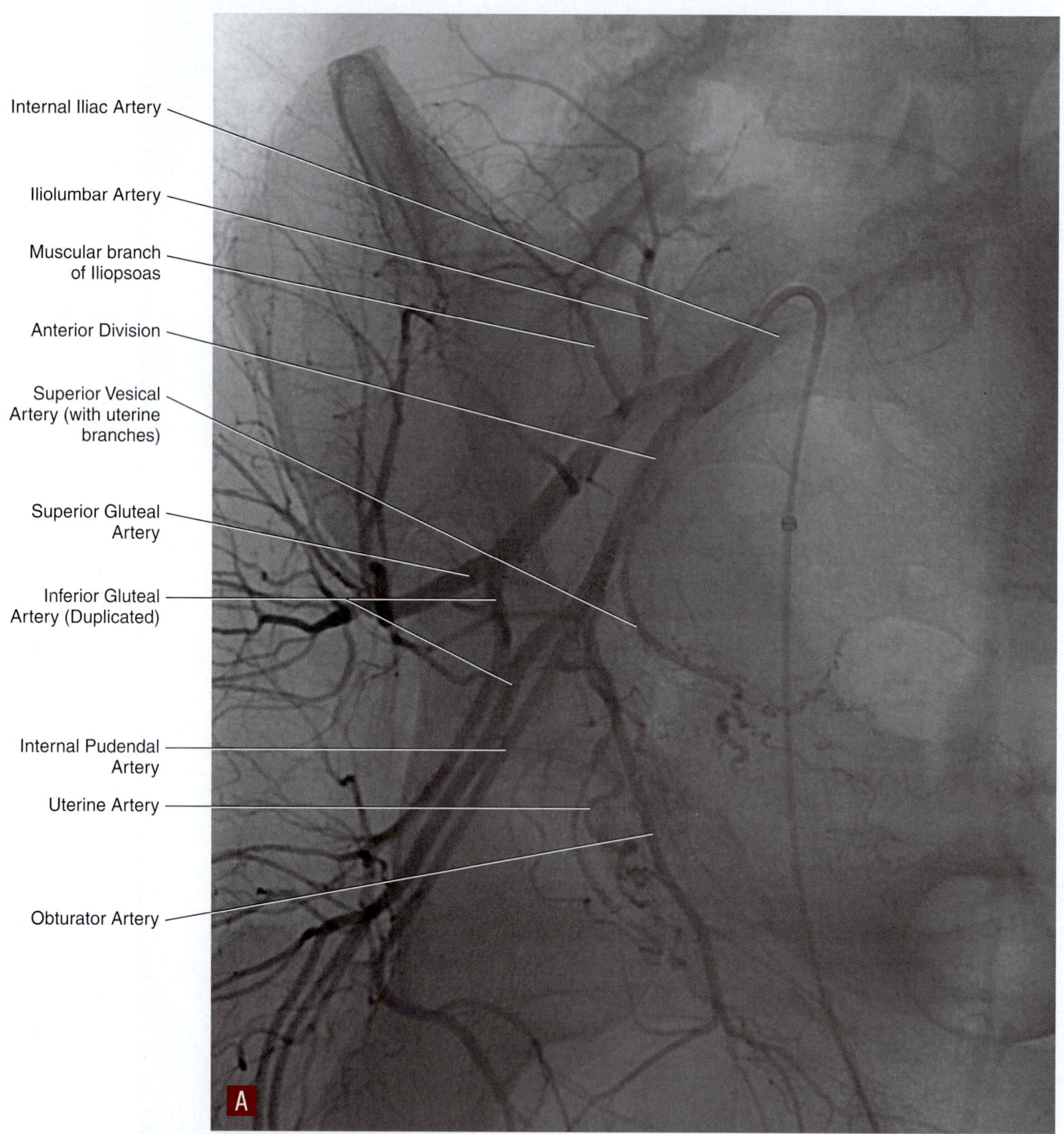

Figure 19.15. Variant origins of uterine blood supply. **A**, Pelvic arteriogram in a female patient with uterine fibroids and a diminutive right uterine artery arising as a common trunk with the superior vesical artery. **B**, Selective angiogram of the right ovarian artery in the same patient showing dominant supply to the fibroid as seen in a type II uterine-ovarian anastomosis. **C**, External iliac artery angiogram in a different patient showing the dominant uterine supply on the left to be from a left artery of the round ligament. The artery arises from the left inferior epigastric artery, which also gives rise to a left aberrant obturator artery.

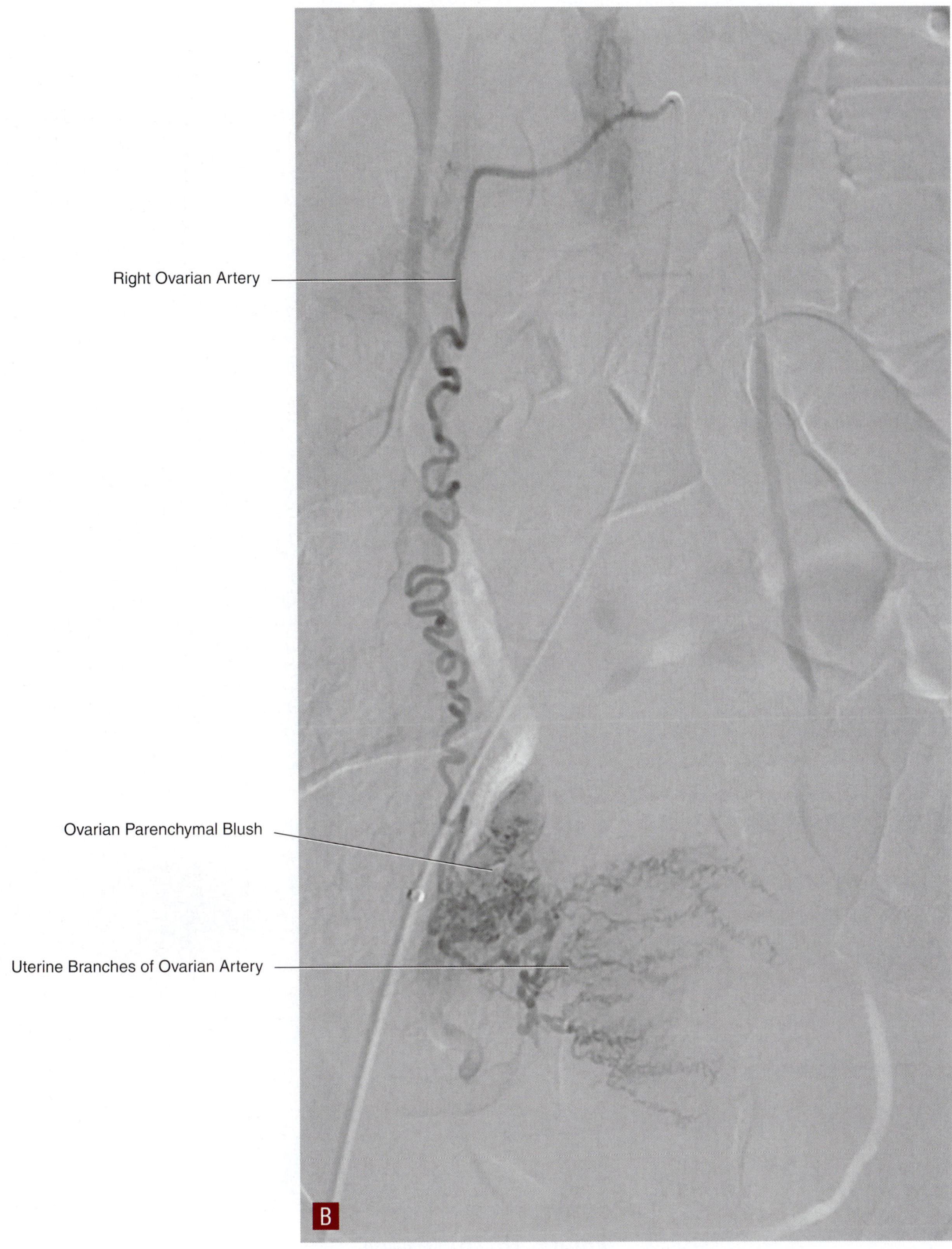

Figure 19.15. *Continued*

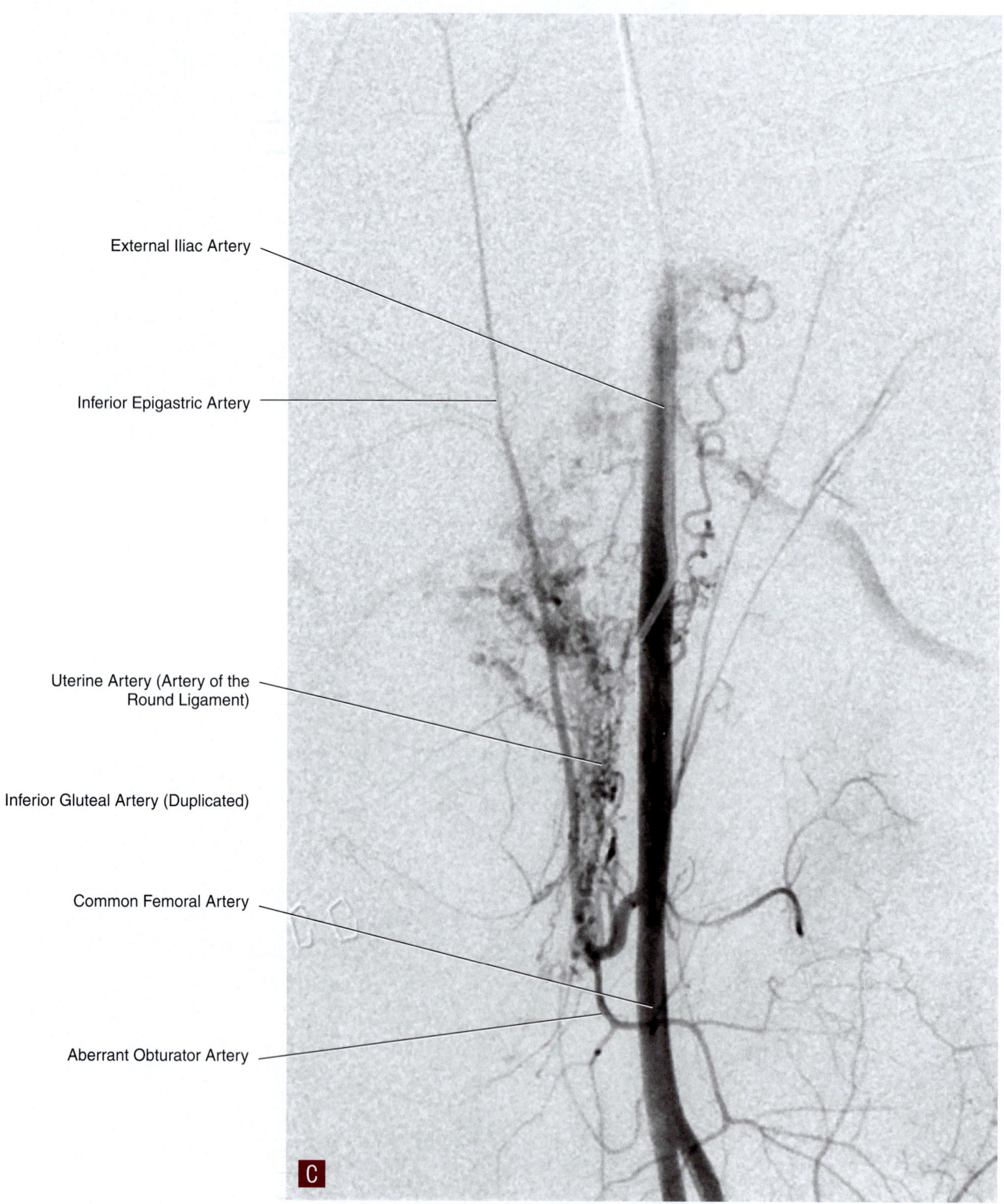

Figure 19.15. *Continued*

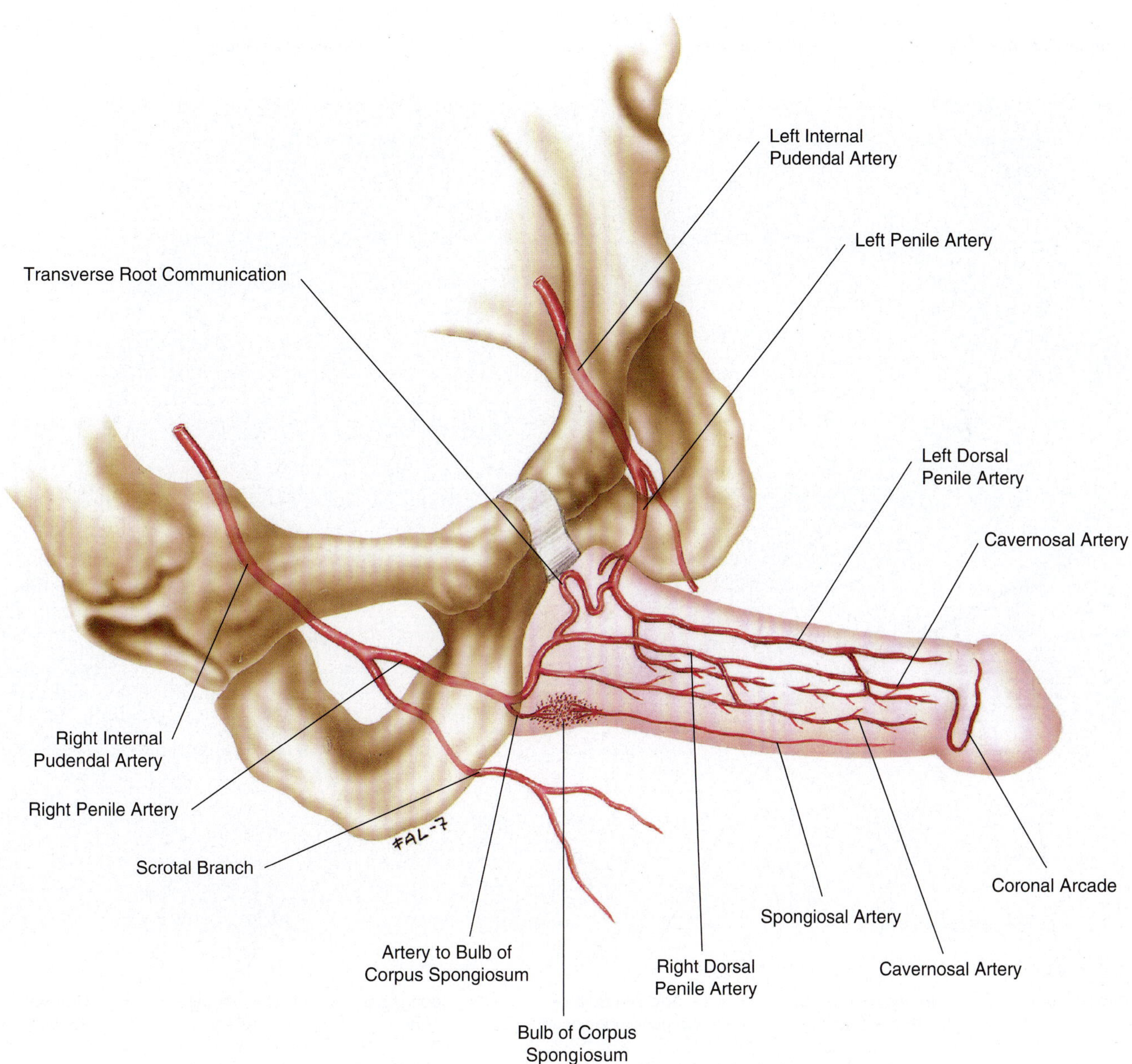

Figure 19.16. Schematic diagram of the penile arterial anatomy in an oblique projection. Not all arteries are always visible in the angiograms. The cavernosal artery is also called the deep penile artery. Branches of the cavernosal artery are the helicine arteries. The spongiosal artery is not always visible and the interruption at the bulb of the corpus spongiosum is an angiographic artifact. Sometimes, the spongiosal artery arises independently from the bulbar artery.

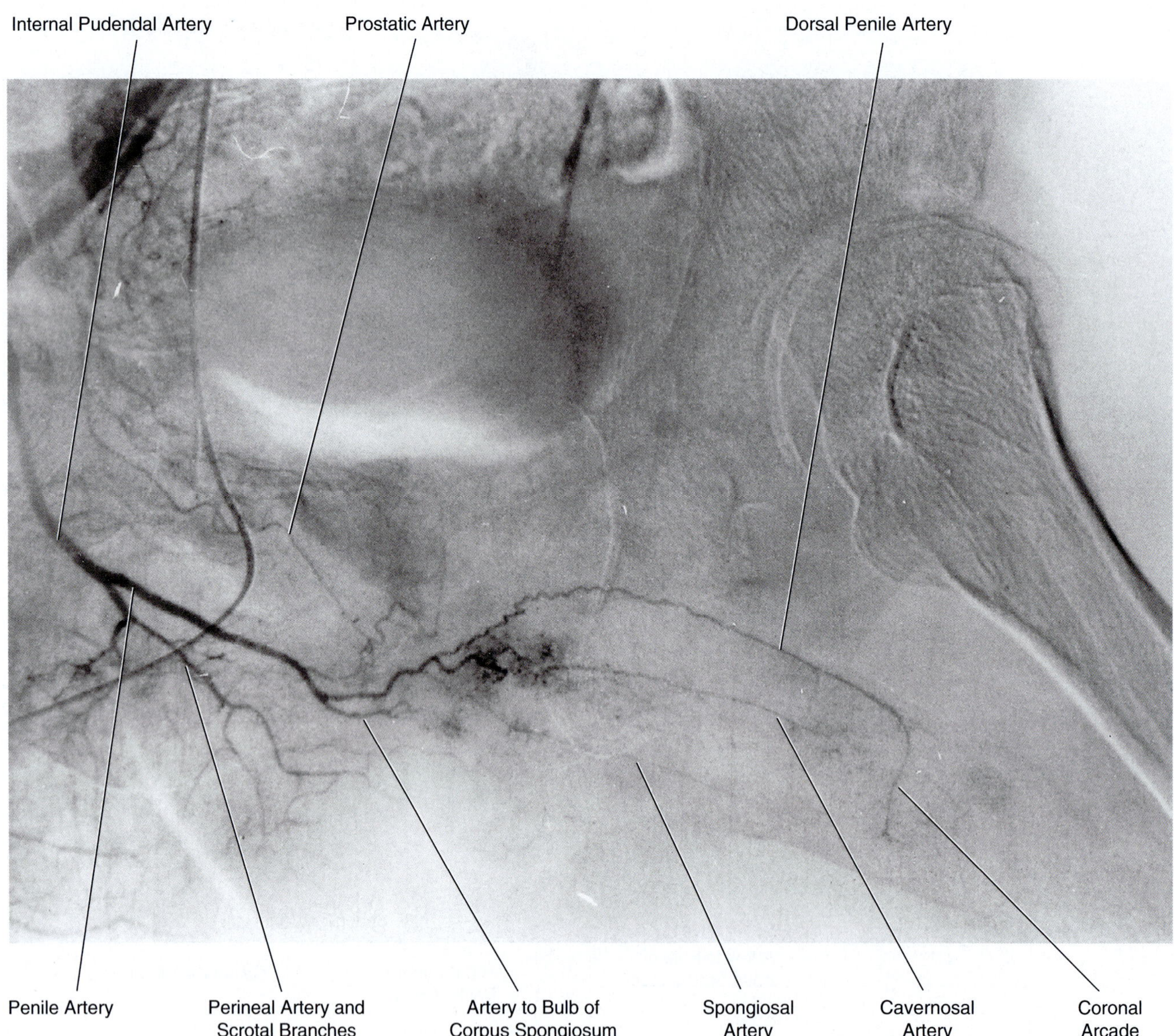

Figure 19.17. Selective right internal pudendal angiogram showing the classic arterial anatomy of the penis in the left posterior projection. The penile artery is the continuation of the internal pudendal artery after it gives origin to the perineal artery, and scrotal branches. Dorsal penile artery is large and long along the dorsum of the penis. Note the coronal arcade. Cavernosal artery is thinner and follows a path inside the corpus cavernosum. The artery to bulb of the corpus spongiosum is the first branch of the penile artery.

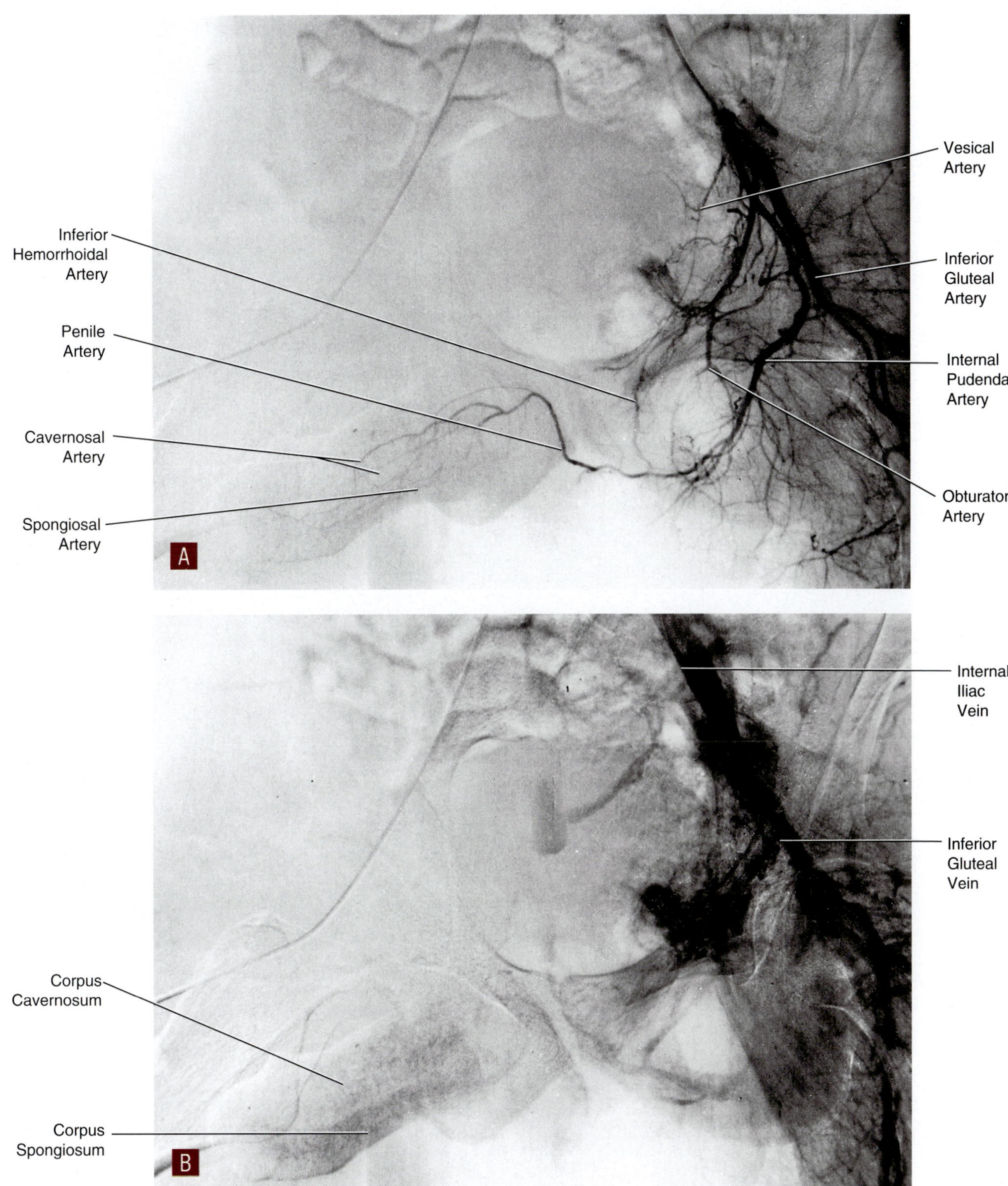

Figure 19.18. **A**, Selective left internal iliac angiogram showing the penile arterial anatomy. Right posterior projection. Note small size of the dorsal penile artery in this patient. The cavernosal artery is larger than usual and freely anastomoses with segments of the dorsal penile artery. **B**, Late phase of the angiogram showing the corpus cavernosum and corpus spongiosum.

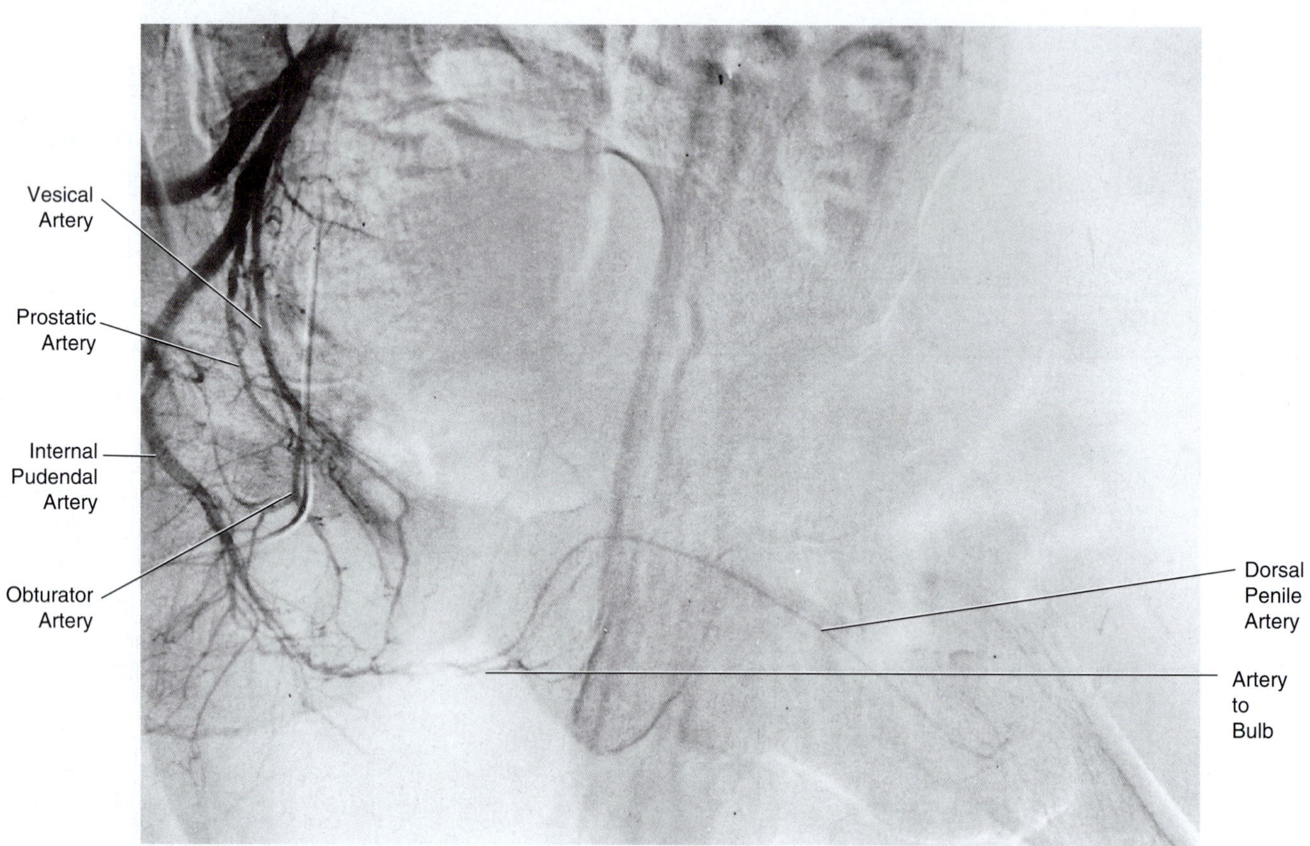

Figure 19.19. Selective angiography of the right internal iliac artery showing only the dorsal penile artery. The cavernosal artery either may be occluded or originate from the left side.

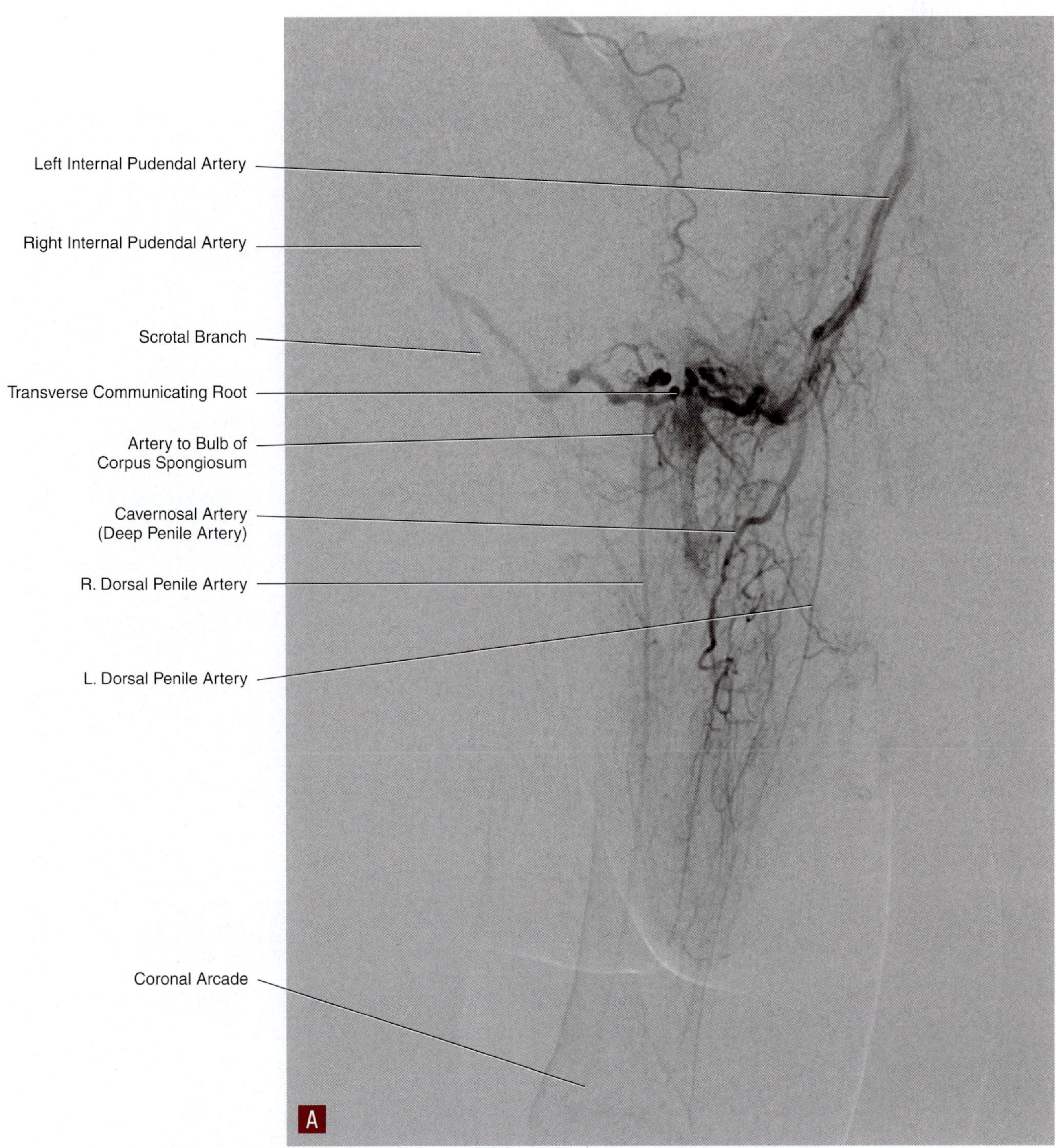

Figure 19.20. A, Selective angiography of the left internal pudendal artery in an anterior-posterior projection. The right dorsal penile artery is visualized filling via the transverse communicating root with reflux into the right internal pudendal artery and prostatic branches. The left dorsal penile artery is diminutive. The left spongiosal and cavernosal arteries are well visualized on the left. The bulbar artery is small. B, Selective angiogram of the right internal pudendal artery in the same patient showing the dorsal penile artery and the cavernosal, spongiosal, and bulbar arteries. Scrotal and perineal branches of the internal pudendal artery are also visualized as is the coronal arcade.

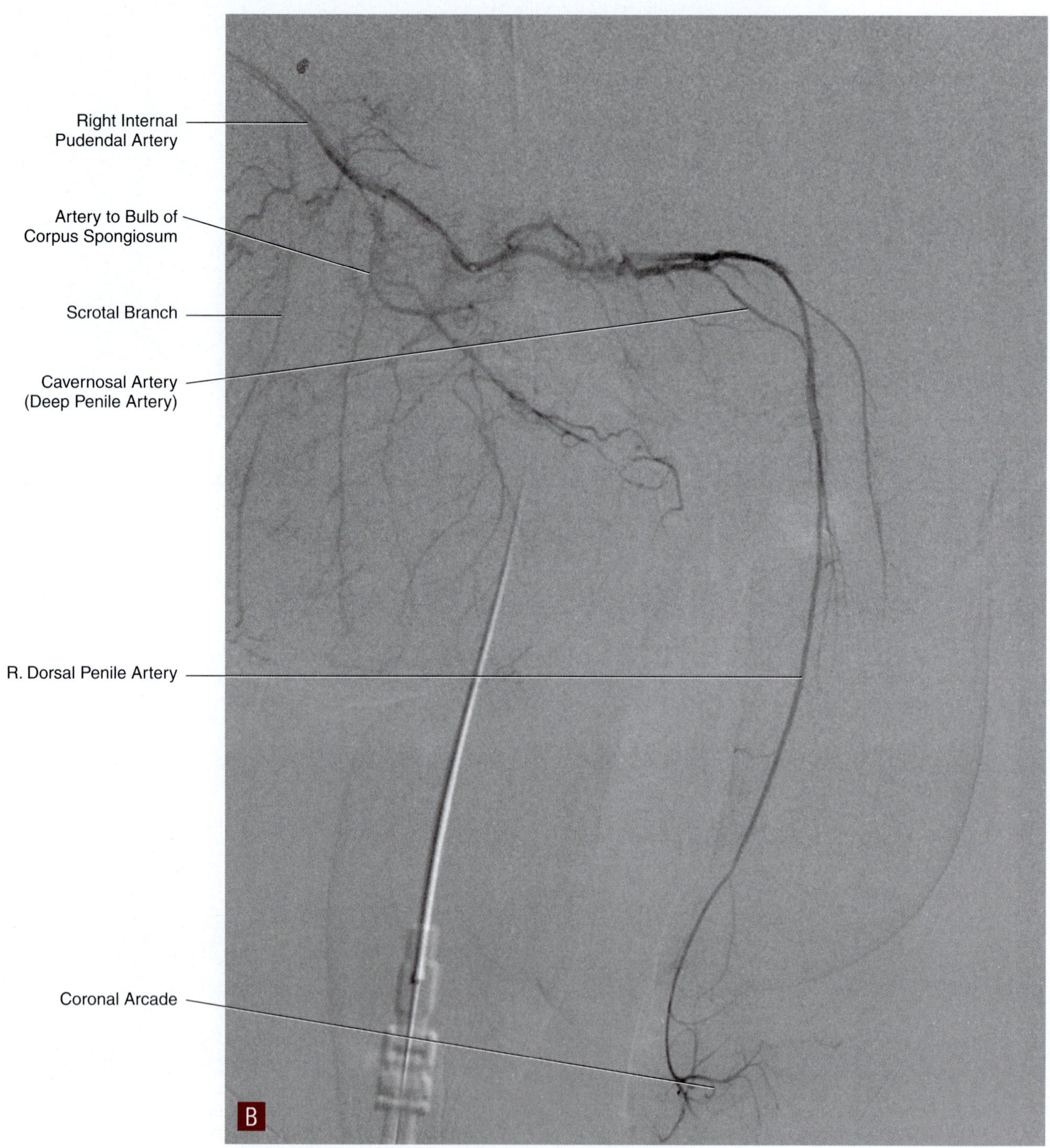

Figure 19.20. *Continued*

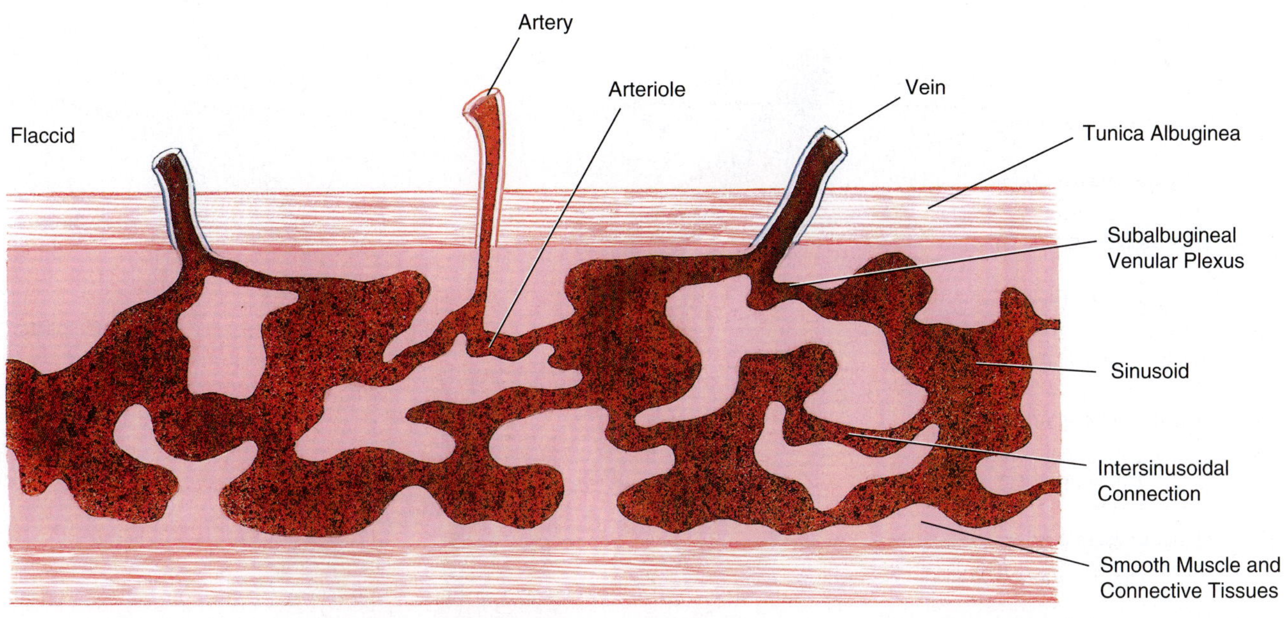

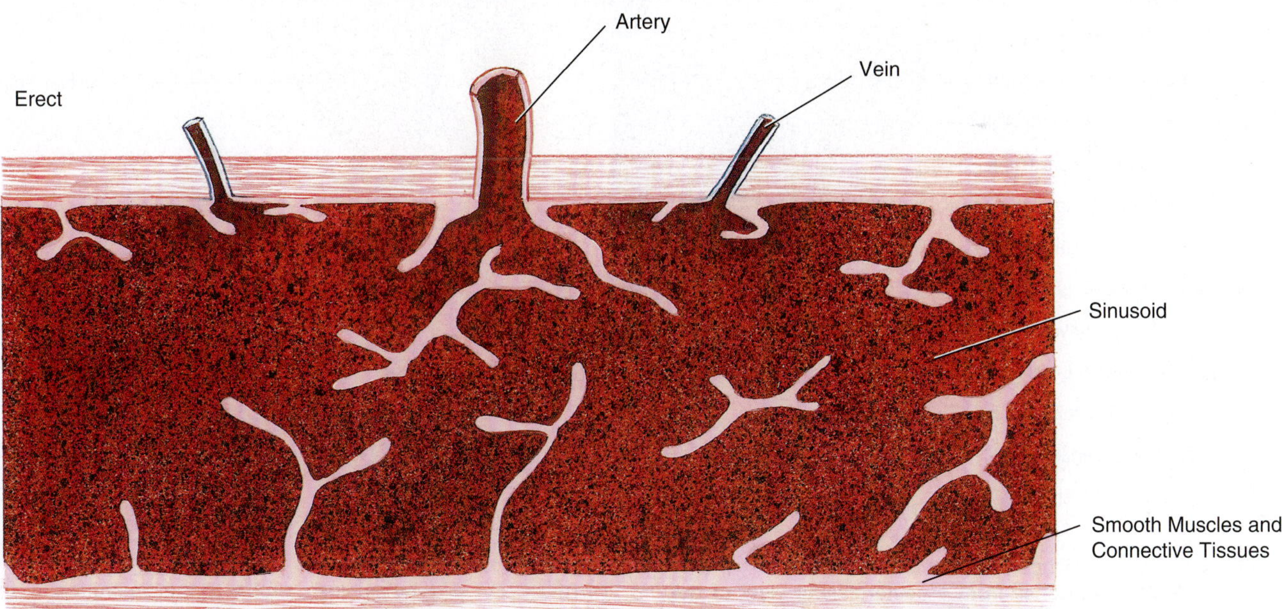

Figure 19.21. Schematic diagram of the cavernosal smooth muscle and sinusoids. When flaccid, the sinusoids are smaller in capacity and the muscle has a high tonus, limiting arterial inflow. Venous outflow is normally unrestricted. After stimulation, the sinusoidal smooth muscle relaxes and the sinusoids distend, reducing resistance to arterial flow and obstructing the venous outflow by compressing the peripheral venules against the tunica albuginea, raising the cavernosal pressure close to systolic pressure.

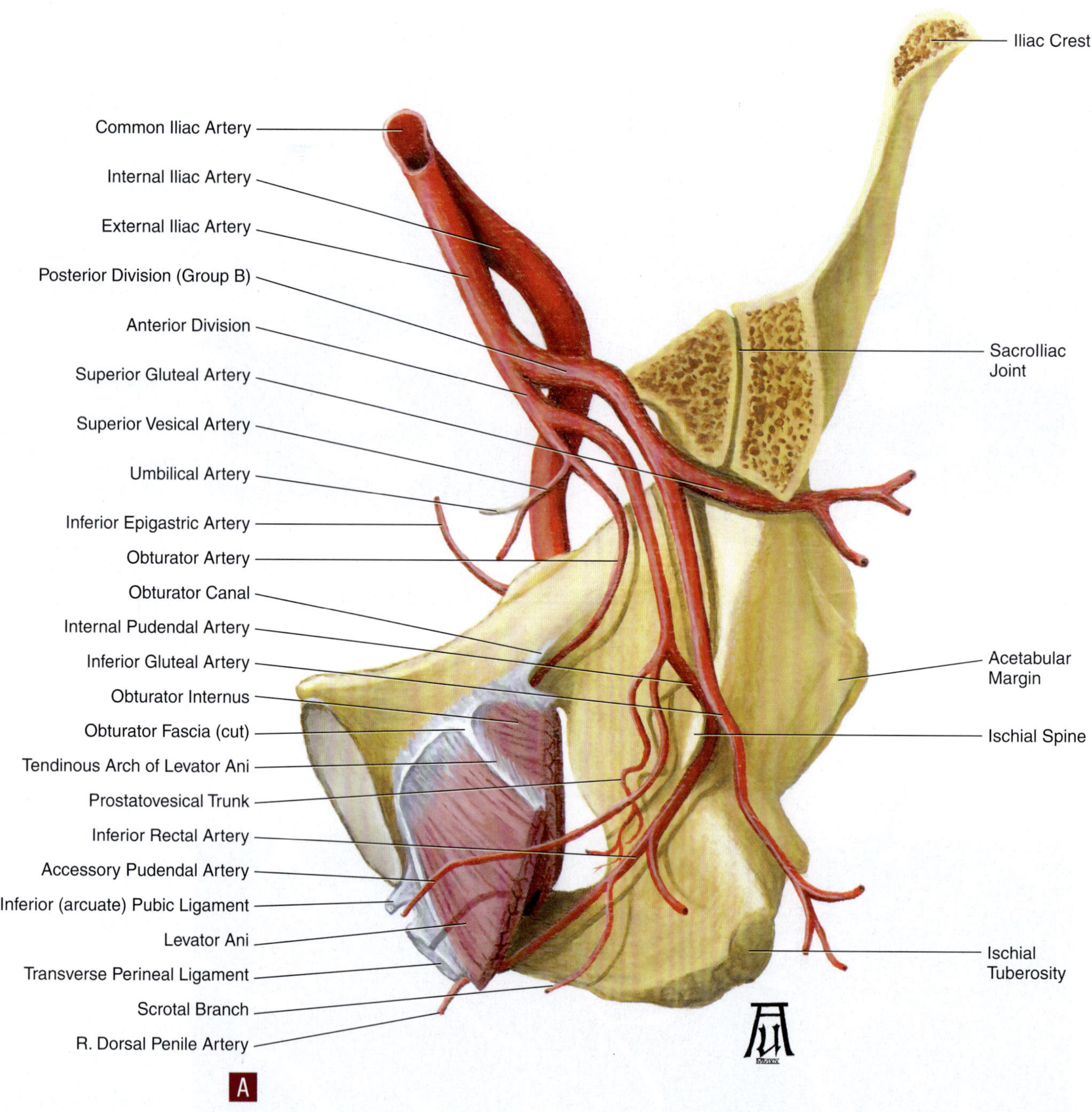

Figure 19.22. Schematic diagram showing four types of accessory pudendal arteries from a posterolateral view of the pelvis with angiographic views. **A**, Lateral accessory pudendal artery arising from the anterior division in a group B internal iliac bifurcation. The artery courses in the groove between the prostate, bladder, and pelvic wall. **B**, Apical accessory pudendal artery arising from the internal pudendal artery. The artery courses laterally and inferior to the puboprostatic ligament along the anterolateral surface of the prostatic apex before entering the dorsal vascular complex. **C**, Lateral accessory pudendal artery arising from an aberrant obturator artery. **D**, Aberrant pudendal artery arising from the obturator artery. In this variant, the aberrant pudendal artery is the main supply to the dorsal vascular complex in the involved pelvic half. **E**, Right anterior oblique view of an aberrant pudendal artery arising (solid black arrows) from the obturator artery (dashed arrows), supplying the dorsal vascular complex with cavernosal blush, similar to the illustration in (**D**). **F**, Aberrant pudendal artery (solid black arrows) arising from the obturator artery (dashed arrows) in the same patient as (**F**) in left anterior oblique view. Prostatic branches (curved dashed arrow) are seen as well as cavernosal blush at the penile hilum (curved solid black arrow). **G**, 3D volume-rendered reconstruction in the sagittal plane of a right hemi pelvis showing a group B internal iliac artery bifurcation with the superior and inferior gluteal arteries arising from the posterior division (curved dashed arrows). The internal pudendal artery (curved solid arrows) arises as a large trunk with the obturator artery (straight dashed arrows) which gives rise to an accessory pudendal artery (solid straight arrows). (Image 22E, 22F, and 22G courtesy of Dr. Tiago Bilhim, MD and João Martins Pisco, MD.)

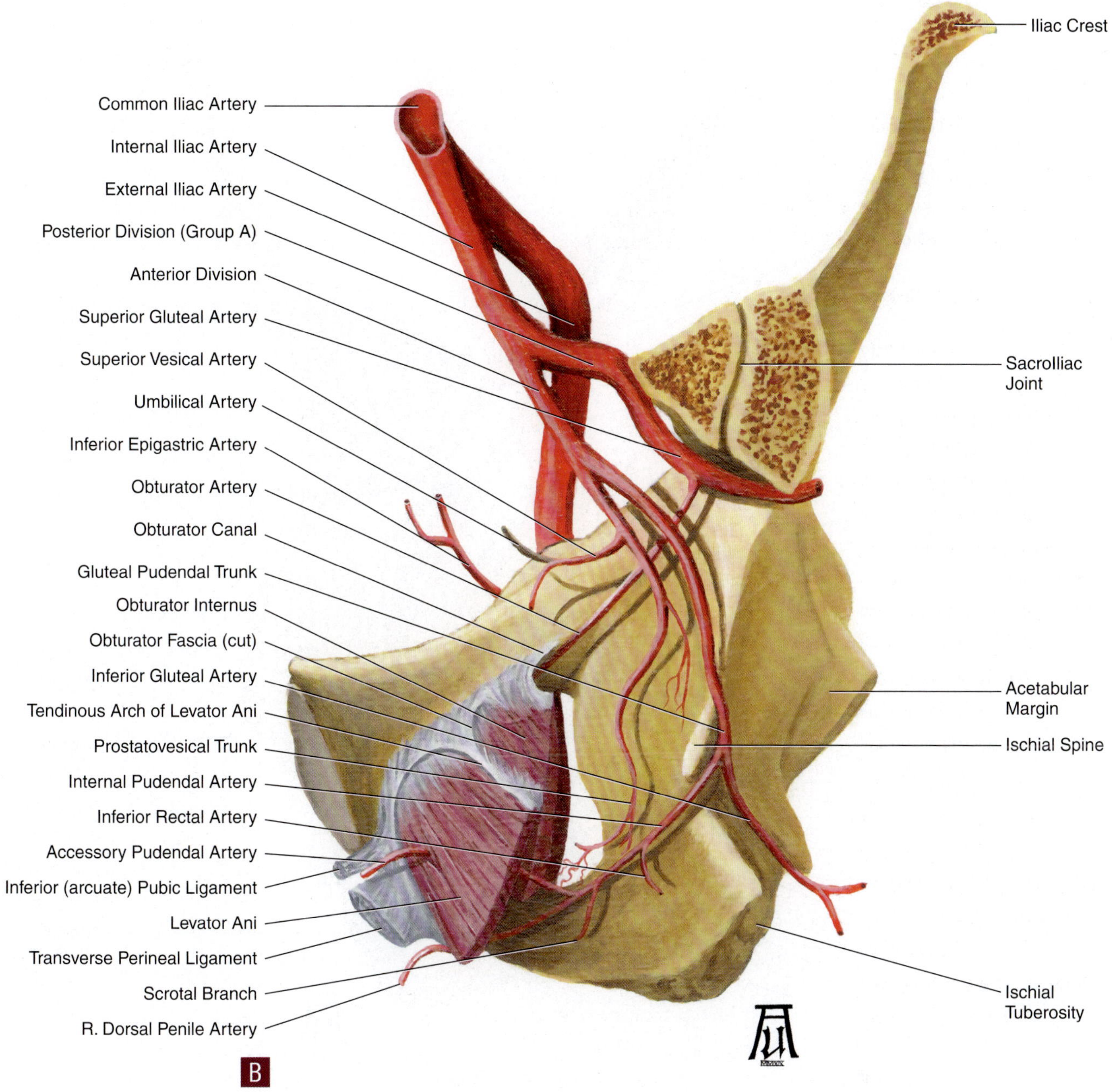

Iliac Crest
Common Iliac Artery
Internal Iliac Artery
External Iliac Artery
Posterior Division (Group A)
Anterior Division
Superior Gluteal Artery
Superior Vesical Artery
Umbilical Artery
Inferior Epigastric Artery
Obturator Artery
Obturator Canal
Gluteal Pudendal Trunk
Obturator Internus
Obturator Fascia (cut)
Inferior Gluteal Artery
Tendinous Arch of Levator Ani
Prostatovesical Trunk
Internal Pudendal Artery
Inferior Rectal Artery
Accessory Pudendal Artery
Inferior (arcuate) Pubic Ligament
Levator Ani
Transverse Perineal Ligament
Scrotal Branch
R. Dorsal Penile Artery
SacroIliac Joint
Acetabular Margin
Ischial Spine
Ischial Tuberosity
B

Figure 19.22. *Continued*

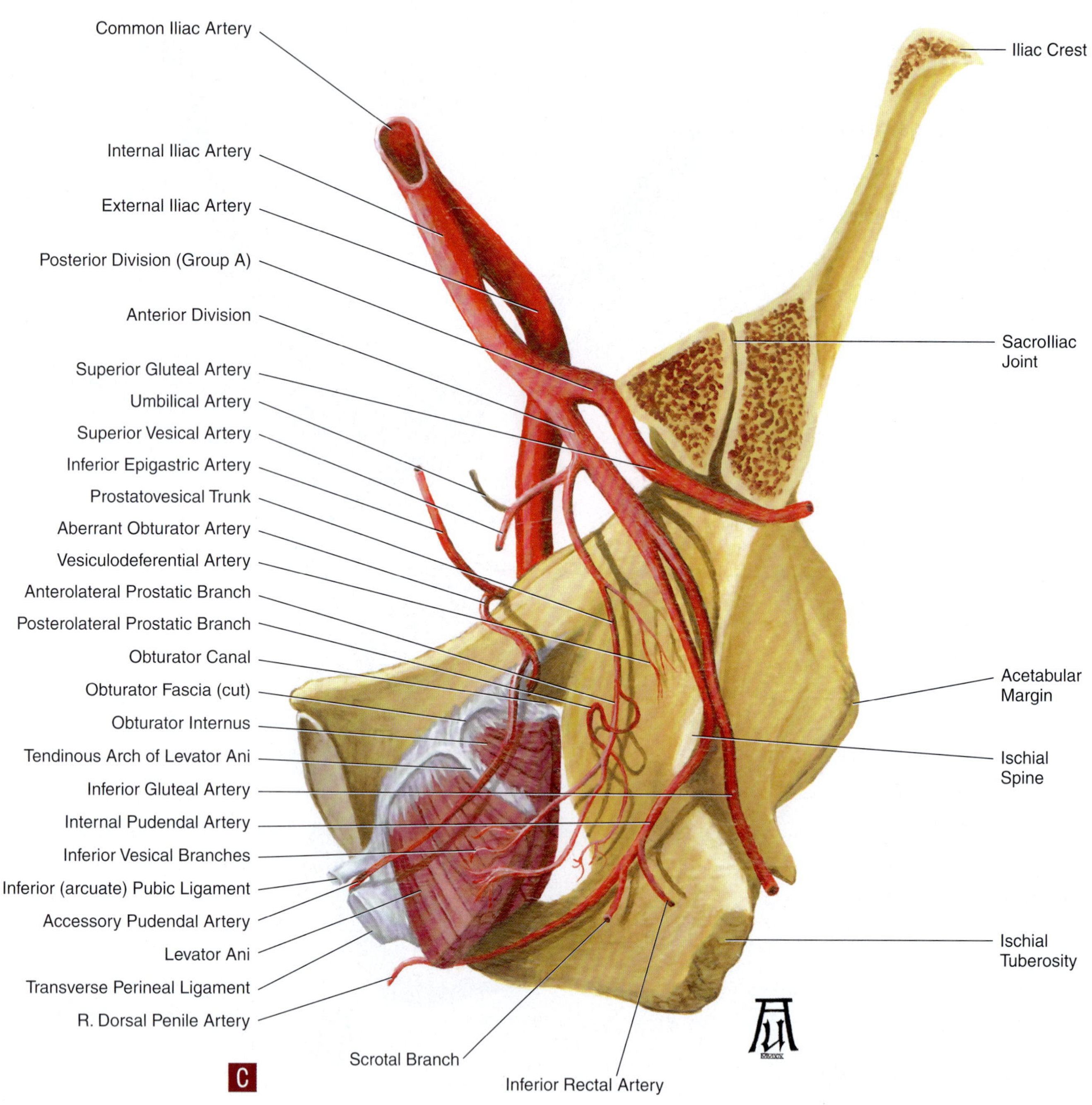

Figure 19.22. *Continued*

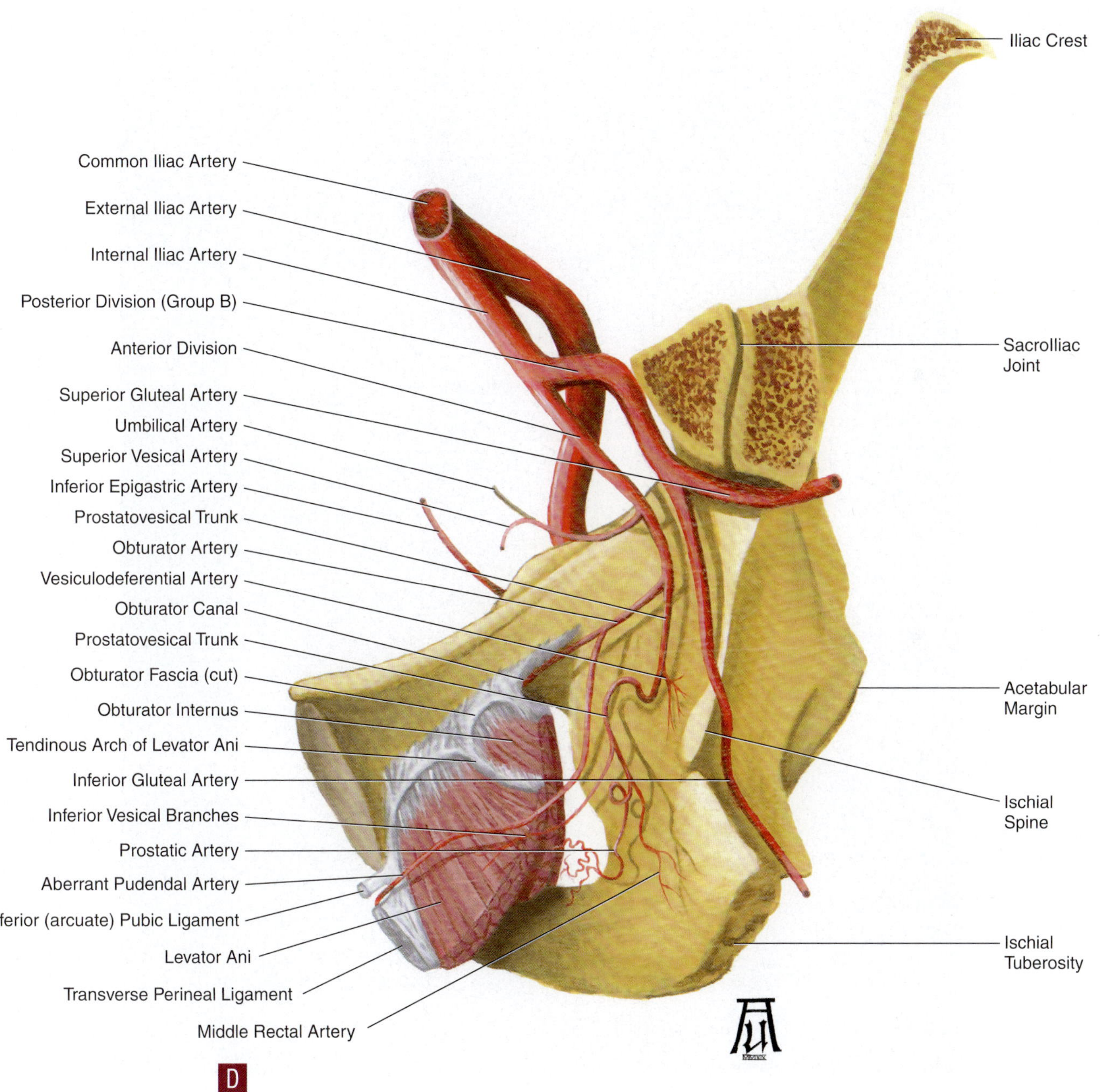

Figure 19.22. *Continued*

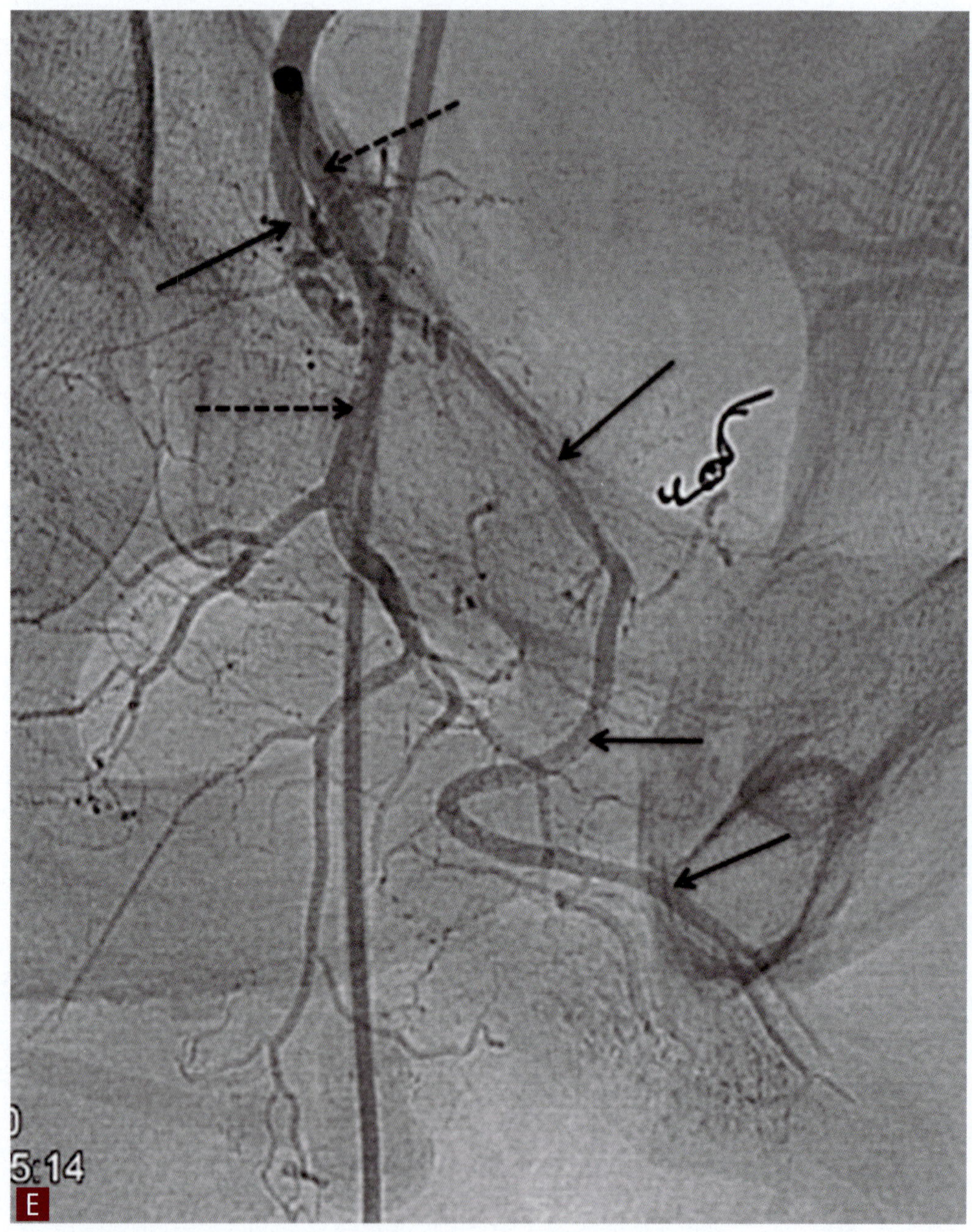

Figure 19.22. *Continued*

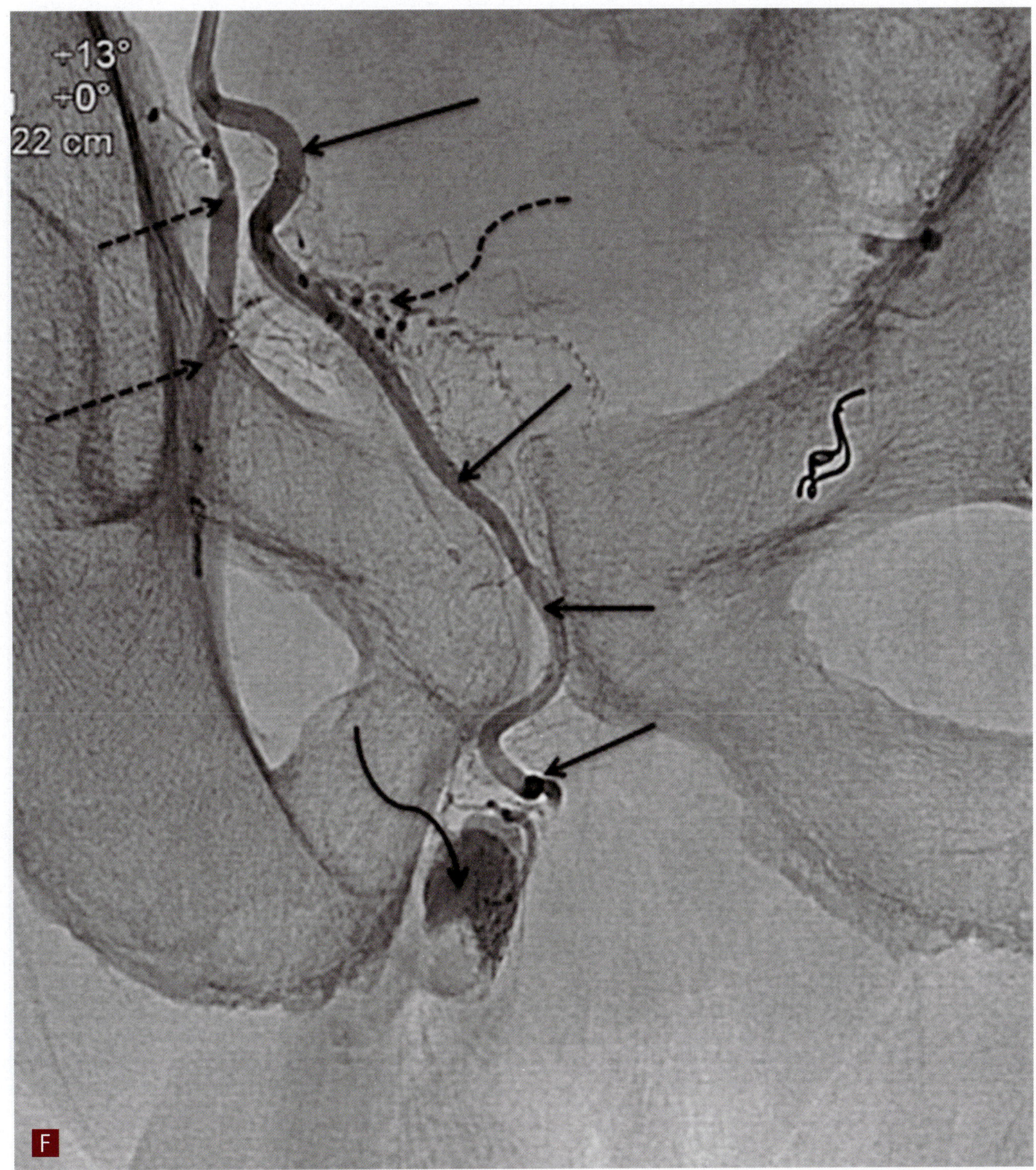

Figure 19.22. *Continued*

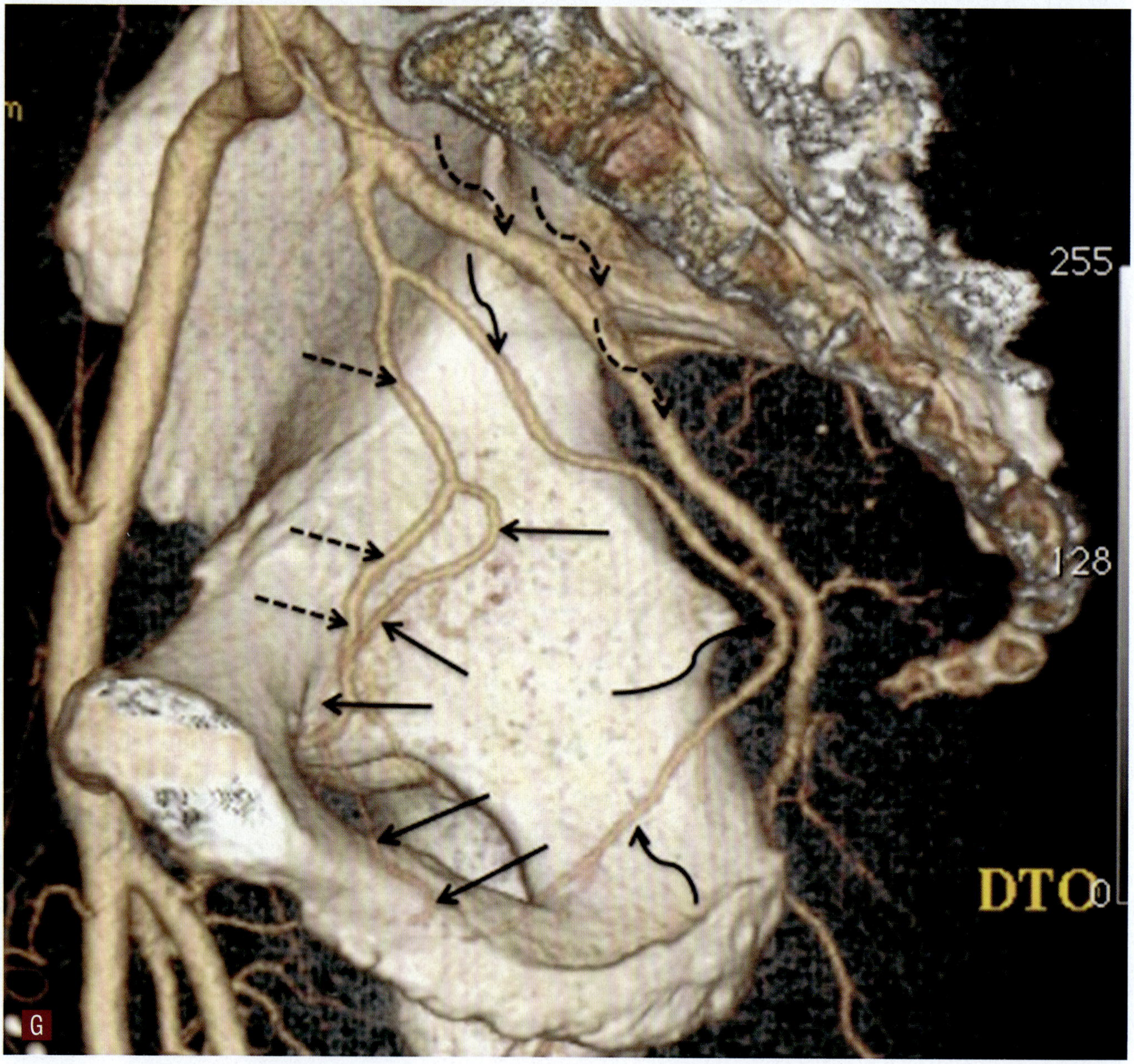

Figure 19.22. *Continued*

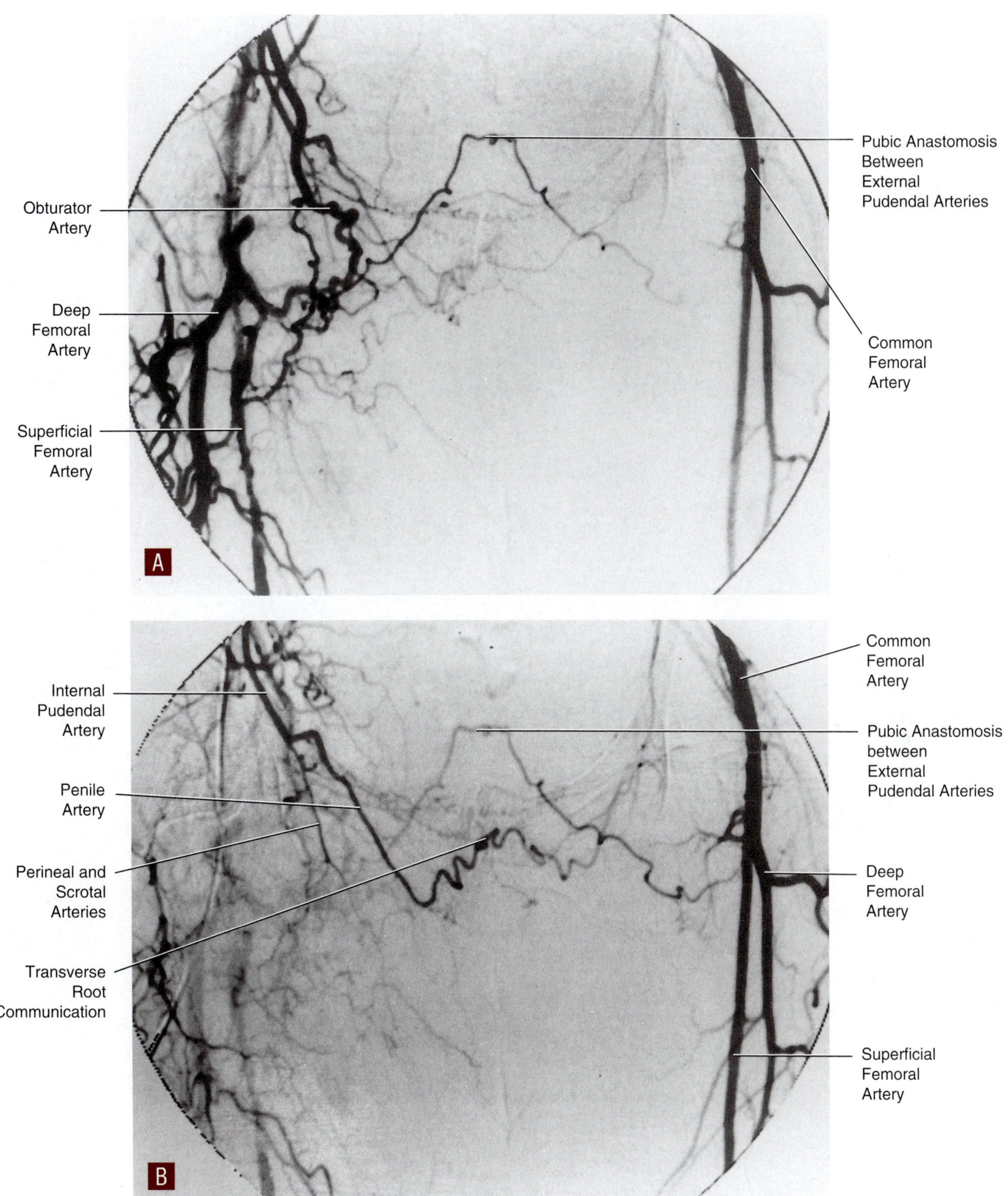

Figure 19.23. Pelvic angiography showing the communications between the right and left arterial systems through the transverse root communication (A) and between medial femoral circumflex arteries or external pudendal arteries (B) in a patient with vascular disease. C, Superselective angiogram of the left obturator artery showing a supply to the transverse root communication.

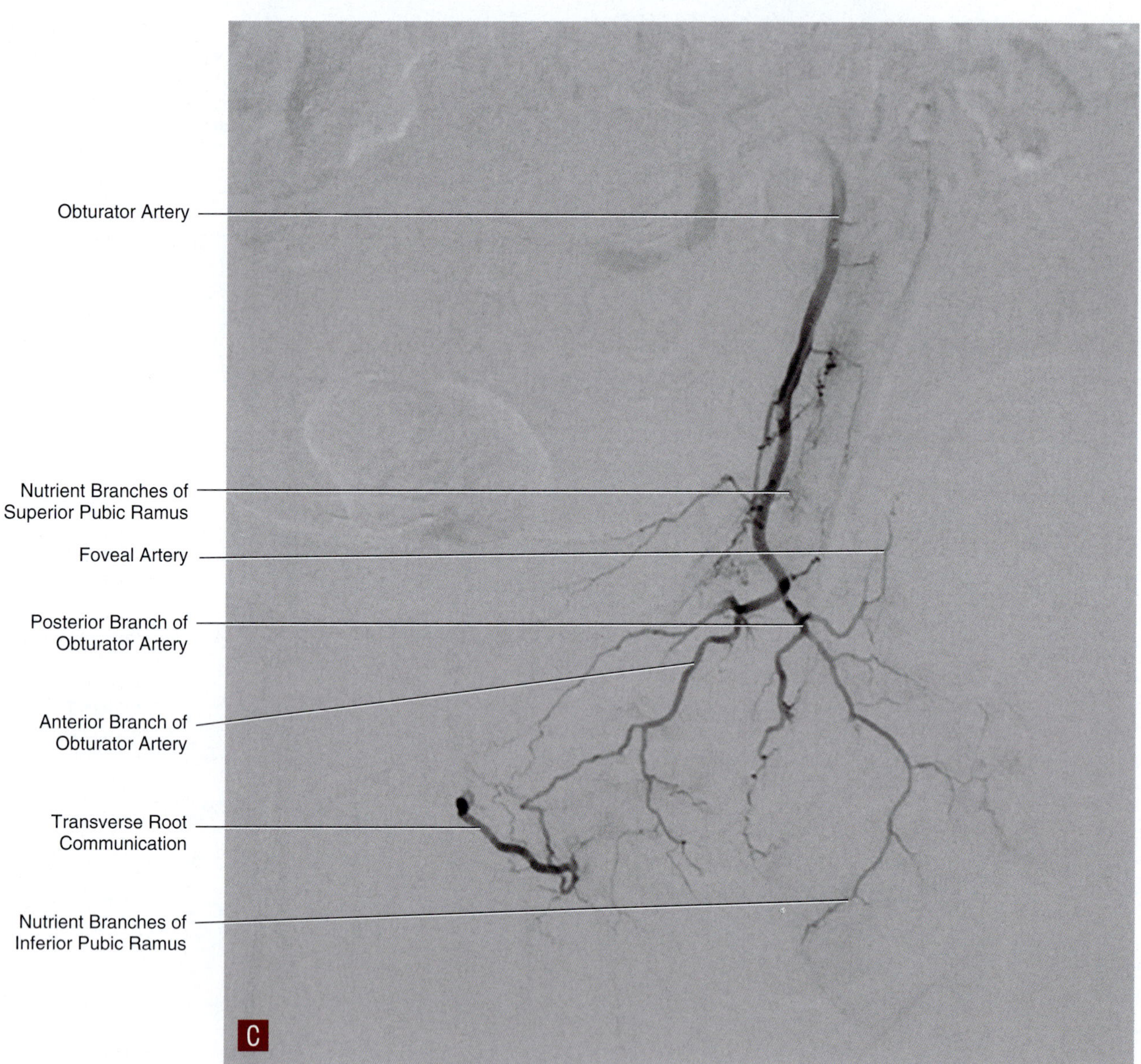

Figure 19.23. *Continued*

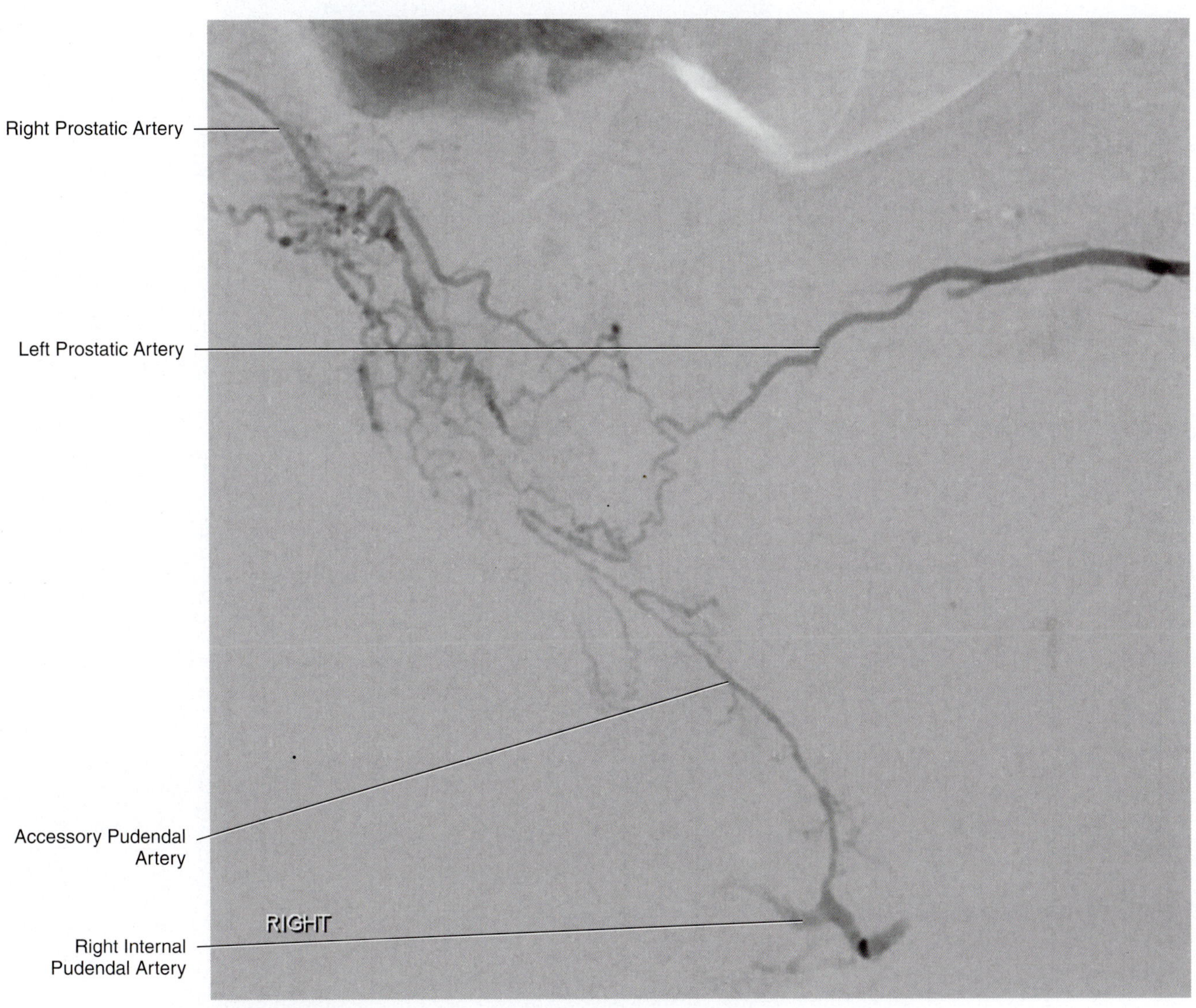

Figure 19.24. Superselective angiogram of the right prostatic artery showing an accessory pudendal artery anastomosing with the right internal pudendal artery.

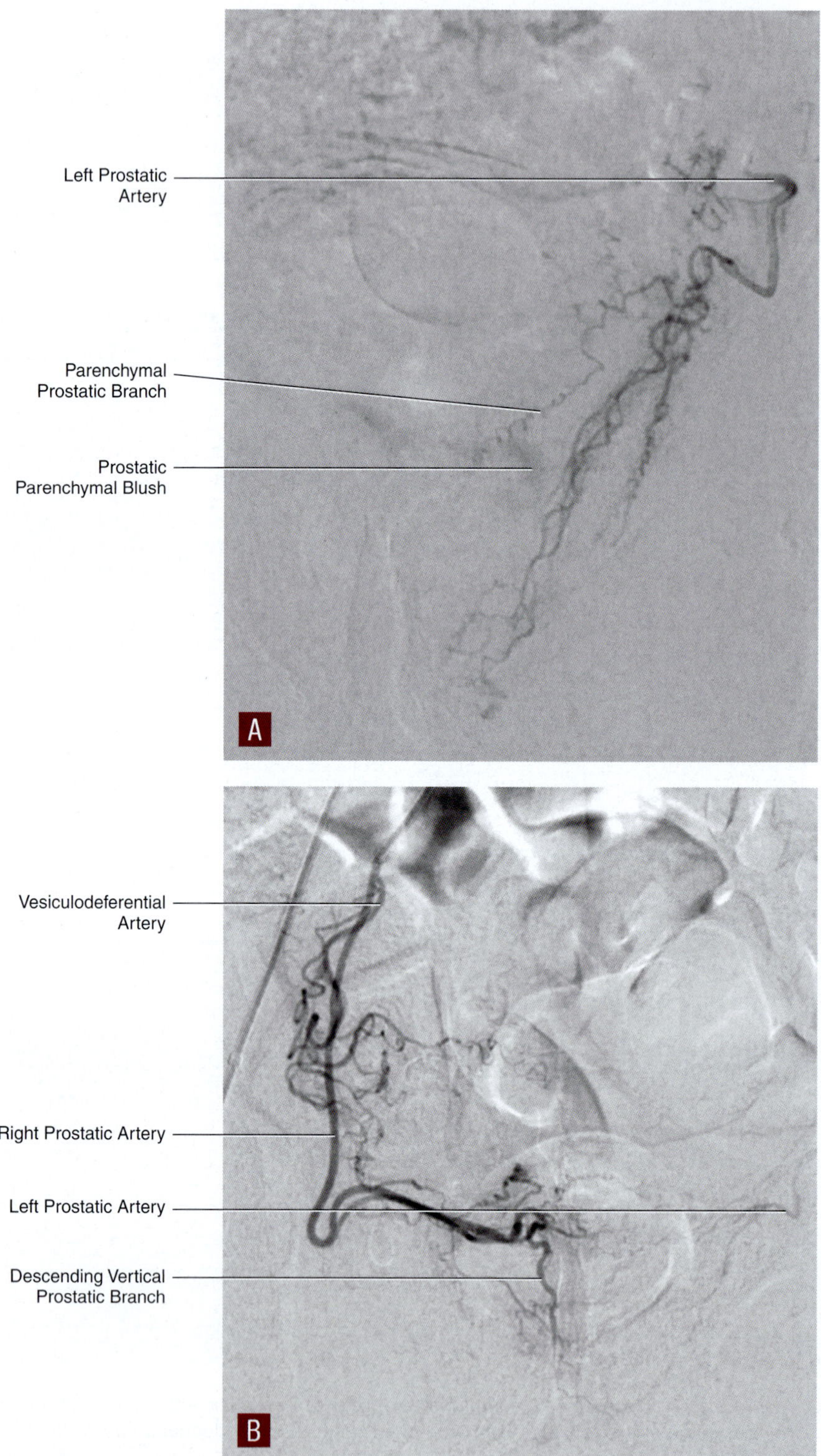

Figure 19.25. Angiographic appearance of the prostatic artery. A, Superselective left prostatic arteriogram showing early parenchymal enhancement and the characteristic spiral prostatic parenchymal branches. B, Right prostatic angiogram with inferior vesical branches, and vesiculodeferential arteries arising from the right prostatic artery. This injection shows a prominent central prostatic arterial communicating branch through which there is retrograde filling of the contralateral prostatic artery. C, Late phase of a superselective prostatic arteriogram showing parenchymal blush and filling of contralateral prostatic branches. D, Late phase superselective prostatic arteriogram showing parenchymal blush, enhancement of the bladder wall, and the median lobe prostatic branch. E, Superselective prostatic arteriogram showing communicating branches to a middle rectal artery. Note the mucosal blush in the lower left part of the figure. F, Filling of the contralateral internal pudendal artery and prostatovesical trunk and a prominent central prostatic arterial communicating branch similar to (B). G, Superselective angiogram of a left middle rectal artery (solid straight arrows) with communicating rectal branches to the superior rectal artery (curved solid arrows) from the inferior mesenteric artery. Anal blush is seen in the inferior aspect of the image (straight dashed arrow) as well as prostatic branches. (Image courtesy of Dr. Tiago Bilhim, MD and João Martins Pisco, MD.)

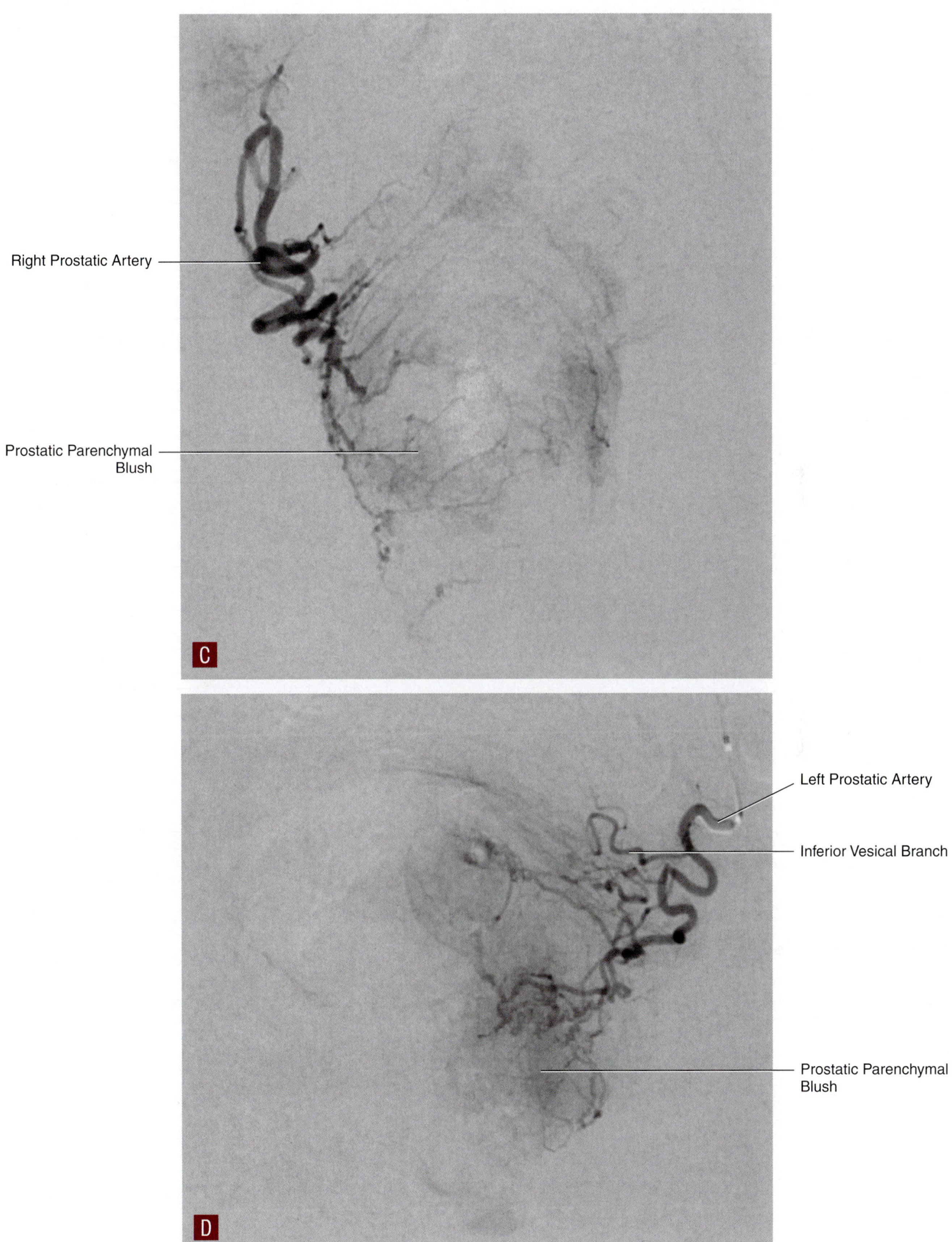

Figure 19.25. *Continued*

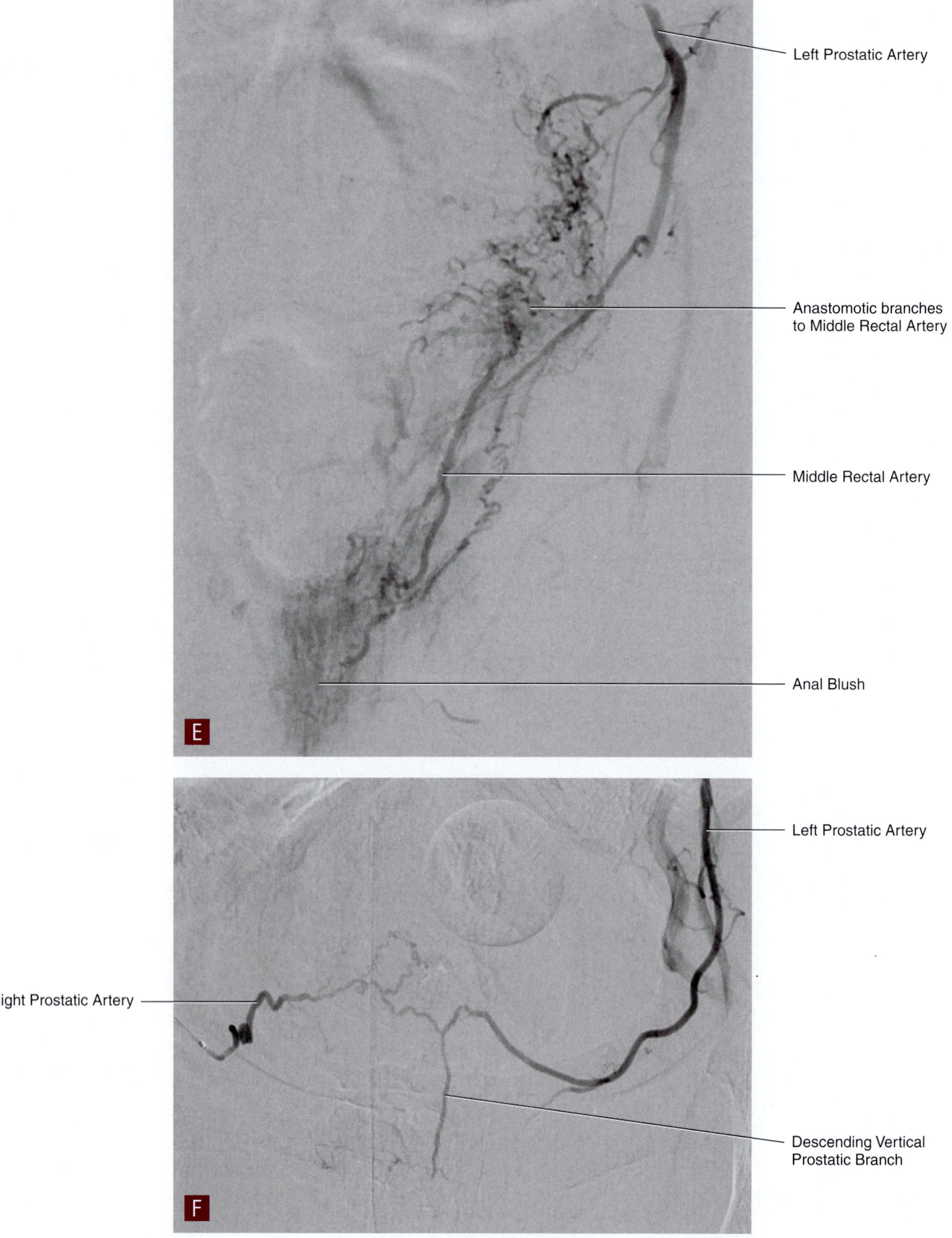

Figure 19.25. *Continued*

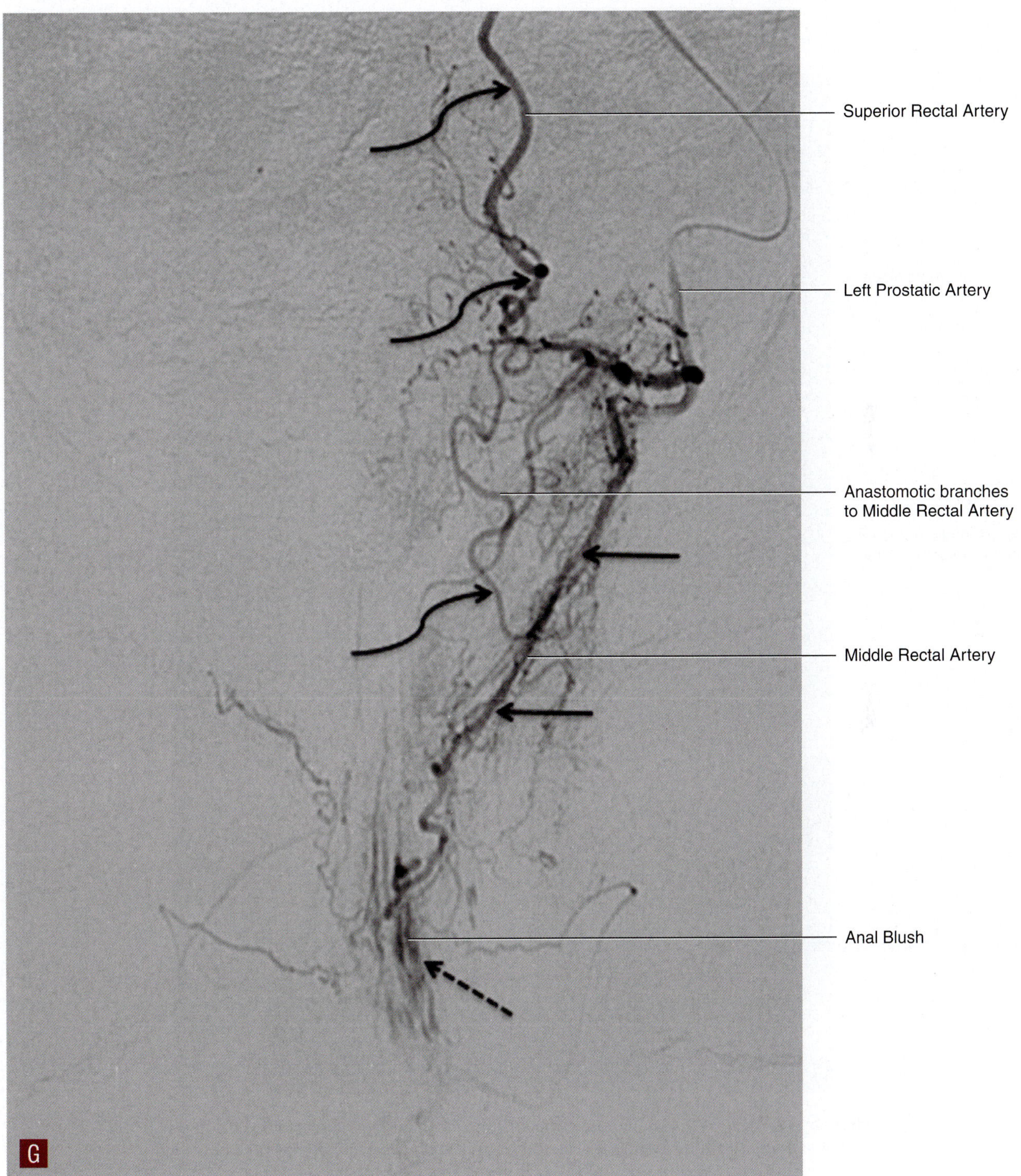

Figure 19.25. *Continued*

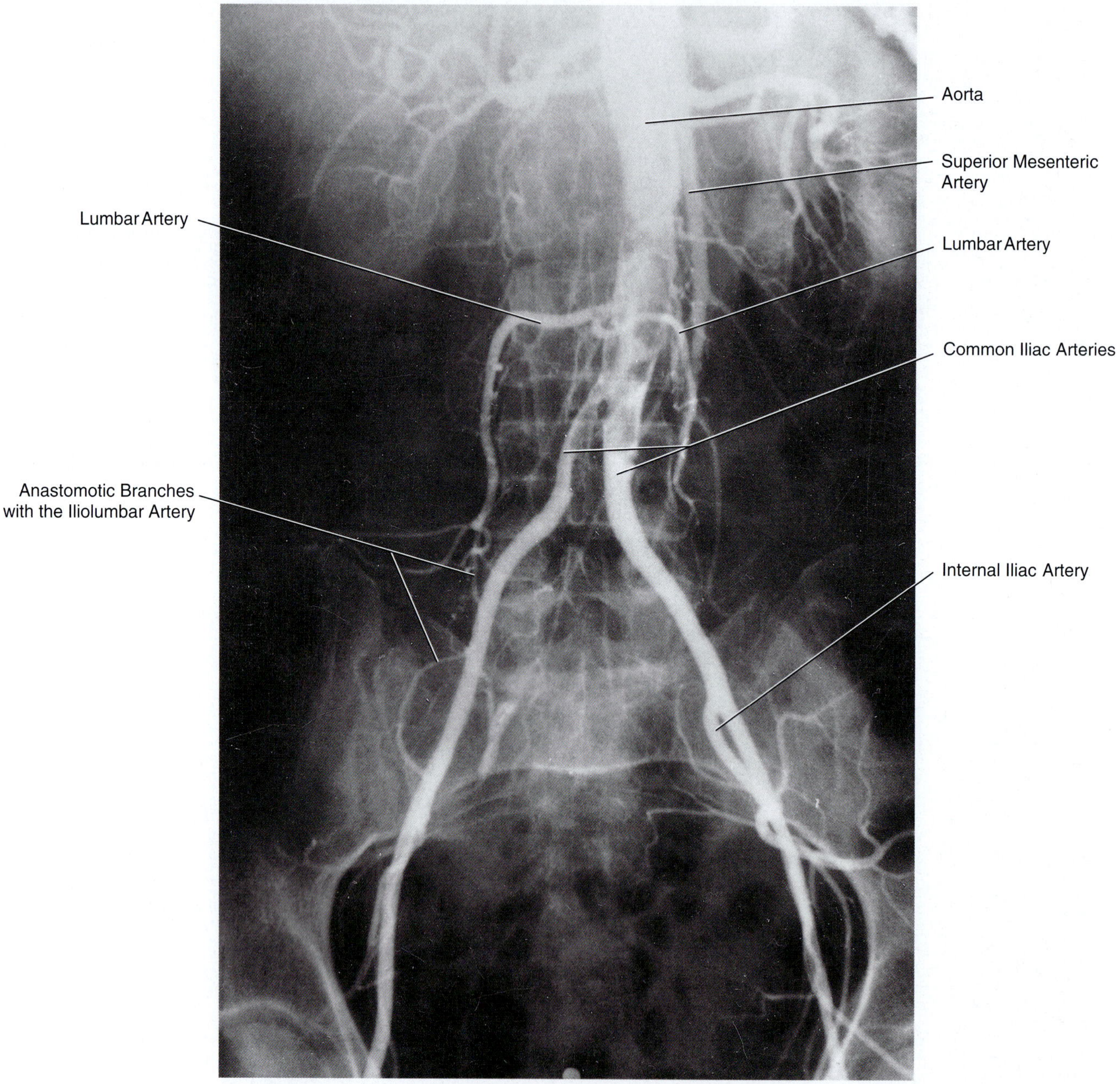

Figure 19.26. Pelvic angiography showing the development of anastomosis between the lumbar arteries and the internal iliac branches, due to an occlusion at the aortic bifurcation.

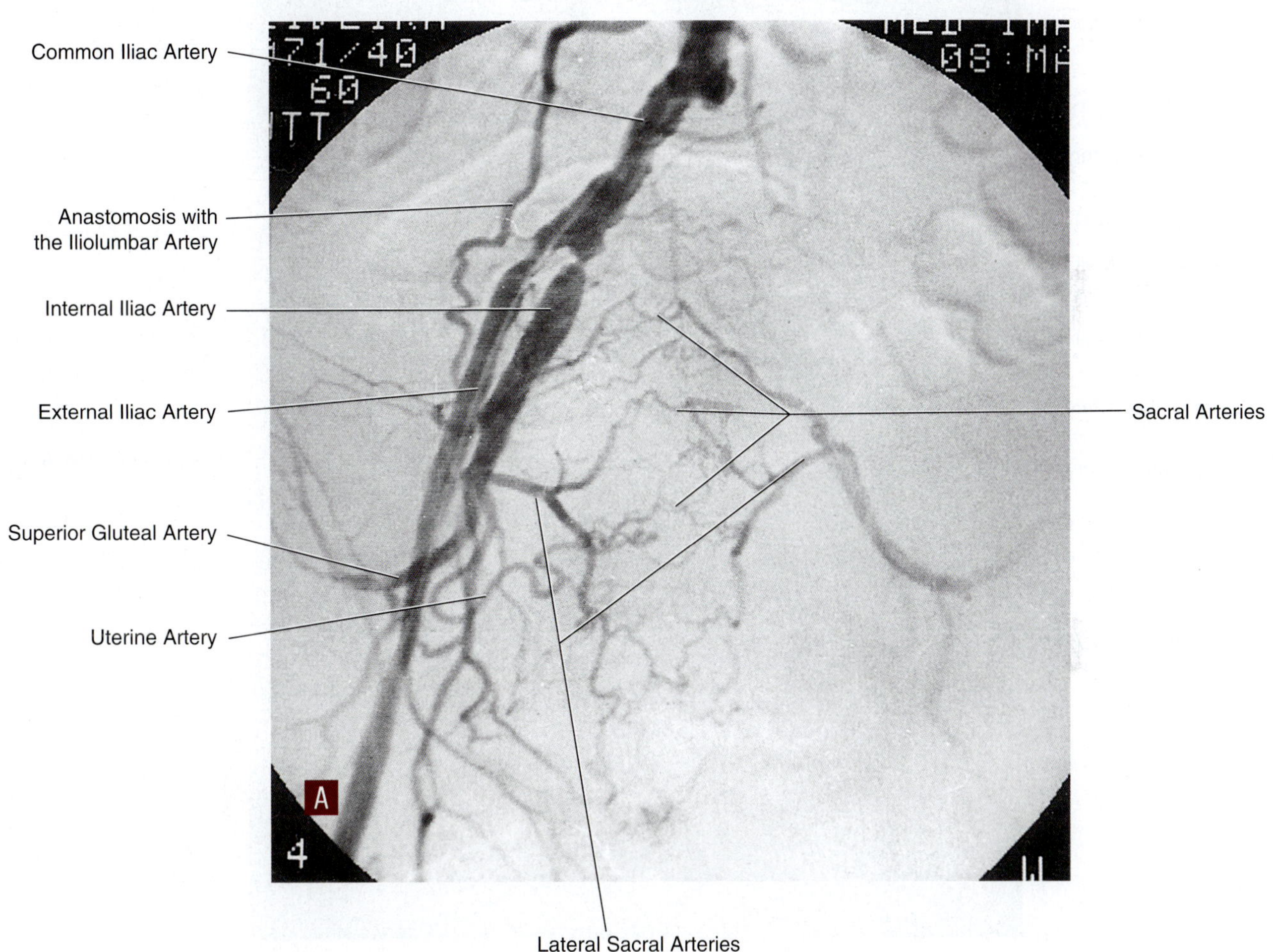

Figure 19.27. A, Pelvic angiography in a patient with arterial occlusive disease in the proximal right internal iliac artery shows development of the lateral sacral arteries and the gluteal arteries. B, Late phase of the same pelvic angiography.

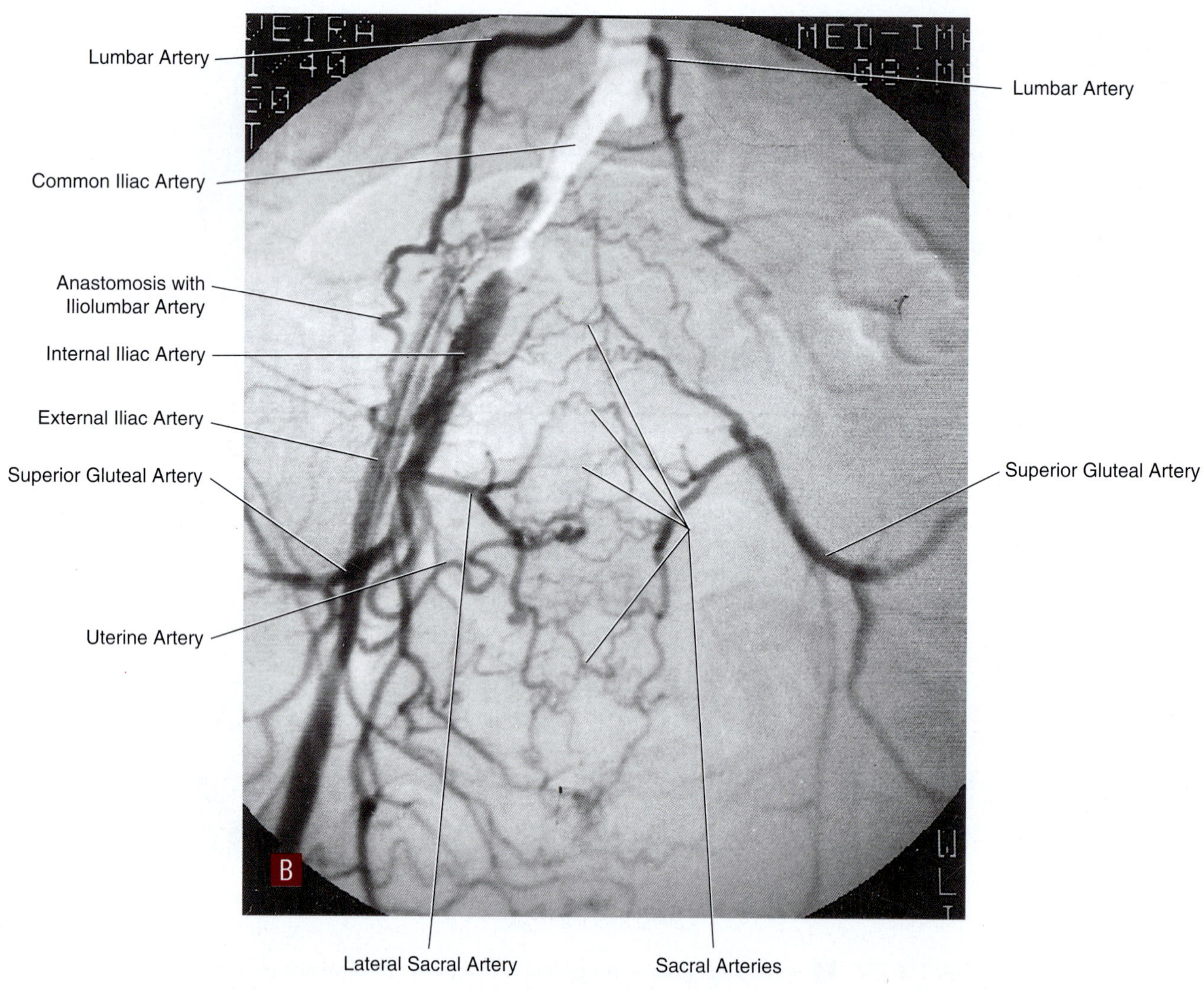

Figure 19.27. *Continued*

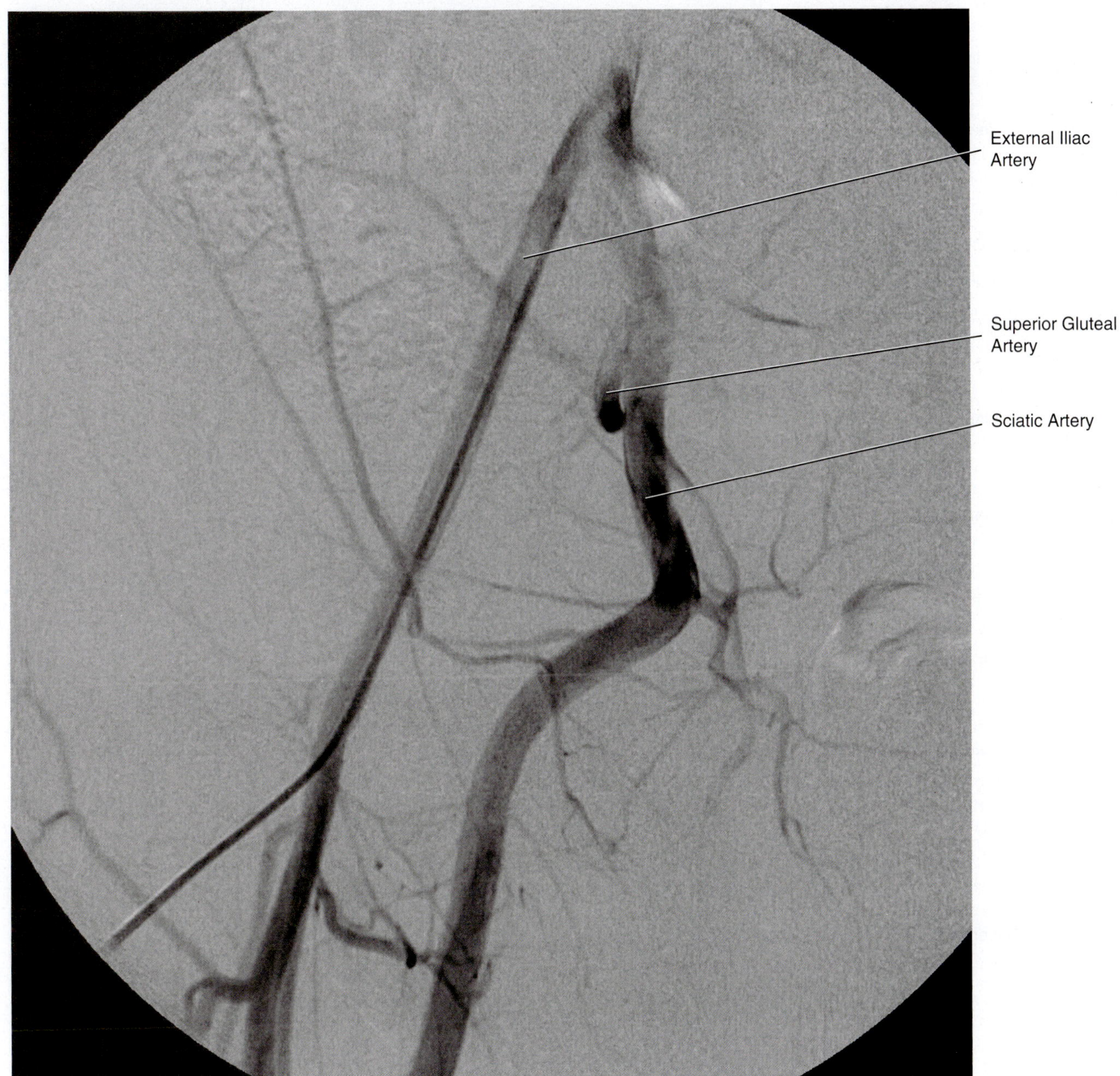

Figure 19.28. Right internal iliac arteriogram showing the persistent sciatic artery instead of the inferior gluteal artery.

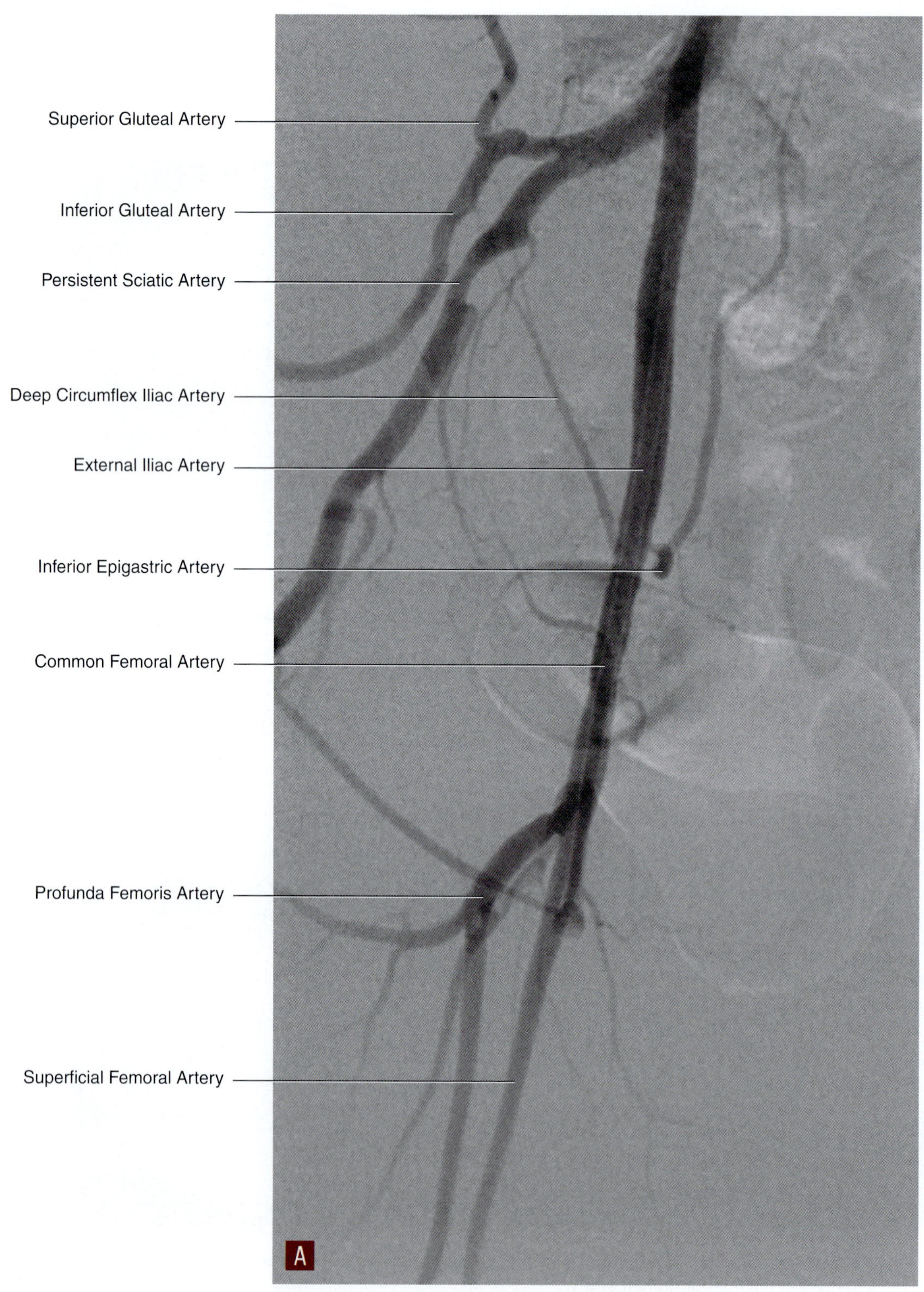

Figure 19.29. **A**, Right external iliac artery angiogram with reflux into the common iliac artery in a right anterior oblique projection showing a persistent sciatic artery, in addition to the superficial femoral artery. The inferior gluteal artery is seen just superior to the persistent sciatic artery. **B**, Right external iliac artery angiogram with reflux into the common iliac artery in an AP projection in the same patient. The stenosis is seen en face in the projection and not apparent.

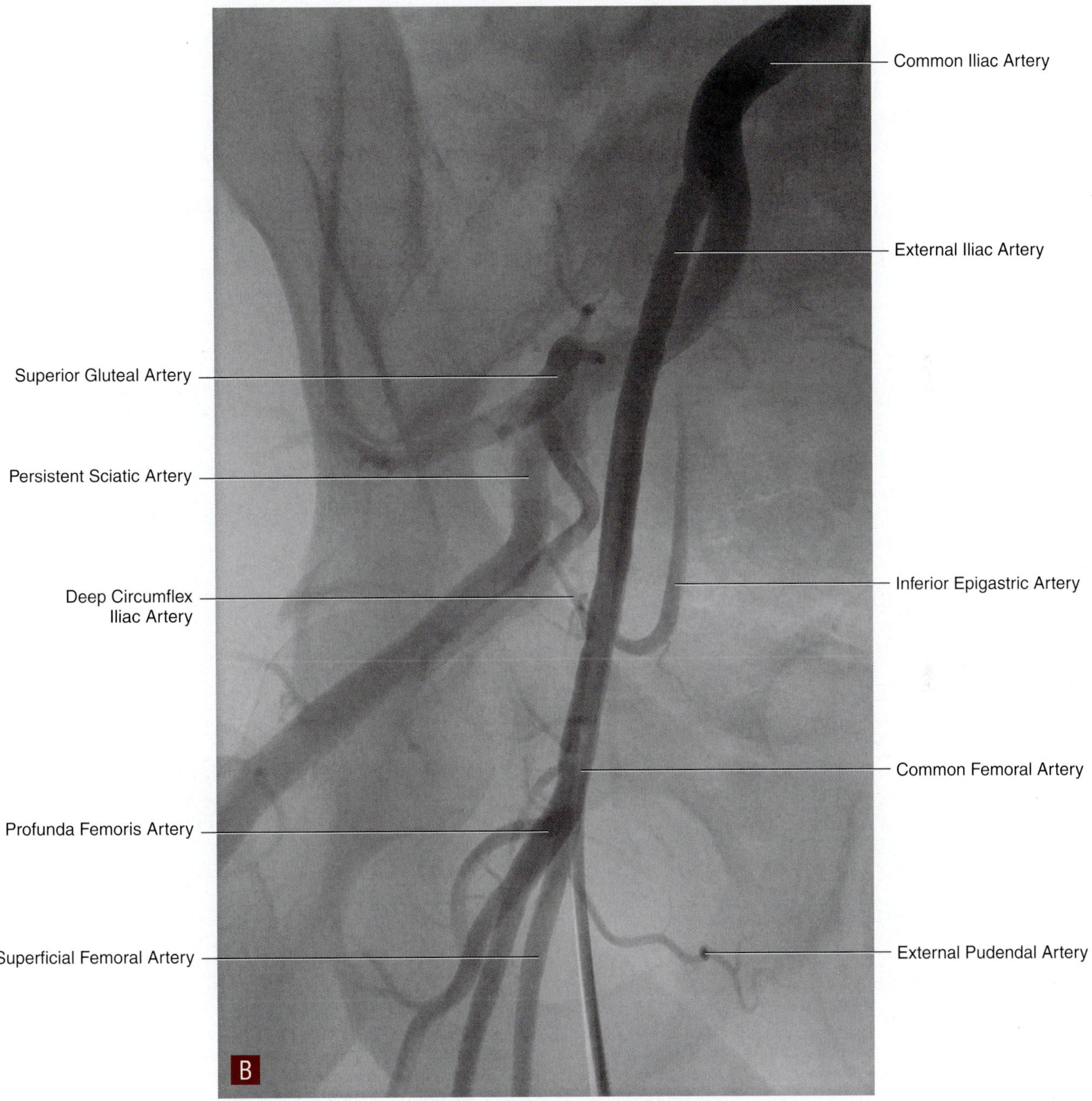

Figure 19.29. *Continued*

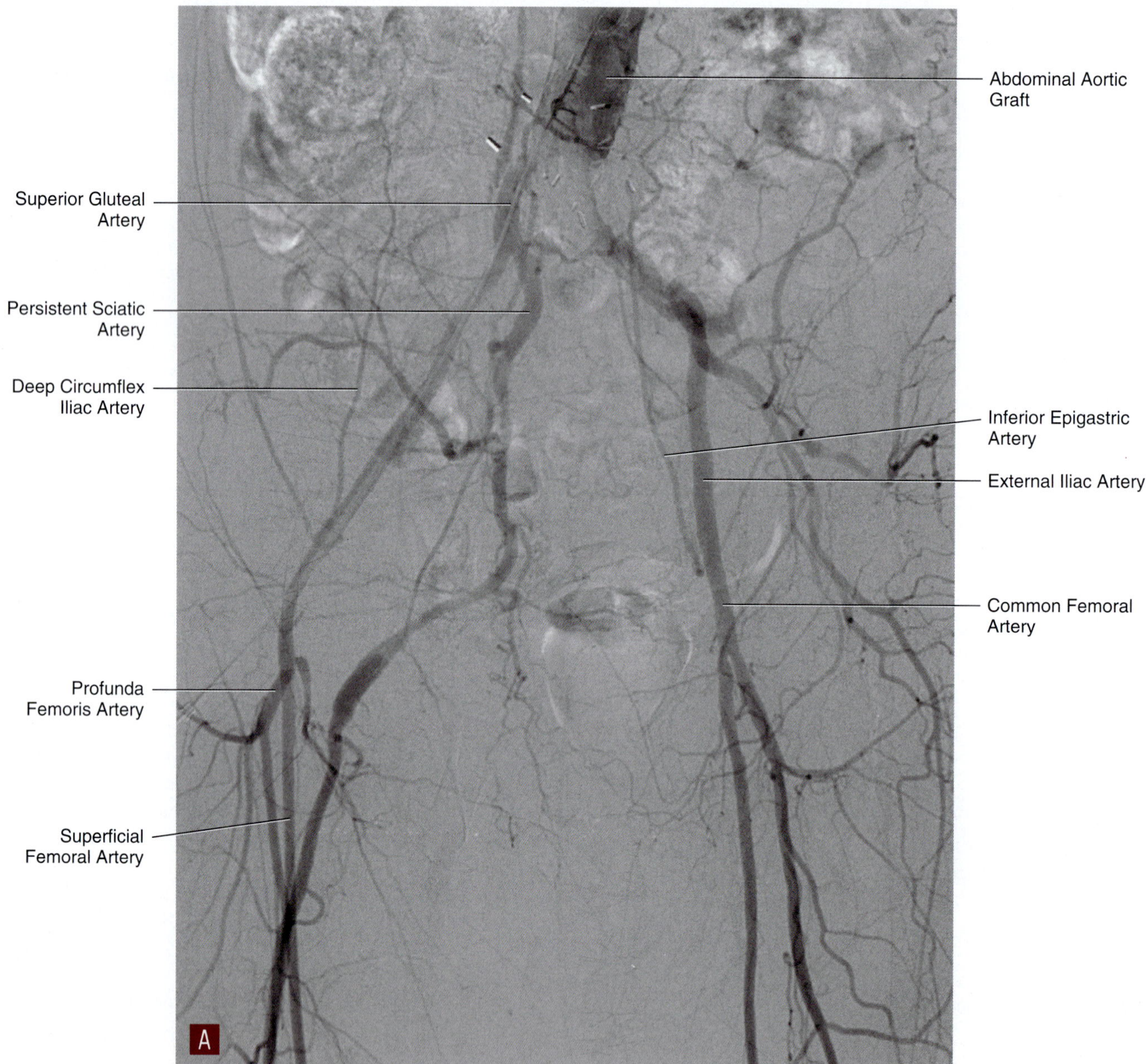

Figure 19.30. Angiographic appearance of a persistent sciatic artery in a patient with an aortobiiliac bypass. **A**, Aortogram in a left anterior oblique projection showing a persistent sciatic artery in addition to the superficial femoral artery. **B**, Aortogram in the same patient, in a right anterior oblique projection. **C**, Aortogram in the same patient, demonstrating the persistent sciatic artery in the arterial outflow of the right lower extremity.

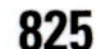

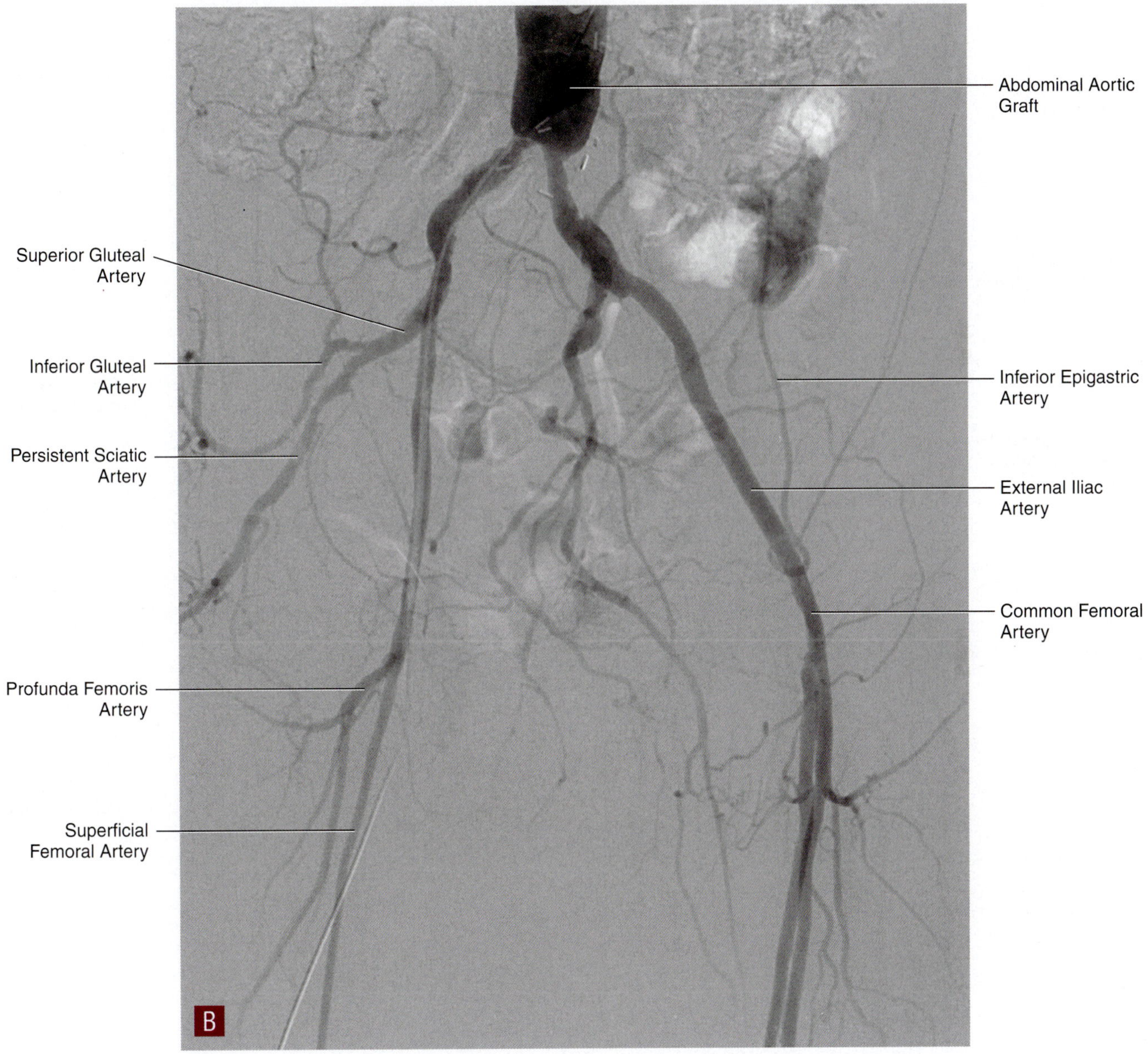

Abdominal Aortic Graft

Superior Gluteal Artery

Inferior Gluteal Artery

Inferior Epigastric Artery

Persistent Sciatic Artery

External Iliac Artery

Common Femoral Artery

Profunda Femoris Artery

Superficial Femoral Artery

B

Figure 19.30. *Continued*

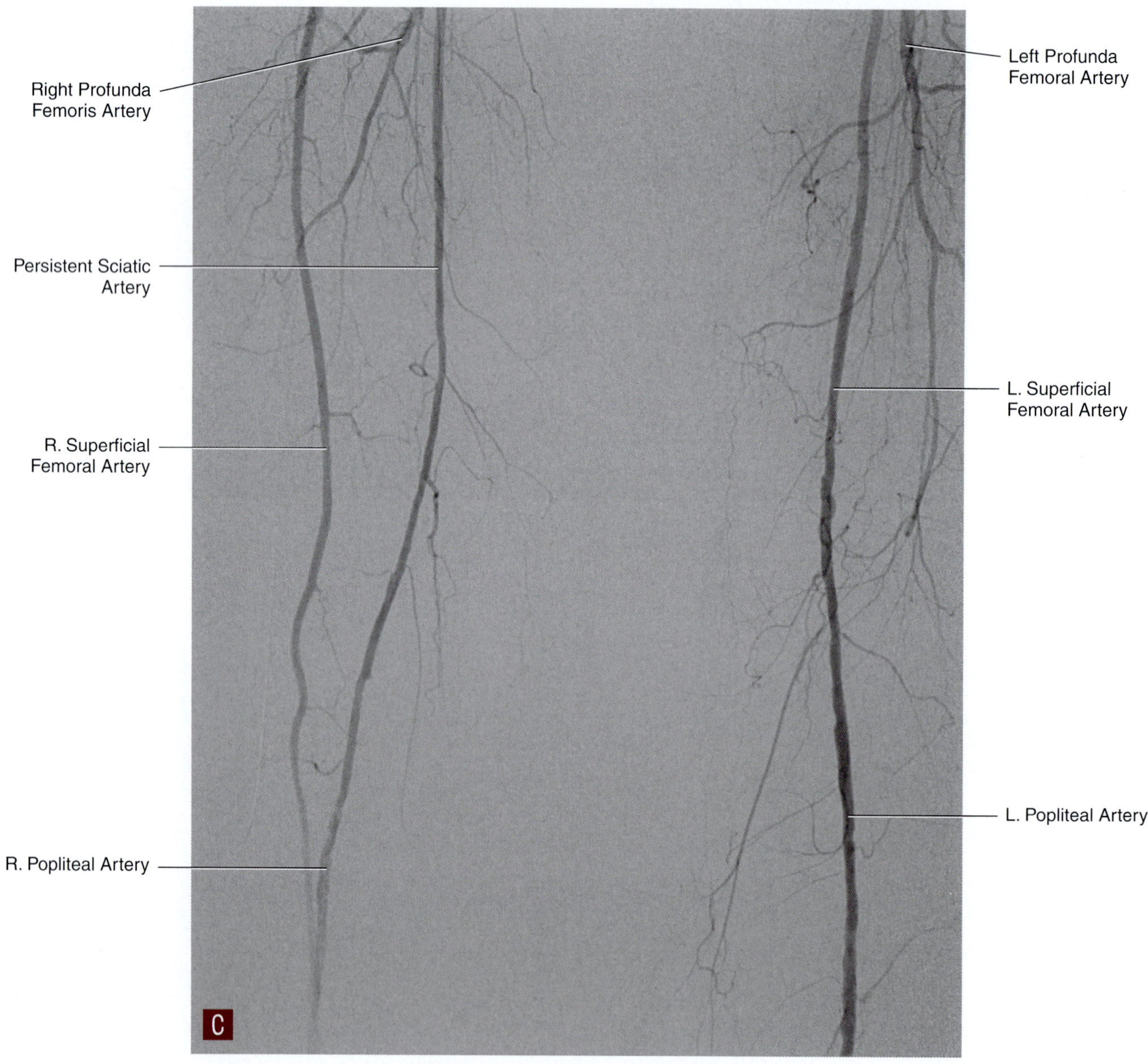

Figure 19.30. *Continued*

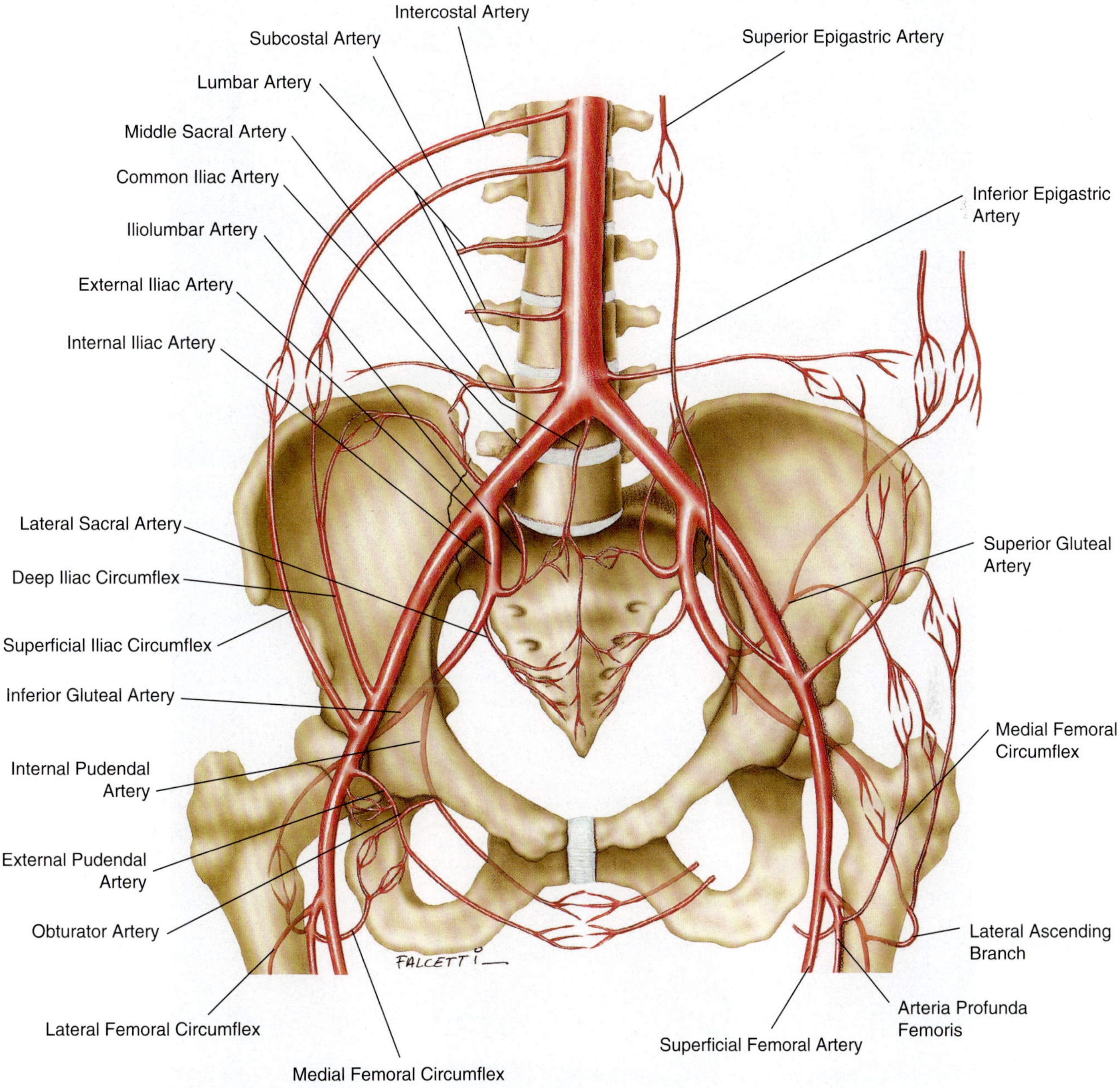

Figure 19.31. Schematic diagram of the major potential parietal pathways of collateral circulation encountered in chronic obstructive vascular disease at the abdominal and pelvic levels.

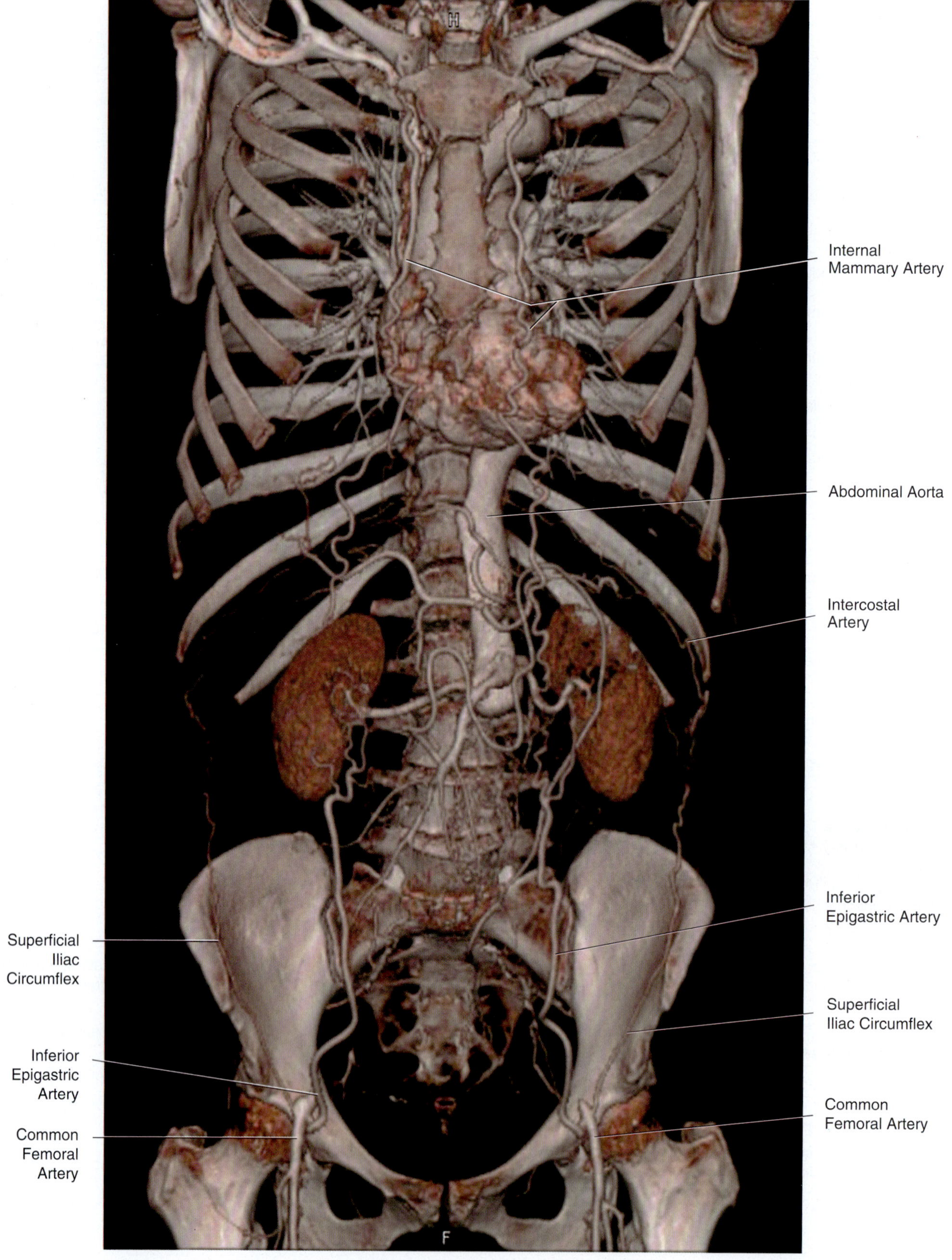

Figure 19.32. Computerized tomographic (CT) angiogram of the thorax and abdomen showing the thoracoabdominal arterial anastomoses through the superior epigastric arteries and the inferior epigastric arteries, connecting with the common femoral arteries through the retiform anastomosis between the two systems. Note the occluded abdominal aorta, which caused the development of the collateral circulation. Anteroposterior view of the 3D reconstruction.

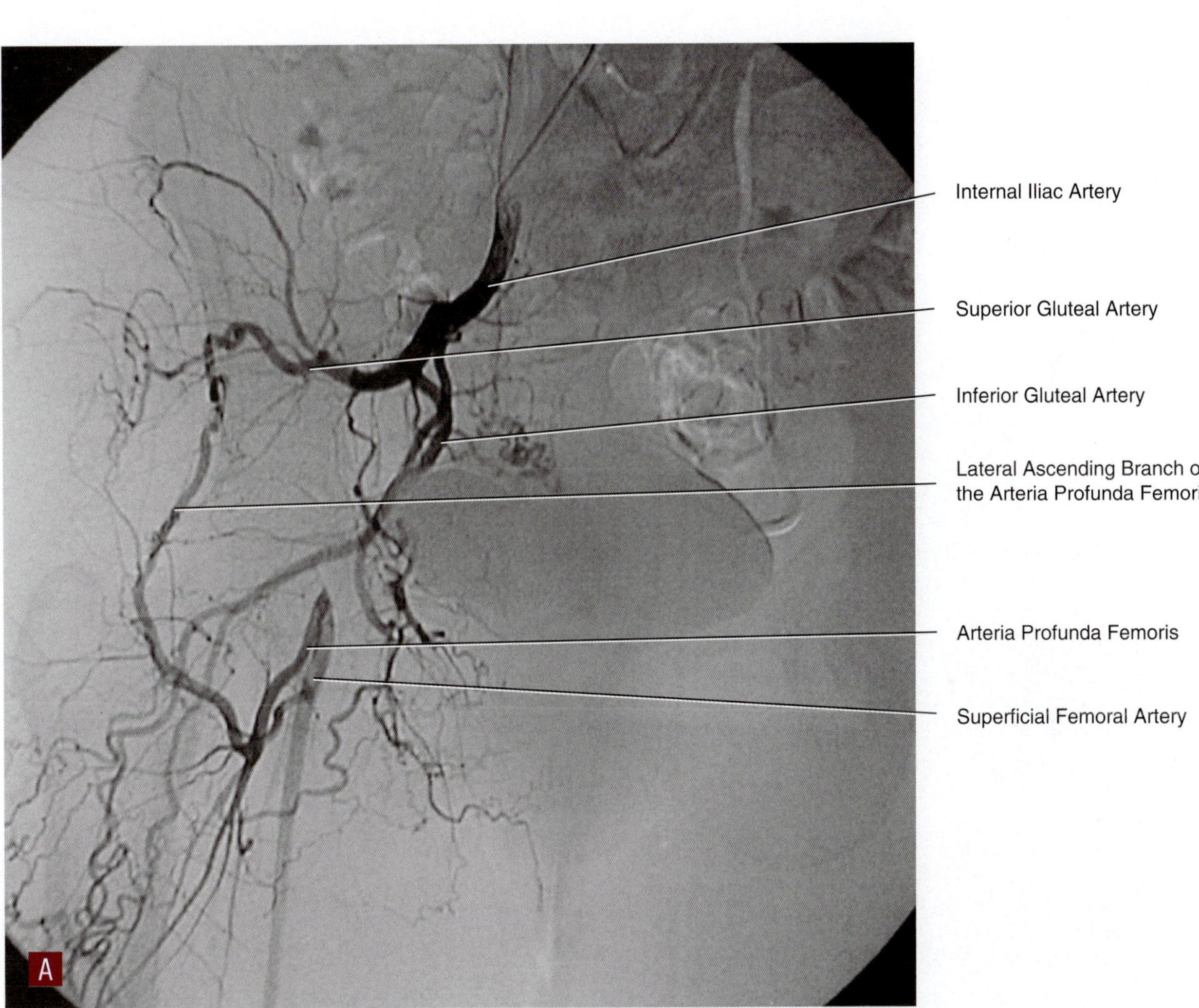

Figure 19.33. A, Anteroposterior view of a right internal iliac arteriogram in an individual with occluded right external iliac artery, with reconstitution of the arteria profunda femoris and superficial femoral artery through collateral anastomosis from lateral branches of the superior gluteal artery and lateral ascending branch of the arteria profunda femoris. Note the continuous line between the two arterial systems called inosculation. B, Lateral view of the same arteriogram showing the continuation between the two systems.

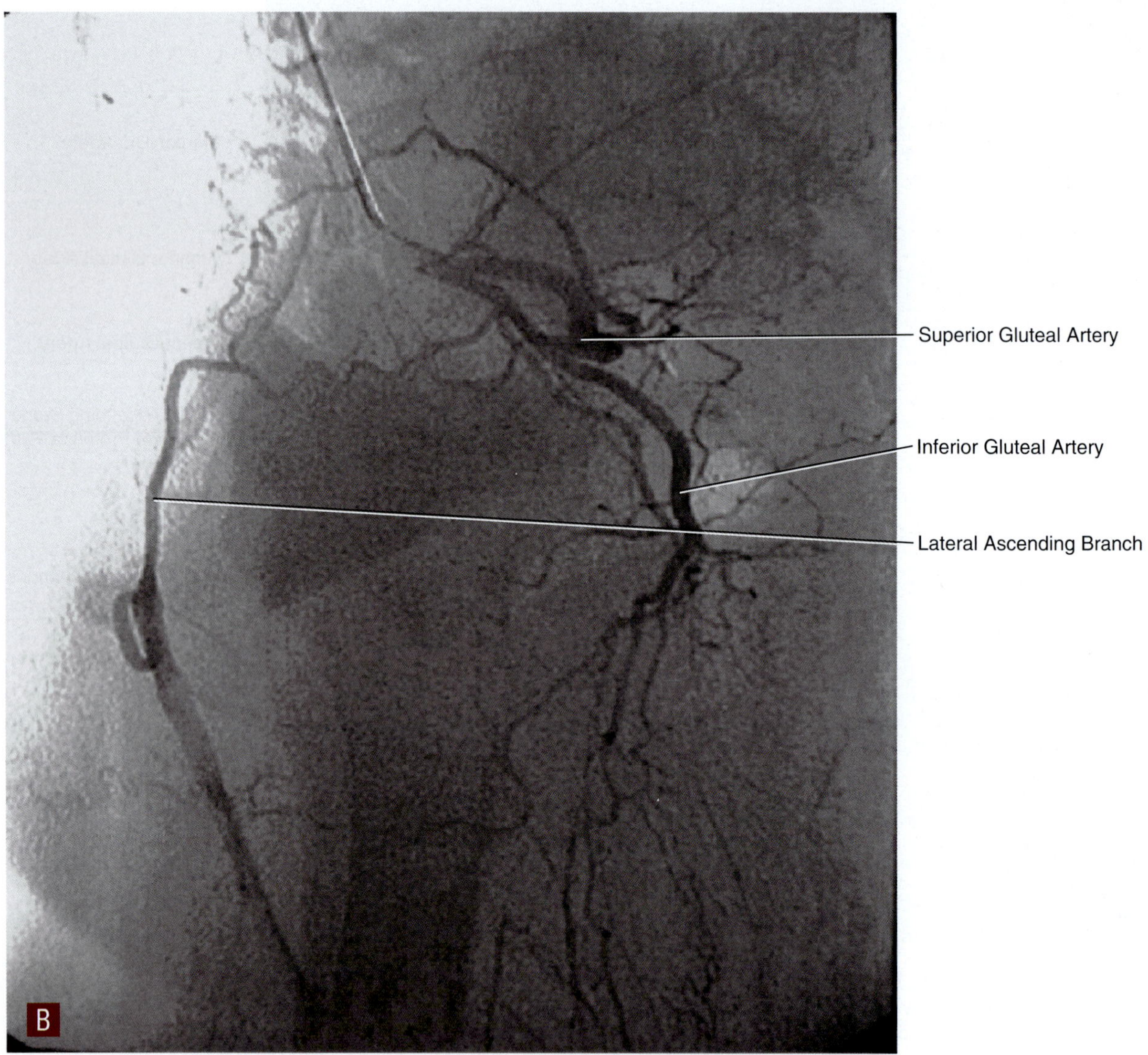

Figure 19.33. *Continued*

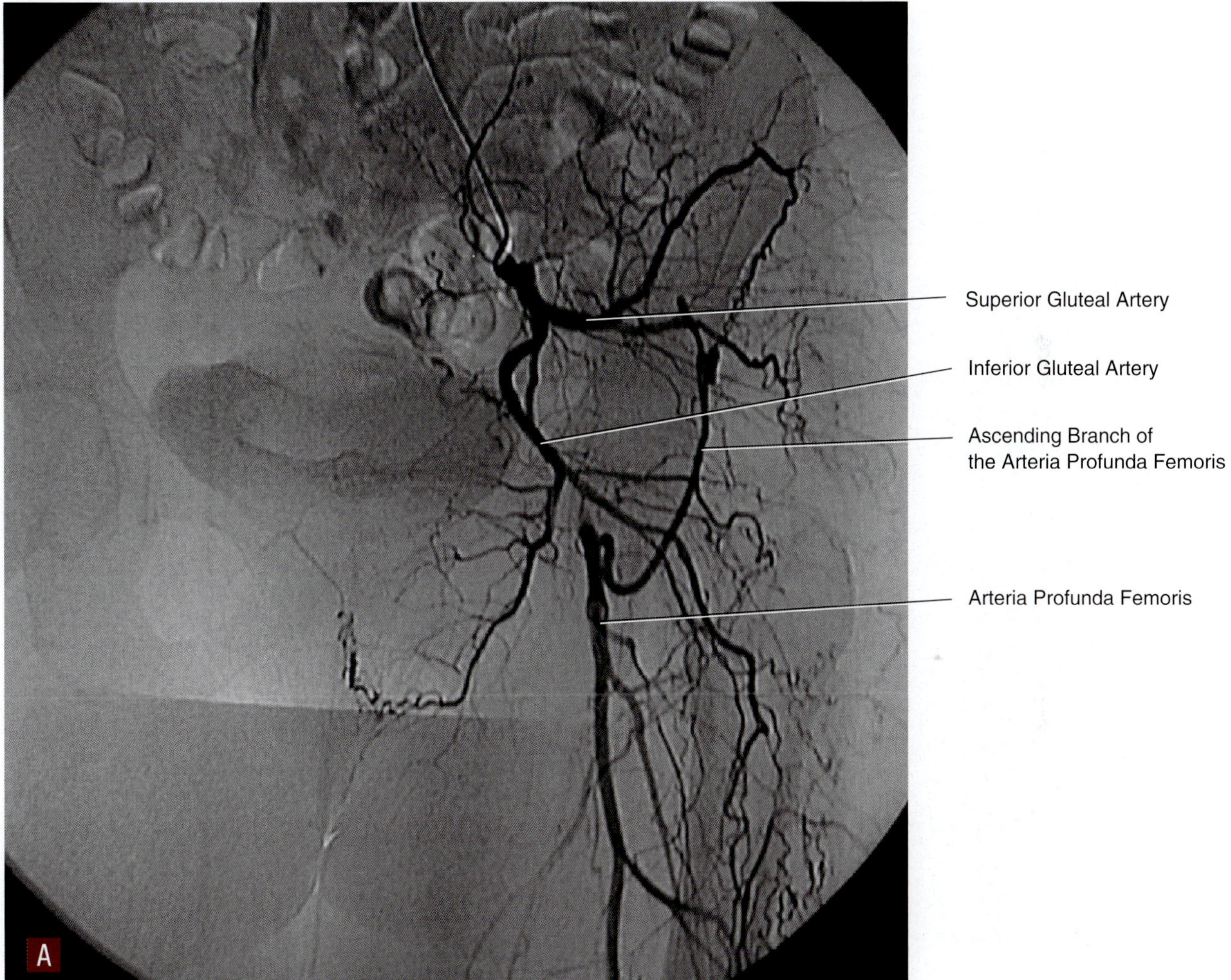

Figure 19.34. **A**, Anteroposterior view of a left internal iliac arteriogram in an individual with occluded left external iliac artery, with reconstitution of the arteria profunda femoris and the superficial femoral artery through collateral anastomosis from lateral branches of the superior gluteal artery and lateral ascending branch of the arteria profunda femoris. Note the type of anastomosis is inosculation. **B**, Lateral view of the same arteriogram showing the continuation of the two systems.

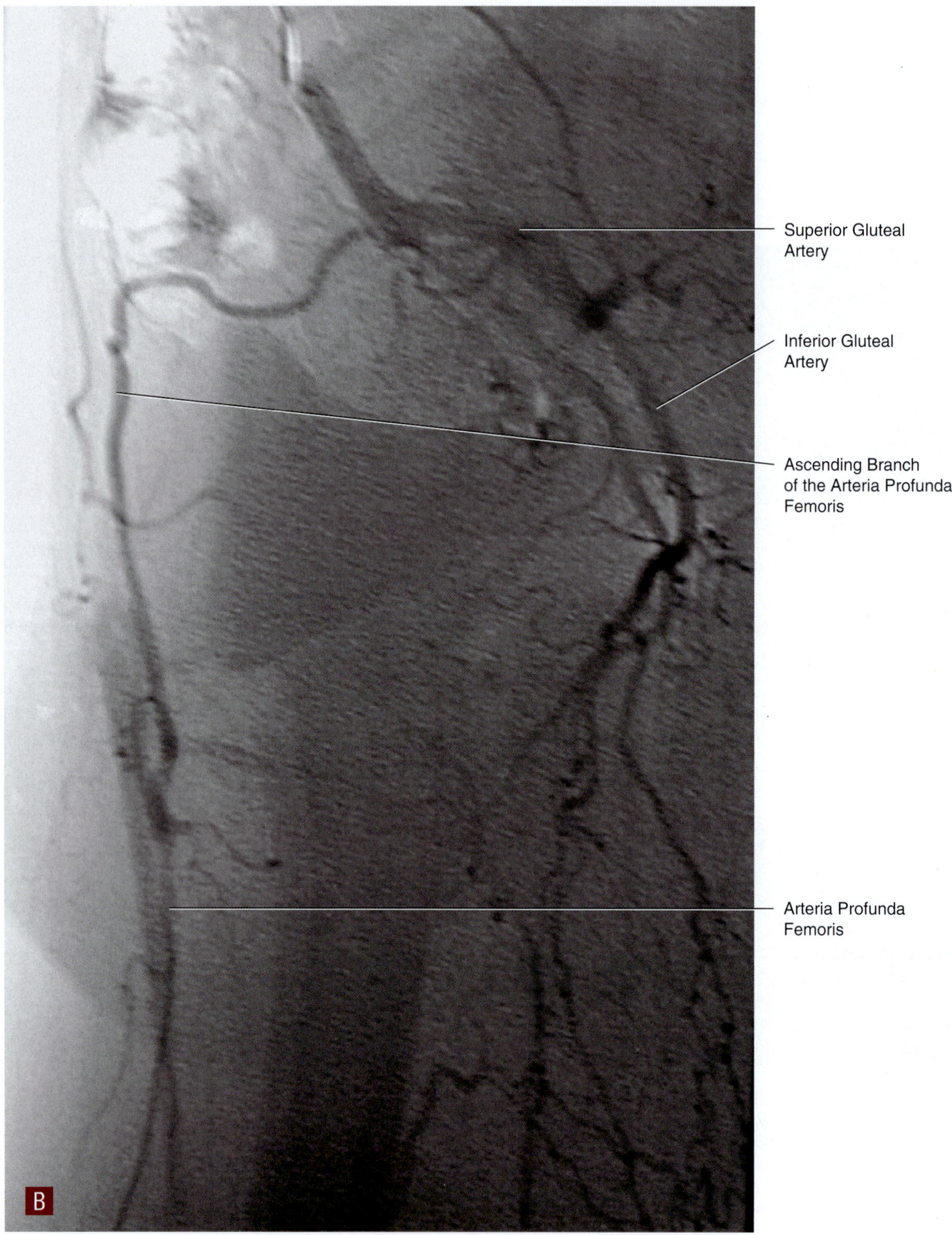

Figure 19.34. *Continued*

20

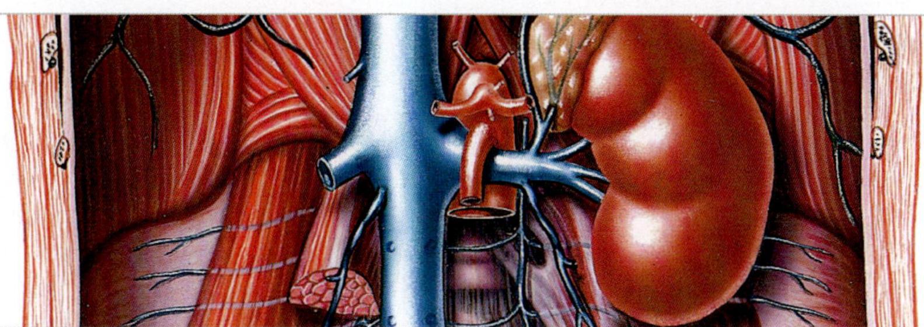

Veins of the Abdomen and Pelvis

The external iliac vein is the continuation of the femoral vein; it begins at the inguinal ligament and joins the internal iliac vein, thereby forming the common iliac vein. The external iliac vein is medial to the iliac artery. This vein is usually valveless.

Veins of the Pelvis (Figs. 20.1 and 20.2)

External Iliac Vein

Tributaries

Inferior epigastric vein
Deep circumflex iliac vein
Pubic vein

Internal Iliac Vein (Figs. 20.3, 20.4, and 20.6)

Several veins converge superiorly in the great sciatic foramen to form the internal iliac vein, to join the external iliac vein, forming the common iliac vein anterior to the sacroiliac joint. Rarely, the internal iliac veins may form a common confluence at the level of the common iliac vein confluence to form the inferior vena cava (IVC) or drain into the contralateral common iliac vein (Fig. 20.4).

Tributaries

- Origin outside the pelvis
  - Superior gluteal veins
  - Inferior gluteal veins
  - Internal pudendal veins
  - Obturator vein
- Anterior to the sacrum
  - Lateral sacral veins
- Origin in visceral venous plexus
  - Middle rectal veins
  - Rectal venous plexus
  - Prostatic venous plexus
  - Vesical plexus
  - Dorsal veins of the penis and penile venous plexus
  - Uterine plexuses
  - Vaginal plexuses

Superior Gluteal Veins (Fig. 20.4). Venae comitantes of the superior gluteal artery. These veins enter the pelvis through the greater sciatic foramen, above the piriformis muscle and join the internal iliac vein as a single trunk.

Inferior Gluteal Veins. Venae comitantes of the inferior gluteal artery. These veins arise proximal and posteriorly in the thigh and anastomose with the medial circumflex femoral and first perforating veins. They enter low in the greater sciatic foramen, joining the internal iliac vein, and connect with the superficial gluteal veins through the gluteal perforating veins.

Internal Pudendal Veins (Fig. 20.5). Venae comitantes of the internal pudendal artery, commencing in the prostatic venous plexus and ending in the internal iliac vein. These receive veins from the penile bulb and the scrotal (or labial) and inferior rectal veins. The deep dorsal vein of the penis ends in the prostatic plexus but is connected through that plexus to the internal pudendal veins.

Obturator Vein. This vein commences in the proximal adductor region and enters the pelvis through the obturator foramen, coursing a retroperitoneal path, passing between the ureter and the internal iliac artery to join the internal iliac vein.

Lateral Sacral Veins (Figs. 20.1, 20.3, and 20.4). These veins are interconnected by the sacral venous plexus and follow the lateral sacral arteries.

Middle Rectal Vein. This vein arises from the rectal venous plexus, receiving tributaries from the bladder, prostate, and seminal vesicle.

Rectal Venous Plexus (Chapter 18, Figs. 18.126, 18.127, 18.132). The rectal venous plexus surrounds the rectum and is connected anteriorly to the vesical plexus in males and to the uterovaginal plexus in females. It has an internal rectal plexus, under the rectal and anal epithelium, and an external rectal plexus outside the muscular layer. In the anal canal, the internal plexus has longitudinal dilations, most prominent in the left lateral, right anterolateral, and right posterolateral sectors. These veins are apt to become varicose and will be known as internal hemorrhoids. The internal plexus drains mostly to the superior rectal vein but connects extensively with the external rectal plexus.

The external rectal plexus drains inferiorly by the inferior rectal veins, a tributary of the internal pudendal vein. The external rectal plexus drains in the middle to a middle rectal vein, a tributary of the internal iliac vein. The superior rectal vein is the beginning of the inferior mesenteric vein and drains the superior part of the external rectal plexus. The veins in the subcutaneous part of the external rectal plexus may thrombose and form the so-called external hemorrhoids. Wide anastomoses between the rectal venous plexus and the internal iliac vein, as well as with the inferior mesenteric vein, establish communication between the portal and systemic venous systems.

Prostatic Venous Plexus. The periprostatic venous plexus is composed of a superficial and a deep plexus. The deep plexus is popularly known as the Santorini plexus. The periprostatic plexus originates from the deep dorsal vein of the penis, when this vessel leaves the penis under the Buck fascia and penetrates the pelvis passing under the symphysis pubis. After penetrating the pelvis, the vein divides into three major branches: the superficial branch and the right and left deep lateral venous plexuses (Figs. 20.6 and 20.7). The superficial branch is centrally located and emerges in the retropubic adipose tissue between the pubic-prostatic ligaments, overlying the bladder neck and the prostate (Figs. 20.8 and 20.9). This vein often has communicating branches over the bladder and into the endopelvic fascia (Fig. 20.8). In 80% of cases, the superficial branch vein is a single midline vessel, presenting early or late bifurcation in the remaining 20% of cases. In 10% of cases, this superficial vein may be double or may have other anatomic variations. In 10% of cases, the superficial vein is absent.

The lateral venous plexuses (deep plexus, Santorini) pass posterolaterally, beneath the visceral or preprostatic fascia (Figs. 20.10-20.12) and communicate freely with the internal iliac vein (hypogastric vein) through the pudendal, obturator, and vesical venous plexuses. The deep venous plexus (Santorini plexus) can be visualized in dissected specimens only after opening the endopelvic fascia and its right and left condensations, which unite the prostate to the dorsal surface of the pubis (the so-called "pubic-prostatic ligaments") (Figs. 20.10-20.12).

Because the lateral plexuses (deep plexus) anastomose freely with other pelvic plexuses, any laceration of this structure can lead to considerable blood loss during any kind of retropubic surgery. In addition, the periprostatic plexus communicates with the paravertebral venous network (Batson plexus), and osseous metastases constitute the most common form of hematogenous metastasis of prostatic carcinoma. The most frequent sites involved are the pelvic bone, lumbar spine, the femur, thoracic spine, and ribs.

Vesical Plexus. The vesical plexus covers the lower bladder and the prostatic base in males and is connected to the prostatic venous plexus in males and to the vaginal venous plexus in females. It is drained by several vesical veins, tributaries of the internal iliac vein.

Dorsal Veins of the Penis and Penile Venous Anatomy (Figs. 20.13-20.17). There is a superficial and a deep dorsal vein of the penis. The superficial dorsal vein of the penis drains the prepuce and skin and is positioned longitudinally along the penis, draining into the external pudendal veins. The superficial dorsal vein of the penis receives, along its course, flow from the corpora cavernosa penis through circumflex veins. The deep dorsal vein of the penis runs backward in the midline, under the fibrous penile sheath. It receives blood flow from the glans penis and corpora cavernosa penis, through the circumflex veins. It reaches the prostatic venous plexus after dividing into right and left branches but has also communications with the internal pudendal veins (Figs. 20.11, 20.18-20.24). The deep dorsal vein of the penis has a venous valve beneath the symphysis pubis. The superficial venous system of the penis including the superficial dorsal vein drains into the superficial femoral vein through the external pudendal vein and the saphenous vein (Figs. 20.25-20.28).

The corpora cavernosa penis is formed by sinusoids surrounded by smooth muscle and connective tissues with high wall tonus. The sinusoidal vascular space and arterial inflow are limited in the flaccid state. The venous outflow is unimpeded. During erection, after neurostimulation or intracavernosal papaverine injection, the sinusoidal smooth muscle relaxes, and distended sinusoids compress and obstruct peripheral venules against tunica albuginea. Simultaneously, resistance to arterial flow decreases until cavernosal pressure approaches systolic pressure (Chapter 19, Fig. 19.18). The crura of the corpora cavernosa penis are drained by crural perforating veins, which are tributaries of the internal pudendal veins (Fig. 20.13).

Uterine Plexuses. The uterine venous plexus extends laterally in the broad ligaments, communicating with the ovarian and vaginal plexuses. The uterine plexus is drained by the uterine vein, which is a tributary of the internal iliac vein (Figs. 20.29 and 20.30). The uterine plexus typically communicates with the ovarian vein.

Vaginal Plexuses. The vaginal plexuses connect with the uterine, vesical, and rectal plexuses and are drained by vaginal veins to the internal iliac veins.

Common Iliac Veins

The common iliac vein arises from the junction of the external and the internal iliac veins at the level of the sacroiliac joint. The common iliac vein follows an oblique direction ending at the level of the fifth lumbar vertebra, joining the contralateral common iliac vein to form the IVC. The right common iliac vein is almost vertical, whereas the left is oblique and longer. The left common iliac vein crosses behind the right common iliac artery and is sometimes compressed by this vessel. The common iliac vein is joined by the iliolumbar and lateral sacral veins (Figs. 20.1 and 20.2).

Variations

The left common iliac vein may ascend left of the aorta to the level of the left renal vein, where it crosses anterior to the aorta to join the IVC.

Median Sacral Veins

The median sacral veins are companions of the median sacral artery, anterior to the sacrum, joining into a single vein and ending in the left common iliac vein or at the junction of the common iliac veins (Figs. 20.1 and 20.4).

Abdominal Veins

Inferior Vena Cava (Figs. 20.1, 20.2, 20.31, and 20.32)

The inferior vena cava carries blood from all the structures and abdominal organs, below the diaphragm, being formed by the confluence of the common iliac veins. It follows an upward direction in front of the lumbar spine to the right of the abdominal aorta. The IVC reaches the liver and has an intrahepatic segment, which may be totally encircled by hepatic parenchyma. It reaches the right atrium of the heart, through the tendinous part of the diaphragm. At the entrance of the inferoposterior part of the right atrium, there is a semilunar valve of the IVC, also known as the Eustachian valve (Fig. 20.32). At this level, a Thebesian valve can also be found covering the coronary sinus ostium where it drains into the right atrium (see Chapter 14).

Variations

A number of anomalies may occur during the development phase of the IVC in fetal life. The vein may be totally replaced by two or more vessels, with failure of interconnection between the common iliac veins and persistence of a longitudinal channel on the left, supracardinal, or subcardinal veins. It may also undergo a complete transposition to the left of the aorta. Chapter 1 has additional details on the formation of the IVC and caval variants.

Collateral Circulation

There is a rich collateral venous network bypassing the IVC in cases of thrombosis, agenesis, or occlusion, either through a superficial or deep venous network. The superficial system includes the epigastric, the circumflex iliac, the lateral thoracic, the thoracoepigastric, the internal thoracic, the posterior intercostal, the external pudendal, and lumbovertebral anastomotic veins. The deep system includes the azygos vein, the hemiazygos, and the lumbar veins. The vertebral venous plexus, including the Batson venous plexus, is also in the collateral venous circuit (Figs. 20.33 and 20.34).

Tributaries

- Lumbar veins
- Ascending lumbar veins
- Gonadal veins
- Renal veins
- Suprarenal veins
- Inferior phrenic veins

Lumbar Veins. There are four pairs of lumbar veins, draining the lumbar muscles and skin from the abdominal wall. The lumbar veins also drain the vertebral venous plexuses and are connected by the ascending lumbar veins. The left-side lumbar veins are longer and cross behind the abdominal aorta. The first and second lumbar veins may connect to the IVC, the ascending lumbar veins, or the lumbar azygos vein (Figs. 20.1, 20.33, and 20.35).

Ascending Lumbar Veins. The ascending lumbar veins originate from the common iliac veins and make connections between the common iliac veins to the iliolumbar and lumbar veins. They ascend behind the psoas major muscles and in front of the vertebral transverse processes. Cranially, they join the subcostal veins and turn medially, forming the azygos vein in the right side and the hemiazygos vein on the left (Fig. 20.35).

Gonadal Veins (Figs. 20.36 and 20.37). Testicular veins: These veins arise from the posterior aspect of the testis and drain the epididymis to form the pampiniform plexus. They follow the spermatic cord, anteriorly to the ductus deferens, crossing the inguinal ring and the inguinal canal, ascending retroperitoneally close to the ureter, anterior to the psoas major as two or more veins with abundant collaterals and anastomoses, in both sides of the testicular artery. The left testicular vein joins in a single vessel and opens into the left renal vein to form a right angle. The right testicular vein joins in a single vessel and opens in the IVC just below the right renal vein, forming an acute angle. The testicular veins have several valves that may be nonfunctioning and cause varicoceles on the testis, mainly on the left side.

Ovarian veins: There is a venous plexus in the broad ligament of the uterus, which communicates with the uterine plexus, from which originate the two ovarian veins in each side, following the path of the ovarian artery and coursing together in each side of the artery, opening at the IVC on the right and on the left renal vein on the left. These veins have valves, and the valvular incompetence may lead to pelvic varices (Figs. 20.30, 20.36, and 20.37).

Renal Veins. **Intrarenal veins:** In contrast to the arteries, there is free circulation throughout the venous system, and, therefore, the veins do not have a segmental model. Nevertheless, the renal venous system presents some anatomic characteristics that are reasonably constant and should be known during angiographic examinations.

Material of investigation: Fifty-two 3-dimensional endocasts of the kidney collecting system together with the intrarenal veins were obtained from 26 fresh cadavers of both sexes of patients, who died of causes not related to the urinary tract.

A blue polyester resin (volume approximately 15.0 mL) was injected into the main trunk of the renal vein to fill in the kidney venous tree and a yellow resin into the ureter (about 5.0 mL) to fill in the collecting system, according to the proportions and technique described previously.

Findings: The intrarenal venous arrangement demonstrates free anastomoses between the veins. The small veins of the cortex, called stellate veins, drain into the interlobular veins, which form a series of arches (Figs. 20.38 and 20.39). Within the kidney substance, these arches are arranged in arcades, which lie mainly in the longitudinal axis. There are usually three systems of longitudinal anastomotic arcades and the anastomoses occur at different levels: between the stellate veins (more peripherally), between the arcuate veins (at the base of the pyramids), and between the interlobar (infundibular) veins (close to the renal sinus) (Figs. 20.38 and 20.39). These anastomoses are named as first order, second order, and third order, from the periphery to the center (Fig. 20.40).

Around the calyceal necks, there are large venous anastomoses (collarlike), formed mainly when the veins draining the posterior half of the kidney cross over at the necks of the minor calices to join the anterior main trunks (Fig. 20.41). There were also horizontal arches, crossing over the calyces to link the anterior and posterior veins, as well as the longitudinal systems at different levels (Fig. 20.42). The venous arcades join one another in both the longitudinal and horizontal planes to produce larger veins that unite to form large trunks. The main renal vein was formed by these trunks, which course toward the hilum where they unite prior to emptying into the vena cava.

In one series, three trunks (28 of 52 casts, 53.8%) and two trunks (15 of 52 casts, 28.8%) joining each other to form the main renal vein were found (Fig. 20.43). Less frequently, four trunks (8 of 52 casts, 15.4%) or five trunks (1 of 52 casts, 1.9%) were found.

Dorsal kidney: In 36 of 52 casts (69.2%), there was a posterior (retropelvic) vein that coursed on the back of the kidney collecting system, either to drain into the renal vein or directly into the vena cava. In 25 of 52 casts (48.1%), the retropelvic vein had a close relationship with the upper infundibulum or to the junction of the pelvis with the upper calix (Fig. 20.44A). In the other 11 of 52 casts (21.1%), the retropelvic vein crossed and was related to the middle posterior surface of the renal pelvis (Fig. 20.44B). In 16 of 52 casts (30.8%), there were no veins on the posterior aspect of the renal pelvis because the veins draining the posterior region crossed anteriorly to join the main anterior trunks of the renal vein (Fig. 20.44C).

Relationship to ureteropelvic junction: In 40.4% of the cases (21 of 52 casts), we found a close relationship between an important tributary of the renal vein and the anterior aspect of the ureteropelvic junction (UPJ) (Fig. 20.45A). Among these cases, there was one vein anterior and another vein posterior to the UPJ, simultaneously (Fig. 20.46A and B). In the other 59.6% of cases (31 of 52 casts), the UPJ was not related to veins, either anteriorly or posteriorly (Fig. 20.45B).

Extrarenal veins: Mostly, the renal vein is formed by the union of two (53.8% of cases) or three intrarenal trunks (28.8%). Less frequently, there were four trunks (15.4%) or five trunks (1.9%) joining to form the main renal vein. After leaving the renal hilum on each side, both renal veins drain into the IVC. The left renal vein is longer than the right vein and usually has a higher penetration into the vena cava. The left renal vein has a ventral course in relation to the abdominal aorta and is caudally located in relation to the origin of the superior mesenteric artery.

The right renal vein does not have tributaries. In contrast, the left renal vein drains an extensive area and usually receives the left inferior suprarenal vein, the left inferior diaphragmatic vein, the left gonadal vein, and the left second lumbar vein. Anatomic variations of the renal veins are less common than the arterial variations. Also, when anatomic variations do exist, they are more frequent in the right side (Fig. 20.47). The renal vein may course posterior to the aorta (retroaortic renal vein) and occasionally may encircle the aorta with an anterior and a posterior division, known as a circumaortic renal vein. When there is a single retroaortic left renal vein, it typically drains into the vena cava more inferiorly than when the vein courses anteriorly.

Material of investigation: The extrarenal veins in 88 "in situ" kidneys were analyzed; these organs were dissected from 44 formalin-fixed cadavers of adult patients, of both sexes, who died of causes unrelated to the urinary tract.

Findings: The left renal vein was single in all of the 44 left kidneys that were analyzed. Considering the right side, in three cases, two renal veins draining to the IVC were present (7.0% of right kidneys or 3.5% of the total kidneys). Among these, in one case, the two veins had similar calibers; the inferior vein was slightly greater in diameter. In the other two cases, the caliber of the inferior vein was less than one-half that of the superior vein caliber.

Capsular and Perirenal Veins. There is a rich venous network around the kidneys, draining the renal capsule and with anastomoses between the intrarenal venous system and the capsular veins. The perirenal veins drain into the gonadal vein, inferior phrenic vein, and suprarenal veins. There are direct anastomoses directly with the main renal vein and with the ureteric veins (Figs. 20.1 and 20.47).

Suprarenal Veins (See Chapter 18, Fig. 18.140). There is only one draining adrenal vein for each adrenal hilum. The right adrenal vein is short and small and opens directly and horizontally into the lateroposterior aspect of the IVC, above the right renal vein (Figs. 20.48-20.50). The left adrenal vein is longer and larger and descends from the adrenal gland posteriorly to the body of the pancreas to open into the left renal vein, joined by a branch of the left inferior phrenic vein, about 1 cm from the IVC (Figs. 20.50-20.52). Angiographically, the hepatic veins of the lower group may be mistakenly identified as the right adrenal vein (Fig. 20.53). Occasionally the right adrenal vein drains into one of the small hepatic veins of the lower group.

Inferior Phrenic Veins. The inferior phrenic veins follow the same distribution as that of the companion inferior phrenic arteries on the lower diaphragmatic surface. The right inferior phrenic vein ends in the IVC, above or together with the right hepatic vein. The left is frequently double, and one branch opens in the IVC or together with the left hepatic vein, whereas the other may join the left adrenal vein or the left renal vein (Fig. 20.54, and Chapter 18, 18.138, 18.139).

Hepatic Veins and Portal Venous System

- Hepatic veins
  - Distribution of the hepatic veins
  - Variations of the hepatic veins
  - Collateral channels
- Portal vein
  - Left gastric vein
  - Right gastric vein
  - Paraumbilical veins
  - Cystic veins
- Splenic vein
  - Short gastric veins
  - Left gastroepiploic vein
  - Pancreatic veins
  - Inferior mesenteric vein
  - Superior rectal veins
  - Sigmoid veins
  - Left colic vein
- Superior mesenteric vein
  - Jejunal and ileal veins
  - Ileocolic veins
  - Right colic vein
  - Middle colic vein
  - Right gastroepiploic
  - Pancreaticoduodenal veins
- Anastomoses between the portal and the systemic circulations
- Pancreatic venous system

Hepatic Veins

Distribution of the Hepatic Veins

The hepatic veins drain the liver parenchyma and start as interlobular veins, draining the sinusoids of the hepatic lobules. According to the classical description, the sinusoids end at the sublobular veins, which will drain into the hepatic veins. The hepatic veins are valveless and are contiguous with the hepatic tissue.

There are three main hepatic veins emerging from the upper, posterior surface of the liver, opening at the IVC, and an individual vein from the caudate lobe (Figs. 20.55-20.57). These are called the upper group, which consists of the large, right, middle, and left hepatic veins, and the smaller caudate lobe vein, delineating four well-defined territories of drainage (Figs. 20.55-20.58).

The right hepatic veins run at the right hepatic fissure, which divides the right hepatic lobe in the anterior and the posterior sectors. The right hepatic vein drains both the anterior (segments VIII and V) and the posterior (segments VI and VII) sectors of the right hepatic lobe (Fig. 20.55).

In 16 of 25 casts of liver specimens, there was only one right hepatic vein of large diameter receiving several tributaries from the several segments of the right lobe (Figs. 20.59-20.64). There is a direct relationship between the right hepatic vein and the bifurcation of the main portal vein and the right branch of the portal vein (Fig. 20.65). Outside the liver, the portal vein crosses over the IVC, and the superior mesenteric vein (SMV) follows a relatively parallel pathway along the IVC (Fig. 20.66).

In two cases, the tributaries from segment VIII were large and reached the right hepatic vein near the IVC. One cast showed two right hepatic veins, parallel to each other and with similar sizes. In two cases, the right hepatic vein had a single short trunk of about 1 cm but was bifid with two parallel veins peripherally. Six livers showed an accessory right hepatic vein, caudal and distal, but parallel to the main vein and posterior to the portal vein bifurcation. In two casts, the right hepatic vein was extremely underdeveloped. In 1.6% of the cases (out of a series of 60 cases), three right hepatic veins were identified, and the most anterior one was located anterior to the portal vein bifurcation and to the anterior branch of the right portal trunk (Fig. 20.67).

The distance from the anterior aspect of the right hepatic vein, at 1 cm from the IVC and the posterior aspect of the portal bifurcation, was measured in a straight line. This distance ranged from 2.7 to 5.4 cm, with a mean distance of 4.41 cm. In the cases in which there were two right hepatic veins, the distance was 1.8 cm from the medial branch and 4.2 cm from the lateral branch. The accessory right hepatic veins and the portal bifurcation were very close (Figs. 20.60-20.62). The distance between the anterior aspect of the accessory right hepatic veins measured at 1 cm from the IVC and the portal bifurcation was 2.2 to 4.3 cm with a mean distance of 3.1 cm (Figs. 20.65 and 20.66).

The middle hepatic vein runs at the middle hepatic fissure, dividing the right hepatic lobe from the left hepatic lobe, and drains most of the medial aspect of the left liver lobe (segment IV) but ,in general, receives a large tributary from the right hepatic lobe (segment V), crossing from the right to the left hepatic lobes. The middle hepatic vein joins the left hepatic vein to form a single venous trunk ending in the anterolateral aspect of the IVC.

There was only one middle hepatic vein in all 25 cases of the series analyzed; this vein joined the IVC directly in about 20% of cases and formed a common trunk with the left hepatic vein in 80% of cases.

The distance between the inferior aspect of the middle hepatic vein, at 1 cm from the IVC and the superior posterior aspect of the portal bifurcation and left portal trunk, was measured in a straight line. This distance ranged from 2.4 to 4.5 cm, with a mean distance of 3.9 cm (Fig. 20.67).

The left hepatic vein runs partially at the fissure for the ligamentum teres and at the left hepatic fissure, between segments II and III, and drains preferentially the lateral sector (segments II and III) of the left hepatic lobe, but also receives tributaries from segment IV (Fig. 20.68). The left hepatic vein is always anterior to the left portal vein.

The caudate lobe vein is an independent tributary of the IVC and opens in the cava in a much lower position, in relation to the three main hepatic veins (Fig. 20.57).

The lower group of hepatic veins are smaller and numerous and drain liver parenchyma directly to the IVC, from the right liver lobe and the caudate lobe.

Variations of the Hepatic Veins

There may be several large accessory hepatic veins draining the upper (diaphragmatic) part of the right and left liver lobes, joining the main hepatic veins, close to the outlet ring at the IVC. Several additional draining veins, from territories not usually drained by the three main veins, may be tributaries of the right, middle, and left hepatic veins (Fig. 20.61).

Accessory hepatic veins may also be encountered in the lower group, draining a variable amount of parenchyma from the right liver lobe, with an incidence of up to 15% of the population (Fig. 20.69).

Venous Collateral Channels

When obstruction of the hepatic veins or the suprahepatic segment of the IVC occurs, several collateral pathways develop and may be divided into three types.

1. Extrahepatic

   Collaterals developed through the liver capsule toward retroperitoneal and intercostal veins (Fig. 20.70).

2. Intrahepatic-interlobar

   Collaterals developed from the hepatic segment with venous obstruction to adjacent patent hepatic veins (Figs. 20.69 and 20.71).

3. Indeterminate type ("Spiderweb" appearance)

   Fine and/or coarse collateral networks emanating from the occluded vein (at phlebography), without certain flow direction (Fig. 20.72).

Portal Vein

The portal vein is about 7 to 8 cm in length and carries visceral blood to the liver, where it ramifies following the segmental pattern, like the hepatic artery, reaching the sinusoids, from which the blood again converges to drain into the IVC through the hepatic veins. There are no valves at the portal vein during the adult life. The portal vein results from the confluence of the splenic vein and the SMV and follows a path posteriorly to the pancreatic head and anteriorly to the IVC, reaching the liver through the lesser omentum and anterior to the epiploic foramen (Figs. 20.55, 20.73-20.79). Inside the lesser omentum and at the porta hepatis, it is posterior to the bile duct and the hepatic artery. The bile duct is parallel, but lateral, whereas the hepatic artery is parallel, but medial (Fig. 20.80).

At the porta hepatis, the portal vein divides into the right and left branches. The right portal branch enters the right hepatic lobe after receiving the cystic vein. It branches into the four segments of the right hepatic lobe (hepatic segments V, VI, VII, and VIII) and in some cases also branches to the caudate lobe (segment I). The left portal branch enters the right hepatic lobe; it is longer and with a smaller diameter, and branches into the four segments of the left lobe (hepatic segments I, IV, II, and III (Figs. 20.55, 20.81, and 20.82). At the left lobe of the liver, it is joined by the paraumbilical veins and the ligamentum teres (residuum of the obliterated left umbilical vein). There is also a connection with the IVC by the ligamentum venosum (remnant of the occluded ductus venosus).

Anatomy of the Portal Bifurcation

The anatomy of the portal vein at the bifurcation is variable, and the bifurcation can be extrahepatic in about 25% of the cases (Fig. 20.83). In 24 livers studied, the portal vein presented a very short and thin right trunk and a long left trunk. In almost every specimen, branches to the caudate lobe were seen arising from the bifurcation of the portal vein or from the first centimeter of the left trunk (Fig. 20.82A and B). One liver presented an anomalous variation at the portal bifurcation. The portal vein bifurcated in a larger left trunk and a smaller right trunk. The left trunk divided further into a real left trunk and branches to segments V and VIII of the right lobe.

In one liver, the artery crossed posteriorly to the origin of the portal trunk to segments V and VIII and followed a joint path close to the posterosuperior aspect of the portal branch to segments VI and VII. In another liver, the hepatic artery bifurcated proximally and to the left of the portal bifurcation, giving off one large anterior branch and a smaller branch, which crossed posterior to the portal bifurcation and followed a path on the posterosuperior aspect of the right trunk for the portal vein. In one case, there was a posterior arterial branch in the first 2 cm of the left portal trunk. In nine specimens, there were arterial and/or biliary structures in between the first 1 cm of the right hepatic vein and the portal bifurcation (Figs. 20.59-20.61). These biliary and arterial branches were oriented toward the segment VIII or segments VI and VII. In these cases, there was an intimate relationship between these two bilioarterial structures, but, overall, the biliary branches were posterior. In general, the biliary and arterial structures are close to the superior aspect of the portal trunks and more frequently are anterosuperior.

Tributaries: Besides the splenic and the SMVs, other tributaries are the left gastric, right gastric, the paraumbilical, and cystic veins (Figs. 20.78 and 20.84).

Right Gastric Vein

The right gastric vein runs to the right along the lesser curvature of the stomach, draining both faces of the stomach, eventually reaching the portal vein. The vein forms a loop with the LGV (Fig. 20.85).

Left Gastric Vein (Coronary Vein)

The left gastric vein drains the gastric wall along the lesser curvature and courses through the letter omentum to reach the portal vein. There are several anastomoses between the esophageal veins and the LGV, representing an important site of portosystemic shunting (Figs. 20.86-20.89).

Paraumbilical Veins

These are small veins, in variable number, extending along the ligamentum teres and median umbilical ligament, connecting veins of the anterior abdominal wall to the left branch of the portal vein. Because the paraumbilical veins connect the portal venous system to the systemic venous system, they form a direct potential portosystemic shunt (Fig. 20.90). The umbilical vein remnant (Baumgarten recess) shows no visible lumen in normal patients. The ligamentum teres shows no lumen even in cirrhotic patients with portal hypertension.

Venous Drainage of the Biliary Tract (Figs. 20.87 and 20.89)

The common bile duct's venous drainage occurs through two interconnected venous plexuses known as the epicholedochal plexus and the paracholedochal venous plexus of Petren. The epicholedochal plexus is the most superficial and consists of a fine reticular network of veins which communicate with a subepithelial venous plexus and an intramural venous plexus via perforators in the duct wall. The paracholedochal venous plexus of Petren usually forms two parallel marginal veins at the 3 o'clock and 9 o'clock positions, while a vein in the posterior surface of the duct at the 6 o'clock position is less frequent. These veins communicate with gastric veins and posterior superior pancreaticoduodenal (PSPD) veins and bring hepatopedal flow of portal venous blood to the hilar venous plexus which drains into portal vein branches in the caudate lobe and segment IV. Cavernous transformation of the portal vein, also known as a cavernoma, is caused by compensatory hypertrophy of the veins in the epicholedochal and paracholedochal venous plexus.

Cystic Veins

There are two types of cystic veins. The first type includes veins originated at the superior surface of the gallbladder, entering the liver parenchyma directly or joining the bile duct vein system. The second, and rarer type, is a single or a double cystic vein joining the right portal branch. The cystic vein typically drains into the 9 o'clock marginal vein.

Variations and Anomalies of the Portal Vein

The normal anatomy of the portal vein is consistent, and the variations and anomalies are relatively uncommon. The variations of the portal vein are related mostly to the different arrangement of the tributaries. The LGV may enter at the junction of the splenic and the portal vein or join the splenic vein. The inferior mesenteric vein may enter the SMV and high intestinal veins may enter directly at the portal vein. The anomalies of the portal vein are related mostly to anomalies of position: portal vein anterior to the head of the pancreas and first part of the duodenum; portal vein entering the IVC; pulmonary vein entering the portal vein; or congenital stricture of the portal vein. A rare variation is the duplication of the portal vein, which may also be related to recanalized occlusion (Fig. 20.91).

Splenic Vein

The splenic vein is one of the two larger tributaries of the portal vein, and its confluence with the SMV actually forms the portal vein. It is a large vein, about 1 cm in diameter, enlarging as it reaches the portal vein. Normally, it is a relatively straight vein but may get very tortuous due to portal hypertension. The main splenic vein is formed by the union of two veins in 76% of the cases, by three branches in 20% of the cases, and by four branches in 4% of the 50 specimens studied. The spleen has a venous segmentation that varies in number but makes totally independent compartments, as visualized in the corrosion endocasts obtained of the intrasplenic venous vasculature (Figs. 20.92 and 20.93). It is originated from the splenic hilum and follows a path from left to right behind the tail and body of the pancreas, receiving several pancreatic venous branches. There is a close correspondence with respect to number and path between the hilar splenic veins and the hilar splenic arteries in 80.6% of the cases. There is no correspondence in 19.4% of the cases. The analysis of 25 casts injected with polyester resin showed two venous segments in 85.0% of cases and three venous segments in 11.0% of cases. There is also a correspondence between splenic venous segments and splenic arterial segments, in which each trabecular artery corresponds to a trabecular vein. The splenic venous segments are entirely independent at the venous or arterial circulation (Figs. 20.92 and 20.93).

Tributaries

Short gastric veins: There are four or five short gastric veins draining the gastric fundus and part of the greater gastric curvature, reaching the splenic vein or one of its large tributaries. These veins are also in communication with the lower esophageal veins and may enlarge markedly when submitted to portal hypertension, thereby reversing the blood flow (Figs. 20.86, 20.94, and 20.95).

Left gastroepiploic vein: This vein runs along the greater gastric curvature, from right to left, draining the walls of the stomach and the greater omentum, reaching the initial part of the splenic vein (Figs. 20.94 and 20.95).

Pancreatic veins: There is a variable number of pancreatic veins draining the body and tail of the pancreas. These veins may be small, draining directly into the splenic vein, or larger and few resulting from the confluence of smaller tributaries, eventually draining into the splenic vein. The full description of the pancreatic vein drainage follows.

Inferior mesenteric vein (Fig. 20.96): The inferior mesenteric vein drains the rectum, the sigmoid colon, and the left colon, joining the splenic vein distally, close to the confluence with the inferior mesenteric vein, posterior to the body of the pancreas. Occasionally it ends at the union of the splenic and SMV and sometimes at the SMV itself.

Tributaries

Superior rectal vein
Sigmoid veins
Left colic vein

The inferior mesenteric vein begins as the superior rectal vein, arising from the rectal plexus, having connections with the middle and inferior rectal veins. It ascends posterior to the peritoneum and receives the sigmoid veins and the left colic vein. The left colic vein continues with the middle colic vein (MCV) at the splenic flexure of the colon.

Superior Mesenteric Vein

The superior mesenteric vein is the largest tributary to the portal vein. It drains the small intestine, cecum, and ascending and transverse parts of the colon, carrying blood to enter the portal circulation. This vein passes behind the pancreatic head and horizontal part of the duodenum; it is anterior to the IVC and joins the splenic vein, forming the portal vein. The SMV is formed by the union of the tributaries from the terminal ileum, the cecum, and the appendix, receiving several other tributaries along its length (Figs. 20.97-20.99).

Tributaries

Jejunal and ileal veins: These are the most numerous tributaries of the SMV. They are named after the respective arteries and conform with the arcade distribution, placed, as a rule, on the left side of the SMVs, from the duodenojejunal junction to the vicinity of the ileocecal junction where ends the ileocolic vein. The first and sometimes the first and second jejunal veins are joined by the inferior pancreaticoduodenal vein, either as a trunk or as separate vessels (Figs. 20.100-20.102).

Ileocolic vein: The ileocolic vein is formed by the union of the anterior and posterior cecal veins, plus the appendicular veins, the last ileal vein, and a colic vein, eventually joining the SMV on its right aspect. It anastomoses freely with the ileal veins and the right colic vein (Fig. 20.100).

Right colic vein: This vein drains the right colon and results from the junction of the several venous arcades of the right colon wall and from the marginal vein. It anastomoses freely with the ileocolic vein and the MCV. It is retroperitoneal and joins the SMV at the level where it crosses over the third part of the duodenum (Fig. 20.97).

Middle colic vein: The middle colic vein drains the transverse colon and has a right and left branch. The right MCV anastomoses with the right colic vein, whereas the left anastomoses with the left colic vein (tributary of the inferior mesenteric vein) at the splenic flexure of the colon. The MCV joins the SMV through the gastrocolic trunk in the majority of cases but may end directly into the SMV itself.

Right gastroepiploic vein: This vein drains the greater omentum and the distal part of the body and the antrum of the stomach. It is a long vein and runs from left to right along the greater gastric curvature. It anastomoses freely with the left gastroepiploic vein and is a major collateral path to drain the spleen when the splenic vein is occluded. The right gastroepiploic (RGE) vein ends at the gastrocolic trunk, tributary of the SMV, joining the middle colic and anterior pancreaticoduodenal veins. It may occasionally end directly at the SMV (Figs. 20.103 and 20.104).

Pancreaticoduodenal veins. The pancreaticoduodenal veins drain the head of the pancreas and the duodenal wall and follow similar anatomic architecture to its arterial structure. There is a posterior pancreaticoduodenal venous arcade and an anterior pancreaticoduodenal venous arcade between the superior and inferior pancreaticoduodenal veins. The posterior superior ends at the portal vein and the anterior superior ends at the gastrocolic trunk, whereas both posterior and anterior inferior end at the SMV, through the first jejunal vein (Fig. 20.105).

Anastomoses Between the Portal and Systemic Circulations

In portal vein obstruction or portal vein hypertension due to liver disease, anastomosis between the portal vein and systemic veins may develop, carrying portal blood into the systemic circulation (Fig. 20.106).

There are four main groups of portal systemic collaterals.

Group I

Where protective mucosal epithelium adjoins absorptive mucosal epithelium.

Group I (A)

At the cardia of the stomach, where the LGV and short gastric veins of the portal system anastomoses with the intercostal, diaphragm-esophageal, and azygos tributaries, veins of the caval system, creating esophageal and gastric fundus varices.

Group I (B)

At the anal canal the superior rectal (hemorrhoidal) vein, tributary of the inferior mesenteric vein (portal system), anastomoses with the middle and inferior rectal (hemorrhoidal) veins of the IVC system, creating hemorrhoids.

Group II

In the falciform ligament through the paraumbilical veins, vestiges of the umbilical circulation of fetal life. Enlargement of these connections, in the presence of portal hypertension, may produce varices of veins radiating from the umbilicus, the caput medusae (part of the Cruveilhier-Baumgarten syndrome). The umbilical vein remnant does not recanalize within the ligamentum teres.

Group III

Where the abdominal organs are in contact with retroperitoneal tissues or adherent to the abdominal wall (intercostal veins, lumbar veins). Includes veins from the liver to the diaphragm (veins of Sappey), veins in the lienorenal ligament and omentum, lumbar veins (veins of Retzius), and veins developed in adhesions and scars of previous surgeries.

Group IV

Connections between the portal system and the left renal vein. This may be through communications directly from the splenic vein or via diaphragmatic, pancreatic, left adrenal, gonadal, or gastric veins.

Other Collaterals

The communications from the gastroesophageal collaterals, retroperitoneal, and venous systems of the abdomen eventually reach the superior vena cava via the azygos or hemiazygos systems. Very rarely a patent ductus venosus connects the left branch of the portal vein to the IVC. In cases of extrahepatic portal venous obstruction, additional collaterals develop toward the liver, entering the liver through the portal vein in the porta hepatis. These collaterals include the veins at the hilum, venae comitantes of the portal vein and hepatic arteries, veins in the suspensory ligaments of the liver, unnamed veins around the gallbladder, and diaphragmatic and omental veins.

Distinct patterns of portosystemic shunting draining through gastric varices have been described (Fig. 20.106). These patterns can be classified based on venous inflow or by venous drainage. When considering venous inflow patterns, there are three basic types. Type 1 consists of a single afferent vein from the LGV, which is the most common type. Type 2 consists of multiple afferent gastric veins, with type 3 being multiple gastric veins which are contiguous with the shunt but do not significantly contribute to the variceal complex. The classification based on venous drainage is composed of four types. Type A being a shunt with a single draining vein, typically the left adrenal vein into the left renal vein. Type B consists of a type A shunt with multiple collateral draining veins. Type C is defined as a gastrocaval and a gastrorenal shunt, and type D having multiple small draining veins without a gastrorenal shunt.

Pancreatic Venous System

The anatomy of the pancreatic veins corresponds roughly to the distribution of the pancreatic arteries (Fig. 20.107).

The head of the pancreas has the venous drainage related to the main stem of the portal vein and to the SMV. The venous drainage of the head of the pancreas is constituted by four main veins, forming two arcades: one posterior and one anterior. The posterior aspect of the pancreas head is drained by one or several PSPD veins directly connected to the dorsal aspect of the portal vein (PV), usually about 2 cm from the point of confluence of the splenic, the superior mesenteric, and the PVs. The posterior arcade also empties into the first jejunal vein or directly into the SMV via the posterior inferior pancreaticoduodenal (PIPD) vein. This arcade runs posteriorly to the pancreatic head in the pancreaticoduodenal sulcus, receiving tributaries from the pancreas and duodenum. The anterior aspect of the pancreas head is drained by the anterior superior pancreaticoduodenal (ASPD) vein, emptying directly into the gastrocolic trunk (GT) beside several smaller veins. The GT receives the RGE vein and the MCV and empties itself into the right aspect of the SMV, from 1 to 3 cm from the junction of the SMV, splenic vein (SV), and PV.

The lower ventral aspect of the head of the pancreas is drained by the anterior inferior pancreaticoduodenal (AIPD) vein, which drains into the first jejunal vein or, in some cases, into the SMV. The AIPD vein is usually joined by the PIPD vein in the last few centimeters before emptying into the first jejunal vein.

The ventral aspect of the pancreas head may be occasionally drained by a vein emptying in the ventral surface of the PV, near the confluence or up to 3 or 4 cm from that point. The larger pancreatic veins draining the pancreas head run on the surface of the organ and not within the parenchyma itself (Figs. 20.108-20.114).

The venous drainage of the pancreas head is usually connected through collaterals to the dorsal pancreatic (DP) vein, which drains part of the mediodorsal part of the head and empties in the dorsal aspect of the portal confluence wall (Figs. 20.115-20.118).

The body of the pancreas is drained by the transverse pancreatic (TP) vein, which empties into either the inferior mesenteric vein, SMV or SV (Figs. 20.119 and 20.120). The TP vein runs along the inferior border of the pancreatic body, parallel to the SV, and receives a large number of small branches from the pancreas body and may be connected to the LGV (Fig. 20.121). Several of the smaller veins draining the body of the pancreas empty into the PSPD vein, the LGV, or directly into the large venous trunks near the confluence (Figs. 20.119 and 20.120).

The tail of the pancreas is drained by a large number of small and short veins that are usually connected to the caudal aspect of the SV. These are mainly intrapancreatic veins that are part of a rich anastomotic venous bed connecting the TP vein and the SV. Some of the lower polar veins of the spleen may also participate in the distal caudal pancreatic venous drainage (Figs. 20.122-20.125).

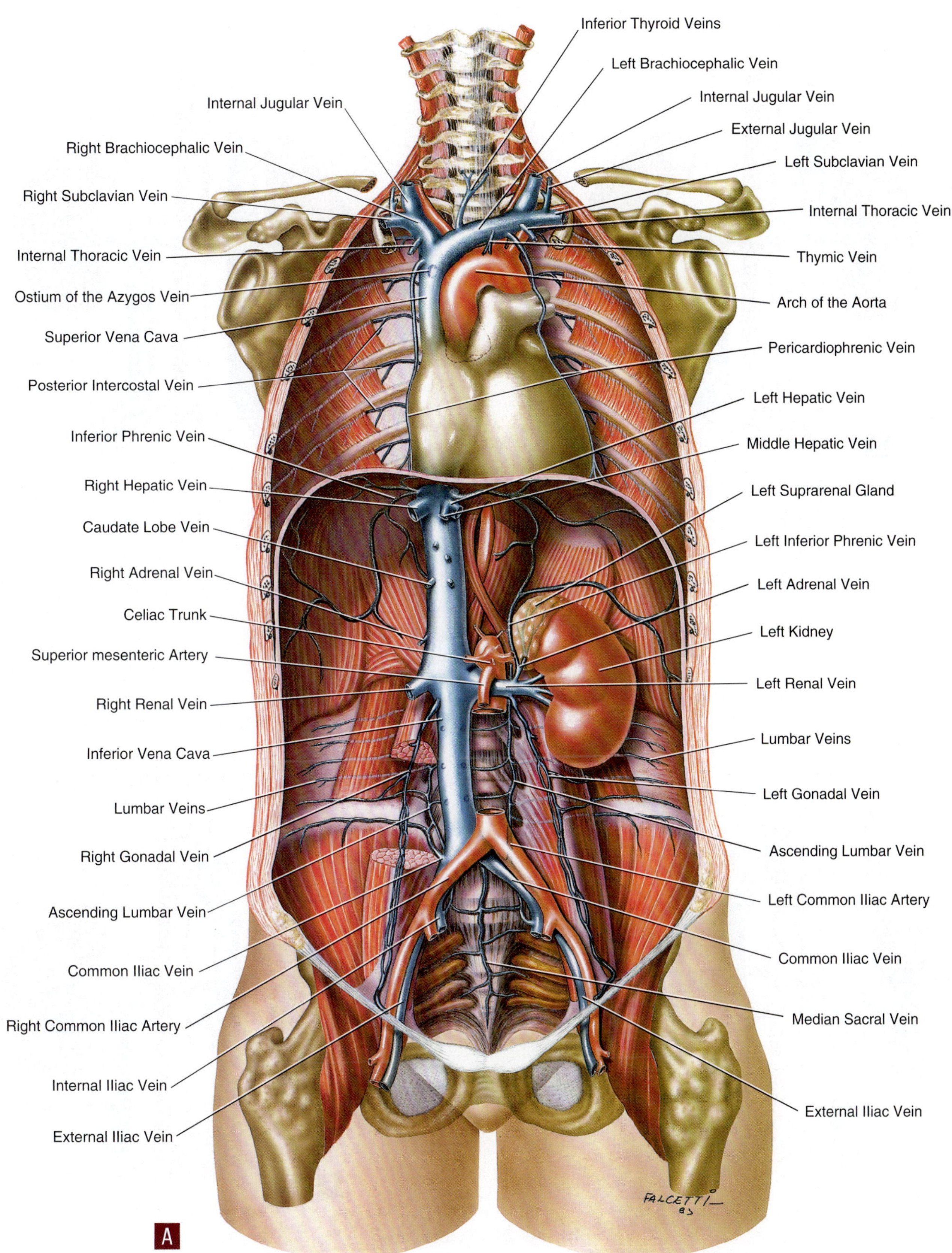

Figure 20.1. **A**, Schematic diagram of the inferior vena cava (IVC), tributary veins of the abdomen and pelvis, as well as the superior vena cava and main venous tributaries of the chest. **B**, Schematic diagram of a left-sided IVC variant. **C**, Duplicated IVC. **D**, Azygos continuation of the IVC. **E**, Hemiazygos continuation of the IVC. **F**, Duplicated IVC with azygos continuation.

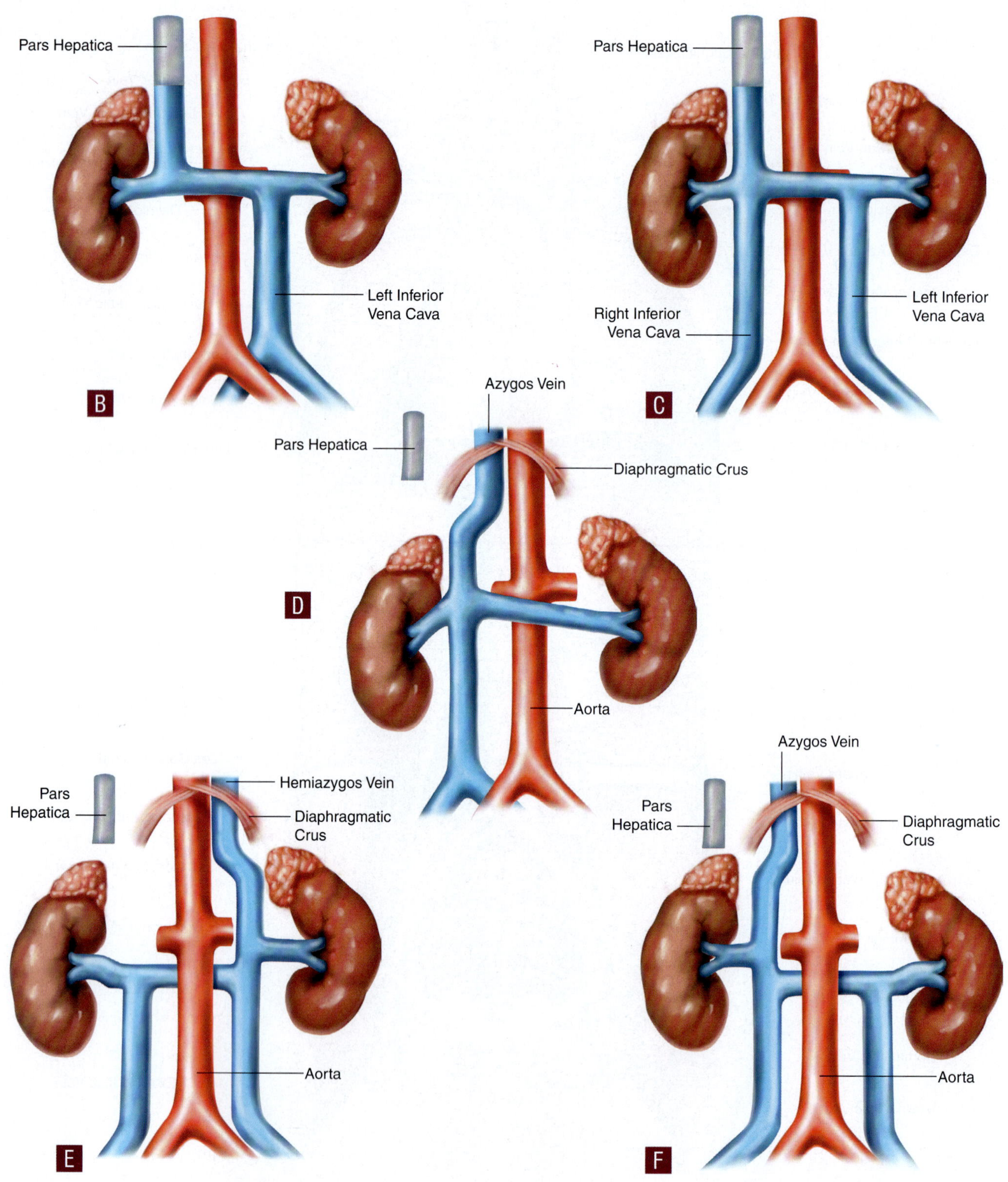

Figure 20.1. *Continued*

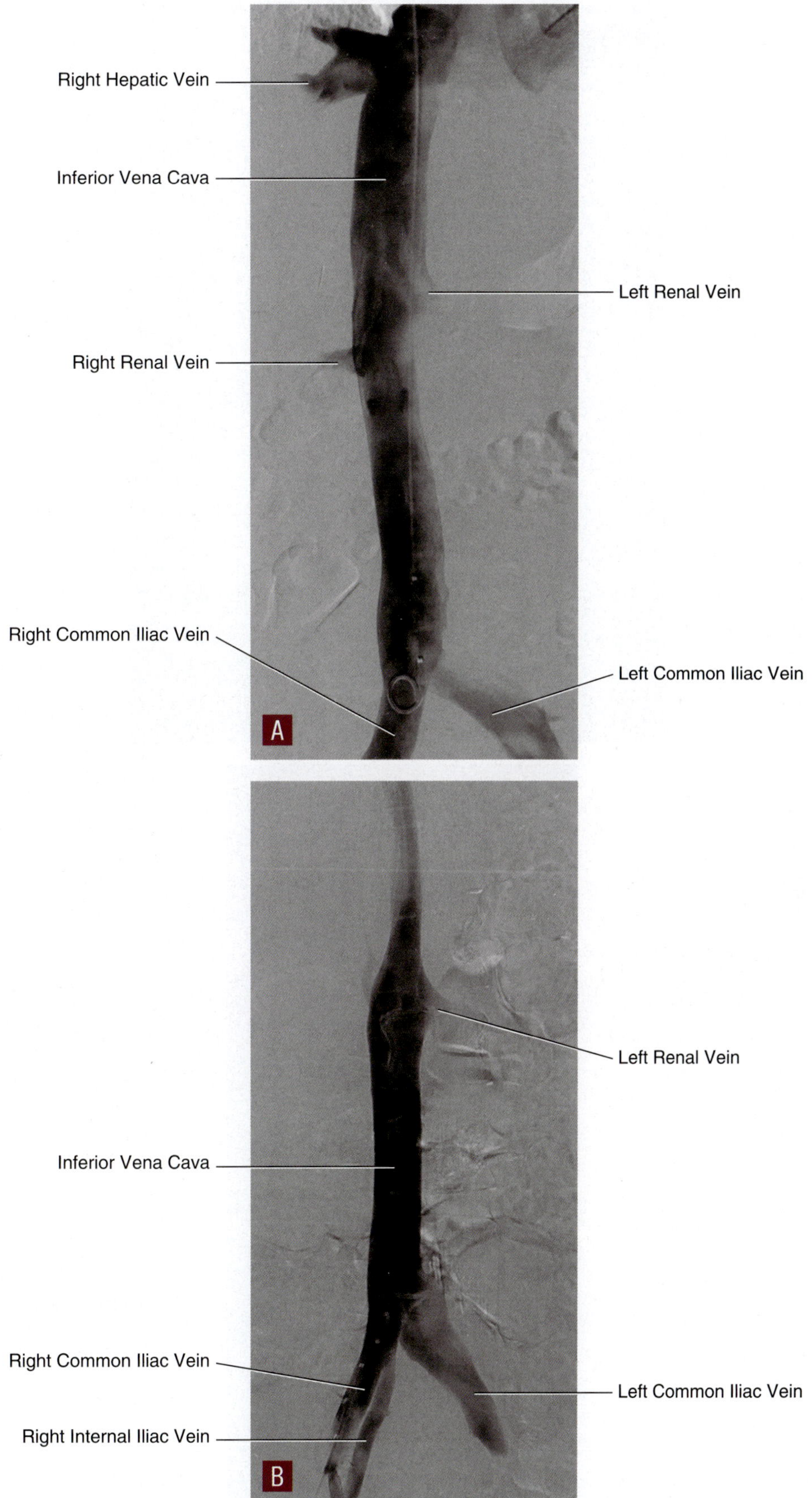

Figure 20.2. **Venography of the iliac veins and inferior vena cava.** A, Normal cavogram with reflux into the hepatic veins and renal veins. B, Normal cavogram. The liver causes some constriction of the vena cava. There is high insertion of the right internal iliac vein.

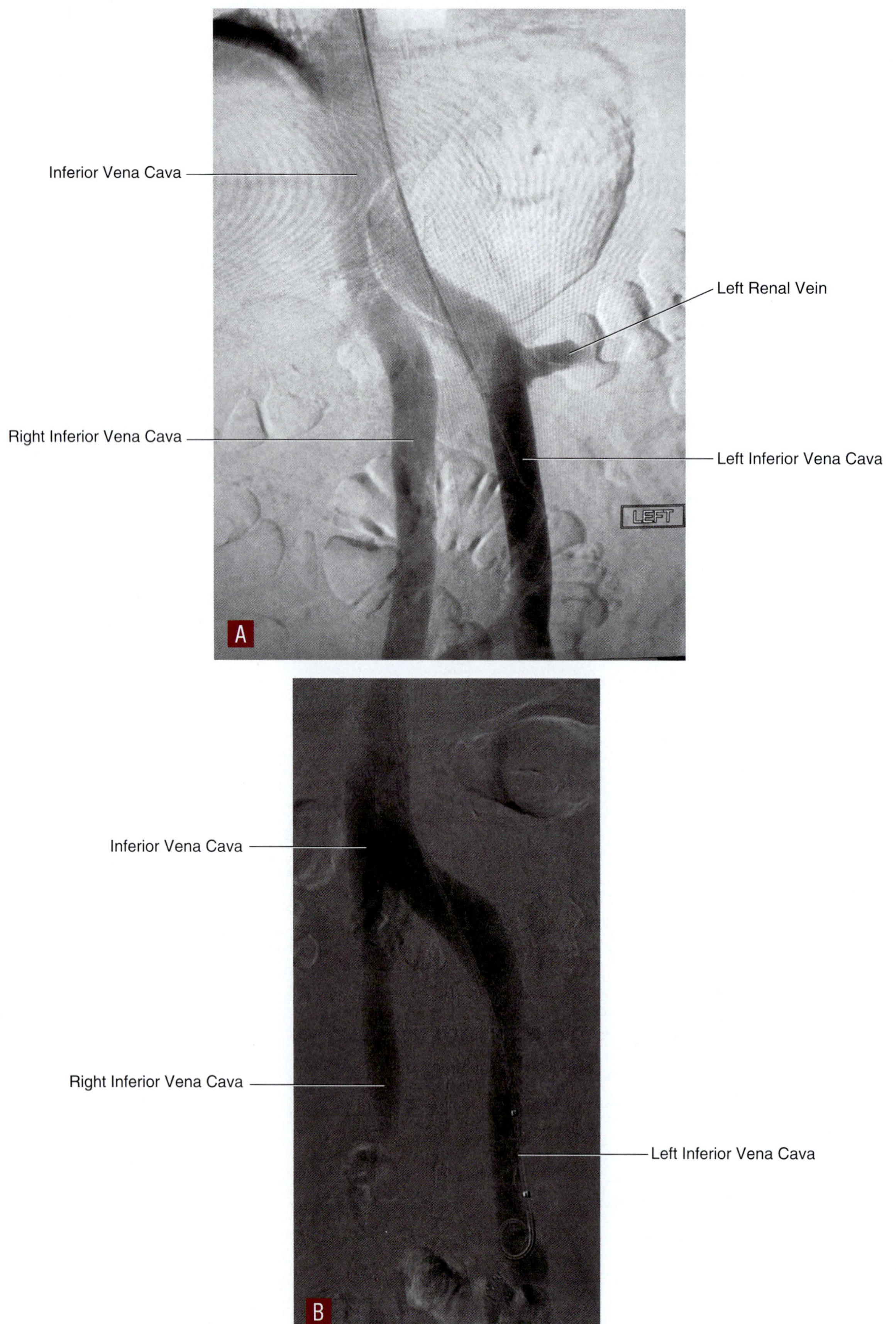

Figure 20.3. A and B, Venography demonstrating two samples of duplicated inferior vena cava.

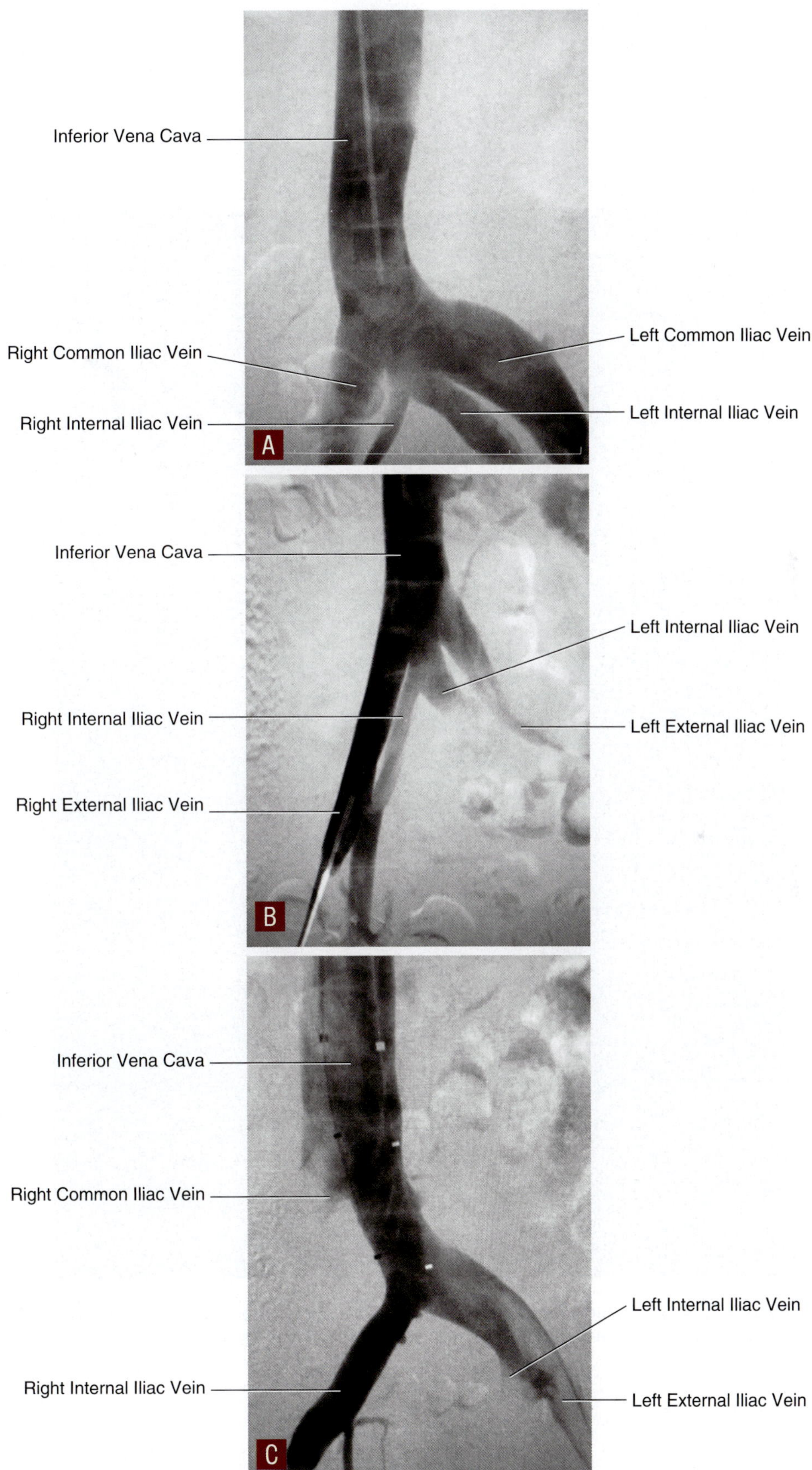

Figure 20.4. A and B, Digital subtraction cavagrams showing a common confluence of the internal iliac veins which drain into the confluence of the common iliac veins to form the inferior vena cava. C, Venogram of the iliac veins and IVC shows a right internal iliac vein draining into the left common iliac vein.

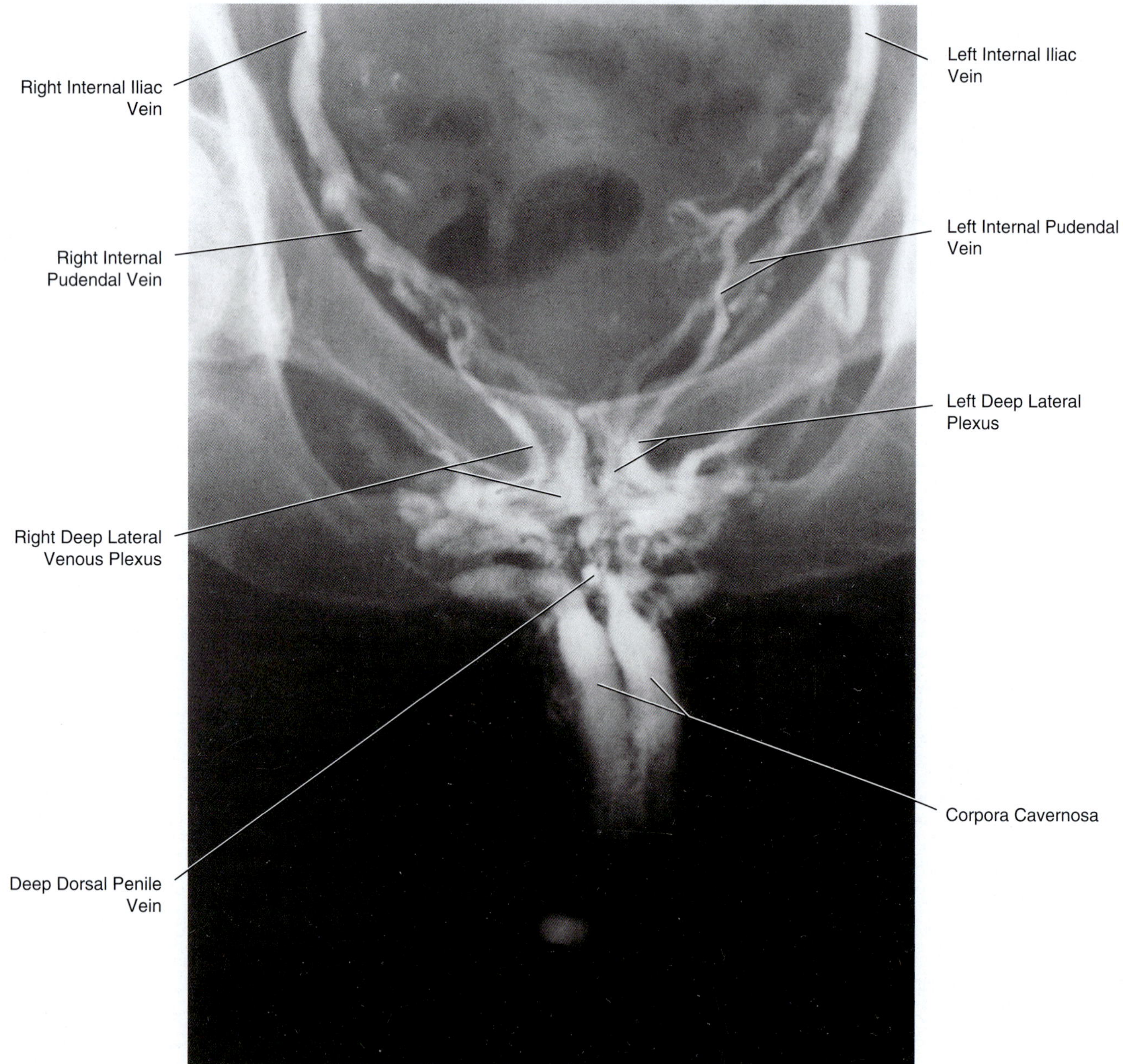

Figure 20.5. Percutaneous cavernosogram showing the corpora cavernosa, the prostatic venous plexus, the internal pudendal veins, and the internal iliac veins.

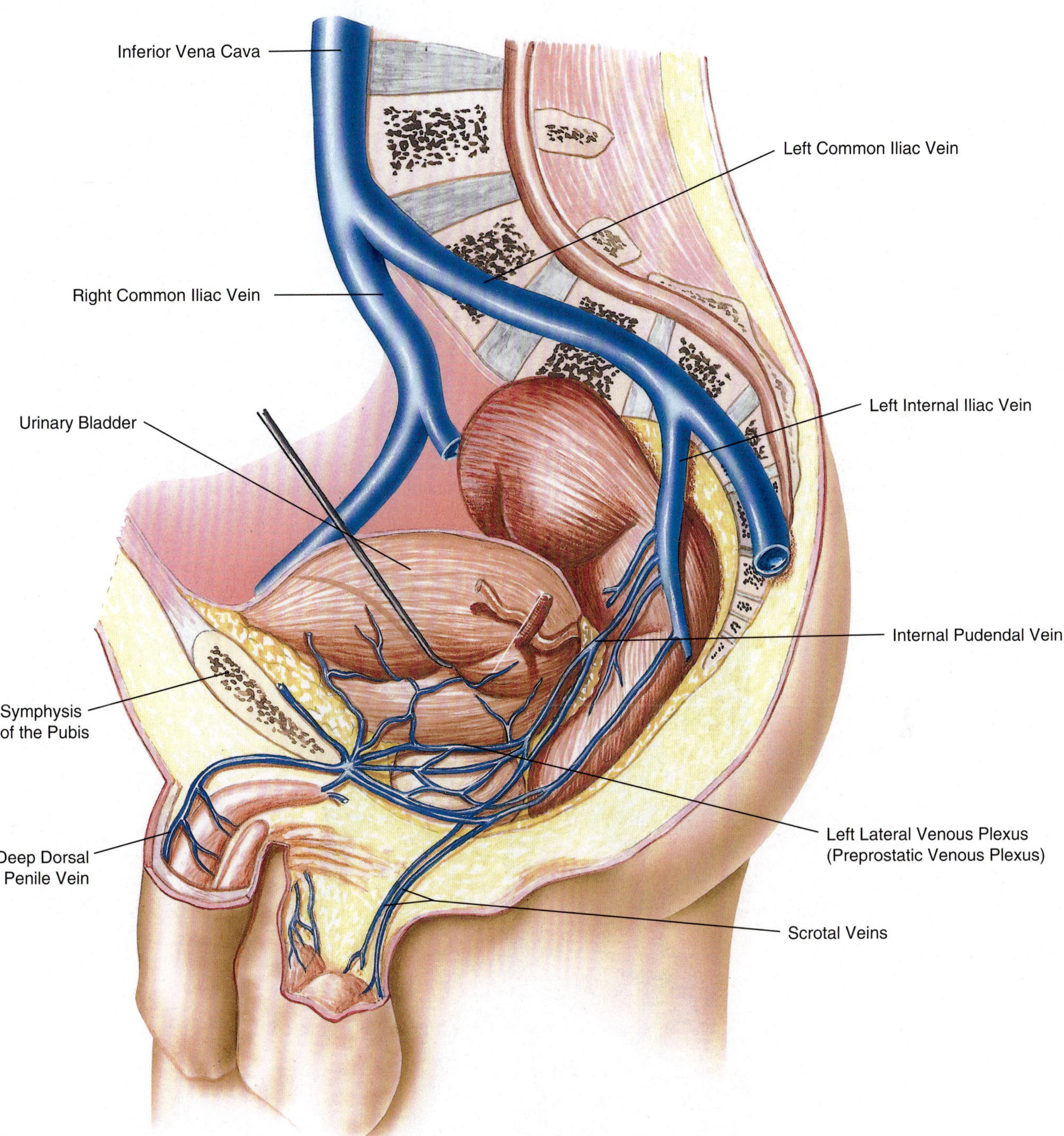

Figure 20.6. Schematic diagram of the male pelvis on a lateral view. It reveals the deep dorsal vein of the penis penetrating the pelvis under the symphysis of the pubis. The left lateral plexus is also seen.

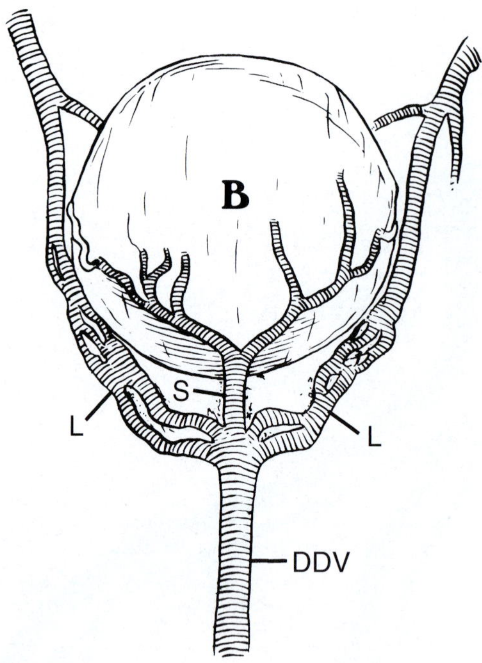

Figure 20.7. Schematic drawing from a superior view of the deep dorsal vein (DDV) of the penis dividing into three major branches; the superficial branch (S) and the right and left deep lateral plexuses (L). B, urinary bladder.

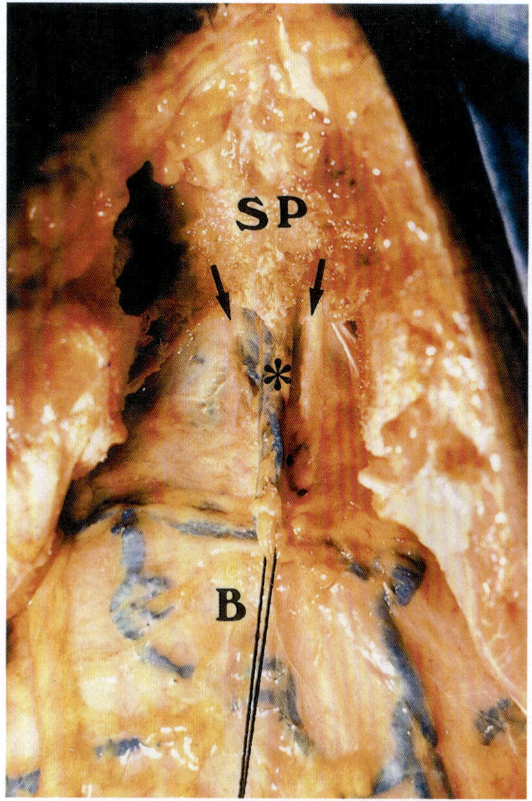

Figure 20.8. Specimen injected with blue latex through the deep dorsal vein of the penis. Superior view of the retropubic space reveals the right and left puboprostatic ligaments (arrows) and the superficial branch of the periprostatic plexus (superficial plexus) centrally located (asterisk) and emerging above the endopelvic fascia, between the puboprostatic ligaments. Note the communication venous branches over the bladder. B, urinary bladder; SP, symphysis pubis.

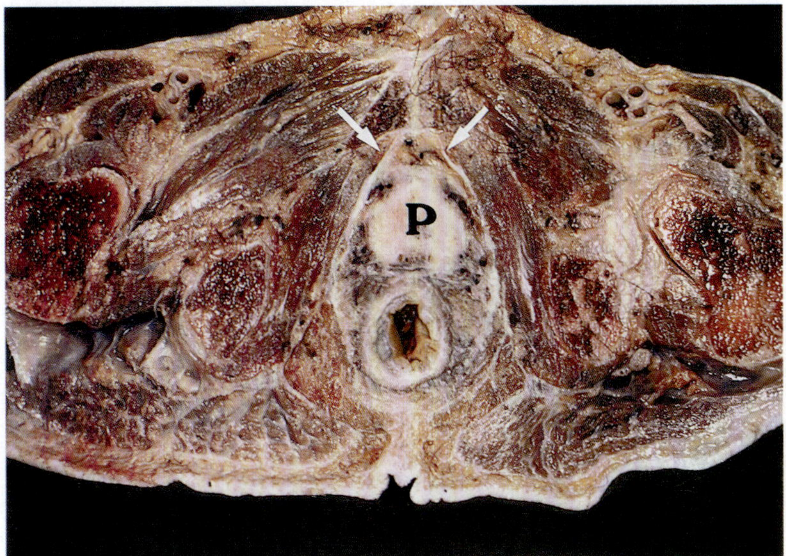

Figure 20.9. Transverse section through the pelvis of a male specimen, reveals the prostate (P) involved by the lateral deep venous plexuses. The whitish band embracing the prostate, the plexuses, and the rectum is the endopelvic fascia. The arrows point out the anterior condensations of the endopelvic fascia, attached to the posterior surface of the symphysis pubis (puboprostatic ligaments). Note the superficial branch (superficial plexus) in the retropubic adipose tissue, between the puboprostatic ligaments.

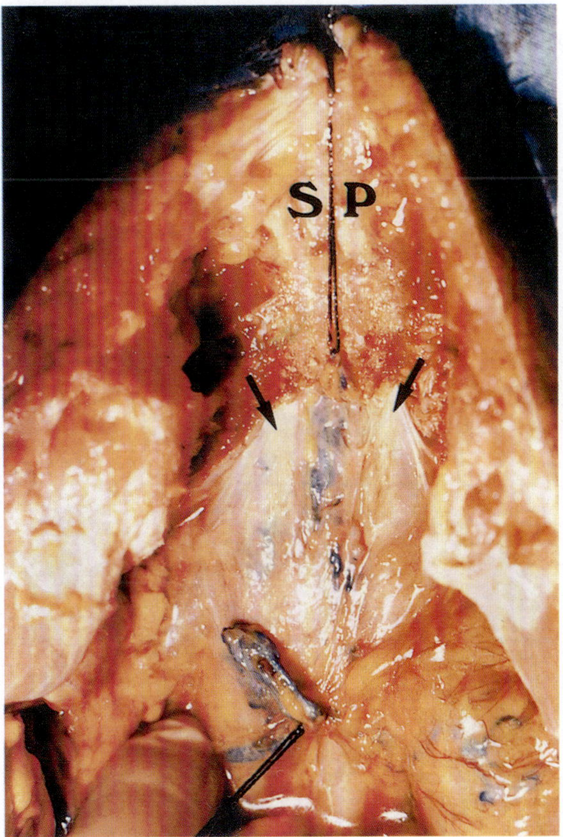

Figure 20.10. Same specimen shown in Fig. 20.8. The superficial branch of the deep dorsal vein (superficial plexus) was divided. Note the endopelvic fascia and the puboprostatic ligaments (arrows). The lateral venous plexuses (deep plexus) are located on the right and left sides, beneath the endopelvic fascia (preprostatic fascia). SP, symphysis pubis.

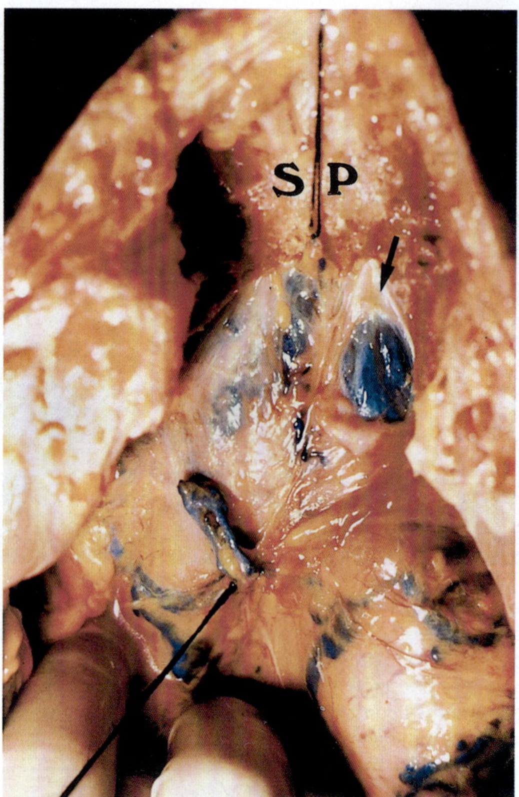

Figure 20.11. Same specimen shown in Fig. 20.10. The right puboprostatic ligament was divided (arrow), and the endopelvic fascia was opened in the right side. Note the right deep lateral plexus injected with blue latex. SP, symphysis pubis.

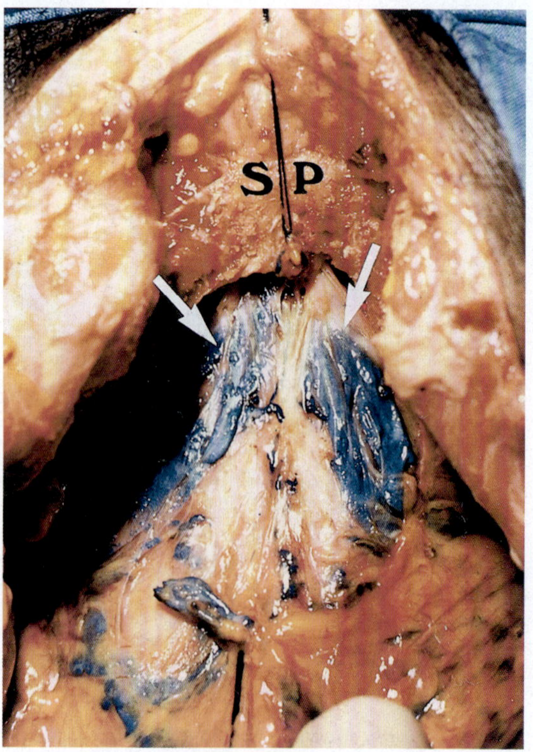

Figure 20.12. Same specimen shown in Fig. 20.11. The left puboprostatic ligament was also divided and the endopelvic fascia was completely opened, exposing the right and left deep venous plexuses (deep plexus, Santorini) (arrows). SP, symphysis pubis.

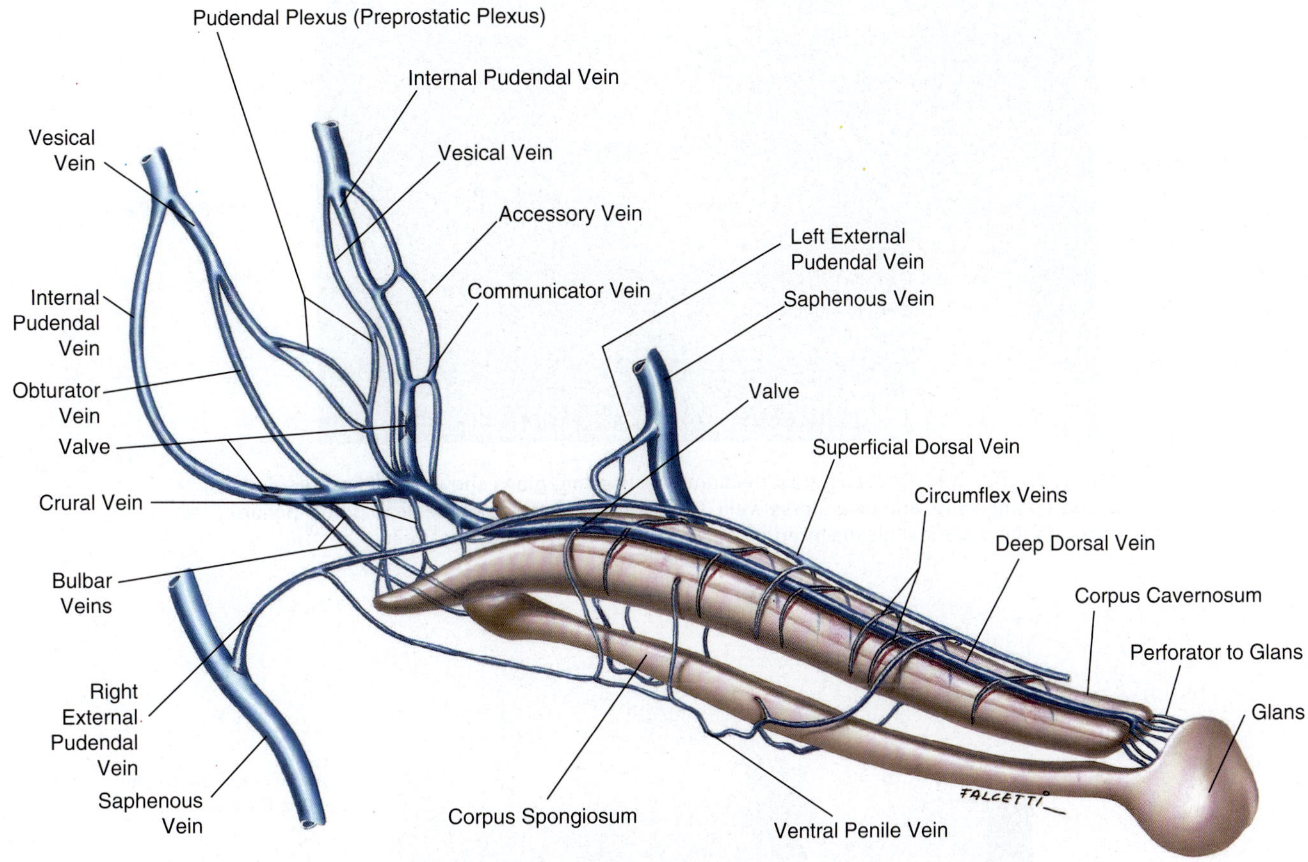

Figure 20.13. Diagrammatic demonstration of the penile venous anatomy draining the corpora cavernosa, as observed on an oblique view. It is noteworthy to observe crural drainage into internal pudendal veins and bulbar drainage via several veins into the internal pudendal vein. There are few communications, or none at all, between the deep and superficial dorsal veins. The drainage of the glans is predominantly into the deep dorsal penile vein; there are, however, direct communications between the glans and corpus cavernosum. The circumflex veins from corpora cavernosa drain into the deep dorsal penile vein but also into superficial dorsal penile vein. The drainage of the deep dorsal penile vein is into the preprostatic plexus and internal pudendal veins. The drainage of the superficial dorsal penile vein is into the external pudendal and then into the saphenous veins.

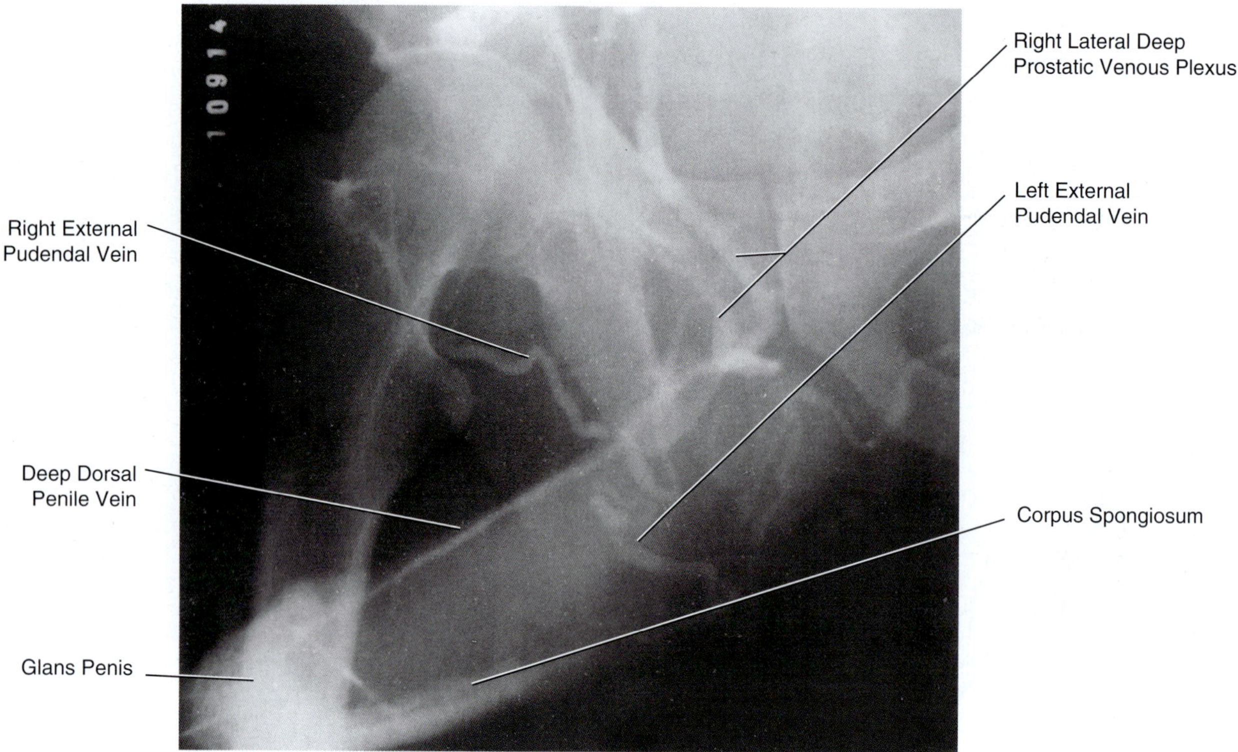

Figure 20.14. Direct contrast medium injection into glans shows opacification of glans, corpus spongiosum, and deep dorsal vein. Note communications of the deep dorsal penile vein with the pudendal plexus (preprostatic) and the external pudendal veins.

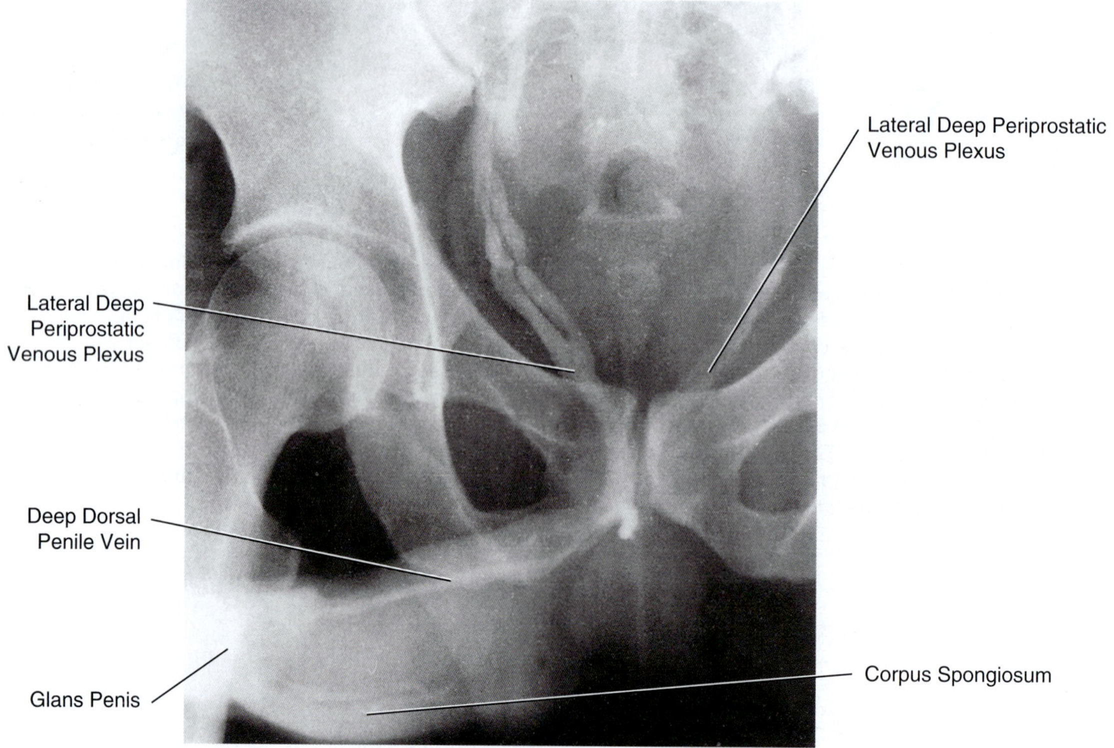

Figure 20.15. Direct contrast injection into glans shows opacification of glans, corpus spongiosum, and deep dorsal vein. The deep dorsal vein drains into the periprostatic plexus.

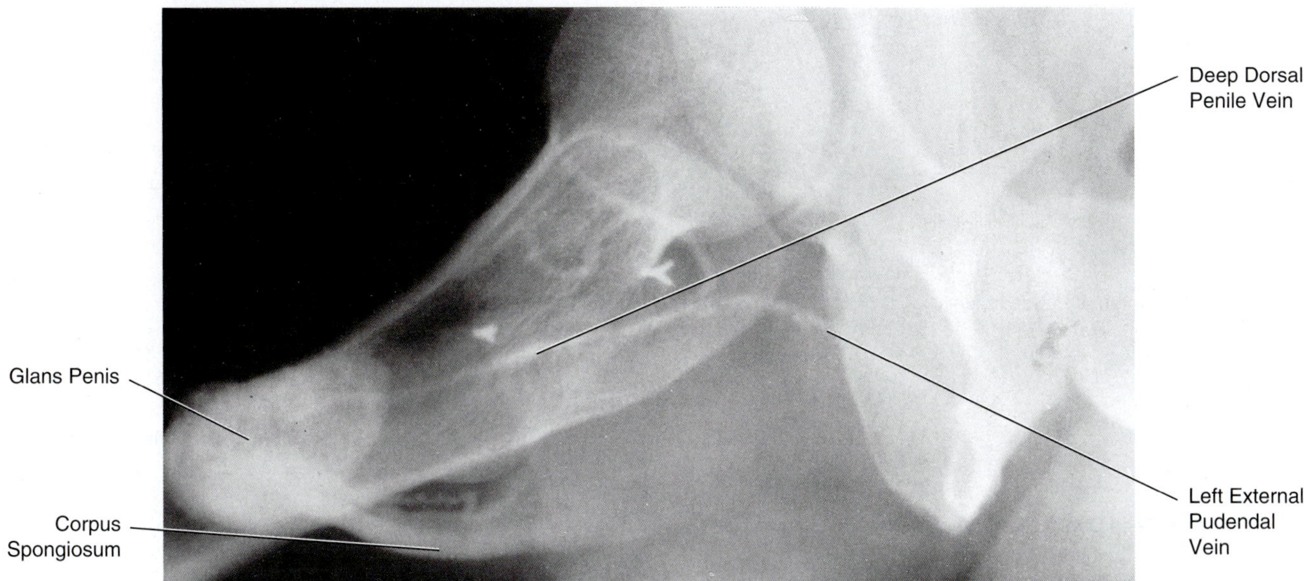

Figure 20.16. Contrast injection into glans shows opacification of glans, corpus spongiosum, and deep dorsal vein. There is communication with the right external pudendal. No communication with the preprostatic plexus is observed.

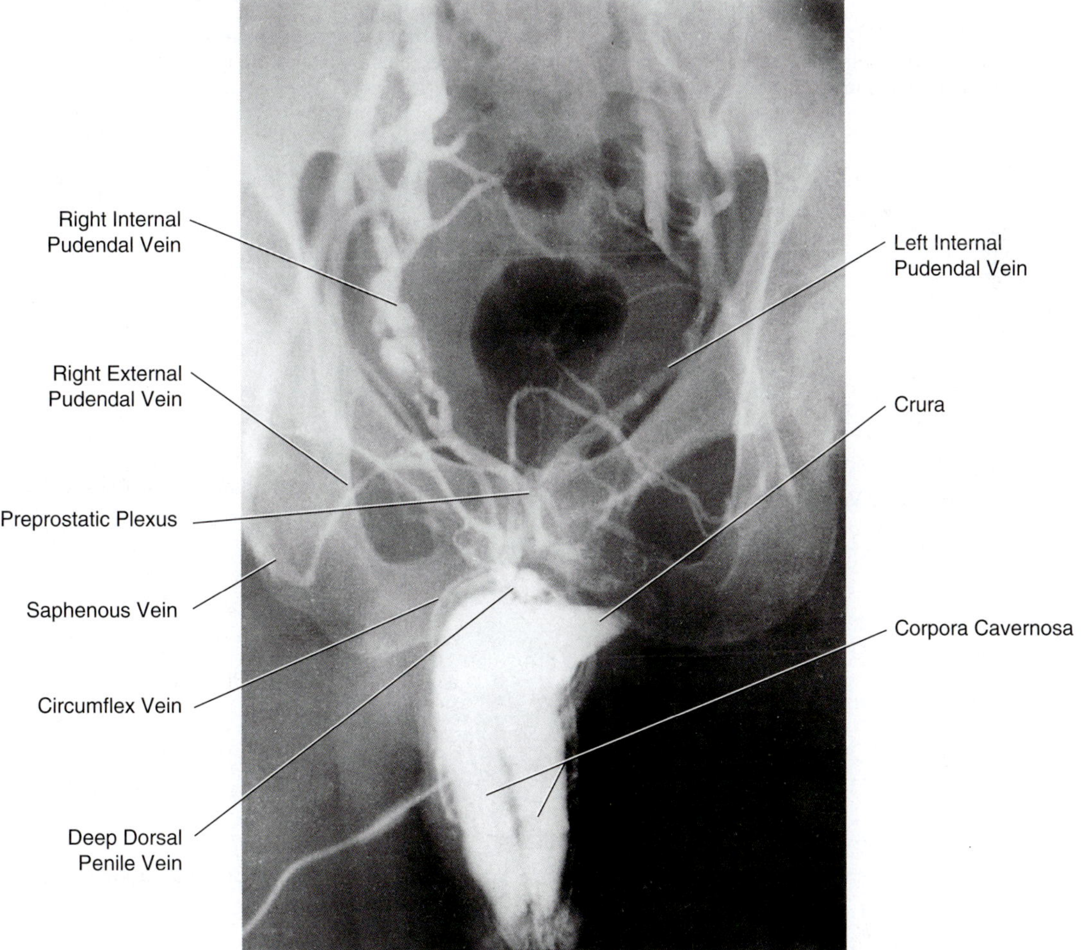

Figure 20.17. Cavernosogram showing opacification of the corpora cavernosa, the deep dorsal vein, the circumflex veins, and the communications with the pudendal plexus and the external pudendal veins, with subsequent opacification of the femoral veins.

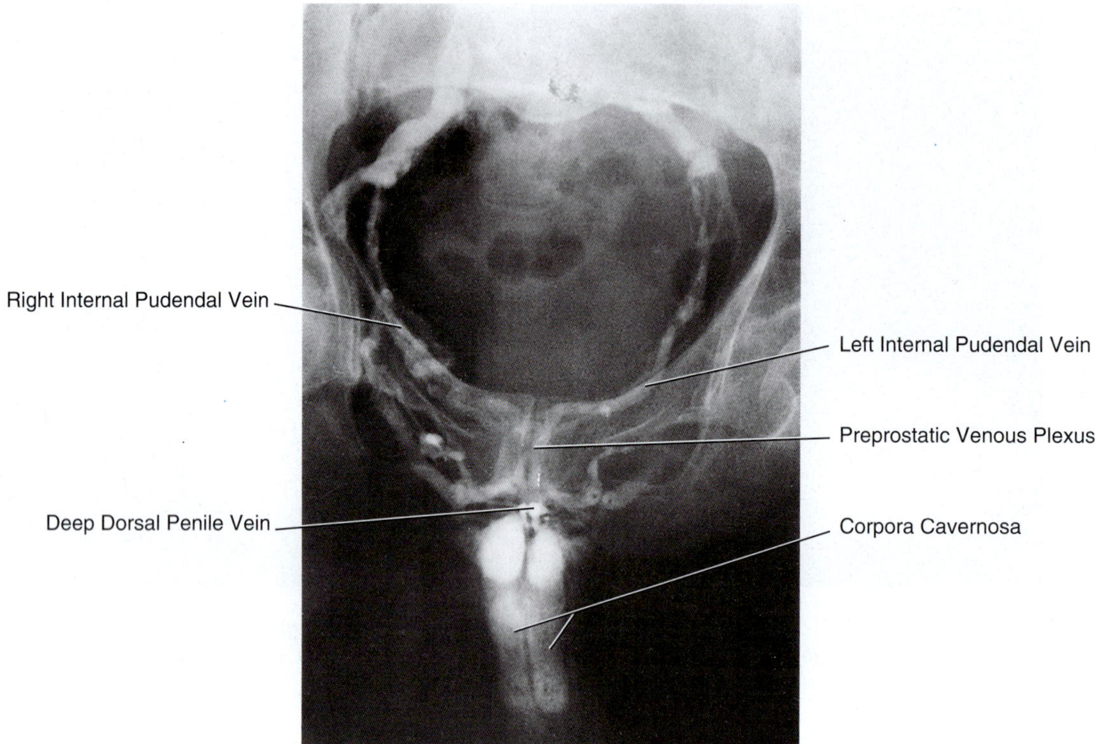

Figure 20.18. Cavernosogram showing opacification of the corpora cavernosa, the deep dorsal vein, and the communication with the preprostatic plexus and the internal pudendal and internal iliac veins.

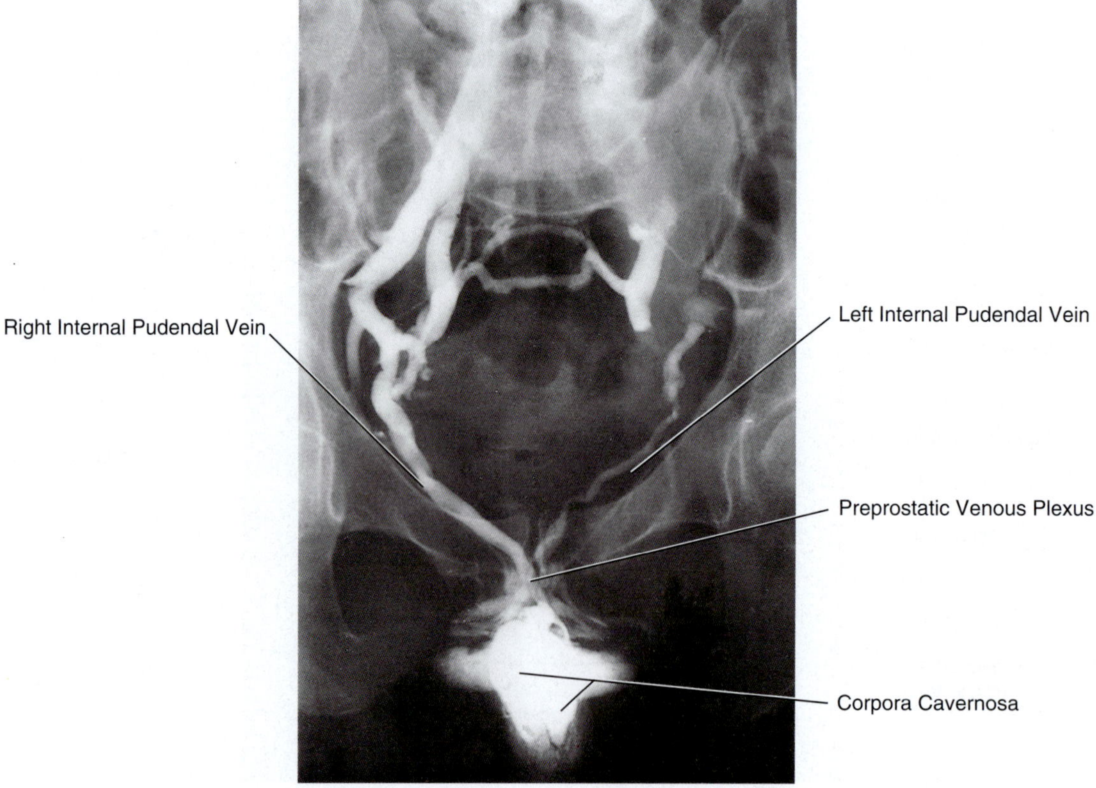

Figure 20.19. Cavernosogram showing opacification of the corpora cavernosa, the deep dorsal vein and the crura of the corpora cavernosa, and the drainage of the penis to the prostatic venous plexus with right and left branches. Note the direct communication with the internal pudendal veins and the internal iliac veins.

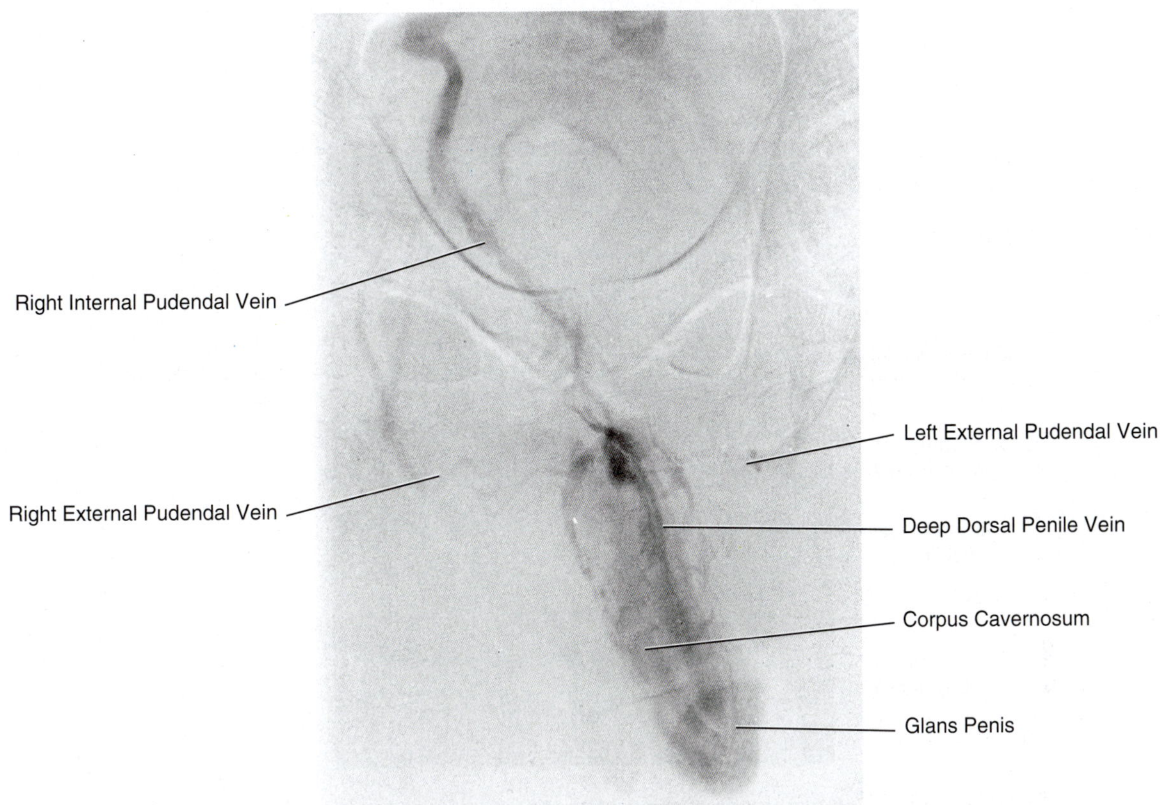

Figure 20.20. Photographic subtraction of the cavernosogram showing opacification of the corpora cavernosa of the penis and the deep and superficial dorsal penile veins. The drainage to the internal pudendal vein on the right is noted.

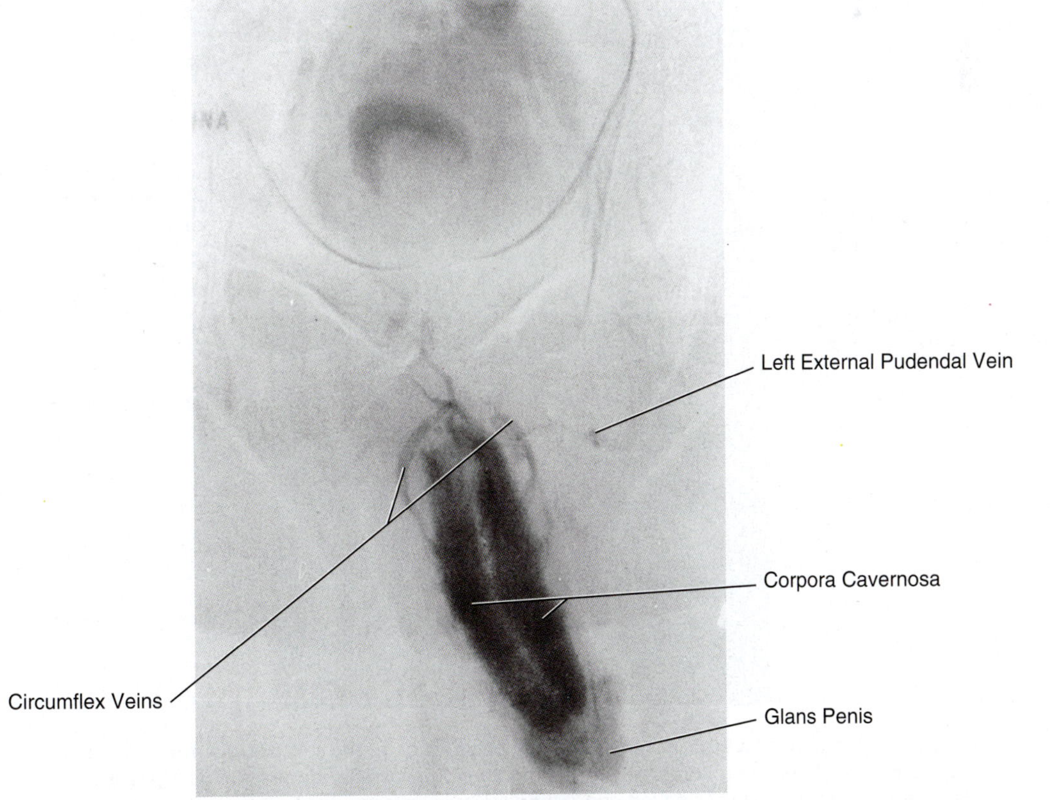

Figure 20.21. Cavernosogram showing opacification of the corpora cavernosa and the drainage through the circumflex veins into the deep dorsal penile vein. Note very faint opacification of the external pudendal vein on the left.

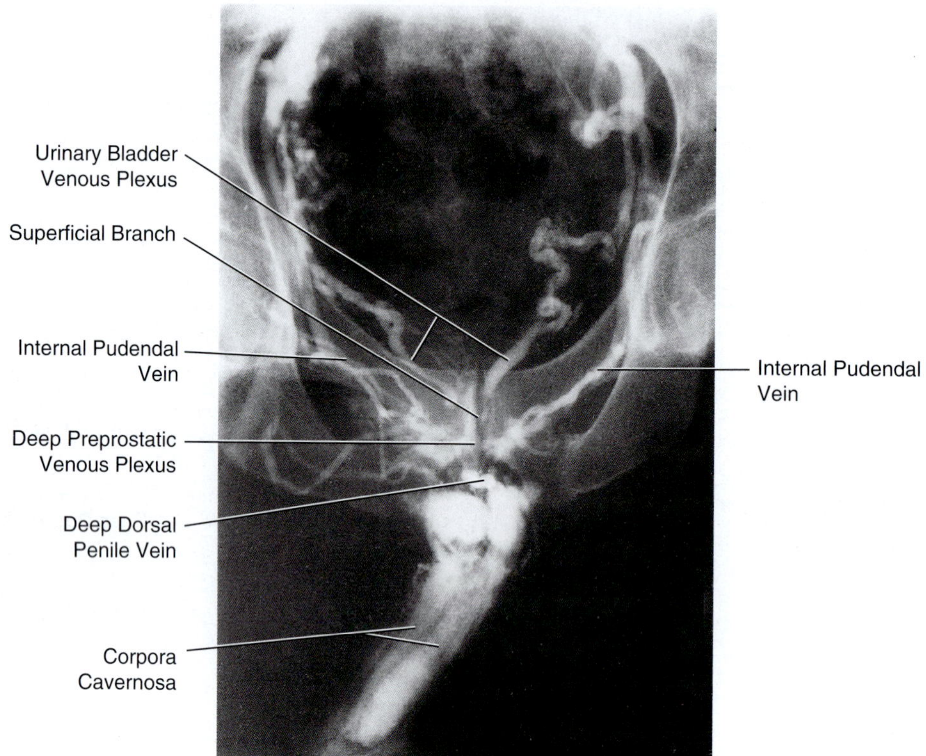

Figure 20.22. Cavernosogram showing opacification of the corpora cavernosa and the drainage through the deep dorsal penile vein and preprostatic venous plexus. The prostatic venous plexus drains into the internal pudendal veins and internal iliac veins.

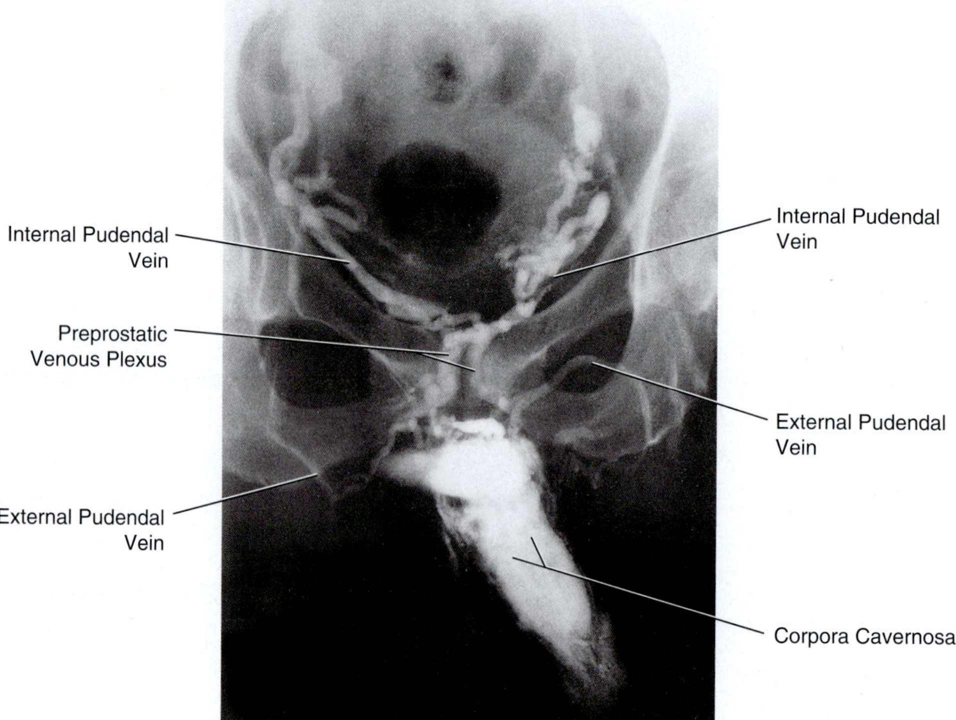

Figure 20.23. Cavernosogram showing opacification of the corpora cavernosa and the drainage through the deep dorsal penile vein and the preprostatic venous plexus. There is a deep venous plexus divided into left and right plexuses. Note the opacification of the external pudendal veins.

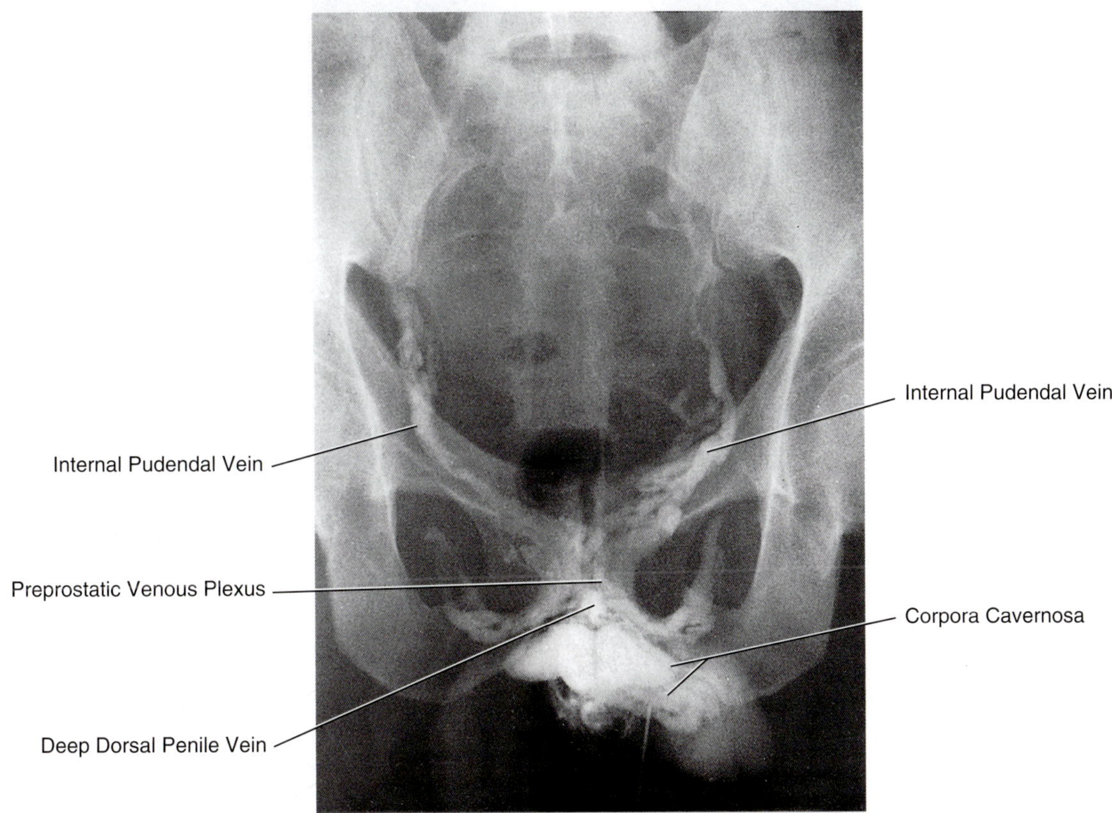

Figure 20.24. Cavernosogram showing the lateral venous plexuses (Santorini deep venous plexus) and the free communications with other pelvic venous plexuses. Note the drainage through the internal pudendal veins. The deep dorsal penile vein is seen.

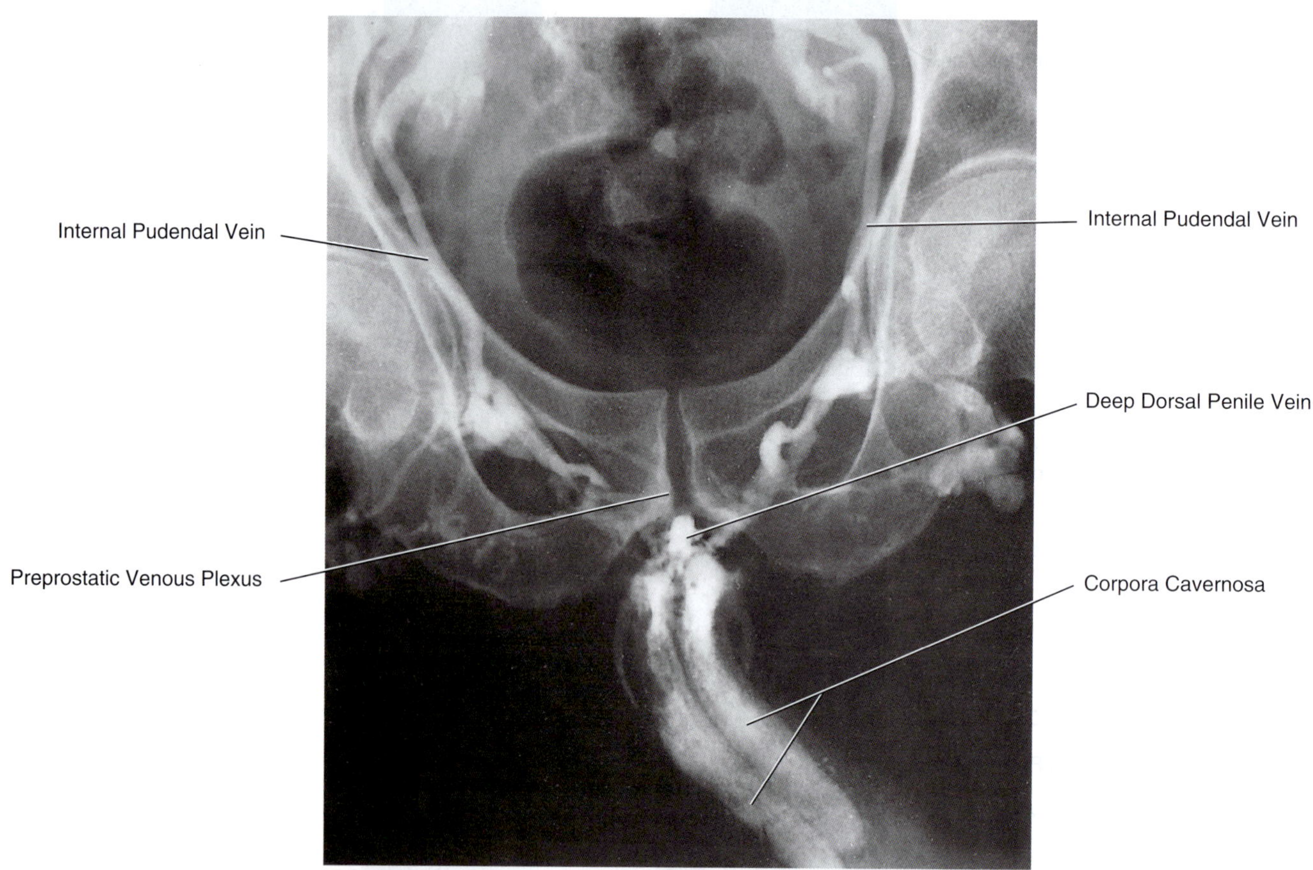

Figure 20.28. Cavernosogram showing the corpora cavernosa and the drainage through the deep venous plexus (preprostatic plexus) and the external pudendal veins.

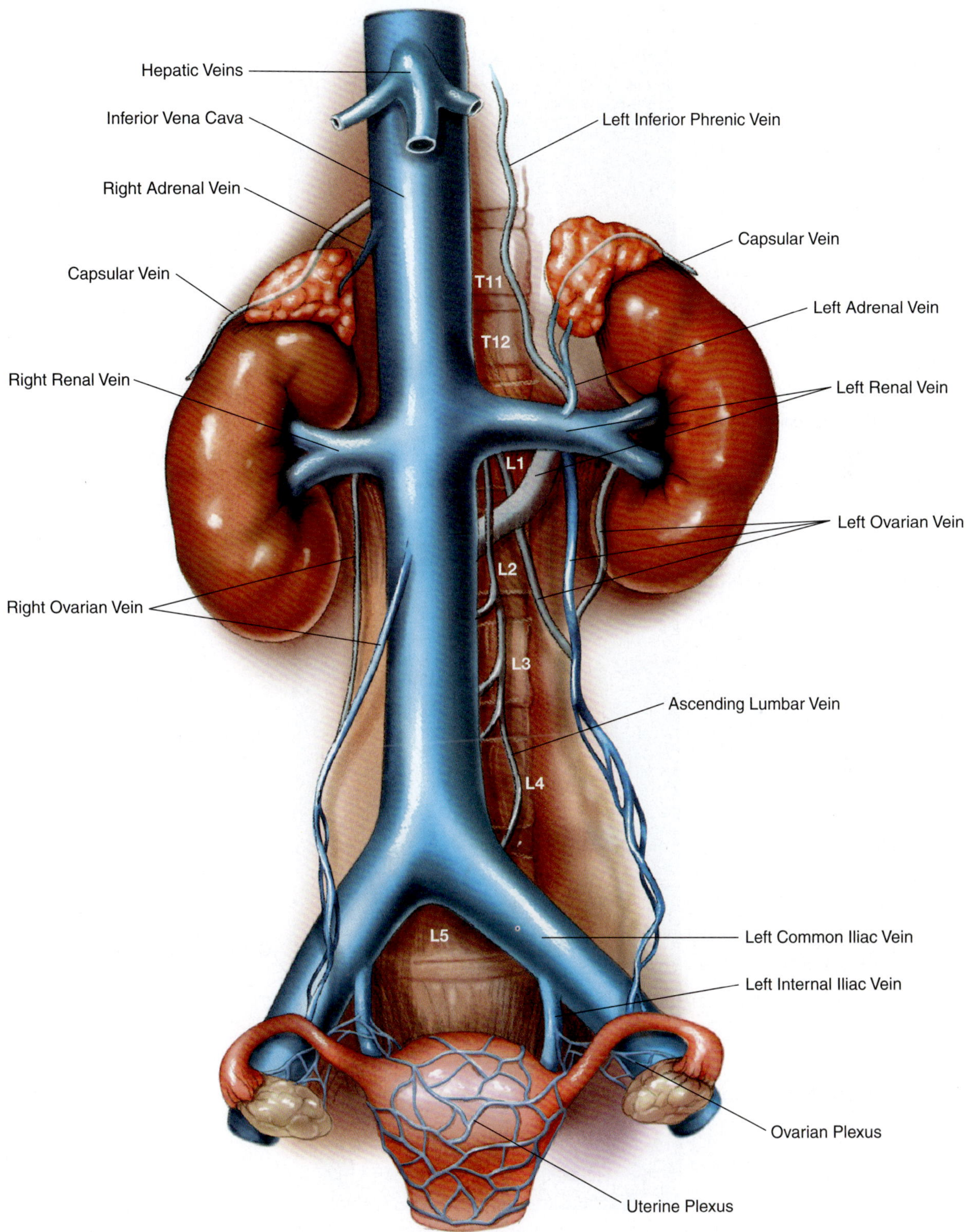

Figure 20.29. Schematic diagram of the uterine, ovarian, and vaginal venous plexuses, showing also the ovarian veins. Note the possible variations in position of the ovarian veins, renal veins, adrenal veins, and the multiple possible anastomoses and relationships.

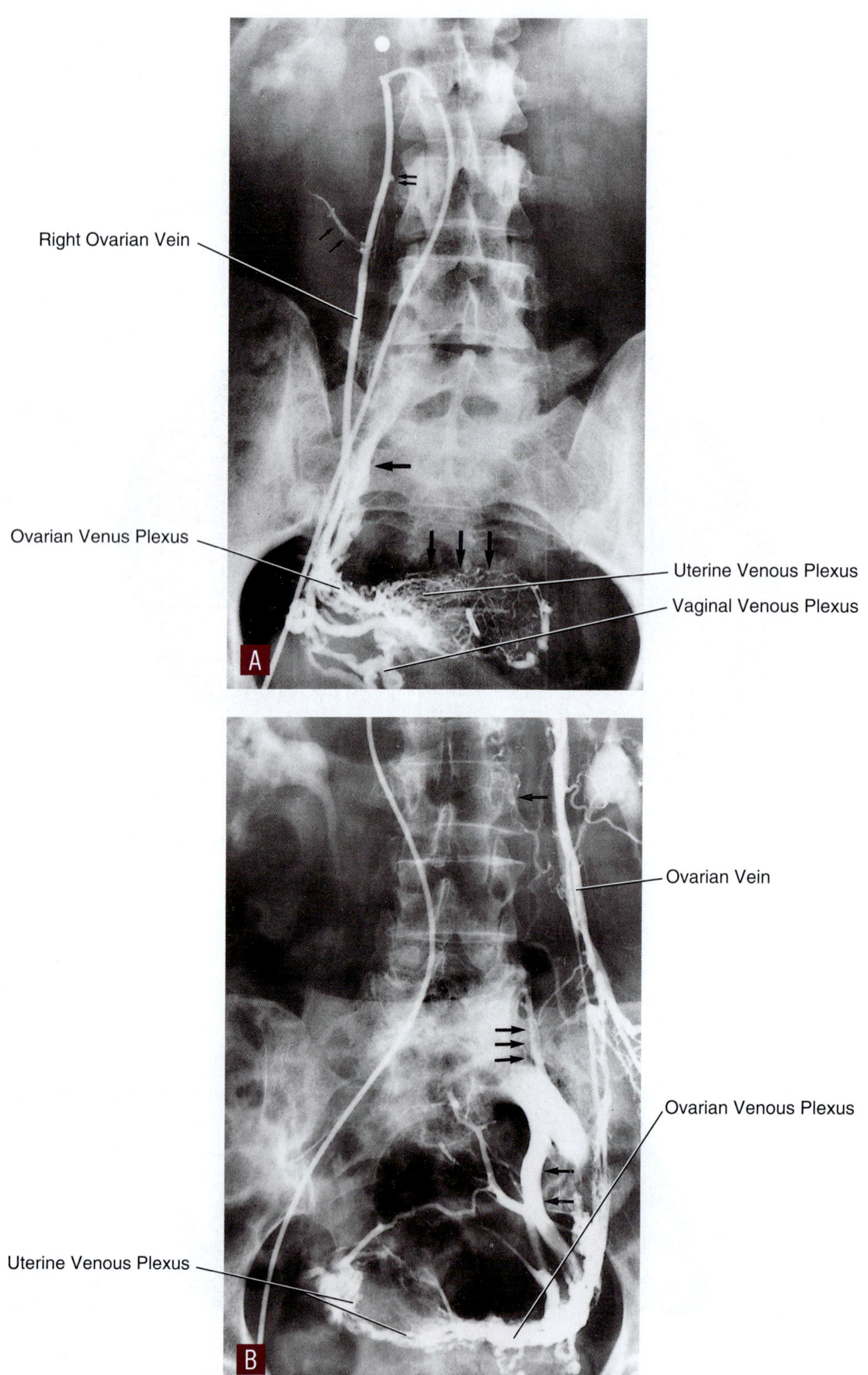

Figure 20.30. **A**, Selective angiography of the right ovarian vein. Note the filling of the uterine venous plexus (three arrows). The ovarian plexus and partial filling of the vaginal plexus are seen. The right internal and common iliac veins are visualized (single arrow). Note the multiple anastomoses of the right ovarian vein with retroperitoneal veins (small arrows). **B**, Selective angiography of the left ovarian vein. Note filling of the uterine venous plexus. This system has wide anastomosis with the internal iliac vein (two arrows) and with the common iliac vein. Note filling of the ascending lumbar vein on the left (three arrows). Note also the multiple anastomoses of the left ovarian vein with the retroperitoneal veins. **C**, Selective venogram of the left gonadal vein showing contrast drainage into the ipsilateral internal iliac vein. There is cross over of contrast material into the right uterine plexus with subsequent drainage into the right internal iliac vein. **D**, Left gonadal vein venogram with balloon occlusion of the left internal iliac vein, showing contrast drainage into the right gonadal and right internal iliac veins.

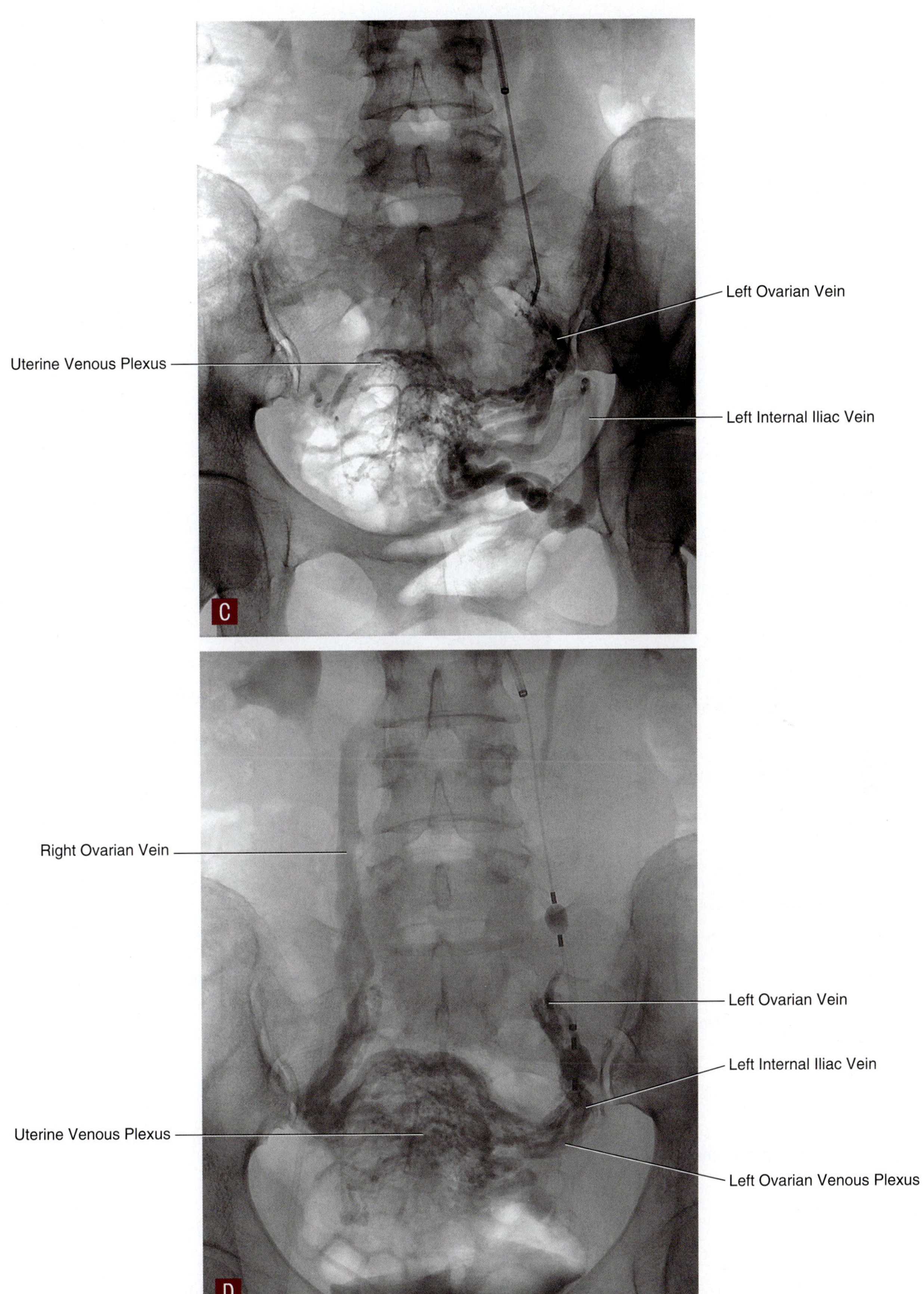

Figure 20.30. *Continued*

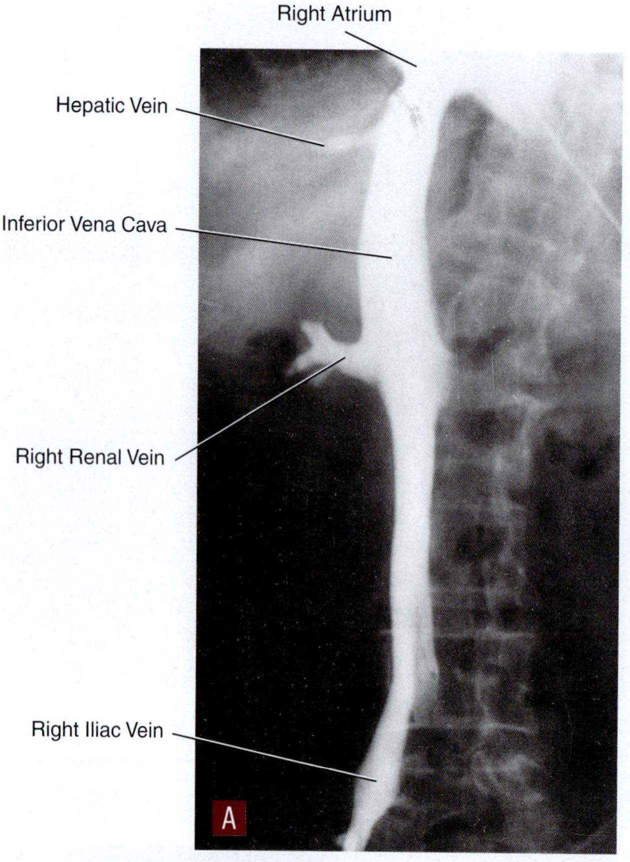

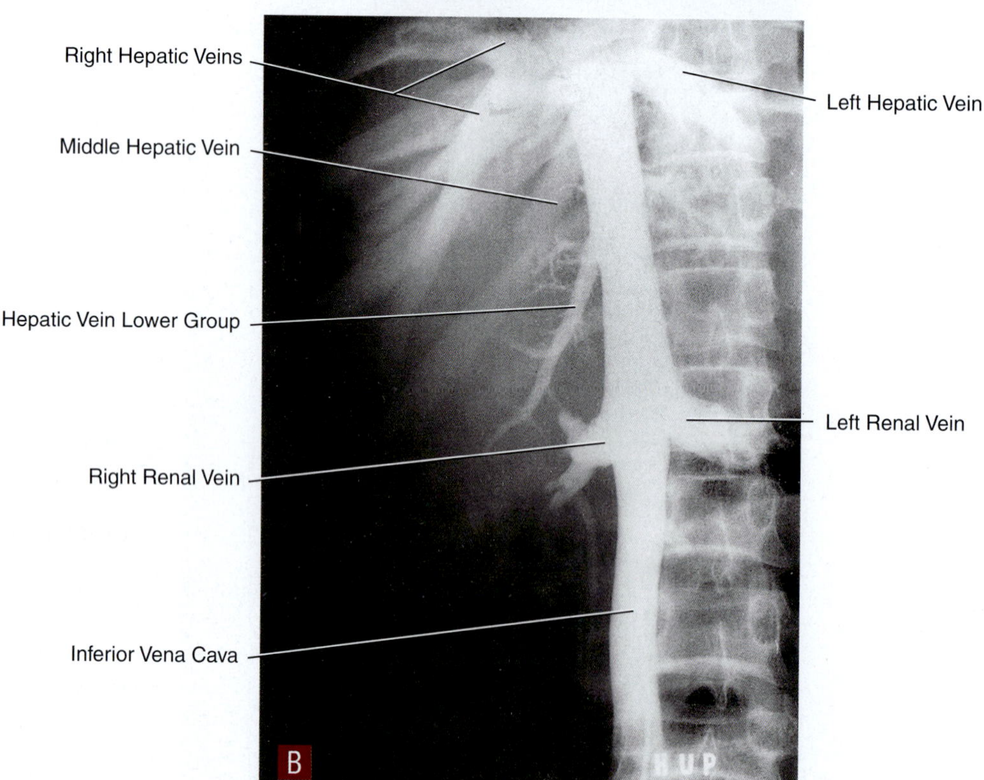

Figure 20.31. **A**, **Venogram of the iliac veins and inferior vena cava.** Note reflux of the contrast medium into the right renal vein and into a hepatic vein. The right atrium is filled with contrast medium. **B**, **Cavagram.** Note the reflux of contrast medium into the renal veins and into the hepatic veins. The hepatic veins are large and the inferior one is well visualized.

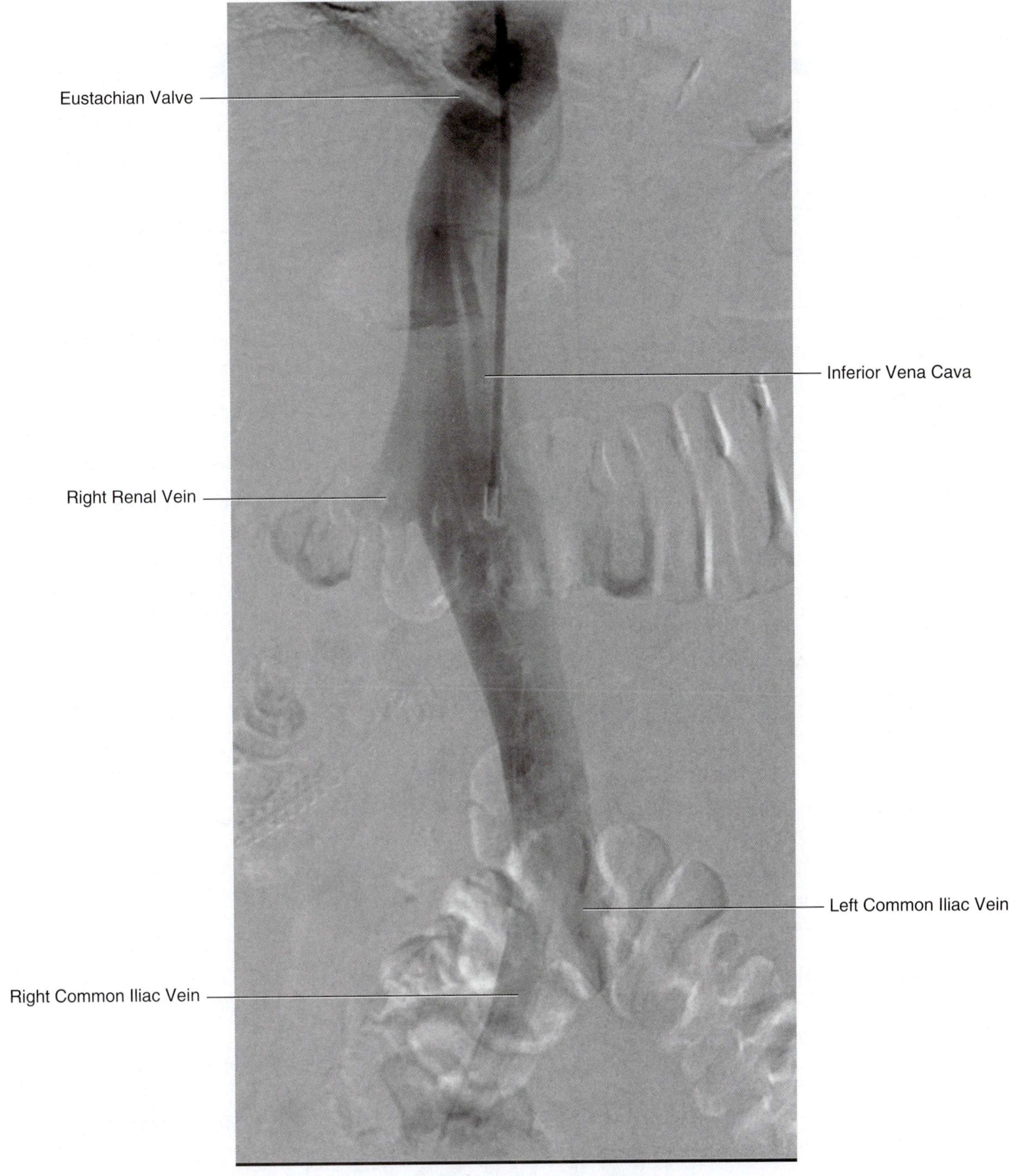

Figure 20.32. Digital subtraction cavagram showing the iliac veins, the right renal vein, and the Eustachian valve at the confluence of the inferior vena cava with the right atrium.

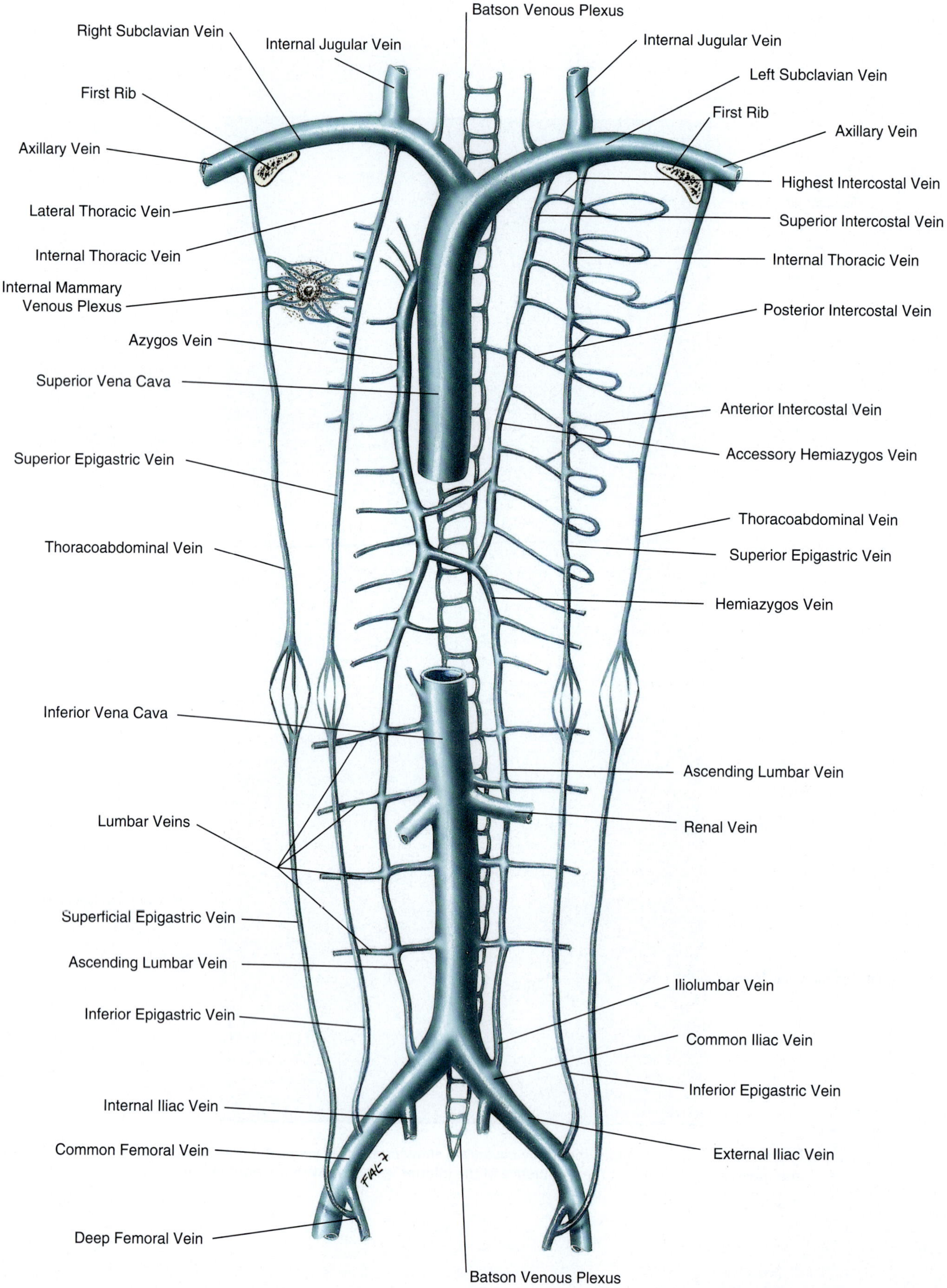

Figure 20.33. Diagram depicting the venous collateral pathways available between the thorax and the abdomen.

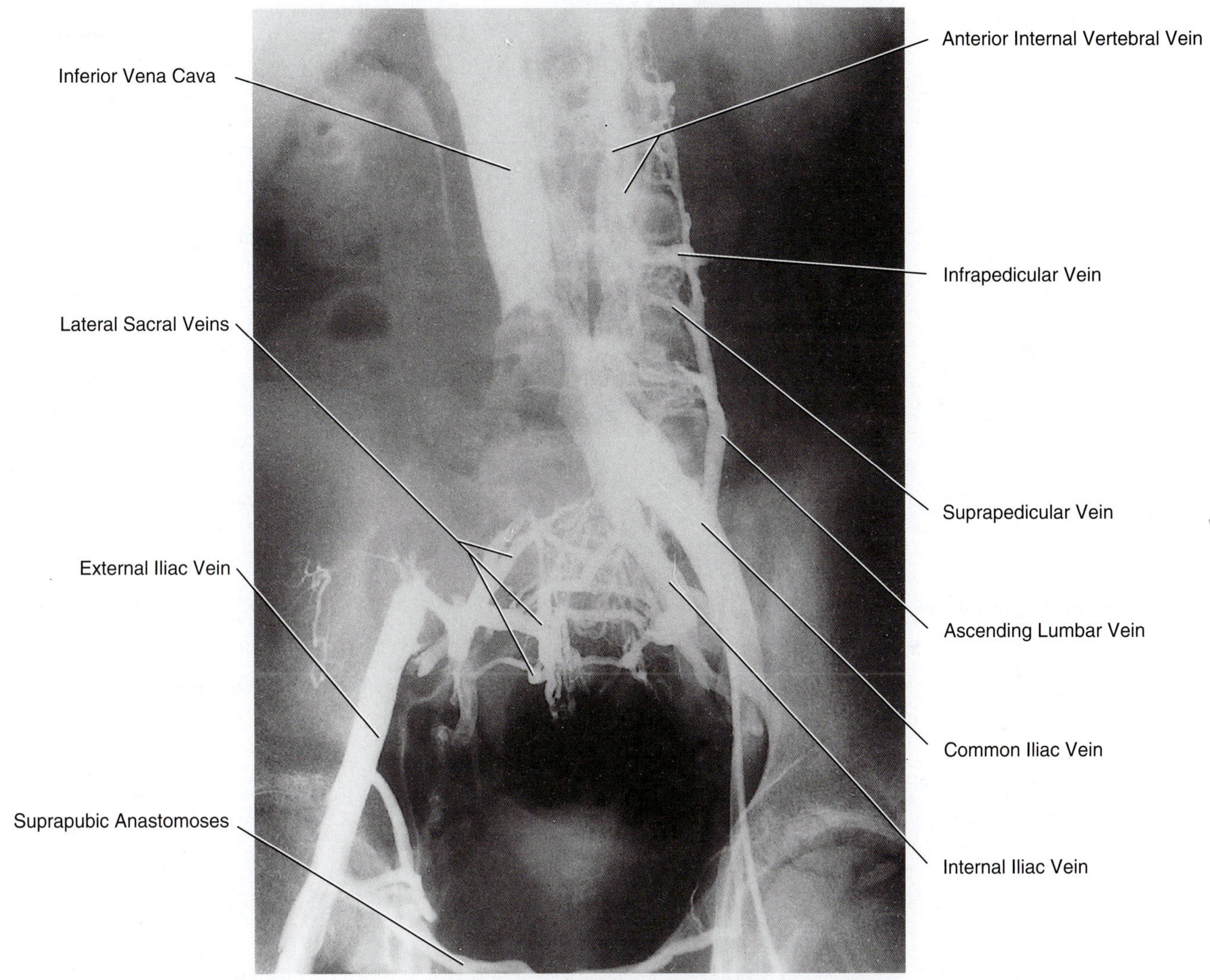

Figure 20.34. Angiogram of the iliac veins and inferior vena cava showing the collateralization into the pelvis and perilumbar veins. Due to the occlusion of the right common iliac and inferior vena cava, there is development of the collaterals. Note the anastomosis between the two iliac veins through the lateral sacral veins. The left ascending lumbar vein is clearly seen and the anastomosis with the epidural plexus is observed through the suprapedicular and infrapedicular veins. The lateral and medial anterior internal vertebral veins also seem as a plexus along the medullar canal.

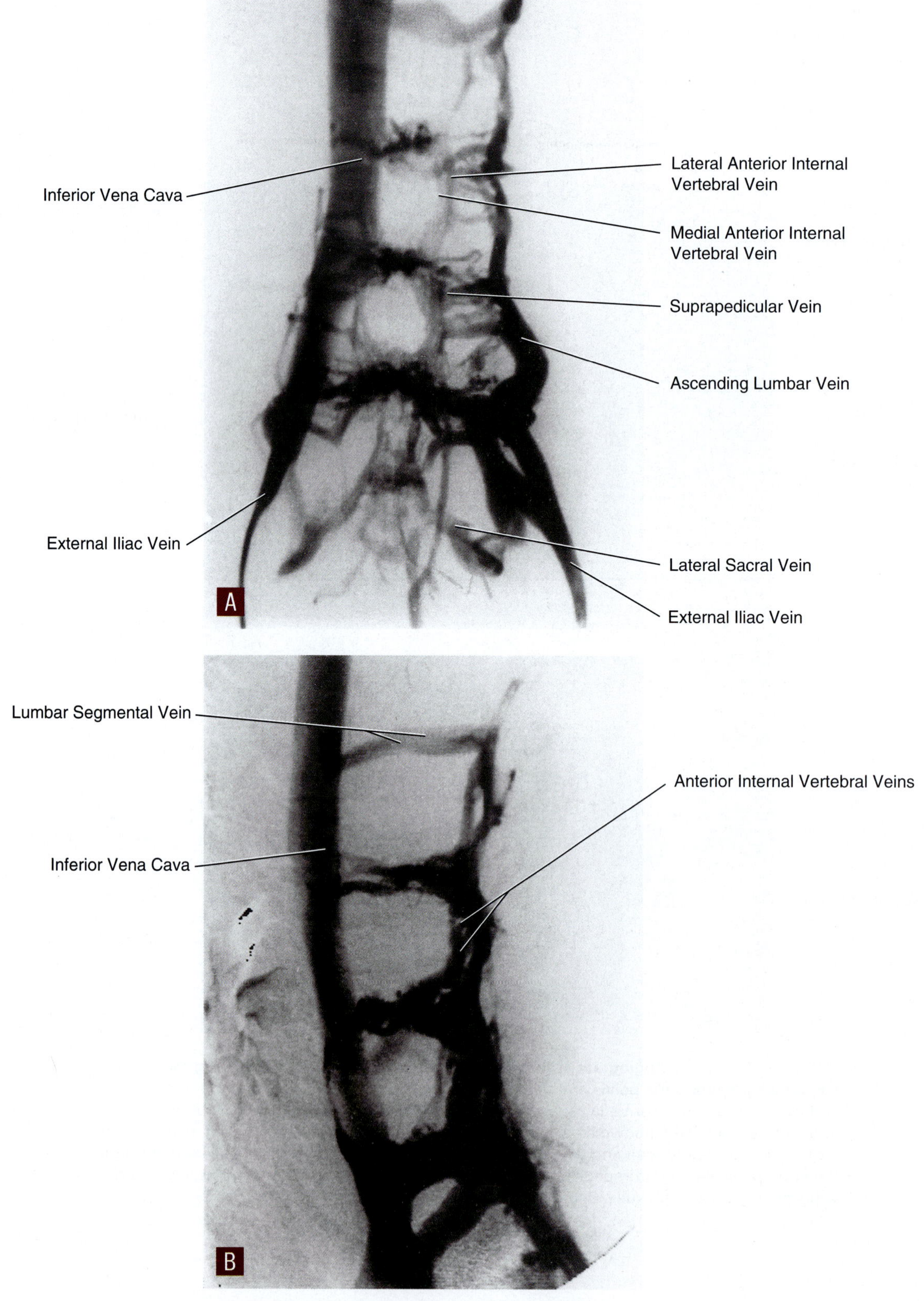

Figure 20.35. **A**, Anterior view of an angiogram of the iliac veins and inferior vena cava showing the vertebral venous plexus. **B**, Lateral view of the angiogram showing the inferior vena cava and the communications through the lumbar segmental veins. Posteriorly, the epidural venous plexus is observed as a dense venous plexus.

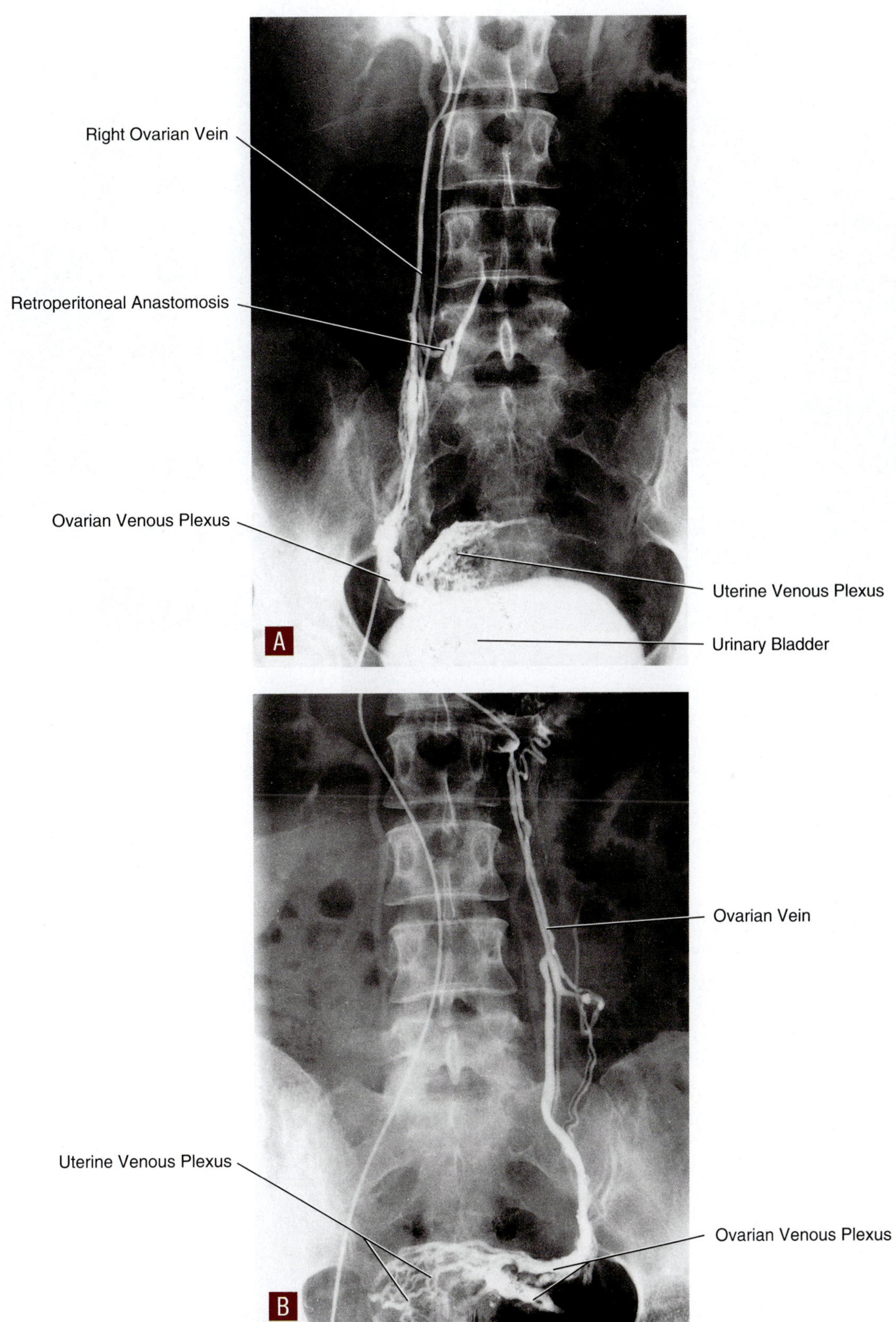

Figure 20.36. **A**, Selective angiography of the right ovarian vein. Note the filling of the ovarian plexus and part of the uterine plexus. Anastomosis with retroperitoneal veins is observed. **B**, Selective angiography of the left ovarian vein. Note the duplication of the vein and the anastomosis with retroperitoneal veins. The uterine venous plexus is also seen.

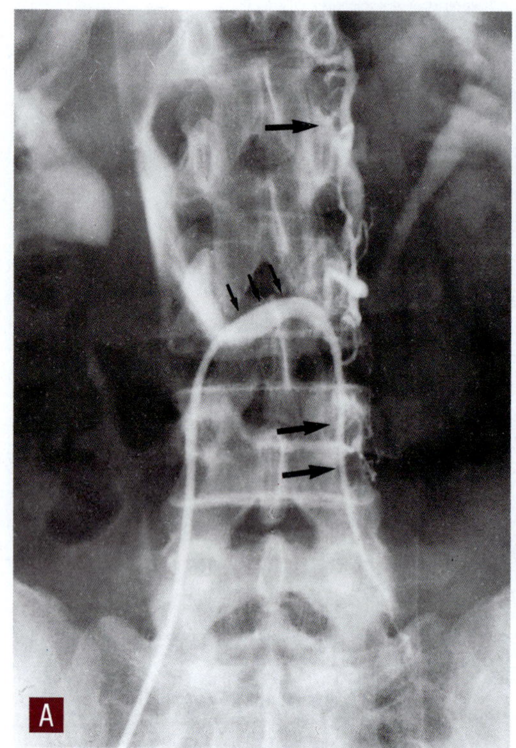

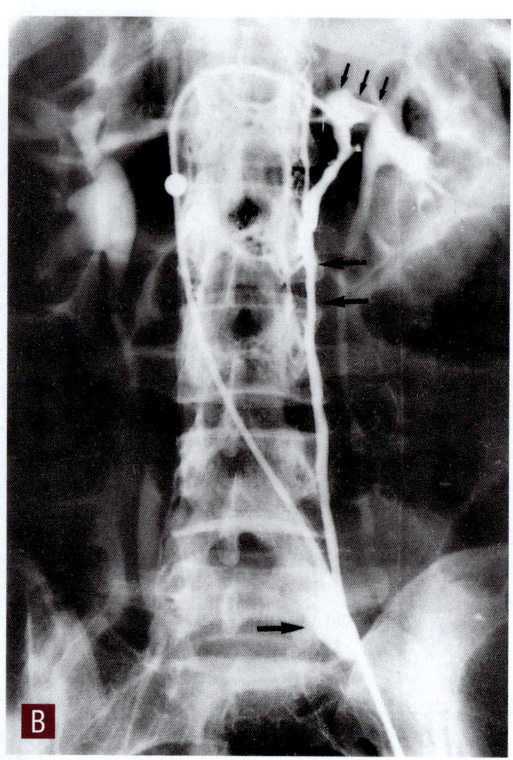

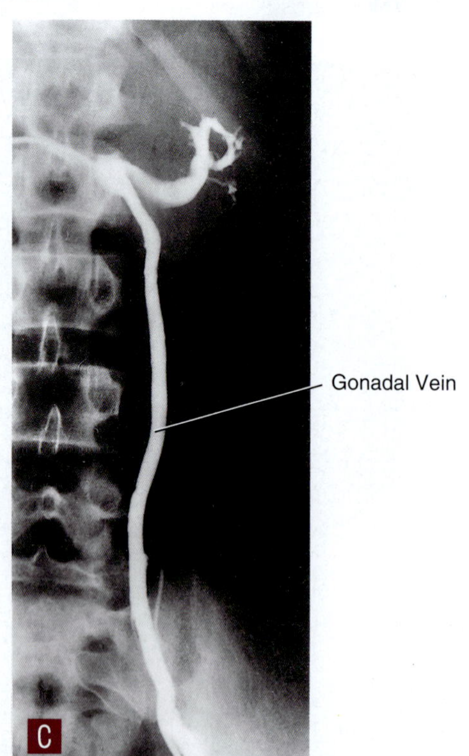

Figure 20.37. **A**, Injection into a segmental lumbar vein (three small arrows). Note opacification of part of the left ovarian vein (one large arrow) and partial opacification of the ascending lumbar vein (two large arrows). **B**, Selective injection into the left ovarian vein (two large arrows). The left renal vein is partially opacified (three arrows). The left common iliac vein is also opacified (one arrow). **C**, Selective injection into the left ovarian vein. There is partial filling of the left renal vein.

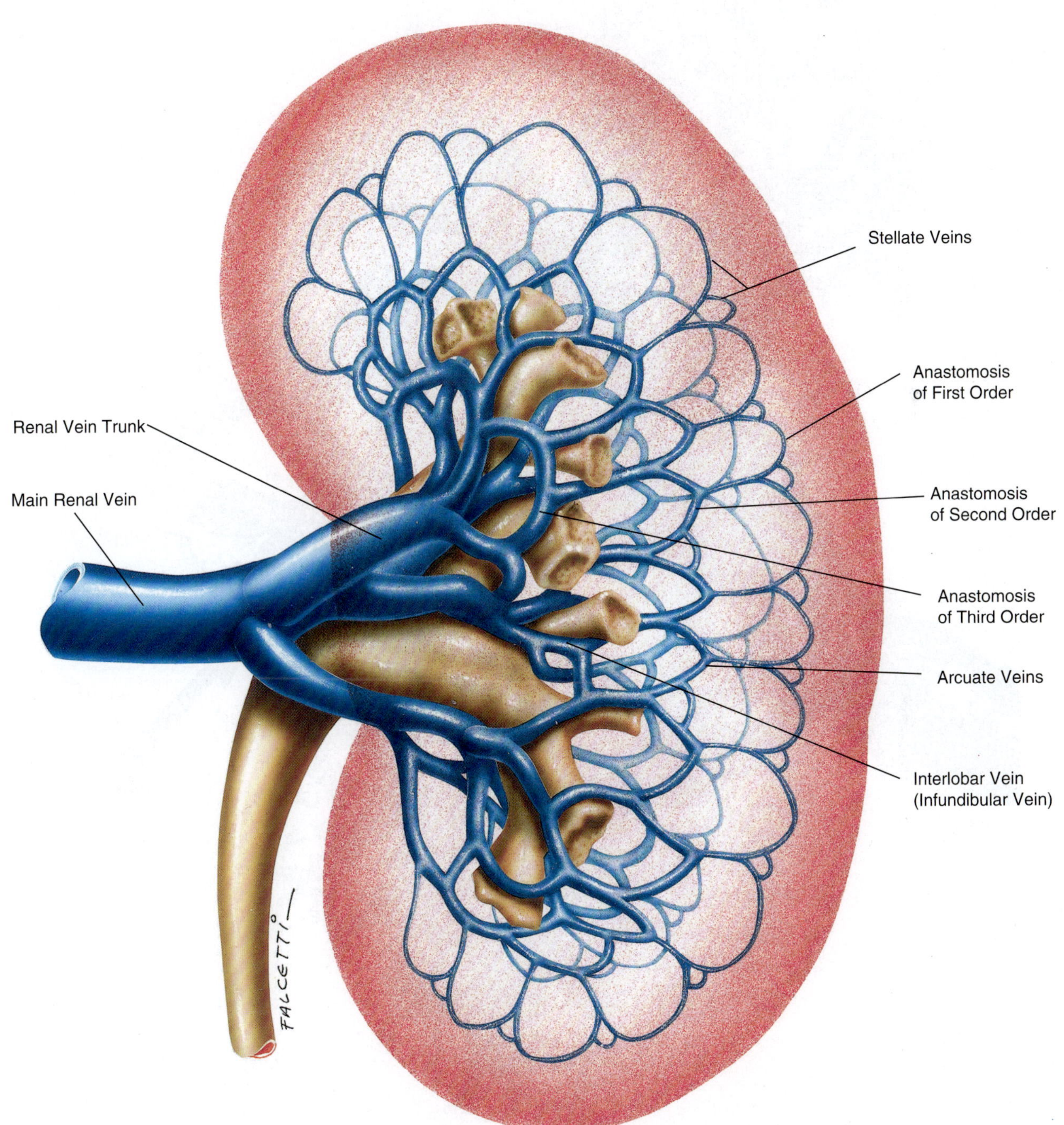

Figure 20.38. Schematic drawing showing the three orders of venous arcades; anastomosis of first order, anastomosis of second order, and anastomosis of third order.

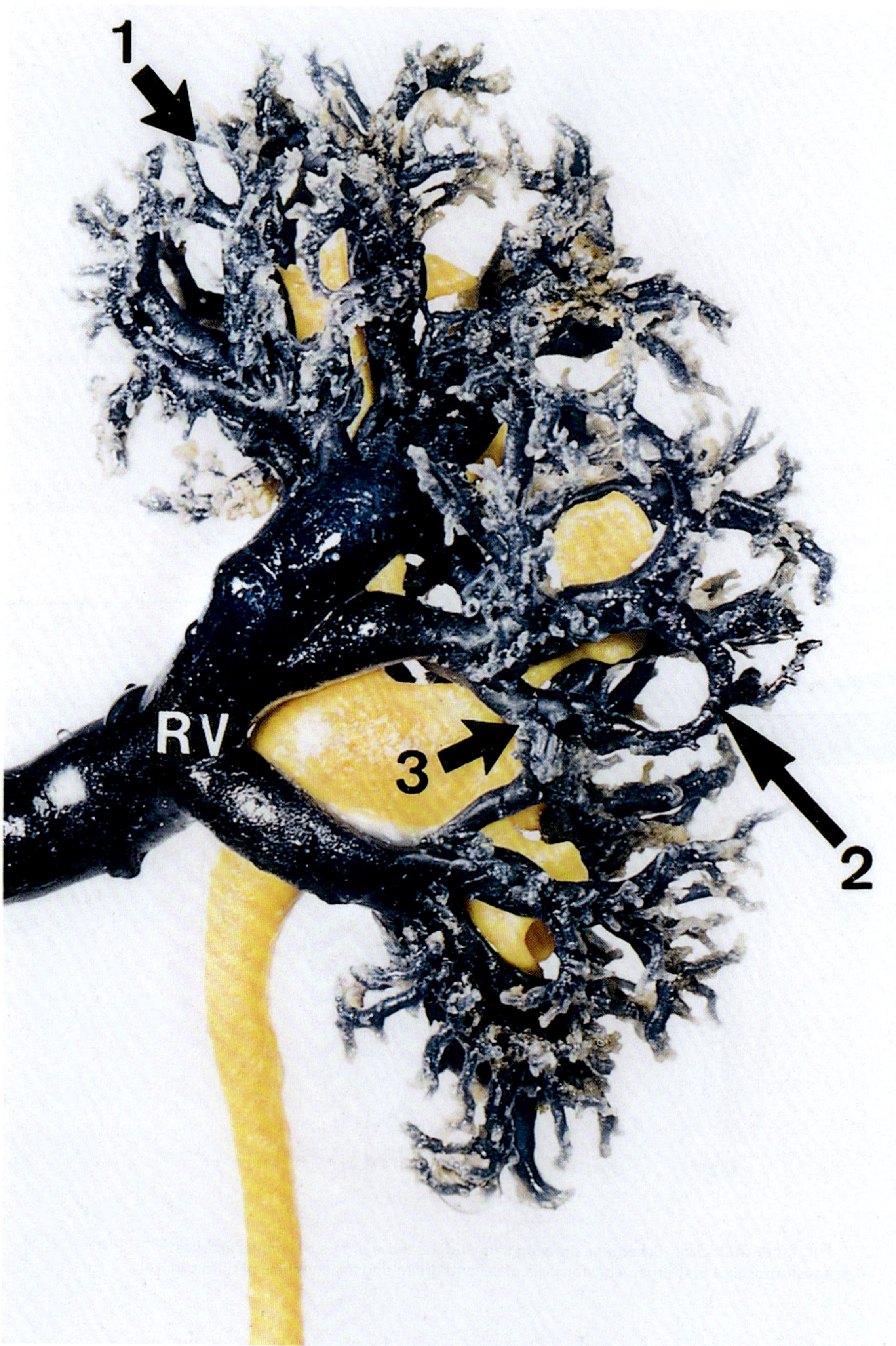

Figure 20.39. Anterior view of a left kidney endocast of the pelvicalyceal system together with the venous vascular tree shows the three systems or longitudinal anastomotic arcades; from lateral (periphery) to medial (hilar): stellate veins (1), arcuate veins (2), and interlobar veins (3). RV, renal vein.

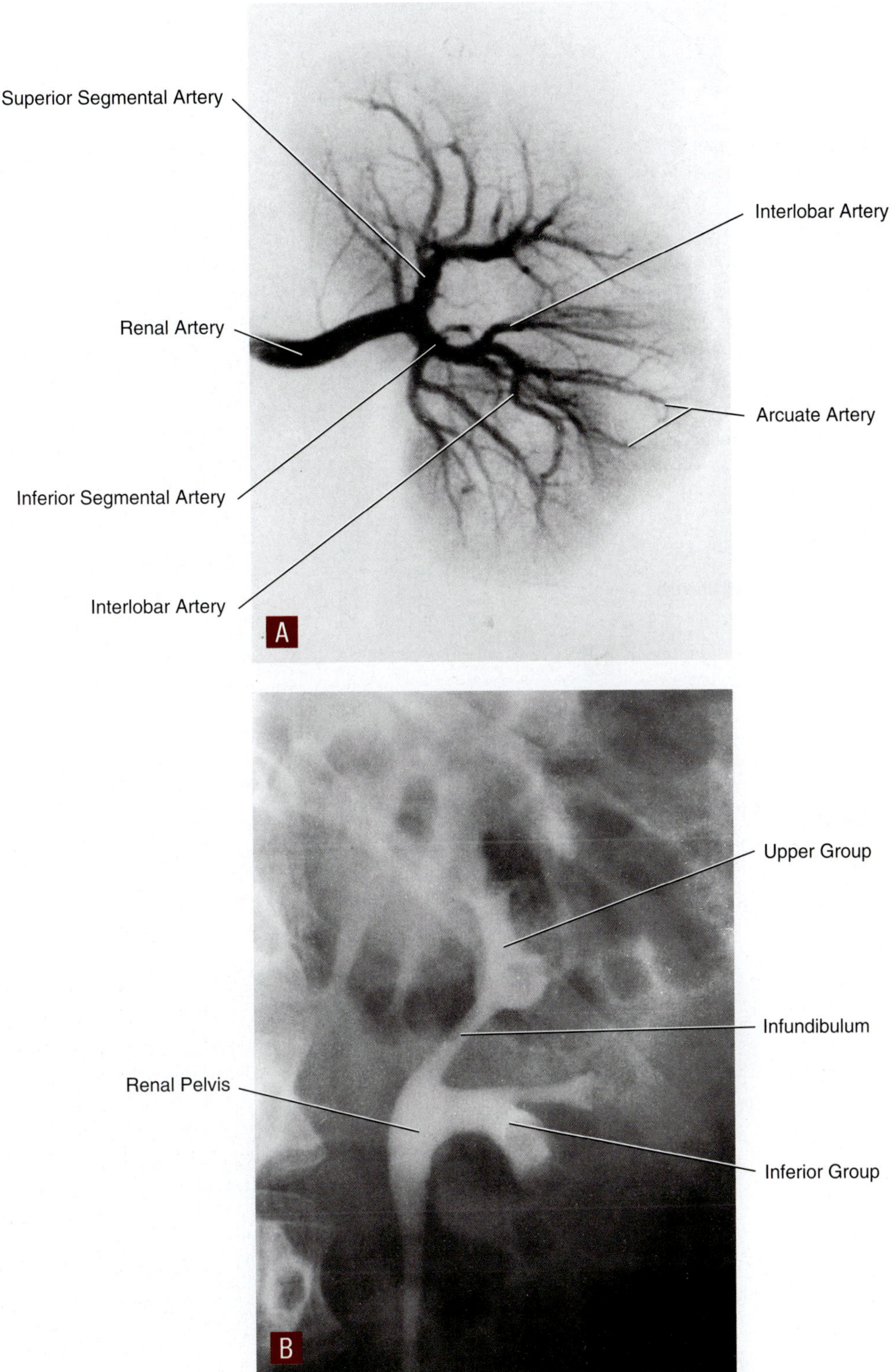

Figure 20.40. **A**, Renal angiogram showing the arterial phase. **B**, Intravenous pyelogram showing the calyceal system in the same subject. **C**, Renal venogram showing the intra- and extrarenal veins. **D**, More peripheral venogram showing the medial, stellate, and arcuate veins.

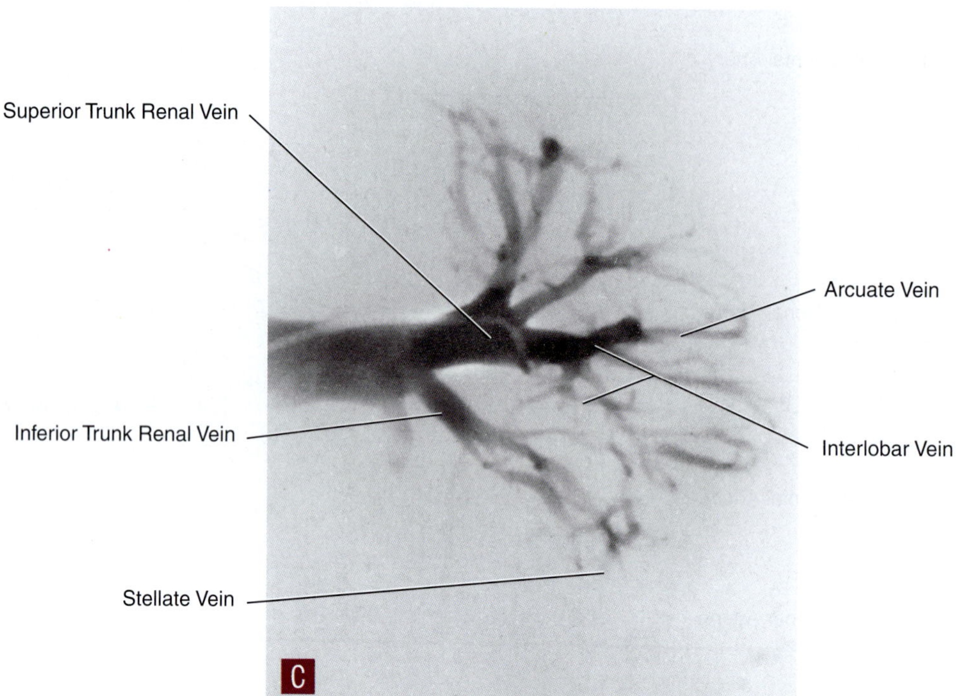

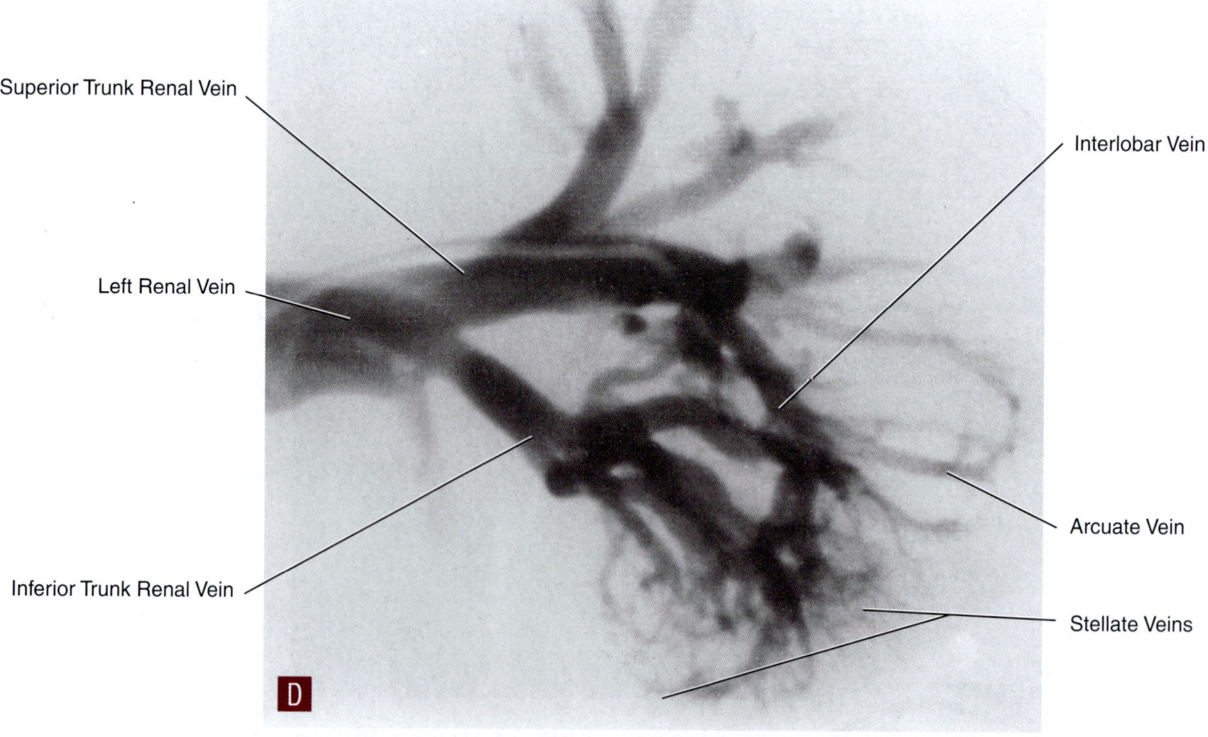

Figure 20.40. *Continued*

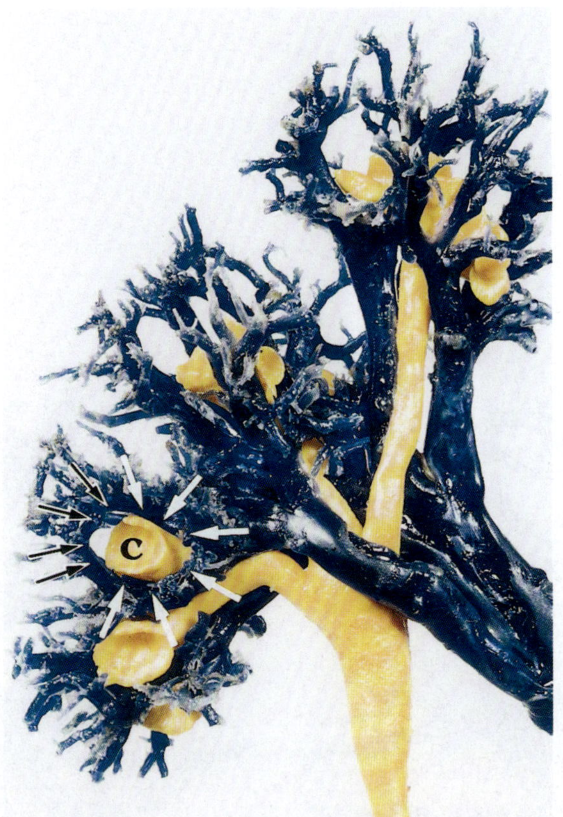

Figure 20.41. Posterior view of an endocast from the left kidney shows large venous anastomosis like a collar (arrows) around the neck of a calix (C).

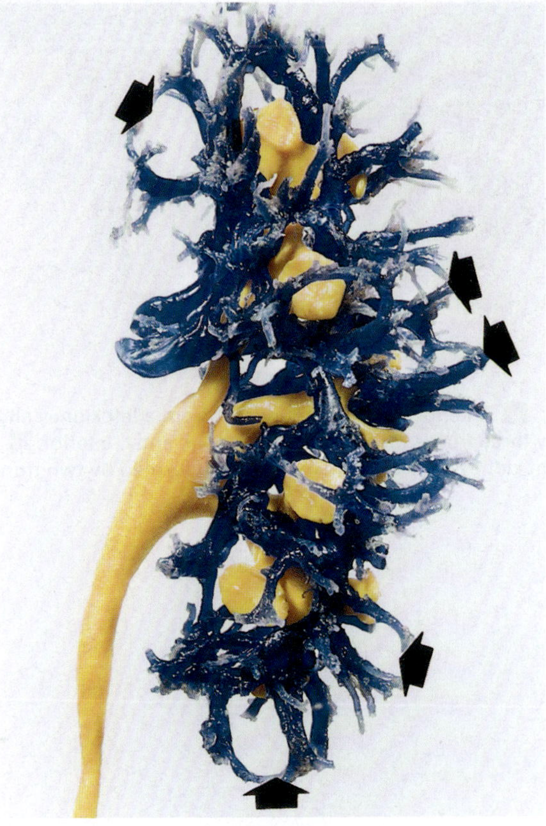

Figure 20.42. Posterior oblique view of an endocast from a right kidney shows horizontal arches linking the anterior and posterior veins, as well as the longitudinal system (arrows).

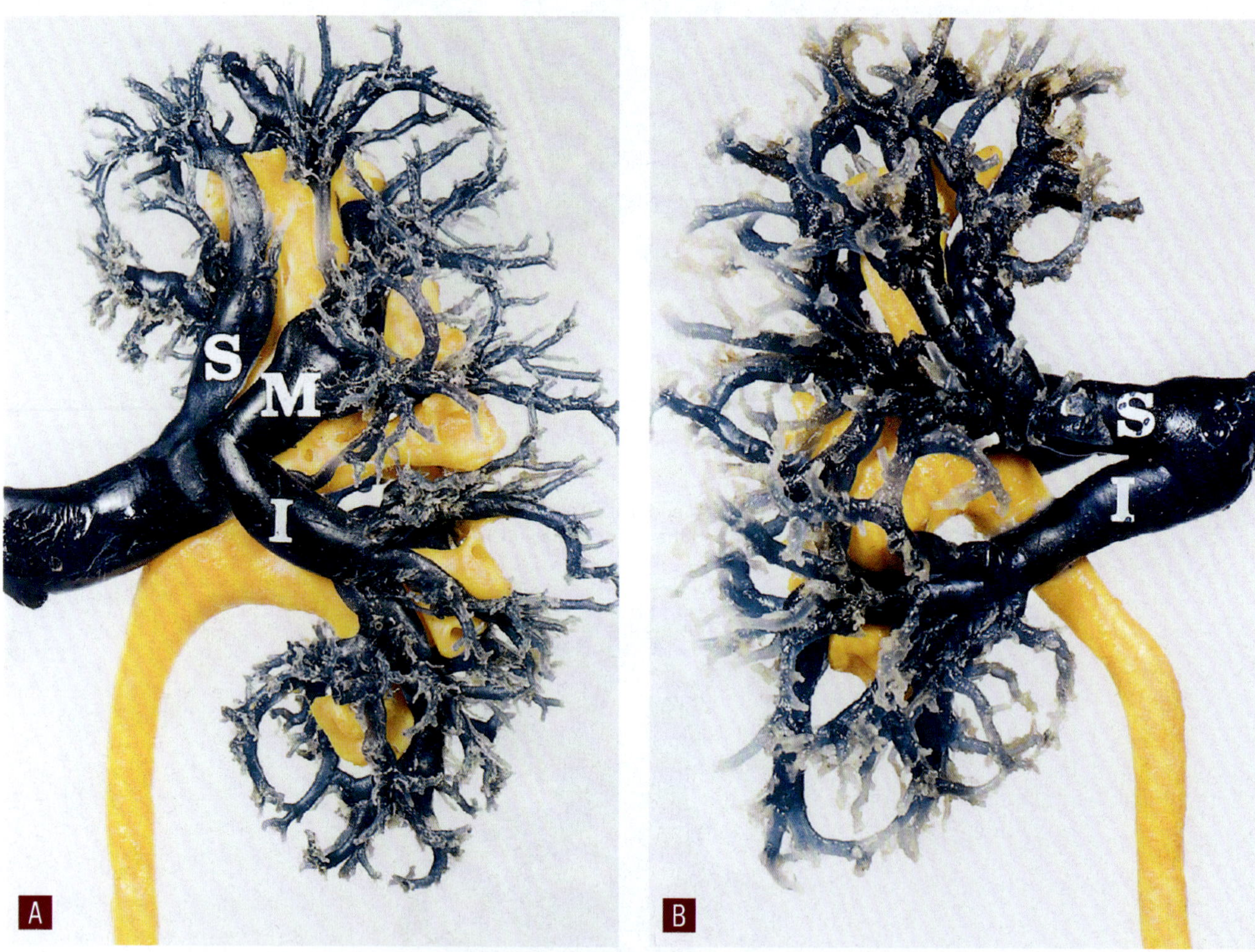

Figure 20.43. A, Anterior view of an endocast from a left kidney shows the main renal vein formed by three trunks. S, superior; M, middle; and I, inferior. B, Anterior view of endocast from a right kidney shows the main renal vein formed by two trunks. S, superior and I, inferior.

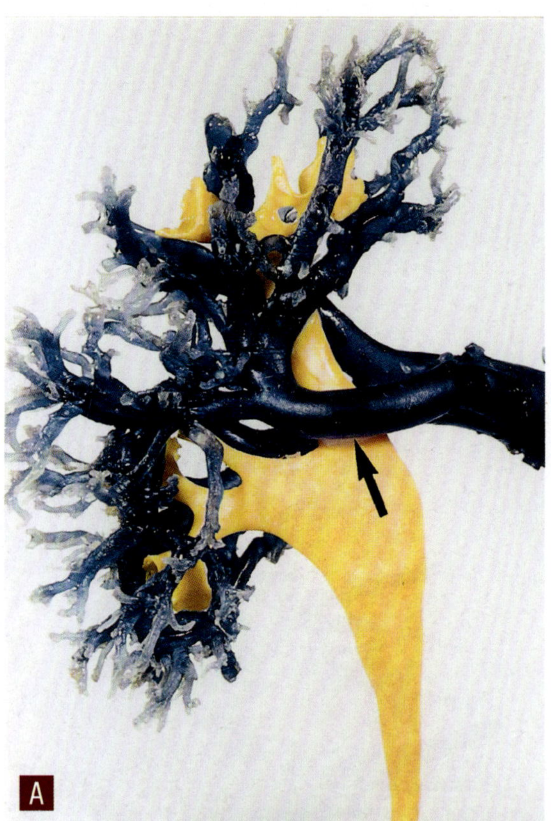

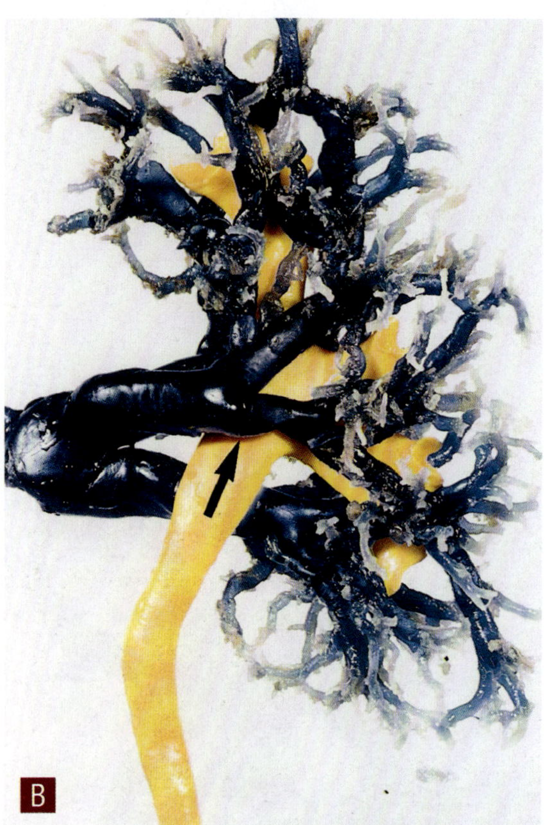

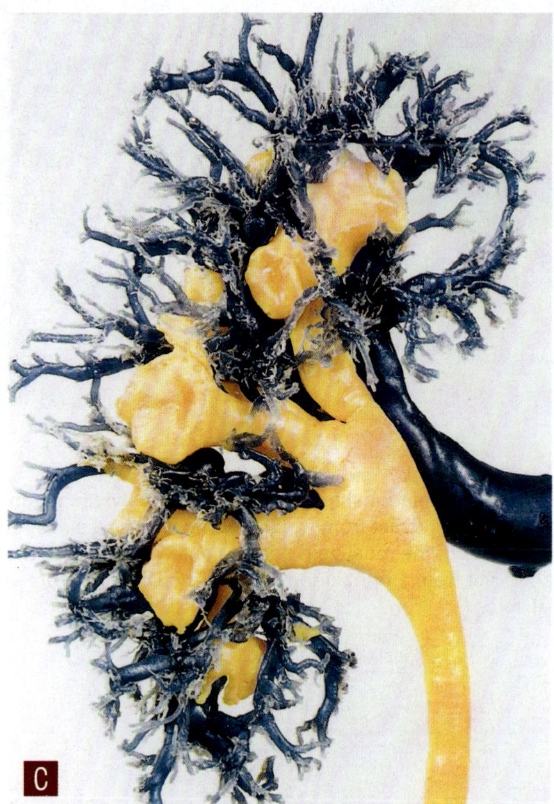

Figure 20.44. A, Posterior view of an endocast from a left kidney reveals a close relationship between a retropelvic vein (arrow) and the junction of renal pelvis with upper calix. B, Posterior view of an endocast from a right kidney shows a prominent retropelvic vein (arrow) crossing the middle posterior aspect of the renal pelvis. C, Posterior view of an endocast from the left kidney reveals that there are no veins on the posterior aspect of the renal pelvis.

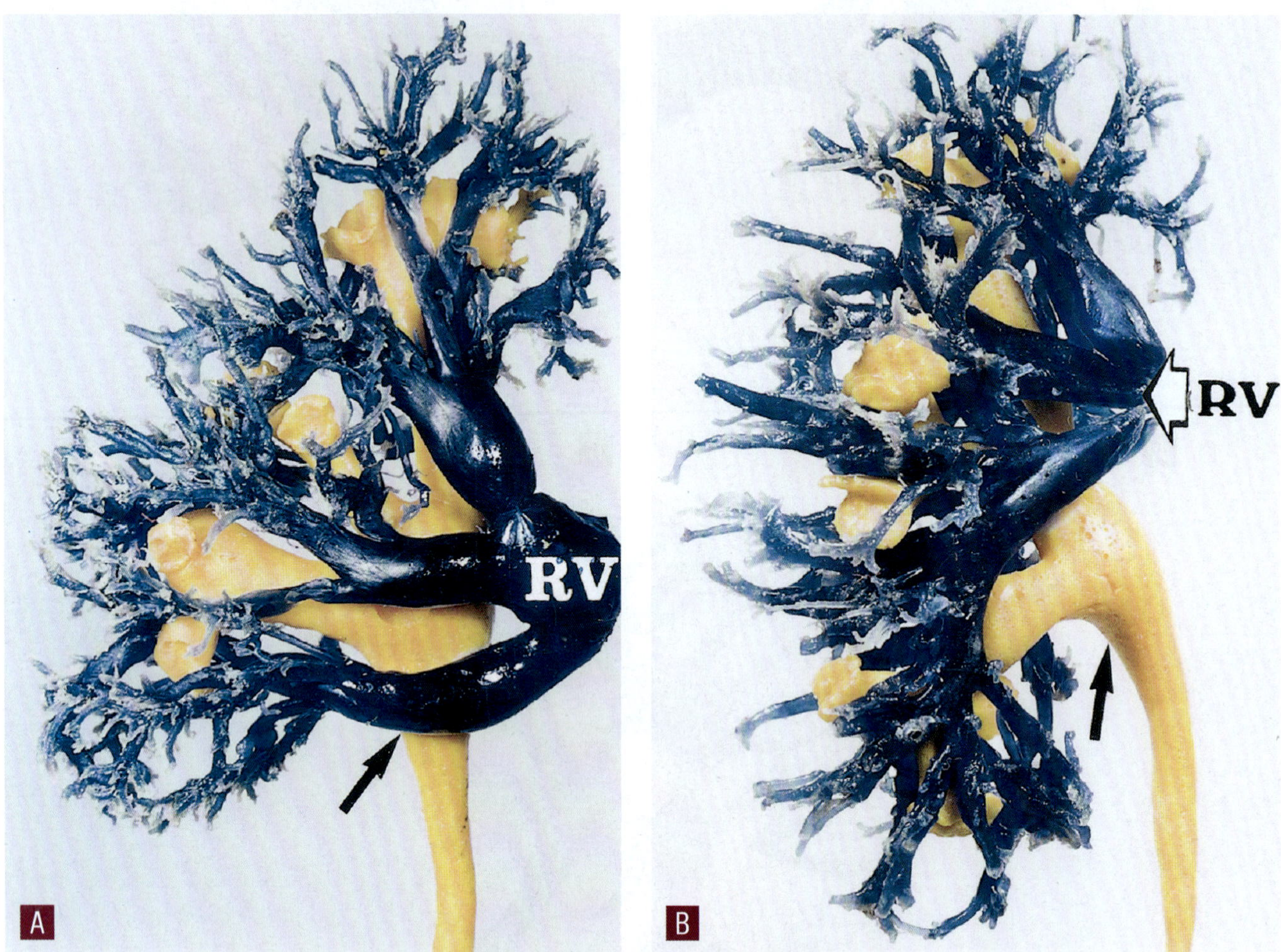

Figure 20.45. Anatomic relationship between ureteropelvic junction (UPJ) and renal veins. A, Anterior view of an endocast from a right kidney shows a close relationship between a prominent inferior tributary of the renal vein and the anterior aspect of the UPJ (arrow). B, Anterior view of an endocast from a right kidney shows the UPJ free from veins (nonvascular area, arrow). RV, renal vein.

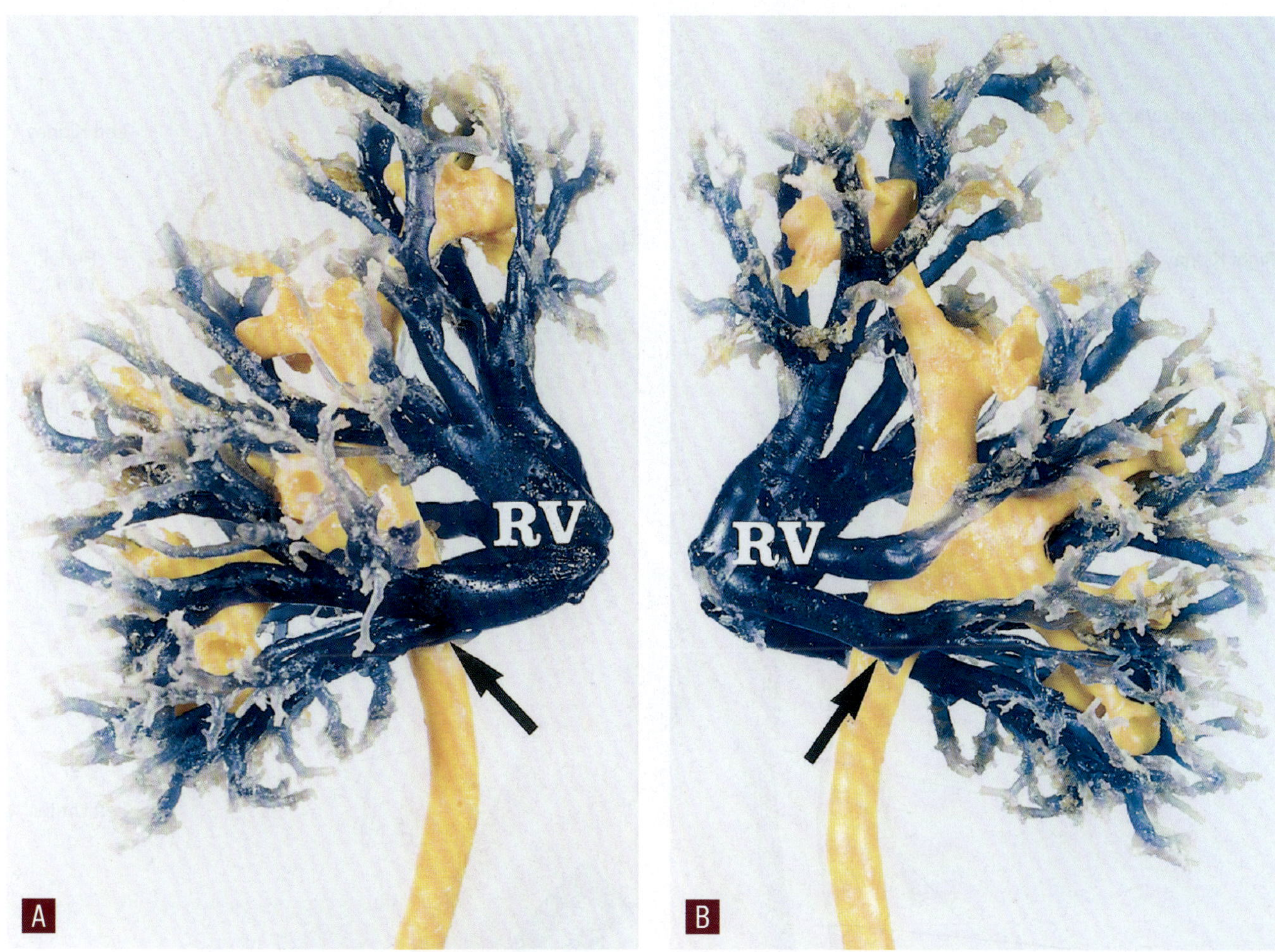

Figure 20.46. **Anatomic relationships between the UPJ and the renal vein.** A, Anterior view of an endocast of a right kidney shows a close relationship between an anterior tributary of the renal vein and the UPJ (arrow). B, Posterior view of the endocast shown in (A) reveals the UPJ in close relationship to a retropelvic vein (arrow). RV, renal vein; UPJ, ureteropelvic junction.

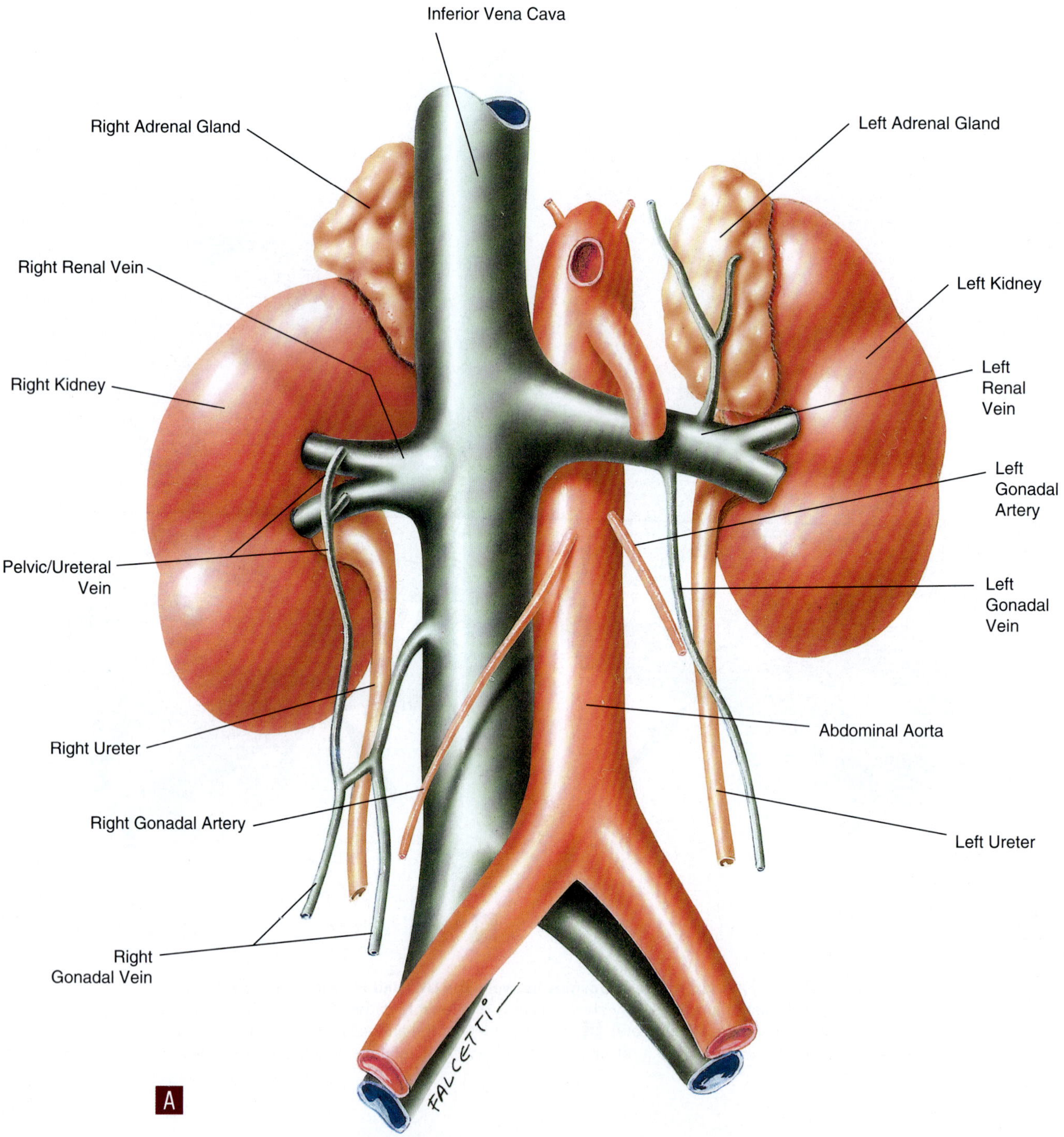

Figure 20.47. **A**, Schematic diagram showing the right and left kidneys and the relationships of the renal veins and the gonadal veins and variations. The renal veins may be partially or totally duplicated. **B**, Schematic diagram showing a retroaortic renal vein with low insertion into the inferior vena cava. **C**, Circumaortic renal vein. **D**, Left common iliac insertion of the left iliac vein.

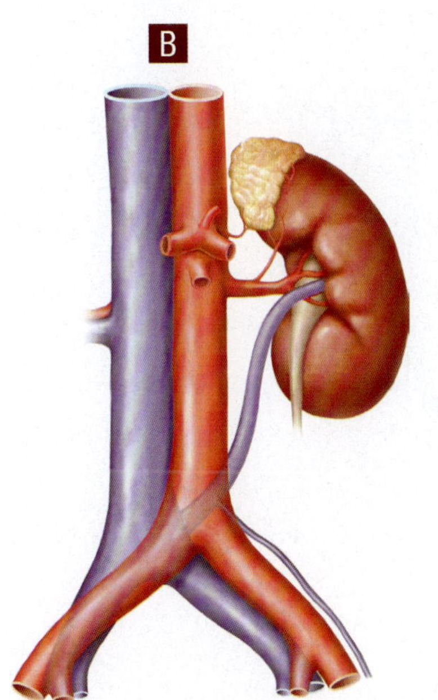

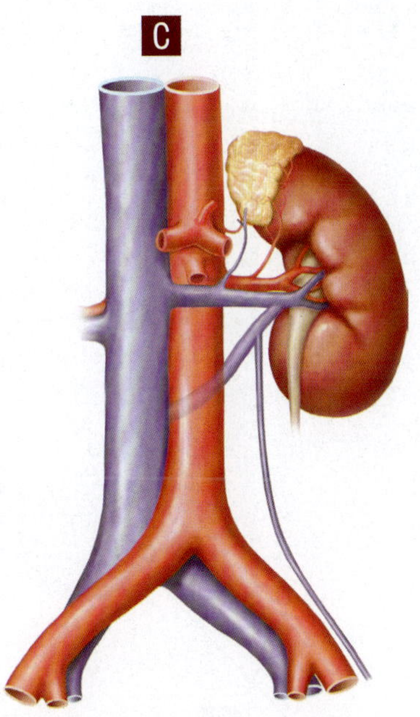

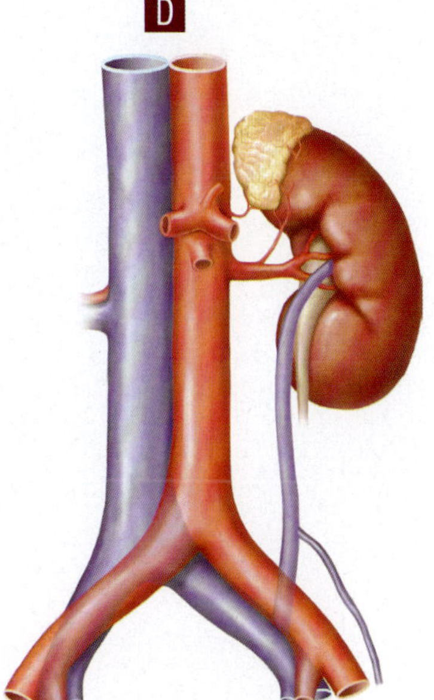

Figure 20.47. *Continued*

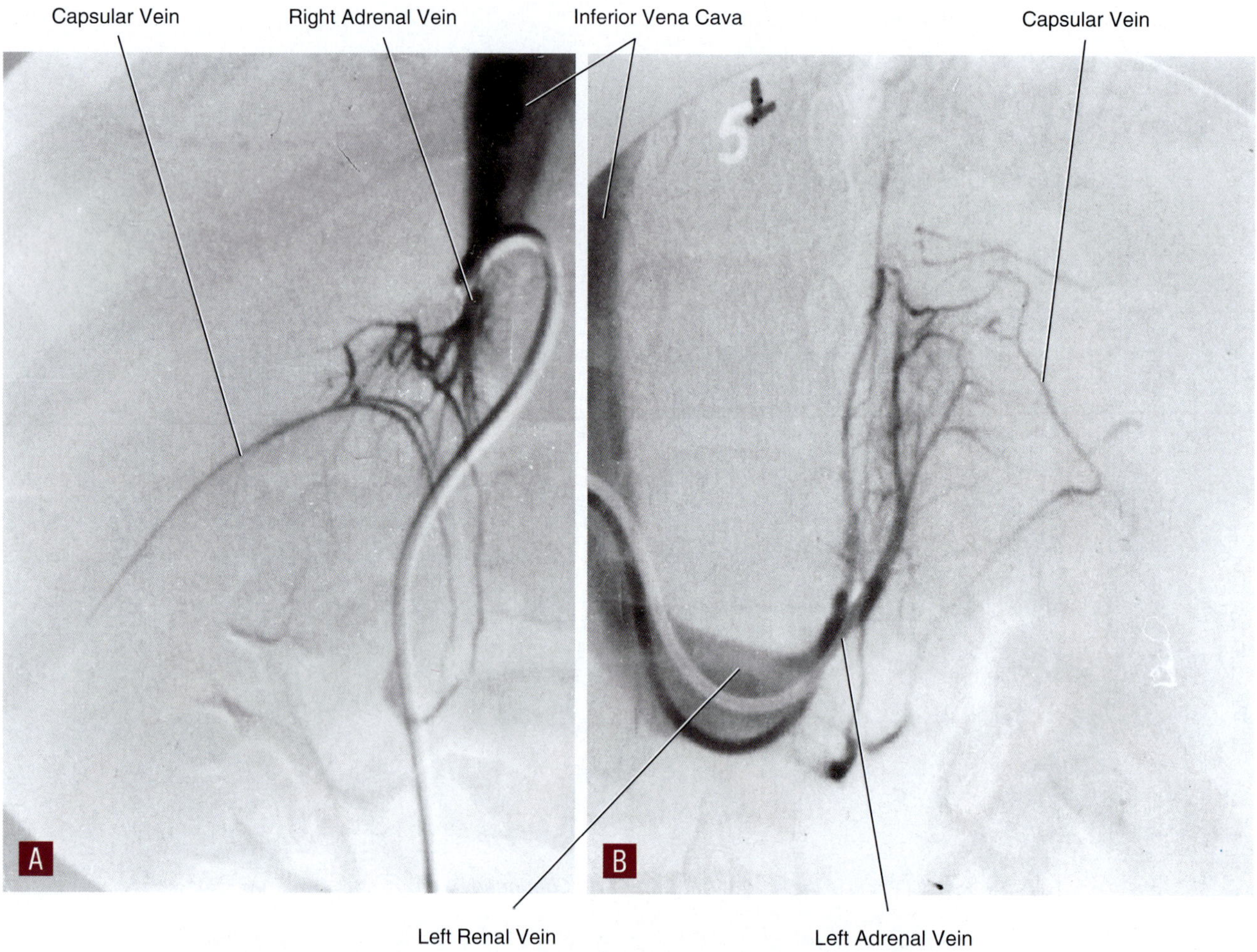

Figure 20.48. Selective venography of the right and left adrenal veins. A, The right adrenal vein ends in the posterolateral aspect of the inferior vena cava. Note the anastomosis with the renal capsular veins. The gland is triangular and small. B, On the left, the adrenal vein is longer and ends in the superior aspect of the left renal vein. Note anastomosis with renal capsular veins and with inferior phrenic veins. The gland is longer and located medially to the kidney. C, Schematic diagram showing the adrenal veins.

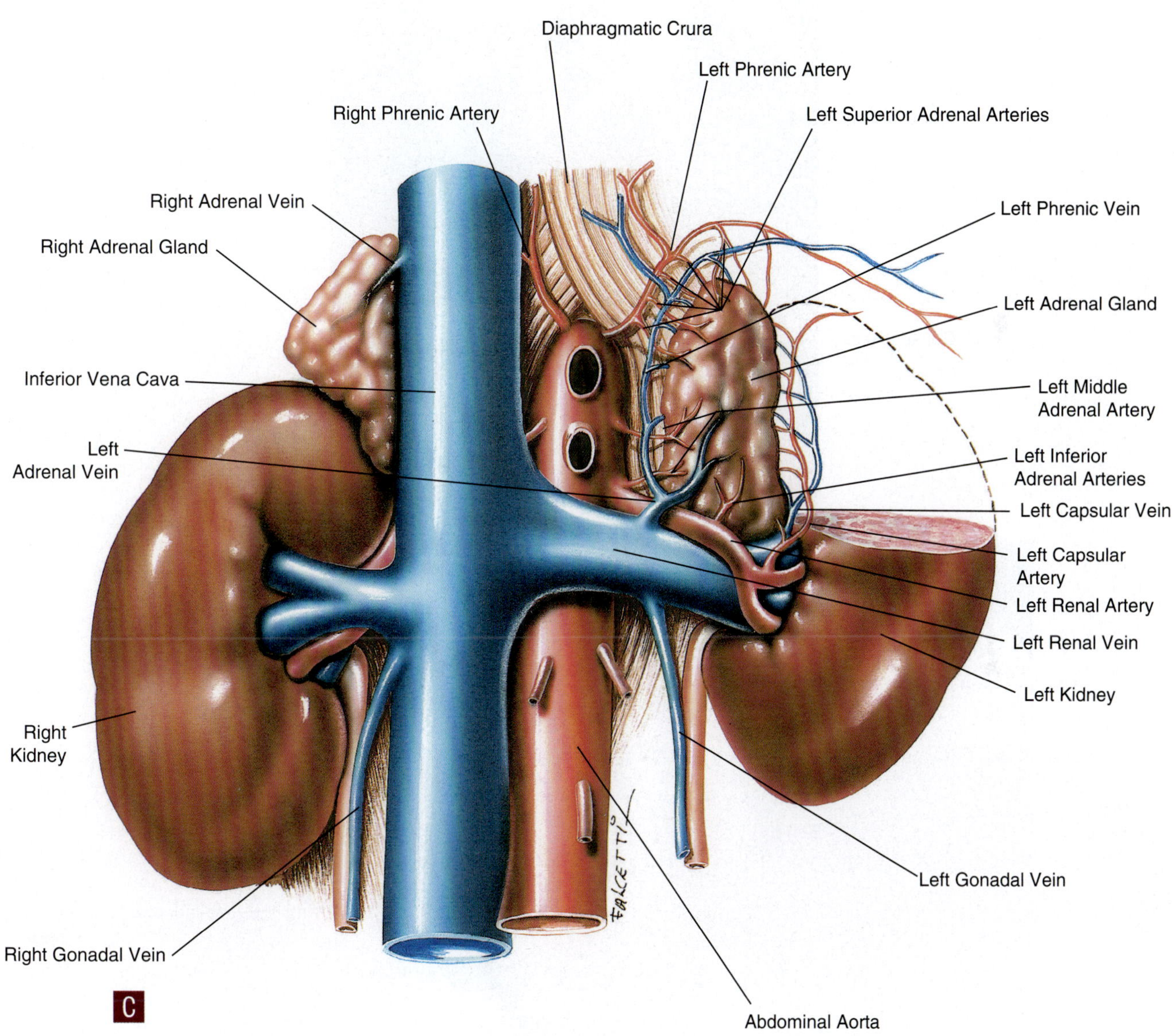

Figure 20.48. *Continued*

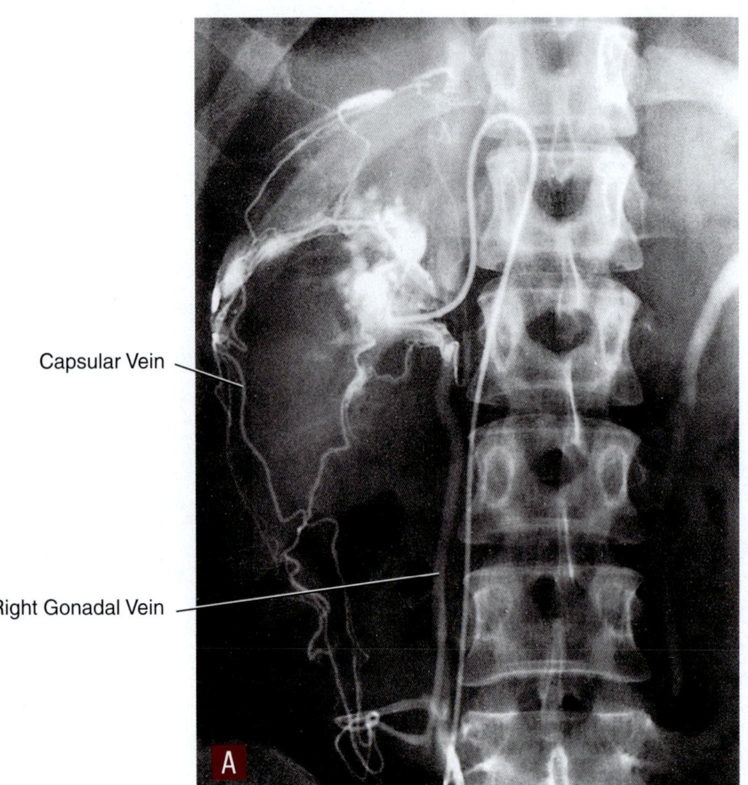

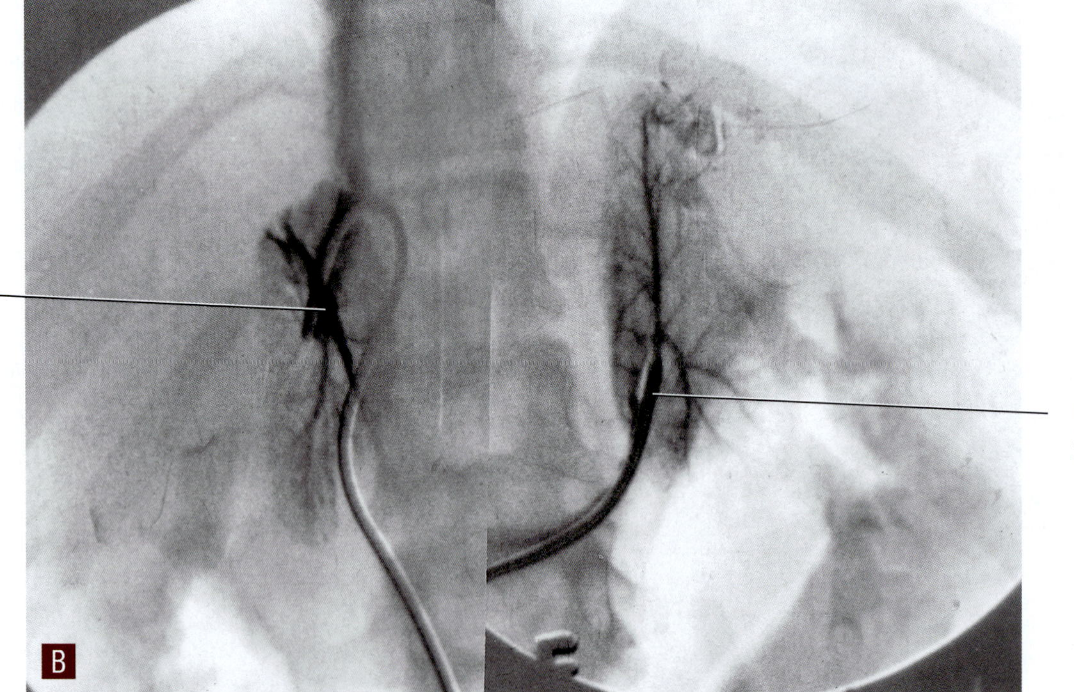

Figure 20.49. A, Selective injection into a renal capsular vein, showing retrograde staining of soft tissues and filling of retroperitoneal veins and gonadal vein. B, Selective injection at the right and left adrenal veins showing the enlarged right and left adrenal glands. Again the right adrenal vein ends in the inferior vena cava, and the left adrenal vein ends in the left renal vein.

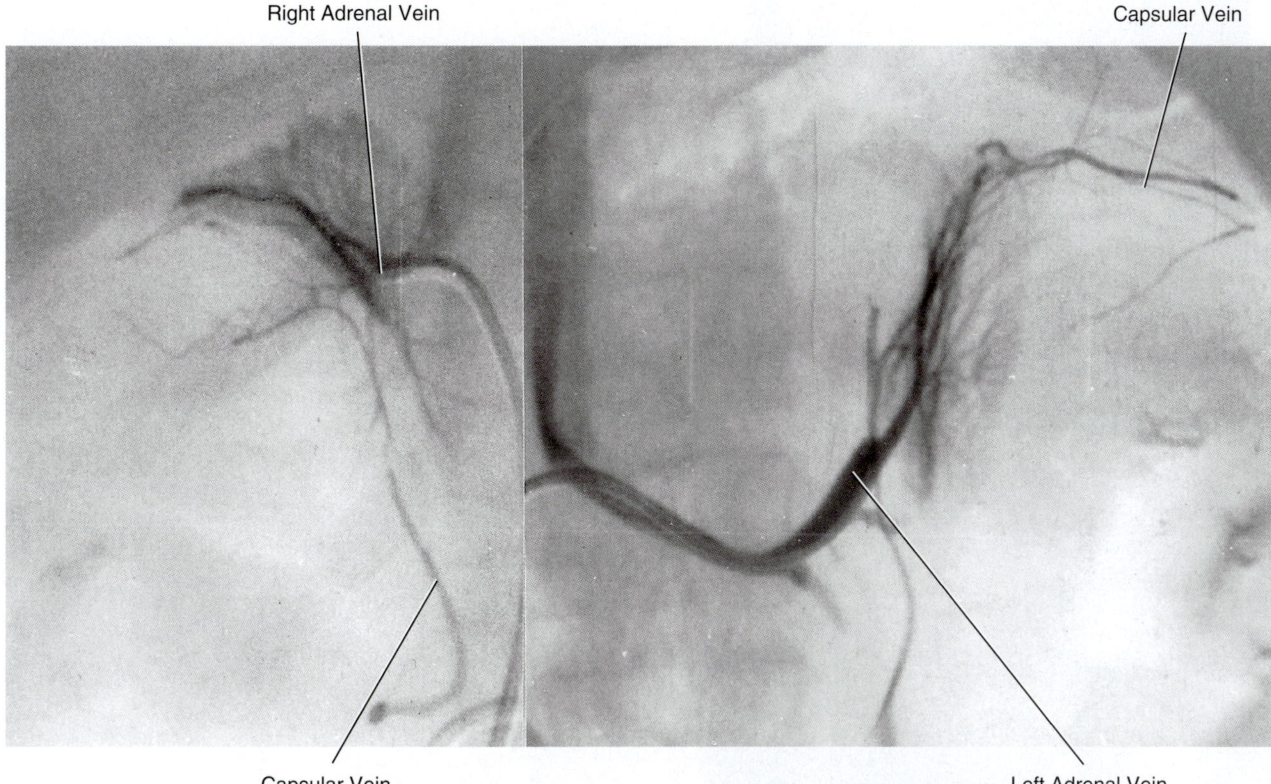

Figure 20.50. Selective injection into the right and left adrenal veins showing the small triangular right adrenal gland riding the upper pole of the kidney and the left longer adrenal gland draining into the left renal vein, located medially to the left kidney.

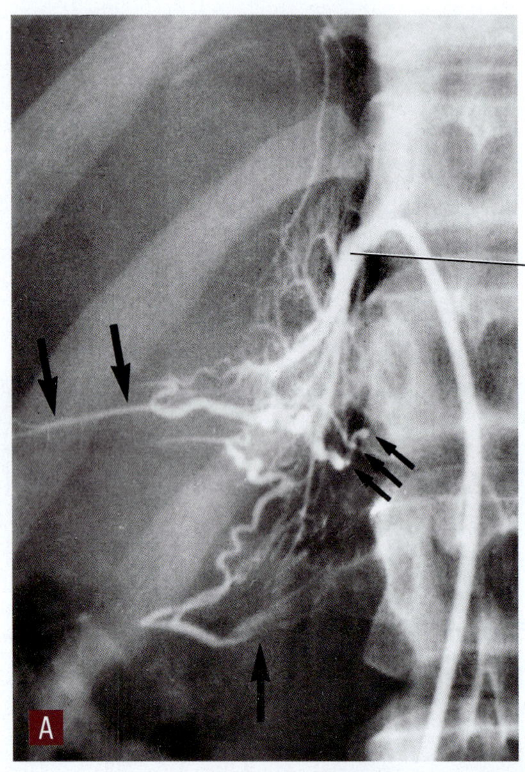

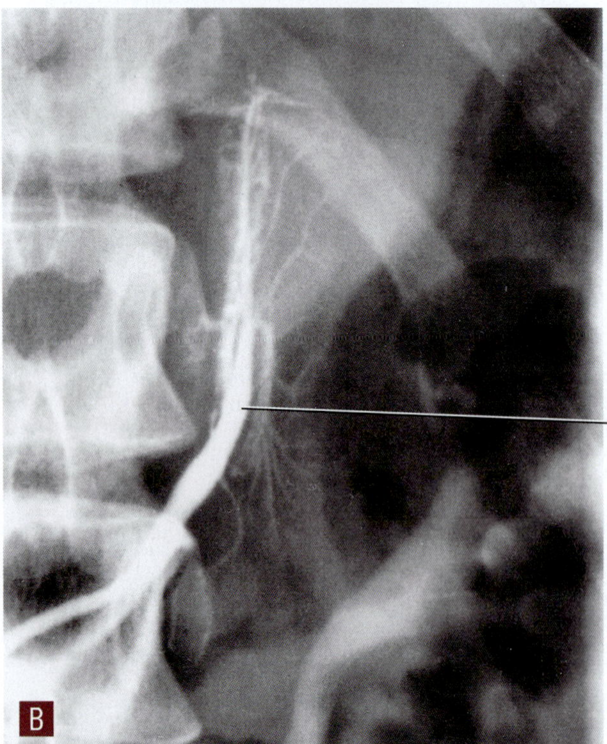

Figure 20.51. A, Selective injection into the right adrenal vein showing the small triangular gland. The arrows point to collaterals and anastomosis with the capsular veins. B, Selective injection into the left adrenal vein showing the long vein and gland. The left adrenal vein drains into the left renal vein.

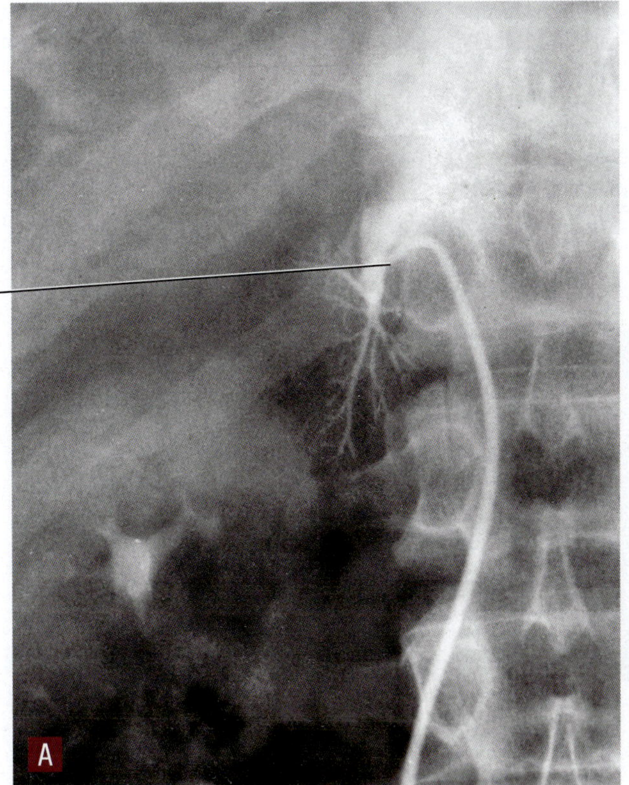

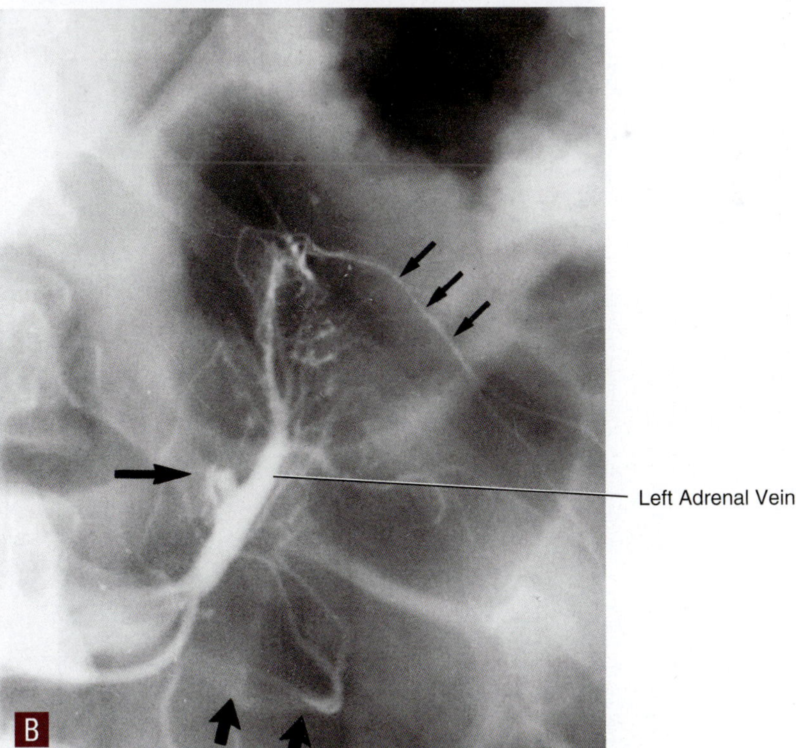

Figure 20.52. A, Selective injection into the right adrenal vein showing the small triangular gland. The right adrenal vein ends into the posterolateral aspect of the inferior vena cava. B, Selective injection into the left adrenal vein. The large arrow shows the stump of the left inferior phrenic vein. The three small arrows show a capsular vein anastomosed with the adrenal vein circulation. The two small arrows show anastomosis with the intrarenal veins.

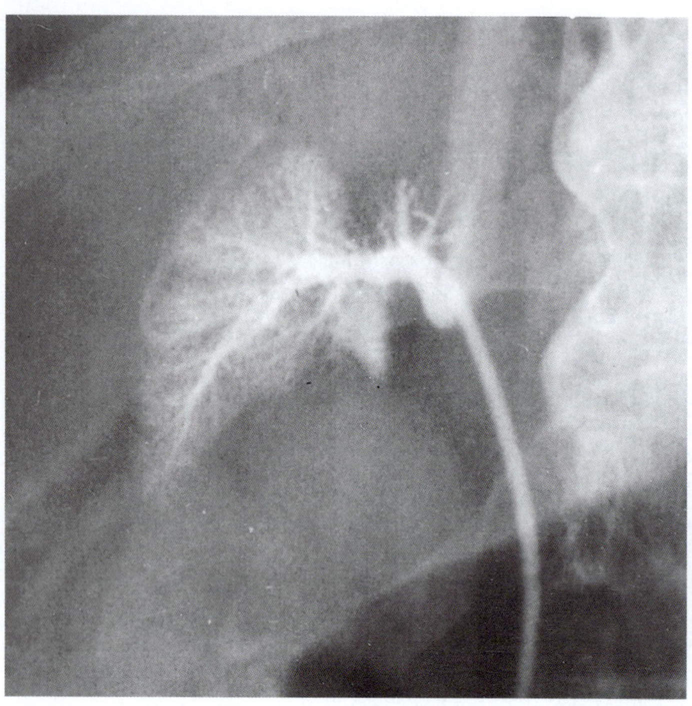

Figure 20.53. Selective injection into one hepatic vein of the inferior group. This vein may mimic the right adrenal vein when an angiographic search is performed.

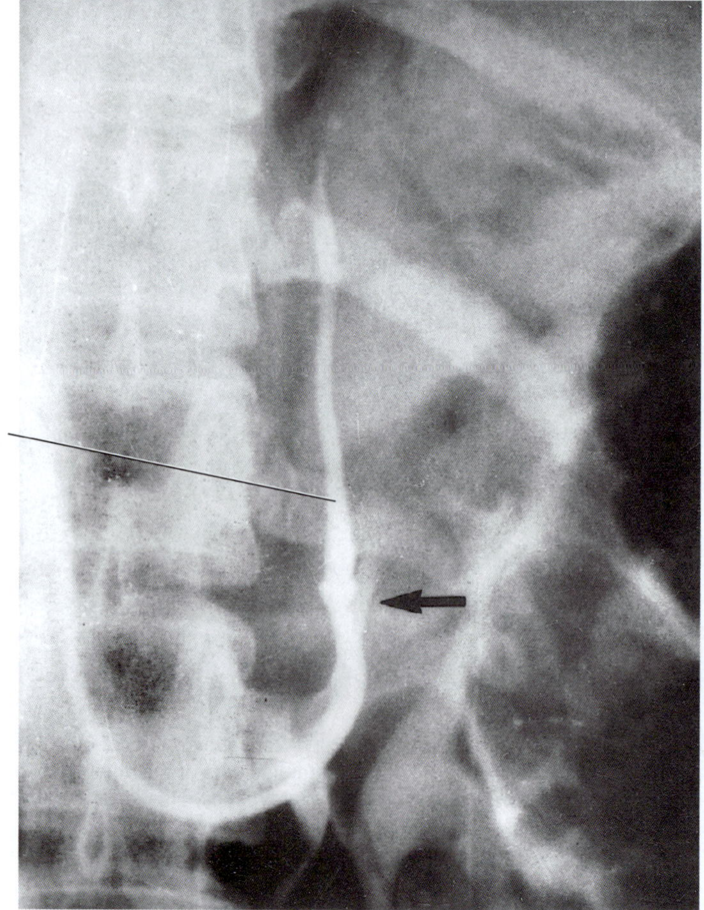

Figure 20.54. Selective injection into a left adrenal vein showing only the left inferior phrenic vein. The arrow shows the real left adrenal vein.

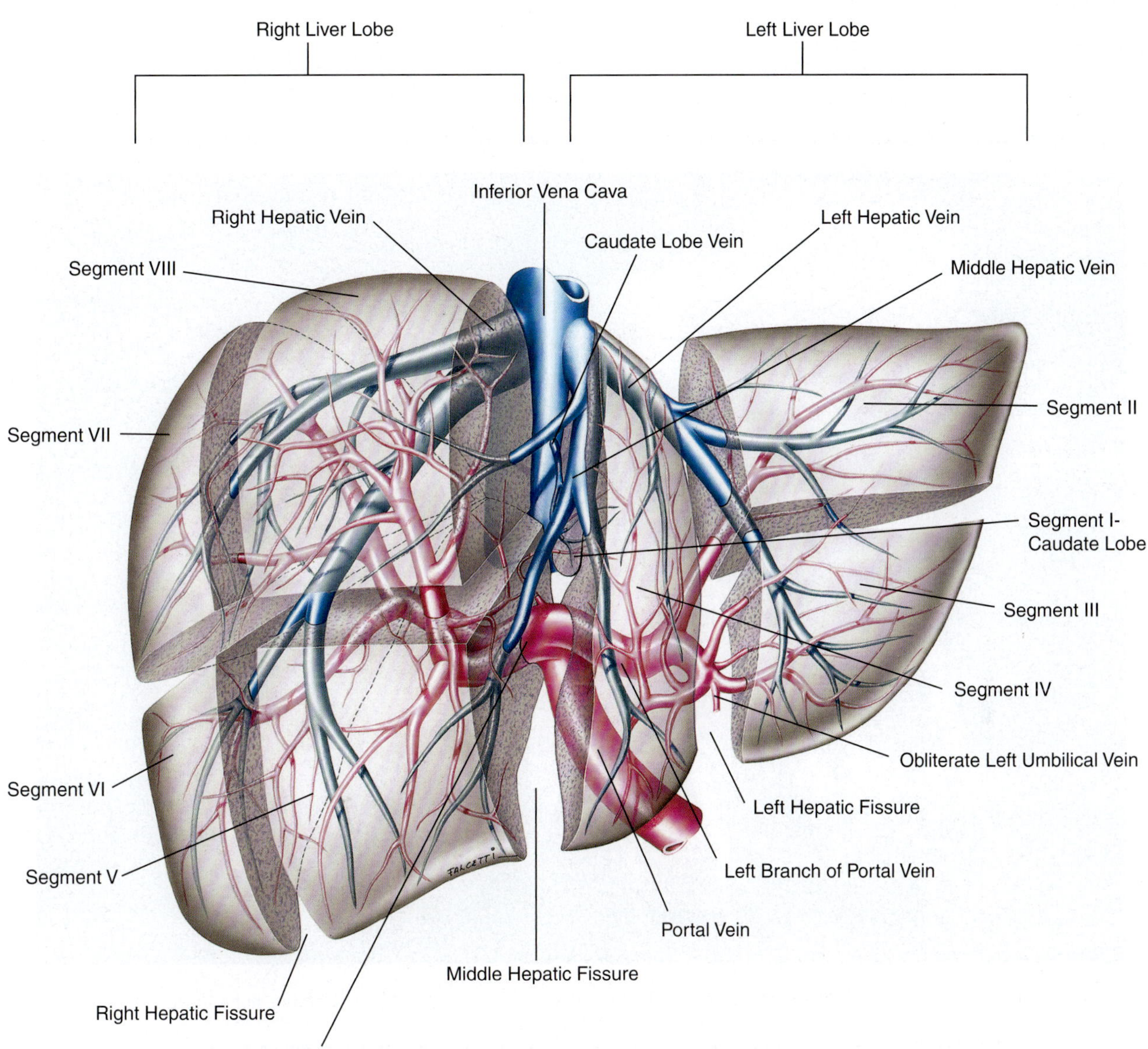

Figure 20.55. Schematic drawing showing the anatomy of the hepatic veins, the portal vein, and the Couinaud segments. The right hepatic vein runs into the right hepatic fissure, while the middle hepatic vein runs into the middle hepatic fissure. The right branch of the middle hepatic vein drains part of the right liver lobe.

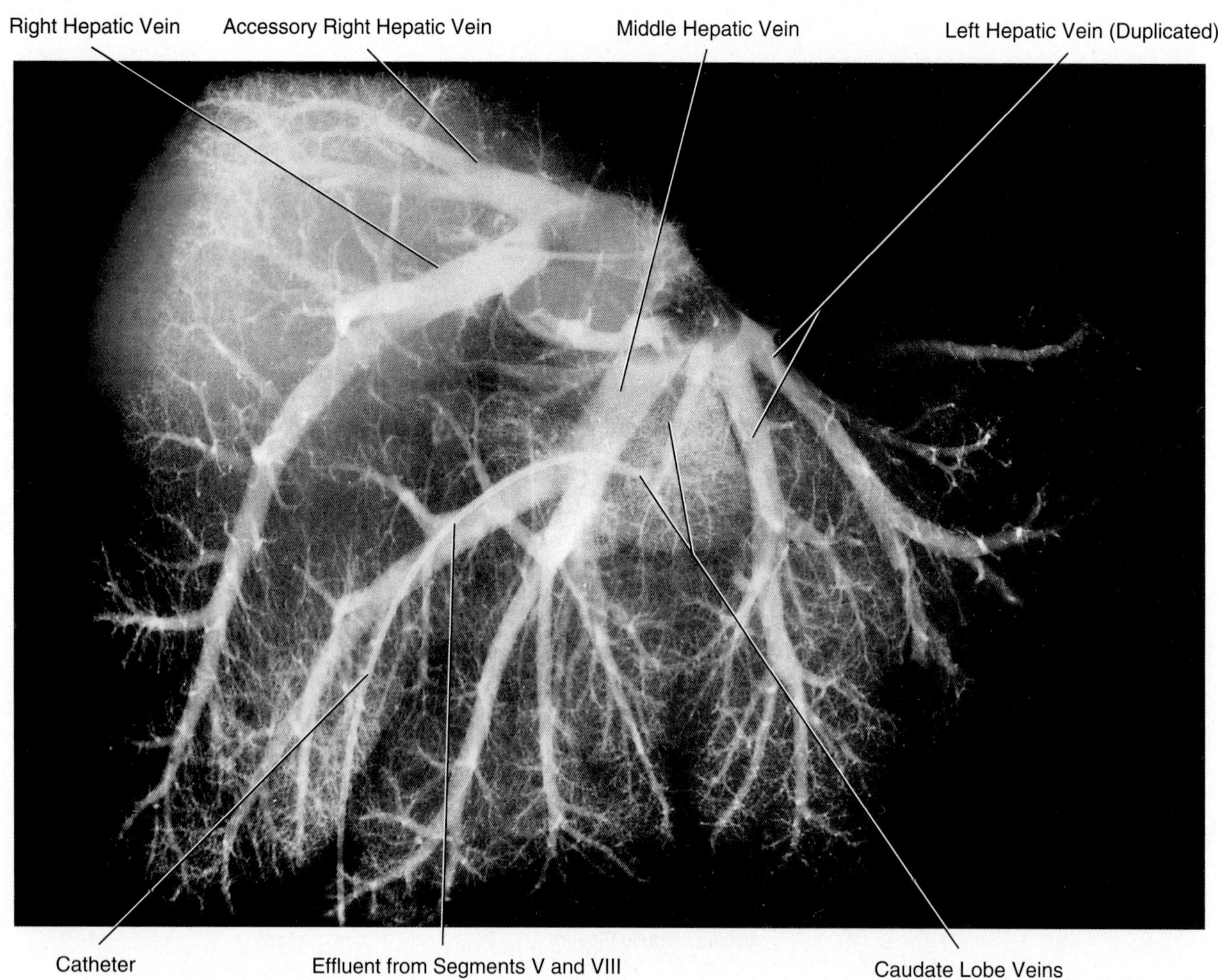

Figure 20.56. Angiography in a liver specimen showing the classic distribution of the hepatic veins. Note the catheter into the caudate lobe vein.

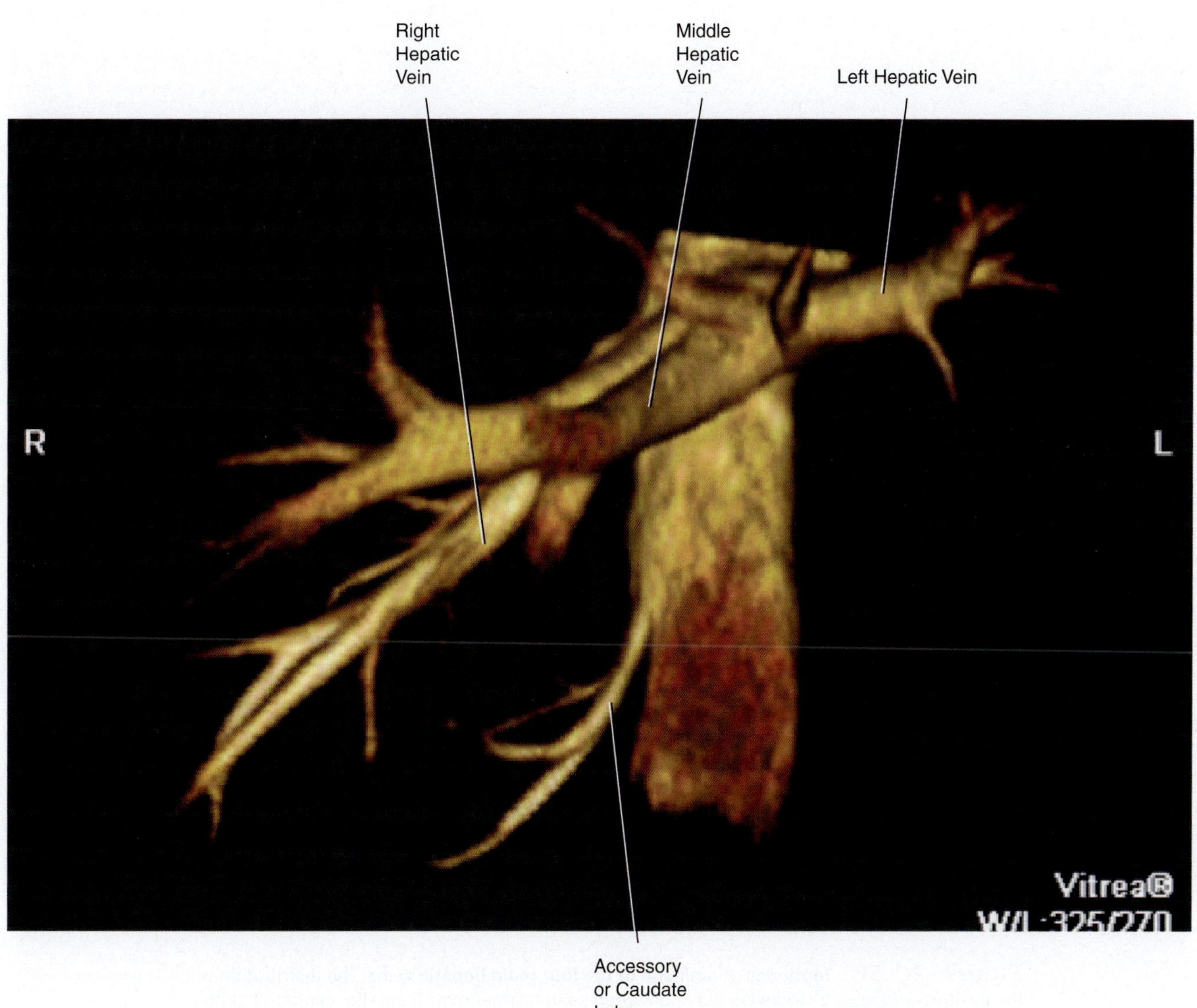

Figure 20.57. Computerized tomographic (CT) angiography with three-dimensional (3D) reconstruction of the hepatic veins and inferior vena cava. Note an accessory right hepatic vein draining direct to the inferior vena cava, or a caudate lobe vein.

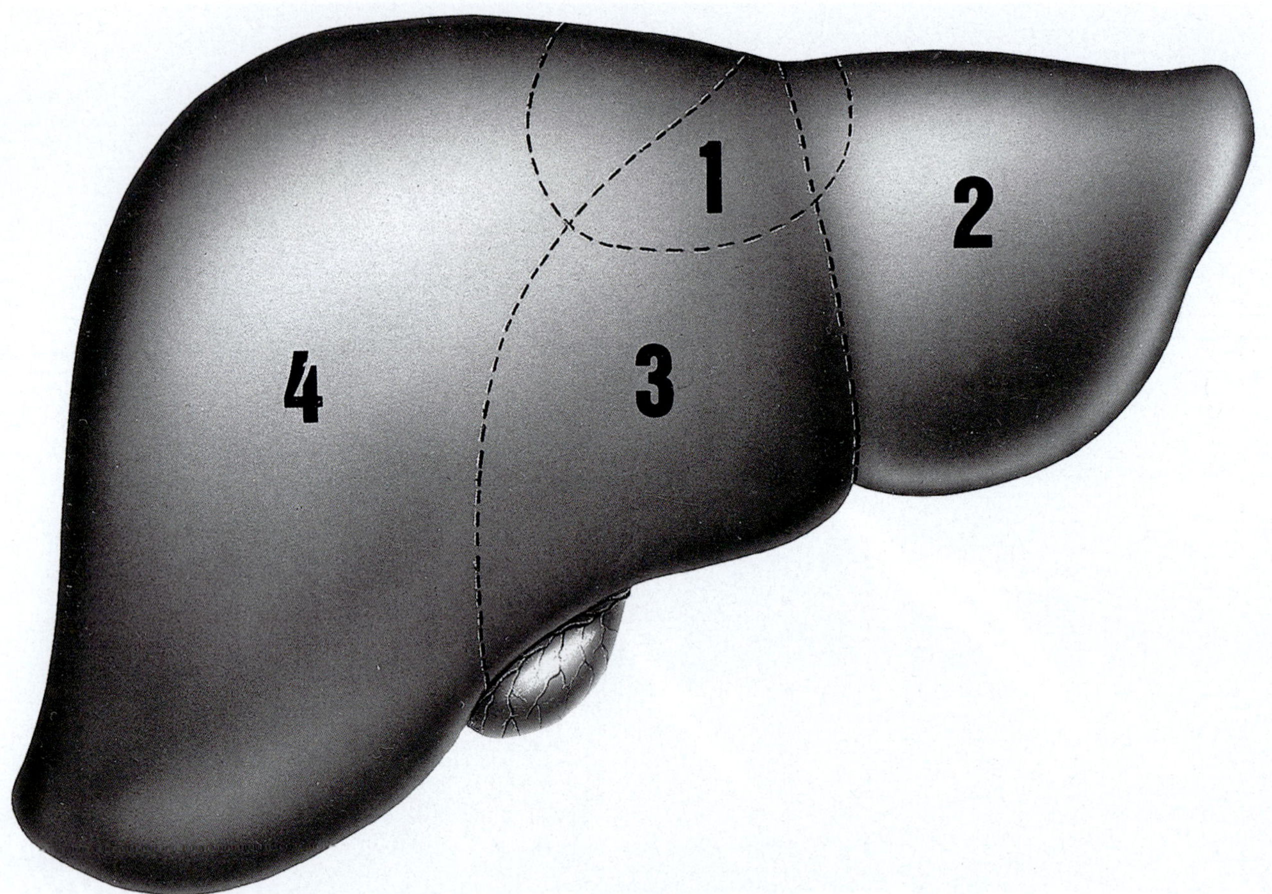

Figure 20.58. Territories of drainage of the four main hepatic veins. The distribution of the territories follows a clockwise direction when seen from above. 1, smaller caudate hepatic vein; 2, left hepatic vein; 3, middle hepatic vein; 4, large right hepatic vein.

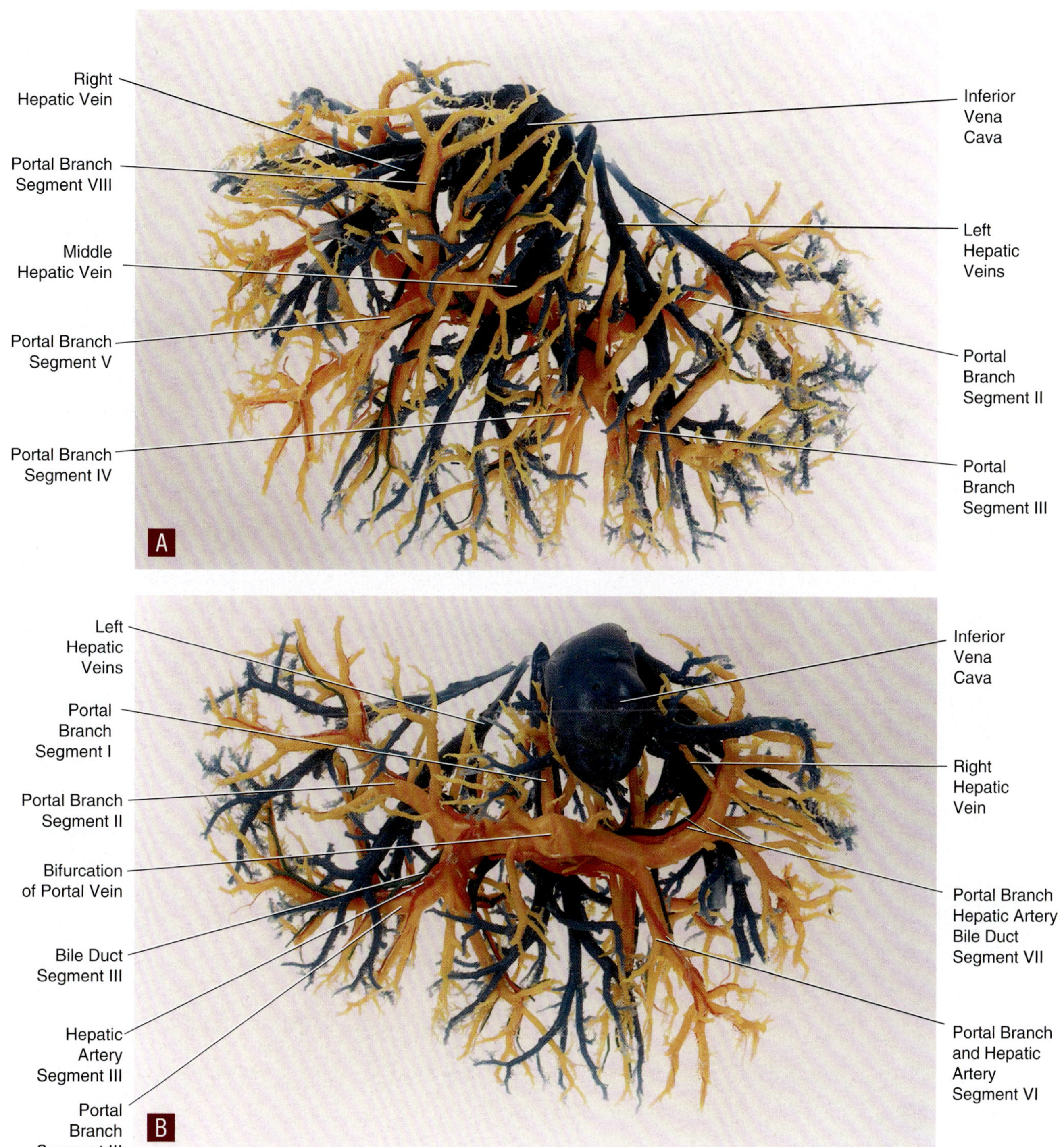

Figure 20.59. **A**, Anterior view of a plastic endocast of a liver specimen. The hepatic veins and inferior vena cava are blue. The portal vein is yellow. The hepatic artery is red and the bile duct is green. **B**, Posterior view of the endocast shows the relationship of the right hepatic artery and right bile duct with the right portal vein.

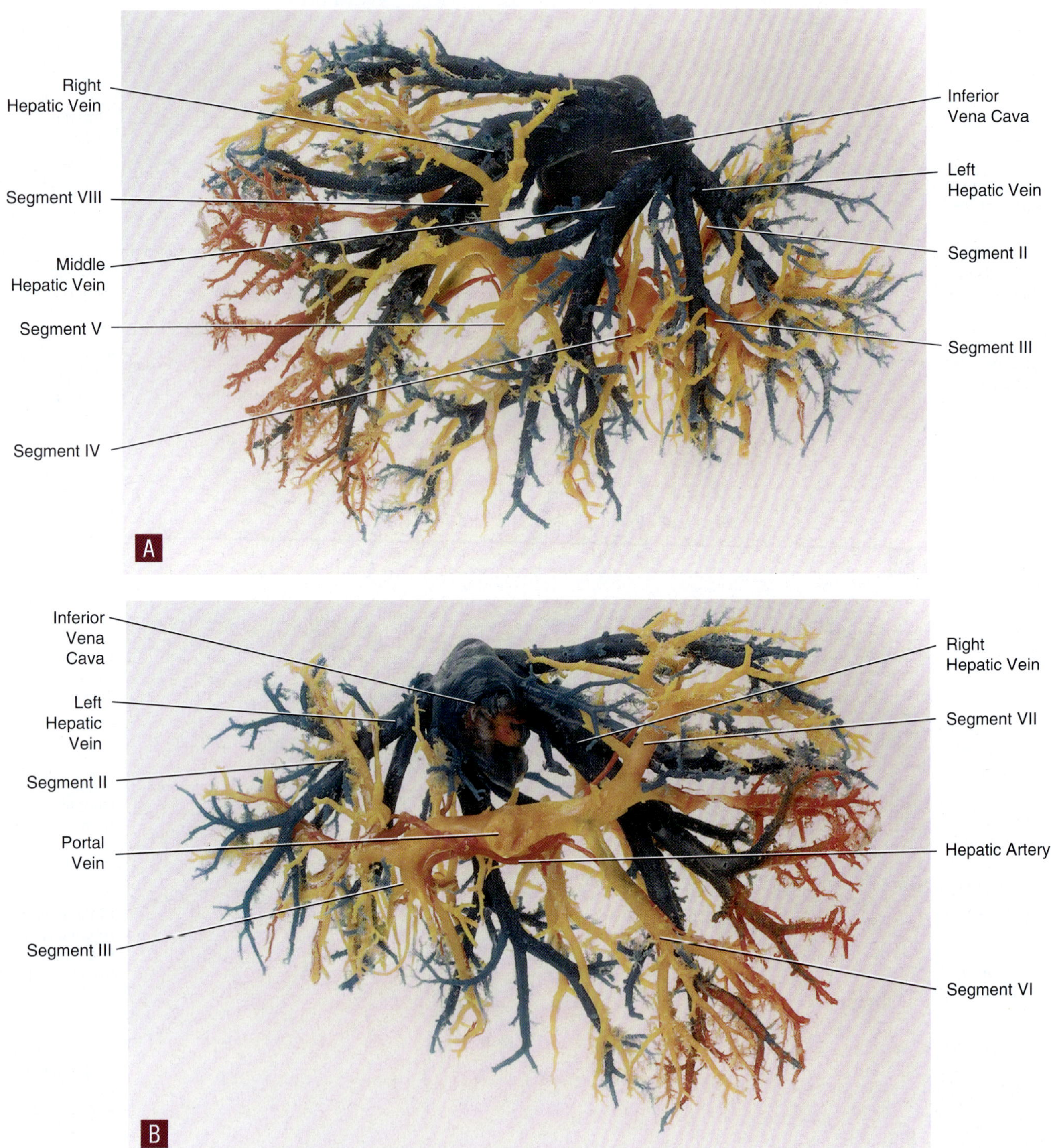

Figure 20.60. **A**, Anterior view of a plastic endocast of a liver specimen. The hepatic veins and inferior vena cava are blue. The portal vein is yellow. The hepatic artery is red and the bile duct is green. In the periphery of the right lobe, the portal vein is red due to mixture of the plastic material from the portal vein with the arterial injection, due to occlusion of the peripheral portal vein. **B**, Posterior view of the plastic endocast of the liver. Note the position of the hepatic artery in relation to the portal vein. The bile duct is less visible.

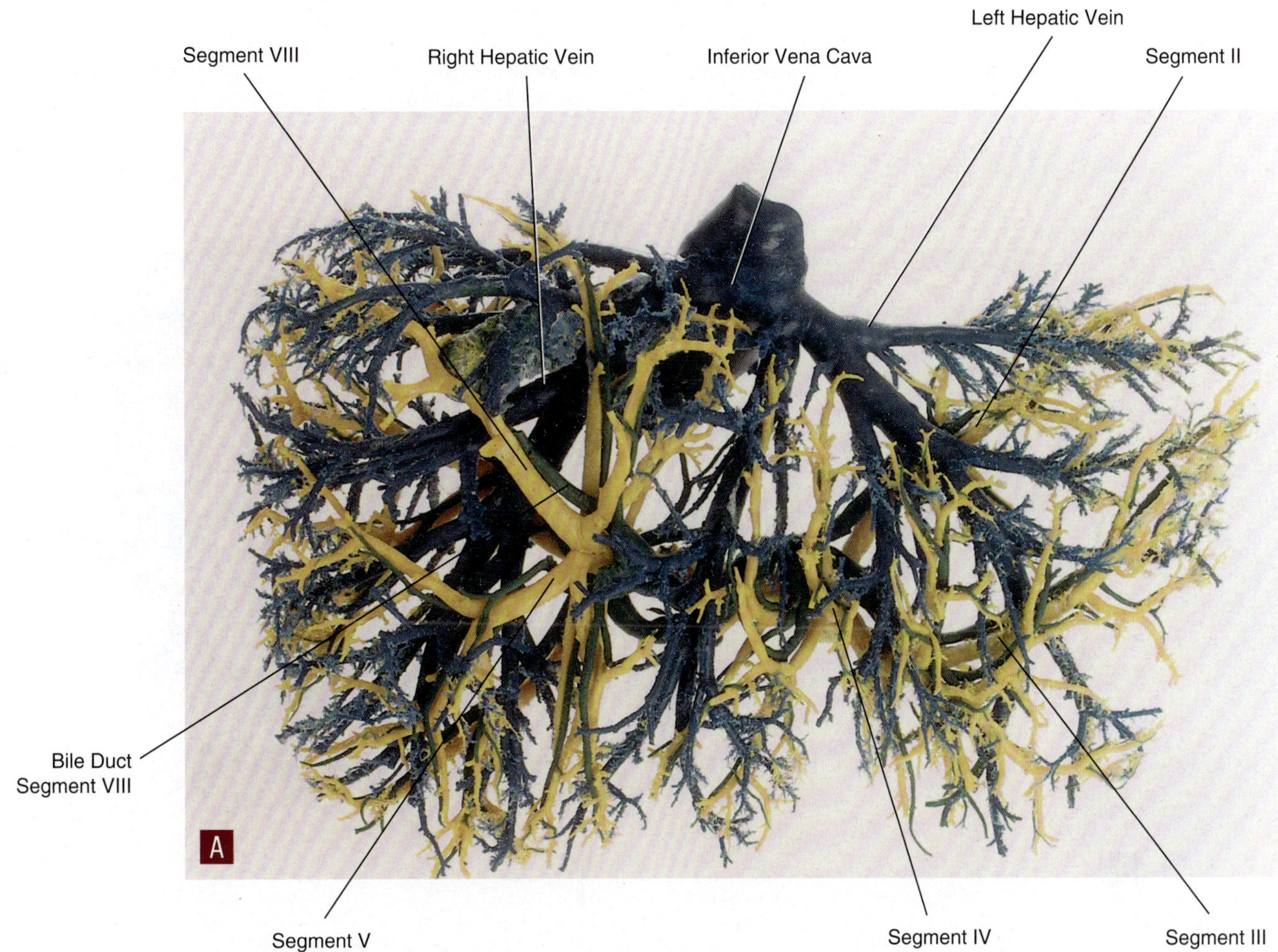

Figure 20.61. A, Anterior view of a plastic endocast of a liver specimen. The hepatic veins and inferior vena cava are blue. The portal vein is yellow. The bile duct is green. Note the relationship of the bile duct with the right portal vein. B, Posterior view of the endocast. Note the relationship of the bile duct with the portal vein.

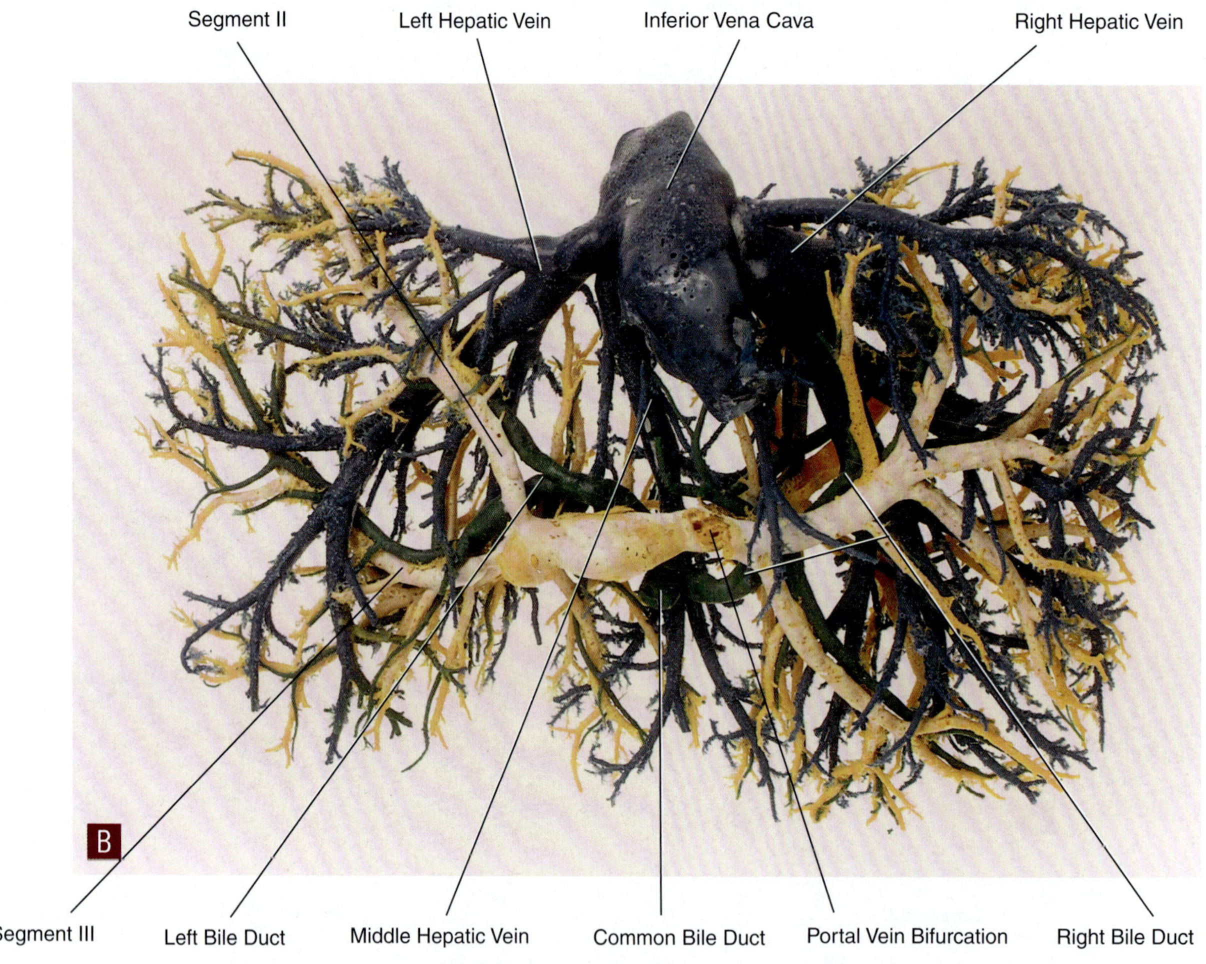

Figure 20.61. *Continued*

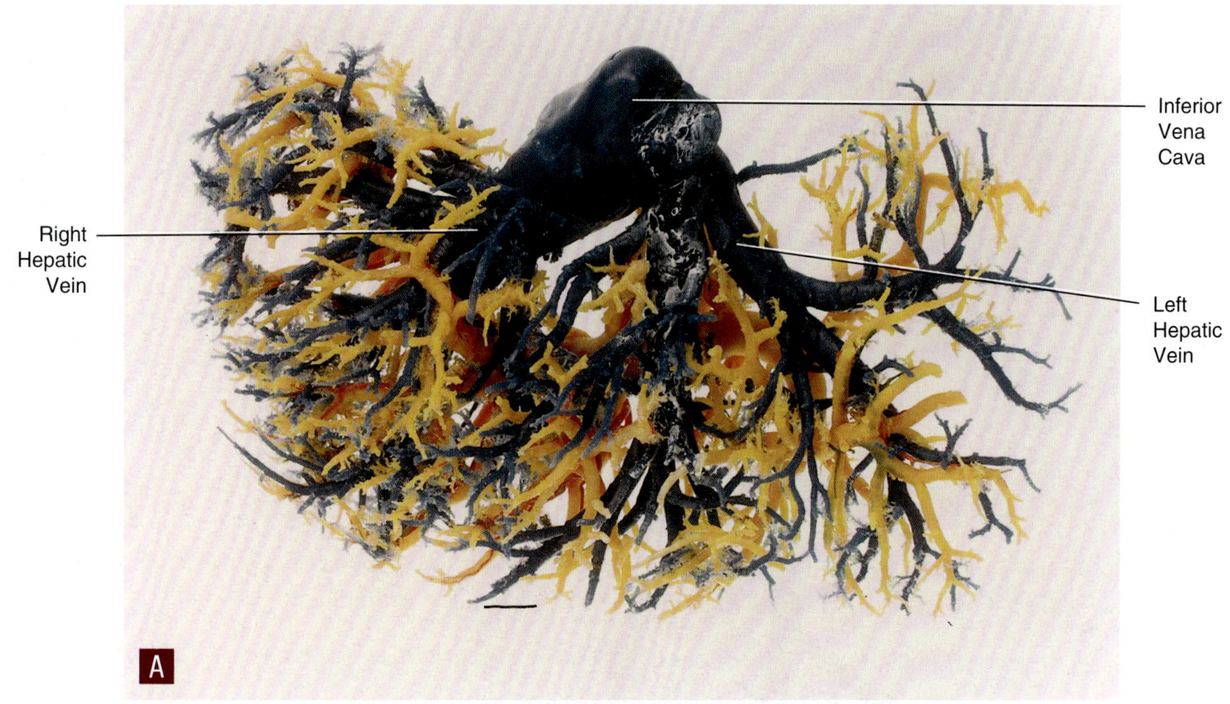

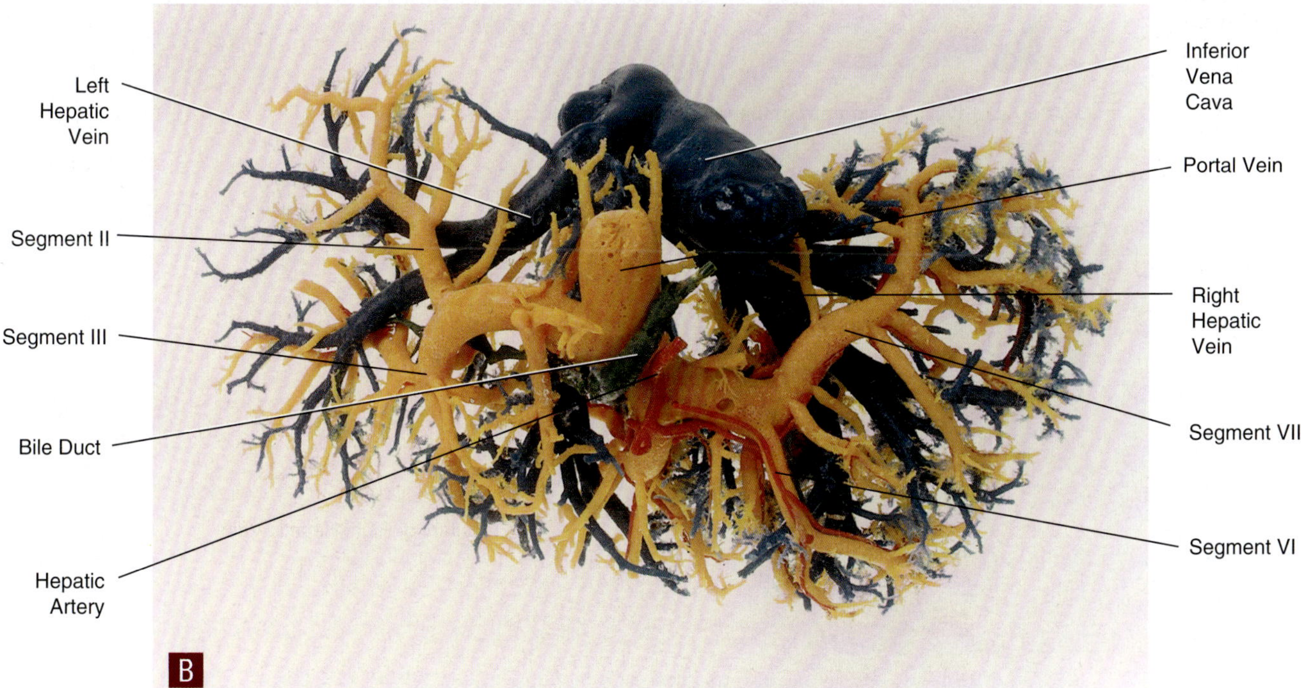

Figure 20.62. **A**, Anterior view of a plastic endocast of a liver specimen. The hepatic veins and inferior vena cava are blue. The portal vein is yellow. The bile duct is green. The hepatic artery is red. Note the relationship of the hepatic artery and bile duct with the portal vein. **B**, Posterior view of the endocast. Note the relationship of the hepatic artery and the bile duct with the portal vein.

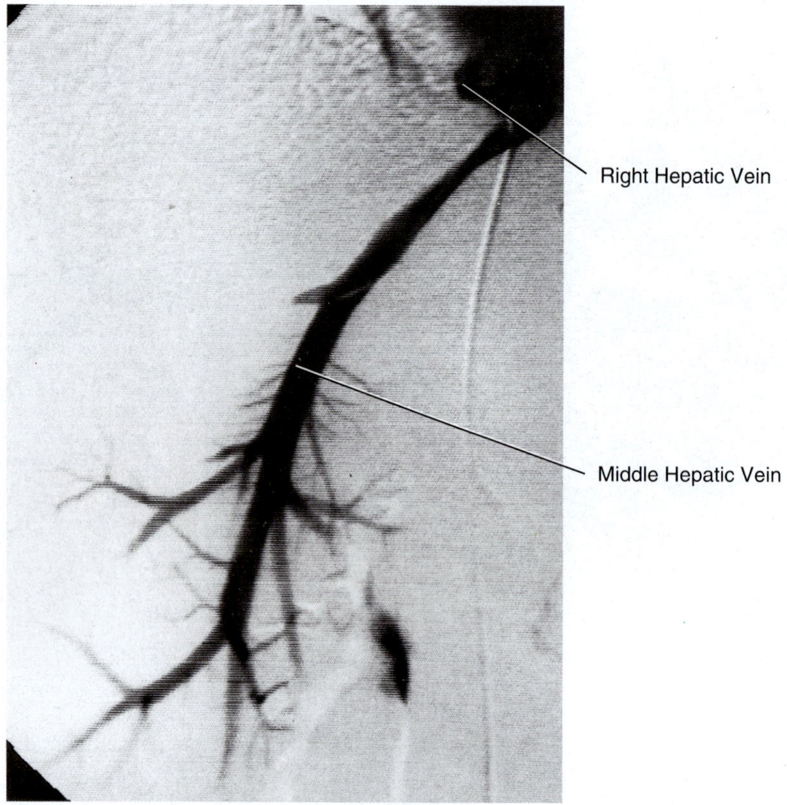

Figure 20.63. Angiogram of the middle hepatic vein.

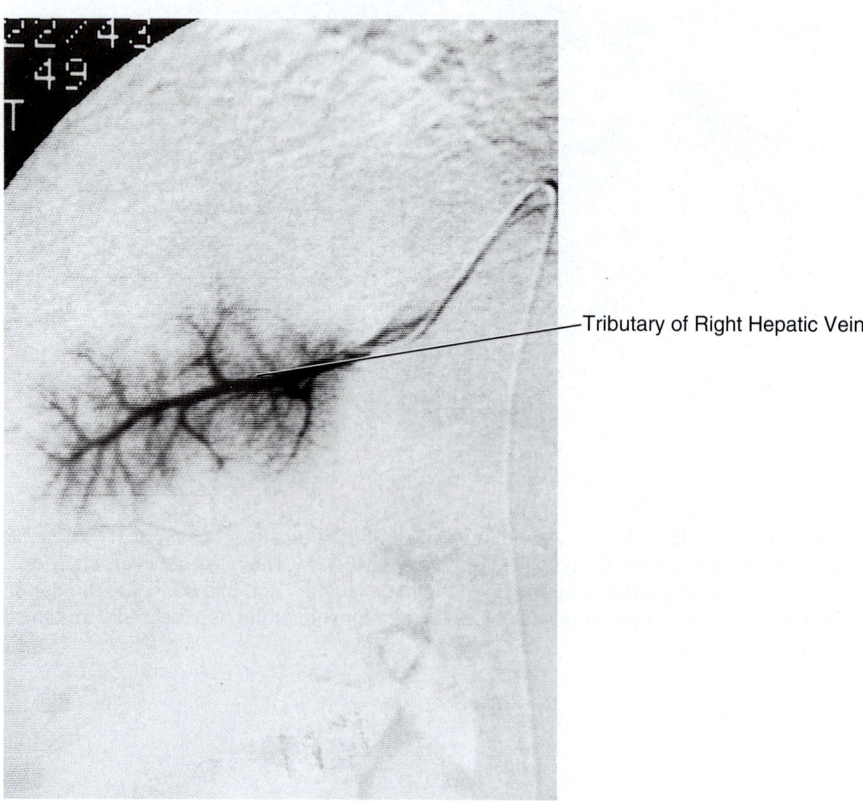

Figure 20.64. Angiogram of the right hepatic vein.

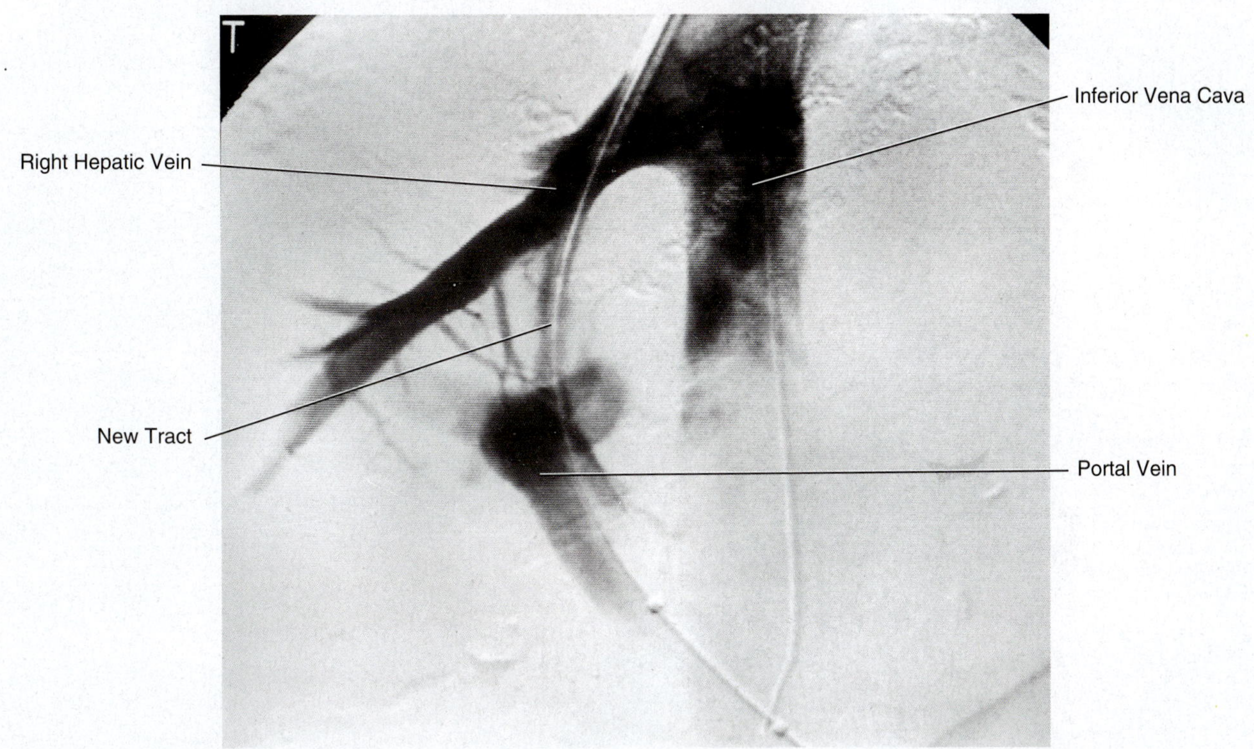

Figure 20.65. Angiogram during a transjugular intrahepatic portosystemic shunt (TIPS) procedure showing the relationships of the right hepatic vein, the portal vein, and the inferior vena cava. There is a tract created by the puncture.

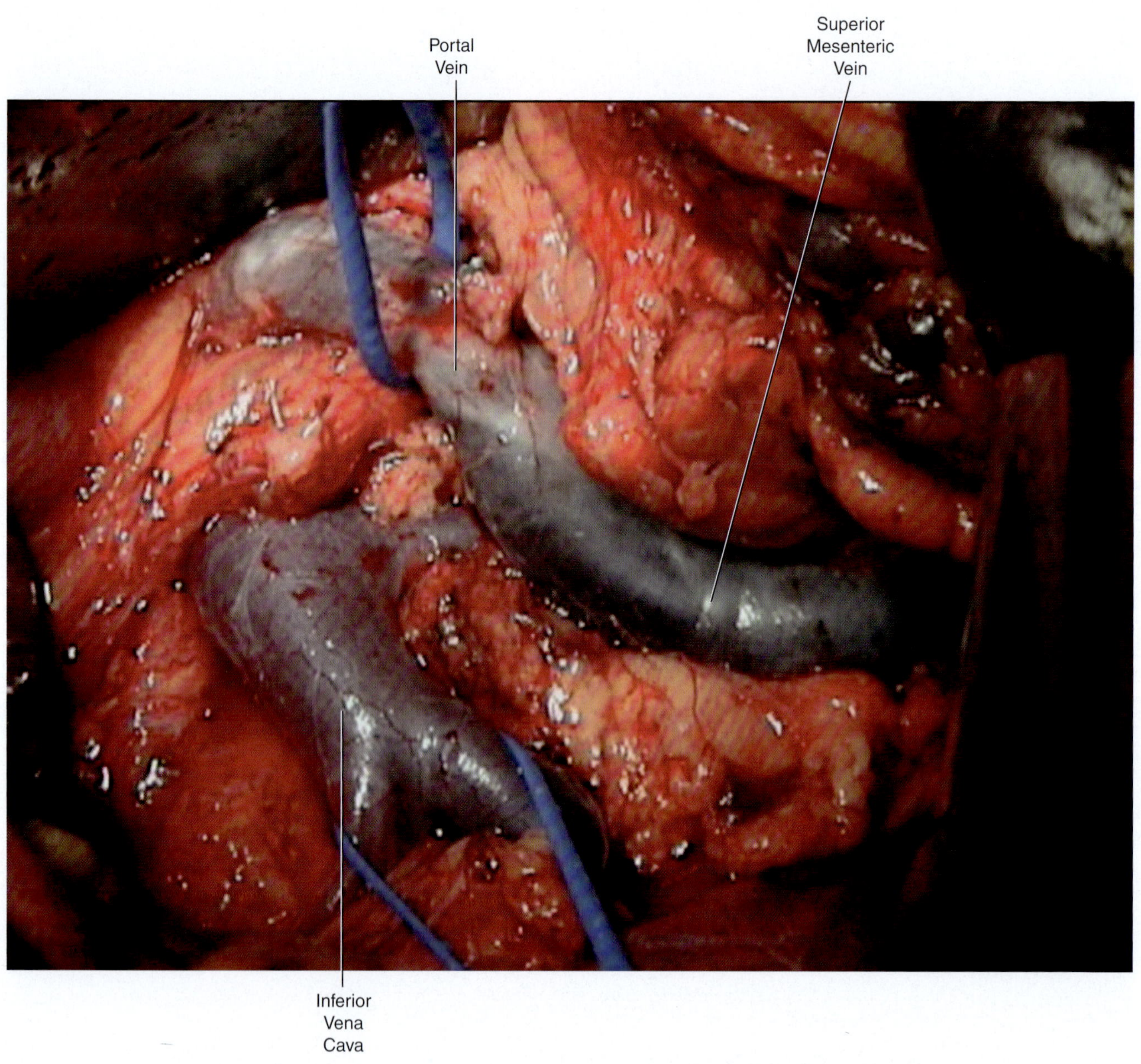

Figure 20.66. Surgical exposure of the inferior vena cava and tributaries, and portal vein and superior mesenteric vein, just before a mesocaval shunt. The upper blue-vessel loop is around the portal vein just after the confluence of the splenic vein (not shown) and the inferior mesenteric vein. The lower blue-vessel loop is around the inferior vena cava.

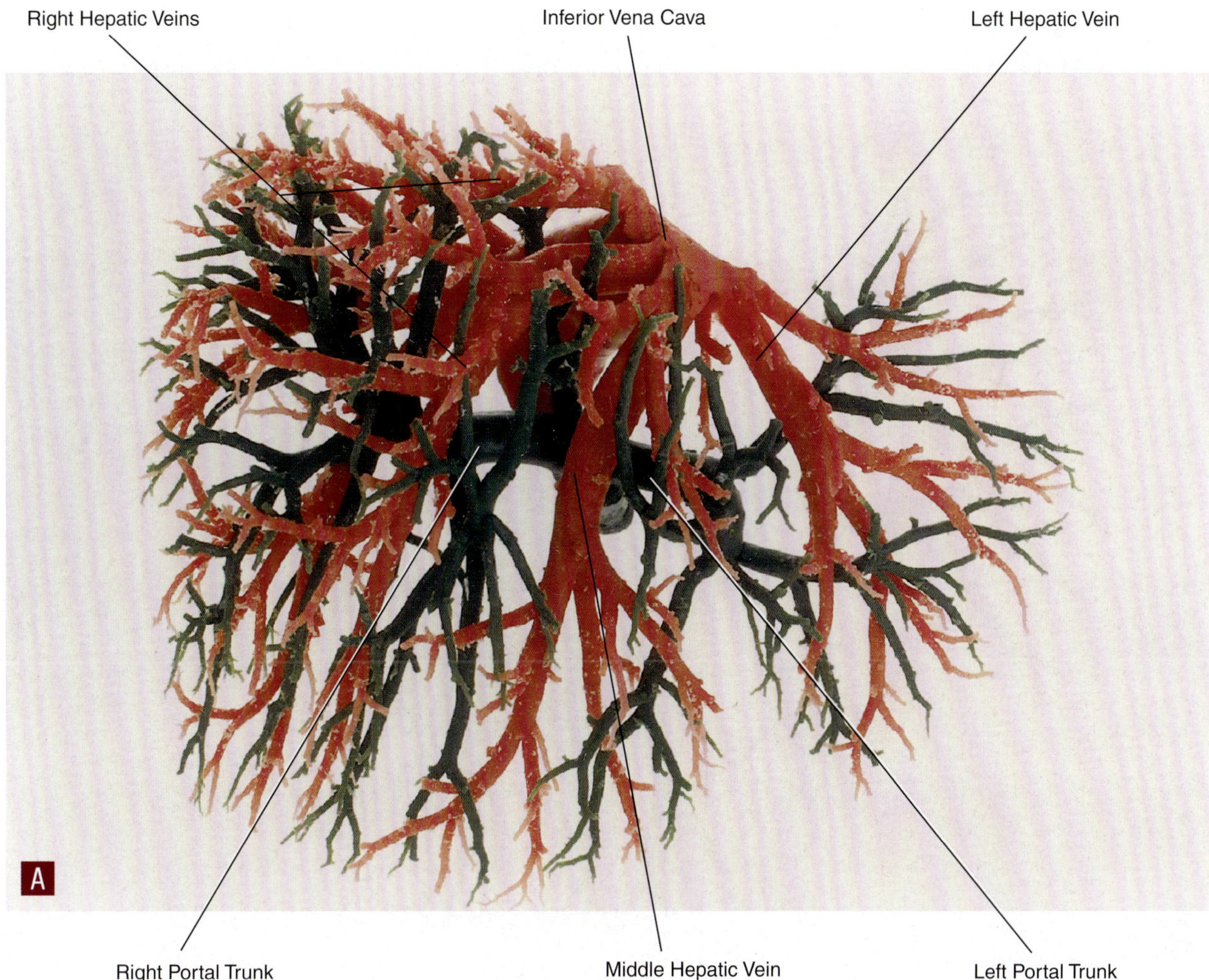

Figure 20.67. A, Anterior view of a plastic endocast of a liver specimen. The hepatic veins and inferior vena cava are red. The portal vein is green. There are three right hepatic veins as an anatomic variation. The most anterior hepatic vein is anterior to the right portal vein. B, Posterior view of the plastic endocast. Note the relationship of the hepatic veins with the portal vein.

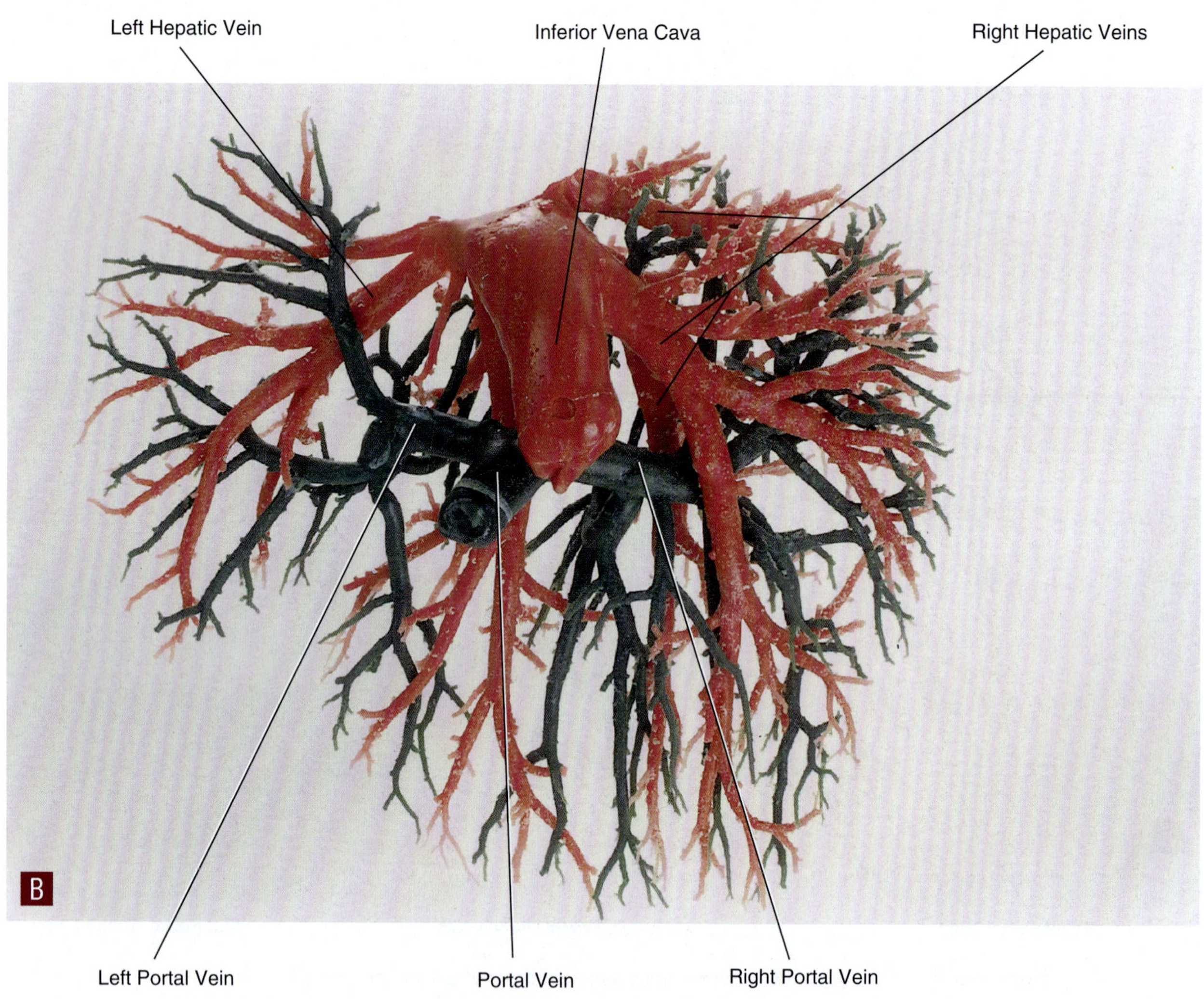

Figure 20.67. *Continued*

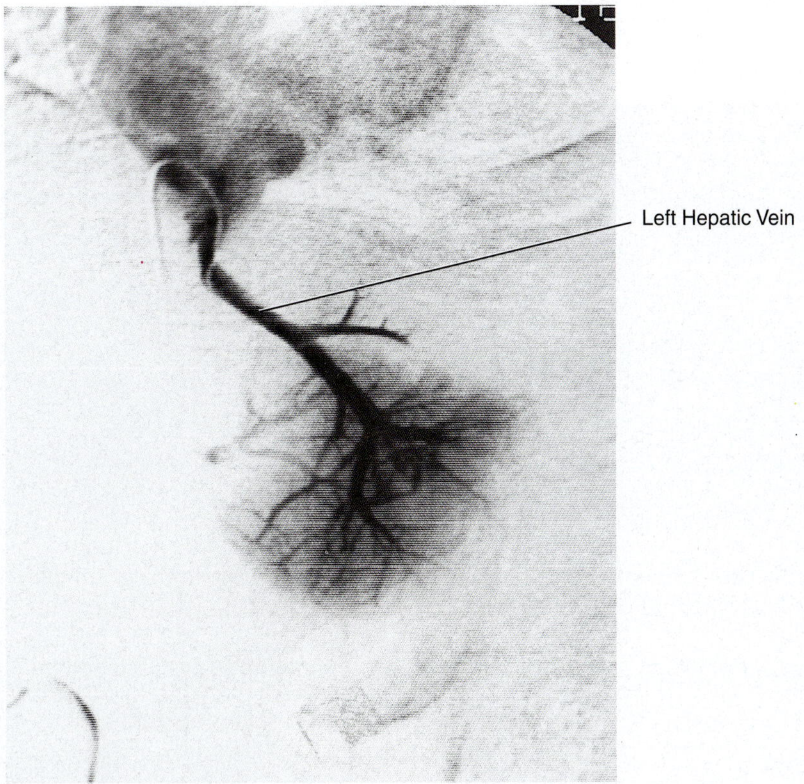

Figure 20.68. Angiogram of the left hepatic vein.

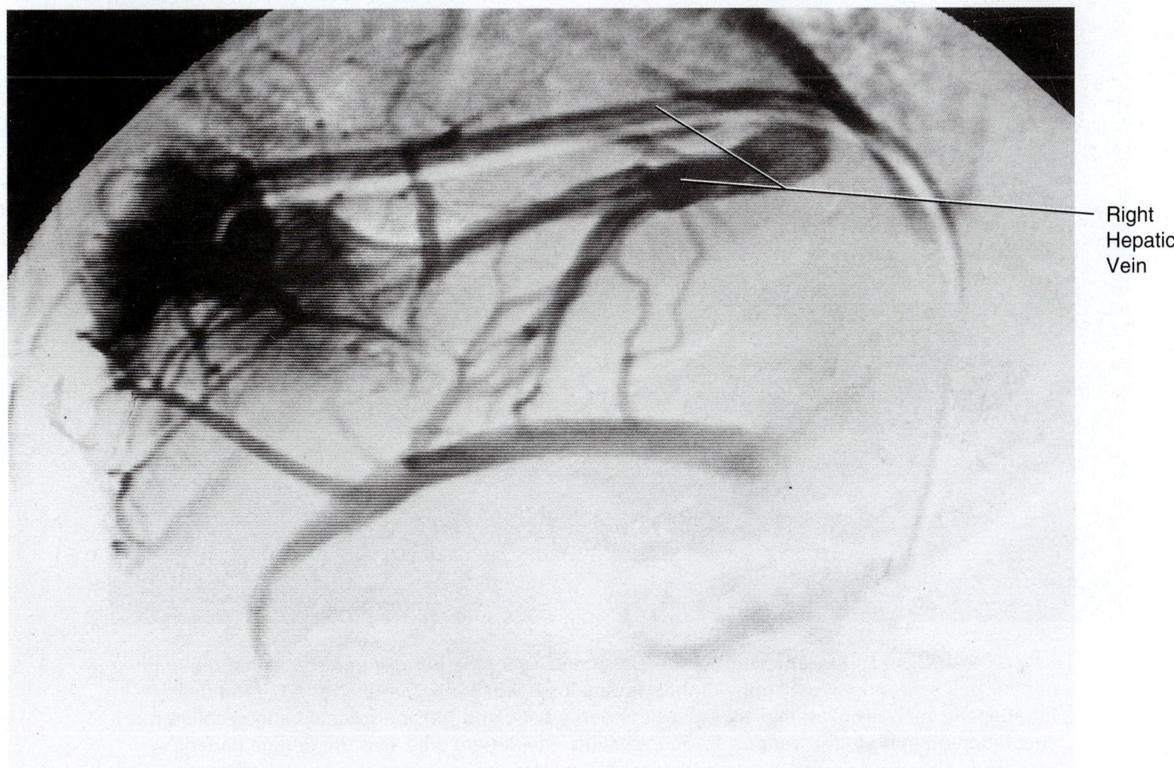

Figure 20.69. Wedged angiogram of the right hepatic vein. Note the reflux of contrast medium into other branches of the right hepatic vein through the intrahepatic collaterals within the same lobe.

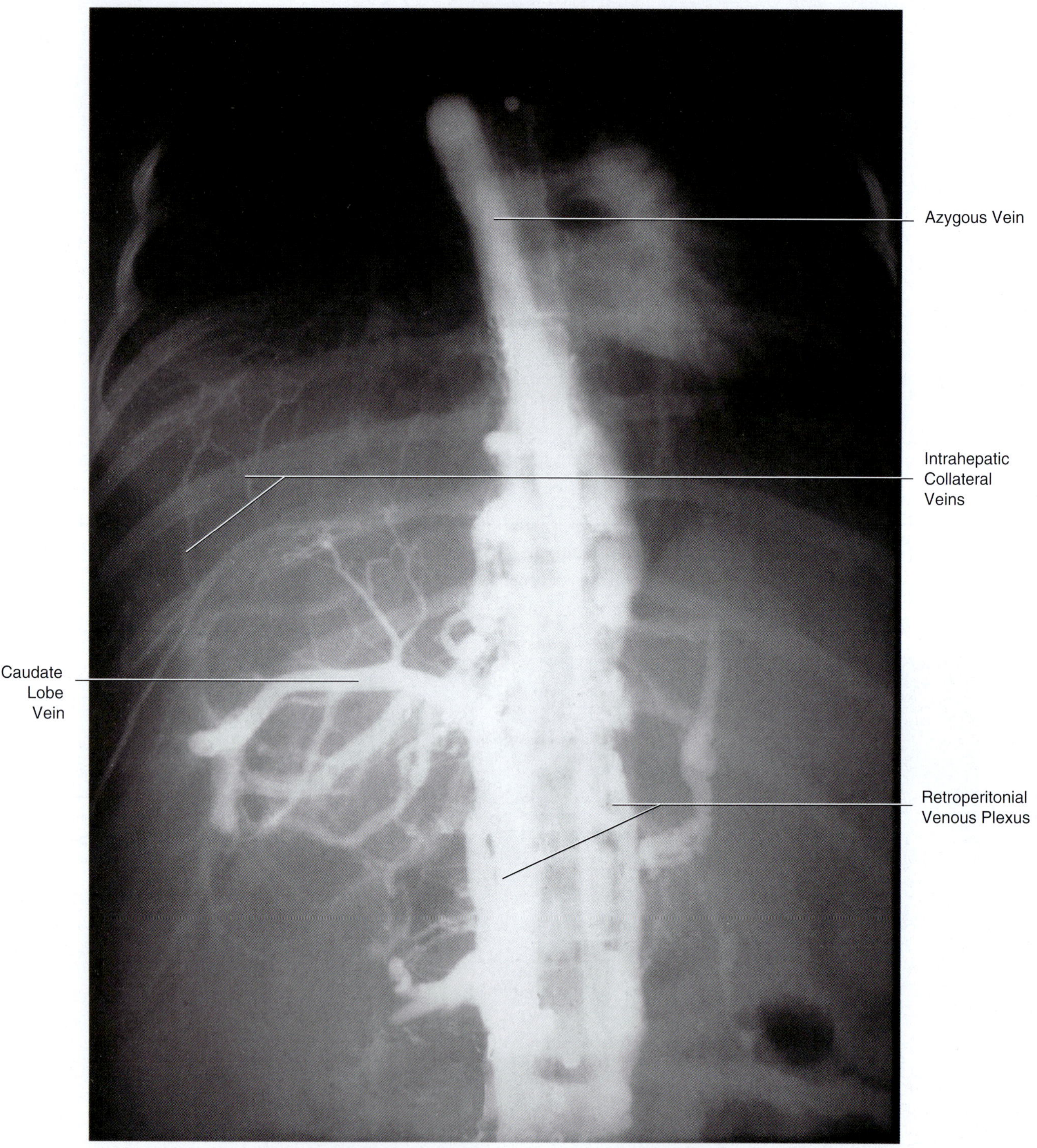

Figure 20.70. Extrahepatic collaterals. Occlusion of the inferior vena cava and the main hepatic veins causing hypertrophy of the caudate lobe vein, with demonstration of multiple intrahepatic venous collaterals, as well as the perihepatic and retroperitoneal venous collateral circulation draining to the venous azygous system. The patient was a young female patient with Budd-Chiari syndrome due to occlusion of the inferior vena cava by a large hepatic cyst.

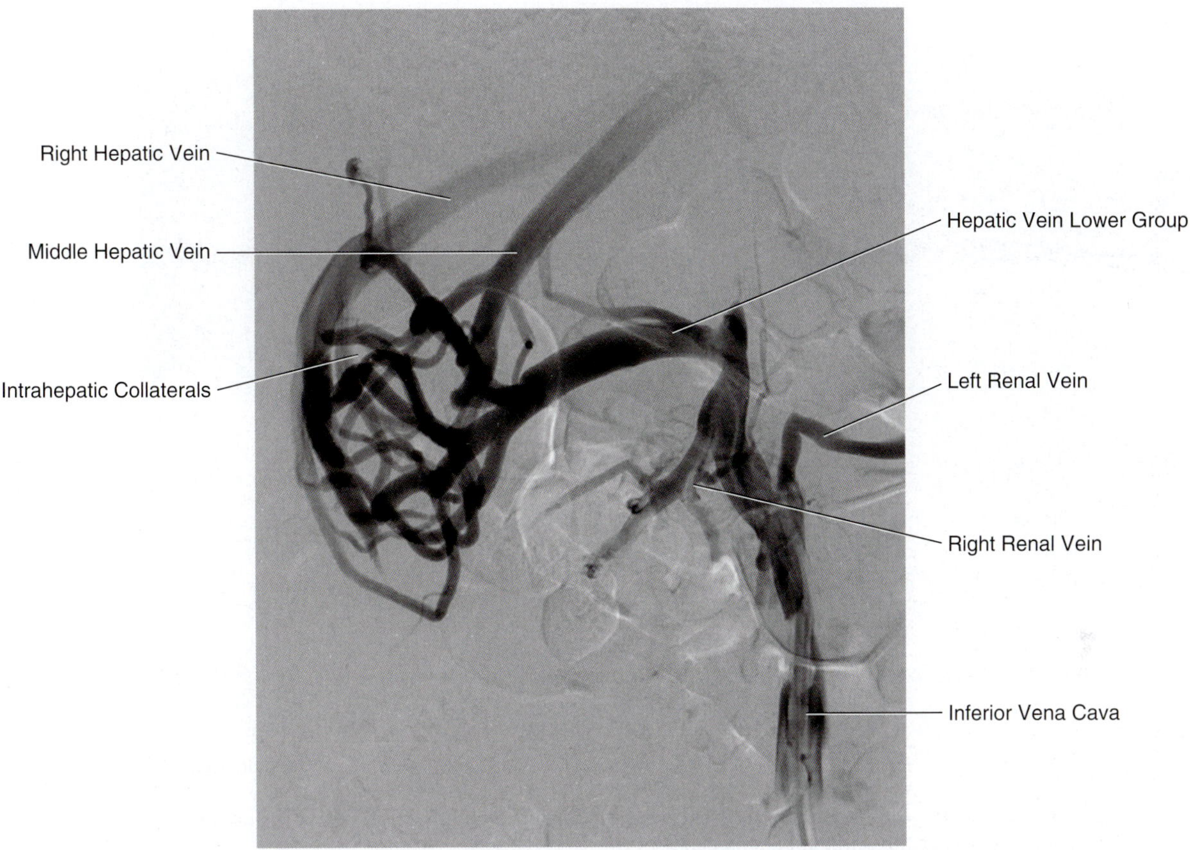

Figure 20.71. Intrahepatic-interlobar collaterals. Cavogram performed through a left femoral hemodialysis catheter on a patient with chronic central venous occlusion of the intrahepatic segment of the inferior vena cava. The drainage pathway depends upon the hepatic vein lower group, which has hypertrophied anastomoses in the hepatic parenchyma with the right and middle hepatic veins. The left and right renal veins are also visualized.

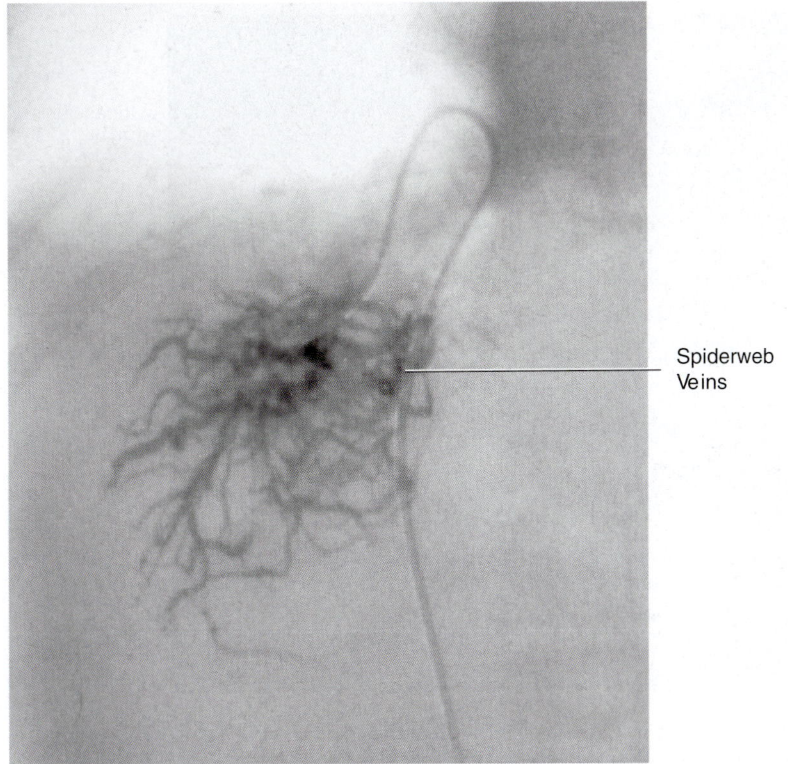

Figure 20.72. Indeterminate type (spiderweb appearance). Fine and coarse collateral network connecting the occluded hepatic vein and the distal intrahepatic vessel segments. "Spiderweb appearance" as encountered in Budd-Chiari syndrome.

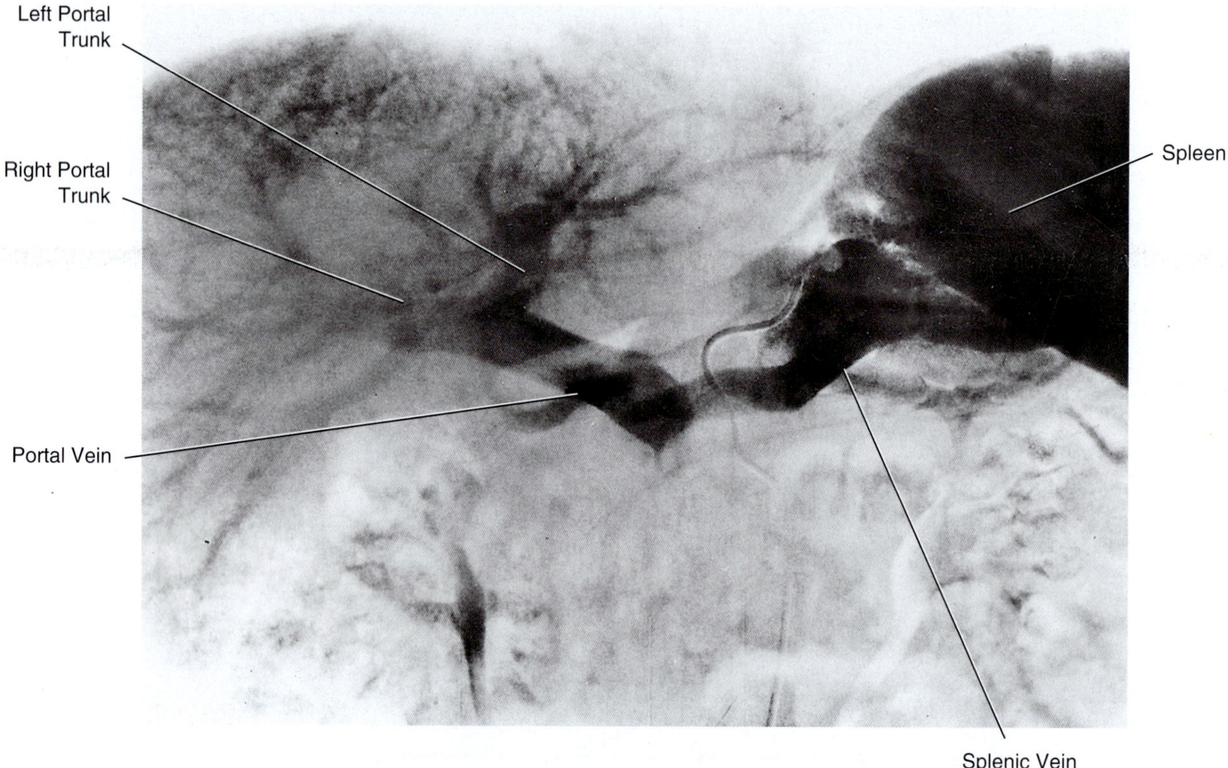

Figure 20.73. Arterial portography showing the opacification of the splenic vein and the portal vein as well as the intrahepatic radicles.

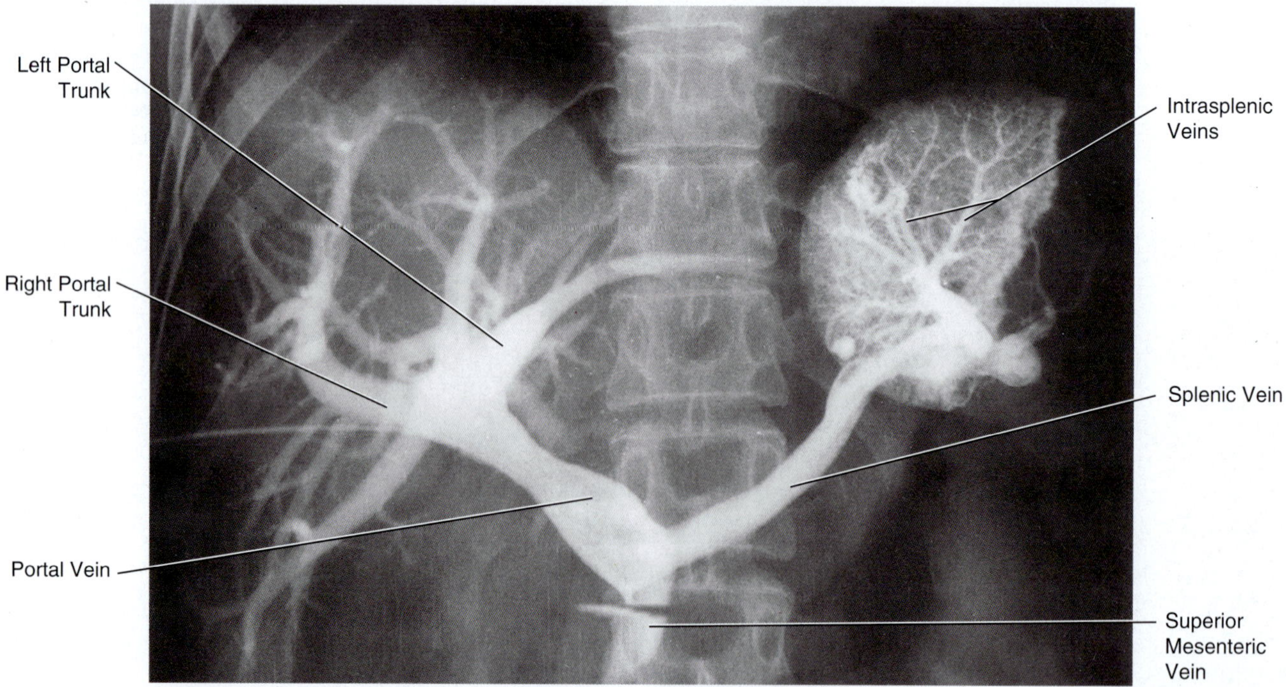

Figure 20.74. Transhepatic portography shows the opacification of the splenic vein, intrasplenic venous branches, and filling of the portal vein and intrahepatic radicles.

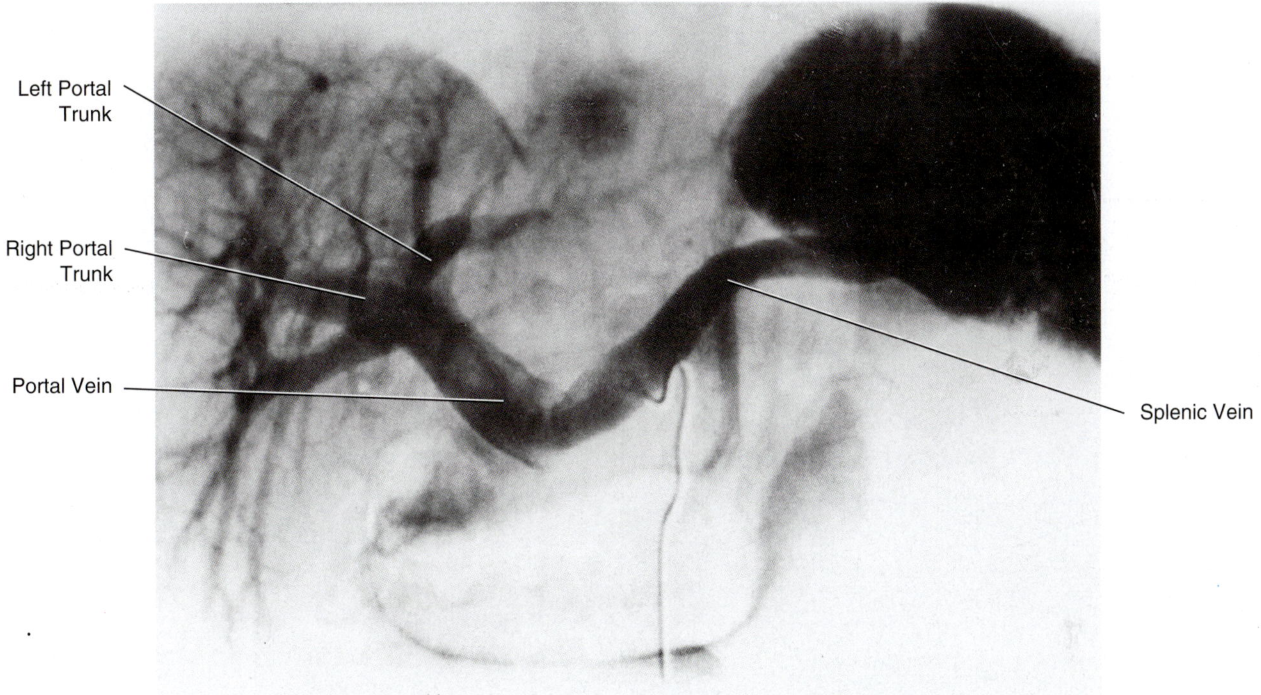

Figure 20.75. Arterial portography shows the splenic blush, the splenic vein opacification, and the portal vein filling.

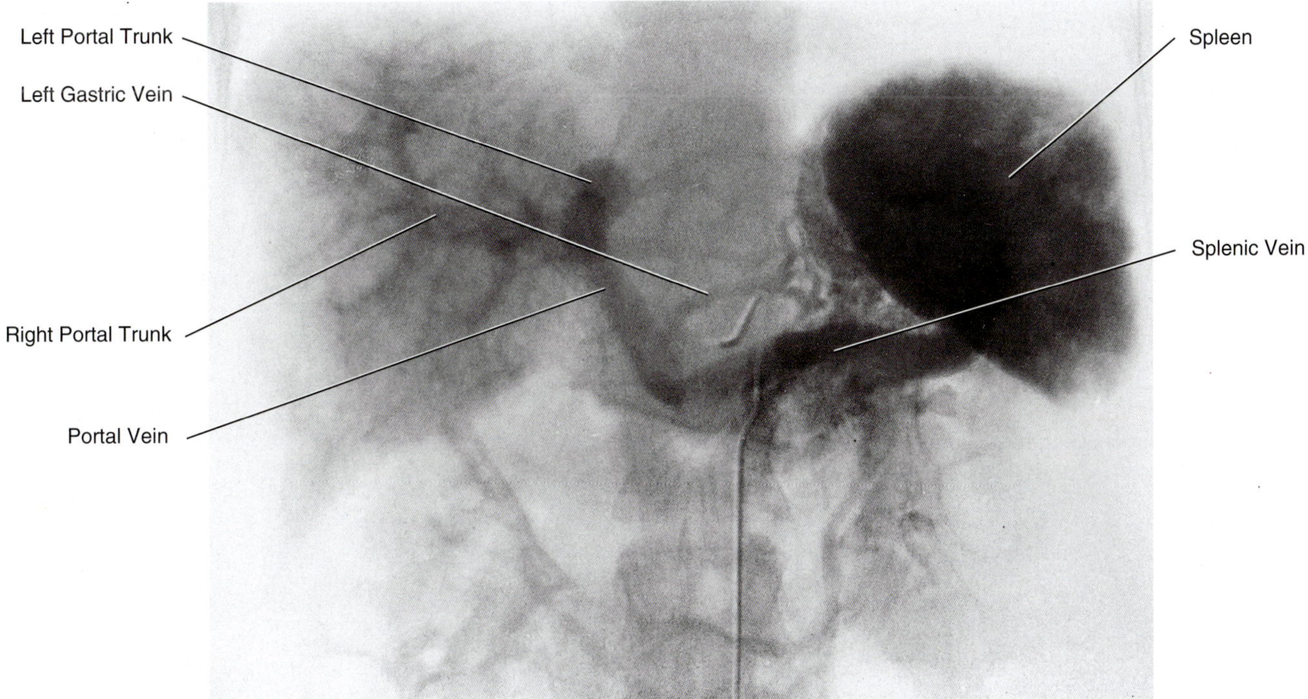

Figure 20.76. Arterial portography shows the splenic blush, the splenic vein opacification and, the portal vein filling.

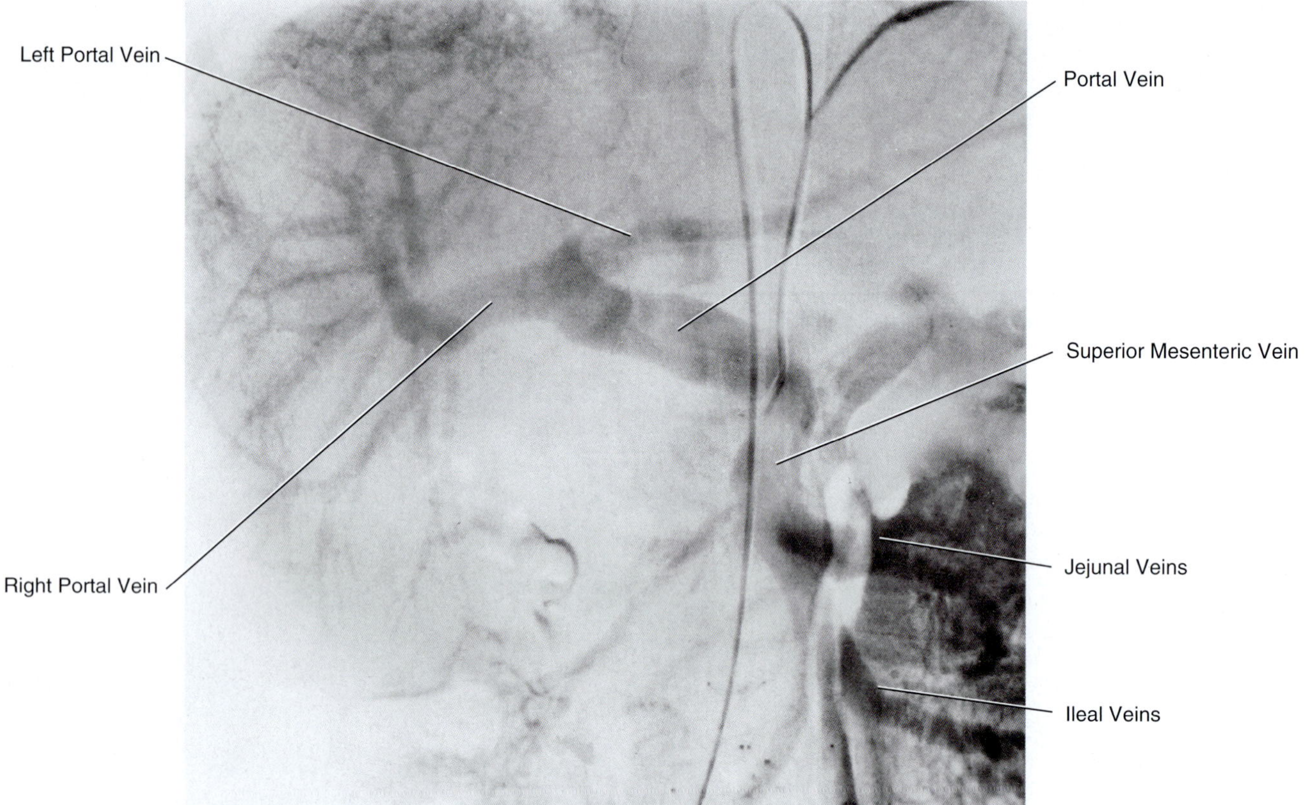

Figure 20.77. Arterial portography with injection into the superior mesenteric artery, showing the superior mesenteric artery, and the portal vein.

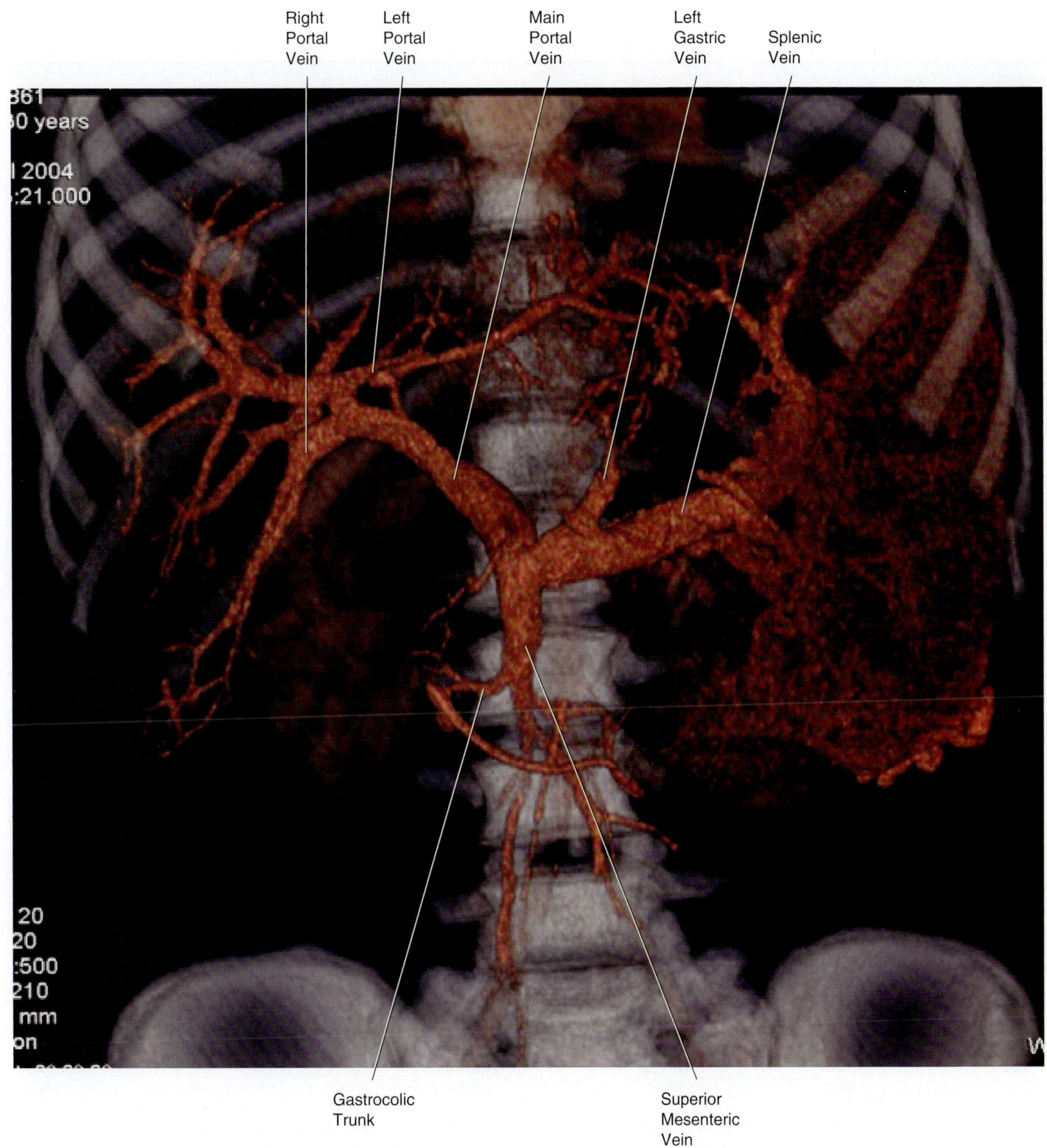

Figure 20.78. CT angiogram with 3D reconstruction of the portal system. Note an enlarged spleen and varices arising from the splenic vein. The splenic vein is patent, as is the superior mesenteric vein. The portal vein is of normal caliber, and the intrahepatic perfusion is unchanged.

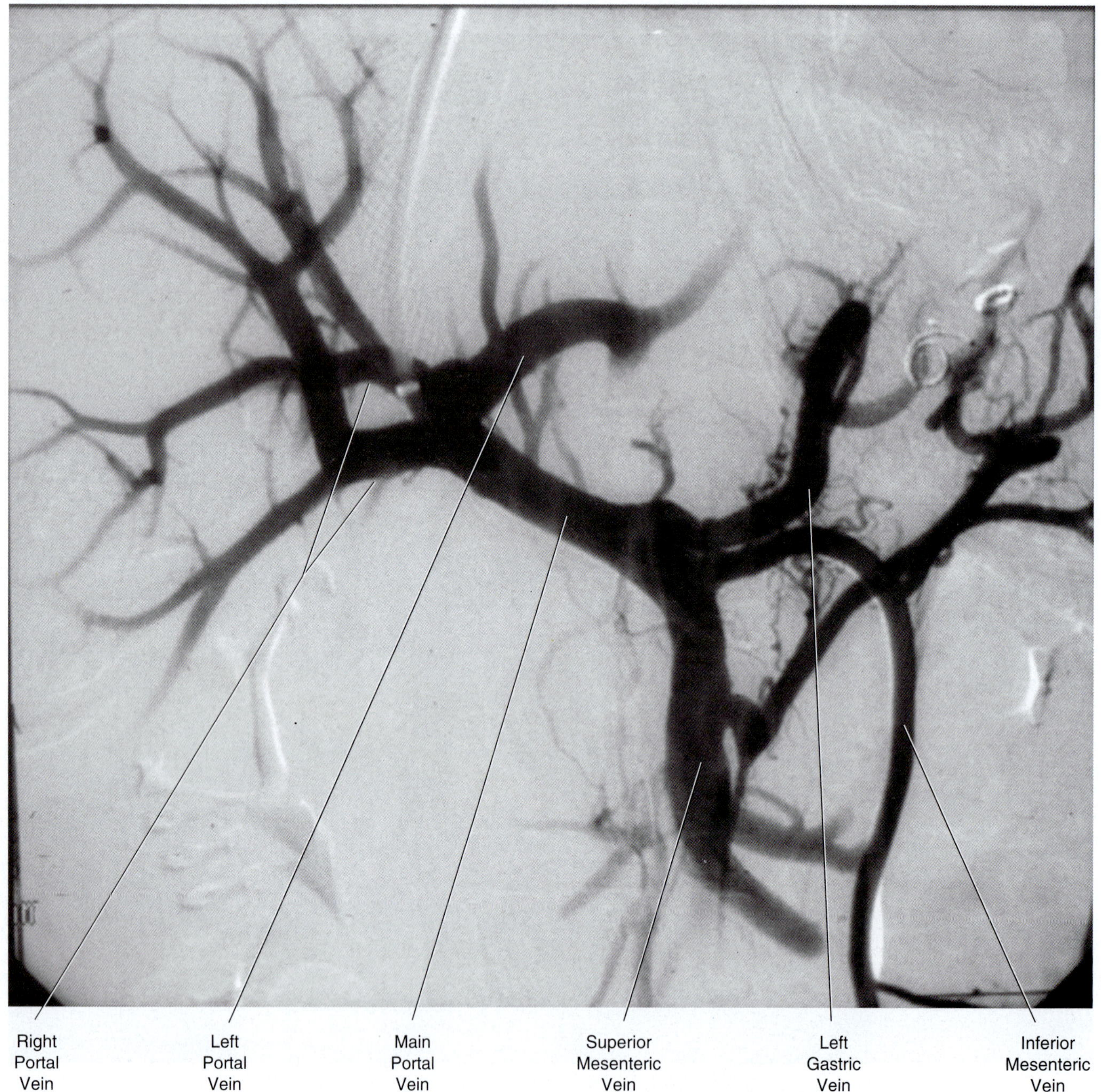

Figure 20.79. Digital subtraction portogram using a transjugular approach in a patient with an occluded TIPS (the stent is barely visible). The splenic vein is absent, but there is a large left gastric vein as well as a patent inferior mesenteric vein with inverted flow. The superior mesenteric vein is partially visible. TIPS, transjugular intrahepatic portosystemic shunt.

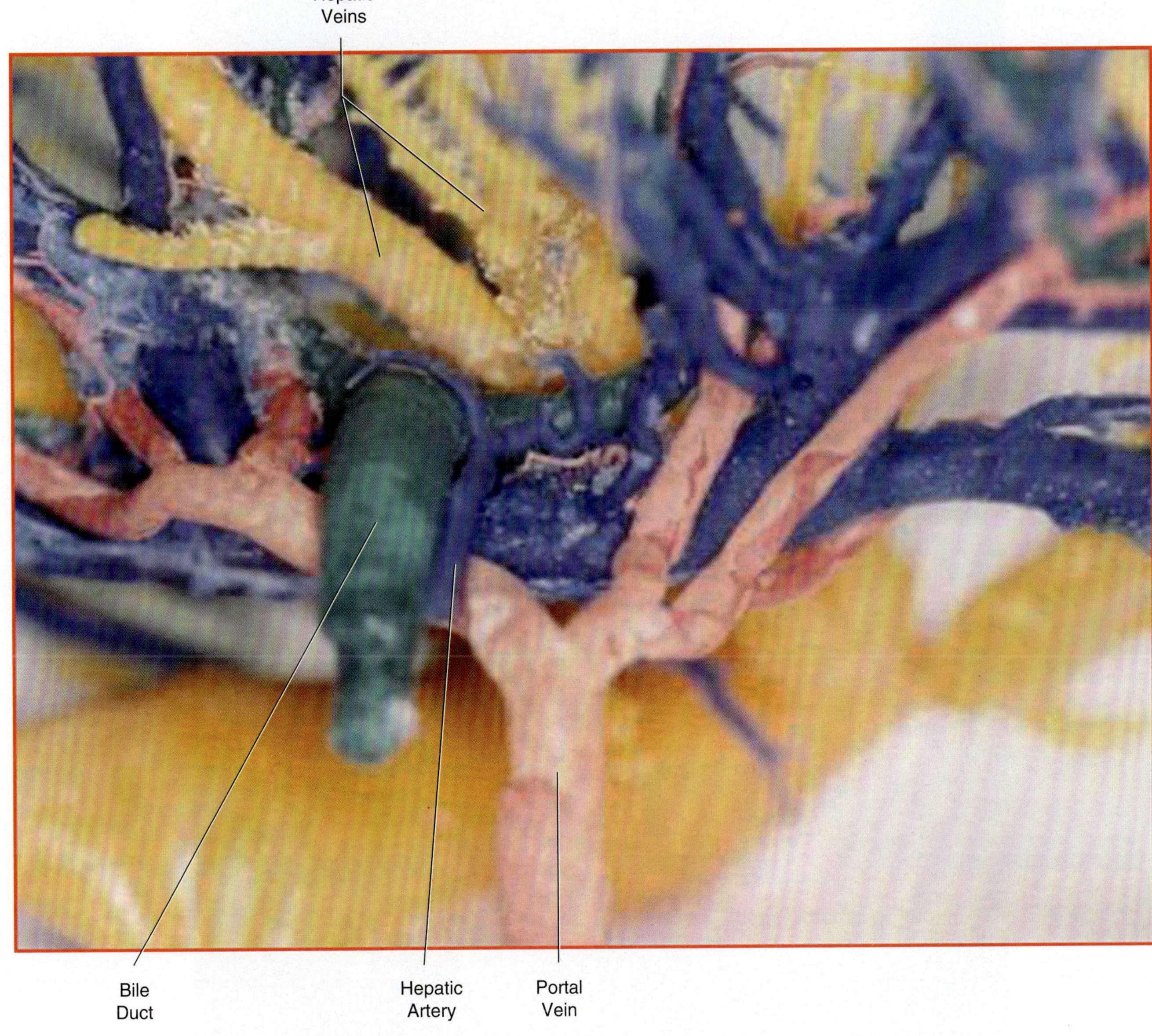

Figure 20.80. Relationship of the three elements in the porta hepatis. The segment of the portal vein located within the lesser omentum and at the porta hepatis is located behind the bile duct and the hepatic artery. The bile duct is parallel to the portal vein and lateral (green), while the hepatic artery is medial (blue). The portal vein is relatively small in this specimen (pink) and the hepatic veins are also visible (yellow).

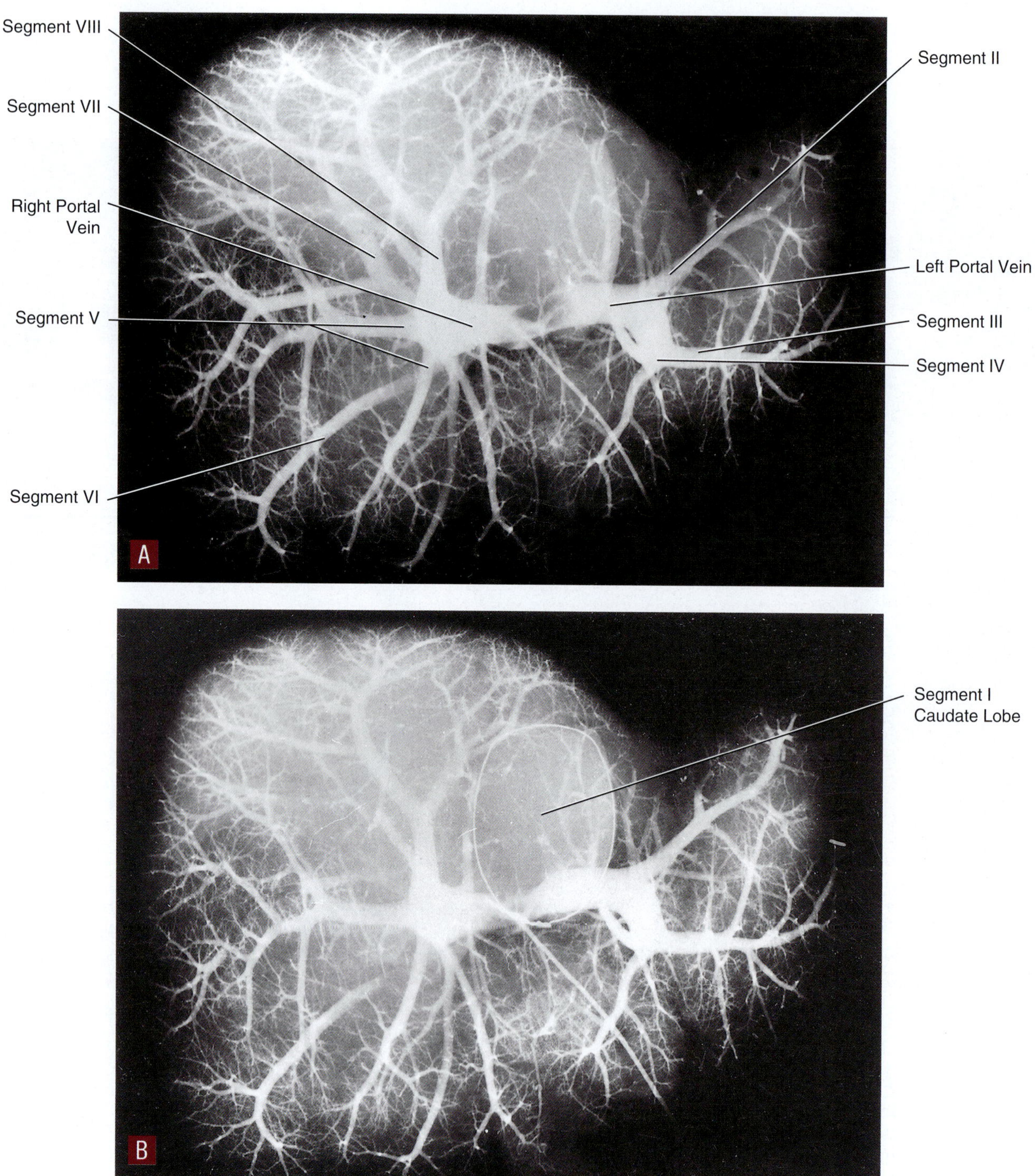

Figure 20.81. A, Specimen of the liver injected into the portal vein. Note the segmental distribution of the portal vein. B, Note the radiopaque mark around the caudate lobe.

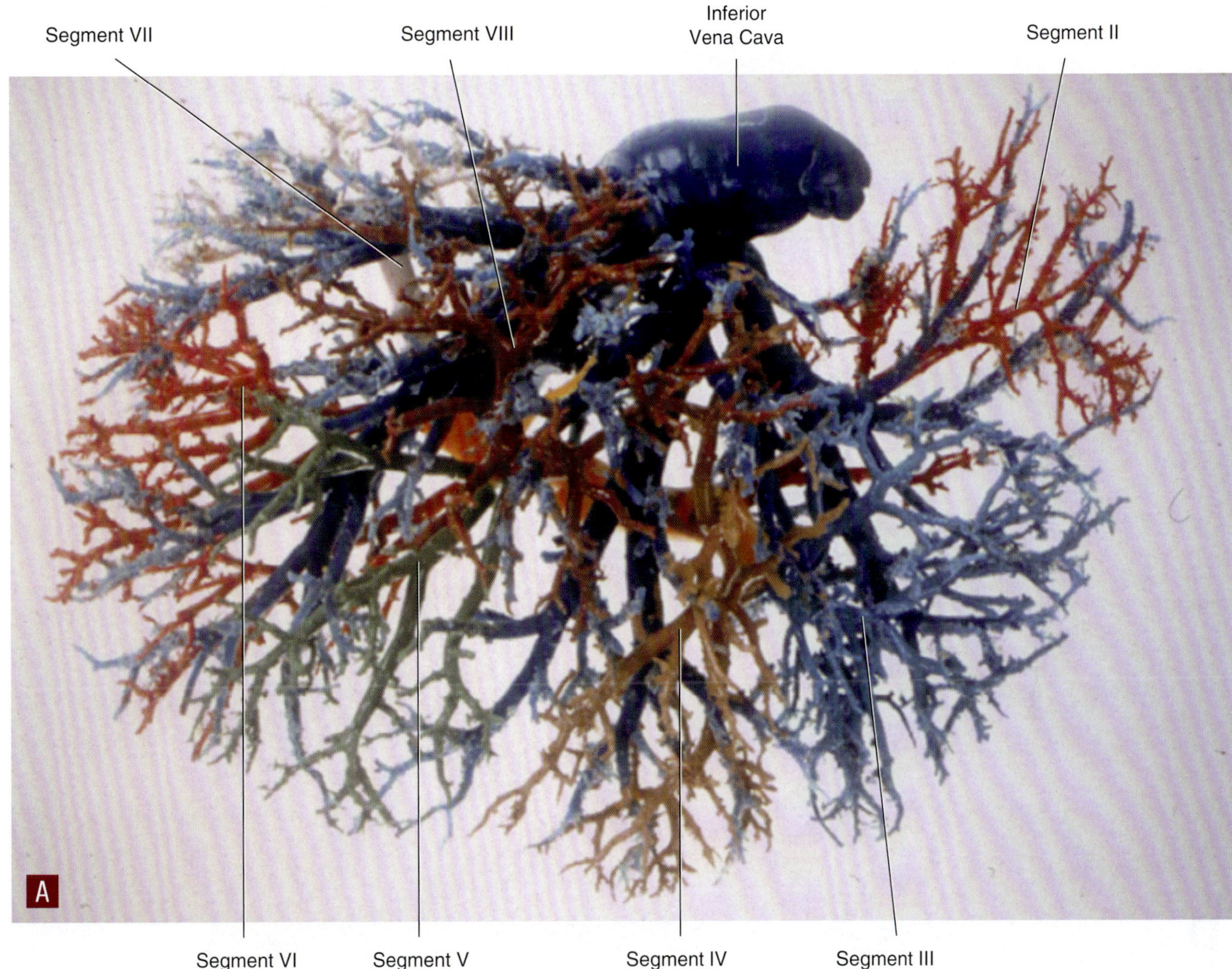

Figure 20.82. Injection cast of a liver specimen with filling of the portal vein and the inferior vena cava and hepatic veins (navy blue). Segment I (caudate lobe) is in light blue. Segment II is in red. Segment III is in dark blue. The segment IV or medial portion of the left lobe is in light brown. Segment V is depicted in green. Segment VI is in red. Segment VII is in white. Segment VIII is in dark brown. A, Anterior view of the injection cast of the portal circulation showing the liver segments in different colors. B, Posterior view of the injection cast of the portal circulation showing the liver segments in different colors.

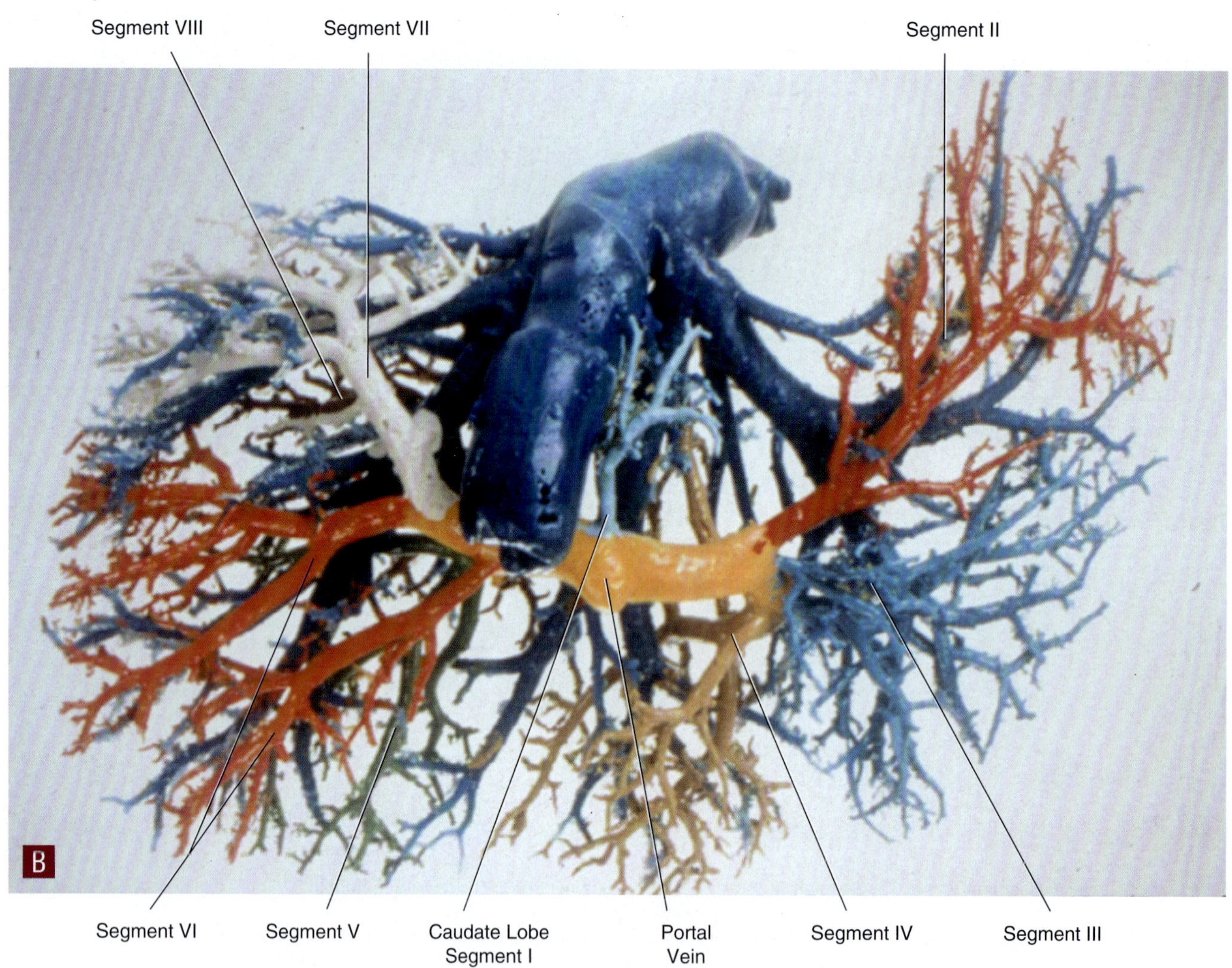

Figure 20.82. *Continued*

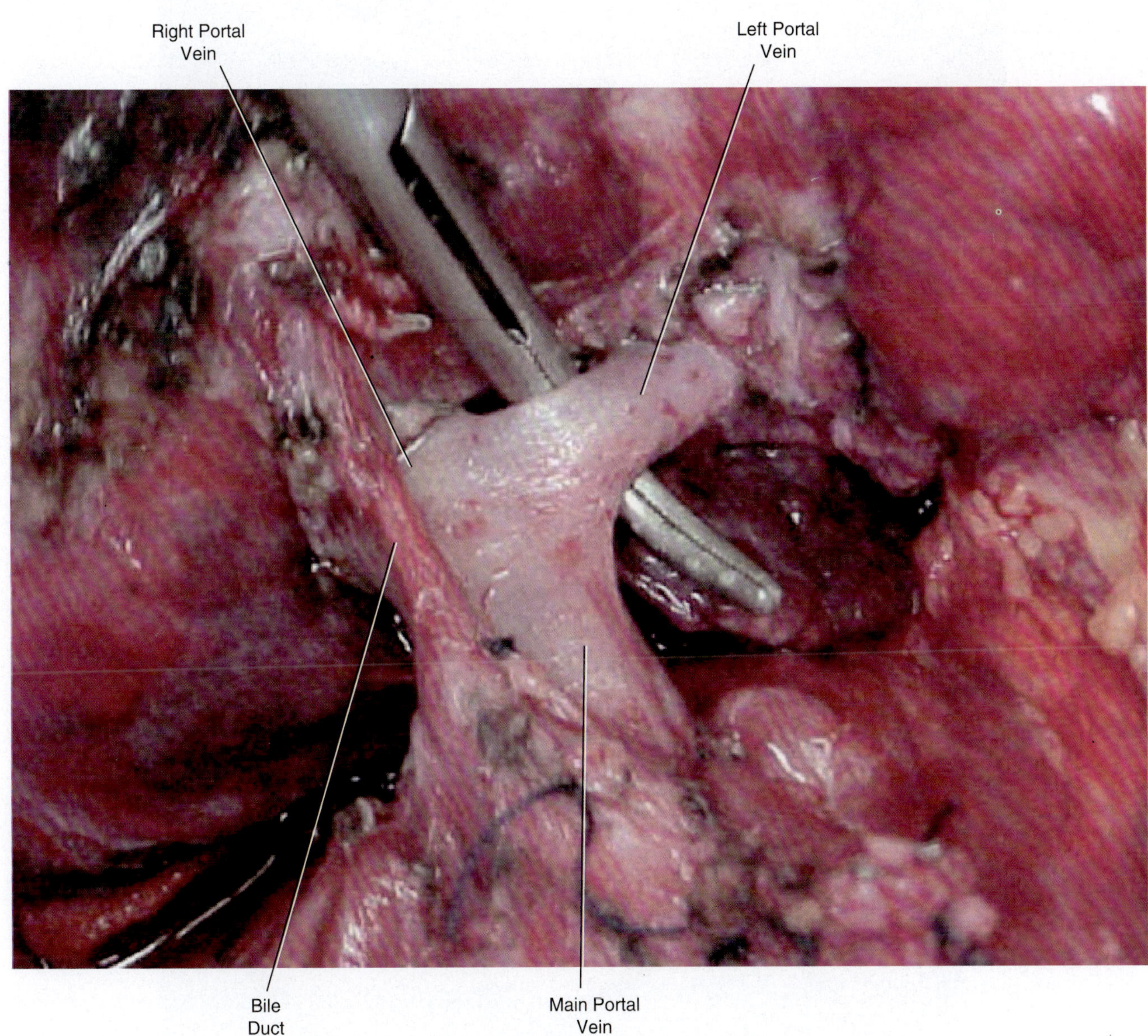

Figure 20.83. Portal vein bifurcation. The open surgery preparation shows the extrahepatic bifurcation of the portal vein (the forceps is located across the bifurcation and behind the left portal vein. Note the bile duct anterior and lateral (on the right of the patient) to the portal vein. The hepatic artery has been ligated and is not shown.

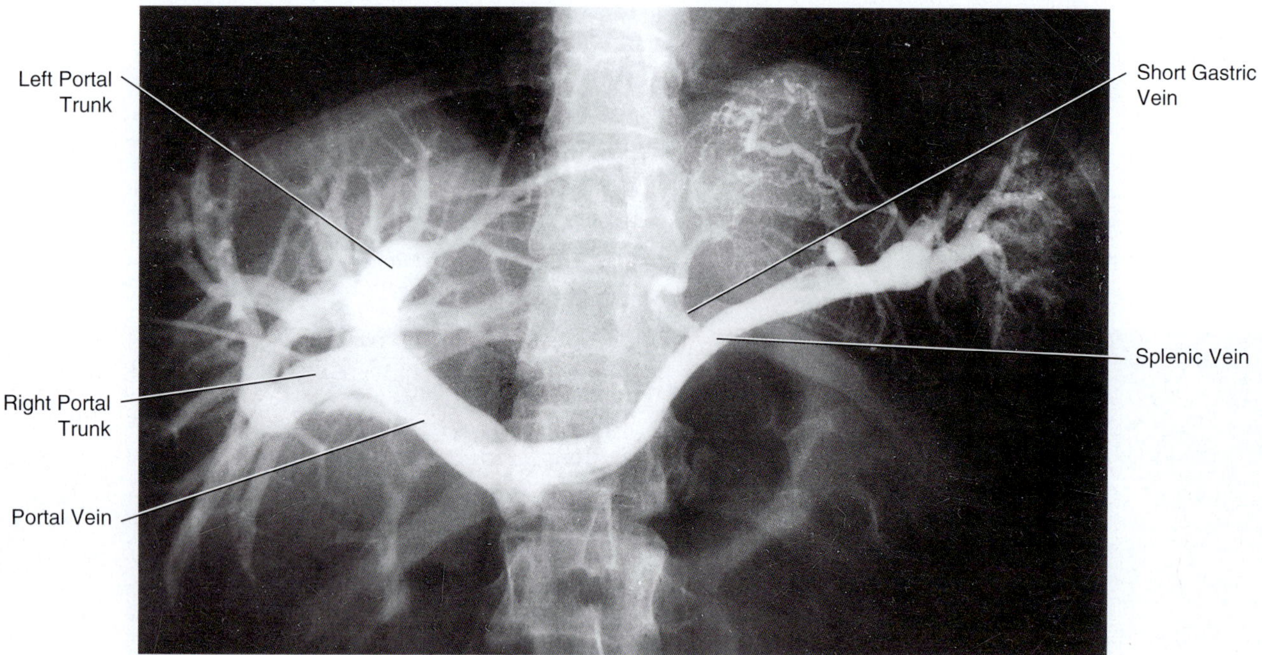

Figure 20.84. Transhepatic portography shows the splenic vein and portal vein densely opacified.

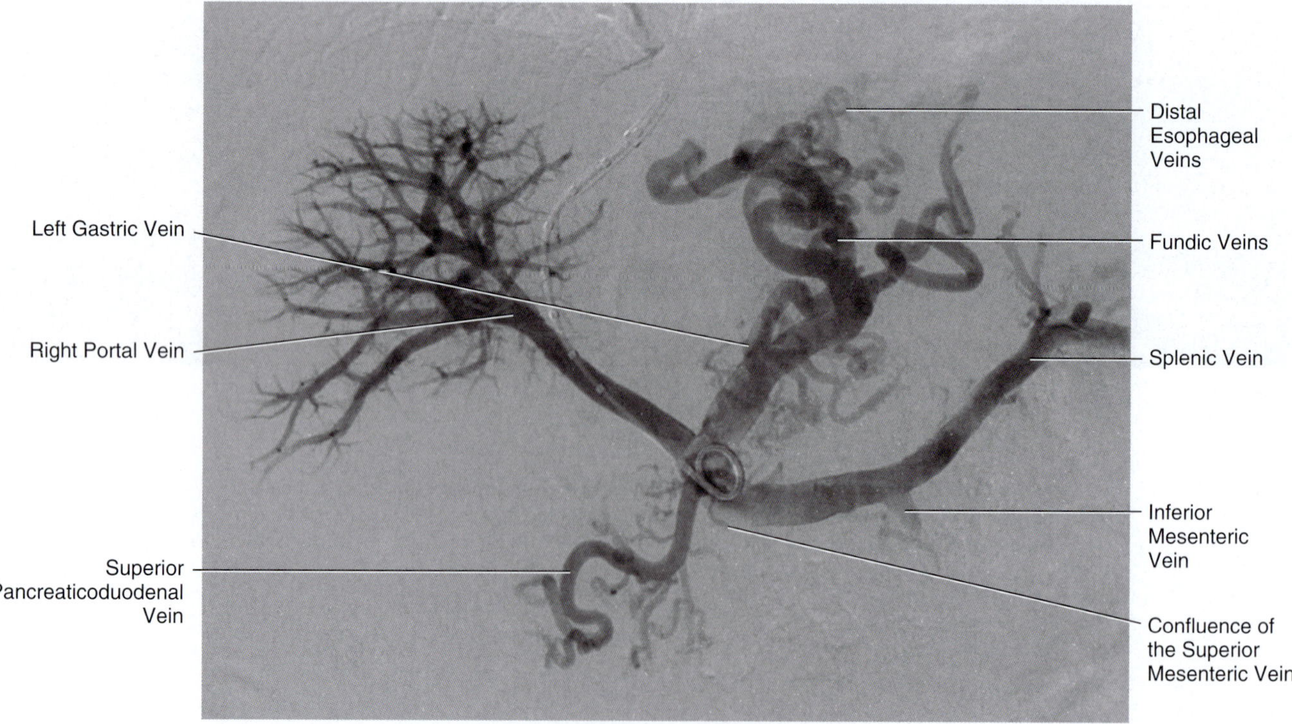

Figure 20.85. Selective injection angiography, by transjugular intrahepatic approach, into the main portal vein showing an enlarged left gastric vein, esophageal varices, and the superior pancreaticoduodenal vein.

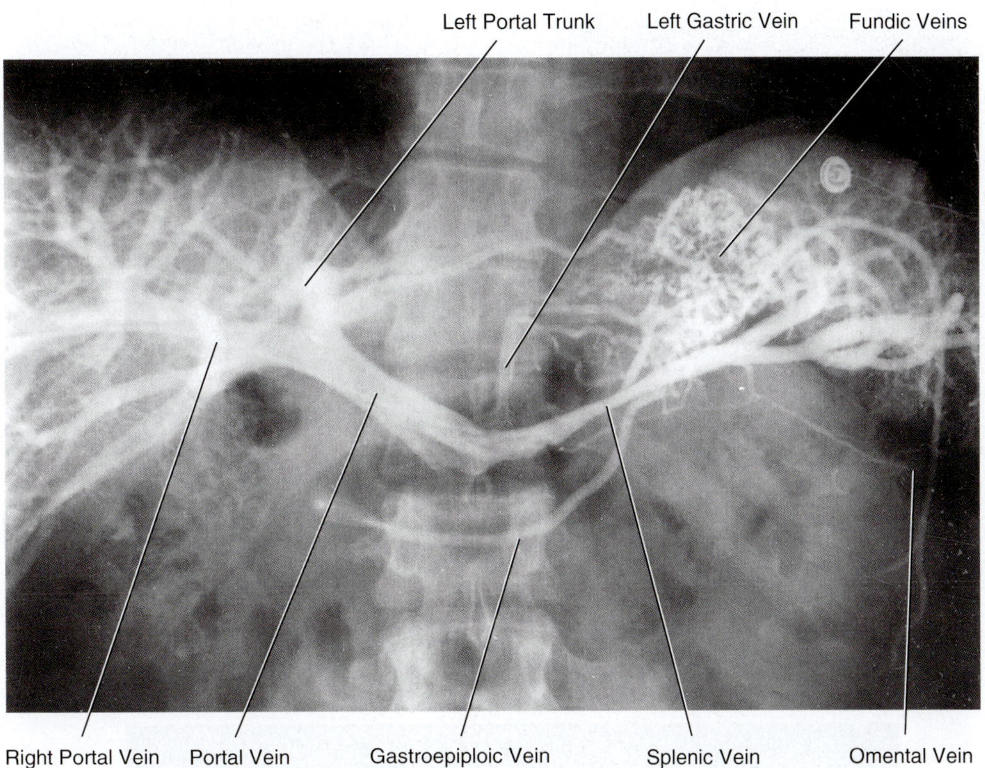

Figure 20.86. Transhepatic portography shows the retrograde filling of the left gastric vein, filling of the short gastric veins, and filling of the left gastroepiploic vein.

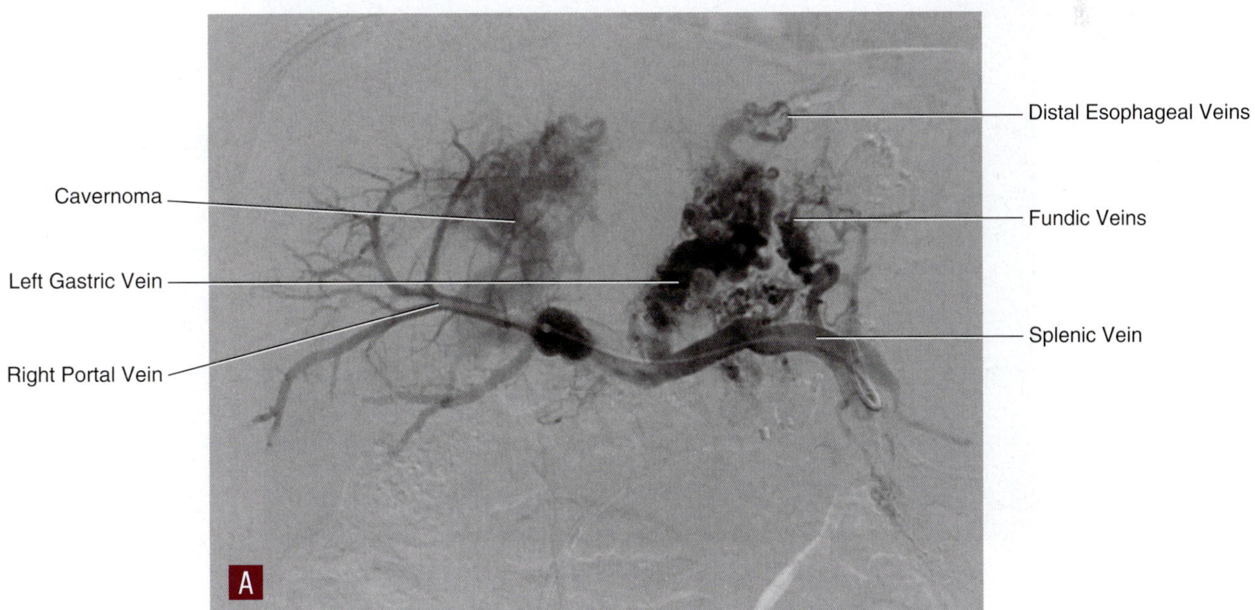

Figure 20.87. **A**, Transhepatic portogram showing occlusion of the main portal vein. Dilated veins arising from the porta hepatis are consistent with cavernous transformation, sometimes termed a "cavernoma." **B**, Later phase during the same injection showing enhancement of esophageal veins, gastric veins, and a gastrorenal shunt. **C**, Axial CT maximum intensity projection during the portal venous phase showing cavernous transformation of the portal vein in the same patient.

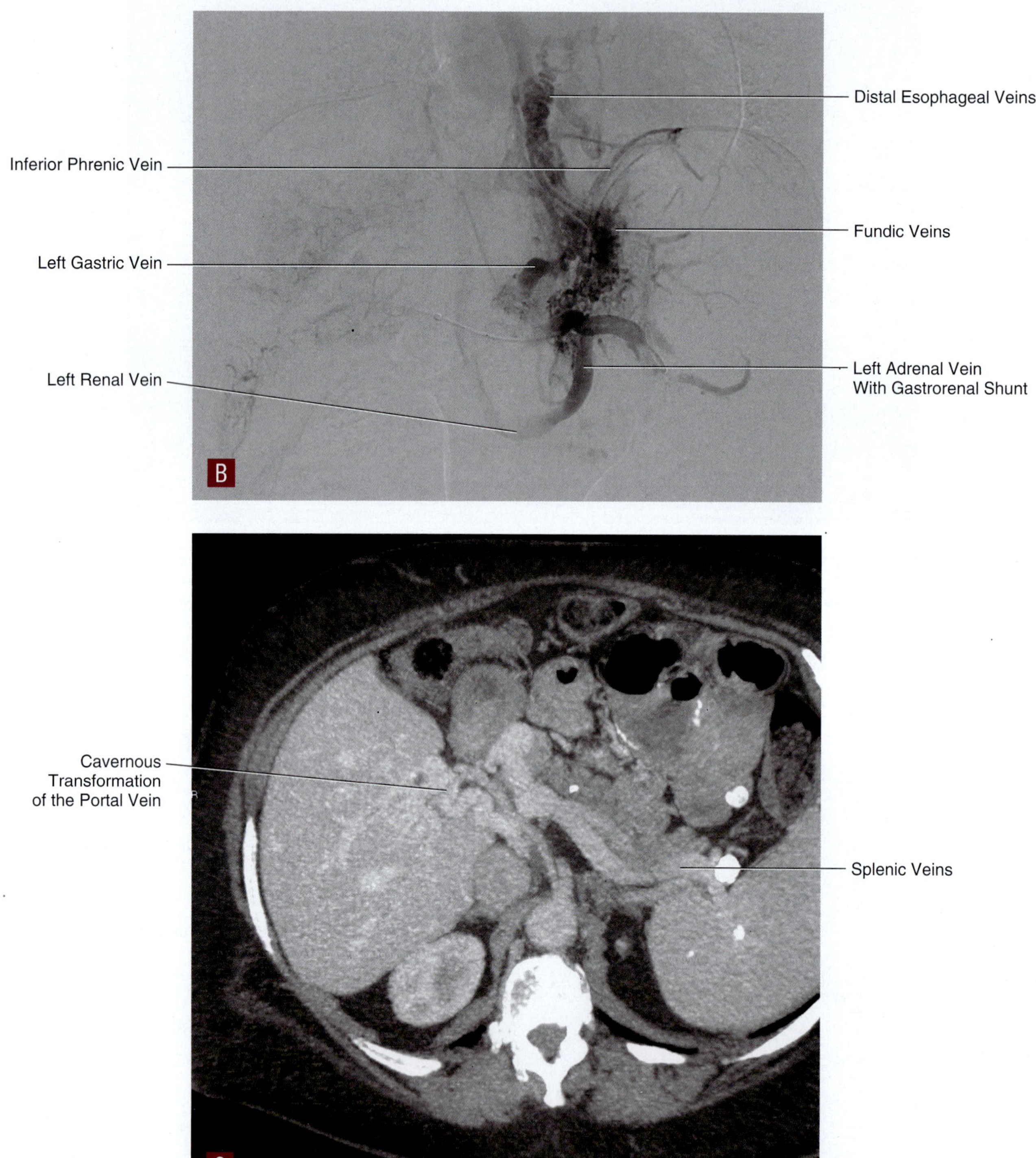

Figure 20.87. *Continued*

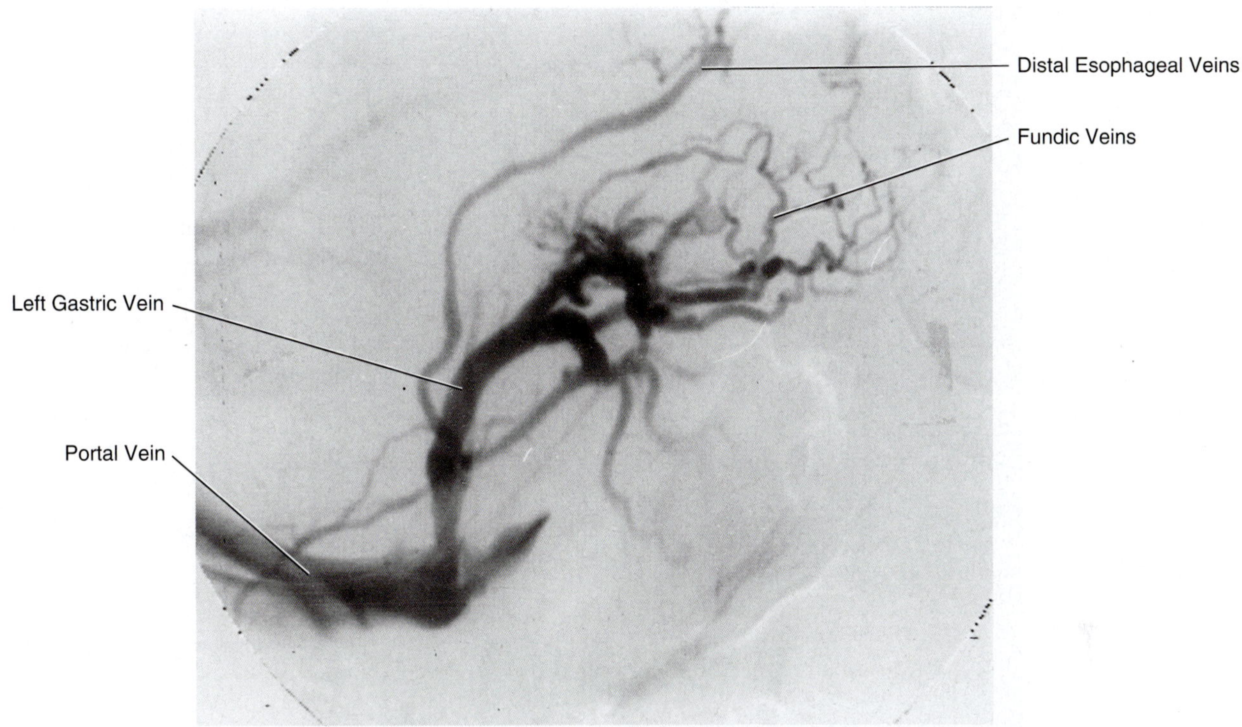

Figure 20.88. Selective injection into the left gastric vein showing filling of the fundic gastric veins and distal esophageal veins.

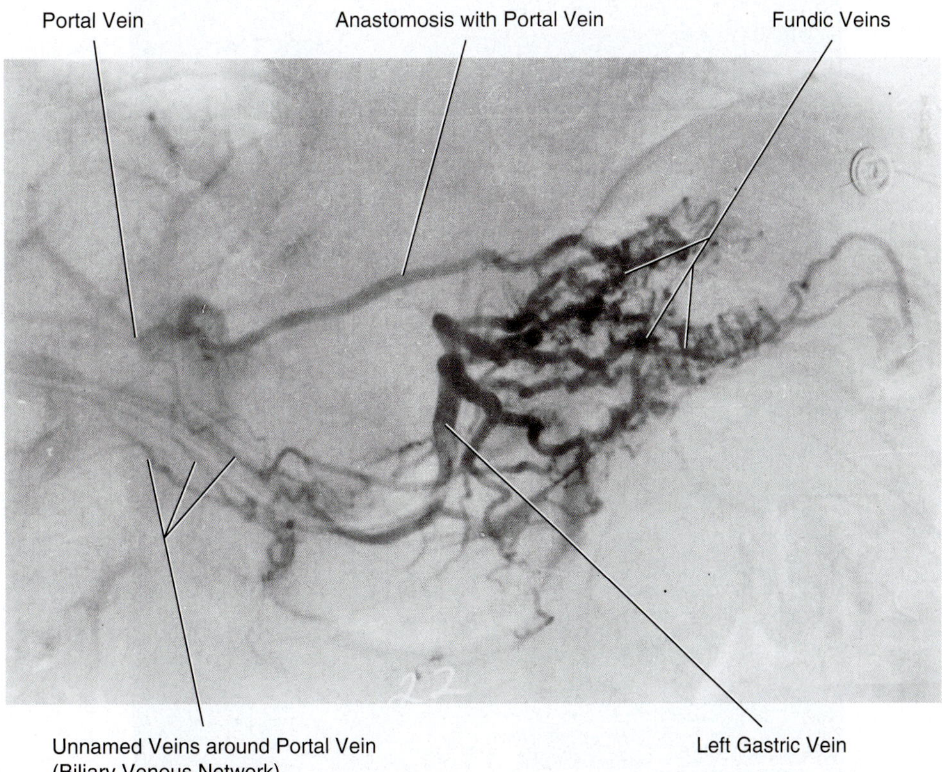

Figure 20.89. Selective injection into the left gastric vein showing filling of the fundic gastric veins and multiple collaterals and anastomoses in the gastric wall. Note the unnamed veins around the portal vein. There is also an anastomosis between the left gastric vein and the intrahepatic portal vein.

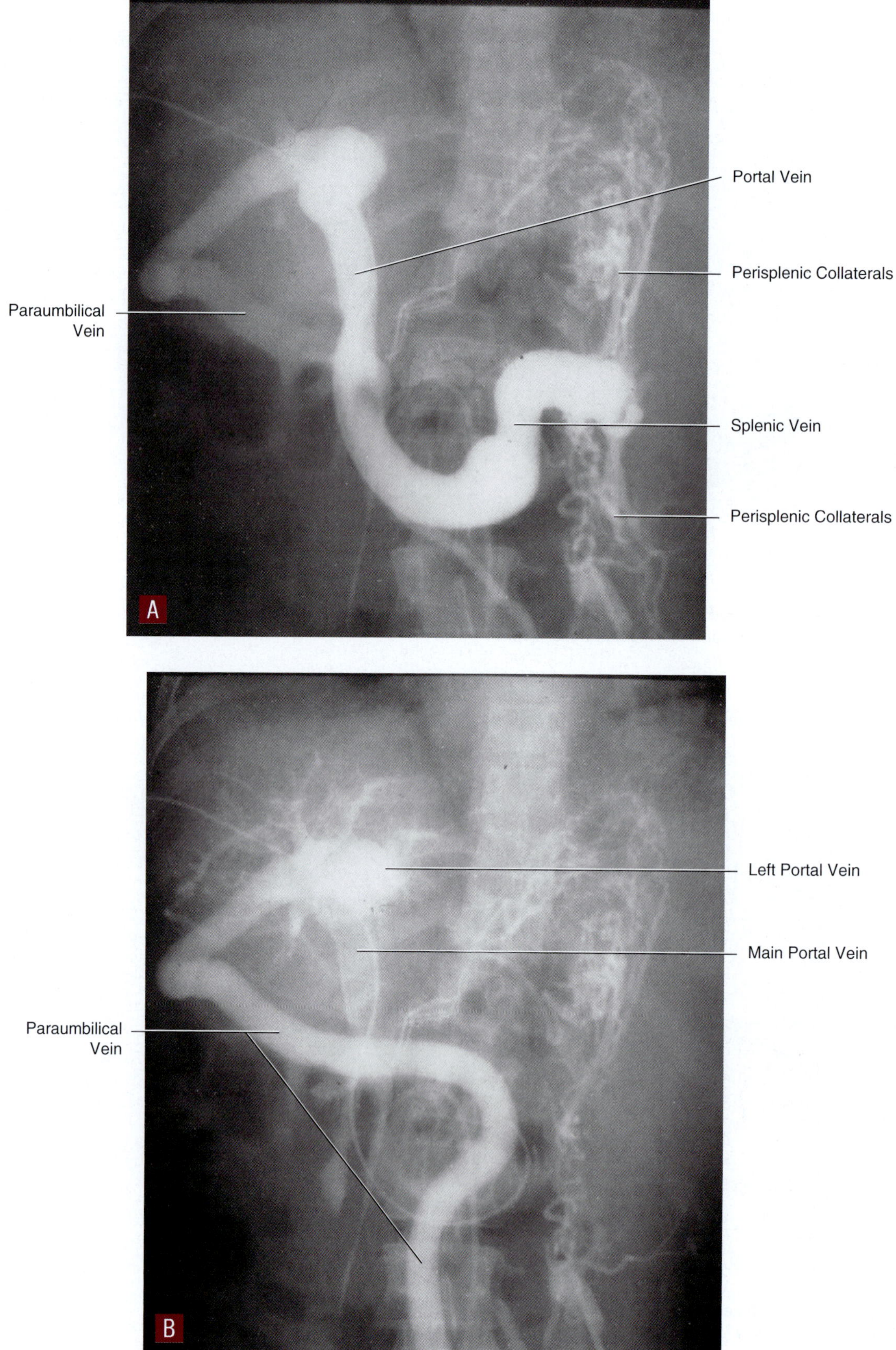

Figure 20.90. A and B. **Paraumbilical vein.** Transhepatic portogram showing a large splenic vein, a relatively reduced portal vein, and the whole system draining directly into a paraumbilical vein. The paraumbilical vein originates from the left hepatic vein and follows the course of the umbilical ligament, connecting to the anterior abdominal wall in an anterior and medial direction. From the abdominal wall, it extends caudally and reaches the umbilical region, where the vein may become superficial causing the "caput medusae." In normal livers, it is very unusual to identify the paraumbilical vein.

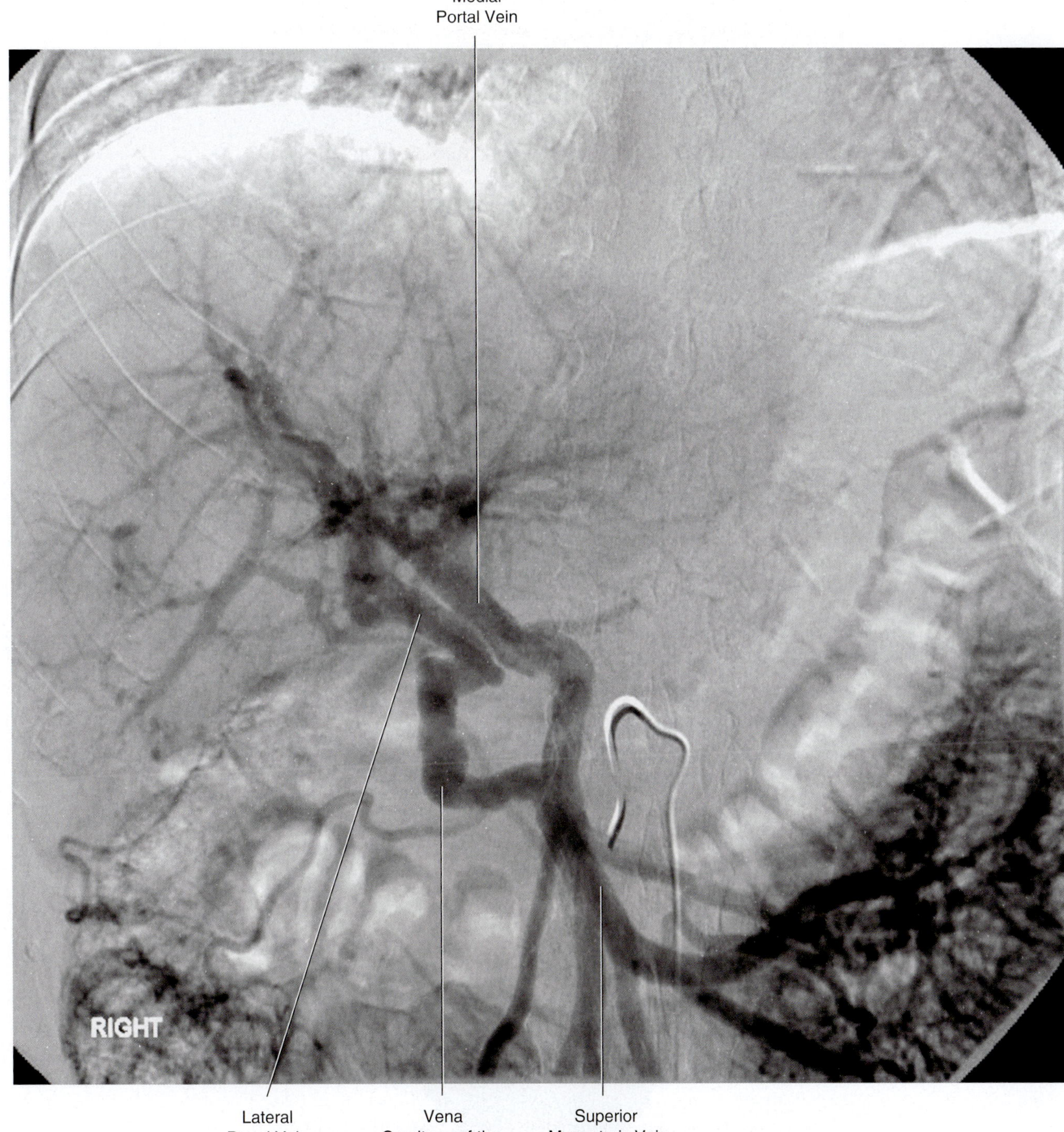

Figure 20.91. Variation of the portal vein. The superior mesenteric angiogram performed with vasodilator enhancement, shows a patent superior mesenteric vein draining into an apparent duplicated portal vein. There are two independent channels going into the liver. The main mesenteric vein drains into what appears to be the main portal vein (medial) and the lateral portal vein seems to receive flow from a collateral from the gastrocolic trunk and possibly into a vena comitans of the portal vein reaching a right-side portal branch. The possibility of a congenital duplication of the portal vein is also possible in this case, since there was no history of portal thrombosis or portal hypertension.

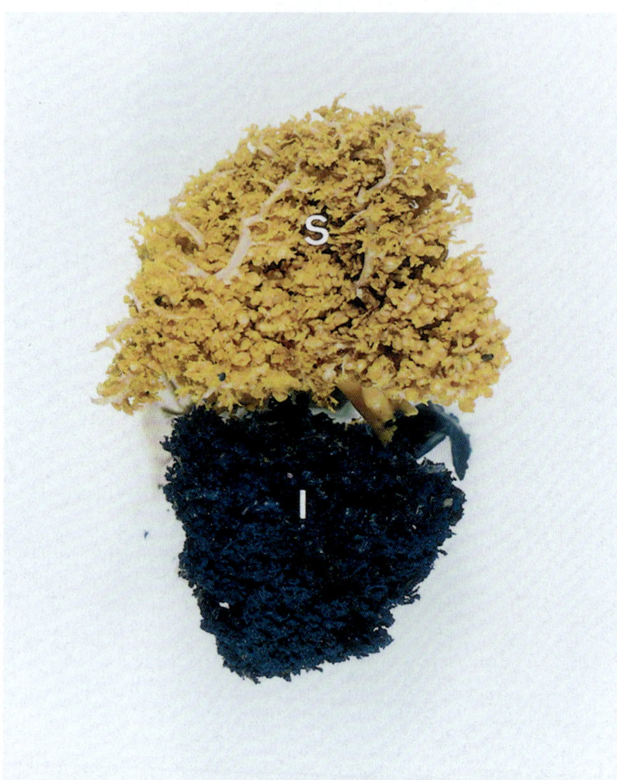

Figure 20.92. Vinilite resin corrosion endocast of the intrasplenic venous vasculature. View of the parietal surface shows two venous segments injected with different colors. S, superior venous segment and I, inferior venous segment.

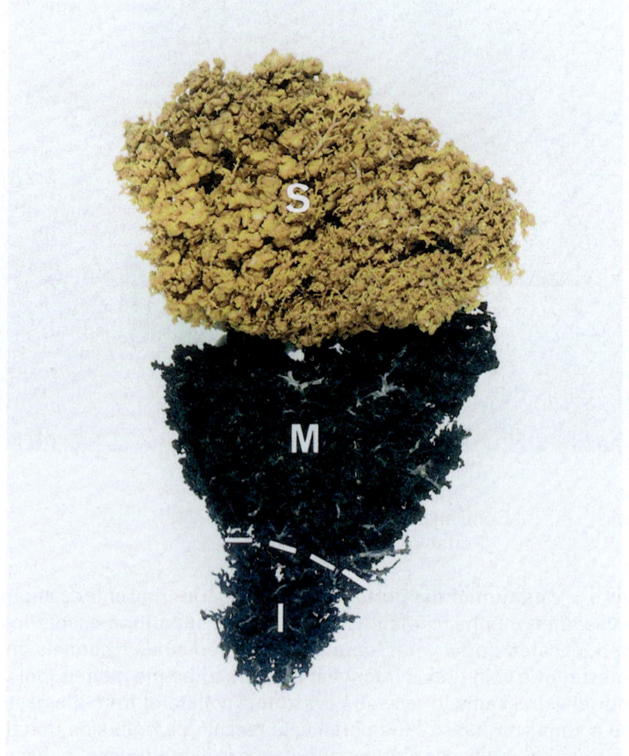

Figure 20.93. Vinilite resin corrosion endocast of the intrasplenic venous vasculature. View of the parietal surface shows three venous segments injected with different colors. S, superior venous segment; M, middle venous segment; and I, inferior venous segment.

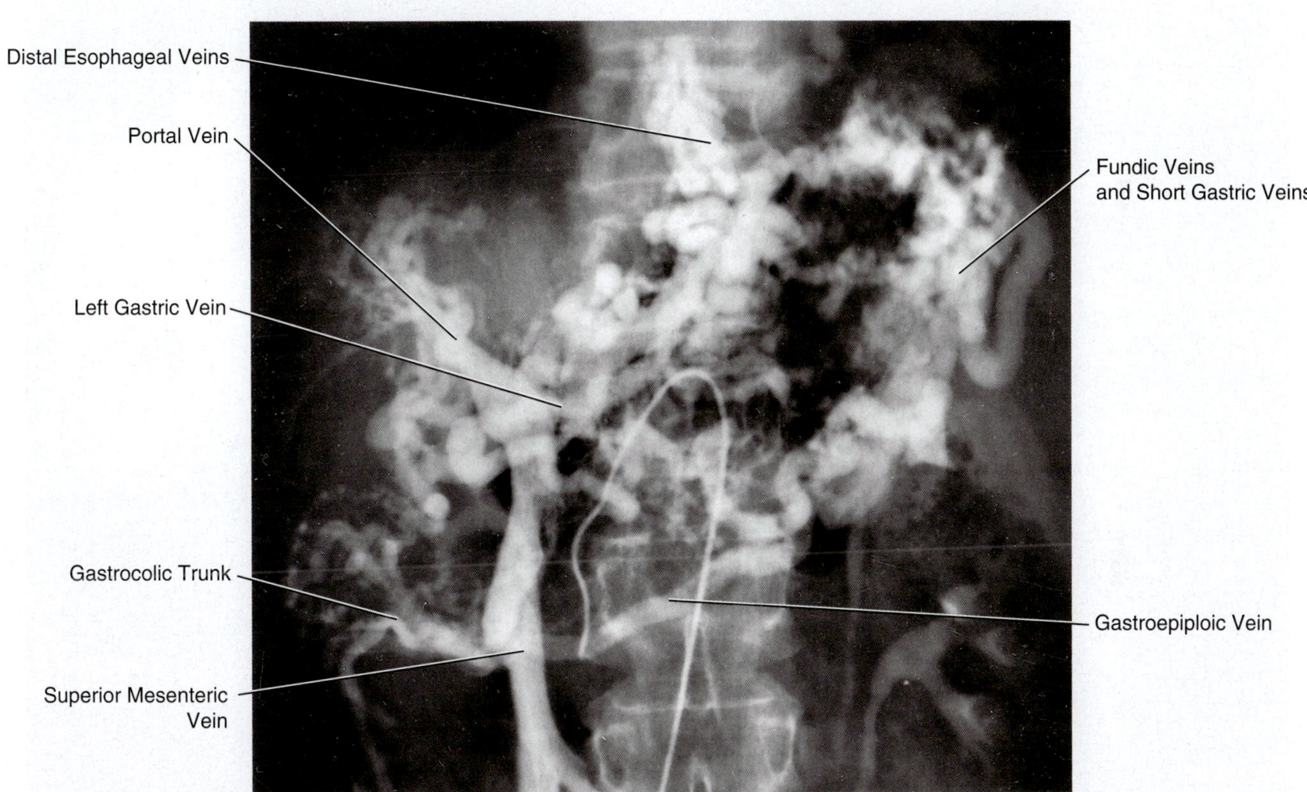

Figure 20.94. Late phase of a superior mesenteric arteriogram showing the opacification of the superior mesenteric vein, portal vein and short gastric veins, and left and right gastroepiploic veins.

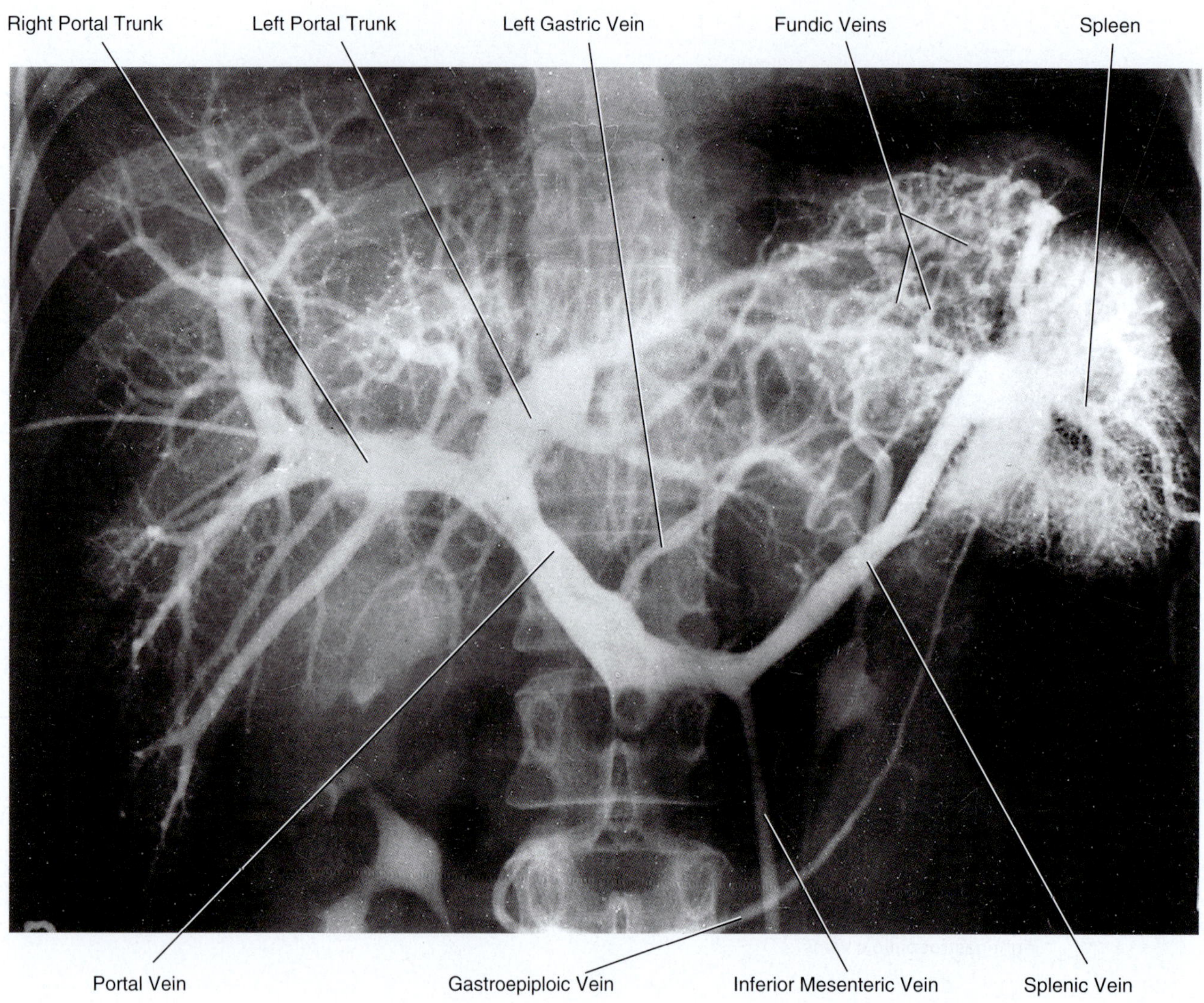

Figure 20.95. Direct transhepatic portography showing the splenic vein, left gastric vein and short gastric veins, and the fundic veins in the stomach. The portal vein is well filled.

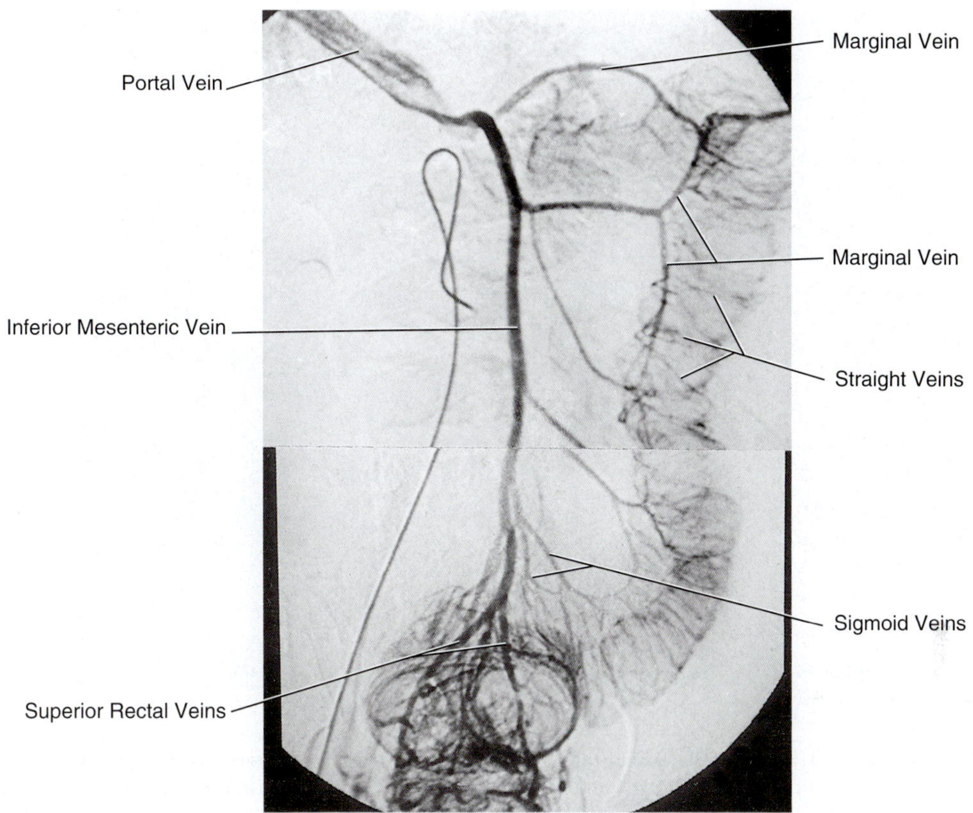

Figure 20.96. Late phase of inferior mesenteric angiogram showing the inferior mesenteric vein and tributaries. Note portal vein filling.

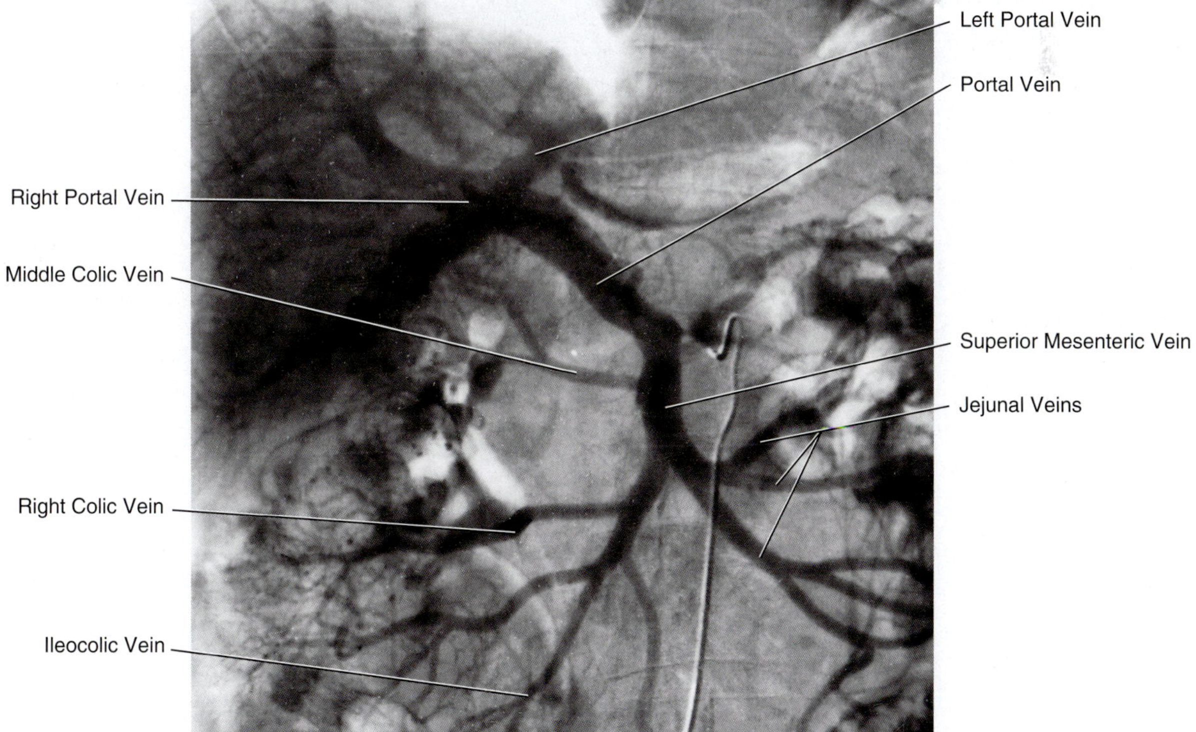

Figure 20.97. Arterial portography obtained through superior mesenteric artery injection. Excellent filling of the superior mesenteric vein and tributaries. The portal vein is also opacified.

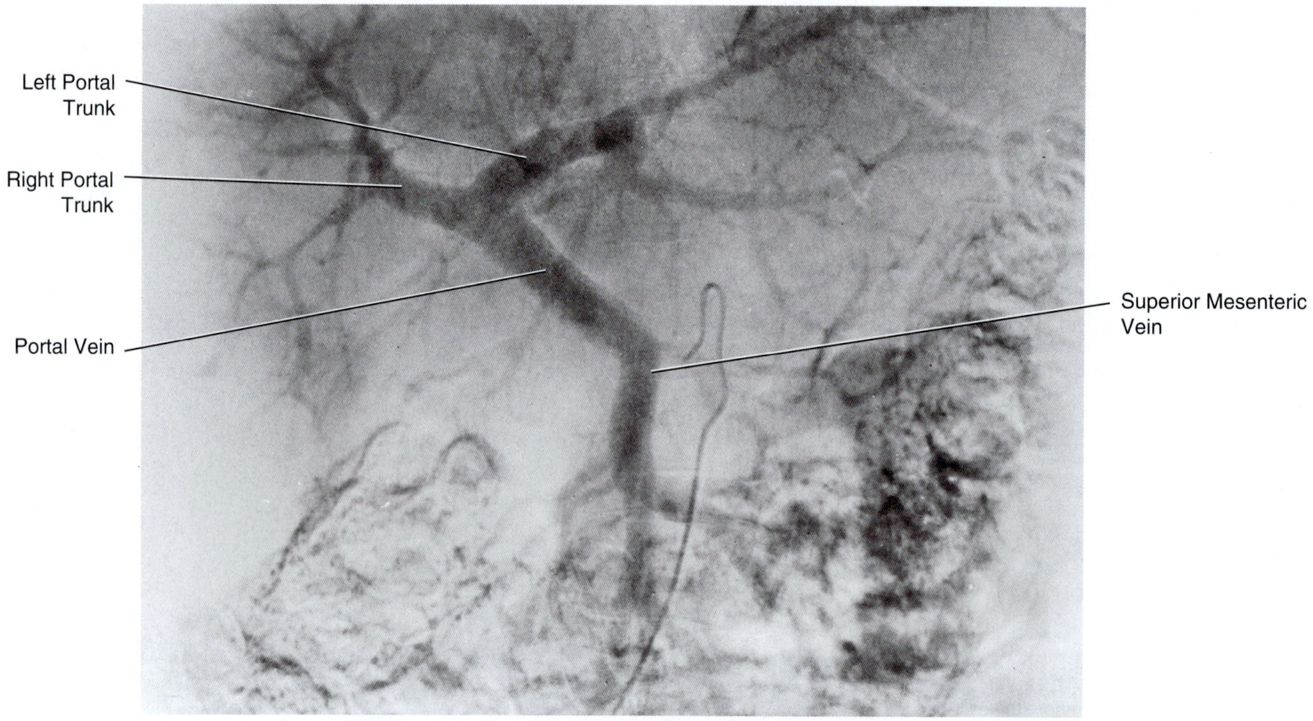

Figure 20.98. Arterial portography obtained by superior mesenteric artery injection. Filling of the superior mesenteric vein and tributaries. The portal vein is also opacified.

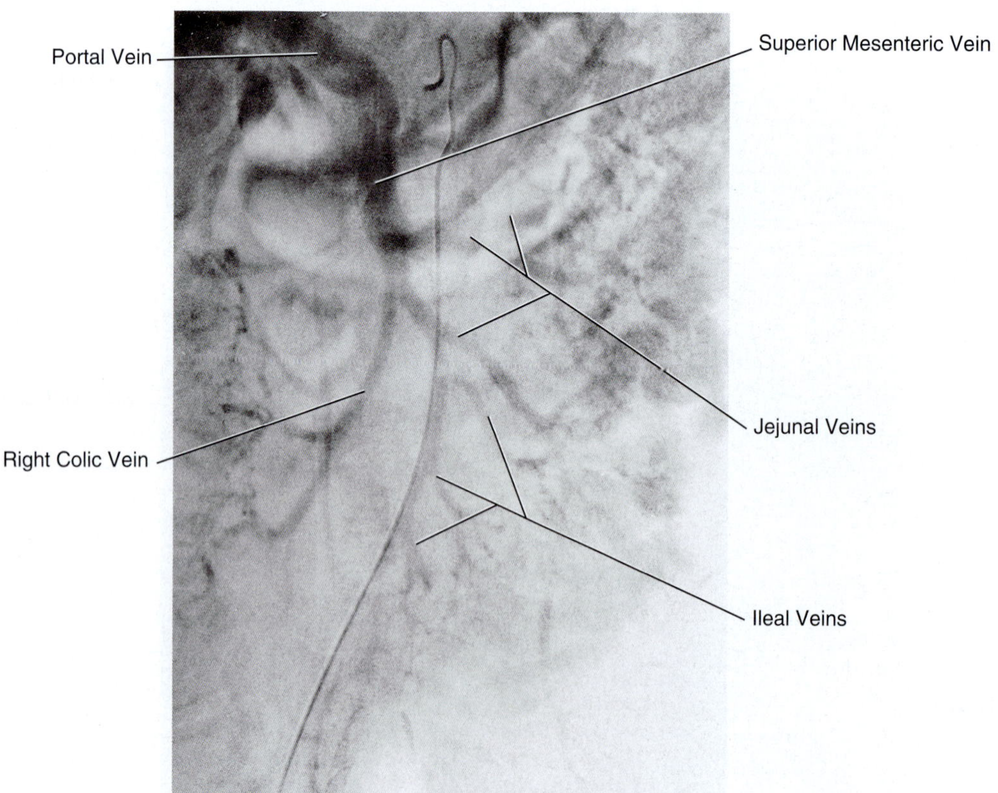

Figure 20.99. Arterial portography showing the superior mesenteric vein.

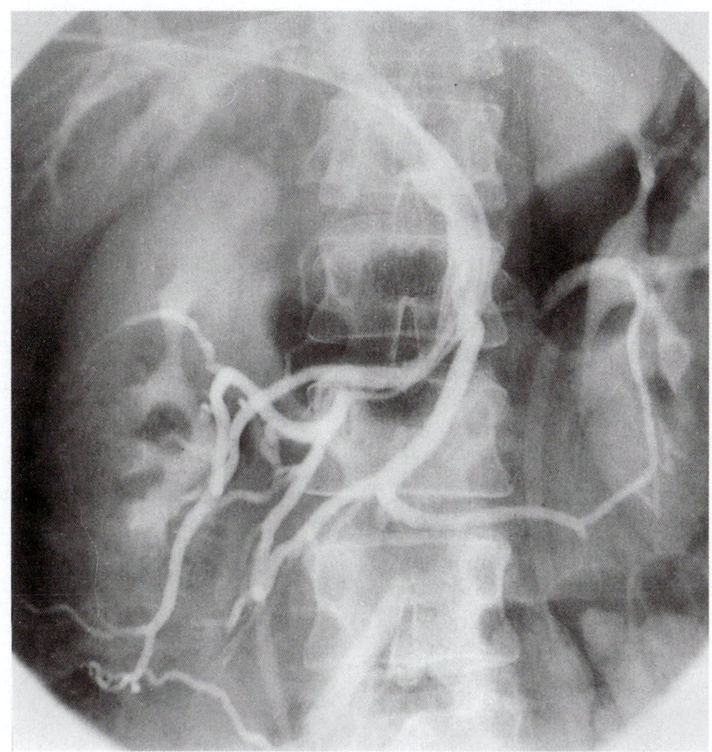

Figure 20.100. Selective injection at the right colic vein. Some of the ileal veins are also opacified.

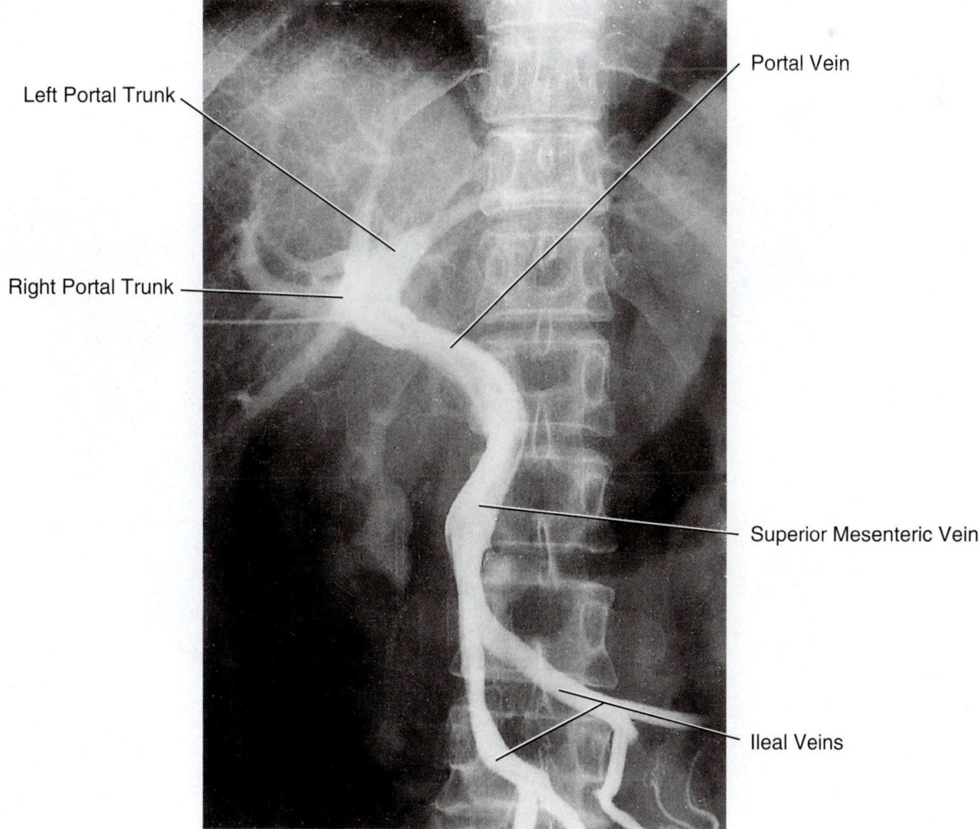

Figure 20.101. **Selective injection at ileal veins.**

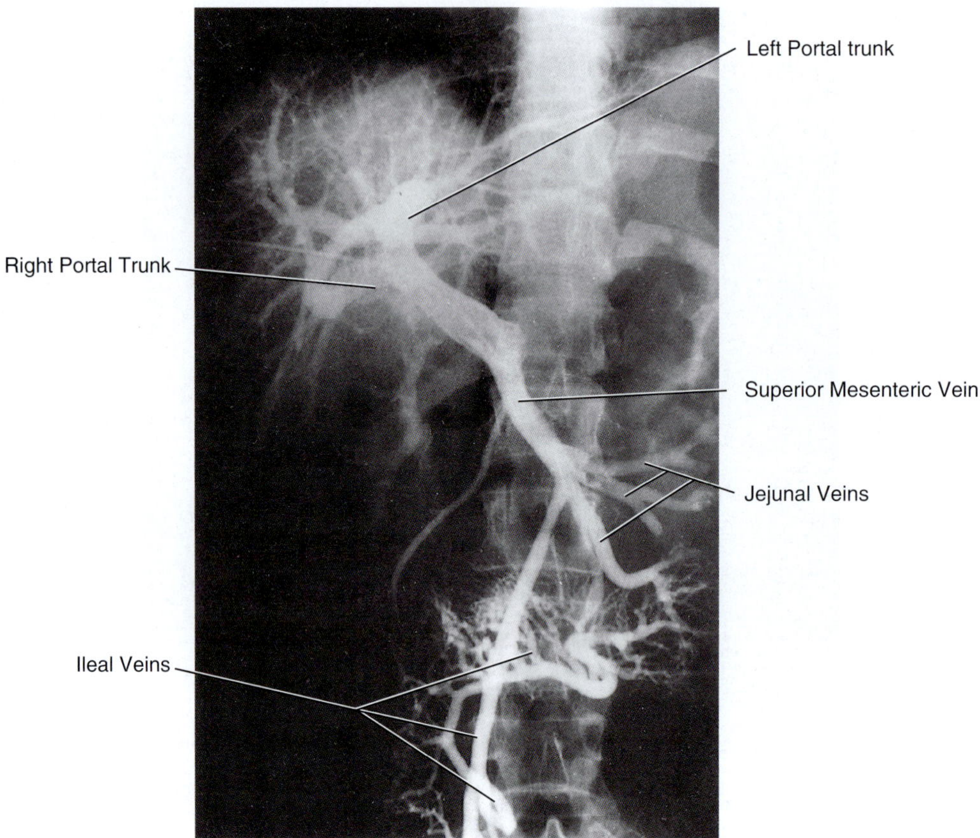

Figure 20.102. **Selective injection at jejunal and ileal veins.**

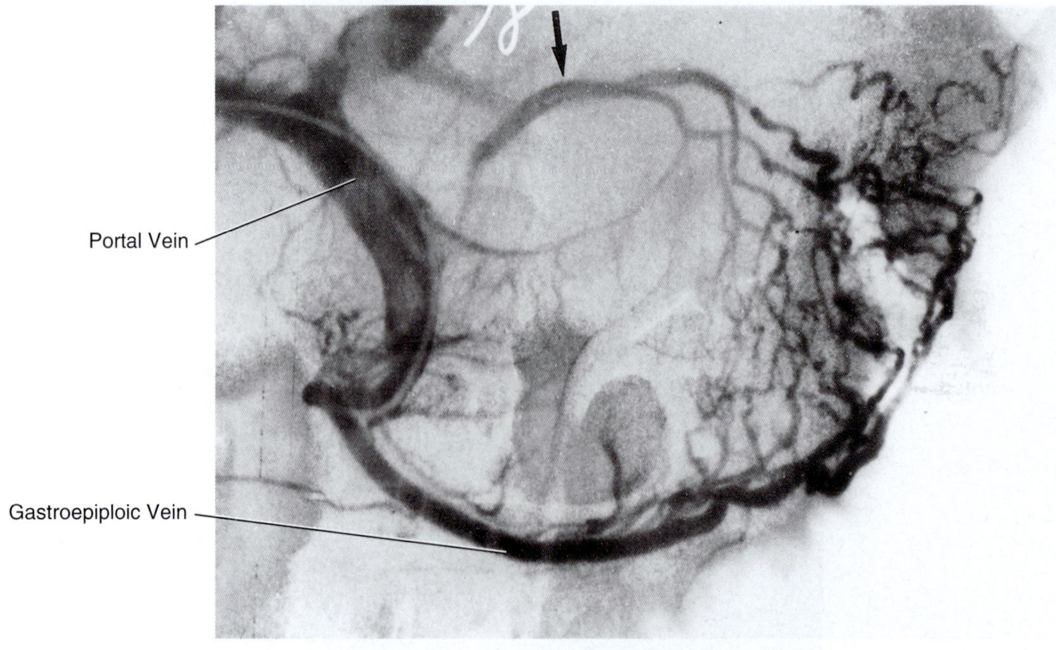

Figure 20.103. Selective injection into the right gastroepiploic vein, shows filling of the gastric wall veins and opacification of the left gastric vein (arrow). The portal vein is opacified.

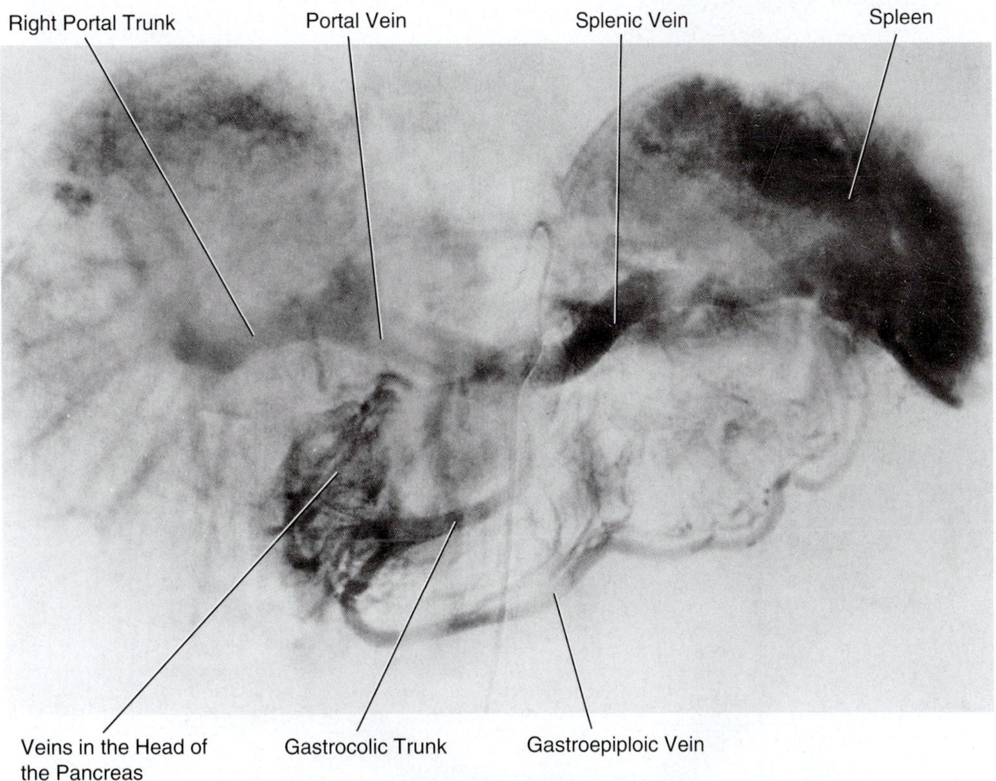

Figure 20.104. Late phase of a selective injection in the celiac trunk. Note filling of the right and left gastroepiploic veins. Note visualization of the gastrocolic trunk with opacification of the pancreatic head veins. The portal vein and splenic vein are well opacified.

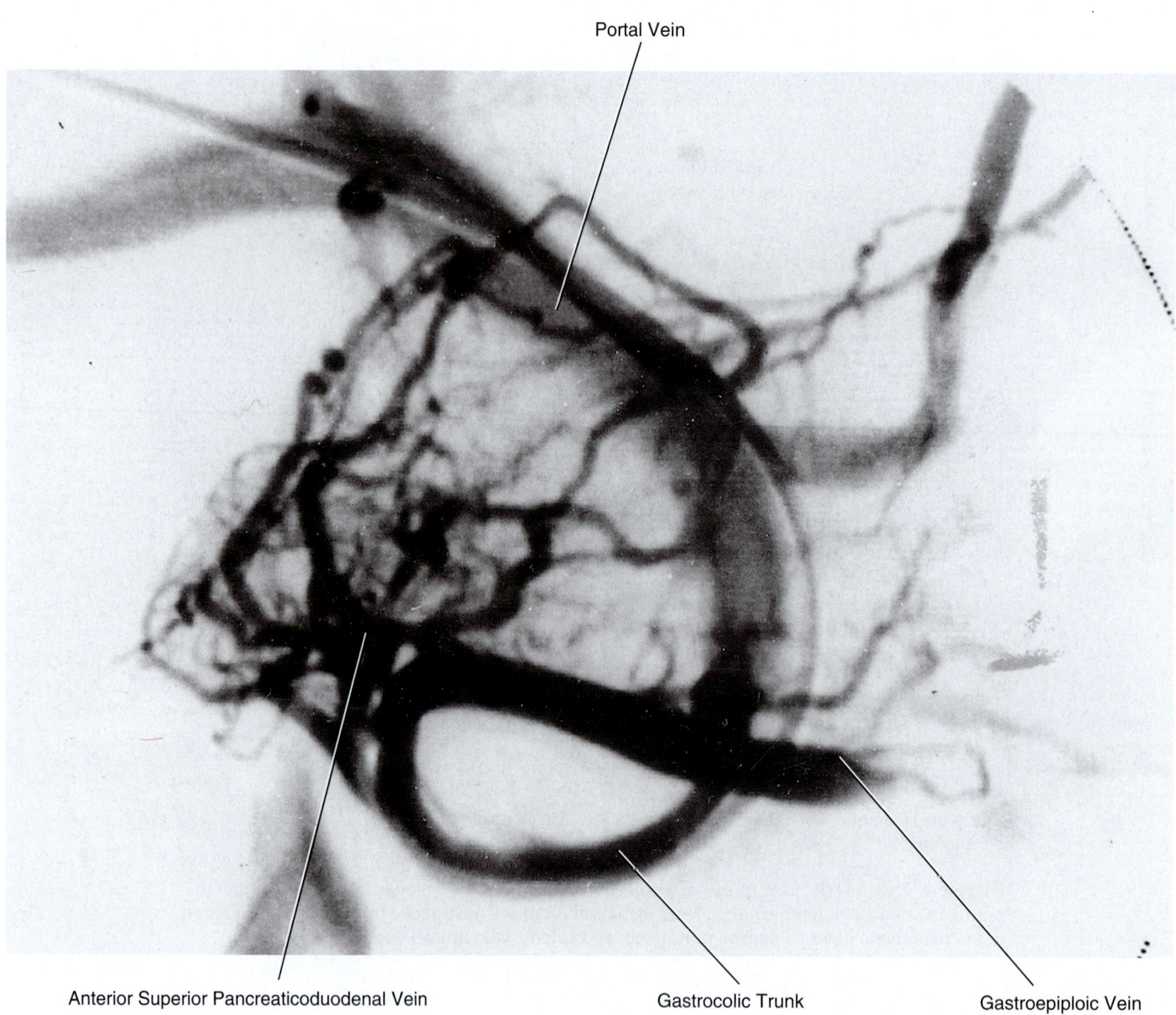

Figure 20.105. Selective injection at the gastrocolic trunk with filling of the pancreatic head veins and the right gastroepiploic vein.

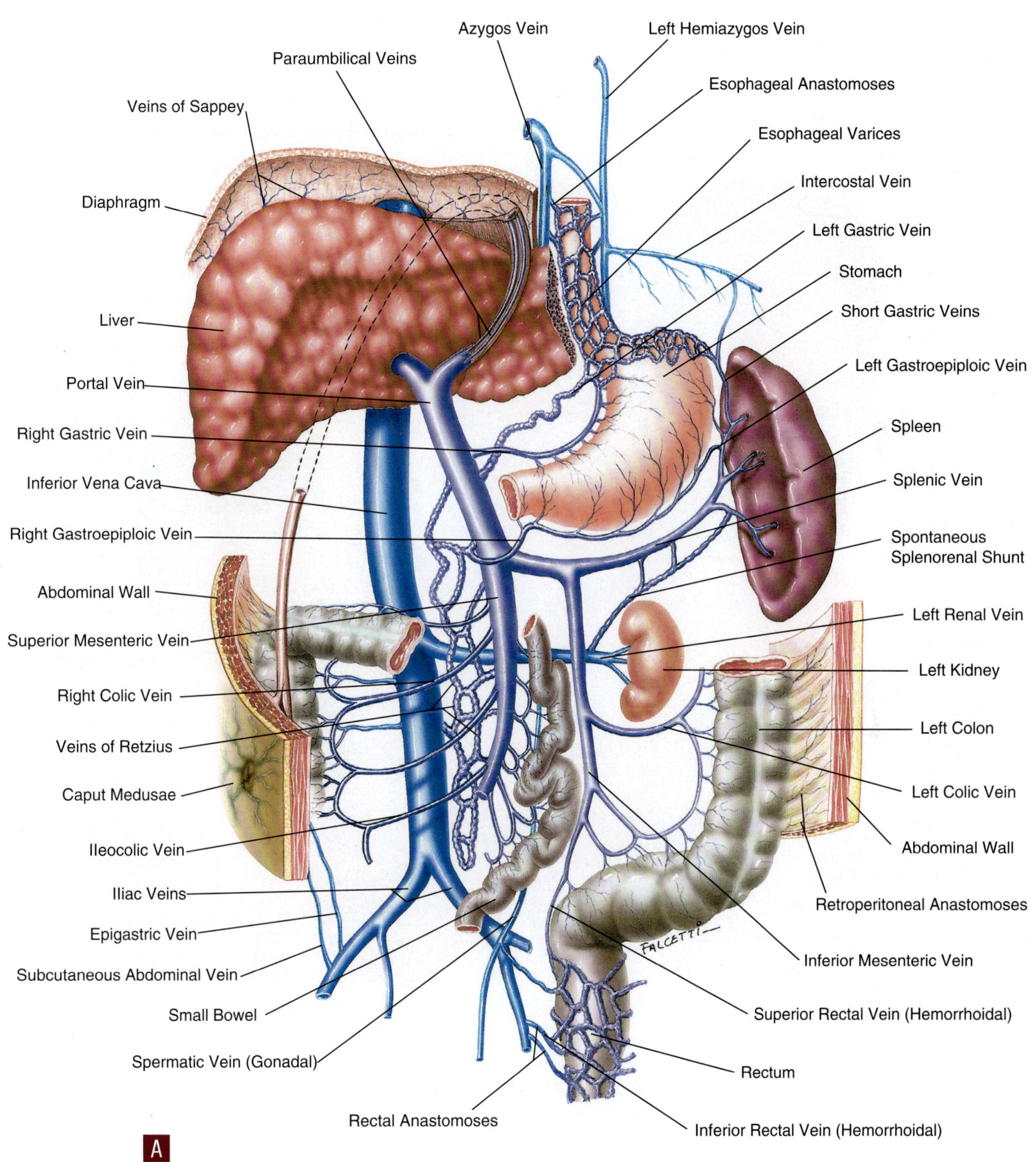

Figure 20.106. A, Sites of portosystemic collaterals and communications. B, Diagram showing the anatomy of the possible gastrorenal and gastrocaval shunts. C, Venous inflow classification of gastrorenal shunts. D, Venous drainage classification of gastrorenal shunts.

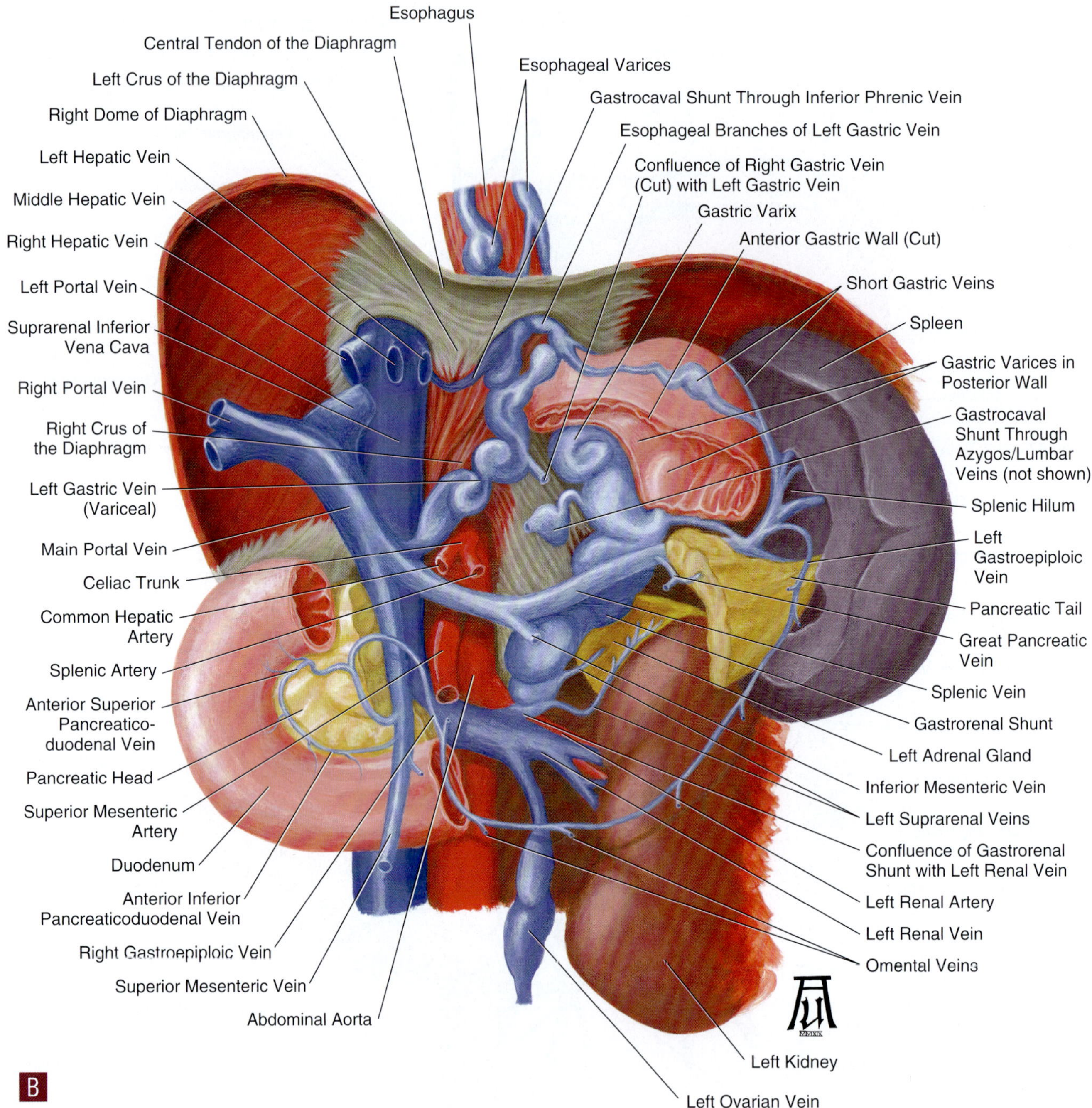

Figure 20.106. *Continued*

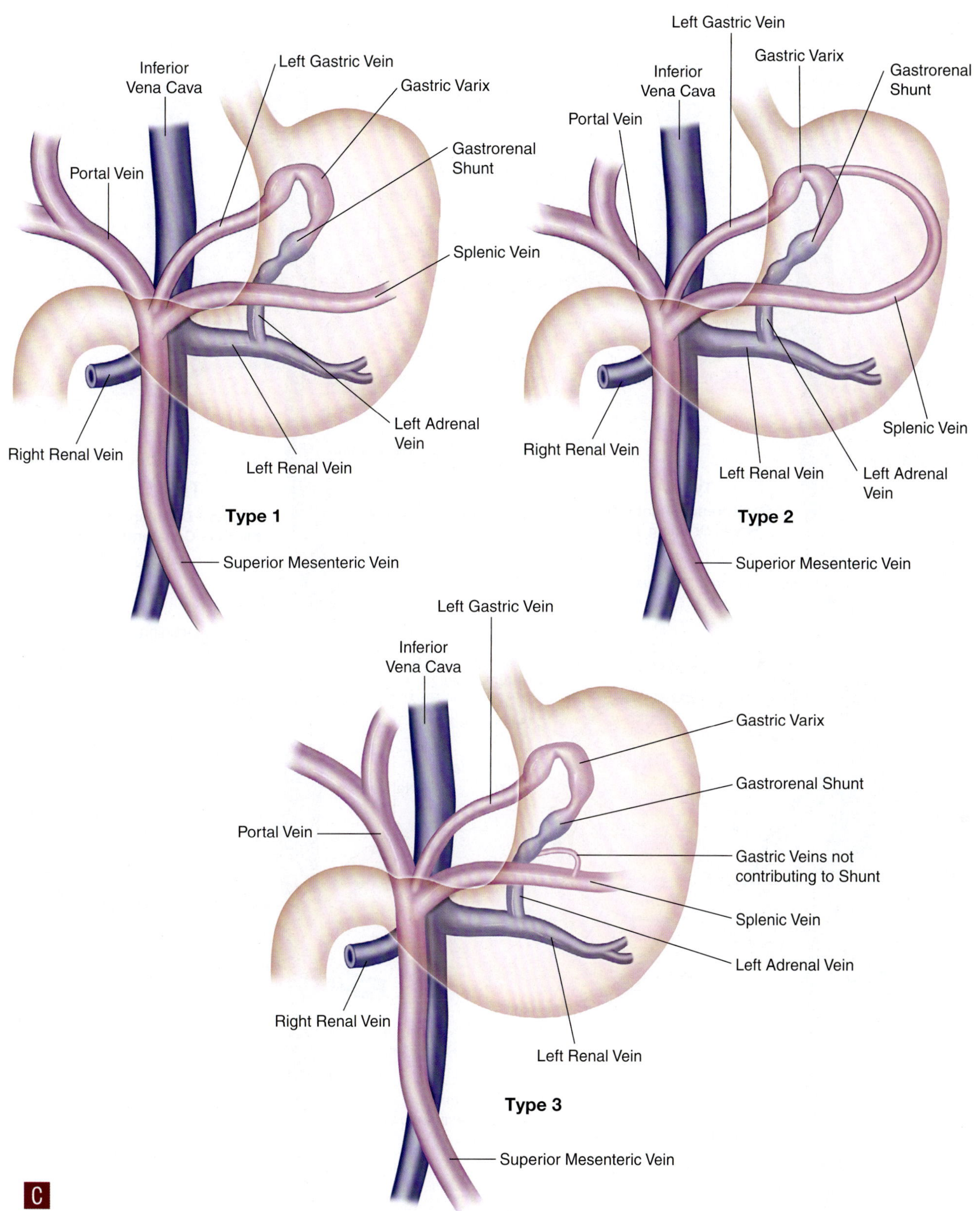

Figure 20.106. *Continued*

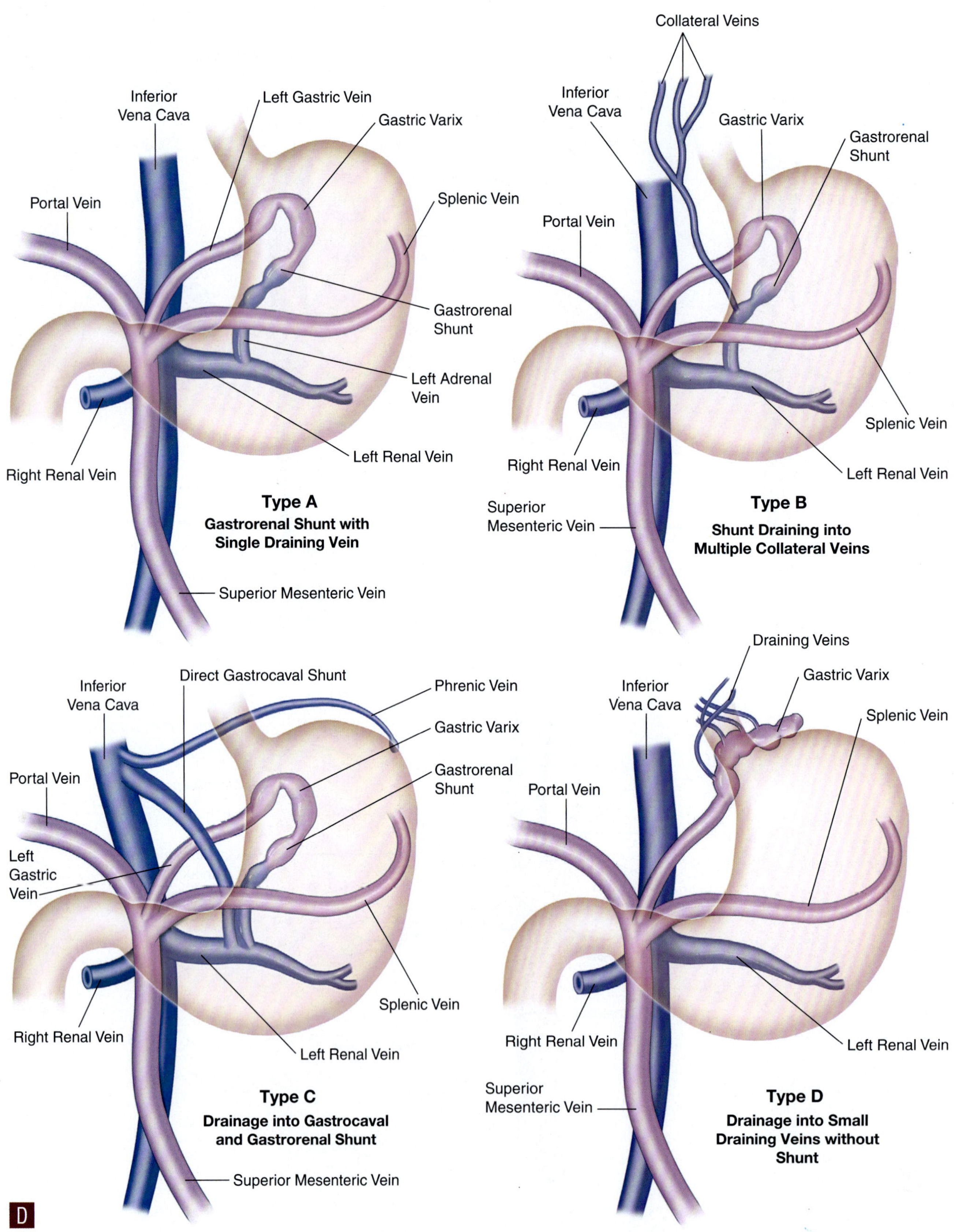

Figure 20.106. *Continued*

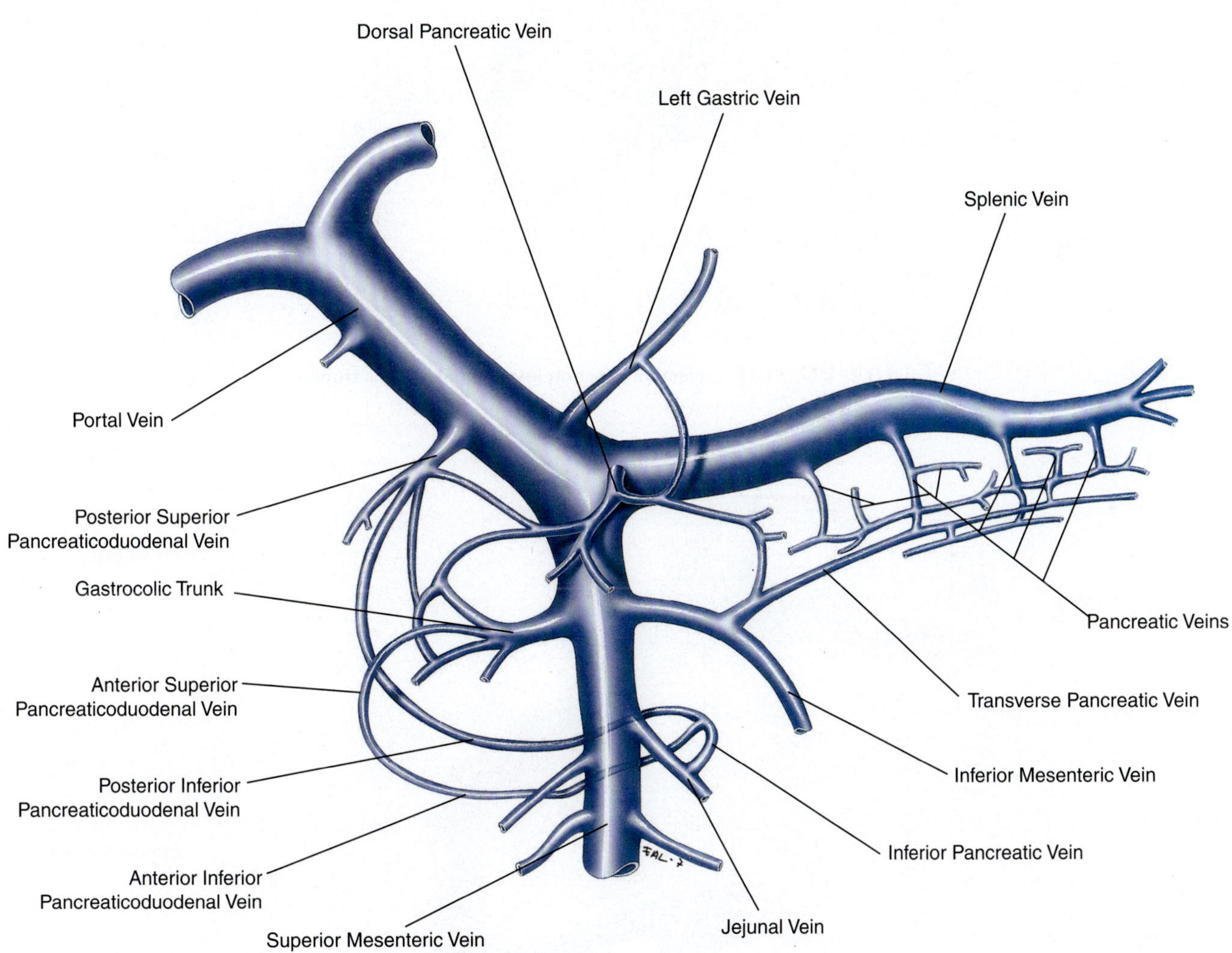

Figure 20.107. **Schematic drawing showing the pancreatic venous drainage.**

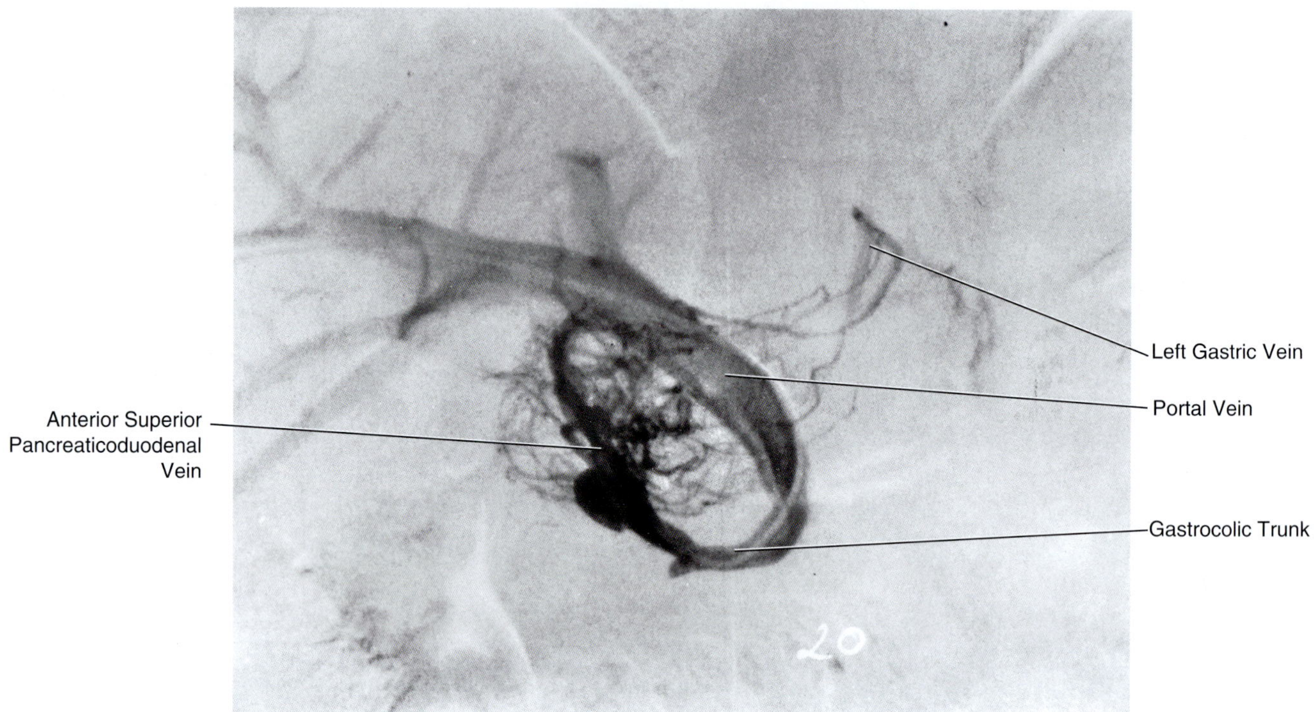

Figure 20.108. Selective injection into the gastrocolic trunk.

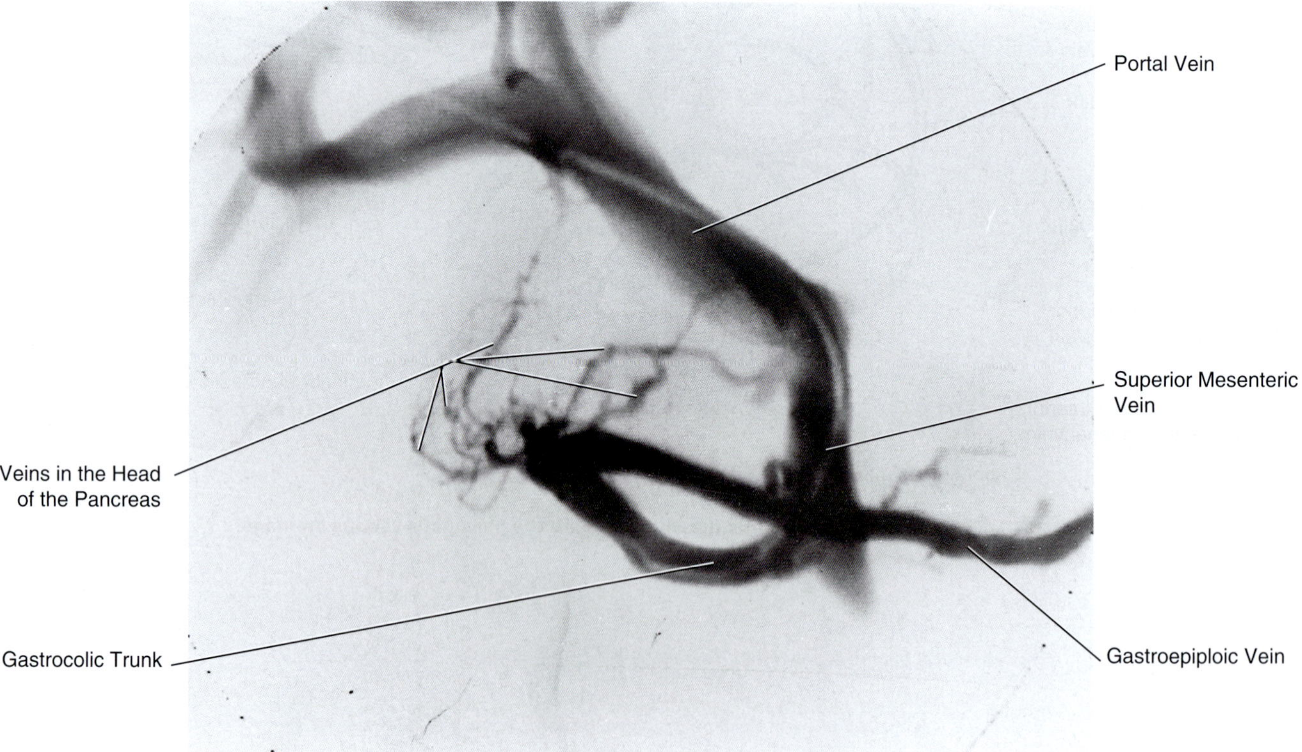

Figure 20.109. Selective injection into the gastrocolic trunk.

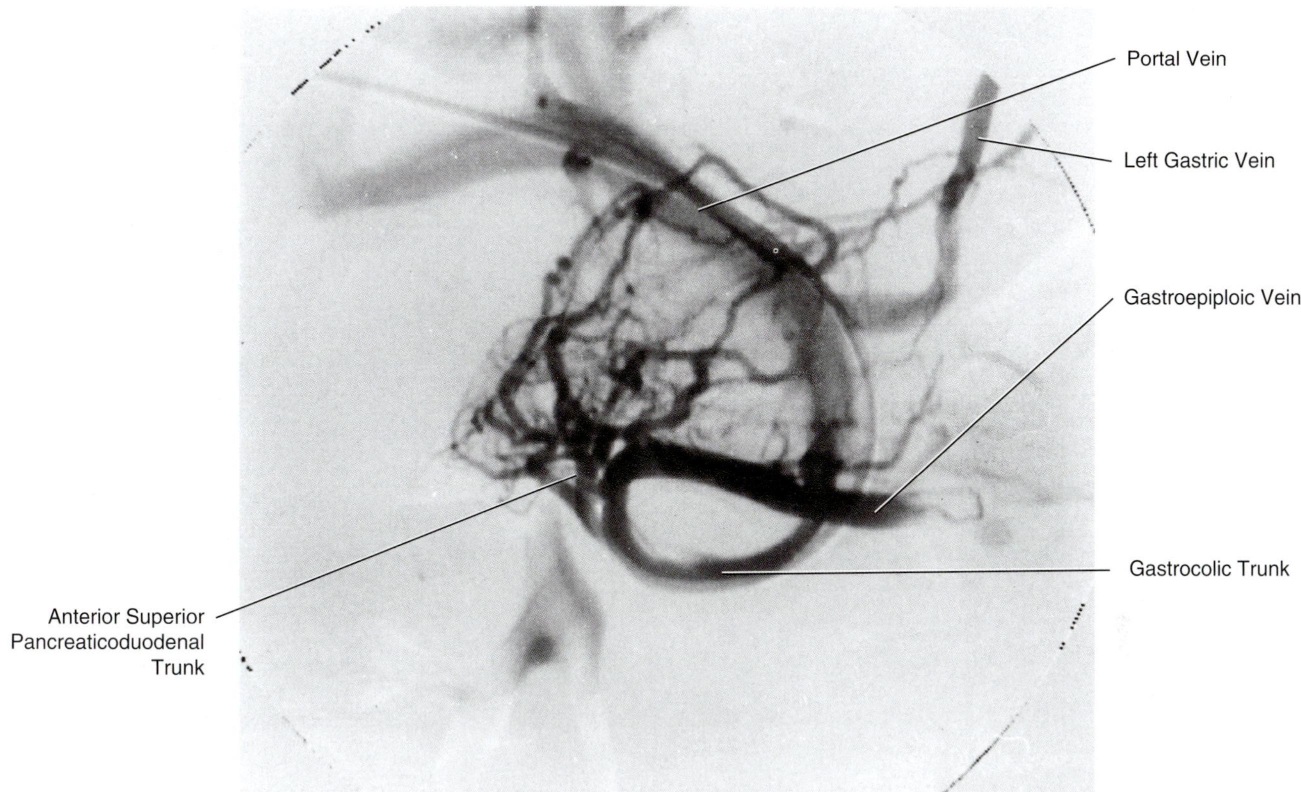

Figure 20.110. **Selective injection into the gastrocolic trunk.**

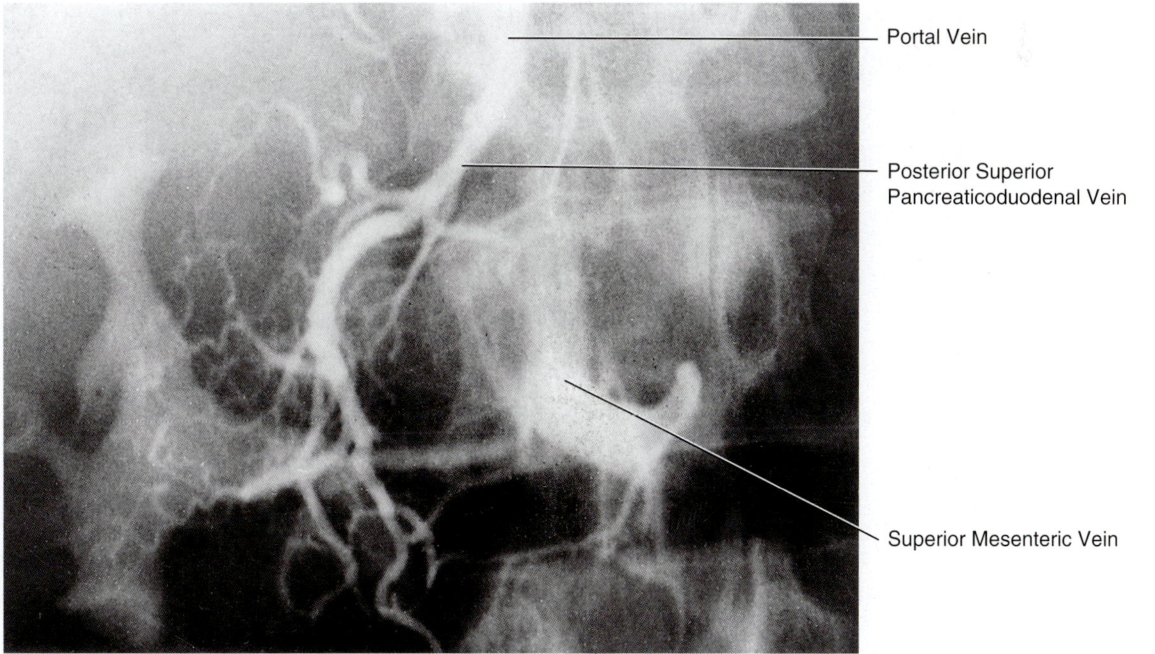

Figure 20.111. **Selective injection into the posterior superior pancreaticoduodenal vein.**

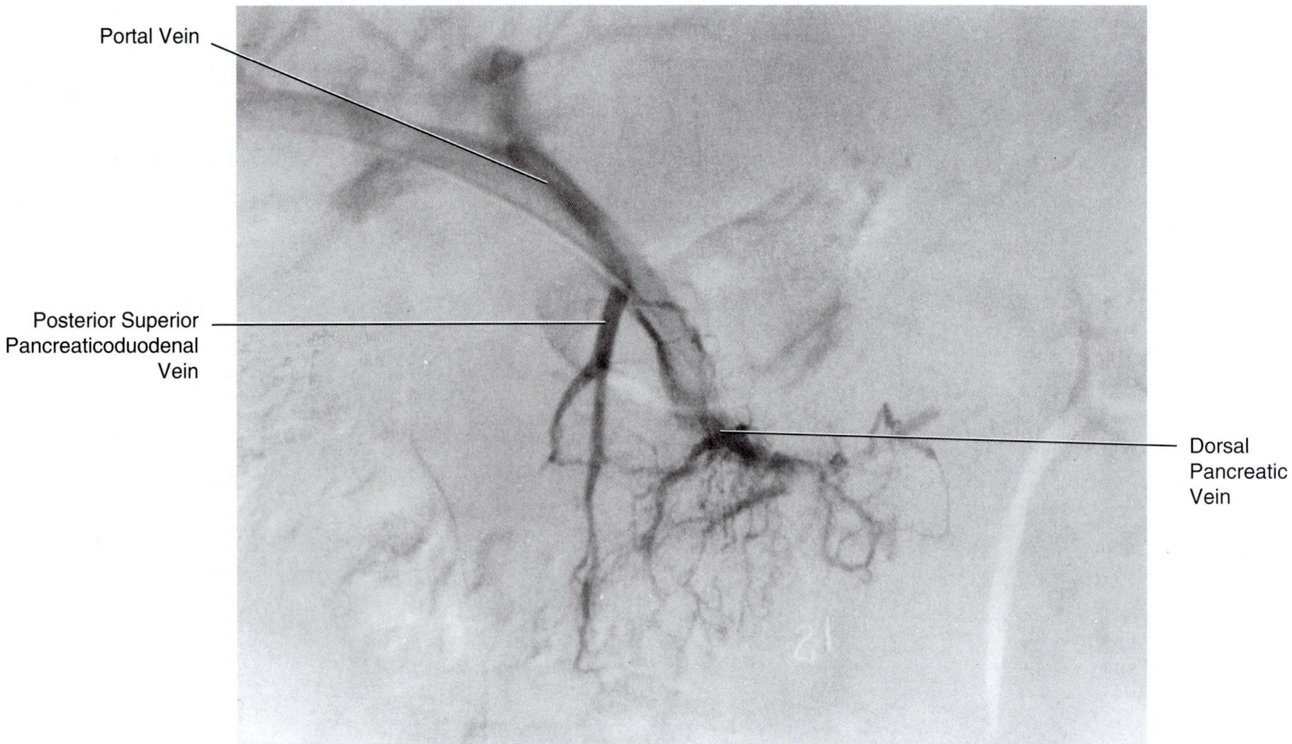

Figure 20.112. Selective injection into the dorsal pancreatic vein with simultaneous opacification of the posterior superior pancreaticoduodenal vein.

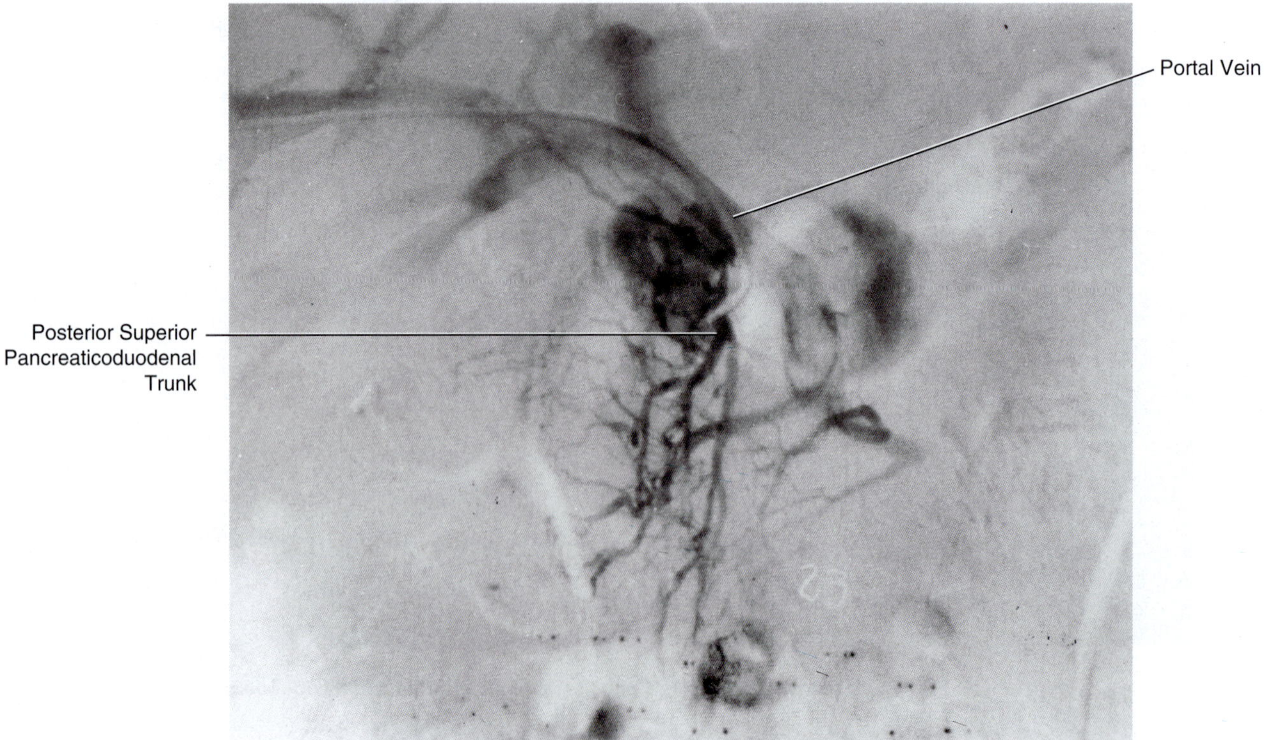

Figure 20.113. Selective injection into the posterior superior pancreaticoduodenal vein.

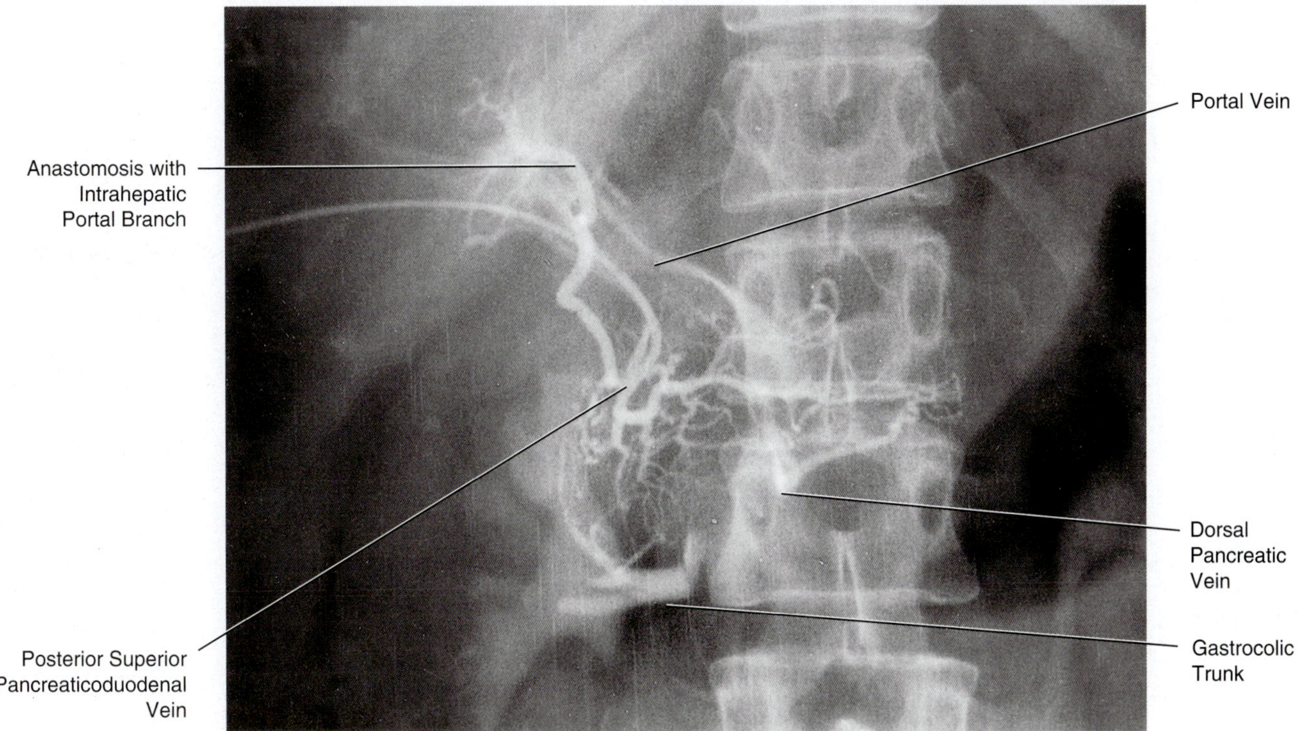

Figure 20.114. Selective venogram at the posterior superior pancreaticoduodenal vein.

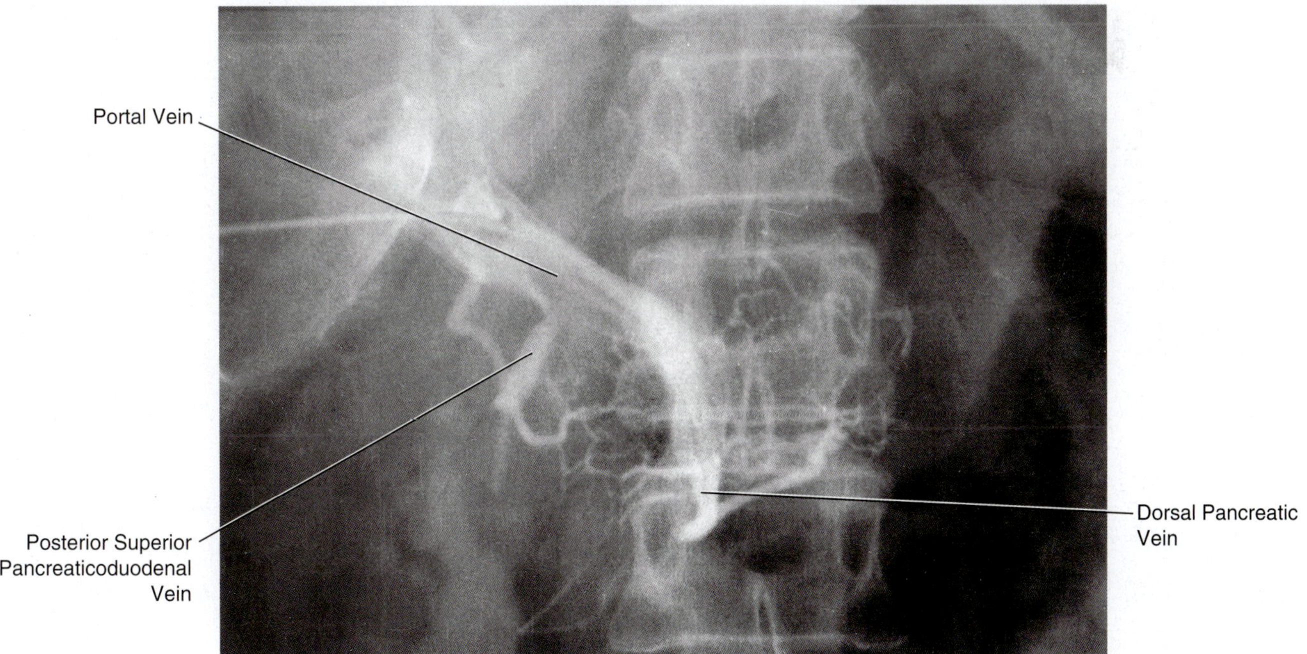

Figure 20.115. Selective venogram of the dorsal pancreatic vein.

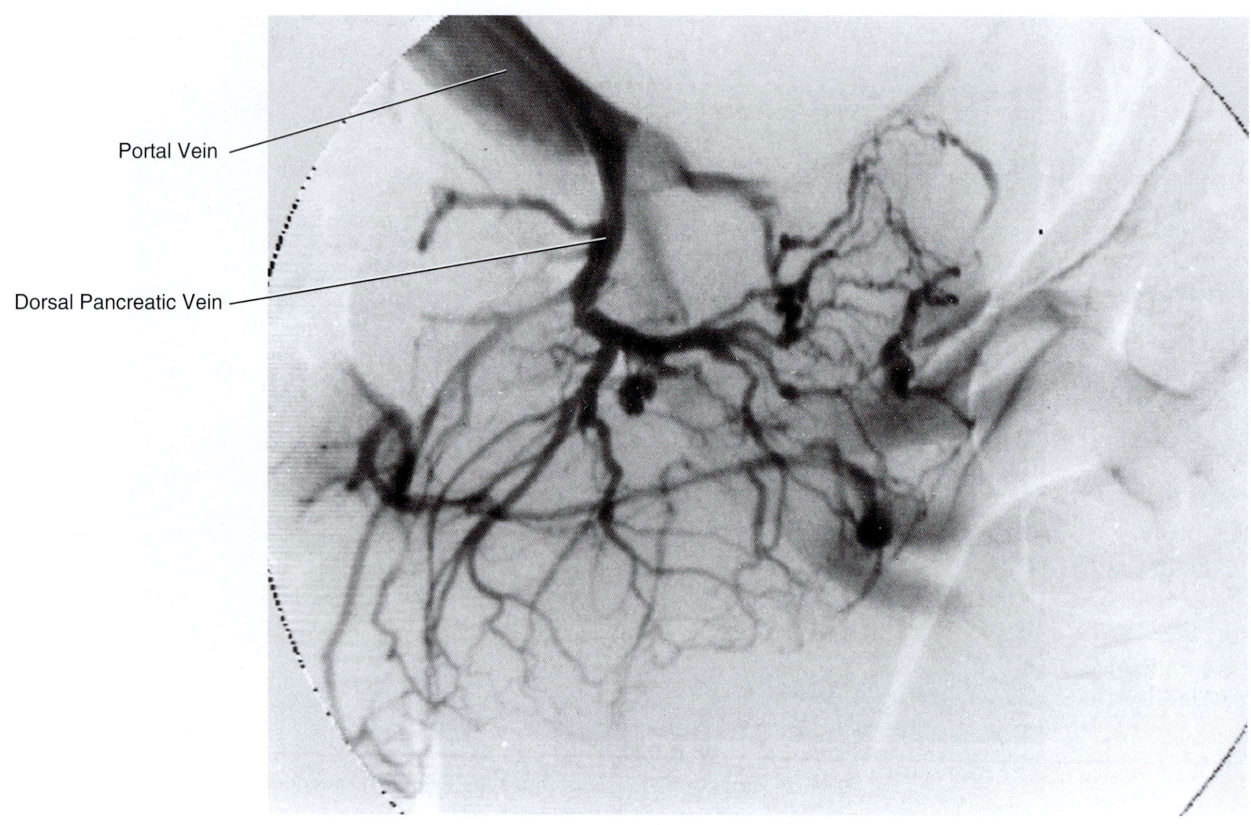

Figure 20.116. Selective venogram of the dorsal pancreatic vein. Note the large size of this vein and the wide anastomotic network with opacification of veins from the head to the pancreatic body. A few venous aneurysms are also seen.

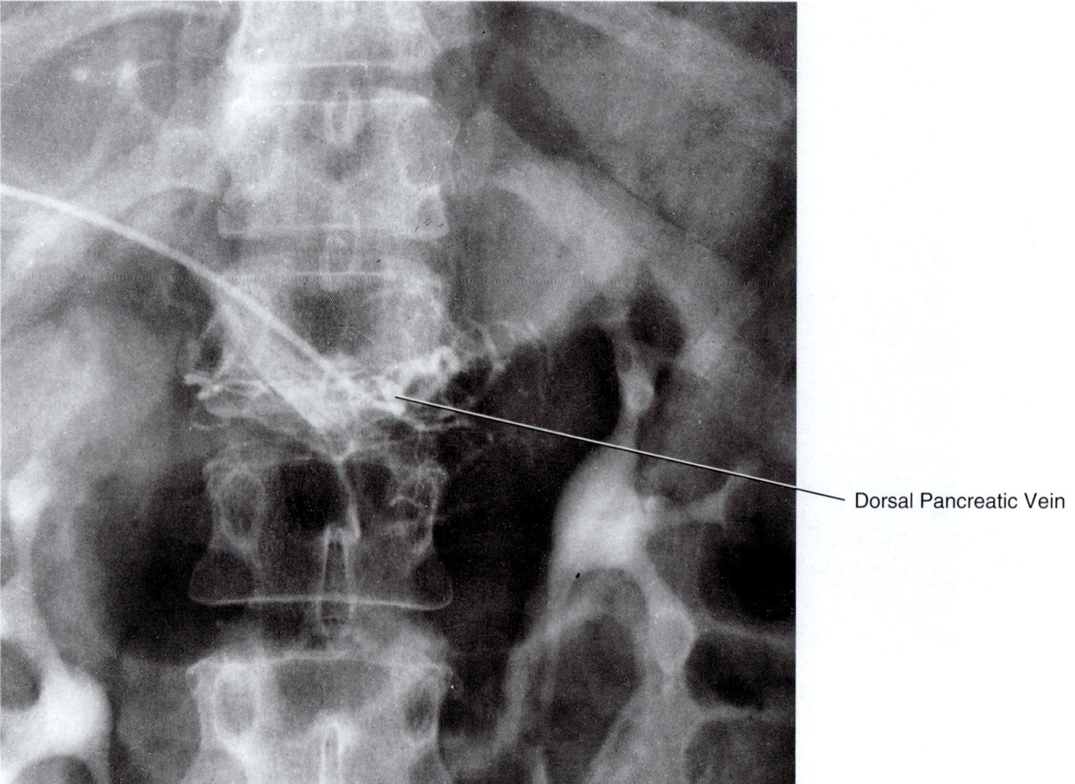

Figure 20.117. Selective venogram of the dorsal pancreatic vein. Note the small size of this vein.

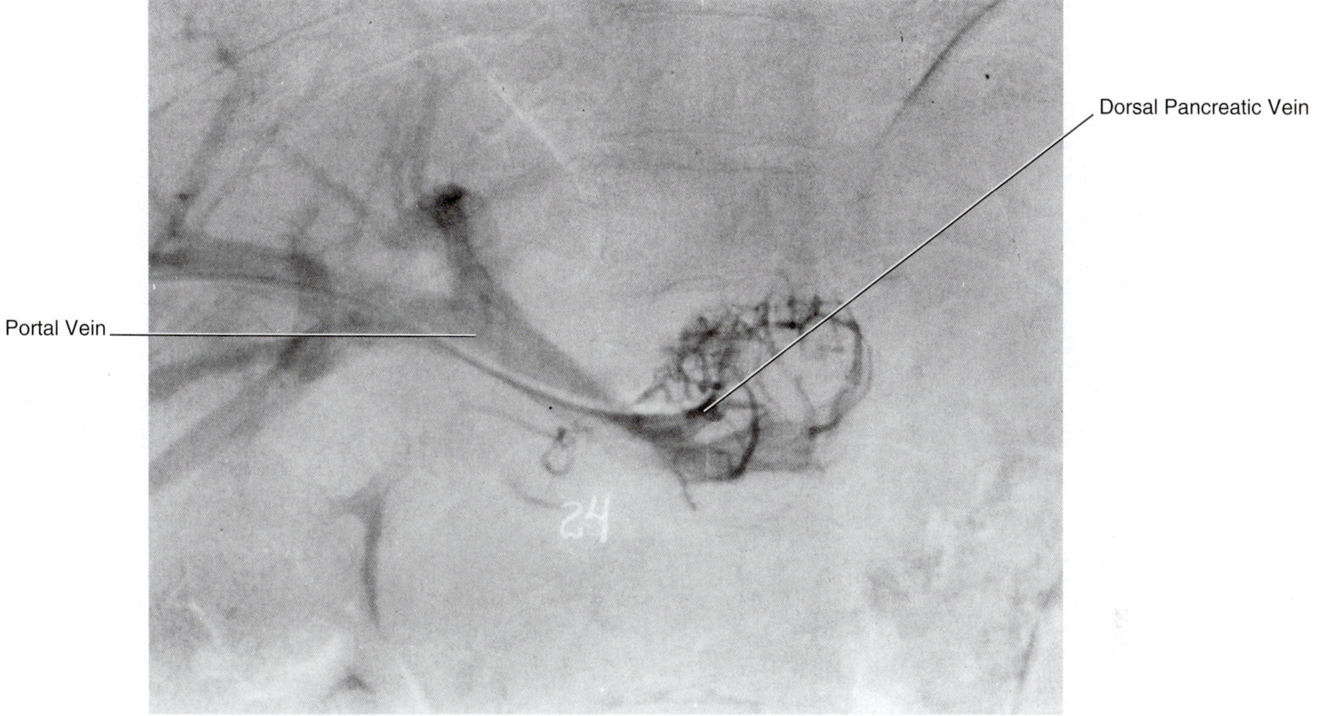

Figure 20.118. Selective venogram of the dorsal pancreatic vein, in an unusual position.

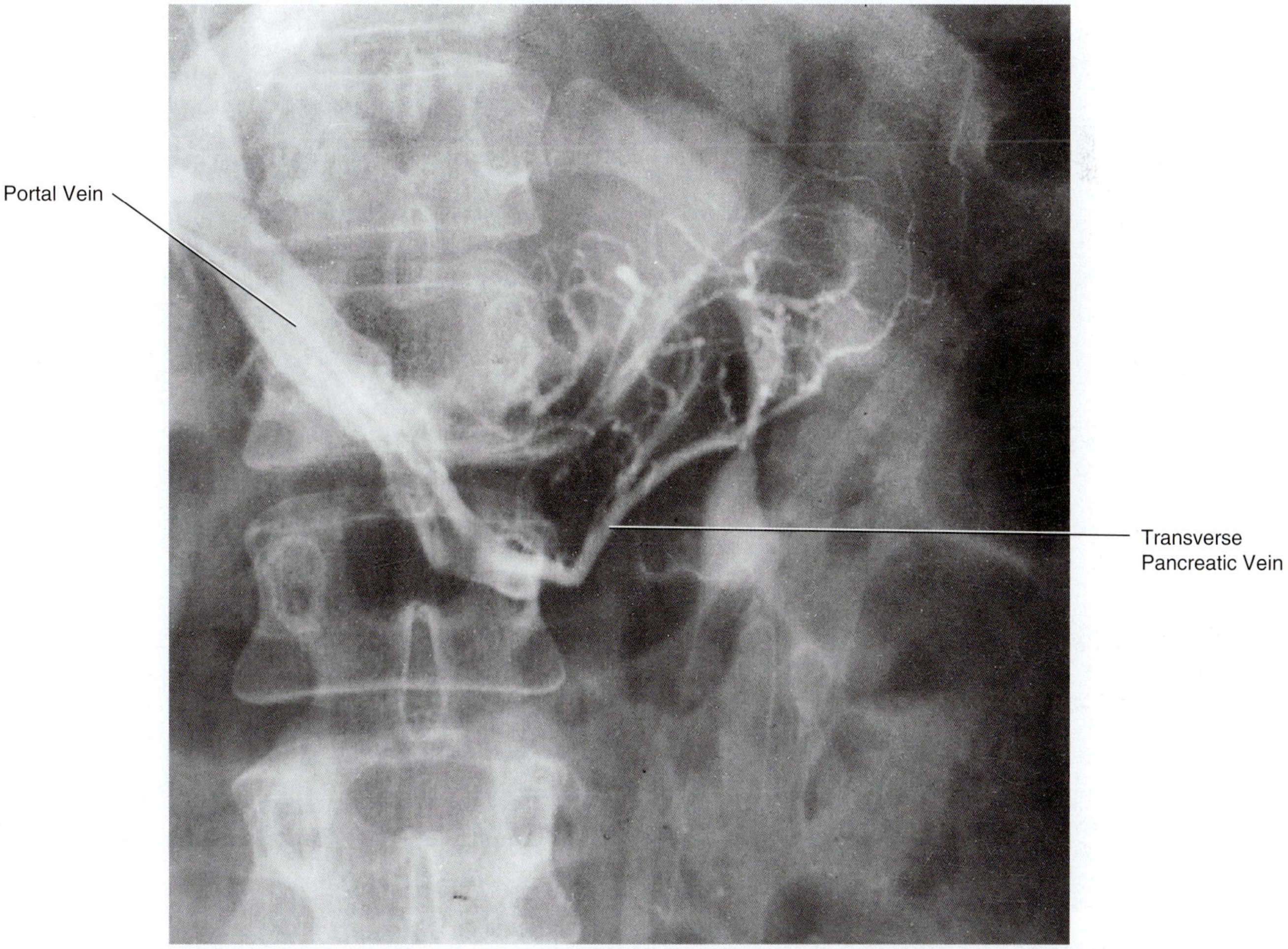

Portal Vein

Transverse Pancreatic Vein

Figure 20.119. Selective venogram of the transverse pancreatic vein.

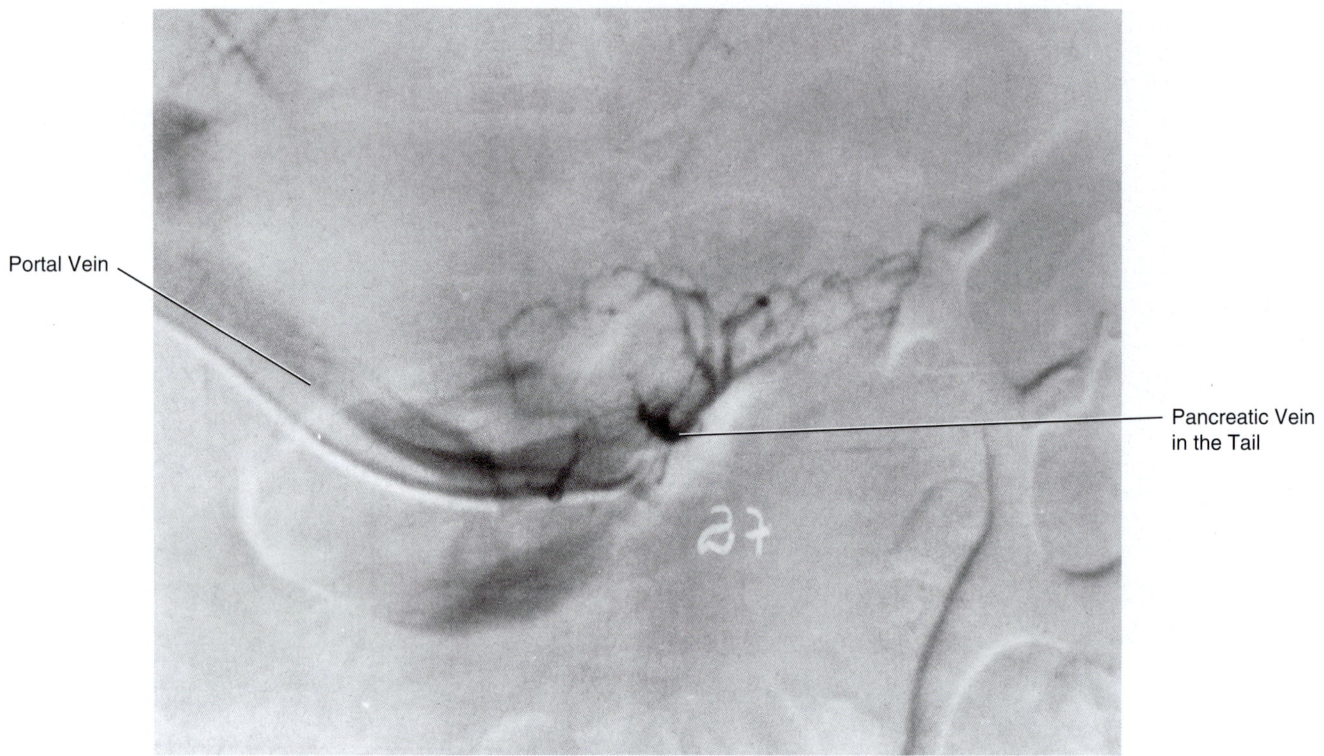

Figure 20.120. Selective venogram of the transverse pancreatic vein.

Left Gastric Vein
Fundic Veins
Transverse Pancreatic Vein

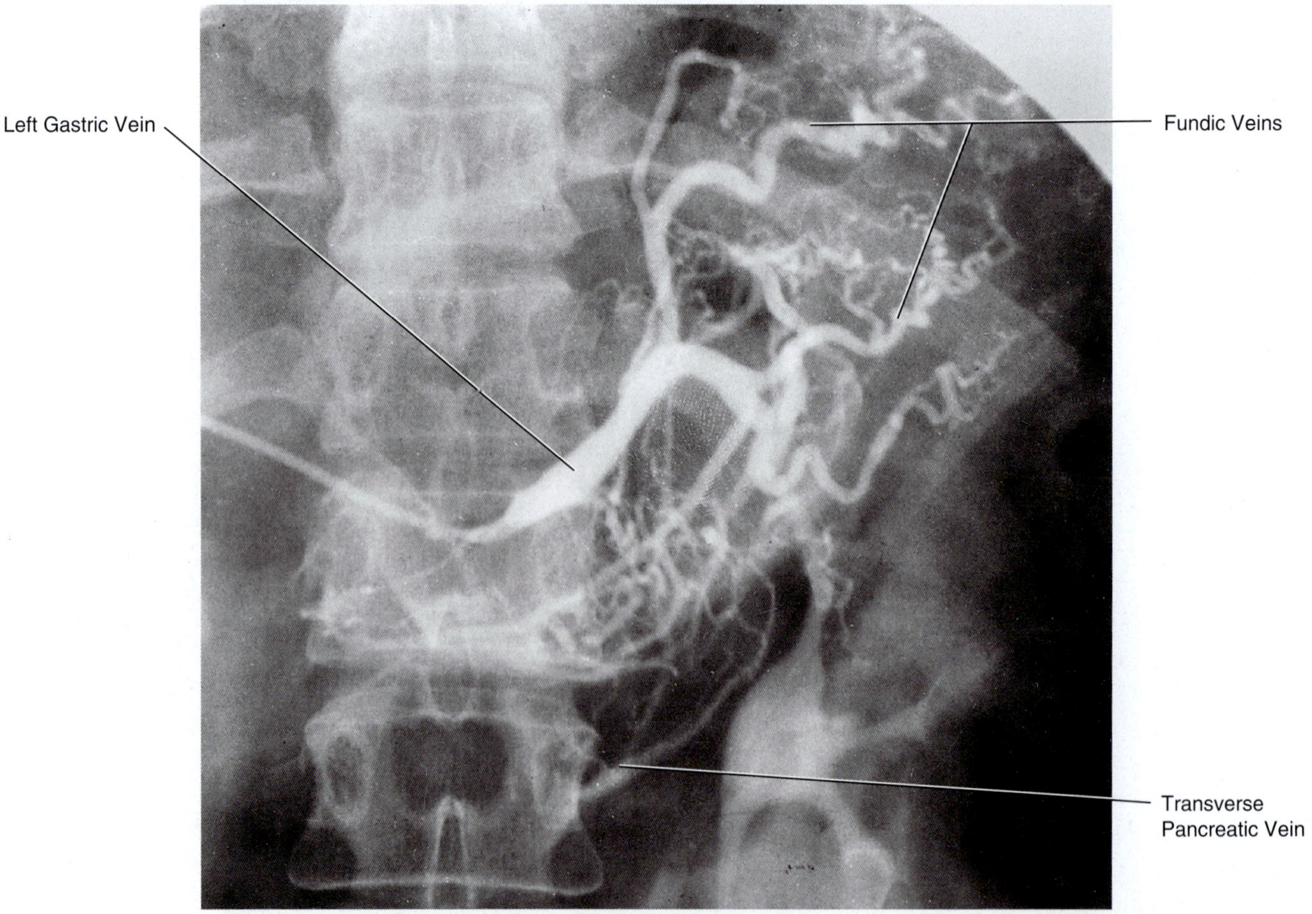

Figure 20.121. Selective venogram of the left gastric vein. Note the anastomosis with the gastric veins and pancreatic veins.

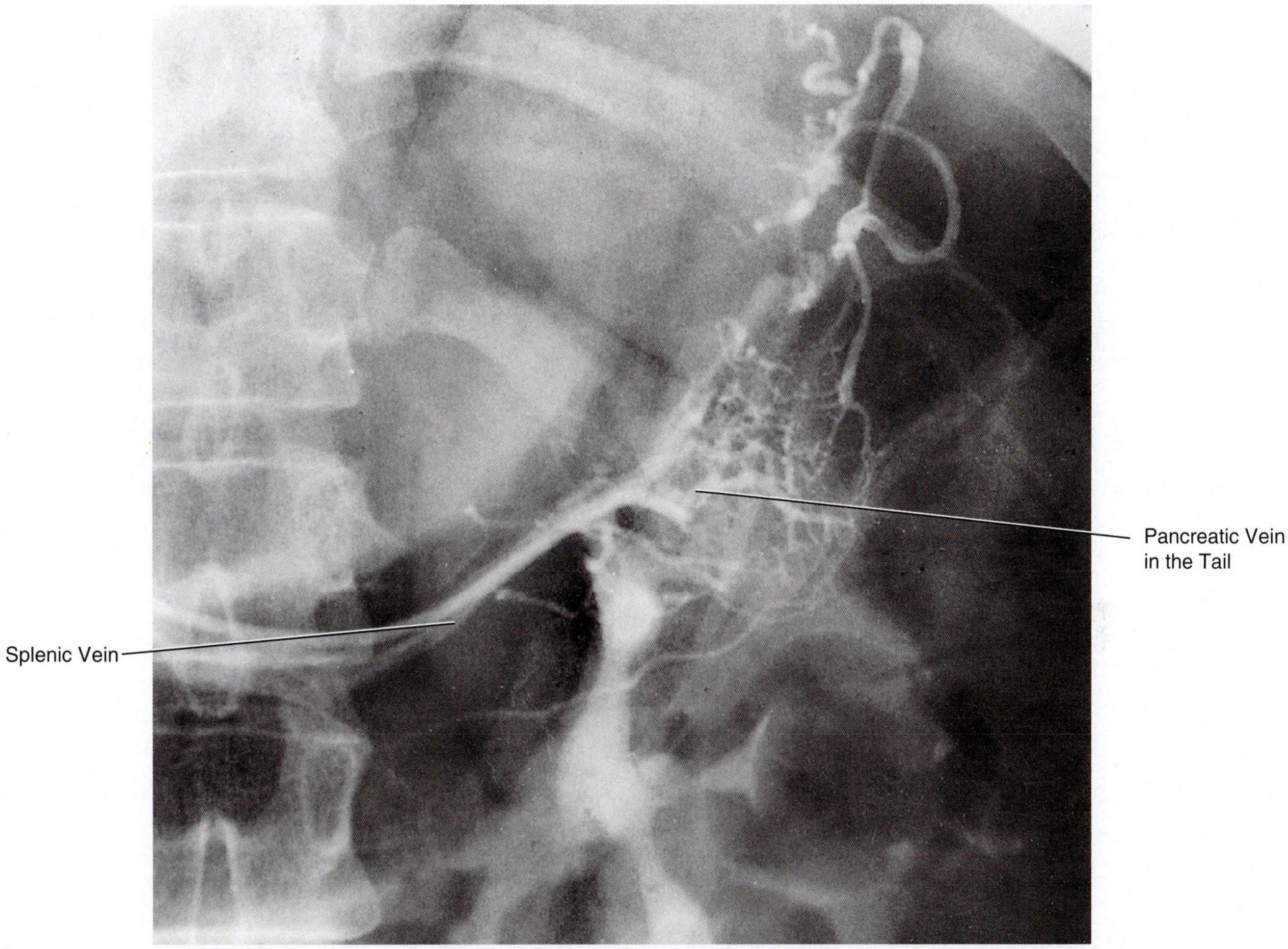

Figure 20.122. Selective venogram of pancreatic veins of the tail.

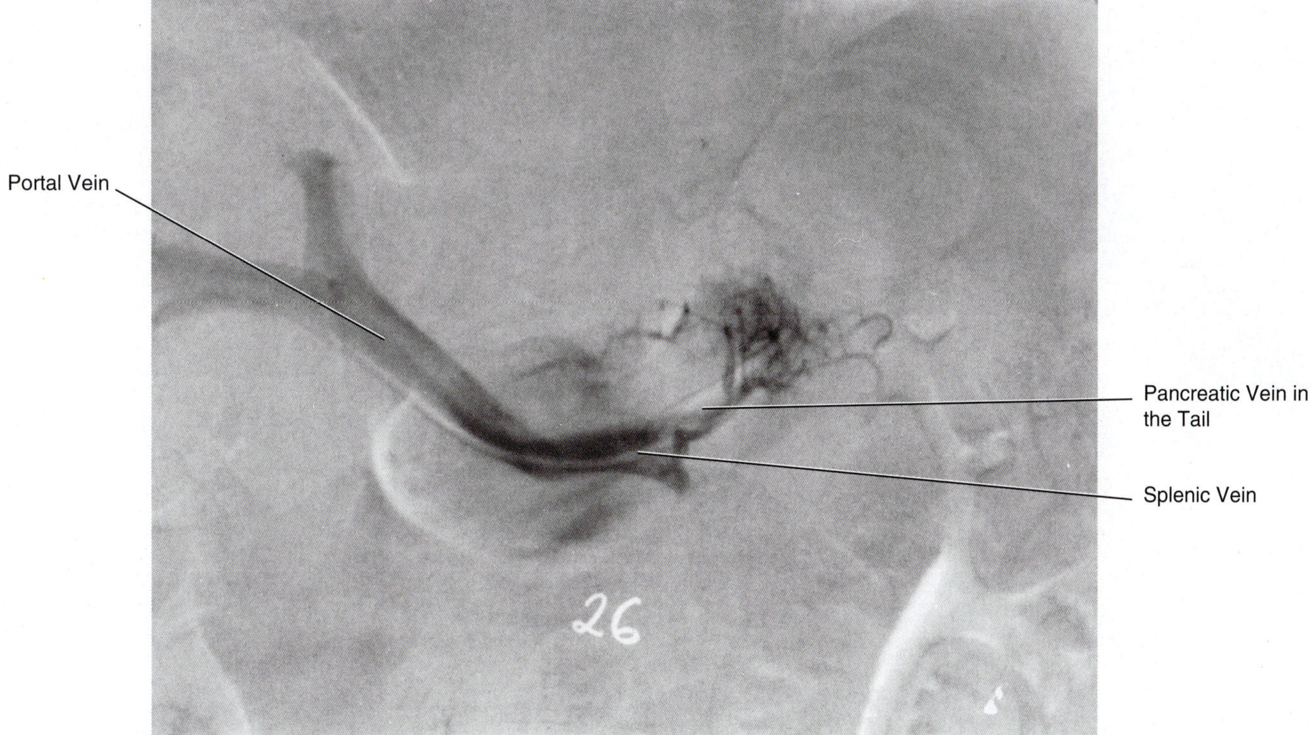

Figure 20.123. Selective venogram of pancreatic veins of the tail.

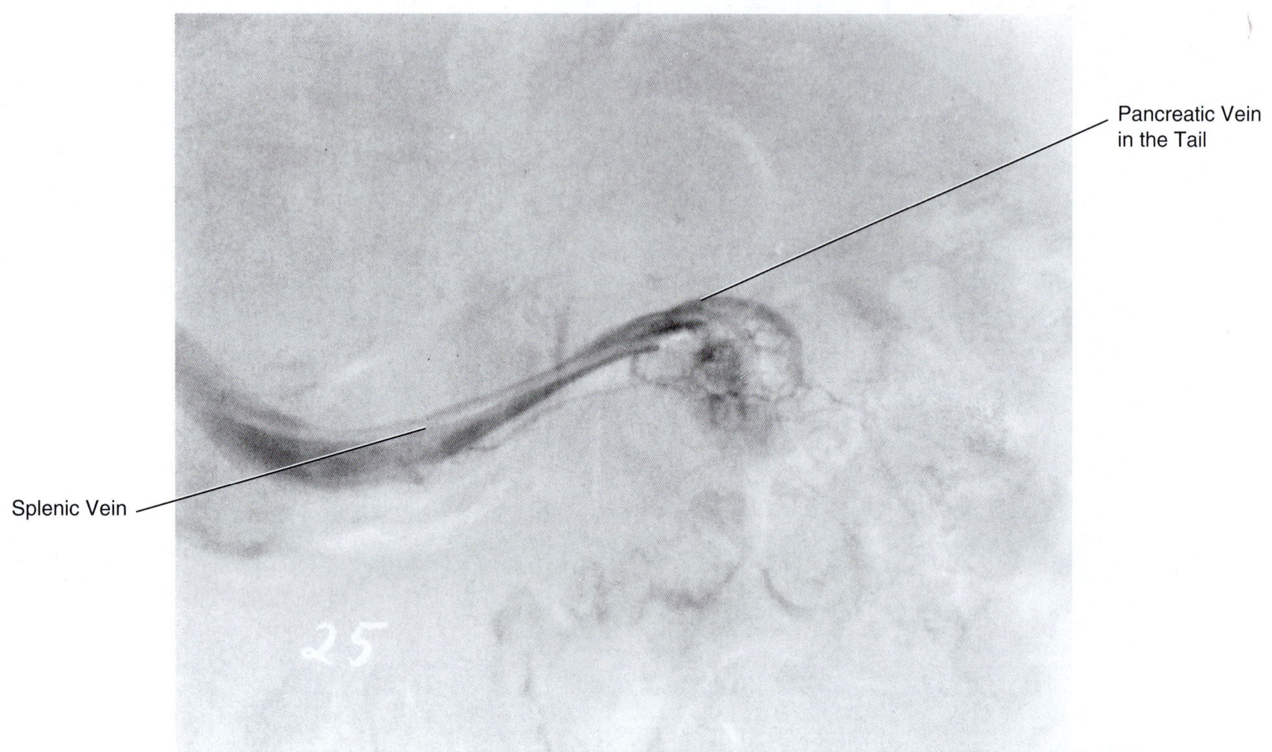

Figure 20.124. Selective venogram of the pancreatic veins of the tail.

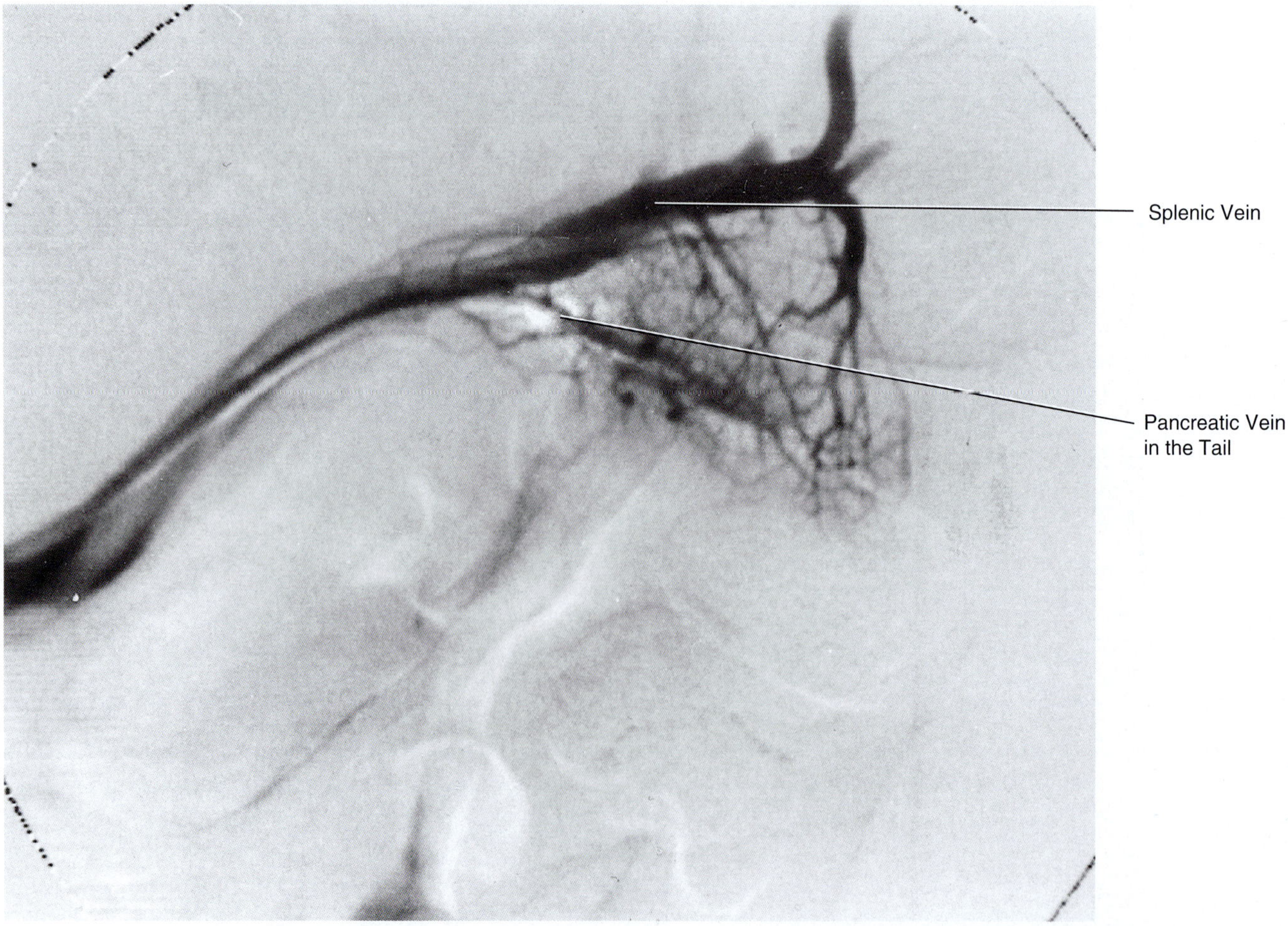

Figure 20.125. Selective venogram of the pancreatic veins of the tail.

21

Lymphatic System of the Abdomen and Pelvis

There are three main groups of lumbar lymph nodes: the preaortic, lateral aortic (right and left), and retroaortic. The preaortic receives drainage from the ventral splanchnic vessels; the lateral aortic drains the viscera supplied by the lateral splanchnic and dorsolateral somatic vessels. The retroaortic lymph nodes drain no specific territory but are mainly an interconnection of the other groups (Figs. 21.1 and 21.2). The intestinal lymph trunks coalesce and join the right and left lumbar lymph trunks to form the highly variable abdominal confluence of lymph trunks, the cranial end of which is the cisterna chyli in 54% or less of the individuals or the thoracic duct per se (Fig. 21.2). The cisterna chyli has variable morphologic characteristics and sizes. It is located to the right of aorta, usually at the level of L1-L2, posterior to the right diaphragmatic crus (Fig. 21.3). Frequently, the cisterna is absent, but when present, it can be multilocular or plexiform. A well-formed cisterna chyli can have a square, triangular, or sigmoid form (Fig. 21.4).

Lumbar Lymph Nodes

Preaortic Lymph Nodes

The preaortic lymph nodes comprise the group located anterior to the abdominal aorta and receive the intestinal trunks, named after the arteries with which they are companions: celiac lymph nodes, superior mesenteric lymph nodes, and inferior mesenteric lymph nodes.

Celiac Lymph Nodes

There are three main groups of lymph nodes sending afferents to the celiac lymph nodes: from gastric lymphatic vessels and nodes (from left gastric nodes, right gastroepiploic nodes, and pyloric nodes) (Fig. 21.5) from hepatic lymphatic vessels and nodes (Fig. 21.6) (from the stomach, duodenum, liver, gallbladder, bile ducts, and head of the pancreas), and from splenopancreatic lymphatic vessels and nodes (from stomach, spleen, and pancreas) (Fig. 21.5).

Superior and Inferior Mesenteric Lymph Nodes

The superior and inferior mesenteric lymph nodes are located close to the origin of the corresponding arteries. They collect lymphatic drainage from the duodenojejunal flexure to the upper anal canal, including the mesenteric, ileocolic, colonic, and pararectal lymph nodes, discharging into the celiac lymph nodes. There are hundreds of lymph nodes in the territory comprising the mesentery. The lymphatic drainage of the rectum and anal canal has a duplicated path. The upper half of the rectum drains to the pararectal nodes and subsequently to the superior mesenteric lymph nodes, whereas the lower half of the rectum and the anal canal drains to the internal iliac lymph nodes. Lymphatic vessels of the mucocutaneous junction reach the medial superficial inguinal nodes (Fig. 21.8).

Lateral Aortic Lymph Nodes

The lateral aortic lymph nodes comprise the group of lymph nodes flanking the abdominal aorta and the inferior vena cava. Several afferents reach those nodes, from the kidney, suprarenal gland, abdominal ureter, posterior abdominal wall, testis, and ovary. The lymph of the pelvic organs reaches the lateral aortic lymph nodes, after passing through regional groups as the internal iliac nodes, external iliac nodes, and common iliac nodes (Fig. 21.9). The internal iliac group receives deep gluteal lymph, and the external iliac group receives the efferents from the inguinal lymph nodes, whereas the common iliac nodes are grouped around the common iliac artery, draining the external and internal iliac nodes and sending efferents to the lateral aortic nodes.

Lymphatic Drainage of the Liver

The liver's lymph originates in the hepatic sinusoids, flowing into the space of Disse that is in communication with the periportal space (of Mall). Hepatic lymphatic flow contributes about half of the flow into the thoracic duct and increases dramatically during hepatic congestion, in states like right heart failure, or portal hypertension. Hepatic lymphatics are divided into a deep and a superficial system (Fig. 21.6). The deep hepatic lymphatic system follows the portal and hepatic veins, whereas the superficial system drains the subcapsular area directly into the mediastinal vessels. About 70% to 80% of hepatic lymph is drained by the deep system. In cases of congestion, the deep lymphatic system undergoes significant distention to accommodate a marked increase in lymphatic flow, causing enlargement of the periportal lymphatic channels. Dilation of the periportal lymphatic system in cases of congestion is responsible for periportal edema which can be seen in cross-sectional imaging (Fig. 21.7).

Lymphatic Drainage of the Urinary and Reproductive Organs

From the Kidney. The intrarenal lymphatics of the kidney are divided into a superficial plexus and a deep plexus. The superficial plexus is located immediately below the renal capsule and is connected with cortical lymphatics. In pathologic conditions (pyelonephritis, for example), this plexus may communicate with an extrarenal plexus located in the perirenal fat, which drains into the lumbo-aortic lymph nodes.

The deep plexus is subcortical, perivascular and reaches the pyramids draining along the arcuate and interlobar vessels, converging to the renal hilus. The collecting channels emerge from the renal hilus, and, if a polar artery is present, a lymphatic channel typically follows it. There are one to four lymphatic channels that emerge from the renal hilus, either anteriorly or posteriorly to the renal vein. These lymphatics may contain multiple anastomoses, giving a plexiform aspect. The lymphatics are usually periarterial, forming an anterior plexus when they come from the kidney's ventral surface or a posterior plexus when they come from the kidney's dorsal surface. In some cases, the lymphatic channels may connect to their lymph nodes directly, without following arterial branches. The drainage of the lymphatic vessels differs in some respects between right and left sides:

Right side. The lymphatic channels of the right kidney may be divided into posterior, anterior, and middle. The posterior lymphatic vessels follow the renal artery, posteriorly to the inferior vena cava. These lymphatics reach the lumbo-aortic lymph nodes, which are located just below the origin of the right renal artery. These drain into the retrocaval nodes, interaortocaval nodes (L1 to L3), and lateral caval nodes, and surrounding the deep surface of the renal artery, they follow the right diaphragmatic crura to reach the right abdominal lymphatic channel. The anterior lymphatic channels, running above the vessels, drain into the posterior lymphatics or, when running medially, end in the precaval nodes. Sometimes, they can cross the inferior vena cava to reach the superior interaortocaval nodes. The middle lymphatics run between the renal vein and the renal artery to reach the anterior and posterior lymphatic groups (Figs. 21.10 and 21.11).

Left side. The lymphatic vessels of the left kidney may be divided into posterior and anterior. The posterior channels leave the renal hilum and run behind the renal vessels to reach the lymphatic nodes of the diaphragmatic crus. The anterior channels run ventrally to the renal vein; they reach the lymph nodes located above or below the renal artery origin, when draining the superior pole or the inferior pole, respectively. There are also lymphatics that come from the inferior pole to reach the lymph nodes that are located in the spermatic artery origin on the lateral surface of the aorta (Figs. 21.10 and 21.12).

On both sides, the lymphatic drainage of the kidney's dorsal surface reaches the lymph nodes of the diaphragmatic crus directly, in contact with the hiatus of the splanchnic nerve. From this point, through the diaphragm, these lymphatics drain into the retroaortic nodes, from T11 to L1 (mediastinal lymphatics) (Fig. 21.10). This detail is very important to be remembered when assessing the spread of renal cell carcinoma metastases.

From the Ureter. The draining lymphatic vessels of the ureter begin in the submucosal, intramuscular, and adventitial plexuses with intercommunications. The lymphatic vessels from the pelvic part of the ureter drain to the common, internal, and external iliac nodes. The lower abdominal part of the ureter drains directly to the common iliac nodes, whereas the proximal ureter drains to the renal collecting vessels or passes directly to the lateral aortic nodes.

From the Bladder. Lymphatic drainage originates at the mucosal, intramuscular, and extramuscular plexuses. The collecting vessels end in the external iliac lymph nodes (Fig. 21.13).

From the Urethra. The lymphatic vessels from the prostatic and membranous urethra in the male and the female drain to the internal iliac nodes. The lymphatic vessels of the anterior male urethra drain to the deep inguinal nodes.

From the Testis. The testis has a superficial plexus that lies deep to the tunica vaginalis and a deep plexus within the testicular parenchyma and epididymis. Four to eight collecting lymphatic trunks ascend at the spermatic cord following the testicular vessels, draining to the lateral and preaortic lymph nodes. The drainage of the ovary is, like the testicular, made by lymphatic trunks, which ascend with the ovarian vessels to the lateral and preaortic lymph nodes.

From the Ductus Deferens, Seminal Vesicle, and Prostate Gland. The lymphatic vessels from the ductus deferens drain to the external iliac nodes. Those from the seminal vesicle drain to the internal and external iliac nodes, and the prostatic lymphatic vessels drain to the internal iliac and sacral nodes.

From the Scrotum and Penis. The scrotal and penile lymphatic drainage goes to the superficial inguinal nodes.

From the Uterus and Uterine Tubes. Lymphatics from the cervix pass laterally to the parametrium and the external iliac nodes, to the internal iliac nodes, and to the rectal and sacral nodes. Lymphatic vessels from the lower part of the uterine body drain mostly to the external iliac nodes, following those from the cervix. The lymphatic vessels from the upper part of the uterine body, the fundus and the tubes, accompany the ovarian lymphatics with the ovarian vessels (Fig. 21.13).

From the Vagina. The lymphatic vessels from the vagina join the lymphatics of the cervix, rectum, and vulva (Fig. 21.13).

Retroaortic Lymph Nodes

The retroaortic lymph nodes have no special area of drainage; they are mostly regarded with the drainage of the posterior abdominal wall, to comprise the periphery of the lateral aortic groups and to participate in the interconnection of the surrounding groups.

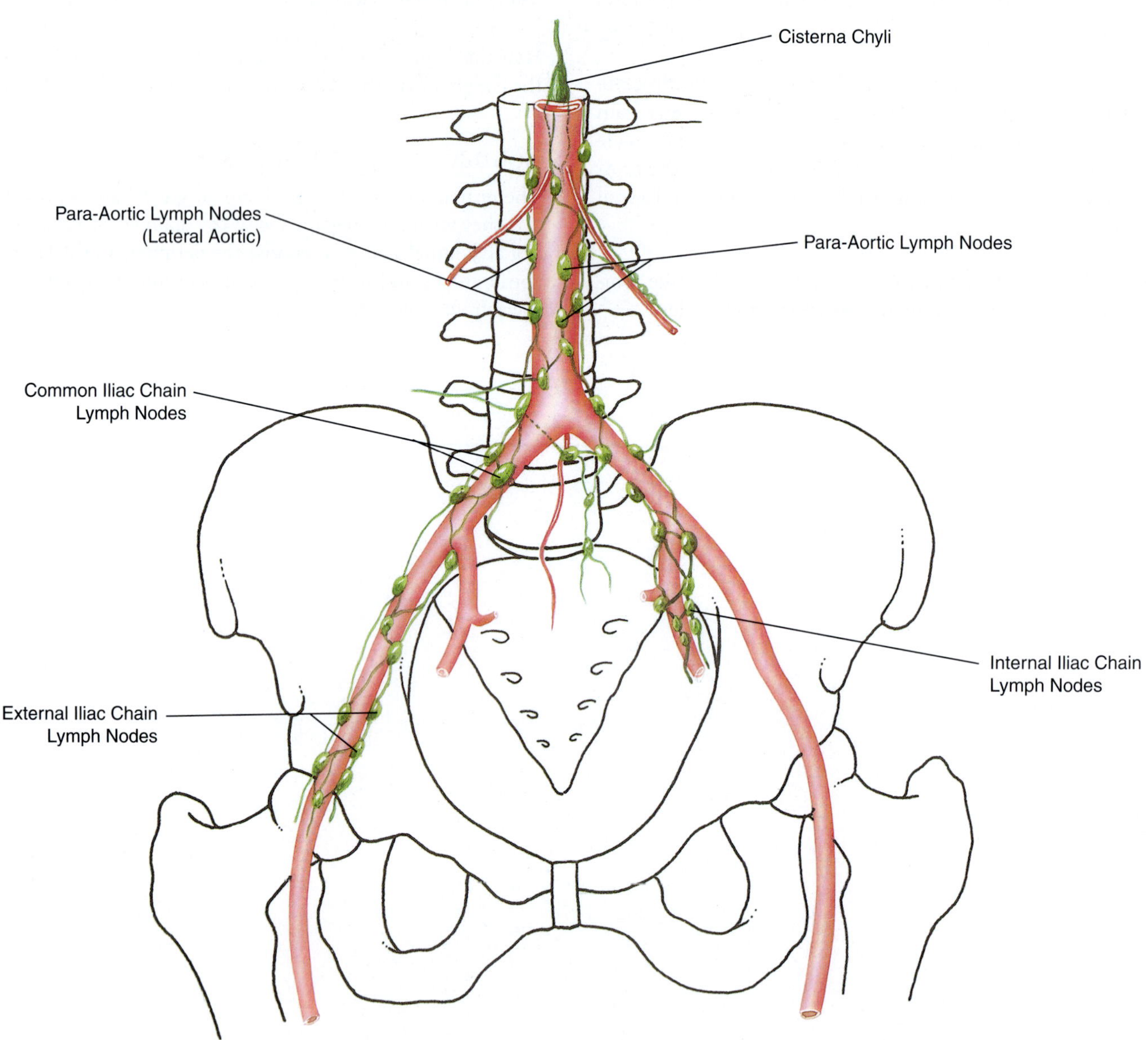

Figure 21.1. Schematic drawing showing the lymphatic drainage of the pelvis and abdomen through the internal iliac, external iliac, and para-aortic lymphatics and lymph nodes. Note the cisterna chyli behind the aorta.

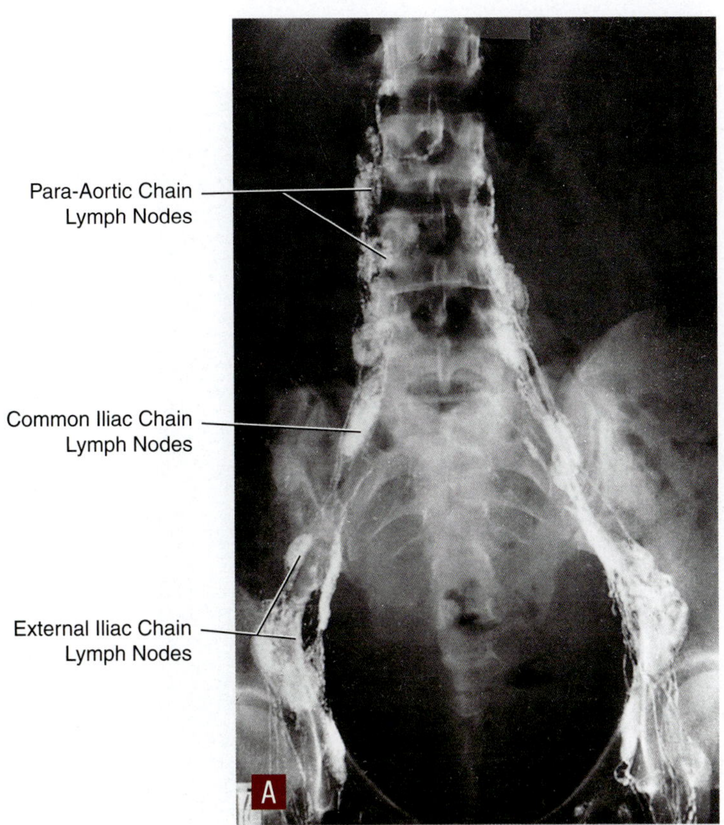

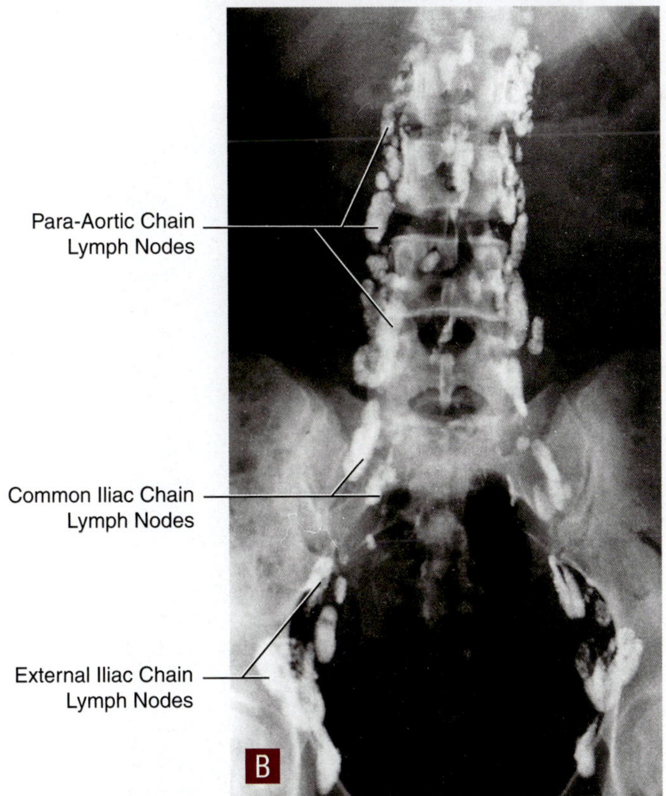

Figure 21.2. A, Early phase of a bilateral lymphangiogram showing the external iliac lymph nodes and the para-aortic lymphatics. B, Late phase of the lymphangiogram showing the lymph nodes of the external iliac and para-aortic groups. C, Early phase of bilateral lymphangiogram with the external and common iliac chain lymph ducts. D, Triangular configuration of the cisterna chyli at the level of T11. There is very early enhancement of the thoracic duct with lipiodol.

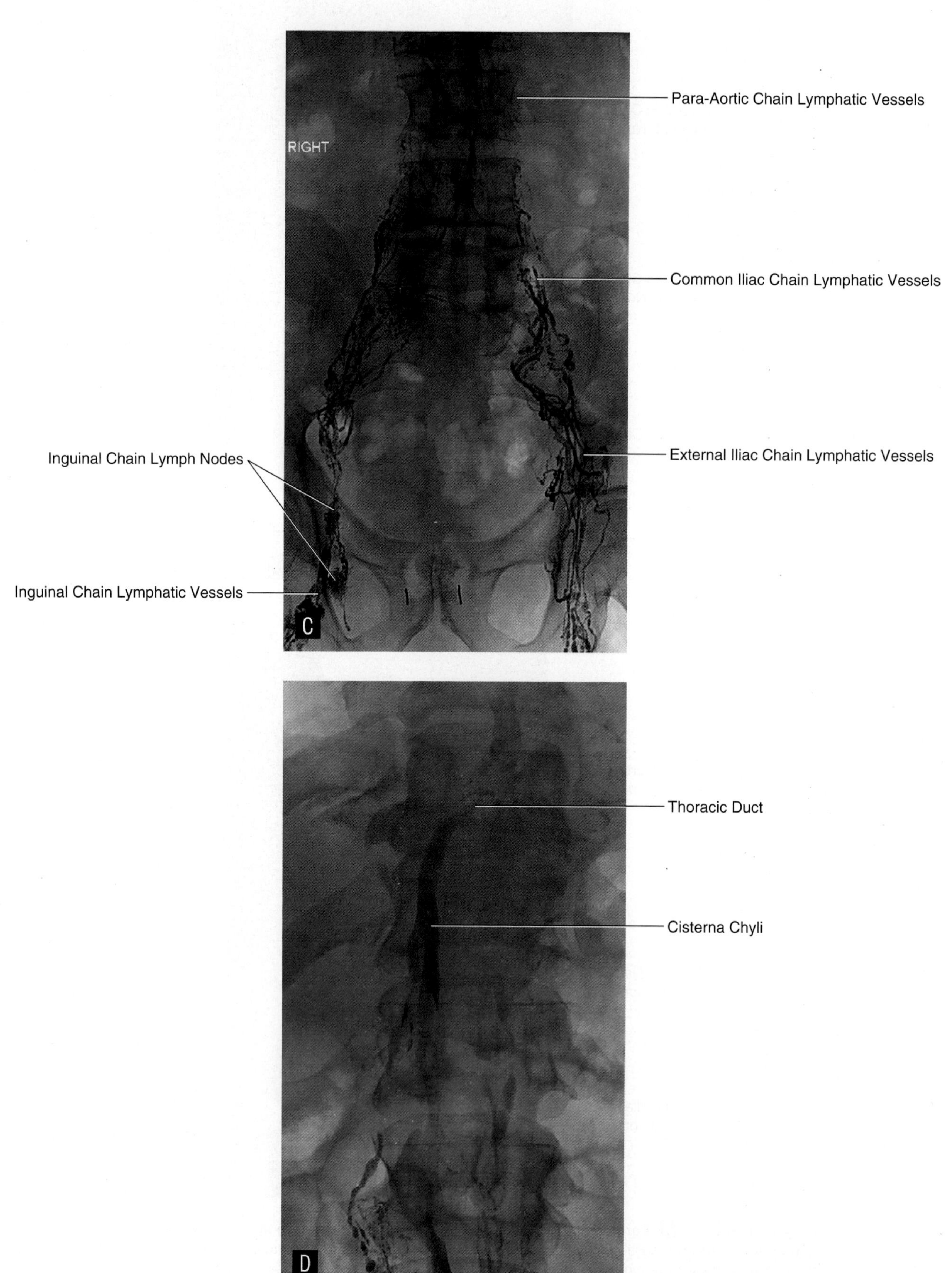

Figure 21.2. *Continued*

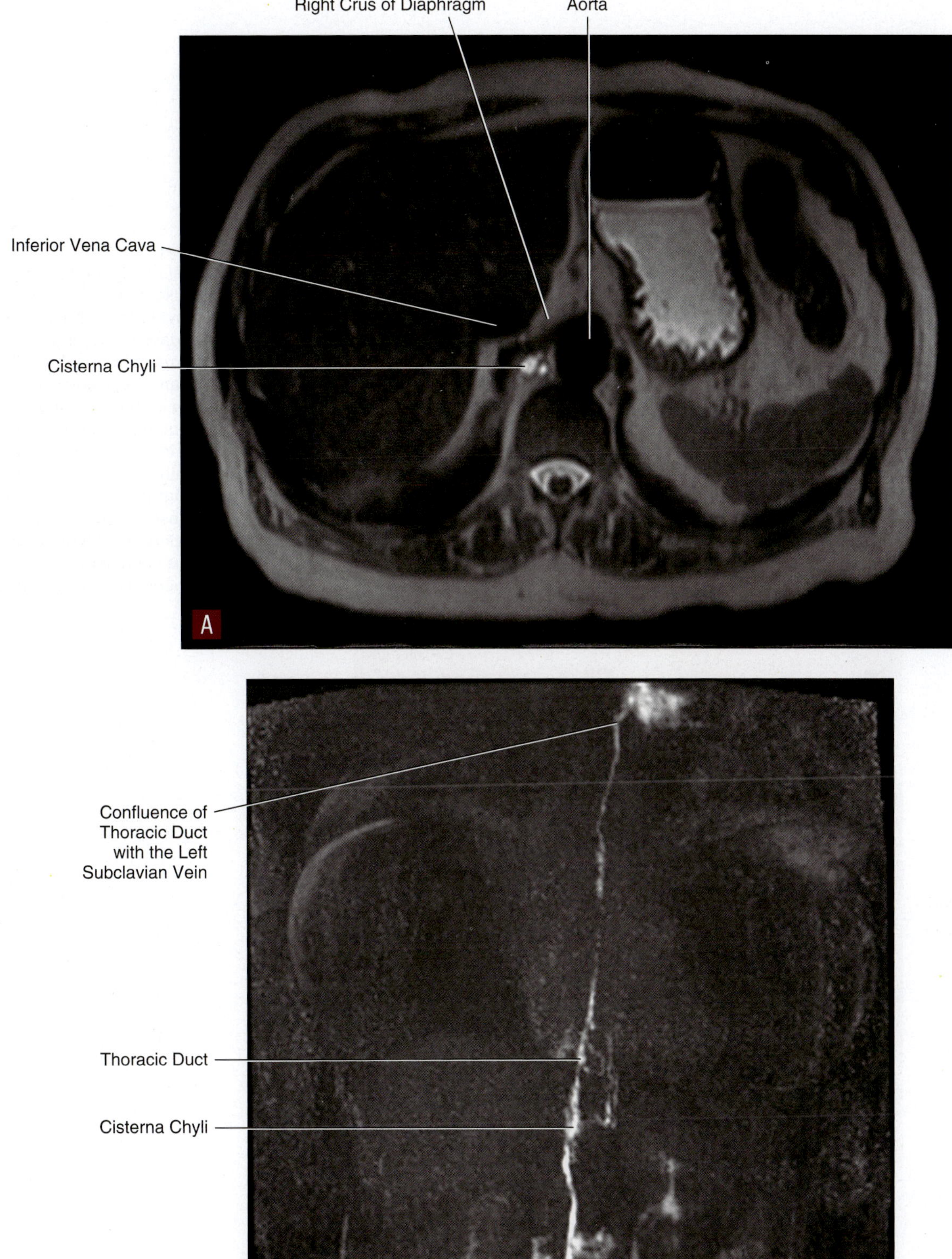

Figure 21.3. **A**, Axial T2-weighed magnetic resonance image at the level of the aortic hiatus with the cisterna chyli visible to the right of the aorta. **B**, MRI lymphangiogram of a normal cisterna chyli, thoracic duct, and confluence with the left subclavian vein.

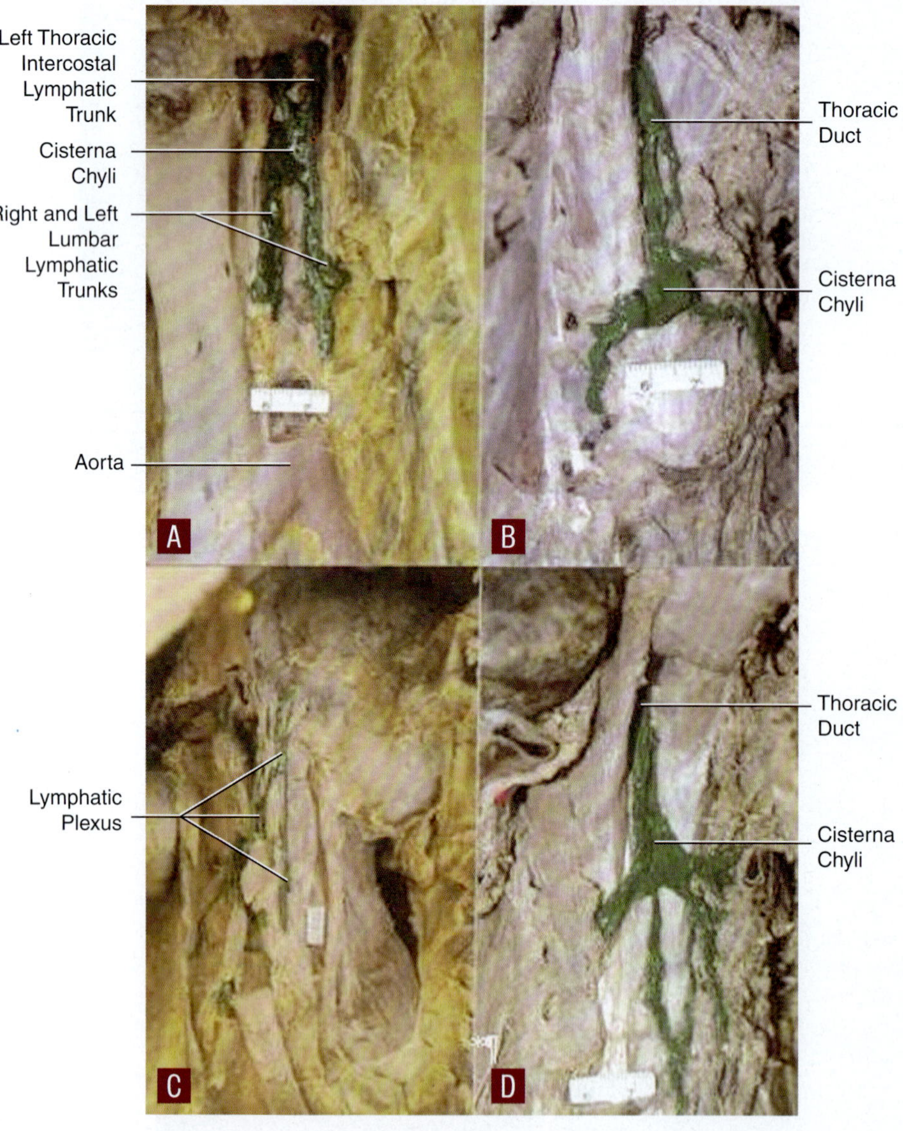

Figure 21.4. Lymphatic vessels of the lumbar region and cisterna chyli depicted after removal of the abdominal aorta in cadaveric preparations. The cisterna chyli may have several formats and is colorized in green in the illustrations. **A**, Square configuration. Note a left intercostal lymphatic trunk reaching the cisterna directly. **B**, Sigmoid configuration. **C**, Absent cisterna. Only a retroperitoneal lymphatic plexus is present. **D**, Triangular configuration.

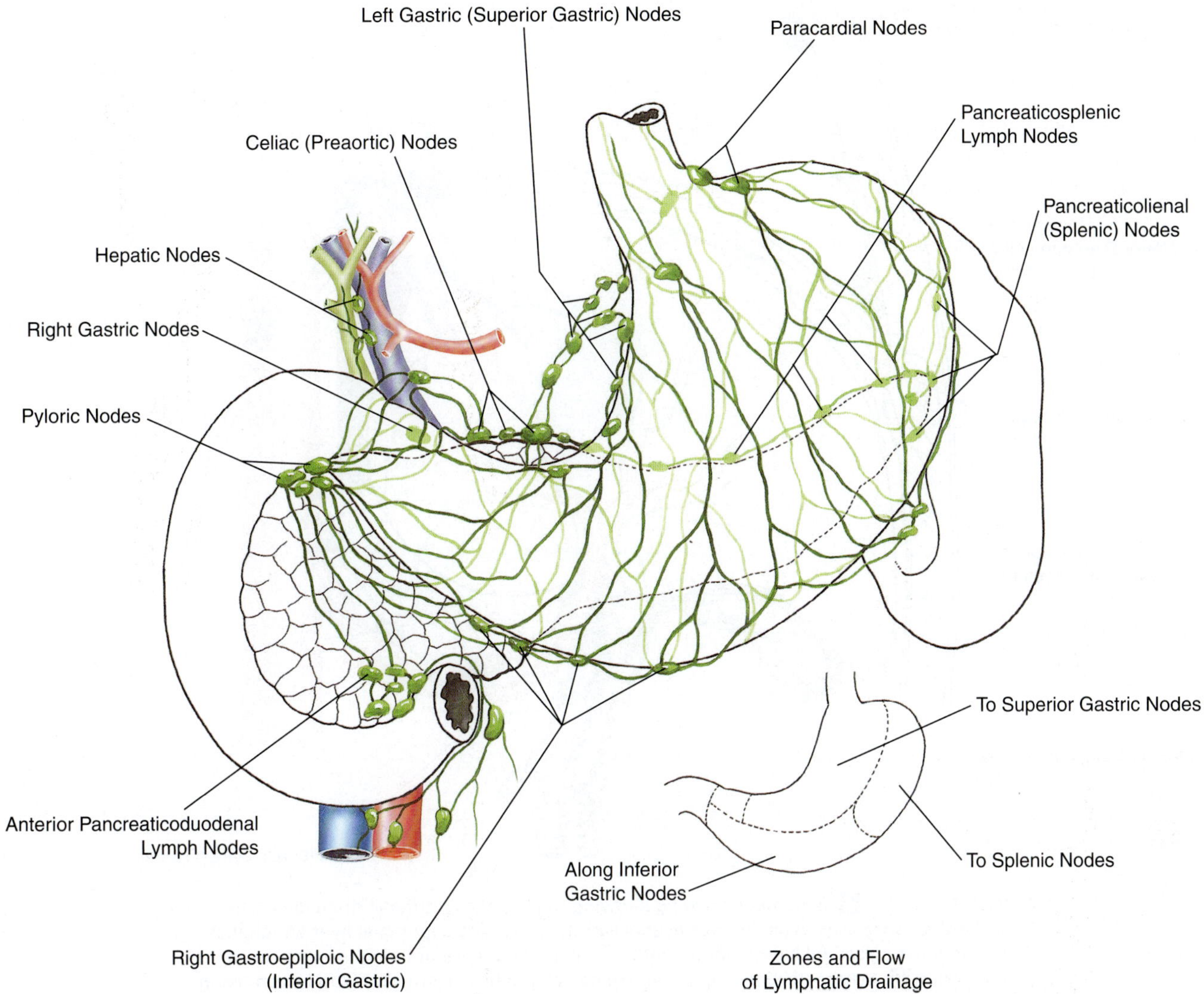

Figure 21.5. Schematic drawing showing the lymphatic drainage of the stomach, pancreas, spleen, and duodenum. Note in the insert the zones and flow of lymphatic drainage of the stomach.

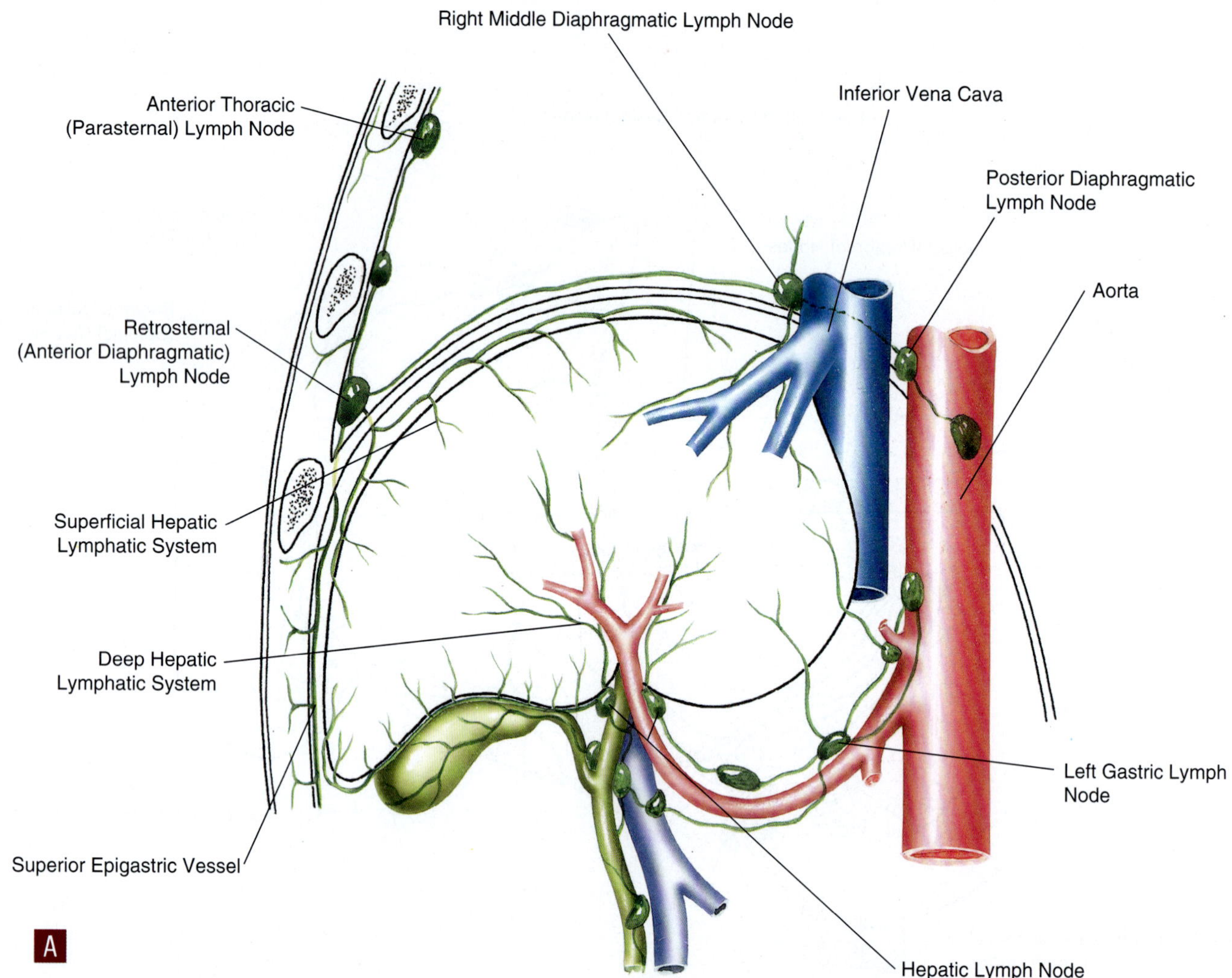

Figure 21.6. **A**, Schematic drawing showing the hepatic lymphatic drainage to the celiac lymph nodes as well as the mediastinal lymph nodes. The superficial liver lymphatics drain into the mediastinal lymph nodes, with the deep lymphatics draining into the celiac lymph nodes. **B**, Schematic drawing of the hepatic lymphatic system, showing lymph being produced in the space of Disse between hepatocytes and sinusoids. Lymph then drains into the network of vessels in the periportal space, known as the space of Mall. **C**, Direct puncture of the hepatic internal lymphatic system with a lipiodol lymphangiogram showing lymphatic hepatic channels flowing toward the porta hepatis. The portal vein lies between the two blue lines. **D**, Later phase of the same lymphangiogram showing extravasation of lipiodol into the duodenum. (B, Reprinted by permission from Springer Nature Itkin MG, Nadolski GJ. Modern techniques of lymphangiography and interventions: Current status and future development. *Cardiovasc Intervent Radiol*. 2017. C and D, courtesy of Maxim Itkin, MD.)

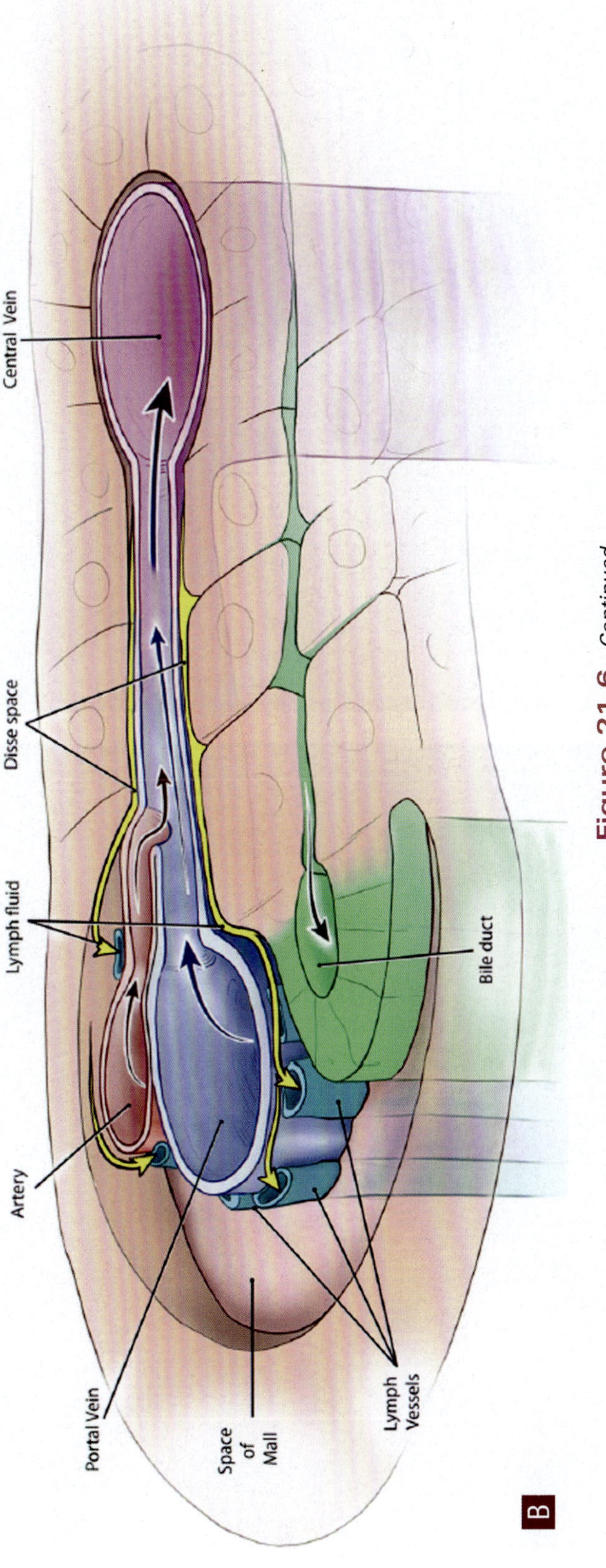

Figure 21.6. *Continued*

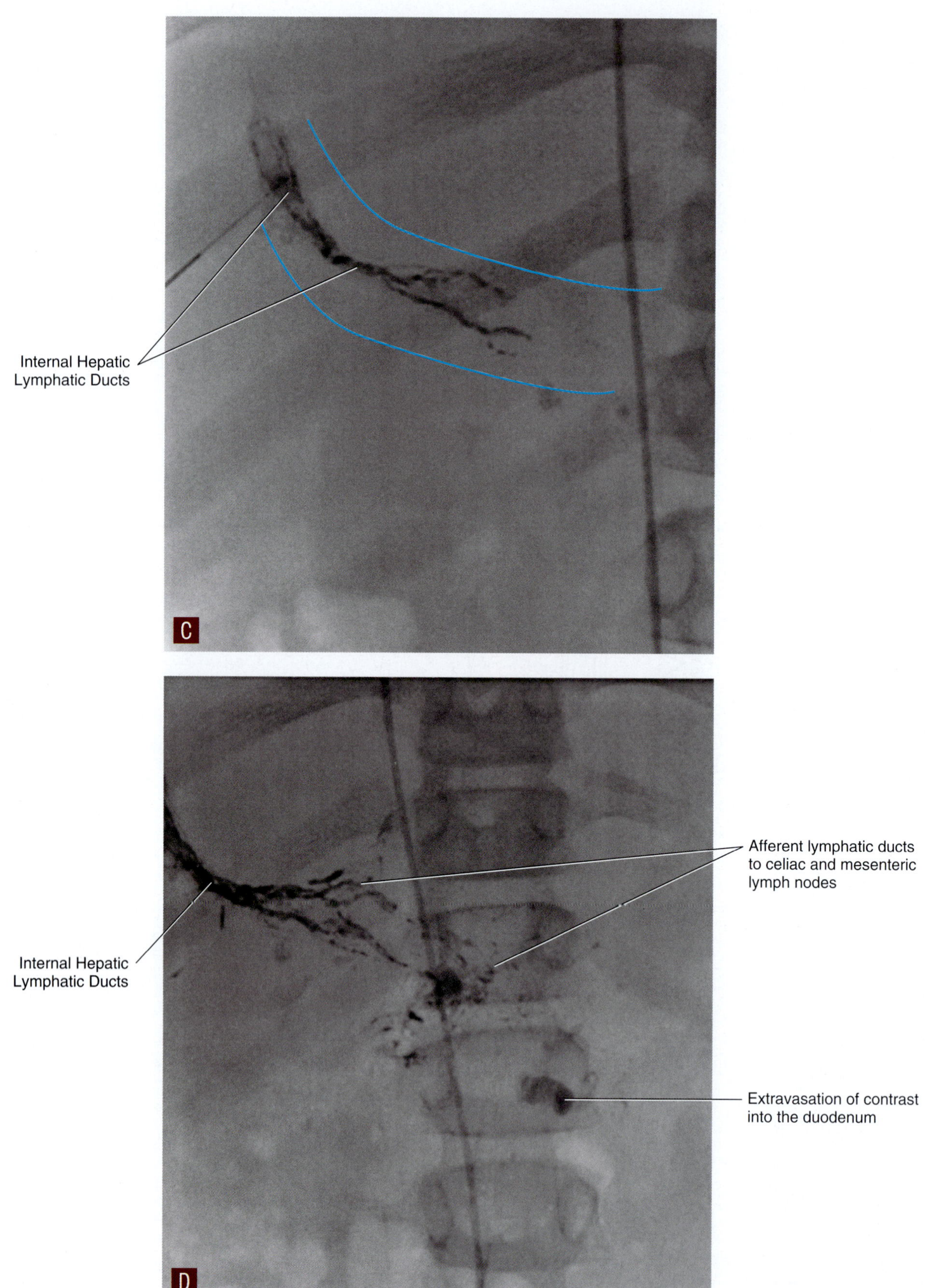

Figure 21.6. *Continued*

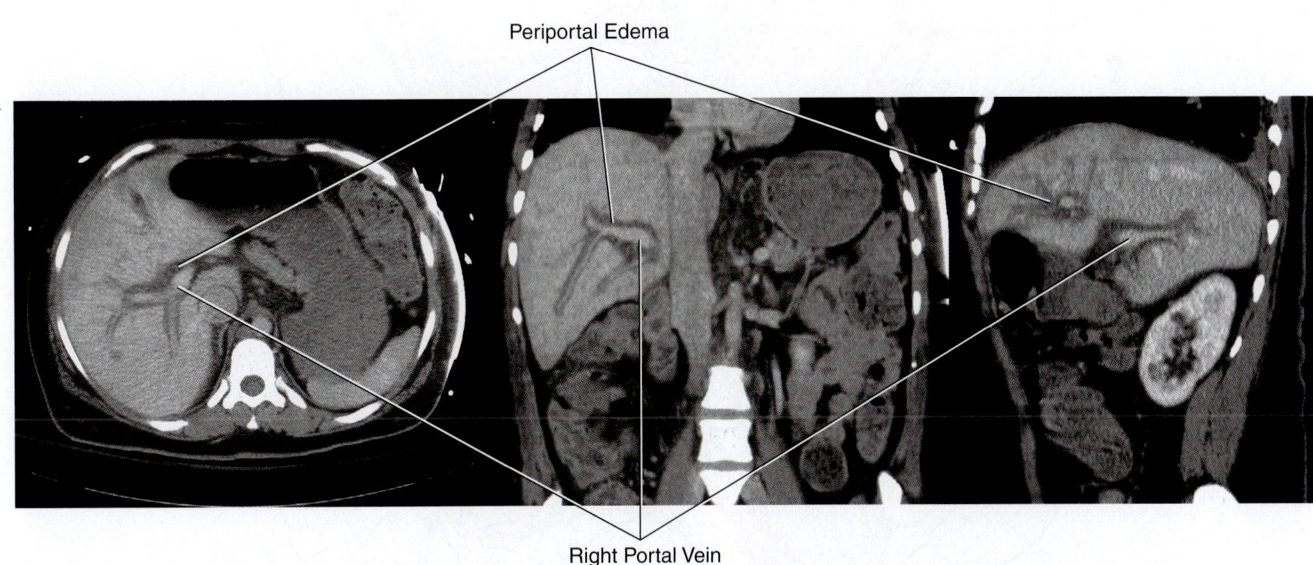

Figure 21.7. Axial, coronal, and sagittal contrast-enhanced CT in the portal venous phase showing periportal edema as hypoattenuation around the portal vein branches.

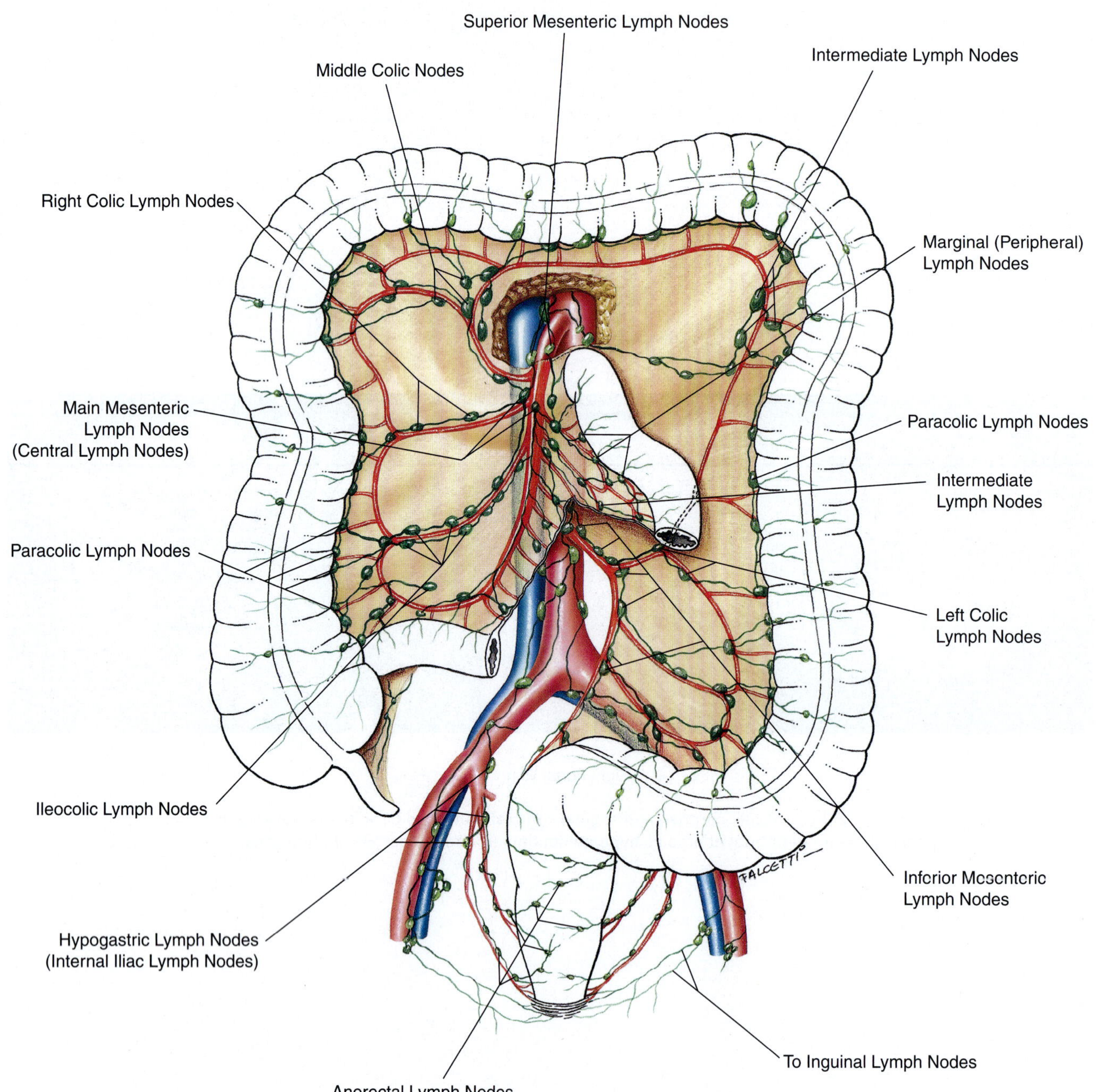

Figure 21.8. Schematic drawing showing the superior and inferior mesenteric lymphatic drainage. Note also the rectal lymphatic drainage demonstrated.

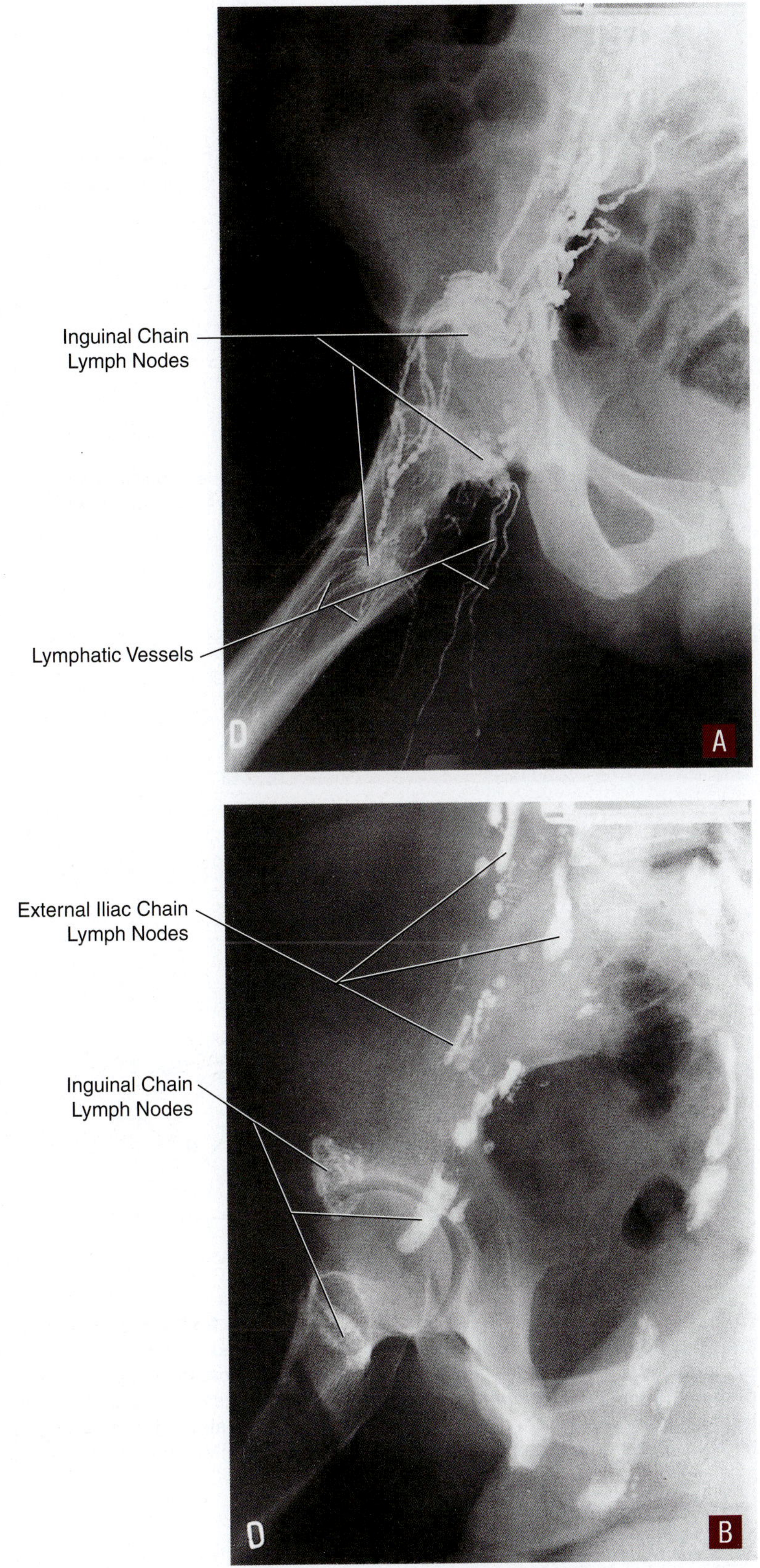

Figure 21.9. **A**, Lymphangiogram of the inguinal group of lymphatics and nodes draining into the external iliac group. **B**, Late phase of a lymphangiogram showing both sides of the external iliac lymph nodes in right oblique. **C**, Late phase of a lymphangiogram showing both sides of the external iliac lymph nodes in left oblique.

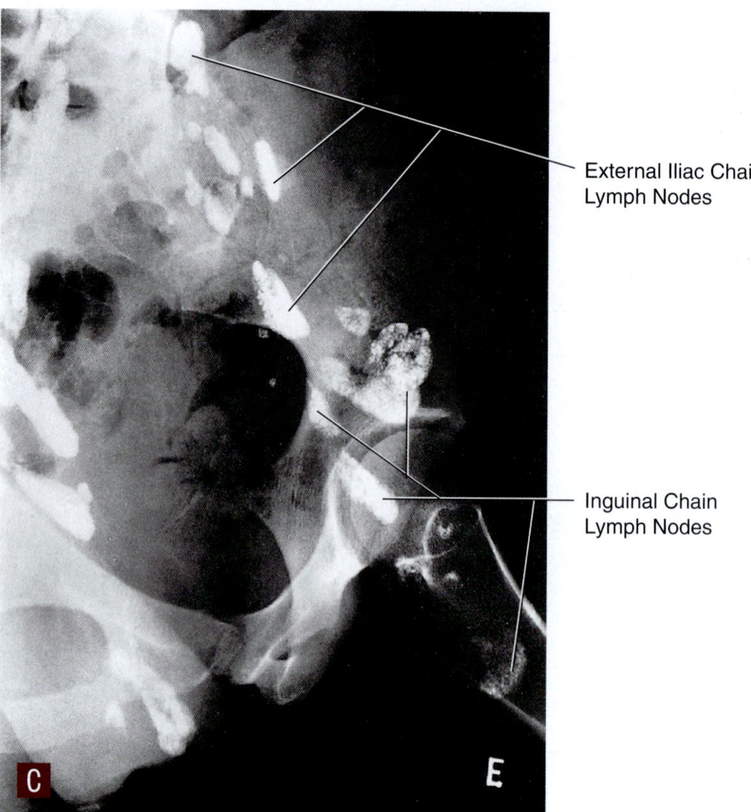

Figure 21.9. *Continued*

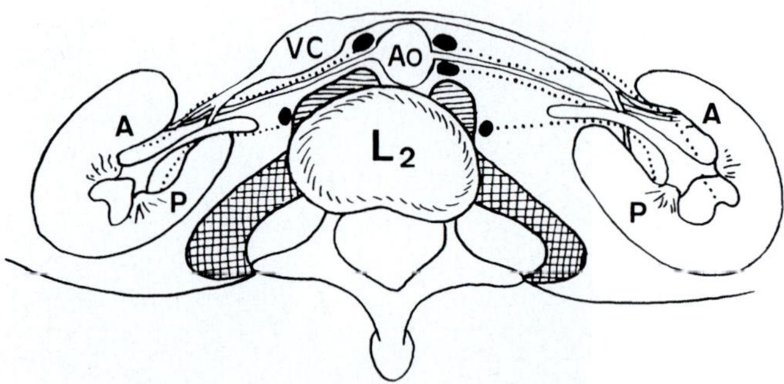

Figure 21.10. Inferior view of a schematic drawing from a transverse section in the retroperitoneal region. The collecting lymphatics are demonstrated with dotted lines. They run to the lateral aortic lymph nodes, in the renal artery origin. Note the lymphatics of the posterior region running to the diaphragmatic crux, from there they can reach the mediastinal lymphatics. A, anterior region of the kidney (ventral surface); Ao, abdominal aorta; L_2, second lumbar vertebra; P, posterior region of the kidney (dorsal surface); VC, inferior vena cava.

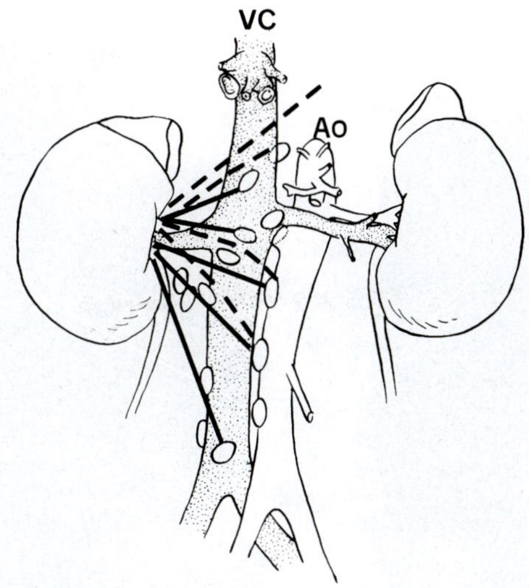

Figure 21.11. Lymphatic drainage of the right kidney. The anterior lymphatic channels are shown with the continuous lines; the posterior channels are shown with the dashed lines. Ao, abdominal aorta; VC, inferior vena cava.

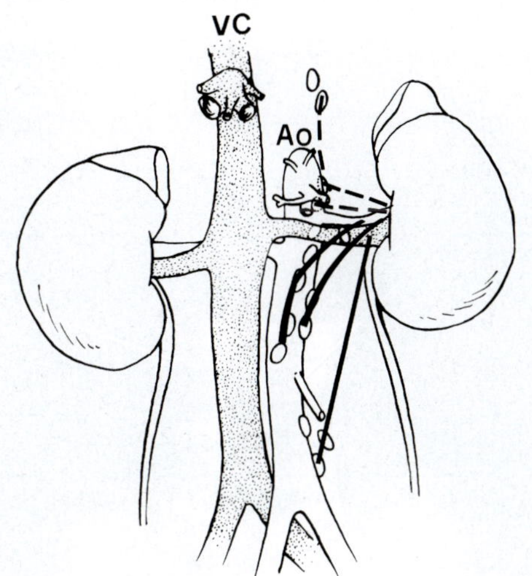

Figure 21.12. Lymphatic drainage of the left kidney. The anterior lymphatic channels are shown with the continuous line; the posterior channels are shown with the dashed line. Ao, abdominal aorta; VC, inferior vena cava.

22

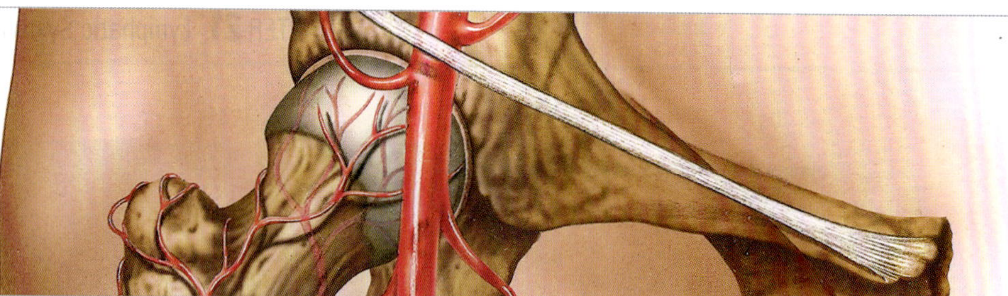

Arteries of the Lower Extremity

The common femoral artery is the continuation of the external iliac artery. It begins at the level of the inguinal ligament and ends at the origin of the deep femoral artery. The continuation of the common femoral artery is then called the superficial femoral artery (SFA). The SFA extends down the leg, where it passes through the adductor canal, giving origin to the popliteal artery (Figs. 22.1-22.3).

Knowledge of the vascular anatomy of the vessels in the groin and the relationship of the vessels with the femoral nerve is relevant. The common femoral artery is a common access to the thoracic and abdominal aorta and their branches. The femoral nerve (most lateral), the common femoral artery (in the center), and the common femoral vein (most medial) have a constant relationship when they pass under the inguinal ligament and reach the inguinal compartment, surrounded by muscles forming a bundle (Fig. 22.2). The common femoral artery is best palpated in the deepest fossa at the level of the inguinal crease. This is a very consistent landmark as the inguinal ligament does not alter its position regardless the patient's weight or body habitus.

Common Femoral Artery

Intravascular Ultrasound of the Common Femoral Artery

Intravascular ultrasound (IVUS) of a large artery such as the femoral artery shows the arterial wall structure in three layers: an inner echogenic layer, a middle hypoechoic layer, and an outer echogenic layer, histopathologically corresponding to the tunica intima, the tunica media, and the tunica adventitia. Next to the artery, the common femoral vein can be seen with a larger diameter and less well-defined layers (Fig. 22.4).

Branches

- Superficial epigastric artery
- Superficial circumflex iliac artery
- Superficial external pudendal artery
- Deep external pudendal artery
- Arteria profunda femoris
- Superficial femoral artery
- Muscular branches
- Descending genicular arteries

Superficial Epigastric Artery

This artery arises about 1 cm below the inguinal ligament and anastomoses with branches of the inferior epigastric artery and the opposite vessels (See Chapter 19, Fig. 19.1).

Superficial Circumflex Iliac Artery (Figs. 22.1 and 22.5)

Superficial External Pudendal Artery (Figs. 22.1 and 22.5)

Deep External Pudendal Artery (Figs. 22.1 and 22.5)

Muscular Branches

Deep Femoral Artery (Arteria Profunda Femoris) (Fig. 22.6)

It is the largest branch of the femoral artery, with an origin about 3.5 cm from the inguinal ligament. It arises laterally and posteriorly from the femoral artery (Figs. 22.7-22.11, 22.13, and 22.14). The deep femoral artery plays an important role in the blood supply of the femoral head. The medial and lateral femoral circumflex arteries supply the femoral head, together with the foveal artery, a branch of the obturator artery.

Branches

- Lateral circumflex femoral artery
  - Ascending branch
  - Descending branch
- Medial circumflex femoral artery
- Perforating arteries. There are usually four (Fig. 22.7)
  - First perforating artery
  - Second perforating artery
  - Femoral nutrient artery
  - Third perforating artery

The end of the deep femoral artery is called the fourth perforating—numerous muscular branches are present at that level.

Anastomoses

- Gluteal arteries—with terminal branches of the medial circumflex femoral artery
- Circumflex femoral arteries—with first perforating artery
- Perforating arteries—communicating with each other
- Fourth perforating artery—with superior muscular branches of popliteal arteries

Descending Genicular Artery (Figs. 22.1 and 22.15)

This artery branches from the SFA before the adductor's canal and anastomoses with the medial superior genicular artery.

Branches

- Saphenous branch—anastomoses with medial inferior genicular artery
- Muscular branches, articular branches

Superficial Femoral Artery (Figs. 22.1, 22.3, 22.5, 22.6, 22.10, 22.12-22.14)

The common femoral artery becomes the SFA distal to the origin of the deep femoral artery. Although some have advocated for a change in nomenclature by calling the SFA the "anterior femoral artery," for the purposes of this chapter, the term "superficial femoral artery" will be used to refer to the femoral artery distal to the deep femoral origin, up to the adductor hiatus. Its diameter averages about 5 mm, ranging widely between approximately 2.5 and 9.0 mm.

The SFA courses through the adductor canal surrounded by the sartorius, the vastus medialis, and the adductor longus, where it gives small muscular branches. Just proximal to the adductor hiatus, the descending geniculate artery arises and branches into the saphenous artery and the articular branch of the descending geniculate artery. A separate origin of the descending geniculate artery and the saphenous artery can also be seen in about half of cases.

The SFA is exposed to significant mechanical stresses during knee flexion, including foreshortening, radial compression, bending, torsion, axial tension, and axial compression. The effects of leg flexion on the SFA are not fully understood and remain a subject of investigation. However, an in-vivo study of the conformational changes of the SFA on flexion has shown that it usually foreshortens by approximately 13% and twists by 60°. Left-sided SFAs usually twist in a counterclockwise direction, whereas right SFAs usually twist in a clockwise direction.

Branches

Descending genicular artery (Figs. 22.1 and 22.15)

- Muscular branches

Popliteal Artery

The popliteal artery is the continuation of the SFA passing the adductor's canal, continuing until branching into anterior and posterior tibial arteries (Figs. 22.15-22.19).

Branches

- Cutaneous branches
- Superior muscular branches
- Sural arteries
- Superior genicular arteries
- Middle genicular artery
- Inferior genicular arteries

Cutaneous Branches

Superior Muscular Branches (Figs. 22.15, 22.18, and 22.19)

Two or three branches.

Sural Arteries (Figs. 22.15, 22.16, and 22.20)

Two arteries as a rule.

Superior Genicular Arteries (Figs. 22.15, 22.16, 22.18, and 22.21)

Branches

- Medial superior genicular artery
- Anastomoses with the descending genicular artery and medial inferior genicular artery
- Lateral superior genicular artery
- Anastomoses with the descending lateral circumflex, with the lateral inferior genicular artery, descending genicular artery, and medial superior genicular artery

Middle Genicular Artery (Figs. 22.15, 22.16, 22.18, and 22.21)

This artery is small and not always recognizable.

Inferior Genicular Arteries (Figs. 22.15, 22.16, 22.18, 22.21, and 22.22)

Branches

- Medial inferior genicular artery
  - Anastomoses with the lateral inferior genicular artery, the medial superior genicular artery, the anterior tibial recurrent artery and the saphenous branch, and the descending genicular artery.
- Lateral inferior genicular artery
  - Anastomoses with the medial inferior genicular artery, the lateral superior genicular artery, and anterior and posterior tibial recurrent and circumflex peroneal arteries.

Genicular Anastomoses (Figs. 22.15 and 22.22)

Superficial Network

- Fascia
- Skin
- Fat

Deep Network

- Articular surface
- Bone
- Marrow
- Capsule
- Synovial membrane

Participating Vessels

- Medial genicular artery
- Lateral genicular artery
- Descending genicular artery
- Descending branch of lateral circumflex femoral
- Circumflex peroneal
- Anterior tibial recurrent arteries
- Posterior tibial recurrent arteries

The popliteal artery most commonly branches into the anterior tibial artery and the tibioperoneal trunk. It is also called the trifurcation of the popliteal artery. The tibioperoneal trunk branches into the posterior tibial artery and peroneal arteries (Figs. 22.23 and 22.24). Some variations in the popliteal trifurcation are encountered (Figs. 22.25 and 22.26B).

Anterior Tibial Artery

This artery is one of the terminal branches of the popliteal artery. It originates in the back of the leg and passes forward between the two heads of tibialis posterior muscle and through the upper part of the interosseous membrane to the front of the leg, medial to the neck of the fibula, descending to the ankle and continuing to the dorsum of the foot, where it is named arteria dorsalis pedis (dorsal artery of the foot). Sometimes the anterior tibial artery originates high in the middle of the popliteal artery.

Branches (Figs. 22.26 and 22.27)

- Posterior tibial recurrent artery
- Anterior tibial recurrent artery
- Muscular branches
- Anterior medial malleolar artery
- Anterior lateral malleolar artery

Posterior Tibial Recurrent Artery (Fig. 22.23)

This inconstant branch arises before crossing the interosseous membrane.

Anterior Tibial Recurrent Artery (Figs. 22.23 and 22.24)

This artery arises from the frontal part of the anterior tibial artery, after crossing the interosseous membrane.

Muscular Branches (Fig. 22.24)

Muscular branches are numerous and anastomose with the posterior tibial and peroneal arteries.

Anterior Medial Malleolar Artery (Figs. 22.28 and 22.29)

This artery anastomoses with the posterior tibial artery and medial plantar arteries.

Anterior Lateral Malleolar Artery (Fig. 22.29)

The anterior lateral malleolar artery anastomoses with the perforating branch of the peroneal artery and ascending twigs from lateral tarsal artery.

Anastomosis at the Ankle Level (Fig. 22.26)

- Medial malleolar network
  - Anterior medial malleolar branch of anterior tibial artery
  - Medial tarsal branch of dorsalis pedis
  - Malleolar-calcaneal branches of posterior tibial arteries
  - Branches from the medial plantar artery

- Lateral malleolar network
  - Anterior lateral malleolar branch of anterior tibial artery
  - Lateral tarsal branch of dorsalis pedis
  - Perforating and calcaneal branch of peroneal and rami from the lateral plantar artery

Arteries of the Foot

The anterior arteries of the foot are distal branches of the anterior tibial artery. The angiosomes supplied by the anterior tibial artery can be seen in Fig. 22.28.

Anterior Tibial Branches in the Foot (Figs. 22.30-22.34)

Arteria Dorsalis Pedis (Dorsal Artery of the Foot)

Extension of the anterior tibial artery on the dorsal aspect of the foot.

Branches

- Tarsal arteries
  - Laterals
  - Medials—join the medial malleolar network
- Arcuate artery
  - Anastomoses with the lateral tarsal and lateral plantar arteries; gives off the second, third, and fourth dorsal metatarsal arteries
- Dorsal metatarsal arteries

Joined by the proximal and distal perforating arteries from the plantar arch, and plantar metatarsal arteries, respectively. The dorsal metatarsal arteries divide distally into two dorsal digital branches for the sides of adjoining toes. The fourth dorsal metatarsal artery gives off a lateral branch to the fifth toe. The first dorsal metatarsal artery arises from the dorsal artery of the foot before it passes into the sole, branching distally to the great toe and to the adjoining sides of the first and second toes.

Posterior Tibial Artery

This artery arises from the tibioperoneal trunk, which is the continuity of the popliteal artery after the origin of the anterior tibial artery. The posterior tibial artery passes downward on the back of the leg, reaching the foot, and passes in the back of the medial malleolus. It divides into the medial and lateral plantar arteries (Figs. 22.24, 22.26-22.28, 22.30, and 22.31).

Branches

- Circumflex fibular artery
- Nutrient artery
- Muscular branches
- Communicating branch
- Medial malleolar branches

Circumflex Fibular Artery

The circumflex fibular artery may arise from the anterior tibial artery.

Peroneal Artery (Fibular Artery) (Figs. 22.23-22.28, 22.35-22.38)

The peroneal artery is positioned between the tibia and fibula. This artery arises from the tibioperoneal trunk a few centimeters after the origin of the posterior tibial artery. The angiosomes supplied by the peroneal artery can be seen in Fig. 22.28.

Branches

- Muscular branches
- Nutrient artery of the fibula
- Perforating branch (through interosseous membrane)
  - Arises 5 cm above the lateral malleolus. Anastomoses with the anterior lateral malleolar artery. May take the place of the arteria dorsalis pedis.
  - Communicating branch (anastomoses with the communicating branch of the posterior tibial artery) (Figs. 22.35-22.38).
- Calcaneal (terminal) branches (communicates with the calcaneal branches of the posterior tibial artery and anterior lateral malleolar artery)

Nutrient Artery of the Tibia

The nutrient artery of the tibia is one of the largest nutrient arteries in the body and arises from the proximal posterior tibial artery.

Muscular Branches

These branches provide nutrition to the muscles in the back of the leg.

Communicating Branch

The communicating branch is the transverse artery in the back of the tibia and anastomoses with the communicating branch of the peroneal artery.

Medial Malleolar Branches

The medial malleolar branches are part of the malleolar network.

Arteries of the Foot

The arteries of the foot are distal branches of the posterior tibial artery. The angiosomes supplied by the posterior tibial artery can be seen in Fig. 22.28.

Posterior Tibial Branches in the Foot (Figs. 22.28, 22.30, 22.39-22.42)

Calcaneal Branches

These branches anastomose with the medial malleolar arteries and calcaneal branches of the peroneal artery.

Medial Plantar Artery

It is the smaller terminal plantar branch of the posterior artery. It passes along the base of the first metatarsal bone and the medial border of the first toe, anastomosing with a branch of the first metatarsal artery. This artery supplies three small superficial digital branches, joining the first, second, and third plantar arteries.

Lateral Plantar Artery

This artery is the largest terminal plantar branch of the posterior tibial artery. It runs lateral and distal to the base of the fifth metatarsal bone and turns medially to the area between the base of the first and second metatarsal bones, connecting with the distal aspect of the dorsal artery of the foot, completing the plantar arch.

Branches

- Muscular branches
- Superficial branches
- Anastomotic branches—to the lateral tarsal and arcuate arteries
- Calcaneal branch—occasionally present

Plantar Arch

Branches

- Three perforating branches
  - Anastomoses with the dorsal metacarpal arteries
- Four plantar metatarsal arteries
  - Each divides into two plantar digital arteries: distal perforating branch joining the dorsal metatarsal artery; first plantar metatarsal artery springs from the junction of the lateral plantar and dorsal artery of the foot; the digital branch for the lateral side of the fifth toe arises from the lateral plantar artery

Variations in the Arteries of the Foot

There are about six variations described for the plantar arteries of the foot (Fig. 22.43): types Ia and Ib; types IIa, IIb, and IIe; and type III.

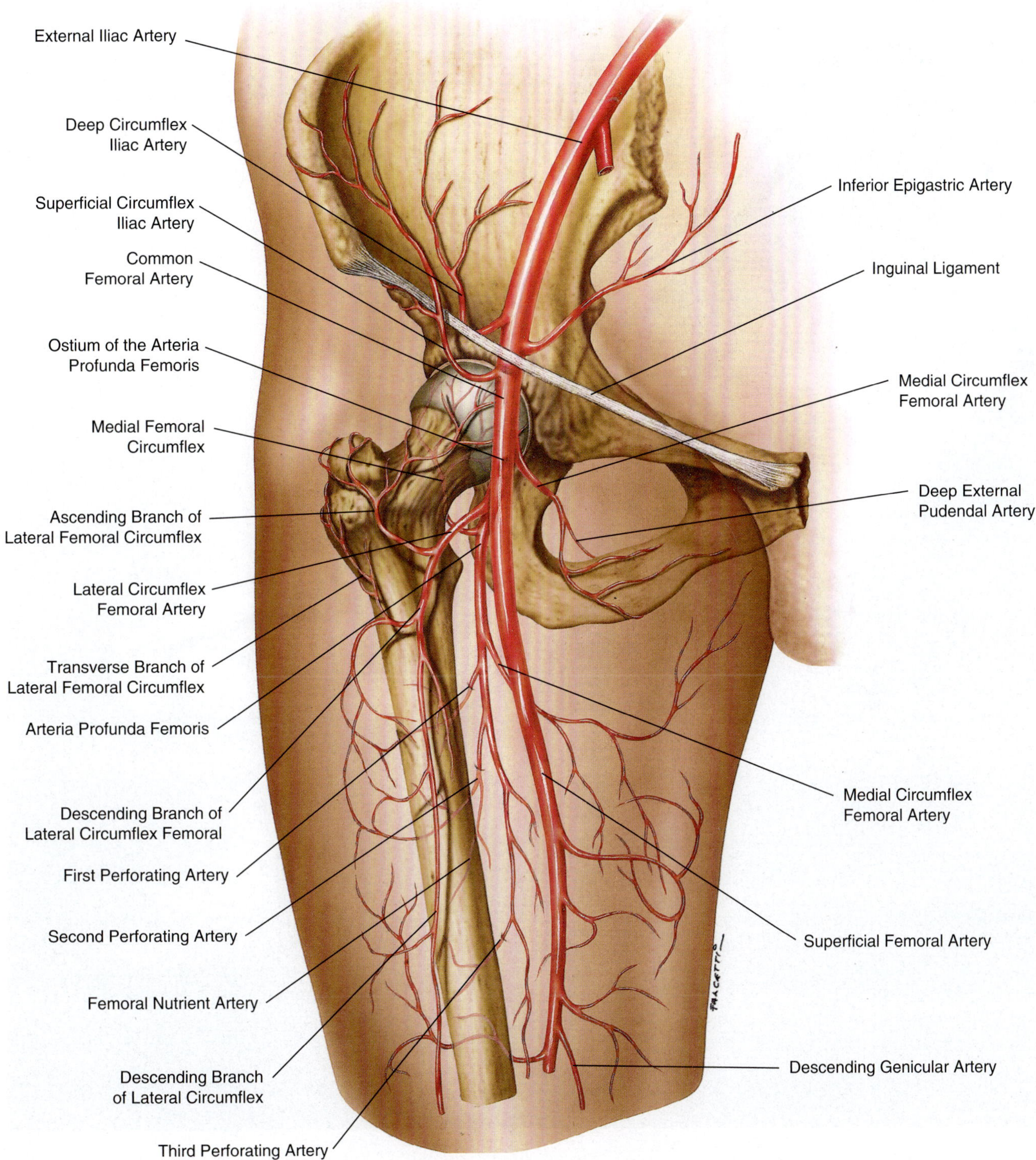

Figure 22.1. Schematic drawing demonstrating the right femoral artery and main branches. Note the perforating arteries, branches of the deep femoral artery.

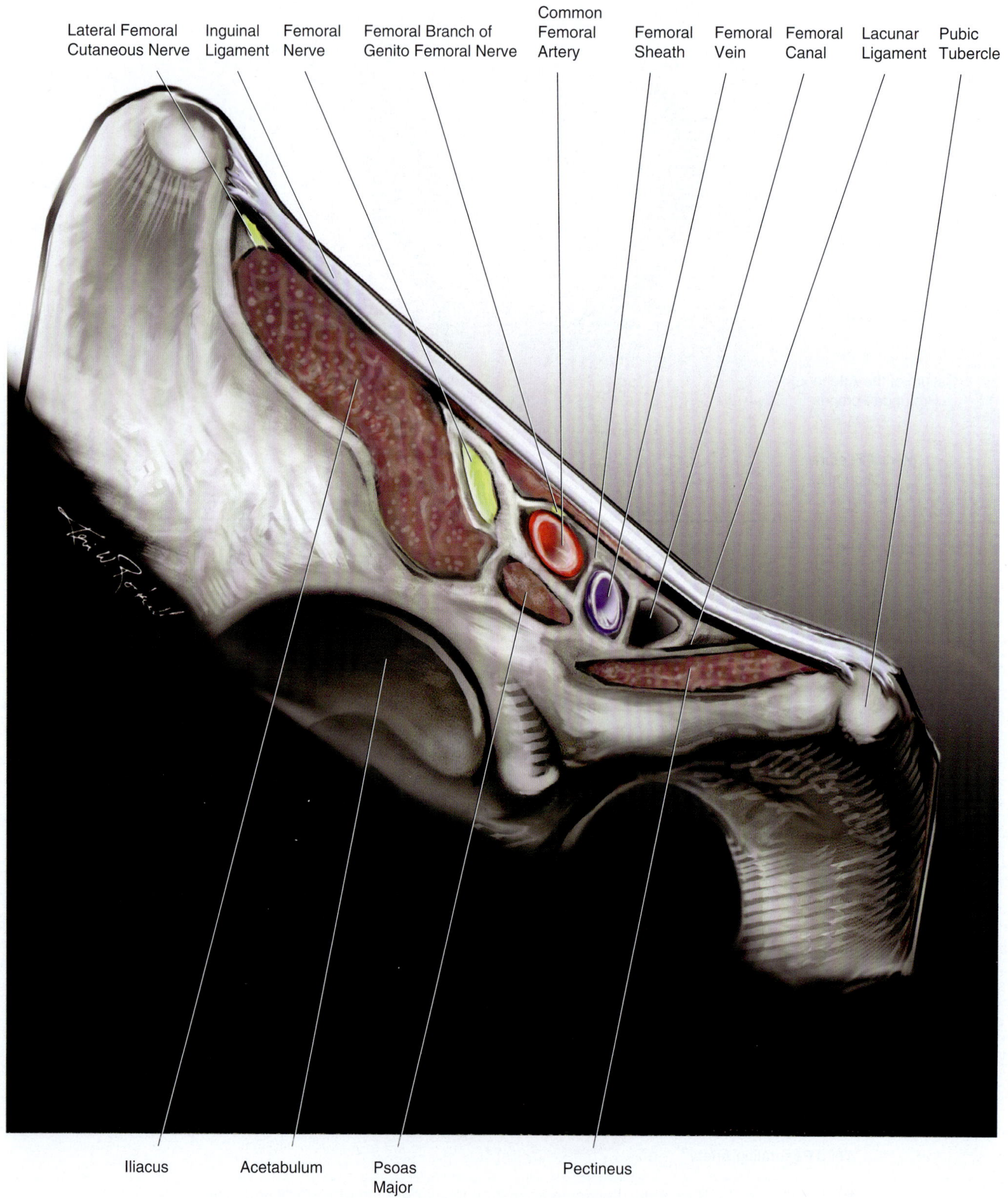

Figure 22.2. Schematic drawing demonstrating the vascular and nerve structures passing under the inguinal ligament through the right inguinal canal. View from below.

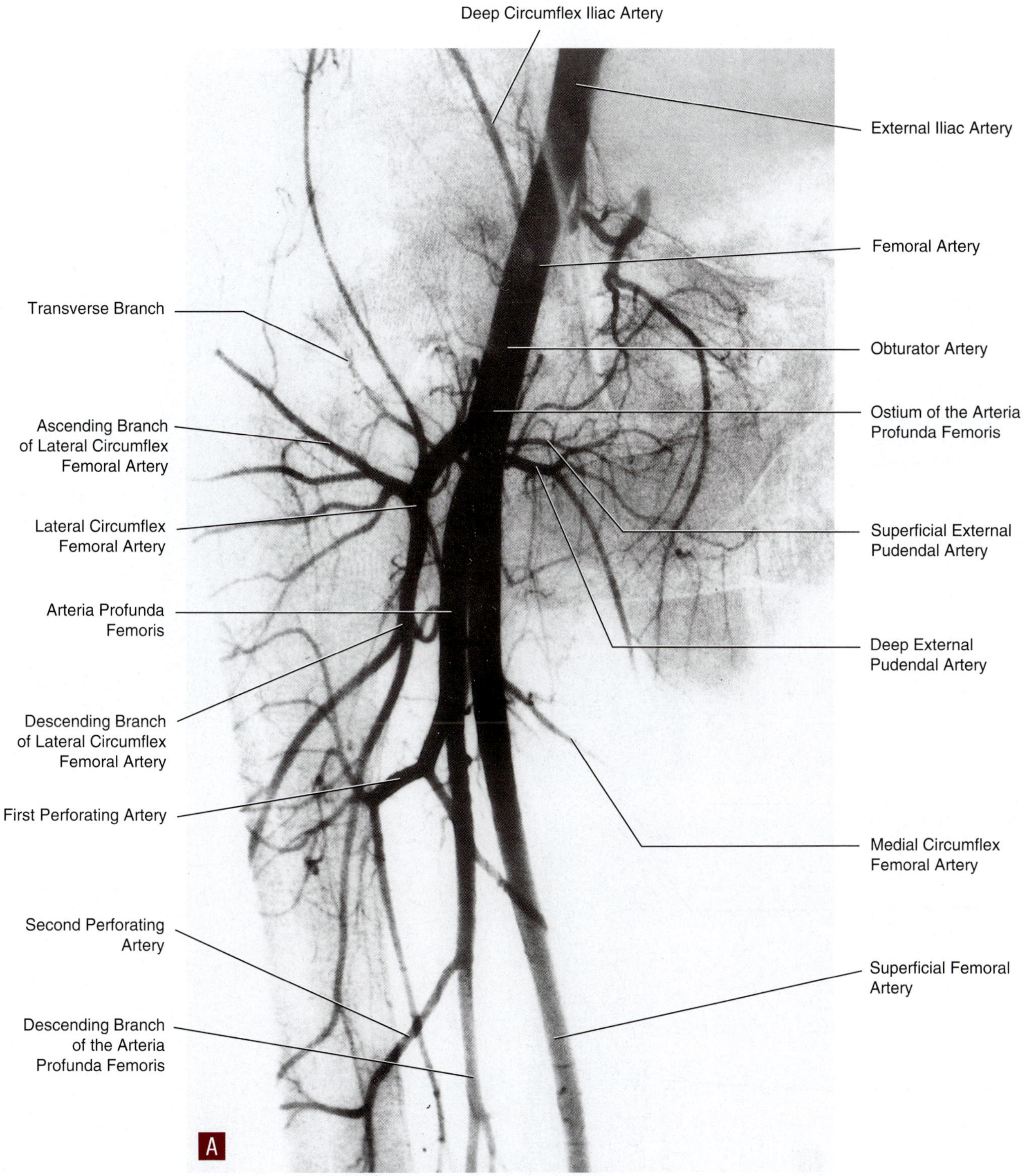

Deep Circumflex Iliac Artery
External Iliac Artery
Femoral Artery
Transverse Branch
Obturator Artery
Ascending Branch of Lateral Circumflex Femoral Artery
Ostium of the Arteria Profunda Femoris
Lateral Circumflex Femoral Artery
Superficial External Pudendal Artery
Arteria Profunda Femoris
Deep External Pudendal Artery
Descending Branch of Lateral Circumflex Femoral Artery
First Perforating Artery
Medial Circumflex Femoral Artery
Second Perforating Artery
Superficial Femoral Artery
Descending Branch of the Arteria Profunda Femoris
A

Figure 22.3. **A**, Angiography of the right femoral artery and main branches. **B**, Late phase of the femoral arteriography showing the companion veins of the femoral artery and branches. **C**, Angiography of the left femoral artery shows patency of all femoral branches.

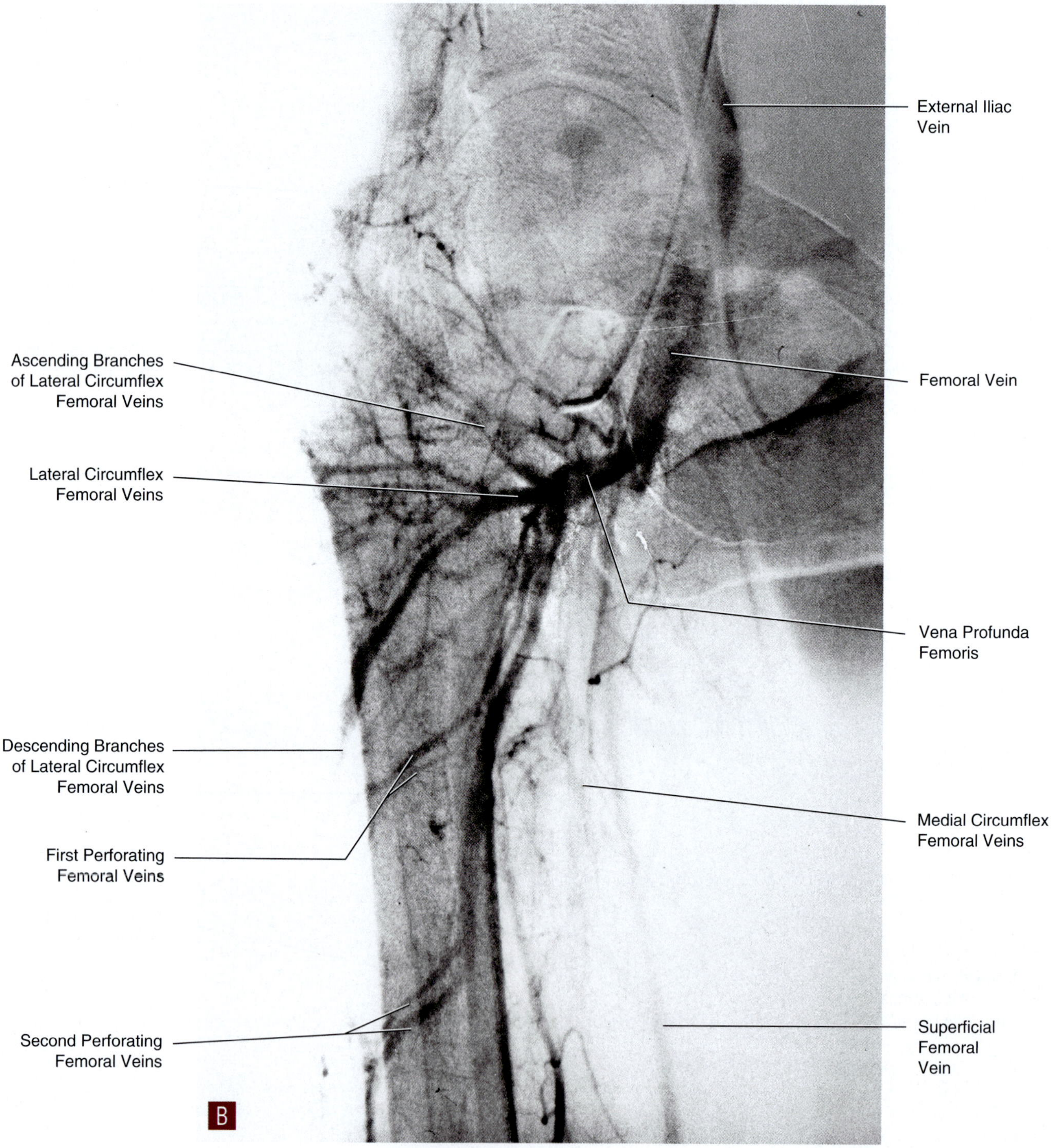

External Iliac Vein
Ascending Branches of Lateral Circumflex Femoral Veins
Femoral Vein
Lateral Circumflex Femoral Veins
Vena Profunda Femoris
Descending Branches of Lateral Circumflex Femoral Veins
Medial Circumflex Femoral Veins
First Perforating Femoral Veins
Second Perforating Femoral Veins
Superficial Femoral Vein
B

Figure 22.3. *Continued*

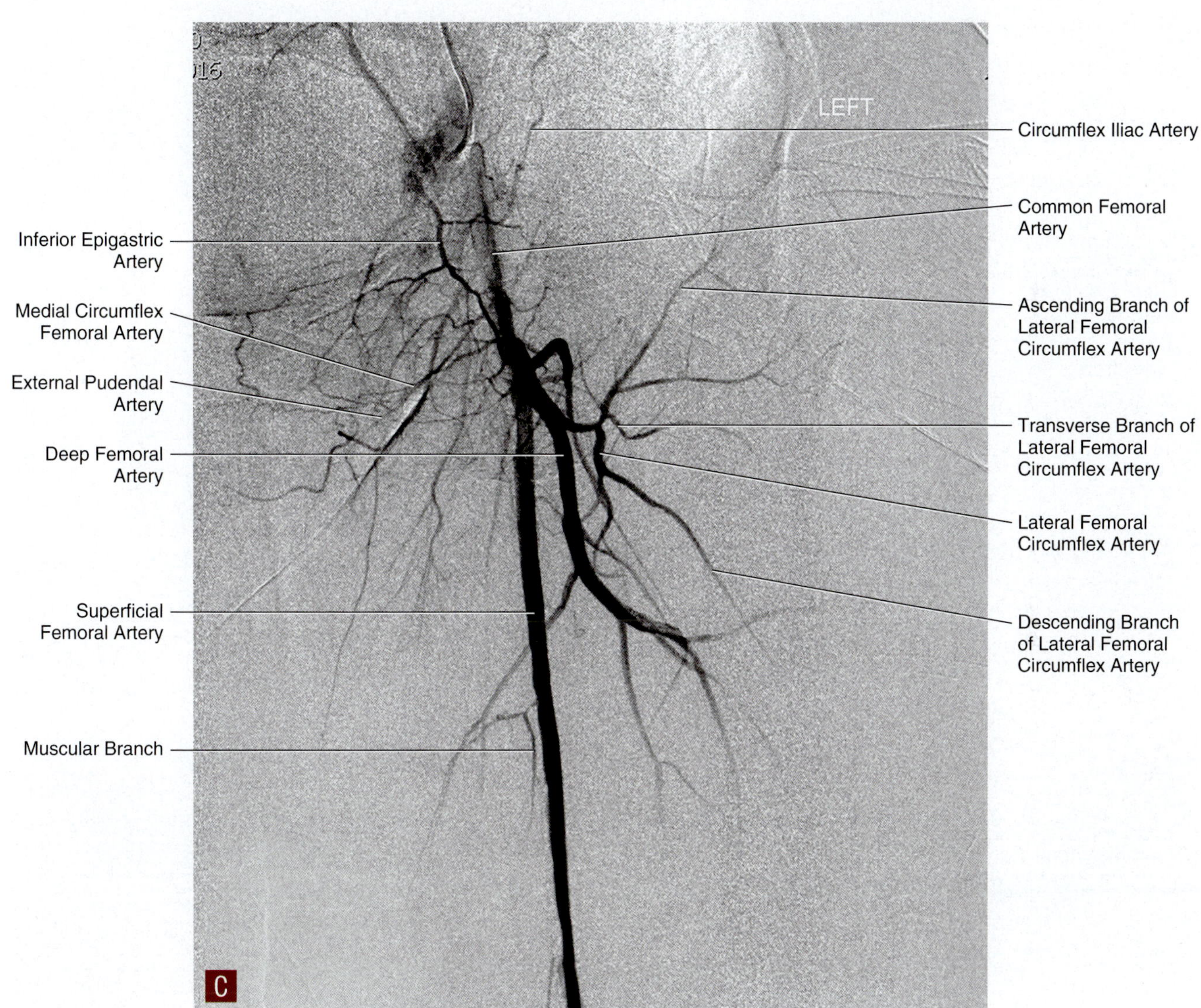

Figure 22.3. *Continued*

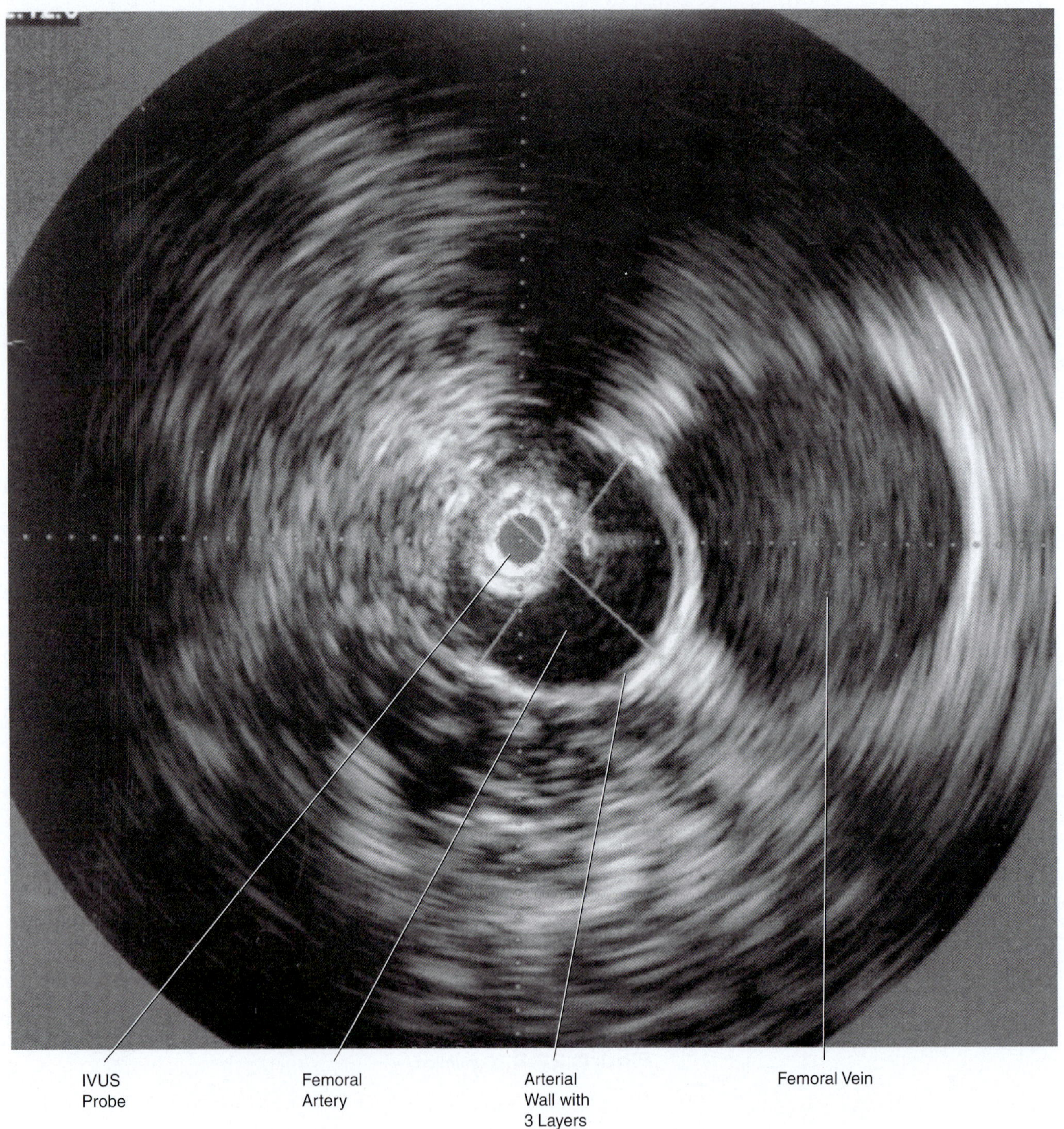

Figure 22.4. IVUS demonstrating the femoral artery and the femoral vein. Note the three layers of the arterial wall; the most internal hyperechoic, a middle layer hypoechoic, and an external hyperechoic layer fusing with the surrounding tissues. IVUS, intravascular ultrasound.

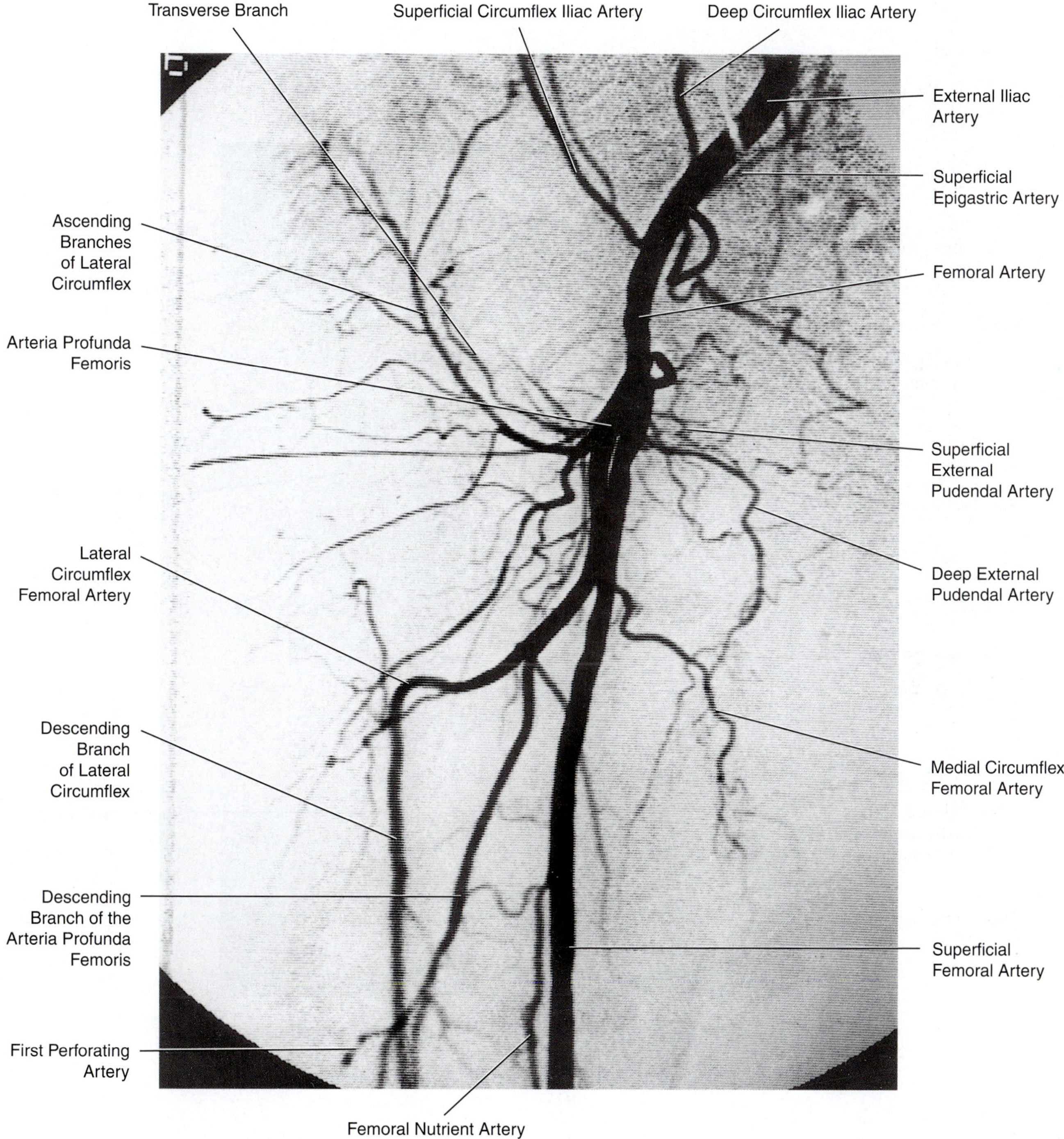

Figure 22.5. Angiogram of the right femoral artery and main branches.

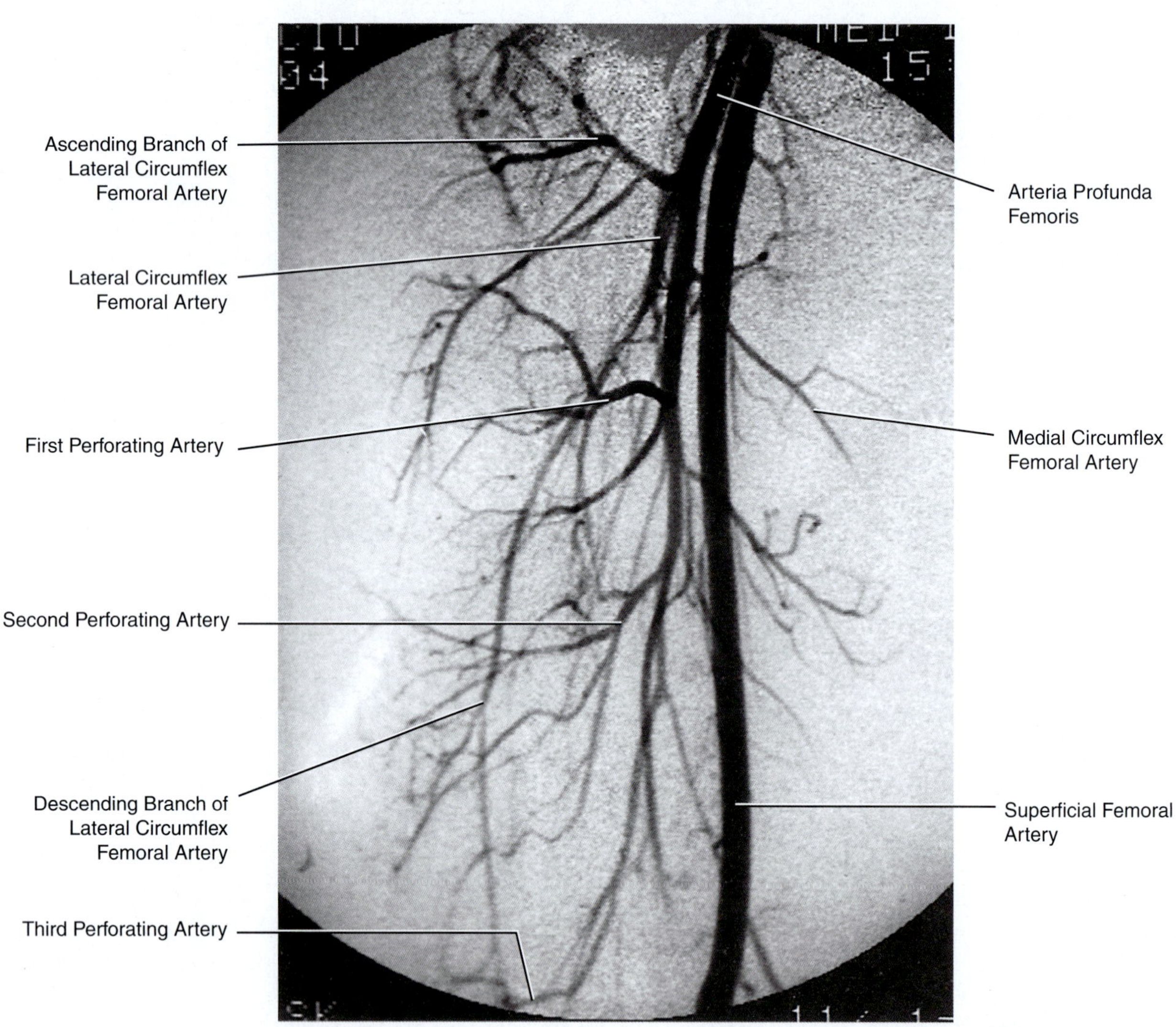

Figure 22.6. Angiogram of the right femoral artery and main branches.

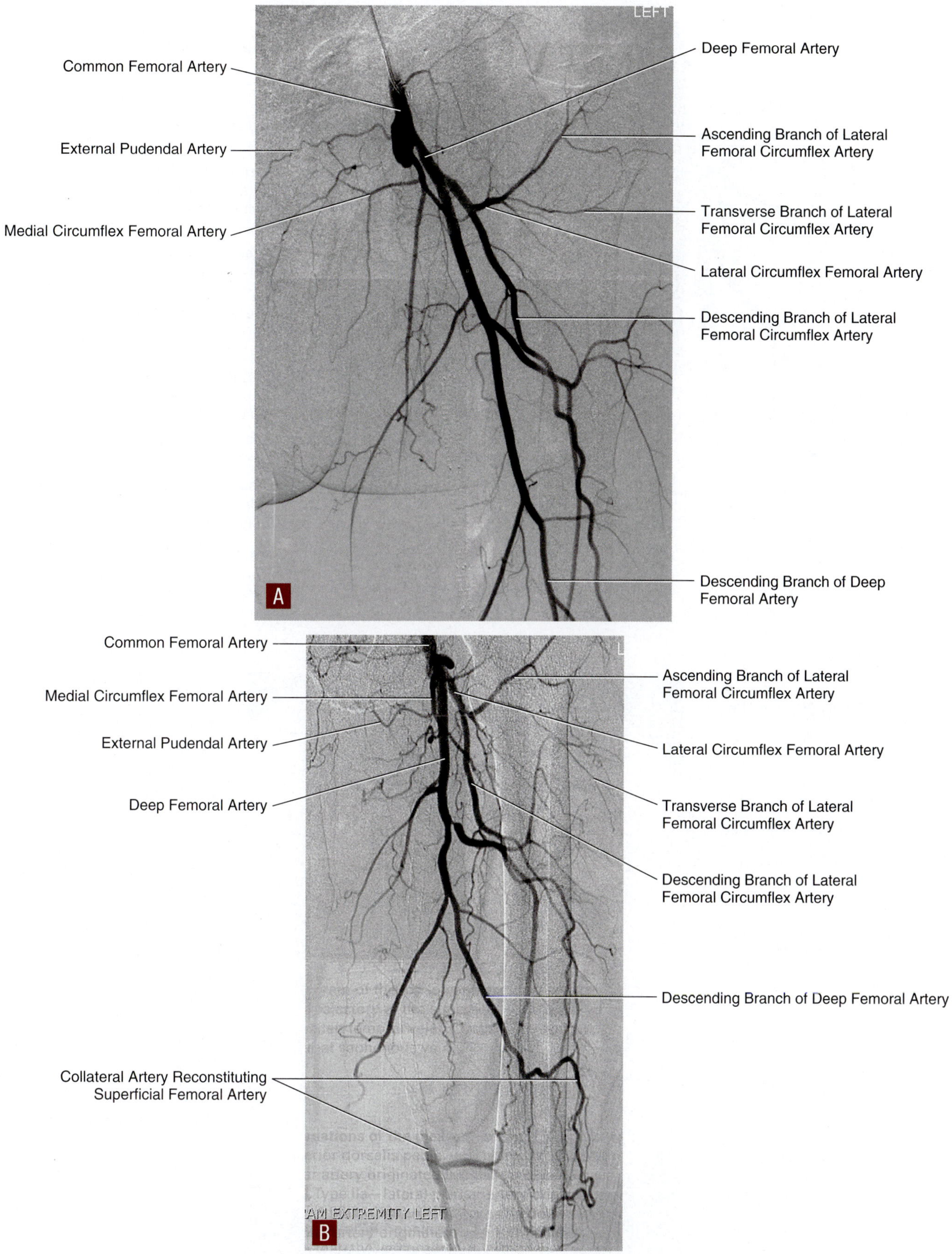

Figure 22.7. Angiogram of the left lower extremity at level of the thigh. **A**, Left profunda femoral artery and branches are patent. The left SFA is occluded at the origin. **B**, Long occlusion of the left SFA. Note the collateral circulation between the deep femoral artery muscular branches and the distal SFA at the level of the adductor canal. SFA, superficial femoral artery.

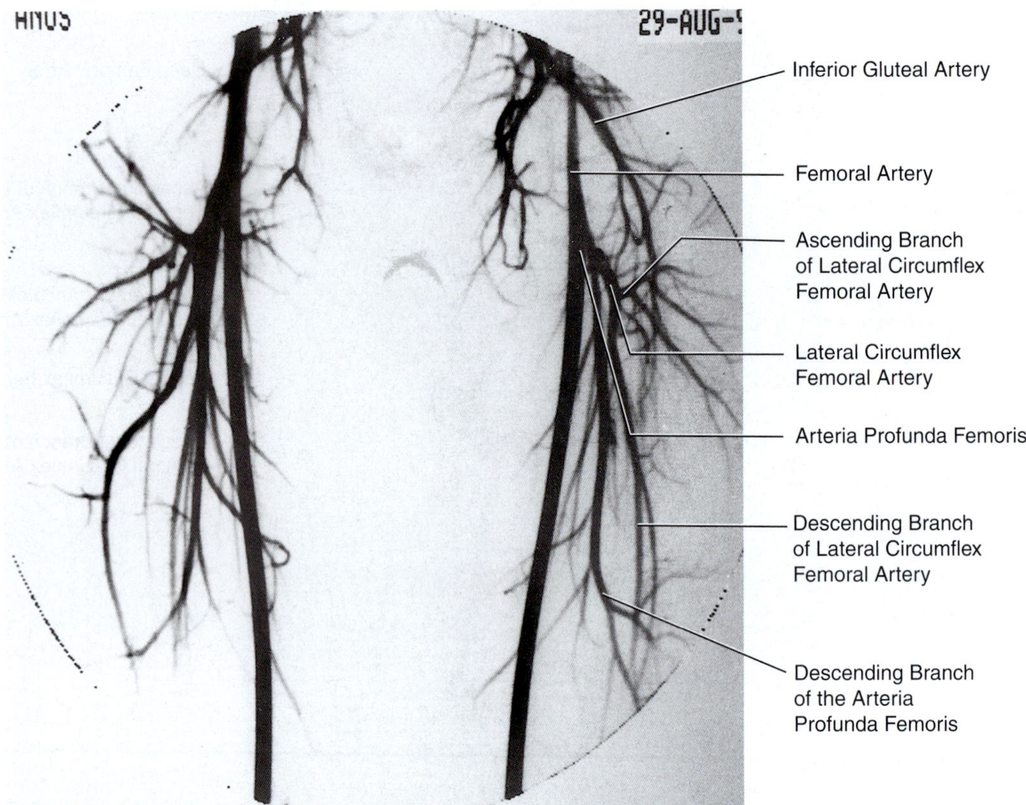

Figure 22.8. Angiogram of both femoral arteries.

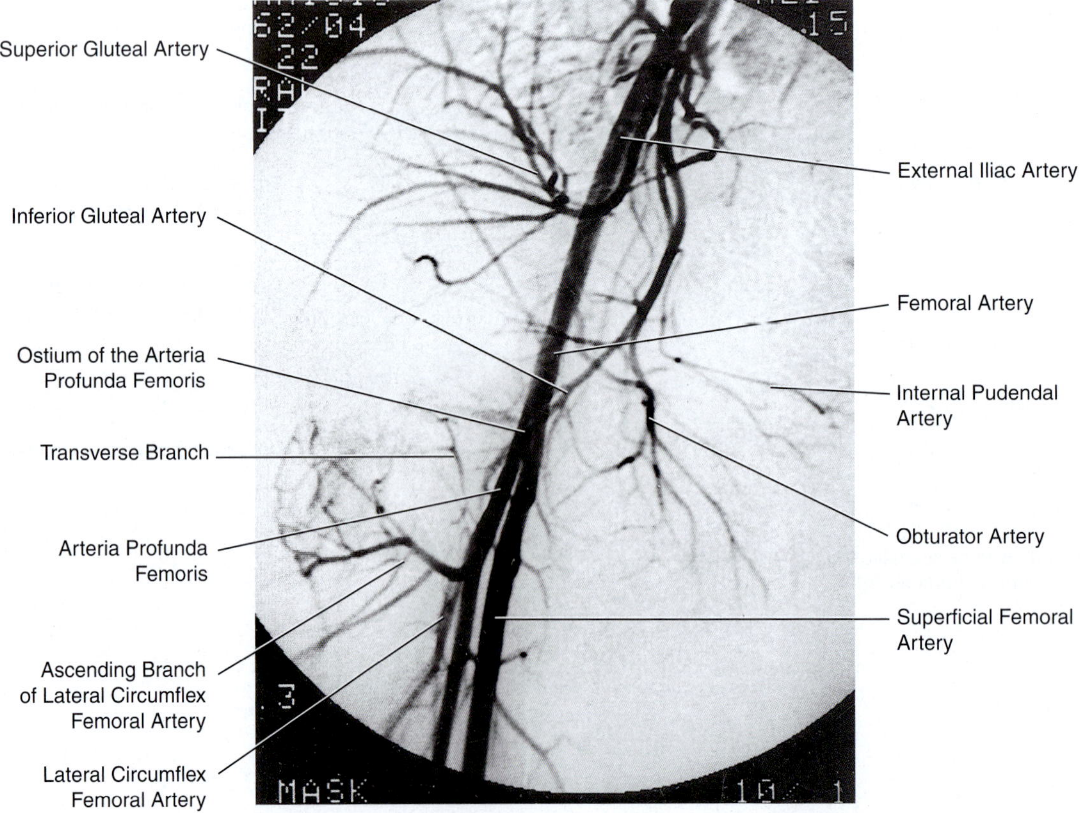

Figure 22.9. Angiogram of the right femoral artery and branches.

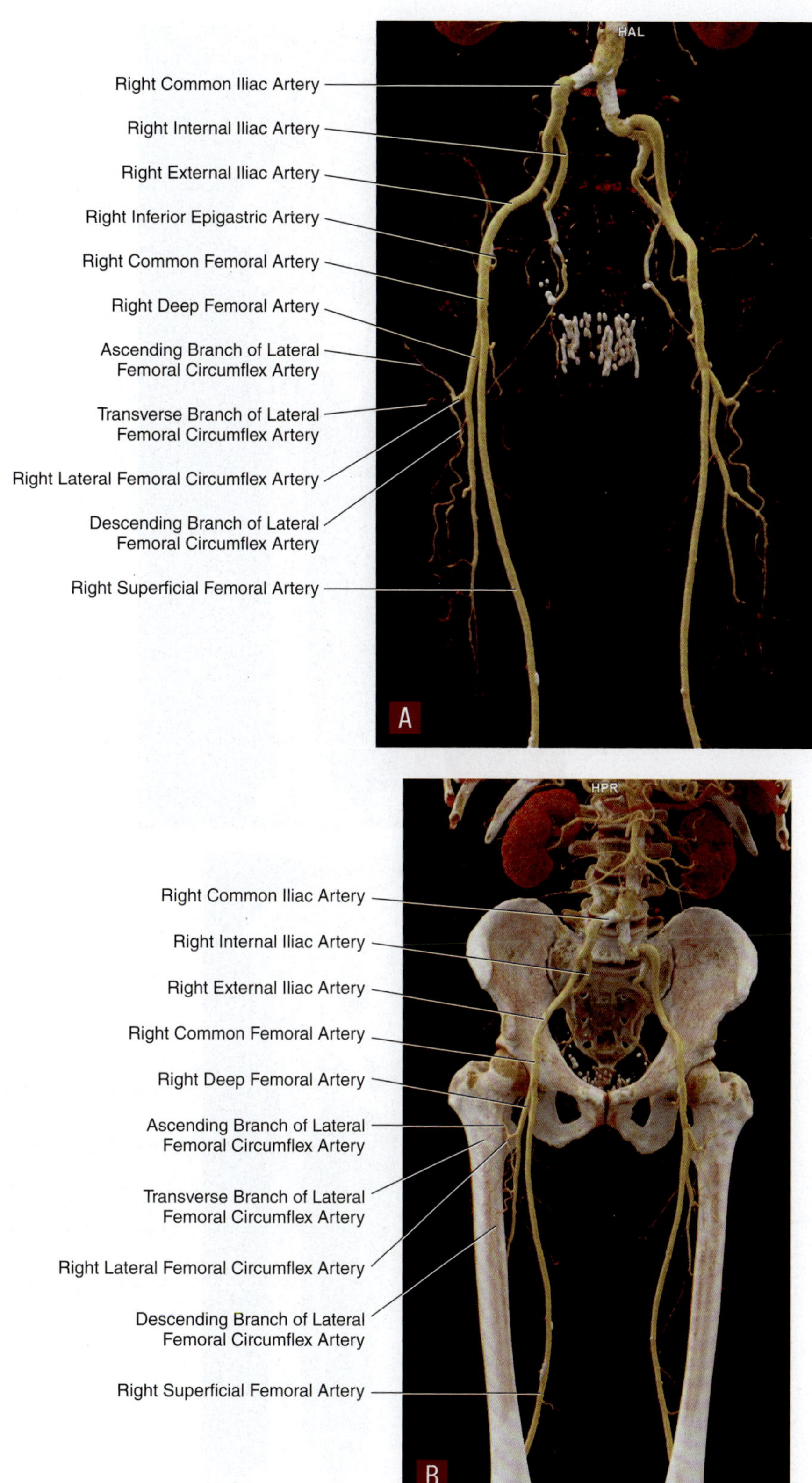

Figure 22.10. **A**, Cinematic 3D reconstructions of a computed tomography angiogram (CTA) of the pelvis and proximal lower extremities. Note the calcifications in both common iliac arteries. **B** to **D**, CTA with cinematic 3D reconstruction of the pelvis and thighs showed in AP, RAO, and LAO views. **E** and **F**, Similar reconstructions in lateral-oblique and true lateral views. Note the trajectory of the superficial femoral artery from a cranial anterior position in relation to the femur to a more caudal and posterior position at the level of the transition to the popliteal artery (posterior to the popliteal fossa). AP, anteroposterior; LAO, left anterior oblique; RAO, right anterior oblique.

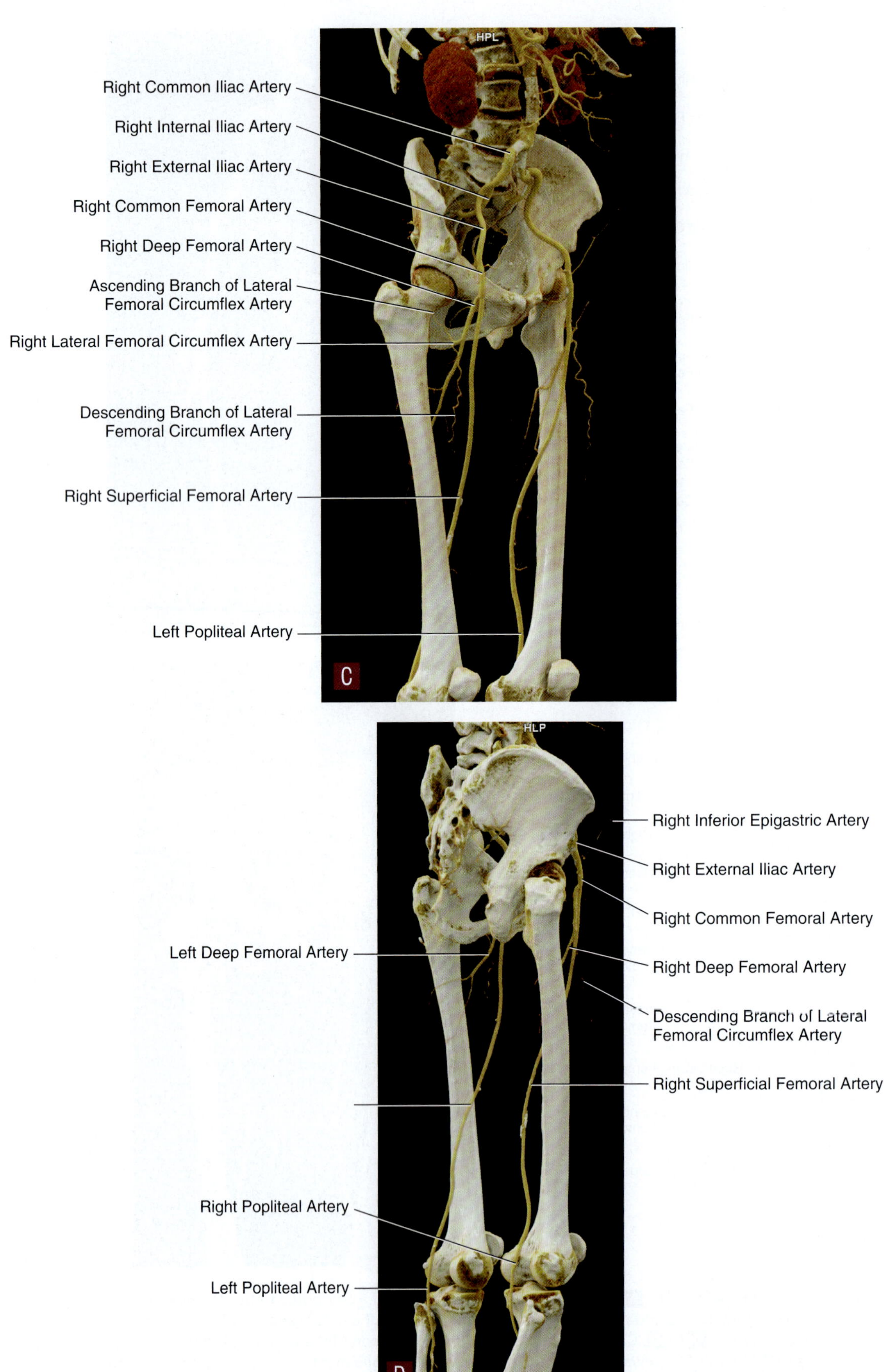

Figure 22.10. *Continued*

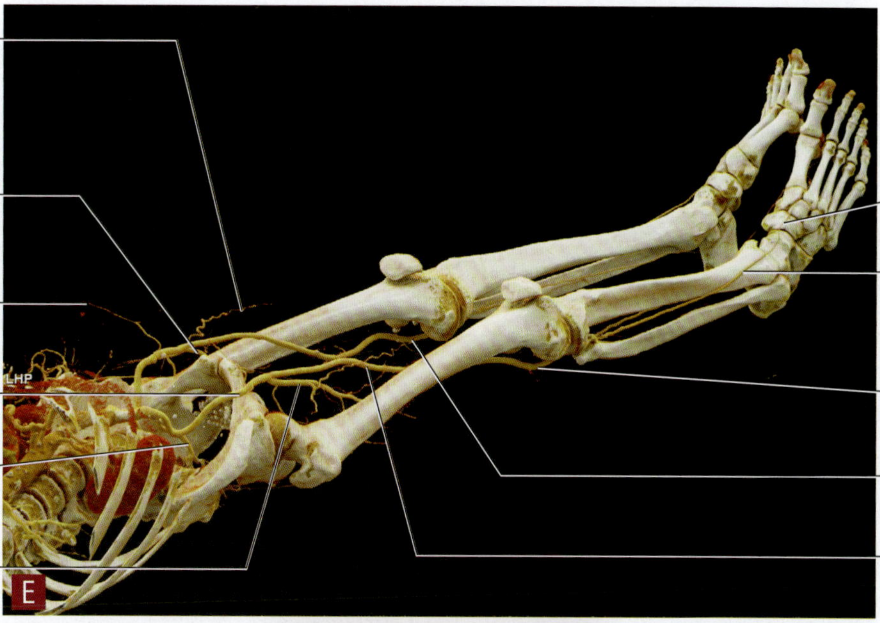

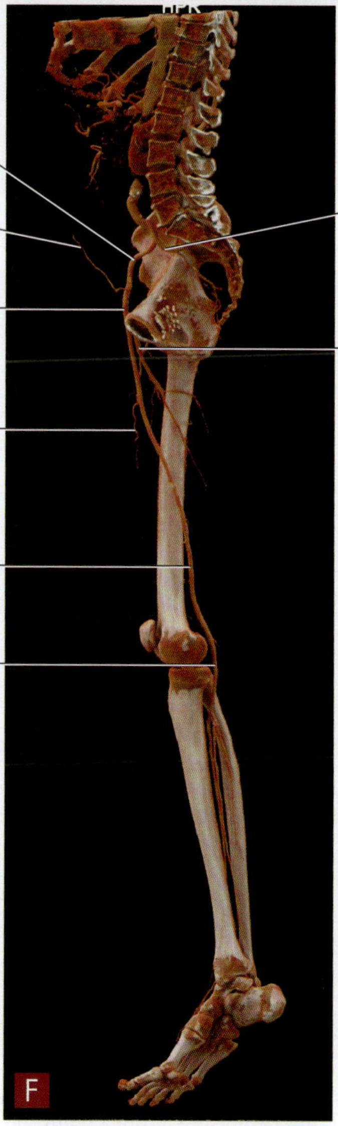

Figure 22.10. *Continued*

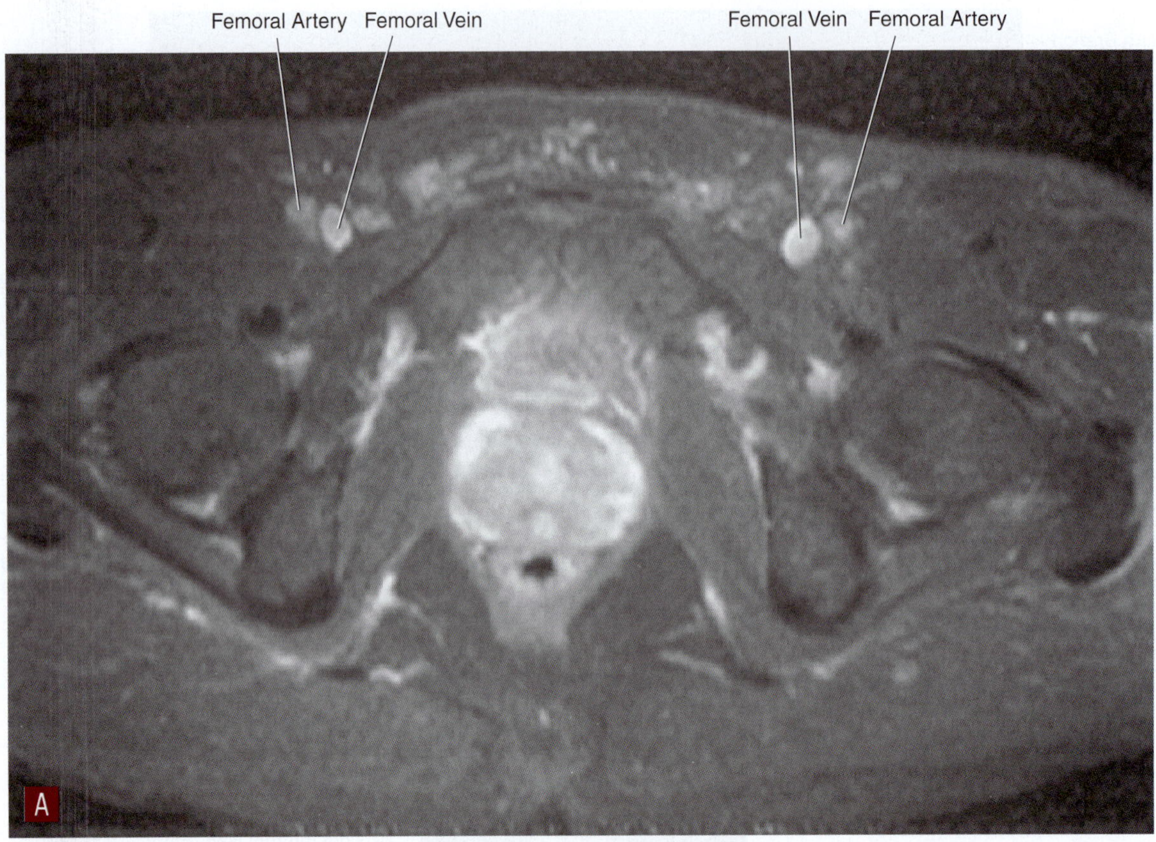

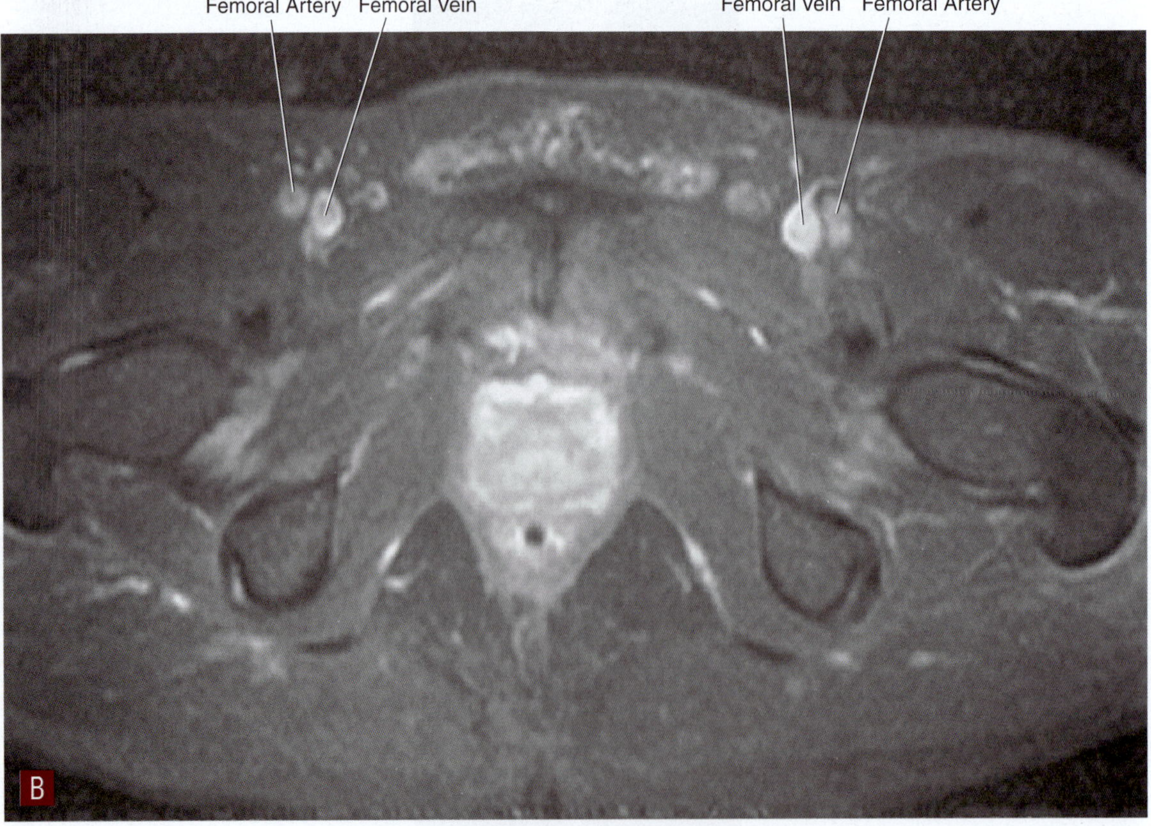

Figure 22.11. A to F, Axial magnetic resonance angiogram (MRA) of the inguinal vessels. Note the prominence of the corpora cavernosa penis in the most distal images.

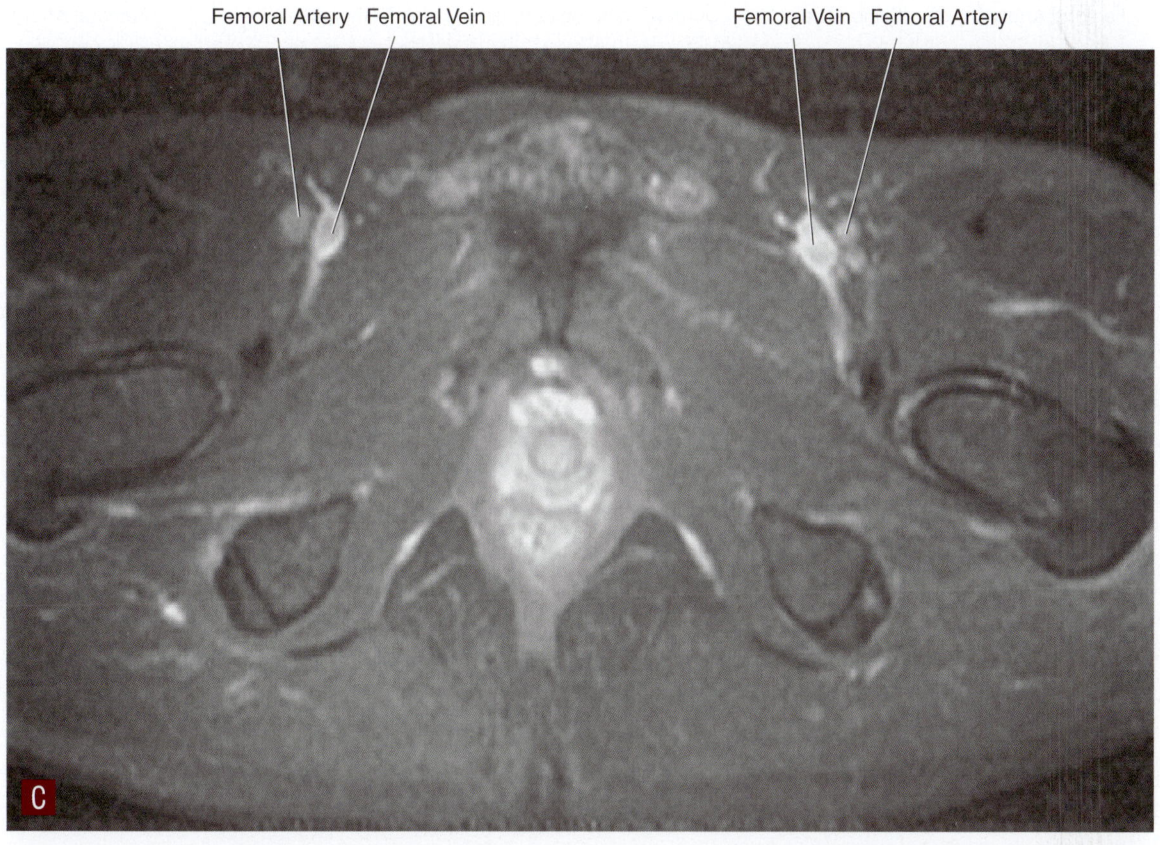

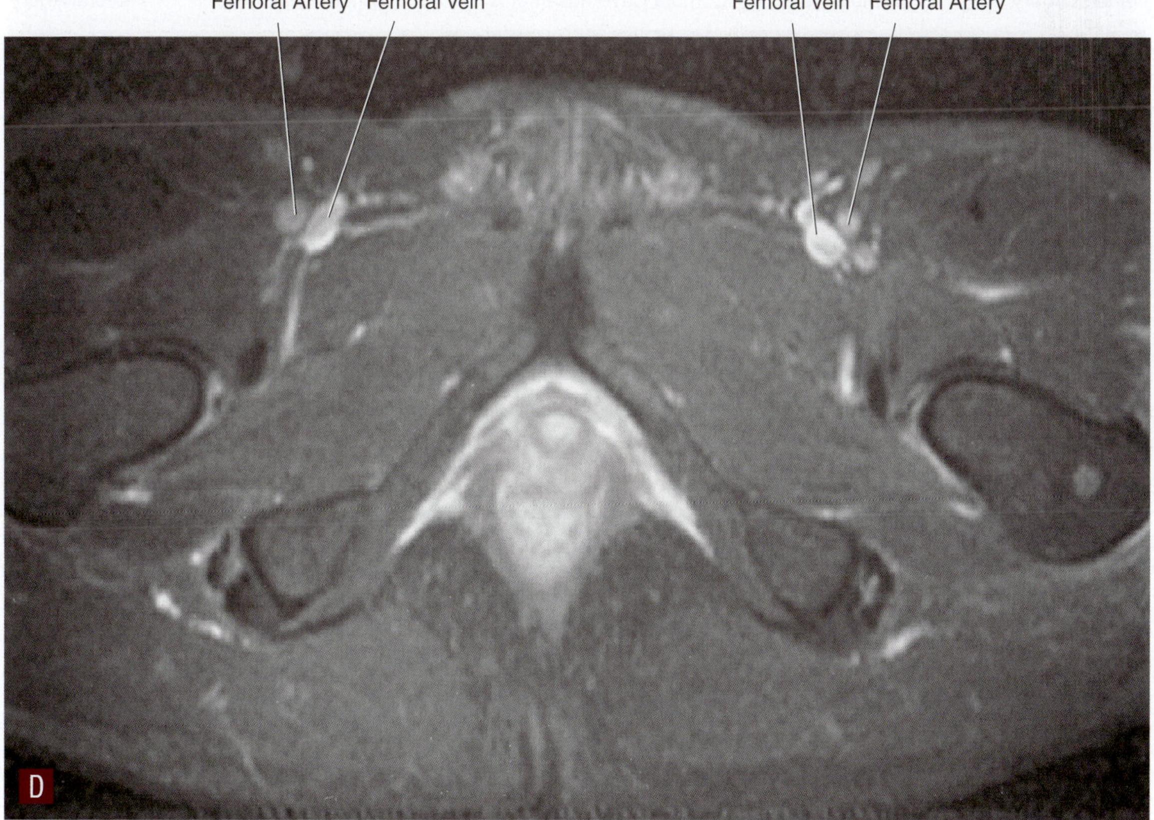

Figure 22.11. *Continued*

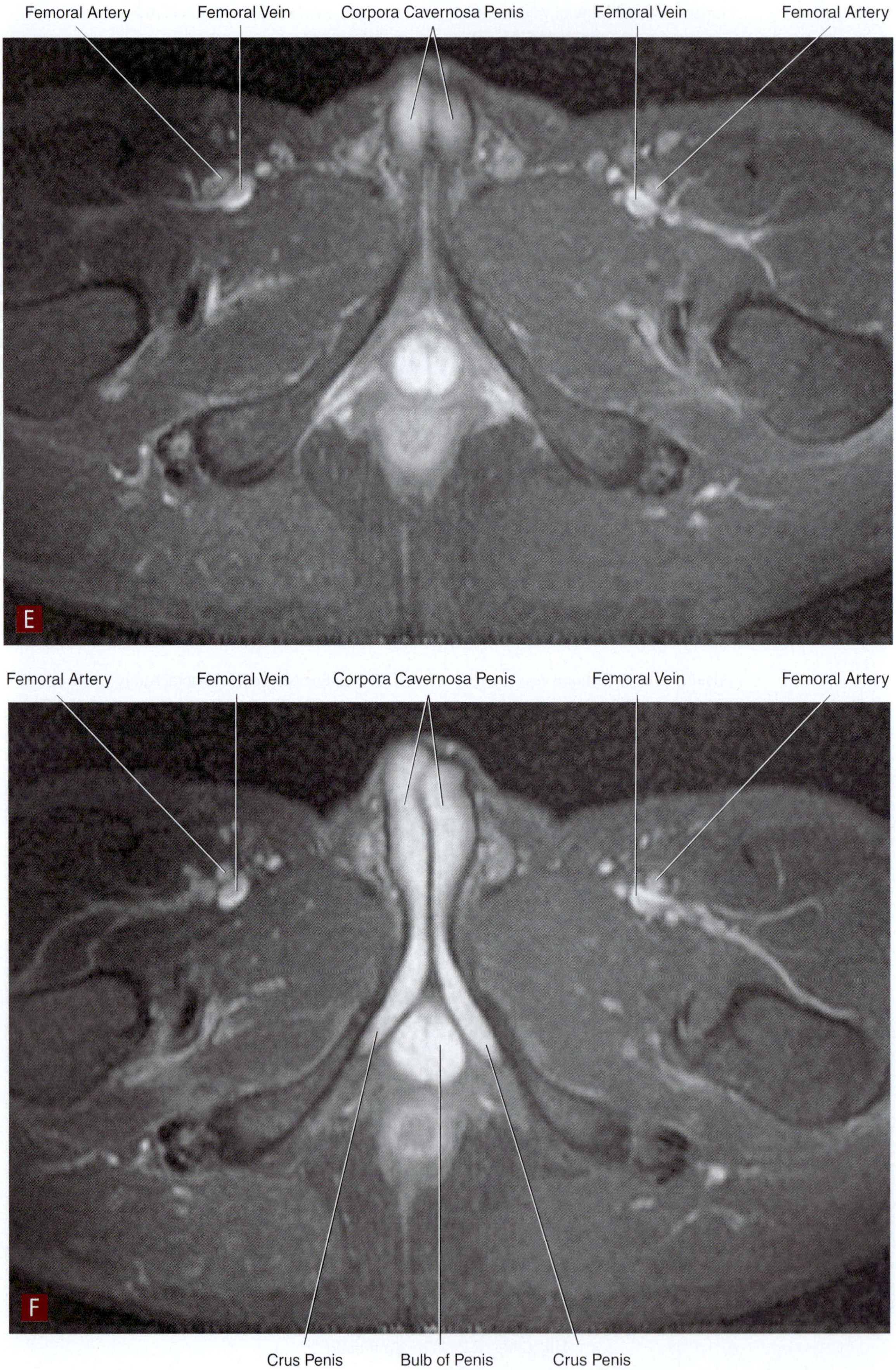

Femoral Artery
Femoral Vein
Corpora Cavernosa Penis
Femoral Vein
Femoral Artery
E
Femoral Artery
Femoral Vein
Corpora Cavernosa Penis
Femoral Vein
Femoral Artery
F
Crus Penis
Bulb of Penis
Crus Penis

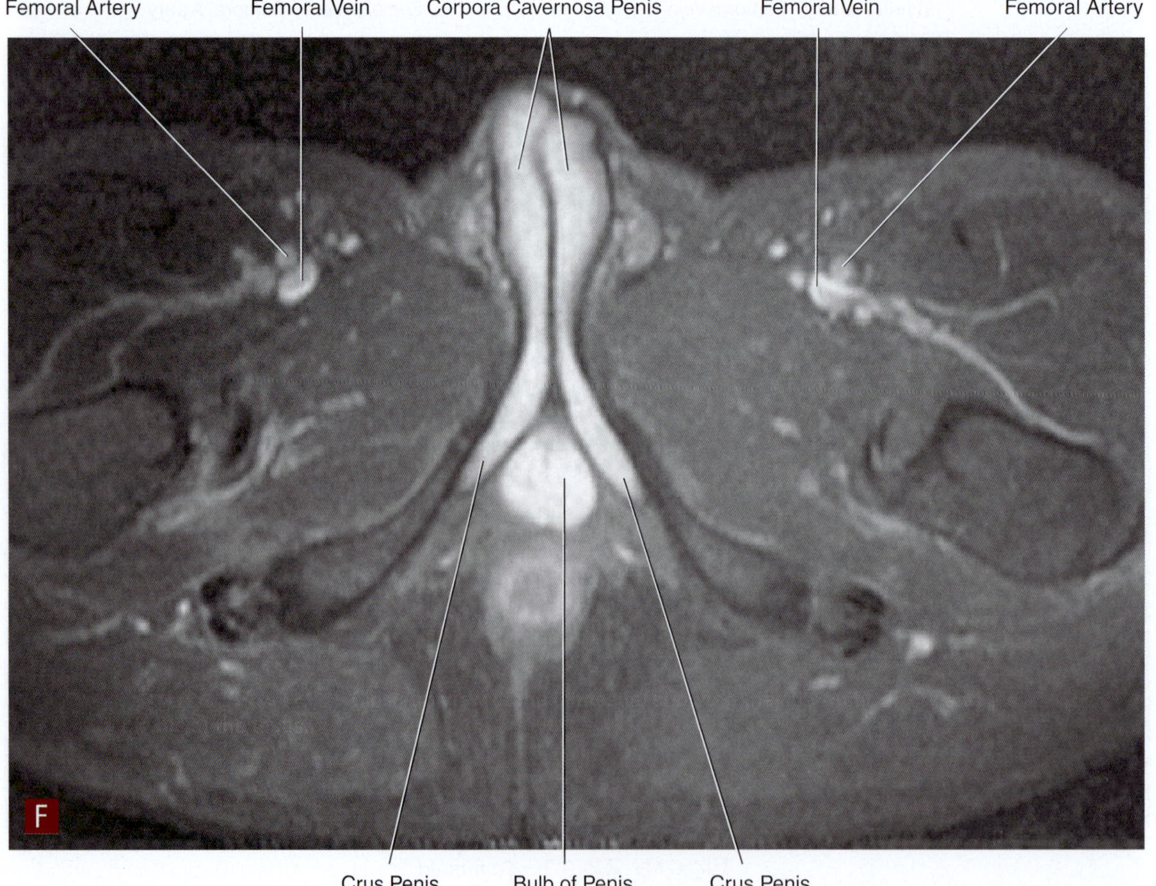

Figure 22.11. *Continued*

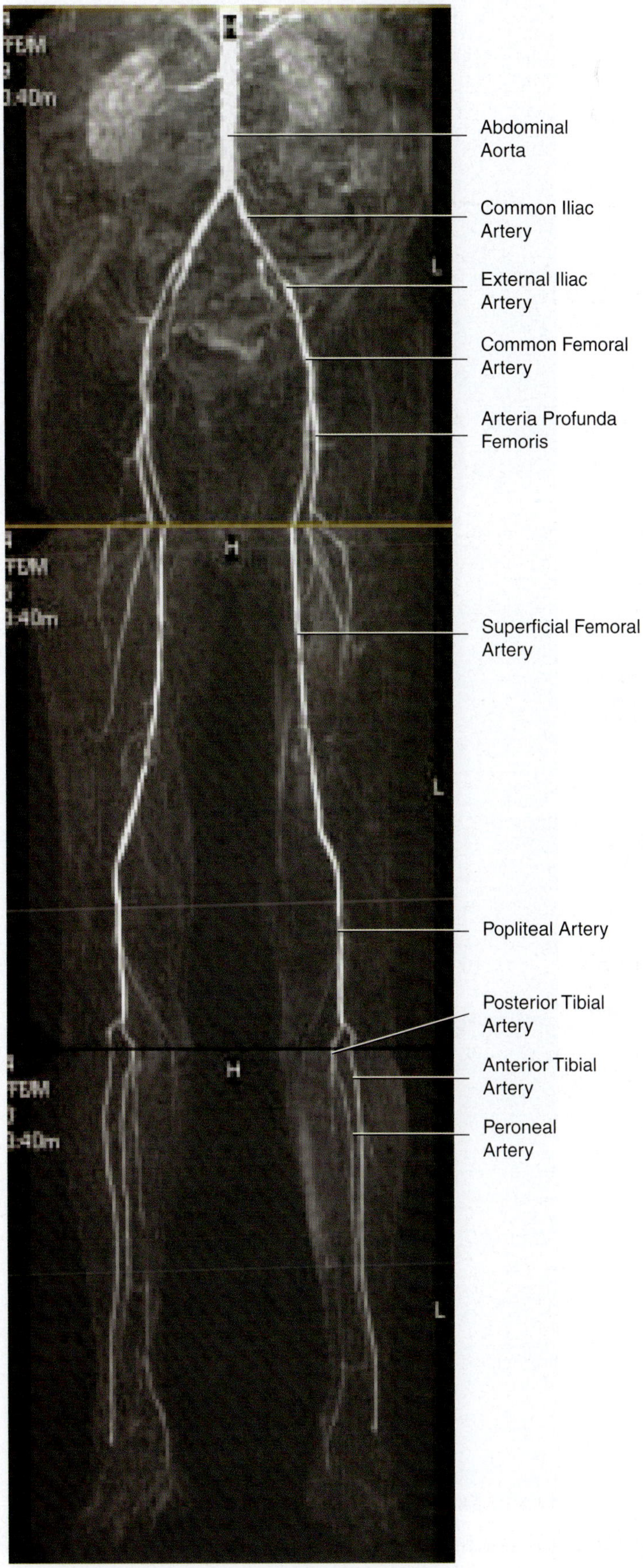

Abdominal Aorta

Common Iliac Artery

External Iliac Artery

Common Femoral Artery

Arteria Profunda Femoris

Superficial Femoral Artery

Popliteal Artery

Posterior Tibial Artery

Anterior Tibial Artery

Peroneal Artery

Figure 22.12. MRA of the circulation of the lower extremities. Note the degradation of the image in the transition of the images. MRA, magnetic resonance angiogram.

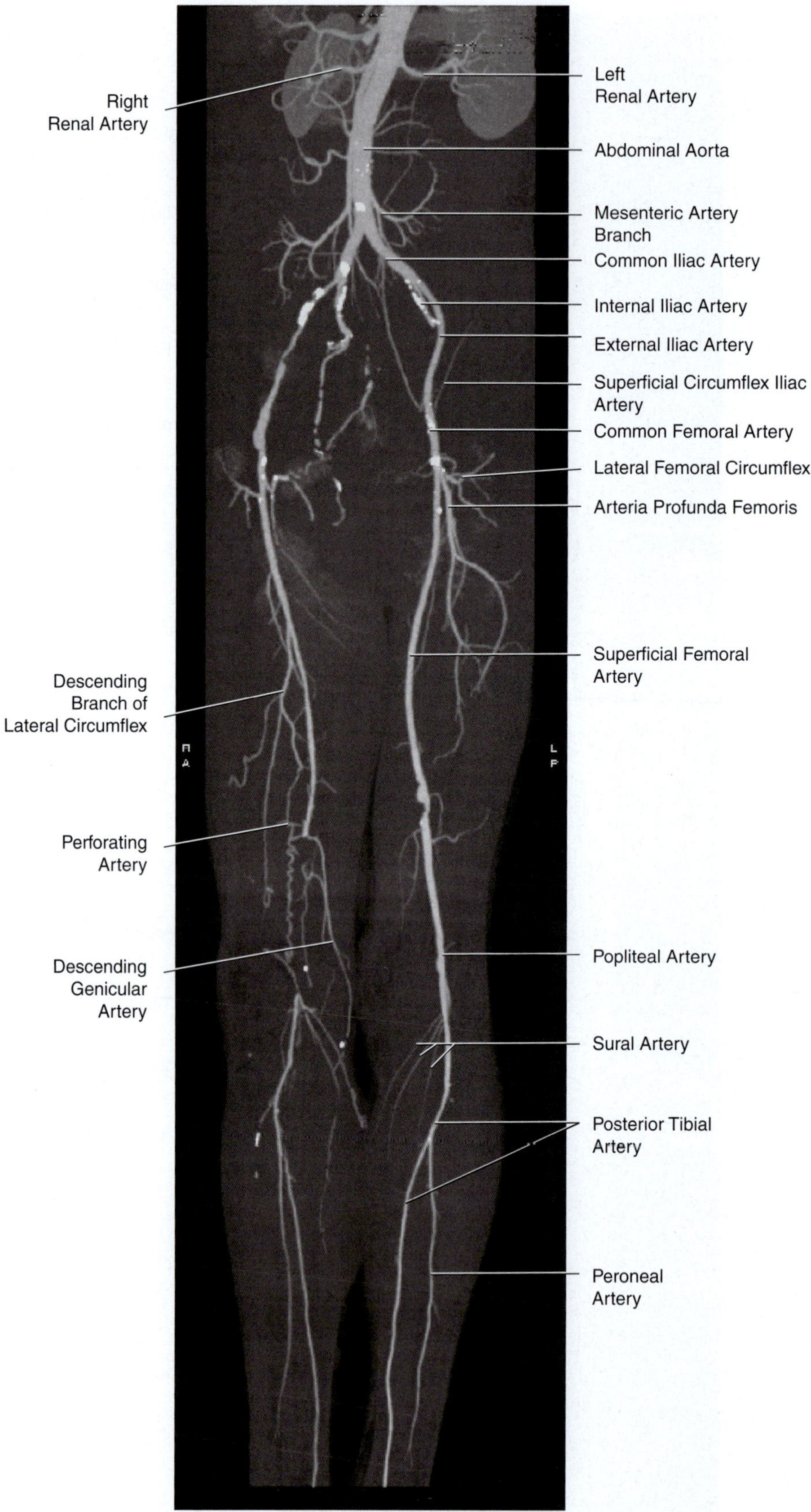

Figure 22.13. CTA with maximum intensity projection (MIP) reconstruction of the abdominal aorta and arteries of the pelvis and lower extremities. Note extensive calcification of the iliac vessels and occlusion of the right distal superficial femoral and popliteal arteries. CTA, computed tomography angiography.

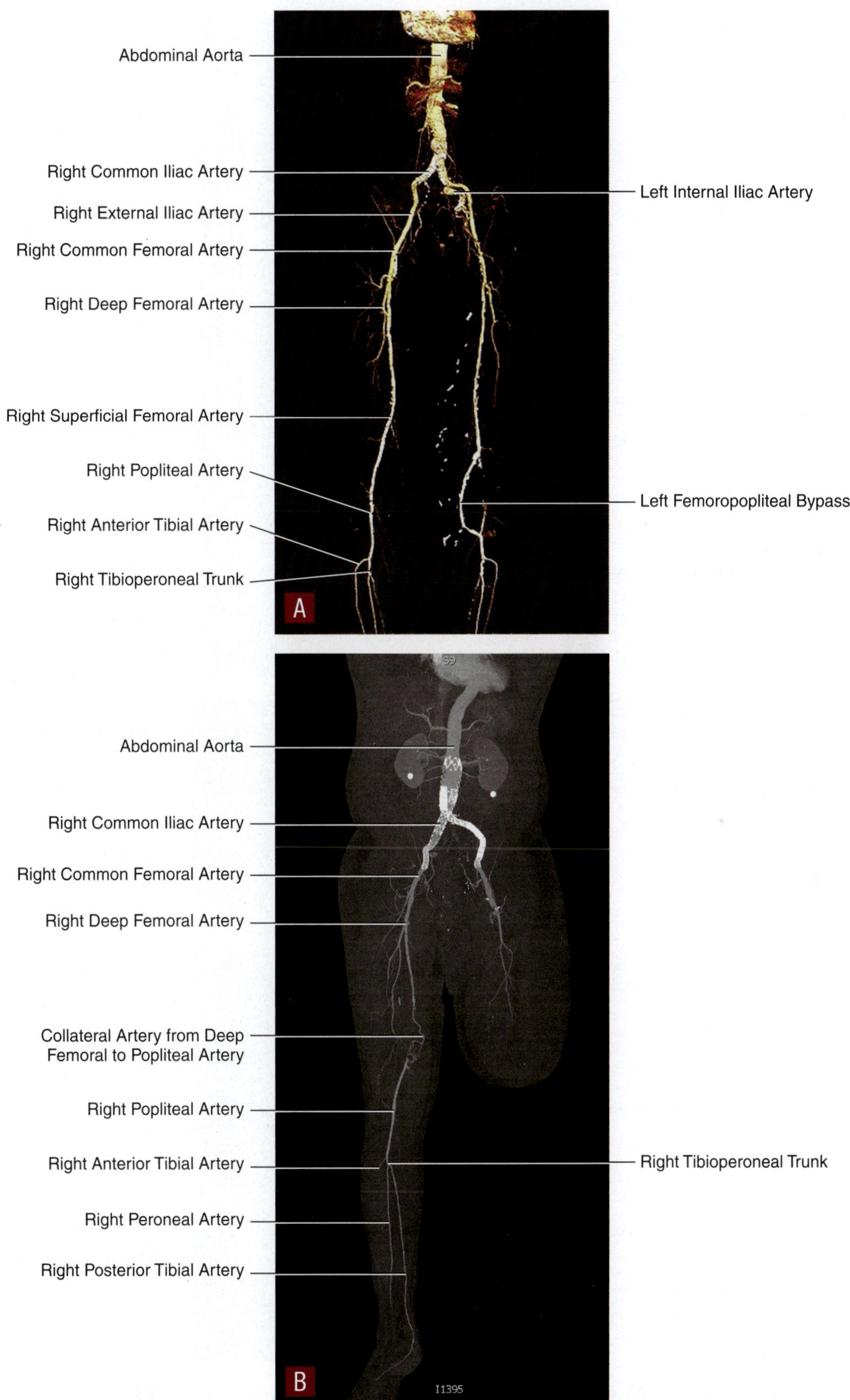

Figure 22.14. **A**, 3D reconstruction of the abdominal aorta and lower extremities CTA. Note the left popliteal artery occlusion and the patency of the distal SFA-popliteal bypass. **B**, MIP of CTA of the abdominal aorta and of the lower extremities. Note the patent AAA stent-graft, associated with bilateral SFA occlusive disease and left above the knee amputation. CTA, computed tomography angiography; MIP, maximum intensity projection; SFA, superficial femoral artery.

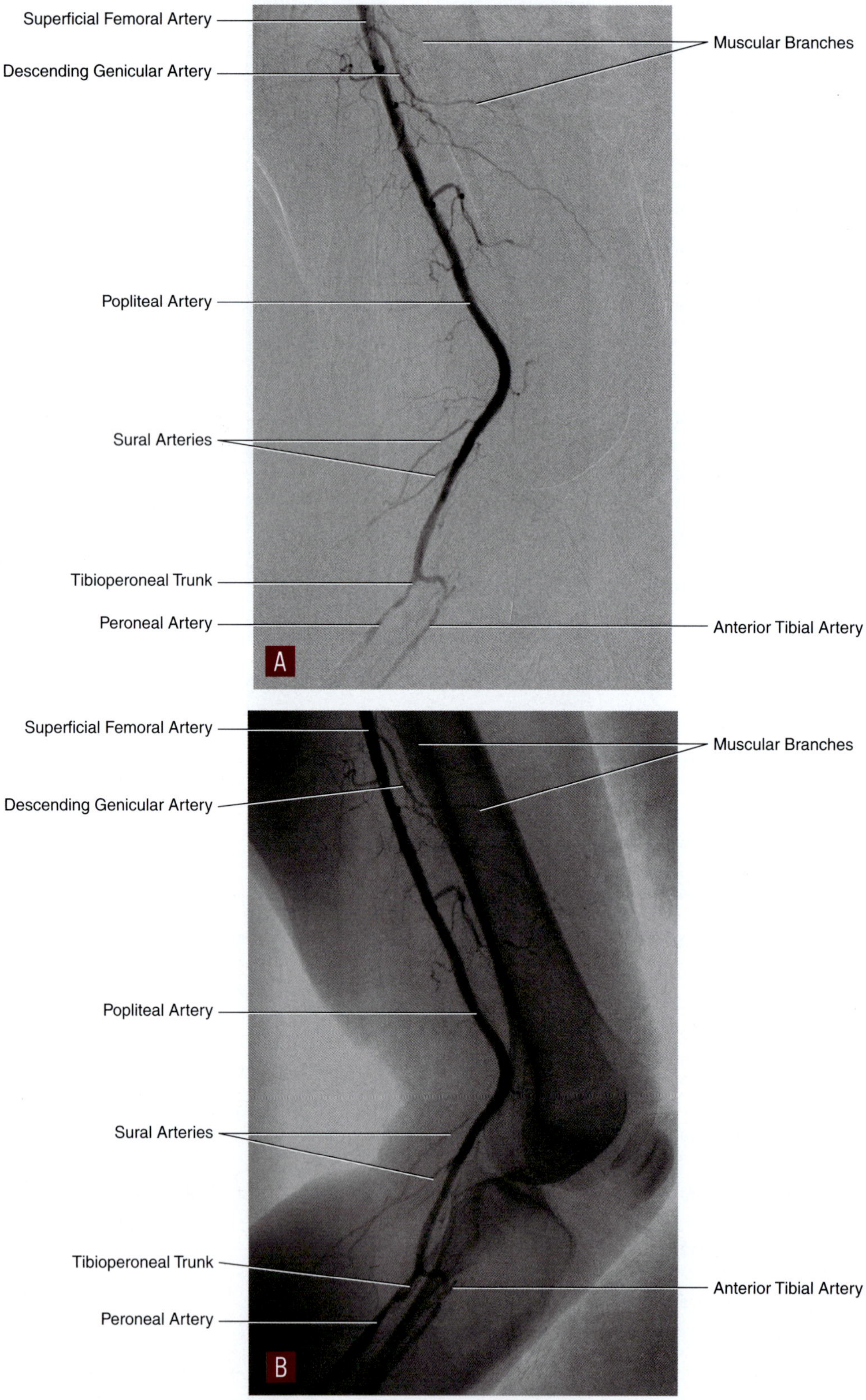

Superficial Femoral Artery
Descending Genicular Artery
Popliteal Artery
Sural Arteries
Tibioperoneal Trunk
Peroneal Artery
Muscular Branches
Anterior Tibial Artery
A

Superficial Femoral Artery
Descending Genicular Artery
Popliteal Artery
Sural Arteries
Tibioperoneal Trunk
Peroneal Artery
Muscular Branches
Anterior Tibial Artery
B

Figure 22.15. A and B, Left lower extremity angiograms in subtraction (A) and in native (B) shows the changes in the distal SFA and popliteal arteries with partial knee flexion. C, Right lower extremity angiograms in subtraction with the knee in partial flexion. D, Right lower extremity angiograms in native with the knee in full flexion. Note the the patent stent in the SFA-popliteal artery transition and the consequent accordion (kinking) effect on these arteries. E to G, Angiograms of the right distal SFA and popliteal arteries with the leg straight (E) and on flexion (F and G). Note the patent popliteal stent and the arterial kinking and rotation when the knee is flexed. SFA, superficial femoral artery.

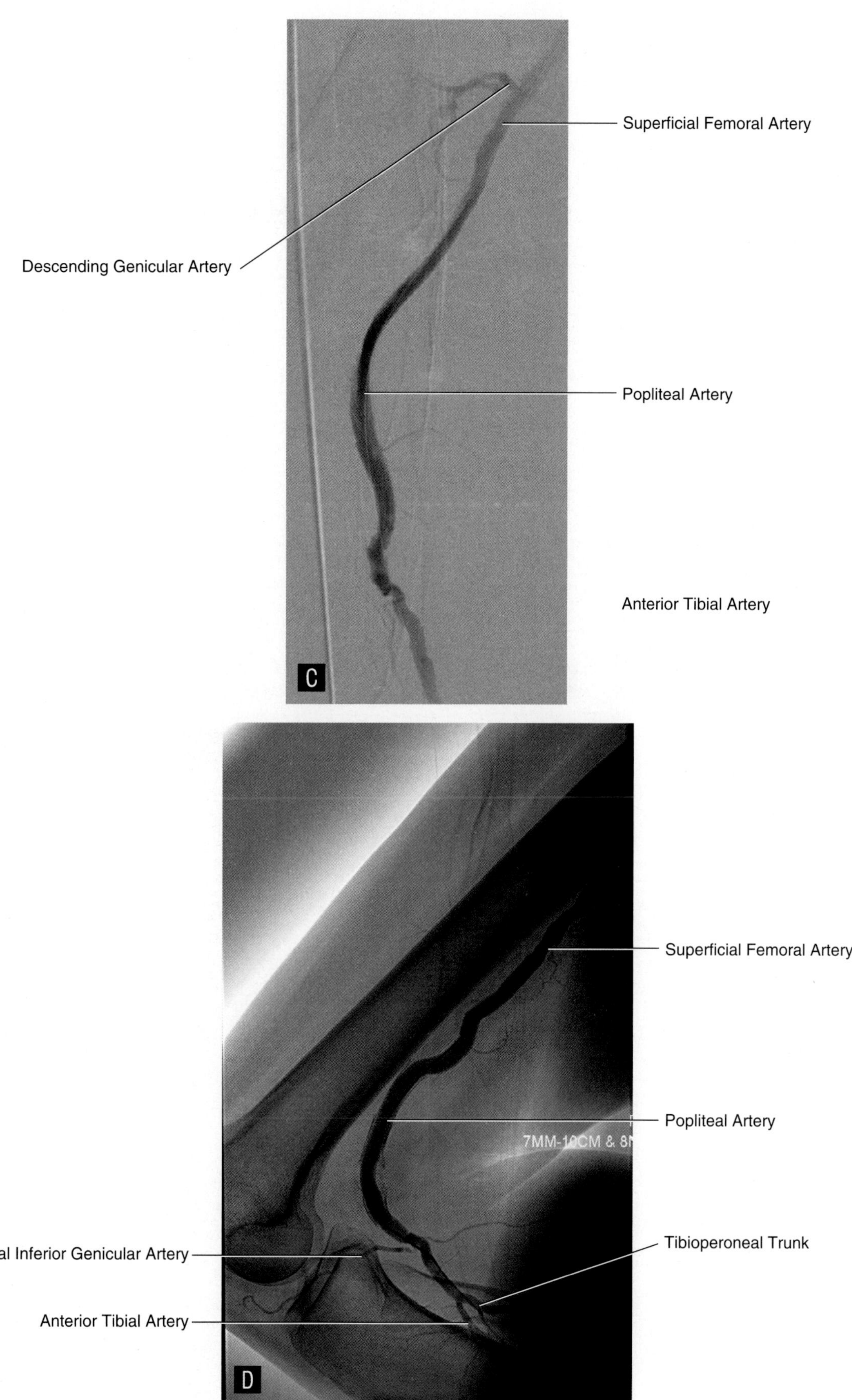

Figure 22.15. *Continued*

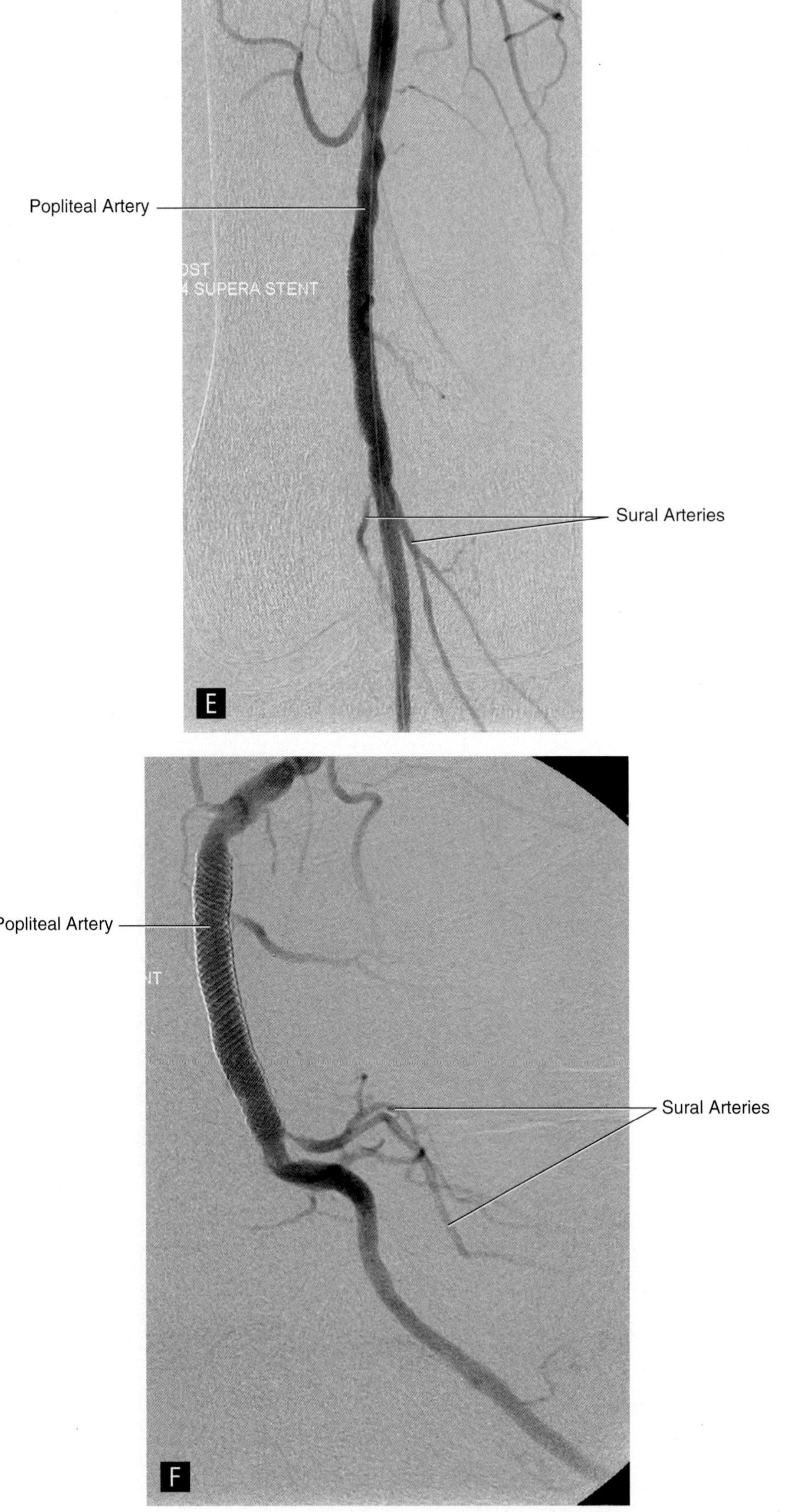

Figure 22.15. *Continued*

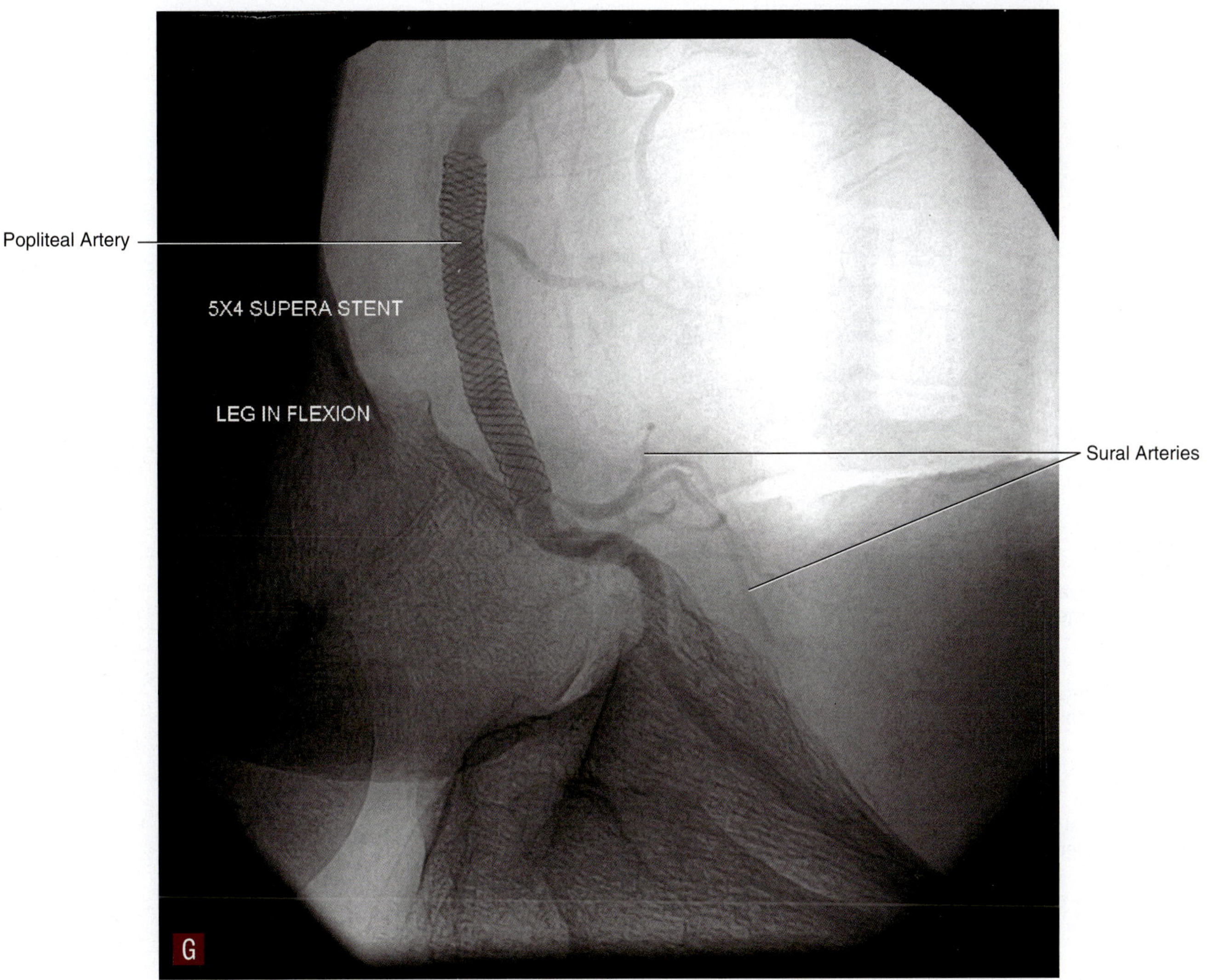

Figure 22.15. *Continued*

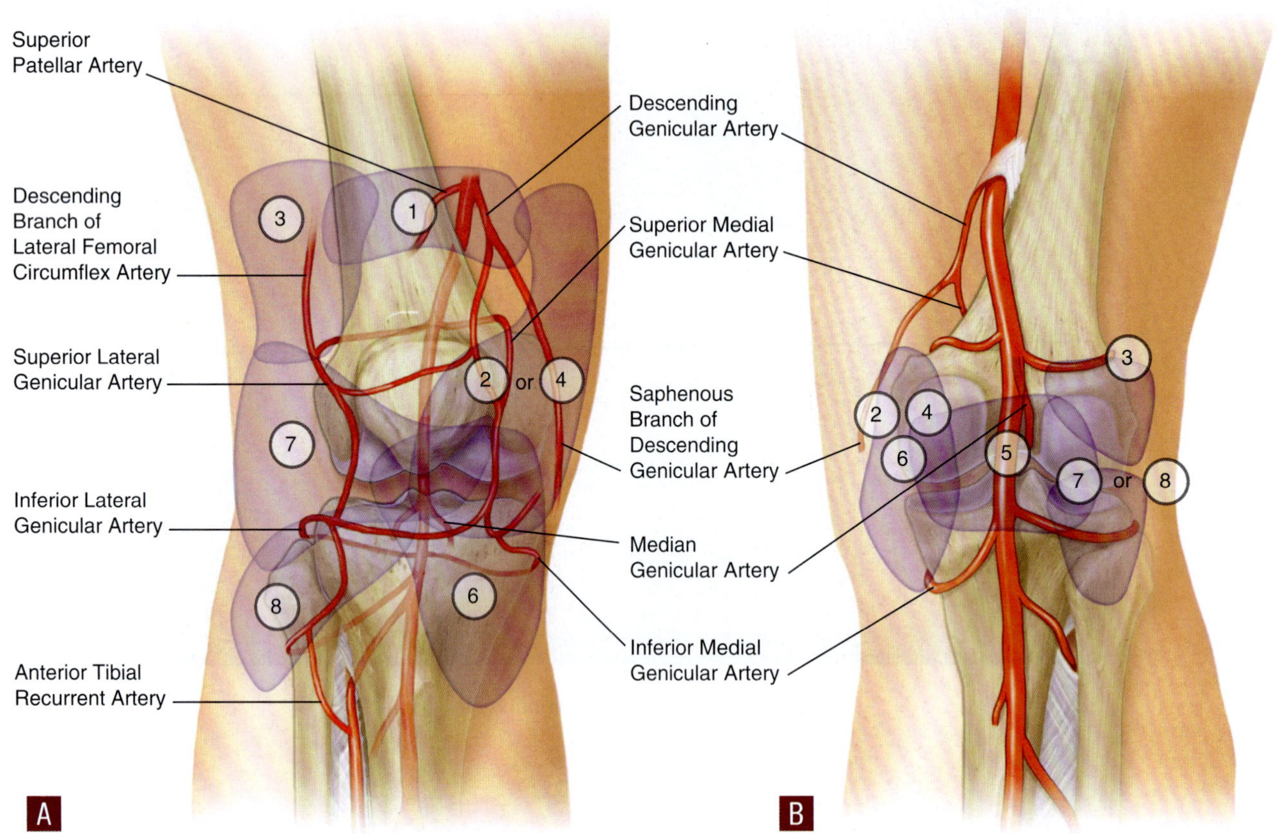

Figure 22.16. Schematic drawing of the popliteal artery branches to the knee joint in the anterior view (A), and posterior view (B) and the corresponding territories of genicular artery distribution. 1, superior patellar artery; 2, descending genicular artery; 3, superior lateral genicular artery; 4, superior medial genicular artery; 5, median genicular artery; 6, inferior medial genicular artery; 7, inferior lateral genicular artery; 8, anterior tibial recurrent artery.

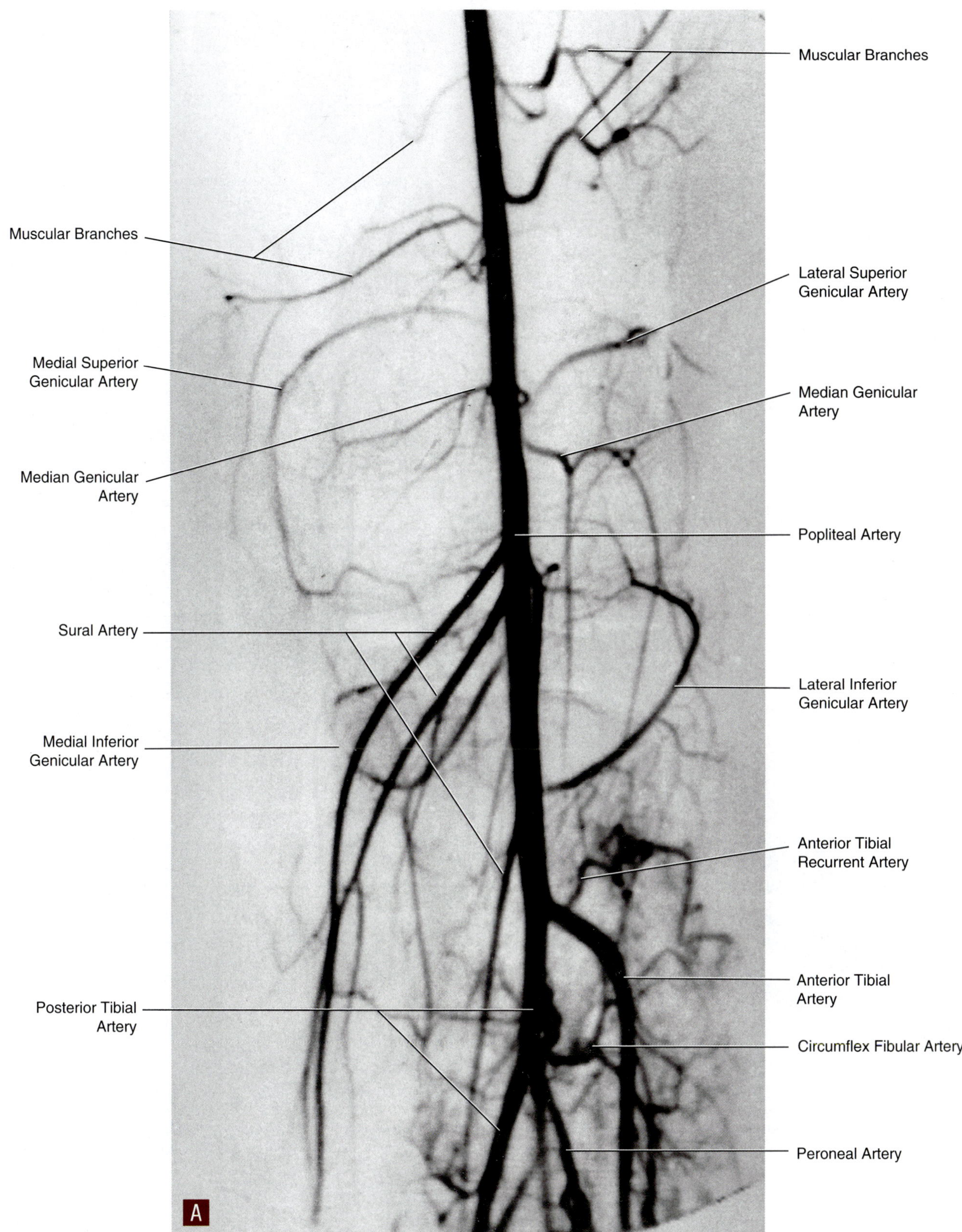

Figure 22.17. **A**, Anterior view of an angiogram of the popliteal artery and branches. **B**, Lateral view of the popliteal artery, showing the main branches. Note that the circumflex fibular artery supplies a hypervascular lesion in the popliteal fossa. **C**, Normal left lower extremity arteriogram at the level of the knee. Note a long popliteal artery and some geniculate branches. Variation of the anatomy. **D**, Left lower extremity arteriogram at the level of the knee. Note the geniculate branches and the sural artery. PT and AT are occluded proximally. **E**, Right lower extremity arteriogram at the level of the knee and proximal calf. Note the geniculate arteries. AT, anterior tibial; PT, posterior tibial.

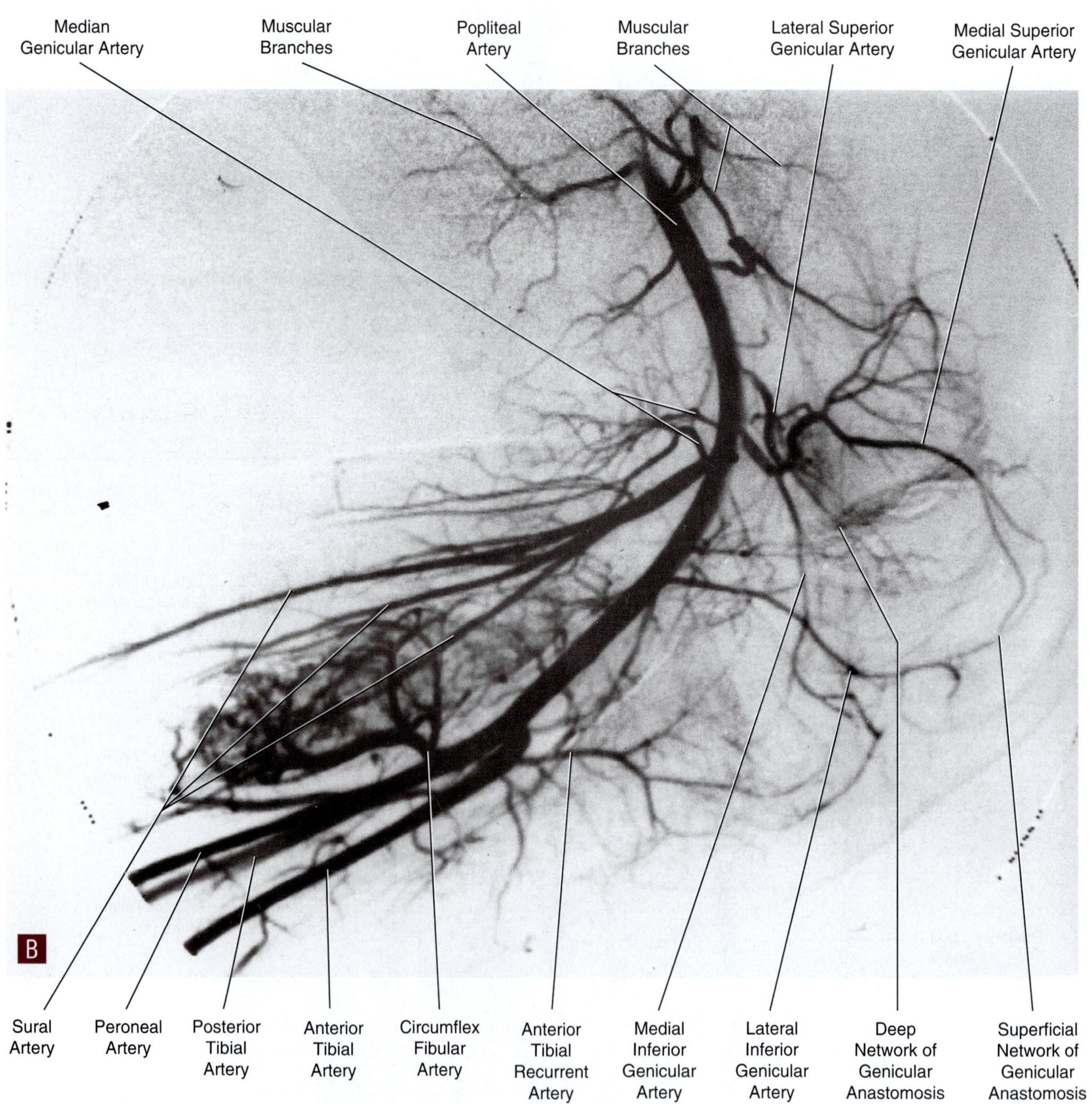

Figure 22.17. *Continued*

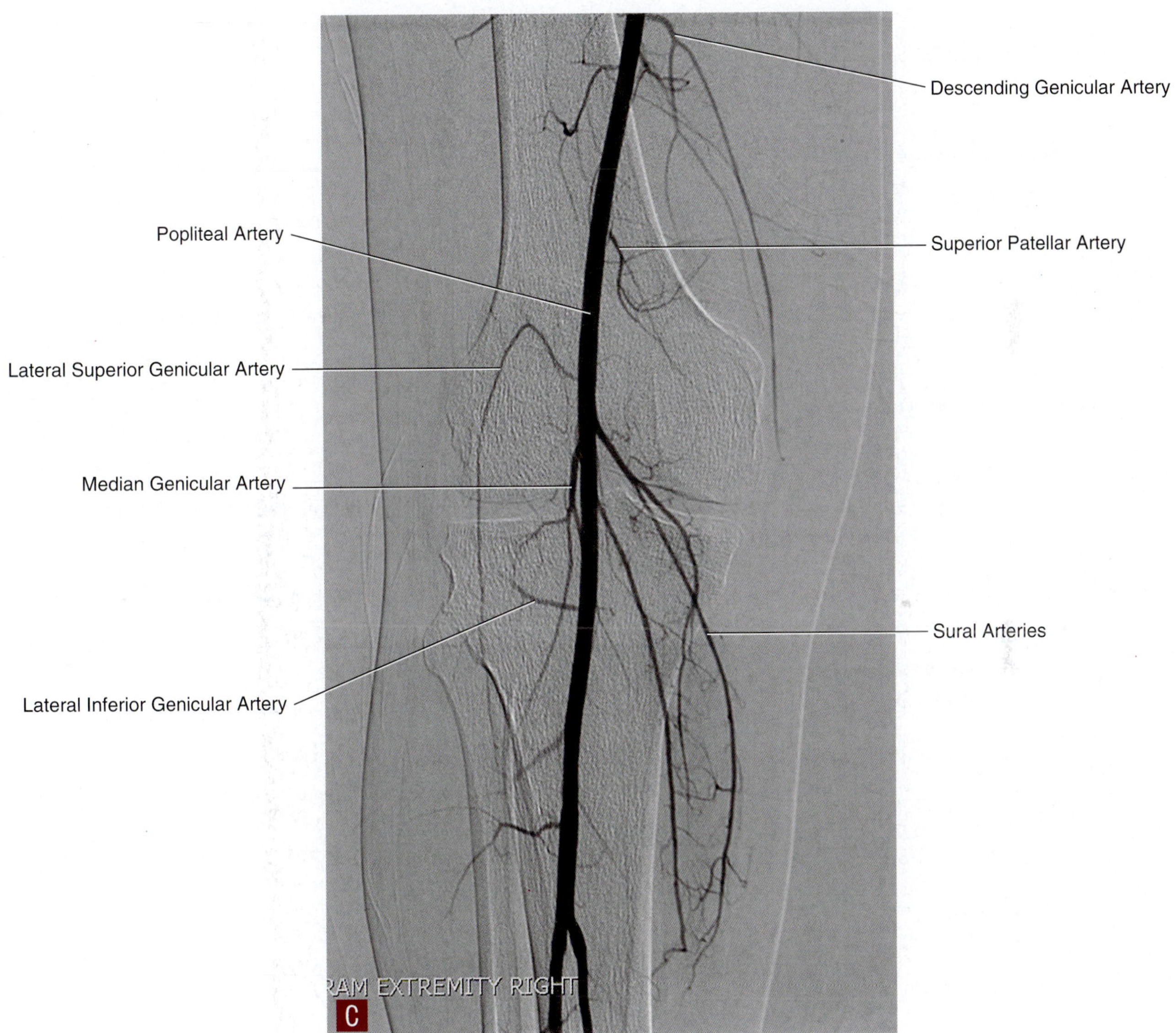

Figure 22.17. *Continued*

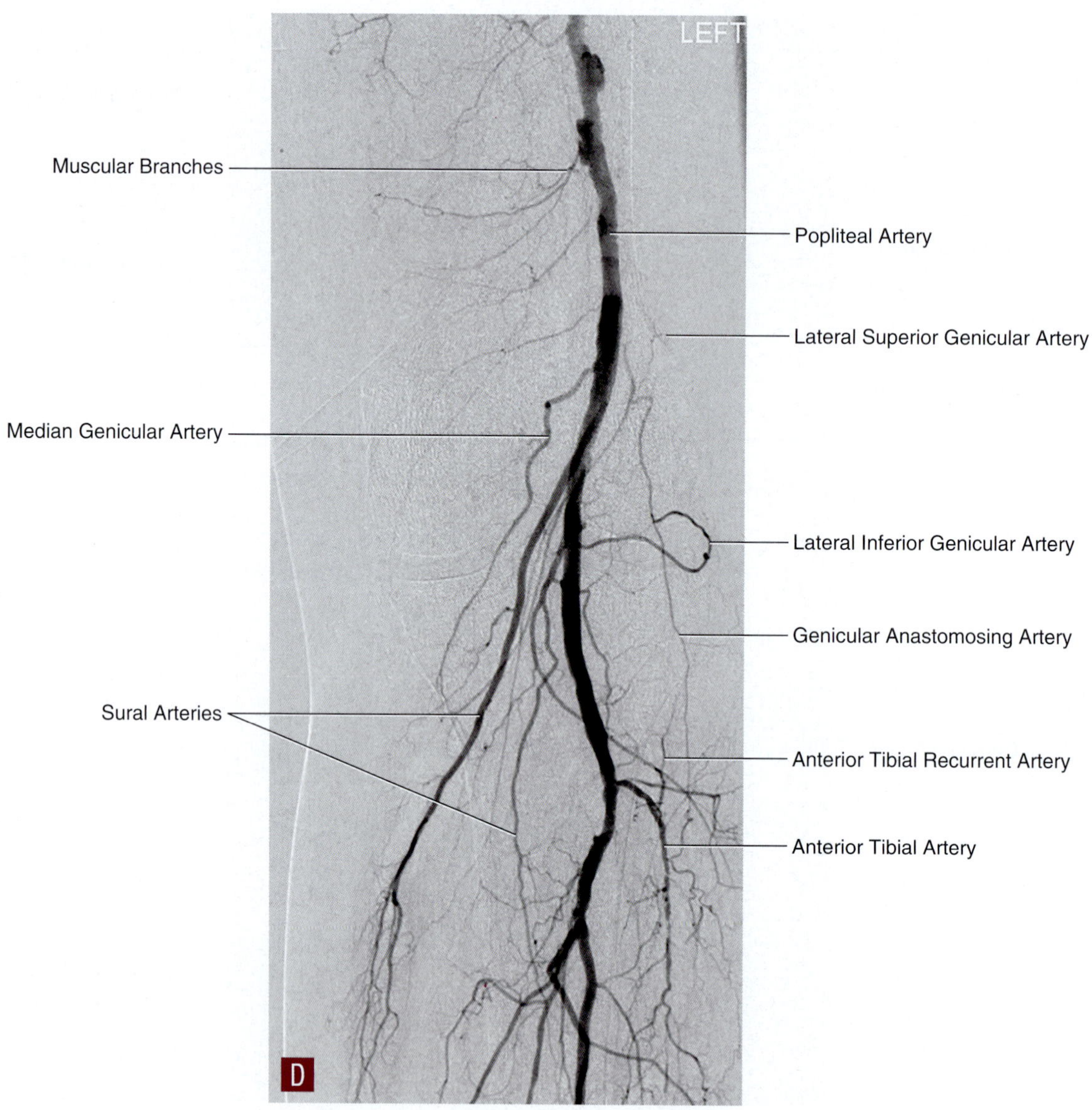

Figure 22.17. *Continued*

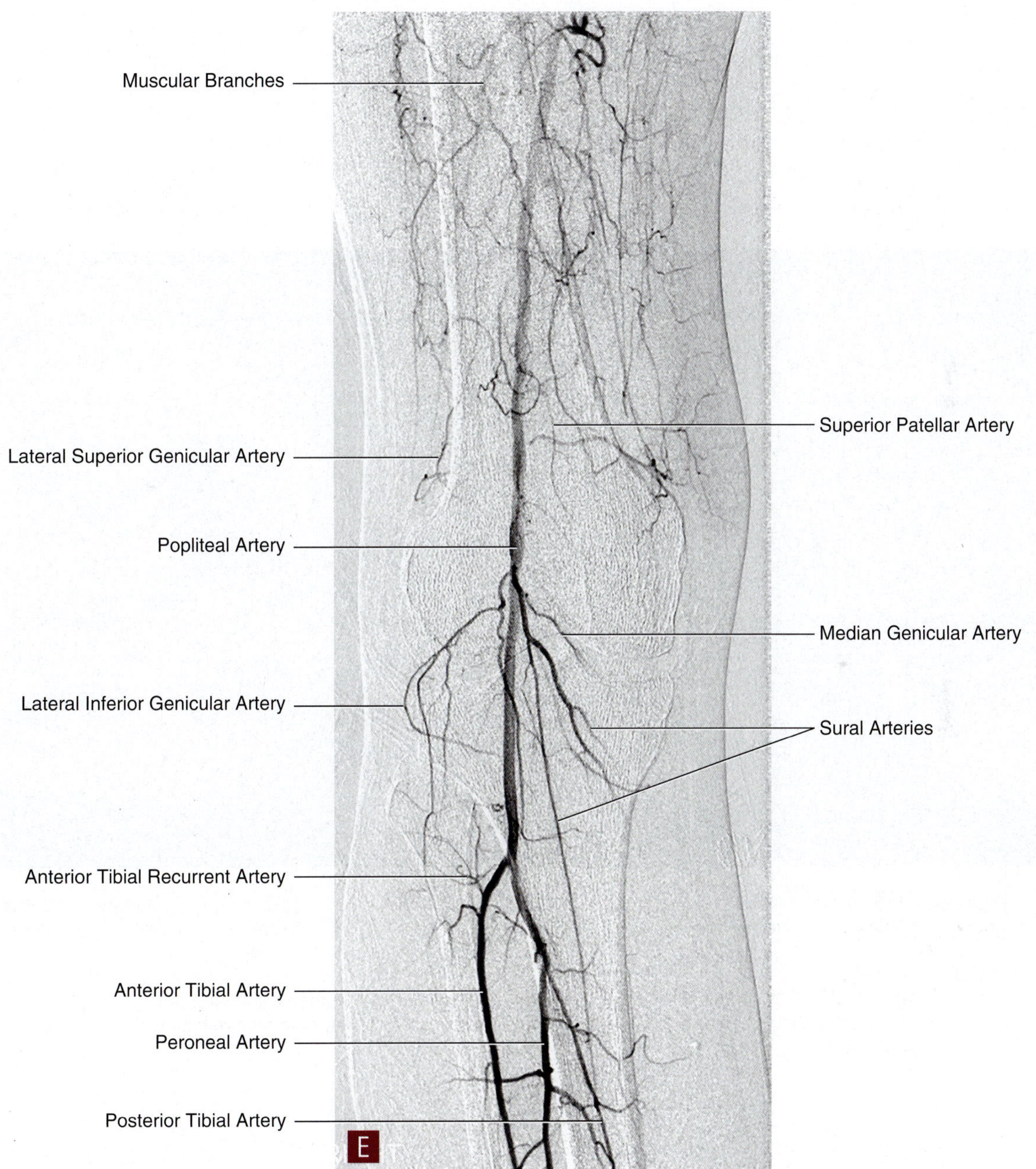

Figure 22.17. *Continued*

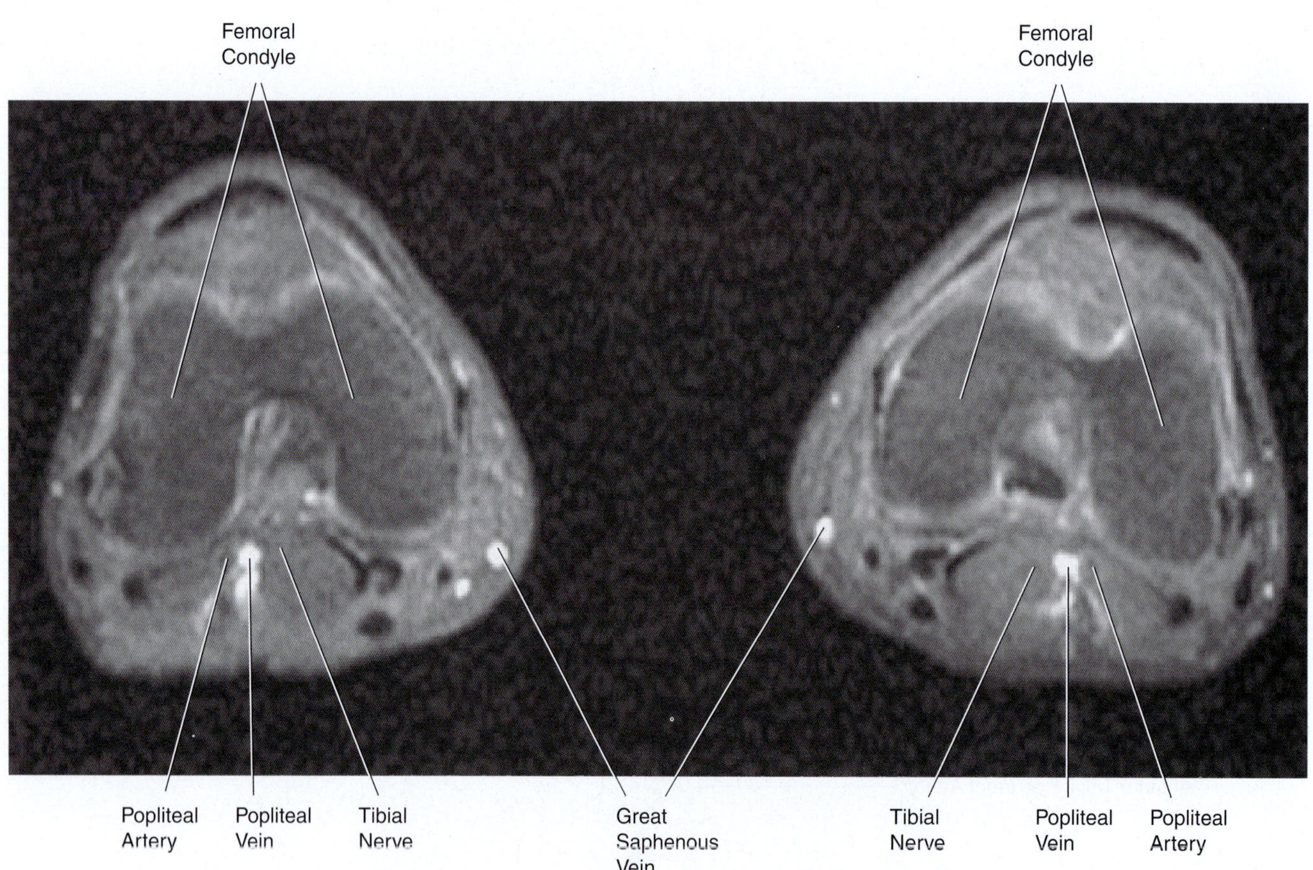

Figure 22.18. **Axial** MRA of the leg vessels at the level of the knees, showing the popliteal arteries and veins, and the relationship of the vessels. MRA, magnetic resonance angiogram.

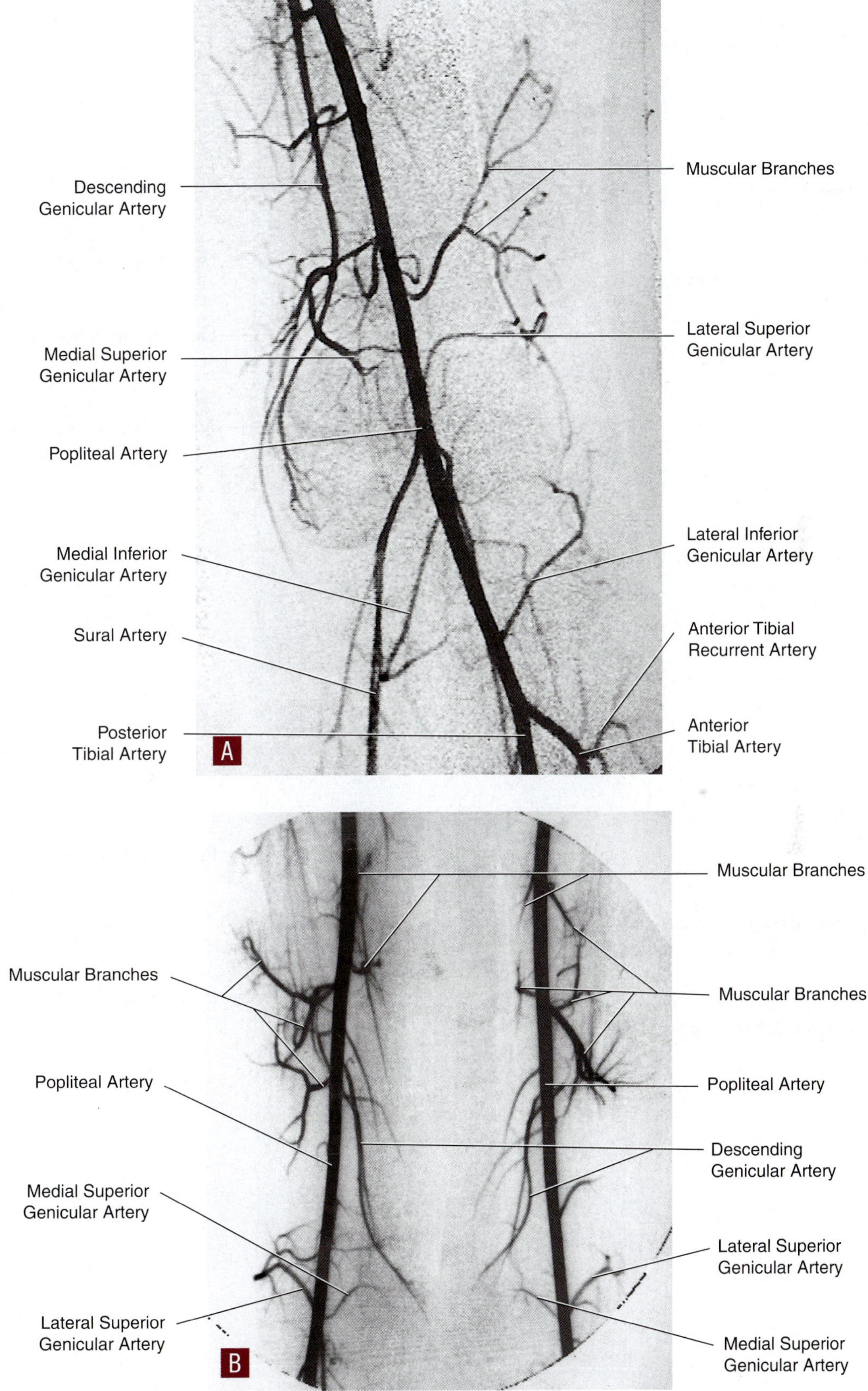

Figure 22.19. A, Anterior view DSA of a popliteal artery and main branches. B, Anterior view of DSA of bilateral popliteal arteries and main branches. DSA, digital subtraction angiography.

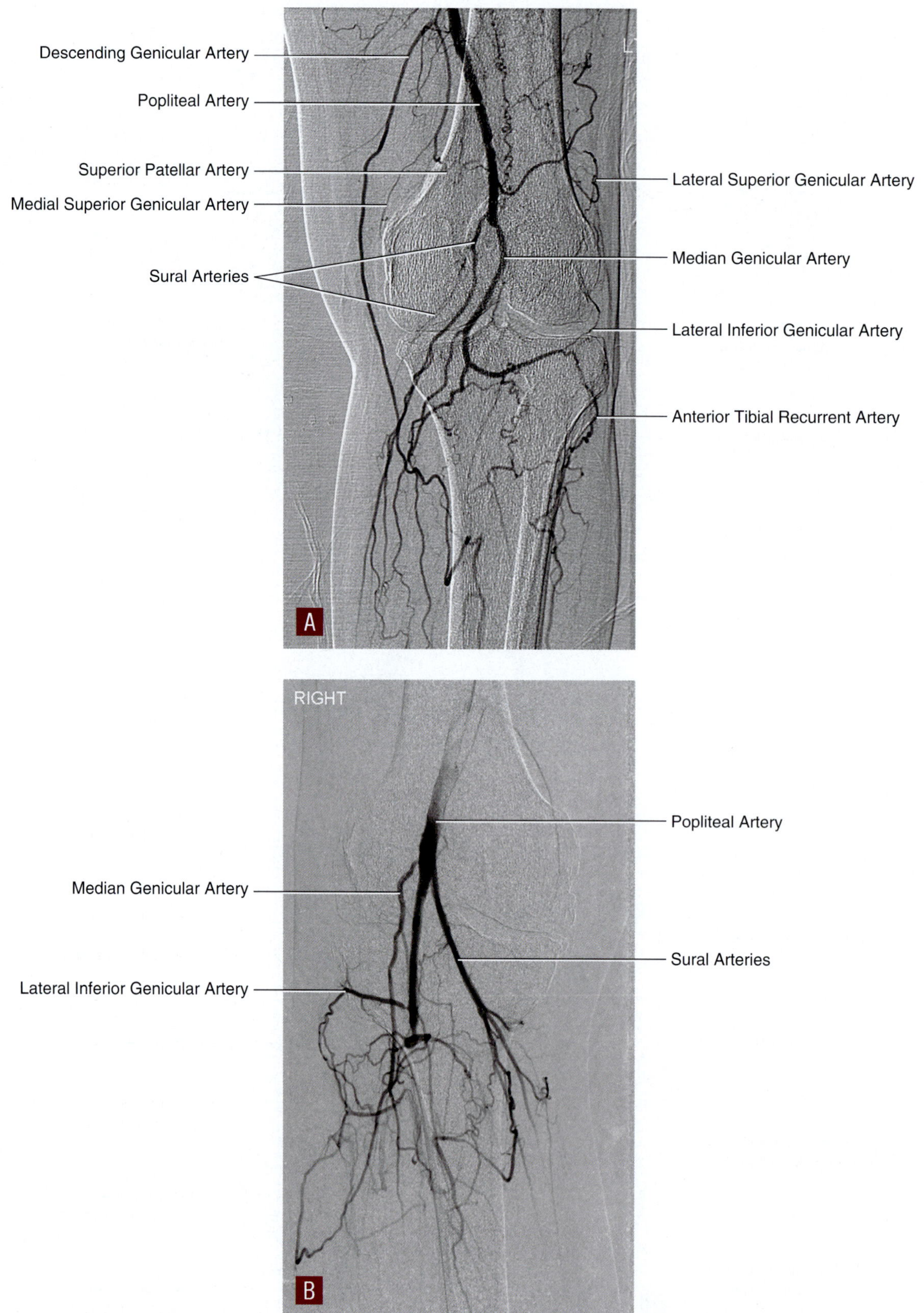

Figure 22.20. **A**, Right lower extremity arteriogram at the level of the knee and proximal calf. Note the occlusion of the tibioperoneal trunk and the extensive collaterals through muscular branches. **B**, Left lower extremities arteriogram. Note the chronic occlusion of the popliteal artery and the collateral circulation to the calf.

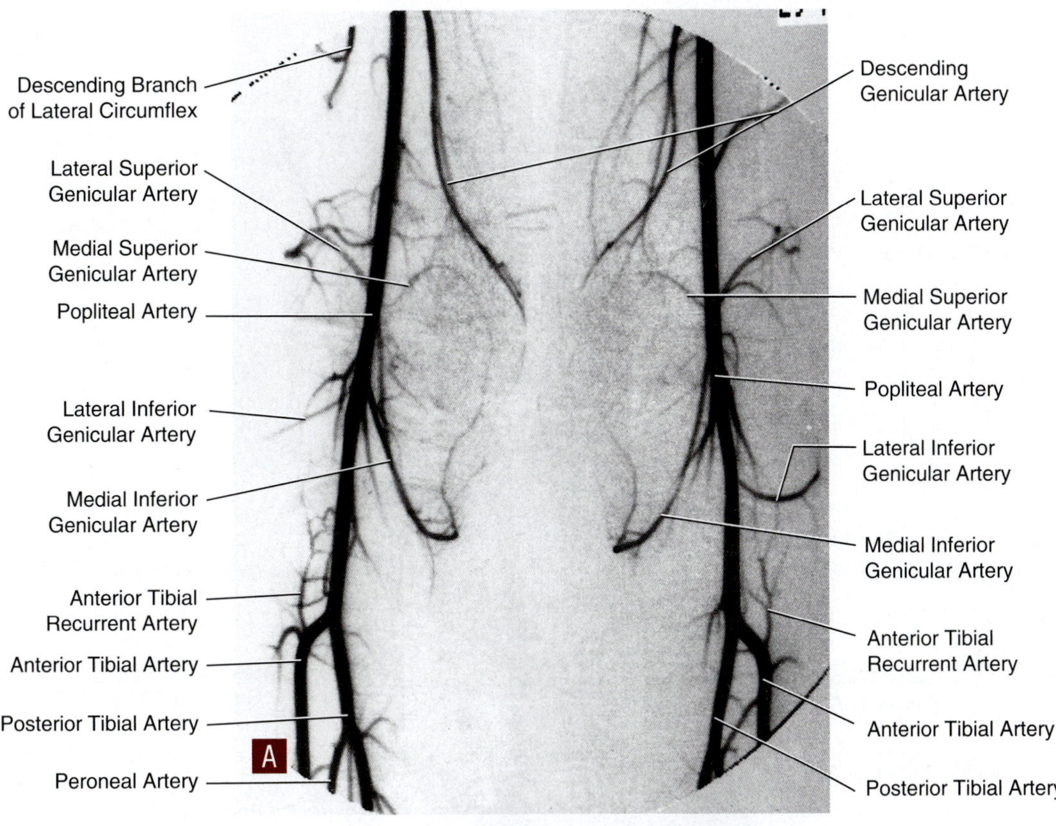

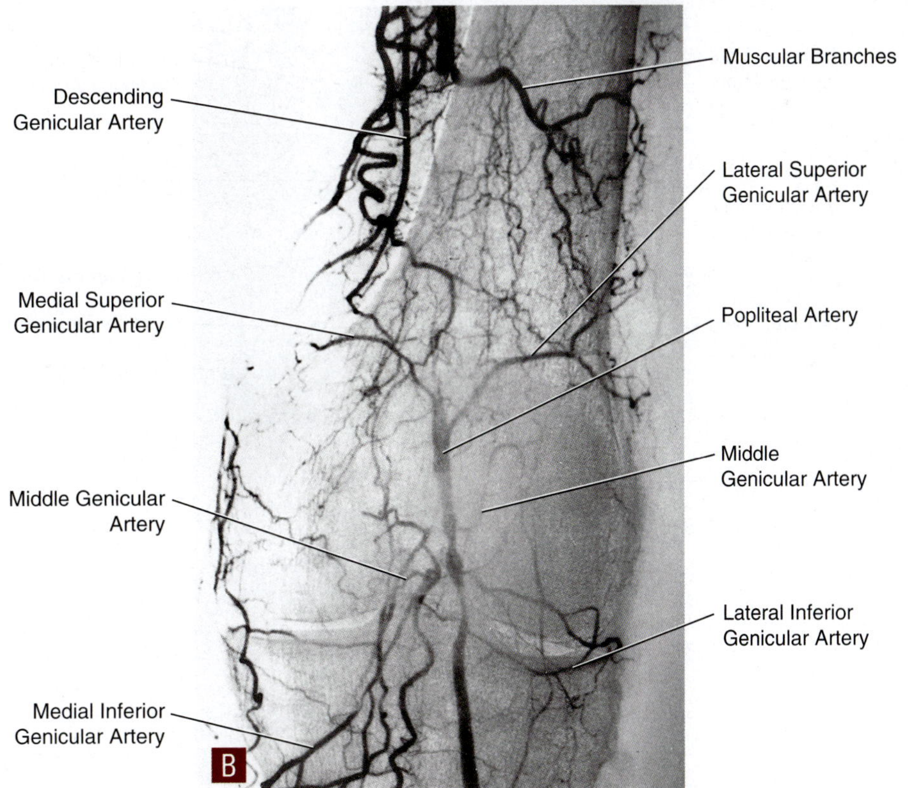

Figure 22.21. **A**, Anterior view DSA of the popliteal artery showing the main branches. **B**, DSA of the distal SFA and popliteal artery shows occlusion of the SFA/popliteal artery transition with extensive collateral network between the muscular branches and the medial and lateral genicular arteries. **C**, Anterior view DSA popliteal artery trifurcation showing the origins of the anterior tibial artery, posterior tibial artery, and peroneal artery. DSA, digital subtraction angiography; SFA, superficial femoral artery.

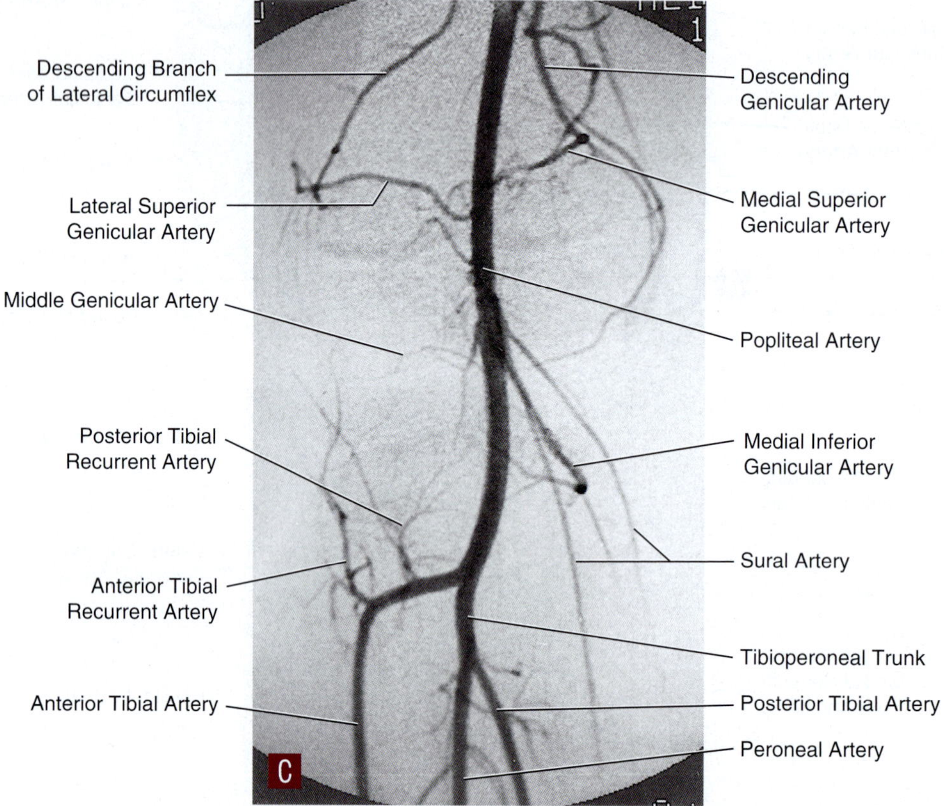

Figure 22.21. *Continued*

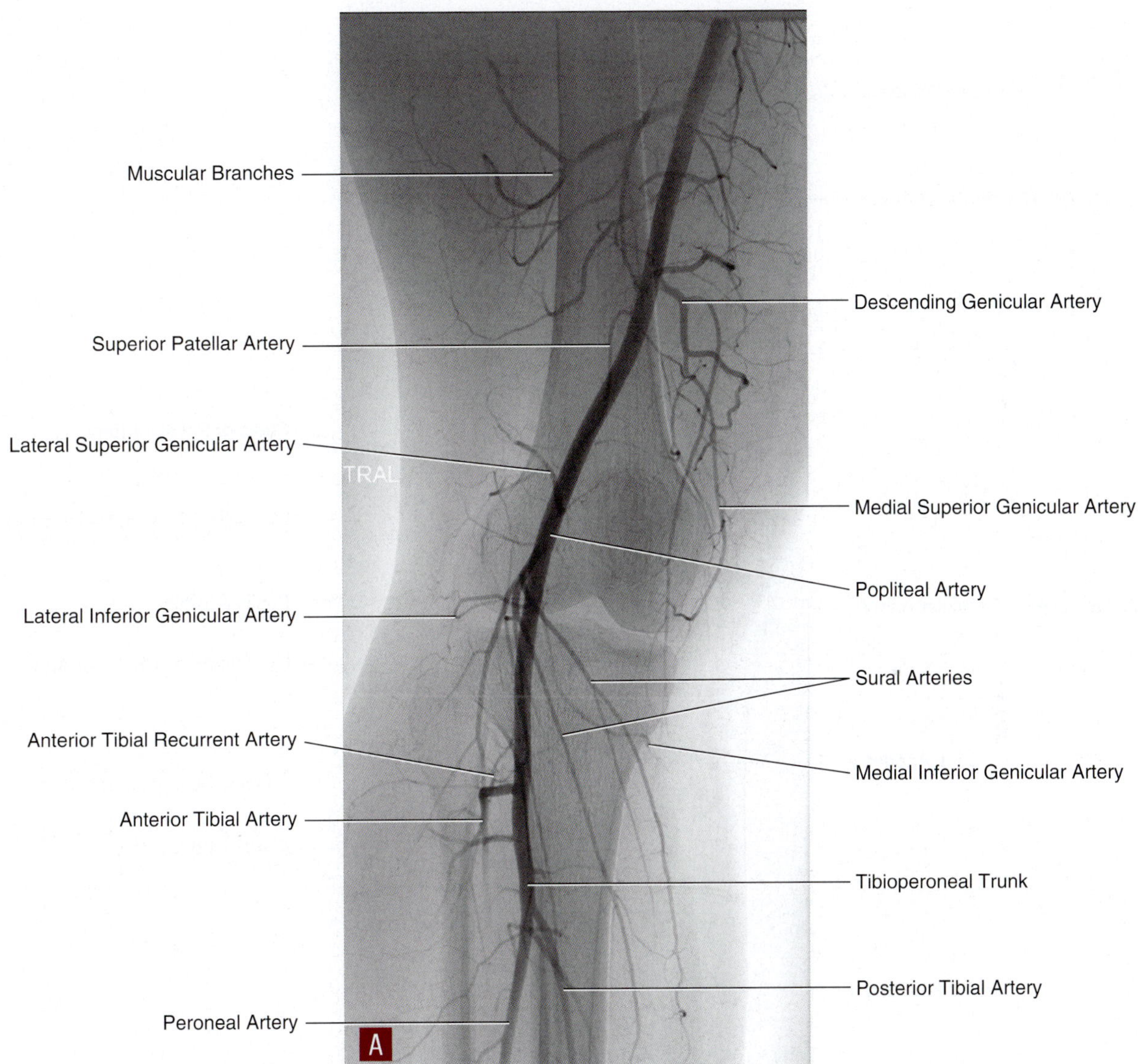

Figure 22.22. A to E, DSA and native angiograms of the right lower extremity at the level of the knee. Observe the correlation between popliteal arteries and the medial and lateral superior geniculate arteries and the medial and lateral inferior geniculate arteries. The anastomosis between these arteries may play an important role in chronic popliteal artery occlusions. DSA, digital subtraction angiography.

Muscular Branches

Descending Genicular Artery

Superior Patellar Artery

Lateral Superior Genicular Artery

Medial Superior Genicular Artery

Popliteal Artery

Lateral Inferior Genicular Artery

Sural Arteries

Anterior Tibial Recurrent Artery

Anterior Tibial Artery

Peroneal Artery

Posterior Tibial Artery

B

Figure 22.22. *Continued*

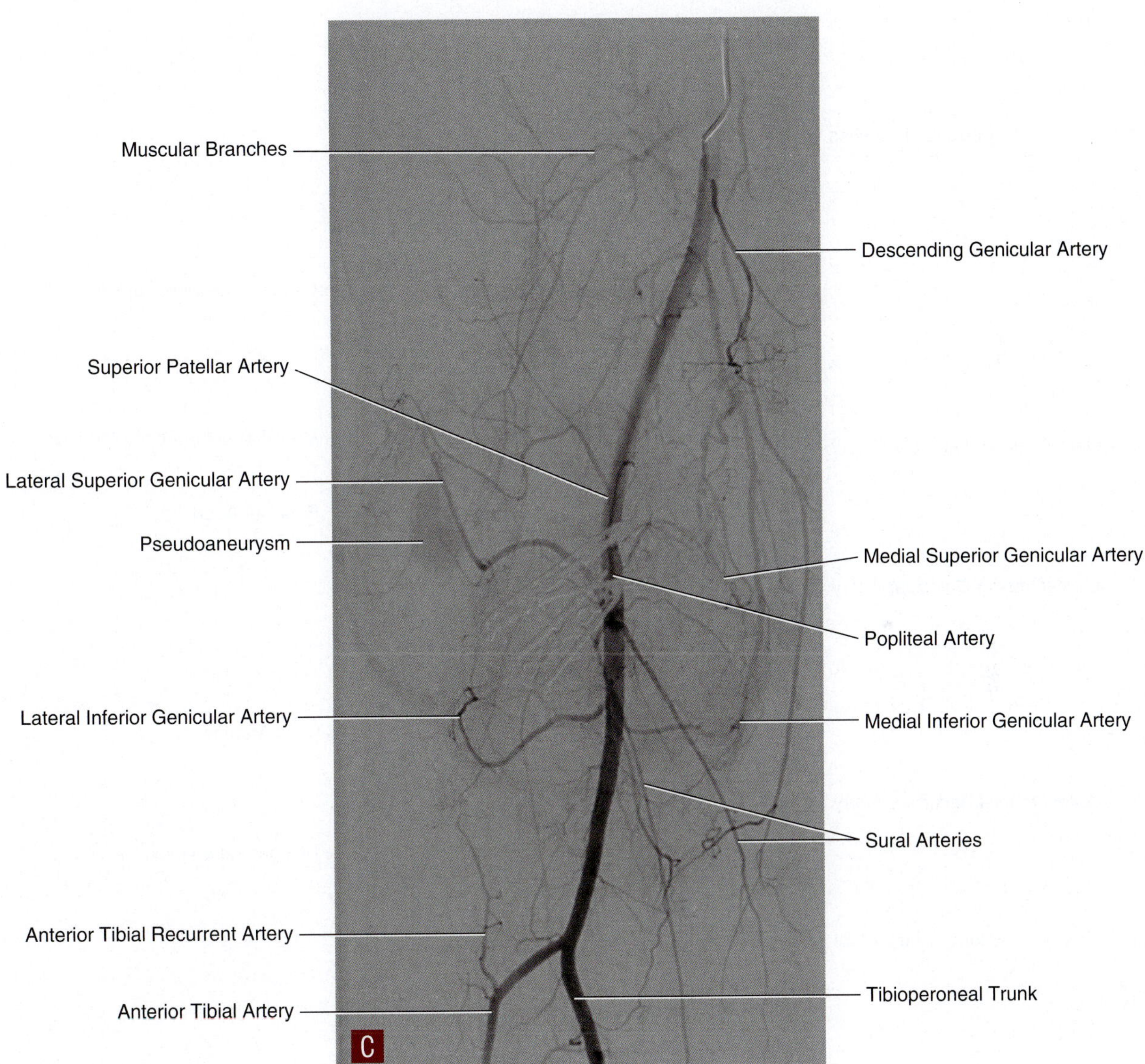

Figure 22.22. *Continued*

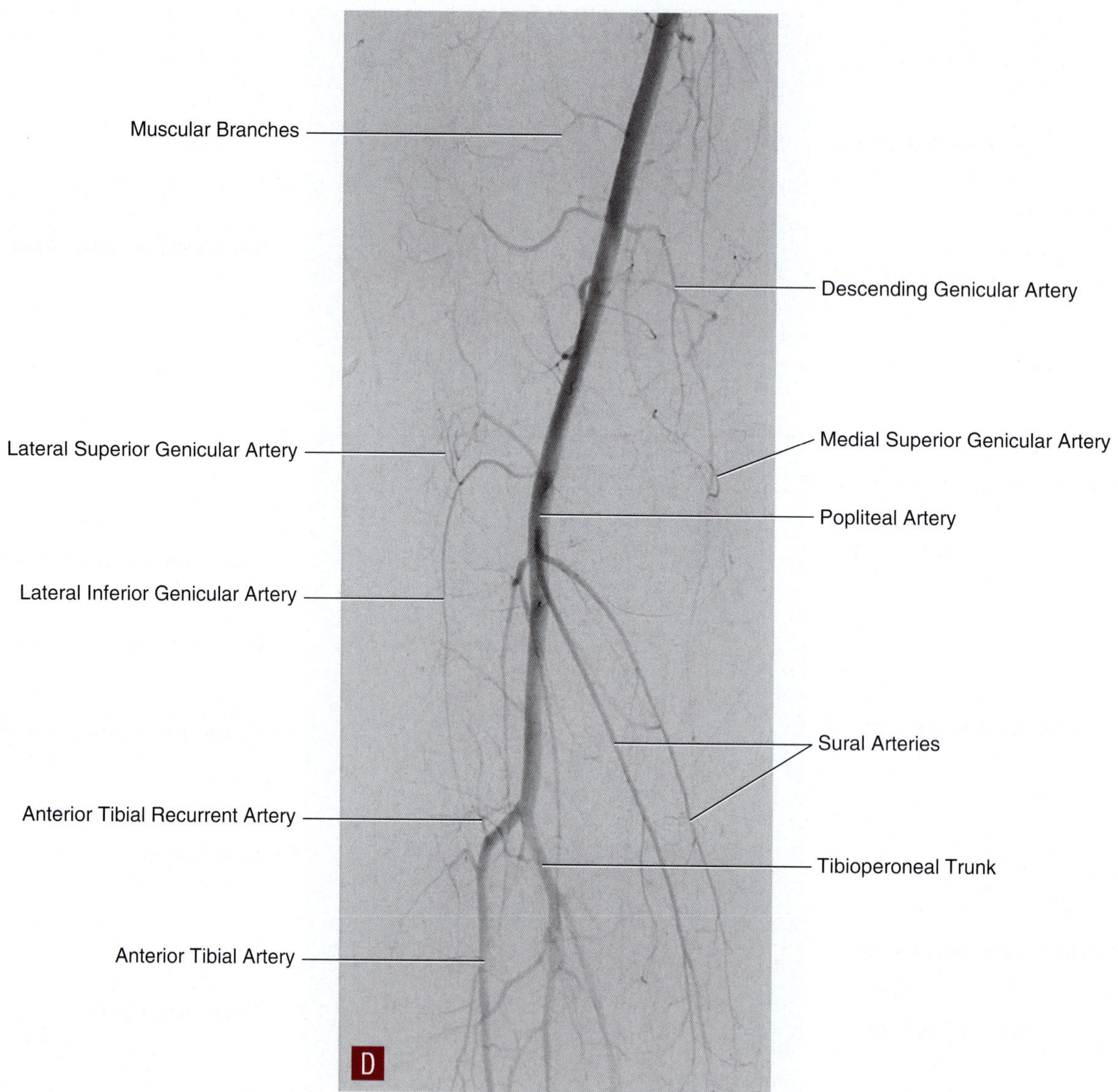

Figure 22.22. *Continued*

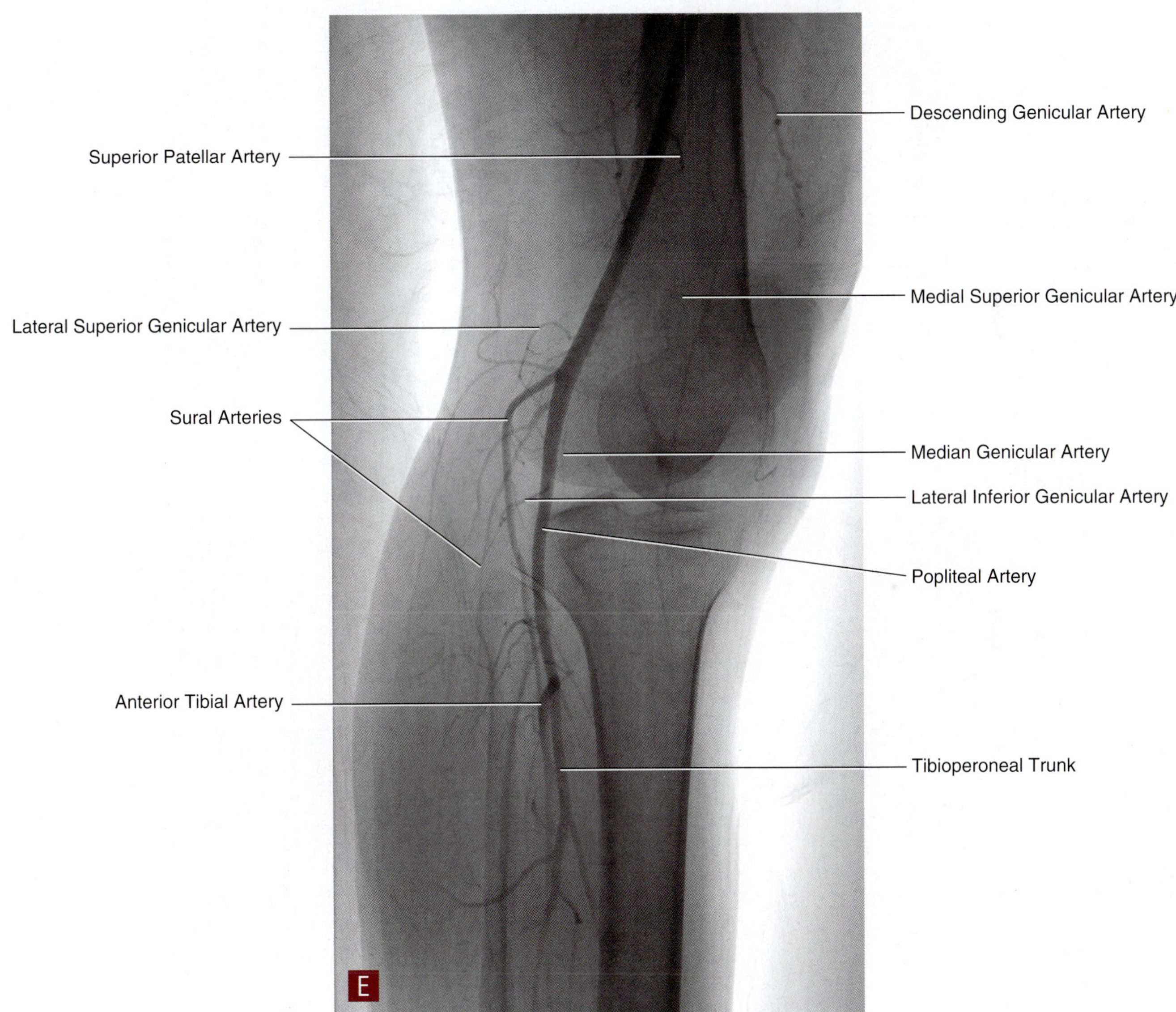

Figure 22.22. *Continued*

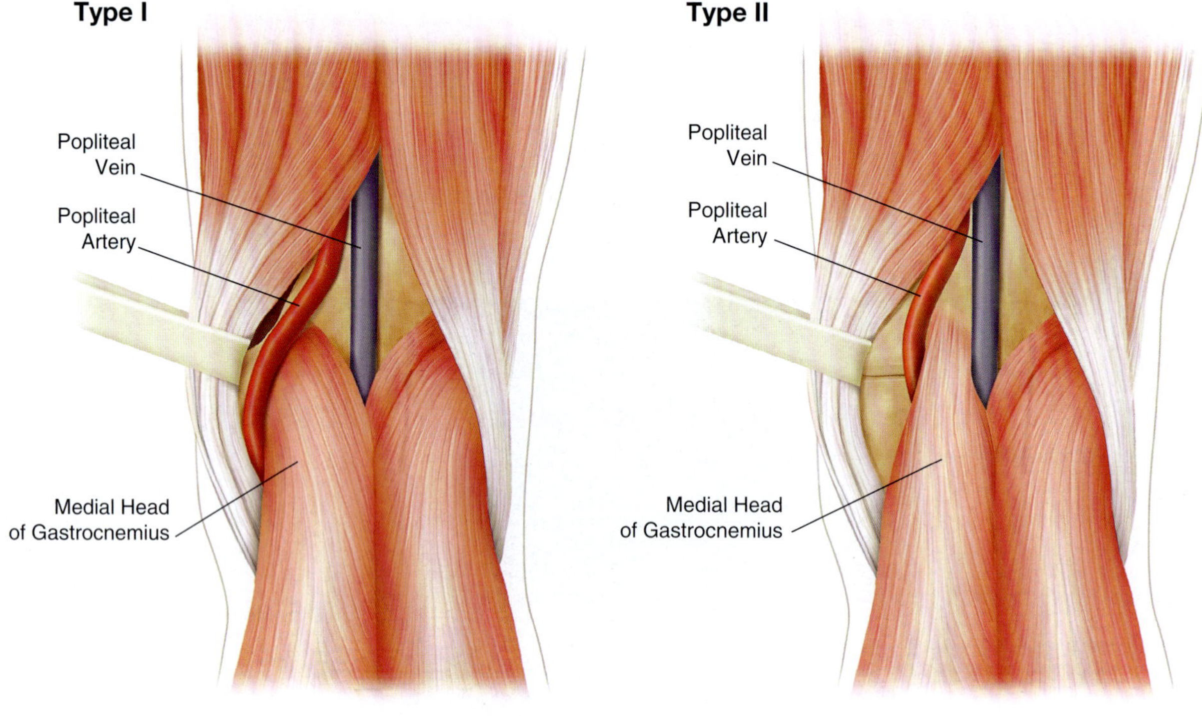

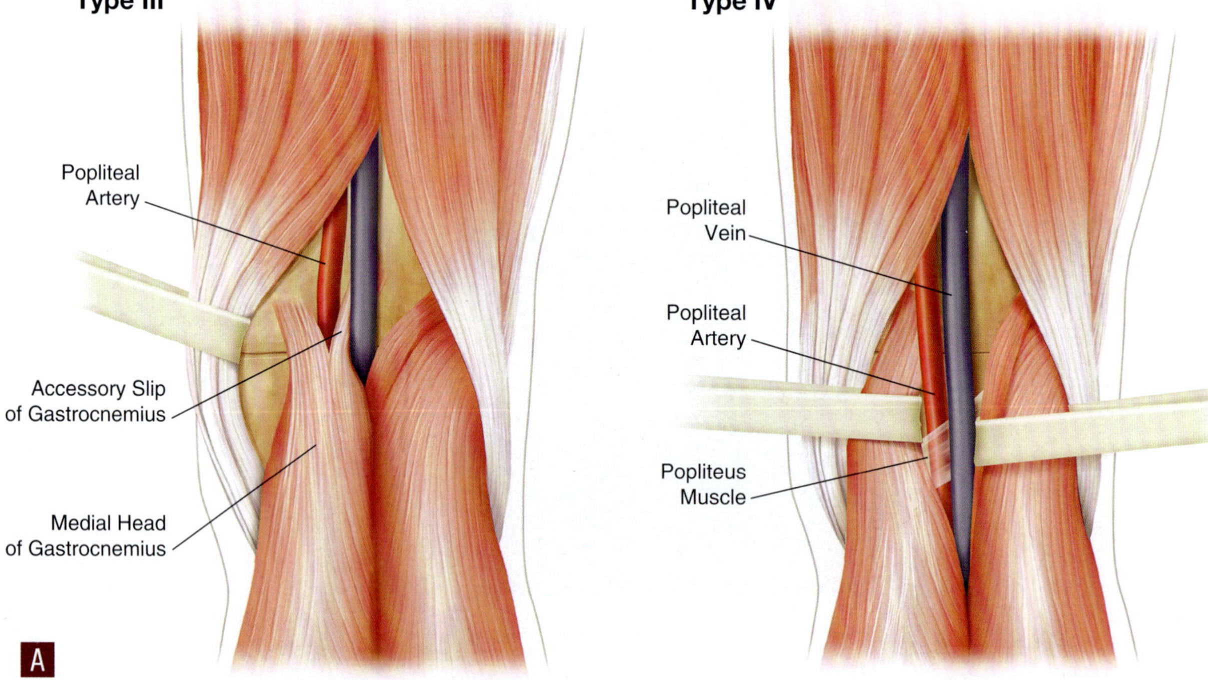

Figure 22.23. **A**, Schematic drawings, posterior view of the popliteal fossa. Note the four types of popliteal artery entrapment. Type I, the medial head of the gastrocnemius is normal, but the popliteal artery runs in an aberrant course. Type II, the medial head of the gastrocnemius is located laterally, no deviation of popliteal artery. Type III, there is an abnormal muscle bundle from the medial head of the gastrocnemius that surrounds and constricts the popliteal artery. Type IV, the popliteal artery is entrapped by the popliteus muscle. **B** and **C**, DSA of the lower extremities at the level of the knees (during plantar flexion of the feet) shows temporary occlusion of both right (B) and left (C) popliteal arteries. DSA, digital subtraction angiography.

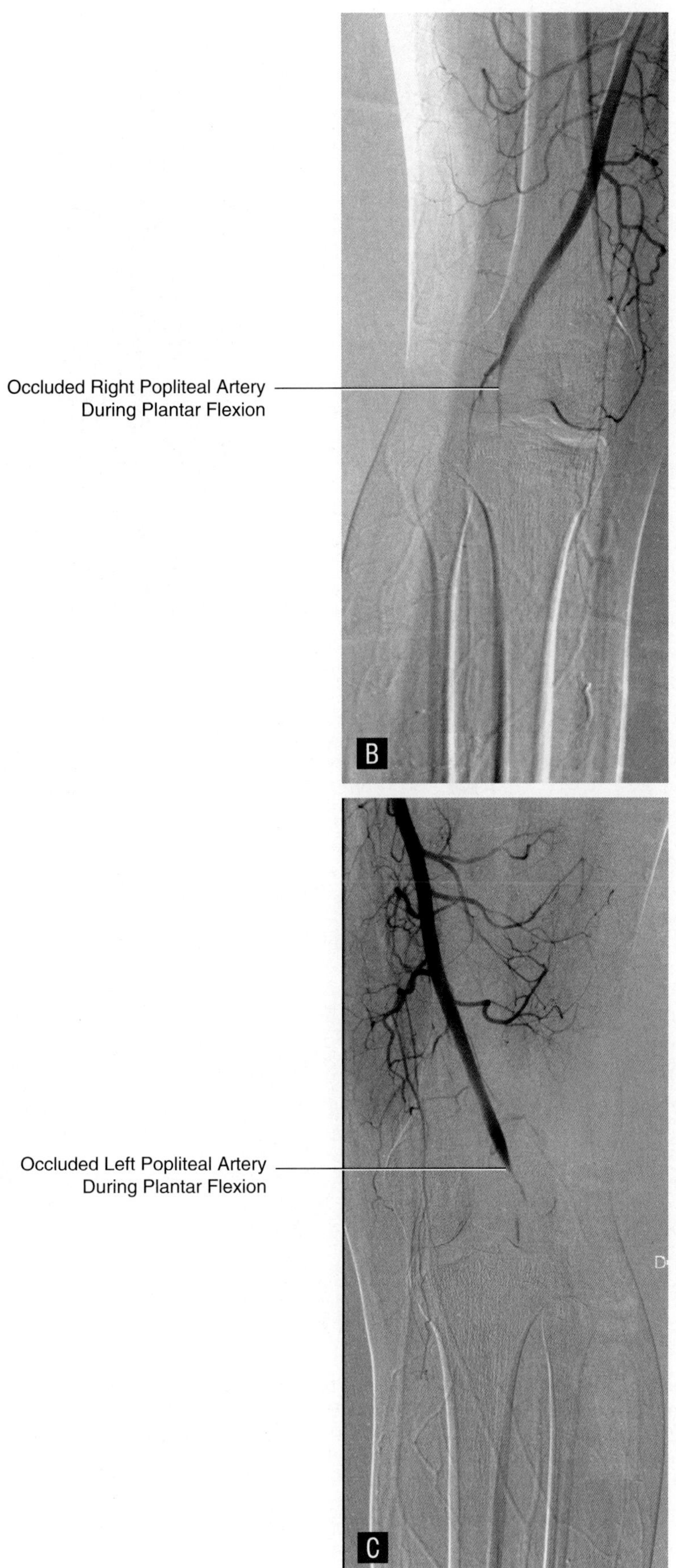

Figure 22.23. *Continued*

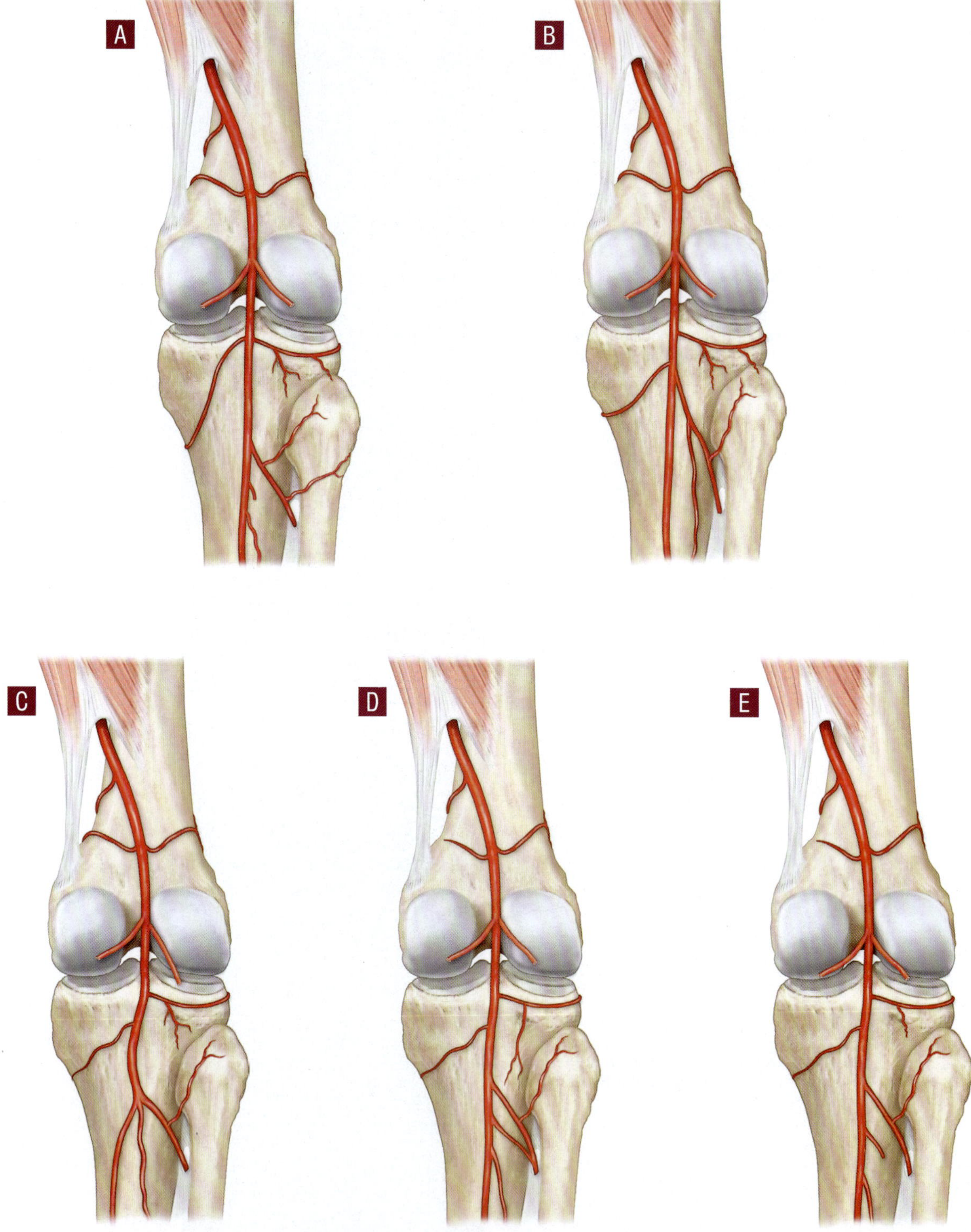

Figure 22.24. Variations of the popliteal bifurcation. A, Regular most frequent trifurcation. B, Tibioperoneal trunk with the anterior tibial artery. C, Trifurcation of the three main arteries at the same level. D, Anastomosis of the anterior tibial artery and tibioperoneal trunk. E, Long tibioperoneal trunk.

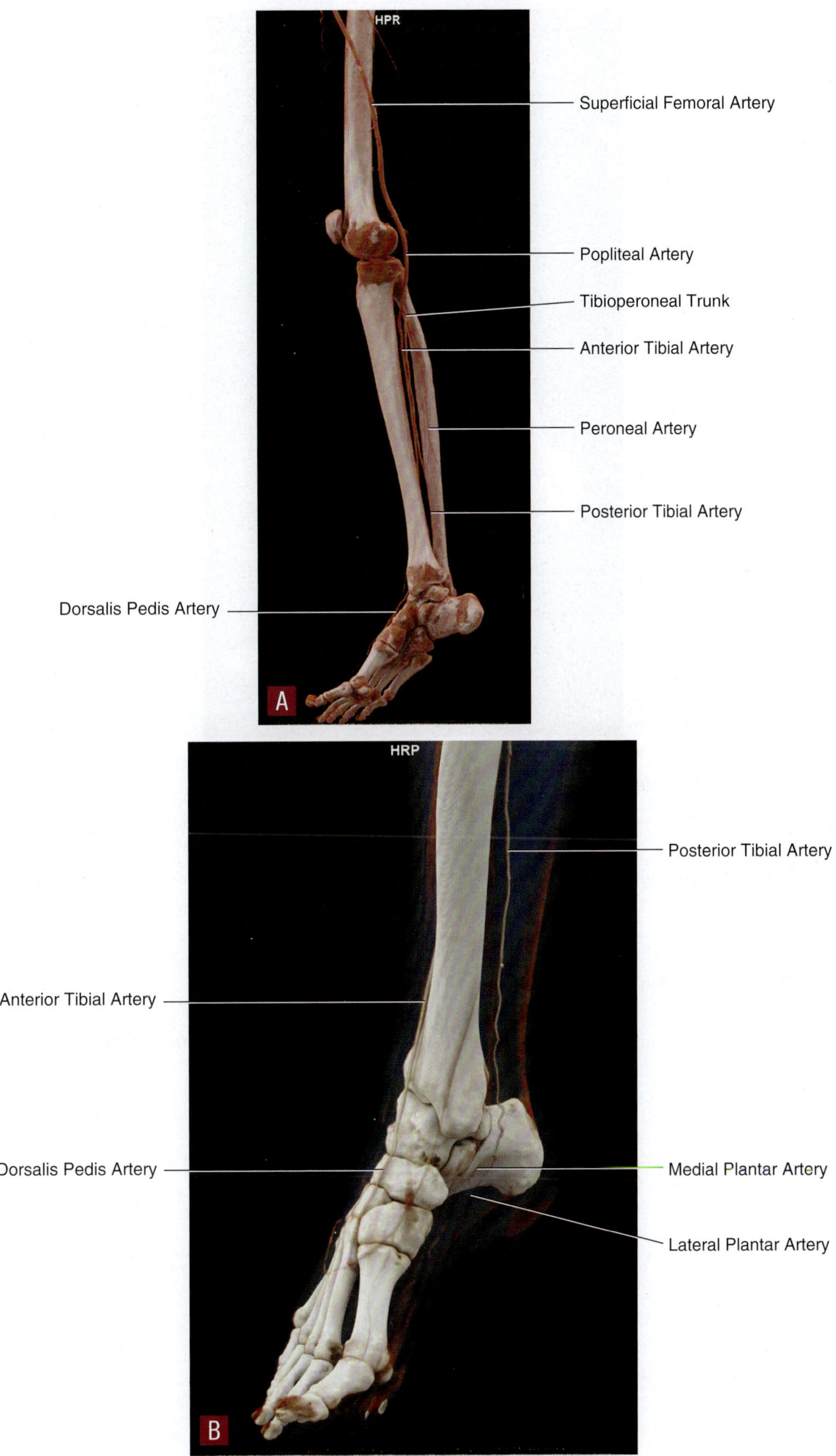

Figure 22.25. A to D, Cinematic 3D reconstructions of distal lower extremity CTA from multiples views. Note the correlation between anterior and posterior tibial arteries and their branches at the level of the ankle and foot. CTA, computed tomography angiography.

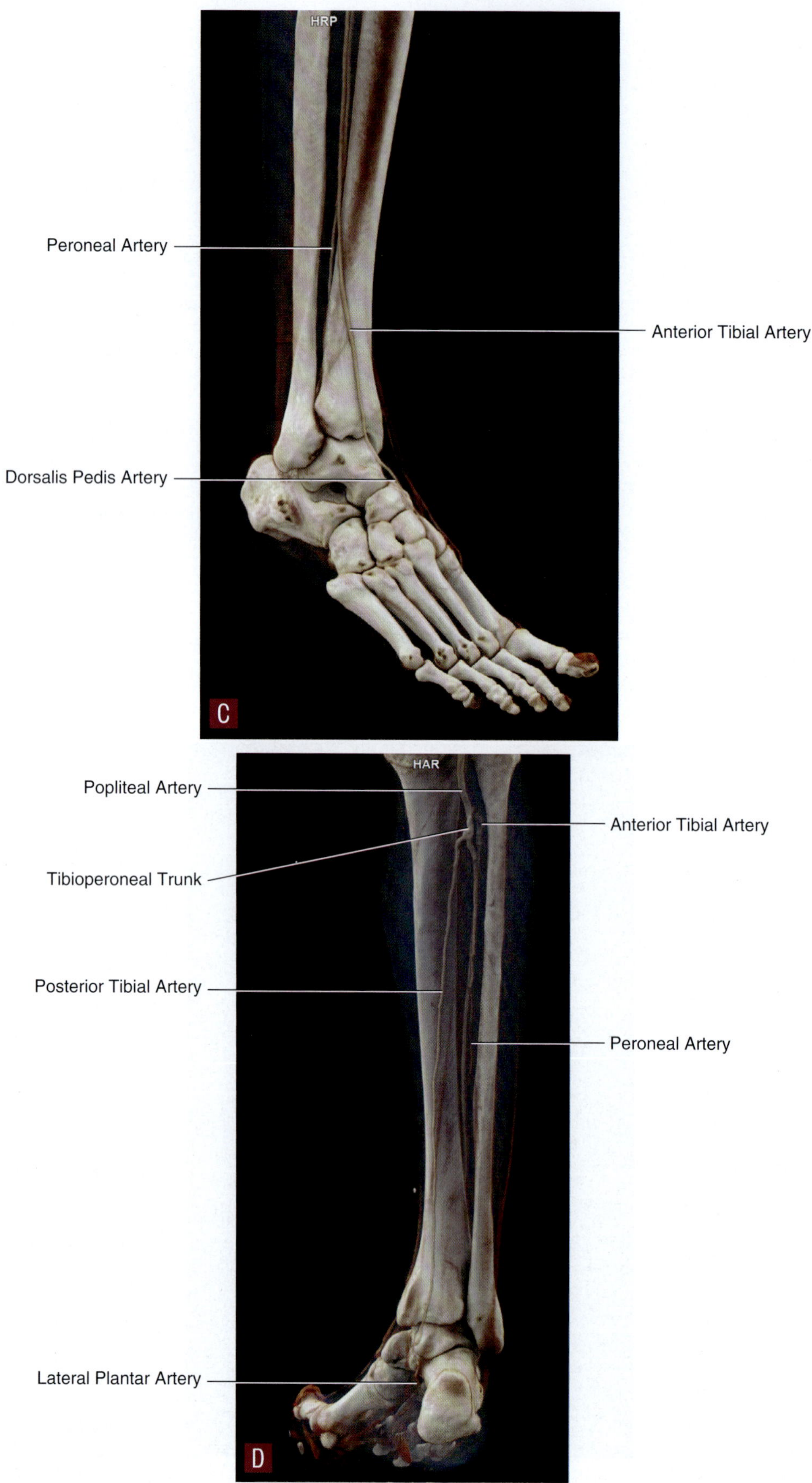

Figure 22.25. *Continued*

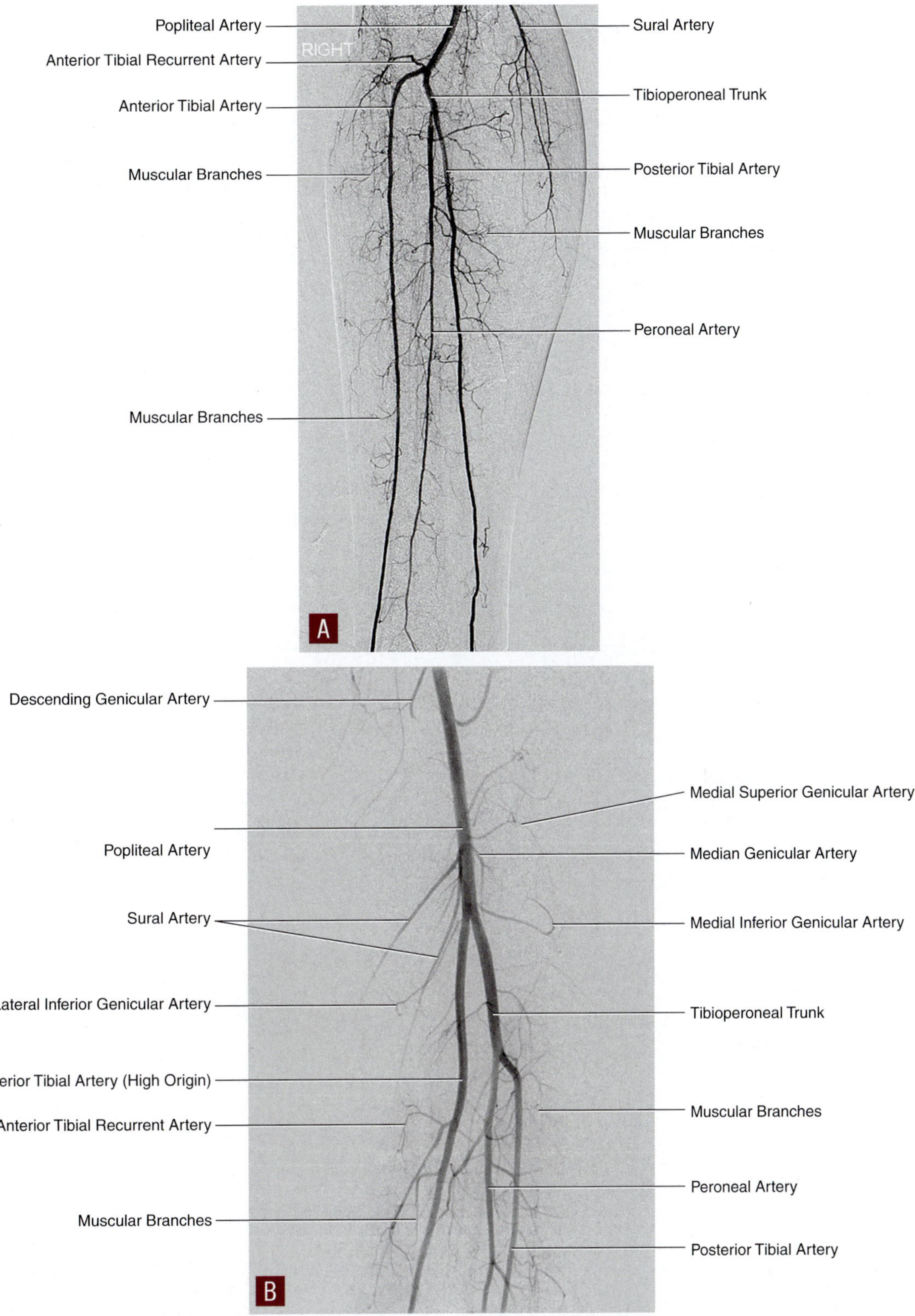

Figure 22.26. **A** to **F**, Right lower extremity DSAs at the level of the calf. **A**, Typical anatomy of the popliteal artery bifurcation into AT artery and tibioperoneal trunk. Short tibioperoneal trunk bifurcates into PT and peroneal arteries. **B**, Observe the high AT artery origin from the popliteal artery at the level of the popliteal fossa. **C**, Normal arteriogram at the level of left knee and proximal calf. Note the geniculate and muscular branches. **D**, Left lower extremity arteriogram. Note the long tibioperoneal trunk. Variation of the anatomy. There are multisegmental stenosis in the posterior tibial artery. **E**, Bilateral DSA of lower extremities at the level of the knees and calves. All vessels are normal. E1, Left lower extremity arteriograms at the level of the calf. The AT is patent proximally. The peroneal is occluded, as well as the proximal PT. There is collateral circulation through the muscular branches. E2, Delayed phase of the same angiogram. **F**, Corkscrew aspect of the peroneal artery typical of Buerger disease, also called thromboangiitis obliterans. This finding typically represents hypertrophy of the vasa vasora of the involved vessel. AT, anterior tibial; DSA, digital subtraction angiography; PT, posterior tibial; PTA, percutaneous transluminal angioplasty.

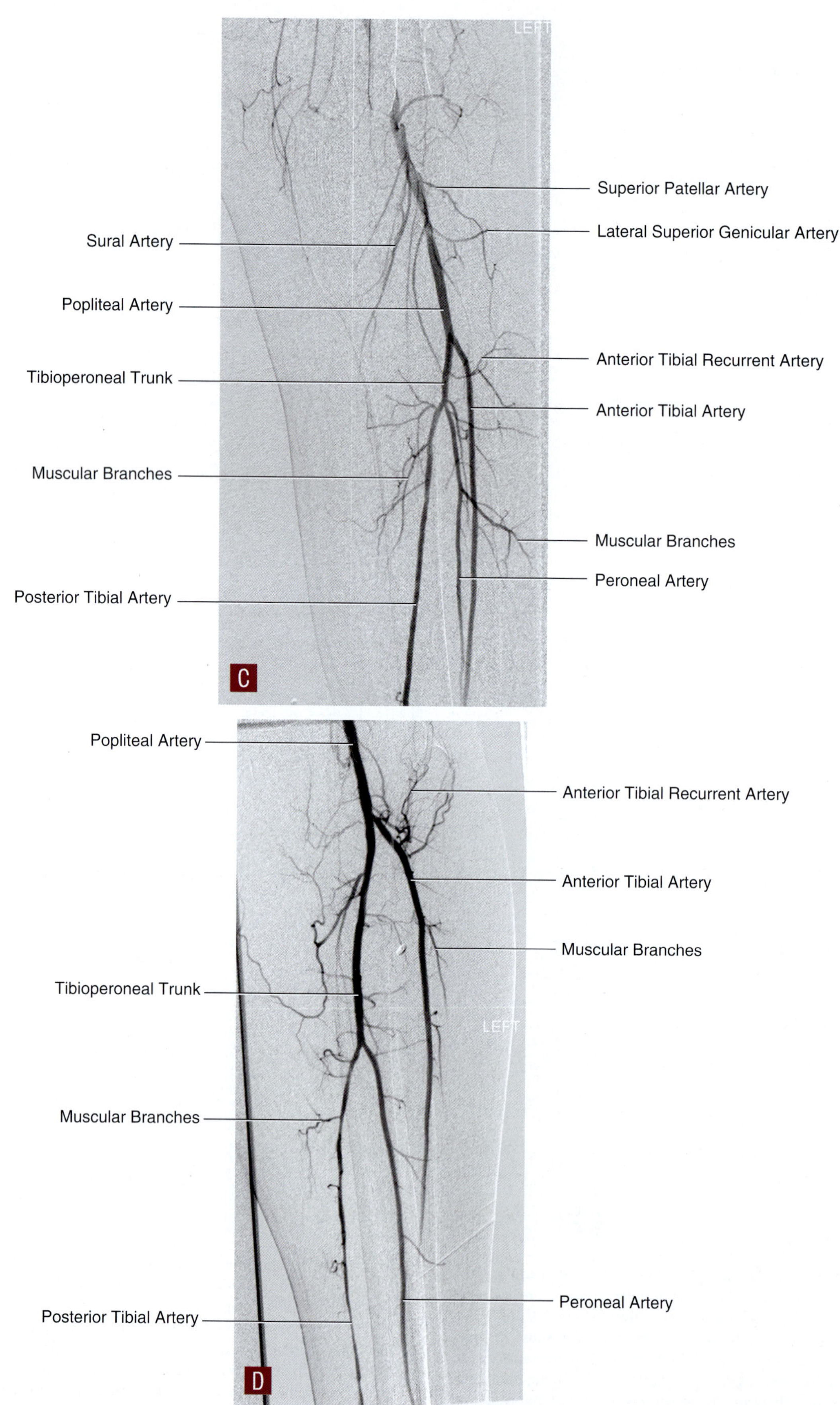

Figure 22.26. *Continued*

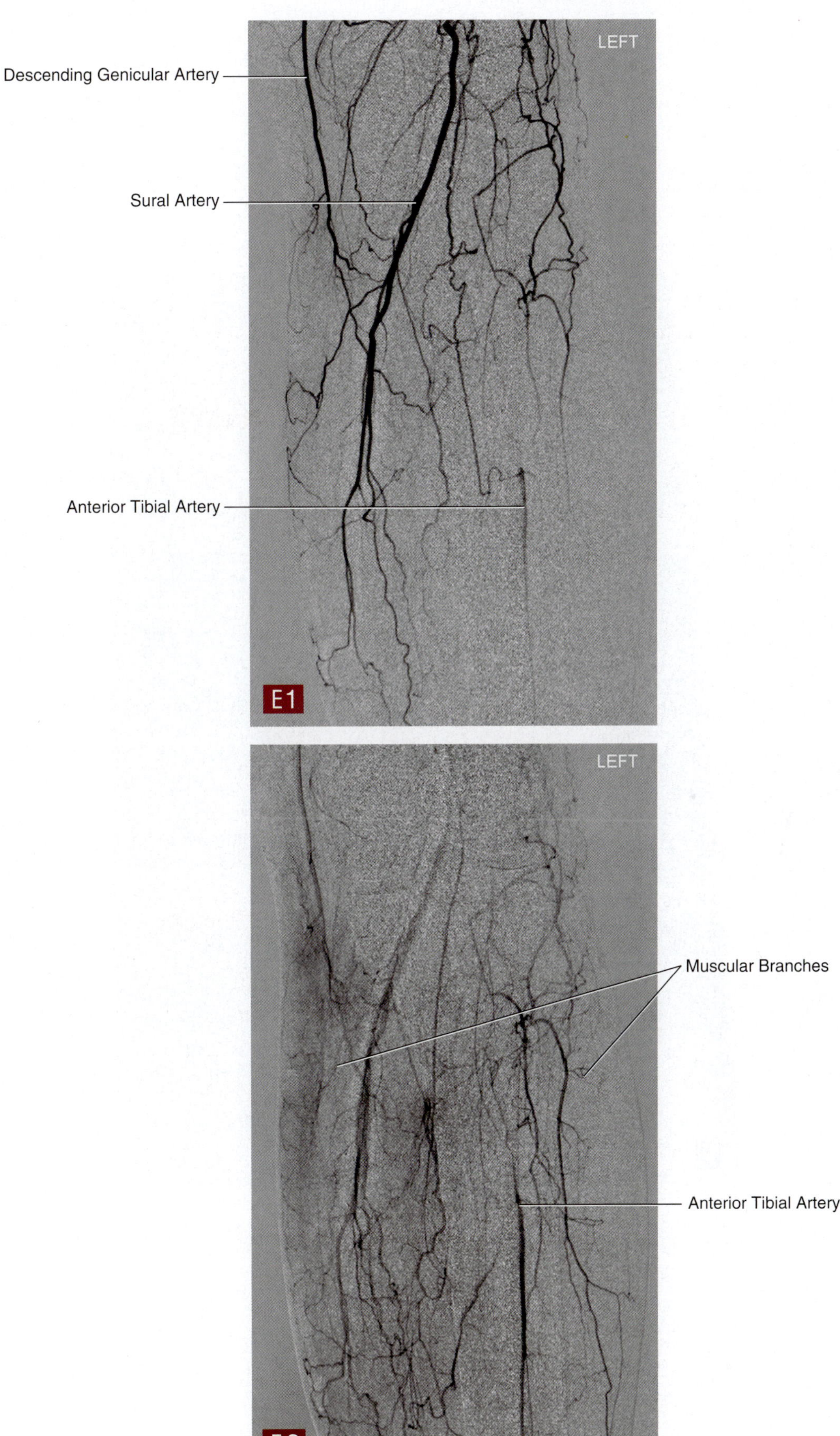

Figure 22.26. *Continued*

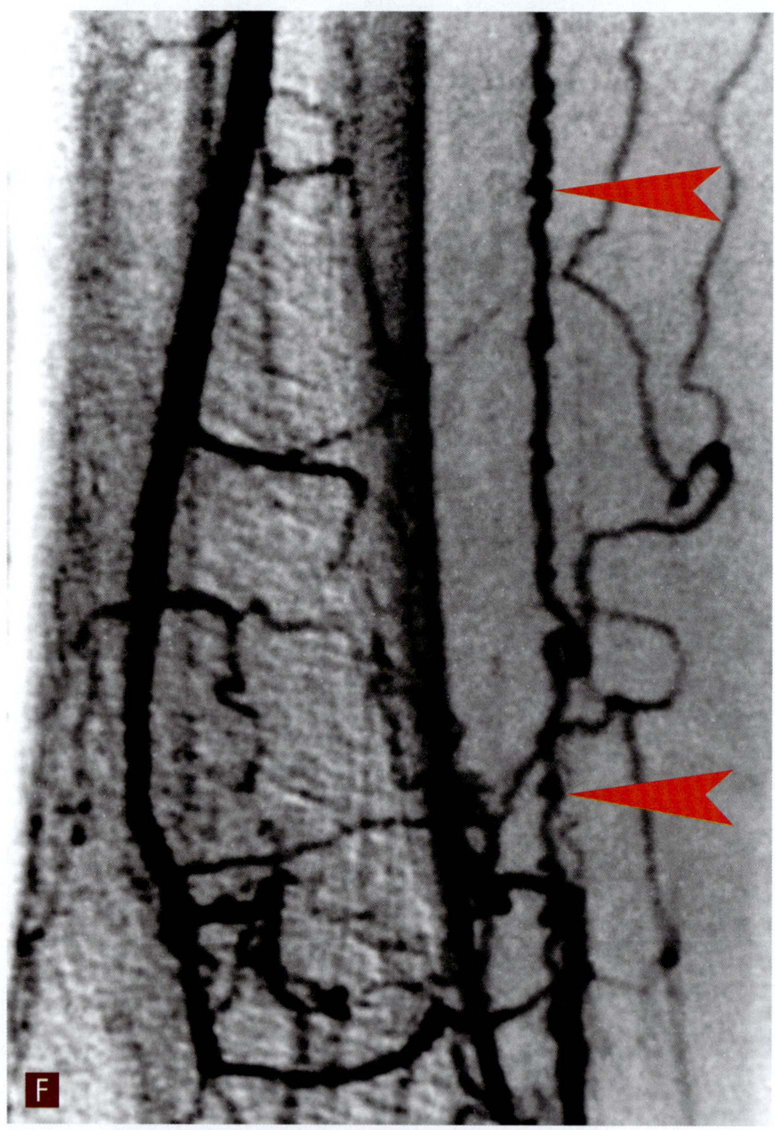

Figure 22.26. *Continued*

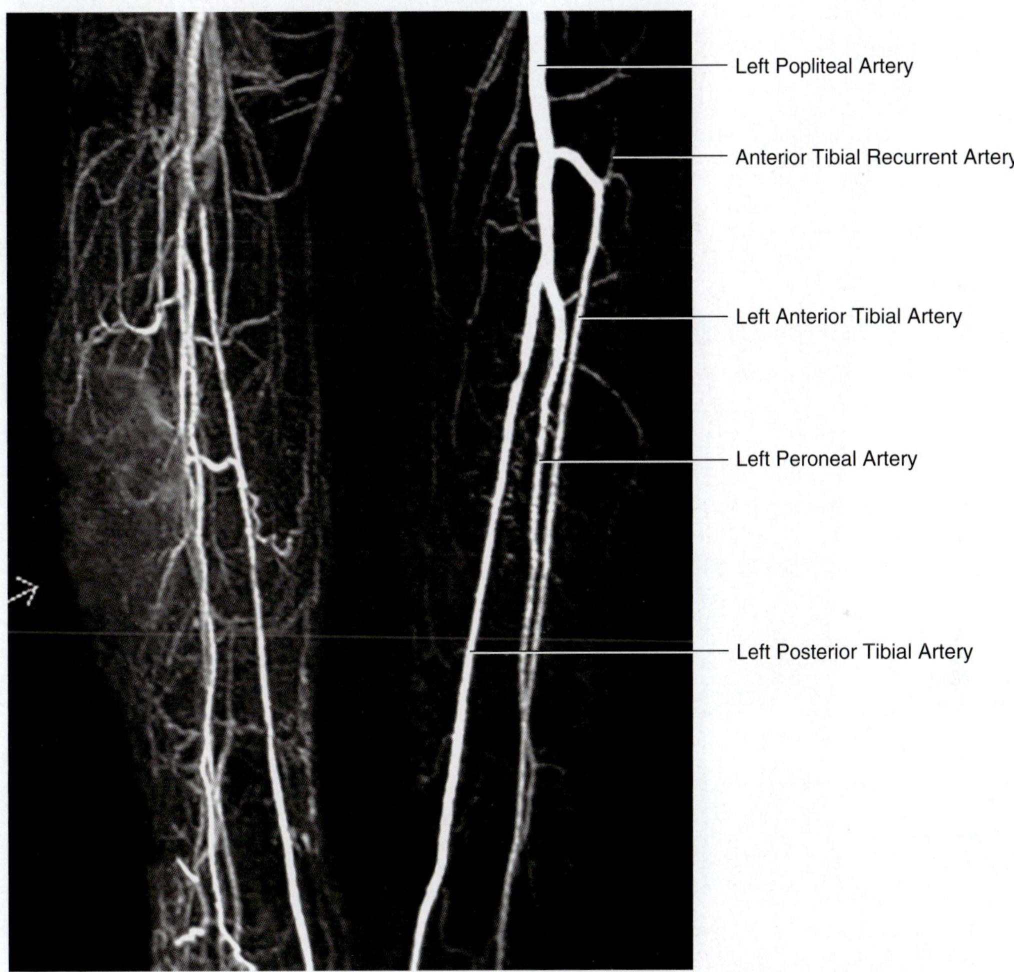

Figure 22.27. Bilateral lower extremities MRA. Note the hypervascular mass in the lateral aspect of the right calf and early opacification of the venous system in comparison with the left calf. Findings are consistent with an arteriovenous malformation in the right calf. MRA, magnetic resonance angiogram.

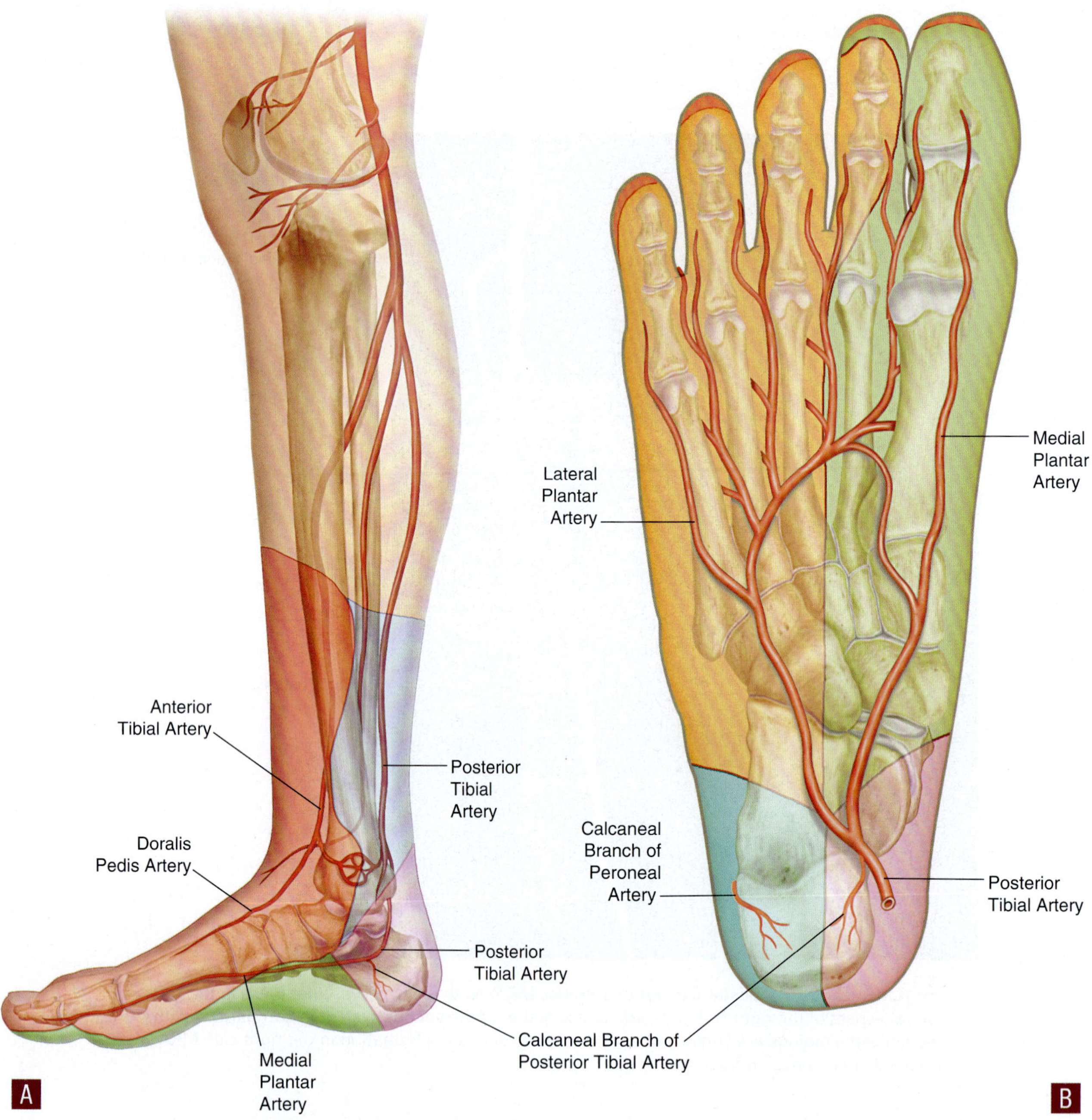

Figure 22.28. A, Schematic drawing of the arterial circulation and corresponding angiosomes of the right ankle and foot in a lateral view. B, Schematic drawing of the angiosome concept showing the five angiosomes and their respective supplying artery.

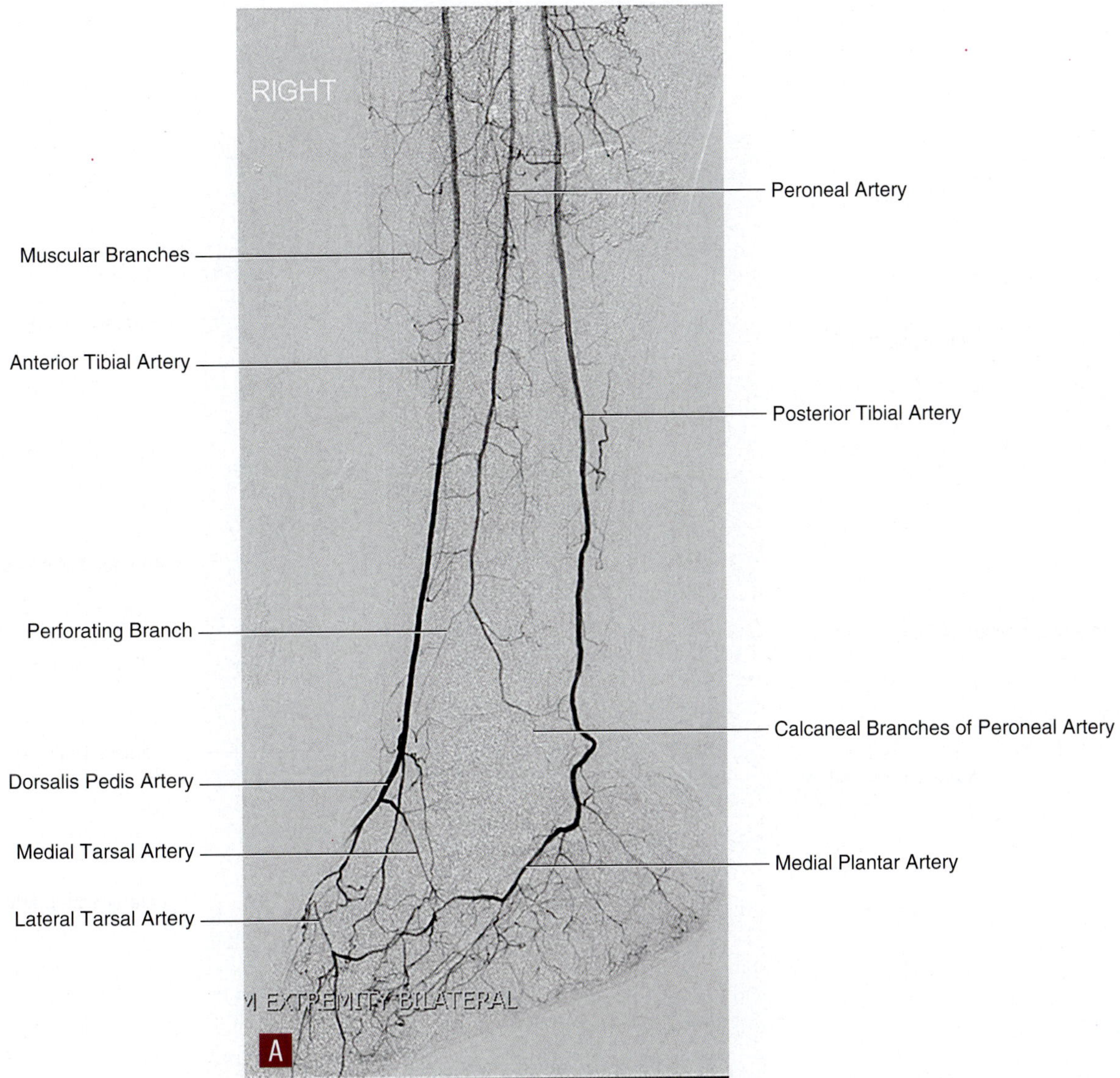

Figure 22.29. **A**, Right lower extremity arteriogram at the level of the calf. Patent AT, PT, and peroneal arteries. At the level of the foot, note the occlusion of the dorsalis pedis artery and patency of the lateral plantas artery. **B**, Left lower extremity arteriogram at the level of the ankle. Note the chronically occluded AT and PT. Peroneal artery is patent. Small anastomotic branch is responsible for the vascularization of the distal forefoot. **C**, Left lower extremity arteriogram at the level of the ankle. Single vessel run-off. The patent AT and a short segment of the dorsalis pedis. There is poor perfusion to the forefoot. **D**, Left lower extremity arteriogram at the level of the foot. Note the chronically occluded AT and PT. Peroneal artery is patent. Through an anastomotic branch, the medial and lateral plantar branches vascularize the distal forefoot. **E**, Anterior view of an angiogram of the right ankle. AT, anterior tibial; PT, posterior tibial.

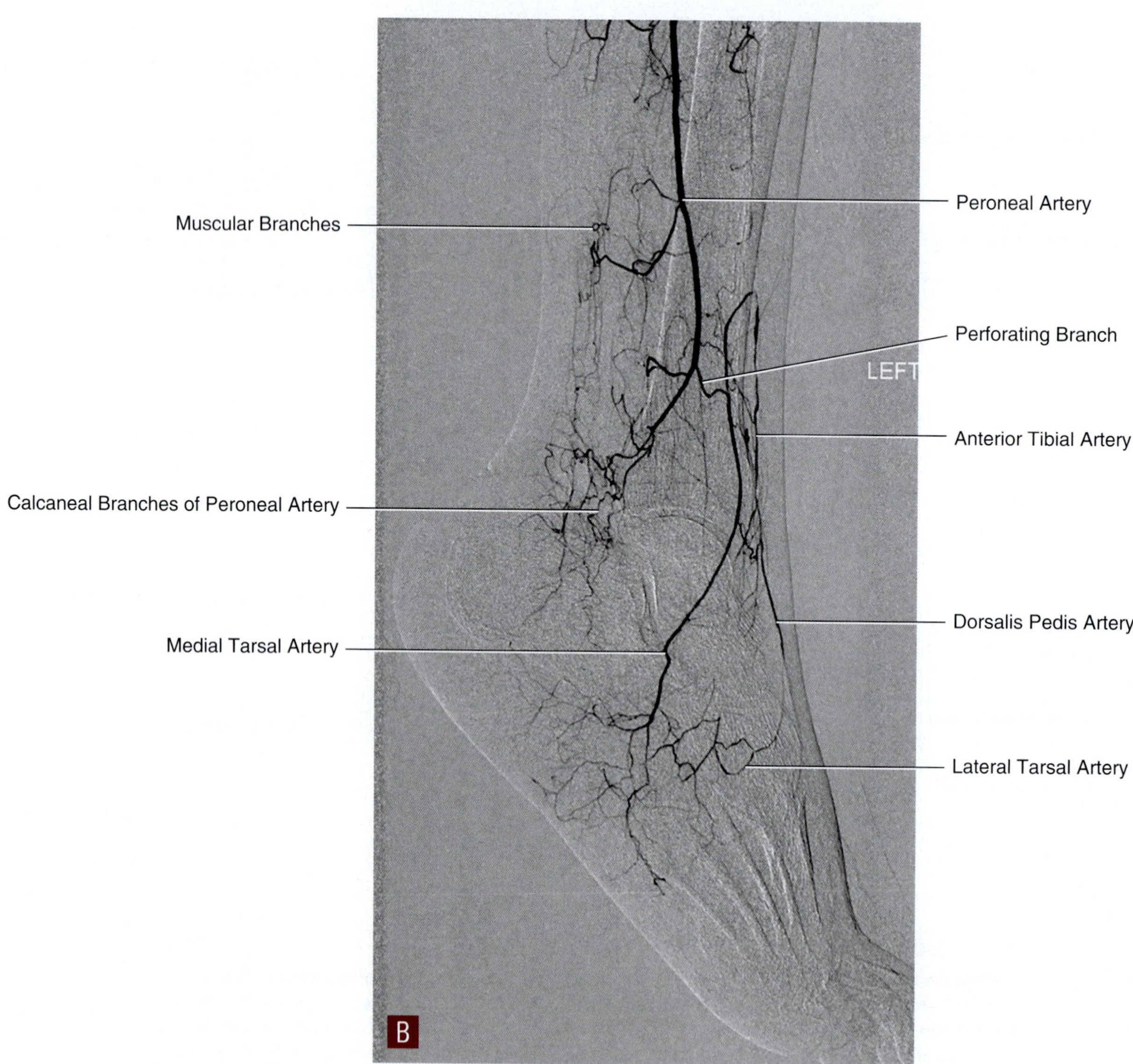

Figure 22.29. *Continued*

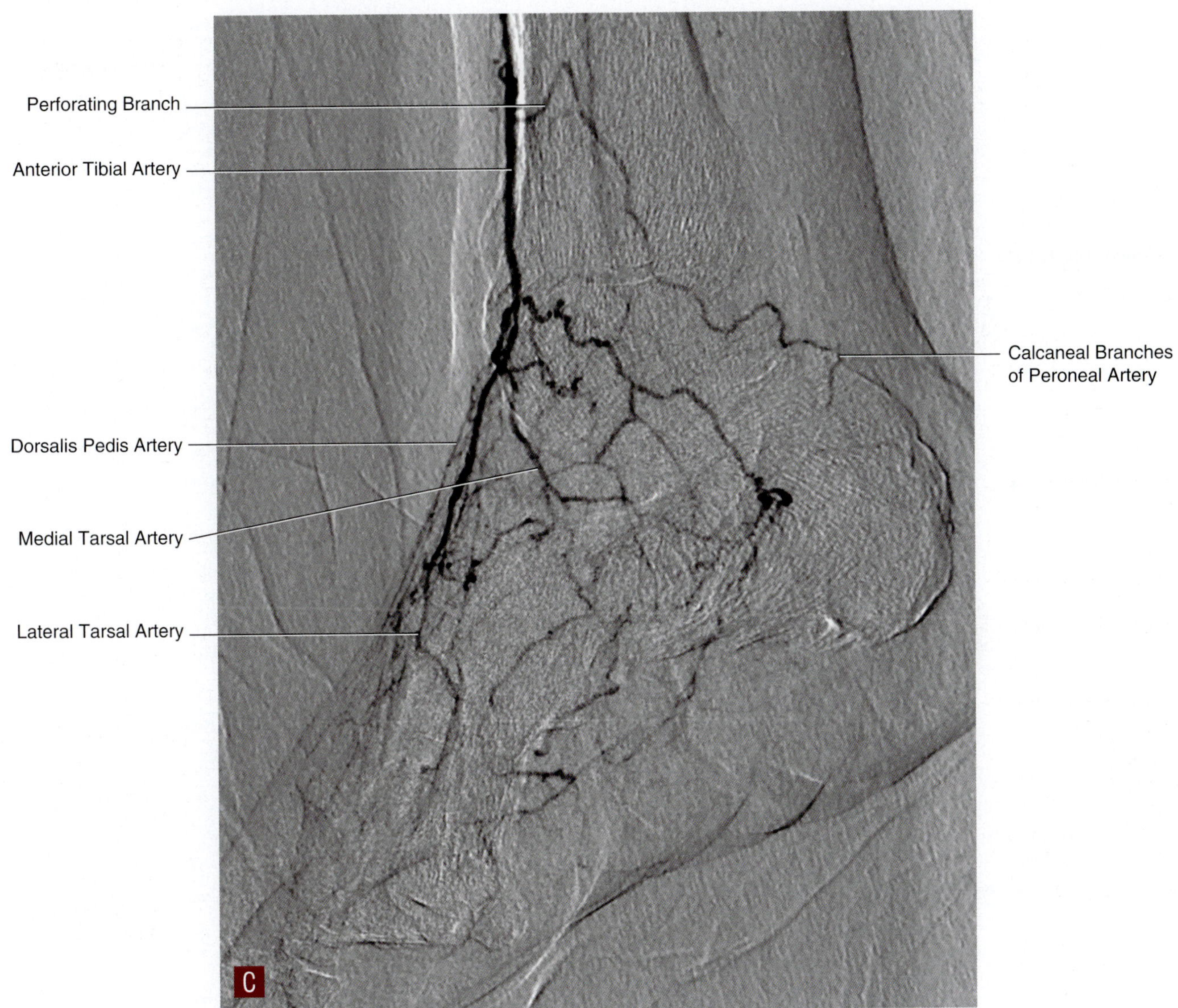

Figure 22.29. *Continued*

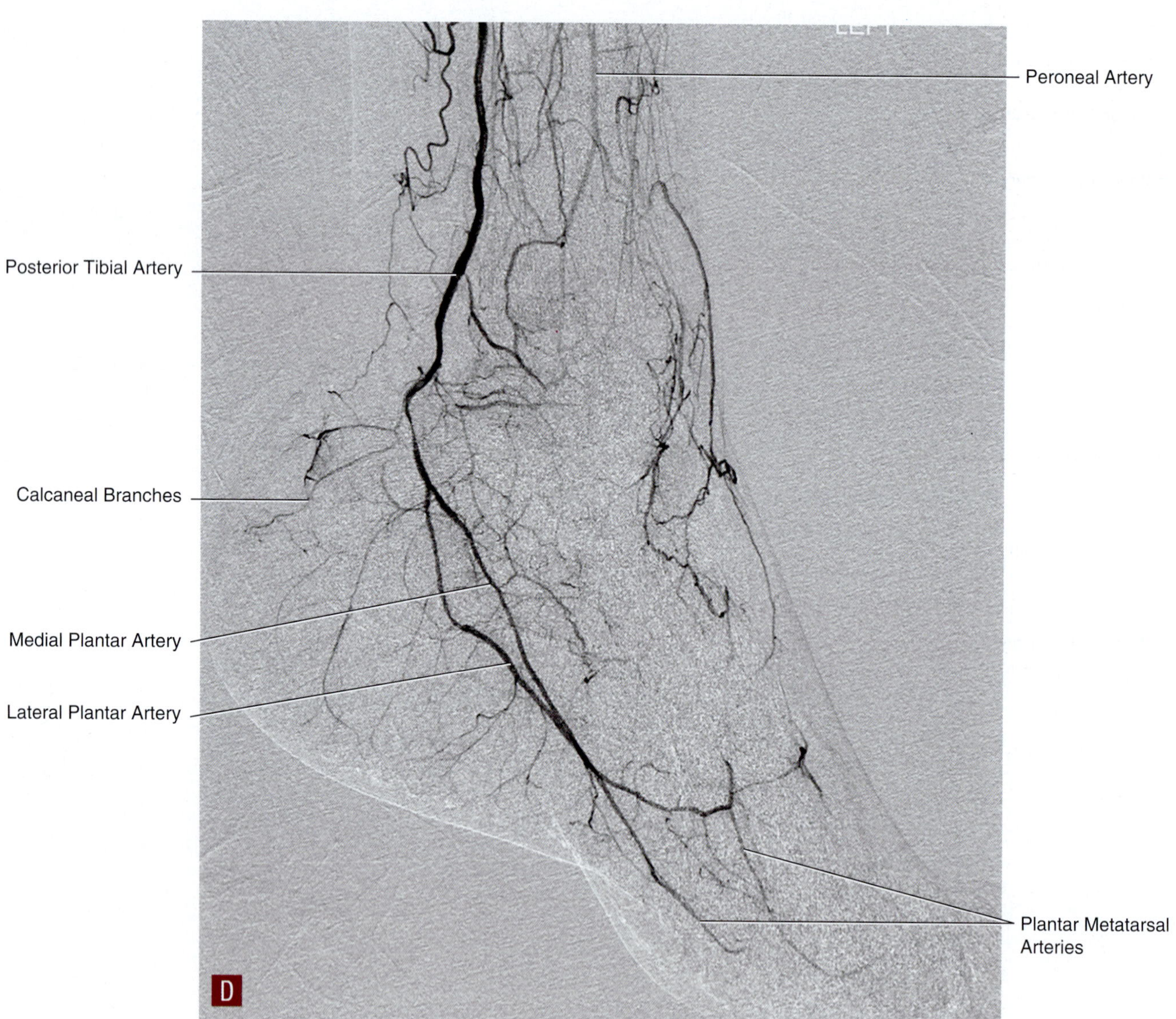

Figure 22.29. *Continued*

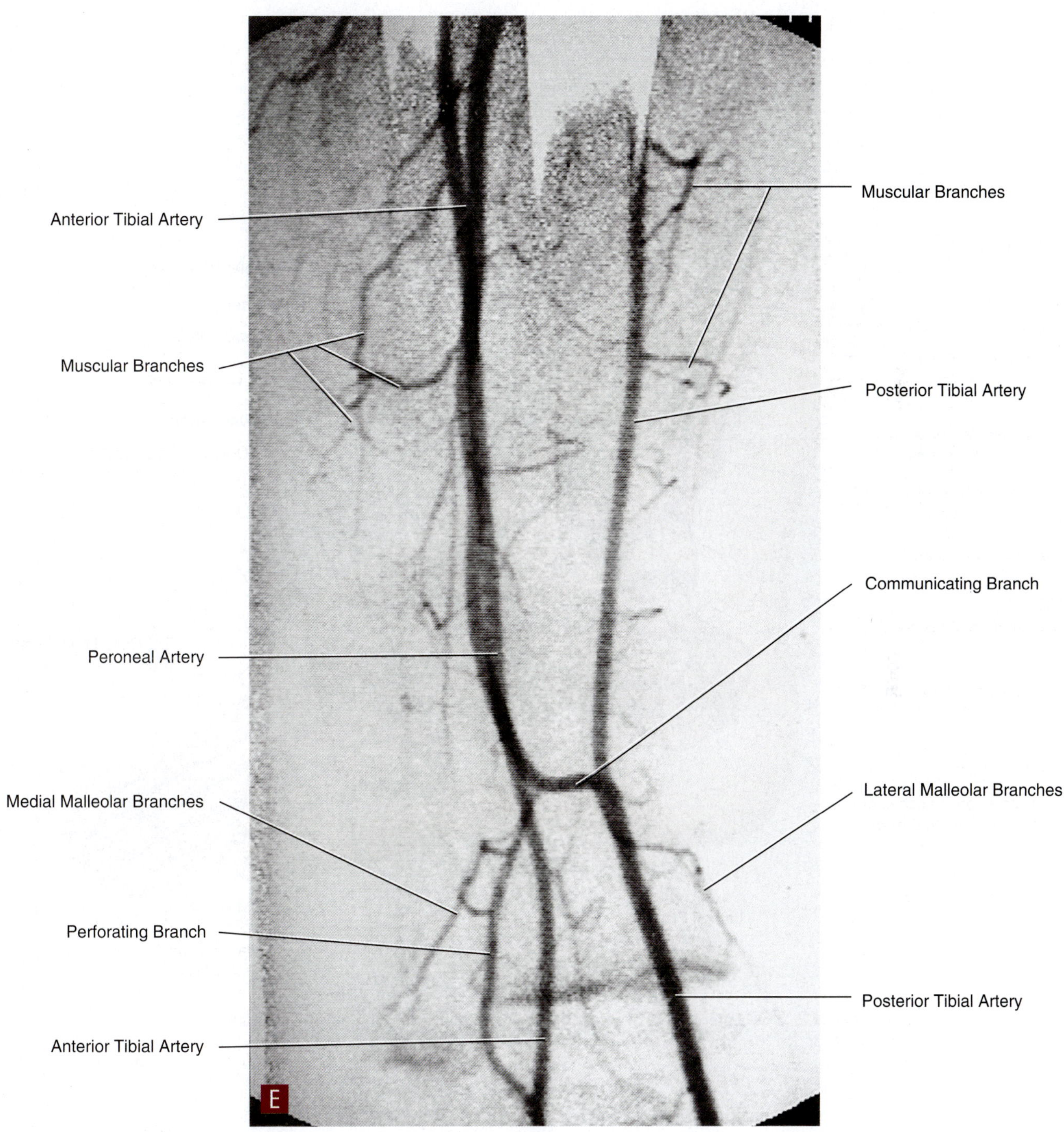

Figure 22.29. *Continued*

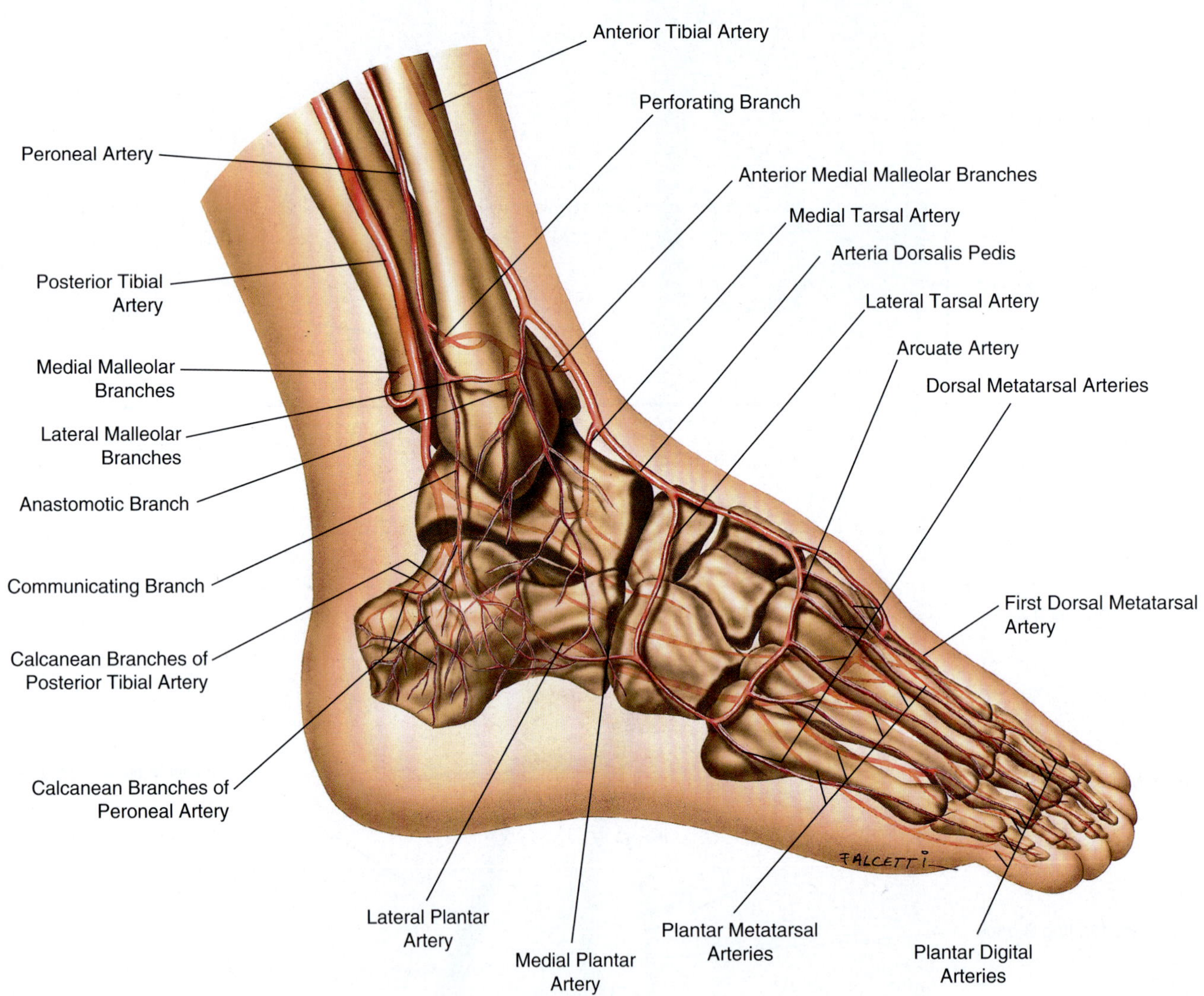

Figure 22.30. Lateral view of a schematic drawing showing the arterial circulation of the right foot.

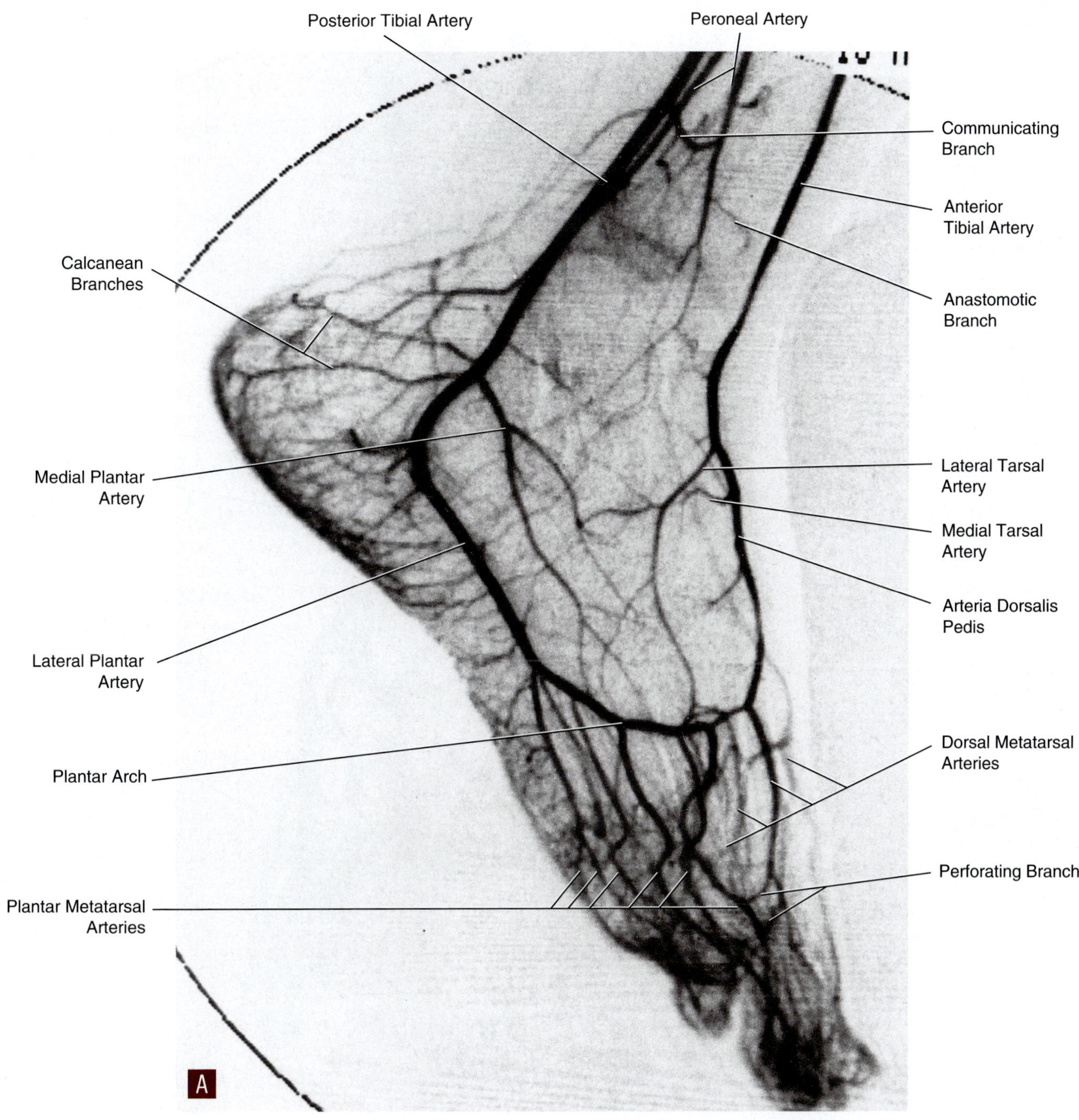

Figure 22.31. **A**, Early phase of a lateral view of an angiogram of the right foot. **B**, Late phase of the foot angiogram showing the venous drainage of the foot.

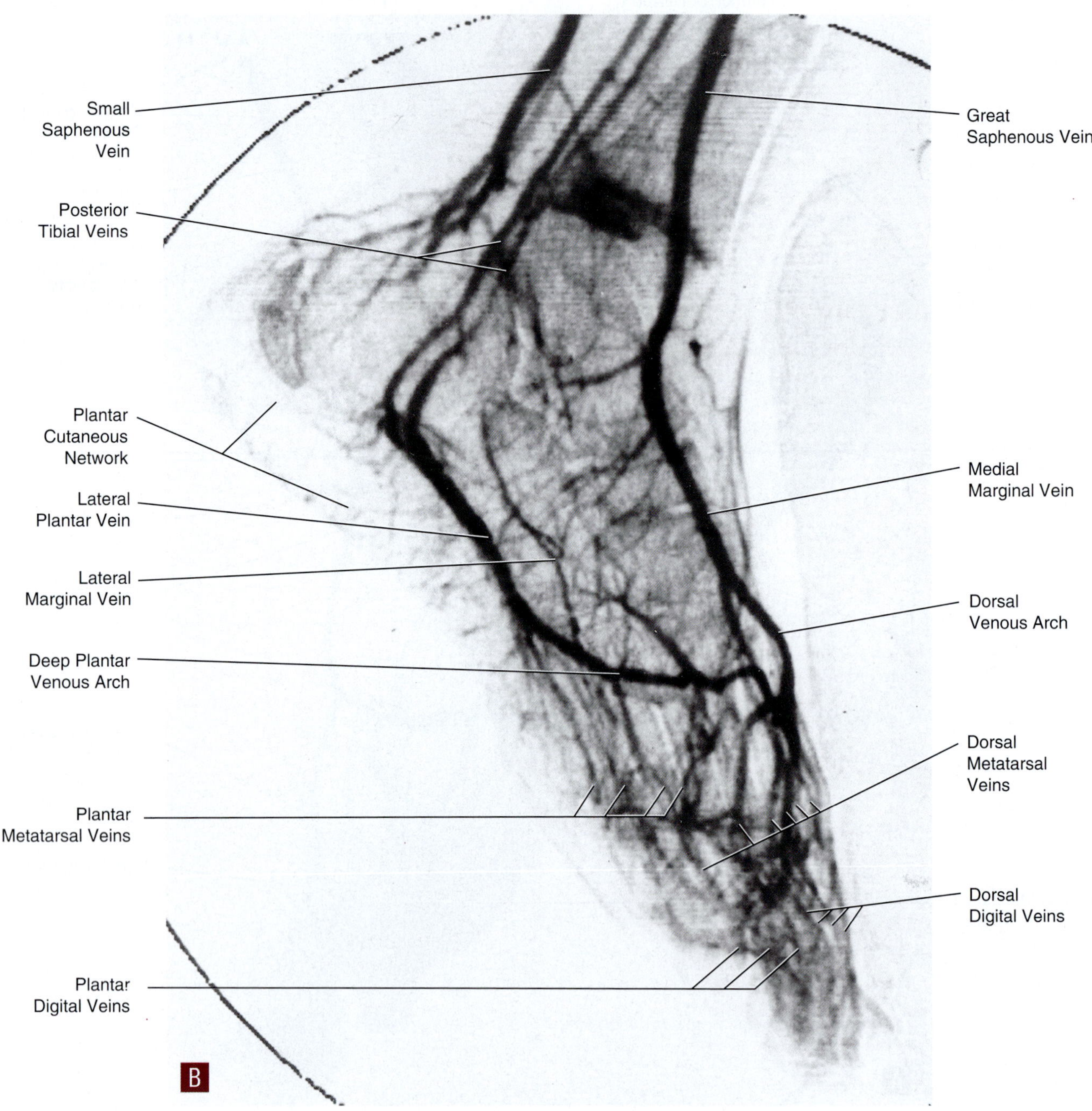

Figure 22.31. *Continued*

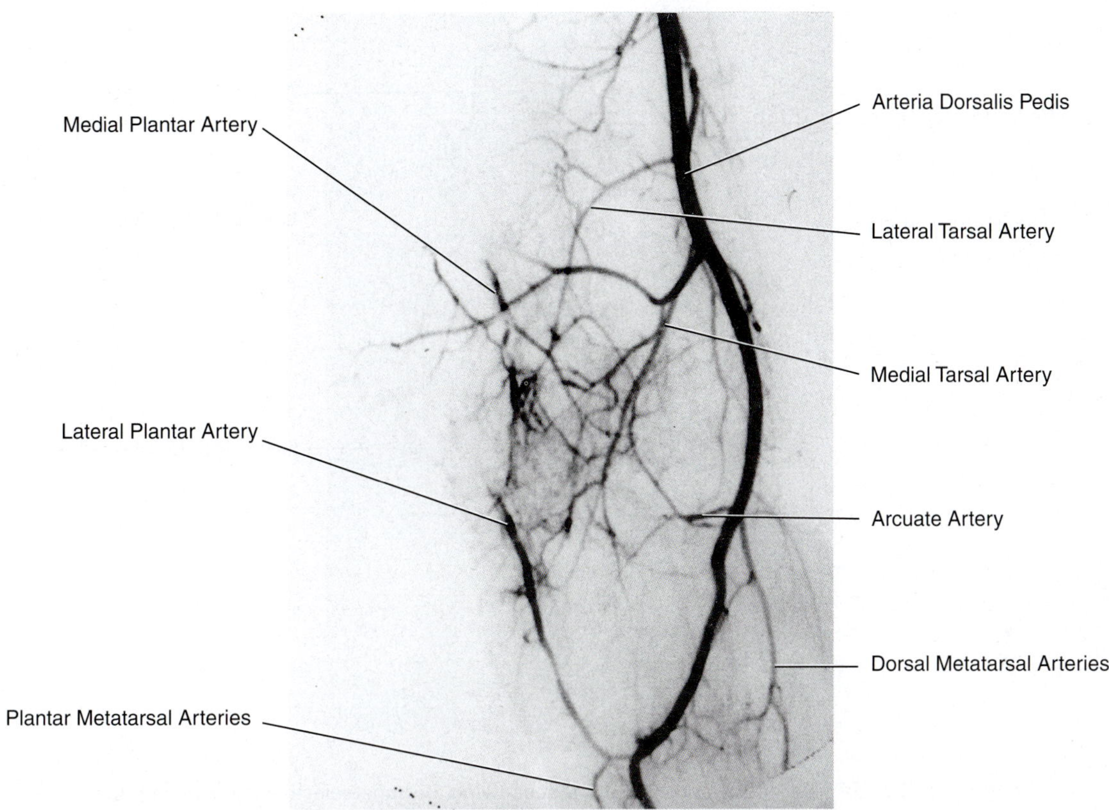

Figure 22.32. Lateral view of a superselective angiogram of the arteria dorsalis pedis and branches.

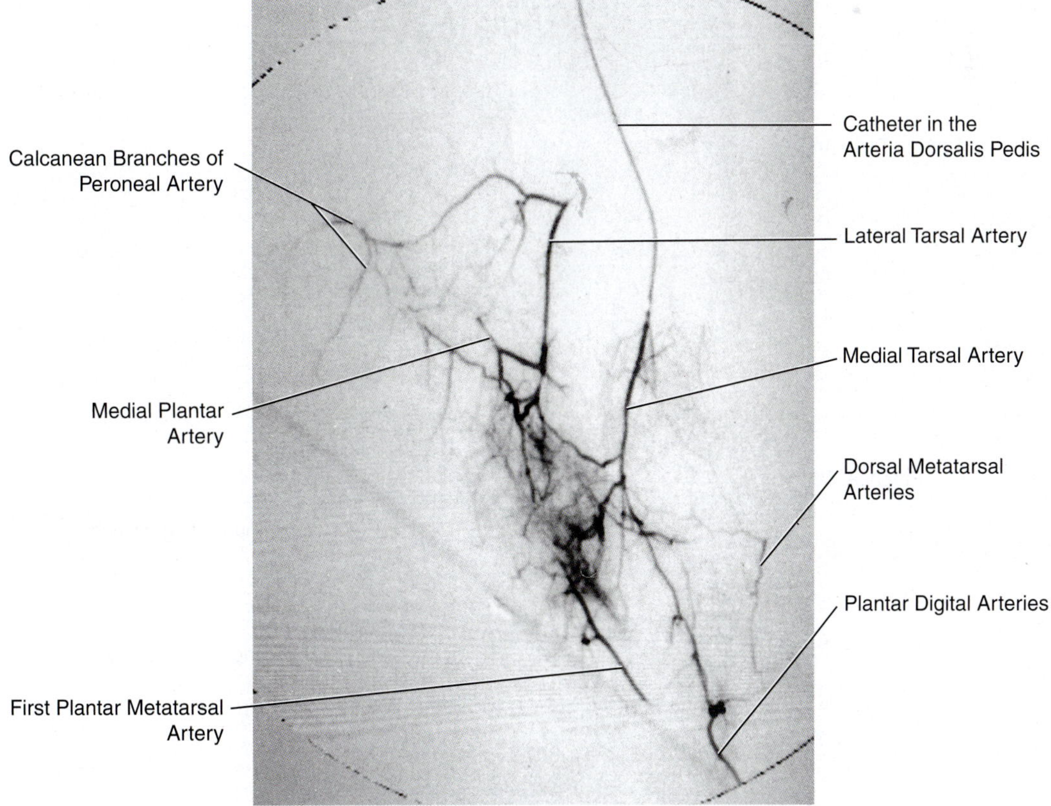

Figure 22.33. Lateral view of a superselective angiogram of the medial tarsal artery, branch of the arteria dorsalis pedis.

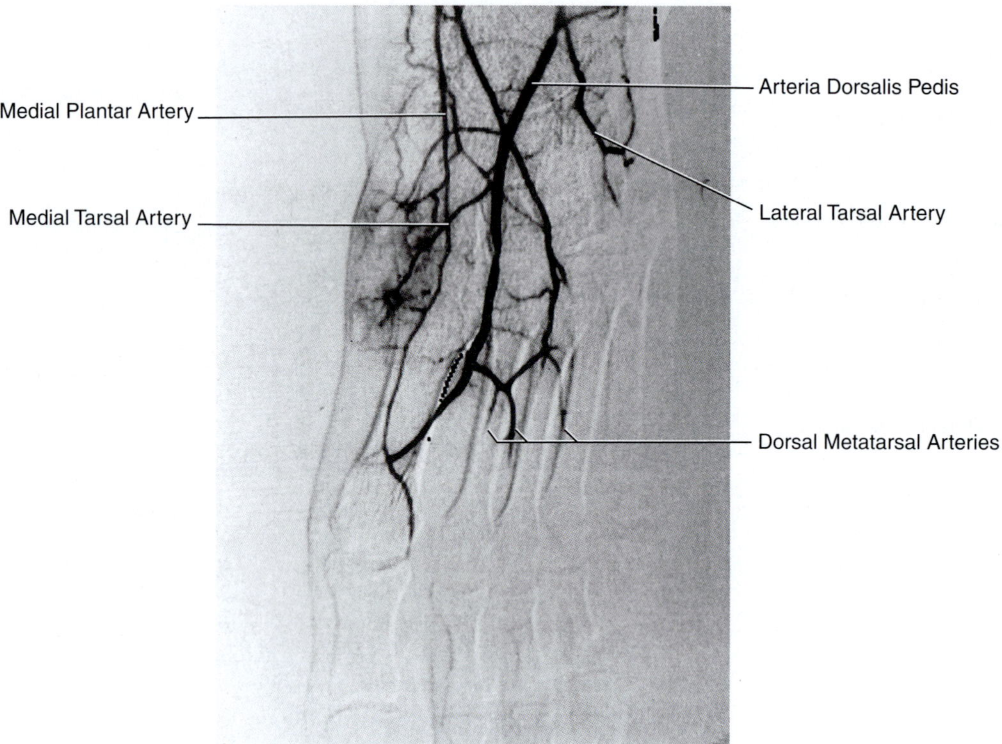

Figure 22.34. Anterior view of the left foot showing the superselective injection into the arteria dorsalis pedis and main branches.

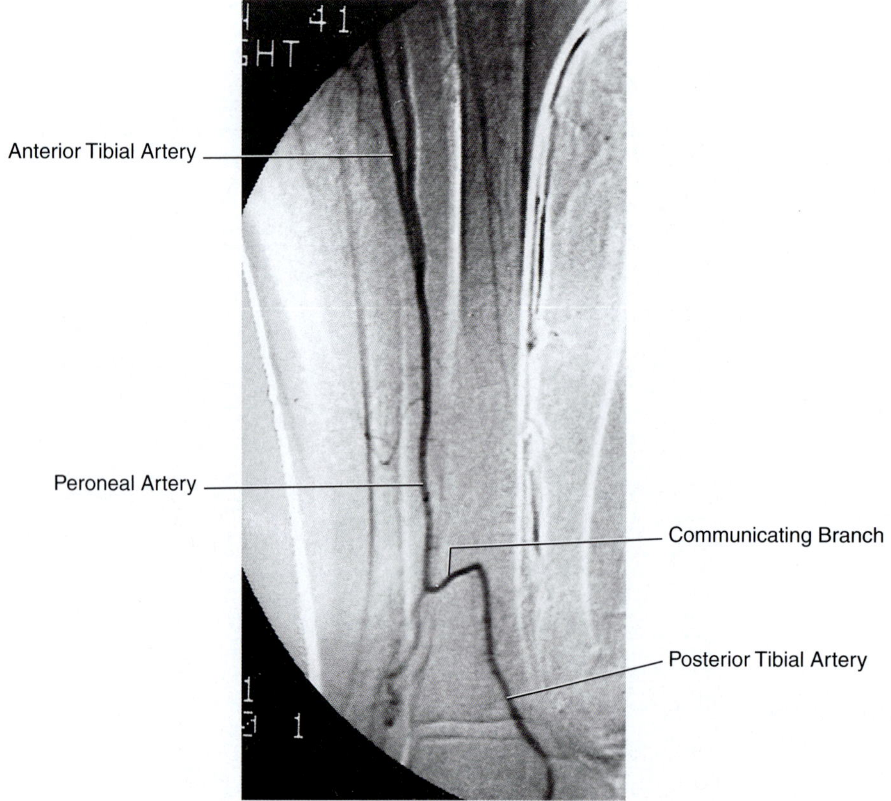

Figure 22.35. Anterior view of an angiogram of the arterial circulation of the right ankle.

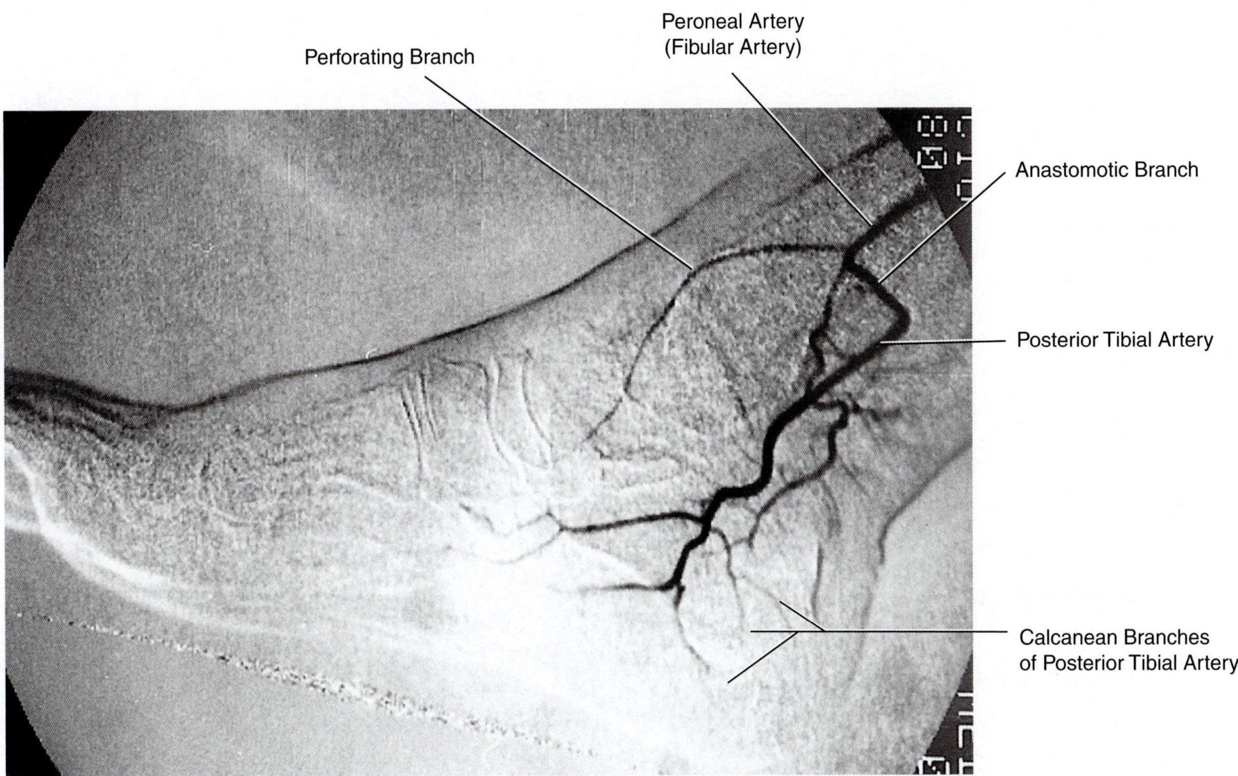

Figure 22.36. Lateral view of the angiogram of the arterial circulation of the peroneal artery and anastomotic branches with the posterior tibial artery.

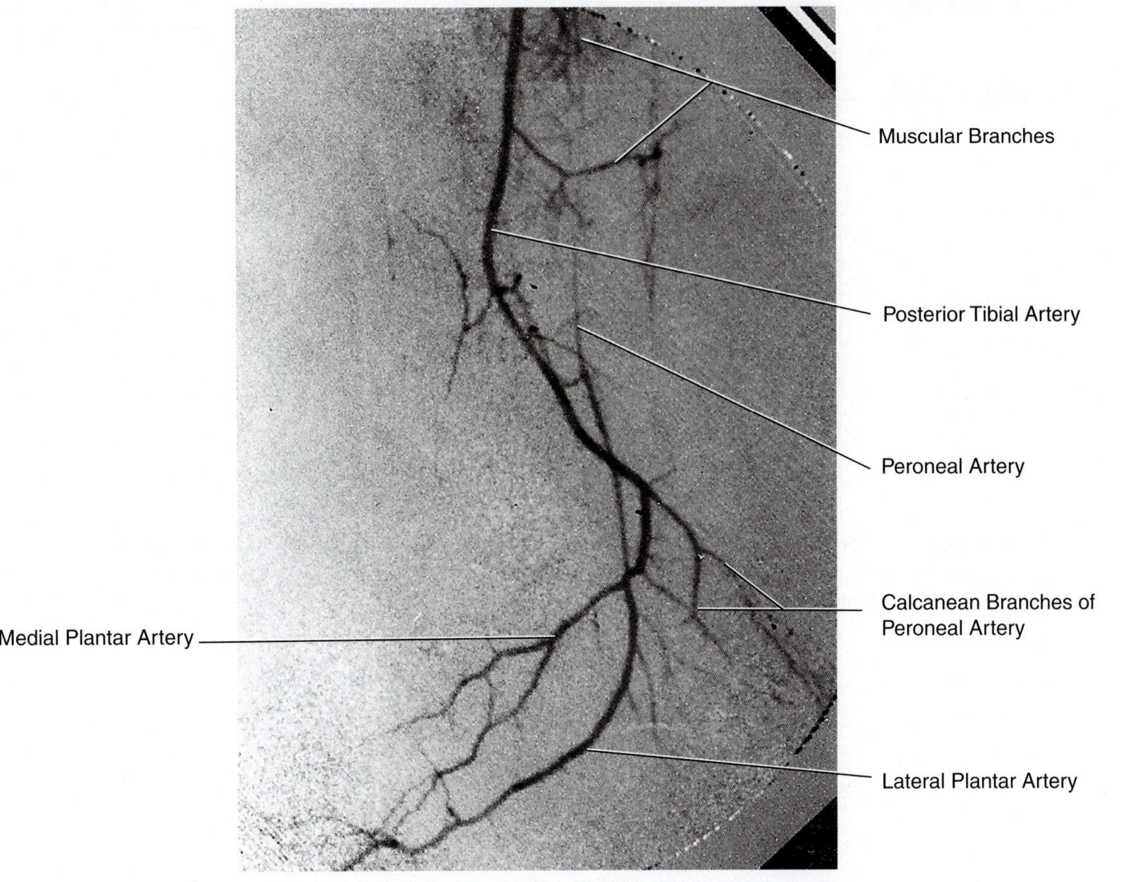

Figure 22.37. Lateral view of the angiogram of the arterial circulation of the posterior tibial artery and the calcanean branches and plantar arteries.

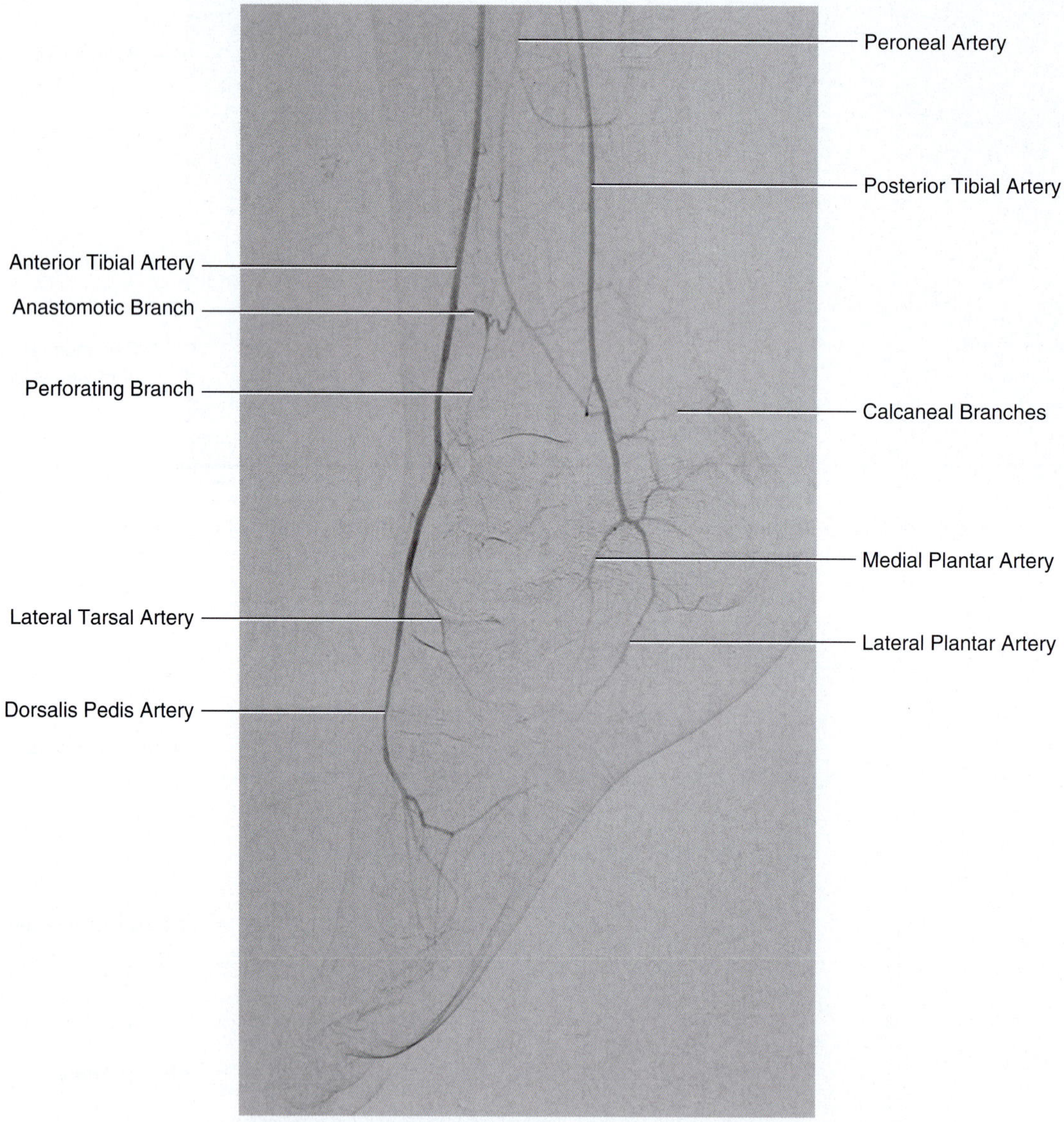

Peroneal Artery
Posterior Tibial Artery
Anterior Tibial Artery
Anastomotic Branch
Perforating Branch
Calcaneal Branches
Medial Plantar Artery
Lateral Tarsal Artery
Lateral Plantar Artery
Dorsalis Pedis Artery

Figure 22.38. Lateral view of the angiogram of the right foot, showing the arterial circulation of the posterior tibial artery and anastomotic branches with the anterior tibial artery and arteria dorsalis pedis.

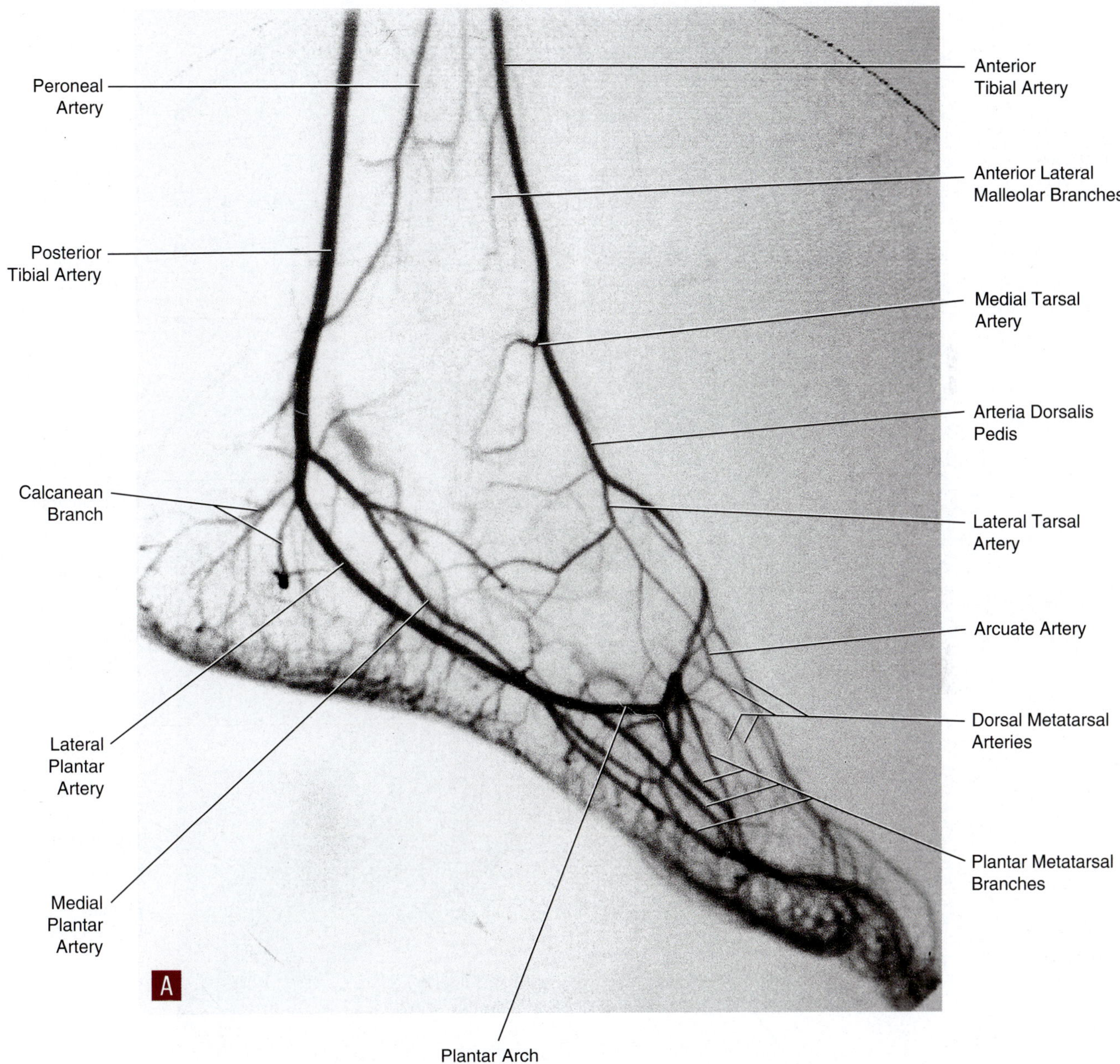

Figure 22.39. A, Lateral view of an angiogram of the arterial circulation of the foot. B, Late phase of the angiogram of the left foot showing the venous drainage. Note that there is a venous malformation in the plantar veins of the foot.

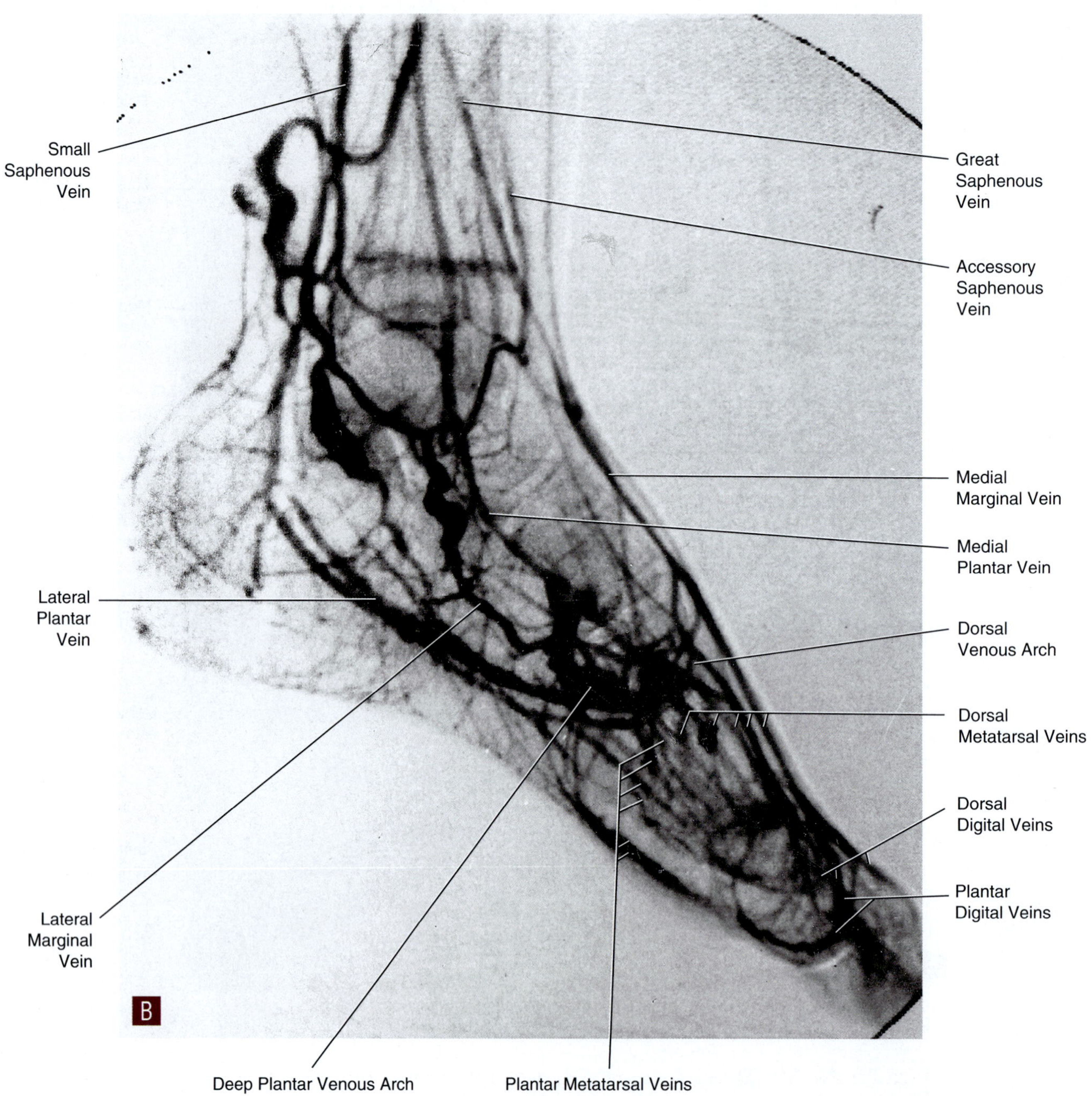

Figure 22.39. *Continued*

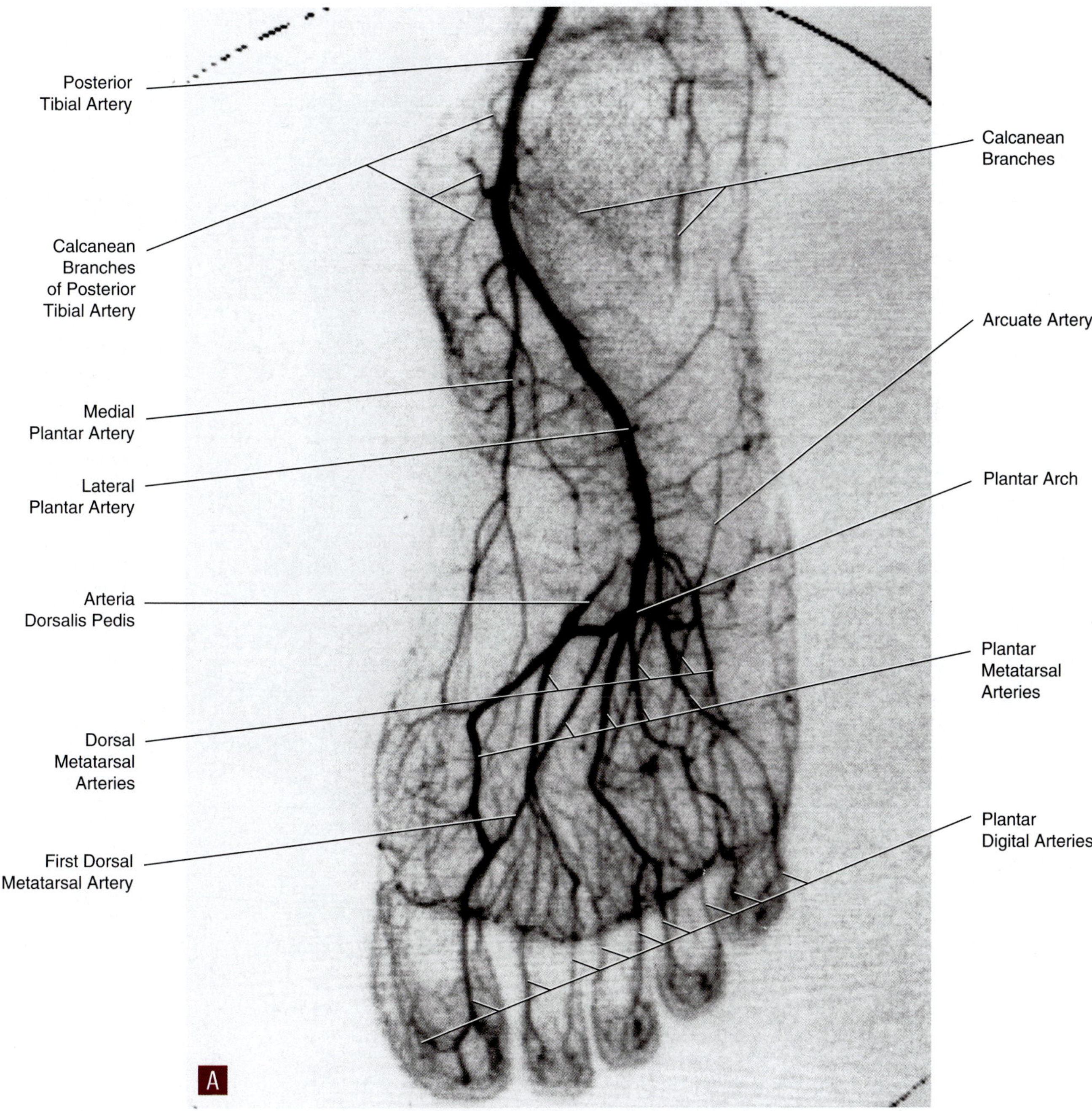

Figure 22.40. A, Anterior view of the angiogram of the left foot with a selective injection in the posterior tibial artery, showing the plantar and metatarsal arteries as well as the plantar arch. B, Late phase of the angiogram of the foot showing the venous drainage and the deep plantar venous arch. C, Late phase of the angiogram showing the plantar cutaneous arch.

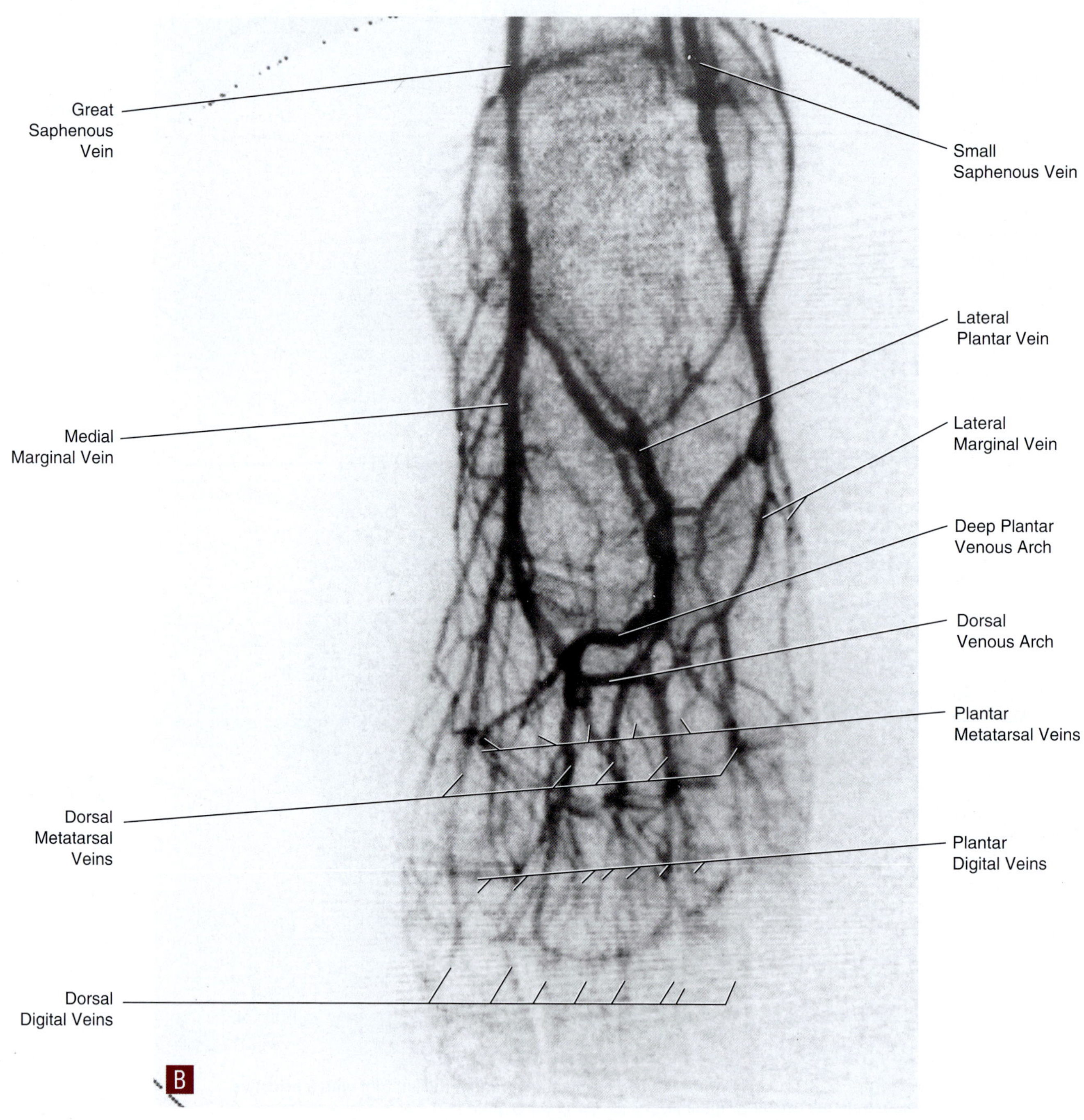

Figure 22.40. *Continued*

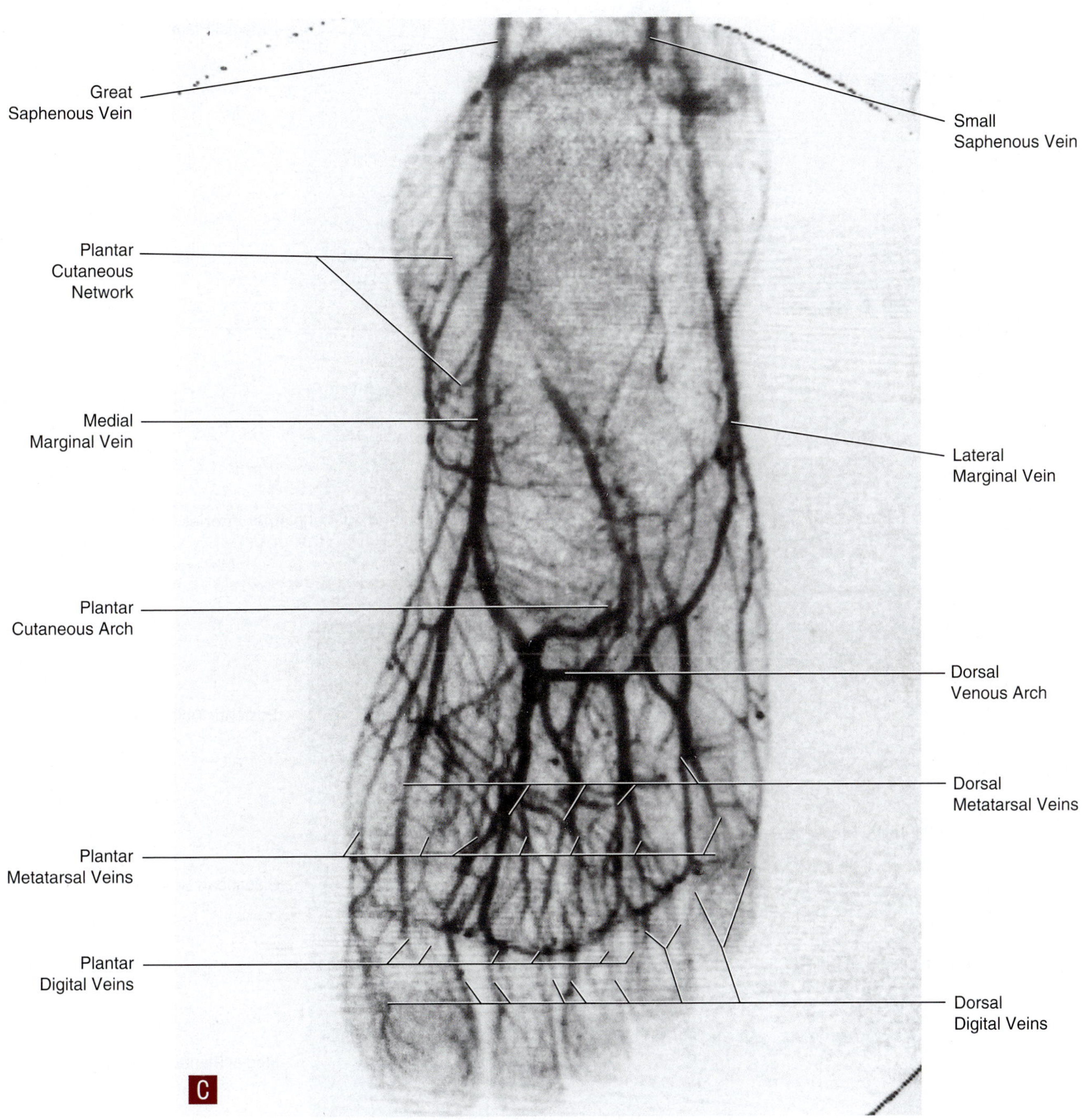

Figure 22.40. *Continued*

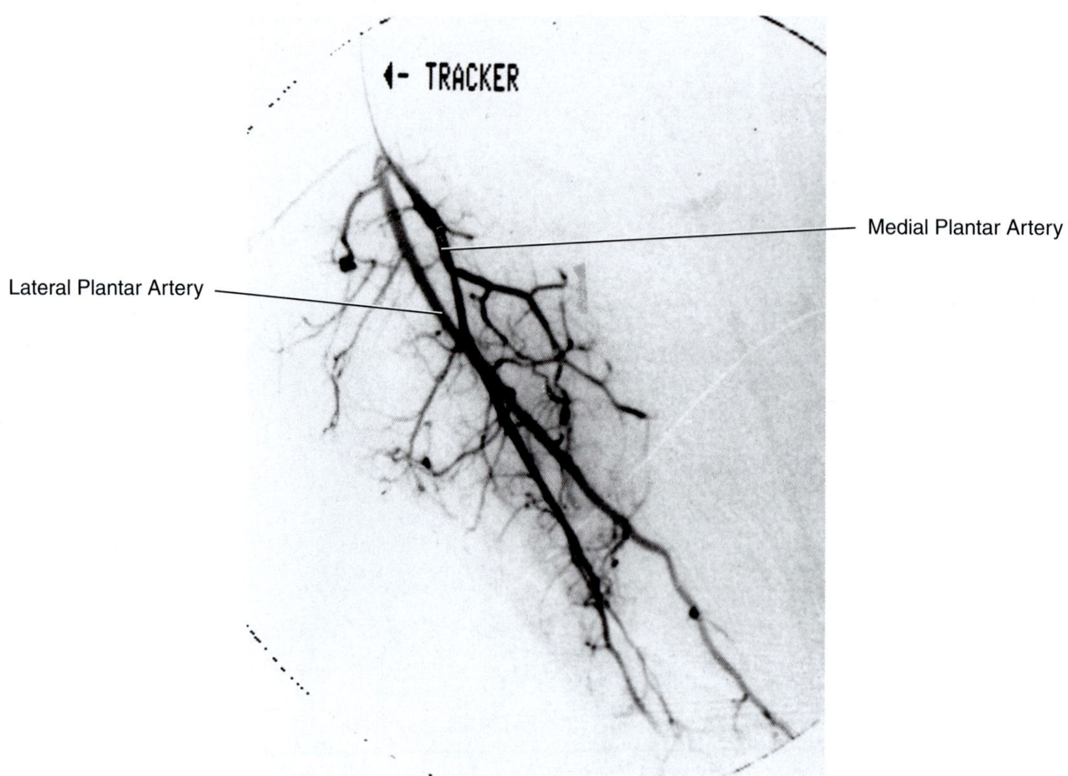

Figure 22.41. Superselective angiography of the lateral and medial plantar arteries.

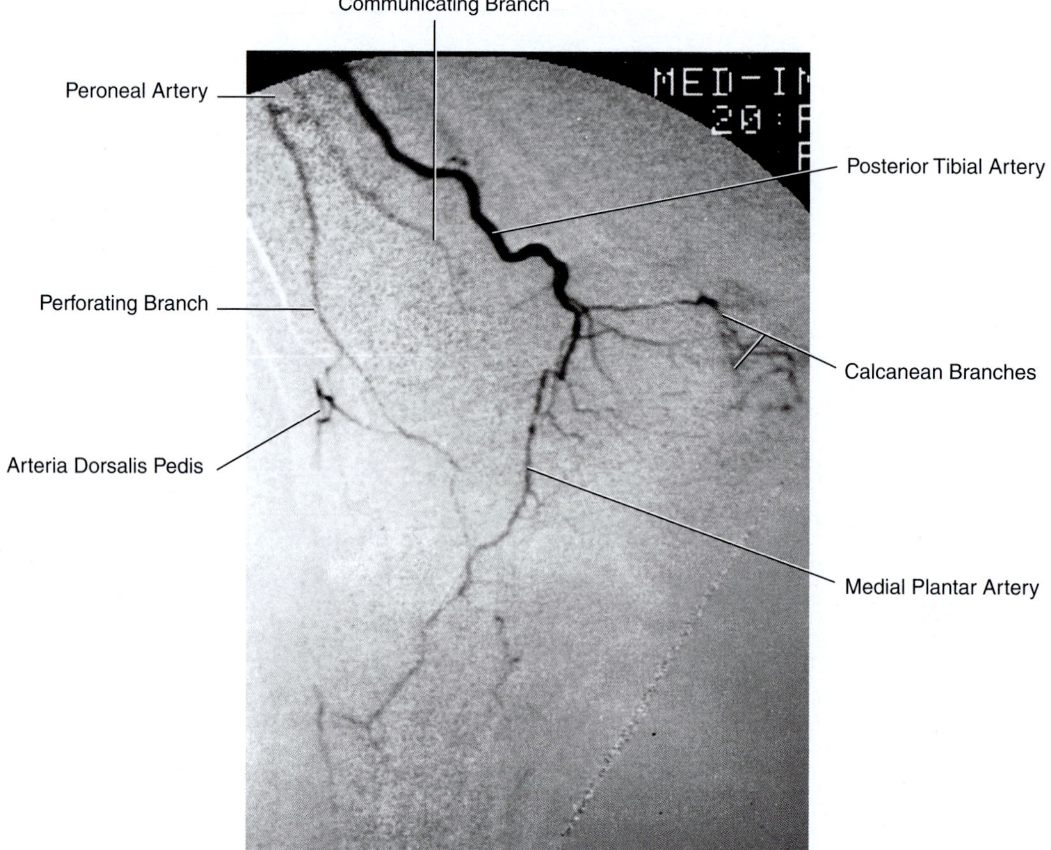

Figure 22.42. Lateral view of the foot with occlusion of the anterior tibial artery, showing the anastomosis between the anterior and posterior systems.

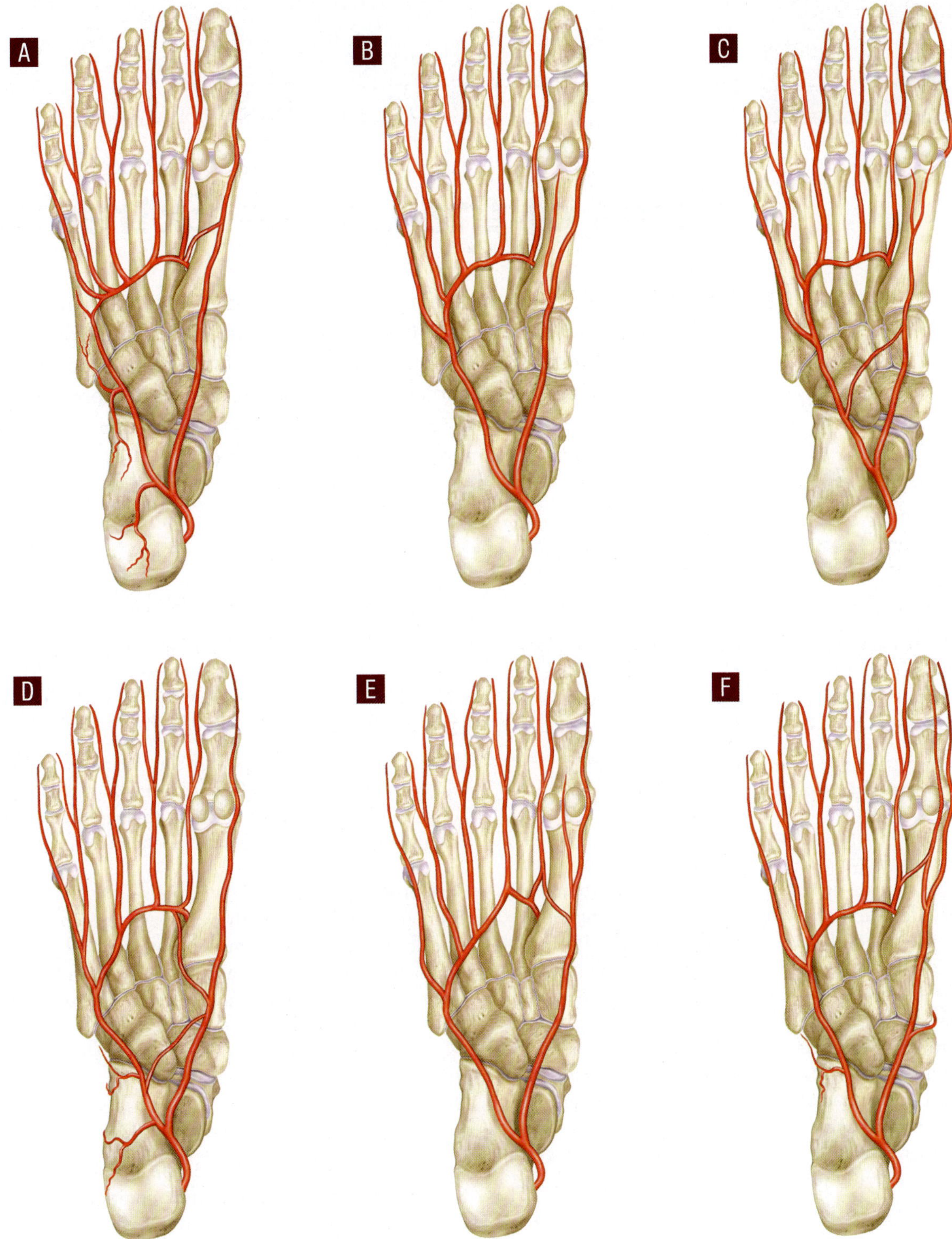

Figure 22.43. Variations of the plantar arteries. A, Type Ia—deep plantar artery originated from the anterior dorsalis pedis, which gives origin to all the metatarsal arteries. B, Type Ib—deep plantar artery originated from the arteria dorsalis pedis and partially from the lateral plantar artery. C, Type IIa—lateral plantar artery originates the fourth space metatarsal artery. D, Type IIb—lateral plantar artery originates the fourth and third metatarsal arteries. E, Type IIc—lateral plantar artery originates the fourth, third, and second metatarsal arteries. F, Type III—lateral plantar artery after originating the metatarsal arteries goes to the dorsal aspect of the foot and communicates with the arteria dorsalis pedis.

23

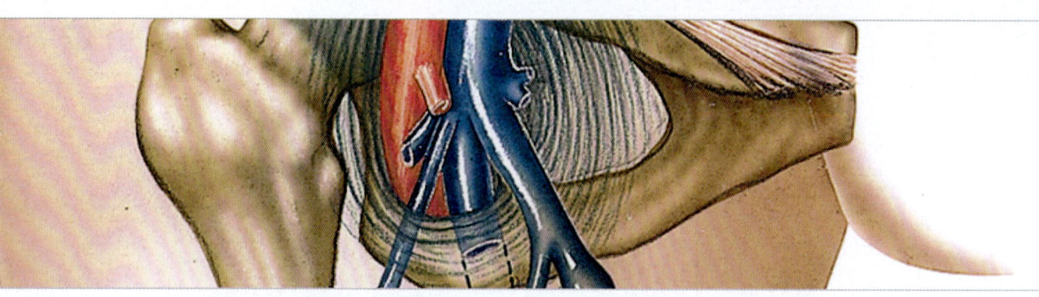

Veins of the Lower Extremity

The veins of the lower extremities may be divided into two main groups, deep and superficial. The superficial veins are found between the skin and the superficial fascia. The deep venous system accompanies the arteries, are under the superficial fascia, and are distributed among the four muscular fascia compartments. Valves are present in the superficial and deep systems but are more numerous in the deep veins (Fig. 23.10).

Superficial Veins of the Lower Limb

The main named superficial veins are the great (long, greater, magna) and small (lesser, parva) saphenous veins. Most of the tributaries to this system are unnamed (Figs. 23.1 and 23.2).

Great (Long, Magna, Internal) Saphenous Vein

The great saphenous vein is the longest vein in the human body. This vein begins in the medial marginal vein of the foot and end joining, through the saphenous opening, the femoral vein below the inguinal ligament (Figs. 23.2-23.4). The great saphenous is often duplicated below the knee, and it is often connected to the small saphenous vein through a long superficial vein called Giacomini vein (Fig. 23.1). The great saphenous vein ascends anterior to the tibial malleolus and crosses the distal third of the medial surface of the tibia obliquely to its medial border. From there, it ascends posteromedial to the border of the knee, then to the medial aspect of the thigh and finally joins the femoral vein through the saphenous opening.

Tributaries

At the ankle—medial marginal vein (Fig. 23.7)
In the leg—free communications with the small saphenous vein and deep veins, perforating veins, frontal vein, tibial malleolus vein, and from the calf
In the thigh—from the medial and posterior aspect, may form the accessory saphenous vein
Superficial epigastric
Superficial circumflex iliac
Superficial external pudendal vein
Thoracoepigastric vein

Small (Short, Parva, External, Lesser) Saphenous Vein

This vein is a continuation of the lateral marginal vein of the foot, at the back of the leg, ending in the popliteal vein (Fig. 23.9). It receives numerous cutaneous tributaries and communicates with the great saphenous vein.

Perforating Veins

The great and lesser saphenous veins are connected with the deep veins through the perforating veins. The perforating veins have valves arranged so that normally they prevent the flow of blood from the deep to the superficial veins (Figs. 23.2 and 23.3).

The perforating veins are found in the foot, leg, and thigh.

In the Foot

There are usually four perforating veins.

- One 2.5 cm below the medial malleolus
- One 3.5 cm below and anterior to the medial malleolus
- Two 3.0 cm below and anterior to the lateral malleolus

In the Leg

There are usually 16 constant perforating veins (Fig. 23.8A).

- 8 drain into the posterior tibial veins (Cockett and Boyd veins)

- 4 drain into the peroneal veins
- 4 drain into the soleal and gemelar veins

In the Thigh

There are two constant perforating veins (Dodd Group or perforating veins of Hunter) (Fig. 23.3C.)

Deep Veins of the Lower Limb

These veins are companions of the arteries and their branches.

In the Foot (Figs. 23.1 and 23.9)

The plantar digital veins arise from plexuses on the surface of the digits and communicate with the dorsal digital veins and join to form four plantar metatarsal veins.

The plantar metatarsal veins communicate through perforating veins with the veins of the dorsum of the foot forming the deep plantar venous arch, accompanying the plantar arterial arch.

The medial and lateral plantar veins run backwards, arising from the deep plantar venous arch, following the corresponding tract of the arteries. After communicating with the great and small saphenous veins, they join behind the medial malleolus to form the posterior tibial veins.

In the Leg

Posterior Tibial Veins (Figs. 23.8B, C and 9)

These veins are companions of the posterior tibial artery. Major effluents are peroneal veins (companions of the peroneal artery) and perforating veins from the superficial system.

Anterior Tibial Vein (Figs. 23.8B, C and 9)

The anterior tibial veins are companions of the anterior tibial artery and dorsal artery of the foot. They cross the interosseous membrane and join the posterior tibial veins to form the popliteal veins.

Popliteal Vein (Figs. 23.6B, 23.8B and C, 11)

This vein follows an upward direction through the popliteal fossa and the adductor canal, where it is named femoral vein. Tributaries are the small saphenous vein, gastrocnemius and sural veins, and other muscular veins.

In the Thigh

Femoral Vein (Superficial Femoral Vein) (Figs. 23.5A-C, 6A, and 11F)

Tributaries are the popliteal and muscular veins. The femoral vein may be duplicated for a long or short segment (Figs. 23.5C and 23.11F).

Deep Femoral (Profunda Femoris) Vein (Figs. 23.7 and 23.8D)

The deep femoral vein is anterior to the deep femoral artery and receives muscular tributaries and perforating branches, establishing anastomoses with the popliteal vein (below it) and inferior gluteal vein.

Common Femoral Vein (Figs. 23.1-3A, 5C)

This vein is short in length; it follows the tract of the common femoral artery as the continuation of the popliteal and femoral (also called superficial femoral) veins, ending about the level of the inguinal ligament, becoming the external iliac vein. The lateral and medial circumflex femoral veins and the superficial epigastric veins are also usual tributaries.

At the inguinal ligament, the common femoral vein is medial to the corresponding artery, occupying the middle compartment of the femoral sheath. Through the saphenous opening, the great saphenous vein joins the common femoral vein.

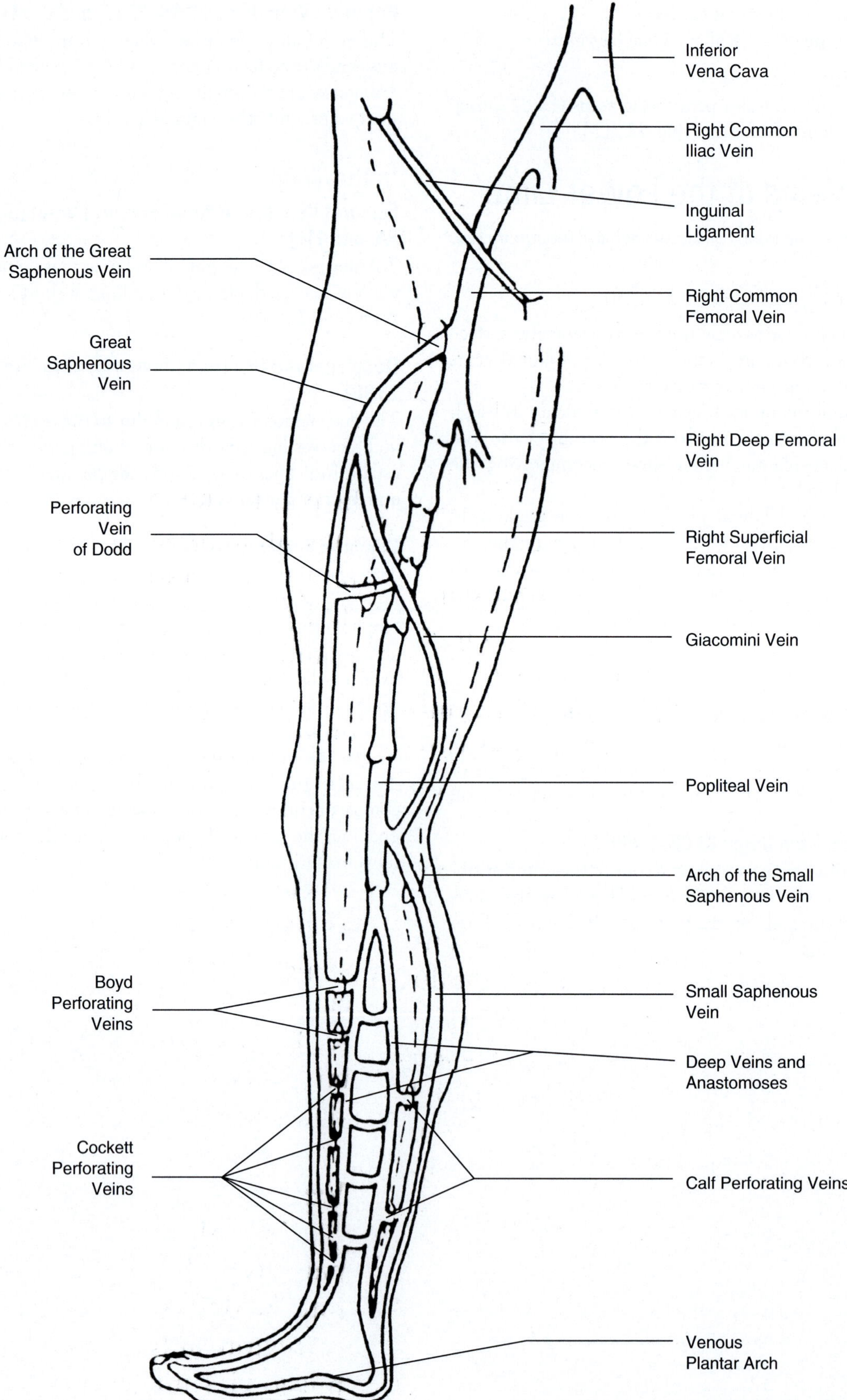

Figure 23.1. Schematic drawing of the lower extremity deep and superficial venous system. Note the perforating or communicating veins.

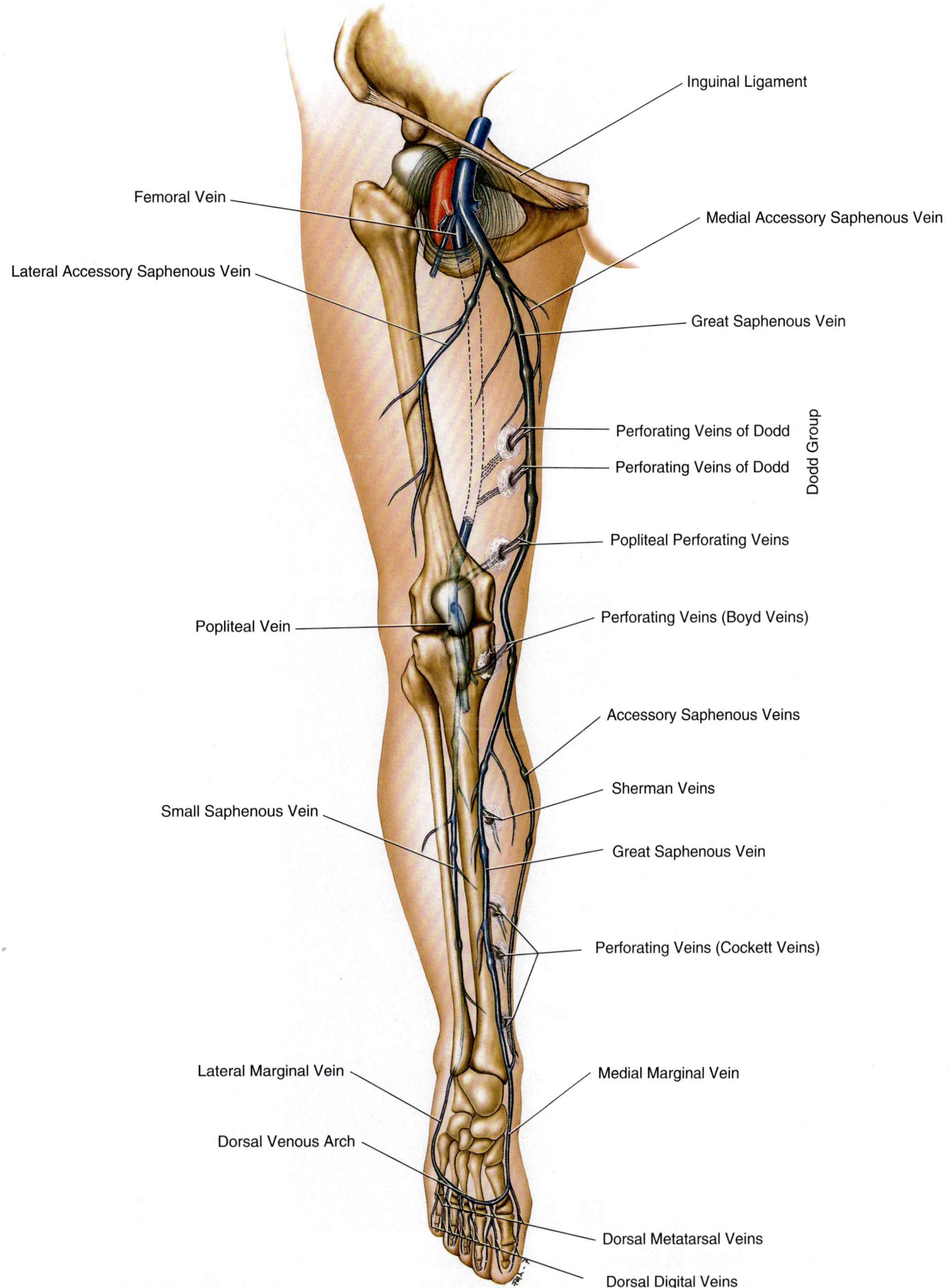

Figure 23.2. Schematic drawing showing the superficial venous system of the right lower extremity.

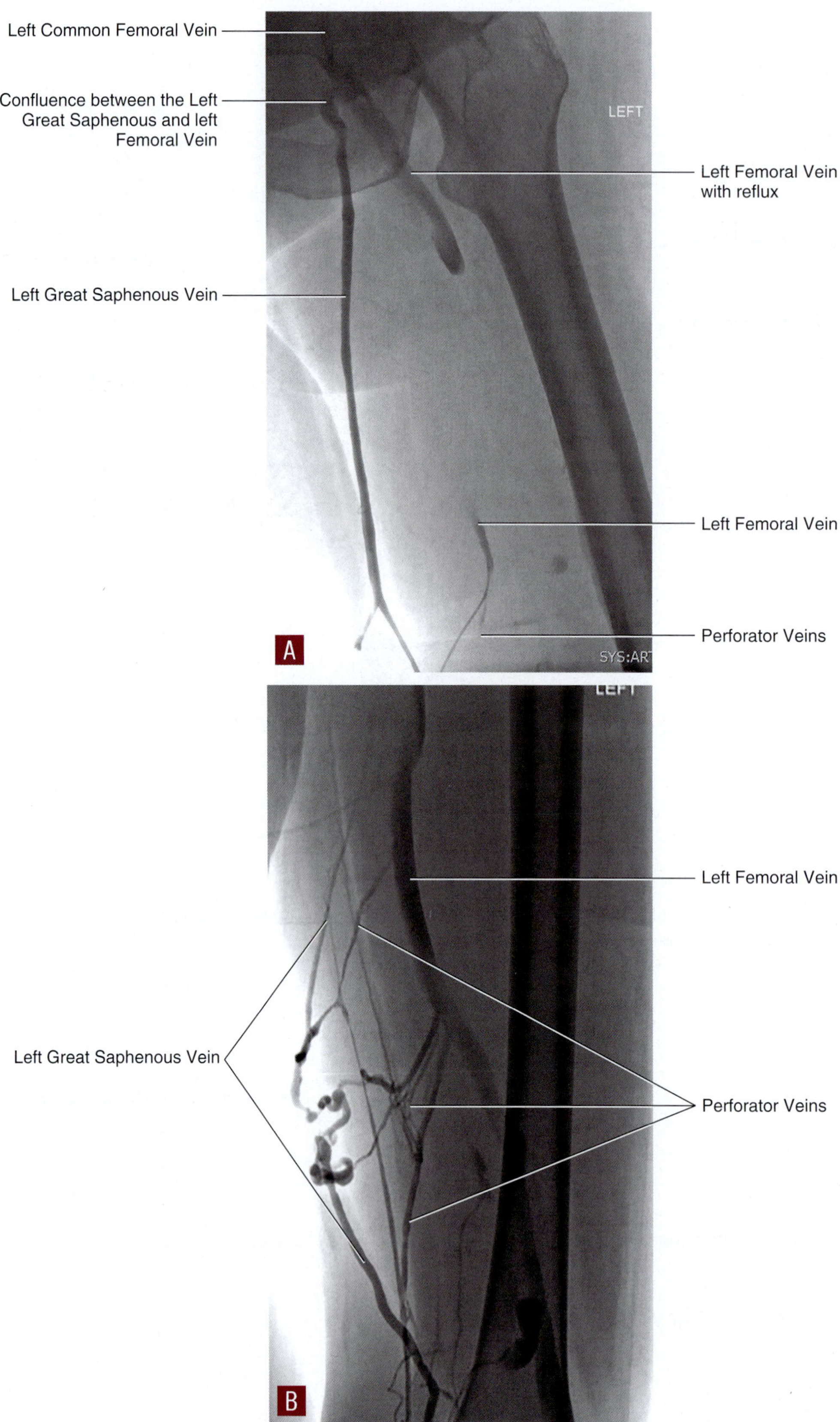

Figure 23.3. **A**, Venogram of the left lower extremity Patent confluence of the left great saphenous vein (GSV) and the femoral vein forming the left common femoral vein. **B**, Patent left GSV and perforator veins. **C**, Tortuous but patent left GSV. **D**, Patent GSV at the level of the calf. **E**, Anatomical variations at the junction of the great saphenous vein and the relationship of the tributaries at the level of the saphenous opening. EP, superficial external pudendal vein; GSV, great saphenous vein; SE, superficial epigastric vein; SIC, superficial iliac circumflex vein.

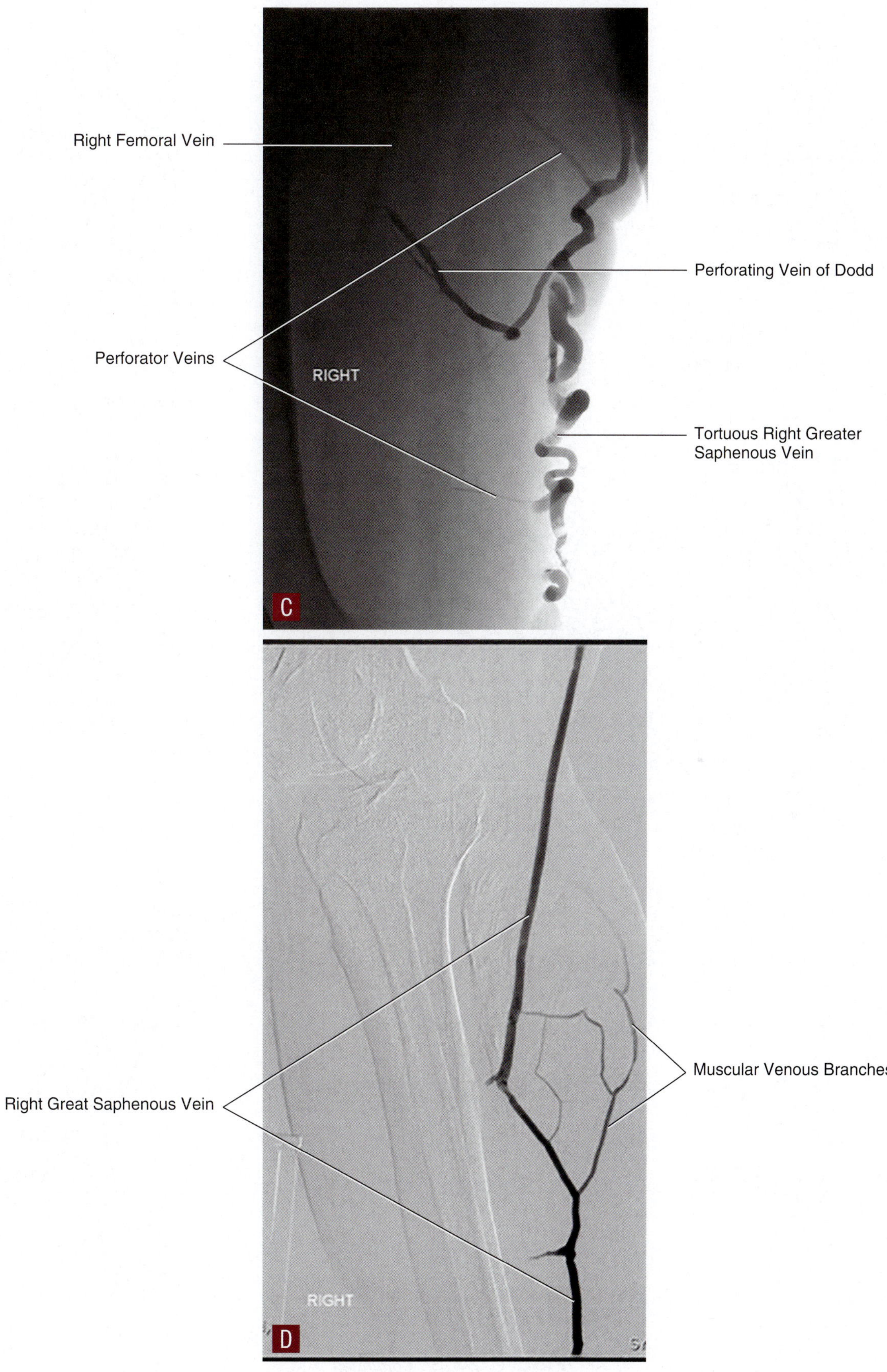

Figure 23.3. *Continued*

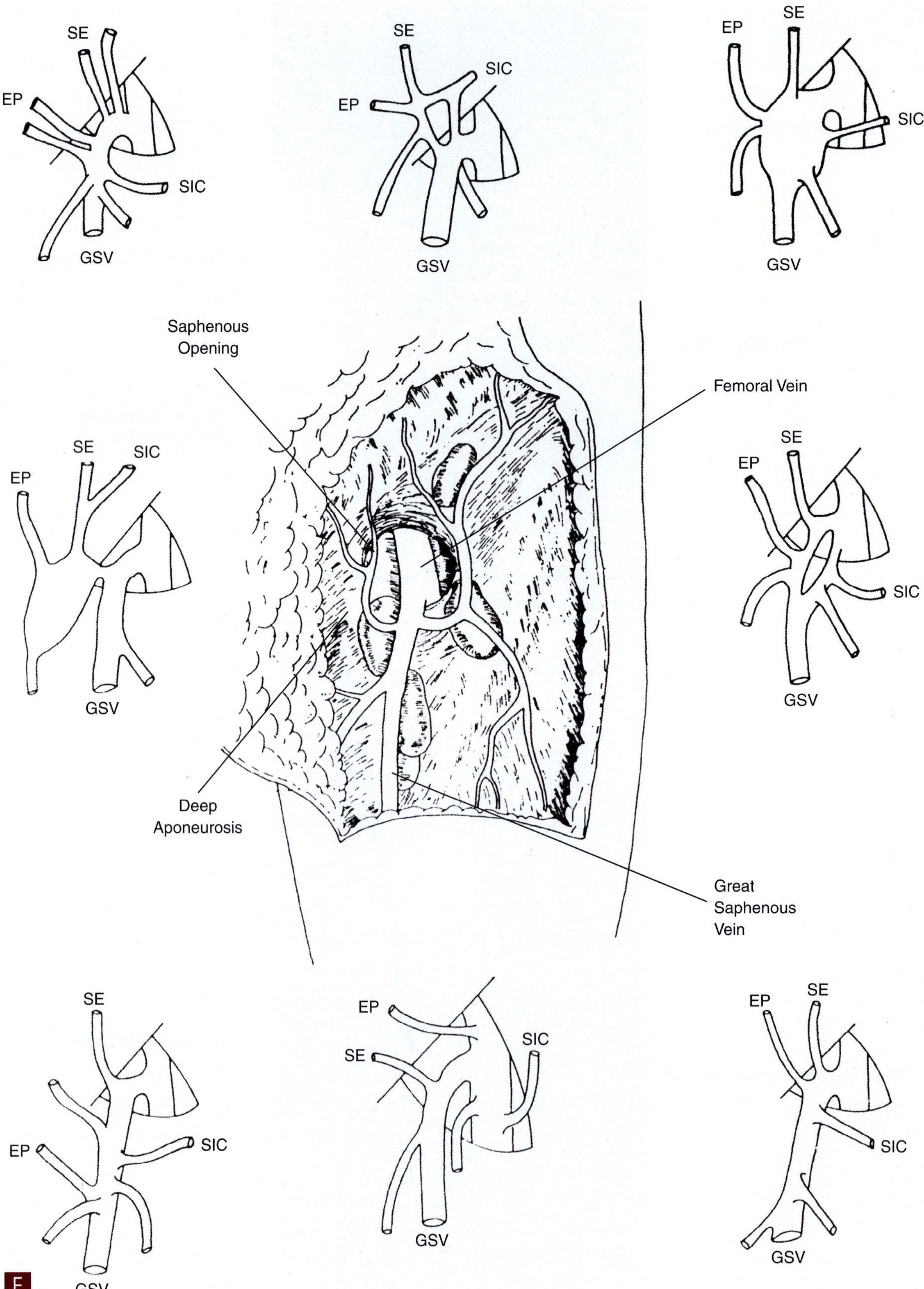

Figure 23.3. *Continued*

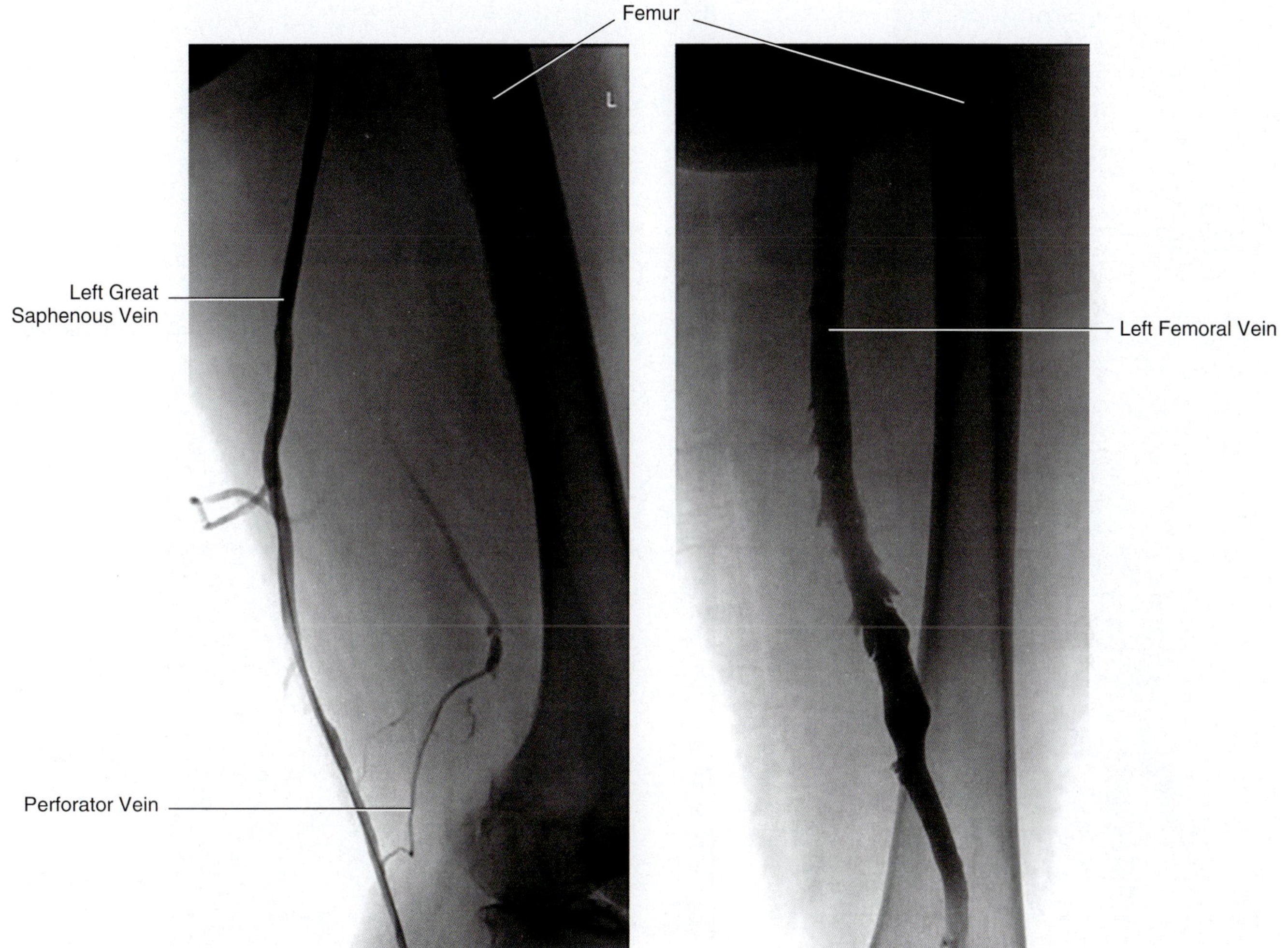

Figure 23.4. Venogram of the left lower extremity. In relation to the left femur, note the typical distance and the trajectory of the superficial venous system (left GSV) in comparison to the deep venous system (left femoral vein). Observe the typical difference in caliber between these two veins. GSV, great saphenous vein.

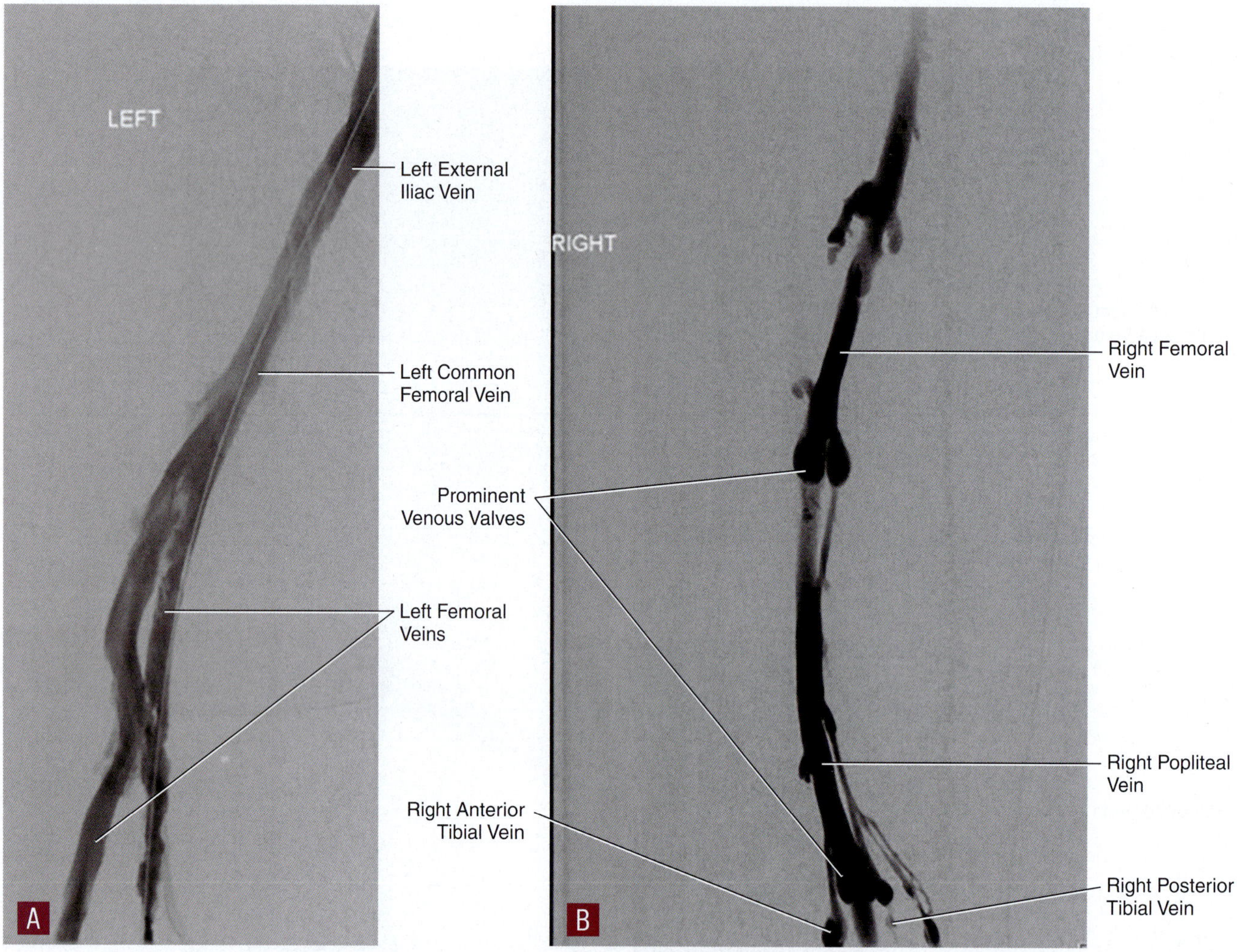

Figure 23.5. Venograms of the deep venous system of the right lower extremity. **A**, Patent external iliac and common femoral veins, as well as the confluence of two femoral veins. **B**, Patent right femoral vein. Note the prominent valves. **C**, Patent pair right femoral veins (patient is on the angiography table in prone position). **D**, Note multiple patent femoral veins.

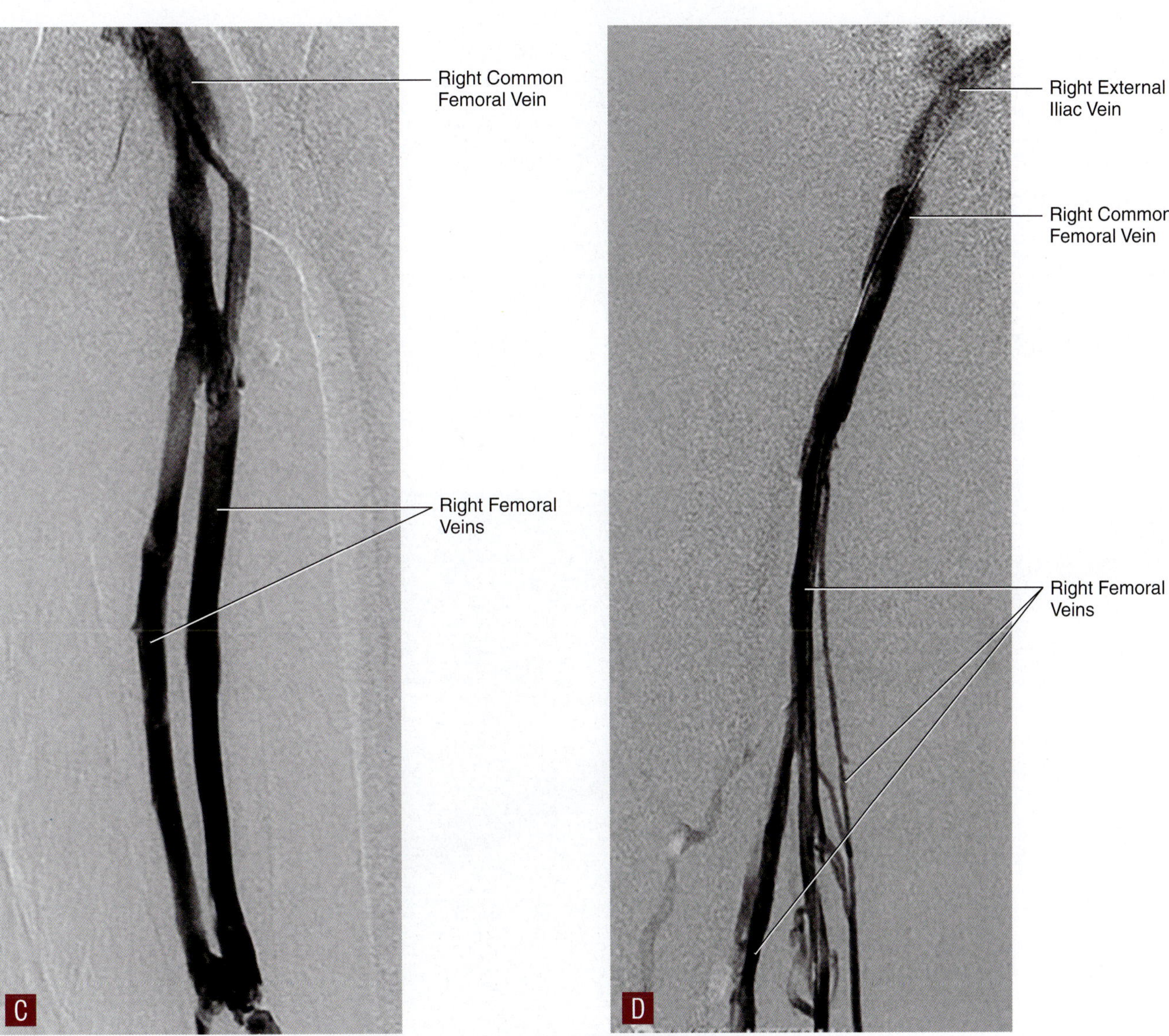

Figure 23.5. *Continued*

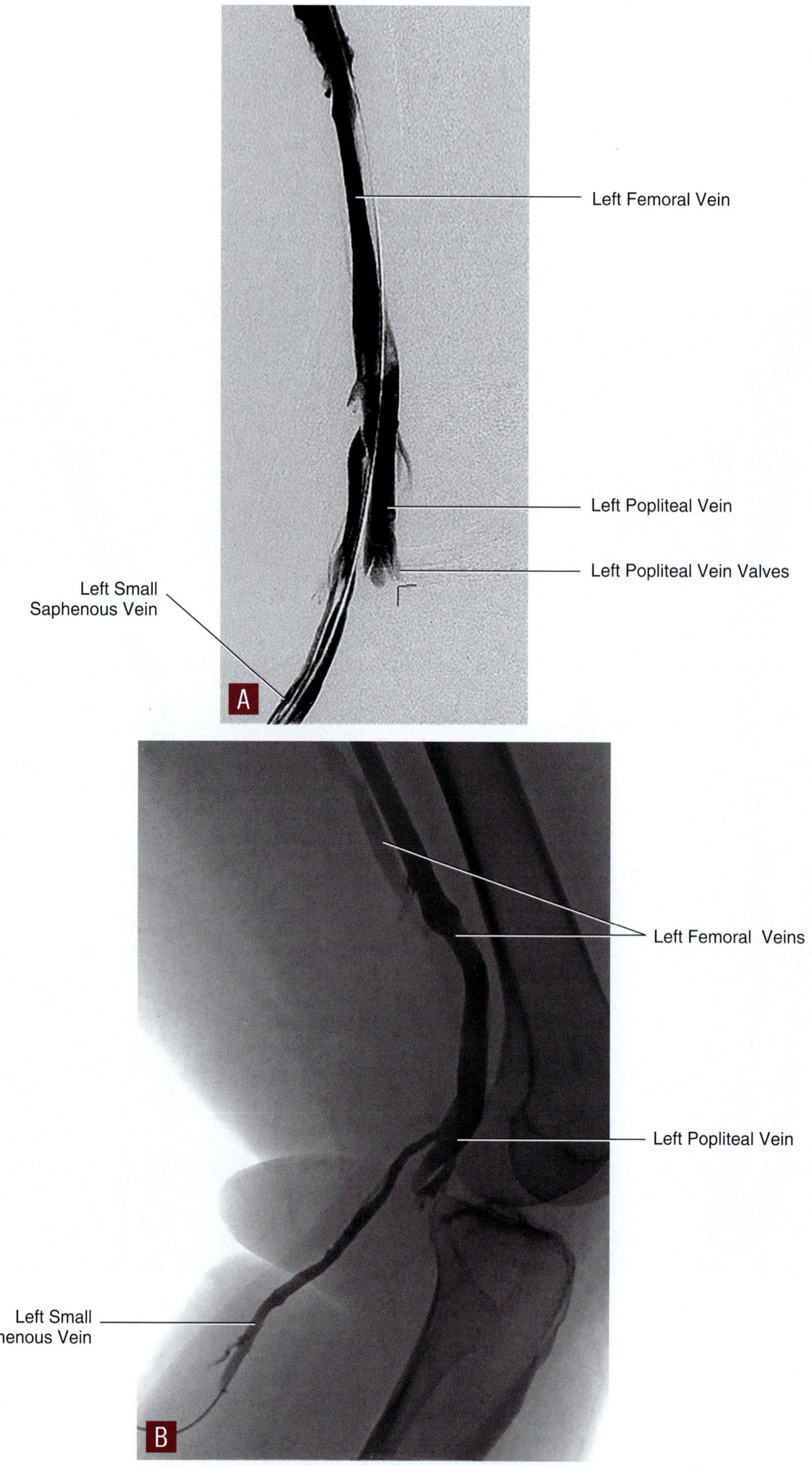

Figure 23.6. A, Venogram performed through the left small saphenous vein during the closure of the popliteal vein valve leaflets (arrowhead). The popliteal and femoral veins are patent post pharmacomechanical thrombectomy to treat acute DVT. Access through the left small (lesser) saphenous vein allows direct access to the popliteal vein, and the DVT treatment can be performed with the patient in supine ("frog leg") position. At the end of the case, compressive hemostasis is performed on the small saphenous vein and not on the popliteal vein. B, Patent small saphenous vein draining into the popliteal vein. DVT, deep vein thrombosis.

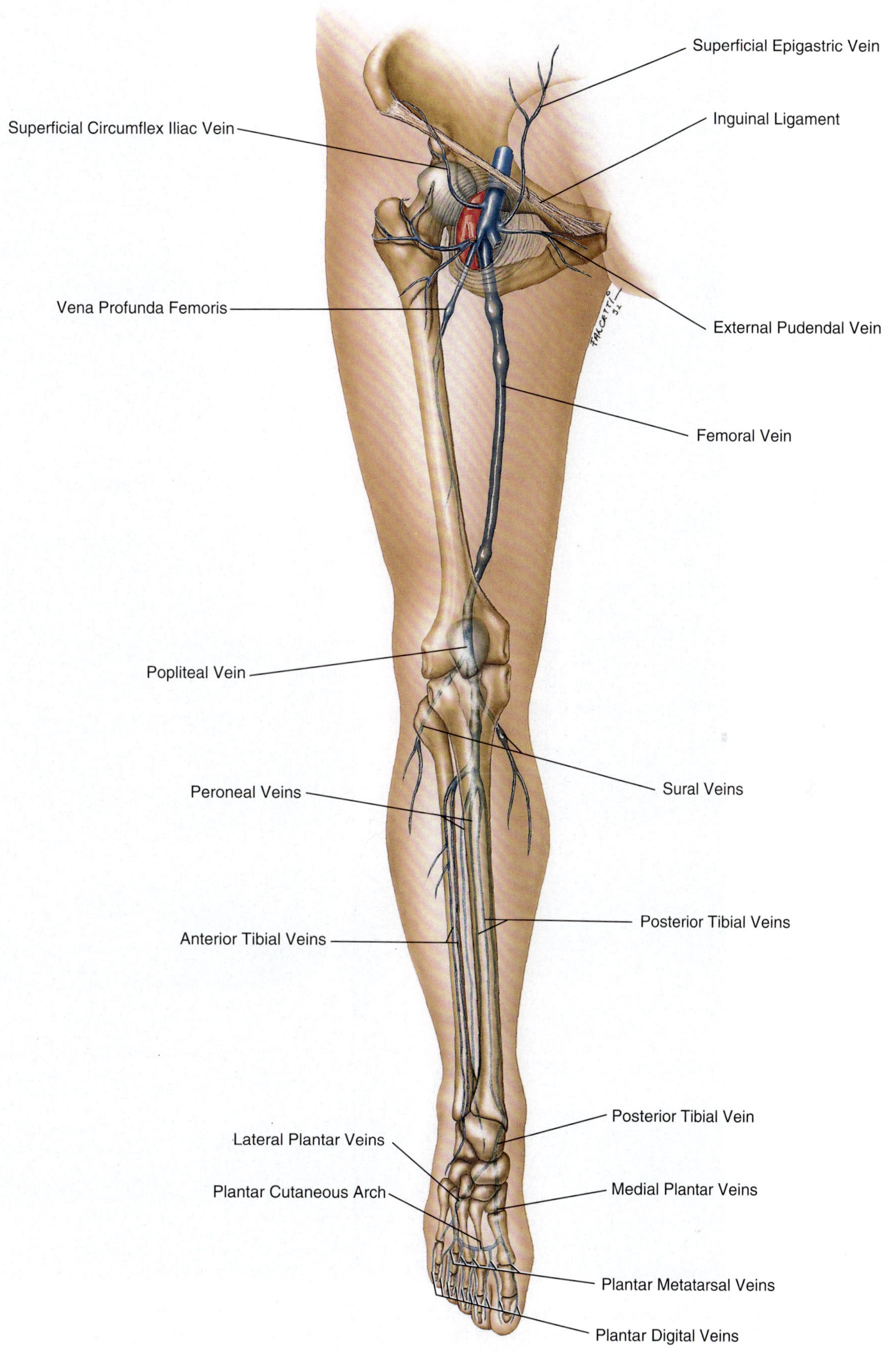

Figure 23.7. **Schematic drawing of the deep venous system of the right lower extremity.**

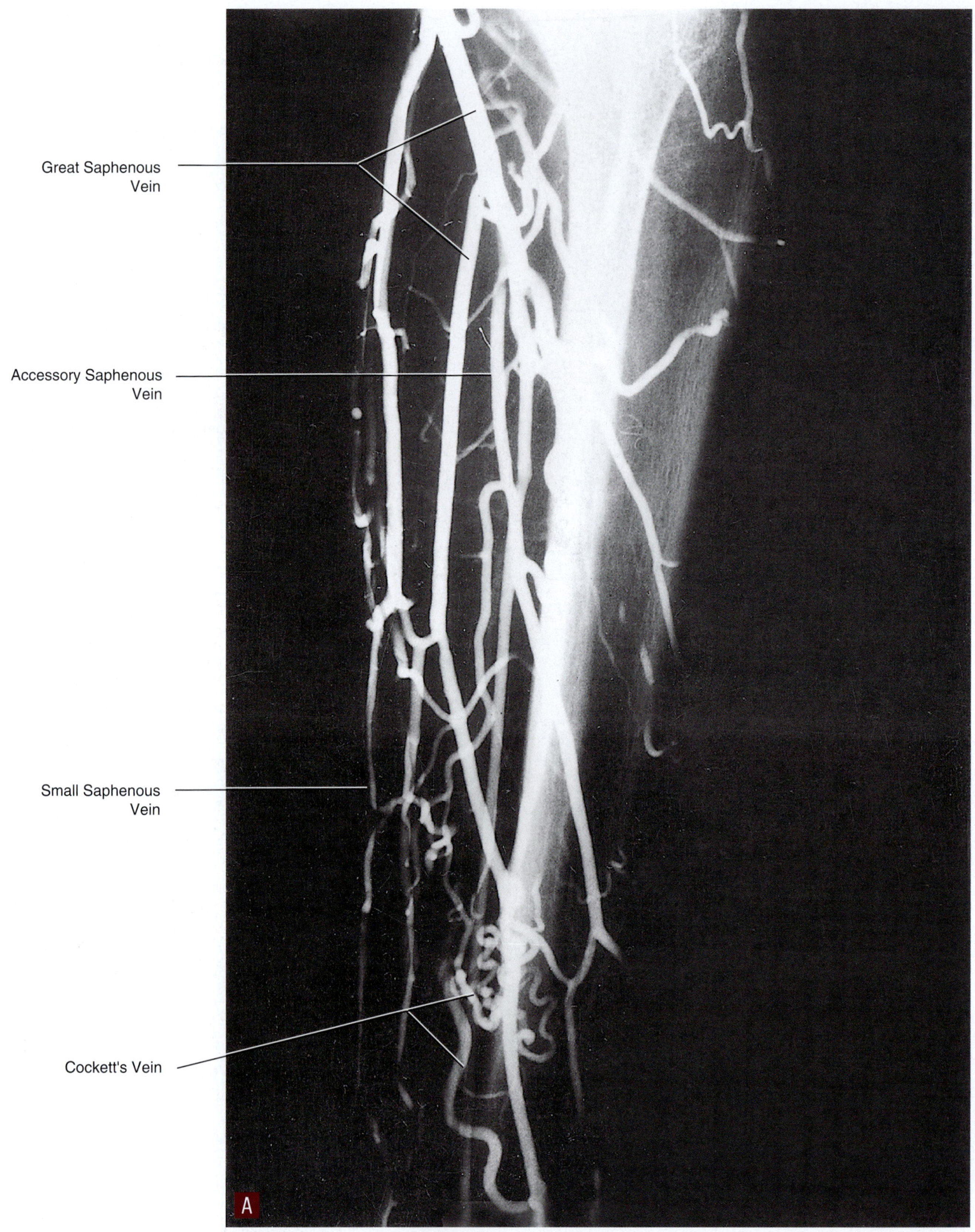

Figure 23.8. Lower extremity venograms. Note the (A) superficial venous system and the (B) deep venous systems at the level of the calves. C, Venogram shows the left deep and superficial venous systems at the level of the thigh and calf. D, Venogram shows the right deep venous systems at the level of the thigh and proximal calf. E, Venogram shows the left deep venous systems at the level of the pelvis and thigh.

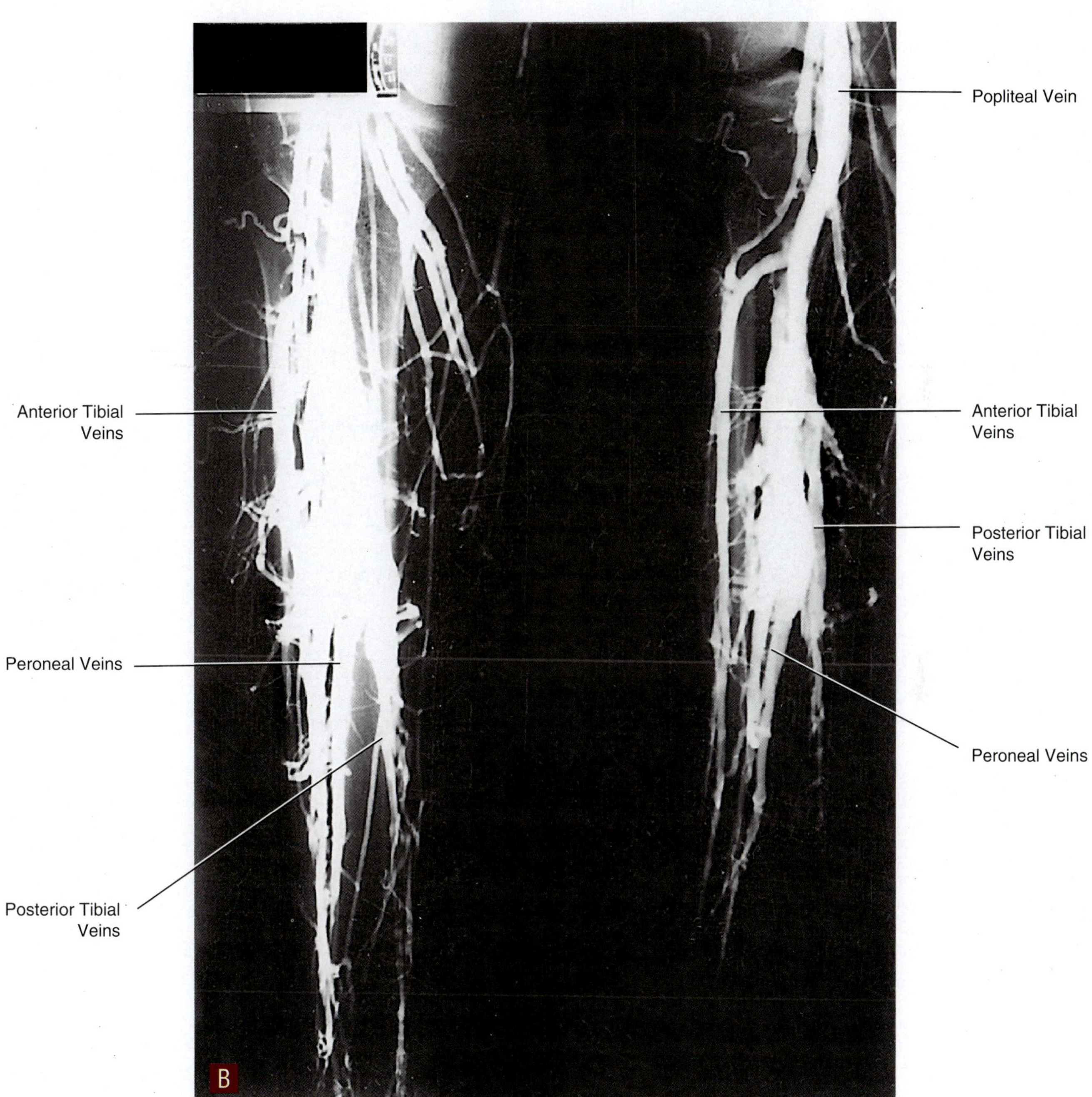

Figure 23.8. *Continued*

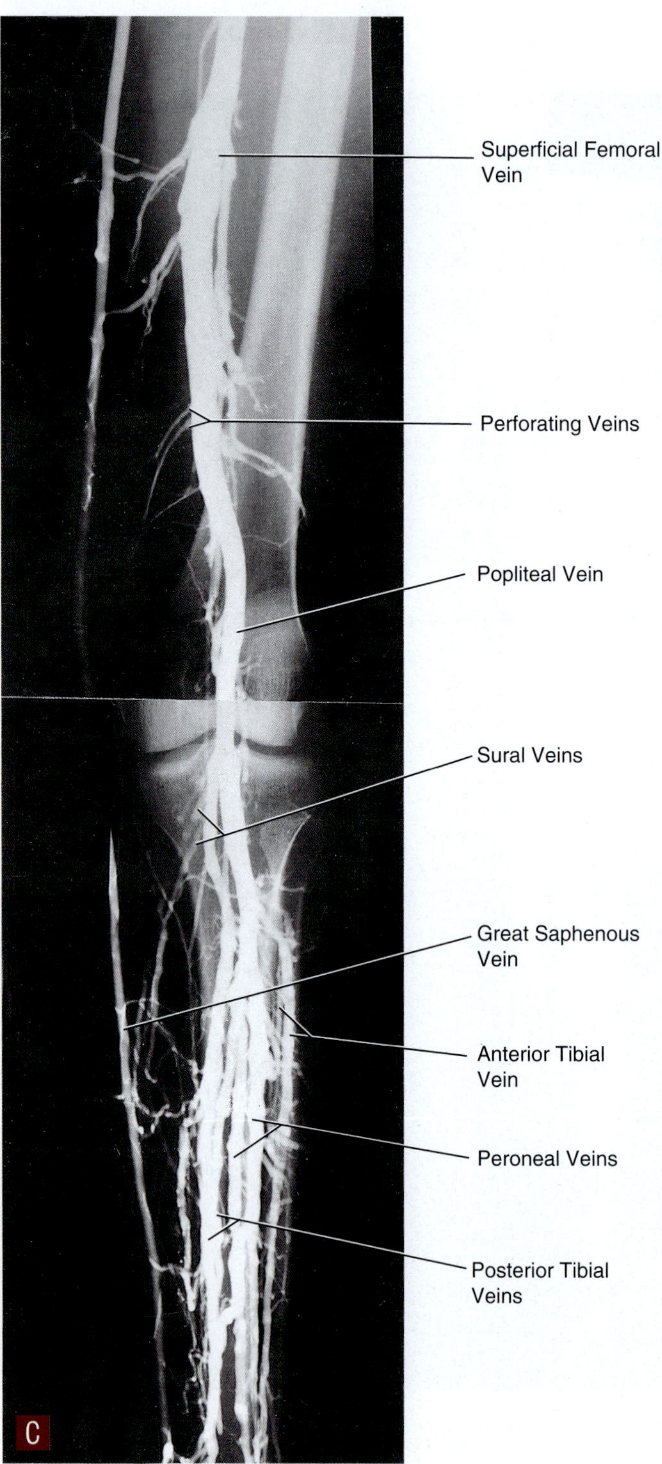

Figure 23.8. *Continued*

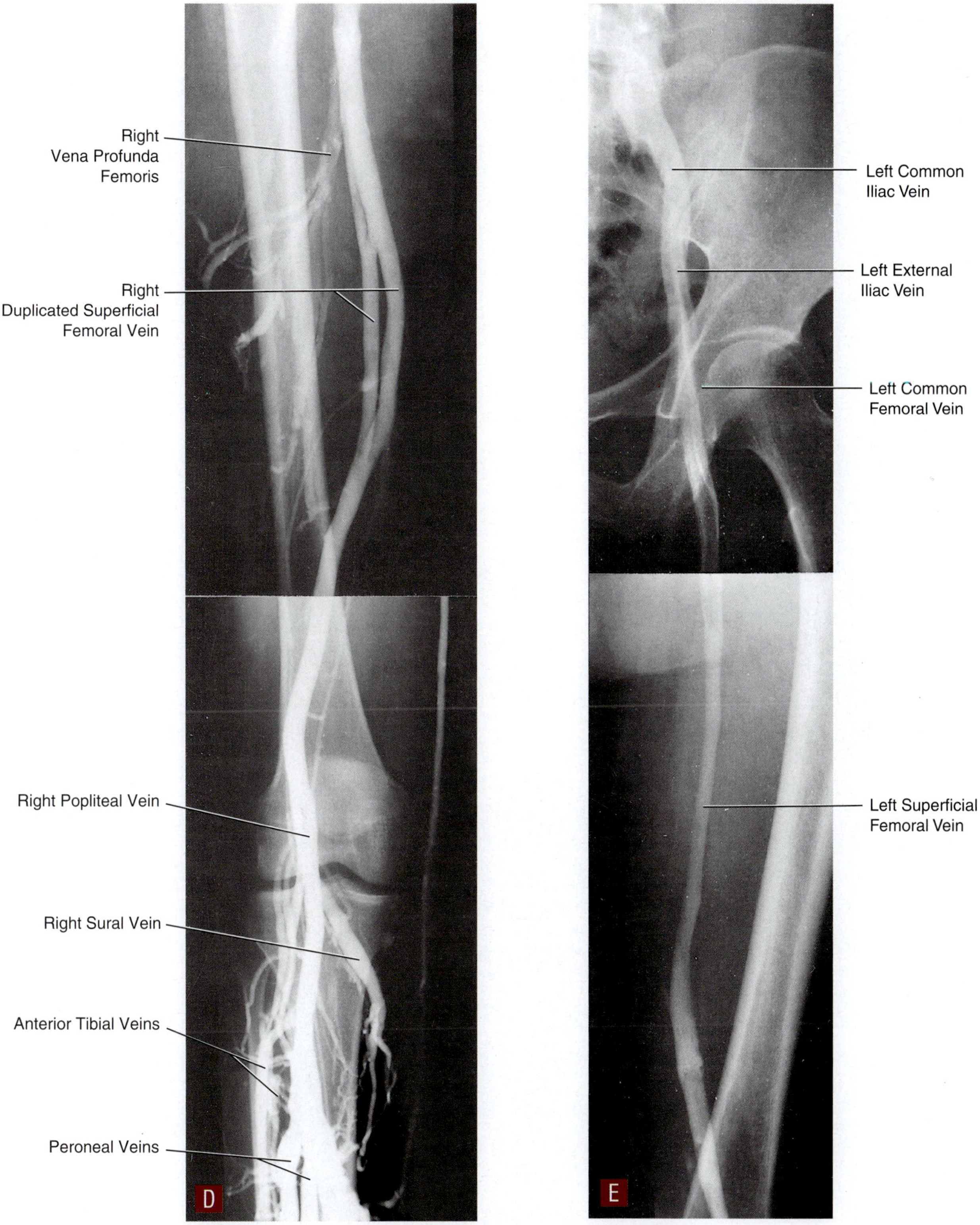

Right Vena Profunda Femoris

Right Duplicated Superficial Femoral Vein

Right Popliteal Vein

Right Sural Vein

Anterior Tibial Veins

Peroneal Veins

D

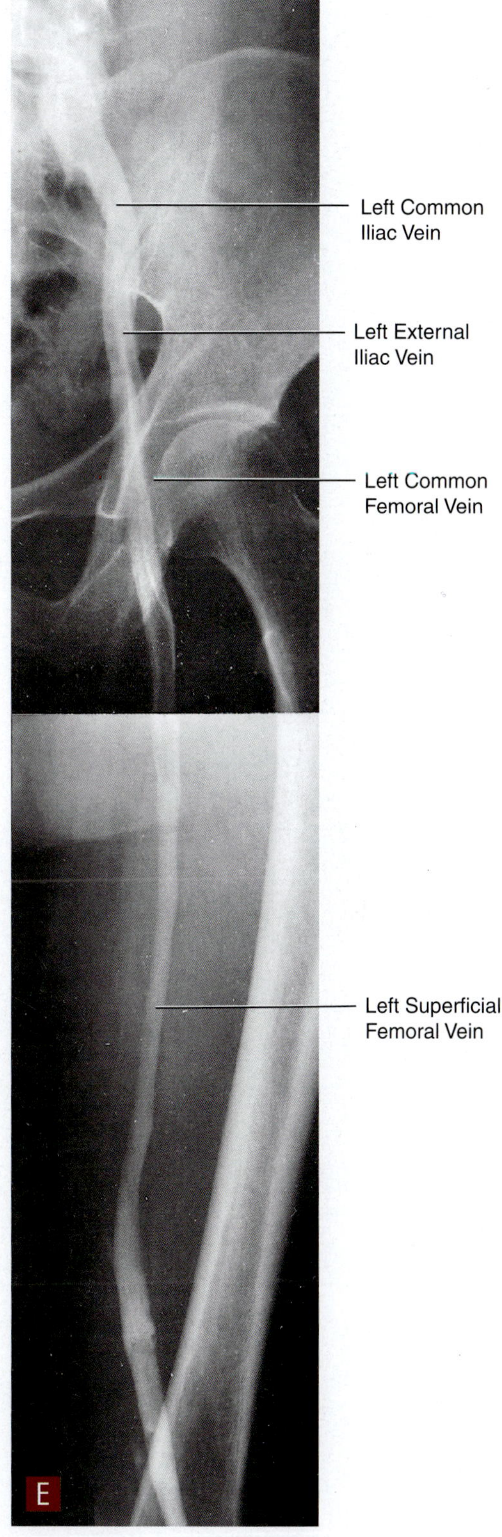

Figure 23.8. *Continued*

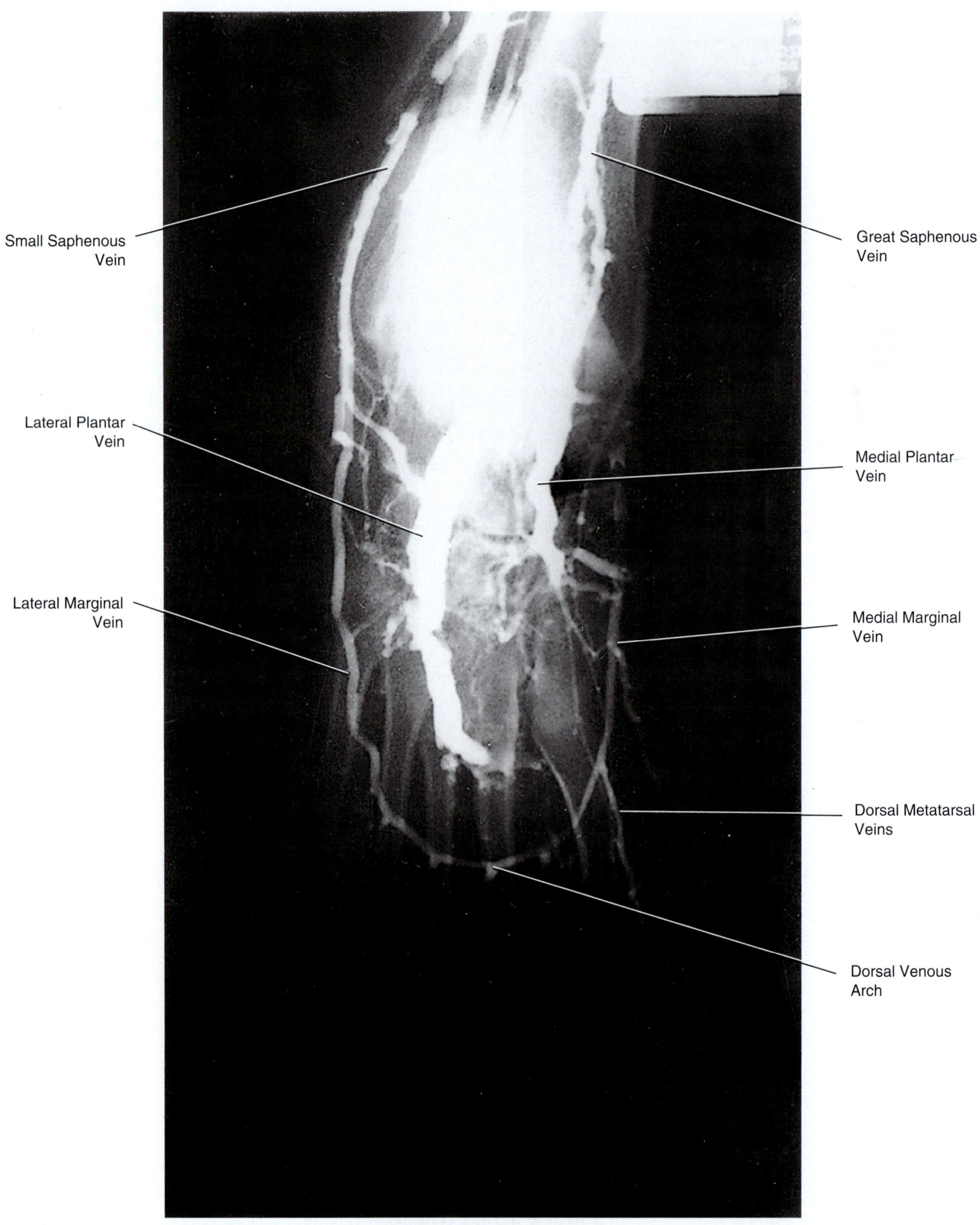

Figure 23.9. Venogram of the right foot.

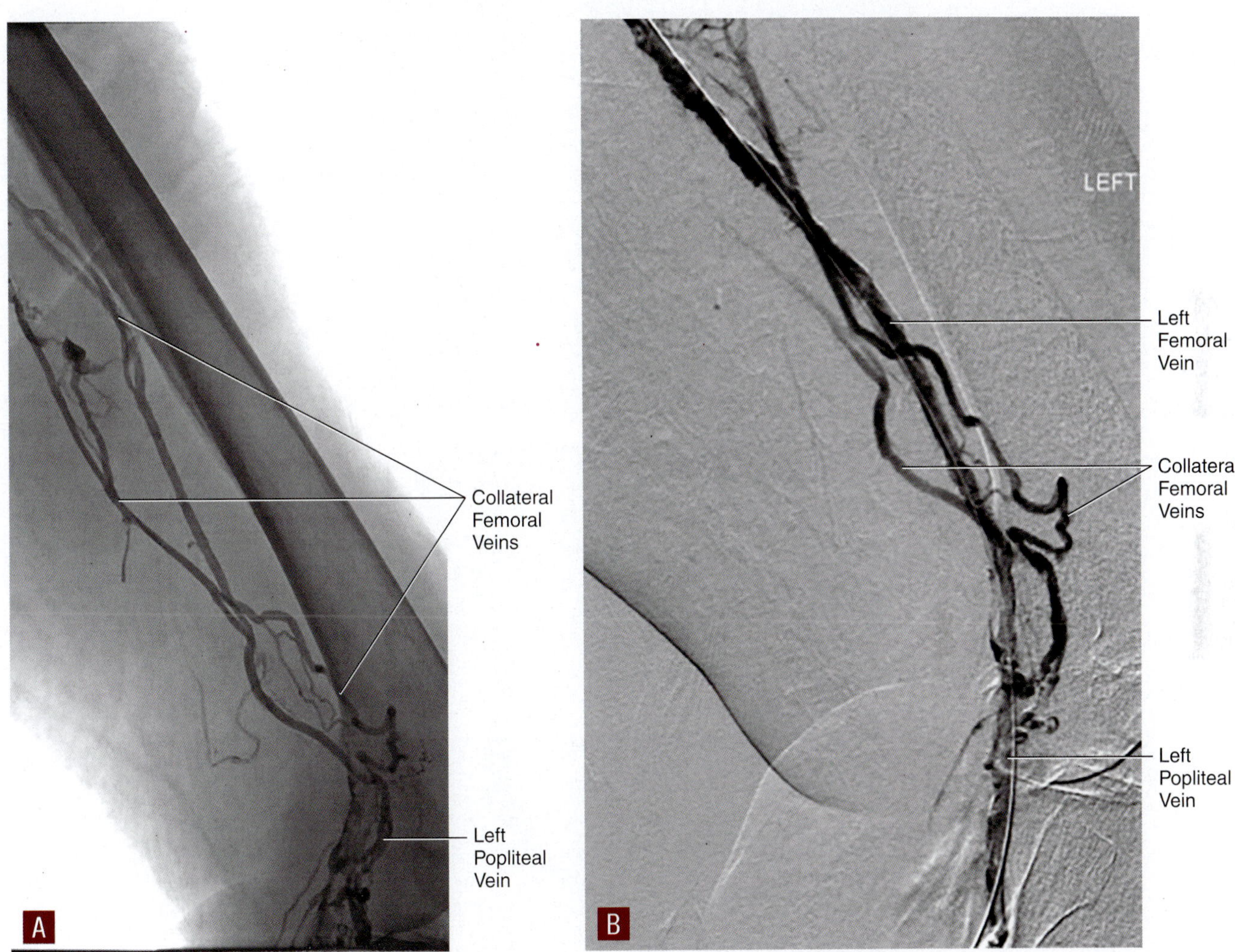

Figure 23.10. Venogram of the deep venous system of the left lower extremity. A, Patient with acute deep venous thrombosis (DVT). Note collaterals pre (A) and post (B) pharmacomechanical thrombectomy.

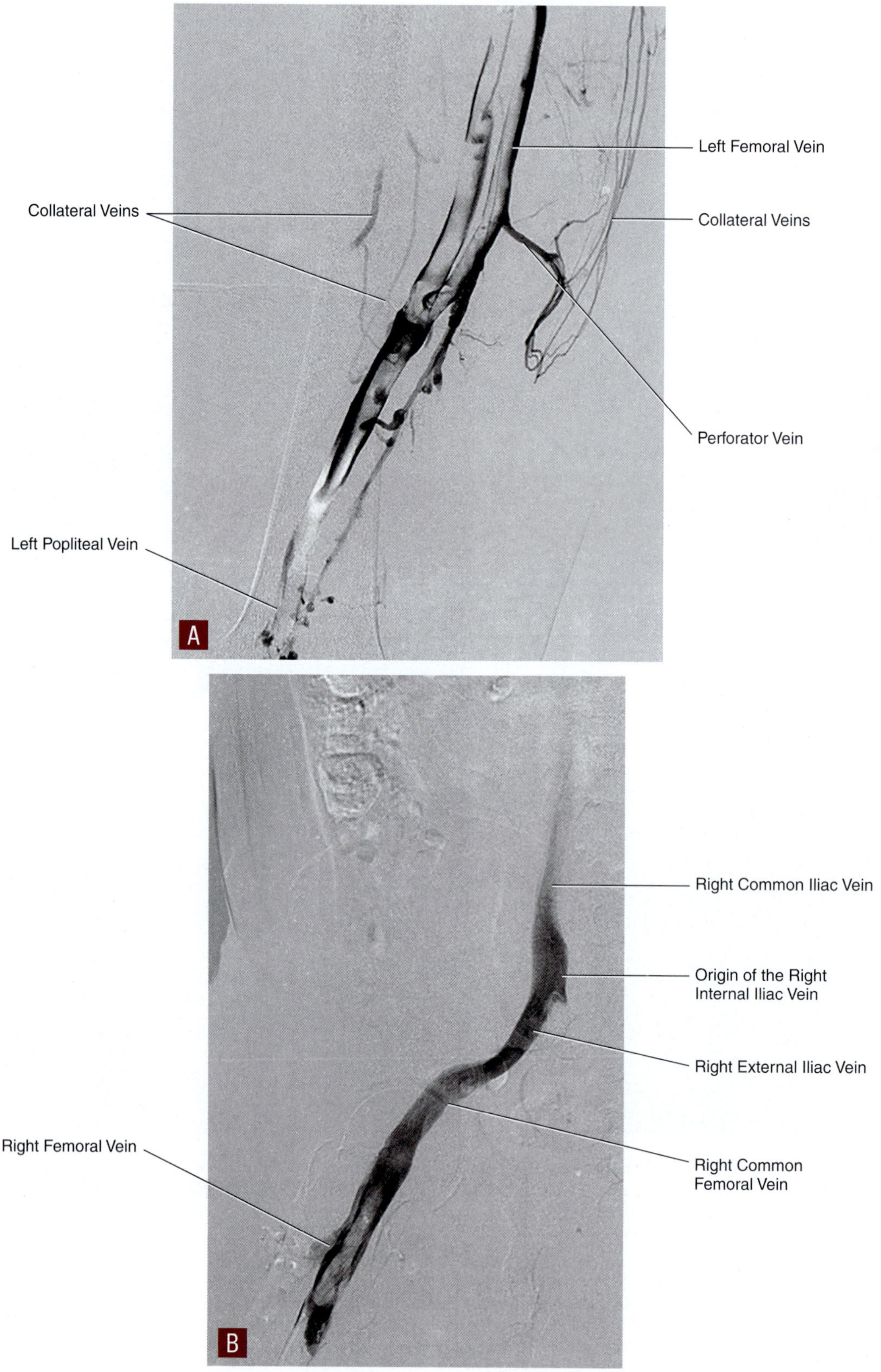

Left Femoral Vein

Collateral Veins

Collateral Veins

Perforator Vein

Left Popliteal Vein

A

Right Common Iliac Vein

Origin of the Right Internal Iliac Vein

Right External Iliac Vein

Right Common Femoral Vein

Right Femoral Vein

B

Figure 23.11. Lower extremity venograms in patients with DVT. **A**, Extensive DVT in the left femoral veins. Patient is in prone position. **B**, Acute DVT with a "floating clot" in the right femoral vein, note the patient is supine position. **C**, Acute DVT with a clot in the transition between the right common femoral and right external iliac veins. Note the drainage through the right inferior epigastric vein. Patient is in prone position. **D**, Chronic DVT in the left common femoral and external iliac veins. Note several collaterals. Patient is in prone position. **E**, Acute DVT with clots in the anterior and posterior tibial, peroneal, and popliteal veins. **F**, Acute left femoral DVT, patient in prone position. Note the difference between both femoral veins: one normally patent and the most medial with clots (acute DVT). DVT, deep vein thrombosis.

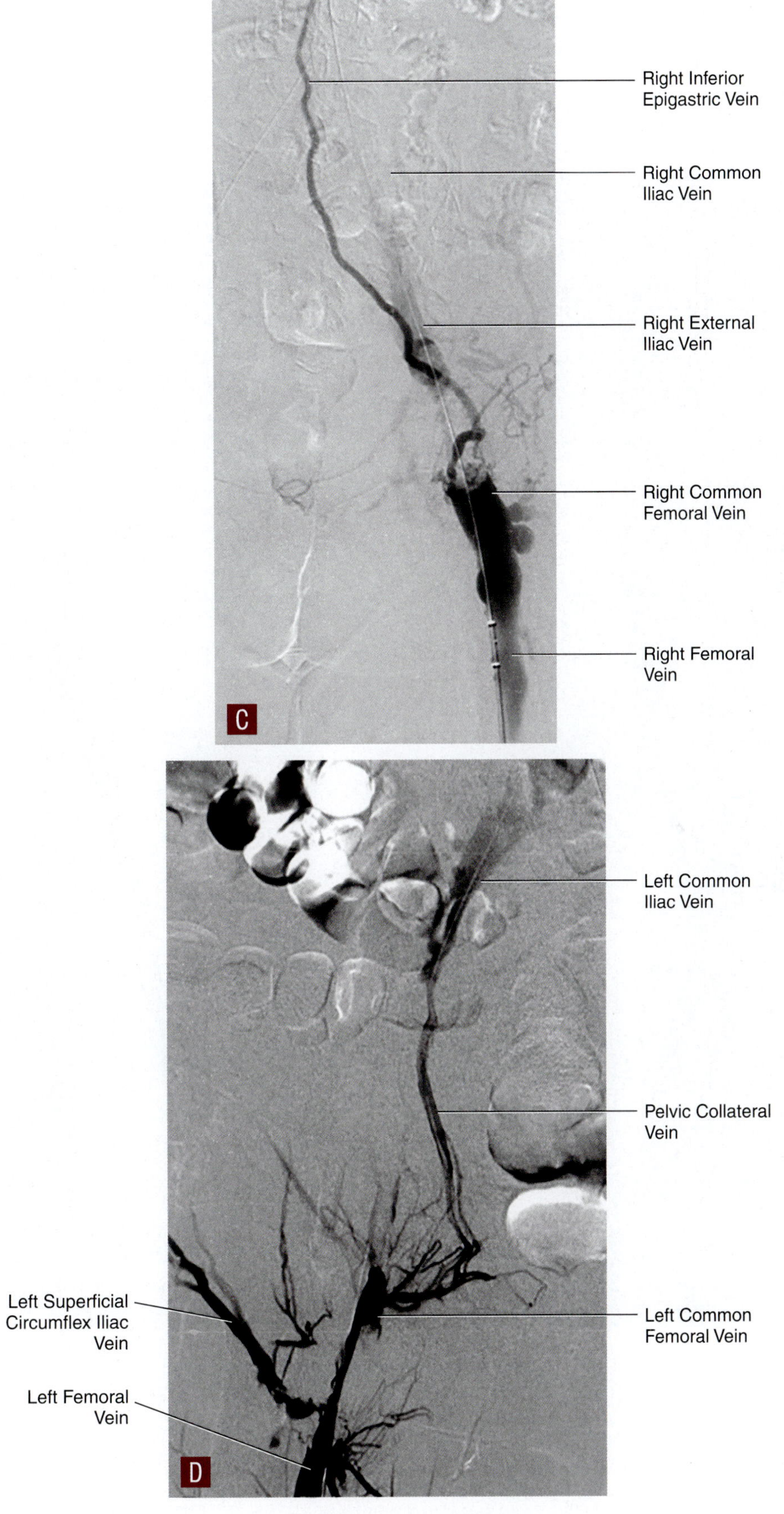

Figure 23.11. *Continued*

Right Popliteal Vein
Right Anterior Tibial Vein
Right Posterior Tibial Vein
Right Peroneal Vein
E

Left Common Femoral Vein
LEFT
Left Femoral Veins
F

Figure 23.11. *Continued*

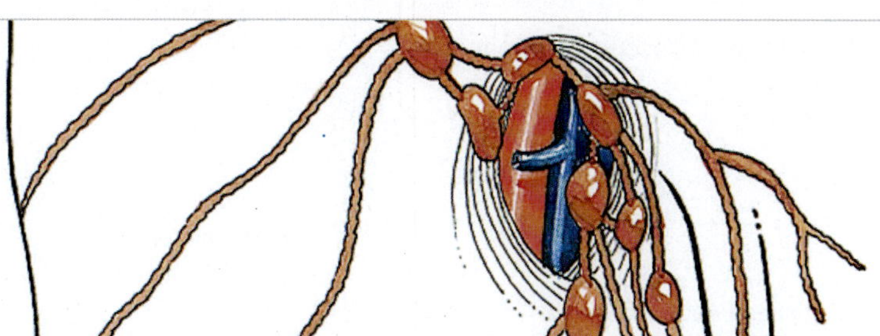

24

Lymphatic System of the Lower Extremity

The superficial lymphatic vessels drain the superficial tissues, beginning in lymphatic plexuses beneath the skin. The foot is drained by a group of larger medial vessels following the path of the great saphenous vein and a lateral group of smaller vessels that follows the small saphenous vein in the calf and thigh (Fig. 24.1).

The lymphatics of the medial group follow the great saphenous vein up to the groin, ending in the lower group of the superficial inguinal lymph nodes (Fig. 24.2). The lateral group of lymphatic vessels follows the small saphenous vein, ending in the popliteal lymph nodes. Some of these lymphatic vessels, however, will cross to the front of the leg, joining the medial group. The buttock lymphatic drainage is oriented to the upper group of the superficial inguinal lymph nodes.

Superficial Lymphatic Drainage

Deep Lymphatic Drainage

The lymphatic vessels of the deep group follow the main blood vessels and are divided into several groups, named after the related artery and veins, such as: anterior tibial, posterior tibial, peroneal, popliteal, and femoral. The deep lymphatic vessels of the foot and leg reach the popliteal lymph nodes, whereas the drainage of the thigh reaches the deep inguinal lymph nodes. The deep lymphatic drainage of the gluteal and ischial regions follows the blood vessels and is named after them. The superior gluteal lymphatics drain to a lymph node at the greater sciatic foramen, and the inferior gluteal lymphatics drain to the internal iliac lymph nodes after passing through a couple of small lymph nodes close to the piriformis muscle.

Popliteal Lymph Nodes

There are typically six or seven small popliteal lymph nodes in the popliteal fossa. They receive lymphatic drainage from the small saphenous vein territory, knee joint, genicular artery territory, and the trunks from the tibial vessels (Fig. 24.1).

Deep Inguinal Lymph Nodes

The deep inguinal lymph nodes are two or three in number and are medial to the femoral vein. They receive the deep lymphatic afferents from the femoral vessels group and from the penis or clitoris. They may also receive the superficial lymphatics from the superficial inguinal lymph nodes. The efferents drain to the external iliac lymph nodes.

Superficial Inguinal Lymph Nodes

There are two groups of superficial inguinal lymph nodes: upper and lower groups (Figs. 24.3 and 24.4). The upper group forms a chain below the inguinal ligament. Laterally, they receive afferents, which drain the gluteal tissues and abdominal wall. Medially, they receive the superficial lymphatics from the external genitalia, anal canal and perineal region, uterine vessels, and abdominal wall. The lower group forms a chain along the terminal great saphenous vein. They receive the superficial lymphatic vessels of the lower extremity, except from the back and lateral side of the calf (Fig. 24.1). The drainage of the superficial inguinal lymph nodes (Fig. 24.5) is directly to the external iliac lymph nodes.

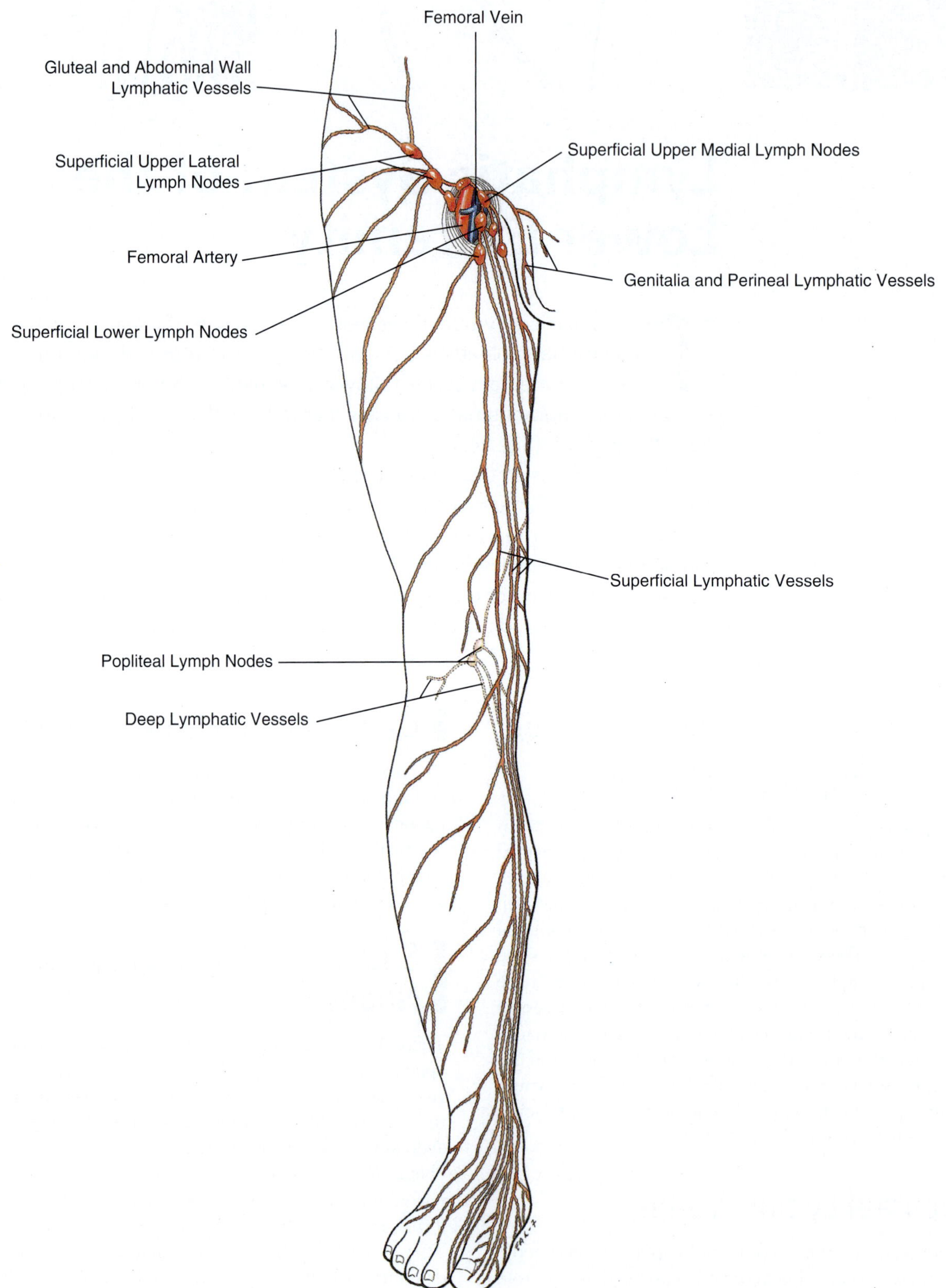

Figure 24.1. Schematic diagram of the lymphatic drainage of the lower extremity.

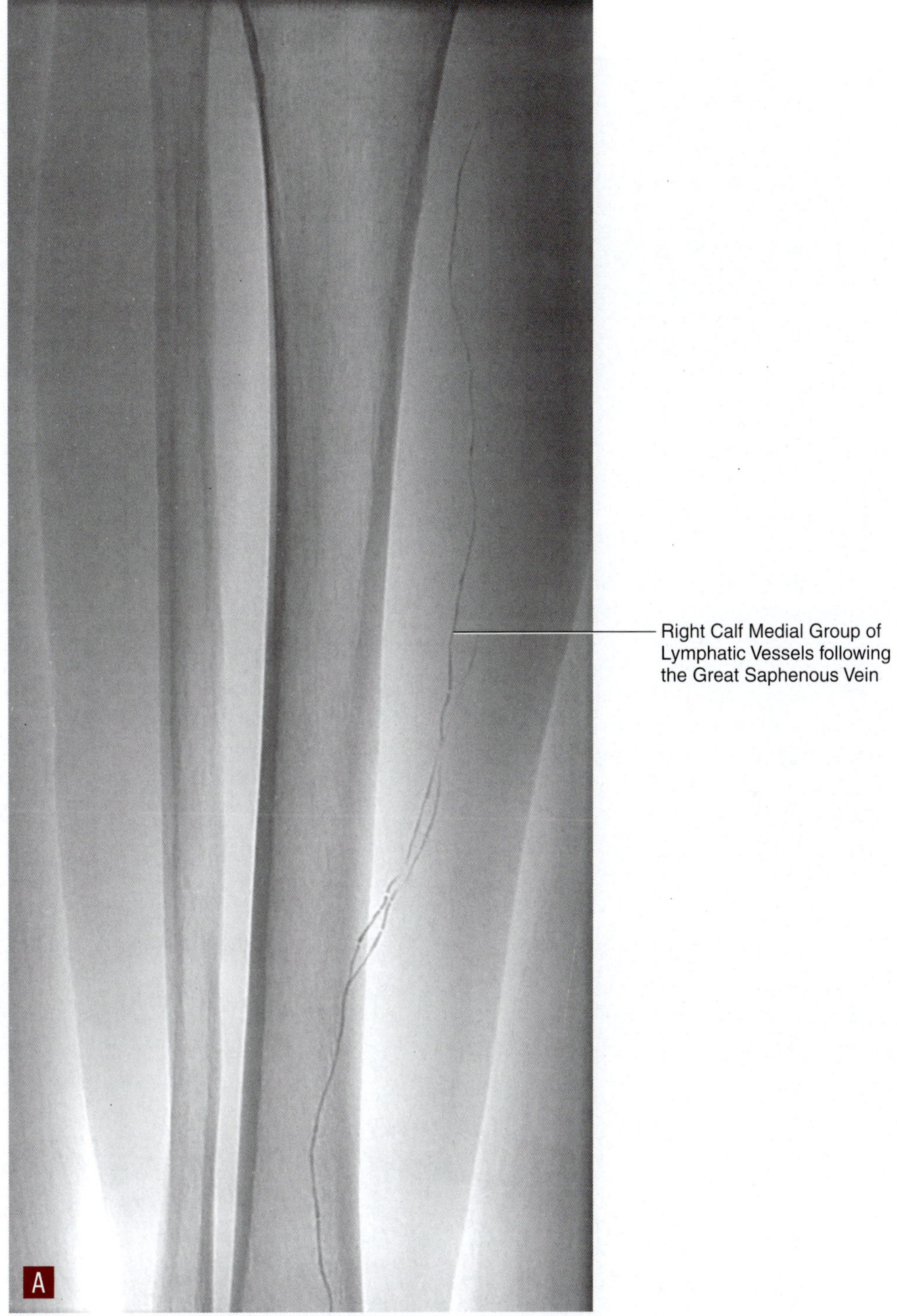

Figure 24.2. **A**, Right calf lymphatic vessels. **B**, Right calf lymphatic vessels at the knee. The medial group of lymphatic vessels depicted here follows the path of the great saphenous vein all the way from the ankle to the groin. Normal lymphatics are very small in diameter and poorly visualized in the lymphangiogram. **C**, Right thigh lymphatic vessels following the great saphenous vein. **D**, Right thigh lymphatic vessels with a common confluence into a right superficial lower lymph node.

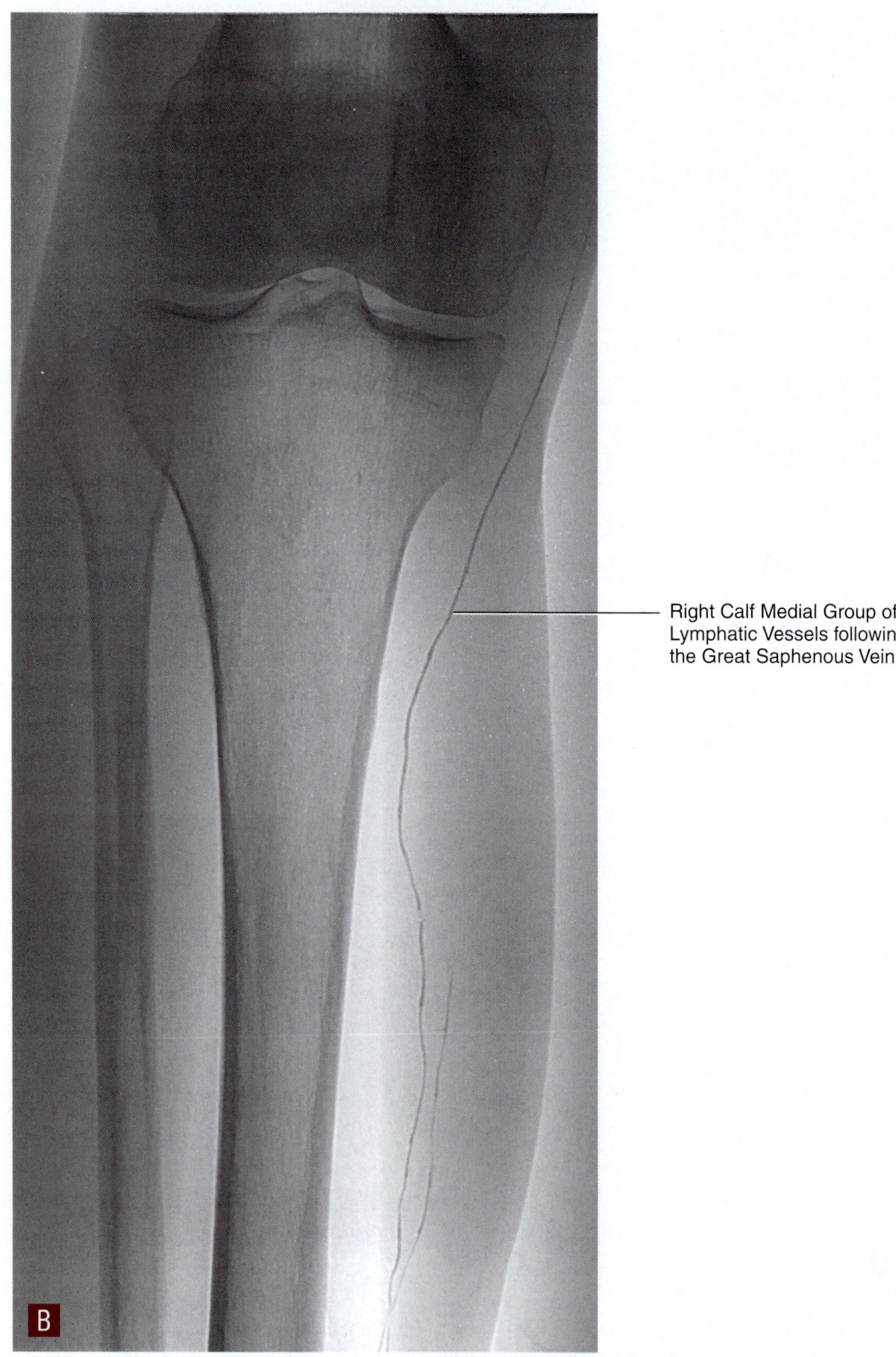

Figure 24.2. *Continued*

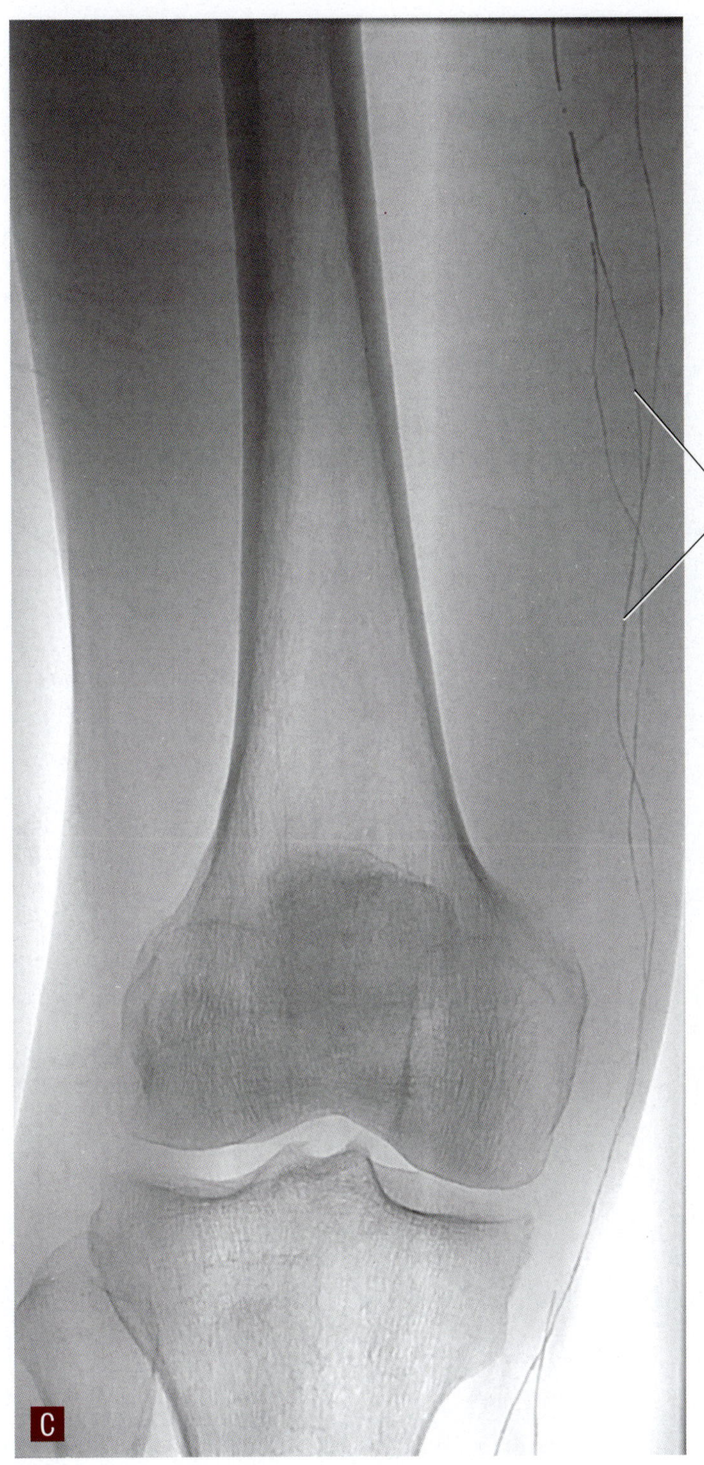

Figure 24.2. *Continued*

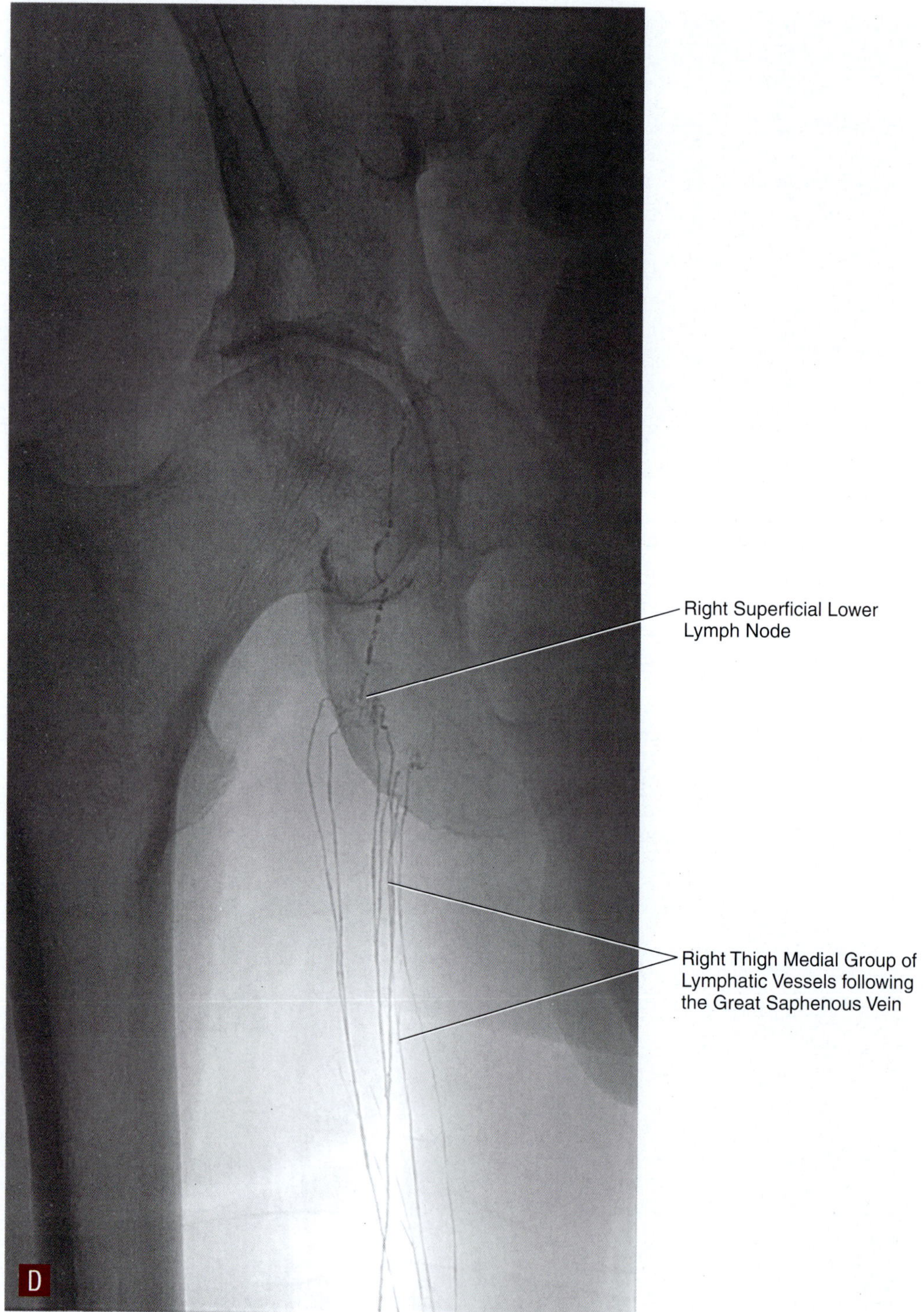

Figure 24.2. *Continued*

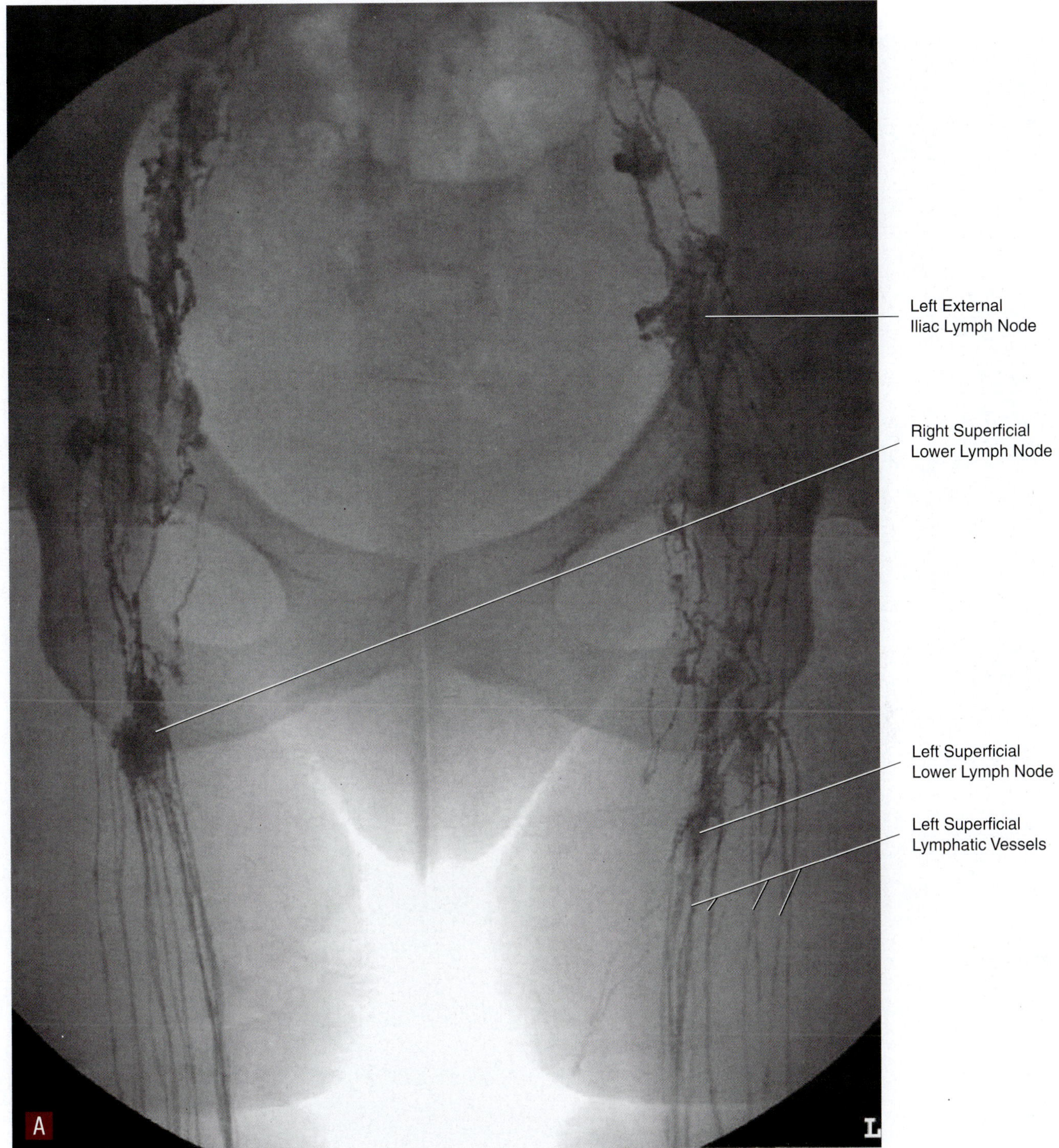

Figure 24.3. **A**, Bilateral inguinal lymphangiogram, vascular phase, showing the lymphatic vessels in both groins reaching the superficial groin lymph nodes. The inguinal lymph nodes connect to the external iliac lymph nodes and lymphatic vessels. **B**, Late-phase lymphangiogram (storage phase) showing mostly the lymph nodes in the groins and iliac chains, and a few lymphatic vessels.

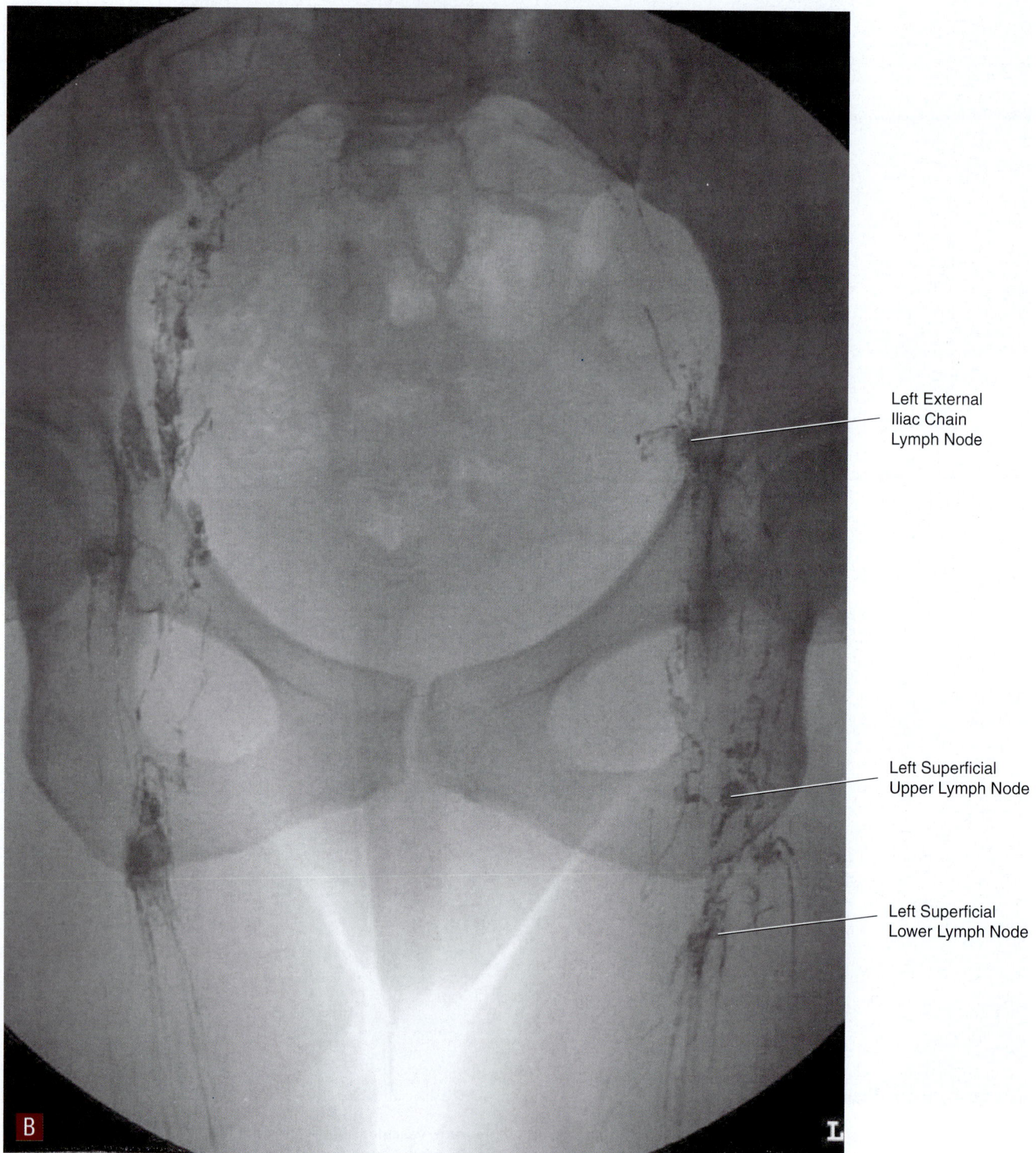

Figure 24.3. *Continued*

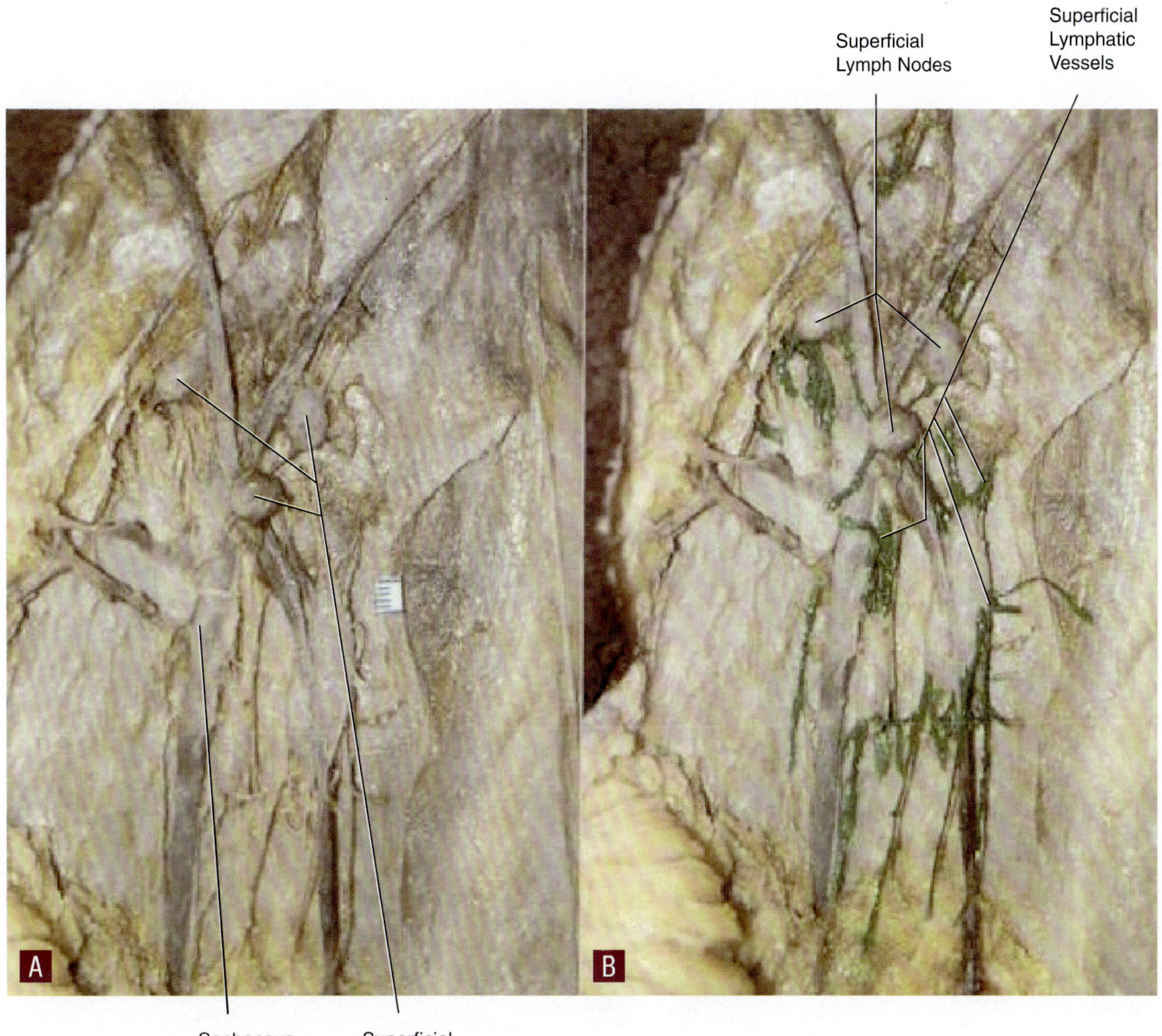

Figure 24.4. Lymphatic vessels and superficial lymph nodes of the left inguinal region depicted after removal of the skin in a cadaveric preparation. **A**, Unenhanced dissection of the left groin showing the great saphenous vein and some tributaries. The lymphatic vessels are barely visible. The superficial lymph nodes are visible. **B**, The inguinal lymphatic vessels are colorized in green in the illustration. The superficial lymphatic vessels join the superficial lower and upper lymph nodes. Superficial lateral lymphatic vessels are also visible. (From Souza-Rodrigues CF.)

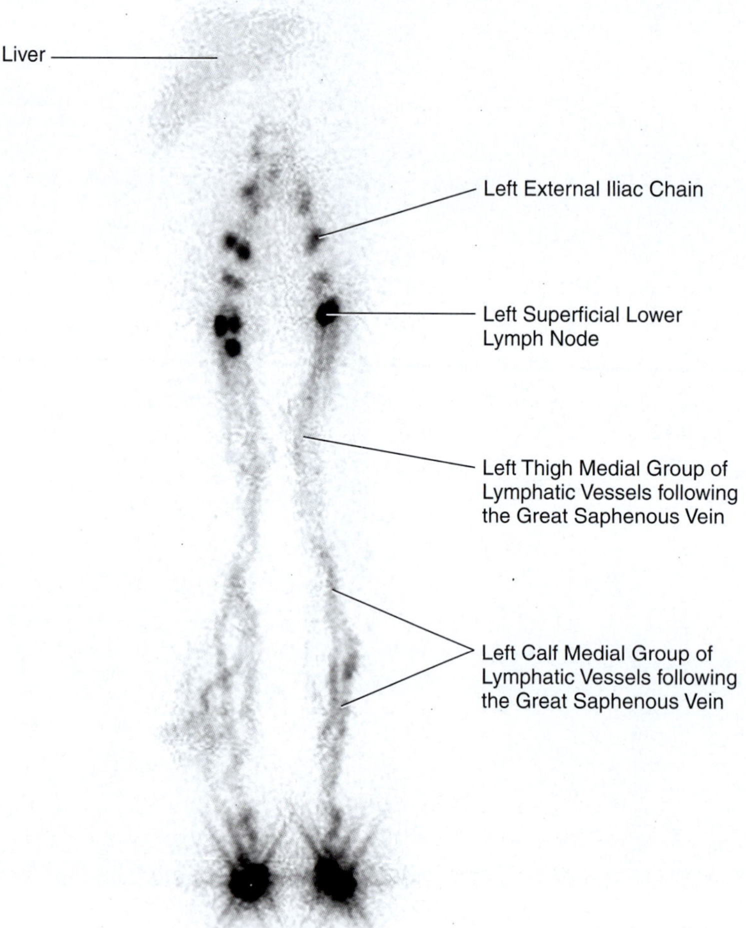

Figure 24.5. Lymphoscintigram showing the bilateral lower extremity lymphatic vessels, popliteal lymph nodes, and inguinal lymph nodes.

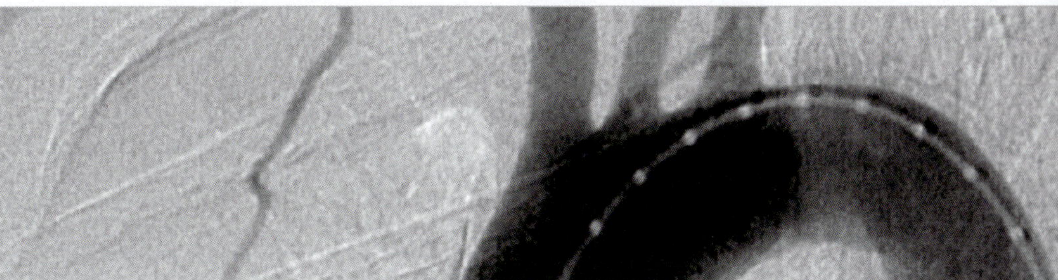

25

Suggested Readings

1. Fetal Circulation

Bautch VL, James JM. Neurovascular development: the beginning of a beautiful friendship. *Cell Adhes Migr*. 2009;3:199-204.

Carlson BM. *The cardiovascular system*. In: *Human Embryology and Developmental Biology*. St. Louis: Mosby; 1994:372-406.

Collardeau-Frachon S, Scoazec J-Y. Vascular development and differentiation during human liver organogenesis. *Anat Rec Adv Integr Anat Evol Biol*. 2008;291:614-627.

Corliss CE. *The circulatory system*. In: *Patten's Human Embryology. Elements of Clinical Development*. New York: McGraw-Hill; 1976:389-452.

Gregg L, Gailloud P. The role of the primitive lateral basilovertebral anastomosis of padget in variations of the vertebrobasilar arterial system: the primitive lateral basilovertebral anastomosis. *Anat Rec*. 2017;300:2025-2038.

Kau T, Sinzig M, Gasser J, et al. aortic development and anomalies. *Semin Interv Radiol*. 2007;24:141-152.

Obel W. The umbilical vein in different periods of life in man. *Folia Morphol*. 1976;35:173-179.

Rudolph AM. Hepatic and ductus venous blood flows during fetal life. *Hepatology*. 1983;3:254-258.

2. Arteries of the Head and Neck

Al-Rafiah A, El-Haggagy AA, Aal IH, Zaki AI. Anatomical study of the carotid bifurcation and origin variations of the ascending pharyngeal and superior thyroid arteries. *Folia morphologica*. 2011;70(1):47-55.

SJDimmick, KCFaulder. Normal variants of the cerebral circulation at multidetectory CT angiography. *Radiographics*. 2009;29:1027-1043.

Djindjian R, Merland JJ. *Super-Selective Arteriography of the External Carotid Artery*. 1st ed. Berlin: Springer-Verlag; 1978:1-550.

Lasjaunias P, Berenstein A. *Functional anatomy of craniofacial arteries*. In: *Surgical Neuroangiography*. Vol 1. New York: Springer-Verlag; 1987:1-426.

Lasjaunias P, Berenstein A. *Functional vascular anatomy of brain, spinal cord and spine*. In: *Surgical Neuroangiography*. Vol 3. New York: Springer-Verlag; 1990:1-337.

Layton KF, Kallmes DF, Cloft HJ, Lindell EP, Cox VS. Bovine aortic arch variant in humans: clarification of a common misnomer. *Am J Neuroradiol*. 2006;27(7):1541-1542.

Newton TH, Potts DG. *Radiology of the skull and brain*. In: *Angiography*. Vol 2. St. Louis: CV Mosby; 1974.

Osborn AG. *The aortic arch and great vessels*. In: *Diagnostic Cerebral Angiography*. 2nd ed. Philadelphia, PA: Lippincott Williams & Wilkins; 1999:3-29.

Osborn AG. *Osbourn's Brain: Imaging, Pathology, and Anatomy*. 1st ed. Philadelphia, PA: Lippincott, Williams & Wilkins; 2013.

3. Veins of the Head and Neck

Krayenbühl H, Yaşargil MG, Huber P, et al. *Cerebral Angiography*. Stuttgart: Thieme Publishing Group; 1982.

Lasjaunias P, Berenstein A. *Functional vascular anatomy of brain, spinal cord and spine*. In: *Surgical Neuroangiography*. Vol 3. New York: Springer-Verlag; 1990:1-337.

McMinn RMH. *Last's Anatomy: Regional and Applied*. Edinburgh: Elsevier; 2003.

Newton TH, Potts DG. *Radiology of the skull and brain*. In: *Angiography*. Vol 2. St. Louis: CV Mosby; 1974.

Osborn AG. *Diagnostic Cerebral Angiography*. 2nd ed. Philadelphia, PA: Lippincott Williams & Wilkins; 1999.

Osborn AG. *Osbourn's Brain: Imaging, Pathology, and Anatomy*. 1st ed. Philadelphia, PA: Lippincott, Williams & Wilkins; 2013.

Rhoton AL. *Rhoton Cranial Anatomy and Surgical Approaches*. Philadelphia: Lippincott Williams & Wilkins; 2003.

Schild HH, Strack TR. Selective simultaneous bilateral sampling from the inferior petrosal sinuses. In: Uflacker R, Sorensen R, eds. *Percutaneous Venous Blood Sampling in Endocrine Diseases*. New York: Springer-Verlag; 1992:48-74.

Suzuki Y, Matsumoto K. Variations of the superficial middle cerebral vein: classification using three-dimensional CT angiography. *AJNR Am J Neuroradiol*. 2000;21(5):932-938.

Williams PL, Warwick R, Dyson M, Bannister LH. *Angiology*. In: *Gray's Anatomy*. 37th ed. Edinburgh: Churchill Livingstone; 1989:661-858:chap 6.

4. Lymphatic System of the Head and Neck

Fischer HW, Lawrence MS, Thornbury JR. Lymphography of the normal adult male: observations and their relation to the diagnosis of metastatic neoplasm. *Radiology*. 1962;78:399-406.

Fischer HW, Zimmerman GR. Roentgenographic visualization of lymph nodes and lymphatic channels. *MR*. 1959;81:517-534.

Williams PL, Warwick R, Dyson M, Bannister LH. *Angiology*. In: *Gray's Anatomy*. 37th ed. Edinburgh: Churchill Livingstone; 1989:661-858:chap 6.

5. Arteries of the Spinal Cord and Spine

Doppman JL, Di Chiro G, Ommaya AK. *Selective Arteriography of the Spinal Cord*. 1st ed. St. Louis: Warren II. Green, Inc.; 1969:3-16.

Lasjaunias P, Berenstein A. *Functional vascular anatomy of brain, spinal cord and spine*. In: *Surgical Neuroangiography*. Vol 3. New York: Springer-Verlag; 1990:1-337.

Rodesch G, Lasjaunias P, Berenstein A. Functional vascular anatomy of the spine and spinal cord. *Rivista Neuroradiologia*. 1992;5(suppl 2):63-66.

Santillan A, Nacarino V, Greenberg E, Riina HA, Gobin YP, Patsalides A. Vascular anatomy of the spinal cord. *J Neurointerventional Surg*. 2012;4:67-74.

Tveten L. Spinal cord vascularity. I. Extraspinal sources of spinal cord arteries in man. *Acta Radiol (Diagn)*. 1976;17:1-16.

Tveten L. Spinal cord vascularity. III. The spinal cord arteries in man. *Acta Radiol (Diagn)*. 1976;17:257-273.

6. Veins of the Spinal Cord and Spine

Batson OV. The function of the vertebral veins and their role in the spread of metastases. *Ann Surg*. 1940;112:138-148.

Drasin GF, Daffner RH, Sexton RF, Cheatham WC. Epidural venography: diagnosis of herniated lumbar intervertebral disc and other disease of the epidural space. *AJR Am J Roentgenol*. 1976;126:1010-1016.

Gershater R, Holgate RC. Lumbar epidural venography in the diagnosis of disc herniations. *AJR Am J Roentgenol*. 1976;126:992-1002.

Gershater R, St Louis EL. Lumbar epidural venography. Review of 1,200 cases. *Radiology*. 1979;131:409-421.

Pearce JMS. The craniospinal venous system. *Eur Neurol*. 2006;56:136-138.

Tveten L. Spinal cord vascularity. I. Extraspinal sources of spinal cord arteries in man. *Acta Radiol (Diagn)*. 1976;17:1-16.

Tveten L. Spinal cord vascularity. III. The spinal cord arteries in man. *Acta Radiol (Diagn)*. 1976;17:257-273.

7. Thoracic Aorta and Arteries of the Trunk

Balm R, Reekers JA, Jacobs MJ. Classification of endovascular procedures for treating thoracic aortic aneurysms. In: Jacobs MJ, Branchereau A, eds. *Surgical and Endovascular Treatment of Aortic Aneurysms*. Armonk, NY: Futura Publishing Company; 2000:19-26.

Blake HA, Manion WC. Thoracic arterial arch anomalies. *Circulation*. 1962;26:251-265.

Botenga ASJ. *Selective Bronchial and Intercostal Arteriography*. Baltimore: The Williams and Wilkins Co.; 1970:1-159.

Caix M, Descottes B, Rousseay DG, Rousseau D. The arterial vascularization of the middle thoracic and lower esophagus. *Anat Clin*. 1982;3:95-106.

Cauldwell EW, Siekert RG, Lininger RE, Anson J. The bronchial arteries: an anatomic study of 150 cadavers. *Surg Gynecol Obstet*. 1948;86:395-412.

Fisher RG, Whighan CJ, Trinh C. Diverticula of Kommerell and aberrant subclavian arteries complicated by aneurysms. *Cardiovasc Intervent Radiol*. 2005;28:553-560.

Free K, Low VHS. The aberrant subclavian artery. *AJR Am J Roentgenol*. 1997;168:481-484.

Hellekant C. *Bronchial Angiography and Intra-arterial Chemotherapy in Lung Carcinoma* [thesis]. Malmo, Sweden: University of Lund; 1978:1-100.

Hollinshead WIT. *The thorax, abdomen, and pelvis*. In: *Anatomy for Surgeons*. Vol 2. New York: Harper & Row; 1971.

Ishimaru S. Endografting of the aortic arch. *J Endovasc Ther*. 2004;11(suppl 2):62-71.

Jardin M, Remy J. Control of hemoptysis: systemic angiography and anastomoses of the internal mammary artery. *Radiology*. 1988;168:377-383.

Jesinger RA. Breast anatomy for the interventionalist. *Tech Vasc Interv Radiol*. 2014;17:3-9.

Knight GC, Codd JE. Anomalous right subclavian artery aneurysms. Report of 3 cases, with a review of the literature. *Tex Heart Inst J*. 1991;18:209-218.

Netter FH. Anatomy of the esophagus. In: Netter FH, ed. *Digestive System. Part I: Upper Digestive Tract*. Vol 3. New York: The Ciba Collection of Medical Illustrations; 1966:34-46.

Pisco JBM. *Angioplastia Transluminal Percutanea* [thesis]. Lisboa, Portugal: Universidade Nova de Lisboa; 1990:1-334.

Tan RT, McGahan JP, Link DP, Lantz BMT. Bronchial artery embolization in management of haemoptysis. *J Intery Radiol*. 1991;6:67-76.

Uflacker R, Kaemmerer A. Picon PD, et al. Bronchial artery embolization in the management of hemoptysis: technical aspects and long-term results. *Radiology*. 1985;157:637-644.

8. Veins of the Thorax

Abrams HL. The vertebral and azygos venous systems and some variations in systemic venous return. *Radiology*. 1957;69:508-525.

Drane WE, Watt AC, Marks DS. Obstruction of the superior vena cava or its major tributaries demonstrated by bolus-injection excretory urography. *Radiology*. 1982;144:499-504.

Fritzsche P, Andersen C, Smith DC. Collateral circulation secondary to upper extremity venous thrombosis visualized during excretory urography. *Radiology*. 1982;144:495-498.

Sonavane SK, Milner DM, Singh SP, Abdel Aal AK, Shahir KS, Chaturvedi A. Comprehensive imaging review of the superior cena cava. *RadioGraphics*. 2015;35:1873-1892.

Sorensen R. Selective venous sampling for parathyroid hormone excess. In: Uflacker R, Sorensen R, eds. *Percutaneous Venous Blood Sampling in Endocrine Diseases*. New York: Springer-Verlag; 1992:125-150.

Thomas ML. Phlebography. *Arch Surg*. 1972;104:145-151.

Williams PL, Warwick R, Dyson M, Bannister LH. *Angiology*. In: *Gray's Anatomy*. 37th ed. Edinburgh: Churchill Livingstone; 1989;661-858:chap 6.

Yune HY, Klatte EC. Mediastinal venography. *AJR Am J Roentgenol*. 1986;147:674-684.

9. Lymphatic System of the Thorax

Fischer HW, Lawrence MS, Thornbury JR. Lymphography of the normal adult male: observations and their relation to the diagnosis of metastatic neoplasm. *Radiology*. 1962;78:399-406.

Fischer HW, Zimmerman GR. Roentgenographic visualization of lymph nodes and lymphatic channels. *AJR Am J Roentgenol*. 1959;81:517-534.

Fraser RG, Pare JAP, Pare PD, Fraser RS, Genereux GP. The normal chest. In: Fraser RG, Pare JAP, Pare PD, Fraser RS, Genereux GE, eds. *Diagnosis of Diseases of the Chest*. 3rd ed. Philadelphia: W.B. Saunders Co.; 1988:1-314.

Hollinshead WH. *The thorax, abdomen, and pelvis*. In: *Anatomy for Surgeons*. Vol 2. New York: Harper & Row; 1971.

10. Pulmonary Arterial Circulation

Anand SH. Proximal interruption of the pulmonary artery: a case series. *J Clin Diagn Res*. 2015;9(12):TD04-TD06.

Boyden EA. *Segmental Anatomy of the Lungs*. New York: McGraw-Hill; 1955.

Carter BW, Lichtenberger JP, Wu CC. Congenital abnormalities of the pulmonary arteries in adults. *Am J Roentgenol*. 2014;202:W308-W313.

Castañer E, Gallardo X, Rimola J, et al. Congenital and acquired pulmonary artery anomalies in the adult: radiologic overview. *RadioGraphics*. 2006;26:349-371.

Dotter CT. The normal pulmonary arteriogram. In: Abrams HL, ed. *Abrams Angiography. Vascular and Interventional Radiology*. 3rd ed. Boston: Little, Brown and Co.; 1983:715-722.

Fraser RG, Pare JAP, Pare PD, Fraser RS, Genereux GP. The normal chest. In: Fraser RG, Pare JAP, Pare PD, Fraser RS, Genereux GE, eds. *Diagnosis of Diseases of the Chest*. 3rd ed. Philadelphia: W.B. Saunders Co.; 1988:1-314.

Murata K, Itoh H, Todo G, et al. Bronchial venous plexus and its communication with pulmonary circulation. *Invest Radiol*. 1986;21:24-30.

Nagaishi C. *Functional Anatomy and Histology of the Lung*. Baltimore: University Park Press; 1972.

11. Pulmonary Venous Circulation

Dotter CT. The normal pulmonary arteriogram. In: Abrams HL, ed. *Abrams Angiography. Vascular and Interventional Radiology*. 3rd ed. Boston: Little, Brown and Co.; 1983:715-722.

Fraser RG, Pare JAP, Pare PD, Fraser RS, Genereux GP. The normal chest. In: Fraser RG, Pare JAP, Pare PD, Fraser RS, Genereux GP, eds. *Diagnosis of Diseases of the Chest*. 3rd ed. Philadelphia: W.B. Saunders Co.; 1988:1-314.

Murata K, Itoh H, Todo G, Itoh T, Kanaoka M, Furuta M, Torizuka K. Bronchial venous plexus and its communication with pulmonary circulation. *Invest Radiol*. 1986;21:24-30.

Nagaishi C. *Functional Anatomy and Histology of the Lung*. Baltimore: University Park Press; 1972.

12. Pulmonary and Thoracic Lymphatic System

El-Sherief AH, Lau CT, Wu CC, Drake RL, Abbott GF, Rice TW. International association for the study of lung cancer (IASLC) lymph node map: radiologic review with CT illustration. *RadioGraphics*. 2014;34:1680-1691.

Fraser RG, Pare JAP, Pare PD, Fraser RS, Genereux GP. The normal chest. In: Fraser RG, Pare JAP, Pare PD, Fraser RS, Genereux GP, eds. *Diagnosis of Diseases of the Chest*. 3rd ed. Philadelphia: W.B. Saunders Co.; 1988:1-314.

Nagaishi C. *Functional Anatomy and Histology of the Lung*. Baltimore: University Park Press; 1972.

13. Heart and Coronary Arteries

Abuchaim DCS, Spera CA, Faraco DL, RibasFilho JM, Malafaia O. Dominância coronariana em corações humanos em moldes por corrosão. *Rev Bras Cir Cardiovasc*. 2009;24(4):514-518.

Agarwal PP, Dennie C, Pena E, et al. Anomalous coronary arteries that need intervention: review of pre- and postoperative imaging appearances. *RadioGraphics*. 2017;37:740-757.

Chen JJ, Manning MA, Frazier AA, Jeudy J, White CS. CT Angiography of the cardiac valves: normal, diseased, and postoperative appearances. *RadioGraphics*. 2009;29:1393-1412.

Goldberg A, Southern DA, Galbraith PD, Traboulsi M, Knudtson ML, Ghali WA. Coronary dominance and prognosis of patients with acute coronary syndrome. *Am Heart J*. 2007;154:1116-1122.

Gupta T, Saini A, Sahni D. Terminal branching pattern of the right coronary artery in left-dominant hearts: a cadaveric study. *Cardiovasc Pathol*. 2013;22:179-182.

Kini S, Bis KG, Weaver L. Normal and variant coronary arterial and venous anatomy on high-resolution CT angiography. *Am J Roentgenol*. 2007;188:1665-1674.

Litmanovich DE, Kirsch J. Computed tomography of cardiac valves. *Radiol Clin North Am*. 2019;57:141-164.

Netter FH. Heart. In: Netter FH, ed. *The Netter Collection of Medical Illustrations: The CIBA Collection of Medical Illustrations*. 1st ed. Vol 5. New York: The Ciba Collection of Medical Illustrations; 1969:1-293.

Netter FH. *Atlas of Human Anatomy*. Summit, New Jersey: Ciba-Geigy Corporation; 1989.

Pansky B, House EL. *Review of Gross Anatomy*. 2nd ed. London: The Macmillan Co.; 1971:1-493.

Saremi F, Sánchez-Quintana D, Mori S, et al. Fibrous skeleton of the heart: anatomic overview and evaluation of pathologic conditions with CT and MR Imaging. *RadioGraphics*. 2017;37:1330-1351.

Shah SS, Teague SD, Lu JC, Dorfman AL, Kazerooni EA, Agarwal PP. Imaging of the coronary sinus: normal anatomy and congenital abnormalities. *RadioGraphics*. 2012;32:991-1008.

Shriki JE, Shinbane JS, Rashid MA, et al. Identifying, characterizing, and classifying congenital anomalies of the coronary arteries. *RadioGraphics*. 2012;32:453-468.

Williams PL, Warwick R, Dyson M, Bannister LH. *Angiology*. In: *Gray's Anatomy*. 37th ed. Edinburgh: Churchill Livingstone; 1989:661-858:chap 6.

14. Cardiac Veins

Ho SY, Sánchez-Quintana D, Becker AE. A review of the coronary venous system: a road less travelled. *Heart Rhythm*. 2004;1:107-112.

Klimek-Piotrowska W, Hołda MK, Koziej M, Strona M. Anatomical barriers in the right atrium to the coronary sinus cannulation. *PeerJ*. 2016;3:e1548.

Netter FH. Heart. In: Netter FIT, ed. *The Netter Collection of Medical Illustrations: The CIBA Collection of Medical Illustrations*. 1st ed. Vol 5. New York: The Ciba Collection of Medical Illustrations; 1969:1-293.

Williams PL, Warwick R, Dyson M, Bannister LH. *Angiology*. In: *Gray's Anatomy*. 37th ed. Edinburgh: Churchill Livingstone; 1989:661-858:chap 6.

15. Arteries of the Upper Extremity

Coleman SS, Anson BJ. Arterial patterns in the hand. Based upon a study of 650 specimens. *Surg Gynecol Obstet*. 1961;113:409-424.

Daseler EH, Anson BJ. Surgical anatomy of the subclavian artery and its branches. *Surg Gynecol Obstet*. 1959;108:149-174.

Ikeda A, Ugawa A, Kazihara Y, Hamada N. Arterial patterns in the hand based on a three dimensional analysis of 220 cadaver hands. *J Hand Surg*. 1988;13A:501-509.

Janevski BK. *Angiography of the Upper Extremity*. The Hague: Martinus Nijhoff Publishers; 1982:37-122.

Jesinger RA. Breast anatomy for the interventionalist. *Tech Vasc Interv Radiol*. 2014;17:3-9.

Netter FH. Anatomy. Upper limb. In: Netter F II, ed. *Musculoskeletal System. Part I: Anatomy, Physiology and Metabolic Disorders*. Vol 8. New York: The Ciba Collection of Medical Illustrations; 1987:20-74.

van Deventer PV, Graewe FR. The blood supply of the breast revisited. *Plast Reconstr Surg*. 2016;137:1388-1397.

16. Veins of the Upper Extremity

Janevski BK. *Angiography of the Upper Extremity*. The Hague: Martinus Nijhoff Publishers; 1982:37-122.

Netter FH. Anatomy. Upper limb. In: Netter F II, ed. *Musculoskeletal System. Part I: Anatomy, Physiology and Metabolic Disorders*. Vol 8. New York: The Ciba Collection of Medical Illustrations; 1987:20-74.

Netter FH. *Atlas of Human Anatomy*. Summit, New Jersey: Ciba-Geigy Corporation; 1989.

Thomas ML. Phlebography. *Arch Surg*. 1972;104:145-151.

17. Lymphatic System of the Upper Extremity

Fischer HW, Lawrence MS, Thombury JR. Lymphography of the normal adult male: observations and their relation to the diagnosis of metastatic neoplasm. *Radiology*. 1962;78:399-406.

Fischer HW, Zimmerman GR. Roentgenographic visualization of lymph nodes and lymphatic channels. *AJR Am J Roentgenol*. 1959;81:517-534.

Netter FH. Anatomy. Upper limb. In: Netter FH, ed. *Musculoskeletal System. Part I: Anatomy, Physiology and Metabolic Disorders*. Vol 8. New York: The Ciba Collection of Medical Illustrations; 1987:20-74.

18. Abdominal Aorta and Branches

Adams DB. The importance of extrahepatic biliary anatomy in preventing complications at laparoscopic cholecystectomy. *Surg Clin North Am*. 1993;73:861-871.

Anson BJ, Cauldwell EW, Pick JW, Beaton LE. The blood supply of the kidney, suprarenal gland, and associated structures. *Surg Gynecol Obstet*. 1947;84:313.

Arora R, Soulen MC, Haskal ZJ. Cutaneous complications of hepatic chemoembolization via extrahepatic collaterals. *J Vasc Interv Radiol*. 1999;10:1351-1356.

Baba Y, Miyazono N, Ueno K, et al. Hepatic falciform artery: angiographic findings in 25 patients. *Acta Radiol.* 2000;41:329-333.

Baum S. Normal anatomy and collateral pathways of the mesenteric circulation. In: Boley SJ, ed. *Vascular Disorders of the Intestine.* 1st ed. New York: Apple-Century-Crofts; 1971:1-18.

Bianchi HF, Albanese EF. The supraduodenal artery. *Surg Radiol Anat.* 1989;11:37-40.

Bismuth H. Surgical anatomy and anatomical surgery of the liver. *World J Surg.* 1982;6:3-9.

Boijsen E. Angiographic studies of the anatomy of single and multiple renal arteries. *Acta Radiol Suppl.* 1959;183:1-135.

Charnsangavej C, Chuang VP, Wallace S, Soo C-S, Bowers T. Angiographic classification of hepatic arterial collaterals. *Radiology.* 1982;144:485-494.

Chen WJ, Ying DJ, Liu ZJ, et al. Analysis of the arterial supply of the extrahepatic bile ducts and its clinical significance. *Clin Anat.* 1999;12:245-249.

Cho KJ, Lunderquist A. The peribiliary plexus: the microvascular architecture of the bile duct in the rabbit and in clinical cases. *Radiology.* 1983;147:357-364.

Clark HP, Carson WF, Kavanagh PV, et al. Staging and current treatment of hepatocellular carcinoma. *Radiographics.* 2005;25:S3-S23.

Couinaud C. *Le foie: Etudes anatomiques et chirurgicales.* 1st ed. Paris: Masson & Cie; 1957:1-530.

Daseler EH, Anson BJ, Hambley WC, Reiman AF. The cystic artery and constituents of the hepatic pedicle: a study of 500 specimens. *Surg Gynecol Obstet.* 1947;85:47-63.

da Silva Filho AR. *Vascularizaçao arterial do baeo: Estudo da independência e análise proporcional dos seus segmentos* [thesis]. Sao Paulo, Brazil: Escola Paulista de Medicina; 1991:1-63.

Demachi H, Matsui O, Takashima T. Scanning electron microscopy of intrahepatic microvasculature casts following experimental hepatic artery embolization. *Cardiovasc Intervent Radiol.* 1991;14:158-162.

Douglas TC, Cutter W. Arterial blood supply to the common duct. *Arch Surg.* 1948;57:599-612.

Ekataksin W, Zou Z, Wake K. A new look at the "hepatic" artery: intrahepatic arterial compartmentation in mammalian livers. *Hepatology.* 1995;22:159A.

Ekataksin W, Wake K. Liver units in three dimensions. I. Organization of argyrophilic connective tissue skeleton in porcine liver with particular reference to the "compound hepatic lobule". *Am J Anat.* 1991;191:113-153.

Fine H, Keen EN. The arteries of the human kidney. *J Anat.* 1966;100:881-894.

Flint ER. Abnormalities of the right hepatic, cystic and gastroduodenal arteries, and of the bile ducts. *Br J Surg.* 1923;10:509-512.

Garti I, Meiraz D. Ectopic origin of main renal artery. *Urology.* 1980;15:627-629.

Gazelle GS, Haaga JR. Hepatic neoplasms: surgically relevant segmental anatomy and imaging techniques. *AJR Am J Roentgenol.* 1992;158:1015-1018.

Gibo M, Hasuo K, Inoue A, et al. Hepatic falciform artery: angiographic observations and significance. *Abdom Imaging.* 2001;26:515-519.

Gruttadauria S, Foglieni CS, Doria C, et al. The hepatic artery in liver transplantation and surgery: vascular anomalies in 701 cases. *Clin Transpl.* 2001;15:359-363.

Hashimoto M, Heianna J, Tate E, et al. The feasibility of retrograde catheterization of the right gastric artery via the left gastric artery. *J Vasc Interv Radiol.* 2001;12:1103-1106.

Healey JE Jr. Vascular anatomy of the liver. *Ann NY Acad Sci.* 1970;170:8-17.

Healey JE Jr, Schroy PC, Sorensen RJ. The intrahepatic distribution of the hepatic artery in man. *J Int Coll Surg.* 1953; 20:133-148.

Hentati N, Fournier HD, Papon X, et al. Arterial supply of the duodenal bulb: an anatomoclinical study. *Surg Radiol Anat.* 1999;21:159-164.

Ibukuro K, Tsukiyama T, Mori K, et al. The congenital anastomoses between hepatic arteries: angiographic appearance. *Surg Radiol Anat.* 2000;22:41-45.

Ibukuro K, Tsukiyama T, Mori K, et al. Hepatic falciform ligament artery: angiographic anatomy and clinical importance. *Surg Radiol Anat.* 1998;20:367-371.

Kan Z, Invacev K, Lunderquist. Peribiliary plexa—important pathways for shunting of iodized oil and silicon rubber solution from the hepatic artery to the portal vein: and experimental study in rats. *Invest Radiol.* 1994;29:671-676.

Kan Z, Ivancev K, Lunderquist A, et al. In vivo microscopy of hepatic tumors in animal models: a dynamic investigation of blood supply to hepatic metastases. *Radiology.* 1993;187:621-626.

Kardon RH, Kessel RG. Three–dimensional organization of the hepatic microcirculation in the rodent as observed by scanning electron microscopy of corrosion casts. *Gastroenterology.* 1980;79:72-81.

Kim H-C, Chung JW, Lee W, et al. Recognizing extrahepatic collateral vessels that supply hepatocellular carcinoma to avoid complications of transcatheter arterial chemoembolization. *Radiographics.* 2005;25:S25-S39.

Kim HK, Chung JW, Song BC, et al. Ischemic bile duct injury as a serious complication after transarterial chemoembolization in patients with hepatocellular carcinoma. *J Clin Gastroenterol.* 2001;32:423-427.

Kinnunem J, Totterman S, Tervahartiala P. Ten renal arteries. *Eur J Radiol.* 1985;5:300-301.

Koehler RE, Korobkin M, Lewis F. Arteriographic demonstration of collateral arterial supply to the liver after hepatic artery ligation. *Radiology.* 1975;117:49-53.

Lafortune M, Madore F, Patriquin H, Breton G. Segmental anatomy of the liver: a sonographic approach to the Couinaud nomenclature. *Radiology.* 1991;181:443-448.

Le Bail B, Balaubaud C, Bioulac-Sage P. Anatomy and structure of the liver and biliary tree. In: Prieto J, Rodes J, Shafritz DA, eds. *Hepatobiliary Diseases.* Berlin: Springer-Verlag; 1992:1-38.

Liu DM, Salem R, Bui JT, et al. Angiographic considerations in patients undergoing liver-direct therapy. *J Vasc Interv Radiol.* 2005;16:911-935.

Lunderquist A. Angiography in carcinoma of the pancreas. *Acta Radiol.* 1965;suppl 235:1-143.

Lunderquist A. Arterial segmental supply of the liver. *Acta Radiol.* 1967;suppl 272:1-86.

MacSween RNM, Scothorne RJ. Developmental anatomy and normal structure. In: MacSween RNM, Anthony PP, Scheuer PJ, eds. *Pathology of the Liver.* 2nd ed. Edinburgh: Churchill Livingstone; 1987:1-45.

Machalek L, Holibkova A, Tuma J, Houserkova D. The size of the splenic hilus, diameter of the splenic artery and its branches in the human spleen. *Acta Univ Palacki Olomuc.* 1998;141:45-48.

Manso JC, DiDio LJ. Anatomical variations of the human suprarenal arteries. *Ann Anat.* 2000;182:483-488.

Marston A. *Intestinal Ischaemia.* 1st ed. London: Edward Arnold Publisher Ltd; 1977:1-190.

Merklin RJ. Arterial supply of the suprarenal gland. *Anat Rec.* 1962:141:359.

Merklin RJ, Michels NA. The variant renal and suprarenal blood supply with data on inferior phrenic, ureteral and gonadal arteries. A statistical analysis based on 185 dissections and review of the literature. *J Int Coll Surg.* 1958;29:41.

Michels NA. The ever varied blood supply of the liver and its collateral circulation. *J Int Coll Surg.* 1957;27:1-17.

Michels NA. *Blood Supply and Anatomy of the Upper Abdominal Organs With a Descriptive Atlas*. Philadelphia: J. B. Lippincott Co.; 1955.

Michels NA. The hepatic, cystic and retroduodenal arteries and their relations to the biliary ducts. *Ann Surg*. 1951;133:503-524.

Michels NA. The variational anatomy of the spleen and splenic artery. *Am J Anat*. 1942;70:21-26.

Millward-Sadler GH, Jezequel A-M. Normal histology and ultrastructure. In: Millward-Sadler GH, Wright R, Arthur MJP, eds. *Wright's—Liver and Biliary Disease*. 3rd ed. Vol 1. London: WB Saunders; 1992:3-11.

Mizumoto R, Suzuki H. Surgical anatomy of the hepatic hilum with special reference to the caudate lobe. *World J Surg*. 1988;12:2-10.

Miyazaki M, Ito H, Nakagawa K, et al. Unilateral hepatic arterial reconstruction is unnecessary in biliary tract carcinomas involving lobar hepatic artery: implications of interlobar hepatic artery and its prevention. *Hepatogastroenterology*. 2000;47:1526-1530.

Moar JJ, Tobias PV. Multiple renal arteries. *S Afr Med J*. 1958;67:399.

Motta PM. Scanning electron microscopy of the liver. In: Popper H, Schaffner F, eds. *Progress in Liver Diseases*. Vol 7. New York: Grime & Stratton; 1982:1-16.

Myers MA. Normal anatomic relationships and variants. In: Myers MA, ed. *Dynamic Radiology of the Abdomen*. New York: Springer-Verlag; 1992.

Nery JR, Frasson E, Rilo HLR, et al. Surgical anatomy and blood supply of the left biliary tree pertaining to partial liver grafts from living donors. *Transpl Proc*. 1990;22:1492-1496.

Netter FH. Anatomy of the abdomen. In: Netter FH, ed. *Digestive system. Part II: Lower Digestive Tract*. 1st ed. Vol 3. New York: The Ciba Collection of Medical Illustrations; 1969:10-44.

Netter FH. Anatomy of the lower digestive tract. In: Netter FH, ed. *Digestive System. Part II: Lower Digestive Tract*. 1st ed. Vol 3. New York: The Ciba Collection of Medical Illustrations; 1969:47-81.

Netter FH. Normal anatomy of the liver, biliary tract and pancreas. In: Netter FH, ed. *Digestive System. Part III: Liver, Biliary Tract and Pancreas*. Vol 3. New York: The Ciba Collection of Medical Illustrations; 1967:2-31.

Netter FH. Anatomy of the stomach and duodenum. In: Netter FH, ed. *Digestive System. Part I: Upper Digestive Tract*. Vol 3. New York: The Ciba Collection of Medical Illustrations; 1966:49-65.

Nordmark L. Angiography of the testicular artery. *Acta Radiol [Diagn]*. 1977;18:25-32.

Northover JMA, Terblanche J. A new look at the arterial supply of the bile duct in man and its surgical implications. *Br J Surg*. 1979;66:379-384.

Notkovich H. Variations of the testicular and ovarian arteries in relation to the renal pedicle. *Surg Gynecol Obstet*. 1956;103:487-495.

Parke WW, Michels NA, Ghosh GM. Blood supply of the common bile duct. *Surg Gynecol Obstet*. 1963;117:47-55.

Pennington N, Soames RW. The anterior visceral branches of the abdominal aorta and their relationship to the renal arteries. *Surg Radiol Anat*. 2005;22:1-9.

Pick JW, Anson BJ. The inferior phrenic artery: origin and suprarenal branches. *Anat Rec*. 1940;78:413.

Pierson JM. The arterial blood supply of the pancreas. *Surg Gynecol Obstet*. 1943;77:426-430.

Redman HC, Reuter SR. Arterial collaterals in the liver hilus. *Radiology*. 1970;94:575-579.

Sampaio FJB. Renal arterial pedicle: anatomic analysis applied to urologic and radiologic procedures. In: Sampaio FJB, Uflacker R, eds. *Renal Anatomy Applied to Urology, Endourology and Interventional Radiology*. 1st ed. New York: Thieme Medical Publishers; 1993:47-53.

Sampaio FJB. Anatomic study and proportional analysis of the kidney arterial segments. In: Sampaio FJB, Uflacker R, eds. *Renal Anatomy Applied to Urology, Endourology and Interventional Radiology*. 1st ed. New York: Thieme Medical Publishers; 1993:39-46.

Sampaio FJB. Relationships of intrarenal arteries and the kidney collecting system. In: Sampaio FJB, Uflacker R, eds. *Renal Anatomy Applied to Urology, Endourology and Interventional Radiology*. 1st ed. New York: Thieme Medical Publishers; 1993:23-32.

Sampaio FJB. Arterial and venous anatomic relationships to the ureteropelvic junction. In: Sampaio FJB, Uflacker R, eds. *Renal Anatomy Applied to Urology, Endourology and Interventional Radiology*. 1st ed. New York: Thieme Medical Publishers; 1993;77-81.

Sampaio FJB. Anatomical background for nephron-sparing surgery in renal cell carcinoma. *J Urol*. 1992;147:999-1005.

Sampaio FJB, Aragao AHM. Anatomical relationship between the intrarenal arteries and the kidney collecting system. *J Urol*. 1990;143:679-681.

Sampaio FJB, Favorito LA. Endopyélotomie. Etude anatomique des rapports vasculaires de la jonction pyélouréterale (JPU). *J d'Urol*. 1991;97:73-77.

Sampaio FJB, Mandarin-de-Lacerda CA. 3-Dimensional and radiological pelvicaliceal anatomy for endourology. *J Urol*. 1988a; 140:1352-1355.

Sampaio FJB, Mandarin-de-Lacerda CA. Anatomical classification of the kidney collecting system for endourological procedures. *J Endourol*. 1988b;2:247-251.

Sampaio FJ, Passos MA. Renal arteries: anatomic study for surgical and radiological practice. *Surg Radiol Anat*. 1992;14:113-117.

Sarkar AK, Roy TS. Anatomy of the cystic artery arising from the gastroduodenal artery and its choledochal branch–a case report. *J Anat*. 2000;197:503-506.

Segall H. An experimental anatomical investigation of blood and bile channels of the liver. *Surg Gynecol Obstet*. 1923;37:152-178.

Sherlock S. *Diseases of the Liver and Biliary System*. 8th ed. Oxford: Blackwell Scientific Publications; 1992:1-578.

Song SY, Chung JW, Kwon JW, et al. Collateral pathways in patients with celiac axis stenosis: angiographic-spiral CT correlation. *Radiographics*. 2002;22:881-893.

Soo CS, Chuang VP, Wallace S, et al. Treatment of hepatic neoplasm through extrahepatic collaterals. *Radiology*. 1983;147:45-49.

Soyer P, Roche A. Three-dimensional imaging of the liver. *Acta Radiol*. 1991;32:432-435.

Stapleton GN, Hickman R, Terblanche J. Blood supply of the right and left hepatic ducts. *Br J Surg*. 1998;85:202-207.

Sugarbaker PH, Nelson RC, Murray DR, Chezmar JL, Bernardino ME. A segmental approach to computerized tomographic portography for hepatic resection. *Surg Gynecol Obstet*. 1990; 171:189-195.

Sundgren R. Selective angiography of the left gastric artery. *Acta Radiol*. 1970;suppl 299:1-100.

Terblanche J, Allison HF, Northover JMA. An ischemic basis for biliary strictures. *Surgery*. 1983;94:52-57.

Terblanche J, Worthley CS, Spence RAJ, et al. High or low hepaticojejunostomy for bile duct strictures. *Surgery*. 1990;108:828-834.

Tohma T, Cho A, Okazumi S, et al. Communicating arcade between the right and left hepatic arteries: evaluation with CT and angiography during temporary balloon occlusion of the right or left hepatic artery. *Radiology*. 2005;237:361-365.

Ueno K, Miyazono N, Inoue H, et al. Embolization of the hepatic falciform artery to prevent supraumbilical skin rash during transcatheter arterial chemoembolization for hepatocellular carcinoma. *Cardiovasc Intervent Radiol*. 1995;18:183-185.

Uflacker R, Reichert P, D'Albuquerque LC, Oliveira e Silva A. Liver anatomy applied to the placement of transjugular intrahepatic portosystemic shunt (TIPS). *Radiology*. 1994;191:705-712.

VanDamme J-P, Bonte J. *Vascular Anatomy in Abdominal Surgery*. 1st ed. New York: Thieme Medical Publishers; 1990:1-142.

Vellar ID. The blood supply of the biliary ductal system and its relevance to vasculobiliary injuries following cholecystectomy. *Aust NZ J Surg*. 1999;69:816-820.

Vellar ID. Preliminary study of the anatomy of the venous drainage of the intrahepatic and extrahepatic bile ducts and its relevance to the practice of hepatobiliary surgery. *Aust NZ J Surg.* 2001;71:418-422.

Yamagami T, Kato K, Tanaka O, et al. Influence of hepatopetal flow of the retroportal artery on efficiency of repeated hepatic arterial infusion chemotherapy. *J Vasc Interv Radiol.* 2005;16:1391-1395.

Yamauchi T, Furth S, Ohtomo K, Itai Y. Stereoscopic digital subtraction angiography of hepatic artery and vein. *MR.* 1987;148:825-826.

Yule E. The arterial supply of the duodenum. *J Anat.* 1927;61:344-348.

Wilkie DP. The blood supply to the duodenum with special reference to the supra-duodenal artery. *Surg Gynecol Obstet.* 1911;13:399-405.

Wind P, Chevallier JM, Sarcy JJ, et al. The infrapyloric artery and cephalic pancreatoduodenectomy with pylorus preservation: preliminary study. *Surg Radiol Anat.* 1994;16:165-172.

Zanier JFC. *Acesso percutanco ao rim em endourologia* [thesis]. Rio de Janeiro, Brazil: Universidade Federal do Rio de Janeiro; 1990:1-109.

19. Arteries of the Pelvis

Bilhim T, Pereira JA, Fernandes L, Rio Tinto H, Pisco JM. Angiographic anatomy of the male pelvic arteries. *AJR.* 2014;203:W373-W382.

Bilhim T, Rio Tinto H, Fernandes L, Pisco JM. Radiological anatomy of prostatic arteries. *Tech Vasc Interv Radiol.* 2012;15:276-285.

Bilhim T, Pisco JM, Furtado A, et al. Prostatic arterial supply: demonstration by multirow detector angio CT and catheter angiography. *Eur Radiol.* 2011;21:1119-1126.

Bookstein JJ. Penile angiography: the last angiographic frontier. *AJR Am J Roentgenol.* 1988;150:47-54.

Bookstein JJ, Lang EV. Penile magnification pharmacoarteriography: details of intrapenile arterial anatomy. *AJR Am J Roentgenol.* 1987:148:883-888.

Borell U, Fernstrom I. The ovarian artery. An arteriographic study in human subjects. *Acta Radiol.* 1954;42:253-265.

Clegg EJ. The arterial supply of the human prostate and seminal vesicles. *J Anat.* 1955;89:209-216.

de Assis AM, Moreira AM, de Paula Rodrigues VC, et al. Pelvic arterial anatomy relevant to prostatic artery embolisation and proposal for angiographic classification. *Cardiovasc Intervent Radiol.* 2015;38:855-861.

Delcour C, Vandenbosch G, Delatte, et al. Penile arteriography: technical advances. *AJR Am J Roentgenol.* 1988;150:803-804.

Erturk SM, Tatli S. Persistent sciatic artery aneurysm. *JVIR.* 2005;16:1407-1408.

Fernstrom I. Arteriography of the uterine artery. *Acta Radiol Suppl.* 1955;20:1-100.

Gomez-Jorge J, Keyoung A, Levy EB, Spies JB. Uterine artery anatomy relevant to uterine leiomyomata embolization. *Cardiovasc Intervent Radiol.* 2003;26:522-527.

Hassen-Khodja R, Batt M, Michetti C, et al. Radiologic anatomy of the anastomotic systems of the internal iliac artery. *Surg Radiol Anat.* 1987;9:135-140.

Mandell VS, Jaques PF, Delany DJ, Oberheu V. Persistent sciatic artery: clinical, embryologic, and angiographic features. *AJR Am J Roentgenol.* 1985;144:245-249.

Pelage JP, Cazejust J, Pluot E, et al. Uterine fibroid vascularization and clinical relevance to uterine fibroid embolization. *RadioGraphics.* 2005; 25:S99-S117.

Pelage JP, Le Dref O, Soyer P, et al. Arterial anatomy of the female genital tract: variations and relevance to transcatheter embolization of the uterus. *AJR.* 1999;172:989-994.

Razavi MK, Wolanske KA, Hwang GL, et al. Angiographic classification of ovarian artery-to-uterine artery anastomoses: initial observations in uterine fibroid embolization. *Radiology.* 2002;224:707-712.

Soyer P, Boudiaf M, Jacob D, et al. Bilateral persistent sciatic artery: a potential risk in pelvic arterial embolization for primary postpartum hemorrhage. *Acta Obstet Gynecol Scand.* 2005;84:604-605.

VanDamme J-P, Bonte J. *Vascular Anatomy in Abdominal Surgery.* 1st ed. New York: Thieme Medical Publishers; 1990:1-142.

Walsh PC. *Radical retropubic prostatectomy.* In: *Campbell's Urology.* Vol 3. Philadelphia: WB Saunders; 1986:2754-2775.

Williams PL, Warwick R, Dyson M, Bannister LH. *Angiology.* In: *Gray's Anatomy.* 37th ed. Edinburgh: Churchill Livingstone; 1989:661-858:chap 6.

Williams PL, Warwick R, Dyson M, Bannister LH. *Splanchnology.* In: *Gray's Anatomy.* 37th ed. Edinburgh: Churchill Livingstone; 1989:1245-1475:chap 7.

20. Veins of the Abdomen and Pelvis

Anderson RC, Adams P, Burke B. Anomalous inferior vena cava with azygos continuation (infrahepatic interruption of the inferior vena cava). Report of 15 new cases. *J Pediatr.* 1961;59:370-383.

Bass J, Redwine M, Kramer L, Huynh P, Harris J. Spectrum of congenital anomalies of the inferior vena cava: cross-sectional imaging findings. *RadioGraphics.* 2000;20:639-652.

Ramesh Babu CS, Sharma M. Biliary tract anatomy and its relationship with venous drainage. *J Clin Exp Hepatol.* 2014;4:S18-S26.

Bergstrand I, Eckman CA. Portal circulation in portal hypertension. *Acta Radiol [Diagn] (stock).* 1957;47:1-22.

Bookstein JJ. Penile angiography: the last angiographic frontier. *MR.* 1988;150:47-54.

Bookstein JJ. Cavernosal venoocclusive insufficiency in male impotence: evaluation of degree and location. *Radiology.* 1987; 164:175-178.

Bookstein JJ, Lurie AL. Selective penile venography: anatomical and hemodynamic observations. *J Urol.* 1988;140:55-60.

Chermet J, Bigot JM. *Venography of The Inferior Vena Cava and Its Branches.* New York: Springer-Verlag; 1980:1-232.

Cho KJ, Geisinger KR, Shields JJ, Forrest ME. Collateral channels and histopathology in hepatic vein occlusion. *AJR Am J Roentgenol.* 1982;139:703-709.

Coolsaet BLRA. The varicocele syndrome: venography determining the optimal level for surgical management. *J Urol.* 1980;124:833-839.

Couinaud C. The parabiliary venous system. *Surg Radiol Anat.* 1988;10:311-316.

da Silva Filho AR. *Vascularizacao venosa do baço: Estudo morfológico da formaçao da veia esplênica e análise segmentar intraparenquimatosa* [thesis]. Fortaleza, Brazil: Universidade Federal do Ceará; 1992:1-46.

Delcour C, Wespes E, Schulman CC, et al. Investigation of the venous system in impotence of vascular origin. *Urol Radiol.* 1984;6:190-193.

Doehner GA. The hepatic venous system. Its pathologic roentgen anatomy. *Radiology.* 1968;90:1124-1131.

Doehner GA. The hepatic venous system. Its normal roentgen anatomy. *Radiology.* 1968;90:1119-1123.

Doehner GA, Ruzicka FF, Hoffman G, Rousselot LM. The portal venous system: its roentgen anatomy. *Radiology.* 1955;64:675-687.

Göthlin J, Lunderquist A, Lylen U. Selective phlebography of the pancreas. *Acta Radiol.* 1974;15:474-480.

Healey JE Jr. Vascular anatomy of the liver. *Ann NY Acad Sci.* 1970;170:8-17.

Helander CG, Lindblon A. retrograde pelvic venography. ACTA *Radiol (Diagn).* 1959;51:401-414.

Johnstone FRC. The suprarenal veins. *Am J Surg.* 1957;94:615.

Juttner HU, Jenney JM, Rails PW, Goldstein LI, Reynolds TB. Ultrasound demonstration of portosystemic collaterals in cirrhosis and portal hypertension. *Radiology.* 1982;142:459-463.

Kardon RH, Kessel RG. Three-dimensional organization of the hepatic microcirculation in the rodent as observed by scanning electron microscopy of corrosion casts. *Gastroenterology*. 1980;79:72-81.

Keller FS, Niles NR, Rosch J, et al. Retrograde pancreatic venography: autopsy study. *Radiology*. 1980;135;285-293.

Lafortune M, Constantin A, Breton G, Legare AG, Lavoie P. The recanalized umbilical vein in portal hypertension: a myth. *AJR Am J Roentgenol*. 1985;144:549-553.

Lavoie P. Legare AG, Viallet A. Portal catheterization via the round ligament of the liver. *Am J Surg*. 1967;144:822-830.

Leger L, Lenriot JP, Lemaigre G. Physiopathology of portal hypertension. Circulatory neophysiology after portacaval shunt. In: Child CG, ed. *Portal Hypertension. Major Problems in Clinical Surgery*. Philadelphia: W.B. Saunders Co.; 1974:165-195.

Le Bail B, Balaubaud C, Bioulac-Sage P. Anatomy and structure of the liver and biliary tree. In: Prieto J, Rodes J, Shafritz DA, eds. *Hepatobiliary Diseases*. Berlin: Springer-Verlag; 1992:1-38.

MacSween RNM, Scothorne RJ. Developmental anatomy and normal structure. In: MacSween RNM, Anthony PP, Scheuer PJ, eds. *Pathology of the Liver*. 2nd ed. Edinburgh: Churchill Livingstone; 1987:1-45.

Madrazo B, Jafri SZ, Shirkhoda A, Roberts JL, Ellwood RA. Portosystemic collaterals: evaluation with color Doppler imaging and correlation with CT and MRI. *Semin Intery Radiol*. 1990;7:169-184.

Merklin RJ, Eger SA. The adrenal venous system in man. *J Int Coll Surg*. 1961;35:572.

Michels NA. *Blood Supply and Anatomy of the Upper Abdominal Organs With a Descriptive Atlas*. Philadelphia: J.B. Lippincott Co.; 1955.

Mikaelsson CG. Venous communications of the adrenal glands. *Acta Radiol (stock)*. 1970;10:369.

Millward-Sadler GH, Jezequel A-M. Normal histology and ultrastructure. In: Millward-Sadler GH, Wright R, Arthur MJP, eds. *Wright's—Liver and Biliary Disease*. 3rd ed. Vol 1. London: WB Saunders; 1992:3-11.

Moltz L, Sorensen R. Selective venous sampling for the differential diagnosis of female hyperandrogenemia. In: Uflacker R, Sorensen R, eds. *Percutaneous Venous Blood Sampling in Endocrine Diseases*. New York: Springer-Verlag; 1992:1-27.

Morin C, Lafortune M, Pomier G, Robin M, Breton G. Patent paraumbilical vein: anatomic and hemodynamic variants and their clinical importance. *Radiology*. 1992;185:253-256.

Motta PM. Scanning electron microscopy of the liver. In: Popper H, Schaffner F, ed. *Progress in Liver Diseases*. Vol 7. New York: Grune & Stratton; 1982:1-16.

Myers MA. Normal anatomic relationships and variants. In: Myers MA, ed. *Dynamic Radiology of the Abdomen*. New York: Springer-Verlag; 1992.

Myers RP. Anatomical variation of the superficial preprostatic veins in respect to radical retropubic prostatectomy. *J Urol*. 1991;145:992-993.

Netter FH. Anatomy of the abdomen. In: Netter FH, ed. *Digestive System. Part II: Lower Digestive Tract*. 1st ed. Vol 3. New York: The Ciba Collection of Medical Illustrations; 1969:10-44.

Netter FH. Anatomy of the lower digestive tract. In: Netter FH, ed. *Digestive System. Part II: Lower Digestive Tract*. 1st ed. Vol 3. New York: The Ciba Collection of Medical Illustrations; 1969:47-81.

Netter FH. Anatomy of the stomach and duodenum. In: Netter FH, ed. *Digestive System. Part I: Upper Digestive Tract*. Vol 3. New York: The Ciba Collection of Medical Illustrations; 1966:49-65.

Netter FH. Normal anatomy of the liver, biliary tract and pancreas. In: Netter FH, ed. *Digestive System. Part III: Liver, Biliary Tract and Pancreas*. Vol 3. New York: The Ciba Collection of Medical Illustrations; 1967:2-31.

Obel W. The umbilical vein in different periods of life in man. *Folia Morphol*. 1976;35:173-179.

Petik B. Inferior vena cava anomalies and variations: imaging and rare clinical findings. *Insights Imaging*. 2015;6:631-639.

Reiner WG, Walsh PC. An anatomical approach to the surgical management of the dorsal vein and Santorini's plexus during radical retropubic surgery. *J Urol*. 1979;121:198-200.

Sabri S, Saad WEA. Anatomy and classification of gastrorenal and gastrocaval shunts. *Semin Interv Radiol*. 2011;28:296-302.

Sampaio and Aragao, 1990 Sampaio FJB, Aragao AIIM. Anatomical relationship between the renal venous arrangement and the kidney collecting system. *J Urol*. 1990;144:1089-1093.

Sampaio FJB. Arterial and venous anatomic relationships to the ureteropelvic junction. In: Sampaio FJB, Uflacker R, eds. *Renal Anatomy Applied to Urology, Endourology and Interventional Radiology*. 1st ed. New York: Thieme Medical Publishers; 1993:77-81.

Sano A, Kuroda Y, Moriyasu F, et al. Portopulmonary venous anastomosis in portal hypertension demonstrated by percutaneous transhepatic cineportography. *Radiology*. 1982;114(3):479-484.

Saint JH. The epicholedochal venous plexus and its importance as a means of identifying the common duct during operations on the extrahepatic biliary tract. *Br J Surg*. 1961;48:489-498.

Sherlock S. *Diseases of the Liver and Biliary System*. 8th ed. Oxford: Blackwell Scientific Publications; 1992:1-578.

Soyer P, Roche A. Three-dimensional imaging of the liver. *Acta Radiol*. 1991;32:432-435.

Sugarbaker PH, Nelson RC, Murray DR, Chezmar JL, Bernardino ME. A segmental approach to computerized tomographic portography for hepatic resection. *Surg Gynecol Obstet*. 1990;171:189-195.

Uflacker R. Pancreatic venous sampling. In: Uflacker R, Sorensen R, eds. *Percutaneous Venous Blood Sampling in Endocrine Diseases*. New York: Springer-Verlag; 1992:75-118.

Uflacker R, Reichert P, D'Albuquerque LC, Oliveira e Silva A. Liver anatomy applied to the placement of transjugular intrahepatic portosystemic shunt (TIPS). *Radiology*. 1994;191:705-712.

VanDamme J-P, Bonte J. *Vascular Anatomy in Abdominal Surgery*. 1st ed. New York: Thieme Medical Publishers; 1990:1-142.

van Leeuwen MS, Fernandez MA, van Es HW, Stokking R, Dillon EH, Feldberg MAM. Variations in venous and segmental anatomy of the liver: two- and three-dimensional MR imaging in healthy volunteers. *AJR Am J Roentgenol*. 1994;162:1337-1345.

Walsh PC. *Radical retropubic prostatectomy*. In: *Campbell's Urology*. Vol 3. Philadelphia: WB Saunders; 1986:2754-2775.

Williams PL, Warwick R, Dyson M, Bannister LH. *Angiology*. In: *Gray's Anatomy*. 37th ed. Edinburgh: Churchill Livingstone; 1989:661-858:chap 6.

Yamauchi T, Furui S, Ohtomo K, Itai Y. Stereoscopic digital subtraction angiography of hepatic artery and vein. *MR*. 1987;148:825-826.

Zanier JFC. *Acesso percutaneo ao rim em endourologia* [thesis]. Rio de Janeiro, Brazil: Universidade Federal do Rio de Janeiro; 1990:1-109.

21. Lymphatic System of the Abdomen

Delmas V, Hidden G, Dauge MCL. Organisation du drainage lymphatique au niveau de l'appareil urinaire et genital de l'homme. *Bull Soc Anat Paris*. 1989;13:95-103.

Delmas V, Hidden G, Dauge MCL. Remarques sur les lymphatiques du rein: Le premier relais nodal. *Bull Soc Anat Paris*. 1989;13:105-109.

Fischer HW, Lawrence MS, Thornbury JR. Lymphography of the normal adult male: observations and their relation to the diagnosis of metastatic neoplasm. *Radiology*. 1962;78:399-406.

Fischer HW, Zimmerman GR. Roentgenographic visualization of lymph nodes and lymphatic channels. *AJR Am J Roentgenol*. 1959;81:517-534.

Giuliani L, Gilberti C, Martorana G. Lymphadenectomy. Lymphatic drainage of the kidney. In: Giuliani L, Gilberti C, Martorana G, eds. *Atlas of Surgery for Renal Cancer*. 2nd ed. Milan: Grafiche Mazzucchelli; 1989:43-45.

Guez D, Nadolski GJ, Pukenas BA, Itkin M. Transhepatic lymphatic embolization of intractable hepatic lymphorrhea. *J Vasc Interv Radiol.* 2014;25:149-150.

Itkin M, Nadolski GJ. Modern techniques of lymphangiography and interventions: current status and future development. *Cardiovasc Intervent Radiol.* 2018;41:366-376.

Souza-Rodrigues CF. Anatomia aplicada do sistema linfatico. In: Pitta GBB, Castro AA, Burihan E, eds. *Angiologia e cirurgia vascular: Guia ilustrado.* Maceio: UNCISAL/ECMAL & LAVA; 2003.

Tanaka M, Iwakiri Y. The hepatic lymphatic vascular system: structure, function, markers, and lymphangiogenesis. *Cell Mol Gastroenterol Hepatol.* 2016;2:733-749.

VanDamme J-P, Bonte J. *Vascular Anatomy in Abdominal Surgery.* 1st ed. New York: Thieme Medical Publishers; 1990:1-142.

22. Arteries of the Lower Extremity

Golan JF, Garrett WV, Smith BL, et al. Persistent sciatic artery and vein: an unusual case. *J Vasc Surg.* 1986;3:162-165.

Mussbichler H. Arteriographic investigation of the normal hip in adults. Evaluation of methods and vascular findings. *Acta Radiol.* 1971;11:195-215.

Netter FH. Anatomy. Lower limb. In: Netter FH, ed. *Musculoskeletal System. Part I: Anatomy, Physiology and Metabolic Disorders.* Vol 8. New York: The Ciba Collection of Medical Illustrations; 1987:75-121.

23. Veins of the Lower Extremity

Greitz T. Phlebography of the normal leg. *Acta Radiol (Diagn).* 1955;44:1-20.

Jacobsen BH. The venous drainage of the foot. *Surg Gynecol Obstet.* 1970;131:22-24.

Netter FH. Anatomy. Lower limb. In: Netter FH, ed. *Musculoskeletal System. Part I: Anatomy, Physiology and Metabolic Disorders.* Vol 8. New York: The Ciba Collection of Medical Illustrations; 1987:75-121.

Thomas ML. Phlebography. *Arch Surg.* 1972;104:145-151.

24. Lymphatic System of the Lower Extremity

Heman PG, Benninghoff DL, Nelson JH, Mellins HZ. Roentgen anatomy of the ilio-pelvic-aortic lymphatic system. *Radiology.* 1963;80:182-193.

Larson DL, Lewis SR. Deep lymphatic system of the lower extremity. *Am J Surg.* 1967;113:217-220.

Netter FH. Anatomy. Lower limb. In: Netter FH, ed. *Musculoskeletal System. Part I: Anatomy, Physiology and Metabolic Disorders.* Vol 8. New York: The Ciba Collection of Medical Illustrations; 1987:75-121.

Souza-Rodrigues CF. Anatomia aplicada do sistema linfatico. In: Pitta GBB, Castro AA, Burihan E, eds. *Angiologia e cirurgia vascular: Guia ilustrado.* Maceio: UNCISAL/ECMAL & LAVA; 2003.

Vitek J, Kaspar Z. The radiology of the deep lymphatic system of the leg. *Br J Radiol.* 1973;46:120-124.

25. Suggested Readings

Hollinshead WH. *The thorax, abdomen, and pelvis.* In: *Anatomy for Surgeons.* Vol 2. New York: Harper & Row; 1971.

International Anatomic Nomenclature Committee. Nomina anatomica. Warwick R, Brookes M, eds. *Angiologia.* 5th ed. I.A.N.C. Baltimore: Williams & Wilkins; 1983.

Kadin S. *Atlas of Normal and Variant Angiographic Anatomy.* 1st ed. Philadelphia: W.B. Saunders Co.; 1991:1-529.

Netter FH. *Atlas of Human Anatomy.* Summit, New Jersey: Ciba-Geigy Corporation; 1989.

Pansky B, House EL. *Review of Gross Anatomy.* 2nd ed. London: The Macmillan Co.; 1971:1-493.

Williams PL, Warwick R, Dyson M, Bannister LH. *Angiology.* In: *Gray's Anatomy.* 37th ed. Edinburgh: Churchill Livingstone; 1989:661-858:chap 6.

Williams PL, Warwick R, Dyson M, Bannister LH. *Splanchnology.* In: *Gray's Anatomy.* 37th ed. Edinburgh: Churchill Livingstone; 1989:1245-1475:chap 7.

INDEX

Numerals in *italics* indicate a figure, and **bold** indicate a table.

A

B

C

J

K

L

W

Y

Z